FIFTH EDITION

GYNECOLOGIC HEALTH CARE

WITH AN INTRODUCTION TO PRENATAL AND POSTPARTUM CARE

Ellen Solis, DNP, CNM, FACNM
Nurse-Midwifery Specialty Director and Associate Professor
Child, Family, and Population Health Nursing (CFPHN)
University of Washington School of Nursing

Molly Altman, PhD, CNM, MPH, FACNM
PhD Program Director and Associate Professor
School of Nursing and Dental Hygiene
University of Hawai'i at Mānoa

JONES & BARTLETT
LEARNING

World Headquarters
Jones & Bartlett Learning
25 Mall Road
Burlington, MA 01803
978-443-5000
info@jblearning.com
www.jblearning.com

Jones & Bartlett Learning books and products are available through most bookstores and online booksellers. To contact Jones & Bartlett Learning directly, call 800-832-0034, fax 978-443-8000, or visit our website, www.jblearning.com.

Substantial discounts on bulk quantities of Jones & Bartlett Learning publications are available to corporations, professional associations, and other qualified organizations. For details and specific discount information, contact the special sales department at Jones & Bartlett Learning via the above contact information or send an email to specialsales@jblearning.com.

30612-5

Production Credits
Vice President, Innovative Learning and Assessment Solutions: Ada Woo
Senior Director, Content Production and Delivery: Christine Emerton
Director, Product: Melissa Kleeman-Moy
Manager, Content Development: Bill Lawrensen
Content Manager: Christina Freitas
Content Coordinator: Rachelle Soden
Manager, Intellectual Properties and Content Production: Kristen Rogers
Content Production Manager: Madelene Nieman
Senior Intellectual Property Specialist (eBook): Colleen Lamy
Director, Marketing: Andrea DeFronzo
Senior Product Marketing Manager: Lindsay White
Director, Product Fulfillment: Aaron McKinzie
Purchasing Manager: Wendy Kilborn
Composition and Project Management: S4Carlisle Publishing Services
Cover and Text Design: MPS Limited
Media Developer: Faith Brosnan
Intellectual Property Specialist: Lisa Passmore
Cover Image: The symbol on the cover is adapted from The Changer by K Robins and is used with the permission of K Robins Designs. Background: © filo/DigitalVision Vectors/Getty Images
Printing and Binding: The P.A. Hutchison Company

Library of Congress Cataloging-in-Publication Data
Library of Congress Cataloging-in-Publication Data unavailable at time of printing.
LCCN: 2025042307

6048

Printed in the United States of America
30 29 28 27 26 10 9 8 7 6 5 4 3 2 1

Dedication

To my partner in all things, Gabriel—whose steady love, humor, and unwavering belief in me made the early mornings and late nights of this project not only bearable, but meaningful. Thank you for keeping the coffee flowing, the dinners amazing, and the perspective grounded.

To my children, Coleman and Isabella, now forging your own paths—you continue to teach me about integrity, curiosity, and the power of showing up. Thank you for listening to talk of placentas at the dinner table, your opinions, your patience, your insight, and for reminding me that the work we do should reflect the values we live. I'm endlessly proud of who you are and who you're becoming.

To my colleagues, friends, and mentors—especially Liz, Clare, Melicia, Stephanie, Meghan, Signey, Katie, Letitia, Andie, Lauren, Keely, Farrah, Tiffany, Vanessa, Carissa, Amie, Kirstie, Kristy, Ray, James, and Tiffani—you are my brain trust and unwavering supporters. Thank you for your wisdom, encouragement, and the generous exchange of ideas that shaped this work. Also, thank you for teaching me to suture 20 years ago, keeping me humble, and tolerating my "just one more edit" emails.

To my current midwifery students at the University of Washington—your perspectives, questions, and bold ideas directly helped shape the changes in this edition. To my former students at Georgetown University and the University of Illinois, thank you for challenging me, inspiring me, and reminding me that teaching is always a two-way street (and that I should never underestimate the power of a well-placed question).

To the readers of this text—whether you're just beginning your journey or deep in practice—I hope this edition meets you with clarity, compassion, and a sense of possibility.

Finally, to my brilliant co-editor, Molly—you never know where and when you'll find the people who become your lifelong co-conspirators and friends. I'm so glad we found each other. Thank you for your partnership, patience, and shared commitment to making this edition more inclusive, more rigorous, and more human.

—Ellen Solis

I dedicate this text to my pōhaku, my partner-in-crime, and my dear wife, Naomi, who creates space for turmoil while holding me grounded in the moments of uncertainty. I also dedicate this to my wonderfully spunky, kind, and generous child Nai'a, for whom the moments of peeking over my shoulder while reviewing chapters gave way to impromptu anatomy lessons and discussions about puberty, family planning, and bodily autonomy. I should also dedicate this book to her friends' parents, who are now subjected to unexpected conversations at the dinner table after hearing about chlamydia and IUDs at school.

To my friends, colleagues, and mentors across the globe who supported me in numerous ways and encouraged radical thinking as we approached this work—I am so appreciative of how we can come together in a period of regressive and oppressive transition and still push for equity and change. A special call-out to the chaos muppets in my life who challenge me to think and dream bigger, to find solutions to the unsolvable, and to continuously challenge boundaries in my work.

To the contributors, reviewers, and thought partners who wrote and reviewed pieces of this text. It wouldn't be what it is without your input and dedication to the work. A big thank you to all of the students who provided essential feedback on how textbooks in sexual and reproductive health could be improved, serving as the impetus for the changes in this edition.

Lastly, I dedicate this book to my amazing friend and co-editor, Ellen. From our first conversation over Zoom in a parking lot to now, we've been able to move mountains together in collaboration. Your presence in my life has made all of my work more meaningful, and I am grateful to be by your side in this endeavor and for many more.

—Molly Altman

CONTENTS

PREFACE

When we were asked to take on the honor of continuing the legacy of Schuiling and Likis' *Gynecologic Health Care*, we felt a mix of gratitude, dread, and responsibility to the women's health and gynecologic healthcare community. This holistic, feminist-oriented, person-centered textbook has been the cornerstone of advanced practice gynecological education in schools and programs across the country and globe. It has educated thousands of students and shaped evidence-based practice in sexual and reproductive health for over 15 years. Drs. Schuiling and Likis have worked diligently to navigate the complex environment around gendered language, with small yet significant changes throughout the first four editions to adapt to the changing cultural understanding of women's health, including health for transgender, nonbinary, and intersex individuals. When they asked us to assume the editorship, we recognized the importance and the immense responsibility this position entailed. Who are we to assume such an important role?

We want to start by introducing ourselves to you.

I am Ellen Chaney Solis (she/her), and 2026 marks my 19th year as a Certified Nurse Midwife and my 10th year as an educator and researcher. I am a mixed-race (Black/white), queer, cisgender woman, nurse, midwife, and educator from rural California. My perspective is shaped by experiences of racial marginalization and over two decades of clinical practice across diverse regions of the United States. I am the current specialty director of the Nurse-Midwifery Education Program and an associate professor at the University of Washington. I pursued my nursing and midwifery education at the University of Pennsylvania and Frontier Nursing University, receiving my BSN from Penn in 2002, my MSN from FNU in 2007, and my DNP from FNU in 2016. As an early-career midwife, I practiced at a robust midwifery practice in Illinois and taught at the University of Illinois and at Georgetown University. While working toward my doctorate, I moved into clinical leadership, teaching nursing and midwifery students, and using the knowledge and skills I gained through my DNP to educate my students and effect evidence-based change in my clinical practice. As a clinician and leader, I worked toward reducing weight bias and stigma for pregnant people who desire midwifery care, collaborated on policy initiatives to increase access to midwives for rural and underserved people in Illinois, and studied ways to use simulation and technology to enhance midwifery students' educational experiences and confidence. All of my advocacy, research, and leadership has been done with community stakeholders and through the lens of reproductive justice and trauma-informed care. I have used the *Gynecologic Health Care* textbook throughout my career as a resource and as one of the best tools to bring evidence-based information to students. I strongly believe that knowledge of gynecologic care is a crucial foundation for providers to take the best possible care of patients, and I hope the fifth edition of *Gynecologic Health Care* reaches students and providers who desire quality evidence-based information.

I am Molly Altman (she/her), currently an associate professor and the PhD program director at the University of Hawai'i at Mānoa School of Nursing and Dental Hygiene. I am a white, queer, cisgender woman, nurse midwife, educator, and researcher, with ancestors originating from both Western and Eastern Europe. I became a certified nurse midwife in 2005, practiced in various settings across the United States and globally for several years, and then returned for my PhD in nursing science in 2012. At that time, I joined the faculty at the University of Washington and started teaching in the nurse-midwifery program, using the first and then second editions of this very textbook. Upon completion of my PhD, I completed a post-doctoral fellowship and returned to the University of Washington as tenure-track faculty in 2018. In 2020, I assumed the role of the program director of the nurse-midwifery program at a time in which we needed to navigate racialized harms that were occurring. I led our program through a truth and reconciliation process using transformative justice as a framework, which supported numerous other programs in working to create more equitable and inclusive spaces within healthcare education. My research background has focused on reducing bias and discrimination in health care, which also translates seamlessly to education. All students have the right to access quality education to become the types of providers our patients and communities need and deserve. This is why I agreed to assume the torch for *Gynecologic Health Care* alongside Ellen.

For the fifth edition, we have chosen to take the stance of moving the textbook to be as gender inclusive as possible. This decision was not made lightly—women and girls in this country continue to be harmed through sexism and patriarchal systems that create barriers to appropriate education, health care, and resources. We also recognize the immense need to recognize the impacts of excluding our transgender, nonbinary, and intersex communities and the harm that occurs when communities deserving equitable care are erased from our textbooks through gendered language. With this in mind, we have supported our contributing authors to utilize gender-neutral language, when possible, which in most circumstances is easily done using the words "person," "individual," "patient," or "client," terms that apply to women and everyone who would benefit from the care we provide. We have also added a new chapter on trauma-informed care as well as more comprehensive resources around pregnancy diagnosis, decision making, and abortion. Further, there is new content on the history of our professions and recognition of the need for transformative change to ensure we continue to reduce health inequities in every way possible.

We hope to build your trust and hold accountability for ensuring that future generations of advanced practice clinicians have access to high-quality, inclusive, and comprehensive gynecologic healthcare knowledge. Thank you for being a part of this journey and please reach out to us if you have feedback.

Ellen Solis
Molly Altman

FOREWORD

We are alumni and former faculty members of Frontier Nursing University. As Frontier faculty we co-taught a women's health course for nurse-midwifery and nurse practitioner students. While teaching this course, we became aware of the significant need for a book that presented gynecologic health from a woman-centered, health-oriented, feminist viewpoint with an emphasis on the importance of respecting normal physiology and providing evidence-based clinical care. We also wanted a book with language and illustrations that reflected treating the whole person, not just body parts or a condition. We came to the conclusion that we would have to create the book we needed, and this is how the first edition of *Women's Gynecologic Health* came about. Each edition expanded with new chapters and extensive revision of existing chapters to ensure comprehensive content that reflected current standards of care. Over time, the book's content incorporated gender-inclusive gynecologic health care with language fitting for all persons needing this type of care. Our focus broadened from "women" to "persons," and the title of the book changed to *Gynecologic Health Care* to reflect the book's evolution.

When we decided to retire, one of our biggest dilemmas was finding the right persons to take on co-editing our book, *Gynecologic Health Care*. Handing our book off to editors who possessed academic and clinical knowledge, with both practice and teaching experience in gynecologic health care, was critical. It was also essential to find co-editors who were committed to keeping the book's focus of providing holistic gynecologic care that is based in science, is gender inclusive, and uses the most up-to-date practice guidelines. We were thrilled when Ellen Chaney Solis, DNP, CNM, FACNM and Molly Altman, PhD, CNM, MPH, FACNM agreed to become the next co-editors.

Dr. Solis and Dr. Altman are highly respected midwives who are well known for their expertise, having received numerous honors for their work. We knew them and of their many significant contributions to practice, teaching, and research prior to asking if they might be interested in becoming the new co-editors. It was with great pride, respect, and confidence that Francie and I handed off the roles of co-editor to our two colleagues.

We have been looking forward to the publication of the fifth edition of *Gynecologic Health Care* and the fresh perspectives Dr. Solis and Dr. Altman will bring. We thank them for their work and dedication in taking on the very large task of being co-editors, sharing their expertise, and continuing the legacy of our book. We are confident that educators, students, and clinicians will be pleased to read the new and expanded content and how it supports gynecologic care that is inclusive, comprehensive, and evidence-based.

Kerri Durnell Schuiling, PhD, CNM (ret), NP, FACNM, FAAN

Frances E. Likis, DrPH, NP, CNM, FACNM, FAAN

Founding co-editors of Gynecologic Health Care

CONTRIBUTORS

Evelyn Addo-Wallace, DNP, MPH, WHNP-BC
Assistant Professor and Assistant Director of DNP Scholarly Projects
Berkeley School of Nursing
Georgetown University
Washington, DC
I am a Black, heterosexual, cisgender woman, nurse practitioner, educator, and health equity advocate of African descent. My clinical and academic work as a women's health nurse practitioner has been shaped by over a decade of providing care to marginalized communities across the Northeast United States. My content expertise focuses on advancing health equity and reducing racial disparities in gynecologic and reproductive health outcomes for minoritized women and birthing people.

Ivy M. Alexander, PhD, APRN, ANP-BC, FAANP, FAAN
Clinical Professor
Elisabeth DeLuca School of Nursing; School of Medicine
University of Connecticut
Storrs, Connecticut
I am a straight, white woman, mom, partner, sister, daughter, aunt, cousin, and friend, with ancestors originating from Western and Northern Europe. My research, clinical expertise, and program development focus on midlife women's health (especially menopause symptom management; osteoporosis prevention, identification, and management; and disease prevention) and increasing access to high-quality primary care, including sexual and reproductive health care, for medically underserved and disadvantaged persons.

Amy Alspaugh, PhD, CNM, FACNM
Assistant Professor
University of Tennessee, Knoxville
Knoxville, Tennessee
I am a straight, white, cisgender woman, nurse midwife, researcher, and educator from Appalachia. My goal in both research and teaching is ensuring patient-centered, respectful, and holistic care is available to everyone regardless of identity, location, or resources.

Tia Andrighetti, DNP, CNM, CNE, CHSE-A, FACNM
Associate Professor
Innovation Coach-Simulation Coordinator
Frontier Nursing University
Versailles, Kentucky
I am a white, cisgender woman, nurse, midwife, and educator from rural New Hampshire. My perspective is shaped by growing up in a non-ethnically diverse state, then moving to and practicing nursing and midwifery in a very ethnically diverse area. Much of my career has been spent teaching midwifery students and now educating faculty on the use of simulation in the education of various advanced practice nursing specialties.

Kathryn Atkin, DNP, WHNP-BC, ANP-BC
Assistant Professor
Berkeley School of Nursing
Georgetown University
Washington, DC
Beth Israel Deaconess Plymouth OB/GYN and Midwifery
Plymouth, Massachusetts
I am a cisgender woman, nurse practitioner, and educator. My scholarly work explores the intersection of environmental health and reproductive outcomes, with a focus on how climate-related exposures disproportionately affect women and pregnant people and contribute to racial disparities in perinatal health. I am dedicated to advancing health equity by translating research into practice and promoting policies that support safe and equitable care, and I foster a learning environment that prepares students to deliver evidence-based, patient-centered prenatal, sexual, and reproductive health care.

Zahra Amirkhanzadeh Barandouzi, PhD, RN
Assistant Professor
Nell Hodgson Woodruff School of Nursing
Emory University
Atlanta, Georgia
I am a nurse scientist and educator whose personal and professional experiences have been shaped by immigration and cross-cultural perspectives. My work focuses on advancing equity in clinical research and improving outcomes for people with cancer through rigorous science and meaningful community engagement. I bring expertise in cancer symptom assessment and management, biobehavioral research, and interdisciplinary collaboration to support inclusive and person-centered care.

Nicole (Nikki) R. Clark, DNP, APRN, FNP-BC
Specialty Instructor
Oakland University
Rochester, Michigan
I am a white, heterosexual, cisgender woman from Rochester, MI. I practice as a family nurse practitioner, and I am an educator at Oakland University. My clinical expertise includes primary care and preventive medicine. My research interests include quality improvement in primary care and collegiate health.

Desireé Mullis Clement, DNP, APRN, CNM, FNP-BC, FACNM, FAANP, FAAN
Associate Professor
Assistant Dean for Academic Operations
Nell Hodgson Woodruff School of Nursing
Emory University
Atlanta, Georgia
I am a white, cisgender woman, nurse midwife, family nurse practitioner, and nurse educator. I am also a proud Navy Veteran, nurse leader, and educator. I have been a nurse for 30 years, a midwife for 23 years, and a family nurse practitioner for 11 years. Presently, I teach graduate level nursing education across multiple program levels along with being an administrator who helps manage 200+ full-time faculty and researchers at a large urban university within the southeastern United States. My areas of research focus mainly on innovative teaching strategies, simulation development for enhancing student learning, clinical instructor and preceptor skills training, and modernizing state statutes that remove barriers on APRN scope of practice in Georgia. My deep understanding of various pedagogical approaches, along with my experience holding multiple leadership roles within academe and health care, help with fostering my abilities to mentor others in their professional development and assists both faculty and students.

Susanrachel B. Condon, CM, DM, FACNM
Assistant Professor and Interim Program Director, Midwifery, School of Health Professions
SUNY Downstate Health Science University
Brooklyn, New York
I am a certified midwife with a doctorate in midwifery in full-scope clinical practice and a midwifery educator. My research, commitment to reproductive justice, and hands-on approach to didactic and clinical midwifery education is informed by three decades of witnessing nonconsensual examinations and obstetric violence perpetrated on people across the age, socioeconomic, ethnic, and racial spectra in all practice settings. As a midwife, I strive to model an approach to providing respectful, culturally humble reproductive care across the life span. As a didactic educator and clinical preceptor, I endeavor to nurture emerging clinicians, many of whom come from communities of color and/or are immigrants, toward sustainable and fulfilling careers in midwifery.

Katie DePalma, DNP, CNM, WHNP-BC, FACNM
Assistant Professor
Berkeley School of Nursing
Georgetown University
Washington, DC
I am a queer, partnered, nonbinary, able-bodied, neurodiverse white Irish-American. My work as a nurse midwife, nurse practitioner, and educator is grounded in the need to replace oppressive structures and systems with those that are based in self-determination, connectedness, and collective liberation.

Sarah M. Dorsey, MS, CNM
Certified Nurse Midwife
Intermountain Health, St. Vincent Regional Hospital
Billings, Montana
I am a white, heterosexual, cisgender woman, and nurse midwife originally from Boise, Idaho. The focus of my career as a midwife is to improve access to midwifery and mental health care in rural states.

Taneesha Douglas, CNM, MSN, MBA
Clinical Associate Professor of Nursing
Nurse-Midwifery Program
Bethel University
Saint Paul, Minnesota
I am a Black woman, practicing nurse midwife, and educator with over two decades of experience in nursing and midwifery. My perspective is shaped by my experiences as a Black woman providing care in diverse communities and by my years of practice in birth centers since 2010. My professional focus centers on reducing health disparities, advancing equitable and person-centered maternity care, and exploring the intersections of health and spirituality in reproductive health.

Nora Drummond, DNP, CNM, FNP, FACNM
Clinical Assistant Professor
University of Michigan
Ann Arbor, Michigan
My research explores the intersection of chronic disease and pregnancy within today's technology-driven cultural landscape. Drawing from my experiences supporting families as a nurse midwife and family nurse practitioner, I have developed an interest in understanding the ways health information, misinformation, and the development of online cultures influence family health outcomes. Additionally, my perspective as a white mother within a mixed-race family provides both personal and professional insight into the complex realities of embedded advantage and disadvantage in our healthcare system. This combination of lived experience and clinical practice fuels my commitment to advancing more equitable and informed maternal and family health, with an emphasis on navigating and harnessing emerging technologies to support families in today's digital environment.

Meghan Eagen-Torkko, PhD, CNM, FACNM
Associate Dean of Academic and Clinical Affairs and Associate Professor
Wayne State University
Detroit, Michigan
I am a neurodivergent, white, queer, cisgender woman, the daughter of a working-class family, a first-generation college graduate, a wife, a nurse, a midwife, and a mother. I started working in abortion care in 1997, and my scholarship and clinical practice center around identifying and interrogating the relationships between power and sexual and reproductive health. Trauma theory and reproductive justice principles are foundational to my scholarly and clinical work, and I have had the honor to care for patients of all genders in Title X clinics for my entire midwifery career.

Melicia Escobar, DNP, CNM, WHNP-BC, FACNM
Associate Professor and Program Director, Nurse-Midwifery/WHNP & WHNP Programs
Berkeley School of Nursing
Georgetown University
Washington, DC
Midwife
Jefferson Health
East Norris, Pennsylvania
I am a Latina cisgender woman, nurse midwife, WHNP-BC, first-gen college graduate, and educator from Philadelphia, PA with ancestors from Colombia, Western Europe, and the Philippines. My perspective is shaped by the immigrant work ethic, being a first-generation student in higher education, lived and clinical experience in the U.S. health system, and Quaker and Jesuit education. My focus as an educator is to advance midwifery and WHNP education through innovative curriculum design and implementation that promotes health equity, reproductive justice, and person-centered care.

Mara Evans, DNP, CNM
Assistant Professor, Nurse-Midwifery/WHNP and WHNP Programs
Berkeley School of Nursing
Georgetown University
Washington, DC
I am a white, heterosexual, cisgender woman, nurse midwife, and educator born in Madison, Wisconsin and now living in the Blue Ridge Mountains of North Carolina. My perspective is shaped by 15 years of practice in the hospital, birth center, and humanitarian setting. My teaching and scholarship focus on midwifery education, reproductive justice, and equitable global partnerships that strengthen perinatal and newborn health.

Heidi Collins Fantasia, PhD, RN, WHNP-BC, FNAP, FAAN
Professor and Department Chair
Solomont School of Nursing, Zuckerberg College of Health Sciences
University of Massachusetts, Lowell
Lowell, Massachusetts
I am a white, heterosexual, cisgender woman, researcher, academic, and women's health nurse practitioner of Western European ancestry. My perspective is shaped by three decades of providing care to minoritized people and communities. My research focuses on the intersection of violence and the reproductive health of women and individuals.

Wendy R. Gibbons, DNP, CNM, MN, FACNM
Assistant Professor, Clinical Track
Nell Hodgson Woodruff School of Nursing
Emory University
Atlanta, Georgia
I am a multi-race, cisgender woman, nurse, and midwife with ancestral roots in Western Europe and the Northern American Plains. For over three decades, I have practiced in Georgia across birth center and high-risk obstetric settings—experiences that have shaped a comprehensive perspective on reproductive health. My teaching and clinical practice emphasize enhancing the birth and healthcare experience by integrating patient values, cultural contexts, and evidence-based practice, while recognizing that healthcare systems have historically privileged certain voices and marginalized others. As an educator, I am committed to preparing nurses and midwives to engage critically with clinical practice, honor patient autonomy, respect cultural variation, and advance equitable, humanistic, and person-centered care.

Lisa M. Hachey, DNP, APRN-CNM, FACNM
Associate Professor of Clinical Nursing
University of Cincinnati, College of Nursing
Cincinnati, Ohio
I am a nurse midwife, educator, and innovator with more than three decades of clinical practice across diverse care settings. My expertise spans trauma-informed care, midwifery education, and the design of technology-driven solutions—including simulation, patent work, and AI applications—to advance equitable health care and strengthen clinical training through future-oriented innovation.

Hanne S. Harbison, MHSPH, MSN, WHNP-BC
Advanced Senior Lecturer
University of Pennsylvania School of Nursing
Philadelphia, Pennsylvania
I am a white, queer, cisgender woman, wife, mother and women's health gender-related nurse practitioner and educator with ancestors from Western Europe. My practice and research interests are in reducing disparities in sexual and reproductive health through provider education. I have expertise in vaginitis, sexually transmitted diseases, and menopause care.

Paige Hardy, DNP, APRN, CNM
Associate Professor of Nursing
Bethel University
Saint Paul, Minnesota
I am a white, cisgender woman, mom, step-mom, grandma, wife, sister, nurse midwife, and professor. I have been practicing nurse-midwifery in rural Minnesota since 2003. My clinical experience includes working as a full-scope midwife and sexual assault nurse examiner. My career is driven by a commitment to bridging the gap in healthcare access for rural populations. As an educator, my goal is to mentor the next generation of clinicians, modeling the compassionate, evidence-based care that every woman deserves—regardless of her zip code.

Ella T. Heitzler, PhD, WHNP-BC, FNP-BC, RNC-OB, FNPWH
Associate Professor
Berkeley School of Nursing
Georgetown University
Washington, DC
I am a white, straight, cisgender woman, wife, mother, women's health nurse practitioner, educator, and researcher with roots in the Appalachian Mountains. My clinical experience is anchored in gynecologic and sexual health care, while my research explores the screening of cis and transgender patients for a history of sexual violence.

Abigail Howe-Heyman, PhD, CNM, RN, FACNM
Director, Midwifery Track/Practice Associate Professor
University of Pennsylvania School of Nursing
Philadelphia, Pennsylvania
I am a midwife, nurse, educator, and researcher. My clinical experience includes working as a full-scope midwife, a sexual assault nurse examiner, and, currently, as a provider of gynecologic care to undocumented Spanish-speaking patients. These experiences, as well as my experiences working with learners from many walks of life and backgrounds, inform my practice and scholarship.

Annette Jakubisin-Kanicki, PhD, APRN, ANP-BC, FNP-BC, FAANP, FAAN
Clinical Professor
Associate Dean for Graduate Studies
University of Connecticut, Elisabeth DeLuca School of Nursing
Storrs, Connecticut
I am a white woman, wife, mother, and nurse and a first-generation college graduate educated in the foothills of Appalachia. These lived experiences have shaped my understanding of structural inequities, access to education, and the importance of centering diverse perspectives in my professional work. As a certified nurse practitioner and professor with extensive clinical practice and decades of leadership in graduate nursing education, I specialize in clinical practice, curriculum development, and advancing nurse practitioner preparation to meet the needs of diverse populations. My scholarship and practice center on women's health, cardiovascular health promotion for women, and improving access to health care for underserved communities.

Lisa Kane Low, PhD, CNM, FACNM, FAAN
Professor
School of Nursing
Department of Women and Gender Studies
University of Michigan
Ann Arbor, Michigan
I am a midwife, educator, and researcher who has spent her career focusing on creating strategies and models of care to optimize the experience of pregnancy and childbirth for all families. I am a white, cisgender woman, wife, mother, and recently nana who combines my love of family with being an advocate for and ally with diverse individuals and communities to prioritize equity and shared opportunity.

Deborah Brandt Karsnitz, DNP, CNM, CNE, FACNM
Professor
Frontier Nursing University
Versailles, Kentucky
I am a white, cisgender woman, nurse midwife, and advanced practice educator, originally from Pennsylvania and currently residing in Kentucky. My primary focus of expertise and dissemination has focused on the care of women during postpartum, in particular, postpartum complications and perinatal mood and anxiety disorders, as well as maternal morbidity and mortality in the United States.

L'Oréal Kennedy, MD, DNP
Resident
Stanford University
Palo Alto, California
I am a Black, queer, cisgender woman, descendent of the enslaved, first-generation college student, nurse midwife, physician, and current OB/GYN resident. My purpose is rooted in Black resistance, a commitment to reproductive equity and justice among marginalized communities, and an undying dedication to dismantling systemic oppression. As a future gynecologic oncologist, I will continue to center these values and remain devoted to improving cancer prevention and treatment for historically and contemporarily excluded populations.

Sarah K-M. Maguire, DNP, CNM, NP-C
Adjunct Lecturer
University of Michigan
Ann Arbor, Michigan
I am a white, straight, cisgender woman, nurse practitioner, nurse midwife, and educator who was raised in rural northern Michigan. My experience with the foster care system has guided my interest in healthcare access for incarcerated individuals and barriers to care for those who are economically marginalized. I acknowledge my privileged access to education and resources, and I continuously strive to be mindful of my biases as a care provider.

Elizabeth Mayerson, DNP, RN, APRN, FNP-BC, CNE
Assistant Clinical Professor
Director of Prelicensure Programs
Elisabeth DeLuca School of Nursing
University of Connecticut
Storrs, Connecticut
I am a Caucasian, heterosexual, cisgender woman, primary care nurse practitioner, nurse educator, and nurse leader. My content expertise includes primary care, women's health, pharmacology, substance misuse, and nursing education.

Kelly McBroom, PhD, CNM, FACNM
Assistant Professor
Seattle University College of Nursing
Seattle, Washington
I am a white cisgender woman, midwife, educator, and researcher. My firstborn infant died of congenital CMV, leading to my research interests in perinatal palliative care and infectious disease. I have lived and worked extensively in the global South, so I bring sensitivity to issues facing immigrants and indigenous communities and leverage my privilege to center these voices.

Heather McCracken, DNP, APRN-CNP, WHNP-BC
Assistant Professor
University of Cincinnati, College of Nursing
Cincinnati, Ohio
As a women's health nurse practitioner, educator, wife, mother, and daughter, my perspective has been shaped by the stories and experiences of the women I have encountered. These interactions have taught me the importance of listening and advocating for equitable, patient-centered care. I believe every person deserves to be seen and heard. My goal is to create learning environments that foster empathy and prepare providers to deliver compassionate care while improving the healthcare experience for those we serve.

Linda McDaniel, DNP, CNM, WHNP, FACNM, RNFA
Assistant Professor
Frontier Nursing University
Versailles, Kentucky
I am a passionate educator and clinician who serves professionally as an Assistant Professor and Certified Nurse Midwife. I bring over 15 years of clinical practice in women's health, providing me with firsthand insight into the complexities of patient management and care systems. My contribution to this work is informed by this extensive clinical background, ensuring that theoretical concepts are grounded in real-world application.

Joanne Motino Bailey, PhD, CNM
Director, Nurse-Midwifery, Michigan Medicine and Collegiate Lecturer, Women's and Gender Studies
University of Michigan
Ann Arbor, Michigan
I am a straight, white, cisgender woman, director of nurse-midwifery, and lecturer. My expertise is in midwifery care practices and weaving together the social construction of health within a biomedical world.

Elizabeth G. Muñoz, DNP, CNM, FACNM
Assistant Professor of Nursing
The University of Alabama at Birmingham
Birmingham, Alabama
Carle Foundation Hospital
Urbana, Illinois
I am a white, cisgender woman, nurse midwife, and midwifery educator born and raised in rural Alabama, now living in Illinois. My career as a midwife has been shaped by my previous career as an actor and artist, which informs everything from teaching style to how I make connections with those for whom I provide care. My scholarly work has focused on decreasing body size bias and bias toward pregnant individuals with substance use disorders.

Signey M. Olson, DNP, CNM, WHNP-BC, FACNM
Assistant Professor
Berkeley School of Nursing
Georgetown University
Washington, DC
I am a white, queer, partnered, neurodiverse, gender-fluid individual, nurse midwife, nurse practitioner, educator, and gestational parent. In my work and research, I seek to recognize, understand, and dismantle the systemic power dynamics and bias that are deeply intertwined with advancement of health justice and liberation through amplification of community voices with lived experience.

Tamara Pavlik-Maus, MSN, WHNP-BC
Assistant Professor of Clinical Nursing
University of Cincinnati College of Nursing
Cincinnati, Ohio
I am an educator, program director, and doctoral student with over three decades of clinical practice and a continually curious approach to teaching and curriculum development. My perspective is shaped by leading grant-funded simulation initiatives, contributing to technology-driven instructional innovation, and participating in a national multi-site project, work that collectively reflects expertise in clinical simulation, program development, and scholarly collaboration.

Jamie Pelaez, DNP, CNM
Adjunct Faculty
Loyola University New Orleans
New Orleans, LA
As a certified nurse midwife and educator, my perspective is grounded in over 10 years of experience in birthwork. Practicing across diverse regions of the United States as a military spouse has shaped my understanding of how culture, access, and systems of care influence maternal and newborn outcomes. My passion for and experience in community birth further inform my dedication to honoring physiologic birth, autonomy, and health equity.

Keely Robinson, DNP, CNM, ARNP, MA
Clinical Assistant Professor
University of Washington School of Nursing
Seattle, Washington
I am a white, queer, cisgender woman and am proud to be a nurse midwife, advanced practice nurse, and nursing and midwifery educator. I spent the first 10 years of my career in international public health, serving vulnerable communities in Thailand, Haiti, and Eastern Burma. In my current clinical practice, I specialize in complex gynecologic care that is deeply rooted in the tenets of reproductive justice and respect for personal bodily autonomy.

Melissa Romero, PhD, FNP-BC, CNE
Professor and Graduate Program Coordinator
Northern Michigan University
Marquette, Michigan
I am an educator and nurse practitioner from the Upper Peninsula of Michigan. My research and content expertise examines personal growth and grief experiences in caregivers and acute and chronic pelvic pain.

Lee K. Roosevelt, PhD, MPH, CNM, FACNM
Clinical Associate Professor
University of Michigan, School of Nursing
Ann Arbor, Michigan
I am a white, queer, cisgender woman, nurse midwife, educator, researcher, and mother to two neurodiverse children. My work is shaped by more than two decades of clinical practice and a commitment to promoting full-scope midwifery care including abortion and gender-affirming care. As an educator and researcher, I focus on strengthening patient–provider alliance through relational decision making to advance justice-oriented, person-centered care.

Bethany D. Sanders, PhD(c), MSN, CNM
Faculty Attending Nurse Midwife
Vanderbilt University Medical Center
Nashville, Tennessee
I am a white, cisgender, heterosexual woman, nurse midwife, mother, and doctoral candidate with 20 years of experience practicing in full-scope midwifery care in the American South. While I have diverse interests in various aspects of clinical practice, my research focuses on exploring health disparities in maternal health outcomes for Black birthing people, specifically the impact of doula care when patient–provider racial discordance is present. I value patient-centered care with particular weight to patient autonomy.

Christine Alexandra Sargent, DNP, APRN, NP-C
HealthDrive
Middletown, Connecticut
University of Connecticut
Storrs, Connecticut
I am a practicing nurse practitioner with Health Drive Medical Group, seeing patients in the sub-acute, long-term care, and assisted living facility settings. I also hold a doctor of nursing practice degree in which my research and content expertise examines ways to decrease unnecessary polypharmacy through a focus on deprescribing based on patients' individual factors and needs.

Shilpy Sarguru, DNP, WHNP-BC
Nurse Practitioner
Chicago Women's Health Center
Chicago, Illinois

Janell Senda, DNP, CNM, FNP-C
Instructor
Vanderbilt University, Vanderbilt University Medical Center
Nashville, Tennessee
I am a white, straight, cisgender woman, mother, nurse midwife, nurse practitioner, and educator in Nashville, Tennessee. My work has spanned the areas of primary care, gynecologic care, and urgent care. I am currently a proud faculty member at Vanderbilt University School of Nursing.

Stephanie Tillman, PhD, CNM, FACNM
Founder
Feminist Midwife, LLC
I am a white, queer, and genderqueer midwife, ethicist, and educator. My perspectives and scholarship are shaped by sexual assault survivorship, care provision in free clinics and community hospital settings, and feminist and queer ethics. In my career I hope to offer trauma-informed practices for patient empowerment alongside forthright critiques of the healthcare industrial complex.

Jessica Wellette, DNP, APRN, WHNP-BC
Assistant Professor
Vanderbilt University School of Nursing
Nashville, Tennessee
I am a white, heterosexual woman, nurse, women's health nurse practitioner, and nursing educator from Tennessee. My nursing career has focused on improving women's health care and nursing education. My research and content expertise have centered around gynecology, obstetrics, sexual dysfunction, doula care, nursing pedagogy, and simulation.

Bethany Rolfe Witham, DNP, FNP-BC
Associate Teaching Professor
DNP Program Director, School of Nursing DNP Program
University of Washington
Seattle, Washington
Sea Mar Community Health Center
Seattle, WA
I am a white, cisgender woman, family nurse practitioner, and educator. My perspective is shaped by over 20 years of experience working in Federally Qualified Health Centers (FQHCs), and a deep commitment to equitable, culturally responsive, person-centered care. My research centers on designing and implementing culturally grounded interventions that address the unique needs of patients and learners, ensuring care and education are accessible and inclusive.

Matthew Witkovic, DNP, FNP-BC

Katrina Wu, PhD, CNM
Midwife
Twin Cities Birth Center
Saint Paul, Minnesota
I am a white, queer, cisgender woman with over a decade of experience in nurse-midwifery clinical practice and education. My practice and research focus includes community birth practice settings, telemedicine, and improving access to culturally congruent care.

Andrea H. Zengion, ND, CNM, WHNP-BC, LAc, EAMP
Assistant Teaching Professor
University of Washington School of Nursing
Seattle, Washington
I am a white, queer, cisgender woman, midwife, educator, naturopathic doctor, and acupuncturist with ancestors from Eastern and Western Europe. My work centers on providing trauma-informed, bias-informed patient care, and on educating and empowering future providers, with an emphasis on trauma-informed care and pedagogy; fostering compassion; and decreasing bias in educational and clinical spaces.

Ruth E. Zielinski, PhD, CNM
Clinical Professor
University of Michigan School of Nursing – Midwifery Program
Ann Arbor, Michigan
I am a white, cisgender woman who spent my childhood in the Middle East and Pakistan. I have been a midwife for 30 years and faculty in a midwifery program for 12 years. I have had the opportunity to collaborate with midwives, other providers, and community leaders in Sub-saharan Africa, Haiti, Mongolia, Myanmar, and Denmark. The focus of my research and clinical practice is improving maternal health through scholarship and community, pre-service, and continuing education.

SECTION

1

Introduction to Gynecologic Health Care

CHAPTER 1

A Feminist Perspective on Health

Lisa Kane Low
Joanne Motino Bailey

HEALTH CARE AND GYNECOLOGIC HEALTH

The state of health care today reflects the intersections of the varied identities we hold combined with our position in society. Many healthcare advances have been made, yet comprehensive, compassionate healthcare services that address the complexity and diversity of how we live our lives and experience health and disease are still lagging.

This text is based on a feminist framework in an effort to advance the quality of health care, initially aimed at addressing disparities in gynecologic health care in today's society. Using a feminist perspective, the complexity of health is considered by paying attention to one's gender and sex status in society and the potential for unequal access to opportunity and power, while focusing on whole person and gynecologic health and well-being. Not all people with gynecologic needs identify as women. The terms "woman" and "women's health" are often exclusionary of transgender women, transgender men, gender-expansive, and nonbinary-identifying individuals. This perpetuates a silence and invisibility to their lived experience of health and health care.

Language remains imperfect as we continue to search for inclusive ways to describe varied experiences regarding health, particularly gynecologic health. In this text, we are using gender-inclusive language to acknowledge all who deserve to access gynecologic health care. We also acknowledge that sexism remains pervasive and avoiding the use of the term "woman" completely also risks erasure of the historical context and subsequent current policies that lead to ongoing disparities in healthcare delivery, research, and outcomes for women and feminine-presenting people. We use the word "woman" and "women" when it is essential to the context and example being presented.

The purpose of this chapter is to provide an overview of the experience of health using a feminist perspective and gender considerations as a lens for exploring gynecologic health. The glossary in **Box 1-1** offers definitions of key terms that are used throughout this text and are linked to feminist critical analysis of gender and health.

WHAT IS FEMINISM?

The author bell hooks (2000) offers a definition of feminism that is well suited for addressing the context in which people experience health and wellness: "feminism is a perspective that acknowledges the oppression of women/feminine-identifying people within a patriarchal society and struggles toward the elimination of sexist oppression and domination for all human beings." Acknowledging the oppression of women is increasingly difficult because affluence and increased opportunities within some sectors of employment and education are construed as equal access or equity in opportunity. However, hooks defines oppression as "not having a choice" (hooks, 2000). With this definition, many more individuals can recognize constraints in their personal experiences. Examples of such practices include unjust labor practices, lower wages for equal work, lack of maternity leave policies, limited access to a range of contraceptive options, policies that deny access to gender-affirming care, and an inability to access desired healthcare providers. These examples indicate the breadth of experiences within the context of a patriarchal society that seeks to deny equal access to power, resources, and opportunities based on gender.

Characteristics of a feminist perspective include the use of critical analysis to question assumptions about societal expectations and the value of various roles on both sociopolitical and individual levels. The process of critical analysis is accomplished by rejecting conceptualizations of individuals who identify as women as homogeneous and acknowledging the range of experiences and expressions of gender. It acknowledges power imbalances and uses the influence of gender as the foremost consideration in the analysis. Using a gender lens that is informed by feminism permits areas of disparity to be identified both among groups, based on gender, and within groups, based on the recognition of heterogeneity.

A feminist health perspective explores the context of how individuals live their lives both collectively and individually within a patriarchal society. The various social, environmental, and economic aspects, or social drivers of health, become integral to understanding the context in which people are able to achieve health and well-being. Furthermore, feminism requires consideration of health, as influenced by the intersection of sexism, racism, class, nation, and gender, within a framework that acknowledges the role of oppression as it affects those who identify as women and their health as individuals and as a group. **Box 1-2** summarizes the components of a feminist perspective when considering health issues or models of care, which can help reframe one's view of the experience of health from a feminist perspective.

BOX 1-1 Glossary of Key Terms

cisgender: An individual whose gender identity coincides with that individual's birth-assigned sex (e.g., a cisgender man is often referred to as simply "man," and a cisgender woman is often referred to as simply "woman").
classism: Discrimination or prejudice on the basis of social class.
discrimination: The prejudicial treatment of an individual based on that person's actual or perceived membership in a certain group or category (e.g., race, ethnicity, sexual orientation, national origin).
feminism: A movement to end sexism, sexist exploitation, and oppression.
gender: Refers to the socially constructed roles, behaviors, expressions and identities of women, men, and gender-diverse people.
homophobia: Prejudice against individuals who carry sexual minority identities respectively (e.g., part of the LGBTQIA+ community).
intersectionality: The unique combination of multiple identities based on race, class, gender, and other characteristics, and the compounded experience of oppression based on these identities.
medicalization: Defining or treating a physiologic process or behavior as a medical condition or disease.
oppression: Exercise of authority or power in an unjust manner; according to hooks (2000), "not having a choice."
patriarchy: A social system of institutions that privileges cis-men, resulting in male domination over access to power, roles, and positions within society.
power: The ability to do something, act in a particular way, or direct/influence others' behavior or a course of events.
race: Socially constructed categorization of individuals and communities based on a combination of physical attributes and cultural heritage.
racism: Individual and structural practices that create and reinforce oppressive systems of race relations.
sex: Biological classification as female, male, or intersex based on chromosomes, genitalia, and reproductive organs.
sexism: Individual and institutional practices that privilege cisgender men over women and gender-diverse people.
social construction: The process by which societal expectations of behavior become interpreted as innate, biologically determined characteristics.
social drivers of health: The conditions, context, or environments where people live, work, learn, worship, play, and age that affect access to health care and healthcare outcomes (also referred to as social determinants of health).
socioeconomic status: An indicator that encompasses income, education, and occupation.
structural racism: Macro-level systems, social forces, institutions, and processes that reinforce oppressive race relations.
transgender or trans: An individual whose gender identity does not coincide with that individual's assigned sex at birth.
transphobia: Prejudice against individuals who are transgender or trans.

BOX 1-2 Components of a Feminist Perspective on Health

- Works *with* individuals as opposed to *for* individuals
- Uses heterogeneity as an assumption, not homogeneity
- Minimizes or exposes power imbalances
- Rejects androcentric models as normative
- Challenges the medicalization and pathologizing of normal physiologic processes
- Seeks social and political change to address health issues

GENDER

What does gender have to do with the experience of health? Although gynecologic health is focused on the female sex (as determined by chromosomes, genitalia, and sexual organs), its priorities are shaped by what are traditionally considered socially important attributes of being a woman (such as reproductive capacity and feminine appearance). Gender is defined as a person's self-representation as man, woman, nonbinary, and/or other gender identities, and the way in which social institutions respond to that person based on the individual's gender presentation. Gender is often congruent with sex (e.g., a person with female genitalia identifies as being a woman, or cisgender), but it can also be incongruent (e.g., a person with female chromosomes may identify as being a man, or transgender man). Sex and gender are irreducibly entangled from both the research and practice perspectives, as most of the research and practice has either assumed a binary gender (e.g., man, woman) or assumed that gender equals sex (e.g., all women are cisgender women, all men are cisgender men).

Gender is a socially constructed attribute that is shaped by biology, environment, and experience and is expressed through appearance and behavior (Fausto-Sterling, 2019). Social construction is the process by which societal expectations of behavior become interpreted as innate characteristics that are biologically determined. Thus, behaviors associated with femininity become confused with innately determined behaviors rather than being recognized as socially constructed behaviors. As a result, health risks, treatments, and approaches to care are not necessarily biologically based aspects of health, but rather they are determined by social expectations rooted in assumptions about gender differences (Van Anders, 2022). In addition, diagnoses can be influenced by gender assumptions regarding behavior or what is socially constructed as feminine behavior. A significant body of literature has documented such influences on the manner of diagnosis and treatment in mental health (Neitzke, 2016) as well as in the mismanagement of women's cardiovascular risks (Lee et al., 2021; Zhao et al., 2020; Leonard et al., 2024) and inadequate education to prevent cardiovascular disease in women (Hilleary et al., 2019; Depa et al., 2022).

Three primary aspects must be considered when examining the impact of gender on health. The first is the priorities assigned to research, treatment, and outcomes in women's health as compared to men's health (Johnson, 2025). The second is the context of gender, including how it affects the process of providing healthcare services, which encompasses an acknowledgment of power differentials. The third aspect is the social construction of gender, including how it affects health. Each aspect has implications for the way people access, receive, and respond to health care. Collectively, these three aspects provide opportunities for us to better understand healthcare experiences and assist in the identification of underlying factors that influence healthcare disparities based on gender.

Social role expectations based on gender can create undue burdens and may subsequently lead to increased health risks. For example, limited access to all contraceptive options creates reproductive health risks. Extensive cultural preoccupation with dieting and thinness may lead to unsafe dieting practices and precipitate eating disorders. Anorexia and bulimia are more prevalent among individuals who identify as women and sexual- and gender-diverse individuals despite the lack of a clear biologic explanation for this predominance.

Another example of a gender-based health risk is the disproportionate amount of violence that individuals who identify as women or trans women experience (Lutgendorf, 2019; Wirtz et al., 2020). Gender-based violence includes any act that results in physical, sexual, or psychological harm or suffering (United Nations General Assembly, 1993). The multiple health consequences of violence reveal the persistent layers of health consequences associated with a gender-based health risk. Refer to Chapters 15 and 16 for further discussion of this topic.

INTERSECTIONALITY

Gender interacts with many other identities that affect healthcare delivery and outcomes. Intersectionality is the unique combination of multiple identities based on race, socioeconomic status (SES), gender, nation status, ability, and other factors, as well as the experience of oppression based on these identities (Crenshaw, 1989). Disparities in health outcomes are often better explained by considering the intersections of multiple forms of oppression based on identity (Etherington, 2015; Smith, 2021). For example, people of color with low SES often receive different health services and have worse health outcomes compared to more affluent white people. Although low SES is the single most powerful contributor to illness and premature death (Mena & Bolte, 2019), there are numerous examples of worse health outcomes based on race even after controlling for SES (Williams et al., 2019).

Disparities in health outcomes across racial differences are often assumed to be genetic or biologic, referred to as biological determinism. In reality the disparities are significantly driven by social forces of discrimination or racism. Discrimination is unjust treatment that is based on appearance or identity and is often described primarily as an interpersonal construct (e.g., a person expressing racist opinions). Even more damaging than interpersonal discrimination is systemic or structural discrimination; such injustice perpetuates large-scale, often invisible processes, policies, systems, or structures (e.g., underfunded school systems in poor districts, locations of subsidized housing) that are much harder to dismantle than individual opinions. Structural discrimination impacts the social, political, geographic, and economic influences on health, yet it is very difficult to quantify and often is misidentified (Krieger et al., 2022). There are numerous examples of the negative effects of racism and discrimination within health care at the individual, community, and structural levels. Medical racism refers to situations in which a healthcare professional's clinical decision making, treatment decisions and health care encounters are influenced by a patient's race (Davis, 2019) or assumptions about race and biological determinism. This can occur at the level of individual interactions or can be institutionalized in the form of using race as a determinant in health care calculations of risk or benefits for treatments that assume biological determinism (Hernandez-Boussard et al., 2023). An additional example of the interactions between discrimination on an individual pairing with structural discrimination is the concept of "Obstetric Racism" (Davis 2019; Odems et al., 2024). Obstetric racism is the intersection of gender-based obstetric violence, a form of reproductive control and abuse, combined with medical racism (Davis, 2019; Odems et al., 2024).

SOCIAL DRIVERS OF HEALTH

The structural components of where we live, learn, work, and play (social drivers of health) impact health across the lifespan (Lumpkin, 2021; CMS, 2024). Where we live encompasses factors such as access to living space with good air quality, access to safe drinking water, access to green space, a safe environment for spending time outdoors, local grocery stores with high-quality fresh food, neighborhood and community support, and even the distance to a place of employment, which dictates the ability to walk to work versus having a lengthy car commute. Where we learn incorporates factors such as access to well-equipped, safe schools with challenging and engaging curricula that teach skills to prepare students for high-quality employment and future life skills. Where we work reflects access to living wages, safe working conditions, healthcare benefits, and a sense of meaningful work. Where we play includes types of recreation that promote physical activity, community connection, and long-term healthy behaviors such as exercise. Feminist considerations in relation to health disparities in these areas include race, ethnicity, and gender bias in hiring, access to resources, availability of healthcare providers, and contraceptive options. Policies or practices that impose undue stress or limit access based on gender contribute to health disparities and are a form of structural bias.

Understanding access and delivery of gynecologic health requires a grasp of gender-based disparities and the multiple factors such as types of medical care, geographic location, migration, acculturation, sexism, racism, exposure to stress, and access to resources. Only by incorporating these factors into the discussion can we fully and accurately appreciate and begin to address the health disparities people experience.

A MODEL OF CARE BASED ON A FEMINIST PERSPECTIVE

A model of care that is based on a feminist perspective contrasts sharply with a biomedical model, particularly in the areas of power and control, as well as in the definition of what is health compared to pathology. A feminist model supports egalitarian relationships and identifies the person as the expert on their own body. The person is at the center of this healthcare model. The following key points provide further insights into a feminist-based model of care:

- The model of care must focus on *being with*, not *doing for* the person. This frames the model of care as a partnership as opposed to a model of care in which treatment decisions are directed by others and then dictated to the person.
- Heterogeneity, rather than homogeneity, is assumed. Using broad generalizations like "all women," with their inherent exclusionary, gender-based assumptions, essentializes people rather than acknowledging diversity among individuals and across experiences. An assumption of heterogeneity considers people on an individual basis, tailoring health care and services to everyone's unique needs rather than treating all who seek gynecologic health care as a uniform group with the assumption of similarity across all considerations of health.
- The feminist model of care seeks to minimize or expose power imbalances that are inherent in most current healthcare models, especially those based on a biomedical model. Power should be distributed equally within the healthcare interaction, and the interaction should be based on a belief in an individual's right to self-determination and their self-knowledge of their body. Therefore, the role of the clinician focuses on providing support, information, education, and skillful knowledge, as opposed to asserting authority over the decision-making ability of the individual.
- A feminist framework rejects androcentric models of health and disease as normative. The pervasiveness in healthcare research and practice of male-based models being extrapolated to the female body assumes they are merely a biologic variant of men. This misapplication of androcentric models within health also serves to medicalize or pathologize normal physiologic processes, such as menstruation, childbirth, and menopause (Councilor & Fink, 2024; Nisha, 2021). Medicalization is the process of labeling conditions as diseases or disorders as a basis for providing medical treatment. In contrast, the feminist model acknowledges as normal those physiologic changes that occur over an individual's lifespan, such as menarche and menopause.
- The medicalization of biologic functions, such as menstruation, pregnancy, and menopause, is frequently cited as an illustration of both the social construction of disease and the general expansion of medical control into everyday life (Nisha, 2021; Conrad, 1992; Zola, 1972).
- A feminist framework acknowledges the broader context in which individuals live their lives (social drivers of health) and the subsequent challenges to their health as a result of living within a patriarchal society. It argues for a process of social and political change that would eliminate gender bias and sexism. This includes consideration of how the personal health decisions and healthcare interactions a person experiences are influenced by the larger structural and political context in which people live their lives, including access to services and resources.

SOCIAL MODELS VERSUS BIOMEDICAL MODELS OF HEALTH

As the discussion of the social construction of gender and its relationship to health unfolds, it becomes evident that a broader model of health must be employed to address the health consequences of gender bias and sexism and their implications for overall health and well-being. The first step in broadening the model of health requires redefining health itself. Health is predominately biomedically defined as the absence of disease—a narrow definition that does not address the context in which the absence of disease may occur. Considering only the absence of disease fails to address quality of life or the opportunity to reach the individual's potential. To gain a fuller appreciation of the scope of health, the dominance of the medical model as the rubric that defines health must be challenged to broaden the lens of what is health and to expand its definition. Without a broader definition, opportunities to understand the social realities and complexities within the healthcare system and the experiences of health for an individual and the collective community will remain limited. Without a broader perspective, which aspects of health are understood or studied will also be limited to individual characteristics or behaviors devoid of the context in which those behaviors and/or experiences are occurring. The biomedical model, as a conceptualization of health, generally does not address health beyond an individual perspective.

An alternative to the biomedical definition of health is offered by the World Health Organization (WHO), which defines health as "a state of complete physical, mental, and social well-being and not merely the absence of disease or infirmity" (WHO, n.d.). This broader definition is based on assumptions of what must be present to secure health for individuals and the community in which they live. It addresses the social context in which individuals live their lives, including the communities where they live, work, and play. According to WHO, the following prerequisites must be in place before health can occur:

- Freedom from the fear of war
- Equal opportunity for all
- Satisfaction of basic needs for food, water, sanitation, education, and decent housing
- Secure work
- Useful role in society
- Political will
- Public support

Germane to this definition is the commitment to address social injustice, equity, economic development and opportunity, and accessibility of healthcare services as a basic human right for all individuals in any society. WHO's definition of health requires that the community and environment in which people live must also be considered in the same context as a new medical procedure. The constraints of an individualistic biomedical model of health that focuses only on disease become readily apparent when the WHO's broader context and definition of health are considered. Using this definition of health, the social aspects of health and the contributors to health are acknowledged, broadening the lens to include factors that must be addressed to support individual and collective health.

A social model of health is more congruent with a feminist perspective, compared to the biomedical model. The social model of health expands the contributors to health beyond just the individual body, extending them to the family, community, and society. This broader perspective enhances the understanding of health disparities that are rooted in the social and cultural forces that affect how individuals live their lives. Broadly, this model of health is being incorporated more frequently in healthcare delivery as social drivers of health are assessed, such as housing instability, food insecurity, and experiences of violence.

The interconnectedness of working and living conditions, environmental conditions, and access to community-based healthcare services becomes a focus when health and well-being are framed within a social context. Questions about health and well-being for an individual focus on these factors as well as lifestyle decisions and health habits. The prevention of health problems requires social accountability in combination with individual responsibility. This wider emphasis, in turn, forces greater consideration of the various social drivers of health and structural discrimination that can either support or degrade an individual's health.

A social model of health also requires asking questions about the health effects of socially situated factors such as racism, sexism, and other forms of oppression. A whole person-centered model of health is a requirement of the feminist social model of health care. The broader social models do not ignore biologic or genetic components of health, nor is the significance of individual health habits denied. However, the broader social model frames these issues as important to health, but no more so than experiences within everyday life, access to healthcare services, economic disparities, racial or ethnic identity, and membership within a community. The feminist social model of health also acknowledges the structural constraints that are present such as racism, sexism, homophobia, and transphobia that create policy and practice barriers to achieving health.

The health risks associated with the social construction of gender and the inequities associated with gender-based assumptions are essential components of the feminist social model of health. As links are forged among human rights, social justice, social models of health, health disparities, and opportunities to address those disparities, a feminist perspective offers new strategies and ways of thinking or asking questions that can promote expanded approaches to health issues.

FEMINIST STRATEGIES FOR THE ANALYSIS OF HEALTH

Several aspects of analysis are important when considering health from a feminist perspective. The following strategies for analyzing health using a feminist framework were originally adapted from Franz and Stewart's (1994) strategies for conducting feminist research and later updated to integrate contemporary definitions, language, and feminist theoretical perspectives. Each of the strategies listed in **Table 1-1** can be used to form a question one can ask about health issues. Taken together, they constitute a feminist lens that allows for new considerations to arise as health issues are reframed. The following discussion highlights the way some of the strategies can be applied.

Look for What Has Been Left Out or What We Do Not Know

This strategy is particularly applicable to investigations into the scientific basis of gynecologic health. Much of what we know about health needs, outside of reproductive health, is historically based on androcentric models. Until the 1990s almost all medical research that was not related to maternity care or gynecology was conducted using male participants (human and animal), with the findings then being generalized to everyone.

Consumer health advocates, health activists, and members of the scientific community have been instrumental in coming together to address the many limitations concerning women's health care and scientific investigations of women's health issues. In 1993, the National Institutes of Health's (NIH) Revitalization Act was considered a milestone in addressing sex and gender as well as racial representation in science. The Revitalization Act required that females and people of color, and their subpopulations, be included in all NIH-supported biomedical and behavioral research, including phase 3 clinical trials, in numbers adequate to ensure valid analysis of differences in intervention effects; that the cost not be the basis for exclusion from clinical trials; and that outreach programs to recruit these individuals for clinical trials are adequately supported. As a result of this policy change, important progress has been documented in terms of significantly greater inclusion of a wider representation of the population in research investigations.

Consider the Risks and Benefits of Speaking in Terms of Groups Versus Individuals

Reclaiming control of health care to be person-centered and away from clinicians and focusing on a person's role and authority over their own health was initially promoted by well-educated white, straight, cisgender women from middle- and higher-income groups. This limited view within the women's health movement of the 1970s–1980s revealed the problematic underpinnings of presumed homogeneity across all women and was exclusionary in who was actually referred to in the use of the term "women." Essentially, this wave of the women's health movement could be critiqued as assuming homogeneity of women's health issues rather than heterogeneity. It treated women's health as a monolith with equal application of issues and focus across everyone. In response, the National Black Women's Health Project was launched in 1983 by Byllye Avery, with the goal of understanding Black women's health issues in the broader social context. This project, which was eventually renamed the Black Women's Health Imperative, remains the only national organization dedicated to improving the health and wellness of Black women (Black Women's Health Imperative, 2015). Importantly, this organization defines its goal as addressing health and wellness through a framework that includes physical, emotional, and financial aspects, thereby incorporating social considerations and the biological elements of health.

From a practical standpoint, this meant that instead of everyone working within one organization on what presumably are issues for all women's health, individual organizations, representing and defined by various individuals and groups, could organize to address their specific health concerns. However, the various organizations could build alliances and coalitions with one another when issues of common interest were identified

TABLE 1-1 Strategies for Analysis of Health from a Feminist Perspective

Strategies	Questions
Look for what has been left out or what we do not know.	• What do we know, how do we know it, and who knows it? • Why don't we know? What do we want to know and why? • Who determines what is left out or who has access to what we want to know?
Analyze your own role or relationship to the issue or topic.	• Is it personal? What is the meaning of this issue for you as an individual? • Is it political? What is the meaning of this issue for you as a member of an identified group? • Depending on your relationship to the issue, can you be objective in its analysis or are you engaged personally and subjectively? • Are you invested in the outcome or topic or not? • Why do you care about the issue?
Identify a person's agency in the midst of social constraints and the biomedical paradigm.	• Are people really just victims, or are they acting with agency? • Are individuals making choices despite positions of less power or influence? • Are the choices allowing individuals to remain in control, or do they allow individuals to have some form of power in the context of the situation? • By identifying a person's agency in a particular context, can we learn new ways of understanding or approach to the health implications?
Consider the social construction of gender and how its assumptions may be used to define what health is, limit options, or presume which behaviors and/or choices can be made within the context of health.	• Explore gendered assumptions about the value of anatomy such as breasts or facial appearance. • Would this health issue be defined or explored in the same manner if it primarily affected only one sex? • Do socially prescribed gender norms influence how this health condition is understood or defined (e.g., mental health)?
Explore the precise ways in which gender defines or affects power relationships and the implications of those power dynamics in terms of health.	• Physician/nurse • Clinician/patient • Parent/adolescent • Husband/wife • Parent/child • Father/daughter • Partnered or not partnered woman • Heterosexual/queer
Identify other significant aspects of an individual's or group's social position and explore the implications of that position as it relates to health issues.	• Consider examples such as an adolescent who is seeking reproductive healthcare services or a same-sex couple seeking fertility services. • Ask who has access to various forms of healthcare services and resources and who does not. • Consider the intersections of race, class, gender, sexuality, and socioeconomic status. • Who has a choice, what constitutes a choice, and who is able to exercise the right to make choices within the context of health?
Consider the risks and benefits of generalizations and speaking in terms of groups versus individuals.	• Who do we mean when we refer to "women" and who are we including or excluding? • Consider who benefits from generalizations or assumptions of homogeneity versus heterogeneity or what are the risks of treating "all women" as a monolith? • Is value placed on having a coherent understanding of a health issue compared to acknowledging diversity or complexity in how the issue is experienced? • Which reflects reality most accurately—a coherent story or an appreciation for diversity in the understanding of the health issue? • When "grouping" occurs, who is missing from the group or who might not be reflected in the group process?

Data from Franz, C., & Stewart, A. (Eds.). (1994). *Women creating lives: Identities, resilience, and resistance*. Westview Press.

(Hart, 2012). This model of multi-organizational focus and amplifying advocacy efforts regarding health issues has continued to grow with current examples including the work of Black Mamas Matter Alliance. In their alliance model, "existing organizations and individuals whose work is deeply rooted in reproductive justice, respectful maternity care, birth justice, and the human rights frameworks" are included (https://blackmamasmatter.org/our partners/). This matrix model acknowledges the unique contributions of the local individual voices and organizations while also seeking to advance a broader health activism agenda on a national scale.

Explore the Precise Ways in Which Gender Defines Power Relationships and the Implications of Those Power Dynamics on Health

Creating health care from a feminist perspective requires the acknowledgment of power differentials between individuals who are consuming health care and those who provide it (clinicians). It also mandates attempts to minimize power differentials by developing a partnership model of care provision. In this model, rather than invoking a level of authority by virtue of being a clinician, the clinician acknowledges the life experiences and knowledge that the person brings to the interaction. What makes a practice feminist is not who provides the health care, but rather how that care is provided, how the clinician thinks about their work, and which populations the clinician works with.

Hierarchical relationships and structures are typically elements of the traditional healthcare delivery system, but feminist practice requires an active process of action to decrease asymmetrical relationships. Examples of simple actions include not having a person undress prior to meeting the clinician so the individual can greet the clinician as an equal rather than from a vulnerable position (naked and wrapped in an ill-fitting paper gown); and having a person check their own weight, as opposed to having someone else do it, to place some accountability for health on their shoulders. These actions send the message that the person can control aspects of their healthcare experiences. Although these simple changes can be readily made in the healthcare office setting, each demonstrates power sharing rather than placing the person in a dependent position for aspects of their health care that they should rightly control.

Checking power imbalances and addressing them, even simply by means of introduction and the way the clinician sits in relation to the person, can give them greater power in the relationship. Careful use of language and terminology must occur in all discussions and information that is provided. Seeking consent before touching or initiating any component of an exam and assuring the person has control over what is or is not done during an examination is required (LoGiudice et al., 2023; Tillman, 2020).

Each of the strategies provide an opportunity to consider the details and the global aspects of health care and the intersection of gender within health issues. These strategies can be applied both individually and collectively. They are not meant to be an exhaustive checklist to determine whether something is being considered from a feminist perspective but rather are meant to serve as guidelines and considerations that allow for the identification of blind spots in how we are able to think about health issues when we are potentially constrained by the limitations of the biomedical model. Using these strategies, clinicians, policy makers, and people themselves can reframe expectations, approaches, and the focus of health research, healthcare delivery, and receipt of healthcare services.

WHY A TEXT ON GYNECOLOGY?

Taking the same feminist strategies we use for analyzing health and applying them to this text on gynecologic aspects of health creates opportunities. Focusing on gynecology for clinicians is important because reframing and expanding considerations of gynecologic health from a feminist perspective may more accurately reflect the experience of gynecologic health for people in their everyday lives. By offering a feminist perspective throughout the chapters in this text, we seek to dispel myths that pathologize normal gynecologic functioning, and we seek to support physiology as opposed to medicalizing it. We also offer a framework for providing gynecologic health care that considers the social, emotional, and intimate and physical nature of this aspect of health care.

References

Black Mamas Matter Alliance. https://blackmamasmatter.org/our-partners/ Accessed November 19, 2024.

Black Women's Health Imperative. (2015). *Our story.* https://bwhi.org/our-story/

Centers for Medicare & Medicaid Services. (2025). Social drivers of health and health-related social needs. CMS.gov. [cited 2024 Nov 23]. from: https://www.cms.gov/priorities/innovation/key-concepts/social-drivers-health-and-health-related-social-needs#:~:text=At%20a%20community%20level%2C%20these,the%20neighborhood%20and%20built%20environment

Conrad, P. (1992). Medicalization and social control. *Annual Review of Sociology, 18*, 209–232.

Councilor, K. C., & Fink, A. E. (2024, June). Gendered bodies: A graphic medicine commentary. *Social Science & Medicine, 351*(Suppl 1), 116436. https://doi.org/10.1016/j.socscimed.2023.116436. Epub 2024 May 31. PMID: 38825376.

Crenshaw, K. (1989). Demarginalizing the intersection of race and sex: A black feminist critique of antidiscrimination doctrine, feminist theory, and antiracist politics. *University of Chicago Legal Forum,* 139–167. Reprinted in D. Kairys (Ed.), *The politics of law: A progressive critique* (2nd ed., pp. 195–217). Pantheon, 1990.

Davis, D. A. (2019). Obstetric racism: The racial politics of pregnancy, labor, and birthing. *Medical Anthropology, 38*(7), 560–573.

Depa, N., Desai, S., Patel, S., Silvi, S., Hanif, S., Rizvi, S., Rahman, F., Ortega, G., Hsieh, Y. C., Malik, P., Pathrose, R. P. M., Parikh, T., & Mansuri, Z. (2022, August). Mental health disparities amongst sexual-minority adolescents of the US—A national survey study of YRBSS-CDC. *Psychiatry Research, 314,* 114635. https://doi.org/10.1016/j.psychres.2022.114635. Epub 2022 May 14. PMID: 35640323.

Etherington, N. (2015). Race, gender, and the resources that matter: An investigation of intersectionality and health. *Women and Health, 55*(7), 754–777.

Fausto-Sterling, A. (2019). Gender/sex, sexual orientation, and identity are in the body: How did they get there? *Journal of Sex Research, 56*(4–5), 529–555. https://doi.org/10.1080/00224499.2019.1581883

Franz, C., & Stewart, A. (Eds.). (1994). *Women creating lives: Identities, resilience, and resistance.* Westview Press.

Hart, E. (2012). *Building a more inclusive women's health movement: Byllye Avery and the development of the National Black Women's Health Project, 1981–1990* [Doctoral dissertation, University of Cincinnati].

Hernandez-Boussard, T., Siddique, S. M., Bierman, A., Hightower, M., & Burstin, H. (2023). Promoting equity in clinical decision-making: Dismantling race-based medicine. *Health Affairs, 42*(10), 1369–1373.

Hilleary, R. S., Jabusch, S. M., Zheng, B., Jiroutek, M. R., & Carter, C. A. (2019). Gender disparities in patient education provided during patient visits with a diagnosis of coronary heart disease. *Women's Health, 15*. https://doi.org/10.1177/1745506519845591

hooks, b. (2000). *Feminism is for everybody*. South End Press.

Johnson, P. A., Brindis, C. D., Donelan, K., et al. (2025). New directions for women's health: Expanding understanding, improving research, addressing workforce limitations. *Health Affairs Project Hope, 44*(2), 156–162. Published online January 22, 2025. https://doi.org/10.1377/hlthaff.2024.01004

Krieger, N., Rowley, D. L., Herman, A. A., Avery, B., & Phillips M. T. (2022, June). REPRINT OF: Racism, sexism, and social class: Implications for studies of health, disease, and well-being. *American Journal of Preventive Medicine, 62*(6), 816–863. https://doi.org/10.1016/j.amepre.2022.04.001. PMID: 35597564.

Lumpkin, J. R., Perla, R., Onie, R., & Seligson, R. (2021). What we need to be healthy—And how to talk about it. *Health Affairs*. May 3, 2021. Accessed January 29, 2025.

Lee, M. T., Mahtta, D., Ramsey, D. J., et al. (2021). Sex-related disparities in cardiovascular health care among patients with premature atherosclerotic cardiovascular disease. *JAMA Cardiology, 6*(7), 782–790. https://doi.org/10.1001/jamacardio.2021.0683

Leonard, S. I., Sharma, Y., Hughes, T. L., Jackman, K. B., & Bruzzese, J. M. (2024, October). Weight stigma and mental and emotional health among sexual and gender minority individuals: A scoping review. *LGBT Health, 11*(7), 496–513. https://doi.org/10.1089/lgbt.2023.0025. Epub 2023 Nov 10. PMID: 37948558.

LoGiudice, J., Tillman, S., and Sarguru, S. (2023). A midwifery perspective on trauma-informed care clinical recommendations. *Journal of Midwifery & Women's Health, 68*(2), 165–169. https://doi.org/10.1111/jmwh.13462

Lutgendorf, M. A. (2019, September). Intimate partner violence and women's health. *Obstetrics and Gynecology, 134*(3), 470–480. https://doi.org/10.1097/AOG.0000000000003326. PMID: 31403968.

Mena, E., Bolte, G., & ADVANCE GENDER Study Group. (2019, December). Intersectionality-based quantitative health research and sex/gender sensitivity: A scoping review. *International Journal for Equity in Health, 18*(1), 199. https://doi.org/10.1186/s12939-019-1098-8. PMID: 31864366; PMCID: PMC6925460.

Neitzke, A. B. (2016). An illness of power: Gender and the social causes of depression. *Culture, Medicine, and Psychiatry, 40*, 59–73. https://doi.org/10.1007/s11013-015-9466-3

Nisha, Z. (2021, September). The medicalisation of the female body and motherhood: Some biological and existential reflections. *Asian Bioethics Review, 14*(1), 25–40. https://doi.org/10.1007/s41649-021-00185-z. PMID: 34925555; PMCID: PMC8636540.

Odems, D. S., Czaja, E., Vedam, S., Evans, N., Saltzman, B., & Scott, K. A. (2024). "It seemed like she just wanted me to suffer": Acts of obstetric racism and birthing rights violations against Black women. *Qualitative Research in Health*, 6, 100479. https://scholars.uky.edu/en/publications/it-seemed-like-she-just-wanted-me-to-suffer-acts-of-obstetric-rac

Smith, N. C. (2021, September). Black-White disparities in women's physical health: The role of socioeconomic status and racism-related stressors. *Social Science Research, 99*, 102593. https://doi.org/10.1016/j.ssresearch.2021.102593. Epub 2021 Jun 3. PMID: 34429206.

Tillman, S. (2020). Consent in pelvic care. *Journal of Midwifery & Women's Health, Special Issue: Ethics in Midwifery and Health Care, 65*(6), 749–758. https://doi.org/10.1111/jmwh.13189

United Nations General Assembly. (1993). *Declaration on the elimination of violence against women*. https://www.un.org/en/genocideprevention/documents/atrocity-crimes/Doc.21_declaration%20elimination%20vaw.pdf

Van Anders, Sari M. (2022). Gender/sex/ual diversity and biobehavioral research. Psychology of Sexual Orien *tation and Gender Diversity, 11*(3), 471–487. https://doi.org/10.1037/sgd0000609

Williams, D. R., Lawrence, J. A., & Davis, B. A. (2019, April). Racism and health: Evidence and needed research. *Annual Review of Public Health, 40*, 105–125. https://doi.org/10.1146/annurev-publhealth-040218-043750. Epub 2019 Feb 2. PMID: 30601726; PMCID: PMC6532402.

Wirtz, A. L., Poteat, T. C., Malik, M., & Glass, N. (2020, April). Gender-based violence against transgender people in the United States: A call for research and programming. *Trauma Violence Abuse, 21*(2), 227–241. https://doi.org/10.1177/1524838018757749. Epub 2018 Feb 13. PMID: 29439615.

World Health Organization. (n.d.). *What is the WHO definition of health?* https://cdn.ymaws.com/www.safestates.org/resource/resmgr/connections_lab/glossary_citation/WHO_Health_Definition.pdf

Zhao, M., Woodward, M., Vaartjes, I., Millett, E. R. C, et al. (2020, My). Sex differences in cardiovascular medication prescription in primary care: A systematic review and meta-analysis. *Journal of the American Heart Association, 9*(11), e0147426. https://doi.org/10.1161/JAHA.119.014742

Zola, I. (1972). Medicine as an institution of social control. *Sociological Review, 20*, 487–504.

CHAPTER 2

Racism, Colonialism, and Inequities in Sexual and Reproductive Health Care

Ellen Solis

Molly R. Altman

We would like to acknowledge the previous authors of this chapter for their contributions: Elizabeth Donnelly, Kim Dau, Karline Wilson-Mitchell, and Jyesha Isis Wren.

INTRODUCTION

People of color, especially Black and Indigenous people, experience gross inequities in health. These health inequities are the actualization of racism and colonialism. The aim of this chapter is to help clinicians address inequities that are rooted in racism and colonialism by understanding and being prepared to address sources of oppression within health care. The chapter begins with key concepts and definitions, followed by a brief history of the development of racism and colonialism in the United States and the history of structural inequities in sexual and reproductive health care. This is followed by a description of applicable theories, frameworks, and concepts for understanding and addressing oppression and guidance interpreting race-related health disparities data. The final section of the chapter presents key interventions for addressing racism and related inequities.

Orientation of the Chapter

All people have different orientations and understandings of racism, colonialism, and other sources of oppression due to our individual lived experiences and positionalities. For people of color who may experience racism and other sources of oppression on an almost daily basis, having required readings that define and describe these experiences often causes harm and has negative impacts on learners. For this reason, we have clearly delineated the sections in this chapter that highlight material for those who are new to these concepts or who do not carry lived experience of oppression, which should help those who experience racism and/or have lived experiences of the impacts from racism and colonialism navigate content that may be impactful. Further, the appendix includes additional resources (**Appendix 2-A**) that may be helpful for those with different understandings of these concepts. Our hope is that all readers will get the knowledge they need to improve individual healthcare practice and work to dismantle systems and structures that cause harm within healthcare settings.

Author Reflexivity

All people in the United States are born into and grow up with the constructs of racism and colonialism permeating our experience. The authors of this chapter are no different. Even while we hold a collective commitment to antiracism, we both have our own bias and areas for growth. We recognize that dismantling this system requires collective effort. With that in mind, we give thanks to those who supported the development of this chapter, especially the students who shared their perspectives on what is needed to reduce harm to learners within sexual and reproductive health education.

We are the authors of this chapter and the editors of this textbook, and our positionality and lived experiences have influenced the framing that we have chosen to take on this textbook for this edition. As such, we recognize that we do not represent all experiences, nor do we have knowledge of all types and experiences of oppression experienced by the communities we serve as midwives. We recognize that there may be content within this chapter that may unintentionally reinforce the very structures we aim to dismantle. We humbly ask that readers of this chapter keep an open mind and a critical eye. If you recognize room for growth in this chapter, share this with your fellow students and the authors. It is only by working together and bringing each other along that society will dismantle the systems that privilege the few at the expense of the many.

KEY CONCEPTS AND DEFINITIONS

This section is intended to build a shared understanding of terminology used in this chapter and the textbook.

Health Equity, Health Disparities, and Health Inequities

Gross inequities in human society are responsible for preventable death and morbidity of millions of people (DHHS, 2022). Achieving optimal health, reducing unconscionable premature loss of life, and averting preventable health conditions requires working toward equity not just in clinical care, but also in society. This work requires understanding health equity and inequities that influence individual, community, and societal health.

Health equity is defined as the "attainment of the highest level of health for all people. Achieving health equity requires valuing everyone equally with focused and ongoing societal efforts to address avoidable inequalities, historical and contemporary injustices, and the elimination of health and health-care disparities" (Healthy People 2030, n.d.). To achieve health equity, it is critical that healthcare providers understand the social, political, and institutional structures and the interpersonal relationships that impact individuals' and communities' health, values, and relationship to health care. Healthcare providers must also understand how these forces shape their personal life experiences and impact their approach to the provision of health care and how healthcare professions and institutions are shaped by these forces.

Conversely, a *health disparity* is "a particular type of health difference that is closely linked with social, economic, and/or environmental disadvantage. Health disparities adversely affect groups of people who have systematically experienced greater obstacles to health based on their racial or ethnic group; religion; socioeconomic status; gender; age; mental health; cognitive, sensory, or physical disability; sexual orientation or gender identity; geographic location; or other characteristics historically linked to discrimination or exclusion" (Healthy People 2030, n.d.). While the terms health disparity and health inequity are often used interchangeably, health disparity denotes a difference in outcomes between different social groups, while health inequity highlights that the difference is unfair or unjust (National Heart, Lung, Blood Institute, 2024).

Drivers of health inequities often include *social determinants of health*, which are the non-medical conditions in which a person lives, works, and plays that impact health. There are significant racial and ethnic differences in social determinants of health across the United States, such as food and housing insecurity, employment opportunities, and lack of social connectedness (Town et al., 2022). *Structural determinants of health* include larger societal, political, or economic structures that create power imbalances that drive health disparities (Town et al., 2022).

Power, Privilege, Oppression, and Positionality

Individuals from socially, politically, and/or economically disadvantaged communities are not inherently disadvantaged. Instead, their inequality is the result of political and social structures that create and maintain hierarchical relationships among social groups. These hierarchical relationships ensure that individuals from certain social groups, such as people who are cisgender, male, heterosexual, and/or White, have greater access to power. *Power* is the ability to direct or influence the behavior of others, oneself, or a course of events (Givens et al., 2018). When power is unearned and unfairly advantages some people over others, it is called *privilege*. When certain groups are systematically denied access to power, it is called *oppression*. Privilege and oppression grant variable and inequitable access to social, political, and economic resources, such as wages, high-quality education, safe housing and communities, and comprehensive health care, which results in variable and inequitable access to power.

Positionality refers to how a person's individual social identities (i.e., race, gender, class) interact with others in terms of power, privilege, and oppression (Altman et al., 2020). When a person carries a social identity that holds relative societal privilege as compared to another, it creates a power imbalance that may subject those who carry identities that are marginalized to oppression. A common example of this dynamic exists in recognizing *implicit bias*, which is a negative attitude or perception against a specific social group, of which a person is often not aware due to their own social position (American Psychological Association, n.d.). The power associated with different social identities often lies on a spectrum and may change based on context and those with whom a person is interacting, but often the impacts from privilege and oppression are collectively applied to social identities due to structural determinants of health. The Intersectional Wheel of Privilege (Watkins, 2021) provides a good example of how different social identities carry privilege and marginalization based on individual positionality (**Figure 2-1**).

While positionality refers to individual identities and a person's acknowledgment of power related to each social position, it is important to note that this discussion also refers to population-level effects that impact communities and groups. The fact that "some individuals in an excluded or marginalized group may have escaped from some of the disadvantages experienced by most members of that group . . . do[es] not negate the fact that the group as a whole is disadvantaged in ways that can be measured" (Braveman et al., 2018, p. 4). Similarly, the fact that some people from privileged social groups may experience disadvantage does not negate the privilege experienced by the group as a whole.

It is important to also note that positionality, specifically the power that can be attributed to a given identity, can shift based on context. For example, the creation of "affinity" spaces (Pour-Khorshid, 2018), defined as spaces that are specific to people with a given identity, lends to increased power and strength for those who hold shared identities within that affinity space. Those who are not included in these affinity spaces may feel excluded or marginalized; however, the larger power differentials that exist based on collective privilege of a group are driving those feelings, largely feeling entitled to be a part of a space meant for someone else. A social media group or thread specifically meant for Black women is an example of an affinity space that serves to create a space where Black women can be somewhat protected from experiences of racism and oppression. Feelings of exclusion or entitlement to be in that space without holding the specified identity, in this case Black women, should signal a need to examine any implicit bias or privilege that may exist impacting a person's experience and view of others.

Intersectionality

Each individual is a unique mix of social identities and the interactions among those identities (e.g., race, ethnicity, gender, class, sexual orientation, age, disability/ability, migration status, religion) (Motley et al., 2023). In some individuals, a socially privileged identity may moderate the disadvantages of a socially oppressed identity. In other cases, individuals who have multiple socially oppressed identities may experience disparities that are different from those found at the population level of any single disadvantaged group. The compounding effect of having multiple socially oppressed identities is called *intersectionality*. The term was coined by Kimberlé Crenshaw (1994) in her work describing the unique challenges faced by Black women in sex and race discrimination legal cases because they were both Black and women. Black men did not face the same gendered experiences as Black women, and White women did not face the same racialized experiences as Black women. The Black women she was representing experienced unique racialized and gendered discrimination.

Race, Racism, Indigeneity, and Colonialism

Understanding the role racism plays in health inequities requires a shared understanding of the concepts of race, indigeneity, racism, and colonialism. In this chapter, *race* is defined

FIGURE 2-1 **Intersectional Wheel of Privilege.**

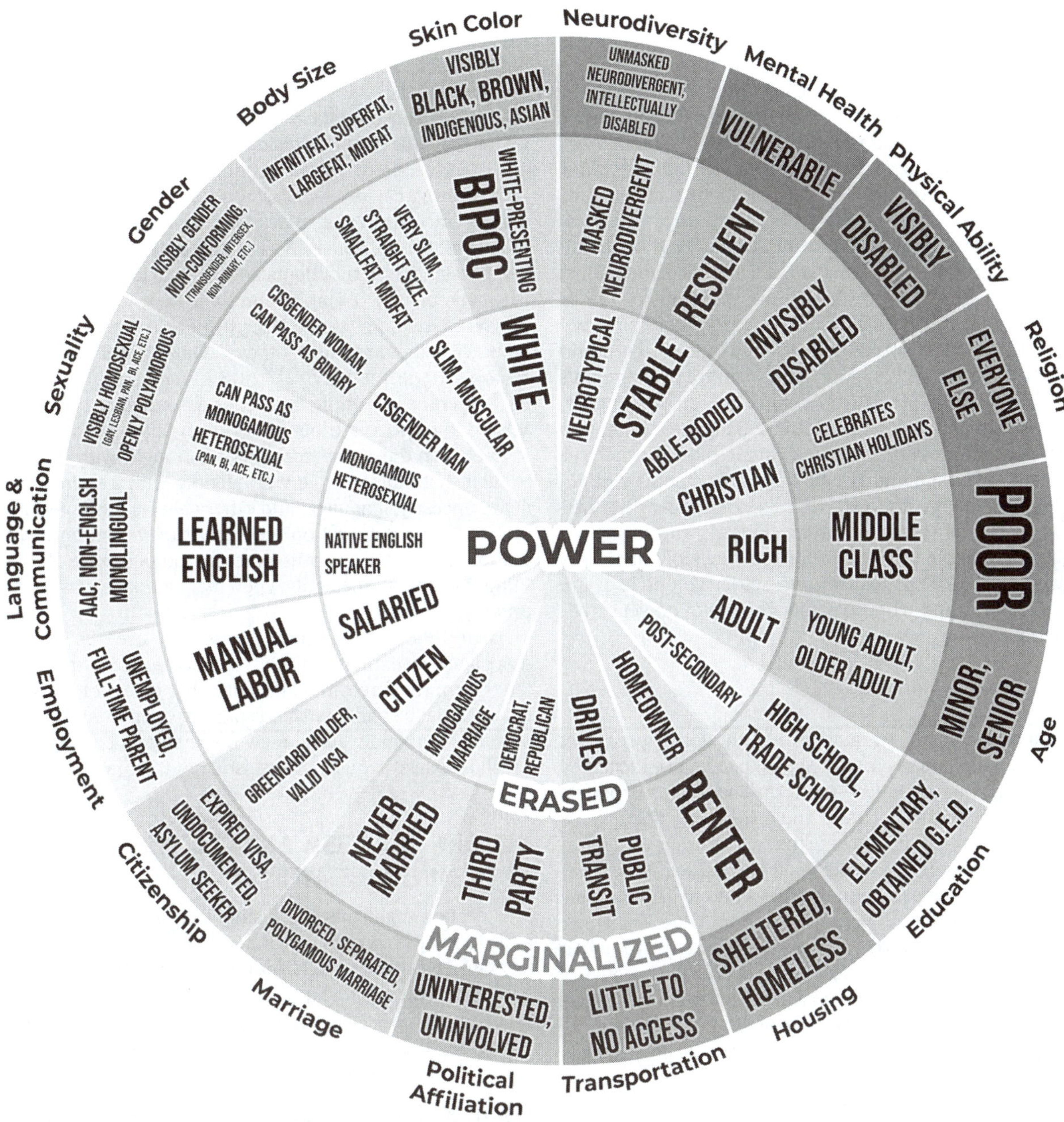

Note: The language noted in this figure may be different than what is commonly used. This is related to the choice for communities to self-identify the language they use for themselves. Given this, please ask what terms a person or community wants you to use, and do not assume that these terms are universal.
Reproduced from Intersectionality Wheel of Privilege: As Observed in the USA, version 2 by Tessa Watkins, Just1Voice.com/wheel-of-privilege. Adapted from Sylvia Duckworth, Canadian Council for Refugees, and Olena Hankivsky, PhD.

as "the social construction and categorization of people based on perceived shared physical traits that result in the maintenance of a sociopolitical hierarchy. The term is also loosely applied to geographic, cultural, religious, or national groups. The significance often accorded to racial categories might suggest that such groups are objectively defined and homogeneous; however, there is much heterogeneity within categories, and the categories themselves differ across groups and cultures" (American Psychological Association, n.d.). This chapter uses the long-standing definition of *racism* described by Dr. Camara Jones (2002): "Racism is a system of structuring opportunity and assigning value based on phenotype ('race'), that unfairly disadvantages some individuals and communities, unfairly advantages other individuals and communities, and undermines realization of the full potential of the whole through the waste of human resources" (p. 10).

When referring to Indigenous peoples or *Indigeneity* as an identity, this chapter uses the following definition: "Indigenous peoples are the descendants of the peoples who inhabited the Americas, the Pacific, and parts of Asia and Africa prior to European colonization" (University of California Los Angeles, 2020). In the United States, the peoples originating within the contiguous part of the country are often referred to as Native American or American Indian collectively, with 574 recognized tribes included in this designation (Bureau of Indian Affairs, 2024). Alaska and Hawaii, the two discontinuous states, have Indigenous people who still reside on their original homelands and are referred to as Alaska Native and Native Hawaiian communities respectively. Indigeneity and race are distinct concepts that warrant differentiation but often are conflated when talking about legal definitions of race. Oppression experienced by Indigenous peoples in the United States is predominantly from *settler colonialism*, defined as "a form of exogenous domination in which the primary goal of the colonial movement is to obtain and stay on the land, seeking the elimination of Indigenous communities—as individuals but especially as peoples with sovereign status and claims" (Wispelwey et al., 2023). Settlers, in this context, seek to bring their own ideologies and structures, which further displace and marginalize Indigenous people through racialized views of superiority (Wispelwey et al., 2023). Racism and settler colonialism are intrinsically linked and work in conjunction with power, privilege, and oppression.

Racial Descriptors

Throughout this chapter the authors use the term "people of color" as an umbrella term to describe all people not racialized as White in the United States. The term encompasses people from a wide range of racial, ethnic, and cultural identities.

Because U.S. society operates within a racial hierarchy that privileges White people above others, it can be helpful to view the experiences of people who are not racialized as White together when describing the impacts of racism generally. However, the term "people of color" completely loses its power when it is used instead of a more precise term (e.g., using "people of color" instead of "Black" or "African American" to describe people who are the American Descendants of Slavery [ADOS]).

As for words that describe specific communities, we intentionally use a variety of terms within this chapter to recognize that racial categorization is challenging and imperfect. Racial categories can be externally imposed, internally developed, or developed through a process that is a combination of social interactions, self-identification, and others' perceptions (Lemelle, 2011). This chapter uses multiple terms for individual racial categories, including African American and Black, Native American and American Indian, and Hispanic, Latiné, and Latinx. The authors recognize that some individuals will identify with multiple terms, while others may self-identify with a single term. The hope is to be inclusive of the wide range of ways that individuals identify and to help demonstrate the challenge of language for describing socially constructed racial groups. In the interest of preserving any terms of self-identification, and in an attempt to offer the richest level of data and information to readers, when applicable this chapter uses terms cited in the primary references. Readers will also note throughout the chapter that "White" is the only racial term that is lowercase, while other ethno-racial terms are capitalized. The authors agree with Kapitan's position that "general editorial standards may call for equal treatment when it comes to the words *Black* and *White*, but until equal treatment exists in our larger society, calls for equal treatment in language only serve to whitewash cultural context, identity and history" (2016, para. 4).

The U.S. census makes a distinction between race and ethnicity for Hispanic people. This distinction is not typically made of any other people when collecting or reporting population-level data. Census categories, also used in health science research, identify race as White, Black or African American, American Indian or Alaska Native, Asian, and Native Hawaiian or Other Pacific Islander. Respondents are asked to identify their ethnicity (Hispanic or non-Hispanic) and their race separately. Ethnicity is typically understood to refer to people who share common ancestry, language, and other cultural attributes (Sáenz & Morales, 2019; Temkin et al., 2018). When a distinction is made between race and ethnicity, race is described as being primarily related to physical attributes. However, attempts at distinguishing between these two concepts are fraught with difficulties; it is clear that many people who identify with a shared race also share ancestry, language, and other cultural attributes. Because this chapter is focused on the impact of racism on health, the authors have chosen to use the language of race throughout. Ethnicity is mentioned only when that language was used by the underlying study.

Lastly, the authors have chosen to use the term "race-associated disparities" instead of "race-based disparities." The latter term reinforces the false idea that race, not racism, is the cause of the disparities. The disparities seen in research are associated with individuals' race, but the basis of this disparity is the individuals' exposure to racism, not their race.

HISTORY OF RACISM AND COLONIALISM IN THE UNITED STATES

This section highlights the history and development of racism and colonialism within the United States, as well as the history of how reproductive coercion impacts sexual and reproductive healthcare access and provision. Additionally, the history of racism within medical research, how racism impacts the criminalization of pregnancy, and the history of racism within gynecologic health professions is described.

The Development of Racism in the United States

"The variable 'race' is not a biological construct that reflects innate differences, but a social construct that precisely captures the impacts of racism" (Jones, 2000, p. 1212).

This section presents an overview of the development and perpetuation of pro-White/anti-Black racism and settler colonialism in the United States. While important, it is beyond the scope of this chapter to provide a complete and in-depth presentation of all people's history with respect to the construction of race and the development of the system of racism in the United States (refer to Appendix 2-A for some further resources). The focus on the development and persistence of anti-Black racism is crucial because it is deeply embedded in how race is more generally constructed in the United States. By beginning to understand anti-Blackness, readers can more deeply grasp other forms of racism; however, a risk of sharing this story alone is that it plays into the perception that racism is something that occurs only to Black people and that it is perpetuated only by White people. Of course, this misses the experiences of wide swaths of people in the United States. It is the authors' hope, however, that sharing this brief introduction to the history of the construction of race for one people can deepen readers' understanding of the environment in which healthcare providers practice and that it will encourage readers to be aware of the need to further their understanding with respect to other communities.

Humans have long identified differences between those who share their own group identity and those who do not (i.e., in-group and out-group) based on cultural practices, geographic location, language, and other identifying factors. Using this framework, the concept of race was used by slave traders to justify and support the African slave trade (Kendi, 2023). Slave traders used the notion of an inferior "Black race" that encompassed all people from the phenotypically, linguistically, geographically, and culturally diverse communities of Africa. With this racial construct in place, they justified slaving expeditions by suggesting that slavery and exposure to Christianity was an improvement over freedom in Africa. Thus, the concept of a "superior White race" was already 200 years in the making when it was brought to the region now called the Americas by early English, French, Spanish, and Dutch colonizers.

Colonialism, Racism, and Health in the United States

The roots of racism in the United States are inseparable from the broader history of European settler colonialism. Settler colonialism, a specific form of colonialism, is characterized by the aim to displace and replace Indigenous populations with a new society of settlers. In the United States, settler colonialism was not merely a political or economic project—it was a cultural and ideological one that imposed European norms, values, and hierarchies on colonized peoples (Veracini, 2024). Settler colonialism facilitated the violent displacement and genocide of Indigenous peoples, the establishment of settler colonies, and the institutionalization of racial hierarchies that privileged whiteness. These hierarchies were embedded in legal systems, religious doctrine, and economic practices, and they continue to shape American society (Gone et al., 2019). Colonial ideologies justified the seizure of Indigenous lands through doctrines such as *"terra nullius"* (land belonging to no one) and the "Doctrine of Discovery," which framed non-European peoples as uncivilized and unworthy of sovereignty. These ideas were codified in U.S. law and policy, including the Indian Removal Act of 1830 and the establishment of the reservation system. The forced assimilation of Indigenous peoples—through boarding schools, religious conversion, and the suppression of native languages and cultures—was a direct extension of colonial logic that sought to erase Indigenous identities and replace them with Euro-American norms (Fish et al., 2024; Stringer, 2024).

The legacy of colonialism is not confined to historical events; it continues to shape contemporary American society in profound and measurable ways. One of the clearest examples is in the U.S. territory of Puerto Rico, where colonial governance has led to systemic underfunding of health care, exclusion from federal health policies such as the Affordable Care Act, and the privatization of essential services. These structural inequities have contributed to disproportionately high rates of chronic illness, maternal mortality, and mental health disorders among Puerto Ricans, arguably making colonialism a sociostructural determinant of health (Martin & Pace, 2025).

The impacts of colonialism continue to manifest in health disparities, particularly among Indigenous and other marginalized communities. Historical trauma, a concept rooted in colonial violence and displacement, is now recognized as a significant determinant of health. It contributes to elevated rates of chronic illness, mental health disorders, and substance use among marginalized populations in the United States (Gone et al., 2019).

Moreover, colonialism's psychological legacy (often referred to as "colonial mentality") is a form of internalized oppression in which individuals from formerly colonized communities devalue their own culture and identity that has been linked to internalized racism, lower self-esteem, and reduced help-seeking behaviors among marginalized communities (Tolentino et al., 2023). Colonial mentality has also been linked to negative mental health outcomes, including depression, anxiety, and low self-esteem. This phenomenon has been documented among Filipino Americans and other ethnic minorities in the United States, where it contributes to reduced help-seeking behavior and cultural disconnection (Tolentino et al., 2023).

In education, colonial legacies persist through curricula (including curricula taught in U.S. schools of nursing) that marginalize Indigenous knowledge systems and histories. Native American students often face educational environments that fail to reflect their cultural identities, contributing to lower academic achievement and higher dropout rates. These disparities are compounded by the historical trauma of boarding schools, where Indigenous children were forcibly removed from their families and subjected to cultural erasure—a practice rooted in colonial ideologies of assimilation and control (Brave Heart et al., 2011).

Within the U.S. colonies and early states, the foundations of settler colonialism were transformed into a system of legally and socially defined categories (Kendi, 2023). Racial categorizations that privileged a "White race" were used to justify and uphold the displacement and genocide of Indigenous peoples as well as the capture and long-term enslavement of African peoples. Colonialization and slavery directly benefited people of European descent, allowing for the acquisition of land, free labor, and corresponding economic resources (Bailey et al., 2017). The racial stereotypes developed to support the legal and civic codes that upheld slavery persist to this day—Black people were represented as lazy, stupid, aggressive, more sexually promiscuous, and having a higher pain tolerance (Bailey et al., 2017; Kendi, 2023; Prather et al., 2018). Belief in the inherent superiority of the White race persisted beyond the dissolution of the institution of slavery. For example, it underpinned the legalized anti-Black racial segregation of the Jim Crow era, it facilitated the state-sanctioned removal of Indigenous children from their homes and forced their assimilation into both the English language and European cultural norms in boarding schools (Bailey et al., 2017), and supported the internment of Japanese people during World War II while White Germans remained free (Yoo et al., 2022).

The interconnected nature of racism and colonialism persist in the structures that develop and maintain the racial inequities seen today. Take, for example, persistent housing segregation and its impacts on African American wealth accumulation.

FIGURE 2-2 **Likelihood of having a bad outcome among African American and White people in the United States.**

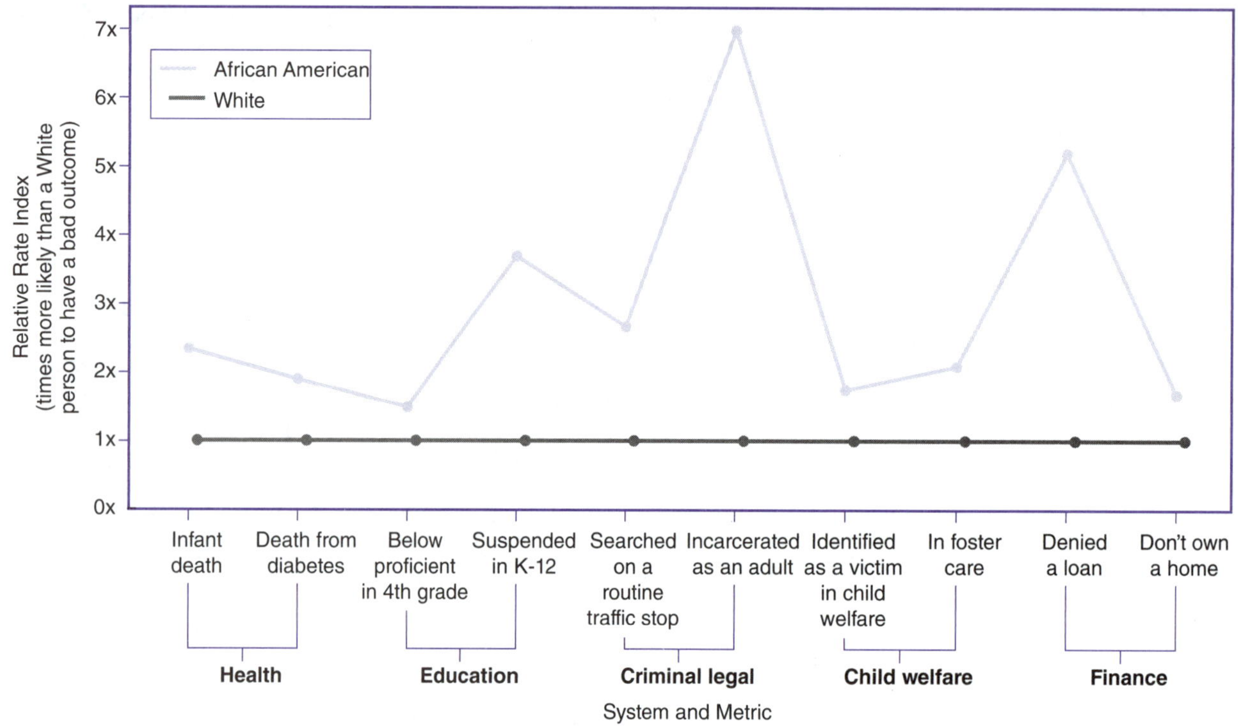

Reproduced from Hayes-Greene, D., & Love, B. P. (2018). The groundwater approach: Building a practical understanding of structural racism. The Racial Equity Institute. https://static1.squarespace.com/static/578fa7e3d482e9af82f8f507/t/5c1b08a50ebbe8eec9f38d21/1545275564106/REI+Groundwater+Approach.pdf.

From the 1930s to the 1960s, the Federal Housing Administration (FHA) subsidized the development of suburban housing while requiring that these homes not be sold to Black people. Simultaneously, in a process known as redlining, the FHA systematically denied insurance on mortgages for homes owned by African Americans. Readers can find their community's historical redlining documents on the University of Richmond's Mapping Inequality website (https://dsl.richmond.edu/panorama/redlining/#loc=4/36.71/-96.93&opacity=0.8). The lack of access to government-insured mortgages meant that Black families were subject to predatory loans (Coates, 2014; Charron-Chénier, 2020) that conferred a higher risk of losing their homes. These families also spent more money on homes that had less resale value, and they were less likely to be able to take out a second mortgage. Collectively these policies ensured ongoing racial segregation and supported the persistence of the wealth gap between African Americans and White Americans (Gross, 2017).

Redlining and the resulting housing segregation and lack of access to home equity as a means toward wealth accumulation is often cited as a primary example of the role of structural racism in the development and maintenance of pro-White/anti-Black racial inequities. However, it is important to note that the nature of structural racism is such that housing segregation does not act alone; it is the fulcrum from which a cascade of inequity operates. For example, residential segregation results in segregated education. Education funding is tied to property values; thus, communities with lower property values almost always have under-resourced schools. Subpar education subsequently limits employment opportunities and access to increasing a community's financial resources. Further, residential segregation results in poor communities of color often living in substandard housing that is overburdened with environmental toxins, has inadequate access to healthy food, and has higher rates of exposure to the criminal justice system, all of which combine to cause poor health.

These factors, and many more, act in concert to create persistent race-associated disparities across multiple axes. An example of this can be seen in The Racial Equity Institute's graphic (refer to **Figure 2-2**) that shows a broad range of disparities faced by African Americans. Understanding the pervasiveness, persistence, and structural nature of the disparities will help clinicians recognize that differences in health outcomes are not due principally to health behaviors, genetics, or cultural factors; rather, health disparities are the physical manifestation of racism. Additional resources about the history and effects of racism in the United States can be found in Appendix 2-A.

Racism and Colonialism in Sexual and Reproductive Health

Every indignity that comes from the denial of reproductive autonomy can be found in slave women's lives—the harms of treating women's wombs as procreative vessels, of policies that pit a mother's welfare against her unborn child, and of government's attempts to manipulate women's childbearing through threats and bribes (Roberts, 1997, p. 23).

Control over enslaved individuals' reproduction, and the destruction of family units in both Black African slave and Native American communities, were key strategies employed to develop and maintain the power of White men in the early United States (Dunbar-Ortiz, 2014; Kendi, 2023; Roberts, 1997). One of the earliest laws codifying the racial categories of slavery was an 1862 Virginia law that ensured any child born of an enslaved woman would be a slave; this law clarified that slaves who were raped by their White owners, or who were forced into sexual relationships with other slaves, would bear children who would be owned by those slave owners (Kendi, 2023; Roberts, 1997).

The White colonialists also employed tactics to control Native American reproduction and family structures. From 1869 into the 1960s, Native American children were stolen from their families and placed in boarding schools with the explicit intent to "Kill the Indian, Save the Man" (Dunbar-Ortiz, 2014; National Native American Boarding School Healing Coalition, n.d.). The children were forbidden to speak their native language, wear traditional clothes, or engage in traditional cultural practices. Sexual and physical abuse was rampant in the schools and persisted well into the 1980s. The violence in boarding schools and the destruction of family and community connections are recognized as the root cause of the grave disparities in sexual and intimate partner violence seen in Native American communities (Smith, 2005; National Native American Boarding School Healing Coalition, n.d.). At the same time, colonial and federal policies targeted Indigenous women's reproductive autonomy. From the 19th century through the 1970s, Indigenous women were subjected to forced sterilizations, often during unrelated medical procedures and/or without full informed consent. These practices were part of broader efforts to assimilate and control Native populations. The Indian Health Service (IHS), a federal agency responsible for providing care to Indigenous communities, has been implicated in numerous cases of coerced sterilization. A 1976 U.S. General Accounting Office report found that four IHS had sterilized 3,406 Native American women without proper consent between 1973 and 1976 (U.S. Government Accountability Office, 1976).

State efforts to control the reproduction and family formation of those deemed unfit found new life in the Eugenics movement from the 1920s to 1940s (Roberts,1997; Stern, 2016). This movement was fueled by fears of White "race suicide" due to lower birth rates among White U.S.-born women, as compared to foreign-born women, and racist ideas that described the moral and intellectual superiority of the White race (Roberts, 1997). During this period, 32 states enacted compulsory sterilization laws (Stern, 2016).

These laws initially focused on incarcerated and institutionalized men, but they were subsequently applied more aggressively to women (Roberts, 1997). Female sterilization laws focused on women who were mentally disabled, poor, and of color (Roberts, 1997; Stern, 2016). Even as the Eugenics movement was debunked and fell out of favor, forced sterilization of people of color, especially women, persisted into the 1970s.

Women of color, especially Black, Latinx, and Native American women, were sterilized without their consent after giving birth, during treatment for other unrelated concerns, or for the purpose of physician resident education (Roberts, 1997; Tajima-Peña, 2015). Meanwhile, White women encountered barriers to accessing sterilization (Roberts, 1997). Activist efforts in the 1970s resulted in sterilization reform that persists today; federally funded programs require informed consent and a 30-day waiting period, hysterectomies may not be performed for sterilization, and sterilization may not be performed on those who are minors, mentally incompetent, or institutionalized. However, even with these protections in place, people are still subject to coercion. In 2010, 146 inmates in California prisons underwent sterilization without required state approval, and many of these individuals were coerced (Johnson, 2013). Additionally, in 2020, the American Civil Liberties Union (ACLU) filed a complaint to the federal Office of the Inspector General in the Department of Homeland Security alleging that a government-paid physician was known to be repeatedly performing sterilization procedures on women in Immigration and Customs Enforcement (ICE) custody (Amiri, 2023).

Reproductive coercion is not limited to sterilization. In the 1990s, many states enacted laws that required women who relied on government aid to use Norplant, a hormonal, long-acting, highly effective, provider-controlled method of contraception and efforts to control poor women's reproduction persist. In 2017, South Dakota Medicaid would not reimburse for the removal of a contraceptive implant if the intent was for the recipient to become pregnant (McKee, 2016).

Beyond government policies, there is strong evidence that clinicians continue to pressure pregnant-capable individuals of color to limit reproduction. Research shows that clinicians are more likely to recommend intrauterine devices to Black and Latinx women with low socioeconomic status than to White women with similar socioeconomic status (Dehlendorf et al., 2010). Women of color and women with low incomes are more likely to report being pressured to use a contraceptive method and limit their family size (Dehlendorf et al., 2016). In a qualitative study of 38 young Black and Latinx women, 71% recounted experiences of pressure in contraceptive care. The authors note that "experiences of implicit pressure influenced participants' uptake and discontinuation of contraception, interactions with providers writ large, and willingness to seek future care" (Gomez & Wapman, 2017, p. 223). Similarly, in a study of 1,783 women from across the United States, women of color were more likely than White women to rate the following features of contraception as extremely important: user control over starting and stopping the method, methods that would not change the user's menstrual cycle, and methods that would not affect return to fertility. The authors note it is probable that the history of reproductive abuse of poor people and people of color underpins some of these preferences (Jackson et al., 2016). Additional resources about reproductive coercion and abuses can be found in Appendix 2-A.

History of Racism within Medical Research

No history of gynecology would be complete without mention of the racist history of medical experimentation on Black and brown bodies. The most well-known example is the Tuskegee Study of Untreated Syphilis, in which the U.S. Public Health Service studied the life course of syphilis in approximately 400 Black men. The men were denied the effective standard treatment of penicillin and advised not to seek treatment elsewhere. The researchers endeavored to ensure that local physicians and clinics would not treat these men if they sought care elsewhere.

Additionally, the men were made to undergo unnecessary phlebotomy, lumbar punctures, and autopsies (Alsan & Wanamaker, 2018; Howell, 2017; Tobin, 2022). The consequences of untreated syphilis were borne not only by the men, but also by entire communities because the men's partners and children were allowed to contract the disease (Washington, 2017). This experimentation was made possible due to racist beliefs about biological differences between the races; the researchers were interested to learn if neurosyphilis would manifest differently in "primitive" and "underdeveloped" Black brains (Howell, 2017).

This study continued for 40 years and was stopped only after a journalist broke the story in 1972 (Alsan & Wanamaker, 2018; Howell, 2017; Tobin, 2022). Awareness of the Tuskegee Study of Untreated Syphilis has been demonstrated to reduce Black men's utilization of both inpatient and outpatient medical care (Alsan & Wanamaker, 2018).

Lesser known is the 1946 to 1948 study by the U.S. Public Health Service in which vulnerable people (children, orphans, sex workers, Indigenous people, people with leprosy, people with mental illness, prisoners, and soldiers) in Guatemala were intentionally infected with syphilis, gonorrhea, and chancroid without their consent (Rodriguez & García, 2013; Spector-Bagdady & Lombardo, 2019). **Box 2-1** contains an explicit and graphic description of the experience of one woman who was subjected to this study. This description is included to humanize the individuals upon whom this research was perpetrated and to encourage readers to fully face the complex history upon which current scientific knowledge and practices are based.

BOX 2-1 Experience of Berta, a Woman in the Guatemala Sexually Transmitted Disease Experiments

Berta was a female patient in the psychiatric hospital. Her age and the illness that brought her to the hospital are unknown. In February 1948, Berta was injected in her left arm with syphilis. A month later, she developed scabies (an itchy skin infection caused by a mite). Several weeks later, [lead investigator Dr. John] Cutler noted that she had also developed red bumps where he had injected her arm, lesions on her arms and legs, and her skin was beginning to waste away from her body. Berta was not treated for syphilis until three months after her injection. Soon after, on August 23, Dr. Cutler wrote that Berta appeared as if she was going to die, but he did not specify why. That same day he put gonorrheal pus from another male subject into both of Berta's eyes, as well as in her urethra and rectum. He also re-infected her with syphilis. Several days later, Berta's eyes were filled with gonorrheal pus, and she was bleeding from her urethra. On August 27, Berta died.

Reproduced from Rodriguez, M. A., & García, R. (2013). First, do no harm: The US sexually transmitted disease experiments in Guatemala. *American Journal of Public Health, 103*(12), 2122–2126. https://doi.org/10.2105/AJPH.2013.301520

Well before these studies/experiments, J. Marion Sims, often called the "father of modern gynecology," performed much of his research on the repair of vesicovaginal fistulas and the development of the Sims speculum on Anarcha, Lucy, and Betsey, enslaved Black women who were forced to undergo repeated unanesthetized surgeries (Owens, 2017; Prunty, Bukavina, & Hallman, 2021). Similarly, the first large-scale study on oral hormonal contraceptives, funded by Margaret Sanger, was performed on women in Puerto Rico who were not informed that the pill was experimental (PBS, n.d.; White Junod & Marks, 2002; Liao & Dollin, 2012). Reframing education to center those who were subjected to these abuses is a necessary step toward reconciling the harmful history within gynecology.

History of Racism within Gynecologic Health Professions

From the earliest days of European colonization through the 21st century, gynecologic care and outcomes have been shaped by racial hierarchies that privilege White women while subjecting Indigenous, Black, immigrant, and other marginalized people to coercion, neglect, and abuse. This is particularly evident in the erasure of Black, immigrant, and Indigenous midwives. Prior to the 20th century, midwifery was a respected and essential practice in the United States, particularly in Black, Indigenous, and immigrant communities. These midwives not only provided culturally competent care but also served as vital community health leaders (Niles & Drew, 2020). However, the rise of the medical profession—dominated by White, male physicians—systematically displaced these traditional practitioners under the guise of safety, professionalization, and public health reform. This displacement was not merely incidental but part of a broader strategy to consolidate medical authority and marginalize non-White knowledge systems. Black midwives in the American South, often referred to as "granny" or preferably "grand" midwives, were targeted by public health campaigns that framed them as unclean, untrained, and dangerous, despite their extensive experience and community trust. Similarly, Indigenous midwives were undermined by colonial policies that sought to assimilate Native populations and dismantle traditional practices, including birth work. The medicalization of birth—shifting childbirth from homes to hospitals—was a key mechanism in this erasure. By the mid-20th century, childbirth had become a highly medicalized event, with obstetricians replacing midwives as the primary birth attendants. This transition was not neutral; it was shaped by racialized narratives that devalued the expertise of individuals and communities of, positioning White male physicians as the sole arbiters of safe and modern care (Niles & Drew, 2020). This shift had profound consequences. The removal of culturally grounded midwifery care disrupted community-based safety nets and contributed to the growing mistrust of the medical system among communities of color. Moreover, it laid the groundwork for ongoing reproductive injustices and systematic abuse justified by racist assumptions about the intelligence and reproductive fitness of non-White individuals (Luke, 2018; Dawley, 2000).

The legacy of this history is evident in today's stark racial disparities in maternal and reproductive health outcomes. Individuals of color continue to experience higher rates of maternal mortality, preterm birth, and inadequate pain management compared to their White counterparts. Implicit bias among healthcare providers contributes to disparities in patient counseling and care provision (Saluja & Bryant, 2021).

These experiences reflect a broader pattern of reproductive coercion rooted in historical abuses and ongoing structural inequities. Addressing the history of racism in gynecologic health professions requires more than acknowledgment—it demands systemic change. Professional organizations such as the American College of Obstetricians and Gynecologists (ACOG); the American College of Nurse Midwives (ACNM); the American Nurses Association (ANA); the Association of Women's Health, Obstetric and Neonatal Nurses (AWHONN); and Nurse Practitioners in Women's Health (NPWH) have called for an honest reckoning with the field's racist past and a commitment to equity in care delivery. This includes integrating antiracist education into medical and nursing curricula, promoting culturally safe care, and ensuring that marginalized communities have a voice in shaping reproductive health policy and practice (ACOG, 2022; ACNM, 2021; ANA, 2022; AWHON, 2021; NPWH, 2020). Understanding the historical roots of racism in gynecologic care is not only an ethical imperative—it is a clinical one. The persistent disparities in maternal health outcomes, reproductive autonomy, and patient trust are direct consequences of this legacy. By confronting and learning from this history, clinicians can begin to dismantle the structural inequities that continue to harm patients today. Only through this critical reflection and commitment to justice can the United States build a healthcare system that is truly equitable, evidence-based, and centered on the dignity and well-being of all people.

The Criminalization of Pregnancy

The criminalization of pregnancy in the United States is a deeply racialized phenomenon, rooted in a long history of surveillance and punishment of marginalized communities. In her 2024 book *The Pregnancy Police: Conceiving Crime, Arresting Personhood*, legal scholar Grace Howard documents how pregnant people—particularly those who are Black, Indigenous, poor, or otherwise marginalized—are increasingly treated as criminal suspects rather than patients. Drawing on over a thousand arrest records, Howard reveals how the state, through a network of healthcare providers, social workers, and law enforcement, polices pregnancy under the guise of protecting fetal life.

Earlier research by Paltrow and Flavin (2013) found that in 413 cases where pregnancy was a necessary factor in depriving someone of their physical liberty, over half involved Black women. Nearly half (48%) of these Black women were reported by healthcare providers, compared to just 27% of White women. These deprivations included arrests, incarceration, forced medical interventions, and involuntary confinement in hospitals or treatment programs. The majority of these cases (84%) involved allegations of recreational drug use (Roberts, 1997). As Howard and others argue, the racialized panic over "crack babies" in the 1980s laid the groundwork for punitive policies that disproportionately target Black and Brown pregnant people. These narratives, rooted in White supremacist ideologies, cast certain pregnant bodies as inherently dangerous and morally suspect (Howard, 2024). Howard emphasizes that the criminalization of pregnancy is not just about individual bias—it is systemic. Healthcare providers often act as gatekeepers to the carceral system, disproportionately drug testing and reporting patients of color. These actions are shaped by institutional policies and cultural narratives that equate poverty and nonconformity with parental unfitness.

Since the U.S. Supreme Court's decision in *Dobbs v. Jackson Women's Health Organization* (2022), which overturned *Roe v. Wade*, the legal landscape has become even more hostile to pregnant people (Baden et al., 2024). In the 2 years following the ruling, multiple cases have emerged in which individuals were arrested, detained, or prosecuted for actions related to their pregnancies. These include people criminalized for seeking abortion care, experiencing pregnancy loss, or allegedly self-managing abortions in states with restrictive laws. For example, in states enforcing total abortion bans, individuals have been investigated for miscarriages or stillbirths, with law enforcement seizing medical records and interrogating patients about their pregnancy outcomes. In some cases, people have been charged with crimes such as "abuse of a corpse" or "fetal homicide" based on unproven allegations of self -managed abortion. These prosecutions disproportionately affect people of color, immigrants, and those living in poverty—communities already over-policed and under-protected by the healthcare system.

The consequences of this criminalization are devastating. Individuals may not seek abortions and be forced to carry a pregnancy due to fear of prosecution; pregnant people may avoid prenatal care for fear of being reported, leading to worse health outcomes; parents may be incarcerated or lose custody of their children based on unproven allegations. As Howard argues, dismantling the pregnancy policing apparatus requires a fundamental rethinking of how society values bodily autonomy, reproductive justice, and racial equity. Additional resources on this topic can be found in Appendix 2-A.

HOW RACISM IMPACTS PHYSIOLOGY

Exposure to racism, whether it is structural or interpersonal, causes chronic, cumulative, biological stress. This stress negatively impacts both the individual and their offspring. It is critical to understand that the physiologic effects of racism are not due to underlying race-linked genetic differences, nor are they due to behavioral differences. This section reviews what is currently understood about the physiologic mechanisms whereby racism manifests in the body.

"Weathering" is the umbrella term used to describe earlier onset of negative health conditions and normal aging that results from chronic exposure to social and economic disadvantage (Forde et al., 2019). The concept was first proposed by Dr. Arlene Geronimus (1992, 1996) to explain why infants born to Black mothers tend to fare better when their mother is in her teens and infant outcomes worsen as maternal age increases into the 20s and early 30s. This contrasts with infants born to White mothers, whose outcomes are best when their mothers are in their 20s and early 30s.

Subsequent research has demonstrated the weathering effect on a wide range of outcomes including body mass index, diabetes, hypertension, stroke, and longevity (Forde et al., 2019). A number of underlying mechanisms, described in this section, have been proposed as contributors to the pattern of weathering.

Allostatic load is an objective measurement of chronic stress (McEwen & Seeman, 2009; Rodriquez et al., 2019; Riggan et al., 2021). Under conditions that promote health, the body is responsive to external stressors and is able to maintain homeostasis. The ability to maintain homeostasis in the face of acute stressors is called allostasis (McEwen & Seeman, 2009). When exposed to cumulative or chronic stressors, this normal healthful mechanism can be disrupted. The effects of this dysregulation are termed allostatic load (or overload). Dysregulation involves multiple interconnected systems and affects cellular, metabolic, and cardiovascular function (McEwen, 2018).

There are four mechanisms by which allostatic load is proposed to operate: (1) repeated activation, where the body does not have the time to return to homeostasis between exposures; (2) lack of adaptation, where the body does not adapt to a recurrent stress and learn to manage it more effectively; (3) prolonged exposure, where the body mounts an appropriate stress response but does not return to homeostasis in a timely manner; and (4) inadequate response, where the body mounts an insufficient response to the stressor (McEwen, 2018). For example, the catecholamines, which include epinephrine (adrenaline), norepinephrine (noradrenaline), and dopamine, are involved in regulating heart rate and blood pressure, allowing an individual to transition among sleep, restful waking, and physical exertion while maintaining homeostasis.

These chemicals can be beneficial in managing short-term stressors as well, providing oxygenation to the brain during stressful events. However, chronic exposure to stress-induced surges of blood pressure (repeated activation) or a body that is no longer able to downregulate blood pressure (prolonged exposure) is at higher risk for atherosclerosis and resulting coronary artery disease, stroke, peripheral artery disease, kidney problems, and type 2 diabetes (McEwen & Seeman, 2009; McEwen, 2018).

Numerous studies have found increased allostatic load in Black people as compared to White people (Chyu & Upchurch, 2011; Geronimus et al., 2006; Rodriquez et al., 2018; Seeman et al., 2008; Tavares et al., 2022). This difference persists when wealth and exposure to discrimination is taken into account (Chyu & Upchurch, 2011; Cuevas et al., 2024). In fact, the largest racial disparity in allostatic load is seen within middle/upper class individuals, alluding to the impact of racism rather than socioeconomic status as a main driver (Cuevas et al., 2024). Exposure to racial discrimination explains the majority of the difference in allostatic load between Black and White individuals (Cuevas et al., 2024; Miller et al., 2021).

While research is scant, there is evidence of higher allostatic load among Latinx people (Rodriguez et al., 2018), and there's a growing body of evidence highlighting that recent migration to the United States is actually protective against higher allostatic load, likely due to the decreased exposure to racism (Chyu & Upchurch, 2018; Cedillo et al., 2021; Touma & Hummer, 2022). In fact, a study examining the protective nature of recent immigration status found that it took 20 years of living in the United States for foreign-born Hispanic people to have a similar allostatic load compared to U.S.-born Hispanic people (Yellow Horse & Santos-Lozada, 2019). Research examining the impacts of chronic stress among Indigenous, Latinx, and Asian communities living in the United States is complicated by the heterogeneity of these populations, given the wide range of racial identities and diverse countries/locales of origin encompassed within these groups.

Data from Canada, however, indicates a dose-response increase in allostatic load from exposure to structural inequities and discrimination among First Nations people (Currie et al., 2020), which could likely be applied to Indigenous communities in the United States as well. The shortening of telomeres is another mechanism by which chronic stress may contribute to weathering. Telomeres are noncoding nucleotide sequences found on the ends of chromosomes. Telomeres help protect the genetic code of the chromosome during transcription. During each transcription event, a chromosome loses some of the nucleotides at the end of the chromosome. While telomerase helps to rebuild the telomeres, they shorten over time. Shorter telomeres are correlated with a number of age-related and chronic-stress-related diseases (Mathur et al., 2016). Premature shortening of the telomeres has been documented in response to exposure to racism and discrimination (Chae et al., 2020). In particular, established coping mechanisms to gender-mediated racism have been linked to shorter telomeres among Black women (Thomas et al., 2022).

Epigenetics describes the mechanisms by which gene expression is turned on or off, or whether it is upregulated or downregulated, in response to environmental factors. For example, when chronic stress occurs, the genes responsible for inflammatory response are upregulated, while those responsible for antiviral and antibody production are downregulated. Chronic inflammation is implicated in a number of chronic diseases, such as hypertension, diabetes, obesity, and depression. Epigenetic changes have been proposed as a mechanism for increased weathering both in the individual and in their children (Conching & Thayer, 2019; Ohm, 2019). Clearly stated, chronic stress can lead to epigenetic changes that impact children in utero, which explains how we see weathering effects persist through generations.

UNDERSTANDING INEQUITY IN GYNECOLOGIC HEALTH

One of the most profound consequences of racism is its effect on individual and population health. Across a variety of health conditions and indicators, people of color, especially Black and Indigenous people, have a greater incidence of disease and more frequent unfavorable outcomes than White people (National Academies of Sciences, Engineering, and Medicine, 2017). While increasing attention is being paid to the significant racial and ethnic disparities in maternal morbidity and mortality (Jain et al., 2018), there are also pervasive and persistent race-associated disparities across gynecologic health and health care. For example, endometrial cancer, fibroids, and endometriosis rates are consistently higher among Black women (Doll, 2023; Katon et al., 2023). Further, the risk of death from reproductive cancers such as endometrial and breast cancer is higher for Black women than White women (Doll, 2023; Pederson et al., 2024). While statistics demonstrate the scope of the problem of race-associated disparities, knowing this information is only a small step toward health equity.

The more important work is understanding why these disparities exist and designing effective interventions to remedy them. Unfortunately, research to date has often fallen short. There has been a resurgence of research during the COVID-19 pandemic attributing racial disparities in mortality to biologic differences in susceptibility rather than recognizing the impacts of social determinants of health and structural racism on health outcomes (Elias et al., 2021; Kimani, 2023). Researchers and clinicians must stop concentrating on biological conceptualizations of race and instead focus on the effects of racism on health and health outcomes. As Dr. Joia Crear-Perry states, "Black isn't the risk factor, racism is" (Muse, 2018, p. 24).

Understanding race-associated disparities through the lens of racism rather than a biological conceptualization of race is complex and requires intentional focus on the drivers and consequences of racism as impacts on health inequities. Most research uses participant race as a proxy for racism, which may miss the mark on understanding possible avenues for decreasing disparities (Collaboratory for Health Justice, 2021).

Using race as a proxy variable ignores the compounding impacts from other sources of oppression, such as economic/social class, gender, nationality, and/or ethnicity, making it hard to attribute disparities to racism alone (Collaboratory for Health Justice, 2021). More appropriately, studies should also examine the specific drivers of racism, which can include such things as discrimination, implicit bias, mistreatment, disrespectful care, and social determinants of health stemming from structural racism. These drivers can influence potential interventions to decrease race-associated disparities from racism (Bailey et al., 2017). Inclusion of structural determinants of health that capture structural racism are also essential; for example, discriminatory laws and policies, housing segregation, police violence, and mass incarceration (Alson et al., 2021). Further, studies could utilize measures that capture the consequences of racism, such as toxic stress markers, allostatic load, and mental health outcomes to use with studies testing potential interventions so that change can be assessed.

Interpreting existing evidence within the framing of racism is essential to understanding race-associated disparities data. When studies describe inequities in care experiences and health outcomes based on race, several questions should be critically considered (refer to **Box 2-2**).

BOX 2-2 Approach to Critically Analyzing Race-Based Data

Introduction/Purpose/Aims

1. How is race being considered in this study? Is it used as a social or biological construct? Was the intention clear in the research questions and/or aims?

Methods

2. How was race measured? Were participants able to self-identify? Was there sufficient disaggregation of race to have meaningful results?
3. Was race clearly noted as being a proxy for racism or other social inequity? Was there discussion about the relationship of race as a measure of racism or similar?
4. How was data analysis conducted in relation to race? Was there clear rationale for inclusion of a race variable? Was it clear that it was considered a social variable (instead of a biological variable)?

Results

1. Did the study only report race-associated statistics or was there further interpretation as to the social factors that could have influenced the findings (e.g., social determinants of health, economic impacts, discrimination)?

Discussion/Conclusion

2. Was a framework such as critical race theory (or others) used in interpreting findings from the study?

Data from Ross, PT, Hart-Johnson T, Santen SA, Zaidi NLB. Considerations for using race and ethnicity as quantitative variables in medical education research. Perspect Med Educ. 2020 Oct;9(5): 318-323. https://doi.org/10.1007/s40037-020-00602-3. PMID: 32789666; PMCID: PMC7550522; Collaboratory for Health Justice (2021). Best Practices for Using Race in Public Health Research. University of Illinois Chicago. Report. https://doi.org/10.25417/uic.15159393.v1 and Yale School of Medicine Office of Health Equity Research. Best Practices for Collecting and Analyzing Race and Ethnicity Data. 2025. Accessed June 18, 2025 at https://files- profile.medicine.yale.edu/documents/33d77238-3851-441c-ab14-fcd1ac49a0ef.

ADDRESSING RACISM AND RACE-ASSOCIATED DISPARITIES

The preceding sections have provided an overview of the history and current manifestations of racism. This background is needed for healthcare providers and scientists to have a clear understanding about what racism is and how it operates to shift thinking, research, and interventions away from race and toward racism. This section highlights how individuals, healthcare teams, and communities are taking steps to improve race-associated disparities by confronting racism, including key theories and frameworks to guide understanding, and actions to address, racism and health disparities.

Theories and Frameworks

A number of scholars and theorists have proposed a variety of mechanisms and models for understanding the causes of health disparities as well as tools and techniques for effective interventions. This section presents a brief introduction to these theories, frameworks, and related concepts, which are summarized in **Table 2-1** and explicitly focus on structural and systemic understanding and solutions. Theories and concepts that focus on individual choices, health behaviors, lifestyle, and culture are not included. This focus is intentional; the root cause of race-associated disparities is racism.

Because racism is socially constructed and maintained by institutions, theories that describe the problem and define the interventions must also be structural and systemic (Harvey & McGladrey, 2019).

Critical Race Theory

Critical race theory (CRT) emerged out of legal scholarship in the 1970s. Its development was informed by radical feminism, critical legal theory, the Black power and Chicano movements, philosophy, and works by American antiracism leaders such as W. E. B. Du Bois, Martin Luther King Jr., and Cesar Chavez (Flores, 2017). Since the 1970s, CRT has become "a collection of activists and scholars engaged in studying and transforming the relationship among race, racism and power" (Delgado & Stefancic, 2017, p. 3) in fields as varied and diverse as education, psychology, communications, political science, and public health.

TABLE 2-1 Definitions of Theories and Frameworks Used to Understand and Address Health Disparities

Theory	Definition
Critical race theory	A theoretical framework organized around the following concepts: • Race consciousness (awareness that race is a social construct) • Contemporary orientation (change efforts are oriented toward contemporary manifestations of racism) • Centering the margins (change efforts are focused on and guided by the perspective, experience, and voices of people from marginalized communities) • Praxis (taking action is required to make change) (Zewude & Sharma, 2021; Ford & Airhihenbuwa, 2010)
Reproductive justice	Reproductive justice is "the human right to maintain personal bodily autonomy, have children, not have children, and parent the children we have in safe and sustainable communities. To achieve reproductive justice, we must analyze power systems, address intersecting oppressions, center the most marginalized, and join together across issues and identities" (SisterSong, n.d., para. 1).
Cultural safety	Cultural safety "encompasses a critical consciousness where healthcare professionals and healthcare organizations engage in ongoing self-reflection and self-awareness and hold themselves accountable for providing culturally safe care, as defined by the patient and their communities, and as measured through progress towards acheiving health equity. Cultural safety requires healthcare professionals and their associated healthcare organisations to influence healthcare to reduce bias and achieve equity within the workforce and working environment" (Curtis et al., 2019).
Structural competency	Structural competency is the trained ability to understand how symptoms, attitudes, or diseases represent downstream implications of a wide variety of upstream structural systems (Metzl & Hansen, 2014).

The core tenets of CRT hold that (1) racism is a common and everyday experience for people of color, (2) racism preferentially benefits White people over people of color, and (3) race is a social construct. CRT is grounded in a commitment to taking action to make changes to dismantle racism. The theory recognizes that the manifestation of racism changes over time, as does the racialization of different groups, and orients change efforts toward contemporary manifestations of racism. CRT holds that the key to dismantling racism is to center at the margins and uplift and share counter-stories. Centering from the margins means that perspective, experience, and voices from marginalized communities guide the work. Counter-stories describes the important role that storytelling, especially personal narratives and allegory, holds for shifting the dominant culture toward antiracism.

Ford and Airhihenbuwa (2010, 2018) have made important contributions to the public health literature demonstrating the importance of CRT to public health discourse and research, and they have demonstrated how to apply CRT to public health research. They note that CRT provides "tools [that] help researchers illuminate racial biases embedded in a field or in a study's aims, methods, conclusions, etc., and develop strategies to address them" (2018, p. 224). One tool that is used within public health to support anti-racist interventions is the Public Health Critical Race Praxis, which operationalizes CRT within research while recognizing the impact utilizing race and ethnicity has in racializing results and impacting the biological misconception of race (Ford and Airihenbuwa, 2010; Ford & Pirtle, 2025).

Reproductive Justice

Reproductive justice is a human rights framework, a theory, and a sociopolitical movement that identifies the fundamental human right of reproductive autonomy (Ross, 2007; Ross & Solinger, 2017; Ross, 2020). The core principles recognize the fundamental human rights of reproductive autonomy, including (1) the right to not have a child, (2) the right to have a child, and (3) the right to parent children in safe and healthy environments (Ross, 2007; Ross & Solinger, 2017; Ross, 2020). The term "reproductive justice" was coined in 1994 by a group of African American women soon after attending the International Conference for Population and Development in Cairo, Egypt (Ross & Solinger, 2017). The analysis and movement were developed, in part, in reaction to the limited framework of choice presented by the pro-choice movement. The pro-choice movement, led by middle- and upper-class White, cisgender women, frequently ignored the reproductive health concerns of women of color, women who were poor, transgender people, and others. For example, the pro-choice movement has continued to focus on personal and individual choice in abortion care despite the fact that the Hyde Amendment, passed in 1976 just 3 years after *Roe v. Wade*, bans Medicaid coverage for abortion, disproportionately reducing access to abortion for people who are poor and people of color. In 1997, the SisterSong Women of Color Reproductive Justice Collective was formed by members of the original group, in coalition with 16 organizations representing women from Native American, African American, Latinx, and

Asian American communities. Since that time, the movement has grown, and a large number of organizations and individuals work collectively to realize reproductive justice.

The Reproductive Justice framework not only applies to abortion rights and reproductive autonomy; it expands to the right to health and wellness in all aspects of a person's life (Grady et al., 2019). Having the ability to choose whether to, and when to if desired, build a family has impact on a person's economic, educational, professional, and personal journey (Paltrow et al., 2022). Reproductive justice applies to all health care—reproductive autonomy and limitations thereof can impact other health conditions, the ability to maintain wellness, and the ability to manage existing health concerns. Lastly, the last tenet of reproductive justice—"the right to parent children in safe and healthy environments"—is a direct reference to the need to identify and address social and structural determinants of health that impact the health of individuals and families (Liddell & Kington, 2021; Hayes et al., 2020). As a human rights framework, reproductive justice asserts the right for all individuals to have autonomy over their life and well-being individually and within community.

Cultural Safety—Moving Beyond Cultural Competency and Cultural Humility

The concept of cultural competency was first described in the health science literature by Cross et al. (1989). Since then, cultural competency has become the dominant approach to training healthcare providers to care for diverse populations and reduce healthcare disparities (Alizadeh & Chavan, 2016; Metzl et al., 2018; Shen, 2018). The theory underlying cultural competency is that improving healthcare provider familiarity with the values, customs, and belief models of various racial and ethnic groups will improve provider–client communication and thus mitigate health disparities, with having knowledge about cultural practice being enough to be considered "competent."

In 1998, Tervalon and Murray-García described cultural humility as a counterpoint to cultural competence. They define cultural humility as "incorporat[ing] a lifelong commitment to self-evaluation and critique, to redressing the power imbalances in the physician–patient dynamic, and to developing mutually beneficial and non-paternalistic partnerships with communities on behalf of individuals and defined populations" (Tervalon & Murray-García, 1998, p. 123). In their call for cultural humility, they make explicit the need to recognize and redress interpersonal, institutional, and systemic power imbalances. However, this too missed the mark in operationalization of the concept of cultural humility, creating a static expectation of awareness being enough without direct action (Curtis et al., 2019).

Cultural safety as a concept was first developed in the 1990s by Dr. Irihapeti Ramsden and Māori nurses, in response to harms to Indigenous communities within healthcare practice (Ramsden, 2015). Cultural safety centers the patient experience within the healthcare setting, holding the clinician responsible for acknowledging their own biases, assumptions, and privilege that may influence the quality of the healthcare experience (Curtis et al., 2019). Rather than focusing on the patient's culture, which creates a perspective of "othering," cultural safety focuses on the clinician's own culture (e.g., identity, positionality, power, values) as the main driver of quality within health care.

Further, cultural safety uses an action-oriented framework, with the active practice of critical self-reflection as a requirement to high-quality care provision. Further, cultural safety, specifically a culturally safe environment, is defined by the person or community, not by the clinician or healthcare system. To actualize cultural safety within health care, both the individual clinicians and the larger healthcare systems and structures need to center the needs, experience, and knowledge of those most impacted by racism, colonialism, and other sources of oppression. **Figure 2-3** and **Table 2-2** depict and describe the five principles of cultural safety (Ball, 2025).

Structural Competency

Structural competency, originally presented as a framework to expand and replace cultural competency in medical schools (Metzl & Hansen, 2014), quickly found utility in a wide range of disciplines for students and current providers alike. Structural competency is the trained ability to understand how symptoms, attitudes, or diseases represent downstream implications of a wide variety of upstream structural systems. It is defined by the development of five core skills: (1) recognize the structures that shape clinical interactions, (2) develop an extra-clinical language of structure, (3) rearticulate cultural presentations in structural terms, (4) imagine structural interventions, and (5) develop structural humility (refer to **Table 2-3**). The structural competency framework has been used to improve clinicians' knowledge and skills in addressing racism and race-associated disparities in health care (Metzl & Hansen, 2014; Metzl et al., 2018).

Actions to Address and Mitigate Racism in Health Care

A number of health science scholars (Eichelberger et al., 2016; Hardeman et al., 2016; Jones, 2002; Metzl & Roberts, 2014; Kimani, 2023) have considered what healthcare providers can do to address racism and mitigate race-associated disparities in health. Key themes that emerge are the importance of understanding the history and current manifestations of racism, the ability to identify and describe racism, and taking concrete action to address racism (refer to **Box 2-3**).

Reducing Implicit Bias

Maina et al.'s 2018 systematic review into research on implicit racial and ethnic bias in healthcare providers found only two studies that looked at interventions to reduce implicit bias in healthcare providers (Maina et al., 2018). One study found that participation in a multicultural training course reduced pro-White/anti-Black implicit bias; the other study found no impact for providers who did a virtual cultural competency immersion training. While more studies have examined implicit bias training since that review, few have shown these training programs to be effective (Sabin et al., 2022; Gopal et al., 2021; Mavis et al., 2022). However, strategies have been identified to support healthcare providers and institutions to become aware of implicit biases and work to decrease the impact of biases on health care. **Table 2-4** highlights several ways that providers can act to recognize and reduce their biases.

Studies have shown that high levels of cognitive stressors increase implicit bias, and the impact of cognitive load on worsening implicit bias has been demonstrated to impact healthcare providers (Maina et al., 2018). Other techniques for reducing

FIGURE 2-3 Five principles of cultural safety.

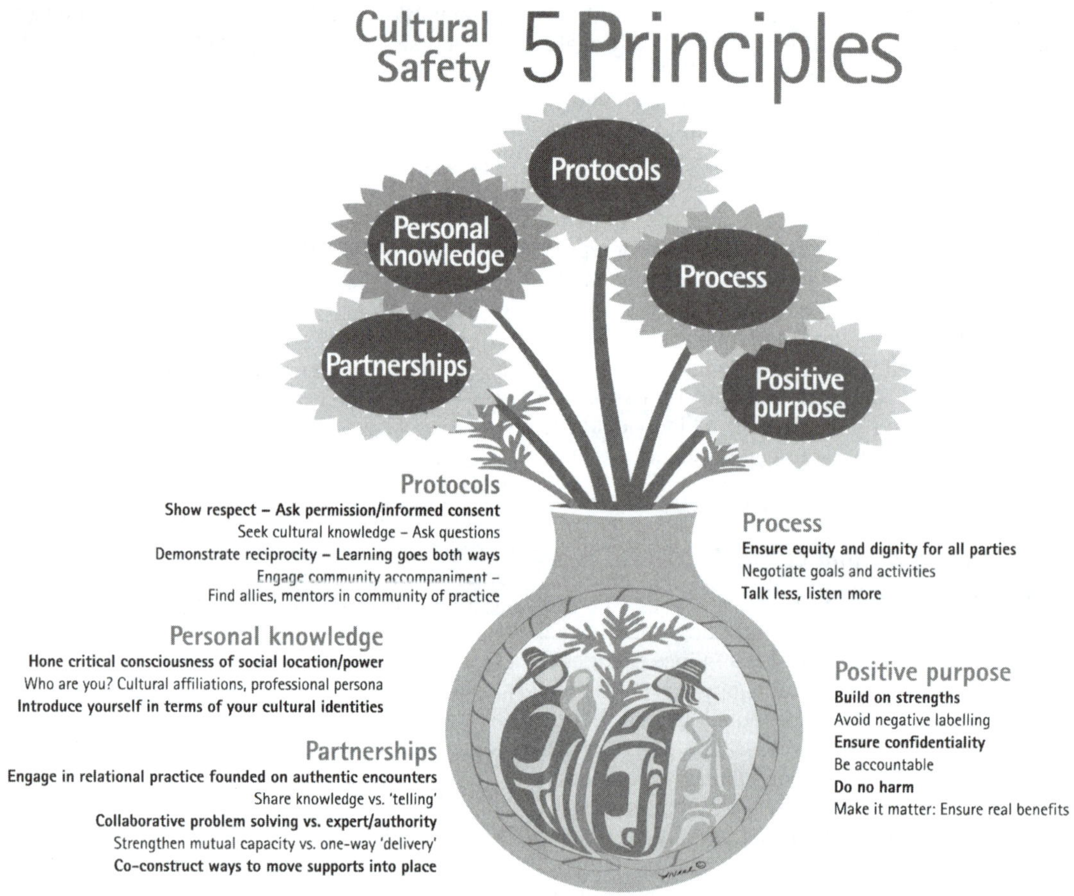

Reproduced from Ball, J. Cultural Safety 5 Principles. Early Childhood Development Intercultural Partnership. 2025. Accessed June 14, 2025 at https://ecdip.org/cultural-safety/

TABLE 2-2 Five Principles of Cultural Safety

1.	Personal knowledge	Need for personal, critical self-reflection of own personal background, biases and assumptions, and how these may influence interactions with patients.
2.	Partnership	Need for relationship building and partnerships between providers and community members to identify unmet needs, cultural influences impacting care, shared decision making, and centering community experiences.
3.	Protocols	Understanding cultural practices and diverse forms of engagement in health care, and ensuring healthcare interactions are shaped in ways that are culturally congruent and respectful.
4.	Process	Ongoing self-reflection and assessment of practice, with adaptations to meet individual patient needs.
5.	Positive purpose	Assuring that the process and experiences of care have positive outcomes, as defined by patients, prioritizing the needs, values, and desires of patients throughout the entire care experience.

Data from Ball, J. Cultural Safety 5 Principles. Early Childhood Development Intercultural Partnership. 2025. Accessed June 14, 2025 at https://ecdip.org/cultural-safety/

TABLE 2-3 Five Skill Sets of Structural Competency

Skill	Description
Recognize the structures that shape clinical interactions	Consider how economic, social, and political forces impact the patient's presentation and health history and the interaction between the patient and clinician.
Develop an extra-clinical language of structure	Utilize an interdisciplinary approach to study and understand how social structures impact the health of communities. Relevant disciplines include critical race theory, medical anthropology, sociology, economics, political science, and urban planning.
Rearticulate cultural presentations in structural terms	Develop the capacity to recognize and describe a clinical presentation in structural terms, especially when faced with a presentation that would typically be framed as cultural.
Imagine structural interventions	Conceive of structural interventions to address structural barriers to optimal health.
Develop structural humility	Recognize that one can never fully understand how economic, social, and political forces impact another's life and thus approach all efforts to address structural inequality with an open mind and humility.

Reproduced from Serbin, J. W., & Donnelly, E. (2016). The impact of racism and midwifery's lack of racial diversity: A literature review. *Journal of Midwifery & Women's Health, 61*(6), 694–706. https://doi.org/10.1111/jmwh.12572

BOX 2-3 Interventions for Addressing Racism and Race-Associated Disparities

Awareness

- Define and name racism.
- Learn about, understand, and accept the racist roots of the United States.
- Understand how racism has shaped our narrative about disparities.
- Recognize how racism operates within healthcare structures and systems.
- Be more aware of the ways racism is embedded in institutions and operates apart from blatant acts of individual bias.

Acknowledgment

- Critically reflect on our own biases and assumptions that contribute to racism.
- Identify how our positionality impacts how we interact with patients, families, and communities.
- Be skeptical of race-based differences in diagnosis.
- Interrogate the use of race in clinical algorithms and base clinical decision making on individual needs and circumstances.
- Learn lessons from other professions that have taken active steps toward addressing structural racism.

Action

- "Center at the margins"; specifically, diversify the workforce, develop community-driven programs and research, and help to ensure that oppressed and under-resourced people and communities gain positions of power.
- Be more politically vocal about structural issues that impact patients.
- Institute place-based, multisector, equity-oriented initiatives.
- Advocate for policy reform.
- Train the next generation of health professionals to ensure a diverse workforce.
- Support increasing racial diversity of leadership within institutions.
- Make racial disparities a key focus for quality improvement projects.
- Modify interventions with the goal that they are successful only when they show racially equitable improvements.

cognitive load include decreasing patient–provider ratios, improving insurance access for patients, integrating care so that referrals are more seamless, and other structural changes that would reduce the stress of providing modern health care. Most importantly, research into techniques for reducing implicit bias shows that motivation is a key to successful reduction in implicit bias. By committing to reducing your own implicit bias, you are setting yourself up for successful reduction in implicit bias.

Workforce Diversification

The most important intervention to address race-associated health disparities is to increase the racial diversity of those

TABLE 2-4 **Combatting Implicit Bias and Stereotypes**

Strategy	Description
Stereotype replacement	Become aware of the stereotype you hold and create non-stereotypical alternatives to them.
Counter-stereotypic imaging	Remember or imagine someone from a stereotyped group who does not fit the stereotype.
Individuating	See each person as an individual, not a group member. Pay attention to things about them besides the stereotypes of their group.
Perspective-taking	Imagine the perspective of someone from a group different than your own ("Put yourself in the other person's shoes").
Contact	Seek ways to get to know people from different social groups. Build your confidence in interacting with people who are different than you. Seek opportunities to engage in discussions in safe environments, spend time outside your usual social groups, or volunteer in a community different than your own.
Emotional regulation	Reflect on your "gut" feelings and negative reactions to people from different social groups. Be aware that positive emotions during a clinical encounter make stereotyping less likely.
Mindfulness	Keep your attention on the present moment so you can recognize a stereotypic thought before you act on it.

Reproduced from Think Cultural Health Education. Combating implicit bias and stereotypes. Accessed June 21, 2025 at https://thinkculturalhealth.hhs.gov/maternal-health-care/assets/pdfs/Combating_implicit_bias_and_stereotypes.pdf

providing care (Boyd, 2019; Serbin & Donnelly, 2016; Alspaugh et al., 2023; Shen et al., 2018; Altman et al., 2023; American College of Nurse-Midwives [ACNM], 2024; Guglielminotti et al., 2022). By increasing the racial diversity of the professions that provide health care, the problem is tackled along multiple axes. Diversifying the healthcare workforce increases opportunity for racial concordance between patients and providers, increases understanding of the intersectional impacts of racism and discrimination, and creates opportunity for shifting awareness of structures and systems that better support racialized communities (Serbin & Donnelly, 2016; ACNM, 2024; Alspaugh et al., 2023). It is not only the presence of racially diverse clinicians that impacts health disparities, but the inherent models of care and lived experiences of these clinicians that create a culturally safe clinical environment (Jeffers et al., 2023).

Given the choice, people of color are more likely to choose healthcare providers who share their racial and ethnic identity (Jang et al., 2018; Alspaugh et al., 2023; Serbin & Donnelly, 2016). Clients with racially and linguistically concordant healthcare providers are more likely to receive better interpersonal care and be more satisfied with their care (Shen et al., 2018; Wusu et al., 2019; Altman et al., 2023). It is important to note that the setting in which racial concordant care is provided is equally important, particularly in bridging the gap between healthcare institutions and community structures—"larger institutional transformations [are needed]—for example, greater access to resources, more flexible institutional regulations, and an organizational culture committed to diversifying biomedical norms" (Lo & Nguyen, 2018, p. 165). This can look like creating wraparound services within clinic structures including social work, mental health, and care coordination support, or possibly weaving in traditional or cultural mechanisms of support within the healthcare system (De Ornelas et al., 2025; Nijagal et al., 2025).

Providers of color are also healthcare recipients of color and members of communities of color. Addressing the social and structural barriers that people of color face in accessing higher education, secure and well-paying jobs, positions of leadership, and roles that promote personal and community power are powerful antiracism interventions (Cuellar & Cheshire, 2018; Serbin & Donnelly, 2016).

Access to education for health-related professions is a significant part of the equation. Aspiring clinicians seek education to advance their professional capacity and role; however, the majority of educational programs for nurse practitioners, nurse-midwives, and physician associates utilize a predominantly White lens. This often excludes diverse perspectives and knowledge based in cultural and community expertise, leading to harmful environments for students of color (Mehra et al., 2023; Altman et al., 2024; Hamzavi & Brown, 2023). Increasing racial and ethnic diversity of faculty within these programs is a crucial step toward improving educational experiences for students of color; however, there is more to be done. Recent work highlighted community-driven priorities for ways in which clinician education can be transformed to better support students of color—these priorities included incorporating the real history of racism within health care; centering the voices and experiences of communities of color; and building structures to support recruitment, retention, and successful graduation of students of color (Altman et al., 2025).

The rationale for workforce diversification is clear and compelling. There is quite a bit published about increasing the pipeline and improving the numbers of people of color in health worker educational pathways. Little is written, however, about effective methods for supporting people of color within healthcare education and the healthcare workforce. Just increasing recruitment efforts for training clinicians of color is not enough;

experiences of burnout are significantly higher for clinicians of color when entering the workforce, often due to institutions not addressing racism and discrimination effectively (Johnson et al., 2019). There is much work to be done to change the culture of the healthcare delivery systems so that all providers are fully respected and able to bring the full force of their talents to bear on addressing race-associated disparities.

CONCLUSION

Racism in the United States privileges people identified as White at the expense of those identified as people of color, especially Black and Indigenous people of color. Racism, not race, is the cause of the pervasive and persistent race-associated disparities across gynecologic health and health in general. Racism also underpins the lack of racial diversity found in healthcare providers. Racism is socioculturally pervasive and persistent; it is woven throughout the social, political, and economic fabric of the United States.

Race-associated health disparities are the physical manifestation of racism, which is responsible for the unconscionable preventable death and morbidity of millions of people. Healthcare providers in specific, and people who live in the United States in general, bear the moral imperative to address racism by shifting power balances toward equity. Dismantling racist systems and structures requires collective effort. Each individual must determine where and how they will best contribute to the collective effort. This effort is a lifelong commitment, and the role an individual plays will necessarily change based on context and personal growth. The reader is invited to consider this question: What steps can I personally commit to take toward dismantling racism?

References

Alizadeh, S., & Chavan, M. (2016). Cultural competence dimensions and outcomes: A systematic review of the literature. *Health & Social Care in the Community, 24*(6), e117- e130. https://doi.org/10.1111/hsc.12293

Alsan, M., & Wanamaker, M. (2018). Tuskegee and the health of black men. *The Quarterly Journal of Economics, 133*(1), 407–455. https://doi.org/10.1093/qje /qjx029

Alson, J. G., Robinson, W. R., Pittman, L., & Doll, K. M. (2021). Incorporating measures of structural racism into population studies of reproductive health in the United States: A narrative review. *Health Equity, 5*(1), 49–58.

Alspaugh, A., Suárez-Baquero, D. F. M., & Mehra, R., et al. (2023, June 1). "Patients want to see people that look like them": Aspiring midwives of color as resistance to racism through concordant care in the United States. *SSM—Qualitative Research in Health, 3,* 100226.

Altman, M. R., Afulani, P. A., Melbourne, D., & Kuppermann, M. (2023, June). Factors associated with person-centered care during pregnancy and birth for Black women and birthing people in California. Birth, 50(2), 329–338. https://doi .org/10.1111/birt.12675

Altman, M. R., Kantrowitz-Gordon, I., & Moise, E., et al. (2020). Addressing positionality within case-based learning to mitigate systemic racism in health care. Nurse Educator, 46(5), 284–289. https://doi.org/10.1097/NNE.0000000000000937

Altman, M. R., Sherley, C., Lazarus, J., Kantrowitz-Gordon, I., & Ward, T. M. (2024, October). Transformative justice to support truth and reconciliation within nurse-midwifery education. *Nursing Inquiry, 31*(4), e12660. https://doi.org/10.1111 /nin.12660

Altman, M. R., Uthmaan, S., Washington, T., Niang, B., Gilmore, C., Fletcher, V., Salazar Monk, L., Kennedy, L. O., & Community Accountability Council. (2025). Community-led priorities for re-envisioning midwifery education to better support Black and Indigenous learners. *Journal of Midwifery and Women's Health* doi:10.1111 /jmwh.70014.

American College of Nurse-Midwives. (2024). How to recruit and retain more midwives of color. Accessed February 17, 2025, https://midwife.org/wp-content /uploads/2024/08/UPDATED_031324_ACNM_Landscape-Analysis-and-Strategic -Plan-for-Education-Report_hiRes-1.pdf

American College of Nurse-Midwives. (2021, March 10). Position statement: Against racism and racial bias. https://legacy.midwife.org/acnm/files/cclibraryfiles/filename /000000008243/ACNM%20Position%20Statement%20Against%20Racism%20 and%20Racial%20Bias%203.10.2021.pdf

American College of Obstetricians and Gynecologists. (2022). Racism in obstetrics and gynecology [Statement of policy]. https://midwife.org/wp-content/uploads/2024 /10/Racism-and-Racial-Bias.pdf

American Nurses Association. (2022). Racial reckoning statement. https://www .nursingworld.org/~4a4e56/globalassets/docs/ana/ana-racial-reckoning -statement-2022.pdf

American Psychological Association. Implicit bias. Accessed December 26, 2024 at https://www.apa.org/topics/implicit-bias

American Psychological Association. Race. Accessed December 26, 2024 at https:// dictionary.apa.org/race

Amiri, B. (2023, February 27). Reproductive abuse is rampant in the immigration detention system: ACLU. American Civil Liberties Union. https://www .aclu.org/news/immigrants-rights/reproductive-abuse-is-rampant-in-the -immigration-detention-system

Anarcha, Lucy, Betsey, Mothers of Gynecology: Montgomery: More up campus. (n.d.). https://www.anarchalucybetsey.org/

Association of Women's Health, Obstetric and Neonatal Nurses. (2021). Racism and bias in maternity care settings [Position statement]. https://www .awhonn.org/resources-and-information/published-resources/awhonn- position -statements/

Baden, K., Dreweke, J., & Gibson, C. (2024, May). Clear and growing evidence that Dobbs is harming reproductive health and freedom. Guttmacher Institute. https:// www.guttmacher.org/2024/05/clear-and-growing-evidence-dobbs-harming -reproductive-health-and-freedom

Bailey, Z. D., Krieger, N., Agénor, M., Graves, J., Linos, N., & Bassett, M. T. (2017). Structural racism and health inequities in the USA: Evidence and interventions. *The Lancet* (British Edition), *389*(10077), 1453–1463. https://doi.org/10.1016 /S0140- 6736(17)30569-X

Ball, J. (2025). *Cultural Safety 5 Principles.* Early Childhood Development Intercultural Partnership. Accessed June 14, 2025 at https://ecdip.org/cultural-safety/

Boyd, R. W. (2019). The case for desegregation. *Lancet, 393*(10190), 2484–2485. https:// doi.org/10.1016/S0140-6736(19)31353-4

Brave Heart, M. Y. H., Chase, J., Elkins, J., & Altschul, D. B. (2011). Historical trauma among indigenous peoples of the Americas: Concepts, research, and clinical considerations. *Journal of Psychoactive Drugs, 43*(4), 282–290. https://doi.org/10.1080 /02791072.2011.628913

Braveman, P., Arkin, E., Orleans, T., Proctor, D., Acker, J., & Plough, A. (2018). What is health equity? *Behavioral Science & Policy, 4*(1), 1–14. https://doi.org/10.1353/bsp.2018.0000

Bureau of Indian Affairs. 2024. Accessed January 14, 2025 at https://www.bia.gov/ service/tribal-leaders-directory

Campbell, N. D. (2018). When should screening and surveillance be used during pregnancy? *AMA Journal of Ethics, 20*(1), 288–295. https://doi.org/10.1001 /journalofethics.2018.20.3.msoc1-1803

Cedillo, Y. E., Bertrand, B., Baker, E., Cherrington, A. L., Beasley, T. M. , & Fernández, J. R. (2021, February). Assimilation, acculturation, and allostatic load in u.s.- and foreign-born hispanics. *Journal of Immigrant and Minority Health, 23*(1), 35–44. https://doi .org/10.1007/s10903-020-01012-7. PMID: 32333289; PMCID: PMC8543841.

Chae, D. H., Wang, Y., Martz, C. D., Slopen, N., Yip, T., Adler, N. E., Fuller-Rowell, T. E., Lin, J., Matthews, K. A., Brody, G, H., Spears, E. C., Puterman, E., & Epel, E. S. (2020, March). Racial discrimination and telomere shortening among African Americans: The Coronary Artery Risk Development in Young Adults (CARDIA) Study. *Health Psychology, 39*(3), 209–219. https://doi.org/10.1037/hea0000832. Epub 2020 Jan 13. PMID: 31928029; PMCID: PMC7373166.

Charron-Chénier, R. (2020). Predatory inclusion in consumer credit: Explaining Black and White disparities in payday loan use. *Sociological Forum* (Randolph, N.J.), *35*(2), 370–392. https://doi.org/10.1111/socf.12586

Chyu, L., & Upchurch, D. M. (2011). Racial and ethnic patterns of allostatic load among adult women in the United States: Findings from the National Health and Nutrition Examination Survey 1999–2004. *Journal of Women's Health, 20*(4), 575–583. https://doi.org/10.1089/jwh.2010.2170

Chyu, L., & Upchurch, D. M. (2018). A longitudinal analysis of allostatic load among a multi-ethnic sample of midlife women: Findings from the Study of Women's Health Across the Nation. *Women's Health Issues, 28*(3), 258–266. https://doi .org/10.1016/j.whi.2017.11.002

Clarke, E. (2021). Indigenous women and the risk of reproductive healthcare: Forced sterilization, genocide, and contemporary population control. *Journal of Human Rights and Social Work, 6*(2), 144–147. https://doi.org/10.1007/s41134-020-00139-9

Coates, T.-N. (2014, June). The case for reparations. *The Atlantic*. https://www.theatlantic.com/magazine/archive/2014/06/the-case-for-reparations/361631/

Collaboratory for Health Justice. (2021). Best Practices for Using Race in Public Health Research. University of Illinois Chicago. Report. https://publichealth.uic.edu/community-engagement/collaboratory-for-health-justice/best-practices-race-public-health-research/#:~:text=Best%20practices%20to%20address%20concerns%20with%20using%20%22race%22&text=Show%20that%20you%20have%20thoughtfully,your%20study%20design%20and%20interpretation.&text=If%20you%20are%20using%20race,race%20as%20a%20demographic%20variable.

Conching, A. K. S., & Thayer, Z. (2019). Biological pathways for historical trauma to affect health: A conceptual model focusing on epigenetic modifications. *Social Science & Medicine, 230*, 74–82. https://doi.org/10.1016/j.socscimed.2019.04.001

Crenshaw, K. W. (1994). Mapping the margins: Intersectionality, identity politics, and violence against women of color. In M. A. Fineman & R. Mykitiuk (Eds.), *The public nature of private violence* (pp. 93–118). Routledge.

Cross, T. L., Bazron, B., Dennis, K., & Isaacs, M. (1989). *Towards a culturally competent system of care: A monograph on effective services for minority children who are severely emotionally disturbed.* Georgetown University Child Development Center. https://files.eric.ed.gov/fulltext/ED330171.pdf

Cuellar, N. G., & Cheshire, M. (2018). Leadership challenges in building a Hispanic nursing workforce. *Nurse Leader, 16*(1), 43–47. https://doi.org/10.1016/j.mnl.2017.11.007

Cuevas, A. G., McSorley, A. M., Lyngdoh, A., Kaba-Diakité, F., Harris, A., Rhodes-Bratton, B., & Rouhani, S. (2024, July). Education, income, wealth, and discrimination in Black-White allostatic load disparities. *American Journal of Preventive Medicine, 67*(1), 97–104. https://doi.org/10.1016/j.amepre.2024.02.021. Epub 2024 Mar 6. PMID: 38458268; PMCID: PMC12034296.

Currie, C. L., Copeland, J. L., Metz, G. A., Chief Moon-Riley, K., & Davies, C. M. (2020, January). Past-year racial discrimination and allostatic load among indigenous adults in Canada: The role of cultural continuity. *Psychosomatic Medicine, 82*(1), 99–107. https://doi.org/10.1097/PSY.0000000000000754. PMID: 31609919; PMCID: PMC6946095.

Curtis, E., Jones, R., Tipene-Leach, D. et al. (2019). Why cultural safety rather than cultural competency is required to achieve health equity: A literature review and recommended definition. *International Journal for Equity in Health, 18*, 174. https://doi.org/10.1186/s12939-019-1082-3

Dawley, K. (2000). The campaign to eliminate the midwife. *American Journal of Nursing, 100*(10), 50 –56. https://doi.org/10.1097/00000446-200010000-0002

De Ornelas, M., Harley, K. G., Davis, D., Gruver, A., Santana, D. C., Hayes, K., Tesfalul, M., & Wren, J. A. (2025, May–June). Community-centered and antiracist model of whole-person perinatal care: Beloved birth Black centering. *Journal of Midwifery and Women's Health, 70*(3), 468–475. https://doi.org/10.1111/jmwh.13761. Epub 2025 May 21. PMID: 40396192; PMCID: PMC12172577.

Dehlendorf, C., Mengesha, B., & Ti, A. (2016). *Improving contraceptive counseling through shared decision-making curriculum.* Innovating Education in Reproductive Health. https://www.innovating-education.org/2016/03/2743/

Dehlendorf, C., Ruskin, R., Grumbach, K., Vittinghoff, E., Bibbins-Domingo, K., Schillinger, D., & Steinauer, J. (2010). Recommendations for intrauterine contraception: A randomized trial of the effects of patients' race/ethnicity and socioeconomic status. *American Journal of Obstetrics & Gynecology, 203*(4), 319.e1–319.e8. https://doi.org/10.1016/j.ajog.2010.05.009

Delgado, R., & Stefancic, J. (2017). *Critical race theory: An introduction* (3rd ed.). NYU Press.

Doll, K. M. (2023, September). Endometrial cancer and reproductive justice. *Obstetrics and Gynecology, 142*(3), 477–480. https://doi.org/10.1097/AOG.0000000000005305. Epub 2023 Aug 3. PMID:37590979.

Dunbar-Ortiz, R. (2014). *An indigenous peoples' history of the United States.* Beacon Press.

Eichelberger, K. Y., Doll, K., Ekpo, G. E., & Zerden, M. L. (2016). Black lives matter: Claiming a space for evidence-based outrage in obstetrics and gynecology. *American Journal of Public Health, 106*(10), 1771–1772. https://doi.org/10.2105/AJPH.2016.303313

Elias, A., Ben, J., Mansouri, F., & Paradies, Y. (2021). Racism and nationalism during and beyond the COVID-19 pandemic. *Ethnic and Racial Studies*, 44(5), 783–793.

Fish, J., Ansloos, J., O'Keefe, V. M., & Gone, J. P. (2024). Truth and reconciliation for whom? Transitional justice for Indigenous peoples in American psychology. *American Psychologist, 79*(4), 618–630. https://doi.org/10.1037/amp0001234

Flores, L. A. (2017). Critical race theory. In Y. Y. Kim & K. McKay-Semmler (Eds.), *The international encyclopedia of intercultural communication* (pp. 1–5). John Wiley & Sons.

Ford, C. L., & Airhihenbuwa, C. O. (2010, October). The public health critical race methodology: Praxis for antiracism research. *Social Science & Medicine, 71*(8), 1390–1398. https://doi.org/10.1016/j.socscimed.2010.07.030. Epub 2010 Aug 11. PMID: 20822840.

Ford, C. L., & Airhihenbuwa, C. O. (2018). Commentary: Just what is critical race theory and what's it doing in a progressive field like public health? [Suppl. 1]. *Ethnicity & Disease, 28*, 223–230. https://doi.org/10.18865/ed.28.S1.223

Ford, C. L., & Pirtle, W. (2025, April). Invited commentary: Race, ethnicity, and racism in epidemiologic research—perspectives from Public Health Critical Race Praxis (PHCRP). *American Journal of Epidemiology, 194*(4), 927–935.

Forde, A. T., Crookes, D. M., Suglia, S. F., & Demmer, R. T. (2019, May). The weathering hypothesis as an explanation for racial disparities in health: A systematic review. *Annals of Epidemiology, 33*, 1–18.e3. https://doi.org/10.1016/j.annepidem.2019.02.011

Geronimus, A. T. (1992). The weathering hypothesis and the health of African-American women and infants: Evidence and speculations. *Ethnicity & Disease, 2*(3), 207–221.

Geronimus, A. T. (1996). Black/White differences in the relationship of maternal age to birthweight: A population-based test of the weathering hypothesis. *Social Science & Medicine, 42*(4), 589–597. https://doi.org/10.1016/0277-9536(95)00159-X

Geronimus, A. T., Hicken, M., Keene, D., & Bound, J. (2006). "Weathering" and age patterns of allostatic load scores among blacks and whites in the United States. *American Journal of Public Health, 96*(5), 826–833. https://doi.org/10.2105/AJPH.2004.060749

Givens, M., Kindig, D., Inzeo, P. T., & Faust, V. (2018, February 1). *Power: The most fundamental abuse of health inequity?* Health Affairs. https://www.healthaffairs.org/do/10.1377/hblog20180129.731387/full/

Gomez, A. M., & Wapman, M. (2017). Under (implicit) pressure: Young Black and Latina women's perceptions of contraceptive care. *Contraception, 96*(4), 221–226. https://doi.org/10.1016/j.contraception.2017.07.007

Gone, J. P., Hartmann, W. E., Pomerville, A., Wendt, D. C., Klem, S. H., & Burrage, R. L. (2019). The impact of historical trauma on health outcomes for Indigenous populations in the USA and Canada: A systematic review. *The American Psychologist, 74*(1), 20–35. https://doi.org/10.1037/amp0000338

Gopal, D. P., Chetty, U., O'Donnell, P., Gajria, C., & Blackadder-Weinstein, J. (2021, March). Implicit bias in healthcare: Clinical practice, research and decision making. *Future Healthcare Journal, 8*(1), 40–48. https://doi.org/10.7861/fhj.2020-0233. PMID: 33791459; PMCID: PMC8004354.

Grady, G., Hinshaw-Fuselier, S., & Friar, N. (2019, September). Expanding perspectives: A social inequities lens on intimate partner violence, reproductive justice, and infant mental health. *Infant Mental Health Journal, 40*(5), 624–639. https://doi.org/10.1002/imhj.21809. Epub 2019 Jul 17. PMID: 31314924; PMCID: PMC6972627

Gross, T. (2017). *A "forgotten history" of how the US government segregated America.* NPR. https://www.npr.org/2017/05/03/526655831/a-forgotten-history-of-how-the-u-s-government-segregated-america

Guglielminotti, J., Samari, G., Friedman, A. M., Lee, A., Landau, R., & Li, G. Nurse workforce diversity and reduced risk of severe adverse maternal outcomes. *American Journal of Obstetrics & Gynecology MFM, 4*(5), 100689. https://doi.org/10.1016/j.ajogmf.2022.100689. Epub 2022 Jul 10. PMID: 35830955; PMCID: PMC9872864.

Hamzavi, N., & Brown, H. (2023, October). "Who has been here that looks like me?": A narrative inquiry into Black, Indigenous, and People of Color graduate nursing students' experiences of White academic spaces. *Nursing Inquiry, 30*(4), e12568. https://doi.org/10.1111/nin.12568

Hardeman, R. R., Medina, E. M., & Kozhimannil, K. B. (2016). Structural racism and supporting Black lives—the role of health professionals. *New England Journal of Medicine, 375*(22), 2113–2115. https://doi.org/10.1056/NEJMp1609535

Harvey, M., & McGladrey, M. (2019). Explaining the origins and distribution of health and disease: An analysis of epidemiologic theory in core Master of Public Health coursework in the United States. *Critical Public Health, 29*(1), 5–17. https://doi.org/10.1080/09581596.2018.1535698

Hayes, C. M., Sufrin, C., & Perritt, J. B. (2020, January). Reproductive justice disrupted: Mass incarceration as a driver of reproductive oppression. *American Journal of Public Health, 110*(S1), S21–S24. https://doi.org/10.2105/AJPH.2019.305407. PMID: 31967889; PMCID: PMC6987912.

Hayes-Greene, D., & Love, B. P. (2018). The groundwater approach: Building a practical understanding of structural racism. The Racial Equity Institute. https://racialequityinstitute.org/groundwater-approach/

Healthy People 2030. Priority Areas. Accessed January 14, 2025 at https://odphp.health.gov/healthypeople/priority-areas/health-equity-healthy-people-2030

Howard, G. (2024). *The pregnancy police : conceiving crime, arresting personhood.* University of California Press.

Howell, J. (2017). Race and U.S. medical experimentation: The case of Tuskegee [Suppl. 1]. *Reports in Public Health, 33*(33), e00168016. https://doi.org/10.1590/0102-311x00168016

Jackson, A. V., Karasek, D., Dehlendorf, C., & Foster, D. G. (2016). Racial and ethnic differences in women's preferences for features of contraceptive methods. *Contraception, 93*(5), 406–411. https://doi.org/10.1016/j.contraception.2015.12.010

Jain, J. A., Temming, L. A., D'Alton, M. E., Gyamfi-Bannerman, C., Tuuli, M., Louis, J. M., Srinivas, S. K., Caughey, A. B., Grobman, W. A., Hehir, M., Howell, E., Saade, G. R., Tita, A. T. N., & Riley, L. E. (2018). SMFM special report: Putting the "M" back in MFM: Reducing racial and ethnic disparities in maternal morbidity and mortality: A call to action. *American Journal of Obstetrics and Gynecology, 218*(2), B9–B17. https://doi.org/10.1016/j.ajog.2017.11.591

Jang, Y., Yoon, H., Kim, M. T., Park, N. S., & Chiriboga, D. A. (2018). Preference for patient–provider ethnic concordance in Asian Americans. *Ethnicity & Health*, 1–12. https://doi.org/10.1080/13557858.2018.1514457

Jeffers, N. K., Canty, L., Drew, M., Grayson, N., Amani, J., Marcelle, E., & Amore A. D. (2023, June). Beyond "patient-provider race matching." Black midwives clarify a vision for race-concordant care to achieve equity in Black perinatal health: A commentary on "Do Black birthing persons prefer a Black health care provider during birth? Race concordance in birth." *Birth, 50*(2), 267–272. https://doi.org/10.1111/birt.12720. Epub 2023 Apr 23. PMID: 37088917.

Johnson, C. G. (2013). *Female inmates sterilized in California prisons without approval.* Reveal, from the Center for Investigative Reporting. https://www.revealnews.org/article/female-inmates-sterilized-in-california-prisons-without-approval/

Johnson, J., Cameron, L., Mitchinson, L., et al. (2019, December). An investigation into the relationships between bullying, discrimination, burnout and patient safety in nurses and midwives: Is burnout a mediator? *Journal of Research in Nursing, 24*(8), 604–619. https://doi.org/10.1177/1744987119880329

Jones, C. P. (2000). Levels of racism: A theoretic framework and a gardener's tale. *American Journal of Public Health, 90*(8), 1212–1215. https://doi.org/10.2105/AJPH.90.8.1212

Jones, C. P. (2002). Confronting institutionalized racism. *Phylon, 50*(1/2), 7–22. https://doi.org/10.2307/4149999

Kapitan, A. (2016, September 21). *Ask a radical copyeditor: Black with a capital "B."* Radical Copyeditor. https://radicalcopyeditor.com/2016/09/21/black-with-a-capital-b/

Katon, J. G., Plowden, T. C., & Marsh, E. E. (2023, March). Racial disparities in uterine fibroids and endometriosis: A systematic review and application of social, structural, and political context. *Fertility and Sterility, 119*(3), 355–363. https://doi.org/10.1016/j.fertnstert.2023.01.022. Epub 2023 Jan 20. PMID: 36682686; PMCID: PMC9992263.

Kendi, I. X. (2023). *Stamped from the beginning: The definitive history of racist ideas in America.* Perseus Books, LLC.

Kimani, R. W. (2023, May). Racism, colonialism and the implications for nursing scholarship: A discussion paper. *Journal of Advanced Nursing, 79*(5), 1745–1753. https://doi.org/10.1111/jan.15634. Epub 2023 Mar 7. PMID: 36882970; PMCID: PMC10389119.

Lawrence, J. (2000). The Indian Health Service and the sterilization of Native American women. *American Indian Quarterly, 24*(3), 400–419. https://www.jstor.org/stable/1185911

Lemelle, A. J. (2011). Conceptual, operational, and theoretical overview of African American health related disparities for social and behavioral interventions. In A. Lemelle, W. Reed, & S. Taylor (Eds.), *Handbook of African American health: Social and behavioral interventions* (pp. 3–33). Springer. https://doi .org/10.1007/978-1-4419-9616- 9_1

Liao, P. V., & Dollin, J. (2021, December). Half a century of the oral contraceptive pill: Historical review and view to the future. *Canadian Family Physician, 58*(12), e757–e760. PMID: 23242907; PMCID: PMC3520685.

Liddell, J. L., & Kington, S. G. (2021, January). "Something was attacking them and their reproductive organs": Environmental reproductive justice in an Indigenous tribe in the United States Gulf Coast. *International Journal of Environmental Research and Public Health, 18*(2), 666. https://doi.org/10.3390/ijerph18020666. PMID: 33466865; PMCID: PMC7830890.

Lo, M. C. M., & Nguyen, E. T. (2018). Caring and carrying the cost: Bicultural Latina nurses' challenges and strategies for working with coethnic patients. *The Russell Sage Foundation Journal of the Social Sciences, 4*(1), 149–171. https://doi.org/10.7758/rsf.2018.4.1.09

Luke, J. M. (2018). *Delivered by midwives: African American midwifery in the twentieth-century South.* University Press of Mississippi.

Maina, I. W., Belton, T. D., Ginzberg, S., Singh, A., & Johnson, T. J. (2018). A decade of studying implicit racial/ethnic bias in healthcare providers using the implicit association test. *Social Science & Medicine, 199*, 219–229. https://doi.org/10.1016/j.socscimed.2017.05.009

Martin, J. N., & Pace, T. W. W. (2025). Colonialism as a social determinant of health in Puerto Rico: Using the socioecological model to examine how the Jones Act impacted health after Hurricane María. *Journal of Transcultural Nursing, 36*(1), 8–15. https://doi.org/10.1177/10436596241274123

Mathur, M. B., Epel, E., Kind, S., Desai, M., Parks, C. G., Sandler, D. P., & Khazeni, N. (2016). Perceived stress and telomere length: A systematic review, meta-analysis, and methodologic considerations for advancing the field. *Brain, Behavior, and Immunity, 54*, 158–169. https://doi.org/10.1016/j.bbi.2016.02.002

McEwen, B., & Seeman, T. (with Allostatic Load Working Group). (2009). *Allostatic load and allostasis.* University of California, San Francisco. https://pubmed.ncbi.nlm.nih.gov/10649824/

McEwen, B. S. (2018). Redefining neuroendocrinology: Epigenetics of brain -body communication over the life course. *Frontiers in Neuroendocrinology, 49*, 8–30.

McKee, C. (2016). *CMS highlights state policies to improve access to long-acting reversible contraceptive methods.* National Health Law Program. https://healthlaw.org/wp-content/uploads/2016/04/2016_04_12_Improving_Access_LARCs.pdf

Mehra, R., Alspaugh, A., Joseph, J., et al. (2023, February). Racism is a motivator and a barrier for people of color aspiring to become midwives in the United States. *Health Services Research, 58*(1), 40–50. https://doi.org/10.1111/1475-6773.14037

Metzl, J. M., & Hansen, H. (2014). Structural competency: Theorizing a new medical engagement with stigma and inequality. *Social Science and Medicine, 103*, 126–33.

Metzl, J. M., Petty, J., & Olowojoba, O. V. (2018). Using a structural competency framework to teach structural racism in pre-health education. *Social Science & Medicine, 199*, 189–201. https://doi.org/10.1016/j.socscimed.2017.06.029

Metzl, J. M., & Roberts, D. E. (2014). Structural competency meets structural racism: Race, politics, and the structure of medical knowledge. *AMA Journal of Ethics, 16*(9), 674–690.

Miller, H. N., LaFave, S., Marineau, L., Stephens, J., & Thorpe, R. J., Jr. (2021, July). The impact of discrimination on allostatic load in adults: An integrative review of literature. *Journal of Psychosomatic Research, 146*, 110434. https://doi.org/10.1016/j.jpsychores.2021.110434. Epub 2021 Mar 24. PMID: 33810863; PMCID: PMC8172431.

Motley, D. N., Victorian, J., Denis, K., & Brooks, B. D. (2023, December). Applying an intersectionality framework to health services research. *Family Systems & Health, 41*(4), 417–424. https://doi.org/10.1037/fsh0000859. PMID: 38284973.

Muse, S. (2018). *Setting the standard for holistic care of and for Black women.* Black Mamas Matter Alliance. http://blackmamasmatter.org/wp-content/uploads/2018/04/BMMA_BlackPaper_April-2018.pdf

National Academies of Sciences, Engineering, and Medicine. (2017). *Communities in action: Pathways to health equity.* National Academies Press.

National Association of Nurse Practitioners in Women's Health. (2020, October). Structural racism and implicit bias in women's healthcare [Position statement]. https://cdn.ymaws.com/npwh.org/resource/resmgr/positionstatement/npwh-ps-102020-structuralrac.pdf

National Heart, Lung, and Blood Institute. (2024). Health Disparities and Inequities. Accessed January 14, 2025 at https://www.nhlbi.nih.gov/science/health-disparities

National Native American Boarding School Healing Coalition. (n.d.). *US Indian boarding school history.* https://boardingschoolhealing.org/education/us-indian-boarding-school-history/

National Women's Health Network. (2019). *Policy issues: Long-acting reversible contraceptives (LARCs).*

Nijagal, M. A., Odiase, O. J., Bell, A. J., El Ayadi, A. M., Williams, S., Nicolaisen, C., Jacobs, G., Mack, B., LaSerre, M., Stewart, C., Crockett, K., & Afulani, P. A. (2025, March). The Family and Pregnancy Pop-Up Village: Developing a one-stop shop of services to reduce pregnancy care-related inequities in San Francisco. *Birth, 52*(1), 66–77. https://doi.org/10.1111/birt.12839. Epub 2024 Jun 17. PMID: 38887141; PMCID: PMC11829268.

Niles, P. M., & Drew, M. (2020, October 22). Constructing the modern American midwife: White supremacy and White feminism collide. Nursing Clio. https://nursingclio.org/2020/10/22/constructing-the-modern-american-midwife-white-supremacy-and-white-feminism-collide/

Ohm, J. E. (2019). Environmental exposures, the epigenome, and African American women's health. *Journal of Urban Health, 96*, 50–56. https://doi.org/10.1007 /s11524-018-00332-2

Owens, D. C. (2017). *Medical bondage: Race, gender, and the origins of American gynecology.* University of Georgia Press. https://doi.org/10.2307/j.ctt1pwt69x

Paltrow, L. M., & Flavin, J. (2013). Arrests of and forced interventions on pregnant women in the United States, 1973–2005: Implications for women's legal status and public health. *Journal of Health Politics, Policy and Law, 38*(2), 299–343. https://doi.org/10.1215/03616878-1966324

Paltrow, L. M., Harris, L. H., & Marshall, M. F. (2022, August). Beyond abortion: The consequences of overturning *Roe*. *American Journal of Bioethics, 22*(8), 3–15. https://doi.org/10.1080/15265161.2022.2075965. Epub 2022 Jun 2. PMID: 35652910.

PBS. *The Puerto Rico pill trials.* (n.d.). American Experience. https://www.pbs.org/wgbh/americanexperience/features/pill-puerto-rico-pill-trials/

Pederson, H. J., Al-Hilli, Z., & Kurian, A. W. (2024, June). Racial disparities in breast cancer risk factors and risk management. *Maturitas, 184*, 107949. https://doi.org/10.1016/j.maturitas.2024.107949. Epub 2024 Feb 29. PMID: 38652937.

Petrella, C., & Begley, J. (2013). The color of corporate corrections: The overrepresentation of people of color in the for-profit corrections industry. *Radical Criminology, 2*(2013), 139–148.

Pour-Khorshid, F. (2018). Cultivating sacred spaces: A racial affinity group approach to support critical educators of color. *Teaching Education, 29*(4), 318–329.

Prather, C., Fuller, T. R., Jeffries, W. L., Marshall, K. J., Howell, A. V., Belyue-Umole, A., & King, W. (2018). Racism, African American women, and their sexual and reproductive health: A review of historical and contemporary evidence and implications for health equity. *Health Equity, 2*(1), 249–259. https://doi.org/10.1089/heq.2017.0045

Prunty, M., Bukavina, L., & Hallman, J. C. (2021, November). Anarcha, Lucy, and Betsey: The mothers of modern gynecology. *Urology, 157*, 1–4. https://doi.org/10.1016/j.urology.2021.06.048. Epub 2021 Aug 23. PMID: 34437896.

Ramsden, I., (2015). Towards cultural safety. In D. Wepa (Ed.), *Cultural Safety in Aotearoa New Zealand* (2nd ed., pp. 5–25). Cambridge University Press: Melbourne.

Riggan, K. A., Gilbert, A., & Allyse, M. A. (2021, February). Acknowledging and addressing allostatic load in pregnancy care. *Journal of Racial and Ethnic Health Disparities, 8*(1), 69–79. https://doi.org/10.1007/s40615-020-00757-z. Epub 2020 May 7. PMID: 32383045; PMCID: PMC7647942.

Roberts, D. E. (1997). *Killing the black body: Race, reproduction, and the meaning of liberty.* Pantheon Books.

Rodriquez, E. J., Kim, E. N., Sumner, A. E., Nápoles, A. M., & Pérez-Stable, E. J. (2019). Allostatic load: Importance, markers, and score determination in minority and disparity populations [Suppl. 1]. *Journal of Urban Health, 96*, 3–11. https://doi.org/10.1007/s11524-019-00345-5

Rodriguez, M. A., & García, R. (2013). First, do no harm: The US sexually transmitted disease experiments in Guatemala. *American Journal of Public Health, 103*(12), 2122–2126. https://doi.org/10.2105/AJPH.2013.301520

Rodriquez, E. J., Livaudais-Toman, J., Gregorich, S. E., Jackson, J. S., Nápoles, A. M., & Pérez-Stable, E. J. (2018). Relationships between allostatic load, unhealthy behaviors, and depressive disorder in US adults, 2005–2012 NHANES. *Preventive Medicine, 110*, 9–15. https://doi.org/10.1016/j.ypmed.2018.02.002

Ross, L. (2007). What is reproductive justice? In *Reproductive justice briefing book: A primer on reproductive justice and social change* (pp. 4–5). https://www.protectchoice.org/downloads/Reproductive%20Justice%20Briefing%20Book.pdf

Ross, L. (2021). Understanding reproductive justice. In *Feminist Theory Reader* (pp. 77–82). Routledge.

Ross, L., & Solinger, R. (2017). *Reproductive justice: An introduction*. University of California Press.

Ross, P. T., Hart-Johnson, T., Santen, S. A., & Zaidi, N. L. B. (2020, October). Considerations for using race and ethnicity as quantitative variables in medical education research. *Perspectives on Medical Education, 9*(5), 318–323. https://doi.org/10.1007/s40037-020-00602-3. PMID: 32789666; PMCID: PMC7550522.

Sabin, J., Guenther, G., Ornelas, I. J., Patterson, D. G., Andrilla, C. H. A., Morales, L., Gurjal, K., & Frogner, B. K. (2022, December). Brief online implicit bias education increases bias awareness among clinical teaching faculty. *Medical Education Online, 27*(1), 2025307. https://doi.org/10.1080/10872981.2021.2025307. PMID: 35037585; PMCID: PMC8765255.

Sáenz, R., & Morales, M. C. (2019). Demography of race and ethnicity. In D. L. Poston (Ed.), *Handbook of population* (2nd ed., pp. 163–207). Springer Nature Switzerland. https://doi.org/10.1007/978-3-030-10910-3_7

Saluja, B., & Bryant, Z. (2021). How implicit bias contributes to racial disparities in maternal morbidity and mortality in the United States. Journal of Women's Health, 30(2), 270–273. https://doi.org/10.1089/jwh.2020.8874

Seeman, T., Merkin, S. S., Crimmins, E., Koretz, B., Charette, S., & Karlamangla, A. (2008). Education, income and ethnic differences in cumulative biological risk profiles in a national sample of US adults: NHANES III (1988–1994). *Social Science & Medicine, 66*(1), 72–87. https://doi.org/10.1016/j.socscimed.2007.08.027

Serbin, J. W., & Donnelly, E. (2016). The impact of racism and midwifery's lack of racial diversity: A literature review. *Journal of Midwifery & Women's Health, 61*(6), 694–706. https://doi.org/10.1111/jmwh.12572

Shen, M. J., Peterson, E. B., Costas-Muñiz, R., Hernandez, M. H., Jewell, S. T., Matsoukas, K., & Bylund, C. L. (2018). The effects of race and racial concordance on patient-physician communication: A systematic review of the literature. *Journal of Racial and Ethnic Health Disparities, 5*(1), 117–140. https://doi.org/10.1007/s40615- 017-0350-4

SisterSong. (n.d.). Reproductive justice. https://www.sistersong.net/reproductive-justice

Smith, A. (2005). Native American feminism, sovereignty, and social change. *Feminist Studies, 31*(1), 116–132. https://doi.org/10.2307/20459010

Spector-Bagdady, K., & Lombardo, P. A. (2019, March). U.S. Public Health Service STD experiments in Guatemala (1946–1948) and their aftermath. *Ethics and Human Research, 41*(2), 29–34. https://doi.org/10.1002/eahr.500010. PMID: 30895754.

Stern, A. M. (2016, January 7). That time the United States sterilized 60,000 of its citizens. *Huffington Post*. http://www.huffingtonpost.com/entry/sterilization-united-states_us_568f35f2e4b0c8beacf68713

Stringer, H. (2024, June 1). The journey of reconciliation continues: Impact of APA's apology to Indigenous Peoples. *Monitor on Psychology*. https://www.apa.org/monitor/2024/06/indigenous-apology-reconciliation

Tajima-Peña, R. (Director). (2015). *No más bebés* [Film]. Moon Canyon Films.

Tervalon, M., & Murray-García, J. (1998). Cultural humility versus cultural competence: a critical distinction in defining physician training outcomes in multicultural education. *Journal of Health Care for the Poor and Underserved 9*(2), 117–125. https://dx.doi.org/10.1353/hpu.2010.0233.

Tavares, C. D., Bell, C. N., Zare, H., Hudson, D., & Thorpe, R. J., Jr. (2022, March–April). Allostatic load, income, and race among Black and White men in the United States. *American Journal of Men's Health, 16*(2), 15579883221092290. https://doi.org/10.1177/15579883221092290. PMID: 35466781; PMCID: PMC9036348.

Temkin, S. M., Rimel, B. J., Bruegl, A. S., Gunderson, C. C., Beavis, A. L., & Doll, K. M. (2018). A contemporary framework of health equity applied to gynecologic cancer care: A Society of Gynecologic Oncology evidenced-based review. *Gynecologic Oncology, 149*(1), 70–77. https://doi.org/10.1016/j.ygyno.2017.11.013

Think Cultural Health Education. (n.d.). Combating implicit bias and stereotypes. Accessed June 21, 2025 at https://thinkculturalhealth.hhs.gov/maternal-health - care/assets/pdfs/Combating_implicit_bias_and_stereotypes.pdf

Thomas, M. D., Mendez, R. M., Zhang, Y., Wang, Y., Sohail, S., Chae, D. H., Márquez-Magaña, L., Sellers, R., Woods-Giscombé, C. L., & Allen, A. M. (2022, May). Superwoman Schema, racial identity, and cellular aging among African American women. *Gerontologist, 62*(5), 762–772. https://doi.org/10.1093/geront/gnac005. PMID: 35084030; PMCID: PMC9154235.

Tobin, M. J. (2022, May). Fiftieth anniversary of uncovering the Tuskegee syphilis study: The story and timeless lessons. *American Journal of Respiratory and Critical Care Medicine, 205*(10), 1145–1158. https://doi.org/10.1164/rccm.202201-0136SO. PMID: 35500908; PMCID: PMC9872801.

Tolentino, D. A., Roca, R. P. E., Yang, J., Itchon, J., & Byrnes, M. E. (2023). Experiences of Filipino Americans with Type 2 diabetes during COVID-19: A qualitative study. *Western Journal of Nursing Research, 45*(6), 562–570. https://doi.org/10.1177/01939459231162917

Touma, F., Hummer, R. A. (2022, December). Race/ethnicity, immigrant generation, and physiological dysregulation among U.S. adults entering midlife. *Social Science and Medicine, 314*, 115423. https://doi.org/10.1016/j.socscimed.2022.115423. Epub 2022 Oct 4. PMID: 36283331; PMCID: PMC10112471.

Town, M., Eke, P., Zhao, G., et al. (2024). Racial and ethnic differences in social determinants of health and health-related social needs among adults—Behavioral risk factor surveillance system, United States, 2022. *Morbidity and Mortality Weekly Report, 73*, 204–208. http://dx.doi.org/10.15585/mmwr.mm7309a3.

Tervalon, M., & Murray-García, J. (1998). Cultural humility versus cultural competence: A critical distinction in defining physician training outcomes in multicultural education. *Journal of Health Care for the Poor and Underserved, 9*(2), 117–125. https://doi.org/10.1353/hpu.2010.0233

United Negro College Fund. (n.d.). *K-12 disparity facts and statistics*. https://www.uncf.org/pages/k-12-disparity-facts-and-stats

University of California Los Angeles Office of Equity, Diversity, and Inclusion. (2020). Resources on Native American and Indigenous Peoples. Accessed on June 18, 2025 at https://equity.ucla.edu/know/resources-on-native-american-and-indigenous-affairs/native american-and-indigenous-peoples-faqs

University of Richmond. (2025). Mapping Inequality: Redlining in New Deal America. Accessed June 22, 2025 at https://dsl.richmond.edu/panorama/redlining

U.S. Department of Health and Human Services. (2022). *Health equity and health disparities environmental scan*. Rockville, MD: U.S. Department of Health and Human Services, Office of the Assistant Secretary for Health, Office of Disease Prevention and Health Promotion.

U.S. General Accounting Office. (1976, September). *Answers to frequently asked questions*. Washington, D.C.: U.S. General Accounting Office.

Veracini, L. (2024). *Settler colonialism: A theoretical overview* (2nd ed.). Palgrave Macmillan.

Wailoo, K. (2018). Historical aspects of race and medicine: The case of J. Marion Sims. *JAMA: The Journal of the American Medical Association, 320*(15), 1529–1530. https://doi.org/10.1001/jama.2018.11944

Watkins T. (2021). Intersectional Wheel of Privilege. Accessed May 24, 2025 at https://just1voice.com/advocacy/wheel-of- privilege/?srsltid=AfmBOorNULZzsZOBht2sB9m7vZNRg6kpE642xRbPwKdoqvRIBdB7 QL9N

White Junod, S., & Marks, L. (2002, April). Women's trials: The approval of the first oral contraceptive pill in the United States and Great Britain. *Journal of the History of Medicine and Allied Sciences, 57*(2), 117–160. https://doi.org/10.1093/jhmas/57.2.117

Wispelwey, B., Tanous, O., Asi, Y., Hammoudeh, W., & Mills, D. (2023, July). Because its power remains naturalized: introducing the settler colonial determinants of health. *Frontiers in Public Health, 11*, 1137428. https://doi.org/10.3389/fpubh.2023.1137428. PMID: 37533522; PMCID: PMC10393129.

Wusu, M. H., Tepperberg, S., Weinberg, J. M., & Saper, R. B. (2019). Matching our mission: A strategic plan to create a diverse family medicine residency. *Family Medicine, 51*(1), 31–36. https://doi.org/10.22454/FamMed.2019.955445

Yale School of Medicine Office of Health Equity Research. (2025). Best Practices for Collecting and Analyzing Race and Ethnicity Data. Accessed June 18, 2025 at https://files-profile.medicine.yale.edu/documents/33d77238-3851-441c-ab14-fcd1ac49a0ef

Yellow Horse, A. J., & Santos-Lozada, A. R. (2019). Foreign-born Hispanic women's health patterns in allostatic load converge to US-born Hispanic women at a slower tempo compared with men. *Women's Health Issues, 29*(3), 222–230. https://doi.org/10.1016/j.whi.2019.01.001

Yoo, D., Grieman, P., Villaseñor Black, C., Dupuy, D., & Pan, A. (2022). *Knowledge for justice: An ethnic studies reader.* UCLA American Indian Studies Center Publications, Asian American Studies Center Press, Chicano Studies Research Center Press, and the Ralph J. Bunche Center for African American Studies.

Zewude, R., & Sharma, M. Critical race theory in medicine. *CMAJ, 193*(20), E739–E741. https://doi.org/10.1503/cmaj.210178. PMID: 34001553; PMCID: PMC8177947.

APPENDIX 2-A

Additional Resources

DEVELOPMENT AND EFFECTS OF RACISM IN THE UNITED STATES

Books:

A People's History of the United States by Howard Zinn
An Indigenous Peoples' History of the United States by Roxanne Dunbar-Ortiz
The New Jim Crow: Mass Incarceration in the Age of Colorblindness by Michelle Alexander
Racial Formation in the United States (3rd ed.) by Michael Omi and Howard Winant
Stamped from the Beginning: The Definitive History of Racist Ideas in America by Ibram X. Kendi

Movies:

13th by Ava DuVernay
Race: The Power of an Illusion (three-part series) by California Newsreel
Racism: A History (three-part series) by the British Broadcasting Corporation

Podcasts:

Scene on Radio, "Seeing White" (https://www.sceneonradio.org/seeing-white/)
Serial, Season 3, "A Year Inside a Typical American Courthouse" (https://serialpodcast.org/season-three)

REPRODUCTIVE COERCION AND ABUSES

Books:

Killing the Black Body by Dorothy E. Roberts
Medical Apartheid: The Dark History of Medical Experimentation on Black Americans from Colonial Times to the Present by Harriet Washington
Medical Bondage: Race, Gender and the Origins of American Gynecology by Deidre Cooper Owens

Journal articles:

Gomez, A. M., Fuentes, L., & Allina, A. (2014). Women or LARC first? Reproductive autonomy and the promotion of long-acting reversible contraceptive methods. *Perspectives on Sexual and Reproductive Health, 46*(3), 171–175.

Gubrium, A. C., Mann, E. S., Borrero, S., Dehlendorf, C., Fields, J., Geronimus, A. T., Gómez, A. M., Harris, L. H., Higgins, J. A., Kimport, K., Luker, K., Luna, Z., Mamo, L., Roberts, D., Romero, D., & Sisson, G. (2016). Realizing reproductive health equity needs more than long-acting reversible contraception (LARC). *American Journal of Public Health, 106*(1), 18–19.

Movie:

No Más Bebés by Renee Tajima-Peña

CRIMINALIZATION OF PREGNANCY

Books:

The Pregnancy Police: Conceiving Crime, Arresting Personhood by Grace Howard

Movie:

Birthright: A War Story by Civia Tamarkin

News series:

New York Times Editorial Board. (2018). *A woman's rights.* https://www.nytimes.com/interactive/2018/12/28/opinion/pregnancy-women-pro-life-abortion.html

CHAPTER 3

Growth and Development Across the Lifespan

Lee Roosevelt
Lisa Kane Low

Understanding growth and development across the lifespan is essential to comprehending health and well-being, as these processes are deeply intertwined with biologic health. While this text uses growth and development as a framework for discussing variations from what is considered normative, it acknowledges the limitations of a purely biomedical perspective. A biomedical context often reduces individuals' bodies to biological components and physiological processes. Although this approach allows for the quantification of growth, it overlooks the qualitative aspects of how individuals live their lives and how these lived experiences influence their growth and development (Kane Low & Bailey, 2022).

The biomedical model of health is individualist and disease oriented. In contrast, a feminist and social model of health acknowledges the influence of the culture in which people live, their economic status, the social interactions they experience, and the context in which they access and receive health care. A feminist model acknowledges the many other facets of life beyond the physiologic functioning of people and the genetic inheritance that affects their growth and development. Feminism provides a framework to explore the complex interplay between sex and gender while simultaneously challenging biological essentialism, patriarchy, and sexism and addressing power imbalances. As a result, even the manner in which we understand and explain what is included in normative growth and development changes in the expanded framework of a feminist perspective, thereby allowing for a clearer understanding of the complexity inherent in human growth and development.

As a first step in considering life course development (cognitive, psychosocial, and functional behaviors), it is important to acknowledge that traditional models were developed from research about cisgender men. For example, psychoanalyst Erik Erikson (1950) expanded developmental theory beyond the years of adolescence to offer a grand theory of human development (**Table 3-1**). The expansion of this theory was viewed as transformational at the time because no one else had pushed the boundaries of psychosocial theory quite so far (Maree, 2021). Erikson identified eight general stages of development, each of which is the sequential focus of psychological energy. Erikson describes the psychological life of adulthood as centrally organized by four of these themes (Table 3-1) (Maree, 2021). The eight virtues that are the goals of the stages are trust, autonomy, initiative, industry, identity, intimacy, generativity, and integrity.

By explicating a process of resolving eight developmental crises that are sequentially confronted, Erikson's theory offers a comprehensive account of individual development throughout the lifespan that, until recently, was applied to both males and females. However, a critical distinction is that Erikson's stages of psychosocial development are based on studies of white middle-class males; in fact, his initial work on identity was conducted with returning war veterans in the 1950s (Erikson, 1968; Gilligan, 1986). Nevertheless, his model has been universally applied to all people with some gendered assumptions. These underlying assumptions within Erikson's grand theory of development are important because his theory assumes homogeneity of all individuals, with minimal attention paid to gender, socioeconomic, or racial and ethnic variability (Alberts & Durrheim, 2018; de Carvalho & Veiga, 2022; Gilligan, 1993). These assumptions include a normative linear pattern of identity followed by marriage (intimacy) and then childbearing (generativity) in adulthood. Erikson's theory assumes the need for a woman to first develop an intimate relationship with another before she can complete her sense of self as an individual. Interestingly, men (according to his theory) do not have the same requirement. Thus, while the larger context of the theory assumes the desirability of autonomy and distancing oneself from the family of origin, autonomy for women is defined as being dependent on another within the context of a relationship, with a primary focus on caretaking. Erikson grounded his work within normative gendered expectations. Erikson's human development model also posits concepts of gender role identification in traditionally gendered, biologically based constructions that fail to allow for the creation of healthy, nonstigmatized models of LGBTQ+ identities (Owen, 2020).

Other examples of grand theories that are misapplied to all people, regardless of gender identity, include those developed by Kohlberg and Power (1981) and Perry (1968). Kohlberg's levels of moral development are based on interviews with only cisgender men, while Perry actually discarded interviews he had with cisgender women and used only data from interviews with cisgender men to formulate his model of intellectual development. The difficulty that arises when these scales are applied to assess developmental level is that they assume universality in development and treat all genders as a monolith, not acknowledging the multiple variables that can affect progress through the stages (Belenky, 1986; Kane Low, 2001). The use of these androcentric models constrains the manner in which psychosocial

TABLE 3-1 Erikson's Epigenetic Model

Age Period for Crisis	STAGES 1	2	3	4	5	6	7	8
Infancy	Trust versus mistrust							
Early childhood		Autonomy versus shame and doubt						
Play age			Initiative versus guilt					
School age				Industry versus inferiority				
Adolescence					Identity versus identity diffusion			
Young adult						Intimacy versus isolation		
Adulthood							Generativity versus self-absorption	
Mature age								Integrity versus despair

Reproduced from from Low, L. K. (2001). *Adolescents' experiences of childbirth: Nothing is simple*. Unpublished doctoral dissertation, University of Michigan, Ann Arbor, MI.

development is framed. White, cisgender male development is held up as the standard in which other paths through growth and development are viewed as aberrations.

This chapter discusses growth and development by contrasting traditional patriarchal theoretical constructs with feminist theories that challenge some of the basic assumptions about growth and development. Alternative theories of development that focus on relationship and connection have been offered by feminist theorists, queer theorists, psychologists, and researchers (particularly those connected with the Stone Center (Wellesley College) since the 1970s (Deanow, 2011; Miller & Scholnick, 2015; C. Taylor et al., 1994). Although there is substantial variation in the emphasis of feminist scholars, a primary focus is the self in relation to, or in connection with, others (family and peers) as a means of further development. Viewing growth and development through a relational framework stands in stark contrast to theorists such as Kohlberg who argued that to be concerned with relationships and emotions was to sound like "women" and indicated a lower stage of moral development (Gilligan, 2018). Through a feminist perspective, development is construed as broader than the traditional process of individualization and includes the value of maintaining connection and continuity within relationships, which are viewed as primary sources for support and identity development (Deanow, 2011; Gilchrist, 1997; Tummala-Narra, 2013).

The definition of relationships within this model incorporates not just the self in relation to others, but also inner constructions of relationships that form the sense of self and identity development (H. B. Kaplan, 1991; Tummala-Narra, 2013). These relationships contain progressively more conflict, and it is through resolution of this conflict that the relationships become more complex, requiring flexibility that allows connections and relationships to be maintained (Baker Miller, 1987). This view stands in opposition to traditional theories of development, which emphasize conflict resolution as entailing greater disconnection and the development of distinct boundaries around identity formation, characterized as the process of "becoming one's own man" (Baker Miller, 1987).

Deanow (2011) proposed a newer model of development that highlights relationship developmental tasks and obstacles throughout the life cycle (refer to **Appendix 3-A**) (Collins, 2022; Macleod et al., 2020). Previous relational development models were not placed into a chronological framework to compare or contrast them with the age-related stages of other theories. Additionally, the relational development models focused on relational processes between adults and do not address what occurs relationally in childhood or adolescence. Deanow's model identifies two poles—normative relational growth at one end, and age-relational disconnection within age-related stages at the other end—thereby incorporating a chronological relational model of development into a theoretical base that can assist clinicians' understanding of their clients.

Feminist theories are primarily offered in contrast to Erikson's theory of psychosocial development. Gilligan (1982) was an early feminist scholar who offered critiques of his work as being descriptive not only of male development in general, but also of primarily white, privileged male development. Black feminist scholarship has furthered this to include limitations in contrasting models offered by early feminist theorists. A key limitation of early feminist models is that they were developed by white, middle-class, Euro-American cisgender women who interpret relationships and connection as being similar across all people, regardless of intersectional identities or the influence of oppressions (Collins, 2022; Macleod et al., 2020). The process of developing an ethnic-racial identity within the sociocultural context of historical enslavement, racial stigmatization, and discrimination is a crucial task of development that has been historically absent from developmental theorists (Mims & Williams, 2020). The complexity and growth of an ethnic-racial identity mirrors traditionally identified developmental processes, where advancing cognitive capacity enables youth to think more abstractly about who they are in relation to race and ethnicity. The development of an ethnic-racial identity is integrated into all other identities and is shaped by context and experience. However, the intersectionality of identities has little to no representation in psychological research that primarily focuses on race or gender, but not their intersection (Carter & Seaton, 2024; Crenshaw, 1997).

Transgender and gender-diverse people face similar struggles in finding a place for themselves in theories of human growth and development. Although research on this topic remains sparse, it is essential to include current understandings of gender identity development, as well as social reactions to what is termed nonconforming, nonbinary, or gender-diverse expression. Additionally, it is important to explore ways to support transgender youth as they navigate cultural expectations of gender expression and work toward achieving balance, fulfillment, and comfort with their own gender identity (Roosevelt et al., 2024).

Subscription to a model that delineates gender differences versus a model that identifies gender similarities and provides an explanation for differences based on gender is a key philosophical dilemma for developmental theorists. The emphasis on difference, rather than similarity, evokes a debate about the risk of essentializing development by sex and assigning socially constructed gender roles and assumes that the developmental process is chronologic and starts from birth, which therefore ignores the process of identity development experienced by people who do not subscribe to binary gender identities. The controversy arises because the gender differences described by these theories are ascribed to biologic or innate characteristics rather than considering the social and cultural context that can create these differences. The differences described within the theories are wrongly assumed to be biologic in origin, instead of reflecting social constructs of femininity (Crenshaw, 1997). While lauding the work of Gilligan and other early feminist theorists who argue that women have a "different voice" through which they develop and speak, there is the risk of describing a uniquely female experience that is likely based primarily on the social construction of gender roles.

This perspective, which results in differing expectations at different times based on gender, is consistent with the model proposed by Erikson (1950). He argued that the particular developmental crisis is not necessarily chronologically driven, but rather is driven by social expectations for behavior. Thus, expectations for caregiving and consideration as feminine traits may have more to do with socially prescribed gender roles of femininity than with biologically differing pathways for development. More similarities than differences between people may become evident when gender boundaries are broken down. While transformations in gender roles, relational development, and caretaking are in progress, contrasting developmental models with an emphasis on differences that are primarily socially constructed have generally prevailed and, therefore, will inform the perspectives presented in this chapter.

The intention of newer feminist models is not to replace male generalist models of development with feminist generalist models of development, but rather to offer alternatives to the constrained models that were previously misapplied across all people. This chapter provides an overview of growth and development within the linear stages of adolescence through older age using a feminist perspective while also recognizing that despite theories of development being organized chronologically, actual development of a person is a nonlinear and iterative process over time. Emphasis is placed on contrasting models of development outside the traditional biomedical focus.

ADOLESCENCE

The adolescent years are generally described as the time of transition from childhood to young adulthood and are biologically defined as beginning with the onset of puberty and lasting until young adulthood (Alderman et al., 2019). In a chronological sense, this generally encompasses the ages of 11–21 years, although some clinicians may refer to ages 9–12 as the "tween" years and may consider late adolescence as extending to 25 years old (Arnett, 2024; McArthur et al., 2021).

Visible physical changes occur during adolescence, such as breast development and menarche; many additional developmental processes occur during this period that are not outwardly visible but are nonetheless critically important for a healthy transition to adulthood. For example, the brains of adolescents are continuing to develop, which results in increased cognitive skills that enhance their ability to reason and think abstractly. The changes that occur in the adolescent brain are both structural and functional, and they support cerebral maturation (Jansen & Kiefer, 2020). Although the changes that occur during this period are discussed here in the contexts of biology and physiology, there are also qualitative aspects of adolescence that must be considered from a healthcare standpoint. Indeed, it is important to appreciate the context of the adolescent's lived experience to fully understand the adolescent for whom you are providing health care. Their family, neighborhood, workplace, and community are factors that are just as important as their gender, race, sexual orientation, disability or chronic disease, and religious beliefs.

The Biology and Physiology of Adolescent Growth and Development for Those Assigned Female at Birth

The cause of the onset of puberty remains unknown; however, it is known to be influenced by genetics, overall health, social environment, and environmental exposures (H. S. Taylor et al., 2019). Research also continues to suggest that the onset of puberty and its progression is related to weight and body fat mass (H. S. Taylor et al., 2019). Consequently, puberty marks the beginning of a tension between biologic development and the social context in which it occurs. Cultural narratives demand perfection, which causes many young people to suffer great anxiety about their bodies. The challenges faced by young people vary based on race, ethnicity, self-esteem, the social environment, and the contrast between the individual adolescent's sense of themself and society's perceived standard for beauty. In addition, many of the changes during puberty are framed within the social context of sexual development. As their physical sexual characteristics develop, many young people are challenged by a potential mismatch between their socially perceived sexual development and their interpersonal level of maturity and development. Clinicians can be an important source of support and information during what is often framed culturally as a tumultuous phase of development.

Significant changes occur as an adolescent reaches puberty. Probably most significant to many young people, however, are the physical changes associated with puberty, especially the development of secondary sex characteristics. For adolescents assigned female at birth, rapid skeletal growth precedes thelarche (breast development) and pubarche (the appearance of pubic hair) and is mediated by an increase in gonadotropin secretion, which occurs as a result of stimulation from sex steroids (H. S. Taylor et al., 2019). The rising sex steroids ultimately limit bone growth as the epiphyseal closure occurs. It is believed that individuals acquire the majority of their bone mass during early adolescence; thus, this critical period lays the groundwork for prevention of osteoporosis in later years of life.

As estradiol concentrations gradually increase, thelarche is stimulated (H. S. Taylor et al., 2019). Breast development and other pubertal changes follow a specific sequence of events (refer to the stages within the Tanner scale in **Figure 3-1**).

The onset of menses, which occurs when a positive feedback of estrogen on the pituitary and hypothalamus stimulates a surge of luteinizing hormone at midcycle, is critical to ovulation (H. S. Taylor et al., 2019). The age of the onset of puberty has been significantly declining in the United States. The changes that occur during puberty usually happen in an ordered sequence, beginning with thelarche at around age 10 or 11, followed by adrenarche (growth of pubic hair due to androgen stimulation), peak height velocity, and finally menarche (onset of menses), which usually occurs around age 12 or 13. Peak height velocity usually occurs about 2 years after breast budding and about 1 year prior to menarche (H. S. Taylor et al., 2019). Generally, American girls who are Black begin puberty earlier than American girls who are white—8 to 9 years versus 9 years, respectively (H. S. Taylor et al., 2019).

The timing of the growth spurt or peak height velocity in young girls occurs approximately 2 years earlier in puberty than it does for boys (H. S. Taylor et al., 2019). Thelarche normally occurs between the ages of 8 and 13 years. Adrenarche generally begins within 6 months of the advent of thelarche, usually between ages 11 and 12. The general time frame from thelarche to menarche is 2–3 years. As the first several menstrual cycles

FIGURE 3-1 Stages within the Tanner scale.

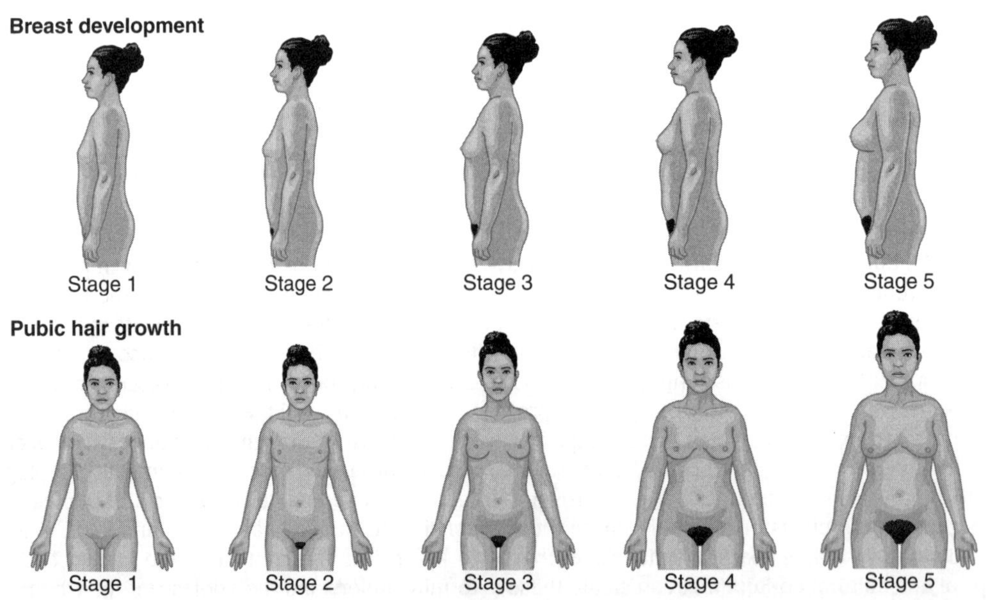

usually do not result in ovulation, an adolescent's first-year experience of menstruating is often characterized by irregular anovulatory cycles and heavy bleeding (H. S. Taylor et al., 2019).

The median age for the onset of menstruation has remained stable despite variations in well-nourished populations in highly resourced countries worldwide, including the United States at 12.8 years, with a range from age 9 to 17 (American College of Obstetrics & Gynecology, 2015, reaffirmed 2021). Compared with Black American girls, Hispanic American girls were more likely to have menarche earlier, whereas white and Asian American girls were more likely to have their first period later (Biro et al., 2018). Asian American, Native Hawaiian, and Pacific Islander (AANHPI) American girls have historically been excluded from research looking at puberty development so very little is known about how pubertal development differs for AANHPI girls as an aggregate or subgroups (Kubo et al., 2024).

The differences in pubertal timing have been fairly consistent over the past 30 years. However, these differences are rooted in social determinants of health and epigenetics. Determinants such as economic stability and neighborhood and built environment are correlated with earlier menarche (Srikanth et al., 2023). Epigentics refers to the way behaviors and environment can cause changes that affect the ways genes work (U.S. Centers for Disease Control and Prevention, 2024). Additionally, exposure to childhood adversity, such as systemic and individually mediated racism, may act through epigentic changes, inflammation, and other biological processes to accelerate biological aging and the onset of pubertal changes (Hamlat et al., 2023).

It is important to remind young people that there is a range for when puberty begins and that the timing varies from one person to another. Adolescents often worry about being on time for the advent of puberty and need to be reassured of the variations in the normal timing of breast development and menarche.

Adolescents assigned female at birth who have not reached puberty by the age of 13 or who have not had menarche by the age of 15 should be evaluated by a clinician to assess the pubertal delay. Even though such a delay may be due to heredity, it is important to rule out other factors that may be impacting their health, such as poor nutrition or eating disorders, involvement in sports/athletics, or genetic and medical conditions. While participation in sports has been linked to later onset of menarche, this link has not been found to be causal; that is, many other confounding factors contribute to this relationship (American College of Obstetrics & Gynecology, 2013, reaffirmed 2024).

Menarche is often a pivotal milestone event with implications for an adolescent's sense of self. It is probably also the most anticipated, feared, and socially misconstrued aspect of female adolescent development. Menarche is often viewed as a significant life event that carries physical, social, and emotional consequences that are important for clinicians to understand so they can promote adolescent health.

Menarche has many layers of social meaning. It is an event that establishes reproductive and sexual potential (H. S. Taylor et al., 2019); thus, it is important both as a physiologic marker of transitioning to adulthood (albeit framed by biomedical metaphors of scientific knowledge) and as one of the social and cultural junctures at which gender identity and gender relations may be shaped (do Amaral et al., 2011; Lee, 2008).

Contemporary U.S. society continues to view menstruation as a taboo subject, and the dominant discourses remain highly negative, suggesting that menstruation and menarche should be kept a secret and are a source of shame and secrecy (Gottlieb, 2020). Unfortunately, the continued systemic perpetuation of the negative discourses around menstruation, womanhood, and the female body have the potential to set adolescents on a highly problematic trajectory that will influence their affective and behavioral experiences across the lifespan (Winkler, 2020). It is important for clinicians who care for adolescents to carefully explore an adolescent's sense of self, body image, and feelings about their transition to young adulthood.

Clinicians can educate adolescents and their parents (or guardians) about what to expect with the experience of puberty and menarche. Experts suggest that adolescents who have been educated about what to expect during puberty and menarche will be much more comfortable with its onset than those who are not. ACOG (2015, reaffirmed 2021) identifies the menstrual cycle as a vital sign and, as such, makes the following recommendations:

- Educate young adolescents and their family about what to expect of a first menses.
- Educate young adolescents and their family about the variations of normal, as well as what might signal a problem and require a clinical visit.
- Ask about the menses at each clinical visit; identify abnormal problems and treat them early to offset potential health concerns that may arise during adulthood.
- Have an understanding of the menstrual patterns of adolescents, be able to differentiate between normal and abnormal, and have the skill to accurately assess and evaluate the adolescent patient.

The Tanner scale is commonly used for assessing sexual maturity and pubertal development. For young people assigned female at birth, it relies on development of the breasts and growth of pubic hair and divides sexual physical maturity into five stages that extend from preadolescence to adult (Figure 3-1). The Tanner scale is widely accepted for staging sexual maturity, but it is not appropriate to use for determining chronological age (Oliván-Gonzalvo et al., 2021).

Adolescence can be particularly challenging because growth in one area may not match growth in another, and both may be mismatched with chronological age. An adolescent's entire body, mind, and relationships are shifting during puberty. These changes can be particularly difficult for young people to navigate because they are striving to conform and not appear different from their peers. Significant amounts of time are spent on appearance and fitting in with group norms. It is important for parents of adolescents to listen when their child expresses dissatisfaction or concerns related to their body or pubertal changes. They need both reassurance that the changes are normal and adult help in keeping their concerns in perspective.

Neurodevelopment

Adolescence is a time of important morphological and functional transformations of the brain. These transformations interact with hormones and other biologic changes in addition to the impact of cultural, economic, and psychosocial forces to shape how an adolescent thinks, feels, and behaves. The prolonged nature of adolescence in human beings creates a period of intense developmental plasticity but also significant vulnerability to internal and external inputs (Ponzi et al., 2020). The adolescent brain is not an immature version of adult brain; instead, it is a unique structure that exhibits specific functional adaptations suited for the demands of growth and development (Opendak & Sullivan, 2019). Extensive proliferation of neurons and synapses occur during the preteen years, followed by pruning of synaptic connections over the next 5–10 years to ensure connectivity while many neurons and synapses are lost (Laricchiuta et al., 2023). Cerebral maturation, or neurodevelopment, and reorganization are both structural and functional in nature (Laricchiuta et al., 2023). Genetic disposition, hormonal influence, and experience affect which neural pathways are developed and retained; clearly, epigenetics plays an important role in the maturation of the adolescent brain (Manotas et al., 2021).

As the adolescent grows older, education, experience, and role models continue to impact brain development. By late adolescence, the prefrontal cortex is more developed, which enables the adolescent to have better abilities at planning, strategizing, and thinking before acting. Thus, the older adolescent is more able to control their impulses (Laricchiuta et al., 2023).

The enhanced understanding and recognition of brain development that occurs during adolescence has pushed clinicians to pay more attention to how adolescents act and react, and to why it is more difficult for an individual to make sound judgments earlier in adolescence. This is particularly important as clinicians teach adolescents about preventive health measures, such as wearing a helmet during activities where there is a risk of a blow to the head (e.g., skiing or bike riding).

Psychosocial and Cognitive Development

The traditional developmental task of adolescence is to develop a sense of identity and autonomy before progressing toward adulthood. The role of peers tends to increase in importance, and it is normal during this time to observe a distancing from parents and other adults as the adolescent tries to find their own separate identity. The interaction between an adolescent's behavior and role performance may either promote or confuse their sense of identity, depending on the social context in which it occurs. Through a process of trial and experimentation, individuals develop their own set of values and beliefs, as well as a sense of themselves as they formalize or commit to their own identity. Initiation of sexual activity, pregnancy, childbearing, and parenting are all gendered roles and experiences that any one individual adolescent may conceptualize differently based on the social, cultural, and historical definitions associated with these behaviors and roles, as well as their peers' and family's perceptions of these events.

In contrast, a feminist perspective of adolescent development emphasizes the young person's relationship with others instead of distancing from others in the process of individuation. Theorists argue that the hallmark of healthy identity development is developing a sense of connection to others, with a primary task being the ability to participate in mutual relationships in which the individual feels active and effective, not lost within the relationship (A. Kaplan et al., 1991). The self-in-relation model of adolescent development proposed by Baker Miller (1991) and her colleagues at the Wellesley College Stone Center defines a woman's sense of self as emerging out of experience with a relational process that begins in infancy. From initial interactions with caregivers through the process of becoming caretakers, the self-in-relation theory argues that women are socialized to care more and more about the development of relationships.

Laurel Silber (2012), along with other feminist scholars such as Carol Gilligan, posits that girls risk "losing their voice" during adolescence and that to stay connected and further develop an authentic sense of self they need to gain the ability to resist cultural norms. This is a monumental task for an adolescent because it requires that they identify their sense of self and be comfortable enough with it that they can simultaneously identify their agency, construct their own boundaries, and speak up. Few, if any, cultures support this developmental challenge (Silber, 2012). As much as the adolescent wants and works toward individuation, they also want and need to feel connected. Herein lies the struggle, which further underscores "the importance of working within the intergenerational relational context in which adolescent girls' struggles are embedded" (p. 132).

Reasoning changes as a child matures. As an individual goes through adolescence, their cognitive development expands from being a very concrete thinker to gaining the ability to think abstractly, reason more effectively, problem solve, and involve themselves in planning for their future (Ponzi et al., 2020). By comparison, cognitive competence develops more slowly over time. As a consequence, adolescents still require guidance in some of their decision making; they are prone to jumping to conclusions and making poor decisions, which can lead to risky behavior (Andrews et al., 2021). For example, older adolescents are usually able to connect intercourse with the potential for pregnancy, but younger adolescents might not be able to appreciate the logical sequencing of these events. Adolescents are particularly influenced by their peers, so it is important for adults to understand the importance of peer pressure and provide the support the adolescent needs to make healthy decisions about risky behaviors, such as consuming alcohol, having unprotected intercourse, and driving too fast. Additionally, using their newly developed hypothetical and deductive reasoning skills to make decisions can be especially difficult when the adolescent is confronting their peers. Maturation in thinking behavior is supported by understanding family members, an emotionally stable environment, appropriate parental discipline, and positive life experiences. The cognitive development of adolescents helps to lay the groundwork for their development of moral reasoning, honesty, and willingness to help and care for others (Andrews et al., 2021). Role modeling by caring adults is important because it reinforces positive behaviors.

Identity Development Among LGBTQ+ Adolescents

Few would argue that adolescents face many demanding challenges as they transition to adulthood. Exploring identity is a normal process for all adolescents. In fact, Erikson (1968) suggests that forming an individual identity is one of the most pressing tasks of adolescence. Youth who do not identify within the traditional binary gender identities of man or woman and/or heterosexuality experience the additional challenges of navigating a gender and sexual identity in a society that discriminates against LGBTQ+ people and a youth culture that remains largely homophobic (Andrews et al., 2021). Generally, an awareness of feeling different or being attracted to someone who is the same gender is what brings an adolescent to recognize that they may have a sexual and/or gender identity that is different from many of their peers. This realization can be frightening, exhilarating, and complex. While navigation of this complexity is aided by a supportive environment at home and in their peer relationships, clinicians can also assist in the process by creating a welcoming and affirming clinical environment (Roosevelt et al., 2024). Helping LGBTQ+ adolescents find ways to increase connectedness in multiple environments such as school, family, home, and peer networks helps them to build resilience and reduces the potential damaging effects of social isolation (Garcia et al., 2020).

The Cass identity model was one of the first theoretical models about lesbian and gay identity development (Cass, 1979). Although this model encompasses six sequential stages of identity development, a person may go back and forth among stages as they navigate the process. The Cass model was based on gay and lesbian identified people, and more cisgender men than cisgender women participated in the research undergirding its development. Later, Kaufman and Johnson (2004) argued that the Cass model is probably less valid today because (1) it did not take sociocultural factors that impact identity into account; (2) there have been many changes in the social stigma associated with LGBTQ+ identity since the model was first developed; and (3) the linear nature of the model suggests that if a person does not go through all the stages, then that person could not become well adjusted (Kaufman & Johnson, 2004). Another, perhaps more obvious, concern with the Cass model is that it does not address gender identity and therefore does not offer a framework for understanding individuals who are transgender or gender diverse.

There are many more models of LGBTQ+ identity formation available today and a central theme in many of them is a socially connected element in the development process as a means of coping with their identity (Cass, 1979; Rosario et al., 2008; Scroggs & Vennum, 2021). Feeling this sense of group identification, or shared identity with a group, can serve as a critical buffer against the negative effect on well-being of marginalized experiences for LGBTQ+ adolescents (Scroggs & Vennum, 2021). The challenge with many of the historical models is that, once again, research on cisgender men has been used to describe outcomes in all populations. Additionally, the development descriptors exist within the binary constructs of gender and sexuality. Early models of sexual identity development also assumed a linear process in which individuals experience increasing self-acceptance as they move through identified milestones (Cass, 1979; Scroggs & Vennum, 2021). This lack of flexibility assumes that the end point is a static identity. Instead, it appears that the timing and sequence of sexuality identity is nonlinear and continually emerging (Chazan & Baldwin, 2021). For all these reasons, expanded models are needed to appreciate identity development, inclusive of LGBTQ+ identity development.

Clinical Application

Almost from birth, children being raised as girls are socialized to be highly oriented to others, so it is not surprising that risky behaviors and conditions such as depression or early sexual activity are more likely to be influenced by the nature of an adolescent girl's relational experiences with significant others, family, and peers. Risk taking can also be a result of a young adolescent's environment, exposure to bullying, expression of symptoms of depression, or even a response to a stigmatized developing identity (Bozzini et al., 2021). There is also a very gendered difference in the motivation behind risk-taking behavior in adolescents. Adolescents socialized as girls are more often influenced by a desire to maintain important relationships than a desire to take on adult behaviors when it comes to risk behaviors (Saint-Eloi Cadely et al., 2020).

The developmental self-in-relation model offered by feminist scholars can be extended into the healthcare visit for adolescents. Trust is a key component of any therapeutic relationship—a fact that cannot be emphasized enough for providers caring for adolescents. Additional time is often needed to establish a trusting relationship with an adolescent.

A relational approach can be very helpful when providing healthcare services to adolescents because it takes into consideration the human relations that influence how they define their health. For example, "Tell me about your friends or who you hang out with," and, "How would you describe yourself in relation to your friends?" are the types of questions that can be asked of adolescents during a healthcare visit to assess who influences them and how they see themselves in relationship to others. The relational assets approach merges developmental assets frameworks and the voice-centered relational work of feminist psychologists (Bertrand, 2021).

The goal is not to isolate the behavior from the relational context in which it occurs, but rather to acknowledge the health implications of behaviors. This enables a more effective approach to risk reduction because the behavior is addressed along with the context in which it occurs. This relational model can be extended throughout all healthcare interactions across the lifespan.

EARLY ADULTHOOD

Young adulthood is generally accepted as spanning the time from late adolescence to the beginning of the perimenopausal years. This period is often referred to as the reproductive years, almost exclusively for people socialized as women, reflecting a societal valuing of reproductive capacities. Chronologically, young adulthood is typically framed as 18–35 years of age. Health care during the young adulthood years traditionally focuses on health promotion and maintenance, with a primary emphasis on reproductive capacity rather than a broader, comprehensive focus on health promotion throughout the lifespan.

Biology and Physiology

The years between ages 18 and 35 are considered biomedically optimal for reproduction. Generally, most people capable of pregnancy experience regular menstrual cycles that are ovulatory, providing opportunity for pregnancy. The biologic changes that accompany a pregnancy and affect parenthood and aging also have a psychological impact in our youth-oriented culture. Contraception can be an important health consideration for people who might not want a pregnancy during these years.

Physical health in young adulthood is promoted by consumption of an adequate diet, exercise, and monitoring of overall well-being. The need for health promotion and maintenance is best met when a person lives within a social context that is conducive to health (Hepburn, 2018). Optimal health is more readily achievable when a person does not have to confront racism, sexism, or classism, but instead has access to quality health care, economic stability, and other resources (Rosenthal & Lobel, 2020). In reality, most people have lives that incorporate intersectional identities, multiple and competing demands related to work, economics, childbearing, and childrearing.

Psychosocial Development

Erikson's (1968) model identifies two crises that occur during early adulthood. The first is the development of intimacy versus isolation—the process of entering into a life partnership with another individual. It is during this developmental phase that gender assumptions about behavior become more typically defined. According to Erikson, women are assumed to require intimacy as a prerequisite for the completion of their identity development, whereas men may progress into this phase without any prior development related to their ability to participate in relationships.

It is this contrast of what is described as normative that challenged Franz and White (1985) to offer an expansion of Erikson's theory of development. Using a feminist lens, Franz and White discourage the use of a single pathway of development that primarily focuses on individuation; instead, they encourage the consideration of a two-pathway process that includes both individuation and attachment. They argue that Erikson does not conceptualize being a woman as somehow inferior or lacking in purpose, nor simply as a vehicle for childbearing and caretaking. Instead, they describe his work as not attending to the process by which attachment occurs through intimacy and relationships with others. Franz and White also posit that Erikson does not provide adequate opportunity in his traditional framework for men to develop the capacity for intimacy and attachment (Franz & White, 1985).

The expanded model that Franz and White (1985) propose includes two processes of development: individuation combined with an attachment pathway in a double-helix model. This model allows for two separate strands to be interconnected, depicting the relationship between psychological individuation and attachment as ascending in a spiral that represents the human life span. The strand representing individuation is essentially the same as it is in Erikson's model, but the attachment strand addresses the neglected relational dimension of human development. **Table 3-2** represents the individuation and attachment strands as described by Franz and White. The authors argue the following point:

> *With changing times and mores, [if] attachment processes were to undergo fuller development in men and individuation processes were to undergo fuller development in women, sex differences might become more elusive than ever, but individuation and attachment would retain their power as psychological variables associated with psychological value in important nomological nets. (Franz & White, 1985, p. 254)*

The second crisis of early adulthood is acquiring the ability to become generative versus stagnant. Here, "generative" is defined as acting on one's concern for the welfare of the next generation. Reproduction and parenting may accomplish this goal, as can service to others. Stagnation occurs when people are unable to step outside of themselves and be generative.

During the young adulthood years, psychosocial development may involve a variety of factors, such as accepting responsibilities (parenting, caring for others), creating a career, forming enduring relationships, caring for older parents, and deciding whether to become a parent. Although all these factors influence psychosocial development, they cannot be understood as generalities that are applied to all people, nor should each be assessed in isolation. Instead, each person's relationship to these factors—to themself and others, to the social context of their life, and to their lived experience—provides insight into their level of psychosocial development.

Clinical Application

There are many transitional periods from age 18 to 35. For people who can become pregnant, contraceptive decisions are of paramount importance, and it is critical for them to have access to and receive information and education about contraceptive options. Decisions related to raising children (or not) are also prominent and frame much of the healthcare services that people assigned female at birth traditionally receive during this phase of their lives. Many lifestyle-related health problems may become apparent during this time. Substance abuse, intimate partner violence, and stress related to their life or those they care for can all negatively affect a person's health during early adulthood. Psychiatric illnesses that may become apparent during these years include bipolar disorder, schizophrenia, and psychosis, independent of perinatal mood disorders.

TABLE 3-2 Franz and White's Adaptation of Erikson's Theory of Development to a Two-Path Model

Pathway	Infancy	Early Childhood	Play Age	School Age	Adolescence	Young Adulthood	Adulthood	Old Age
Individuation pathway	Trust versus mistrust	Autonomy versus shame and doubt	Initiative versus guilt	Industry versus inferiority	Identity versus identity diffusion	Career, lifestyle exploration versus drifting	Lifestyle consolidation versus emptiness	Integrity versus despair
Attachment pathway	Trust versus mistrust	Object and self-constancy versus loneliness and helplessness	Playfulness versus passivity or aggression	Empathy and collaboration versus excessive caution or power	Mutuality interdependence versus alienation	Intimacy versus isolation	Generativity versus self-absorption	Integrity versus despair

Reproduced from Low, L. K. (2001). *Adolescents' experiences of childbirth: Nothing is simple.* Unpublished doctoral dissertation, University of Michigan, Ann Arbor, MI.

Early adulthood also presents a challenging space for many people when considering the gendered division of labor within the home. While an inequitable distribution of unpaid labor can impact any family structure, it tends to be a more common experience in heterosexual relationships where cisgender women end up taking on a disproportionate amount of the domestic labor and childcare in the house (Beban & Roberts, 2024; Haney & Barber, 2022; Tornello, 2020). This increased, unpaid labor in the home tends to occur for women who work outside of the home and leads to what has been coined "the second shift," where women come home from paid work to manage the household (Hochschild & Machung, 2012). While there has been more discussion about "the second shift" and there have been some slow transitions toward a more egalitarian distribution of household tasks in heterosexual relationships, women still tend to bear the burden of the "mental load" in a family unit. The mental load refers to the combination of the cognitive labor of family life, such as thinking, planning, scheduling, and organizing family members. It also encompasses the emotional labor associated with this work (Dean et al., 2022). The mental load has a particularly deleterious impact on health and well-being as it is invisible labor that is uncompensated; rarely negotiated; seeps into work, sleep, and leisure time; and has no start or end date (Dean et al., 2022).

Although young adults are primarily healthy, it is evident there are many opportunities for life events to negatively affect their health. Health promotion and maintenance during this period are critical to ensure optimal health in later years of life.

MIDLIFE

Midlife generally encompass the ages of 40 to 60, plus or minus 10 years, making it a relative approximation (Infurna et al., 2020). Midlife is actually a transition more than a phase of the human life cycle, and during this time many people experience a recognition that their lives are changing irrevocably. Some people will pursue goals and dreams they may have deferred while dealing with the greater life demands they faced in younger adulthood. If they were parenting during their earlier adulthood, transitions into other aspects of their lives may be prompted by their children leaving home. Others may be in the active phases of parenting, as more people delay childbearing decisions until later into the early phases of midlife. During this phase of the life span, Erikson (1950) would continue to identify the phases of generativity versus stagnation as a continuing process.

Biology and Physiology

Perimenopause and menopause are biologic markers of the transition from young adult to midlife. Neither is a syndrome or a disease, but instead, both demonstrate a natural maturing of the reproductive system. Social constructions of perimenopause and menopause abound. Martin (2001) encourages us to reframe them so that our ideas of a "single purpose" for the menstrual cycle can be reconstructed into images of healthy transitions.

During the perimenopausal years, people may experience physical changes associated with decreasing estrogen levels, such as the vasomotor symptoms of hot flashes and flushes. Other changes associated with aging include a decrease in the size of genitalia, changes in breast structure, and decreased skin elasticity. These changes are more fully described in Chapter 14.

Although for many years it was believed a preponderance of midlife people suffered mood changes caused by a deficiency of estrogen during this time of life, more recent studies suggest that psychosocial factors have a much greater effect on mood than do the physiologic transitions of menopause (Kuck & Hogervorst, 2024; O'Reilly et al., 2024).

Psychosocial Development

Midlife is a dynamic period of ongoing transition. During this time, people often experience increased feelings of physical and emotional well-being and greater control over their lives (Infurna et al., 2020). They may pursue new interests, acquire new skills, and enjoy more time with friends and family. Conversely, Gilligan (1982) suggests that midlife may be a time of risk for people precisely because of their embeddedness in relationships, orientation to interdependence, ability to subordinate achievement to care, and conflicts over competitive success.

Midlife can be a time to enjoy hard earned rewards in areas such as earnings, career, family structure, decision-making abilities, self-confidence, control beliefs, and contributions to the community (Infurna et al., 2020). However, people in midlife often experience significant challenges that, while not novel to this age, become more magnified. Because of how caregiving is gendered, women often face an increased stress from the care of aging parents, care for growing children, and balancing careers. This is also the point in time where chronic diseases begin to emerge and changes in metabolism and joint health lead to increased need for access to consistent healthcare resources. The balancing of these myriad of stressors and changes take place within the context of a shrinking social safety net in the form of rising healthcare cost and insufficient family leave policies (Infurna et al., 2020).

Clinical Application

Approaching midlife people in the spirit of valuing self-care and centering their own needs and well-being can have an impact on how they age. Interventions focused on promoting physical activity, engagement in positive social relationships, and creating positive nutritional changes can help people reach an older age with fewer chronic illnesses and positive physical and mental health (An et al., 2020).

Ageism or bias based on age are common in Western society. For the clinician, it is important to provide supportive care throughout a person's lifespan and not assume that their health concerns are entirely related to their age. Healthcare providers are not immune to the deleterious effects of ageism. It permeates the attitudes of providers, the mindset of aging people, and the structure of the healthcare system, and it has a potentially profound influence on the type and amount of care offered, requested, and received (Nemiroff, 2022).

OLDER AGE

Between 2010 and 2020, the population 65 years and over saw the largest and fastest growth in any decade since 1880 to 1890, reaching 55.8 million or 16.8% of the total population in 2020 (Caplan & Rabe, 2023). Many older people are living on limited and fixed incomes, and Medicare reimbursement is either poor or nonexistent for many of the healthcare services needed by this population. The aging process is frequently associated with a number of problematic issues, including chronic medical conditions and challenges related to autonomy and independence.

However, it is important that narratives also dispel myths that aging is synonymous with illness, depression, social isolation, pain, and fatigue. Changing the narrative to include models of healthy aging is an important component of supportive and age-appropriate health care and is critical to maintaining health and quality of life for this population. Another challenge that arises when examining the study of older people is how the successful aging paradigm is framed. Although success in later life is not necessarily a definition grounded in systems of oppression, the narrow conceptualization of success in this paradigm ignores the diversity of the aging experience and how structural influences of homophobia, racism, classism, and so forth create a cumulative life burden that may have a deleterious effect on the health of older people (Simons et al., 2021).

Biology and Physiology

Theories abound about the cause of aging and its biologic and physiologic impacts, but more research is needed to produce definitive findings. What is known is that normal aging can be distinguished from disease. As bodies age and change, and sometimes decline, due to age, the changes do not inevitably lead to chronic diseases such as diabetes, hypertension, and dementia (National Institute on Aging, 2024). Additionally, there is no chronological timetable for human aging. People age differently, and factors such as genetics, lifestyle, and disease processes all affect the aging process. Nevertheless, research has identified some factors that support healthy aging (National Institute on Aging, 2024):

- Exercise and physical activity, especially when it is done regularly
- Maintaining a healthy weight
- Maintaining good nutrition

Overall, many more studies on aging are needed.

Psychosocial Development

Research suggests that older people are often caregivers for ailing spouses or partners, and many end up living alone (because they outlive their partners), but they continue to maintain a connectedness to other family members. There is a dearth of research examining the caregiver issue for LGBTQ+ older adults and their families, because sexual orientation and gender identity as research variables are typically missing in the major studies of gerontology (Candrian & Cloyes, 2021). As LGBTQ+ people grow older and become more reliant on social services and programs, they have less independence from heterosexist institutions. The fear of facing insensitivity and discrimination can reinforce social isolation and lead to avoidance of needed healthcare and social services (Lampe et al., 2024). It is important, therefore, that studies focusing on psychosocial development and the aging process include LGBTQ+ people as participants.

There is also a specific gap in the knowledge about gender-related distinctions and aging. The economic and social conditions in which people live has a significant impact on an individual's health and well-being. In addition to social determinants of health, the capacity of people to actively be part of the decision-making process and their access to the resources needed to maintain health and well-being can have a critical impact on their likelihood of healthy aging (McMaughan et al., 2020). As people age and experience adjustments in mobility, increased risk of chronic health conditions, and a changing capacity for self-care and autonomy in daily activities, some may begin to disengage in society and make unwelcome adjustments to lifelong patterns. This experience of disengagement should not be construed as an inevitable consequence of aging, but instead should be viewed through the lens of what accommodations may be required to support housing, healthcare resources, social support, and transportation to encourage older adults to maintain autonomy, support social interaction, and encourage continued engagement in their communities.

Clinical Application

Ageism is a negative stereotype, prejudice, and/or act of discrimination directed toward elderly people (Jackson et al., 2019). It is endemic in Western societies and is escalating (Cecil et al., 2022). The gendered nature of ageism is especially apparent in the matter of appearance and social visibility. Gender invisibility and erasure has a particularly deleterious impact on women and their feeling of having an equal place in society, socially, economically, and politically (Demos & Segal, 2022). Being culturally and socially visible, valued, and seen as equal to others is central to the tenets of social justice. Yet older women often report not seeing themselves represented in media, being ignored in a range of contexts, being seen for something they are not or only through a single dimension of their identity, and being seen as incapable and undesirable (Westwood, 2023). This creates a scenario where women can feel conflicted between wanting to age authentically and feel the need to mask the signs of aging to counteract lowered social status and cultural invisibility (Cecil et al., 2022).

While all people are living longer and overcoming many of the negative impacts of communicable and chronic conditions, the health issues of older people are still substantial. For some people, older age brings social isolation and, in many cases, economic adversity (Lampe et al., 2024). The impact of this pattern on the aging population and on the well-being of people is in need of further study. Engagement is an important construct in theories of aging that emphasize strengths. A focus on engagement shifts the balance from the deficit and decline approach, which has characterized the study of aging for decades, to a strengths and resilience orientation. The productive aspects of social engagement include such things as work, volunteering, caring for small children, and caregiving. However, engagement can also be an internal, creative, and reflective process for many people. This model of engagement challenges the gendered, racial, and ethnic assumptions that older people will be the sources of caretaking within their families (Westwood, 2023). Longitudinal research that includes a focus on engagement, the influence of social drivers of health, and intersectionality across diverse communities of aging populations is required to inform optimal policy and practice.

CONCLUSION

Other chapters within this text present more detailed discussions of the clinical assessment and management of gynecologic health. Through the continued use of a feminist framework, an expanded model of gynecologic health includes great opportunity to both affect change and improve health outcomes for people.

References

Alberts, C., & Durrheim, K. (2018). Future direction of identity research in a context of political struggle: A critical appraisal of Erikson. *Identity*, *18*(4), 295–305. https://doi.org/10.1080/15283488.2018.1523727

Alderman, E. M., Breuner, C. C., COMMITTEE ON ADOLESCENCE, Grubb, L. K., Powers, M. E., Upadhya, K., & Wallace, S. B. (2019). Unique needs of the adolescent. *Pediatrics*, *144*(6), e20193150. https://doi.org/10.1542/peds.2019-3150

American College of Obstetrics & Gynecology. (2013). ACOG Practice Bulletin No. 136: Management of abnormal uterine bleeding associated with ovulatory dysfunction. *Obstetrics & Gynecology*, *122*(1), 176–185.

American College of Obstetrics & Gynecology. (2015). Committee Opinion No 651: Menstruation in girls and adolescents: Using the menstrual cycle as a vital sign. *Obstetrics & Gynecology*, *126*(6), e143–e146.

An, H.-Y., Chen, W., Wang, C.-W., Yang, H.-F., Huang, W.-T., & Fan, S.-Y. (2020). The relationships between physical activity and life satisfaction and happiness among young, middle-aged, and older adults. *International Journal of Environmental Research and Public Health*, *17*(13), Article 13. https://doi.org/10.3390/ijerph17134817

Andrews, J. L., Ahmed, S. P., & Blakemore, S.-J. (2021). Navigating the social environment in adolescence: The role of social brain development. *Biological Psychiatry*, *89*(2), 109–118. https://doi.org/10.1016/j.biopsych.2020.09.012

Arnett, J. J. (2024). *Emerging Adulthood: The Winding Road From the Late Teens Through the Twenties* (3rd ed.). Oxford University Press.

Baker Miller, J. (1987). Women and power. *Women & Therapy*, *6*(1–2), 1–10. https://doi.org/10.1300/J015V06N01_01

Baker Miller, J. (1991). The development of women's sense of self. In J. Jordan, A. Kaplan, J. B. Miller, I. Stiver, & J. Surrey (Eds.), *Women's growth in connection: Writings from the Stone Center* (pp. 11–26). Guilford Press.

Beban, A., & Roberts, G. (2024). Fair but not equal: Negotiating the division of unpaid labour in same-sex couples in Aotearoa New Zealand and Australia. *LGBTQ+ Family: An Interdisciplinary Journal*, *20*(1), 74–91. https://doi.org/10.1080/27703371.2023.2285276

Belenky, M. (1986). *Women's ways of knowing: The development of self, voice, and mind.* Harper Collins.

Bertrand, M. (2021). Toward a voice-centered relational anti-racist listening praxis in counselor education. *Teaching and Supervision in Counseling*, *3*(2).

Biro, F. M., Pajak, A., Wolff, M. S., Pinney, S. M., Windham, G. C., Galvez, M. P., Greenspan, L. C., Kushi, L. H., & Teitelbaum, S. L. (2018). Age of menarche in a longitudinal US cohort. *Journal of Pediatric and Adolescent Gynecology*, *31*(4), 339–345. https://doi.org/10.1016/j.jpag.2018.05.002

Bozzini, A. B., Bauer, A., Maruyama, J., Simões, R., & Matijasevich, A. (2021). Factors associated with risk behaviors in adolescence: A systematic review. *Brazilian Journal of Psychiatry*, *43*(2), 210–221. https://doi.org/10.1590/1516-4446-2019-0835

Candrian, C., & Cloyes, K. G. (2021). "She's dying and i can't say we're married?": End-of-life care for LGBT older adults. *The Gerontologist*, *61*(8), 1197–1201. https://doi.org/10.1093/geront/gnaa186

Caplan, Z., & Rabe, M. (2023). *The Older Population: 2020* (Nos. C2020BR-07; pp. 1–20). United States Census Bureau.

Carter, R., & Seaton, E. K. (2024). Rethinking pubertal research: Embracing intersectionality. *Child Development Perspectives*. https://doi.org/10.1111/cdep.12527

Cass, V. (1979). Homosexual identity formation: A theoretical model. *Journal of Homosexuality*, *4*(4), 219–235.

Cecil, V., Pendry, L. F., Salvatore, J., Mycroft, H., & Kurz, T. (2022). Gendered ageism and gray hair: Must older women choose between feeling authentic and looking competent? *Journal of Women & Aging*, *34*(2), 210–225. https://doi.org/10.1080/08952841.2021.1899744

Chazan, M., & Baldwin, M. (2021). Queering generativity and futurity: LGBTQ2IA+ stories of resistance, resurgence, and resilience. *International Journal of Ageing and Later Life*, 1–30. https://doi.org/10.3384/ijal.1652-8670.1574

Collins, P. H. (2022). *Black feminist thought, 30th Anniversary Edition: Knowledge, consciousness, and the politics of empowerment.* Routledge. https://doi.org/10.4324/9781003245650

Crenshaw, K. (1997). Demarginalizing the intersection of race and sex: A Black feminist critique of antidiscrimination doctrine, feminist theory and antiracist politics. In *Feminist Legal Theories*. Routledge.

de Carvalho, N. A., & Veiga, F. H. (2022). Psychosocial development research in adolescence: A scoping review. *Trends in Psychology*, *30*(4), 640–669. https://doi.org/10.1007/s43076-022-00143-0

Dean, L., Churchill, B., & Ruppanner, L. (2022). The mental load: Building a deeper theoretical understanding of how cognitive and emotional labor overload women and mothers. *Community, Work & Family*, *25*(1), 13–29. https://doi.org/10.1080/13668803.2021.2002813

Deanow, C. G. (2011). Relational development through the life cycle: Capacities, opportunities, challenges, and obstacles. *Affilia*, *26*(2), 125–138. https://doi.org/10.1177/0886109911405485

Demos, V. P., & Segal, M. T. (Eds.). (2022). *Gender visibility and erasure*. Emerald Publishing.

do Amaral, M. C. E., Hardy, E., & Hebling, E. M. (2011). Menarche among Brazilian women: Memories of experiences. *Midwifery, 27*(2), 203-208. http://doi.org/10.1016/j.midw.2009.05.008.

Erikson, E. H. (1950). *Childhood and Society*. W. W. Norton & Company.

Erikson, E. H. (1968). *Identity Youth and Crisis*. W. W. Norton & Company.

Franz, C. E., & White, K. M. (1985). Individuation and attachment in personality development: Extending Erikson's theory. *Journal of Personality*, *53*(2), 224–256. https://doi.org/10.1111/j.1467-6494.1985.tb00365.x

Garcia, J., Vargas, N., Clark, J. L., Magaña Álvarez, M., Nelons, D. A., & Parker, R. G. (2020). Social isolation and connectedness as determinants of well-being: Global evidence mapping focused on LGBTQ youth. *Global Public Health*, *15*(4), 497–519. https://doi.org/10.1080/17441692.2019.1682028

Gilchrist, K. (1997). *Penelope: A study in the manipulation of myth* [PhD Thesis]. Oxford University.

Gilligan, C. (1982). In a different voice: Psychological theory and women's development. Harvard University Press

Gilligan, C. (1986). Reply by Carol Gilligan. *Signs: Journal of Women in Culture and Society*, *11*(2), 324–333. https://doi.org/10.1086/494226

Gilligan, C. (1993). *In a different voice: psychological theory and women's development*. Harvard University Press.

Gilligan, C. (2018). Revisiting "In a different voice." *LEARNing Landscapes*, *11*(2), 25–30.

Gottlieb, A. (2020). Menstrual taboos: Moving beyond the curse. In C. Bobel, I. T. Winkler, B. Fahs, K. A. Hasson, E. A. Kissling, & T.-A. Roberts (Eds.), *The Palgrave handbook of critical menstruation studies* (pp. 143–162). Springer Singapore. https://doi.org/10.1007/978-981-15-0614-7

Hamlat, E. J., Neilands, T. B., Laraia, B., Zhang, J., Lu, A. T., Lin, J., Horvath, S., & Epel, E. S. (2023). Early life adversity predicts an accelerated cellular aging phenotype through early timing of puberty. *Psychological Medicine*, *53*(16), 7720–7728. https://doi.org/10.1017/S0033291723001629

Haney, T. J., & Barber, K. (2022). The extreme gendering of COVID−19: Household tasks and division of labour satisfaction during the pandemic. *Canadian Review of Sociology/Revue Canadienne de Sociologie*, *59*(S1), 26–47. https://doi.org/10.1111/cars.12391

Hepburn, M. (2018). The variables associated with health promotion behaviors among urban Black women. *Journal of Nursing Scholarship*, *50*(4), 353–366. https://doi.org/10.1111/jnu.12387

Hochschild, A., & Machung, A. (2012). *The second shift: Working families and the revolution at home.* Penguin.

Infurna, F. J., Gerstorf, D., & Lachman, M. E. (2020). Midlife in the 2020s: Opportunities and challenges. *The American Psychologist*, *75*(4), 470–485. https://doi.org/10.1037/amp0000591

Jackson, S. E., Hackett, R. A., & Steptoe, A. (2019). Associations between age discrimination and health and wellbeing: Cross-sectional and prospective analysis of the English Longitudinal Study of Ageing. *The Lancet Public Health*, *4*(4), e200–e208. https://doi.org/10.1016/S2468-2667(19)30035-0

Jansen, K., & Kiefer, S. M. (2020). Understanding brain development: Investing in young adolescents' cognitive and social-emotional development. *Middle School Journal*, *51*(4), 18–25. https://doi.org/10.1080/00940771.2020.1787749

Kane Low, L. (2001). Adolescents' experiences of childbirth: Nothing is simple. [Doctoral Dissertation]. https://deepblue.lib.umich.edu/handle/2027.42/123214

Kane Low, L., & Bailey, J. (2022). A feminist perspective in women's health. In *Gynecologic health care* (4th ed., pp. 3–11). Jones & Bartlett Learning.

Kaplan, A., Klein, R., & Gleason, N. (1991). Women's self development in late adolescence. In *Women's growth in connection: Writings from the Stone Center* (pp. 122–140). Guilford Press.

Kaplan, H. B. (1991). Social psychology of the immune system: A conceptual framework and review of the literature. *Social Science & Medicine*, *33*(8), 909–923. https://doi.org/10.1016/0277-9536(91)90262-B

Kaufman, J. M., & Johnson, C. (2004). Stigmatized individuals and the process of identity. *The Sociological Quarterly*, *45*(4), 807–833. https://doi.org/10.1111/j.1533-8525.2004.tb02315.x

Kohlberg, L., & Power, C. (1981). Moral development, religious thinking, and the question of a seventh stage. *Zygon: Journal of Religion and Science, 16*(3).

Kubo, A., Acker, J., Aghaee, S., Kushi, L. H., Quesenberry, C. P., Jr., Greenspan, L. C., Srinivasan, S., Kanaya, A. M., & Deardorff, J. (2024). Pubertal timing across Asian American, Native Hawaiian, and Pacific Islander subgroups. *JAMA Network Open*, *7*(5), e2410253. https://doi.org/10.1001/jamanetworkopen.2024.10253

Kuck, M. J., & Hogervorst, E. (2024). Stress, depression, and anxiety: Psychological complaints across menopausal stages. *Frontiers in Psychiatry*, *15*. https://doi.org/10.3389/fpsyt.2024.1323743

Lampe, N. M., Barbee, H., Tran, N. M., Bastow, S., & McKay, T. (2024). Health disparities among lesbian, gay, bisexual, transgender, and queer older adults: A structural competency approach. *The International Journal of Aging and Human Development, 98*(1), 39–55. https://doi.org/10.1177/00914150231171838

Laricchiuta, D., Panuccio, A., Picerni, E., Biondo, D., Genovesi, B., & Petrosini, L. (2023). The body keeps the score: The neurobiological profile of traumatized adolescents. *Neuroscience & Biobehavioral Reviews, 145*, 105033. https://doi.org/10.1016/j.neubiorev.2023.105033

Lee. J. (2008). "A Kotex and a smile": Mothers and daughters at menarche. *Journal of Family Issues, 29*(10), 1325–1347. https://doi.org/10.1177/0192513X08316117.

Macleod, C. I., Bhatia, S., & Liu, W. (2020). Feminisms and decolonising psychology: Possibilities and challenges. *Feminism & Psychology, 30*(3), 287–305. https://doi.org/10.1177/0959353520932810

Manotas, M. C., González, D. M., Céspedes, C., Forero, C., & Rojas Moreno, A. P. (2021). Genetic and epigenetic control of puberty. *Sexual Development, 16*(1), 1–10. https://doi.org/10.1159/000519039

Maree, J. (2021). The psychosocial development theory of Erik Erikson: Critical overview. *Early Child Development and Care, 191*(7–8), 1107–1121. https://doi.org/10.1080/03004430.2020.1845163

Martin, E. (2001). *The woman in the body: A cultural analysis of reproduction*. Beacon Press.

McArthur, B. A., Madigan, S., & Korczak, D. J. (2021). Tweens are not teens: The problem of amalgamating broad age groups when making pandemic recommendations. *Canadian Journal of Public Health, 112*(6), 984–987. https://doi.org/10.17269/s41997-021-00585-6

McMaughan, D. J., Oloruntoba, O., & Smith, M. L. (2020). Socioeconomic status and access to healthcare: Interrelated drivers for healthy aging. *Frontiers in Public Health, 8*. https://doi.org/10.3389/fpubh.2020.00231

Miller, P. H., & Scholnick, E. K. (2015). Feminist theory and contemporary developmental psychology: The case of children's executive function. *Feminism & Psychology, 25*(3), 266–283. https://doi.org/10.1177/0959353514552023

Mims, L. C., & Williams, J. L. (2020). "They told me what I was before I could tell them what I was": Black girls' ethnic-racial identity development within multiple worlds. *Journal of Adolescent Research, 35*(6), 754–779. https://doi.org/10.1177/0743558420913483

National Institute on Aging. (2024, April 10). *Healthy aging*. National Institute on Aging. https://www.nia.nih.gov/health/healthy-aging/10-common-misconceptions-about-aging

Nemiroff, L. (2022). We can do better: Addressing ageism against older adults in healthcare. *Healthcare Management Forum, 35*(2), 118–122. https://doi.org/10.1177/08404704221080882

Oliván-Gonzalvo, G., Sanchez-Quiroz, P. L., & De La Parte-Serna, A. C. (2021). Use of Tanner stages to estimate chronological age in alleged child pornography cases: A systematic review. *Andes Pediatrica, 92*(3), 470–477. https://doi.org/10.32641/andespediatr.v92i3.3374

Opendak, M., & Sullivan, R. M. (2019). Unique infant neurobiology produces distinctive trauma processing. *Developmental Cognitive Neuroscience, 36*, 100637. https://doi.org/10.1016/j.dcn.2019.100637

O'Reilly, K., McDermid, F., McInnes, S., & Peters, K. (2024). "I was just a shell": Mental health concerns for women in perimenopause and menopause. *International Journal of Mental Health Nursing, 33*(3), 693–702. https://doi.org/10.1111/inm.13271

Owen, G. (2020). *A queer history of adolescence: Developmental pasts, relational futures*. The University of Georgia Press.

Perry, W. (1968). *Patterns of development in thought and values of students in a liberal arts college: A validation of a scheme. Final Report.* (p. 143). https://eric.ed.gov/?id=ED024315

Ponzi, D., Flinn, M. V., Muehlenbein, M. P., & Nepomnaschy, P. A. (2020). Hormones and human developmental plasticity. *Molecular and Cellular Endocrinology, 505*, 110721. https://doi.org/10.1016/j.mce.2020.110721

Roosevelt, L. K., Kattari, L., & Yingling, C. (2024). Affirming care for transgender and gender-diverse youth. *MCN: The American Journal of Maternal/Child Nursing, 49*(2), 66. https://doi.org/10.1097/NMC.0000000000000981

Rosario, M., Schrimshaw, E. W., & Hunter, J. (2008). Predicting different patterns of sexual identity development over time among lesbian, gay, and bisexual youths: A cluster analytic approach. *American Journal of Community Psychology, 42*(3–4), 266–282. https://doi.org/10.1007/s10464-008-9207-7

Rosenthal, L., & Lobel, M. (2020). Gendered racism and the sexual and reproductive health of Black and Latina women. *Ethnicity & Health, 25*(3), 367–392. https://doi.org/10.1080/13557858.2018.1439896

Saint-Eloi Cadely, H., Finnegan, V., Spears, E. C., & Kerpelman, J. L. (2020). Adolescents and sexual risk-taking: The interplay of constraining relationship beliefs, healthy sex attitudes, and romantic attachment insecurity. *Journal of Adolescence, 84*(1), 136–148. https://doi.org/10.1016/j.adolescence.2020.08.010

Scroggs, B., & Vennum, A. (2021). Gender and sexual minority group identification as a process of identity development during emerging adulthood. *Journal of LGBT Youth, 18*(3), 287–304. https://doi.org/10.1080/19361653.2020.1722780

Silber, L. M. (2012). Adolescent girls and the transgenerational relational catch. *Journal of Infant, Child, and Adolescent Psychotherapy, 11*(2), 121–132. https://doi.org/10.1080/15289168.2012.675821

Simons, R. L., Lei, M.-K., Klopack, E., Beach, S. R. H., Gibbons, F. X., & Philibert, R. A. (2021). The effects of social adversity, discrimination, and health risk behaviors on the accelerated aging of African Americans: Further support for the weathering hypothesis. *Social Science & Medicine, 282*, 113169. https://doi.org/10.1016/j.socscimed.2020.113169

Srikanth, N., Xie, L., Francis, J., & Messiah, S. E. (2023). Association of social determinants of health, race and ethnicity, and age of menarche among US women over 2 decades. *Journal of Pediatric and Adolescent Gynecology, 36*(5), 442–448. https://doi.org/10.1016/j.jpag.2023.05.003

Taylor, C., Gutmann, A., & Taylor, C. (1994). *Multiculturalism: Examining the politics of recognition*. Princeton University Press.

Taylor, H. S., Pal, L., & Sell, E. (2019). *Speroff's clinical gynecologic endocrinology and infertility*. Lippincott Williams & Wilkins.

Tornello, S. L. (2020). Division of labor among transgender and gender non-binary parents: Association with individual, couple, and children's behavioral outcomes. *Frontiers in Psychology, 11*. https://doi.org/10.3389/fpsyg.2020.00015

Tummala-Narra, P. (2013). Psychotherapy with South Asian women: Dilemmas of the immigrant and first generations. *Women & Therapy, 36*(3–4), 176–197. https://doi.org/10.1080/02703149.2013.797853

U.S. Centers for Disease Control and Prevention. (2024, November 13). Genomics and your health. *Epigenetics, Health, and Disease*. https://www.cdc.gov/genomics-and-health/epigenetics/index.html

Westwood, S. (2023). "It's the not being seen that is most tiresome": Older women, invisibility and social (in)justice. *Journal of Women & Aging, 35*(6), 557–572. https://doi.org/10.1080/08952841.2023.2197658

Winkler, I. (2020). Introduction: Menstruation as fundamental. In C. Bobel, I. T. Winkler, B. Fahs, K. A. Hasson, E. A. Kissling, & T.-A. Roberts (Eds.), *The Palgrave Handbook of Critical Menstruation Studies* (pp. 9–13). Springer Singapore. https://doi.org/10.1007/978-981-15-0614-7

APPENDIX 3-A

Deanow's Model of Development Highlighting Relational Tasks and Obstacles Throughout the Lifespan

Age Clusters	Roles	Capacities/Opportunities	Obstacles/Challenges[a]
Infancy: 0–18 months[b]	Primary empathy/ nonresponsive	Learns primary empathy Bonds with caregivers A two-person dynamic Girls may be more encouraged to develop primary empathy, although boys are permitted to learn empathy and satisfaction of relationships	Nonresponsiveness to caregivers Disconnection to caregivers Could be due to biology (autism spectrum) or to neglect and abuse by a caregiver
Toddler: 18 months to 2–3 years[c]	Relational differentiation/ unworthiness	Little girls learn who they are, what they think and feel More attuned to feelings of others Relational differentiation occurs: differentiated from others but more connected in other ways	Develops sense of unworthiness Learns that self is not acceptable Learns not to expect satisfaction in relationships
Preschool: 3–6 years[d]	Caretaking/ diminishment	Begin to engage in authentic mutual relationships with other children Little girls are socialized to become caretakers and to take care of the relationship itself (most of the toys for girls at this age emphasize this)	Danger is that girls may begin to learn to keep aspects of themselves out of relationships if they fear it will negatively impact the relationship Girls may learn that caring about themselves first is selfish Girls may learn the father has more power than the mother This period is complex for little boys, as they begin to become involved in "boy culture," which is evidenced by distancing from their mothers and disengaging from feelings except for anger Little boys may be shamed for crying or other activities viewed as feminine
School age: 7–12 years	Chumship/hurt	Continue to develop relationships at home but also invest a lot of energy into relational development with same-sex peers	Learn that disconnections and conflicts in relationships always cause hurt May develop bullying behaviors; especially noted in boys, as the boy culture emphasizes winning at all costs If unsuccessful in developing positive relationships with peers, the social support for positive relational conflict and engagement is hurt
Adolescence: 12–25 years	Authenticity/ voicelessness	Bringing the evolving sense of self into relationships with parents, other adults, friends, and romantic partners Parents remain important but child begins to redefine the relationship	Very difficult for adolescent girls to bring full self to relationships, which creates a relational paradox—without authenticity, there is no real relationship; in essence, the girl "loses her voice" Growing awareness of sexuality and viewing self as a sexual being For boys, the boy culture continues to have a tight hold, often resulting in a locker-room mentality; physical and sexual dominance develop, and may include violence and risk-taking behaviors

Age Clusters	Roles	Capacities/Opportunities	Obstacles/Challenges[a]
Early adulthood and may be repeated throughout adulthood	Mutuality/ subordination or domination	Physical and societal push to "find a mate" Relationships become a major focus; goal is to achieve a true relational mutuality	Regardless of whether the relationship is same or different sexes, if one partner is male, the relational work is often distorted by the man's inability or lack of desire to be involved wholly in the relationship Dilemma is that while women usually want something to happen in the relationship, men fear it will The difference in relational skill development between men and women is very evident and creates major challenges If male domination is extreme, domestic violence may result
Throughout adulthood (ongoing)	Dexterity/imbalance	Greater opportunities for mutually enhancing relationships (e.g., spouse, partner, children, friends, colleagues) Men at this stage tend to have left the boy culture and are now more into family relationships Relationships at work are especially important for women at this stage	Real challenge for women is finding time to engage in all the relationships and still have a balance in their lives Danger for men at this stage is to adhere to the belief that they need to be the breadwinner and invest in work at the expense of family and friends Men at this age often have few adult male friendships and may be jealous of the friendships their female partners have
Aging/elders	Sustainment/ abandonment or withdrawal	Opportunities for sustaining relationships are strong Relational growth at this age may involve asking for and accepting help due to their decreasing abilities to care for themselves	Diminished capacities and energies along with inevitable disconnections or loss of some friends challenge the relational lives of seniors Some may not want to start new relationships due to fear of loss

Data from Deanow, C. G. (2011). Relational development through the life cycle: Capacities, opportunities, challenges, and obstacles. *Journal of Women and Social Work, 26*(2), 125–138. https://doi.org/10.1177/0886109911405485

[a]Occur when things do not go well for the child/person.
[b]In this age cluster, there is the least difference in the expected relational behavior between boys and girls.
[c]Gender identity is thought to begin at this stage; this should not be confused with gender socialization, which occurs throughout the life cycle.
[d]Relational work takes place at home and in a variety of preschool settings.

CHAPTER 4

Using Evidence to Support Quality Clinical Practice

Bethany Rolfe Witham

The editors acknowledge Katherine Camacho Carr, Holly Powell Kennedy, Sascha James-Conterelli, and Rachel Blatt, who were coauthors of the previous edition of this chapter.

WHAT IS EVIDENCE-BASED PRACTICE?

The elements of evidence-based practice (EBP) were initially defined by Sackett, Strauss, et al. (2000) as "the integration of the best research evidence with clinical expertise and patient values" (p. 1). EBP emphasizes the application of high-quality scientific evidence at every decision-making point in a person's care, encouraging clinicians to engage with research to ensure optimal outcomes for all patients. Since its introduction, the influence of EBP has become increasingly evident in the identification of best clinical practices, the education of clinicians, the development of health policy, and in organizational management and quality improvement (Vetter & Zavotsky, 2025).

EBP begins with a clinical question or query about best practice and then proceeds to identify and evaluate the best research available to find the answer. To comprehensively and accurately answer the question, clinical experience and patient preferences must be integrated with the research evidence. Evidence generated by other researchers that has been preappraised and synthesized by agencies or organizations such as the National Guideline Clearinghouse of the Agency for Healthcare Research and Quality or the Cochrane Database of Systematic Reviews is often used to aid clinicians and patients in decision making. The synthesis of evidence can provide guidelines for practice, diagnostic testing, changes in procedures, treatment plans, or policies. Evidence-based pathways eliminate wide variations in care that may not be efficacious or safe, are superfluous, or are unnecessarily costly. Examination of the evidence can also assist with the development of clinical benchmarking and process- or outcome-based performance measures and provide a rationale for the elimination of unnecessary processes or procedures. The use of evidence complements the clinician's expertise and the patient's personal desires in their health care.

At times, clinicians conduct their own research to generate an answer to a clinical question and identify the most effective therapies or the best way to control costs. For some clinicians, conducting research may entail a small study to develop a clinical protocol. For others, it may involve synthesizing and translating the evidence and developing an implementation plan to make a change in practice. Still others may supervise a clinical trial. Regardless of the scope of the research, the underlying principles are the same. This chapter reviews research principles, methods, and critique techniques to assist clinicians in developing skills in practice-based research so they can provide care that is truly evidence-based.

We recognize that not all people assigned female at birth identify as female or women; however, these terms are occasionally used in this chapter. The use of the words "woman" and "women" is not meant to exclude people who do not identify as women. The research methods, case studies, and resources outlined in this chapter reflect our commitment to inclusive evidence-based care for all individuals.

A FEMINIST AND QUALITY PERSPECTIVE ON RESEARCH

This chapter is founded on feminist and quality frameworks. Clinicians using a feminist framework recognize that hierarchies are an oppressive reality in health care. These hierarchies are implicated in women's health disparities and in the historical lack of research devoted to women's health issues (Doyal, 1995). Feminist theories provide a platform to expose gender inequities, ensure social understanding of women's perspectives, and offer "critiques of the assumptions, biases, and consequences of androcentric philosophies and practices" (Brisolara, 2014, p. 4). Most feminists would agree that science is not acontextual or ahistorical; rather, it must understand a person's history and the context of their life.

Brisolara (2014) outlines eight evaluation principles that are critical to the conduct and translation of gynecologic research:

1. Knowledge is culturally, socially, and temporally contingent.
2. Knowledge is a powerful resource that serves an explicit or implicit purpose.
3. Evaluation is a political activity; evaluators' [researchers'] personal experiences, perspectives, and characteristics come from and lead to a particular political stance.
4. Research methods, institutions, and practices are social constructs.
5. There are multiple ways of knowing.
6. Gender inequities are one manifestation of social injustice. Discrimination cuts across race, class, and culture and is inextricably linked to all three.
7. Discrimination based on gender is systemic and structural.
8. Action and advocacy are considered to be morally and ethically appropriate responses of an engaged feminist evaluator. (pp. 23–31)

Quality in health care implies a degree of excellence, with benchmarks and measures, in the provision of services. There are multiple strategies for assessing quality health care as identified by the Agency for Healthcare Research and Quality (n.d.-b), but it is important to consider context and social constructs, as suggested in a feminist approach. The second framework for this chapter is quality—specifically the Quality Maternal & Newborn Care (QMNC) framework (**Figure 4-1**).

Although the framework context is maternal and newborn health, it is also appropriate for contextualizing evidence in the care of all individuals. The top row of the framework represents what clinicians do in practice—how they screen, provide care, educate, promote health, manage complications, and refer to specialty care when needed. Practice is grounded on the following factors:

- Organization of care: Is care acceptable, accessible, and integrated within the community?
- Values: Is care respectful and tailored to the individual's needs?
- Philosophy: Does care optimize the individual's capabilities? Are interventions used only when necessary?
- Care providers: Who provides care? Are the caregivers competent? Are their roles clearly defined? Do they practice shared decision making?

When evaluating evidence for practice, it is essential for clinicians to consider all components of the evidence-based practice framework, recognizing that research does not exist in isolation. Each of the components is drawn from research and reflects the inherent complexity of healthcare systems and the multifaceted nature of patient care. For example, when comparing different models of care, clinicians must ask: What accounts for differences in outcomes? Are differences due to the preparation of the provider, the provider's philosophy, or both? Alternatively, do differences occur because some models include continuity of care, which may be more important than who provides the care?

THE HISTORY OF EVIDENCE-BASED PRACTICE

The initiation of the modern EBP movement in health care is attributed to British epidemiologist Dr. Archie Cochrane, who was concerned that clinicians often failed to evaluate the effectiveness of their own care and did not have widespread access to the scientific literature (Smith & Rennie, 2014). His initial work in the 1970s led to the review of all randomized controlled trials (RCTs) in perinatal medicine and ultimately to the establishment of the Cochrane Collaboration in 1992, which covers reviews in many fields of health care. The Cochrane Database of Systematic Reviews (Cochrane, 2025), an electronic database that is part of the Cochrane Library, remains one of the largest, most comprehensive reviews of evidence available.

The EBP movement is often described as a paradigm change in health care, moving from reliance on expert opinion and experience to reliance on scientific evidence as the basis for practice (Eisenberg, 2001; Kuhn, 1970). The present paradigm shift to evidence-based care has focused on the identification of the best drugs, clinical practices, and surgical procedures through rigorous study, with RCTs, meta-analyses, and systematic reviews of the scientific literature forming the primary evidence base for patient care (Straus et al., 2019). In response to this shift away from expert opinion, there has been a proliferation of articles, books, and websites instructing clinicians on how to conduct,

FIGURE 4-1 Framework for quality maternal and newborn care.

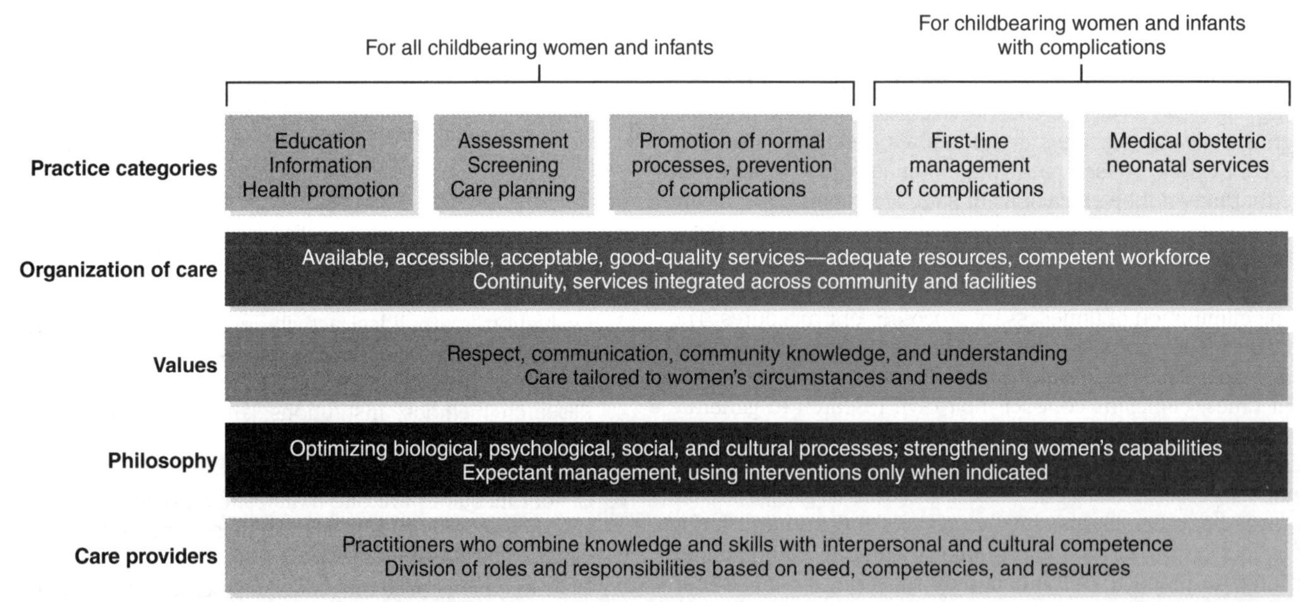

Reproduced from Renfrew, M. J., McFadden, A., Bastos, M. H., Campbell, J., Channon, A. A., Cheung, N. F., Audebert Delage Silva, D. R., Downe, S., Kennedy, H. P., Malata, A., McCormick, F., Wick, L., & Declercq, E. (2014). Midwifery and quality care: Findings from a new evidence-informed framework for maternal and newborn care. *The Lancet, 384*(9948), 1129–1145. https://doi.org/10.1016/S0140-6736(14). Used with permission from Elsevier.

evaluate, interpret, and apply the medical literature (Melnyk & Fineout-Overholt, 2023; The Oxford Review, 2023). Marckmann et al. (2015) present a useful framework for the application of evidence using a public health perspective (**Box 4-1**).

An examination of the state of the EBP movement, the philosophy of science, and the current state of nursing science suggests that the use of evidence is not a new or revolutionary paradigm shift but rather a continuation of long-standing scientific inquiry and clinical reasoning (Sehon & Stanley, 2003). Quine (1952), a philosopher of science, describes scientific knowledge as a web of beliefs, like a spider web, with an exterior edge or frame secured to an existing structure and an interconnected interior of radii and connecting points. Using this metaphor, the web of scientific beliefs encompasses sensory information and new, untested theories that now exist on the evolving periphery of the web. Foundational theories, such as the laws of nature, logic, or mathematics, form the center of the web. The interconnections between the center and the periphery are composed of well-proven hypotheses about health and clinical practice. According to Quine's metaphor, clinical decision making relies on this intricate web of interconnected knowledge and healthcare beliefs, which integrates logical and evidential relationships, research findings, intuition, and professional experience to determine best practices (Quine, 1952).

The sciences of medicine and nursing are similarly composed of a vast network of beliefs, scientific observations, practices, hypothetical relationships, and theories existing in specific contexts. For example, in clinical practice, we encounter observations (e.g., blood pressure), hypotheses (e.g., the need to repeat a measurement to ensure accuracy), and theoretical frameworks (e.g., the psychophysiology of blood pressure regulation), as well as how the blood pressure varies depending on the environment and other influences. Quine (1952) also suggests that scientific observations should not be viewed in isolation but rather examined as part of an integrated whole within the greater body of scientific knowledge. This perspective underscores the value of a multiple-method approach in exploring complex healthcare phenomena, recognizing that clinical decision making is informed by a dynamic interplay of evidence, theory, and contextual factors. The QMNC framework (Renfrew et al., 2014) captures the complexity of factors that influence how people receive care and who provides it.

Bias in interpreting research evidence presents a significant challenge in EBP, as it can distort findings, mislead clinical decision making, and ultimately compromise patient care. Various cognitive biases, such as confirmation bias, preference bias, and motivated reasoning, influence how researchers and clinicians assess and apply evidence (Florczak, 2022). For example, selective reporting and publication bias often lead to an overrepresentation of positive findings, while methodological biases can result in misleading conclusions regarding treatment efficacy. Additionally, financial and ideological influences may affect study design, data interpretation, and the dissemination of research, further skewing the perceived reliability and applicability of scientific findings (Fernández Pinto, 2023). These biases contribute to inconsistencies in clinical guidelines, challenges in translating research into practice, and the potential for suboptimal patient outcomes. To mitigate the impact of bias, clinicians and researchers must employ rigorous critical appraisal skills, uphold transparent research practices, and integrate diverse perspectives (Ratnani et al., 2023). By fostering a more nuanced and reflective approach to evidence interpretation, healthcare professionals can ensure that clinical decisions are guided by the most accurate, comprehensive, and contextually relevant evidence available.

Managers of healthcare settings increasingly recognize that clinicians are not the only ones who should consider the importance of evidence in the provision of quality care and innovative workforce redesign in terms of both quality and cost (Palazzo, 2015). Specifically, management has a key role in preventing the overuse of interventions shown to be ineffective, the underuse of interventions that are effective, and misuse when the evidence is unclear (Kohn et al., 1999). Managers must work in concert with clinicians and patients to provide evidence-based programs and an environment of care that is highly conducive to quality outcomes that are both efficient and cost-effective. Buse (2008) specifically calls for prospective policy analysis using research and the best information relevant to stakeholders in care to provide effective and efficient healthcare systems. A critical aspect of evidence-based management is the integration of quality improvement (QI) and quality assurance (QA) initiatives to foster institutional adoption of evidence-based practices. Quality improvement focuses on systematically refining processes and outcomes through continuous assessment and iterative changes, often using models such as Plan-Do-Study-Act (PDSA) cycles or Lean Six Sigma (Lachman, 2024). In contrast, quality assurance ensures adherence to established standards and guidelines, emphasizing accountability and regulatory compliance (Klein et al., 2023). Both QI and QA frameworks rely on evidence-based strategies to enhance patient safety, reduce variability in care, and optimize resource utilization. Additionally, healthcare institutions are increasingly participating in quality collaboratives—multisite initiatives that bring together organizations to share data, best practices, and implementation strategies to accelerate the adoption of EBPs. These collaboratives, such as the Institute for Healthcare Improvement (IHI) Breakthrough Series or the Agency for Healthcare Research and Quality (AHRQ) EvidenceNOW initiative, serve as powerful mechanisms for scaling evidence-based interventions, fostering interprofessional learning, and driving system-wide improvements (The Breakthrough Series, 2023; EvidenceNOW, 2023). By leveraging these

BOX 4-1 EBP Through a Public Health Lens

- What are the expected health benefits of the intervention for the target population?
- What are the potential burdens and harms of the intervention?
- How does the intervention affect the autonomy of the individuals in the target population?
- Impact on equity: How are benefits and burden distributed?
- Expected efficacy: What are the costs and opportunity costs of the intervention?

Reproduced from Marckmann G., Schmidt, H., & Strech, D. (2015). Putting public health ethics into practice: A systematic framework. *Frontiers in Public Health, 3*, 1-7.

evidence-based management approaches, healthcare leaders can create sustainable structures that enhance patient outcomes while maintaining operational efficiency.

Decisions about which evidence and outcomes are most important should not be made in a vacuum. Studies indicate that the clinical settings most effective in EBP implementation foster a culture that emphasizes adaptability to change and encourages strong nursing and obstetric leadership and collaboration (Furtado et al., 2024). The California Pregnancy-Associated Mortality Review (CA-PAMR), the New York State Task Force on Maternal Mortality and Racial Disparities, and the Washington State Maternal Mortality Review Panel are excellent examples of multidisciplinary groups assisting a state with analyzing causes of maternal mortality and translating those findings into improved care (Morton et al., 2019; New York State Department of Health, 2024; Washington State Maternal Mortality Review Panel, 2023). Resources to improve quality care through EBP can be found at the end of this chapter in **Appendix 4-A**.

Much of the existing scientific knowledge in medicine and nursing comes from a variety of sources, not all of which are evidence-based. There is not always one best way to obtain scientific information about clinical practice. For this reason, we must remain open to and creative about research methods that will give us the best answer or help us better define the interconnected web of knowledge related to the phenomena of interest. Meta-synthesis provides a systematic and scientifically rigorous method for synthesizing qualitative research by integrating patient experiences and contextual factors into the broader evidence base. By systematically reviewing and critically appraising qualitative studies, meta-synthesis strengthens evidence-based practice, offering deeper insights into patient-centered care, healthcare decision making, and the interconnected web of knowledge that informs clinical and policy interventions (Bowden & Bowden, 2022).

RESEARCH AND CLINICAL DECISION MAKING

The dimensions of EBP are multifaceted and often influenced by the discipline in which EBP is applied. Despite these variabilities, EBP consistently serves as a cornerstone of healthcare decision making (Melnyk & Fineout-Overholt, 2023). The educational preparation of clinicians usually includes core content on the research process, which can range from actual participation in research studies to the development of a plan to apply research findings to practice. Unfortunately, the word "research" can provoke anxiety in many clinicians who are years removed from their educational experience. Research, like any skill, must be used on a regular basis to be effective. In today's healthcare landscape, the growing availability of digital resources, professional guidelines, and regulatory mandates has increased clinicians' responsibilities to engage with research. Clinicians are expected to access, appraise, translate, apply, and evaluate the evidence and the expected patient outcomes to guide their practice (Brignardello-Petersen et al., 2021).

One basic strategy to help clinicians overcome hesitation about conducting research or integrating research findings into clinical practice is to reframe their perspective on the subject. By shifting the focus from viewing research as an abstract or daunting academic exercise to recognizing it as a practical tool for improving patient outcomes and solving real-world clinical problems, clinicians can approach research with greater confidence and purpose. Research follows the exact same principles that any good clinician follows in everyday clinical management. These principles are ongoing and often circular in nature. One step usually leads to another and can also raise new questions that take the clinician either back to the beginning or in a new direction. **Table 4-1** compares the steps in the clinical management and research processes and outlines the many similarities.

TYPES OF RESEARCH EVIDENCE

Research evidence comes in many forms. We prefer to call them types of evidence, rather than levels, to dispel the notion that one form is necessarily better than another or to suggest linearity. As previously mentioned, clinical experience and patient preferences are two parts of the clinical decision-making criteria triad. To complete the triad, they are combined with an evaluation of current clinical research.

A randomized clinical trial (RCT) is an experimental study design used to evaluate the effectiveness of an intervention, treatment, or program. In an RCT, participants are randomly assigned to either an experimental group, which receives the intervention, or a control group, which does not receive the intervention (or receives a placebo). This random assignment helps ensure that the groups are comparable, allowing researchers to attribute any differences in outcome to the study intervention. RTCs are often held up as the gold standard in Western medicine because they provide the most reliable evidence on the efficacy of treatments by minimizing bias and confounding factors (Oyelese, 2024). Not all clinical problems lend themselves to this kind of research, though. Whatever research method is used must serve the research question being asked, and the results should be evaluated in terms of the quality of the study, the potential benefit or harm to the patient, and the accumulation of evidence. In the United States, the U.S. Preventive Services Task Force (USPSTF) takes the lead on setting guidelines for evaluating healthcare research evidence (USPSTF, 2018). **Table 4-2** summarizes this approach.

RESEARCH METHODS TO INFORM CLINICAL PRACTICE

The historically defined parameters of science, particularly in the Western tradition, can create tension among researchers and clinicians as to what truly qualifies as scientific evidence. Quantitative, qualitative, and translational research approaches employ a variety of methods and techniques and aim to expand knowledge about a specific phenomenon. Attempting to pinpoint a defining difference among them potentially oversimplifies the complexity of each. Our goal is to help you understand the differences, understand what is credible from each perspective, and decide what is applicable to your practice and research. We do not seek to debate whether one approach is better than another; such a judgment assumes one approach has more truth or value than another. In reality, each approach helps us fill in the web of knowledge where open spaces exist.

Research often begins with a clinical problem or question that needs an answer or needs reevaluation or application in a specific situation or with a specific population or organization. This problem or question usually arises from a broad topical area, so the first task of the researcher is to clearly define the problem. Research questions can be inspired by everyday practice, or they can emerge from other research studies, especially where there

TABLE 4-1 **Alignment of Clinical and Research Processes**

Clinical Management Process	Research Process	Translational Process
Gathering the Data		
Focused on individual clinical scenario. Historical, physical, and laboratory data may be gathered.	Focused on a broader perspective of a health issue. Historical data, a review of literature, and a pilot study may be involved.	Focused on individuals, populations, or systems; examines how evidence applies. A review of the literature and individual or group demographics, culture, and context may be examined.
Identifying the Problem		
An assessment is made of the individual's clinical problem.	A research question and/or hypothesis is generated.	A question is generated related to effectiveness, accessibility/feasibility, cost effectiveness, policy, context, and/or other factors that will promote the uptake or optimal use of best practices.
Development of the Plan		
An evidence-based clinical management plan is used to meet the patient's needs.	A research design is constructed that will best answer the research question.	An implementation plan is developed based on a synthesis of the best scientific information, with consideration of patient or system needs, including contextual factors.
Implementation		
The management plan is implemented.	The research study is conducted.	The implementation stage of translation involves the adoption of interventions that have been demonstrated to improve health, health outcomes, or the healthcare system.
Evaluation of the Results		
Clinical follow-up is conducted to assess the effectiveness of the treatment plan.	Data are analyzed to provide answers to the research questions.	Outcomes are evaluated to assess adoption, change in effectiveness (health outcomes, access to care, usefulness, etc.), cost effectiveness, improvements in safety, quality of care, teamwork and collaboration, and/or patient-centered care.

are discrepancies, inconsistencies, or remaining questions about organizational practices, patient care practices, interventions, or products that are used. Social or policy issues—such as access to care; models of care; effects of racism, gender bias, or other forms of discrimination on health; health disparities; poverty; and violence—can also give rise to important questions.

The question is then translated into aims about what the study proposes to do to meet the gap in our current knowledge and to be significant (Flanagan & Tatano, 2024). This means that an exploration of the literature may reveal either a lack of prior research or an abundance of evidence that has not been incorporated into practice. It also means that the results of the research could make a difference in the healthcare delivery or health outcomes for the population being studied. Translational research, also known as implementation research, also begins with a question and purpose; however, it is aimed at addressing a gap between the availability of existing EBP recommendations and the application of those findings to improve the uptake and use of existing evidence to improve health care, health outcomes, or the healthcare system (Ryder & Jacob, 2022). In other words, translational science addresses healthcare practices that already have an evidence base but may not be a part of routine practice.

Quantitative Research

Experimental research is a rigorous scientific approach used to investigate cause-and-effect relationships by systematically manipulating one or more independent variables and measuring their effects on dependent variables. To enhance the validity of the findings, participants are randomly assigned to either a control group (which does not receive the intervention) or an experimental group (which receives the intervention). This randomization helps minimize bias and ensures that differences in outcomes can be attributed to the manipulated variable rather than other external factors. Researchers carefully control for confounding variables—factors that could otherwise influence the

TABLE 4-2 Recommendations for Using Research Evidence in Clinical Practice[a]

Level of Certainty[b]	Description
High	The available evidence usually includes consistent results from well-designed, well-conducted studies in representative primary care populations. These studies assess the effects of the preventive service on health outcomes. This conclusion is, therefore, unlikely to be strongly affected by the results of future studies.
Moderate	The available evidence is sufficient to determine the effects of the preventive service on health outcomes, but confidence in the estimate is constrained by factors such as: • The number, size, or quality of individual studies • Inconsistency of findings across individual studies • Limited generalizability of findings to routine primary care practice • Lack of coherence in the chain of evidence As more information becomes available, the magnitude or direction of the observed effect could change, and this change may be large enough to alter the conclusion.
Low	The available evidence is insufficient to assess effects on health outcomes. Evidence is insufficient because of: • The limited number or size of studies • Important flaws in study design or methods • Inconsistency of findings across individual studies • Gaps in the chain of evidence • Findings not generalizable to routine primary care practice • Lack of information on important health outcomes More information may allow estimation of effects on health outcomes.

Grade	Definition	Suggestions for Practice
A	The USPSTF recommends the service. There is high certainty that the net benefit is substantial.	Offer or provide this service.
B	The USPSTF recommends the service. There is high certainty that the net benefit is moderate or there is moderate certainty that the net benefit is moderate to substantial.	Offer or provide this service.
C	The USPSTF recommends selectively offering or providing this service to individual patients based on professional judgment and patient preferences. There is at least moderate certainty that the net benefit is small.	Offer or provide this service for selected patients depending on individual circumstances.
D	The USPSTF recommends against the service. There is moderate or high certainty that the service has no net benefit or that the harms outweigh the benefits.	Discourage the use of this service.
I Statement	The USPSTF concludes that the current evidence is insufficient to assess the balance of benefits and harms of the service. Evidence is lacking, of poor quality, or conflicting, and the balance of benefits and harms cannot be determined.	Read the clinical considerations section of USPSTF Recommendation Statement. If the service is offered, patients should understand the uncertainty about the balance of benefits and harms.

Reproduced from U.S. Preventive Services Task Force. (2018). *Methods and processes: Grade definitions.* https://www.uspreventiveservicestaskforce.org/uspstf/about-uspstf/methods-and-processes/grade-definitions

Hierarchy of Research Designs	
I	Evidence obtained from at least one properly conducted, randomized controlled trial.
II-1	Evidence obtained from well-designed controlled trials without randomization.
II-2	Evidence obtained from well-designed cohort or case-control analytic studies, preferably from more than one center or research group.
II-3	Evidence obtained from multiple time series with or without the intervention. Dramatic results in uncontrolled experiments (such as the introduction of penicillin treatment in the 1940s) could be regarded as this type of evidence.
III	Opinions of respected authorities, based on clinical experience, descriptive studies and case reports, or reports of expert committees.

Reproduced from Agency for Healthcare Research and Quality. (n.d.-a). *Agency for Healthcare Research and Quality archive.* http://archive.ahrq.gov/clinic/ajpmsuppl/harris2.htm

[a]The USPSTF grades its recommendations about specific health services or treatments according to one of five classifications that reflect the strength of evidence and magnitude of net benefit (benefits minus harms).

[b]The USPSTF defines certainty as "likelihood that the USPSTF assessment of the net benefit of a preventive service is correct." The net benefit is defined as benefit minus harm of the preventive service as implemented in a general primary care population. The USPSTF assigns a certainty level based on the nature of the overall evidence available to assess the net benefit of a preventive service.

results—by maintaining consistent conditions across all groups. By isolating the independent variable and ensuring controlled conditions, experimental research allows for more precise conclusions about the effectiveness of specific interventions, treatments, or programs (Flanagan & Tatano, 2024). Experimental research is widely used to evaluate new practices and inform evidence-based decision making.

Quasi-experimental research is similar to experimental research, but it does not include random assignment of participants to an experimental or control group for practical, ethical, or other reasons. This weakness prohibits causal inference because it can no longer be assumed that the two groups are equal. Consequently, the findings might be explained by differences among the groups or some other factor. To mitigate these challenges, researchers often implement strategies to control extraneous variables, such as matching groups based on key characteristics or employing statistical techniques to establish group equivalency. Additionally, various quasi-experimental designs, such as nonequivalent control group designs or interrupted time-series analyses, are used to strengthen the validity of the findings (Flanagan & Tatano, 2024). The strength of quasi-experimental research lies in its practicality and feasibility in the real world of health care and informed choice, where research participants often cannot be randomly assigned to groups.

Nonexperimental research is used to answer questions where variable manipulation is neither feasible nor ethical. For example, if we want to study the effects of the death of a child on the parent, the independent variable (the death of a child) is clearly not something that can be manipulated or controlled. However, researchers can identify comparison groups, such as birthing parents who have experienced the naturally occurring death of a child (experimental group) and those who have not (control group). Psychological and physical well-being could still be described, measured, and compared in both groups, but cause and effect cannot be determined. In this kind of study, a wide range of human experiences and factors cannot be manipulated and, therefore, cannot be studied experimentally (Flanagan & Tatano, 2024).

Nonexperimental research provides a way to describe these factors and examine their interrelationships. For example, the New York City Department of Health and Mental Hygiene (NYC DOHMH), in conjunction with the American College of Obstetricians and Gynecologists (2024) have examined trends in maternal mortality data since 2001 (Jiang et al., 2024). NYC DOHMH reviews all deaths of birthing people up to 1 year from the end of pregnancy, regardless of outcome, duration, or site of birth. To improve the accuracy of data collection, mortality information is retrieved from death certificates, the New York Patient Occurrence Reporting and Tracking System (NYPORTS), the Statewide Planning and Research Cooperative System (SPARCS), and birth certificates. This nonexperimental research has revealed vast discrepancies in mortality between birthing individuals who are Black and birthing individuals who are white in New York City. Black non-Hispanic birthing individuals are two and a half times more likely and Hispanic birthing individuals are one and a half times more likely to have a pregnancy-related death than their white counterparts, regardless of education and socioeconomic level (Jiang et al., 2024).

Meta-analyses and systematic reviews are considered highly reliable forms of evidence. A meta-analysis uses a single study as the unit of analysis and statistically combines the findings of several similarly designed studies on the same topic. This method provides a standardized way to compare findings across studies, adding together larger numbers to observe patterns and relationships that might not have otherwise been observed in a single study (Flanagan & Tatano, 2024). A well-conducted meta-analysis allows for a more objective assessment of the evidence obtained in RCTs, especially where findings from multiple studies have produced disagreement or uncertainty. This consideration might be important when testing a new drug, procedure, or intervention that may have different effects in subgroups or varying results in different studies.

Systematic review is the method used to analyze a general body of scientific data using clearly defined criteria. Systematic reviews can include meta-analyses, appraisals of single trials, and other sources of evidence, including gray literature that has been produced by individuals or organizations outside of traditional academic publishing. Great care is taken to find all relevant published and unpublished studies, assess each study, synthesize the findings, present a balanced and unbiased summary of the findings, and consider any flaws that may be present in the evidence. Many high-quality systematic reviews are available in journals and online, most notably the Cochrane Library. The need for rigor in systematic reviews has led to a formal process for their conduct. Although a meta-analysis always uses a quantitative statistical analysis of the findings, a systematic review may include a quantitative meta-analytic combination of study results or a more qualitative summary of the aggregated data (Malterud, 2023).

Rigor in Quantitative Research

Just like clinical practice, quality research depends on adherence to standards to ensure that it is conducted accurately and ethically. The description of the research design must be clear so the reader can fully assess what took place and replicate the study if desired. Errors in any step of the process will invalidate the results. Errors can be minimized through careful attention to the accuracy of the instruments used for measurement, appropriate sample selection, and understanding how to apply the findings in the acceptance or rejection of the research hypotheses.

Variables must be clearly defined to ensure a thorough understanding of what is being tested and measured. Validity refers to how well the measurement actually measures the variable. For example, a sphygmomanometer must accurately reflect a blood pressure measurement. Reliability refers to how consistently the measurement performs when repeated. When measurements involve human-operated instruments, reliability also depends on the operator's technique, such as consistently using the correct cuff size and ensuring proper positioning during each measurement (Polit & Beck, 2022).

A research sample must accurately represent the population it is intended to reflect. Minimizing error requires the use of appropriate sampling techniques and, when possible, random assignment to study groups. For example, when studying the prevalence of menopausal symptoms, the results may vary depending on where the sample is drawn from. A sample from a women's clinic may overrepresent individuals seeking treatment, whereas a sample from a supermarket might capture a broader, more representative population. Additionally, the supermarket's location could introduce biases due to socioeconomic or cultural factors, potentially influencing the findings. These sampling considerations directly affect the generalizability of the study—the extent to which its results can be applied to populations beyond the sample group. Another critical factor in research is statistical power. Power refers to the probability of detecting a real effect, difference, or relationship between variables if one exists. Power is largely influenced by sample size. An appropriately sized sample enhances power by reducing variability and increasing result reliability. A sample that is too small may lack the power to detect meaningful differences, leading to inconclusive findings. Conversely, an excessively large sample may produce statistically significant results that are driven by size rather than actual clinical or practical significance (Zhao & Chen, 2021). Ensuring an optimal sample size strengthens the validity of research conclusions and enhances their applicability to real-world settings.

There are two commonly cited types of errors in research: Type I and Type II (Flanagan & Tatano, 2024). A Type I error is made when the researcher concludes that a relationship exists—for example, drug A is effective in treating disease X—when it actually does not (a false positive, in clinical terms). The differences observed between groups in such cases are often due to a sampling error, such as self-selection bias. Random group assignment controls for sampling error and associated Type I error. The level of significance, referred to as alpha (α) and reported as a *p* value, will also influence a Type I error. The most frequently used levels of significance (i.e., alpha levels) are .05 and .01. With a .05 alpha, the researcher accepts the probability that out of 100 samples, a true hypothesis will be falsely rejected only 5 times, and in 95 out of 100 samples a true hypothesis will be correctly accepted. With a .01 alpha, there is only 1 chance out of 100 that the true hypothesis will be falsely rejected, so this level of significance makes the incidence of Type I error lower. Usually, the minimal acceptable level of significance in quantitative research is .05.

A Type II error, also called beta (β), is made when the researcher concludes that no relationship exists when it actually does (a false negative, in clinical terms). As the risk of a Type I error decreases, the risk of a Type II error increases.

Researchers try to avoid both Type I and Type II errors. To do so, they frequently conduct a power analysis of a sample size while taking into account the desired level of significance (alpha value) and the probability of Type II error (beta value). Random sampling, random assignment to groups to avoid selection bias, and adequate sample size are steps that can help researchers avoid these kinds of errors.

Confidence intervals provide more information than *p* values because they give a range of values and allow inference of the true association of a parameter with a population (Zhao & Chen, 2021). The range specifies where the parameter (e.g., the mean) is most likely to lie (Flanagan & Tatano, 2024). Most confidence ranges are set at 95 percent; they provide a statement of the level of confidence the researcher has about the findings.

Qualitative Research

Qualitative research methods use different techniques and answer different questions than quantitative research methods. Guba and Lincoln (1998) proposed that how we perceive reality provides the backdrop for how we conduct science. This sets the stage for understanding the nature between the knower (researcher) and what can be known, commonly called epistemology. Together they form the question asked about method: How does one choose a way to learn about the world?

A person's view of the world shapes the answer to this question and influences their entire approach to science. Our philosophical assumptions about how we create knowledge, for what purpose that knowledge is used, and how we integrate our own values in this process shape our fundamental approach to research and science (Creswell & Poth, 2023). There are many ways to tell and hear a story—to gain knowledge about people and their health. The richness and details of the individual story provide the data we need to extend our knowledge of the world. The individual's point of view within the constraints of everyday life can be known only from the specifics of each case and cannot be controlled. Scientists using qualitative methods believe that the researcher cannot be fully removed from the participants. For this reason, they sometimes call this type of research "naturalistic," referring to the fact that the testing usually takes place in a setting that is not controlled.

These perspectives differ in fundamental ways from the more objectivist stance of traditional Western science, in which quantitative methods—and particularly the RCT—are highly valued. Ultimately, however, the key features are the different language used, and the different perspective assumed. Each has its place and role; each can inform the other. One induces *why* something happens, and the other deduces *how* it happens. A simple example is the development of a hypothesis, from clinical observations and discussions with individuals using contraception, that a specific method of contraception causes weight gain (qualitative findings). To support this hypothesis, a study using quantitative methods can be designed to examine whether this effect actually does occur.

The research questions most appropriate for investigation via qualitative methods are often exploratory in nature: Why do things happen? What does it feel like? What does it mean? How should I interpret this result? All of these questions are excellent candidates for the use of qualitative methods. Such questions can arise from either clinical problems or specific gaps in clinical evidence.

A variety of lenses serve as the underlying basis for the traditions of qualitative research. The term "bricoleur" is often applied to a scientist who can navigate these traditions and lenses to answer the original research question and questions that emerge as the study progresses. A bricoleur is characterized by their ability to "put together a complex array of data, derived from a variety of sources, and using a variety of methods" (Flanagan & Tatano, 2024). Skills required to accomplish this feat include astute observation, reflection, interpretation, and introspection.

Qualitative Research Design and Methods

Qualitative research focuses on exploring, understanding, and interpreting complex social phenomena, behaviors, and experiences. Emphasis is placed on experience, existence, perspective, context, meaning, and subjectivity (Lim, 2024). Data are derived from multiple sources, such as interviews, fieldwork, observations, video, art, media, and other documents, usually in the form of words, images, or observations rather than numerical statistics. The researcher is considered to be the instrument, and their role is closely tied to the collection and interpretation of data. Sometimes the researcher is also a participant, such as in fieldwork where observations of specific clinical practices are being conducted. The researcher's assumption of this role can lead to an increased level of trust between the participants being observed and the researcher.

Qualitative studies are descriptive from the perspective of those who have experienced a particular phenomenon; therefore, samples are "purposive," not random (Flanagan & Tatano, 2024). In other words, specific research participants are sought who can shed the most light on the research question. For example, if you wanted to learn about the experience of postpartum depression, it would be fruitless to interview people who had never been exposed to this phenomenon.

To refine ideas based on emerging findings in the data analysis, the researcher may "theoretically sample" populations to answer specific questions (Holloway & Galvin, 2024). Sample size is usually not predetermined in such a case, and the power of the samples used in qualitative studies reflects the robust richness of the textual data. Data collection usually continues until the researcher observes saturation or redundancy, or until nothing new is coming to light or being observed. Data analysis is conducted in a variety of ways, but it usually produces findings that are richly descriptive in textual or thematic language.

Choosing from among the many qualitative methods available requires that the researcher understand their disciplinary focus. Each area has its own complexity and methodology (a topic that goes beyond the scope of this chapter). For an easier understanding of some of the basic methods, the various qualitative research approaches have been organized here using general categories adapted from Polit and Beck (2022) to reflect the area of knowledge they explore.

Understanding the Experiences and Processes of Health and Illness

Many research questions in the healthcare realm address what it is like to go through a certain health event. The purpose is to help us find ways to improve life for others who have similar experiences. These approaches focus on understanding the basic experiences and processes of how a person moves through the event. The methods used in such investigations come from the traditions of philosophy and sociology.

Phenomenology is derived from a philosophical tradition that provides a "textual reflection on the lived experiences and practical actions of everyday life with the intent to increase one's thoughtfulness and practical resourcefulness or tact" (van Manen, 1990, p. 4). The focus is on understanding what it is like for this person to be in this experience within the context of their life. Such work is interpretative or hermeneutical, and its findings are often presented as paradigm cases or exemplars, creating "a dialogue between practical concerns and lived experience through engaged reasoning and imaginative dwelling in the immediacy of the participant's worlds" (Benner, 1994, p. 99). The results provide a vivid description that can help us better understand the social, political, or historical context of the individual's experience (Flanagan & Tatano, 2024).

Asking questions from the tradition of sociology assists us in understanding how social structures and human interactions affect people's experience of health and illness (Flanagan & Tatano, 2024; Holloway & Galvin, 2024). These approaches range from understanding how people make sense of their social interactions (symbolic interaction) to discovering how social processes are structured and developed (grounded theory). Charon (1992) describes four central foci of symbolic interactionism:

- The nature of the social interaction
- Human action that both causes and results from social interaction
- Present rather than past focus
- Actions of the person who is unpredictable and active in their world

Grounded theory was developed by Glaser and Strauss in the 1960s as a research method that addresses both the chief concern or problem for people and the basic processes available to address that concern (Glaser, 1978, 1992; Strauss & Corbin, 1998). The goal of this approach is to develop theory in a substantive area that is grounded directly in the data. Grounded theories "are likely to offer insight, enhance understanding, and provide a meaningful guide to action" (Strauss & Corbin, 1998, p. 12). One example is a grounded theory study exploring midwives' experiences with a safe childbirth checklist (Skirnisdottir et al., 2023). This study found that a lack of consensus on how to use the checklist and no common understanding of the purpose of the checklist caused variations in when and how the checklist was used and applied. Based on these findings, leadership can work with the midwives to adapt the checklist and develop strategies for effective implementation.

Understanding Human Behavior

The tradition of psychology focuses specifically on how and why people act; its aim is to describe behavior. Studying human behavior can help us understand how behaviors are related to health and illness. Ethology examines the evolution of human behavior in its natural context (Flanagan & Tatano, 2024). With this methodology, observations of human behavior are used to expose structures that are essential to life. This observational approach can also be used from an environmental perspective, as in ecological psychology. Ecological models examine the relationship of environmental influences with specific human attributes (Humpel et al., 2004). For example, studying the ecology of cyberbullying can expose characteristics, patterns, and contexts, which in turn can facilitate the development of preventive and intervention strategies (Patel & Quan-Haase, 2024).

Learning how people communicate is another approach to learning about human behavior. Human communication has many processes and forms. To explore the construction of meaning in the nuances of these processes, researchers use methods derived from both sociology and linguistics. Sociolinguistics is the examination of the forms and rules of conversation through discourse analysis (Flanagan & Tatano, 2024). Mishler (1984) proposes that by examining the dialogue between clinicians and patients, we can encourage the development of noncoercive discourse and humane clinical practice.

Understanding Cultural Traditions and Influences

One of the oldest qualitative traditions comes from the field of anthropology, where scientists strive to understand cultural variations among the many peoples of the world. Although several approaches are used in this disciplinary area, ethnography is the most commonly employed. An ethnographer's goal is to carefully describe a specific culture. Historically, grand ethnographies often explored indigenous peoples. In health-related research, however, smaller specific subsets are often the focus of study and enable us to understand the intimate nature of people's lives. For example, Gyamfi et al. (2021) used ethnography to examine the cultural, health, and sociological promoters and barriers that Black/African American mothers experience when trying to breastfeed.

Synthesizing Qualitative Research Findings

Meta-synthesis is another qualitative method. This research method analyzes, synthesizes, and interprets a specified body of research and holds the potential to provide valuable insight and knowledge about the distinctive aspects of a phenomenon (Bowden & Bowden, 2022). It shares some commonalities with the type of meta-analysis conducted in quantitative research but is distinguished by some important differences. Meta-synthesis provides an organized yet interpretive approach to a specific group of qualitative studies (Bowden & Bowden, 2022). The meta-synthesis method involves identifying similar qualitative studies about a particular phenomenon, determining how they are related, and synthesizing their findings. By systematically examining qualitative findings, meta-synthesis enhances the credibility and trustworthiness of the conclusions drawn, ensuring that they are based on robust and diverse evidence. This process also helps identify patterns and gaps in the existing literature, guiding future research and informing practice and policy decisions (Malterud, 2023).

Rigor in Qualitative Research

Just as in quantitative research, a clearly articulated study design is essential to understanding the purpose and results of any qualitative project. Because qualitative research uses textual rather than numerical data, relative terms such as "trustworthiness" and "dependability" are used to describe results, whereas "error" is used as the corresponding term with quantitative study results (Holloway & Galvin, 2024). Understanding the specific terminology associated with qualitative research can help you assess whether the results of such studies are valid and reliable.

Credibility reflects how much confidence you have in the study results (Flanagan & Tatano, 2024). It is enhanced by complete descriptions of the sample and setting, data collection, analytic procedures, the way in which decisions were made, and the researcher's role in the study. Preparation and experience with the methods and acknowledgment of preconceived ideas, sometimes called bracketing, are helpful in understanding the researcher's perspective and influence on the study. This practice is similar to evaluating whether a specific statistical test is appropriate in a quantitative study.

A qualitative study should provide enough documentation for the results to be confirmed—a characteristic sometimes called confirmability (Flanagan & Tatano, 2024). Confirmability helps to ensure that later researchers can follow the analysis and understand how decisions were made. The findings are strengthened when evidence shows that a team of researchers participated in peer debriefing and actively sought out negative cases to challenge and refine the conclusions. These procedures allow the research team to reflect on their analysis and to check for bias and interpretative errors. In another approach, called member checking, study participants read and react to the researchers' analytic decisions to see if the findings reflect their personal experience with the phenomenon under investigation.

All research findings should make conceptual sense. The investigators should provide enough broad, rich description to prove that the results clearly fit with the data presented. Transferability refers to how well the findings can be applied to another setting and is similar to the concept of generalizability in quantitative research (Flanagan & Tatano, 2024). A study should provide enough descriptive evidence to help you assess whether the findings could apply to your setting.

Mixed Research Methods

Sometimes, the research questions require a mixed methods approach or a combination of quantitative and qualitative methods. There are multiple ways to combine methods. Perhaps one method is more widely used than the other, or perhaps research is conducted sequentially using the various methods (Creswell & Creswell, 2023). A helpful way to think about this issue is to consider how different lenses help you see different things. You might design a study that examines how a specific intervention affects birthing individual's perinatal outcomes and health behaviors (quantitative measures). Yet, within the same study, you could also interview birthing individuals (qualitative methods) about their experience of the intervention and how it affected their lives. Applying these methods, Savory et al. (2022) integrated quantitative and qualitative data to present a comprehensive look at midwives' skills, knowledge, and experiences of supporting women's mental health.

Another term appropriate to this discussion is "triangulation," which refers to the use of multiple referents to capture a more complete and contextualized picture of the phenomenon under investigation (Flanagan & Tatano, 2024). This approach may involve the use of multiple sources of data, time collection points, sites, and samples because they all provide different perspectives on the same research question.

Translational Research

Translational research, a relatively new area of investigation, explores which evidence-based implementation strategies work in which settings, with which populations, and under what conditions. The American Association of Colleges of Nursing identifies translational research as the focus of the Doctor of Nursing Practice program of study, incorporated into a scholarly project demonstrating the essential elements of Doctor of Nursing Practice education (American Association of Colleges of Nursing, 2018; Trautman et al., 2018). According to Pearson et al. (2012), the purposes of translational research are to enhance the utilization of scientific information "in diverse practice settings, among diverse populations, and under diverse payment systems" (para. 19). Translational science expedites the application of the best evidence into real-world settings to improve healthcare delivery, healthcare outcomes, and/or population health. Best evidence includes findings from quantitative and qualitative research and other scientific efforts, such as case reports and scientific principles (Titler, 2018). Translational research is a dynamic, iterative process encompassing the synthesis, dissemination, exchange, and ethically sound application of knowledge to enhance health outcomes, deliver more effective healthcare services and products, and strengthen the overall healthcare system (Ryder & Jacob, 2022).

Multiple theories and frameworks are used to guide translational or implementation science, and many are the same ones that guide quantitative and qualitative research. The purposes of implementation frameworks and theories are to describe or guide the process of translating evidence into practice, to understand and/or explain what influences implementation outcomes, and to evaluate implementation (Roussel & Thomas, 2024). Several theories, frameworks, or models that are commonly used to guide the design of translational research are identified in **Table 4-3**. Although a number of theories, frameworks, or models can guide translational research, common among them are the following principles:

- Acceptance and adoption of best practices is ongoing and iterative; there is no end point.
- There is always a need to examine the strength and quality of new knowledge before adopting change.
- Many stakeholders need to be included.
- The context is important, including culture, leadership styles, decision making, and organizational structures.

TABLE 4-3 Examples of Common Theories, Frameworks, and Models Used in Translation/Implementation Research

Diffusion of Innovations

Diffusion of innovations is a classic change theory, developed by Rogers (2003), that examines the mechanisms of adoption and the use of innovations by groups or individuals. It is commonly used to inform and guide EBP and translational research.
There are five steps in the innovation/decision process:

1. Knowledge: The person becomes aware of new knowledge or innovation and has some idea of what it is.
2. Persuasion: The person actively seeks information about the innovation or new knowledge and forms a favorable or unfavorable opinion about it.
3. Decision: The person engages in activities that lead to a choice, benefit, or risk of adopting the new knowledge or innovation and makes a choice to adopt or reject it.
4. Implementation: The person considers the uses of the innovation or new knowledge and puts it into practice.
5. Confirmation: The person evaluates the results of the innovation/decision process and makes a decision whether or not to continue its use.

Iowa Model of EBP to Improve the Quality of Care

The Iowa model (Titler et al., 2001) outlines a series of activities with three critical decision points:

1. Decide whether the problem is a sufficient priority for the organization and explore possible changes.
2. Decide whether there is a sufficient research base.
3. Decide whether change is appropriate for adoption in the practice setting.

The Iowa model is more focused on organizational change.

Stetler Model

The Stetler model (Stetler, 2001) is an individual practitioner model rather than an organizational model. Its purpose is to help an individual clinician to go through a systematic series of steps involving critical thinking and decision making to facilitate the effective use of research findings.
The model describes five phases of research utilization:

i. Preparation: The search for and selection of research to be evaluated for practice implementation.
ii. Validation: Appraising the findings of the research using a specific methodology.
iii. Comparative evaluation or decision-making phase: A decision about whether a practice change can be made using four applicability criteria: the substantiating evidence; the fit for using the research findings in the setting; the feasibility of implementing the findings in the setting; and the evaluation of the current practice.
iv. Implementation: Begins when the translation or application of the research findings are implemented and the how-to's are considered.
v. Evaluation.

Ottawa Model of Research Use

The Ottawa Model (Logan & Graham, 2010) is an interactive model that depicts research as a dynamic process of interconnected decisions and actions taken by stakeholders. There are three implicit assumptions of knowledge translation:

- Dynamic and interactive processes between research development and use reflect the complex nature of knowledge translation.
- Patients/clients are central throughout knowledge translation processes, since their health outcomes are the main focus of evidence-based practice.
- Knowledge translation processes are affected by external societal and healthcare environments.

The Ottawa Model of Research Use follows a six-step approach to guide the implementation of an innovation.

1. Set the stage
2. Specify the innovation
3. Assess the innovation, potential adopters, and the environment for barriers and facilitators
4. Select and monitor the knowledge translation strategies
5. Monitor innovation adoption
6. Evaluate Outcomes of the Innovation

(*continues*)

TABLE 4-3 Examples of Common Theories, Frameworks, and Models Used in Translation/Implementation Research (*continued*)

Advancing Research and Clinical Practice Through Close Collaboration (ARCC) Model

The ARCC Model (Melnyk & Fineout-Overholt, 2002) is a system-wide framework for implementing and sustaining evidence-based practice in healthcare organizations and systems.
The model includes seven steps of evidence-based practice:

0. Cultivate inquiry
1. Ask a clinical question using PICO(T) format
2. Search and collect high-quality evidence
3. Critically appraise evidence
4. Integrate and apply evidence into practice
5. Evaluate outcomes of the evidence-based practice change
6. Disseminate outcomes of the evidence-based practice change

Lewin's Theory of Change/Force Field Analysis

Lewin's theory of change process has three stages: unfreezing, movement, and refreezing. Lewin's force field analysis views change as a dynamic balance of forces (driving and restraining) working in opposite directions within an organization or field (Shirey, 2013). The phases include the following:

i. Unfreezing the current situation by increasing the driving forces or decreasing the opposing ones.
ii. Moving or changing toward a new equilibrium—a balance between driving forces and restraining forces.
iii. Refreezing—sustains the change within the organization.

Kotter's Model of Change in Organizations

Kotter's model of change in organizations consists of eight steps (Kotter, n.d.):

1. Creating a sense of urgency
2. Creating a guiding coalition
3. Developing a vision and strategy
4. Communicating the change vision
5. Empowering people for broad-based action
6. Generating short-term wins
7. Consolidating gains and producing more change
8. Anchoring new approaches in the culture

Knowledge to Action (KTA) Framework

The Knowledge to Action (KTA) Framework (Graham et al., 2006) is designed to guide the process of translating research knowledge into practical applications. The framework consists of two main components:
- Knowledge Creation: This involves generating, synthesizing, and tailoring knowledge to make it more applicable and accessible for end users.
- Action Cycle: This part of the framework includes seven phases that help implement the knowledge into practice. These phases involve identifying the problem, adapting knowledge to the local context, assessing barriers to knowledge use, selecting and implementing interventions, monitoring knowledge use, evaluating outcomes, and sustaining knowledge use.

The Johns Hopkins Evidence-Based Practice (JHEBP) Model

The Johns Hopkins Evidence-Based Practice (JHEBP) model (Dang et al., 2022) is a comprehensive problem-solving approach designed to support clinical decision making and improve patient outcomes. It is structured around three main phases, often referred to as the PET process:
- Practice Question: This phase involves identifying a specific clinical question using the PICO format (Population, Intervention, Comparison, Outcome).
- Evidence: In this phase, a thorough literature search is conducted, and the evidence is appraised for its strength and quality.
- Translation: The final phase involves synthesizing the findings to develop recommendations for practice, implementing these recommendations, and evaluating their impact.

Context, including the physical setting and operational dynamics and also the dynamics of a practice and social environment, can have a profound impact on the implementation of change and the adoption of EBP changes (Melnyk & Fineout-Overholt, 2023).

Translational Research Design and Methods

Translational research often relies on the integration of multidisciplinary and multiple types of research—including basic quantitative and qualitative research, patient-oriented research, quality improvement studies, and population-based research—all with the long-term aim of improving health outcomes or the healthcare system. It also incorporates clinicians' expertise and patients' preferences when appropriate (Flanagan & Tatano, 2024). Therefore, the approach to designing translational research projects is somewhat flexible to accommodate the specific aims of the researcher, the characteristics and dynamics of the clinical or organizational issue, and the context. Translational research design is guided by the selected framework, theory, or model. Several research designs are useful in translational research, including descriptive pre- and post-test, correlational, case-control (ex post facto), cross-sectional, and program evaluation, to evaluate patient outcomes or to develop quality improvement initiatives (Moran et al., 2023).

The methodology is concentrated on strategies to promote knowledge translation and the movement of best practices into real healthcare settings. The focus is on critical appraisal, synthesis, and evaluation of existing evidence included in primary studies, systematic reviews, meta-analyses, meta-syntheses, mixed methods syntheses, and/or preappraised data such as that contained in the Cochrane review. Outcomes of translational research can include clinical practice guidelines, care bundles, clinical decision tools, policy development, and/or organizational restructuring (Flanagan & Tatano, 2024). The researcher must also consider the implementation potential of the intervention or change, including the feasibility and cost/benefit ratio of any new practice and the development of an implementation plan. An evaluation following implementation will help to identify any additional barriers or resources related to the support of the proposed change or intervention to facilitate sustainability. A step-by-step guide for the development of a translational research project is outlined in a text by Moran et al. (2023).

Rigor in Translational Research

Because the final goal of translational research is to apply best practices that are evidence-based and have the potential to improve health outcomes, the research must be based on a thorough review, critical appraisal, and synthesis of the scientific literature. Just like qualitative and quantitative research, translational or implementation research also depends on quality standards to ensure evidence is clearly and accurately reported. To facilitate the use of best practices for improving health, healthcare outcomes, or the healthcare system, it is essential to report in detail the strategies used to promote change, address the increased utilization of evidence, and assess the effectiveness of an intervention or change in a specific context.

Critical appraisal is essential in translational research and evidence-based practice to ensure that healthcare decisions are based on valid, reliable, and clinically relevant evidence. Appraisal tools provide structured frameworks for assessing the quality of research, identifying potential biases, and determining applicability to patient care (Buccheri & Sharifi, 2017; Haile, 2022). Several widely used critical appraisal tools cater to different study designs. The Joanna Briggs Institute (JBI) checklists (2024) and the Critical Appraisal Skills Program (CASP) (2017) tools support systematic assessment of qualitative and quantitative research. The Cochrane Risk of Bias Tool (2011) is instrumental in evaluating randomized controlled trials, ensuring that results are not distorted by methodological flaws. Tools such as GRADE (2013) aid in synthesizing evidence and making practice recommendations. For clinical guidelines, AGREE II (2010) provides a comprehensive framework to assess rigor and transparency in guideline development. Tools such as the EBPQI critical appraisal tool facilitate the evaluation of both research and quality improvement initiatives, ensuring that practice changes are based on high-quality evidence (Waldrop et al., 2025). Beyond appraising research, effective reporting is crucial for transparency and replicability. Reporting guidelines like PRISMA (2020) for systematic reviews, CONSORT (2012) for randomized trials, and SQUIRE 2.0 (2016) for quality improvement initiatives help ensure quality, safety, transparency, and standardization in research dissemination. By utilizing structured appraisal frameworks and adhering to reporting guidelines, clinicians and researchers can enhance the credibility and impact of translational research, ultimately improving patient outcomes and healthcare quality. Several checklists, critical appraisal tools, and reporting guidelines used to evaluate the evidence are listed in **Table 4-4**.

MOVING FROM BEST EVIDENCE TO BEST PRACTICE

Research can improve practice by providing answers to clinical questions; evaluating the safety, effectiveness, or cost of therapeutics; refining practice guidelines; or testing theories relevant to practice (Melnyk & Fineout-Overholt, 2023). Research evidence that has been reviewed, compiled, and analyzed by a variety of credible resources enhances our ability to obtain and apply research findings. Organizations that fill this role include the Cochrane Collaboration, professional organizations, and government agencies. This information has also been published on the internet, so it is readily available to the busy clinician. Despite this access to best evidence, many clinicians continue to struggle with the issue of how to apply the results of research to practice: How do you actually make it happen?

As clinicians, we must be able to use web-based tools and be familiar with the EBP resources in all fields of health. We must also be cognizant of the criticisms and limitations of EBP, including overreliance on RCT-derived results and systematic reviews, an emphasis on the routinization of practice, a denial of patient preferences and/or diverse views, and the daunting effort required to stay current because today's best evidence may be tomorrow's inappropriate practice.

Clinicians must be able to critically appraise individual studies to determine how much faith they should put into the findings. The strengths and weaknesses of each study must be readily identifiable. Evidence hierarchies rank studies according to the strength of the evidence they provide (Flanagan & Tatano, 2024). Most such hierarchies put meta-analyses of RCTs at the top and opinions of experts at the bottom. As a consequence, such hierarchies inevitably emphasize a scientific and rational focus and assume that causation (the design of the tightly woven web structure) can be identified only by rigorous quantitative

TABLE 4-4 Examples of Critical Appraisal Tools and Reporting Guidelines and the Type of Evidence They Evaluate

Checklist/Tool/ Reporting Guideline	Systematic review	Literature review	Randomized controlled trial	Cohort study	Case-control study	Qualitative study	Evidence-based practice project	Quality improvement project	Clinical practice guideline
AGREE II (Brouwers et al., 2016)	X			X	X				X
CASP Checklist (CASP, 2017)	X		X	X	X	X			
Cochrane Risk of Bias Tool (Higgins et al., 2011)			X						
CONSORT (Turner et al., 2012)			X						
EBPQI (Waldrop et al., 2025)	X	X					X	X	X
EPQA Guidelines (Lee et al., 2013)							X		
GRADE (Dijkers, 2013)	X								X
JBI Checklists (Aromataris et al., 2024)	X	X	X	X	X	X			
Johns Hopkins Research Evidence Appraisal Tool (Dang et al., 2022)	X		X	X	X	X			
Johns Hopkins Non-Research Evidence Appraisal Tool (Dang et al., 2022)	X		X	X	X	X			X
PRISMA (Page et al., 2021)	X		X						
Rapid Critical Appraisal Checklists (Melnyk & Fineout-Overholt, 2023)	X	X	X	X	X		X	X	
SQUIRE 2.0 (Ogrinc et al., 2016)								X	

study. This approach fails to recognize the gaps in the web of knowledge and discounts qualitative research or naturalistic observations that focus on understanding the human experience. EBP attempts to escape this reductionist approach by integrating information from a variety of well-designed studies, clinical experience, existing resources, and the patient's preference. When developing clinical practice guidelines, protocols, or clinical pathways, all of these elements should be included (Guerra-Farfan et al., 2023). Put simply, no single study or group of studies can provide an infallible answer to a clinical question.

Using models such as the ones proposed in Table 4-3 can make EBP more focused and acceptable to clinicians who, when faced with a proposed change, assert that "this is the way we have always done it." Integrating a methodical approach to applying evidence to practice can be effective in overcoming this all-too-frequent mantra.

BARRIERS TO ACHIEVING QUALITY EVIDENCE-BASED PRACTICE

Institutional Barriers to Implementing and Sustaining EBP

Healthcare institutions and systems often struggle to implement evidence-based practice and sustain change due to a combination of organizational and contextual barriers. Organizational culture plays a significant role, as a lack of a supportive environment and poor communication can hinder EBP adoption. Common challenges include organizational resistance, insufficient leadership support, inadequate resources, and deeply ingrained traditional practices. Time constraints, heavy workloads, and staffing shortages limit opportunities for clinicians to engage in continuous learning and implement new evidence-based protocols (Crawford et al., 2023). Hierarchical structures and limited interprofessional collaboration often result in fragmented decision making, further hindering the adoption of EBP. Many institutions also lack formalized training programs, mentorship, and incentives that encourage ongoing engagement with EBP. Furthermore, policy misalignment and inconsistent integration of EBP into standard operating procedures contribute to a failure to sustain change over time (Furtado et al., 2024).

To successfully implement and sustain EBP, healthcare institutions must adopt a multifaceted, systems-level approach. Leadership engagement is critical. Hospital and clinic administrators should actively promote and support EBP initiatives, involve all team members in decision making, and create clear, practical strategies and tools to facilitate implementation (Berthelsen & Holge-Hazelton, 2021). Institutional policies should allow staff protected time to participate in EBP activities, including ongoing education and competency-based training. Healthcare organizations should also embed EBP into clinical workflows, utilizing decision-support tools, electronic health record (EHR) integration, and standardized protocols to streamline evidence-based interventions (Crawford et al., 2023). Interprofessional collaboration must be fostered by creating shared governance structures where all clinicians contribute to policy and practice changes. Performance incentives, professional development opportunities, and mentorship programs can sustain engagement with EBP (Melnyk et al., 2021). Lastly, continuous monitoring and feedback mechanisms should be implemented using quality improvement frameworks to regularly assess and refine EBP strategies. By addressing these structural, cultural, and leadership barriers, healthcare institutions can enhance their capacity to integrate and sustain evidence-based practices.

Individual Barriers to Implementing and Sustaining EBP

The two factors that clinicians and students most commonly cite for their failure to apply the latest research evidence are (1) lack of time to find research studies and (2) lack of confidence in critiquing those studies. We empathize with both concerns, and in this section, we offer some practical strategies to overcome them.

Finding the Relevant Research

Today's information-rich world places the most recent research virtually at your fingertips. It is important to realize, however, that published findings are inevitably outdated the minute they are published. Journal articles can take 1 to 2 years from first submission to reach the printed page, and textbooks take even longer to be published. The internet, however, has substantially improved our ability to keep up with the most recently published research.

Several excellent sources provide the best evidence in a succinct format for the busy clinician:

- The Cochrane Collaboration makes up-to-date, accurate information about the effects of health care readily available worldwide, including via the Cochrane Database of Systematic Reviews. The Cochrane Collaboration produces and disseminates systematic reviews of healthcare interventions and promotes the search for evidence in the form of clinical trials and other well-controlled studies (Cochrane, 2025).
- PubMed provides free access to millions of citations in peer-reviewed biomedical journals and is another excellent source for research findings, although the reader must evaluate most of the studies to determine their scientific merit and clinical applicability.
- The Joanna Briggs Institute, a not-for-profit research and development center within the Faculty of Health and Medical Sciences at the University of Adelaide, South Australia, offers evidence summaries, systematic reviews, and best practice information sheets to support clinicians in the appraisal and application of the latest evidence.

Many other agencies and organizations prepare evidence-based guidelines and protocols that can usually be accessed on the internet. Additional resources for EBP are listed in Appendix 4-A.

Critiquing Research Studies

Critiquing research studies takes practice and some basic knowledge about how research is conducted. We suggest that all clinicians have a basic research text on their bookshelf to look up unfamiliar terms and statistics. We have used *Polit and Beck's Nursing Research: Generating and Assessing Evidence for Nursing Practice* (2024) to provide some structure for this chapter and find it easy to read and practically written. Many other good basic texts are available, such as *Evidence-Based Practice in Nursing & Healthcare: A Guide to Best Practice* (Melnyk & Fineout-Overholt, 2023).

To assess the applicability of any research findings to patient care, clinicians must evaluate the validity of the research; determine the practicality of implementing the findings; weigh any associated risks and benefits to the patient; and consider the ethical issues, available resources, and cost (Melnyk & Fineout-Overholt, 2023; Berkman et al., 2015). When applying EBP guidelines, clinicians must be able to recognize the limitations of the available databases and the limitations of scientific evidence. They must also know how to integrate clinical expertise, ethical considerations, patient individuality, and choice into the decision-making process.

In addition to these considerations, the socially responsible clinician must take into account social and political barriers, racist and patriarchal histories, and constraints on time, skills, training, and resources that impact the research and literature available to us. There is marked underrepresentation of minorities in published clinical research. Several factors contribute to this disparity, including insufficient training in designing and implementing population-based studies of minorities, challenges in recruiting and retaining members of underrepresented communities, and a general lack of partnership between academic medical centers and racial and ethnic minorities (Bentley-Edwards et al., 2022; Boulware et al., 2022). Furthermore, we can point to a lack of diversity among scientists in academic medical centers. In 2020, racial/ethnic minorities comprised 30% of investigators funded by the National Institutes of Health with only 5% identifying as Black or African American (NIH, 2022).

Additional objectives of implementing quality EBP may include cost reduction, a desire to reduce wide variations in healthcare practices, and the desire to include patients as partners in their own care. None of these ideas are novel to clinicians.

Box 4-2 provides a brief summary of important points to consider when evaluating the quality of a research study and determining whether you should apply the findings to your practice.

BOX 4-2 Practical Points in Critiquing Research Studies

Title

Does the title of the article accurately describe the study? Is the language in the title understandable and informative?

Abstract

Does the abstract accurately present the study? It should summarize the purpose of the study, the problems that were investigated, the research questions or hypotheses, the study design and methodology used, the sample, the instruments used, other data collection procedures, and the results or findings.

Research Questions and Purpose of the Study

What are the research questions? Are these questions researchable in the sense that they can be carried out by the investigators? What is the significance of the study in terms of practice, adding to the body of scientific knowledge, or other areas? Are the research questions stated in a concise and precise manner?

Research Variable

If it is a quantitative study, can you delineate the independent and dependent variables? If it is a qualitative study, is the phenomenon of study clear?

Review of the Literature and Conceptual Framework/Model

Is the literature review relevant to the study? Does it include both timely and classic articles that pertain to the study? Does the review provide adequate background information? Do the authors state how this review provides support for their study (i.e., give background information for the identified research problem/question)?

Sample and Setting

Is there a description of how the sample was selected and the location of the study? What are the sources of bias, if any, that are associated with the sample selection process? Were power and effect size calculated for this study? In qualitative studies, was the sample purposive, and when was the sampling stopped?

Ethical Considerations

Do the authors address protection of human study participants? Did they obtain permission to conduct this study in the setting?

Method: The Design

Is the design appropriate for the research questions? Is it described? Which extraneous variables are associated with the design, if any? Are they identified? Is the description adequate to allow replication of the entire study?

Instrumentation and Data Collection Procedures

How are issues of scientific rigor addressed? Are validity and reliability of the instruments described? Was data collection conducted in a standardized manner? In qualitative research, is the researcher as instrument described?

Data Analysis

Are the analytic techniques supportive and appropriate for the research design? Does the article include supportive graphs, tables, or charts? Do these components help describe the results? Are they easy to understand?

Results

Do the results follow logically from the design and method? Do the authors describe the results in a way that is understandable and clear? Do the results answer the research questions or hypotheses?

Summary and Conclusions

What is your overall impression of the study? Does the author convince you about the conclusions that are drawn? Do the conclusions seem logical in light of the method, procedures, and other factors?

Data from Kaplan, L. (n.d.). *Framework for How to Read and Critique a Research Study*. American Nurses Association. https://www.nursingworld.org/globalassets/practiceandpolicy/innovation--evidence/framework-for-how-to-read-and-critique-a-research-study.pdf

CONCLUSION

As a clinician, when considering the issue of research, it is helpful to look at what it means to use evidence in practice. Examples of applying evidence to clinical practice abound—from the use of preexposure prophylaxis (PrEP) to reduce the risk of sexually acquired HIV infection (Centers for Disease Control and Prevention, 2021), to the evidence for offering an intrauterine device as a form of emergency contraception (Turok et al., 2021), to examining whether birthing individuals need continuous electronic fetal monitoring during labor (Arnold & Gawrys, 2020). Every clinical scenario needs to be addressed from the perspective of your personal experience, the patient's desires, and the best evidence to support your recommendations. Your first challenge is to blend these considerations artfully in everyday practice. Your second challenge is to work within the healthcare system to influence administrators and policymakers to use the best information and evidence possible to provide the highest quality of care.

The key takeaway from this chapter is to question everything. Inquiry should not lead to paralysis but rather foster critical thinking about the root causes of clinical problems and how to identify the best available evidence to address them. Too often, obstetric care relies on tradition, convenience, and "standard of care procedures" that lack evidence and disregard patient preferences. Practices such as the artificial rupture of membranes to speed labor, performing unnecessary cervical exams, utilizing continuous electronic fetal monitoring (EFM), administering synthetic oxytocin, restricting food intake during labor, enforcing supine or semi-sitting birth positions, and overusing cesarean delivery all carry risks and harms that can impact both the birthing parent and child (Liese et al., 2021). Growing evidence links excessive medical interventions and failures in quality care to high rates of mortality and morbidity throughout the childbearing continuum, the early postpartum period, and the first few weeks of life. These issues contribute to iatrogenic harm, with potential long-term consequences that may extend across generations (Dahlen et al., 2013).

As clinicians and researchers, we should never be caught wondering, "Why didn't I ask the question about the potential of our actions over time?" Evidence-based practice encourages us to provide quality care that is tailored to individuals, weighs benefits and harms, is person-centered, works across the whole continuum of care, advances equity, and is informed by evidence, including cost-effectiveness (Kennedy et al., 2018). We owe it to our patients and to ourselves to search for the best evidence to support our healthcare practices.

References

Agency for Healthcare Research and Quality. (n.d.-a). *Agency for Healthcare Research and Quality archive.* http://archive.ahrq.gov/clinic/ajpmsuppl/harris2.htm

Agency for Healthcare Research and Quality. (n.d.-b). *Get to know the AHRQ quality indicators.* https://www.qualityindicators.ahrq.gov

Agency for Healthcare Research and Quality. (2023). *EvidenceNOW: Agency for healthcare research and quality.* https://www.ahrq.gov/evidencenow/index.html

American Association of Colleges of Nursing. (2018). *Defining scholarship for academic nursing.* https://www.aacnnursing.org/news-data/position-statements-white-papers/defining-scholarship-for-academic-nursing

American College of Obstetricians and Gynecologists. (2024). Racial and ethnic inequities in obstetrics and gynecology (Committee Statement No. 10). *Obstetrics & Gynecology, 144*(e62–e74). https://www.acog.org/clinical/clinical-guidance/committee-statement/articles/2024/09/racial-and-ethnic-inequities-in-obstetrics-and-gynecology

Arnold, J. J., & Gawrys, B. L. (2020). Intrapartum fetal monitoring. *American Family Physician, 102*(3), 158–167.

Aromataris, E., Lockwood, C., Porritt, K., Pilla, B., & Jordan, Z. (2024). *JBI manual for evidence synthesis.* Available from: https://jbi.global/critical-appraisal-tools

Benner, P. (1994). The tradition and skill of interpretive phenomenology in studying health, illness, and caring practices. In P. Benner (Ed.), *Interpretive phenomenology: Embodiment, caring, and ethics in health and illness* (pp. 99–127). Sage.

Bentley-Edwards, K. L., Jordan Fleming, P., Doherty, I. A., Whicker, D. R., Mervin-Blake, S., & Barrett, N. J. (2022). The 5Ws of racial equity in research: A framework for applying a racial equity lens throughout the research process. *Health Equity, 6*(1), 917–921. https://doi.org/10.1089/heq.2022.0042

Berkman, N. D., Lohr, K. N., Ansari, M. T., Balk, E. M., Kane, R., McDonagh, M., Morton, S. C., Viswanathan, M., Bass, E. B., Butler, M., Gartlehner, G., Hartling, L., McPheeters, M., Morgan, L. C., Reston, J., Sista, P., Whitlock, E., & Chang, S. (2015). Grading the strength of a body of evidence when assessing health care interventions: An EPC update. *Journal of Clinical Epidemiology, 68*(11), 1312–1324. https://doi.org/10.1016/j.jclinepi.2014.11.023

Berthelsen, C., & Hølge-Hazelton, B. (2021). The importance of context and organization culture in the understanding of nurses' barriers against research utilization: A systematic review. *Worldviews on Evidence-Based Nursing, 18*(2), 111–117. https://doi.org/10.1111/wvn.12488

Boulware, L. E., Corbie, G., Aguilar-Gaxiola, S., Wilkins, C. H., Ruiz, R., Vitale, A., & Egede, L. E. (2022). Combating structural inequities—diversity, equity, and inclusion in clinical and translational research. *The New England Journal of Medicine, 386*(3), 201–203. https://doi.org/10.1056/NEJMp2112233

Bowden, V. R., & Bowden, A. G. (2022). Types of reviews—part 2: Meta-analysis and meta-synthesis. *Pediatric Nursing, 48*(1), 43–49. https://doi.org/10.62116/PNJ.2022.48.1.43

Brignardello-Petersen, R., Carrasco-Labra, A., & Guyatt, G. H. (2021). How to interpret and use a clinical practice guideline or recommendation: Users' guides to the medical literature. *JAMA: The Journal of the American Medical Association, 326*(15), 1516–1523. https://doi.org/10.1001/jama.2021.15319

Brisolara, S. (2014). Feminist theory: Its domains and applications. In S. Brisolara, D. Seigart, & S. SenGupta. (Eds.), *Feminist evaluation and research: Theory and practice* (pp. 3–41). Guilford Press.

Brouwers, M. C., Kerkvliet, K., & Spithoff, K. on behalf of the AGREE Next Steps Consortium. (2016). The AGREE Reporting Checklist: A tool to improve reporting of clinical practice guidelines. *British Medical Journal, 352*(3), e1–e2. https://doi.org/10.1136/bmj.i1152

Buccheri, R. K., & Sharifi, C. (2017). Critical appraisal tools and reporting guidelines for evidence-based practice. *Worldviews on Evidence-Based Nursing, 14*(6), 463–472. https://doi.org/10.1111/wvn.12258

Buse, K. (2008). Addressing the theoretical, practical, and ethical challenges inherent in prospective health policy analysis. *Health Policy and Planning, 23*(5), 351–360.

Centers for Disease Control and Prevention. (2021). *Preexposure prophylaxis for the prevention of HIV infection in the United States—2021 update: A clinical practice guideline.* https://stacks.cdc.gov/view/cdc/112360

Charon, J. M. (1992). *Symbolic interactionism: An introduction, an interpretation, an integration* (4th ed.). Prentice Hall.

Cochrane. (2025). *Knowledge Translation.* https://community.cochrane.org/review-development/knowledge-translation

Crawford, C. L., Rondinelli, J., Zuniga, S., Valdez, R. M., Tze-Polo, L., & Titler, M. G. (2023). Barriers and facilitators influencing EBP readiness: Building organizational and nurse capacity. *Worldviews on Evidence-Based Nursing, 20*(1), 27–36. https://doi.org/10.1111/wvn.12618

Creswell, J. W., & Creswell, J. D. (2023). *Research design: Qualitative, quantitative, and mixed methods approaches* (6th ed.). SAGE.

Creswell, J. W., & Poth, C. N. (2023). *Qualitative inquiry & research design: Choosing among five approaches* (5th ed.). SAGE.

Critical Appraisal Skills Programme. (2017). *CASP checklists.* Retrieved from https://casp-uk.net/casp-tools-checklists/

Dahlen, H. G., Kennedy, H. P., Anderson, C. M., Bell, A. F., Clark, A., Foureur, M., Ohm, J. E., Shearman, A. M., Taylor, J. Y., Wright, M. L., & Downe, S. (2013). The EPIIC hypothesis: Intrapartum effects on the neonatal epigenome and consequent health outcomes. *Medical Hypotheses, 80*, 656–662.

Dang, D., Dearholt, S., Bissett, K., Ascenzi, J., & Whalen, M. (2022). *Johns Hopkins evidence-based practice for nurses and healthcare professionals: Model and guidelines* (4th ed.). Sigma Theta Tau International.

Dijkers, M. (2013). Introducing GRADE: A systematic approach to rating evidence in systematic reviews and to guideline development. *Center on Knowledge Translation for Disability and Rehabilitation Research, 1*(5), e1–e9. https://www.ktdrr.org/products/update/v1n5/

Doyal, L. (1995). *What makes women sick? Gender and political economy of health*. Rutgers University Press.

Eisenberg, J. M. (2001). *Evidence-based medicine: Expert voices*. Agency for Healthcare Research and Quality.

Fernández Pinto, M. (2023). Methodological and cognitive biases in science: Issues for current research and ways to counteract them. *Perspectives on Science, 31*(5), 535–554. https://doi.org/10.1162/posc_a_00589

Flanagan, J. M., & Tatano, C. (2024). *Polit and Beck's nursing research: Generating and Assessing Evidence for Nursing Practice* (12th ed.). Wolters Kluwer Health.

Florczak, K. L. (2022). Best available evidence or truth for the moment: Bias in research. *Nursing Science Quarterly, 35*(1), 20–24. https://doi.org/10.1177/08943184211051350

Furtado, L., Coelho, F., Mendonça, N., Soares, H., Gomes, L., Sousa, J. P., Duarte, H., Costeira, C., Santos, C., & Araújo, B. (2024). Exploring professional practice environments and organizational context factors affecting nurses' adoption of evidence-based practice: A scoping review. *Healthcare, 12*(2), 245. https://doi.org/10.3390/healthcare12020245

Glaser, B. G. (1978). *Theoretical sensitivity*. Sociology Press.

Glaser, B. G. (1992). *Basics of grounded theory analysis*. Sociology Press.

Graham, I. D., Logan, J., Harrison, M. B., Straus, S. E., Tetroe, J., Caswell, W., & Robinson, N. (2006). Lost in knowledge translation: Time for a map? *The Journal of Continuing Education in the Health Professions, 26*(1), 13–24. https://doi.org/10.1002/chp.47

Guba, E. G., & Lincoln, N. K. (1998). Competing paradigms in qualitative research. In N. K. Denzin & Y. S. Lincoln (Eds.), *The landscape of qualitative research: Theories and issues* (pp. 195–220). Sage.

Guerra-Farfan, E., Garcia-Sanchez, Y., Jornet-Gibert, M., Nuñez, J. H., Balaguer-Castro, M., & Madden, K. (2023). Clinical practice guidelines: The good, the bad, and the ugly. *Injury, 54*, S26–S29. https://doi.org/10.1016/j.injury.2022.01.047

Gyamfi, A., O'Neill, B., Henderson, W. A., & Lucas, R. (2021). Black/African American breastfeeding experience: Cultural, sociological, and health dimensions through an equity lens. *Breastfeeding Medicine, 16*(2), 103–111. https://doi.org/10.1089/bfm.2020.0312

Haile, Z. T. (2022). Critical appraisal tools and reporting guidelines. *Journal of Human Lactation, 38*(1), 21–27. https://doi.org/10.1177/08903344211058374

Higgins, J. P. T., Altman, D. G., & Sterne, J. A. C. (2011). Assessing risk of bias in included studies. In J. P. T. Higgins & S. Green (Eds.), *Cochrane handbook of systematic reviews of interventions*. Cochrane Collaboration. https://training.cochrane.org/handbook

Holloway, I., & Galvin, K. (2024). *Qualitative research in nursing and healthcare* (5th ed.). Wiley-Blackwell.

Humpel, N., Owen, N., Leslie, E., Marshall, A. L., Bauman, A. E., & Sallis, J. F. (2004). Associations of location and perceived environmental attributes with walking in neighborhoods. *American Journal of Health Promotion, 18*(3), 239–242.

Jiang, Y., Searing, H., & Jessup, J. (2024). *Pregnancy-associated mortality in New York City, 2016-2020*. https://www.nyc.gov/assets/doh/downloads/pdf/ms/pregnancy-associated-mortality-report-2016-2020.pdf

Joanna Briggs Institute. (2024). *Critical appraisal tools*. https://jbi.global/critical-appraisal-tools

Kaplan, L. (n.d.). *Framework for how to read and critique a research study*. American Nurses Association. https://www.nursingworld.org/globalassets/practiceandpolicy/innovation--evidence/framework-for-how-to-read-and-critique-a-research-study.pdf

Kennedy, H. P., Cheyney, M., Dahlen, H. G., Downe, S., Foureur, M. J., Homer, C. S. E., Jefford, E., McFadden, A., Michel-Schuldt, M., Sandall, J., Soltani, H., Speciale, A. M., Stevens, J., Vedam, S., & Renfrew, M. J. (2018). Asking different questions: A call to action for research to improve the quality of care for every woman, every child. *Birth (Berkeley, Calif.), 45*(3), 222–231. https://doi.org/10.1111/birt.12361

Klein, T. A., Seelbach, C. L., & Brannan, G. D. (2023, March 6). *Quality Assurance*. PubMed; StatPearls Publishing. https://www.ncbi.nlm.nih.gov/books/NBK557503/

Kohn, L. T., Corrigan, J. M., & Donaldson, M. S. (Eds.). (1999). *To err is human: Building a safer health system*. Committee on Quality of Health Care in America, Institute of Medicine.

Kotter, J. (n.d.). *8-step process*. Kotter Inc. https://www.kotterinc.com/8-steps-process-for-leading-change/

Kuhn, T. S. (1970). *The structure of scientific revolutions*. University of Chicago Press.

Lachman, P. (2024). *Handbook of quality improvement in healthcare*. Oxford University Press.

Lee, M. C., Johnson, K. L., Newhouse, R. P., & Warren, J. (2013). Evidence-based practice process quality assessment: EPQA guidelines. *Worldviews on Evidence-Based Nursing, 10*(3), 140–149. https://doi.org/10.1111/j.1741-6787.2012.00264.x

Liese, K. L., Davis-Floyd, R., Stewart, K., & Cheyney, M. (2021). Obstetric iatrogenesis in the United States: The spectrum of unintentional harm, disrespect, violence, and abuse. *Anthropology & Medicine, 28*(2), 188–204. https://doi.org/10.1080/13648470.2021.1938510

Lim, W. M. (2024). What is qualitative research? An overview and guidelines. *Australasian Marketing Journal, 33*(2), 199–229. https://doi.org/10.1177/14413582241264619

Logan, J., & Graham, I.D. (2010). The Ottawa Model of Research Use. In J. Rycroft-Malone & t. Bucknall (Eds), *Models and frameworks for implementing evidence-based practice: Evidence to action* (pp. 83–108). Wiley-Blackwell.

Malterud, K. (2023). *Qualitative metasynthesis: A research method for medicine and health sciences*. Routledge.

Marckmann, G., Schmidt, H., Sofaer, N., & Strech, D. (2015). Putting public health ethics into practice: A systematic framework. *Frontiers in Public Health, 3*, 1–7.

Melnyk, B., & Fineout-Overholt, E. (2002). Putting research into practice. *Reflections on Nursing Leadership, 28*, 22–25.

Melnyk, B. M., & Fineout-Overholt, E. (2023). *Evidence-based practice in nursing and healthcare: A guide to best practice* (5th ed.). Wolters Kluwer.

Melnyk, B. M., Tan, A., Hsieh, A. P., & Gallagher-Ford, L. (2021). Evidence-based practice culture and mentorship predict EBP implementation, nurse job satisfaction, and intent to stay: Support for the ARCC© Model. *Worldviews on Evidence-Based Nursing, 18*(4), 272–281. https://doi.org/10.1111/wvn.12524

Mishler, E. G. (1984). *The discourse of medicine: Dialectics of medical interviews*. Ablex.

Moran, K. J., Burson, R., & Conrad, D. (2023). *The Doctor of Nursing Practice project: A framework for success*. Jones & Bartlett Learning.

Morton, C. H., VanOtterloo, L. R., Seacrist, M. J., & Main, E. K. (2019). Translating maternal mortality review into quality improvement opportunities in response to pregnancy-related deaths in California. *Journal of Obstetric, Gynecologic, and Neonatal Nursing, 48*(3), 252–262. https://doi.org/10.1016/j.jogn.2019.03.003

NIH-Funded Research Workforce. (2022, November 14). National Institutes of Health (NIH). https://www.nih.gov/ending-structural-racism/nih-funded-research-workforce

New York State Department of Health (2024). *New York state maternal mortality review report, 2018-2020*. https://www.health.ny.gov/community/adults/women/maternal_mortality/docs/maternal_mortality_review_2018-2020.pdf

Ogrinc, G., Davies, L., Goodman, D., Batalden, P., Davidoff, F., Stevens, D. (2016). SQUIRE 2.0 (Standards for QUality Improvement Reporting Excellence): Revised publication guidelines from a detailed consensus process. *BMJ Quality & Safety, 25*(12), 986–992. https://doi.org/10.1136/bmjqs-2015-004411

Oyelese, Y. (2024). Randomized controlled trials: Not always the "gold standard" for evidence in obstetrics and gynecology. *American Journal of Obstetrics and Gynecology, 230*(4), 417–425. https://doi.org/10.1016/j.ajog.2023.10.015

Page, M. J., McKenzie, J. E., Bossuyt, P. M., Boutron, I., Hoffmann, T. C., Mulrow, C. D., Shamseer, L., Tetzlaff, J. M., Akl, E. A., Brennan, S. E., Chou, R., Glanville, J., Grimshaw, J. M., Hróbjartsson, A., Lalu, M. M., Li, T., Loder, E. W., Mayo-Wilson, E., McDonald, S., McGuinness, L. A., & Moher, D. (2021). The PRISMA 2020 statement: An updated guideline for reporting systematic reviews. *BMJ (Clinical research ed.), 372*, n71. https://doi.org/10.1136/bmj.n71

Palazzo, M. O. (2015). Transformation by design: Nursing workforce innovation and reduction strategies in turbulent times of change. *Nursing Administration Quarterly, 39*(2), 164–171.

Patel, M.-G., & Quan-Haase, A. (2024). The social-ecological model of cyberbullying: Digital media as a predominant ecology in the everyday lives of youth. *New Media & Society, 26*(9), 5507–5528. https://doi.org/10.1177/14614448221136508

Pearson, A., Jordan, Z., & Munn, Z. (2012). Translational science and evidence-based healthcare: A clarification and reconceptualization of how knowledge is generated and used in healthcare. *Nursing Research and Practice, 2012*, Article 792519. https://www.hindawi.com/journals/nrp/2012/792519/

Polit, D. F., & Beck, C. T. (2022). *Essentials of nursing research: Appraising evidence for nursing practice* (10th ed.). Wolters Kluwer.

Polit, D. F., & Beck, C. T. (2024). Polit and Beck's nursing research: Generating and assessing evidence for nursing practice (12th ed.). Wolters Kluwer.

Quine, W. V. (1952). *From a logical point of view* (2nd ed.). Harvard University Press.

Ratnani, I., Fatima, S., Abid, M. M., Surani, Z., & Surani, S. (2023). Evidence-based medicine: History, review, criticisms, and pitfalls. *Cureus, 15*(2), e35266. https://doi.org/10.7759/cureus.35266

Renfrew, M. J., McFadden, A., Bastos, M. H., Campbell, J., Channon, A. A., Cheung, N. F., Audebert Delage Silva, D. R., Downe, S., Kennedy, H. P., Malata, A., McCormick, F., Wick, L., & Declercq, E. (2014). Midwifery and quality care: Findings from a new evidence-informed framework for maternal and newborn care. *The Lancet, 384*(9948), 1129–1145. https://doi.org/10.1016/S0140-6736(14)60789-3

Rogers, E. M. (2003). *Diffusion of innovations* (5th ed.). The Free Press.

Roussel, L., & Thomas, P. (2024). *Implementation science in nursing*. Taylor & Francis.

Ryder, M., & Jacob, E. (2022). A translational research framework for nurse practitioners. *Journal of Nursing Management, 30*(2), 421–427. https://doi.org/10.1111/jonm.13496

Sackett, D. L., Strauss, S. E., Richardson, W. S., Rosenberg, W., & Haynes, R. B. (2000). *Evidence-based medicine: How to practice and teach EBM*. Churchill Livingstone.

Savory, N. A., Sanders, J., & Hannigan, B. (2022). Midwives' experiences of supporting women's mental health: A mixed-method study. *Midwifery, 111*, 103368–103368. https://doi.org/10.1016/j.midw.2022.103368

Sehon, S. R., & Stanley, D. E. (2003). A philosophical analysis of the evidence-based medicine debate. *BMC Health Services Research, 3*(14). http://www.biomedcentral.com/1472-6963/3/14

Shirey, M. (2013). Lewin's theory of planned change as a strategic resource. *Journal of Nursing Administration, 43*(2), 69–72. https://doi.org/10.1097/NNA.0b013e31827f20a9

Skirnisdottir, V. E., Østenfor, M. M., Vika, N. A., & Katrine, A. (2023). Midwives' experiences with a safe childbirth checklist: A grounded theory study. *Midwifery, 122*, 103676–103676. https://doi.org/10.1016/j.midw.2023.103676

Smith, R., & Rennie, D. (2014). Evidence-based medicine: An oral history. *Journal of the American Medical Association, 311*(4), 365–367.

Stetler, C. B. (2001). Updating the Stetler model of research utilization to facilitate evidence-based practice. *Nursing Outlook, 49*, 272–279.

Straus, S. E., Glasziou, P., Richardson, W. S., Warren S., & Haynes, R. B. (2019). *Evidence-based medicine: How to practice and teach EBM* (5th ed.). Elsevier.

Strauss, A., & Corbin, J. (1998). *Basics of qualitative research: Techniques and procedures for developing grounded theory* (2nd ed.). Sage.

The Breakthrough Series: IHI's Collaborative Model for Achieving Breakthrough Improvement. (2023). Institute for Healthcare Improvement. https://www.ihi.org/resources/white-papers/breakthrough-series-ihis-collaborative-model-achieving-breakthrough

The Oxford Review. (2023). *The essential guide to evidence-based practice*. The Oxford Review Briefings. https://oxford-review.com/evidence-based-practice-essential-guide/

Titler, M. (2018). Translation research in practice: An introduction. *Online Journal of Issues in Nursing, 23*(2), 1–16. https://doi.org/10.3912/OJIN.Vol23No02Man01

Titler, M. G., Kleiber, C., Steelman, V. J., Rakel, B. A., Budreau, G., Everett, L. Q., Buckwalter, K. C., Tripp-Reimer, T., & Goode, C. J. (2001). The Iowa model of evidence-based practice to promote quality care. *Critical Care Nursing Clinics of North America, 13*(4), 497–509.

Trautman, D., Idzik, S., Hammersla, M., & Rosseter, R. (2018). Advancing scholarship through translational research: The role of PhD and DNP prepared nurses. *Online Journal of Issues in Nursing, 23*(2), 1–8. https://doi.org/10.3912/OJIN.Vol23No02Man02

Turner, L., Shamseer, L., Altman, D. G., Weeks, L., Peters, J., Kober, T., & Moher, D. (2012). Consolidated standards of reporting trials (CONSORT) and the completeness of reporting of randomized controlled trials (RCTs) published in medical journals. *Cochrane Database Systematic Reviews, 11*, MR000030. https://doi.org/10.1002/14651858.MR000030.pub2

Turok, D. K., Gero, A., Simmons, R. G., Kaiser, J. E., Stoddard, G. J., Sexsmith, C. D., Gawron, L. M., & Sanders, J. N. (2021). Levonorgestrel vs. copper intrauterine devices for emergency contraception. *The New England Journal of Medicine, 384*(4), 335–344. https://doi.org/10.1056/NEJMoa2022141

U.S. Preventive Services Task Force. (2018). *Methods and processes: Grade definitions*. https://www.uspreventiveservicestaskforce.org/uspstf/about-uspstf/methods-and-processes/grade-definitions

van Manen, M. (1990). *Researching lived experience: Human science for an action sensitive pedagogy*. State University of New York Press.

Vetter, M. J., & Zavotsky, K. E. (2025). *Advancing evidence-based practice in nursing and healthcare*. Elsevier Health Sciences.

Waldrop, J. B., Dunlap, J. J., & Reynolds, S. S. (2025). Evidence-based practice quality improvement critical appraisal tool. *Journal of Nursing Care Quality, 40*(1), 15–23. https://doi.org/10.1097/NCQ.0000000000000789

Washington State Maternal Mortality Review Panel. (2023). *Washington State Maternal Mortality Review Panel: Maternal Deaths 2017–2020*. https://doh.wa.gov/sites/default/files/2023-02/141-070-MaternalMortalityReviewPanelReport-2023.pdf

Zhao, Y., & Chen, D. G. (2021). *Modern statistical methods for health research*. Springer.

APPENDIX 4-A

Resources to Improve Quality Care Through Evidence-Based Practice

ONLINE ACCESS TO THE EVIDENCE BASE: DATABASES

Evidence Collection	Contents	Location
PubMed	Free access to more than 24 million citations across biomedical literature, most with abstract access.	http://www.ncbi.nlm.nih.gov/pubmed
Cumulative Index to Nursing and Allied Health Literature (CINAHL)	Nursing and allied health journal citations, available via EBSCOhost with proxy access.	https://www.ebscohost.com/nursing/products/cinahl-databases/cinahl-complete
EMBASE	International biomedical database covering journals and conference publications, available with proxy access.	http://www.elsevier.com/online-tools/embase
Google Scholar	Free search of literature across multiple disciplines and sources. Can coordinate with library proxies to provide full-text links.	http://scholar.google.com
Database of Abstracts of Reviews of Effects (DARE)	Details of systematic reviews covering healthcare interventions and health services organizations. Includes critical commentary on reliability of evidence.	https://www.crd.york.ac.uk/CRDWeb/
Cochrane Library	Full-text collection of databases that contain high-quality, independent evidence to inform healthcare decision making.	http://www.cochranelibrary.com
Joanna Briggs Institute	A database and tools to access, appraise, and apply the best available evidence.	https://jbi.global/
ACCESSS	Conducts searches simultaneously in several evidence-based information services to provide current best evidence for clinical decisions.	https://www.accessss.org/

ONLINE ACCESS TO THE EVIDENCE BASE: PREAPPRAISED EVIDENCE SOURCES

Evidence Collection	Contents	Location
American College of Physicians (ACP) Journal Club	Subscription. International content selected against criteria for scientific merit and relevance to medical practice. Offers commentary on clinical application of findings.	http://www.acpjc.org
DynaMed	Subscription. Point-of-care reference for clinical decision making. Provides summaries, resources, and overall conclusions updated daily.	http://www.ebscohost.com/dynamed/aboutUs.php
UpToDate	Subscription. Clinical decision support reference with summaries, resources, and evidence-based recommendations for a range of clinical topics.	http://www.uptodate.com
TRIP	Free. This meta-search engine includes results from journals, Cochrane reviews, clinical guidelines, and other websites on various clinical topics.	http://www.tripdatabase.com
BMJ Best Practice	Subscription. Online clinical decision support for a range of clinical topics using evidence based methodology and expert opinion.	https://bestpractice.bmj.com/
Medscape eMedicine	Free. Online resource offers information on diseases, treatments, and medical conditions, as well as tools for clinical decision making.	https://emedicine.medscape.com/

CHAPTER 5

Trauma-Informed Care in Sexual and Reproductive Health Care

Meghan Eagen-Torkko

Trauma-informed care has drawn increased attention in both clinical care and in research in recent years. The use of the term "trauma-informed care" and its operationalization have remained challenging for many clinicians, who may associate trauma with a plane crash or the death of a parent. However, this limited definition of trauma is inconsistent with trauma theory and what we know about how trauma affects individuals (Reeves, 2015). This chapter reviews the physiologic and psychological effects of trauma, the relationships between experiencing trauma and health outcomes, and the implications of these for best practices in trauma-informed care in sexual and reproductive health. Without trauma-informed care, clinicians risk (re)traumatizing patients, with implications for their health, their use of the healthcare system, and their trust in their clinician, in addition to the immediate harm of this.

TRAUMA

While trauma as a concept has historically been associated with a single discrete event like a natural disaster or a violent crime, this definition ignores the equally significant impact of chronic daily racism, for example, or the experience of a global pandemic. By focusing on the "three Es" [event, experience, and effect] as interpreted by the individual, the current definition used by the Substance Abuse and Mental Health Services Administration (SAMHSA) instead (1) centers the trauma on the individual rather than the onlooker, and (2) allows the affected individual to reclaim ownership of their experiences rather than accepting the definition of an outside entity (SAMHSA, 2024). It neither assumes that a given event or series of events is traumatic, nor that it is not, and in that, it restores some power to a person who has experienced a potentially traumatic event(s). Trauma can either be individual or collective-generational. For the purposes of this chapter, we focus on individual trauma, because providers are more often caring for a single individual at a time. However, the impact of collective or generational trauma, such as that experienced by American Indians taken from their families or the enslavement of Black Americans, are known to have ongoing implications for both psychological and physical health. The focus on the individual is not intended to discount these, and the reader is reminded to consider each patient within context.

SAMHSA defines individual trauma as an "event or circumstance resulting in physical harm, emotional harm, and/or life-threatening harm . . . that has lasting adverse effects on the individual" (SAMHSA, 2024). Importantly, individuals may experience such events or circumstances with or without lasting adverse effects, and trauma is defined by the individual who experiences it. Those adverse effects can be short and/or long term and may or may not be associated by the individual with the traumatic event.

The prevalence of trauma varies widely based on the definition used, but data collected globally estimates that 70% of adults experience at least one traumatic event during their lifetimes (Benjet et al., 2016), and large-scale survey data supports the broad prevalence of potentially traumatic experiences (Kessler et al., 2017). As an example, the recent COVID-19 pandemic meets the SAMHSA criteria for a potentially traumatizing event for the entirety of the world population, although not all experienced it as such.

While prevalence of trauma generally is consistently high in the research, the type of trauma and the effects of that trauma vary widely by gender, race, age, location, and other factors (Valentine et al., 2019; Soegaard et al., 2021; Mekawi et al., 2021; Mersky et al., 2024). For example, LGBTQ+ people experience disproportionately high levels of family rejection (Palmer & Francis, 2024) and sexual assault (Blackburn et al., 2023), while people in conflict zones may experience more generalized violence (Zasiekina et al., 2024). However, two things can be stated as categorically accurate about trauma: It is a common experience, and it has predictable effects on human physiology.

EFFECTS OF TRAUMA

Immediate Effects

The experience of trauma has well-defined effects on human physiology. Immediately on exposure to the potential trauma, the sympathetic branch (SNS) of the autonomic nervous system (ANS) activates, releasing epinephrine, norepinephrine, and dopamine (Won & Kim, 2016). These hormones are rapid-acting and cause two effects: activation of the SNS and suppression of the parasympathetic (PNS) branch of the ANS. The activation of the SNS increases heart rate, blood pressure, and sensory hyperarousal/hyperfocus. The suppression of the PNS slows or stops smooth muscle function, which reduces gastrointestinal motility and can cause nausea or other somatic symptoms, as well as a decreased sense of relaxation.

The next stage of the trauma–stress response is activation of the hypothalamic-pituitary-adrenal (HPA) axis. This stage releases some key hormones, including adrenocorticotropin-releasing hormone (ACTH), cortisol, and assorted pro-inflammatory cytokines (Won & Kim, 2016). The effects of these increase blood glucose, decrease insulin sensitivity, suppress the immune response, create inflammation throughout the body (including in the vasculature) and promotes clot formation. This response is extremely logical if the threat were a bear attack, for example, or a motor-vehicle accident, which might need the body to quickly stop bleeding, and increased blood glucose for energy. However, in most situations, these responses occur regardless of safety or need for survival.

The post-stressor phase sees the body, in theory, return to homeostasis: heart rate and blood pressure reduce, hyperarousal decreases, gut motility increases, blood glucose falls, and inflammation resolves. However, repeated or ongoing trauma can delay or stop this physiologic response and leave the individual instead in a lowered but still persistent state of physiologic arousal (Tsigos et al., 2020). These effects—increased blood pressure, increased blood glucose, decreased insulin sensitivity, vascular inflammation, and so on—are all well established to contribute to chronic health issues like cardiovascular disease and diabetes (Osborne et al., 2020; Marcovecchio & Chiarelli, 2012). Chronic or severe traumatic stress, particularly when it occurs in childhood, can also dysregulate other hormones, such as oxytocin, that are implicated in poor health outcomes in adulthood (Downey & Crummy, 2022).

FIGURE 5-1 **Sabia Wade, Birthing liberation trauma response diagram.**

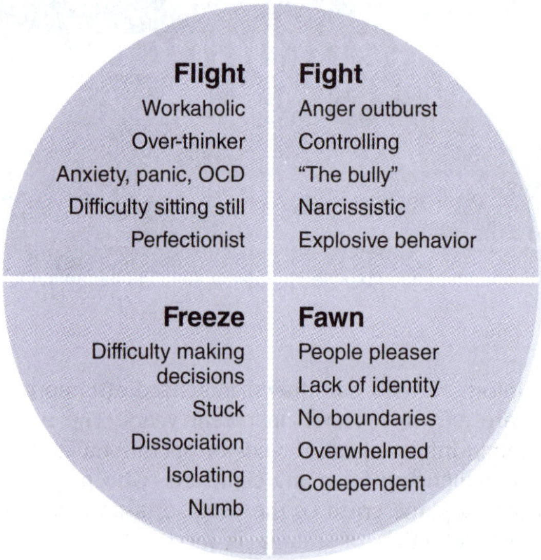

@ Ryan Rose Evans

Long-Term Effects

The long-term effects of trauma vary widely from person to person, and experiencing a traumatic event does not mean the individual will have effects persist past the immediate period. These impacts may or may not apply to any given individual. However, on a population basis, there are patterns of physical and psychological sequelae of trauma, which are striking in their consistency between studies. These sequelae include increased incidence of chronic pelvic pain, migraine, cardiovascular disease, diabetes, anxiety, depression, and difficulty with emotional self-regulation (Magruder et al., 2017; Murchland et al., 2024; Rizeq & McCann, 2023; Ponting et al., 2024; Stubbs & Szoeke, 2022). Because these are chronic conditions, the patients are likely to be seen regularly, and not always successfully, within the healthcare system. Chronic pelvic pain, for example, is common among people who have experienced trauma, and is associated with three times as much use of the emergency department compared to those without it (Green et al., 2022).

The long-term relational and psychological impacts of trauma are also significant for individuals and their children. Many people respond to trauma in one of four ways: fight/flight/freeze/fawn (**Figure 5-1**), which can make responding to stressors in daily life, like parenting or relationships, more challenging. Experiencing pre-pregnancy trauma is associated with less success in breastfeeding (Eagen-Torkko et al., 2017), shortened gestation (Sanjuan et al., 2021), and increased tobacco use (Alhusen et al., 2018), which in turn may reduce self-perception of efficacy as a parent (Bentley & Zamir, 2022) or cause challenges with the dyadic relationship (Lotto et al., 2023). A history of trauma is also associated with poor sleep (de Boer et al., 2020), anxiety and depression (Ter Meulen et al., 2021), and increased substance misuse or abuse (Moustafa et al., 2021), which may represent attempts to manage post-traumatic distress.

Post-Traumatic Stress Disorder (PTSD)

A well-known sequela of trauma, particularly in those who have experienced interpersonal violence or armed conflict, is post-traumatic stress disorder, or PTSD. PTSD is a constellation of symptoms related to hyperarousal/dysregulation of arousal that persist more than six months after the traumatic event, and cause significant distress or difficulty functioning (NIMH, 2024). A more recently recognized variant is complex post-traumatic stress disorder (cPTSD), which is associated with repeated trauma or neglect during childhood and adolescence and often presents somewhat differently from "classic" PTSD (United States Department of Veterans' Affairs, n.d.). Both are categorized as anxiety disorders in the DSM-5 but respond differently to treatments than other anxiety disorders like generalized anxiety or social anxiety. However, both PTSD/cPTSD and PTS (post-traumatic symptoms that do not meet diagnostic criteria but nonetheless cause distress) are treatable disorders, and many patients find significant relief (International Society for Traumatic Stress Studies, n.d.).

Post-Traumatic Growth

A lesser-known phenomenon is post-traumatic growth, in which the individual is able to incorporate and grow from the traumatic experience (Dell'Osso et al., 2022). This is a positive outcome of trauma, and as such is often overlooked by the healthcare system and its focus on pathology. A major goal of both trauma-informed and -specific care is to facilitate and support post-traumatic growth whenever possible. Much of the standards for trauma-informed care, for example, are situations or conditions that support post-traumatic growth (e.g., peer support, collaboration, empowerment), which can provide a powerful base for any trauma-specific work that goes on.

TRAUMA-INFORMED CARE

One of the challenges faced by clinicians caring for people who have experienced trauma is that they often do not disclose that trauma. In one study, 75% of participants would not voluntarily disclose a history of trauma to their healthcare provider due to fear of stigma and shame (Berry & Rutledge, 2016). A second challenge is that much of the care provided in health care, particularly in sexual and reproductive health, relies on bodily contact (e.g., exams, testing) in a way that can retraumatize patients, particularly those who have experienced sexual violence or trauma. Health care providers hold power within the patient–clinician relationship by virtue of the social role accorded to them and the relative vulnerability of patients, and patients tolerating harm from clinicians in order to receive care is well documented in the literature (Selwyn et al., 2021; Lathan et al., 2023). Clinicians may harm patients with the best of intentions, but that does not negate that harm—examples of inadvertent harm may be physical touch without explicit consent, removing or reducing decision-making autonomy, or utilizing language that induces fear of harm. More information on informed consent is in Chapter 8.

Trauma-informed care (TIC) is an approach to patient care that incorporates trauma theory into routine practices without requiring knowledge of a particular patient's trauma history. Much as universal infection precautions are taken with every patient and reduces risk of infection bidirectionally, trauma-informed care reduces the likelihood of retraumatization for patients with a history of trauma, and the likelihood of initial traumatization for those without.

Key Components of TIC

Trauma-informed care begins with a trauma-informed approach. There are four key components of this approach: Realize (understand that trauma is prevalent in society), Recognize (identify potential markers or patterns that can result from previous trauma), Respond (respond to patient needs as they present for the individual), and Resist Retraumatization (avoid inadvertently causing harm, using the understanding of the effects of trauma on individuals) (SAMHSA, 2014). None of these components requires patients to disclose a history of trauma in order for clinicians to implement. Further, TIC must include the following six characteristics: safety; trustworthiness and transparency; peer support; collaboration and mutuality; empowerment, voice, and choice; and cultural, historical, and gender issues (see **Table 5-1**).

In order to provide TIC, we need to meet the requirements of all six characteristics, although they may look different in different circumstances.

The four Rs of TIC require that the clinician realize, recognize, respond, and resist retraumatization, but the process does not start or end there. For example, requiring patients to have a physical exam at the first visit—a common practice in many practice models—does not demonstrate the six characteristics of TIC because it is not transparent (about what the purpose of the exam is for this patient), and it is not a collaborative or mutual decision (about whether to have an exam at all). While the clinician is the one who performs the exam, the medical assistant who rooms the patient and assumes that they will need to disrobe and instructs the patients to do so is also violating the six characteristics (particularly empowerment, voice, and choice). This places both the clinician and the other clinic staff in the position of inadvertently causing harm. Patients often experience waiting for the provider while partially disrobed as disempowering or violative, because cultural norms around nudity are closely linked to power. What does it mean to the patient to be partially disrobed and sitting while the clinician is fully dressed, often in a white coat and/or business attire? What impact does this have on their perceived or actual power to disagree or question the clinician?

Another place this can appear is in routine intake forms, which often include questions about trauma history. This is in keeping with the recommendation that all patients be asked about their history of trauma in order to both recognize that

TABLE 5-1 What Does TIC Mean in Practice?

Six Characteristics of TIC	Things to Ask Yourself
Safety	Are we safe people/institutions?
Trustworthiness and Transparency	Do we do what we say we will? Are we clear about what that is?
Peer Support	Can this person access support from others in similar circumstances or with similar experiences?
Collaboration and Mutuality	Are decisions being made by agreement and discussion between the clinician and the patient/client?
Empowerment, Voice, and Choice	Are we careful to ensure space for patients to express themselves and their decisions? Are we elevating those decisions within the healthcare system?
Cultural, Historical, and Gender Issues	Are we caring for people within their individual contexts and with an awareness of the effects of these?

Data from Substance Abuse and Mental Health Services Administration (SAMHSA). (2014). *SAMHSA's concept of trauma and guidance for a trauma-informed approach.* https://store.samhsa.gov/sites/default/files/sma14-4884.pdf

experience and potentially provide helpful diagnostic information (Owens et al., 2022). However, asking patients/clients to complete history forms that include traumatic events in their past without providing an option to decline, and an alert that some questions may be triggering for some people, likewise may violate the six characteristics and the four Rs by failing to resist potential retraumatization, and therefore their care cannot be considered TIC.

TRAUMA-INFORMED CARE IN SEXUAL AND REPRODUCTIVE HEALTH CARE

Sexual and reproductive health care is a particularly important area in which to provide TIC, in part because the rates of sexual violence are so extraordinarily high. Most research in sexual violence identifies an approximately 25–40% risk of sexual abuse or assault during a cisgender woman's lifetime (Basile et al., 2022), and while the rates are lower in the literature for cisgender men (4–30%) (Basile et al., 2022), these are almost certainly underestimated. Data on sexual violence for LGBTQ+ people is less comprehensive, but suggests higher rates (Atteberry-Ash et al., 2020), with approximately half of trans people experiencing such violence (Abern et al., 2023). Providing Sexual and Reproductive Health (SRH) care requires that the clinician ask questions about topics that may be particularly painful for the patient, as well as often examine parts of the body that may have been involved in past abuse or assault. Using a strategic approach in implementing TIC will ensure clinicians are able to adhere to the four Rs and six characteristics of TIC across all types of care provision (**Table 5-2**).

A first step in trauma-informed care in SRH is for the clinician to consider what they need to do to establish safety for a given patient. While privacy and respectful language can be helpful, asking patients what they need to feel safe can also be a useful strategy. Being explicit that patients can decline to respond to any questions, as well as decline any part of the exam, can be particularly helpful in initial meetings. This, like anything in TIC, can and should be offered to all patients, regardless of stated history.

Transparency with patients about why questions are being asked (e.g., "We ask everyone this question so that we know

TABLE 5-2 Recommendations for Implementing TIC

Recommendation	Questions to Consider
Consider what patients need to establish safety.	"What can I do to help you feel safe/secure in our visits? What has helped you in the past?"
Provide transparency about why certain questions are being asked and why certain tests are being recommended.	"I'm asking these questions in order to find out _____. That will help me understand more about your experience/ recommend a course of action/find out what is going on for you."
Consider whether exams can be deferred to a second visit.	Ask yourself: What will an exam tell me that I need to know right now? Will it change my plan of care or can it wait?
Always ask for consent for anytime touch is required.	"I would like to examine your breast to find out more about the lump you're feeling. Is that okay with you?" "Is it okay if I touch your shoulder/arm?"
Consider a chaperone for exams.	"I offer a chaperone to everyone if they would like to have one for exams. Would you like to have a chaperone today? They are there to support you, so it is your decision."
Avoid using potentially triggering language, such as "victim" or "survivor."	Consider: People who have experienced . . . Other women who have had . . . A history of . . .
Be aware of assumptions regarding the impact of trauma on chronic conditions such as pain.	"Have you noticed anything that makes your pain better or worse? Was there a time in your life when the pain was less? What was different?" Ask yourself: Am I making assumptions about pain because of their history? Would I have a different diagnosis for someone who did not have a history of assault/abuse/trauma?
Ensure all patient interactions include TIC, not just with the clinician.	Consider: Warm handoffs to other providers and clinic staff Ongoing trainings with clinical staff about TIC Checking in with clients about their experiences regularly, either by anonymous survey or directly

you are getting the testing/care/etc. that you need") can help to build trust and increase willingness to share information that may be painful for the patient. Rather than "screening for STIs," consider naming each test and getting permission to send them. If this is the first time to see a patient, consider deferring the exam if this is appropriate—they may be due for a Pap, but does it need to happen on the first visit, or can you discuss contraception or other topics the patient identifies? When you do an exam, discuss what exam you would like to do and why, and be cautious about assuming consent for touch. The widely considered best practice is to ask permission to touch any patient, in any way, whether an "intimate" exam or not, prior to any touch (Tillman, 2020).

The topic of exam chaperones often comes up in the context of trauma. While some people do consider it reassuring to have another person present for an exam, others consider the presence of another person observing the exam to be violative. The American College of Obstetrics & Gynecology (ACOG) recommends the routine use of chaperones for pelvic, breast, and rectal exams, regardless of the gender of the examiner (ACOG, 2020), and the U.S. Veterans' Administration, for example, mandates this. However, while chaperonage may provide protection in some cases, it does not in all, and the patient's preference for the number of people in the room during such an exam must be honored as well. Chaperonage is not, in itself, a trauma-informed practice, but does seek to avoid retraumatization, which is an important principle of TIC. One possible option, if a patient declines a chaperone, is to offer self-collected swabs for HPV and/or infection, for example, or to discuss the purpose of the chaperone and to set boundaries for where they stand in the room. In all circumstances, care should be individualized.

Clinicians should be aware of and cautious about the language used in both written and verbal communication, as well as their nonverbal communication. For example, the language around "survivor" and "victim" is an active topic when describing people who have experienced interpersonal violence. "Survivor" is often recommended as a term that focuses on agency and the success in surviving assault(s), but some people who have experienced interpersonal trauma argue that it implies a success that they do not feel, or that it shifts responsibility from the actions of another person into an impersonal event like a hurricane or earthquake. Both terms are problematic for other people who have experienced intimate partner violence (IPV) or other traumas, who argue that the trauma is only one part of their life-course history, and that they do not want to be defined by the actions of another. All of these perspectives are valid for the people who hold them, and therefore rather than assuming what preferred language would be, the clinician should ask the person what language to use when it is relevant. When it is not known (as in TIC, since it does not require disclosure of previous traumas), the clinician should consider describing events rather than renaming patients as "victims" or "survivors" (e.g., "Some people who have experienced XYZ find this treatment/strategy helpful.").

There is sometimes a tendency for clinicians to assume a history of trauma exists when it may not, or that a known history of trauma accounts for symptoms, particularly difficult to diagnose and/or treat symptoms like chronic pelvic pain. This can lead to symptoms being minimized or not included in a differential diagnosis and can cause delay in diagnosis. While it is important to recognize that a history of trauma is associated with an increased risk of chronic pain, for example, it is equally important for the clinician to recognize that such a history may play little or no role in the health of the individual patient. It is not TIC, for example, to assume that chronic pelvic pain is related to a history of childhood abuse without excluding disorders like endometriosis or pelvic inflammatory disease, and clinicians need to be cautious about generalizing or making assumptions based on a disclosed or suspected history.

Trauma-informed care considerations need to be incorporated into the entirety of the patient care experience, and not limited to the interaction with the healthcare clinician. There are many opportunities for every member of the clinic staff to contribute to a trauma-informed environment. For example, health history forms are often distributed at the front desk for patients to complete, without a content notice about topics or why they are important, or a note clarifying that patients are free to decline to answer any question. Consideration needs to be given to the safety of patients and their information; having a policy of bringing all patients back alone to ask questions about IPV and safety may mitigate suspicions of an abusive partner who has accompanied the patient, for example, if it is "just policy." However, this common practice may also violate the patient's right to always have an advocate or companion with them, so exceptions may be necessary to individualize care.

Access to helpline information in bathrooms or other private spaces is often advocated, since patients who are actively experiencing violence or trauma may have no privacy except in a bathroom, but such material can also be triggering for those who have a history of IPV, for example, and so consideration should be given to visual representations and words that are chosen for the materials. Clinics must be clear with patients that if they are using insurance and they are not the policyholder, the clinic cannot guarantee that the insurer will not send documentation to the policyholder about their care. Additionally, consideration should be given to the physical environment when possible. For example, many people who have experienced trauma prefer to sit with their backs to walls, and softer ambient light may be less activating to a hypersensitive autonomic nervous system than bright fluorescent lights. Ensuring adequately sized and appropriate gowns and sheets for modesty during exams is another important consideration for TIC in sexual and reproductive healthcare.

Because patients often spend significant time with clinic staff other than the clinician, it is important for all members of the staff to understand the basic principles of TIC and their importance, including the potential effects of trauma on interpersonal communication and anxiety levels in settings like health care. These should be included in onboarding and/or continuing development for employees and can be considered as essential as understanding of the principles of Health Insurance Portability and Accountability Act (HIPAA) or blood-borne pathogen transmission, both of which are routinely required of clinic staff. Trauma-informed care requires shifting the frame away from specialty care delivered to people who have experienced specific harms and are seeking treatment for those harms, to the idea that trauma histories are common and that reducing the risk to those with those experiences does not require disclosure of that history. This knowledge of trauma-informed principles benefits both patients and staff, who are then able to better respond to the needs of patients and may find their work both less frustrating and more satisfying.

CONCLUSION

Trauma-informed care is less a set of prescriptive tasks than it is operationalizing principles and norms, with a firm understanding of trauma theory. Potentially traumatic experiences are almost ubiquitous, but the effects of those experiences vary widely, and the right of patients to interpret their own histories is crucial. Post-traumatic growth is also an important goal, and clinicians should maximize support for this whenever possible. Trauma-informed care uses this understanding of trauma to build systems and practices that build trust and avoid creating new or repeated traumas. This is essential in sexual and reproductive health care, in part because it is a socially vulnerable specialty, and in part because of the high rate of sexual violence in the United States, both disclosed and undisclosed. Becoming familiar with TIC and how it can be incorporated into both individual practice and clinic/system processes is crucial to providing safe, effective health care.

References

Abern, L., Diego, D., Krempasky, C., Cook, J., & Maguire, K. (2023). Prevalence of sexual assault in a cohort of transgender and gender diverse individuals. *Journal of General Internal Medicine, 38*(5), 1331–1333.

Alhusen, J. L., Geller, R., Jellig, J., Budhathoki, C., & Decker, M. (2018). Intimate partner violence, small for gestational age birth and cigarette smoking in the pregnancy risk assessment monitoring system. *Journal of Women's Health* (Larchmont, N.Y. 2002), *27*(4), 458–465. https://doi.org/10.1089/jwh.2017.6322

American College of Obstetricians & Gynecologists (ACOG). (2020). *Committee Opinion 796: Sexual Misconduct.* https://www.acog.org/clinical/clinical-guidance/committee-opinion/articles/2020/01/sexual-misconduct

Atteberry-Ash, B., Walls, N. E., Kattari, S. K., Peitzmeier, S. M., Kattari, L., & Langenderfer-Magruder, L. (2020). Forced sex among youth: accrual of risk by gender identity, sexual orientation, mental health and bullying. *Journal of LGBT Youth, 17*(2), 193–213. https://doi.org/10.1080/19361653.2019.1614131

Basile, K. C., Smith, S. G., Kresnow, M., Khatiwada, S., & Leemis, R. W. (2022). *The National Intimate Partner and Sexual Violence Survey: 2016/2017 Report on Sexual Violence.* Atlanta, GA: National Center for Injury Prevention and Control, Centers for Disease Control and Prevention.

Benjet, C., Bromet, E., Karam, E. G., Kessler, R. C., McLaughlin, K. A., Ruscio, A. M., Shahly, V., Stein, D. J., Petukhova, M., Hill, E., Alonso, J., Atwoli, L., Bunting, B., Bruffaerts, R., Caldas-de-Almeida, J. M., de Girolamo, G., Florescu, S., Gureje, O., Huang, Y., Lepine, J. P., ... Koenen, K. C. (2016). The epidemiology of traumatic event exposure worldwide: Results from the World Mental Health Survey Consortium. *Psychological Medicine, 46*(2), 327–343.

Bentley, G., & Zamir, O. (2022). The role of maternal self-efficacy in the link between childhood maltreatment and maternal stress during transition to motherhood. *Journal of Interpersonal Violence, 37*(21–22), NP19576–NP19598.

Berry, K. M., & Rutledge, C. M. (2016). Factors that influence women to disclose sexual assault history to health care clinicians. *Journal of Obstetric, Gynecologic & Neonatal Nursing, 45*(4), 553–564.

Blackburn, A. M., Bystrynski, J. B., Rieger, A., Garthe, R. C., Piasecki, M., & Allen, N. E. (2023). Sexual assault revictimization among sexual minority individuals: A systematic review and meta-analysis. *Psychology of Violence, 13*(4), 286.

de Boer, M., Nijdam, M. J., Jongedijk, R. A., Bangel, K. A., Olff, M., Hofman, W. F., & Talamini, L. M. (2020). The spectral fingerprint of sleep problems in post-traumatic stress disorder. *Sleep, 43*(4), zsz269.

Dell'Osso, L., Lorenzi, P., Nardi, B., Carmassi, C., & Carpita, B. (2022). Post Traumatic Growth (PTG) in the frame of traumatic experiences. *Clinical Neuropsychiatry, 19*(6), 390.

Downey, C., & Crummy, A. (2022). The impact of childhood trauma on children's wellbeing and adult behavior. *European Journal of Trauma & Dissociation, 6*(1), 100237.

Eagen-Torkko, M., Low, L. K., Zielinski, R., & Seng, J. S. (2017). Prevalence and predictors of breastfeeding after childhood abuse. *Journal of Obstetric, Gynecologic & Neonatal Nursing, 46*(3), 465–479.

Green, I., Briggs, M., Soto, D. E., Cole, K., Wygant, J., Burnett, T., . . . & Thao, V. (2022). Health care utilization by patients with chronic pelvic pain. *Obstetrics & Gynecology, 10,* 1097.

International Society for Traumatic Stress Studies (ISTSS). (n.d.). Adult prevention and early treatment for PTSD. https://istss.org/clinical-resources/trauma-treatment/adult-prevention-and-early-treatment-for-ptsd/

Kessler, R. C., Aguilar-Gaxiola, S., Alonso, J., Benjet, C., Bromet, E. J., Cardoso, G., . . . & Koenen, K. C. (2017). Trauma and PTSD in the WHO world mental health surveys. *European Journal of Psychotraumatology, 8*(sup5), 1353383.

Lathan, E. C., Selwyn, C. N., Gigler, M. E., Langhinrichsen-Rohling, J., & Gilmore, A. K. (2023). College students' trust, betrayal, and needs during and after their worst nonassault-related healthcare experiences differ based on sexual violence exposure. *Violence & Victims, 38*(6), 858–878.

Lotto, C. R., Altafim, E. R. P., & Linhares, M. B. M. (2023). Maternal history of childhood adversities and later negative parenting: A systematic review. *Trauma, Violence, & Abuse, 24*(2), 662–683.

Magruder, K. M., McLaughlin, K. A., & Elmore Borbon, D. L. (2017). Trauma is a public health issue. *European Journal of Psychotraumatology, 8*(1), 1375338.

Marcovecchio, M. L., & Chiarelli, F. (2012). The effects of acute and chronic stress on diabetes control. *Science Signaling, 5*(247), pt10.

Mekawi, Y., Carter, S., Brown, B., Martinez de Andino, A., Fani, N., Michopoulos, V., & Powers, A. (2021). Interpersonal trauma and posttraumatic stress disorder among Black women: Does racial discrimination matter? *Journal of Trauma & Dissociation, 22*(2), 154–169.

Mersky, J. P., Lee, C. P., & Hami, D. (2024). Adverse childhood experiences and sexual orientation: An intersectional analysis of nationally representative data. *American Journal of Preventive Medicine, 66*(3), 483–491.

Moustafa, A. A., Parkes, D., Fitzgerald, L., Underhill, D., Garami, J., Levy-Gigi, E., Stramecki, F., Valikhani, A., Frydecka, D., & Misiak, B. (2021). The relationship between childhood trauma, early-life stress, and alcohol and drug use, abuse, and addiction: An integrative review. *Current Psychology, 40*, 579–584.

Murchland, A. R., Koenen, K. C., & Hayes-Larson, E. (2024). The link between traumatic experiences and health in late life: challenges and opportunities for U.S.-based longitudinal aging cohorts. *American Journal of Epidemiology, 194*(3), 565–572.

National Institutes for Mental Health (NIMH). (2024). Post-traumatic stress disorder. https://www.nimh.nih.gov/health/topics/post-traumatic-stress-disorder-ptsd

Osborne, M. T., Shin, L. M., Mehta, N. N., Pitman, R. K., Fayad, Z. A., & Tawakol, A. (2020). Disentangling the links between psychosocial stress and cardiovascular disease. *Circulation: Cardiovascular Imaging, 13*(8), e010931.

Owens, L., Terrell, S., Low, L. K., Loder, C., Rhizal, D., Scheiman, L., & Seng, J. (2022). Universal precautions: The case for consistently trauma-informed reproductive healthcare. *American Journal of Obstetrics and Gynecology, 226*(5), 671–x677.

Palmer, C. W., & Francis, S. E. (2024). The role of family rejection of gender expression on minority stress and mental health of sexual and gender minority adolescents. *Sexuality Research and Social Policy, 21*(3), 998–1013.

Ponting, C., Bond, M., Rogowski, B., Chu, A., & Lieberman, A. F. (2024). Childhood and adulthood trauma exposure: Associations with perinatal mental health and psychotherapy response. *Journal of Traumatic Stress, 37*(1), 178–186.

Reeves, E. (2015). A synthesis of the literature on trauma-informed care. *Issues in Mental Health Nursing, 36*(9), 698–709.

Rizeq, J., & McCann, D. (2023). The cognitive, emotional, and behavioral sequelae of trauma exposure: An integrative approach to examining trauma's effect. *Psychological Trauma: Theory, Research, Practice, and Policy, 15*(2), 313.

Sanjuan, P. M., Fokas, K., Tonigan, J. S., Henry, M. C., Christian, K., Rodriguez, A., Larsen, J., Yonke, N., & Leeman, L. (2021). Prenatal maternal posttraumatic stress disorder as a risk factor for adverse birth weight and gestational age outcomes: A systematic review and meta-analysis. *Journal of Affective Disorders, 295*, 530–540.

Selwyn, C. N., Lathan, E. C., Richie, F., Gigler, M. E., & Langhinrichsen-Rohling, J. (2021). Bitten by the system that cared for them: Towards a trauma-informed understanding of patients' healthcare engagement. *Journal of Trauma & Dissociation, 22*(5), 636–652.

Søegaard, E. G. I, Kan, Z., Koirala, R., Hauff, E., & Thapa, S. B. (2021). Gender differences in a wide range of trauma symptoms after victimization and accidental traumas: A cross-sectional study in a clinical setting. *European Journal of Psychotraumatology, 12*(1). http://doi.org/10.1080/20008198.2021.1975952

Stubbs, A., & Szoeke, C. (2022). The effect of intimate partner violence on the physical health and health-related behaviors of women: A systematic review of the literature. *Trauma, Violence, & Abuse, 23*(4), 1157–1172.

Substance Abuse and Mental Health Services Administration (SAMHSA). (2014). *SAMHSA's concept of trauma and guidance for a trauma-informed approach.* https://store.samhsa.gov/sites/default/files/sma14-4884.pdf

Substance Abuse and Mental Health Services Administration (SAMHSA). (2024). *What is trauma?* https://www.samhsa.gov/find-help/trauma

Ter Meulen, W. G., Draisma, S., van Hemert, A. M., Schoevers, R. A., Kupka, R. W., Beekman, A. T. F., & Penninx, B. W. J. H. (2021). Depressive and anxiety disorders in concert–A synthesis of findings on comorbidity in the NESDA study. *Journal of Affective Disorders*, 284, 85–97. https://doi.org/10.1016/j.jad.2021.02.004

Tillman, S. (2020). Consent in pelvic care. *Journal of Midwifery & Women's Health*, *65*(6), 749–758.

Tsigos, C., Kyrou, I., Kassi, E., & Chrousos, G. P. (2020). Stress: Endocrine physiology and pathophysiology. In K. R. Feingold, B. Anawalt, M. R. Blackman, et al. (Eds.). Endotext [Internet]. South Dartmouth (MA): MDText.com, Inc.; 2000-. Available from: https://www.ncbi.nlm.nih.gov/books/NBK278995/

Valentine, S. E., Marques, L., Wang, Y., Ahles, E. M., Dixon De Silva, L., & Alegría, M. (2019). Gender differences in exposure to potentially traumatic events and diagnosis of posttraumatic stress disorder (PTSD) by racial and ethnic group. *General Hospital Psychiatry, 61,* 60–68. http://doi.org/10.1016/j.genhosppsych.2019.10.008. PMID: 31715388; PMCID: PMC6870874.

U.S. Department of Veterans Affairs (USDVA). (n.d.). *Complex PTSD: History and definitions.* https://www.ptsd.va.gov/professional/treat/essentials/complex_ptsd.asp

Won, E., & Kim, Y. K. (2016). Stress, the autonomic nervous system, and the immune-kynurenine pathway in the etiology of depression. *Current Neuropharmacology*, *14*(7), 665–673. http://doi.org/10.2174/1570159x14666151208113006. PMID: 27640517; PMCID: PMC5050399.

Zasiekina, L., Duchyminska, T., Bifulco, A., & Bignardi, G. (2024). War trauma impacts in Ukrainian combat and civilian populations: Moral injury and associated mental health symptoms. *Military Psychology*, *36*(5), 555–566.

SECTION

2

Health Assessment and Promotion

CHAPTER 6

Health Promotion

Katrina Wu
Sarah Dorsey
The editors acknowledge Kathryn Osborne, who was the author of the previous edition of this chapter.

Health promotion is a foundational component of primary health care. Note that some national recommendations for health promotion counseling and interventions continue to distinguish guidelines according to people's sex assigned at birth, as statistical reporting of sex is often linked to health conditions, risks, and causes of death. Accordingly, some of the terminology in this chapter reflects health promotion strategies based on sex assigned at birth due to the binary gender terms common in this literature. Use of these terms is not meant to exclude people who seek gynecologic care and do not identify as women.

The leading causes of death for adults in the United States are largely related to modifiable, behavioral risk factors, with heart disease being the number one cause of death (Centers for Disease Control and Prevention [CDC], 2024a, 2024h). Although there have been significant reductions in the number of adults who use tobacco over the past three decades, 19.8% of U.S. adults reported current use in 2022, and smoking-related illnesses continue to be the number one preventable cause of death in the United States (CDC, 2024d). The CDC has identified smoking, poor nutrition, physical inactivity, and excessive alcohol use as the primary risk factors for chronic diseases and managing chronic conditions accounts for over $4 billion in annual medical expenditures each year (CDC, 2024a). Health promotion and disease prevention must be priorities to improve the overall health of the nation and to reduce the spending of our limited healthcare dollars on illnesses related to modifiable risk factors.

HEALTH PROMOTION: A NATIONAL INITIATIVE

The 1979 surgeon general's report *Healthy People: The Surgeon General's Report on Health Promotion and Disease Prevention* and its 1990 companion piece *Healthy People 1990: Promoting Health/ Preventing Disease: Objectives for the Nation* set the stage for the development of a national initiative that is founded on scientific evidence and focuses on disease prevention (CDC, 1989). In 1990, the U.S. Department of Health and Human Services released *Healthy People 2000: National Health Promotion and Disease Prevention Objectives*, a health promotion initiative that included 376 health objectives intended to move the U.S. population toward improved levels of wellness by the end of the 20th century. Healthy People was designed to support state and local agencies and private organizations in the development of plans aimed at improving the health status of all Americans (National Center for Health Statistics [NCHS], 2015). Since the 1990 inception of this initiative, the Department of Health and Human Services has identified 10-year national health objectives that are used to measure changes in health status over time. The membership of the Healthy People initiative includes stakeholders from both the private and public sector, including the Department of Health and Human Services, state and local health departments, and hundreds of private-sector groups and organizations. Members of the initiative periodically assess the health status of the nation and evaluate the effectiveness of specific interventions. Progress toward meeting the objectives is monitored by the National Center for Health Statistics and is made available through periodic publication of progress reports during each decade (NCHS, 2020).

As the fifth iteration, Healthy People 2030 was devised using a framework focused on social determinants of health (SDOH) and advancing health equity, citing a vision for "a society in which all people can achieve their full potential for health and well-being across the lifespan" (Healthy People 2030, n.d. -b; NCHS, 2020). SDOH comprise a range of personal, social, economic, and environmental factors that influence health status and fall under several broad categories, including policy making, social factors, health services, individual behavior, biology, and genetics. The overarching goals of Healthy People 2030 are as follows:

- Attain healthy, thriving lives and well-being free of preventable disease, disability, injury, and premature death.
- Eliminate health disparities, achieve health equity, and attain health literacy to improve the health and well-being of all.
- Create social, physical, and economic environments that promote attaining the full potential for health and well-being of all.
- Promote healthy development, healthy behaviors, and well-being across all life stages.
- Engage leadership, key constituents, and the public across multiple sectors to take action and design policies that improve the health and well-being of all (Healthy People 2030, n.d. -b; NCHS, 2020).

In addition to including the final goal focused on health policy, the primary change between 2020 and 2030 was the reduction of the total number of measurable objectives from 1,111 in Healthy People 2020 to 358 in Healthy People 2030 (Healthy People 2030, n.d. -b; Healthy People 2030, n.d. -c). Fewer objectives have reduced redundancy and increased prioritization of the identified objectives. The 2030 objectives are broken down into general topic areas under five larger groupings: (1) health conditions, (2) health behaviors, (3) population groups, (4) settings and systems, and (5) social determinants of health (Healthy People 2030, n.d. -a).

Within the population groups section, there are subtopics and specific objectives listed for both "LGBT" and "Women" that are particularly pertinent for gynecologic health providers and are listed in **Box 6-1**. Clinicians are encouraged to use these objectives to establish local programs aimed at improving the health of communities. More information about these objectives, specifically ways in which they may be applied to the delivery of gynecologic health care, and the ongoing development of Healthy People 2030 can be found at http://www.healthypeople.gov.

As the United States continues to grapple with the financial realities of health care, it is becoming increasingly clear to policy makers, clinicians, and insurance underwriters that allocating healthcare dollars for health promotion and disease prevention has significant benefits. The United States spent $4.5 trillion on health care in 2022, or 17.3% of the nation's gross domestic product (Centers for Medicare & Medicaid Services [CMS], 2024). Healthcare expenditures have tripled over the past two decades, with total spending per person averaging $13,493 in 2022 (CMS, 2024; Kaiser Family Foundation, 2024a). In 2021, half of the total U.S. healthcare budget was spent on just 5% of the population—individuals whose healthcare expenses were largely related to expensive chronic conditions, many of which were preventable (Kaiser Family Foundation, 2024b).

BOX 6-1 Healthy People 2030 Topics Addressed for LGBT Persons and Women

LGBT

- Adolescents
- Cancer
- Drug and Alcohol Use
- Health and Mental Disorders
- Public Health Infrastructure
- Sexually Transmitted Infections
- Tobacco Use

Women

- Iron Deficiency
- Cancer
- Family Planning
- Foodborne Illness
- Osteoporosis
- Pregnancy and Childbirth
- Sexually Transmitted Infections
- Tobacco Use
- Vaccination

Data from Healthy People 2030. (n.d. -f). LGBT. https://odphp.health.gov/healthypeople/objectives-and-data/browse-objectives/lgbt and Healthy People 2030. (n.d. -i). Women. https://odphp.health.gov/healthypeople/objectives-and-data/browse-objectives/women

The Affordable Care Act

The 2010 passage of the Patient Protection and Affordable Care Act (ACA) signaled additional congressional support for health promotion. Key provisions of the ACA established a mandate for every American to carry health insurance, increased access to health insurance through Medicaid expansion, and the creation of health insurance exchanges/marketplaces, where both individuals and employers can purchase lower-cost health insurance policies. Moreover, the ACA includes multiple reforms relative to individual and group health insurance policies that are sold on and off the exchanges. Among those reforms is a mandate that all insurance policies sold on and off an exchange must include, at a minimum, an essential health benefits package. This package includes coverage for preventive health services that are recommended by the U.S. Preventive Services Task Force (USPSTF), with no cost sharing (through deductibles or copayments) to the individual. See Chapter 9 for a more detailed discussion of the USPSTF.

Since its passage in 2010, there have been some changes to the ACA that affected the key provisions and original intent of the law. A 2012 ruling by the Supreme Court upheld the constitutionality of the mandate for every U.S. citizen and legal resident to carry health insurance, but it paved the way for individual states to opt out of the requirement to expand Medicaid (Kaiser Family Foundation, 2012). As of 2024, 14 states have not adopted Medicaid expansion, which has limited the law's ability to improve access to health care, particularly for low-income adults in non-expansion states, where an estimated 1.5 million adults earn too much to qualify for Medicaid but not enough to qualify for marketplace subsidies (Kaiser Family Foundation, 2024b, 2024d). In 2017, President Trump issued an executive order that would, in effect, expand the availability of short-term health insurance policies that are not compliant with the requirements of the ACA—policies that typically exclude coverage of preventive health services and pregnancy care (Kaiser Family Foundation, 2024c; Promoting Healthcare Choice, 2017). The tax reform bill that was signed into law in 2017 then did away with the tax penalty for failing to carry health insurance, which essentially eliminated the individual mandate (Tax Cuts and Jobs Act, 2017). While the public appreciated notable protections for those with pre-existing health conditions, the individual mandate for coverage and challenges in the initial launch of the health insurance marketplaces caused political polarization (Kaiser Family Foundation, 2024c). Since the inception of the Affordable Care Act in 2010, rates of those uninsured in the United States have dropped from approximately 15% to a record-low of 7.7% in 2023 (Kaiser Family Foundation, 2024c). Readers are advised to remain cognizant of changes in health policy that alter insurance coverage of preventive health services and gynecologic health care.

Preventive Health Services for Those Assigned Female at Birth Under the Affordable Care Act

All ACA-compliant policies are required to cover, with no cost sharing to the individual, the screening and counseling services recommended by the USPSTF and the Women's Preventative Services Initiative, under the direction of the American College of Obstetricians and Gynecologists (Kaiser Family Foundation,

2024c; Health Resources and Services Administration, 2024). Regarding preventive health services for adults, the following essential health benefits must be covered:

- Annual preventative visits (with recommended counseling, screening, and immunizations)
- Contraceptives and related services
- Breastfeeding support (including breast pumps and other supplies)
- Maternity and newborn care (Kaiser Family Foundation, 2024c, Health Resources and Services Administration, 2024)

Clinicians should be aware that a small percentage of adults are covered under grandfathered policies that are exempt from the requirement of no cost sharing for these preventive health services. Furthermore, Medicaid is not subject to the same requirements, although the ACA includes incentives for individual states to include the same preventive health services covered under Medicaid at no cost sharing to the individual (Kaiser Family Foundation, 2024c).

Moving away from the traditional medical focus on treating illness to health care that includes health promotion and disease prevention is an important step in the quest for cost containment (Lim et al., 2022). The looming question is, how can a healthcare delivery system that is illness centered undergo a paradigm shift to focus on wellness? At the federal level, implementation of Healthy People 2030 and the ACA has brought about initial changes in the priority placed on health promotion and disease prevention, but much work is yet to be done to achieve this shift in paradigm. Clinicians are taking initial steps in this direction by clarifying the definitions of health and prevention. The multidisciplinary nature of healthcare delivery creates an opportunity for variations in these definitions.

DEFINING HEALTH

Many organizations and specialty groups have their own standard definition of health. Perhaps the broadest of these definitions is that established by the World Health Organization (WHO) in 1948: "Health is a state of complete physical, mental and social well-being and not merely the absence of disease or infirmity" (2024, para. 1). To some, this definition may appear to make health unattainable. Yet, when health is viewed through a holistic lens, this definition begins to make sense. A holistic view of health includes its assessment in the context of physical, mental, and social well-being. Health, as defined in various contexts, can be achieved even in the presence of illness. For example, a young person who has been HIV positive for 5 years may feel a sense of physical, mental, and social well-being if they are being cared for in a healthcare delivery system that addresses their healthcare needs in a holistic fashion. The presence of a disease state does not exclude this individual from being considered healthy according to the WHO definition of health.

Nursing is a discipline that focuses on health and wellness. Consequently, numerous nursing theorists have proposed definitions of health. Perhaps one of the most well known is that developed by Martha Rogers (1970), who theorized that the study of human beings would yield meaningful theories and concepts only when their wholeness is perceived. Rogers's perception has served as a springboard for the development of myriad nursing definitions of health, each of which uses a holistic lens, viewing human beings as whole persons, encompassing mind, body, and spirit.

Madeleine Leininger, expanding on the work of earlier nurse theorists, provided a conceptual framework for nursing care. She proposed that caring is the essence of nursing and described the inextricable relationship between caring and respect for the culture of individual patients (Leininger, 1985). Supporting this theory are the definitions of evidence-based nursing practice that, very early on, included patients' values and preferences as essential components of the evidence upon which to base clinical practice (Melnyk & Fineout-Overholt, 2005). Melnyk and Fineout-Overholt (2023) define evidence-based practice as an approach to clinical decision making that integrates the most relevant research evidence, one's own clinical experience, and patient preferences and values. Including patients' values in clinical decision making recognizes the influence that the individual's values and beliefs have on outcomes of care and situates evidence-based practice within the patient's cultural context.

Applying Leininger's theory of transcultural caring and Melnyk and Fineout-Overholt's definition of evidence-based nursing practice to earlier definitions of health, one could conclude that proper health care requires a consideration of the whole person and must include knowledge and appreciation for the cultural context of the individual. This view provides a definition of health that is patient specific and includes the individual patient's cultural perceptions of health. Health promotion, then, encompasses a wide range of services that are delivered in a culturally congruent manner and that promote the general health and well-being of individuals and the communities in which they live.

DEFINING PREVENTION

The delivery of healthcare services aimed at the prevention of physical and mental illness and disease is defined on three levels:

1. Primary prevention is accomplished with the delivery of services focused on preventing disease in susceptible populations. Health education and counseling, lifestyle modification in healthy individuals, and targeted immunization are examples of primary prevention.
2. Secondary prevention focuses on the early detection of disease and prompt treatment aimed at reducing the severity of the disease and limiting its short- and long-term consequences. Routine laboratory screening and mammograms are examples of secondary prevention.
3. Tertiary prevention is the delivery of health services that limit disability and promote recovery from clinical disease states. Taking insulin to control diabetes and counseling services for those with depression are examples of tertiary prevention.

For over four decades, the USPSTF has been providing evidence-based recommendations regarding the effective use of preventive services to reduce morbidity and mortality rates. After an ongoing examination of the use and effectiveness of hundreds of preventive services, the USPSTF makes recommendations on three categories of preventive health services—screenings, behavioral counseling, and preventive medications—for which evidence supports the realization of significant health benefits (USPSTF, 2021b). The rest of this chapter focuses on behavioral counseling and immunizations as primary preventive efforts in healthcare delivery.

COUNSELING AND EDUCATION AS PREVENTIVE STRATEGIES

Clinicians are in a prime position to offer information that gives their patients tools to maintain a healthy lifestyle and assist in altering behaviors that may cause harm or illness. Patients often seek information during their yearly physical examination that can guide them in making lifestyle changes and confirm that their current practices are an effective means of maintaining health. However, episodic visits may offer more frequent opportunities for providing health promotion and disease prevention information. Many patients seek health care only from providers who specialize in gynecologic health, such as midwives and obstetrician-gynecologists. Given this reality, it is essential that all healthcare providers use each patient encounter as an opportunity to provide preventive health services.

In keeping with the basic tenets of evidence-based practice described by Melnyk and Fineout-Overholt (2023), the USPSTF continues to seek out and appraise the evidence regarding effective counseling interventions using well-established rating schemas. It provides recommendations that are intended to be integrated with the clinician's own expertise and experience, as well as the patient's preference and values, to guide professional decision making and practice (USPSTF, 2018c). Under the revised recommendation schema, the USPSTF (2018c) recommends that decisions to use services for which the balance of benefits is similar to the balance of harm (little or no net benefit) should be made based on professional judgment and patient preference. The USPSTF also recommends that clinicians use every patient interaction as an opportunity to participate in counseling and education. See Chapter 9 for a detailed discussion of the USPSTF.

EFFECTIVE COUNSELING INTERVENTIONS FOR HEALTHY PEOPLE

Patient education and counseling are important components of primary health care and have been identified as a primary responsibility for primary care providers (American Academy of Family Physicians, 2024). Much of this education and counseling is individualized and conducted as part of a plan aimed at managing specific problems or conditions. Described in this section are the USPSTF's counseling recommendations for use in gynecologic health and primary care settings. **Table 6-1** summarizes the recommendations to which the USPSTF has assigned a grade of A or B (high or moderate expected benefit) and which must, therefore, be covered by ACA-compliant insurance policies sold on and off the health insurance exchanges with no cost sharing. Of note, USPSTF guidelines that have been updated more recently consistently use gender-inclusive terms, while gendered language is still present in some of the guidelines set to be updated in the near future. Table 6-1 utilizes the language USPSTF used at the time this chapter was written; however, these recommendations can be applied to all people assigned female at birth, regardless of gender.

Breastfeeding and Chestfeeding

Healthy People 2030 and USPSTF value the benefits and reduced risk for illness inherent in breastfeeding and chestfeeding to both infants and their parents (USPSTF, 2016; Healthy People 2030, n.d. -e). While breastfeeding initiation is high in the United States, with the most recent data indicating 83.2% in 2019 (CDC, 2022), continuation rates are much lower. Based on the 2015 baseline that indicated only 24.9% of infants were exclusively breastfed at 6 months, Healthy People 2030 set a goal of 42.4%; updated data in 2020 showed only minimal improvement at 25.4% (Healthy People 2030, n.d. -e). Healthy People 2030 has a second breastfeeding goal to increase the proportion of infants breastfed at 1 year to 54.1% (Healthy People 2030, n.d. -d). This goal's status is considered to be "improving," having increased from 35.9% in 2015 to 37.6% in 2020 (Healthy People 2030, n.d. -d).

As of 2024, the USPSTF is in the process of updating their recommendations, but their stance as of 2016 was that they strongly encourage interventions in both the prenatal and postpartum period to support breastfeeding (USPSTF, 2016). Providing breastfeeding education and counseling is clearly an established component for support. Chapter 34 will expand on interventions to promote and support breastfeeding and chestfeeding (USPSTF, 2016; Healthy People 2030, n.d. -d).

Falls in Older Adults

Falls among older adults are a serious public health concern. Over a quarter of older adults, or 14 million, report falling each year, with falls leading to over 3 million emergency room visits each year (CDC, 2024e). Those who fall are twice as likely to fall a second time, and falls are the leading cause of traumatic brain injuries (CDC, 2024e). In 2021, falls were the greatest cause for injury-related deaths in adults aged 65 or greater (CDC, 2024e). An estimated 50 billion is spent annually on medical expenditures for the treatment of fall-related injuries (CDC, 2020e). As the population of older adults continues to grow, the costs and suffering associated with falls in older adults will only worsen. Therefore, the USPSTF (2024) recommends providing falls prevention counseling to all community-dwelling adults aged 65 and older who are at increased risk for falls.

Risk factors associated with falls include older age (65 years and older), history of previous falls, difficulty with mobility or balance, vitamin D deficiency, medications like sedatives that could impact stability, vision challenges, foot pain or insufficient footwear, and home hazards like throw rugs or uneven steps (CDC, 2024e; USPSTF, 2024). The CDC has numerous fall prevention resources available for patients and caregivers under their Stopping Elderly Accidents, Death and Injuries (STEADI) initiative, facilitating convenient handouts to provide patients (CDC, 2024e). STEADI encourages clinicians to screen for risk factors and then address modifiable risk factors using both clinical and community strategies (CDC, 2024e).

Counseling for falls prevention should include recommendations for supervised individual or group exercise classes, focused primarily on balance, gait, and functional training; exercises addressing flexibility, endurance, and strength training are also beneficial (USPSTF, 2024). In the previous USPSTF guidelines in 2018, they recommended against routine administration of vitamin D supplementation for the purpose of falls prevention; however, their 2024 guidelines do not address it and state their stance will be communicated in an upcoming updated vitamin D guideline separate from their falls prevention guideline. The American Geriatrics Society recommends that adults at risk for falls maintain a serum hydroxy vitamin D concentration of at least 25–30 ng/mL, and they recommend against routine screening for vitamin D in the absence of risk factors; notably, this recommendation has not been updated since 2014 (American Geriatrics Society, 2014). Lastly, while the USPSTF recommends offering multifactorial interventions for falls prevention to those

TABLE 6-1 Grade A and B Counseling Recommendations of the USPSTF

Topic	Target Population	Recommendation Summary	Grade
BRCA-related cancer	Women with a family history of breast, ovarian, tubal, or peritoneal cancer	Screen those with a family history associated with increased risk and refer those with a positive screen for genetic counseling.	B
Breastfeeding and chestfeeding	All pregnant women and new mothers	Provide counseling interventions during pregnancy and the postpartum period to promote and support breastfeeding.	B
Falls prevention	Community-dwelling adults aged 65 and older at increased risk for falls	Provide falls prevention counseling, including recommendations for exercise or physical therapy.	B
Healthy diet and physical activity for cardiovascular prevention	Adults with cardiovascular risk factors, defined as one or more of the following: hypertension, dyslipidemia, mixed or multiple risk factors such as metabolic syndrome or an estimated 10-year cardiovascular disease risk of 7.5% or greater	Offer or provide a referral for behavioral counseling to promote a healthy diet and physical activity.	B
Healthy weight and weight gain in pregnancy	Pregnant persons	Offer effective behavioral counseling interventions aimed at promoting healthy weight gain and preventing excess gestational weight gain in pregnancy.	B
Intimate partner violence	Women of reproductive age	Screen and then provide or refer women who screen positive to ongoing support services.	B
Perinatal depression	Pregnant and postpartum persons	Screen all pregnant and postpartum persons and then provide or refer those at increased risk to counseling interventions.	B
Sexually transmitted infections	All sexually active adolescents and all adults at increased risk for infection	Provide behavioral counseling to prevent sexually transmitted infections.	B
Skin cancer	Adolescents and young adults up to age 24 who have fair skin types	Provide counseling about minimizing exposure to ultraviolet radiation.	B
Tobacco smoking cessation	All adults, including pregnant persons	Ask all adults about tobacco use and provide cessation counseling and interventions for those who use tobacco. Offer pharmacotherapy approved by the Food and Drug Administration to nonpregnant adults who smoke.	A
Tobacco use in adolescents	School-aged children and adolescents	Provide education and counseling to prevent initiation of tobacco use.	B
Unhealthy alcohol use	All adults aged 18 and older, including pregnant persons	Screen for unhealthy alcohol use and provide those engaged in risky or hazardous drinking with brief behavioral counseling interventions to reduce unhealthy alcohol use.	B
Unhealthy drug use	All adults aged 18 and older	Screen by asking questions (not testing biological specimens) when services for accurate diagnosis, effective treatment, and appropriate care can be offered or referred.	B
Weight loss	Adults with a body mass index of 30 or higher	Offer or provide a referral for intensive, multicomponent behavioral interventions.	B

Data from U.S. Preventive Services Task Force. (2024). *A & B recommendations*. https://www.uspreventiveservicestaskforce.org/uspstf/recommendation-topics/uspstf-a-and-b-recommendations#more with identified, modifiable risks, they do not support routinely offering interventions to all older adults (USPSTF, 2024).

Motor Vehicle Safety

Motor vehicle accidents are a leading cause of death in the United States, with the majority of crash-associated deaths occurring to passengers and drivers. Seat belt use is the best way to decrease injuries and save lives, as it reduces severe crash-related deaths and injuries by approximately half (CDC, 2024f).

Counseling recommendations regarding seat belt use have evolved since the early work of the USPSTF. The earliest recommendations were to advise all people about the proper use and placement of lap and shoulder restraints and to avoid riding with an alcohol-impaired driver or driving while alcohol impaired. Legislative efforts and community-based interventions over the past two decades have resulted in high rates of seat belt use among people of all ages; an estimated 90–92% of all adults in the United States currently use seat belts (CDC, 2024f). The USPSTF found no well-conducted research that evaluated the effect of counseling in the primary care setting on seat belt use (USPSTF, n.d. -b). It also did not find any research addressing the impact of counseling in the primary care setting on driving while under the influence of alcohol or riding with an impaired driver. Consequently, the USPSTF makes no recommendation for or against counseling patients in the primary care setting about seat belt use (USPSTF, n.d. -b). Nevertheless, strong evidence suggests that seat belt laws and enforcement strategies, which include periodic reminders from a healthcare provider, have resulted in increased use of these restraints and a subsequent reduction in serious crash-related injuries and death (CDC, 2024f).

Skin Cancer

The most common type of cancer in the United States is skin cancer, and the deadliest form—melanoma—is usually caused by excessive exposure to ultraviolet (UV) light (USPSTF et al., 2018a). The USPSTF recommends that all fair-skinned adolescents and young adults aged 10 to 24 be counseled to minimize exposure to UV light. A smaller benefit has also been found in educating adults older than 24 (USPSTF et al., 2018a). While the USPSTF note that the majority of skin cancer prevention research has been conducted with fair-skinned individuals, ultimately influencing the population focus of their recommendations (USPSTF, 2018a), UV protection is important and beneficial for preventing sunburn, premature aging, and skin cancer in all skin types for all ages (Passeron et al., 2021; CDC, 2023). Decisions to provide similar counseling to people older than age 24 should be individualized and made based on the presence of risk factors (USPSTF et al., 2018a).

Individuals at increased risk of developing skin cancer include those with light-colored hair and eyes, freckling, and a history of frequent burning when exposed to the sun (USPSTF et al., 2018a). People with a family history of skin cancer and people who are immunocompromised are also at increased risk for skin cancer. Measures to minimize UV exposure include wearing hats, sunglasses, sun-protective clothing, using sunblock with a sun-protection factor (SPF) of at least 15, limiting time in the sun (particularly between the hours of 10 a.m. and 4 p.m.), and avoiding the use of tanning beds. In addition to counseling adolescents and young adults about how to minimize UV exposure, counseling strategies that include a description of the effects of UV light on skin appearance, such as early aging, have also been effective (USPSTF et al., 2018a).

COUNSELING INTERVENTIONS FOR PEOPLE WITH ADDITIONAL RISK FACTORS

The counseling interventions described thus far have been recommended for adults regardless of existing symptoms or risk factors. In addition to establishing these guidelines, the USPSTF has made recommendations regarding counseling interventions for individuals with certain risk factors for disease. See Chapter 8 for an in-depth discussion of recommendations related to screening for risk factors.

BRCA-Related Cancer

Breast cancer is the leading cause of cancer in those assigned female at birth in the United States and the second-leading cause of cancer death (Surveillance, Epidemiology, and End Results program [SEER], 2024). Many of the risk factors for breast cancer, such as sex, age, genetics, and family history, are nonmodifiable; most breast cancers are diagnosed in women over 50 years of age (CDC, 2024c). An estimated 5–10% of breast cancers are related to hereditary mutations in the *BRCA1* and *BRCA2* genes (USPSTF et al., 2019b). In addition to breast cancer, *BRCA1* and *BRCA2* gene mutations are associated with ovarian, fallopian tube, and peritoneal cancers. Screening for *BRCA1* and *BRCA2* gene mutations is recommended only for women with a personal or family history of breast, ovarian, fallopian tube, or peritoneal cancer; the USPSTF recommends against routine risk assessment for women whose personal or family history is not linked with *BRCA1/2* gene mutations (USPSTF et al., 2019b). Be advised that this topic is currently under review; check the USPSTF website for updated recommendations.

There are numerous validated screening tools for assessing breast cancer risk and the likelihood of a *BRCA1/2* mutation briefly outlined in the USPSTF's recommendation; however, they have found insufficient evidence to recommend one screening tool above others (USPSTF, 2019b). For patients with a positive screen on any validated screening tool, the USPSTF (2019b) recommends genetic counseling, and possible testing, with a healthcare provider who is specially trained to conduct such counseling. As a service that is recommended by the USPSTF, genetic counseling for adults at increased risk of *BRCA* mutations should be covered by health insurance with no cost sharing to the patient. However, some may not have health insurance, and some may be covered by insurance that is not ACA compliant. Moreover, those with a positive screen may live in communities where there are no genetic counseling services available. Healthcare providers who screen adults for breast cancer risks are advised to remain cognizant of the availability of, and costs associated with, genetic counseling. Genetic counseling resources for clinicians and patients, including online support and advocacy groups, can be found on the website of the National Institutes of Health's National Human Genome Research Institute (https://www.genome.gov/). A detailed discussion of cancers that affect those assigned female at birth can be found in Chapters 17 and 28.

Healthy Diet and Physical Activity: Interventions for People at Increased Risk for Cardiovascular Disease

The recommendations for diet and exercise counseling have changed over time with the emergence of new evidence. In the second edition of *Guide to Clinical Preventive Services*, the USPSTF (1996) recommended that everyone be counseled to limit the amount of fat and cholesterol in their diet and to devise plans for diet and regular exercise that balance caloric intake with energy expenditures. In 2002, those recommendations were amended following a review of more recent research that revealed there was insufficient evidence to advise either for or against routine dietary counseling or behavioral counseling to promote a healthy diet and physical activity for patients in primary care settings (USPSTF, 2002).

More recently, the USPSTF (2014) identified evidence to support the provision of intensive behavioral counseling interventions for adults who have additional risk factors for cardiovascular disease. For patients without these risk factors, the USPSTF recognized that while there is a strong correlation between diet, physical activity, and cardiovascular health, the benefits associated with routinely counseling all patients in primary care settings about diet and exercise were very small (USPSTF, 2017). Consequently, the latest 2020 USPSTF guidelines, which are currently under review, recommend that rather than incorporating diet and exercise counseling into the care of all patients, clinicians may choose to selectively provide this counseling when appropriate. More specifically, this type of counseling is likely to be most beneficial for patients who have expressed an interest in and a readiness to make behavioral changes (USPSTF, 2017). The potential harms associated with providing this counseling include the missed opportunity to spend time providing other counseling that could have greater benefits.

Heart disease is the leading cause of death for women in the United States; however, only 56% of women are aware of this (CDC, 2024b). In 2021, heart disease accounted for 1 in 5 female deaths. Types of heart disease include heart failure, arrythmias, and coronary artery disease. Several key risk factors for heart disease can be modified with dietary changes. These modifiable risk factors include high levels of low-density lipoprotein (LDL) cholesterol, hypertension, diabetes, tobacco use, alcohol use, physical inactivity, and excess weight (CDC, 2024b).

The USPSTF (2020b) recommends that all adults with risk factors for cardiovascular disease (CVD) be offered or referred for behavioral interventions to promote a healthy diet and physical activity. CVD risk factors in this USPSTF recommendation are defined as people with hypertension or elevated blood pressure, dyslipidemia, and/or mixed risk factors, such as an estimated 10-year CVD risk of ≥7.5% or metabolic syndrome using a screening tool like the Framingham Risk Score or Pooled Cohort Equations. This guideline intentionally excludes elevated blood glucose levels, obesity, and smoking as modifiable risk factors, as these are addressed in other guidelines. The USPSTF defines a healthy diet as one high in fruits, vegetables, whole grains, lean proteins, oils, and non- or low-fat dairy, while also being lower in sodium, saturated or trans fats, and added sugars (USPSTF et al., 2020b). Appropriate physical activity is defined as 75–150 minutes of moderate to vigorous aerobic exercise each week, with strength training twice weekly (USPSTF et al., 2020b). The counseling strategies that appear to be most effective are very intensive, occur in group or individual settings, and require frequent contact (by phone or face to face) over 6 to 18 months. Counseling and education also appear to be most effective when conducted by a team of interventionists alongside the clinician, such as nutritionists, physical therapists or trainers, nurses, and lifestyle coaches (USPSTF et al., 2020b). While it is possible that these services can be provided in primary care settings, when time and additional personnel are not available, patients should be referred for specialty care (USPSTF et al., 2020b).

Perinatal Depression

An estimated 1 out of 7 people who give birth in the United States are affected by perinatal depression, which is a depressive disorder during pregnancy or postpartum (USPSTF et al., 2019a). Perinatal depression can result in poor health outcomes for both birthing people and infants. Counseling interventions offer an effective approach to the prevention of postpartum depression when provided to those at increased risk. As a result, the USPSTF (2019a) recommends that pregnant and postpartum persons who are at increased risk for depression be provided with or referred for counseling interventions. Risk factors for perinatal depression include a history of depression, current symptoms of depression or anxiety that do not reach the threshold for diagnosis, socioeconomic risk factors such as lower income or adolescence, recent intimate partner violence, and a history of significant negative life events. The most effective counseling interventions appear to be interpersonal therapy and cognitive behavioral therapy (USPSTF et al., 2019a). A detailed discussion regarding the screening and management of postpartum mood disorders, including postpartum depression, can be found in Chapter 34.

Sexually Transmitted Infection Screening and Prevention

The USPSTF (2020a) recommends behavioral counseling to prevent sexually transmitted infections (STIs) in all sexually active adolescents and all sexually active adults at increased risk for STIs. Adults at increased risk for STIs include those with current STIs or infections within the past year, individuals with multiple current sexual partners, and inconsistent external or internal condom use. Counseling should be based on individual risk factors, which can be assessed during a sexual history, and on local information about the epidemiologic risks for STIs (USPSTF et al., 2020a). See Chapters 8 and 22 for more information.

Patients identified as being at increased risk for the acquisition of an STI need to receive information about STIs, STI transmission, risk factors, and ways to reduce their likelihood of infection (USPSTFet al., 2020a). Such measures include abstinence, regular use of external or internal condoms, and limiting the number of sexual partners. The USPSTF found little evidence to support the effectiveness of brief individual counseling sessions in the primary care setting and no evidence to support abstinence-only education. In contrast, strong evidence suggests that moderate- to high-intensity counseling, delivered in multiple individual or group sessions (with a total duration of two or more hours), results in a statistically significant reduction in STIs. A single counseling intervention that is less than 30 minutes may also be effective (USPSTF et al., 2020a).

Adults who are at increased risk for STIs should be advised to use barrier methods correctly and consistently with every sexual encounter in accordance with the manufacturer's recommendations (CDC, 2021; USPSTF et al., 2020a). Appropriate barrier methods would include polyurethane or latex condoms during penetrative sex, when using penetrative sex toys, or oral–genital sex; gloves during digital–genital sex; and latex or polyurethane sheets (i.e., dental dams) during oral–genital sex (CDC, 2021). Measures to negotiate condom use and to reduce the chance of infection when a partner will not use a condom should also be discussed; for example, an internal condom for vaginal use can be used to provide more control for receptive partners (CDC, 2021).

Behavioral counseling can include training in condom use and communication about safer sex (USPSTF et al., 2020a).

Pre-exposure vaccination is an effective method for protecting against vaccine preventable STIs (CDC, 2021). All uninfected, unvaccinated individuals who are at increased risk for STIs should be offered screening and counseled to receive a hepatitis B vaccine; in addition, all adolescent and young adults should be counseled about the appropriateness of the human papillomavirus vaccine (HPV). The hepatitis A vaccine is recommended for people who are unhoused (CDC, 2021). For more information on STI screening and prevention, see Chapter 22.

Any discussion regarding counseling patients about sexual behavior would be incomplete without addressing contraceptive counseling. The USPSTF does not address contraceptive counseling in its recommendations for clinical preventive services. However, the CDC (2024i) recommends person-centered contraceptive counseling, and provides contraceptive guidance for clinicians. Moreover, Healthy People 2030 has the goal of decreasing the unintended pregnancy rate from 43% to 36.5% (Healthy People 2030, n.d. -g). Counseling should be based on information obtained from a detailed sexual history. Effective contraceptive methods and approaches used for patient education and counseling aimed at pregnancy prevention are described in detail in Chapter 13.

Tobacco Use

Smoking is the leading preventable cause of death in the United States (USPSTF, 2021a). Lung cancer is the leading cause of cancer death among those assigned female at birth (SEER, 2024). The USPSTF (2021a) strongly recommends that clinicians ask all adults (including all pregnant people) about tobacco use and offer counseling and behavioral interventions that aid in smoking cessation to all patients who use tobacco. Nonpregnant adults who smoke should also be provided with pharmacotherapy approved by the Food and Drug Administration for smoking cessation. Evidence demonstrates that interventions such as behavioral counseling and the use of pharmacotherapeutics, including nicotine replacement therapy, can increase the number of patients who attempt to quit and remain abstinent for 1 year. The USPSTF found insufficient evidence regarding the safe use of pharmacotherapy during pregnancy and was therefore unable to determine the balance of benefits and harms of pharmacotherapy during pregnancy (USPSTF, 2021a).

While a single brief encounter may offer some benefit, repeated sessions of longer duration are more effective. Similar to counseling patients about alcohol misuse, a framework provided by the five A's is an effective way to engage patients who smoke in discussion about cessation:

- Ask about tobacco use.
- Advise to quit through clear personalized messages.
- Assess willingness to quit.
- Assist to quit.
- Arrange follow-up and support. (USPSTF, 2021a)

To prevent initiation of tobacco use, the USPSTF (2020c) also recommends behavioral counseling interventions for all adolescents and school-aged children. Effective strategies include face-to-face individual counseling, group counseling, printed materials, telephone calls and mobile device messaging, and messages sent through the U.S. mail. Regardless of the methods used or the frequency of counseling, the strategies that appear to be most effective include the provision of age-appropriate information about the consequences of tobacco use, the impact of social pressure, warnings about tobacco marketing, and effective ways to say no to tobacco use. Counseling aimed at providing parents with tools to help their children remain tobacco free has also been effective. For adolescents and school age children who already use tobacco, the USPSTF found insufficient evidence to evaluate the balance of benefits and harm of interventions for tobacco use cessation (USPSTF, 2020c).

Unhealthy Alcohol Use: Interventions for People Who Engage in Risky or Hazardous Drinking

Screening patients for risky or hazardous drinking behavior is described in Chapter 9. For adults aged 18 and older who screen positive for alcohol misuse, the USPSTF (2018d) recommends the use of multiple brief (6–15 minutes) behavioral counseling interventions aimed at reducing unhealthy alcohol use. In the absence of sufficient evidence to weigh the balance of benefits against harms, the USPSTF makes no recommendation regarding screening and counseling for adolescents (USPSTF, 2018d). Be advised that this topic is currently under review; check the USPSTF website for updated recommendations.

The brief intervention for at-risk drinkers recommended by the National Institute on Alcohol Abuse and Alcoholism (2023) is based on the five As framework: ask, advise, assess, assist, and arrange follow-up. After the screening identification of someone who engages in risky or hazardous drinking, clinicians should begin the intervention by describing their conclusions and making recommendations for change. Steps should be taken to assess the person's readiness to change and establish plans for follow-up (National Institute on Alcohol Abuse and Alcoholism, 2023).

Weight Loss

More than 40% of those assigned female at birth in the United States are designated by conventional classification systems as obese (USPSTF, 2018b). Obesity, which is defined as a body mass index (BMI) greater than or equal to 30, is linked to disability and other health concerns such as type 2 diabetes, various cancers, and increased risk for cardiovascular disease for some individuals (USPSTF, 2018b). BMI is increasingly known to be an outdated and imprecise measure of health (Olson et al., 2023), and healthcare providers have been found to demonstrate substantial weight-based biases, ranging from inappropriate gestures and language, reduced eye contact and physical touch, beliefs that their patients with obesity are lazy or prone to treatment noncompliance, and attributing the majority of patient health concerns to their weight (Lawrence et al., 2021). Body size is multifactorial, influenced by environmental, genetic, and biological processes, and reducing it to personal responsibility through diet and exercise alone creates an inaccurate clinical picture that can perpetuate psychological and physical harm (Rubino et al., 2020). Experiencing weight stigma and biases in healthcare settings has been shown to increase healthcare avoidance and directly impact the adequacy of care received (Rubino et al., 2020). Providers should actively reflect on their own biases and the weight-based stigma inherent in their workplaces to effect change to promote a supportive and inclusive healthcare experience that is welcoming and person-centered for bodies of all sizes.

The USPSTF recommends offering or referring adults with a BMI of 30 or greater for intensive multicomponent behavioral interventions (USPSTF, 2018b). The most effective interventions provide ongoing support (1 to 2 years in duration) for initiation and maintenance of changes in diet and physical activity (USPSTF, 2018b). Although there is a role for primary care providers in the provision of this counseling and support, there is evidence that the benefits of behavioral interventions may be greater when provided primarily by professionals with specialized training, such as dieticians, behavioral therapists, psychologists, lifestyle coaches, and exercise physiologists (USPSTF, 2018b). This topic is currently under review, refer to the USPSTF website for updated recommendations.

IMMUNIZATION GUIDELINES AND RECOMMENDATIONS

In addition to counseling interventions to assist patients in making healthy lifestyle choices and changes, primary prevention includes the delivery of targeted immunizations. Immunizations play an important role in the prevention of infectious diseases, many of which are debilitating and may be fatal. As has been true since the inception of Healthy People initiatives, Healthy People 2030 recognizes the effectiveness of immunizations as a strategy to significantly reduce the incidence of vaccine-preventable disease and identifies immunization status as one of the leading health indicators by which to measure the health of the nation (Healthy People 2030, n.d. -a). The USPSTF also acknowledges the importance of immunizations as a primary preventive measure. Since 1996, it has deferred to the CDC's Advisory Committee on Immunization Practices regarding evidence-based recommendations and guidelines for clinicians (USPSTF, n.d. -a).

Primary care clinicians are in a key position to implement policies to improve the immunization status of individuals in the United States. However, evidence suggests that many of these clinicians fail to provide appropriate preventive care services, including immunizations, to people in the outpatient setting. Several investigators have examined barriers to initiation and administration of recommended vaccines. Vaccine hesitancy occurs when a person is uncertain about or declines a vaccine despite its availability, and this is a crucial barrier to high levels of immunization coverage (Germann et al., 2022). Another common finding across studies is missed opportunities for vaccination in primary care settings (Kelly et al., 2023; Loskutova et al., 2020; Ryan et al., 2022). Vaccine administration is viewed by many as a preventive health service delivered only at periodic well-patient visits with a primary care provider. However, vaccine coverage can be optimized if every visit to a healthcare provider is viewed as an opportunity to offer and administer recommended vaccines. This includes single-dose vaccines and the initiation or completion of vaccines that require more than one dose, which can be accomplished at episodic or problem-focused visits.

Although the number of children and adults who receive the recommended vaccines has improved over the years, vaccine rates in the United States, particularly for adults, remain suboptimal (Lu et al., 2021). People seek healthcare services for multiple reasons, including contraceptive counseling, yearly physical examinations, prenatal care, preconception care, urgent care, and care for chronic conditions. Each of these encounters should be considered an opportunity to provide preventive health services for patients, including the administration of recommended vaccines.

Current immunization guidelines for people who are considered to have complete vaccine coverage are summarized in **Table 6-2**; catch-up vaccine schedules for individuals who are not fully immunized can be found on the CDC website (http://www.cdc.gov). When considering appropriate vaccination schedules, it is important to note that the measles, mumps, and rubella (MMR), herpes zoster vaccine live (ZVL), live attenuated influenza vaccine (LAIV), and varicella vaccines (VAR) are contraindicated for people who are pregnant or immunocompromised, including some people with HIV infection (CDC, 2024g). When they are indicated, the recombinant zoster vaccine (RZV) and the HPV vaccine should be delayed until after pregnancy (CDC, 2024g). It is also important to note that Table 6-2 is a brief listing of vaccines and does not include the multiple footnotes that are included in the CDC recommendations; this must be taken into consideration when deciding on appropriate vaccine administration for certain at-risk people across the life span.

Vaccines for severe acute respiratory syndrome coronavirus-2 (SARS-CoV-2), respiratory syncytial virus (RSV), and Mpox have been approved since the last edition of this text. Severe acute respiratory syndrome coronavirus-2 causes coronavirus disease 2019 (COVID-19). On March 11, 2020, the World Health Organization (WHO) classified COVID-19 as a pandemic (WHO, 2020). SARS-CoV-2 can cause a range of health problems, from mild symptoms to severe health complications and mortality rates (Yadav et al., 2023). In December 2020, the U.S. Food and Drug Administration (FDA) issued emergency use authorization for the first COVID-19 vaccine (FDA, 2020). Pregnant and lactating people were excluded from the initial COVID-19 vaccines; however, observational data has shown that these vaccines are safe in the peripartum period (Germann et al., 2022). Vaccine formulations and administration recommendations have evolved since the first ones were available to the public and as the virus has mutated; check with the CDC for the most current recommendations.

Respiratory syncytial virus can cause significant morbidity and mortality in infants. In October 2023, the CDC and other organizations endorsed RSV vaccination with Pfizer's bivalent RSVpreF vaccine (trade name Abrysvo) for pregnant patients (American College of Nurse-Midwives, 2024; American College of Obstetricians and Gynecologists, 2023; CDC, 2023). RSV is the main reason U.S. infants are hospitalized, and the Abrysvo vaccine may decrease the risk of infant hospitalization for RSV by 57% during the first six months of life (CDC, 2023). The vaccine is seasonal, administered September through January in most of the continental United States, and available to pregnant individuals between 32 weeks 0 days and 36 weeks 6 days gestation. There is also an RSV vaccine for infants; the majority of newborns will benefit from protection from either infant immunization or maternal RSV vaccination. If a person gives birth less than 2 weeks after being immunized in pregnancy, clinicians should consider recommending infant immunization as well (CDC, 2023).

Mpox is an infection caused by the monkeypox virus and has caused intermittent outbreaks in the past several decades (FDA, 2024). In response to an outbreak in May 2022, emergency use authorization was granted by the FDA for the vaccine JYNNEOS in August 2022, and then it became commercially available in April 2024 (FDA, 2024). Mpox causes a painful, pruritic rash anywhere on the body, and may be accompanied by flu-like symptoms (CDC, 2025a). It spreads through close, skin-to-skin contact or sexual contact, touching contaminated items, and bodily fluids

TABLE 6-2 Recommended Vaccination Schedule

Vaccine	AGE-RELATED RECOMMENDATIONS						
	11–12 Years	**13–18 Years**	**19–26 Years**	**27–49 Years**	**50–59 Years**	**60–64 Years**	**≥ 65 Years**
COVID-19	See CDC recommendations for previously vaccinated and unvaccinated adolescents.		Unvaccinated: one dose of updated Moderna or Pfizer-BioNTech, or two-dose series of updated Novavax. Previously vaccinated with one or more doses of any COVID-19 vaccine: one dose of any updated COVID-19 vaccine administered at least 8 weeks after most recent COVID-19 vaccine dose.				
Hepatitis A	Two doses if not previously immunized.		Two or three doses for anyone not fully vaccinated who requests vaccination, people with risk factors such as chronic liver disease or who receive clotting factor concentrates, those who use illegal drugs, and those who have occupational or travel exposure to hepatitis A. May use three-dose series HepA-HepB when indicated.				
Hepatitis B	Three doses beginning at birth; two or three doses ages 11–18 if not previously immunized.		Two, three, or four doses for people who have not been previously immunized and those with risk factors for infection: end-stage renal disease, HIV infection, chronic liver disease, occupational and/or household exposure, incarceration, travel exposure, IV drug use, increased STI risk.				
Human papillomavirus (HPV)	Two or three doses at age 11–12.	Two or three doses for all persons aged 11–26 and not previously immunized.		Adults age 27–45 years: Use shared clinical decision making; complete two or three dose series depending on age at initial vaccination.			
Influenza	Adolescents and people of all ages should receive one dose of flu vaccine annually during flu season. Live vaccine is contraindicated and should not be administered during pregnancy or to individuals with certain risk factors. See the CDC recommendations for vaccine types to use for people across the life span.						
Measles, mumps, and rubella (MMR)	Two doses for those not previously immunized.		One dose for all adults born in or after 1957 with no evidence of immunity to measles, mumps, or rubella; one or two doses for certain populations at increased risk.[a] Contraindicated in pregnancy.				
Meningococcal	One dose at age 11–12 if not previously immunized, with booster at age 16.		Two doses for adults older than age 18 at increased risk for infection: first-year college students living in dormitories, military recruits, microbiologists exposed to *Neisseria meningitidis*, and people traveling to epidemic areas. See the CDC recommendations for certain adults who may need a second dose.				
Mpox		Minimum age 18 years. Two doses for those at risk for Mpox infection or whose sexual partners are at risk for Mpox.					

Pneumococcal (conjugate or polysaccharide)	One or two doses for people with certain underlying medical conditions or immunocompromised conditions, such as chronic heart/lung/liver disease, diabetes mellitus, chronic asplenia, chronic alcoholism, cochlear implant, HIV infection, cigarette smoking, Hodgkin disease, lymphoma, leukemia, solid organ transplant, hemoglobinopathies. A booster dose may be necessary based on risk factors and type of vaccine administered. See CDC recommendations for guidance on which pneumococcal vaccines a patient needs and when.	One dose for all people aged 65 years or older.
Respiratory syncytial virus (RSV)	During pregnancy 32 weeks 0 days through 36 weeks 6 days gestation: One dose regardless of previous infection, seasonal administration (September–January in most of continental United States). Age 60 years or older: One dose (based on shared decision making); individuals at increased risk for severe RSV most likely to benefit from vaccine.	
Td/Tdap (tetanus, diphtheria/tetanus, diphtheria, pertussis)	One-time dose of Tdap for those who have received the primary immunization series followed by Td or Tdap booster every 10 years. • Pregnant people should receive one dose of Tdap with each pregnancy, preferably at 27–36 weeks gestation.	
Varicella	Two doses for all people born in or after 1980 without evidence of immunity (previous infection or vaccination). Contraindicated in pregnancy.	
Zoster (herpes)	Not recommended.	Two doses of RZV (2–6 months apart for all adults aged 50 years and older).

Data from Centers for Disease Control and Prevention. (2024). *Immunization schedules: For healthcare providers*. https://www.cdc.gov/vaccines/hcp/imz-schedules/index.html

[a]A second dose of MMR is recommended for people who (1) have been exposed to measles or mumps, or who live in an outbreak area; (2) are students in postsecondary education institutions; (3) work in a healthcare facility; (4) plan international travel; (5) close contacts of immunocompromised persons without evidence of immunity to measles, mumps, or rubella. Unvaccinated persons born before 1957 without evidence of mumps immunity and who work in healthcare settings should receive one dose of MMR; administering a second dose during an outbreak should be strongly considered. Rubella immunity should be determined for all people of childbearing age; those without evidence of immunity should receive the MMR vaccine upon completion or termination of pregnancy and before discharge from the healthcare facility. MMR vaccine is contraindicated in pregnancy and severe immunocompromising conditions (see CDC guidance on immunization for people living with HIV).

TABLE 6-3 Resources for Clinicians

Resource	Description	Website
Centers for Disease Control and Prevention	Website of a leading authority on health promotion and disease prevention. Includes resources for patient education on topics addressed in this chapter.	https://www.cdc.gov/
Immunization schedules	Downloadable immunization schedules for healthcare providers.	https://www.cdc.gov/vaccines/schedules/hcp/index.html
U.S. Preventive Services Task Force (USPSTF)	Website of a leading authority on health promotion and disease prevention.	https://www.uspreventiveservicestaskforce.org/
USPSTF A & B recommendations	Published recommendations of the USPSTF with a grade of A or B.	https://www.uspreventiveservicestaskforce.org/uspstf/recommendation-topics/uspstf-a-and-b-recommendations
USPSTF Electronic Preventive Services Selector (ePSS app)	Downloadable app that includes updated recommendations of the USPSTF.	https://epss.ahrq.gov/PDA/index.jsp

like respiratory secretions or through open lesions (CDC, 2025a). The two-dose vaccine is given four weeks apart and is recommended to those at increased risk for infection (CDC, 2025b). While there have been outbreaks in the United States, the greatest regional risk at the time this chapter was written would be for those traveling to several countries in central and east Africa and anticipating having sex with a new partner or at a commercial sex venue (CDC, 2025b). In addition to those traveling, the CDC also recommends the vaccine to anyone with a suspected Mpox exposure, those with an occupational risk (e.g., laboratory technicians or healthcare workers at risk for exposure), those who have sex with gay or bisexual males who have had a new STI diagnosis or more than one partner in the past 6 months, and those who anticipate visiting or have visited a commercial sex venue in the past 6 months (CDC, 2025b). Check the CDC for the most current list of at-risk countries and a detailed list of those for whom the vaccine is recommended (CDC, 2025b).

CONCLUSION

This chapter has examined the definitions of health and prevention and the utilization of those definitions in the provision of primary preventive services, both as a national initiative and for individual clinicians. Readers are encouraged to use this information, in conjunction with frequently updated guidelines from the USPSTF, CDC, and other organizations, in the development of management plans addressing the total healthcare needs of individuals across the lifespan. Links to the websites of the USPSTF, CDC, and additional resources for clinicians are listed in **Table 6-3**. Clinicians may be particularly interested in the USPSTF Electronic Preventive Services Selector (the ePSS app), which can be downloaded to most mobile devices. Given that the recommendations for preventive services are frequently updated in response to the ongoing work of the USPSTF, readers are advised to use ePSS or regularly consult the USPSTF website for changes.

References

American Academy of Family Physicians. (2024). *Primary care.* https://www.aafp.org/about/policies/all/primary-care.html

American College of Nurse-Midwives. (2024). *Position statement: Immunization throughout the life course including in pregnancy and postpartum.* https://midwife.org/wp-content/uploads/2024/10/Immunization-Throughout-the-Life-Course-Including-In-Pregnancy-and-Postpartum.pdf

American College of Obstetricians and Gynecologists. (2023, December 11). *Maternal respiratory syncytial virus vaccination.* https://www.acog.org/clinical/clinical-guidance/practice-advisory/articles/2023/09/maternal-respiratory-syncytial-virus-vaccination#:~:text=AAP's%20Policy%20Statement.-,ACOG%20Recommendations,prevent%20RSV%20LRTI%20in%20infants.

American Geriatrics Society Workgroup on Vitamin D Supplementation for Older Adults. (2014). Recommendations abstracted from the American Geriatrics Society consensus statement on vitamin D for prevention of falls and their consequences. *Journal of the American Geriatric Society, 62*(1), 147-152. https://doi.org/10.1111/jgs.12631

Centers for Disease Control and Prevention. (1989). Health objectives for the nation. *Morbidity and Mortality Weekly Report, 38*(37), 629–633. https://www.cdc.gov/mmwR/preview/mmwrhtml/00001462.htm

Centers for Disease Control and Prevention. (2020). *Cost of older adult falls.* https://stacks.cdc.gov/view/cdc/122747

Centers for Disease Control and Prevention. (2021, July 22). *Sexually transmitted infections treatment guidelines, 2021.* https://www.cdc.gov/std/treatment-guidelines/toc.htm

Centers for Disease Control and Prevention. (2022). *Breastfeeding report card.* https://www.cdc.gov/breastfeeding-data/breastfeeding-report-card/?CDC_AAref_Val=https://www.cdc.gov/breastfeeding/data/reportcard.htm

Centers for Disease Control and Prevention. (2023, September 22). *CDC recommends new vaccine to help protect babies against severe respiratory syncytial virus (RSV) illness after birth.* https://www.cdc.gov/media/releases/2023/p0922-RSV-maternal-vaccine.html#:~:text=On%20September%2022%2C%202023%2C%20members,respiratory%20tract%20infection%20in%20infants

Centers for Disease Control and Prevention. (2023, October 18). *Many older adults don't protect their skin from the sun.* https://www.cdc.gov/cancer/research/many-older-adults-dont-protect-their-skin-from-the-sun.html#:~:text=Background,Wear%20a%20long%2Dsleeved%20shirt.

Centers for Disease Control and Prevention. (2024a, October 4). *About chronic diseases.* https://www.cdc.gov/chronic-disease/about/index.html

Centers for Disease Control and Prevention. (2024b, May 15). *About women and heart disease.* https://www.cdc.gov/heart-disease/about/women-and-heart-disease.html

Centers for Disease Control and Prevention. (2024c, March 11). *Breast cancer risk factors.* https://www.cdc.gov/breast-cancer/risk-factors/index.html

Centers for Disease Control and Prevention. (2024d, September 17). *Current cigarette smoking among adults in the United States.* https://www.cdc.gov/tobacco/php/data-statistics/adult-data-cigarettes/index.html

Centers for Disease Control and Prevention. (2024e, May 16). *Facts about falls.* https://www.cdc.gov/falls/data-research/facts-stats/index.html

Centers for Disease Control and Prevention. (2024f, April 24). *Facts about seat belt use.* https://www.cdc.gov/seat-belts/facts/index.html

Centers for Disease Control and Prevention. (2024g, August 14). *Immunization schedules: For healthcare providers.* https://www.cdc.gov/vaccines/hcp/imz-schedules/index.html

Centers for Disease Control and Prevention, Kochanek, K. D., Murphy, S. L., Xu, J., & Arias, E. (2024h, March). *Mortality in the United States, 2022.* https://www.cdc.gov/nchs/products/databriefs/db492.htm#section_2

Centers for Disease Control and Prevention. (2024i, May 14). *Unintended pregnancy.* https://www.cdc.gov/reproductive-health/hcp/unintended-pregnancy/index.html

Centers for Disease Control and Prevention. (2025a, January 30). *How Mpox spreads.* https://www.cdc.gov/mpox/causes/?CDC_AAref_Val=https://www.cdc.gov/poxvirus/mpox/if-sick/transmission.html

Centers for Disease Control and Prevention. (2025b, February 14). *Mpox vaccination.* https://www.cdc.gov/mpox/vaccines/index.html

Centers for Medicare & Medicaid Services. (2024). *National health expenditure data: Historical.* https://www.cms.gov/data-research/statistics-trends-and-reports/national-health-expenditure-data/historical

Food and Drug Administration. (2020, December 11). *FDA news release: FDA takes key action in fight against COVID-19 by issuing emergency use authorization for first COVID-19 vaccine.* https://www.fda.gov/news-events/press-announcements/fda-takes-key-action-fight-against-covid-19-issuing-emergency-use-authorization-first-covid-19

Food and Drug Administration. (2024, September 11). *Key facts about vaccines to prevent Mpox disease.* https://www.fda.gov/vaccines-blood-biologics/vaccines/key-facts-about-vaccines-prevent-mpox-disease#:~:text=On%20August%209%2C%202022%2C%20FDA,dose%20series%2C%204%20weeks%20apart.

Germann, K., Kiefer, M. K., Rood, K. M., Mehl, R., Wu, J., Pandit, R., Lynch, C. D., Landon, M. B., Grobman, W. A., Costantine, M. M., & Venkatesh, K. K. (2022). Association of initial COVID-19 vaccine hesitancy with subsequent vaccination among pregnant and postpartum individuals. *BJOG: An International Journal of Obstetrics and Gynaecology, 129*(8), 1352–1360. https://doi.org/10.1111/1471-0528.17189

Health Resources and Services Administration. (2024). *Women's preventative services guidelines.* https://www.hrsa.gov/womens-guidelines

Healthy People 2030. (n.d. -a). *Browse objectives by topic.* https://odphp.health.gov/healthypeople/objectives-and-data/browse-objectives

Healthy People 2030. (n.d. -b). *Healthy People 2030 framework.* https://odphp.health.gov/healthypeople/about/healthy-people-2030-framework

Healthy People 2030. (n.d. -c). *How has Healthy People changed?* https://odphp.health.gov/healthypeople/about/how-has-healthy-people-changed

Healthy People 2030. (n.d. -d). *Increase the proportion of infants who are breastfed at 1 year.* https://odphp.health.gov/healthypeople/objectives-and-data/browse-objectives/infants/increase-proportion-infants-who-are-breastfed-1-year-mich-16

Healthy People 2030. (n.d. -e). *Increase the proportion of infants who are breastfed exclusively through age 6 months.* https://odphp.health.gov/healthypeople/objectives-and-data/browse-objectives/infants/increase-proportion-infants-who-are-breastfed-exclusively-through-age-6-months-mich-15

Healthy People 2030. (n.d. -f). *LGBT.* https://odphp.health.gov/healthypeople/objectives-and-data/browse-objectives/lgbt

Healthy People 2030. (n.d. -g). *Reduce the proportion of unintended pregnancies – FP-01.* https://health.gov/healthypeople/objectives-and-data/browse-objectives/family-planning/reduce-proportion-unintended-pregnancies-fp-01

Healthy People 2030. (n.d. -h). *Vaccination.* https://health.gov/healthypeople/objectives-and-data/browse-objectives/vaccination

Healthy People 2030. (n.d. -i). *Women.* https://odphp.health.gov/healthypeople/objectives-and-data/browse-objectives/women

Kaiser Family Foundation. (2012). *A guide to the Supreme Court's decision on the ACA's Medicaid expansion.* https://www.kff.org/health-reform/issue-brief/a-guide-to-the-supreme-courts-decision/

Kaiser Family Foundation. (2024a). *Health care costs and affordability.* https://www.kff.org/health-policy-101-health-care-costs-and-affordability/?entry=table-of-contents-introduction

Kaiser Family Foundation. (2024b). *How do health expenditures vary across the population?* https://www.kff.org/slideshow/how-health-expenditures-vary-across-the-population-slideshow/

Kaiser Family Foundation. (2024c). *The Affordable Care Act 101.* https://www.kff.org/health-policy-101-the-affordable-care-act/?entry=table-of-contents-what-is-the-affordable-care-act

Kaiser Family Foundation. (2024d). *Status of state Medicaid expansion decisions: Interactive* https://www.kff.org/affordable-care-act/issue-brief/status-of-state-medicaid-expansion-decisions-interactive-map/

Kelly, M. K., Stephens-Shields, A. J., Hannan, C., Rand, C. M., Localio, R., Shone, L. P., Steffes, J., Davis, K., Grundmeier, R. W., Humiston, S. G., Albertin, C., McFarland, G., Abney, D. E., Szilagyi, P. G., & Fiks, A. G. (2023). Missed opportunities for adolescent immunizations at well-care visits during the COVID-19 pandemic. *The Journal of Adolescent Health: Official Publication of the Society for Adolescent Medicine, 73*(3), 595–598. https://doi.org/10.1016/j.jadohealth.2023.05.008

Lawrence, B. J., Kerr, D., Pollard, C. M., Theophilus, M., Alexander, E., Haywood, D., & O'Conner, M. (2021) Weight bias among health care professionals: A systematic review and meta-analysis. *Obesity, 29*(11), 1802–1812. https://doi.org/10.1002/oby.23266

Leininger, M. M. (1985). Transcultural care diversity and universality: A theory of nursing. *Nursing and Health Care, 6*, 209–212.

Lim, S. A., Khorrami, A., & Wassersug, R. J. (2022). Twenty years on—has patient-centered care been equally well integrated among medical specialties? *Postgraduate Medical Journal, 134*(1), 20–25. https://doi.org/10.1080/00325481.2021.2009237

Loskutova, N. Y., Smail, C., Callen, E., Staton, E. W., Nazir, N., Webster, B., & Pace, W. D. (2020). Effects of multicomponent primary care-based intervention on immunization rates and missed opportunities to vaccinate adults. *BMC Family Practice, 21*(1), 46. https://doi.org/10.1186/s12875-020-01115-y

Lu, P. J., Hung, M. C., Srivastav, A., Grohskopf, L. A., Kobayashi, M., Harris, A. M., Dooling, K. L., Markowitz, L. E., Rodriguez-Lainz, A., & Williams, W. W. (2021). Surveillance of vaccination coverage among adult populations—United States, 2018. *Morbidity and mortality weekly report. Surveillance summaries, 70*(3), 1–26. https://doi.org/10.15585/mmwr.ss7003a1

Melnyk, B. M., & Fineout-Overholt, E. (2005). *Evidence-based practice in nursing and healthcare: A guide to best practices.* Lippincott, Williams, & Wilkins.

Melnyk, B. M., & Fineout-Overholt, E. (2023). *Evidence-based practice in nursing and healthcare: A guide to best practices* (5th ed.). Wolters Kluwer.

National Center for Health Statistics. (2015). *Healthy People 2000.* https://www.cdc.gov/nchs/healthy_people/hp2000.htm

National Center for Health Statistics. (2020). *Healthy People 2030.* https://www.cdc.gov/nchs/healthy_people/hp2030.htm

National Institute on Alcohol Abuse and Alcoholism. (2023, September 14). *How to apply the NIAAA core resource on alcohol in clinical practice.* https://www.niaaa.nih.gov/sites/default/files/How-to-Apply-the-Core-Resource-on-Alcohol-in-Clinical-Practice.pdf

Olson, S. M., Muñoz, E. G., Solis, E. C., & Bradford, H. M. (2023). Mitigating weight bias in the clinical setting: A new approach to care. *Journal of Midwifery & Women's Health, 69*(2), 180–190. https://doi.org/10.1111/jmwh.13578

Passeron, T., Lim, H. W., Goh, C. L., Kang, H. Y., Ly, F., Morita, A., Ocampo Candiani, J., Puig, S., Schalka, S., Wei, L., Dreno, B. & Krutmann, J. (2021). Photoprotection according to skin phototype and dermatoses: Practical recommendations from an expert panel. *Journal of the European Academy of Dermatology and Venereology, 35*(7), 1460–1469. https://doi.org/10.1111/jdv.17242

Promoting Healthcare Choice and Competition Across the United States, 82 F.R. 48385 (proposed October 17, 2017). https://www.federalregister.gov/documents/2017/10/17/2017-22677/promoting-healthcare-choice-and-competition-across-the-united-states

Rogers, M. E. (1970). *An introduction to the theoretical basis of nursing.* Davis.

Rubino, F., Puhl, R. M., Cummings, D. E., Eckel, R. H., Ryan, D. H., Mechanick, J. I., Nadglowski, J., Ramos Salas, X., Schauer, P. R., Twenefour, D., Apovian, C. M., Aronne, L. J., Batterham, R. L., Berthoud, H. R., Boza, C., Busetto, L., Dicker, D., De Groot, M., Eisenberg, D., . . . Dixon, J. B. (2020) Joint international consensus statement for ending stigma of obesity. *Nature Medicine, 26*, 485–497. https://doi.org/10.1038/s41591-020-0803-x

Ryan, G. W., Perry, S. S., Scherer, A., Charlton, M. E., Ashida, S., Gilbert, P. A., & Askelson, N. (2022). Factors contributing to missed opportunities for human papillomavirus vaccination among adolescents, ages 11 to 13, in Iowa. *Vaccine: X, 11*, 100192. https://doi.org/10.1016/j.jvacx.2022.100192

Surveillance, Epidemiology, and End Results Program. (2024). *Cancer stat facts: Common cancer sites.* https://seer.cancer.gov/statfacts/html/common.html

Tax Cuts and Jobs Act, Pub. L. No. 115-97, Title I Part VIII § 11081 (2017). https://www.congress.gov/bill/115th-congress/house-bill/1

U.S. Preventive Services Task Force. (n.d. -a). *Immunizations for adults.* https://www.uspreventiveservicestaskforce.org/uspstf/recommendation/immunizations-for-adults

U.S. Preventative Services Task Force. (n.d. -b). Motor vehicle occupant restraints: Counseling. https://www.uspreventiveservicestaskforce.org/uspstf/recommendation/motor-vehicle-occupant-restraints-counseling

U.S. Preventive Services Task Force. (1996). *Guide to clinical preventive services* (3nd ed.). Williams & Wilkins. https://www.ncbi.nlm.nih.gov/books/NBK15435/

U.S. Preventive Services Task Force. (2002). *Guide to clinical preventive services* (3rd ed.). https://www.ncbi.nlm.nih.gov/books/NBK15435/

U.S. Preventive Services Task Force. (2014). The guide to clinical preventive services 2014: Recommendations of the U.S. Preventive Services Task Force. Agency for

Healthcare Research and Quality. https://www.ahrq.gov/sites/default/files/wysiwyg/professionals/clinicians-providers/guidelines-recommendations/guide/cpsguide.pdf

U.S. Preventive Services Task Force. (2016). *Final recommendation statement: Breastfeeding: Primary care behavioral counseling interventions.* https://www.uspreventiveservicestaskforce.org/uspstf/recommendation/breastfeeding-primary-care-interventions

U.S. Preventive Services Task Force. (2017). *Healthful diet and physical activity for cardiovascular disease prevention in adults without known risk factors: Behavioral counseling.* https://www.uspreventiveservicestaskforce.org/Page/Document/UpdateSummaryFinal/healthful-diet-and-physical-activity-for-cardiovascular-disease-prevention-in-adults-without-known-risk-factors-behavioral-counseling

U.S. Preventive Services Task Force, Grossman, D. C., Curry, S. J., Owens, D. K., Barry, M. J., Caughey, A. B., Davidson, K. W., Doubeni, C. A., Epling, J. W., Jr., Kemper, A. R., Krist, A. H., Kubik, M., Landefeld, S., Mangione, C. M., Silverstein, M., Simon, M. A., & Tseng, C. W. (2018a). Behavioral counseling to prevent skin cancer: U.S. Preventive Services Task Force recommendation statement. *JAMA, 319*(11), 1134–1142. https://doi.org/10.1001/jama.2018.1623

U.S. Preventive Services Task Force, Curry, S. J., Krist, A. H., Owens, D. K., Barry, M. J., Caughey, A. B., Davidson, K. W., Doubeni, C. A., Epling, J. W., Jr., Grossman, D. C., Kemper, A. R., Kubik, M., Landefeld, C. S., Mangione, C. M., Phipps, M. G., Silverstein, M., Simon, M. A., Tseng, C. W., & Wong, J. B. (2018b). Behavioral weight loss interventions to prevent obesity-related morbidity and mortality in adults: U.S. Preventive Services Task Force recommendation statement. *JAMA, 320*(11), 1163–1171. https://doi.org/10.1001/jama.2018.13022

U.S. Preventive Services Task Force. (2018c). *Grade definitions.* https://www.uspreventiveservicestaskforce.org/uspstf/about-uspstf/methods-and-processes/grade-definitions

U.S. Preventive Services Task Force, Curry, S. J., Krist, A. H., Owens, D. K., Barry, M. J., Caughey, A. B., Davidson, K. W., Doubeni, C. A., Epling, J. W., Jr., Kemper, A. R., Kubik, M., Landefeld, C. S., Mangione, C. M., Silverstein, M., Simon, M. A., Tseng, C. W., & Wong, J. B. (2018d). Screening and behavioral counseling interventions to reduce unhealthy alcohol use in adolescents and adults: U.S. Preventive Services Task Force recommendation statement. *JAMA, 320*(18), 1899–1909. https://doi.org/10.1001/jama.2018.16789

U.S. Preventive Services Task Force, Curry, S. J., Krist, A. H., Owens, D. K., Barry, M. J., Caughey, A. B., Davidson, K. W., Doubeni, C. A., Epling, J. W., Jr., Grossman, D. C., Kemper, A. R., Kubik, M., Landefeld, C. S., Mangione, C. M., Silverstein, M., Simon, M. A., Tseng, C. W., & Wong, J. B. (2019a). Interventions to prevent perinatal depression: U.S. Preventive Services Task Force recommendation statement. *JAMA, 321*(6), 580–587. https://doi.org/10.1001/jama.2019.0007

U.S. Preventive Services Task Force, Owens, D. K., Davidson, K. W., Krist, A. H., Barry, M. J., Cabana, M., Caughey, A. B., Doubeni, C. A., Epling, J. W., Jr, Kubik, M., Landefeld, C. S., Mangione, C. M., Pbert, L., Silverstein, M., Simon, M. A., Tseng, C. W., & Wong, J. B. (2019b). Risk assessment, genetic counseling, and genetic testing for BRCA-related cancer: US Preventive Services Task Force recommendation statement. *JAMA, 322*(7), 652–665. https://doi.org/10.1001/jama.2019.10987

U.S. Preventive Services Task Force, Krist, A. H., Davidson, K. W., Mangione, C. M., Barry, M. J., Cabana, M., Caughey, A. B., Donahue, K., Doubeni, C. A., Epling, J. W., Jr., Kubik, M., Ogedegbe, G., Pbert, L., Silverstein, M., Simon, M. A., Tseng, C. W., & Wong, J. B. (2020a). Behavioral counseling interventions to prevent sexually transmitted infections: U.S. Preventive Services Task Force recommendation statement. *JAMA, 324*(7), 674–681. https://doi.org/10.1001/jama.2020.13095

U.S. Preventive Services Task Force, Krist, A. H., Davidson, K. W., Mangione, C. M., Barry, M. J., Cabana, M., Caughey, A. B., Donahue, K., Doubeni, C. A., Epling, J. W., Jr., Kubik, M., Landefeld, S., Ogedegbe, G., Pbert, L., Silverstein, M., Simon, M. A., Tseng, C. W., & Wong, J. B. (2020b). Behavioral counseling interventions to promote a healthy diet and physical activity for cardiovascular disease prevention in adults with cardiovascular risk factors: U.S. Preventive Services Task Force recommendation statement. *JAMA, 324*(20), 2069–2075. https://doi.org/10.1001/jama.2020.21749

U.S. Preventive Services Task Force, Owens, D. K., Davidson, K. W., Krist, A. H., Barry, M. J., Cabana, M., Caughey, A. B., Curry, S. J., Donahue, K., Doubeni, C. A., Epling, J. W., Jr., Kubik, M., Ogedegbe, G., Pbert, L., Silverstein, M., Simon, M. A., Tseng, C. W., & Wong, J. B. (2020c). Primary care interventions for prevention and cessation of tobacco use in children and adolescents: U.S. Preventive Services Task Force recommendation statement. *JAMA, 323*(16), 1590–1598. https://doi.org/10.1001/jama.2020.4679

U.S. Preventive Services Task Force, Krist, A. H., Davidson, K. W., Mangione, C. M., Barry, M. J., Cabana, M., Caughey, A. B., Donahue, K., Doubeni, C. A., Epling, J. W., Jr., Kubik, M., Ogedegbe, G., Pbert, L., Silverstein, M., Simon, M. A., Tseng, C. W., & Wong, J. B. (2021a). Interventions for tobacco smoking cessation in adults, including pregnant persons: U.S. Preventive Services Task Force recommendation statement. *JAMA, 325*(3), 265–279. https://doi.org/10.1001/jama.2020.25019

U.S. Preventative Services Task Force. (2021b). *USPSTF: An overview.* https://www.uspreventiveservicestaskforce.org/uspstf/about-uspstf/task-force-resources/uspstf-overview

U.S. Preventative Services Task Force. (2024). *Final recommendation statement—Falls prevention in community-dwelling older adults: Interventions.* https://www.uspreventiveservicestaskforce.org/uspstf/recommendation/falls-prevention-community-dwelling-older-adults-interventions

World Health Organization. (2020, March 11). *WHO Director-General's opening remarks at the media briefing on COVID-19 – 11 March 2020.* https://www.who.int/director-general/speeches/detail/who-director-general-s-opening-remarks-at-the-media-briefing-on-covid-19---11-march-2020

World Health Organization. (2024). *What is the WHO definition of health?* https://www.who.int/about/frequently-asked-questions

Yadav, T., Kumar, S., Mishra, G., & Saxena, S. K. (2023). Tracking the COVID-19 vaccines: The global landscape. *Human Vaccines & Immunotherapeutics, 19*(1), 2191577. https://doi.org/10.1080/21645515.2023.2191577

CHAPTER 7

Gynecologic Anatomy and Physiology

Nicole R. Clark

A focus on health encourages everyone to be knowledgeable about their bodies, to appreciate their unique form and function, and to take responsibility for caring and making decisions about their bodies that will positively affect their health. This chapter reviews what has traditionally been labeled female anatomy and physiology and discusses how these body parts and processes directly affect the individual's gynecologic health and well-being. It is important to note that some individuals are born with a genital anatomy that does not appear to fit the standard binary definitions of female or male. The term intersex, also referred to as differences of sex development (DSD), is an umbrella term that refers to a range of congenital variations. The variations can involve many factors, including genital ambiguity, unexpected chromosomal genotype, hormonal variations, or differences in sexual phenotype (Garland et al., 2021).

Since not all people assigned female at birth identify as female or women, it is imperative for clinicians to ensure that the care provided is appropriate for the individual's anatomy and physiology and is provided with respect for the person's gender identity.

PELVIC ANATOMY

Pelvic Bones and Pelvic Joints

The pelvis is composed of (1) two hip bones, also known as coxal bone or pelvic bone; (2) the sacrum; and (3) the coccyx. The hip bones consist of the pubis, the ischium, and the ilium, all of which are fused together at the acetabulum (Hoffman et al., 2020a). The ilium comprises the posterior and upper portion of the hip bone, forming what is known as the iliac crest. It articulates with the sacroiliac joint posteriorly, and together with its ligaments is the major contributor to pelvic stability. The pubic bones articulate anteriorly with the symphysis pubis and, with their inferior angles from the descending rami, form the important bony landmark of the pubic arch (**Figure 7-1**). The ischial spines are bony prominences that are clinically important because they are used as landmarks when performing pudendal blocks and in other medical procedures, such as sacrospinous ligament suspension (Nunziato & Valea, 2022). The ischial spines are also used to assess the progression of fetal descent during childbirth.

The sacrum and the coccyx shape the posterior portion of the pelvis. The sacrum is formed by the fusion of the five sacral vertebrae; it includes the important bony landmark of the sacral promontory and joins the coccyx at the sacrococcygeal symphysis. The coccyx is formed by the fusion of four rudimentary vertebrae, is usually movable, and is itself a key bony landmark. The "true pelvis" constitutes the bony passageway through which a fetus must maneuver to be born vaginally.

The Caldwell-Moloy pelvis classification is widely known, and includes four basic pelvic types: gynecoid, android, anthropoid, and platypelloid (Caldwell & Moloy, 1933) (**Figure 7-2**). Each pelvic type is classified in accordance with the characteristics of the posterior segment of the inlet. However, as research has progressed, it becomes apparent that most pelvises are not pure types, and most individuals do not have pelvises that fit neatly into these categories (VanSickle et al., 2022). Consequently, this classification system is no longer considered reliable or predictive.

Pelvic Support

Pelvic support structures include not only the muscles and connective tissue of the pelvic floor, but also the fibromuscular tissue of the vaginal wall and endopelvic connective tissue (Hoffman et al., 2020a). The piriformis and obturator internus muscles and their fasciae form part of the walls of the pelvic cavity. The piriformis muscle originates at the front of the sacrum, near the third and fourth sacral foramina. This muscle leaves the pelvis by passing laterally through the greater sciatic foramen and inserts in the upper border of the greater trochanter of the femur. The origin of the obturator internus muscle includes the pelvic surfaces of the ilium and ischium and the obturator membrane. It exits the pelvis through the lesser sciatic foramen, where it attaches to the greater trochanter of the hip, enabling it to function in external hip rotation (Hoffman et al., 2020a).

The deep perineal space is a pouch that lies superiorly to the perineal membrane (**Figure 7-3**). The perineal membrane consists of connective tissue also referred to as the parietal fascia, visceral fascia, and extraserosal fascia (Hoffman et al., 2020a). This deep space is continuous with the pelvic cavity and contains the compressor urethrae and urethrovaginal sphincter muscles, the external urethral sphincter, parts of the urethra and vagina, branches of the pudendal artery, and the dorsal nerve and vein of the clitoris (Hoffman et al., 2020a). The perineal membrane (also known as the urogenital diaphragm, although this label is a misnomer) is a sheet made up of dense fibrous tissue that spans the opening of the anterior pelvic outlet. The perineal membrane

FIGURE 7-1 **Pelvic bones.**

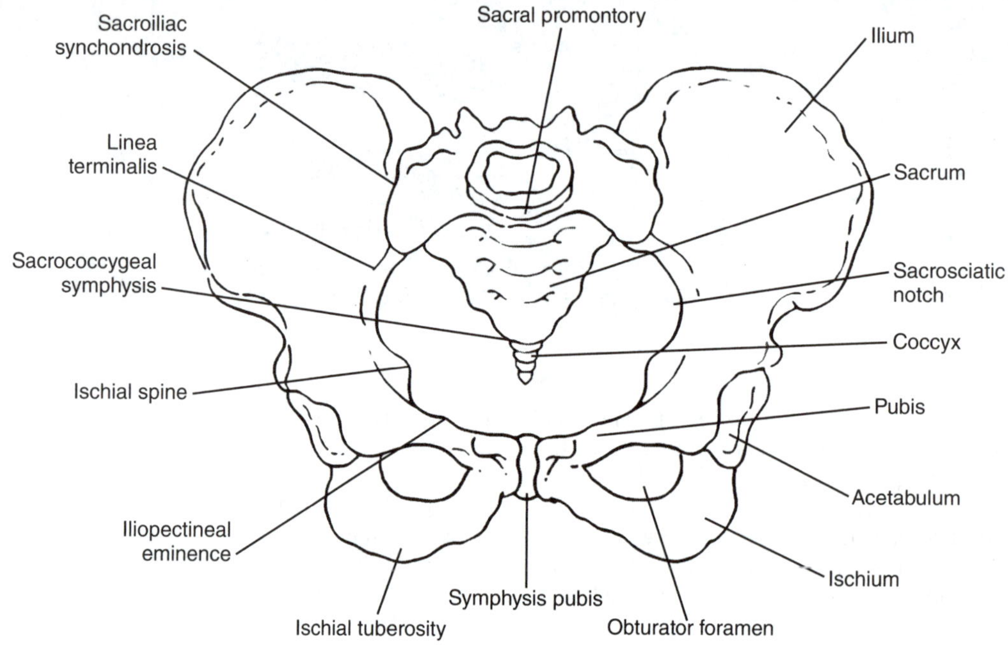

FIGURE 7-2 **Caldwell–Moloy classification of pelvises.**

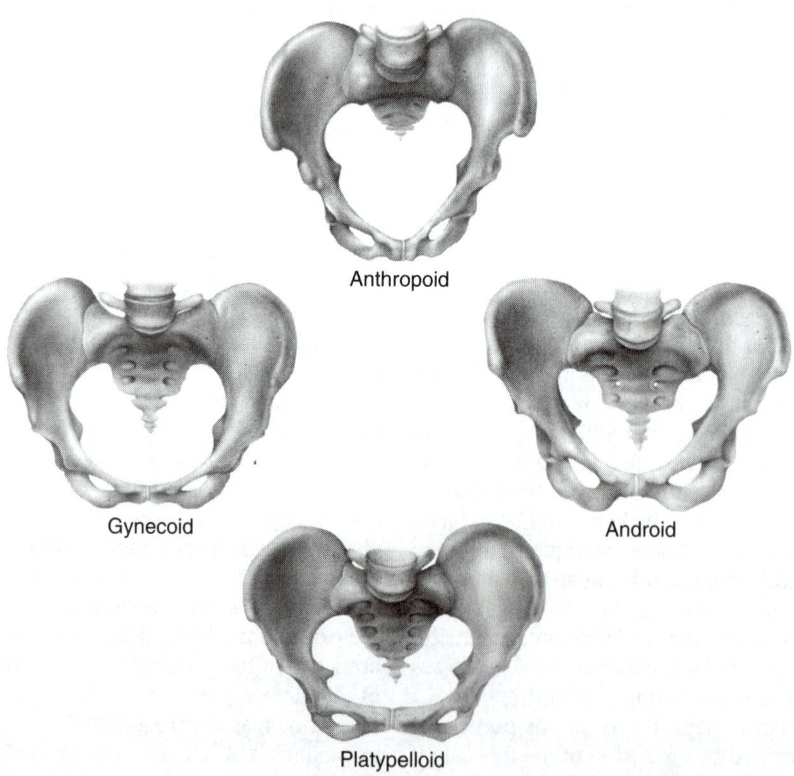

FIGURE 7-3 **Superficial musculature of the perineum.**

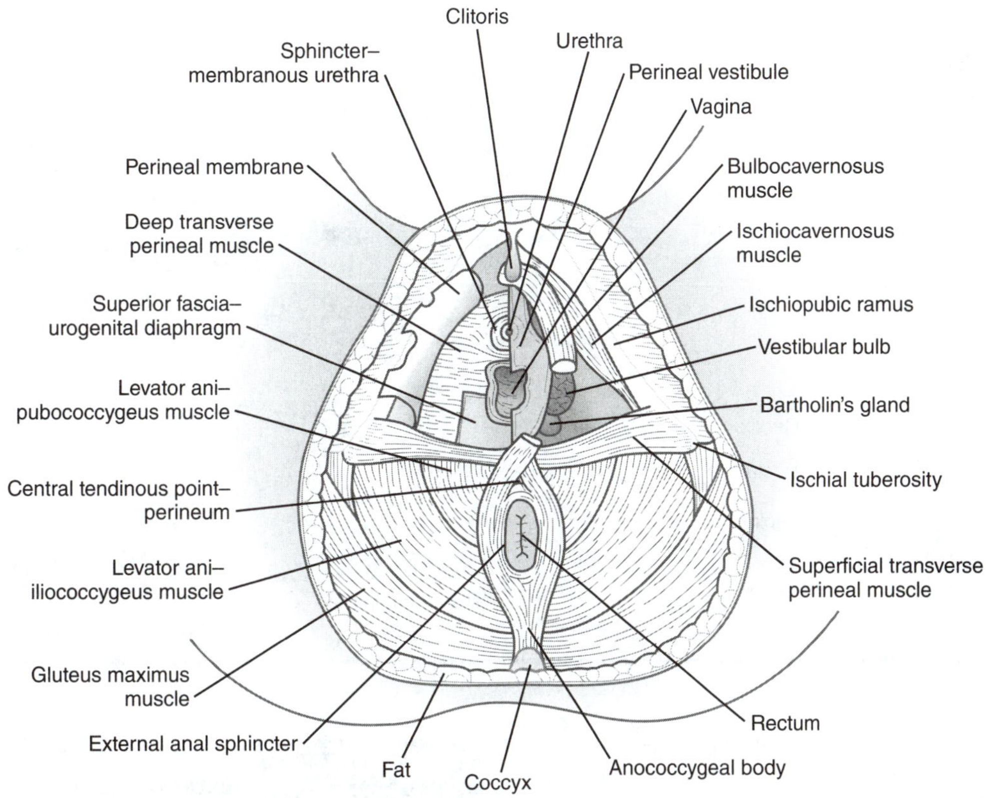

attaches to the side walls of the vagina and provides support to the distal vagina and urethra by attaching these structures to the bony pelvis (Hoffman et al., 2020a).

The levator ani muscle is a critical component of pelvic support; indeed, it is often considered the most important muscle of the pelvic floor (Hoffman et al., 2020a). Normally this muscle is in a constant state of contraction, providing support for all the abdominopelvic contents against intra-abdominal pressures. The levator ani muscle is actually a complex unit of several muscles with different origins, insertions, and functions. The pubococcygeus, puborectalis, and iliococcygeus are the primary components making up this muscle. The pubococcygeus is further divided into the pubovaginalis, puboperinealis, and puboanalis.

The levator ani and coccygeus muscles form the pelvic floor, and the related fascia form a supportive sling for the pelvic contents. The muscle fibers insert at various points in the bony pelvis and form functional sphincters for the vagina, rectum, and urethra. The origin of the levator ani muscle is the pubic bone and the adjacent fascia of the obturator internus muscle. Various portions of this muscular sheet insert on the coccyx (the anococcygeal raphe) and the perineal body, which is a fibrous band lying between the vagina and the rectum. The different sections of the levator ani muscular sheet are subdivided based on the exact origin and insertion of the fibers:

- The levator prostatae or sphincter vaginae fibers form the sling around the vagina and originate from the posterior surface of the pubis; they insert in the perineal body.
- The puborectalis fibers are important in maintaining fecal continence; they originate from the posterior surface of the pubis and form a sling around the rectum.
- The pubococcygeus fibers originate from the posterior surface of the pubis and insert into the anococcygeal raphe.
- The iliococcygeus fibers originate from the obturator internus fascia and the ischium and insert into the anococcygeal raphe.

The fan-shaped coccygeus muscle lies anterior to the sacrospinous ligament, originates from the ischial spine, inserts into the lower part of the sacrum and coccyx, and works synergistically to aid the levator ani muscle. The transverse perinei are small strap-like muscles that help support the pelvic viscera. They originate from the ischial tuberosity, pass by the genitalia, and insert in the central tendon at the midline. The bulbocavernosus muscles aid in strengthening the pelvic diaphragm and in constricting the urinary and vaginal openings. Their muscle fibers originate in the perineal body and surround the vaginal openings as the muscle fibers pass forward to insert into the pubis. The ischiocavernosus muscle contracts to cause erection of the clitoris during sexual arousal. Its muscle fibers originate in the tuberosities of the ischium and continue at an angle to insert next to the bulbocavernosus muscle (Hoffman et al., 2020a).

GENITALIA

This section describes the multiple organs and anatomic structures that constitute a gynecologic anatomy. These are shown in

FIGURE 7-4 **Midsagittal view of the pelvic organs.**

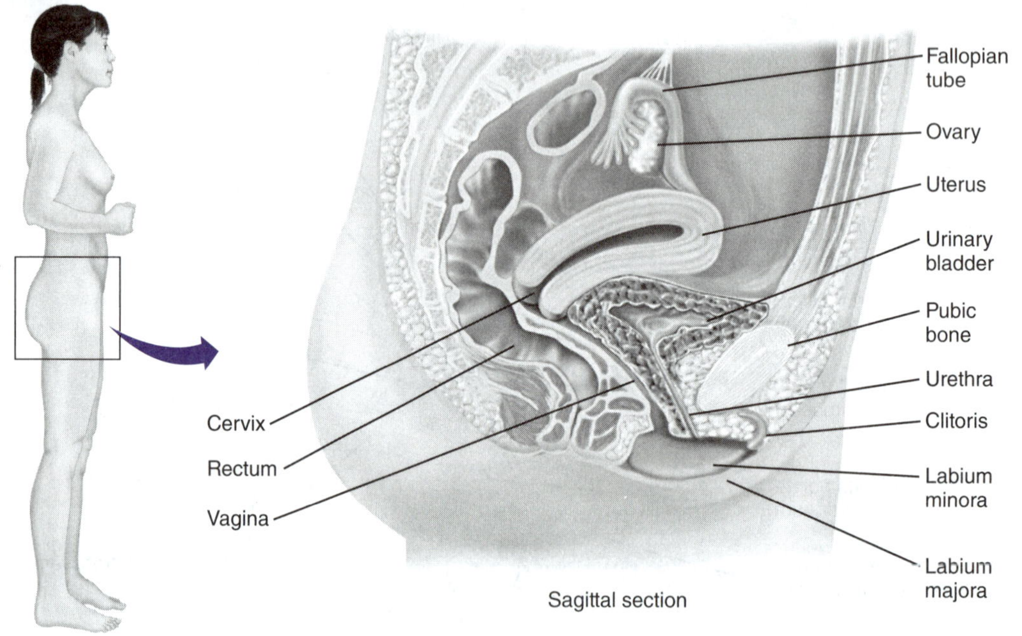

a midsagittal view in **Figure 7-4**. Equally important to the anatomical discussion are the multiple nongenital peripheral anatomic structures involved in sexual responses, such as salivary and sweat glands, cutaneous blood vessels, and breasts.

External Genital Anatomy

Vulva

The vulva is the externally visible outer genitalia (**Figure 7-5**). It includes the mons pubis, labia minora, labia majora, clitoris, urinary meatus, vaginal opening, and corpus spongiosum erectile tissue (vestibular bulbs) of the labia minora and perineum. The vestibule is inside the labia minora and outside the hymen. On each side of the vestibule is a Bartholin gland, which secretes lubricating mucus into the introitus during sexual excitement. The mons pubis is the mound-like fatty tissue that covers and protects the symphysis pubis. During puberty, genital hair growth covers this pad of tissue.

The labia majora are fused anteriorly with the mons veneris (or anterior prominence of the symphysis pubis) and posteriorly with the perineal body (or posterior commissure). They assist in keeping the vaginal introitus closed, which in turn helps prevent infection. The labia minora are surrounded by the labia majora and are smaller, nonfatty folds covered by non-hair-bearing skin laterally and by vaginal mucosa on the medial aspect. The anterior aspect of the labia minora forms the prepuce of the clitoris and also assists in enclosing the opening of the urethra and the vagina.

Vulvae vary in size, related to the amount of adipose tissue, length, and pigmentation of the labia minora or majora, which may be light pink, dark pink, or shades of gray, peach, brown, or black. There is also considerable variation in the size of the labia minora.

FIGURE 7-5 **External genitalia.**

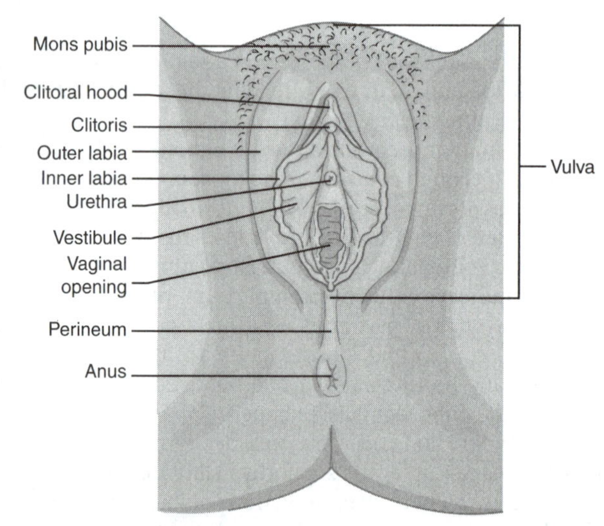

Clitoris

Anatomically, the clitoris is formed from the genital tubercle (Hoffman et al., 2020a). The body measures approximately 2 to 3 cm long, consists of two crura and two corpora cavernosa, and is covered by a sensitive rounded tubercle known as the glans (Nunziato & Valea, 2022). The clitoris is a small, sensitive organ that consists of two paired erectile chambers and is located at the superior portion of the vestibule (Nunziato & Valea, 2022). These chambers are composed of endothelial-lined lacunar spaces, trabecular smooth muscle, and trabecular connective tissue; they are surrounded by a fibrous sheath, the tunica albuginea. The paired corpus spongiosum (bilateral vestibular bulbs) unite ventrally to the urethral orifice to form a thin strand of spongy erectile tissue (pars intermedia) that ends in the clitoris as the glans (Nunziato & Valea, 2022). The clitoris is capped externally by the glans, which is covered by a clitoral hood formed in part by the fusion of the upper part of the two labia minora.

The clitoris has numerous nerve endings and contains tissue that fills with blood with sexual arousal. The blood supply to this organ includes the dorsal and clitoral cavernosal arteries, which arise from the iliohypogastric pudendal bed. The autonomic efferent motor innervation occurs via the cavernosal nerve of the clitoris arising from the pelvic and hypogastric plexus (Hoffman et al., 2020a).

The labia minora, together with the clitoris, play a critical role in sexual activity. Because of their rich nerve and vascular supply, they are easily sensitized and become engorged with blood during sexual arousal. This vascular erectile tissue is capable of becoming significantly enlarged and tense during sexual excitement. In addition to the great quantity of erectile tissue in the clitoris, erectile tissue is found inside the labia majora and minora, around the vulvovaginal opening, and along the lower third of the vagina. A very small quantity of this tissue can also be found in the vaginal walls and along the urethra. Age-associated sexual dysfunction from decreased clitoral sensitivity may be associated with histologic changes in clitoral cavernosal erectile tissue (Cowley et al., 2022).

Periurethral Glands

Two Skene (paraurethral) glands open directly into the vulva and are adjacent to the distal urethra (Nunziato & Valea, 2022). The Skene glands, which release mucus, form a triangular area of mucous membrane surrounding the urethral meatus from the clitoral glans to the vaginal upper rim or caruncle (Hoffman et al., 2020a).

Bartholin or Greater Vestibular Glands

The pea-sized Bartholin glands are located at about the 4 and 8 o'clock positions in the vulvovaginal area, just beneath the fascia. Each gland has an approximately 2 cm duct that opens into a groove between the labia minora and hymen. The glands, which are made of columnar cells that secrete clear or whitish mucus, are stimulated during sexual arousal (Hoffman et al., 2020a). If the Bartholin ducts are blocked, infection can occur, resulting in cyst formation that can lead to the development of an abscess requiring surgical incision and drainage.

Internal Genital Anatomy

Urethra

The urethra is a short conduit, approximately 3.5 to 5 cm long, extending from the base of the bladder and exiting externally to the vestibule (Nunziato & Valea, 2022). The urethral mucosa is composed of stratified transitional epithelium near the urinary bladder; the remaining one-third is lined by a stratified squamous epithelium (Nunziato & Valea, 2022). The urethra passes through the urogenital diaphragm, which is a circular band of skeletal muscle that forms the sphincter urethrae, better known as the external urethral sphincter (Hoffman et al., 2020a). To urinate, this sphincter must be voluntarily relaxed; its typical state is contracted.

Ovaries

The paired ovaries resemble large almonds with their size dependent on age and stage of menstrual cycle; they are located near the lateral walls of the pelvic cavity, and they rest in the ovarian fossa (Hoffman et al., 2020a; Nunziato & Valea, 2022). During reproductive years, each ovary measures approximately 2.5 to 5 cm in length, 1.5 to 3 cm in thickness and 0.7 to 1.5 cm in width (Hoffman et al., 2020a; Nunziato & Valea, 2022). The ovaries become smaller with age (Nunziato & Valea, 2022).

The ovaries produce gametes (also known as ova) and the sex hormones estrogen and progesterone. The color and texture of these organs change with age and reproductive stage. The ovaries in a nulliparous person are situated on a shallow depression called the ovarian fossa, located on either side of the uterus in the upper pelvic cavity. Several ligaments support the ovaries. The broad ligament is the principal supporting membrane of the internal genital organs, including the fallopian tubes and uterus. The remaining ligaments include the mesovarium, a posterior extension of the broad ligament; the ovarian ligament, which is anchored to the uterus; and a suspensory ligament, which is attached to the pelvic wall. The outermost layer of the ovary is composed of a thin layer of cuboidal epithelial cells called the germinal epithelium. Immediately below this epithelial layer is the tunica albuginea, which is made up of collagenous tissue (Nunziato & Valea, 2022).

The ovaries comprise of two parts:

- An outer cortical region (cortex), which is covered by a single layer of cuboidal epithelium contains germinal epithelium, with oogonia and ovarian follicles that number approximately 400,000 at the initiation of puberty (Hoffman et al., 2020a).
- The inner medulla, which consists of fibromuscular tissue, myoid-like contractile cells, and interstitial cells (Hoffman et al., 2020a).

Two ovarian arteries arise from the anterior aorta and descend retroperitoneally. Additional supply arises from ovarian branches of the uterine arteries. (Hoffman et al., 2020a; Nunziato & Valea, 2022). They enter the infundibulopelvic ligaments, finally reaching the mesovarium found in the broad ligament. The ovarian blood supply enters through the hilum, and venous return occurs through a venous plexus, which collects blood from the adnexal region and drains into the vena cava on the right and the renal vein on the left (Hoffman et al., 2020a; Nunziato & Valea, 2022).

Innervation of the ovaries is accomplished by sympathetic and parasympathetic fibers of the ovarian plexus that descend along the ovarian vessels. These nerves supply the ovaries, broad ligaments, and uterine tubes. The parasympathetic fibers in the ovarian plexus arise from the vagus nerves. The nerve fibers to the ovaries innervate only the vascular networks, not the stroma (Nunziato & Valea, 2022). Because the ovaries and surrounding peritoneum are sensitive to pain and pressure, it is important to take great care when examining the ovaries during a bimanual examination.

Fallopian Tubes

The fallopian tubes (also known as oviducts or uterine tubes) are paired narrow muscular tubes that extend approximately 7–12 cm from each cornu of the body of the uterus, outward to their openings near the ovaries (Hoffman et al., 2020a). Each fallopian tube includes four segments:

- The pars interstitialis (intramural portion) penetrates the uterine wall. It contains the fewest mucosal folds, with the myometrium contributing to its muscularis.
- The isthmus, the narrow segment adjacent to the uterine wall, contains few mucosal folds.
- The middle segment, known as the ampulla, is the widest and longest segment. It contains extensive branched mucosal folds and is the most common site of fertilization.
- The infundibulum, the funnel-shaped distal segment, opens near the ovary but is not attached to it. Very fine fingerlike fronds of its mucosal folds, known as fimbriae, project from the opening toward the ovary to help direct the oocyte into the lumen of the fallopian tube (Nunziato & Valea, 2022).

The inner surface of each fallopian tube is covered by fine hairlike structures, called cilia, that help to move ova, when they are released from the ovaries, along the tube and into the cavity of the uterus.

The internal mucosa includes the lamina propria and ciliated columnar epithelium, which consists primarily of three different cell types. On the surface, the abundant ciliated columnar cells beat in waves toward the uterus, aiding in egg transport. Secretory columnar cells comprise 60% of the epithelial lining. Narrow peg cells are interspersed among the ciliated and secretory cells. These cilia propel the film they produce toward the uterus, helping transport the ovum. The muscularis—the middle layer of the fallopian tube wall—contains both inner circular and outer longitudinal smooth muscle layers. Its wavelike contractions move the ovum toward the uterus. The outer covering of the fallopian tubes is the serosa; this lubricative layer is part of the visceral peritoneum (Hoffman et al., 2020a; Nunziato & Valea, 2022).

The ovarian and uterine arteries supply blood to the fallopian tubes. The uterine artery supplies the medial two-thirds of each tube. The uterine veins, which parallel the path of the arteries, provide the venous drainage from this area. Sympathetic and parasympathetic innervation to the fallopian tubes from the hypogastric plexus and pelvic splanchnic nerves regulates the activity of the smooth muscles and blood vessels (Hoffman et al., 2020a; Nunziato & Valea, 2022).

Uterus

The uterus is a fibromuscular, inverted, pear-shaped, hollow, thick-walled organ that opens to the vagina at the cervix and widens toward the top where the uterine tubes enter. Its anatomic regions include the fundus, body, and cervix (**Figure 7-6**). The fundus is the uppermost dome-shaped extension of the uterine body, located above the point of entry of the fallopian tubes. The body is the enlarged main portion. The cervix is the downward constricted extension of the uterus that opens into the vagina.

The uterus lies between the bladder (anteriorly) and the rectum (posteriorly). When the bladder is empty, the uterus angles forward over the bladder. As the bladder fills, the uterus is lifted dorsally and may become retroflexed, pressing against the rectum. The nulliparous uterus is approximately 7 cm long, 5 cm wide, and 2.5 cm thick (Nunziato & Valea, 2022).

The uterine wall of the fundus and body consists of three layers: endometrium, myometrium, and serosa (perimetrium). The uterine mucosa layer consists of a simple columnar epithelium supported by a lamina propria. Simple tubular glands extend from the luminal surface into the lamina propria. The stratum functionale is the temporary layer at the luminal surface that responds to ovarian hormones by undergoing cyclic thickening and shedding. The stratum basale is the deeper, thinner, permanent layer that contains the basal portions of the endometrial glands; this layer is retained during menstruation. The epithelial cells lining these glands divide and cover the raw surface of exposed endometrium during menstruation.

FIGURE 7-6 **Anterior view of internal genital anatomy showing the relationships of the ovaries, fallopian tubes, uterus, cervix, and vagina.**

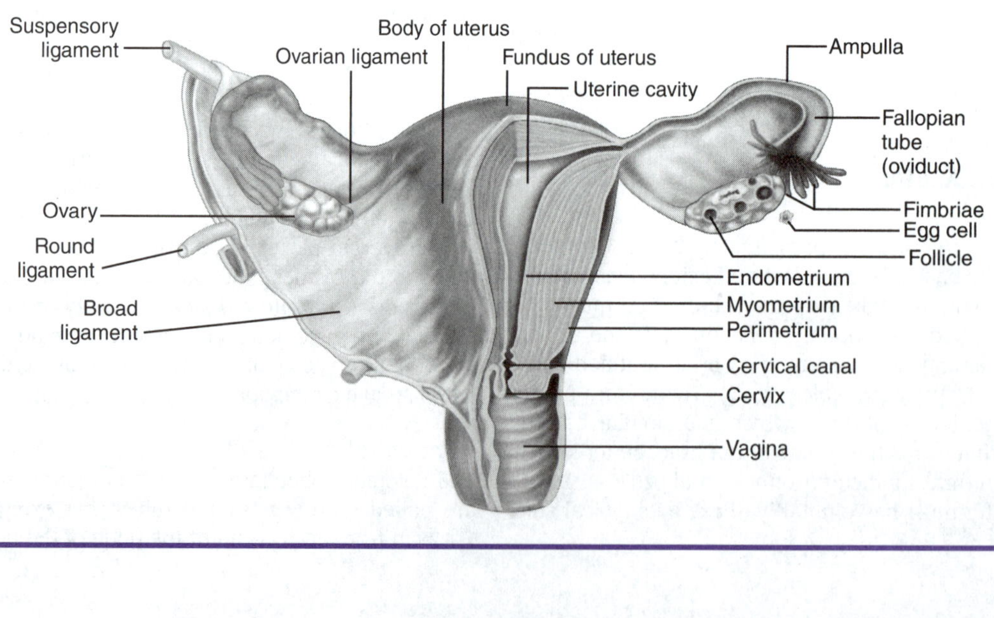

The endometrium receives a double blood supply. In the middle of the myometrium, a pair of uterine arteries branch to form the arcuate arteries. These arteries then bifurcate into two sets of arteries: straight arteries to the stratum basale and coiled arteries to the functionalis. The double blood supply to the endometrium is important in the cyclic shedding of the functionalis; the straight arteries are retained during this process, while the coiled arteries are lost as progesterone levels drop (Hoffman et al., 2020b).

The myometrium is composed of four poorly defined layers of smooth muscle that are thickest at the top of the uterus. The middle layers contain the abundant arcuate arteries. The outer layer of the uterus consists of two types of outer coverings: a cap of serosa covers the fundus and the body is surrounded by an adventitia of loose connective tissue (Hoffman et al., 2020a; Hoffman et al., 2020b).

Structurally, the cervix is made mostly of dense connective tissue, is usually 2.5 to 3 cm in length, and is covered interiorly by a mucus-secreting ciliated epithelium at the upper regions and by stratified squamous epithelium at the vaginal end. The opening of the cervix into the vagina occurs at almost a right angle to the long axis of the vagina. Uterine blood supply is provided via the uterine and ovarian arteries, with venous return traveling via the uterine veins. The hypogastric and ovarian nerve plexuses supply sympathetic and parasympathetic fibers and carry uterine afferent sensory fibers on their way to the spinal cord at T11 and T12 (Hoffman et al., 2020a; Nunziato & Valea, 2022).

Vagina

The vagina is a thin-walled fibromuscular tube extending from the external vulva to the cervix. Its walls are normally in apposition and flattened, but it can extend (stretch) greatly, as observed during childbirth. The length of the vaginal walls varies greatly, but on average the anterior vaginal length is 6 to 9 cm, and the posterior vaginal length is 8 to 12 cm (Hoffman et al., 2020a; Nunziato & Valea, 2022). The upper portion of the vagina encircles the vaginal portion of the cervix. The vagina touches the empty bladder on the ventral and superior surface. Inferiorly, it adheres to the posterior wall of the urethra and opens adjacent to the labia minora.

The internal mucosal layer of the vagina contains transverse known as rugae. This muscular canal extends from the midpoint of the cervix to its opening located between the urethra and the rectum. The mucous membrane lining the vagina and musculature is continuous with the uterus. The vaginal walls can be easily separated because their surfaces are normally moist, lubricated by a basal vaginal fluid.

The vaginal wall is composed of three layers: mucosa, muscle, and adventitia. Vaginal epithelium is stratified squamous epithelium supported by a thick lamina propria. The lamina propria has many thin-walled blood vessels that contribute to diffusion of vaginal fluid across the epithelium. The lamina propria of the mucosa contains many elastic fibers and a dense network of blood vessels, lymph nodes, and a nerve supply. To a much lesser degree than seen in the skin, this epithelium undergoes hormone-related cyclic changes, including slight keratinization of the superficial cells during the menstrual cycle (Hoffman et al., 2020b). The epithelium has no glands, so it does not secrete mucus. Release of estrogen causes the epithelium to thicken, differentiate, and accumulate glycogen. Vaginal bacteria metabolize the glycogen to lactic acid, causing the typically low pH of the vaginal environment.

Loose connective tissue containing many elastic fibers is found underneath the vaginal epithelium, which has a subdermal layer rich in capillaries. This rich vascular supply is the source for vaginal moisture during sexual stimulation (Nunziato & Valea, 2022).

Within the epithelium lie the smooth muscles of the muscularis, which are oriented longitudinally on the outer layer and as circular bundles on the inner layer. The outer layer—the adventitia—consists of dense connective tissue with many elastic fibers, which provides structural support for the vagina. It also contains an extensive nerve supply and venous capillaries. The adventitia is elastic and rich in collagen, provides structural support to the vagina, and allows for expansion of the vagina during intercourse and childbirth.

Some authors describe the vagina wall as having four layers, with the fourth layer consisting of connective tissue housing the large plexus of blood vessels (Nunziato & Valea, 2022). The upper two-thirds of the vagina receive efferent innervation through the uterovaginal plexus, which contains both sympathetic and parasympathetic fibers. The pelvic splanchnic nerves provide the parasympathetic efferent input to the uterovaginal plexus. The proximal two-thirds of the vagina is innervated via the uterovaginal plexus. The lower vagina receives autonomic efferent innervation from the pudendal nerve. The distal one-third of the vagina has primarily somatic sensation; this innervation arises from the pudendal nerve and is carried to the sacral spinal cord (Nunziato & Valea, 2022).

BREAST ANATOMY AND PHYSIOLOGY

The breasts—that is, the mammary glands—are large, modified sebaceous glands contained within the superficial fascia of the chest wall located over the pectoral muscles (Sandadi et al., 2022). Each consists of a nipple, lobes, ducts, and fibrous and fatty tissue. This is shown in **Figure 7-7**. Each breast is composed of 10 to 20 lobes of glandular tissue. The number of lobes

FIGURE 7-7 **Structure of the breast and mammary glands: sagittal section.**

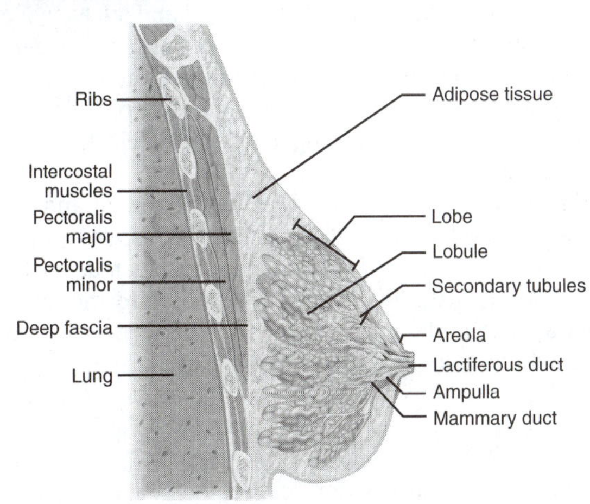

is not related to the size of the breast. The lobes branch to form 10 to 100 lobules per lobe, which are in turn subdivided into many secretory alveoli. These glands are connected together by a series of ducts. The alveoli produce milk and other substances during lactation. Each lobe empties into a single lactiferous duct that travels out through the nipple. As a result, there are 15 to 20 passages through the nipple, resulting in just as many openings in the nipple.

Fatty and connective tissues surround the lobes of glandular tissue. The amount of fatty tissue depends on many factors, including age, the percentage of body fat relative to total body weight, and heredity. Cooper ligaments connect the chest wall to the skin of the breast, giving the breast its shape and elasticity (Sandadi et al., 2022). The size of the breasts in women who are not pregnant reflects the amount of adipose tissue in the breast rather than the amount of glandular tissue. The secretory nature of the breasts develops during pregnancy. After menopause, glandular tissue reverts and is replaced by adipose tissue (Sandadi et al., 2022).

The nipple and areola are located near the center of each breast; the areola is the pigmented area surrounding the nipple. These areas usually have a color and texture that differ from those of the adjacent skin. Notably, the color of the nipple–areolar complex varies and darkens during pregnancy and lactation. The consistency of the nipple and areola may range from very smooth to wrinkled and bumpy. The size of the nipples and areolae also varies a great deal between individuals, and some size variation between an individual's breasts is normal. The nipple and areola are made of smooth muscle fibers and feature a thick network of nerve endings.

The areola is populated by numerous oil-producing Montgomery glands. These glands may form raised bumps and be responsive to the menstrual cycle. They protect and lubricate the nipple during lactation (Sandadi et al., 2022).

The nipple usually protrudes out from the surface of the breast. Some nipples project inward or are flat with the surface of the breast. Neither flat nor inverted nipples appear to affect breastfeeding ability.

Reproductive hormones are vital to the development of the breast during puberty and lactation. Prolactin (PRL) and growth hormone (GH) from the anterior lobe of the pituitary stimulate mammary gland development. These hormones are aided by human placental lactogen from the placenta, which stimulates the mammary gland ducts to become active during pregnancy. Estrogen promotes the growth of the gland and ducts, while progesterone stimulates the development of milk-producing cells. PRL, which is released from the anterior pituitary, stimulates milk production. Oxytocin, which is released from the posterior pituitary in response to suckling, causes milk ejection from the lactating breast.

The lymphatic system in the breast is abundant and empties the breast tissue of excess fluid. Lymph nodes along the pathway of drainage monitor for foreign bodies, such as bacteria or viruses. Although the main flow moves toward the axilla and anterior axillary nodes, lymph drainage has been shown to pass in all directions from the breast (Sandadi et al., 2022).

MENSTRUAL CYCLE PHYSIOLOGY

The initiation of menstruation, called menarche, usually happens between the ages of 12 and 15. Menstrual cycles typically continue until age 45 to 55, when menopause, or the cessation of menstruation, occurs.

Menarche is the most obvious external event that indicates the end of one developmental stage and the beginning of a new one. Widely accepted standards for distinguishing what are regular versus irregular menses, or normal versus abnormal menses, are generally based on what is considered average and not necessarily typical for every individual. According to these standards, the normal menstrual cycle is 21 to 35 days with a menstrual flow lasting 3 to 5 days, although a flow for as few as 2 days or as many as 7 days is still considered normal (Douglas & Lobo, 2022).

The amount of menstrual flow varies, with the average being 50 mL; nevertheless, the volume may be as little as 35 mL or as much as 80 mL. Many people are not aware that anovulatory cycles and abnormal uterine bleeding (changes in bleeding outside of normal) are common after menarche and just prior to menopause (Douglas & Lobo, 2022). See Chapter 25 for more information about abnormal uterine bleeding. Menstrual cycles that occur during the first 1 to 1.5 years after menarche are frequently irregular due to the immaturity of the hypothalamic–pituitary–ovarian axis (Ryntz & Lobo, 2022).

The menstrual cycle is influenced by a complex interaction of hormones. In particular, the monthly rhythmic functioning of the menstrual cycle depends on the changing hormonal concentrations, and numerous patterns in hormone secretion are possible. In fact, it is difficult to find two cycles that are exactly the same. Studies that include women of different ethnicities, occupations, genetics, nutritional status, and age have demonstrated that the length and duration of the menstrual cycle vary widely (Li et al., 2023; Douglas & Lobo, 2022). This variability in menstrual cycle patterns highlights the complex interplay of hormonal regulation controlled by the hypothalamic–pituitary–ovarian (HPO) axis, which regulates the intricate processes underlying reproductive physiology.

The Hypothalamic–Pituitary–Ovarian Axis

Hypothalamus

The hypothalamus controls anterior pituitary functions via the secretion of releasing and inhibiting factors. Together with the pituitary, it manages the production of hormones that serve as chemical messengers for the regulation of the gynecologic system. The hypothalamus initially releases gonadotropin-releasing hormone (GnRH) in a pulsatile manner. On average, the frequency of GnRH secretion is once per 60 to 100 minutes during the early follicular phase, increases to once per 60 to 70 minutes during the middle of the menstrual cycle, then decreases during the luteal phase (Douglas & Lobo, 2022). The release of GnRH stimulates the pituitary gland to produce follicle-stimulating hormone (FSH) and luteinizing hormone (LH). Two other hormones necessary for gynecologic health, estrogen and progesterone, are secreted by the ovaries at the command of FSH and LH.

Pituitary Gland

The oval-shaped, pea-sized pituitary gland is located in a small depression in the sphenoid bone of the skull. It is controlled by the hypothalamus, which secretes releasing factors into a special blood vessel network (hypothalamic–hypophyseal portal system) that feeds the pituicytes (Al-Suhaimi & Khan, 2022). These releasing factors either stimulate or inhibit the release of pituitary hormones that travel via the circulatory system to target organs.

The anterior pituitary synthesizes seven hormones:

- Growth hormone (GH)
- Thyroid-stimulating hormone (TSH)
- Adrenocorticotropin (ACTH)
- Melanocyte-stimulating hormone (MSH)
- Prolactin (PRL)
- Follicle-stimulating hormone (FSH)
- Luteinizing hormone (LH)

FSH and LH (both gonadotropins) are responsible for regulating gynecologic organ activities. FSH targets the ovaries, where it stimulates the growth and development of the primary follicles and results in the production of estrogen and progesterone. The release of FSH from the pituitary is governed by a negative feedback mechanism involving these steroids. In contrast, LH targets the developing follicle within the ovary; it is responsible for ovulation, corpus luteum formation, and hormone production in the ovaries. PRL is responsible for preparing the mammary gland for lactation and brings about the synthesis of milk (Douglas & Lobo, 2022).

Ovaries and Uterus

Complex changes occur in the ovaries and the endometrium as a result of the cyclic fluctuations of gonadotropic hormones. The endometrium emulates the activities of the ovaries; thus, whatever happens in the uterus during the menstrual cycle is precisely correlated with whatever is occurring in the ovaries. The objective of the ovarian cycle is to produce an ovum, while the objective of the endometrial cycle is to prepare a site to nourish and maintain the ovum if it becomes fertilized. The ovarian cycle includes two distinct phases: the follicular phase, and the luteal phase. These two phases are separated by an ovulation period. The endometrial cycle can be divided into the proliferative phase, the secretory phase, and menstruation (Douglas & Lobo, 2022).

Hormonal Feedback System

As mentioned above, the monthly rhythmic functioning of the menstrual cycle depends on the changing concentrations of gonadotropic hormones. The release of LH and FSH from the pituitary depends on the secretion of GnRH from the hypothalamus, which is modulated by the feedback effects of estrogen and progesterone. The hormones LH and FSH, in turn, play important roles in stimulating secretion of estrogen and progesterone.

Almost all hormones are released in short pulses at intervals of 60 to 90 minutes throughout most of the menstrual cycle, with these pulses decreasing in frequency closer to menstruation. Steroid hormones modulate the frequency and amplitude of the pulse, which varies throughout the cycle (Douglas & Lobo, 2022). This is shown in **Figure 7-8**.

Under normal physiologic conditions, GnRH pulses stimulate the release of FSH and LH. As a result of this gonadotropic hormone stimulation, the ovarian follicles develop and produce estrogen. As the amount of estrogen in the circulation increases and reaches the pituitary gland, it affects the amount of FSH and LH secreted, albeit without significantly affecting the pulse frequency (negative feedback).

When the estrogen level becomes high enough, the negative feedback effect on the pituitary is reversed. Now estrogen causes a midcycle positive feedback effect on the pituitary, which results in a surge of LH and FSH and causes ovulation. Under LH influence, the ruptured follicle becomes the corpus luteum and secretes progesterone. Although the presence of progesterone reduces the frequency of the hypothalamic GnRH pulses, the amount of LH released from the pituitary is proportionally increased to sustain the corpus luteum and the production of progesterone. In the absence of pregnancy, the corpus luteum degenerates, progesterone levels decline, and menstruation occurs. The GnRH pulses return to the frequency associated with the beginning of the follicular phase, and a new cycle begins (Douglas & Lobo, 2022).

FIGURE 7-8 Influence of steroid hormones on the ovaries and endometrium.

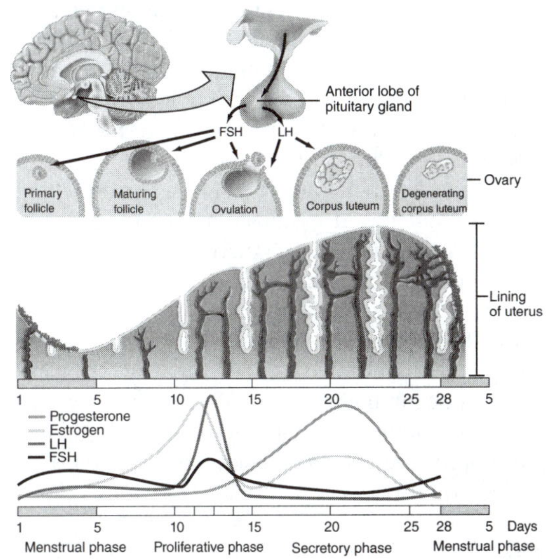

The Ovarian Cycle

The ovarian cycle comprises two phases: follicular and luteal.

Follicular Phase

The follicular phase is characterized by the development of ovarian follicles and usually lasts from day 1 (first day of menses) to day 14 of the ovarian cycle. Folliculogenesis begins during the last few days of the previous menstrual cycle and continues until the release of the mature follicle at ovulation. The decrease in estrogen production by the corpus luteum and the dramatic fall of inhibin levels allow the FSH level to rise during the last few days of the menstrual cycle. During days 2 to 3 of the menstrual cycle, a cohort of primary follicles is recruited from a pool of nonproliferating follicles in response to the increased concentration of FSH (Hoffman et al., 2020b). Follicles that have enough granulosa cells will develop receptors for estrogen and FSH on the cells of the granulosa layers, and LH receptors on the theca cells. The primary role of FSH is to induce the development of increased receptors on the granulosa cells and thereby stimulate estrogen production. The preliminary role of LH is to stimulate the cells' production of androgen that will be converted to estrogen by the granulosa layers.

Between cycle days 5 and 7, only one dominant follicle from the cohort of recruited follicles is destined to ovulate during the next menstrual cycle. As menses progresses, FSH levels decline due to the negative feedback of estrogen and the negative effects of the peptide hormone inhibin, which is secreted by the granulosa and theca cells of the developing follicle (Hoffman et al., 2020b). The decrease in FSH level promotes a more androgenic microenvironment within the adjacent follicles. By the eighth day of the cycle, the dominant follicle (Graafian follicle) is producing more estrogen than the total amount produced by the other developing follicles. In response to the dominant follicle's combined production of estrogen and FSH, LH receptors develop on its outermost granulosa layers. The dominant follicle continues to flourish and gradually moves toward the surface of the ovary. This is shown in **Figure 7-9**. The Graafian follicle contains the ovum and is surrounded by a layer of granulosa cells, which are themselves surrounded by the specialized theca interna and theca externa cells.

When the dominant follicle grows, a cavity forms into which follicular fluid accumulates. This follicular fluid suppresses the final maturation of the dominant follicle until the time of ovulation. The suppressive effects end hours before the LH surge that causes ovulation (Douglas & Lobo, 2022).

Ovulatory Period

Ovulation is the process whereby the mature ovum is released from the follicle (Hoffman et al., 2020b). It occurs approximately 32 hours after the initial rise of the LH surge and about 16 hours after the LH peak; that is, when the highest level of LH is attained (Douglas & Lobo, 2022). Ovulation and the subsequent conversion of the follicle to the corpus luteum are dependent on an increased level of estrogen and the LH surge, which marks the beginning of the rapid rise of LH. During the midfollicular phase, the dominant follicle's FSH levels diminish, but estrogen levels continue to increase. At the end of the follicular phase, estrogen reaches a blood level of approximately 200 picograms per milliliter; this concentration may be maintained for as long as 50 hours (Hoffman et al., 2020b). At this critical time, the high estrogen level initiates a positive feedback of LH, generating the preovulatory LH surge. The LH surge, which begins 34 to 36 hours prior to ovulation and provides a relatively accurate predictor for timing ovulation, is responsible for many changes in the follicle selected for rupture.

Initially the nuclear membrane around the oocyte breaks down, the chromosomes progress through the rest of the first meiotic division, and the egg moves on to the secondary stage. Meiosis ceases at this time and will be initiated again only if the ovum is fertilized. The LH surge stimulates luteinization of the granulosa cells and synthesis of progesterone. Progesterone, in turn, enhances the positive feedback effect of estrogen on the LH surge and is responsible for promoting enzyme activity in the follicular fluid capable of digesting the follicle wall. High levels of LH and progesterone cause the synthesis of prostaglandins and proteolytic enzymes such as collagenase and plasmin. Although the exact mechanism underlying this process is unknown, the activated proteolytic enzymes and prostaglandins digest collagen in the follicular wall, leading to an explosive release of the ovum (oocyte), along with the zona pellucida and corona radiate surrounding it. At ovulation, the ovum is expelled and drawn up by the ciliated fimbriae of the fallopian tube to initiate its migration through the oviduct (Douglas & Lobo, 2022; Hoffman et al., 2020b).

Newer information about the timing of the LH surge and ovulation is available because of the amount of data collected by many clinicians during in vitro fertilization. For example. spontaneous LH surge has a tendency to occur around 3 a.m. in more than two-thirds of individuals, and ovulation has been found to occur primarily in the morning during the spring months and primarily during the evening in autumn and winter (Taylor et al., 2020). In the Northern Hemisphere, from July to February, approximately 90 % of people will ovulate between 4 and 7 p.m., and during the spring, 50 % will ovulate between midnight and 11 a.m. (Taylor et al., 2020). Research studies suggest that ovulation occurs more often from the right ovary than the left, and that oocytes from the right ovary have a higher likelihood for pregnancy than those from the left (Taylor et al., 2020).

FIGURE 7-9 Ovarian phases and endometrial development.

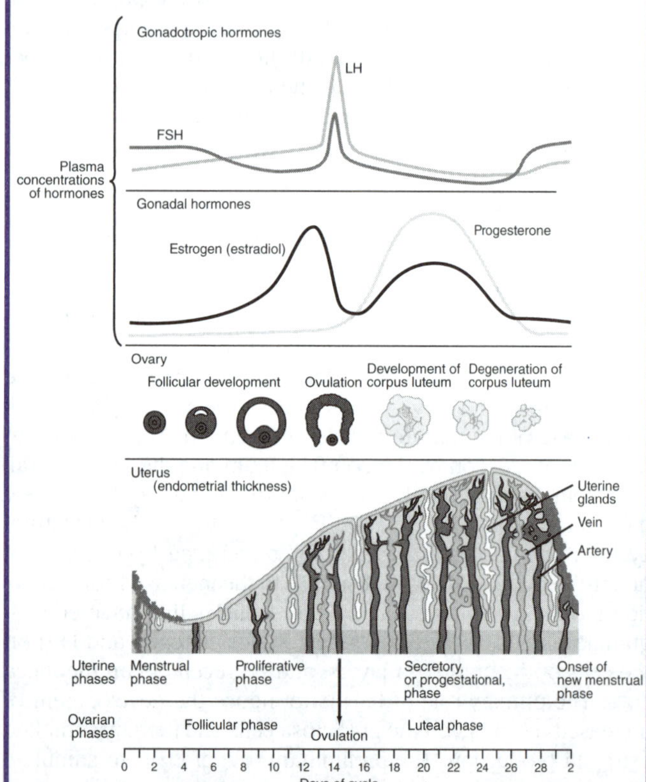

Luteal Phase

Under the influence of LH, the follicle's granulosa cells that are left in the ruptured follicle become enlarged, undergo luteinization, and form the corpus luteum. The corpus luteum continues to function for approximately 8 days after ovulation. It secretes increased progesterone and some estrogen that start the negative feedback loop to the hypothalamus and pituitary gland, preventing further ovulation within the current cycle. In the absence of a fertilized ovum, luteal cells degenerate, causing a decline in estrogen and progesterone levels, and the corpus luteum regresses to become the corpus albicans. As a result of the regression of the corpus luteum, estrogen and progesterone levels decrease rapidly, removing the negative feedback effect. FSH and LH then begin to increase once again to initiate the next menstrual cycle (Douglas & Lobo, 2022).

The Endometrial Cycle

The endometrial cycle has three phases: proliferative, secretory, and menstrual.

Proliferative Phase

The proliferative phase is influenced by estrogen and entails the regrowth of endometrium after the menstrual bleed. It starts on about the fourth or fifth day of the cycle and usually lasts approximately 10 days, ending with the release of the ovum. The proliferative phase involves changes in the endometrium, myometrium, and ovaries. These cyclic changes, which result from fluctuations in gonadotropin and estrogen levels, are characterized by progressive mitotic growth of the decidua functionalis in response to increasing levels of estrogen secreted by the ovary. They occur in preparation for implantation of the fertilized ovum.

At the beginning of the proliferative phase, the endometrium is relatively thin and the endometrial glands are straight, narrow, and short. As the phase progresses, the glands become long and tortuous. The endometrium becomes thicker as a result of the glandular hyperplasia and growth of the stroma. The endometrium proliferates from 4 to 12 mm in height and increases eightfold in thickness in preparation for implantation of the fertilized ovum (Douglas & Lobo, 2022).

Secretory Phase

The secretory phase begins at ovulation. When it is part of a 28-day cycle, it usually lasts from day 15 (the day after ovulation—the exact cycle day will vary with cycle length) to day 28. This phase does not take place if ovulation has not occurred. It tends to be the most constant phase, in terms of time.

During the secretory phase, the glands of the endometrium become more tortuous and dilated and fill with secretions, primarily as a result of increased progesterone production. The endometrium becomes thick, cushiony, and nutritive in preparation for implantation of the fertilized ovum. In the absence of implantation, the corpus luteum shrinks, and progesterone and estrogen levels subsequently decrease. The endometrium begins to regress toward the end of the secretory phase. By days 25 to 26, progesterone and estrogen withdrawal results in increased tortuous coiling and constriction of the spiral arterioles in the thinning layer.

Until the past decade it was believed that decreased blood flow to the superficial endometrial layers resulted in tissue ischemia and resulting menses. The end of menses was believed to be caused, "by longer and more intense waves of vasoconstriction, combined with coagulation mechanisms activated by vascular stasis and endometrial collapse, aided by rapid re-epithelization mediated by estrogen from the emerging new follicular cohort" (Fritz & Speroff, 2011, p. 595). Rather, the current theory suggests that menstruation is initiated by enzymatic autodigestion of the functional layer of the endometrium, which is triggered by estrogen–progesterone withdrawal (Douglas & Lobo, 2022). As estrogen and progesterone levels fall during the days prior to menses, lysosomal membranes become destabilized, such that the enzymes within them are released into the cytoplasm of the epithelial, stromal, and endothelial cells and into the intercellular space. These enzymes are proteolytic: they digest the cells surrounding them as well as surface membranes. Their actions result in platelet deposition, release of prostaglandins, vascular thrombosis, extravasation of red blood cells, and tissue necrosis in the vascular endothelium (Douglas & Lobo, 2022). Enzymatic action progressively degrades the endometrium and eventually disrupts the capillaries and venous system just under the endometrial surface, causing interstitial hemorrhage and dissolution of the surface membrane and allowing blood to escape into the endometrial cavity (Douglas & Lobo, 2022). This degeneration continues and extends to the functional layer of the endometrium, where rupture of the basal arterioles contributes to the bleeding. The concepts about how the menstrual flow ceases remain unchanged.

Menstrual Phase

The menstrual phase begins with the initiation of menses and lasts 3 to 5 days. Historically, it was believed that the initiation of menstruation occurred as a result of a hypoxic event caused by a decrease in estrogen and progesterone, which caused vasoconstriction of the spiral arteries in the basal layer of the endometrium (Taylor et al., 2020). Current studies, however, indicate that the initiation of menstruation is due to enzymatic autodigestion of the functional layer of the endometrium (Taylor et al., 2020). The degradation of the endometrium is progressive and causes interstitial hemorrhage whereby dissolution of the surface membrane allows blood to escape into the endometrial cavity (Taylor et al., 2020). Prostaglandins initiate contractions of the uterine smooth muscle and sloughing of the degraded endometrial tissue, leading to menstruation. The composition of menstrual fluid comprises desquamated endometrial tissue, red blood cells, inflammatory exudates, and proteolytic enzymes. Because some of the clotting factors ordinarily found in blood are lysed by lysosomal enzymes in the uterus, menstrual blood does not clot (Douglas & Lobo, 2022). Plasmin, one of the proteolytic enzymes, has significant fibrinolytic actions that help to prevent clotting of the menstrual fluid (Douglas & Lobo, 2022). For 3 to 5 days, an average of 10 to 80 mL of blood loss occurs. Approximately 2 days after the start of menstruation, estrogen stimulates the regeneration of the surface endometrial epithelium, while concurrent simultaneous endometrial shedding is occurring (Douglas & Lobo, 2022).

Changes in Organs Due to Cyclic Changes

Cervix

After menstruation, the cervical mucus is scant and viscous. During the late follicular phase, it becomes clear, copious, and elastic in response to increased estradiol levels at the end of the follicular phase (Douglas & Lobo, 2022). The quantity of cervical mucus increases, compared to the early follicular phase, and can stretch to at least 6 cm (Douglas & Lobo, 2022). The cervical mucus during this time is clear and stretchable (spinnbarkeit). Microscopic examination reveals that it displays a characteristic ferning appearance during the ovulatory period.

After ovulation, when progesterone levels are high, the amount of cervical mucus once again decreases and becomes thick, viscous, and opaque. This thick mucus is hostile and impenetrable to the sperm. The increased viscosity also reduces the risk of ascending infection at the time of possible implantation.

Increased estrogen levels promote stromal vascularization and edema and relax the myometrial fibers that supply the cervix. Activated collagenase causes the tightly bound collagen bundles to form a loose matrix, triggering the cervix to become softer a few days prior to and at ovulation. In addition, the external cervical os everts prior to ovulation (Hoffman et al., 2022b; Nunziato & Valea, 2022).

Fallopian Tube Mobility

Estrogen stimulates epithelial cell activity, resulting in increased cilia movement and secretions in the uterine tubes. These special effects assist ovum mobility along the fallopian tube following ovulation. Progesterone reverses these effects, thereby inhibiting the peristaltic activity of the fallopian tube smooth muscle.

Vagina

The changes in hormonal levels of estrogen and progesterone have characteristic effects on the vaginal epithelium. This information becomes important when cervical cells are examined under the microscope, as their morphologic differences can be related to specific stages of the menstrual cycle. During the early follicular phase, exfoliated vaginal epithelial cells have vesicular nuclei and are basophilic. They appear flatter than the corresponding cells in the later phases, owing to the influence of progesterone, which causes them to become folded and clumped. The pH of the vagina responds to cyclical changes as estrogen stimulates the growth of lactobacilli. Lactobacilli metabolize glycogen from cervical secretions and produce lactic acid, which decreases the vaginal pH to a level that assists in protecting the gynecologic tract against opportunistic pathogens (Eckert & Lentz, 2022).

CONCLUSION

Gynecological health is a cornerstone of comprehensive care for addressing the unique needs of individuals across the life span. Understanding the anatomy and physiology of the reproductive system provides the foundation for accurate assessment, diagnosis, and treatment of gynecological conditions. By integrating this knowledge with patient-centered care, healthcare providers can empower individuals through education, preventive strategies, and evidence-based interventions.

References

Al-Suhaimi, E. A., & Khan, F. A. (2022). The pituitary gland: Functional relationship with the hypothalamus, structure, and physiology. In E. A. Al-Suhaimi (Ed.), *Emerging concepts in endocrine structure and functions.* Springer. https://doi.org/10.1007/978-981-16-9016-7_4

Caldwell, W. E., & Moloy, H. C. (1933). Anatomical variations in female pelvic bones and their effect on labor with a suggested classification. *American Journal of Obstetrics & Gynecology, 26*, 479–482.

Cowley, D., S., Burke, A., & Lentz, G. M. (2022). Additional considerations in gynecologic care. In D. M. Gershenson, G. M. Lentz, R. A. Lobo, & F. A. Valea (Eds.), *Comprehensive gynecology* (8th ed., pp. 148–187). Elsevier.

Douglas, N. C., & Lobo, R. A. (2022). Reproductive endocrinology: Neuroendocrinology, gonadotropins, sex steroids, prostaglandins, ovulation, menstruation, hormone assay. In D. M. Gershenson, G. M. Lentz, R. A. Lobo, & F. A. Valea (Eds.), *Comprehensive gynecology* (8th ed., pp. 76–105). Elsevier.

Eckert, L. O., & Lentz, G. M. (2022). Genital tract infections: Vulva, vagina, cervix, toxic shock syndrome, endometritis, and salpingitis. In D. M. Gershenson, G. M. Lentz, R. A. Lobo, & F. A. Valea (Eds.), *Comprehensive gynecology* (8th ed., pp. 515–542). Elsevier.

Fritz, M., & Speroff, L. (2011). *Clinical gynecologic endocrinology and infertility.* Lippincott Williams & Wilkins.

Garland, F., Thomson, M., Mitchell, T., & Watrburton, J. (2021). Management of 'disorders of sex development'/intersex variations in children: Results from a freedom of information exercise. Non-therapeutic medical interventions on the bodies of children born with disorders of sex. *Medical Law International, 21*(2) 116–146. https://doi.org/10.1177/09685332211003636

Hoffman B. L., Schorge J. O., Halvorson L. M., Hamid C. A., Corton M. M., Schaffer J. I. (2020a). Anatomy. In B. L. Hoffman, J. O. Schorge, K. D. Bradshaw, L. M. Halvorson, J. I. Schaffer, & M. M. Corton (Eds.), *Williams gynecology (*4th ed., pp. 792–821). McGraw Hill Education. https://accessmedicine-mhmedical-com.huaryu.kl.oakland.edu/content.aspx?bookid=2658&sectionid=223470056

Hoffman B. L., Schorge J. O., Halvorson L. M., Hamid C. A., Corton M. M., & Schaffer J. I. (2020b). Reproductive endocrinology. In B. L. Hoffman, J. O. Schorge, K. D. Bradshaw, L. M. Halvorson, J. I. Schaffer, & M. M. Corton (Eds.), *Williams gynecology (*4th ed., pp. 336–370). McGraw Hill Education. https://accessmedicine-mhmedical-com.huaryu.kl.oakland.edu/content.aspx?bookid=2658&sectionid=241009554

Hoffman, B. L., Schorge, J. O., , Halvorson, L. M., Hamid, C. A., Corton, M. M., & Schaffer, J. I., (2020c). Pediatric and adolescent gynecology. In B. L. Hoffman, J. O. Schorge, K. D., Bradshaw, L. M. Halvorson, J. I. Schaffer, & M. M. Corton (Eds.), *William's gynecology* (4th ed., pp. 320–335). McGraw Hill Education. https://accessmedicine-mhmedical-com.huaryu.kl.oakland.edu/content.aspx?bookid=2658&sectionid=218609057

Li, H., Gibson, E. A., Jukic, A. Z., Baird, D. D., Wilcox, A. J., Curry, C. L., Fischer-Colbrie, T., Onnela, J., Willimas, M. A., Hause, R., Coull, B. A., & Mahalingaiah, S. (2023). Menstrual cycle length variation by demographic characteristics from the Apple Women's Health Study. *Nature Partner Journals Digital Medicine, 6*(1), 1–11. https://doi.org/10.1038/s41746-023-00848-1

Nunziato, J. D., & Valea, F. A. (2022). Reproductive anatomy: Gross and microscopic clinical correlations. In D. M. Gershenson, G. M. Lentz, R. A. Lobo, & F. A. Valea (Eds.), *Comprehensive gynecology* (8th ed., pp. 47–75). Elsevier

Ryntz, T., & Lobo, R. (2022). Abnormal uterine bleeding: Etiology and management of acute and chronic excessive bleeding. In D. M. Gershenson, G. M. Lentz, R. A. Lobo, & F. A. Valea (Eds.), *Comprehensive gynecology* (8th ed., pp. 594–605). Elsevier.

Sandadi, S., Rock, D. T., Orr, J. W., & Valea, F. A. (2022). Breast diseases: Detection, management, and surveillance of breast disease. In D. M. Gershenson, G. M. Lentz, R. A. Lobo, & F. A. Valea (Eds.), *Comprehensive gynecology* (8th ed., pp. 289–322). Elsevier.

Taylor, H. S., Pal, L., & Seli, E. (2020). Regulation of the menstrual cycle. In H. S. Taylor, L. Pal, & E. Seli (Eds.), *Speroff's clinical gynecologic endocrinology and infertility* (9th ed., pp. 137–173). Wolters Kluwer.

VanSickle, C., Liese K. L., & Rutherford J. N. (2022). Textbook typologies: Challenging the myth of the perfect obstetric pelvis. *The Anatomical Record 305*(4), 952–967. https://doi.org/10.1002/ar.24880.

CHAPTER 8

History Taking and Physical Examination in Sexual and Reproductive Care

Stephanie Tillman

Shilpy Sarguru

The editors acknowledge Frances Likis who was a coauthor of the previous edition of this chapter.

Sexual and reproductive care occurs for two main reasons: to maintain or enhance health, and to identify and treat a problem of the sexual and reproductive health system. This chapter presents the core knowledge and skill base for the health history and physical examination related to breast, chest, and pelvic care. Often these examinations are embedded within a clinical visit that has a wider focus on primary care screening and counseling. See Chapters 6 and 9. In other circumstances, it is the base examination for a visit centered on an identified concern, such as vaginal discharge, urinary frequency, a breast lump, heavy menstrual bleeding, sexual assault, and so on which may require further evaluation than is detailed in this chapter. The sexual and reproductive health examination is modifiable and should be individualized to every patient, every time, based on their needs, comfort, and experiences.

This chapter intentionally uses gender-inclusive language because sexual and reproductive health history and physical examination are not performed exclusively for cisgender women (individuals who were assigned female at birth and who identify as women). Healthcare providers working in the field of sexual and reproductive health provide care for people who identify as woman or female, as well as for people who are transgender, nonbinary, and intersex. When caring for transgender, nonbinary, and intersex people, ensure the health history and physical examination are relevant to the anatomy present, regardless of the individual's gender identity (Ellis & Dalke, 2019). See Chapter 11 for further information about providing care for transgender and nonbinary people as well as a more detailed discussion of gender terms and concepts.

CONTEXT AND APPROACH: CONSENT

Healthcare ethics commonly grounds itself in four principles: autonomy, beneficence, non-maleficence, and justice (Beauchamp & Childress, 2019). While these four principles are not all-encompassing, these four are the most identifiable across disciplines within ethical care and will be referred to here. Additional ethical lenses such as feminism, queer theory, and reproductive justice are necessary for a holistic understanding of sexual and reproductive health care. Autonomy in sexual and reproductive health care is importantly delineated into one's autonomy in making decisions impacting their life, such as the type of care they seek from whom, and under what conditions, and in one's autonomy in its bodily form, such as whether to become pregnant or remain pregnant, who to allow to touch one's body, and how one might express their gender. Decisional and bodily autonomy are baseline ethical commitments clinicians engage when collecting a patient's history and conducting a physical examination. At its most basic, this means that patients can consent to or decide against all components of the visit. This includes but is not limited to answering questions, undressing, providing samples for testing, presence of student learners, accompaniment of chaperones, input of family members, and documentation of sensitive information. The provider's recommendation may be related to a line of questioning, such as, "I ask all of my patients a standard line of questioning related to their sexual history so that I can best tailor today's examination and testing to your needs." The recommendation may pertain to a certain type of examination, such as, "I would suggest that I conduct the pelvic examination today rather than you performing a self-swab collection, so that I can visualize internally some of what you are describing." As of this writing, five essential requirements are standard to fulfill ethical and legal obligations of consent, all of which are provider-driven in terms of ensuring the standards are met. See **Figure 8-1**.

Clinicians who are not familiar with ethical or legal requirements in their practice should seek further resources for ensuring their practice aligns with basic requirements. Clinicians should consult their own personal ethic alongside institutional policies, specialty culture, organizational recommendations, as well as state and federal laws. Mandates, expectations of patient compliance, penalization of decisions against care (like risks of reporting to state surveillance) all compromise consent and are unethical. Shared decision making, opt-in and opt-out consent models, and what is or is not covered by "universal" consent documents patients sign when entering a fiduciary relationship with an institution are all worthy of careful thought. Seeking additional learning in what qualifies as coercion in the consent process is important for all clinicians (Tillman, 2020).

CONTEXT AND APPROACH: TRAUMA-INFORMED CARE

Trauma-informed care acknowledges the prevalence of current, recent, and past trauma; emphasizes the range of effects of trauma on a person's physical and mental health; and guides

FIGURE 8-1 **Ethical and legal requirements for informed consent.**

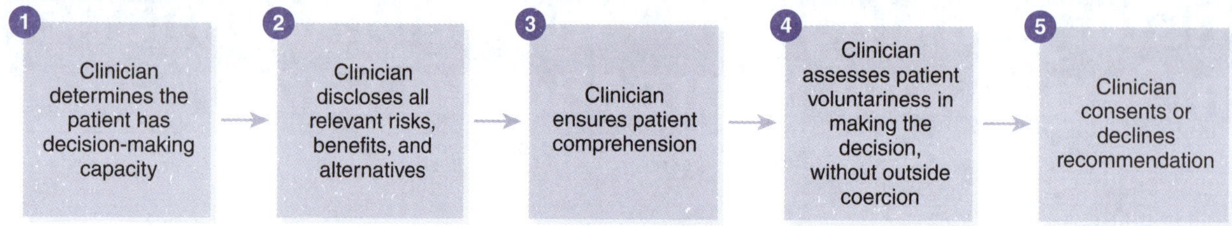

the tone and process of patient care, ideally at both individual and organizational levels (see Chapter 5 for more information on the trauma-informed care framework). For all components of a health history and physical examination, the clinician should state explicitly that at any time the care seeker can accept or decline any offered or recommended evaluation, stop an examination, ask for a change in approach, request a chaperone, or defer care to a future visit (LoGiudice et al., 2023). The provider's language is a key facet of trauma-informed care and is an overt way to express power transfer and emphasize to the patient that they are in control of the visit. Explicit consent, offering words like, "Stop," "Pause," and "Out," for the patient to use during the examination, are all powerful and transparent tools that activate listening and communicating throughout the visit. These types of approaches to ongoing consent acknowledge the patient's control and create space in which the individual knows that their words and bodily responses will be heard and respected. These sample statements in **Box 8-1** offer suggestions for clear verbal transfers of power. Particularly for people with a known sexual assault history and healthcare trauma, providers must take extra caution regarding language, transfer of power, ensuring comfort, validating consent, and considering the presence of a chaperone or a patient advocate for both the patient's comfort and the provider's documentation. Given that many people will experience a sexual assault attempt or rape in their lifetime, but often do not report that event to law enforcement or during the history taking portion of the examination, intentional language and physical examination approaches should be standardized for all patients and sensitive to this issue for every individual regardless of disclosure. The word "stop," so often said during an assault or violation and ignored, is particularly important to hear and respect during a healthcare examination. "Stop" may indicate a check-in is needed, as may have been discussed through the trauma-informed preparation for the exam or may be a patient rescinding consent to continue.

Individuals with a history of sexual assault and healthcare trauma may not and may never report these during history taking, nor should they be required to. Providers may not always know if someone has a history of trauma, even if asked directly in the health history. Some trauma-informed care resources reference the timepoint of patient verbal disclosure of past trauma as the reason to initiate trauma-informed care. This approach is both incorrect and harmful in itself. Disclosure is not a requirement for trauma-informed care and suggesting that providers only engage trauma-informed care for those who disclose is not only antithetical to its premise as a framework, but also lacks reflection on health care itself as a site of trauma and risks causing trauma to patients and providers. If, for example, a patient does not disclose a sexual trauma history, and the provider begins what might be a routine examination that then leads to nonverbal trauma responses, and the provider pushes through that examination not realizing that individualized trauma-informed care would be necessary but rather hurrying through an examination is justified, that approach potentially harms both the patient and the provider. Trauma-informed care is meant for both, and utilized as a standard of care in sexual and reproductive health care, attends to both (Owens et al., 2021). There are signs to be aware of during an examination that could indicate either current or activated trauma, including someone closing or covering their eyes, suddenly grabbing an examination table or an item during the examination, clenching muscles, breathing rapidly, closing legs, crying, or moving away from the provider.

BOX 8-1 Sample Language for Clinicians to Use in Trauma-Informed Care History Taking and Physical Examinations

In the past, how have these examinations been for you? What suggestions might you have for what I can do during today's examination to make it more comfortable?

You are in complete control of this examination. If at any point you feel uncomfortable, want me to pause and wait until you're ready, stop the examination entirely, or have questions, please let me know. I will stop at any point if you ask me to or if I feel that your body is telling me to.

At any point you can ask me to pause and wait for you to let me know when to restart, keep going but slow down, or stop completely and remove all tools or my fingers, and I will follow your direction.

I can understand this [pelvic] examination can be really uncomfortable. My goal is to provide the best care to you that I can. Let me know at any point if I can do anything differently.

Since every person is different, I am ready to modify this examination for every patient. I always check in on what process might work best for you: Would you like for me to explain each step [of the pelvic examination], or would you like to talk about something completely random, like what we did over the weekend or the last movies we saw?

BOX 8-2 Symptom Clusters of PTSD

Re-experiencing/ Intrusion:	Avoidance:	Shifts in cognitions and mood:	Alterations in arousal and emotional reactivity:
Flashbacks, memories, and/or nightmares of the traumatic event	Efforts to evade thoughts, feelings, or reminders of the trauma including dissociation, escapism, or isolation	Numbing, persistent negative feelings, distorted sense of blame, and/or anhedonia	Heightened startle response, hypervigilance, and/or sleep disturbances; outbursts of anger, irritability, aggression, or reckless behavior

Data from American Psychiatric Association (Ed.). (2022). *Diagnostic and Statistical Manual of Mental Disorders: DSM-5-TR* (Fifth edition, text revision). American Psychiatric Association Publishing; and King, D. W., Leskin, G. A., King, L. A., & Weathers, F. W. (1998). Confirmatory factor analysis of the clinician-administered PTSD Scale: Evidence for the dimensionality of posttraumatic stress disorder. *Psychological Assessment, 10*(2), 90–96. https://doi.org/10.1037/1040-3590.10.2.90

Providers should actively monitor for any of these signs, and if they are noted, safely pause or stop the questioning or examination, cover sensitive areas, and discuss concerns with the patient, offering to either modify the process or defer to another visit. People with known trauma, or those who show signs of trauma during an examination, may have established, or can benefit from, coping mechanisms, particularly during healthcare experiences such as sexual and reproductive care that could be activating or retraumatizing. Possible coping mechanisms during a visit, depending on the person's level of distress, include grounding, mental imagery, meditation, breath counting, and progressive muscle relaxation (**Box 8-2**).

Providers should also be cognizant that they can experience secondary trauma (also referred to as trauma exposure response or vicarious trauma) in the healthcare setting. Providers should strive to employ active, empathetic listening when a patient shares about their past experiences with trauma. However, it is important to note that in processing the trauma recalled by the patient, the provider can also feel activated in mind and body. Provision of care can activate one's own prior experiences, which places providers at risk for primary or secondary trauma (LoGiudice et al., 2023, p. 4). The coping skills that would benefit a client who has undergone previous trauma(s) or is currently activated during the history and physical examination could also benefit the provider. It is vital to care for one's own system as well as to maintain self-compassion. Examples of tending to one's own system during a patient visit can include taking a moment to pause, turn the attention to breath and/or to the sensation of feeling both feet on the ground. Other ways one can regulate their nervous system after a patient visit include changing environments outside of the examination room or turning to a trusted colleague to discuss what activation came up for the provider during the exam.

HEALTH HISTORY

The purpose of the health history is to establish a relationship with a person while learning about their health. To a great extent, taking a health history means listening to an individual's story. Both the content and manner of what the patient conveys provide important information for a clinician's understanding of what this individual wants and needs. To optimize health history taking, several social, cultural, environmental, and logistical arrangements should be consistently in place. These include providing a comfortable and private setting, scheduling an appropriate amount of time, and choosing the optimal format and staff member for obtaining the health history.

Privacy is an essential component for obtaining a health history. Ideally, the room or office where the history is taken will have a door that can be closed so no noise or traffic interrupts the interview. A closed door ensures confidentiality and conveys the clinician's intent to offer undivided attention. The patient should remain fully clothed. The clinician and the patient should be seated at a comfortable distance from each other, preferably face to face and at eye level, without furniture or electronics between them. This seating arrangement promotes a conversational, rather than a confrontational or hierarchical, approach. Especially in the age of the electronic health record, each clinician should find a way to minimize computer use during the history taking, as looking primarily at the computer signifies that the interpersonal interaction is not a priority.

Access to health information in the patient's primary or preferred language by a certified medical interpreter is standard of care for all settings and is a requirement for all settings that accept Medicaid or federal funding. When an interpreter is present, they should be seated so that all three persons can see and/or hear one another. If using a video interpreter, the video should be next to or just behind the clinician, facing the patient. Interpretation services provided by non-certified personnel (for example, a provider who speaks some of a patient's language, family members, friends, or staff) should be used only as a last resort or in emergencies when a medical interpreter is not available, because these stand-ins do not meet ethical or legal requirements for healthcare interpretation and cannot be presumed to understand and convey complex medical information.

Traditionally, the optimal way to gather the health history is to interview the patient alone to minimize distractions and ensure privacy, but this presumption that privacy ensures patient security is not always the case and should be evaluated individually. Consider the flow of the visit and try to arrange the initial interaction without any support person present. This allows the clinician to address the patient's preferences as well as their safety with that person or people in attendance. Providers must introduce themselves to each person in the room and ascertain their relationship to the patient, as spouse, partner, family member, and friends may all have different social roles and legal responsibilities during the visit. If the patient prefers to have a support person in the room for a part or the entirety of the visit, affirm this decision. Some patients may bring a patient advocate, guardian, social worker, or caretaker with them, and understanding the legal and clinical implications of those people is an important part of holistic care, including their role in decision making for some or all of the patient's decisions. If young children are present during a patient's visit, ideally a second adult will be available to attend to them to support the patient and the provider's focus during the visit. Realistically, the patient may be the only person in the room able to attend to children or family members for whom they are the caretaker, and clinicians must be supportive and adaptive for these patients. Commend the patient on the work they do to care for their loved ones and ask about what parts of the examination are preferred given the other people present. Providers may offer a follow-up visit if additional support people could make the next visit more comfortable for the patient. It is essential to acknowledge that additional visits may not be feasible, given people's work, transportation, or family circumstances, and accommodations should be made whenever possible to facilitate all necessary or desired care and protect the patient's privacy with coded language or draping during an examination. Providers can also invite children and family members to participate in appropriate components of the examination with patient consent, such as guiding a sibling in hearing a fetal heartbeat or in encouraging a safe partner to understand what changes might be concerning going forward.

If there is another person present during the health history, it is essential that at some point the patient and provider be given the opportunity to speak privately. This practice is advisable for handling topics that may be sensitive. These topics might include gender identity, sexual orientation, sexual health history, safety at home and in relationships, history of trauma, previous diagnoses, prior pregnancies, and mental health concerns. It also allows the clinician to ensure that the choice to have the other person present was made freely and without coercion; for some patients, this may be the first time they understand they can be seen alone, and starting a visit this way can center the patient's autonomy from the beginning. For adolescents accompanied by parents or guardians, this policy is particularly important. When a parent is present, commend their involvement and care, while making space to establish a separate professional relationship with the patient while following state and national guidelines. Research shows that, often, adolescents feel more comfortable disclosing information regarding safety, relationships, sexual activity, and gender identity or expression when their parent is not in the room, and these are critical pieces of information to providing comprehensive health care (Copen et al., 2016; Marcell et al., 2017). Sexual and reproductive health care, mental health care, and substance use and treatment care are often protected ethical and legal categories which grant minors the ability to consent to care without parental notification (Chung et al., 2024). Depending on the state or political climate, however, access to this care or age restrictions may vary. Clinicians should be attentive to these limitations as well as potential loopholes to confidentiality such as a parent's access to the minor's electronic health record or insurance billing statements. Clinicians should stay up to date on state and national guidelines to be transparent with patients and their parents or guardians. Sexual and reproductive care providers may be more aware of these exceptions than other primary care providers the family sees, such as the patient's pediatrician. Therefore, it is essential to be clear with both the patient and the parent about what will and will not be shared during a protected visit. The American Academy of Pediatrics (Marcell et al., 2017; American Academy of Pediatrics, 2021) and the Guttmacher Institute (2023) have additional resources related to minors' consent and access to services.

Schedule an appropriate amount of time for an initial visit to hear the patient's story in an unhurried manner. Structure the interview around standard questions (**Boxes 8-3**, **8-4**, and **8-5**) while allowing the flow to be flexible based on individual responses and needs. Depending on each patient or patient population, these standard questions may be just a starting point into a much more detailed conversation. As much as possible, pose questions that allow open-ended responses, such as, "Tell me about your sexual partners," "Describe your periods," and "How do you feel your overall health is right now?"

When asking patients questions, listen intently; an individual is speaking about their life, and this is an entrusted moment to fully hear them. This involves maintaining eye contact, nodding along with understanding of facts and concerns, asking follow-up questions that pertain specifically to the visit at hand, and responding with words of empathy or excitement as appropriate. During a busy clinic day, the provider's focus may be on many tasks and concerns, and with time each provider discerns how to best manage these competing distractions. Every patient deserves the full attention of the provider during their visit, and providers must find ways to refocus and ensure complete attention during each visit. Whenever possible, utilize a nonverbal or code word system with staff to easily communicate when not to be interrupted, or for the staff to notify of an urgent interruption requiring immediate attention. If support staff calls the provider away from the conversation or there is an emergency that interrupts the examination, the provider must again refocus completely on the patient's concerns. Reassure the patient that they have the provider's attention and intentional focus.

If the topic veers off from the presumed focus, steer the conversation back to the original concern while noting the need to address the additional concern later, including possibly at a separate visit. Interrupt the patient's storytelling flow only for specific clarification or to bring the focus back to the original concern if the conversation seems to be digressing too far. However, if the primary focus ultimately becomes something different than the presumed original concern, allow the patient's storytelling and questions to follow that path as indicated. While history taking in this manner takes time, in many settings, providers may have 15 minutes for an entire visit, including history taking and examination. Each provider finds ways to modify visits and split up history taking and examination as is possible within their clinical setting's constraints. During history taking, the provider should note verbal and nonverbal cues that indicate a patient's preference for or increased safety with an identity concordant provider, questions or examinations that may activate previous trauma, or desire to avoid or focus on sensitive topics like sexuality or reproduction.

A variety of formats may be used for obtaining the health history, ranging from a self-administered questionnaire to an in-person conversation. Any forms or intake processes must be inclusive of all patient populations; available in people's primary or preferred language; and include space for the person's legal name, preferred name, pronouns, gender identity, along with

BOX 8-3 General Health History

Reason for seeking care (chief concern, or "CC")
History of present illness/concern (HPI)
General medical history:
Name, preferred name to use in the care setting, and pronouns
Current health conditions, disabilities

- Previous serious illnesses
- Past hospitalizations
- Prior surgical procedures
- Immunization status

Accidents, injuries
Blood transfusions
Mental health history:

- Current concerns
- Diagnoses and treatments
- Mood changes, including mood disorder screening
- History of, or current concern for, self-harm practices (e.g., cutting) and/or suicidal or homicidal thoughts

Medications and allergies:

- Current medications, including contraceptives and other hormone use
- Over-the-counter medications, including vitamins and supplements
- Medication and other allergies

Substance use:

- Alcohol
- Tobacco, including vaping
- Cannabidiol (CBD) products
- Tetrahydrocannabinol (THC) use, including marijuana products, oral, edible, topical, or inhaled applications
- Unregulated, criminalized, extralegal, and/or illegal substances
- Misuse of over-the-counter, prescribed, or recreational medications

Family health history:

- Physical and mental illnesses

Causes of death of first-degree relatives:

- Congenital malformations, unexplained intellectual and developmental disabilities

Social history:

- Race and ethnicity
- Religion
- Education
- Current activities (e.g., employment, student status, family responsibilities)
- Long-term life plans
- Partner(s)
- Living companions (children, family, roommates)
- Support system

Occupation and finances:

- Current employment
- Occupational safety
- Military service and veteran status
- Financial security
- Insurance status and needs

Safety:

- Personal
- Home
- Community
- Sexual (current and historical)

History of sexual and/or physical abuse, including intimate partner violence (IPV), domestic violence (DV), child sexual abuse (CSA)
Who has access to their chart, billing statements, etc.
Personal habits:

- Health maintenance including exercise, sleep, nutrition, and hydration
- Ongoing health maintenance, such as dental care and eye examinations

BOX 8-4 History of Present Illness/Concern: "OLDCARTS"

- Onset: When did the concern or symptoms begin? What were the circumstances at that time? Have you had this before?
- Location: Where are the symptoms located physically?
- Duration: How long have you had the symptoms?
- Characteristics: Describe the concern or symptoms. In the case of pain, is it sharp, stabbing, dull, radiating, or burning?
- Associated symptoms: What other symptoms happen at the same time as the primary concern? What other symptoms do you believe are connected?
- Relieving factors: What makes your symptoms better or worse? What have you already tried to change or solve the symptoms? How effective have those strategies been?
- Timing: When do the symptoms happen? Are they constant, or do they occur only during certain times or activities (e.g., during particular points in the menstrual cycle, during urination, during exercise, or during sex)?
- Severity: How much is the concern affecting your daily quality of life? In the case of pain, try to rate it on a scale of no pain (0) to the worst pain imaginable (10).

BOX 8-5 Gynecologic Health History

Anatomy inventory

Menstrual history:

- Age at menarche
- Date of last normal menstrual period
- Cycle length, duration, and flow
- Any menstrual irregularities or symptoms associated with menses

Sexual health:

- Sexual orientation
- Gender identity
- Current sexual relationship(s)
- Types of sex, and whether insertive and/or receptive partner: Oral, anal, vaginal, digital, manual, and whether exclusively with other body parts or also with toys, and so on
- Safer sex or harm reduction practices: condoms, dental dams, PrEP/PEP
- Sexual satisfaction, pleasure, and orgasm
- Pain with sex
- Sexual concerns

Contraceptive use (see above for whether patient has engaged/is engaging in type of sex or with partners that could lead to pregnancy for self or others):

- Present contraceptive method: Type, duration used, satisfaction, side effects, and consistency of use
- Previous contraceptive use: Method(s), duration of use, satisfaction, side effects, and reasons for discontinuing

Pregnancy history:

- Gravida and para
- Course of pregnancies: Date, duration, type of birth, complications (pregnancy, birth, and postpartum), newborn's sex assignment, weight, and whether the child is currently alive
- Abortions (induced or spontaneous), ectopic pregnancies, and molar pregnancies: Weeks gestation, management (medical, procedure, surgery), and if any complications

History of genital, pelvic, and sexually transmitted infections:

- Previous vulvar, rectal, vaginal, or pelvic infections and sexually transmitted infections and the number of times and dates for each, if known
- Treatments received, and complications

Genital and breast/chest hygiene (specific questions to ask if there any reported concerns or irritations):

- Cleaning practices (wipes, douching, enemas, specialty soaps or other practices) frequency, medication or solutions used, reasons for use
- Pubic hair removal, bleaching, steaming, herbal applications
- Piercings and tattoos
- Other common hygiene products: Creams, lubricants, scented menstrual products
- Breast/chest binding

Pelvic procedures and surgeries:

- Type of procedure or surgery, date, indication, complications, and outcome

Urologic and rectal health:

- Occurrence and frequency of infections
- Urinary, bowel, or flatus incontinence
- Hemorrhoids, cysts, polyps, varicosities, and any associated bleeding or discharge
- Other abnormal symptoms

Cervical cancer screening:

- Date of last testing, and whether cotesting or HPV-only
- History of an abnormal result; associated testing and procedures, follow-up visits, and results

Abnormal symptoms:

- Pelvic pain, bleeding unrelated to menstruation or with sex, and other symptoms

Sexual trauma history (see Chapter 16, Sexual Assault and Human Trafficking)

- Age(s), assailants (previously safe partners, family members, other known and unknown), whether reported, SANE exam completed

inclusive sexual and relationship histories. Disadvantages to self-administered health questionnaires include the possibilities that answers to items may be omitted, questions may be misunderstood, or terms may be unfamiliar to the respondent. In addition, the entire questionnaire will require visual and verbal review by a nurse or the clinician to fill in missing information and clarify answers. The advantages are that some people may disclose information more freely on sensitive topics in writing than if asked verbally, and the total time for this process may be less than if all information is obtained in an interview. Conversely, open-ended and spontaneous conversation about the health history, and more opportunity for answer clarification alongside development of a patient–provider relationship, is more likely in a verbal interview (Melms et al., 2021). Interviewers must work at the skill required to put a patient at ease, convey respectful attention through their verbal style and behavior, and attend to any miscommunications and misunderstandings in real time. Whenever possible, unhurried conversations can create rapport with patients and achieve complete and effective history taking (Ballard et al., 2024).

All providers should attempt to use common language rather than clinical or textbook terminology when phrasing questions or describing the examination. All attempts must be made to provide resources at the patient's level of understanding, including for consent processes. Interviewers must be attentive to visual cues, such as a furrowed brow, eye squinting, or head tilting, that may indicate the patient did not understand the question. It is appropriate to stop and clarify with questions such as, "I know sometimes healthcare language can be complicated; is there anything I can explain further or differently?" Be careful as to tone during this questioning, intentionally using a compassionate and inviting inflection rather than a neutral or even sharp emphasis. Avoid asking if the patient understood because that approach may pressure them into saying, "yes," partly because in so asking the clinician can imply judgment or shame for not understanding and cause a patient to withhold questions. If unsure as to the patient's comprehension, one possible question might be through a teach- or talk-back method, such as, "Can you tell me what you understand about what I just said?" (Yen & Leasure, 2019).

General Health History

Initially the interviewer makes a brief introduction, states the purposes of the interview, and invites questions at any point during the visit. Following a standard order of questions while obtaining the general health history is helpful for ensuring complete information gathering; however, the interviewer must also consider putting the patient at ease. Initiating the intake with a social history, rather than delving first into health-related history, could facilitate trust in the provider and work toward building a therapeutic relationship.

Reason for Seeking Care/Chief Concern

Asking, "How may I help you today?" or "What brought you here today?" are good ways to begin addressing the chief concern. Encourage the patient to describe the problem or the reason for the visit in their own words.

History of Present Illness/Concern

When the patient has finished describing why they are seeking care, the interviewer will need to obtain additional details about the reason for the visit. To maximize understanding of the concern, the clinician should be sure they have answers to all relevant questions related to the patient's concern. The acronym OLDCARTS (Box 8-4), often used related to pain, covers a full conversation around any reported concern. Historically, the term "history of present illness," or HPI, references the purpose of the visit, though when an individual describes their reason for seeking care it may be related to health maintenance or a concern that might not be defined as illness.

General Medical History

Ask the patient their preferred name and gender pronouns, and use them consistently throughout all interactions. Use a shared decision-making process to decide with the patient what aspects of their reported history feel relevant and safe for those who can access their health record—including any family or other health care team members—to be aware of. Ask if the patient has experienced any significant health conditions, including all hospitalizations and surgical procedures. Many people omit common surgeries, such as cesarean births, tubal ligations, wisdom teeth or tonsil removal, and plastic/cosmetic/aesthetic surgeries such as breast reduction or enhancement. In addition, the interviewer should ask about specific common diagnoses, such as diabetes, hypertension, asthma, and infectious diseases such as a history of tuberculosis or syphilis. A review of adult immunizations is also necessary. Clinicians should be sure to use clear language and avoid innuendo. For communities with particular health risk factors, such as resettled refugees and asylees, seasonal and migrant farm workers, people who live in areas with increased gun violence, or sex workers, specific questions appreciative of their life may best invite the patient to share information specific to their health needs.

Mental Health History

Inquire about any current concerns related to mental health. Employ a gentle approach when speaking about the various contributors to a person's mental health. It is helpful to compassionately inquire about the person's experiences starting from a broader set of questions to ones that become increasingly more specific to assess for their experiences and safety. Offer the context of how larger systems contribute to mental health concerns to comfort the patient with the concept of common humanity. Discuss any current or past diagnoses and treatment related to them, including medications, inpatient care, or outpatient therapy (USPSTF et al., 2023). Ask about coping mechanisms that an individual may not identify as treatment, such as lifestyle modifications that may be healthy (e.g., regular movement practices) or unhealthy (e.g., overuse of substances). Ask specifically about self-harm practices, such as cutting, and past or current suicidal or homicidal thoughts. If a patient reports current suicidal or homicidal ideation, further questioning must follow to elucidate intent, plan, and access to means. As mandated reporters, clinicians then must consider the safest action to care for anyone responding positively to suicidal or homicidal ideation, which, depending on community resources, may include calling emergency services or facilitating direct admission. If the assessment yields that emergency services or direct admission are not urgently needed, be sure to connect the patient with community resources to prevent harm to self or others during times of great distress. Often, a prescreening questionnaire can be helpful in asking specific questions related to daily struggles or general symptoms, such as appetite, hunger, and how others perceive the patient's mental health.

Medications and Allergies

Review all medications the patient is currently taking, including over-the-counter preparations, vitamins, and supplements, and the reasons for their use. If the patient cannot recall the name of a current medication, encourage them to bring the package to the next visit. Hormones, such as contraceptives, including intrauterine devices (IUDs) and implants, are often not included in reported medication lists, so if the patient could become pregnant based on their sexual activity and partners, inquire about current contraceptive use. Specifically inquire about other hormone use, including perimenopausal hormone replacement therapy (HRT) and gender-affirming hormone therapy (GAHT). Obtain information on any allergic responses to medications, foods, the environment, or other substances.

Substance Use

Assess for substance use with a direct yet nonjudgmental style of assessment. Inquire about each substance separately, beginning with legal substances, such as alcohol, tobacco (including vaping), cannabidiol (CBD) products, and, depending on the state, marijuana, and then move to illegal drugs and misuse of over-the-counter and prescribed medications. Ask about the amount and type of each substance used per day or week. Ask about past or current smoking habits, the daily number of cigarettes or joints, the length of time smoked, the number of attempts at quitting, and interest in quitting now. For cannabidiol products and marijuana, ask if the use is recreational or for pain, anxiety, depression, hunger, nausea, or other underlying symptoms, which may be addressed separately or adequately managed with legal cannabis use or other modalities. For illegal drugs, inquire about types, amount, route, and frequency of use. Depending on the community, using common street drug names may provide the patient with additional entrée into the provider's knowledge and comfort base. Asking if there are any medications used outside of their prescription or designation provides information about misuse of accessible medications. People may not automatically disclose a history of substance misuse or abuse, and knowing their current treatment or sobriety status can have an impact on their health. Employ motivational interviewing and assess the patient's level of willingness to reduce or abstain from substance(s). It is vital that the person sets their own goals related to sobriety or decreasing use of substance(s). Encourage self-determination in the patient which can involve setting attainable goals for oneself (Magill et al., 2022). This may be an opportunity to discuss the patient's understanding of the use of Naloxone, often referred to by its brand name, Narcan. Educate the patient on the purpose of Naloxone to quickly reverse the effects of opioids and refer them to community resources, some of which provide this life-saving medication for free to the public (Centers for Disease Control and Prevention [CDC], 2024). See Chapter 9 for further discussion of screening for alcohol misuse and Chapter 6 for how to conduct a brief intervention for individuals who screen positive.

For interviewers who are new to the process, positive answers to these questions may elicit surprise or concern, but these responses must not be visible to the patient. Maintain neutral and supportive facial expressions and tone of voice. As with all information sought during the history taking, specific facts become part of a broader picture of a clinician's approach to care provision; therefore, a nonjudgmental environment is imperative to encourage comfort with sharing the truth, including with legal or illegal substance use.

Family Health History

Gather information about first-degree relatives: parents, grandparents, siblings, and children. A family tree or narrative can be recorded, and information on serious illnesses and causes of death for each of these individuals should be obtained. In addition, occurrences of congenital malformations, unexplained intellectual and developmental disabilities, or other disabilities should be covered to offer clues to possible inherited diseases. Note that for many cancers, such as breast, uterine, and ovarian cancers, and for some acute and chronic conditions, such as myocardial infarctions and hypercholesterolemia, the affected family member's age at diagnosis may impact screening recommendations for the patient.

Social History

Invite the patient to share their social identity categories including race, ethnicity, and religion that may factor into their decision-making framework or care approaches. Never assume based on someone's appearance or language what the answers to social identity questions might be. Ascertain the patient's highest attained educational level, current life activities (e.g., employment or student status), family responsibilities, and long-term life plans. Review relationships, including spouses, partners, sexual relationships, current family or family planning, and current support system. When asking about relationships, never make assumptions about an individual's partner status, partner type(s), and the gender expression and sexuality of the patient and their partner(s). Use open-ended questions, such as "Tell me about your partner or partners" (Savoy et al., 2020). This part of history taking is an excellent opportunity to build patient–provider rapport, so try to allow this conversation to flow organically.

Occupation and Finances

Ask about current employment, concerns about safety or hazardous conditions at work, employment stability, physical safety, and body mechanics. Ask about military service, which is associated with health risks, including post-traumatic stress disorder, traumatic brain injury, and sexual trauma (American Academy of Nursing, 2019). Reviewing financial security, including ability to cover housing and food costs, is imperative to understand the need to connect individuals with further care resources. Further, clarifying an individual's ability to access food and housing separate from their partner can help identify if they are in an economically abusive relationship. Logistics related to healthcare provision are also important, including insurance concerns and barriers to seeking care, the latter of which may range from transportation issues to childcare needs.

Safety

Safety issues are often overlooked during history taking, but they are critical. They range from everyday concerns, such as the use of seat belts in motor vehicles and helmets with bicycle or motorcycle use, to the presence of firearms in the household and whether they are secure from children. Safety in the lived community, including within community housing structures, the presence of gangs, and perceived police safety or threat, are important to address. Immigrant, asylee, and refugee status may be disclosed verbally, but providers should avoid explicitly documenting this information in the health record (Kim et al., 2019). Current or past intimate partner violence, sexual assault, incest, emotional abuse, and/or reproductive coercion are essential components to review so the clinician can fully assess needs around healthy sexual and intimate relationships. All individuals deserve to be asked at every visit about personal and bodily safety.

Inquiring about what to chart for the patient's legal record, and who may have access to that information, is a safety guard clinicians can offer to assure privacy in disclosures. These may include histories of STIs, historical or current partners unaware to a primary partner, or previous pregnancies and outcomes. Additionally, as the visit note becomes a legal record, maintaining awareness of disclosures that can compromise the patient's safety in terms of care sought in other states, such as abortion or gender-affirming care, should be considered alongside institutional, legal, and organizational guidance as laws change. Providers should consider options within electronic record platforms to maintain patient privacy and safety, in collaboration with the patient. As the provider relationship develops, more information may be disclosed with time that was not revealed at the first history-taking session. See Chapters 6, 9, and 15 for more information about intimate partner violence.

Personal Habits

Ask about exercise, sleep patterns, self-care, nutrition, and hydration patterns. A 24-hour dietary recall, including the question "What do you drink when you are thirsty?" can provide a snapshot into common meals, drinks, and snacks. Ongoing health maintenance, such as dental care, eye examinations, and mental health support, can be screened with general questions, such as "What other health or personal-care-related appointments have you had in the past year?"

Mandated Reporting

Many different practice models exist related to the practical use of mandated reporting. Clinicians should be aware of community resources including mutual aid, mental health centers, family support systems, and referral sites within and outside of traditional institutional healthcare systems. Referral to state surveillance models, such as policing, state or national departments for children and families, and other emergency "wellness" checks may offer a form of follow-up but may also put the patient and their family at risk depending on other social and political contexts. Providers should be familiar with trauma-informed referral options for welfare checks and community aid options. Consider legal and licensure requirements to report suicidal or homicidal intent, child or older adult abuse and neglect. When asking questions about current, past, or future health histories including queer care, abortion/miscarriage history, and drug use during pregnancy, for example, be attentive to the legal implications of knowing those answers and documenting in the record. What is legal may not be ethical, and vice versa, and organizational policies related to civil disobedience as well as conscientious objection should be a part of every provider's ethical reflection on care. This may include not reporting immigration or asylee status, patient activities while on probation, and so on without federal warrants or other methods of being compelled by judicial requirements. HIPAA, specialty and licensure codes of ethics, and general privacy measures for patients should be paramount. The clinician's primary role is care and they should not be forced to participate in policing.

Gynecologic Health History

The gynecologic health history elicits significant details that provide the essential background for a concern-focused visit and for a health maintenance visit for an annual or wellness examination. The standard topics for this health history are listed in Box 8-5. Specific points that should be included about each topic follow.

Menstrual History

Menstrual history is usually the first topic in the gynecologic history. It should cover the following information: age at menarche; date when the last normal menstrual period (often referred to as LNMP or LMP) began; length of the cycle, counting from the first day of one menses until the first day of the next menses; average number of days of menses; characteristics of the menstrual flow, such as clotting, color, and consistency; regularity of cycles; and description of any irregularities or accompanying symptoms. In general, cycles range from 24 to 38 days, and menses last from 4 to 7 days (Campbell et al., 2021; Edelman et al., 2022). People can use smartphone apps to track menstrual cycle frequency, length, and symptoms, which help with history taking and can be particularly valuable for people with irregular menses or symptoms that may be connected to hormonal changes. Clinicians should caution patients that these apps may be surveilled at state and national levels, related to the user's fertility and pregnancy outcomes. In perimenopause, document the most recent menstrual cycle and note whether the cycles are regularly irregular (e.g., every 3 months) or irregularly irregular (unpredictable). In menopause, document the month and year of last menses, and note the pertinent negative of "no vaginal bleeding since menopause."

Sexual Health

Ask the patient's sexual orientation and gender identity. Intersex status or traits may be disclosed at this time or in the general health or surgical histories. Ask if the patient is sexually active. If so, ask them to describe their sexual partners. Making partners plural tells patients it is okay to disclose if they have more than one partner. Further questions include types of sex (e.g., oral, vaginal, or anal), including the use of vibrators and sex toys; satisfaction with sexual function; and if the patient or their partners have any shared sexual concerns. Do not presume gender identity, expression, or sexual orientation solely from a description of sexual partners. Follow up these answers as needed with further questions that directly pertain to the patient's healthcare provision and provider understanding (see Chapter 11), rather than probing based on provider interest or lack of understanding. Ask about the number of partners in the recent past or in the patient's lifetime only if it changes the course of their care. Use objective language and standardize history taking for all patients, regardless of presumed sex, gender identity, expression, and sexual orientation. Additional information about assessment of sexual health can be found in Chapter 12.

Contraceptive Use

Inquire about current and past contraceptive use. Do not make assumptions about whether an individual may need to or is currently using contraceptives. Some people use contraception for purposes other than preventing pregnancy, such as menstrual suppression and treatment of health conditions. If the patient or their partner is currently using a contraceptive method, ask if they have questions about their current method and if they are satisfied with the method or desire a change. Discussing methods used in the past may be relevant, depending on the reason for the visit (for example, some methods cause a delay in return to ovulation and thus temporarily impair fertility). Finally, inquiring about the use of emergency contraception, including frequency of use, may provide further information about contraceptive needs.

Pregnancy History

Begin by asking the patient the total number of times they have been pregnant, then ask for a description of each pregnancy in chronological order. The interviewer will use this information to complete the GTPAL five-digit numeric summary description of pregnancies (**Box 8-6**).

Specific information to obtain for each pregnancy includes the year it occurred, its duration, the type of birth (spontaneous vaginal birth, assisted vaginal birth, or cesarean birth), antepartum complications (e.g., gestational diabetes, hypertension),

BOX 8-6 Recording Pregnancy History: GTPAL System

Gravida: The total number of pregnancies, including current pregnancy if applicable

Term: The number of pregnancies that reached 37 0/7 weeks' gestation or greater

Preterm: The number of pregnancies that reached 20 0/7 weeks' gestation to 36 6/7 weeks' gestation, regardless of the number of fetuses or outcomes (i.e., induced abortion, fetal demise, or live birth)

Abortions: The number of spontaneous and induced abortions prior to 20 0/7 weeks' gestation

Living children: The number of living children, which usually equals the total of the term and preterm numbers but may be greater if the patient has had multiple gestations or less if any children have died

Data from American College of Obstetricians and Gynecologists. (2014). *reVITALize obstetric data definitions*. https://www.acog.org/About-ACOG/ACOG-Departments/Patient-Safety-and-Quality-Improvement/reVITALize-Obstetric-Data-Definitions

intrapartum complications (e.g., shoulder dystocia, third- or fourth-degree perineal lacerations, hemorrhage), postpartum complications (e.g., seizure, hospital readmission, depression, anxiety), assigned sex and weight of the newborn, and whether the child is currently alive. The category of abortion includes information about induced abortions, spontaneous abortions, ectopic pregnancies, and molar pregnancies. For these pregnancies, record details of gestational age, management (e.g., spontaneous, medication, or aspiration abortion; dilation and curettage; dilation and evacuation; laparoscopic removal), and any complications. The interviewer should specifically ask for history of abortion or miscarriage to ensure a complete history. Some people will not include all pregnancies in their initial health history interview for their own personal reasons, and they may disclose additional pregnancies at future visits or if they determine it could impact the course of their care. If patients report pregnancies that were not disclosed initially, thank them for providing this additional history and determine how to alert other health providers about this information through the health record.

History of Vaginal and Sexually Transmitted Infections

Ask which types of infections occurred, which treatments were provided, how frequently each infection occurred, and what complications occurred, if any. Naming each infection specifically may promote recall or disclosure. Discuss any known pelvic inflammatory disease (PID) diagnosis. Some people may not know their PID diagnosis by name, so asking about a history of PID symptoms and treatment (significant pelvic pain requiring a few different types of antibiotics) can help with recall. When screening for infection risk, ask only questions needed to determine if sexually transmitted infection (STI) testing and/or recommendations to prevent STIs are warranted. The interviewer will have already ascertained the number of partners and possible risk category in the sexual health history. In this section, it may be appropriate to review some reported history from earlier in the interview, such as "You said you have one current partner; has that been the case over the past 6 months?" Tell the patient why they are being asked about their partners so they know the rationale and can disclose appropriately. Inquire about STI protection use (e.g., condoms, dental dams) and tell them why. Detailed assessment of sexual risk is described in Chapter 22.

Genital and Breast Hygiene

Ask about any concerns related to vaginal hygiene if the patient expresses concern about vulvar or vaginal irritation. Additionally, ask about pubic hair removal and genital piercings if there are any related problems. Review any genital creams, lubricants, menstrual products, wipes, or sprays (namely, scented or dyed products that may increase irritation). In the case of douches or specialty soaps, inquire about the frequency of use, medications or solutions used, and the reasons for douching. For people who bind to flatten or diminish the appearance of their breasts, assess any concerns related to their binding practices (see Chapter 11). Some individuals, especially transgender men and nonbinary people, may refer to their breasts as their chest. See the section on breast examination for additional information.

Gynecologic Procedures and Surgeries

Include information on minor procedures, such as colposcopy, loop electrosurgical excision procedure (LEEP), endometrial biopsy, and cyst or abscess drainage, as well as surgeries, including laparoscopic examination, fibroid resection, tubal ligation, hysterectomy, salpingectomy, and oophorectomy. If serving intersex, transgender, and nonbinary populations, include questions related to any genital procedures or surgeries related to their anatomy at birth. See Chapter 11 for information about gender-affirming surgical procedures. InterACT and Lambda Legal (2018) furnish information about providing care to individuals who are intersex. The information needed includes the year in which the procedure or surgery was performed, indication, significant complications, and outcome. Obtaining pertinent health records may also be useful if detailed information is needed.

If serving populations in which female genital cutting is a known practice, include questions related to this procedure, which is also referred to as female circumcision or female genital mutilation (**Figure 8-2** and **Box 8-7**). For many people affected by cutting, this procedure may be normalized and thus not listed unless specifically asked. Additionally, "mutilation" may not be how the individual identifies with the process or the outcome, and it is a pejorative term about their private anatomy. Thus, asking about being "cut" or "circumcised" is typically more linguistically and culturally appropriate. If vulvovaginal alterations are noted in the examination and were not mentioned in the history, the provider should stop the examination and revisit this section of the history with care.

People may not disclose during the health history that they have been cut for a variety of reasons, including fear that the clinician will disapprove or respond negatively to this information. If a patient does disclose that their genitals were cut, that information may be shared while describing associated complications. A patient may also provide this information in response to an open-ended question, such as "Is there anything else you

FIGURE 8-2 Female genital cutting.

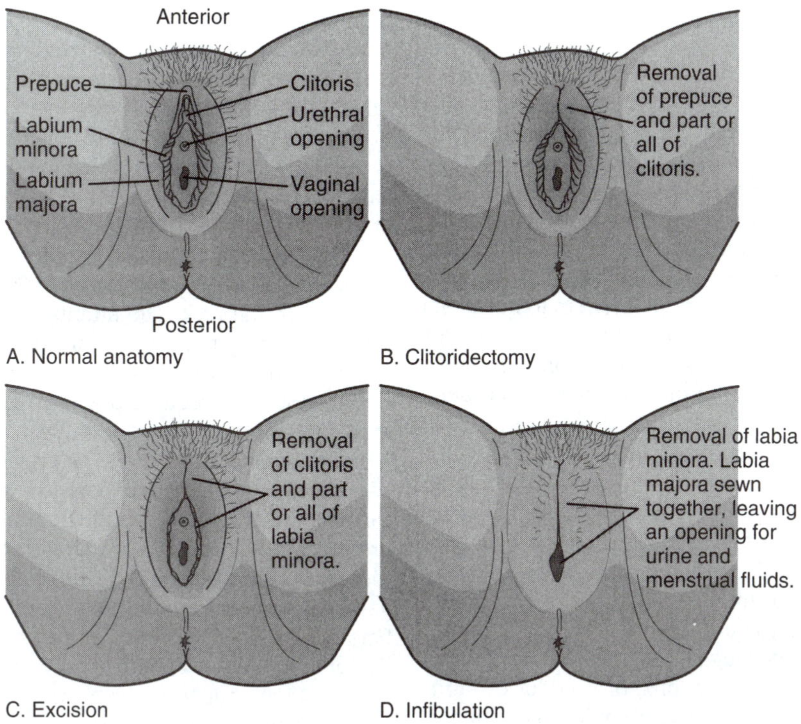

BOX 8-7 Female Genital Cutting

Female genital cutting, also called female circumcision and female genital mutilation, "comprises all procedures that involve partial or total removal of the external female genitalia, or other injury to the female genital organs for nonmedical reasons." There are four major types of female genital cutting:

Type 1, clitoridectomy: Partial or total removal of the clitoris and/or the prepuce.

Type 2, excision: Partial or total removal of the clitoris and the labia minora, with or without excision of the labia majora.

Type 3, infibulation: Narrowing of the vaginal orifice with the creation of a covering seal, accomplished by cutting and repositioning the labia minora and/or the labia majora, with or without excision of the clitoris.

Type 4, other: All other harmful procedures to the female genitalia for nonmedical purposes, such as pricking, piercing, incising, scraping, and cauterizing.

Long-term sequelae of female genital cutting include recurrent urinary tract infections, dermoid cysts, infertility, and obstetric complications.

Reproduced from World Health Organization. (2018). *Female genital mutilation*. https://www.who.int/news-room/fact-sheets/detail/female-genital-mutilation

would like me to know about your health background before we begin your examination?" It is important for the clinician to ask when the cutting occurred, whether the patient has previously had a pelvic examination, and if they are experiencing symptoms of long-term sequelae.

The extent of cutting will be determined during the inspection of the external genitalia. A pediatric speculum and single-digit bimanual examination may be necessary for the pelvic examination. A special form for recording health history and physical findings relevant to female genital cutting can be helpful.

Urologic and Rectal Health

Urologic topics include the occurrence and frequency of urinary tract infections, incontinence, and other abnormal symptoms such as urinary frequency, dysuria, and needing to displace any anatomy (inserting a finger into the vagina) to be able to urinate successfully. Rectal topics include incontinence, constipation, hemorrhoids, bloody stools, pain with defecation, and needing to displace anatomy (putting pressure in vagina) to be able to have a bowel movement.

Cervical Cancer Screening

Review any previous cervical cancer screening history (including anal cancer, if applicable), including the date of the most recent Pap test and human papillomavirus (HPV) test, if applicable, and the date of any abnormal results. With any history of abnormal Pap or HPV test results, ask what subsequent testing occurred. People may not know the name of the test, so give examples that help with recall (e.g., colposcopy, LEEP, or cone). See Chapter 9 for more information on cervical cancer screening.

Abnormal Symptoms

Problems such as pelvic pain and vaginal bleeding not related to menstruation should be fully described. See Chapters 25 and 29, respectively, for detailed information about the assessment of abnormal bleeding and pelvic pain.

Final Steps

The conclusion of the health history should include an invitation for the patient to add comments or ask questions. After the clinician has completed the health history, the next step is to examine, sort, and prioritize the information gathered and decide which further assessment measures, such as physical examination or laboratory tests, are needed. It is often helpful at this time to summarize the findings, offer tentative answers to questions or concerns the patient posed about their health, and discuss recommended screening tests, physical examinations, and laboratory evaluations. This emphasizes the patient–clinician partnership in care. While the patient is dressed, discuss all possible components of the physical examination that may be recommended, such as a breast examination or bimanual examination.

In charting, note pertinent positives and negatives in the review of systems and health history. Clinicians should be cognizant of verbal or documented language that diminishes concerns, devalues presented facts, patronizes emotional or mental health reports, or otherwise calls into question the validity of a report. Documentation should include language such as reports itching, describes pain in certain sexual positions, or no odor or burning, rather than words such as denies or admits, which suggest the patient is not telling the truth or is guilty of something. If, during the history taking, the patient declines some or all of the physical examination, document this as declines breast examination or prefers pelvic examination to be included at a different visit, rather than using words such as refused, which indicates a negative connotation to patient consent to procedures. If there is concern for withheld historical information or a patient's preferred process that differs from a clinician's recommendations, document this in the plan section, detailing education provided, consent process reviewed and the outcomes, and future considerations.

PHYSICAL EXAMINATION FOR A GYNECOLOGIC VISIT

Evaluating a new patient usually includes performing a physical examination. The details and description of the techniques, such as auscultation, are beyond the scope of this chapter. Readers are referred to textbooks on physical examination for a review of maneuvers, equipment, and organization of the examination (Bickley et al., 2024; Jarvis, 2024). This text assumes that the age range for patients will extend from early adolescence beyond menopause. Gynecologic care for children requires specialized pediatric skills that exceed the scope of this chapter.

What constitutes a complete physical examination in the ambulatory gynecology or primary care setting is not standardized. It is customary to evaluate major organ systems briefly and carefully, but not exhaustively. For example, a cardiovascular examination would include complete auscultation of the heart and evaluation of circulation by noting skin color, and it would usually omit other maneuvers, such as checking carotid bruits or palpation of the precordium. When deciding what to include in the physical examination, novice clinicians may want to use the following principle as a guideline: be able to state the rationale for including or excluding any assessment maneuver or particular feature of any organ system. If a rationale for performing a maneuver and obtaining the specific information that maneuver provides can be stated, then including it would be justified.

If family members or partners are present during the history-taking portion of the visit, ask the patient if they would like to proceed with the physical examination portion with or without those individuals present. Keep in mind that evidence of physical violence, identifying past or current experiences of sexual abuse, and an opportunity to speak with the patient alone are all possible components of the physical examination. For people who may currently be experiencing physical or sexual abuse by those in the room, be attentive for deference to questions, positive or negative communications, guarding during physical interactions, or any other sign that might trigger an intuitive response to request others to leave the room during the examination.

Additionally, any patient or provider should be accommodated if they request a chaperone (American College of Obstetricians and Gynecologists, 2020). Chaperones can validate the professional context of care provision, be a support person for the patient if needed during a difficult examination, and offer legal protection for both the patient and the provider. Family members cannot be chaperones. If the chaperone is an employee of the practice, clear confidentiality guidelines should be established. Often chaperones are reserved for cisgender male providers caring for cisgender female patients, but it is reasonable for every patient and provider, regardless of their sex assigned at birth, sexual orientation, or gender identity.

Before beginning any component of the physical examination, providers must consider offering an intentional reflection of power and a verbal acknowledgment and discussion. Inform the patient of their ability to stop or change the examination at any time (see Box 8-1 for suggested language). A patient's mere presence for an evaluation does not indicate consent for every examination component a provider might consider routine. In the outpatient setting, many or all components of the physical examination can be deferred to future visits. Remind the patient that it is okay to be ready for only certain portions of the physical examination at each visit or to decide mid-examination that they are no longer comfortable with continuing the examination that day. Although seeing patients undressed and performing physical examinations on their bodies is routine for clinicians, it is completely out of the range of normal for patients; this must be acknowledged and approached with grace and respect. Finally, it is not always evidence based, nor is it humane, for a physical examination to be required before prescribing requested medications, including contraceptives, and these should not be withheld if an individual declines or defers a physical examination.

General Physical Examination

The order of the examination presented here assumes the patient is sitting up to begin the examination. This description proceeds from head to toe, rather than by system. If someone asks for a certain component of an examination to be first or last, reorder the examination as requested.

1. Physical measurements: Obtain and review blood pressure, pulse, and temperature (if indicated) before performing the

physical examination. Height and blood pressure may be indicated for screening and prevention visits. Weight measurements and associated calculations, such as body mass index (BMI), should only be conducted as needed for the visit or in conjunction with other metrics, and are best chosen through shared decision making with the patient (*AMA Adopts New Policy Clarifying Role of BMI as a Measure in Medicine*, 2023). Historical and contemporary implications of taking weight, recording a body mass based on weight and height, and then making social or moral judgments as well as clinical recommendations for weight loss or restriction to other care opportunities is rooted in racism, the cisgender male form as the presumed default measurement, and disability injustice (Olson et al., 2024). Weight bias has no place in health care. More information can be found through the Association for Size Diversity and Health's resources on Health at Every Size (HAES) (Association for Size Diversity and Health, n.d.). See Chapter 9 for further discussion. Note also that even thoughtful use of body mass index will use body weight, which does not differentiate between muscle and fat mass or identify the distribution of body fat (i.e., visceral vs. other).

2. General appearance: Observe the posture; striking or obvious characteristics or limitations; the general emotional state; and the appropriateness of dress, speech pattern, and social interaction during the visit.
3. Eyes, ears, nose, and throat: Inspect the physical health of the eyes, nose, and ears. Examination of the ears with the otoscope and examination of the eyes with the ophthalmoscope may be performed if indicated. The oropharynx examination includes inspection of the lips, teeth, and gums for dental health, and visualization of the oral cavity for mucosal color, lesions, and tonsillar edema or exudates.
4. Neck: Note the range of motion and palpate lymph nodes in the neck and clavicular area.
5. Thyroid: Palpate the gland and isthmus.
6. Chest and lungs: Auscultate the posterior, lateral, and anterior lobes.
7. Spine: Palpate the vertebral column and inspect the skin.
8. Kidneys: Check for costovertebral tenderness.
9. Reflexes: Elicit patellar and additional reflexes as indicated.
10. Peripheral circulation and varicosities: Inspect the legs and feet.

The patient then reclines, and the examination continues:

11. Heart: Auscultate the heart.
12. Breasts and axillary lymph nodes: See the next section on breast examination.
13. Abdomen: Inspect the skin, palpate superficially and deeply in all quadrants, and palpate the inguinal lymph nodes.
14. Genital and pelvic examination (if indicated): See the following section on pelvic examination.

Breast and Chest Examination

This chapter uses the term "breast" to refer to the mammary glands located over the pectoral muscles, and it uses the term "chest" to refer to the part of the body between the neck and the abdomen. Some individuals refer to breasts as their chest. People who are transgender, nonbinary, or genderqueer may use the term "chest" regardless of whether they have what may be clinically defined as breasts. For people with mastectomy or surgical alteration, "chest" may better define their current chest wall structure.

Despite inconsistent organizational recommendation regarding the efficacy of breast or chest self-examination as well as routine clinical examination for average risk or asymptomatic patients, clinical breast examination performed by health professionals remains a part of the general physical examination. See Chapter 9 for further discussion of breast cancer screening. The breast or chest examination utilizes inspection and palpation, both of which require varying degrees of skin exposure for the patient throughout the examination. Before beginning, providers should discuss why this exposure is needed and employing an approach that is gentle but focused on the examination will convey the clinician's concern and respect. All requests for modifications to exposure should be accommodated when possible. Adequate lighting helps to reveal subtle variations in skin texture and color. Adequate exposure, or having the patient disrobe to the waist, allows simultaneous observation and comparison of both breasts and sides of the chest. As with all physical examinations, wearing gloves during this portion of the examination is not only a universal precaution but reinforces its clinical application for clinical touch in this part of the body. Be conscious of intentional clinical palpation throughout the examination. Utilizing the pads of the second, third, and fourth fingers of the provider's dominant hand at three pressures (light, medium, and deep) will yield the highest sensitivity to changes in tissue. Only one hand should be used to palpate the breast or chest at any time; however, for the patient's comfort and for the provider's ability to adequately palpate larger breasts, the fingertips on the other hand can stabilize tissue during the examination. At no point should the entire hand touch the breast, cup the breast, or slide unnecessarily along the tissue without an explicit clinical purpose. The opposite hand should be used only if the tissue needs to be stabilized; it should not rest unnecessarily on the chest.

Breast and Chest Inspection

The examination begins with the patient in a sitting position, usually on the examining table, with arms relaxed at their sides, and the examiner standing facing them. Start by visually examining the chest. Compare both sides for size, symmetry, contour, skin color, texture, venous patterns, and lesions. Breasts and chests vary in shape, and frequently one side will be slightly larger than the other. The skin texture should be smooth, the contours should be uninterrupted bilaterally, and the venous pattern should be similar bilaterally. Benign lesions, such as nevi, if long-standing, unchanged, and nontender, are considered normal findings. Ask about the history of these skin changes during the examination to clarify as needed.

Next, visually inspect the nipples and areolae. The areolae should be round or oval and nearly equal in configuration bilaterally. The color ranges from pink to black. Areolar sebaceous glands may be seen as slightly raised fleshy protuberances and are a common finding. [Note that in historical anatomy books these may be labeled as "Montgomery" tubercles, so-named for the clinician who first "discovered" them. There is an ongoing effort to utilize correct anatomical nomenclature rather than territorial eponyms, particularly in sexual and reproductive health care. An international comprehensive list of these can be found through the Federative International Programme for Anatomical Terminology (FIPAT) (Federative International Programme for

Anatomical Terminology (FIPAT), 2019)]. Prominent sebaceous glands may be a normal finding if the patient reports no changes. The nipples also should be equal or nearly equal in size. Most nipples are everted. If one or both are inverted, ask if inversion has been a lifelong characteristic. A newly inverted nipple, nipple retraction, or nipple flattening suggests pathology. Surgery for breast reduction, mastectomy for gender affirmation or pathology, or injury may change the presence of or size and shape of the nipple. Look also at the orientation of the nipples. If one points in a different direction from the other, this may be caused by the presence of malignant tissue in the breast or chest. The color of the nipples should be the same as the areolae, while the surface may be smooth or wrinkled. Spontaneous nipple discharge should not be present unless the person is breast- or chestfeeding. Supernumerary or extra nipples may be seen. They are benign, usually small, and commonly mistaken as moles. They may occur anywhere along a vertical line from the axilla to the inner thigh and are usually unilateral.

The last step of inspection in the sitting position is to have the patient change positions slightly so that the contour and symmetry of the breasts or chest can be assessed completely. The three positions for examination while seated are arms over the head, hands pressed against the hips, and leaning forward at the waist. If the patient has noted an abnormality they can only feel when sitting upright, ask them to point to the location while they are still seated and attempt to palpate that specific area.

FIGURE 8-3 **Palpating large breasts.**

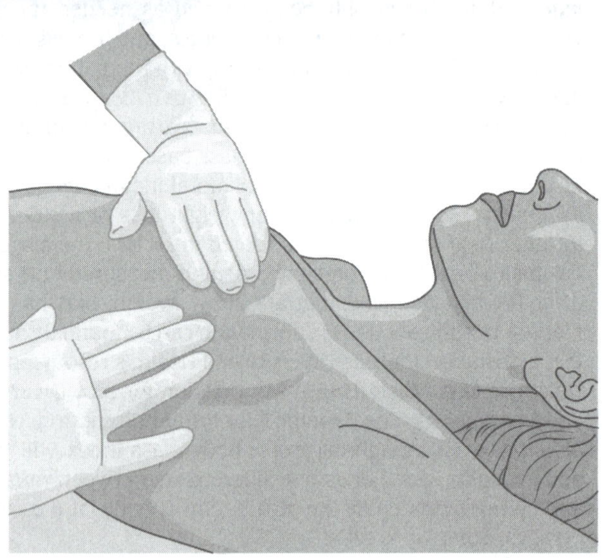

Examination of Lymph Nodes

While the patient is still sitting, evaluate the axillary and supraclavicular lymph nodes. Ask the patient to flex their arm at the elbow. The examiner stands facing the patient but slightly off center. If beginning with the right axilla, use the left hand. Notify the patient that sometimes this deep palpation can cause slight discomfort. Reach deeply into the axillary hollow and press firmly upward with the palmar surfaces of the fingers, then bring the fingers downward to gently roll the soft tissue against the chest wall. Be sure to examine not only the apex, but also the central and medial aspects along the rib cage, the lateral aspect along the medial surface of the arm, the anterior wall along the pectoral muscles, and the posterior wall along the border of the scapula. Repeat this procedure with the other axilla. Axillary lymph nodes are usually not palpable in adults. The supraclavicular area should also be palpated. Hook the fingers over the clavicle and rotate them over the entire supraclavicular area.

Supine Breast Palpation

After the visual inspection and lymph node examination, breast palpation is performed in the supine position. Place a small pillow or folded towel under the shoulder before beginning the examination of the breast on that side. The examiner remains standing facing the patient. Cover the other breast or chest wall with a gown or drape for warmth and comfort. Palpate all four quadrants for nodules and lumps. Use the finger pads because they are more sensitive to touch than the fingertips. Be aware that a firm transverse ridge of compressed tissue is often found along the lower edge of the breast. It comprises the inframammary ridge and is a normal finding. For large breasts or chest walls with dense adipose or muscle tissue, it may be helpful to place one hand beneath the tissue to stabilize it while palpating with the other hand (**Figure 8-3**). Press at three depths—light, medium, and deep—firmly enough to get a good sense of the underlying tissue but not so firmly that the tissue is compressed against the rib cage. Rotate the fingers in a clockwise or counterclockwise direction. Palpate top to bottom in a vertical stripe pattern; a consistent, methodical approach is key to performing a complete examination. Palpate over the nipple in the same pattern and pressure as with the entirety of the breast tissue. Note any discomfort or pain that the patient mentions or responds to physically with a change in facial expression or body movement, stop the examination, and ask how to change the approach to improve comfort.

The axillary process—eponymously referred to as the tail of Spence, tissue that extends from the upper outer quadrant toward the axilla—must also be palpated because most malignancies develop in the upper outer quadrant (VanMeter & Hubert, 2014). This is best done by having the patient raise their arms over their head while the examiner gently compresses the tissue where it enters the axilla between the thumb and fingers (**Figure 8-4**).

Repeat the examination with the patient's arm at their side. This repetition aids in a complete palpation because tissue shifts with different positions. After the entire breast or chest is palpated, notify the patient that the next step is to press the nipple to check for discharge. Compress the nipple between the first finger on each hand to inspect for discharge; avoid compressing with finger and thumb to avoid nonclinical inappropriate touching of the breast or chest. Compression usually causes the nipple to become erect, and it may be momentarily painful. Bilateral clear or white discharge can be normal, depending on the stage of the patient's menstrual cycle or if they have a history of pregnancy. Unilateral discharge, or any green, red, or black discharge, is abnormal and a concern for malignancy.

Breast and chest tissue in adults palpates as dense, firm, and elastic. Prior to and during menstruation, some people experience cyclical tenderness, swelling, and nodularity. If a mass is palpated, note the location, size, shape, consistency, tenderness, mobility, and demarcation of borders. If the mass is then felt equally on the other side, this can be a normal finding given its symmetry.

For the beginning practitioner, explaining the component of each step of the examination while performing it not only ensures a complete review, but it also engages the patient in their care and allows an opportunity to educate them on parts of their anatomy or concerning abnormalities. This step-wise process is also part of ongoing consent and can serve as a reminder that the patient can stop the exam or decline any portion at any time. After this examination becomes second nature, many clinicians simultaneously perform the breast or chest examination while also discussing breast and chest self-awareness, which is knowing how one's breasts or chest normally appear and feel, emphasizing the need to notify the provider of any changes.

An abbreviated form of this examination may include a seated inspection and palpation only in the supine position. Each practitioner modifies the examination according to the individual patient, time per visit, concerning symptoms or history, and if an abnormality is identified by either the patient or the clinician (**Figure 8-5**).

FIGURE 8-4 **Palpating the axillary process.**

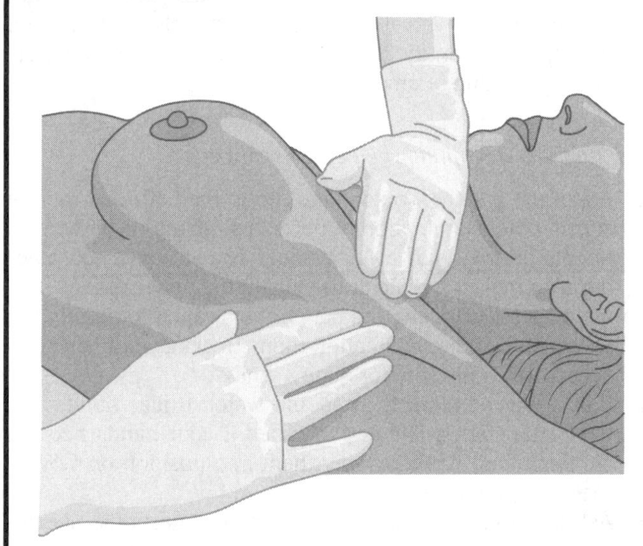

Pelvic Examination

The pelvic examination customarily concludes the sexual and reproductive healthcare examination, but it is not required for an annual well-person examination. The pelvic examination may be included if the patient has questions about their anatomy, is having symptoms externally or internally, is due for cervical or anal cancer screening, or is following up from a prior evaluation. The decision to proceed with this examination is shared between patient and provider (Chor et al., 2019). Additional considerations for the pelvic examination, including whether to include external and/or internal components, should be based on the patient's age, history of coitarche, whether their sexual activity includes penetrative sex, and history of sexual assault (Tillman, 2020). Providers must be clear with patients about the purpose of the examination and how the findings may, or may not, influence the plan of care. Particularly for patients and providers meeting for the first time, it can build rapport for the clinician to offer to defer the pelvic examination for another visit. Further, if patients are asymptomatic, the latest evidence indicates that external and internal examination is unnecessary and should therefore be reserved for symptomatic concerns (U.S. Preventive Services Task Force [USPSTF] et al., 2017; ACOG, 2018 [Reaffirmed 2024]).

At any point in the examination, the patient may experience discomfort or may want the examination to stop for whatever reason. Knowing that this is possible for all patients, providers must discuss this before the examination begins (see Box 8-1 for suggested language). It can be reassuring to patients to know that verbal cues will be respected by the provider. Of utmost importance is following through; if the patient gives a verbal cue to stop the examination and the provider says "almost done" or "just another second," that is a violation of both the patient's trust and body.

The description offered here assumes the reader is familiar with the anatomy of the pelvic structures, particularly the anatomy of the internal and external sexual and reproductive organs (see Chapter 7). A few features of these structures, such as their size, relative locations, and the common findings, are

FIGURE 8-5 **Traditional anatomical nipple, prominent sebaceous glands, mastectomy without nipple.**

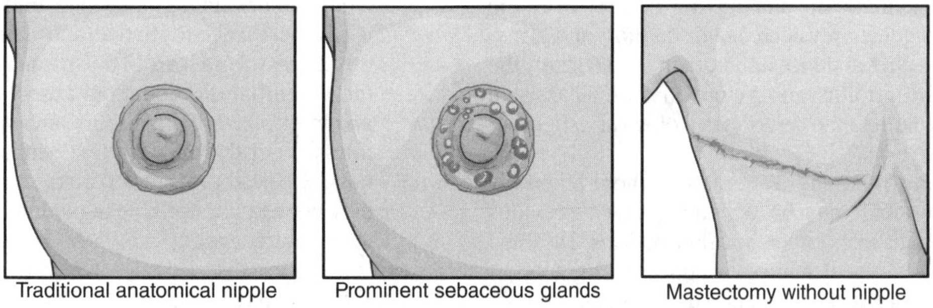

particularly important for easily and successfully performing this examination.

For some patients, the pelvic examination may be the most sensitive or intimate healthcare interaction they experience. This examination is known to be anxiety producing and activating for people with a history of pelvic care trauma, including sexual assault and birth violence. Each individual brings their own experiences and needs to the present examination. The trauma-informed framework reviewed earlier in this chapter is critical during this part of the examination. The full scope of the pelvic examination, including exposing genitalia to a stranger and having tools or the provider's fingers inserted with the potential to cause pain, can itself cause trauma regardless of someone's history, despite all clinician efforts to the contrary. All clinicians who perform this type of examination have the professional responsibility to carry it out proficiently, promptly, and respectfully. Retrospective studies have shown that negative effects from a pelvic speculum examination will cause people to delay or discontinue future care, which is ultimately counterproductive to the intent of the examination (USPSTF et al., 2017; O'Laughlin et al., 2021).

Specific trauma-informed approaches to the pelvic examination that are reasonable to offer in all settings include the following:

- Explicitly state that the examination is in the patient's control and that the provider can completely stop at any time, pause until the patient states they are ready to continue, or defer the examination to another visit.
- Use language that can easily be understood by anyone. Use common words, not medical terms.
- Never talk lightly or make jokes about genitalia or the examination. This is inappropriate. If a patient makes jokes about the examination, gently revert back to professional language (see Box 8-1 for suggestions).
- Ensure privacy for this examination, including closing the door and the curtain, if available. Minimize interruptions from fellow staff members, such as knocking or calling through the closed door.
- Offer a mirror, which can serve multiple purposes. For patients who want to see the clinician's safe and appropriate evaluation, a mirror can be empowering. For people who want to learn more about their own body, the mirror is an opportunity to educate along with the examination. For any new findings or abnormalities, the mirror can help the patient become a partner in the assessment of their body and note any changes or findings for future follow-up.
- Offer speculum self-insertion. For many people, the speculum insertion is the most uncomfortable or traumatic component of the examination and having control over the equipment can significantly decrease discomfort and transfer power. In this circumstance, the patient would insert the speculum past the introitus, and the provider would assist in guiding the speculum to the cervix for cytology and/or other sample collection.
- Offer options for positioning. Patients for whom lithotomy or supine positioning may be activating given previous trauma may benefit from other position options. Disabled patients who use a wheelchair or orthotics for leg support may be most comfortable in a seated, semi-standing, or other supported position that may necessitate additional staff support. Visual examples of these positions can be found in *Table Manners: A Guide to the Pelvic Examination for Disabled Women and Health Care Providers* (Ferreyra & Hughes, 1982; Barbera et al., 2024).
- With speculum self-insertion, or with examinations in positions other than supine, the handle of the speculum may be positioned superior to the introitus. The clinician should guard the handle from causing discomfort to the nearby anatomy, including the clitoris. The speculum should not be rotated for the clinician's comfort unless necessary, as the rotation will be uncomfortable for the patient and potentially cancel out the positive impact of the self-insertion or choosing a position preferable to the patient. Much like learning birth on hands and knees, clinicians should practice and become comfortable with examinations including clinical tools in many patient positions.
- Prepare all materials before getting the patient into position for the examination, including applying gel to the speculum and setting out any swabs or samples the examiner plans to utilize. This minimizes the amount of time the patient is in the lithotomy position and reduces unnecessary exposure. Before the provider leaves the room so that the patient can disrobe, asking whether the patient would prefer to see or not see the tray with all the examination tools can be helpful as, depending on the patient, this level of information may be empowering or anxiety-inducing.

Preparing and Beginning the Pelvic Examination

1. Ask if the patient would like to go to the bathroom before starting the examination. A pelvic examination can be very uncomfortable with a full bladder or rectum. A full bladder also makes it difficult to palpate the pelvic organs. Depending on how long the patient has waited for you in the waiting room or examination room, they may not have had access to a bathroom for quite a while.
2. Wash your hands with soap and water. Utilize hand sanitizer after the patient is positioned if your hands became contaminated while helping them into position or moving the chair and table.
3. Ask if the patient has any concerns or questions. Specifically ask if they prefer to know everything about the process or nothing at all. If they prefer to know about the process, explain the methods used throughout the examination; offer to show all the tools (speculum, collection swabs, etc.) while the patient is still fully clothed and at equal eye level with you. If they prefer to not know the process, cover the examination table and restrict their view of the tools that will be used.
    a. If this is the patient's first genital and pelvic examination, it can be both informative and empowering to review the process from start to finish, including demonstrating the tools that are commonly used, discussing external and internal components, and answering any questions.
    b. If this is not the patient's first genital and pelvic examination, ask about previous examinations and whether they were uncomfortable or painful (see Box 8-1 for suggested language).
4. Offer the option of a drape. It provides some privacy and warmth and may facilitate relaxation, but some people may find it intrusive or unnecessary.

5. Maintain the ability for eye contact during the examination as much as possible, recognizing that individuals may not return eye contact for cultural or other reasons. Raising the head of the examination table slightly and modifying the drape between the legs to not block a face-to-face view, allows visualization if the patient desires and typically does not interfere with the needed positioning for the cervical evaluation.
6. Assist the patient into the discussed position.
7. Offer options for foot placement. Many providers utilize a pull-out examination table, with the patient's knees bent and their feet either flat on the table or the soles of the feet touching with the knees dropped outward. This placement allows patients to modify their body positioning for their own comfort and allows them to easily move if they experience pain or discomfort during the examination. Depending on the type of examination table or the patient's body mechanics, the patient may prefer footrests or knee rests that offer stability and support. Foot pedals can be a form of soft restraint, which keep the patient's pelvis accessible to the provider while preventing the patient from closing their legs as a nonverbal communication method if necessary. For other patients, foot pedals or knee rests might be most comfortable for their body positioning for examinations.
8. Encourage the patient to move to the foot of the examination table until their buttocks are close to or, when necessary, slightly beyond the edge. This positioning is important to allow correct placement of the speculum. Moving down the table can be uncomfortable for the patient if they are already lying back, so encourage them to sit while changing position.
9. Sit on a stool that positions you at eye level with the patient's perineum. Adjust the lighting for the examination so it will not need to be moved again. Don gloves (many clinics have only nonlatex gloves due to provider or patient sensitivities and delayed reactions) and start the examination. Touch the patient and examination materials only after putting on gloves. If you touch other things in the room, such as the seat or the light, change gloves and use clean technique throughout the examination.
10. Ask the patient to drop their knees out to the sides. Never try to force their legs open, even by pressing gently. It is sometimes helpful for the clinician to position their hands outside of the patient's knees or thighs and ask them to drop their legs toward your hands. It is essential to avoid saying "relax" because this word is commonly used by sexual assailants and can be activating for those with an assault history. It is important for each clinician to find language that works for them, such as "drop your legs to the sides" or "let your legs fall open." Saying "I will know that you are ready once you are in position; take your time, and let me know if you have any questions" lets the patient know you will not start until they are ready. This can be a good time to talk about something more casual and move to the side of the table to face the patient until they indicate they are ready to begin the examination.
11. With the patient's consent, tell them that the examination will begin.
12. During the examination, if the patient becomes tense, clenches their pelvic muscles, closes their legs, or becomes upset, conveyed with a change in breathing or expression of concern, stop immediately. Ask if there is anything they need or anything you can do differently. Tell them the examination will not continue until they are ready. Make any adjustments that will ensure comfort before continuing. Some people, whether due to a history of sexual assault or a history of forced or painful pelvic examinations, may request that the examiner "just get it over with" or ignore their responses and hurry through the examination. If this happens, acknowledge and discuss these comments with the patient. Some language could include statements such as "I will go as quickly as possible but do not want to cause you pain in the process." Individualizing this conversation and patient care is critical to a trauma-informed approach and to create a trusting and empowering rapport with the patient.
13. If, during the external examination, the patient has significant discomfort or pain, or if you see the pelvic muscles clamping closed in the absence of a known assault history (perhaps the patient indicates that this happens with intercourse or tampon use), this raises concern for vulvodynia, pelvic pain, or a history of forced vaginal entry. Consider delaying further examination until another visit. If the examination is for general health maintenance rather than for a specific concern, or if further evaluation and testing can be done without vaginal entry, consider adjusting the examination appropriately (e.g., performing urine rather than cervical chlamydia and gonorrhea testing).
14. If you encounter an unexpected finding, avoid expressing surprise in both facial expression and voice. If additional testing is needed, calmly explain that an additional sample is needed based on the examination. If assistance is needed from another health professional to evaluate an abnormal or unexpected finding before the completion of the current examination, briefly explain the finding and the reason for a second examiner's assessment prior to their involvement, then discuss the finding more fully at the end of the examination.

Inspection and Palpation of External Genitalia, Vaginal Orifice, and Accessory Glands

1. Proceed with inspection in an orderly manner so as not to unnecessarily repeat touching. Many clinicians use a one-handed, top-to-bottom approach to ensure a complete examination and minimize repetition. Utilize a consistent pressure throughout the examination to avoid light touch or a poking sensation.
2. Inspect the mons pubis, labia majora, and perineum, noting the pattern of hair distribution, size and shape of the labia, and presence of lesions, scars, rashes, erythema, discharge, discoloration, or piercings (Figure 8-8, Vulvar Anatomy).
3. Start with a firm touch with the back of one gloved hand on one lower thigh, then move the examining hand along the thigh toward the external genitalia. If the patient has indicated that they prefer the examination to be described throughout, helpful language might include, "You will feel my hand on your thigh, then on the outside of your labia. I will be examining just on the outside first, beginning at the top and moving toward the bottom. Let me know if anything is uncomfortable or painful."
4. With the hand that had touched the inner thigh, separate the anterior portion of the labia majora, inspect and palpate the

labia minora, and inspect the urethral orifice and clitoris, moving posteriorly with consistent pressure and using the same fingers (e.g., thumb and first finger, thumb and fourth finger). Note the anatomic placement of the urethral opening and inspect for clitoral enlargement. There is no need to palpate the exposed head of the clitoris or the underlying clitoral body as part of this examination. Do not use both hands to separate the labia on each side; use two fingers of one hand to complete the visual and palpation components of the external examination.

5. Inspect the vaginal introitus for presence or absence of the hymen and hymenal tags and shape of the opening; note swelling, discharge, irregular growths, nevi, or lesions. Be careful not to mistake a hymen for a vaginal septum. If a septum is noted, a bimanual examination must be considered prior to speculum examination to determine the extent of the septum; if there are two complete vaginal canals, cervices, or uteri that may need evaluation; and whether consultation is necessary. Avoid removing the examining fingers and replacing them, poking, or moving the fingers in a stroking manner during the inspection or palpation portions of the examination. Consistent pressure is important for clinical evaluation.
6. This section of the pelvic examination may conclude at this point, or you may continue with one or more of the assessments outlined in steps 7 through 10. Although examination for pelvic organ prolapse, vaginal tone, and gland abnormalities may be considered components of a comprehensive pelvic examination, they are not necessarily performed routinely. Providers often omit these assessments unless there is a specific indication to perform them for an individual patient; therefore, the descriptions of these assessments include specific indications for performing them. You may choose to perform steps 7 through 10 during the bimanual examination, rather than with the external genitalia inspection, according to your preference and patient comfort.
7. If there is a concern for pelvic organ prolapse, maintain labial separation at the anterior aspect of the perineum and visualize the immediate introitus. Ask the patient to cough or bear down. If there is a cystocele (**Figure 8-6**), the anterior vaginal wall will bulge with this maneuver. Observe also for a rectocele (**Figure 8-7**), or bulging of the posterior vaginal wall; this is a far less common finding. Cystoceles, rectoceles, and uterine prolapse are typically graded on their position in the vagina as related to the hymenal ring or the vaginal introitus (**Box 8-8**). Early stages of pelvic organ prolapse, including of the uterus, may not be symptomatic and thus are undetected by history taking. It is important to detail changes in vaginal tone and appropriate pelvic organ suspension in the visit documentation to evaluate for a stable or worsening condition during future evaluations.
8. If there is a concern related to vaginal tone, assess the perineal muscles by asking the patient to tighten their muscles around your fingers in the vagina. This maneuver also ensures appropriate pelvic muscle exercises. If you palpate the patient pushing outward, instruct them to try to grasp your fingers to facilitate understanding of pulling the pelvic floor upward.
9. If there is concern for a greater vestibular gland cyst, eponymously referred to as a Bartholin cyst, or a history of recurrent cysts or abscesses, palpate the glands by inserting the index finger of the examining hand about 2 cm into the vagina near the perineum, turning the hand laterally, and gently palpating the tissue behind the vaginal wall between the thumb and index finger on one side; then, after rotating the examining hand, palpate in the same manner on the

FIGURE 8-6 Cystocele.

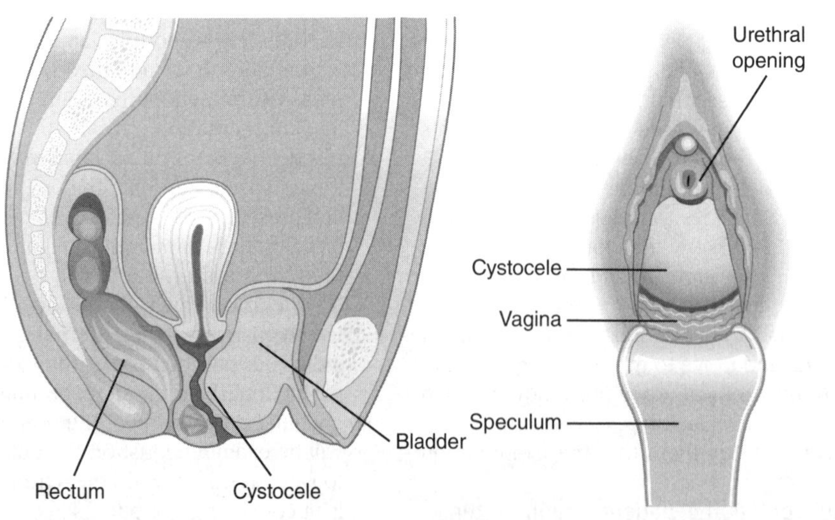

FIGURE 8-7 **Rectocele.**

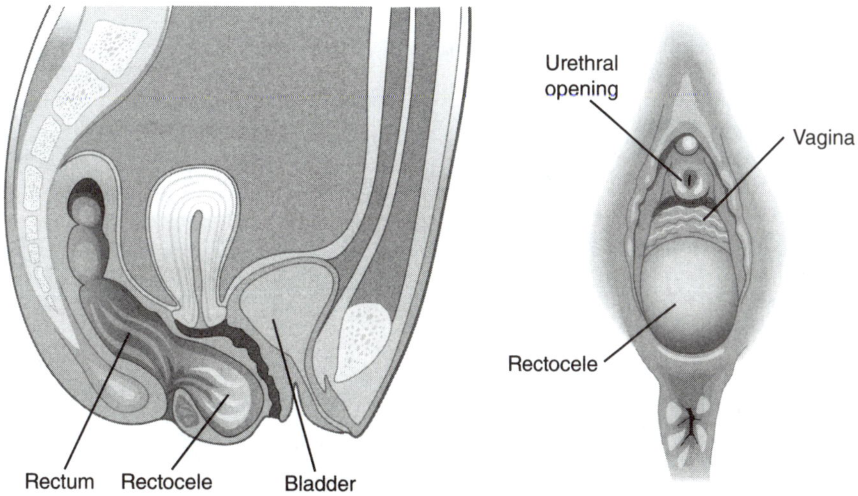

BOX 8-8 Quantification (POP-Q)[a]

Stage 0: No prolapse

Stage I: Most distal portion of the prolapse is more than 1 cm above the level of the hymen.

Stage II: Most distal portion of the prolapse is between 1 cm above the hymen and 1 cm below the hymen.

Stage III: Most distal portion of the prolapse is more than 1 cm below the plane of the hymen but everted ≥ 2 cm less than the total vaginal length.

Stage IV: Complete eversion, or eversion at least within 2 cm of the total length of the lower genital tract.

These initial stages are specified even further based on the stage of prolapse related to the anterior or posterior vaginal wall and the vaginal apex. For more information about additional staging, see Madhu, C., Swift, S., Moloney-Geany, S., & Drake, M. J. (2018). How to use the Pelvic Organ Prolapse Quantification (POP-Q) system? *Neurourology and Urodynamics, 37*(S6). https://doi.org/10.1002/nau.23740

[a]The assessment is performed while the patient strains as if having a bowel movement.

Data from Madhu, C., Swift, S., Moloney-Geany, S., & Drake, M. J. (2018). How to use the Pelvic Organ Prolapse Quantification (POP-Q) system? *Neurourology and Urodynamics, 37*(S6). https://doi.org/10.1002/nau.23740

other side of the vagina. Healthy greater vestibular glands are not palpable, but if they are inflamed this maneuver will elicit notable pain. If a cyst is present, a fluctuant, nontender mass will be palpable. If an abscess is present, the site of the mass will be tender and warm.

10. If there is a concern related to infection, particularly gonorrhea, you may palpate the periurethral glands, eponymously referred to as Skene glands, which lie immediately lateral to the urethral meatus, by turning the examining hand upward, inserting the index finger into the vagina to the second knuckle, pressing gently upward, then pulling this finger outward while pressing against the vaginal tissue. Discharge at the urethral meatus with palpation of the periurethral glands usually indicates infection. This examination lasts only about 10 seconds, but it usually causes pain regardless of the presence of infection. With modern laboratory testing requiring only a few days for results, many clinicians omit this portion of the examination even if there is concern that the patient has an infection because assessment of the periurethral glands is not diagnostic for an STI and would not change management.

Speculum Examination

It is essential that clinicians become familiar with how the speculum operates before performing this examination. This preparation ensures the clinician does not inadvertently cause pain due to incorrect use. Each clinician must also decide which hand to use for holding the speculum—a decision that is based entirely on personal preference. One hand is used to reach for tools and specimens, and it should not touch the patient. The other hand is used solely for examination. These can be distinguished as the room hand and patient hand, respectively. If the hands become cross-contaminated, the clinician should replace one or both gloves before the examination proceeds.

A speculum examination should be utilized as needed, such as for evaluation of vaginal or pelvic pain or cervical cytology screening. This examination is not required annually, nor is it a necessary component of every pelvic examination for symptomatic evaluation if there is no concern or symptom for which a speculum examination would provide further information.

FIGURE 8-8 **Types of specula. A. Top and side views of Graves and Pederson specula. B. Specula are available in metal and plastic.**

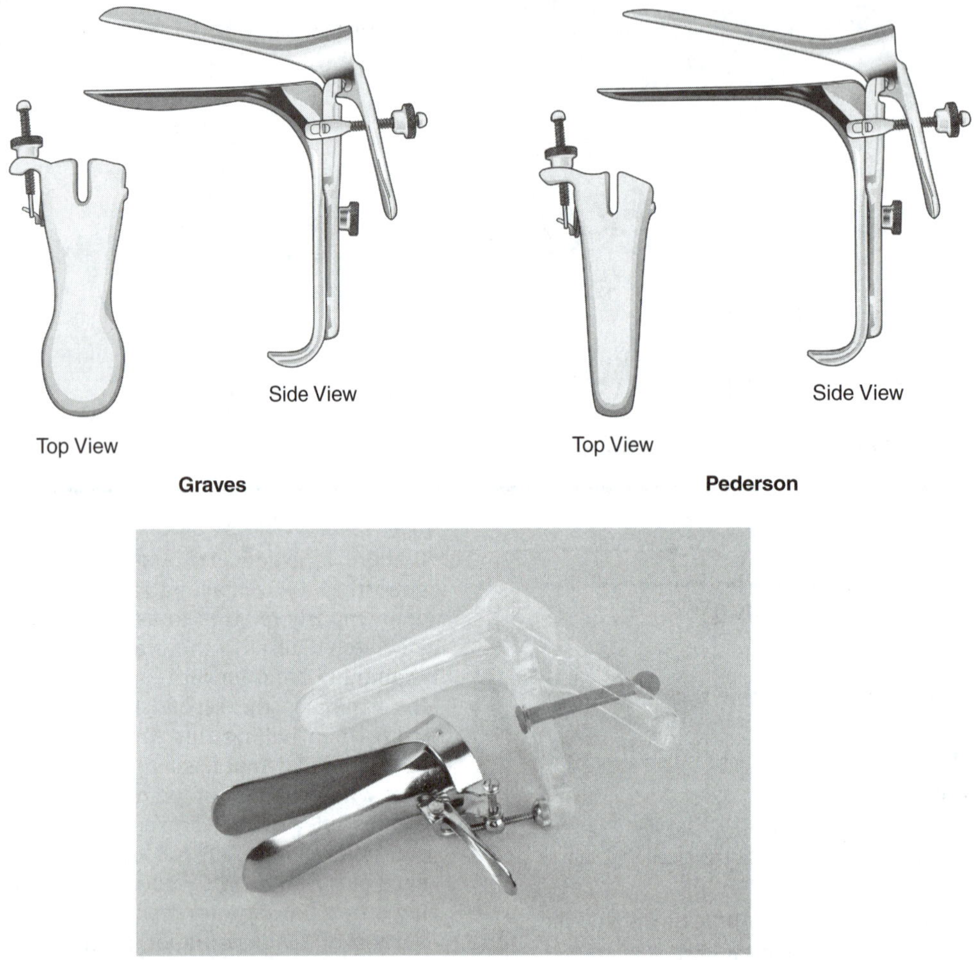

Vaginal swabs for microscopy or STI testing can be obtained without speculum insertion, or patients can self-swab. Speculum examination, as with all components of any examination, should be used intentionally and to garner specific information and assist in overall health determination.

1. Select the appropriate type (Graves or Pederson) and size (pediatric, small, medium or standard, or large) of speculum (**Figure 8-8**). (Eponymous naming of clinical instruments persist, and while these may not carry the same significance as naming anatomy, their use in these populations with that naming must also be recognized.) For parous individuals, the standard Graves speculum is often used. For individuals with significant pelvic or genital adipose tissue, lax vaginal walls, or grand multiparity, the large Graves speculum may allow the best visualization and may also be more comfortable. The wider blade size of the large Graves speculum more effectively holds the vaginal walls open, permitting visualization of the cervix. For individuals who do not engage in vaginal penetration nor use internal menstrual products, but still require an internal examination, individuals who are nulliparous, postmenopausal people, transgender men or nonbinary people on testosterone, and transgender women with neovaginas, the Pederson speculum is the usual choice. Its blades are the same length as those of the Graves speculum, but they are narrower and flat rather than curved. A pediatric speculum may also be considered for these individuals. This shape and size minimizes pressure on the anterior and posterior vaginal walls, promoting a more comfortable examination. Plastic and metal speculums are equally clean and effective, and their availability is often according to provider or clinic preference (Figure 8-8).
2. Warm the speculum by running it under warm tap water or equip the examination table drawer with a heating pad where specula can be stored. The speculum blades can be held in your gloved hand to quickly warm it if there are no other warming options. Lubricate the end of the speculum blades with water-soluble gel. Using a small amount of gel on the speculum does not interfere with cervical cytology

specimens or results, and it decreases the discomfort of speculum insertion (Ilika et al., 2024).

3. If the speculum examination occurs immediately after the external vulvar examination, maintain the same examining hand at the posterior area of the introitus to visualize the anterior aspect of the perineum (i.e., avoid removing the hand and reapplying and reopening the labia whenever possible). The thumb and fourth finger should separate the labia majora to visualize the introitus. This maneuver allows for good visualization of the opening of the vagina. Use the other gloved hand to grasp the speculum, tell the patient they will feel the speculum on the outside of their vagina, and place the blades at an angle on the perineum. Gently press down against the posterior vaginal wall, encouraging the patient to drop their perineal muscle downward to assist with comfort during the examination and visualization of the vaginal orifice. Providers may use language like "drop" or "release" or "soften" to talk the patient through how to adjust anatomy for their comfort during the exam. For some individuals, placement of the speculum at the immediate introitus may unintentionally be on the hymenal ring and increase discomfort. If so, advance the pressure internally by 1 cm, press downward, and encourage the patient to drop their perineal muscle down a second time. Be sure to completely visualize the perineum and the introitus before placing the speculum rather than running the blades of the speculum along the inside of the labia in search of the vaginal orifice. The very close proximity of the urethra and the pubic bone to the anterior vaginal wall can lead to distinct discomfort when the speculum or examining fingers enter and exit the vagina blindly.
4. With the other hand, grasp the speculum with your index finger over the top of the proximal end of the anterior blade and your other fingers around the handle. This position allows control of the blades as the speculum is inserted. Insert the speculum into the vagina at an oblique angle. Remove the fingers that have held the labia open. Keeping the blades closed, let them advance internally, following the direction of the vagina until the blades are all the way in the vagina, pressing posteriorly throughout insertion (**Figure 8-9** and **Figure 8-10**). The length of the blades is 6 to 7 inches, which matches the average length of the vagina. Remember that when lying supine, the vagina typically inclines posteriorly about 45° downward from the vaginal opening toward the sacrum. Keeping the blades at this angle also avoids pressure on the urethra and pubic bone, thereby minimizing discomfort.
5. Rotate the speculum horizontally and insert it completely into the posterior fornix. Note if the labia on either side have pulled inward and gently reposition them away from the speculum. Open the blades by pressing firmly and steadily on the thumbpiece, which should open the top blade upward while maintaining the bottom blade in a posterior position. The cervix should come into view between the blades at the end of the vagina. If it is not immediately visible with the blades wide open, relax the pressure on the thumbpiece, allowing the blades to close. Then reposition the speculum. Retract the speculum partially away from the posterior fornix, redirect the blades at a slightly different angle, and reinsert it obliquely. Open the blades; the cervix should now come into view. Adequate cervical visualization is essential for obtaining any specimens from the cervix. Depending on the position of the uterus, the position of the cervix may be very posterior or anterior. With a clear plastic speculum, if the os is visualized during speculum insertion, continue to insert the speculum to the posterior fornix to visualize the vaginal walls as part of the examination, but retract the speculum and direct the opening of the blades toward the os to avoid discomfort and unnecessary repositioning with the blades already opened.
6. When the cervix is visualized, manipulate the speculum a little farther into the vagina so the cervix is well exposed. If using a metal speculum, tighten the screw on the thumbpiece. If using a plastic speculum, click the upper blade onto the notch of the handle. Describing the noise the speculum might make before starting the insertion may comfort the patient because the noise of the screw or the clicking of the plastic might be disconcerting. The speculum should remain in place so that both hands can be removed, making it possible for you to handle other equipment. Depending on the individual's anatomy and vaginal tone, this may or may not be possible, and a clinical assistant may help in maintaining the speculum's position.

Inspect the cervix for color, position, size, surface characteristics, shape of the os, and discharge. The cervix is remarkable for the vast variety of shapes, sizes, and appearances that are within the range of health. The color should be pink. Symmetric, circumscribed erythema around the os is a normal finding caused by exposing, or everting, the columnar epithelium lining of the endocervical canal. This eversion results from pressure of the speculum blades against the anterior and posterior fornices. Knowledge of cervical anatomy is important so that normal findings versus abnormalities can be documented, including presence of the squamocolumnar junction, ectropion, and transformation zone based on age, phase of the menstrual cycle, pregnancy, menarche, menopause, and malignancy.

The position of the cervix correlates to the position of the uterus. The most common position of the cervix is posterior, indicating an anteverted uterus. The cervix should be located in the midline; significant deviation may indicate a pelvic mass or adhesions. The diameter of the cervix is approximately 2 to 3 cm, and its length is approximately 3 cm. The os of a person who is nulliparous is small and round, while a multiparous os is usually a horizontal slit or may be irregular or stellate (**Figure 8-11**). The surface should be smooth. Cervical cysts, eponymously named Nabothian cysts, may be seen as small white or yellow raised areas; these retention cysts of endocervical glands are a normal variation. See Chapter 27 for more information on benign cervical lesions. Note any friable tissue; a strawberry appearance; abnormal coloration, such as a blue or purple tinge; granular areas; or red or white patchy areas. Note any discharge, and determine if its source is vaginal, which is far more common than a cervical origin. Note the color and consistency of the discharge. Normal vaginal discharge has a neutral odor, is creamy or clear, and is thick or thin, depending on the phase of the menstrual cycle.

Three types of specimens are frequently collected at this point in the speculum examination: cervical cells for cytology screening; a vaginal or endocervical sample for gonorrhea, chlamydia, and trichomoniasis testing; and vaginal

FIGURE 8-9 A. Speculum insertion. B. Speculum placement.

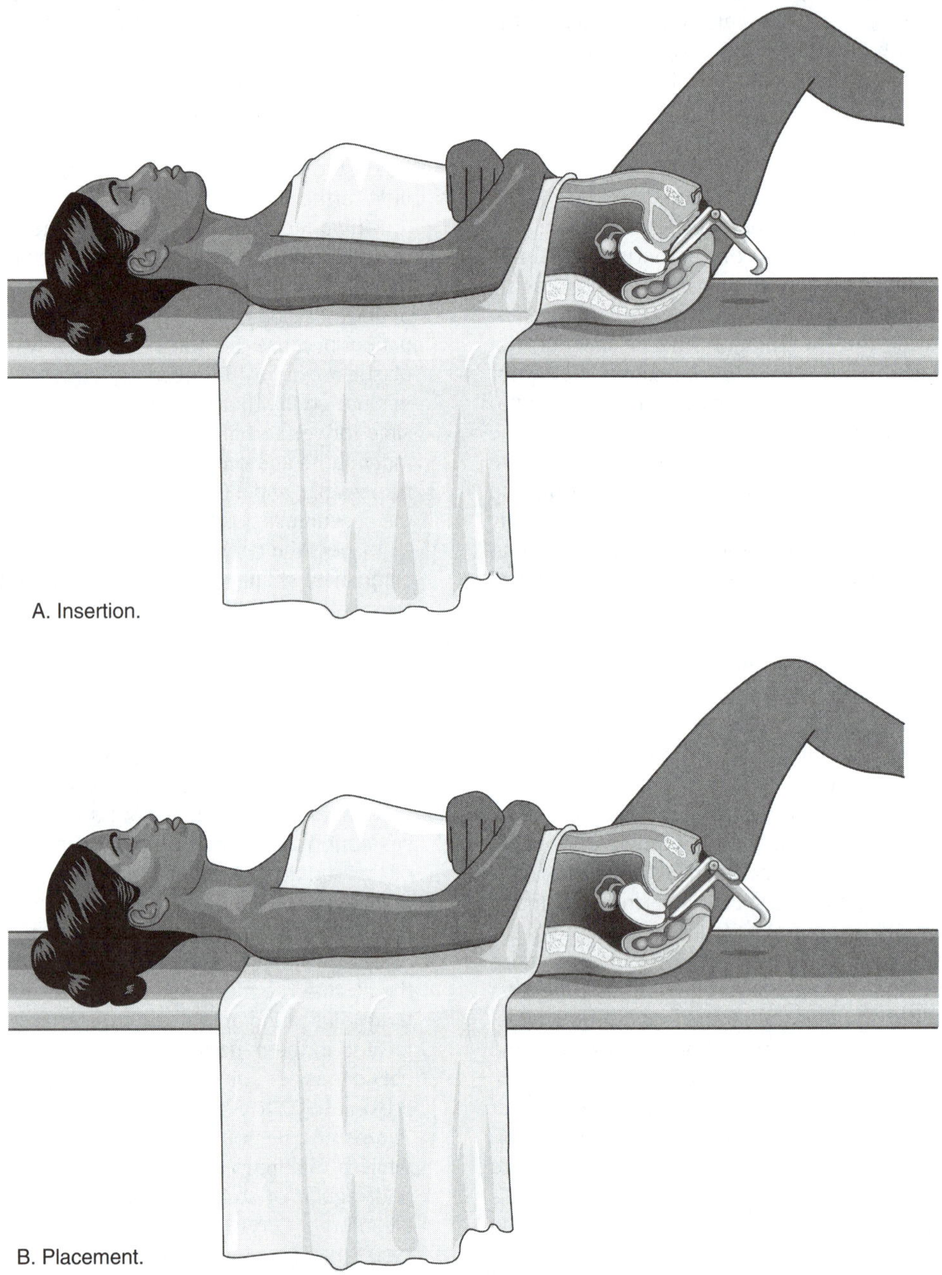

secretions for microscopy (see the chapter appendices for information on these procedures). In some laboratories, the same cervical sample is used for cytology screening and gonorrhea, chlamydia, and trichomoniasis testing. If separate cervical samples are collected for these tests, the optimal order for collecting these specimens is unknown because no evidence exists to guide this choice. Vaginal swabs are the preferred specimen type for such testing, even when a full pelvic examination is performed (Aaron et al., 2023). Urine tests are also an option for STI screening and are reasonable when no vulvar or pelvic examination is otherwise indicated.

7. To begin removing a metal speculum, press on the thumbpiece to keep the blades open, loosen the screw, and withdraw the speculum from around the cervix. To remove a plastic speculum, press on the thumbpiece to release it from the notch that has kept the anterior blade open. When the cervix is no longer within the speculum blades, release most of the pressure on the thumbpiece, rotate the speculum back to the oblique angle, and allow the vaginal walls to close the speculum naturally. Depending on the internal anatomy, the cervix may not release easily from within the blades. If this occurs, use the speculum handle as a lever and gently lift and lower the speculum body while slowly

FIGURE 8-10 **Positioning options for speculum examination.**

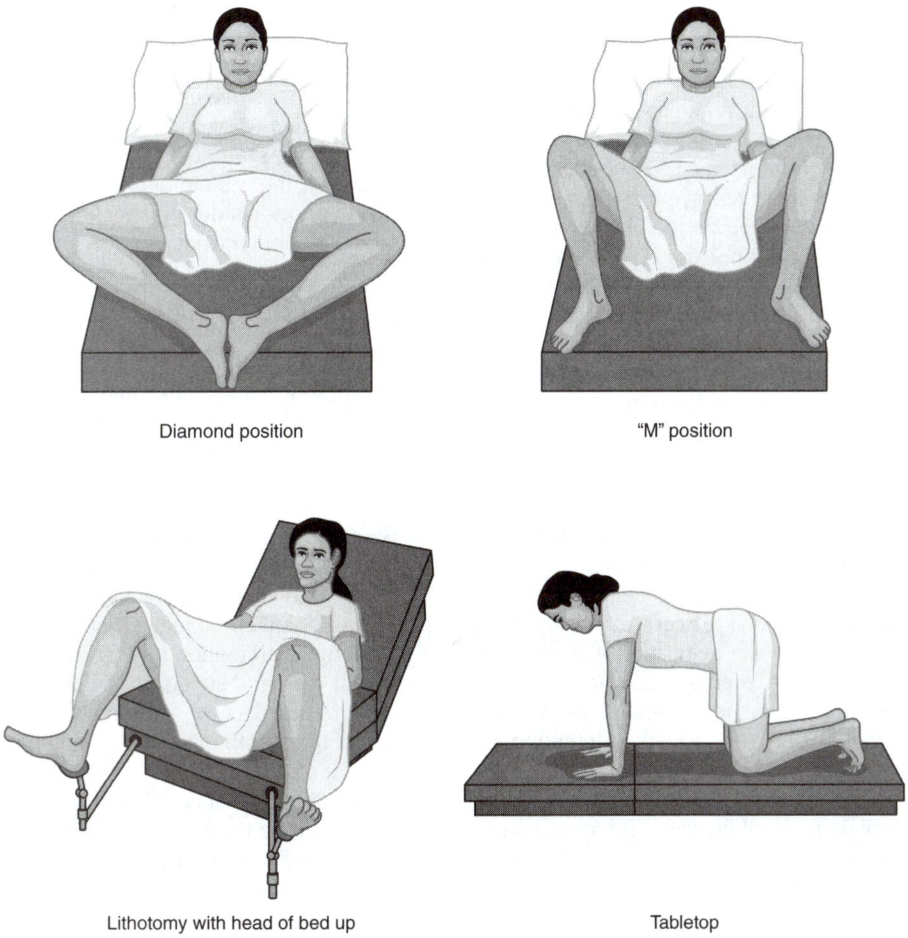

FIGURE 8-11 **Variations of the cervical os.**

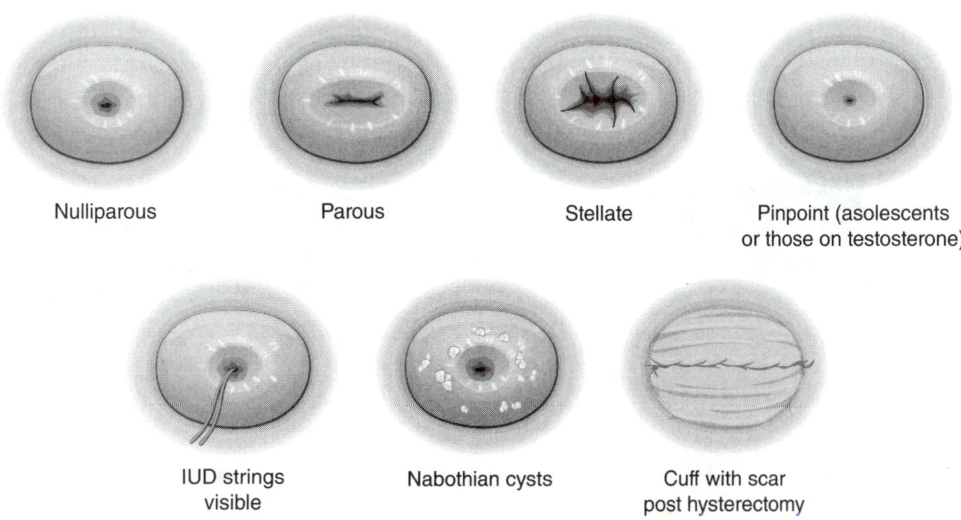

retracting the blades until the cervix releases. The pulling and compression of the cervix into the vaginal canal as the speculum is removed often causes significant discomfort if speculum removal is not performed with careful attention and patience.

As the speculum is withdrawn, inspect the vaginal walls. Note the color, surface characteristics, and secretions. Vaginal mucosa should be almost the same color as the cervix, and the surface should be moist and smooth or rugaed. Normal discharge will appear as previously described.

After inspection, continue to remove the speculum. Release all pressure on the thumbpiece; the blades will close themselves. Taking care not to pinch the vaginal mucosa or labia, quickly and completely withdraw the speculum in an upward direction but with downward pressure, similar to that used during insertion. This maneuver is most comfortable for the patient and avoids unintentional and unnecessary pressure against the urethra and suprapubic bone.

8. Deposit the speculum in an appropriate container.

Bimanual Examination

As with the speculum examination, the bimanual component of the examination is included for specific clinical reasons. This examination is not required annually for pelvic health screening for asymptomatic individuals, nor is it a necessary component of every examination for symptomatic evaluation if there is no concern or symptom for which an internal examination would provide further information. The bimanual examination, as with all components of any examination, should be used intentionally and to garner specific information and assist in overall health determination. Plans for a possible bimanual examination should be discussed while the patient is still dressed. If during the external or speculum examination, the provider determines that a bimanual examination is recommended, a separate explanation and full consent for the bimanual examination should occur with the patient in a comfortable position.

1. Inform the patient that the next step is examining their internal sexual and reproductive organs (**Figure 8-12**). This examination is most easily done with the clinician standing.
2. After the speculum is removed, remove the glove from one hand, and lubricate the index and middle fingers of the gloved hand. Generally, the dominant hand is gloved and used for the internal examination, but this is a clinician preference. If the remaining gloved hand was used for instruments and tools during specimen collection, put on a new glove to avoid introducing foreign bacteria into the vaginal canal. Let the patient know they will feel you touch them on the inside of their thigh, and then on their labia. Using the thumb and fourth finger, separate the labia to visualize the vaginal introitus. Let the patient know they will feel pressure similar to the speculum examination. Ask if it is okay to proceed with the internal examination and await a response. Place the index and third fingers just inside the vaginal orifice, press downward, and encourage the patient to drop or release their perineum downward as much as possible. Gently insert the fingers, maintaining posterior pressure, to the posterior fornix. If the patient reports pain or clenches down with their vaginal muscles, pause the examination and ask what could make them more comfortable or if they want the examination to stop completely.
3. Rotate the hand superiorly, or palm up, maintaining posterior pressure. As the examination continues, be careful of where the thumb of the examining hand is resting. After the hand is rotated superiorly, extend the thumb as far laterally as possible to avoid folding it medially and resting it on the clitoris during the examination.
4. Locate and palpate the end of the cervix with the palmar surface of the examining fingers, then run the examining

FIGURE 8-12 **Bimanual examination.**

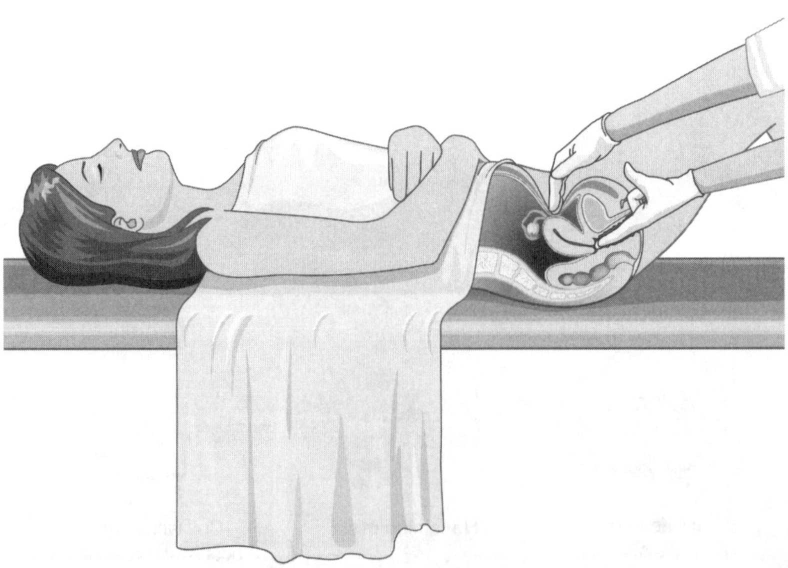

fingers around the circumference of the cervix to feel its size, length, shape, and consistency. A nonpregnant cervix will be firm, like the tip of the nose; during pregnancy it is softer. A multiparous cervix may allow easy palpation inside the external os. Note nodules, surface texture, and position.

5. Assess for cervical motion tenderness by gently grasping the cervix between the fingers, moving it from side to side once, and observing the patient's face for any expression of pain or discomfort while also asking them if this component of the examination is painful. The cervix should move 1 to 2 cm laterally without discomfort. Painful cervical movement suggests a pelvic inflammatory process.
6. Begin palpation of the uterus by placing the non-examining hand on the abdomen, halfway between the umbilicus and the pubis at the midline. Place the fingers in the vagina on the anterior aspect of the cervix. The palms should be facing each other, with one internally on the anterior vaginal wall and the other externally on the abdomen. Notify the patient that it is normal to feel pressure or a strange sensation of movement during this part of the evaluation, to normalize the sensation and aid the patient in differentiating it from pain, which must be noted if present. Slowly slide the abdominal hand down toward the pubis, pressing downward and forward with the flat surface of all four fingers. At the same time, press upward with the fingers inside the vagina. This combination of abdominal and vaginal pressure will feel as if the two hands are pressing against each other. The uterus is relatively mobile, usually inclines forward at about 45°, and is essentially flat. It measures approximately 5 to 8 cm long, 3.5 to 5 cm wide, and 2 to 3 cm thick. If the uterus is anteflexed or anteverted (**Figure 8-13**), the fundus will be palpable between the fingers of the two hands at the level of the pubis. Movement of the uterus during palpation may cause discomfort.
7. If the uterus cannot be palpated with the maneuver described in step 5, alert the patient that a deeper palpation may be necessary to complete the evaluation. Keeping the internalized hand palm up, place the fingers in the vagina together in the posterior fornix with the abdominal hand at the pubis. Press firmly downward with the abdominal fingers. With the fingers in the vagina turned upward, press them up against the cervix, moving it inward. If the uterus

FIGURE 8-13 Variations in uterine position.

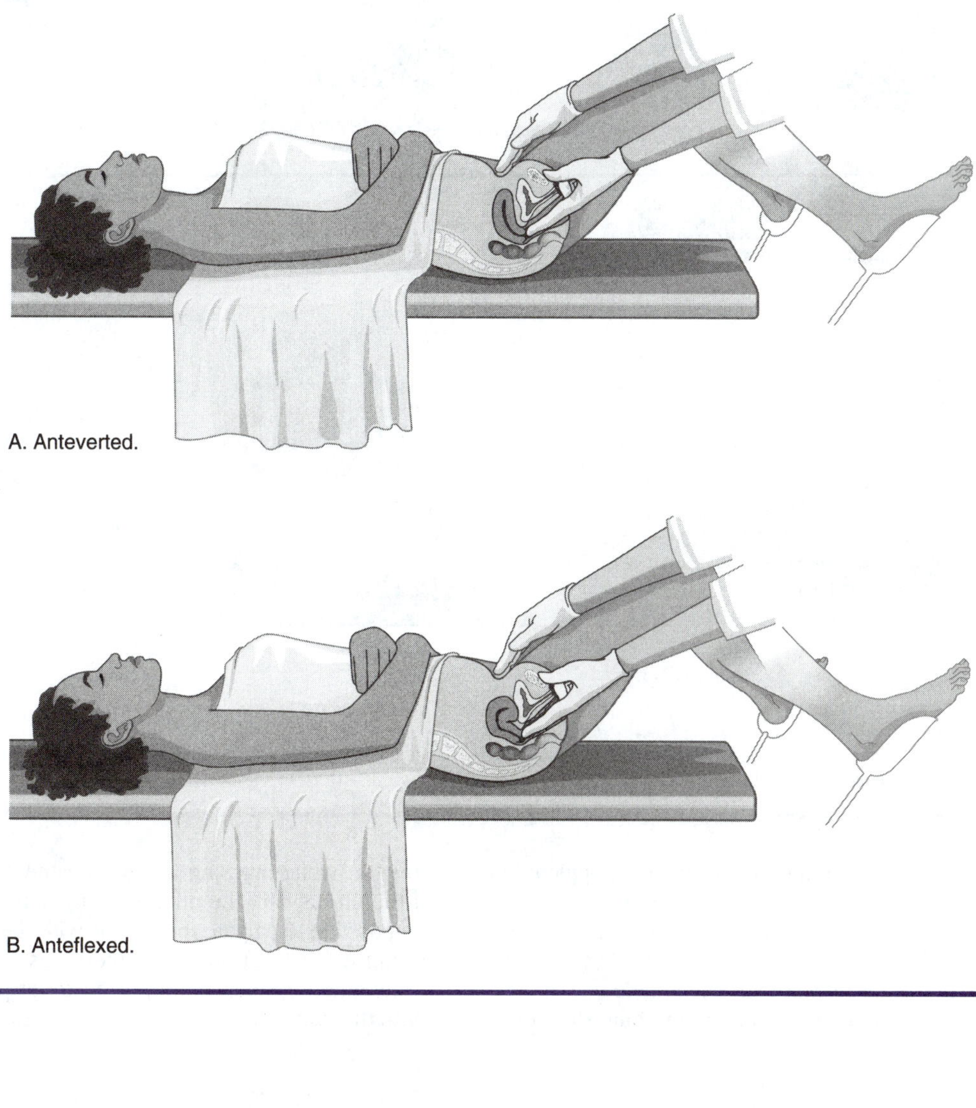

A. Anteverted.

B. Anteflexed.

(continues)

FIGURE 8-13 **Variations in uterine position. (*continued*)**

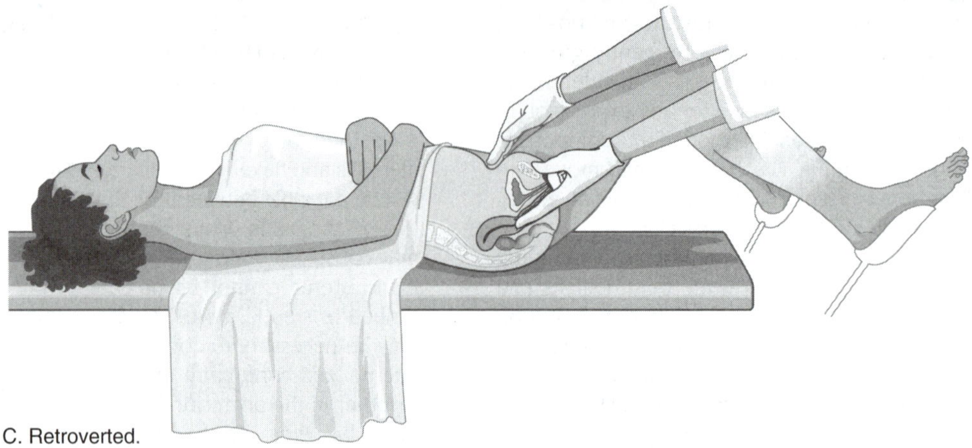

C. Retroverted.

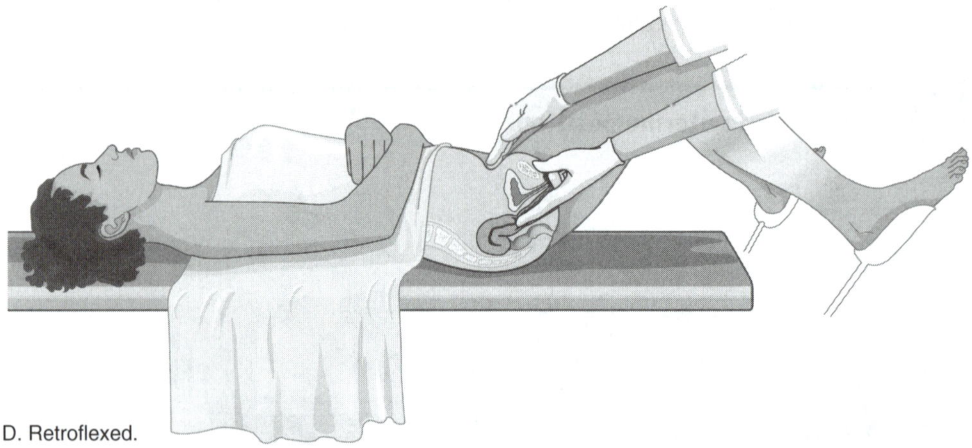

D. Retroflexed.

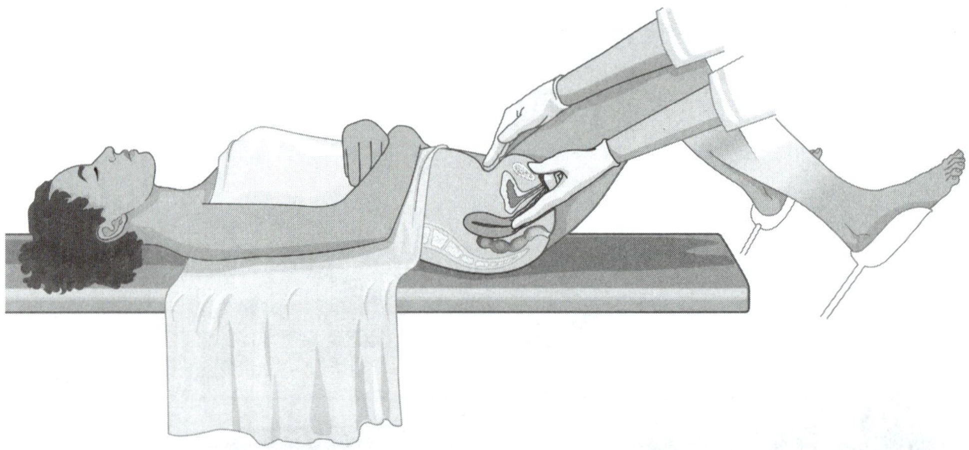

E. Midposition of the uterus.

is retroverted (Figure 8-13), the fundus should be palpable with this maneuver.

8. If the uterus still is not palpated, move the fingers in the vagina to the sides of the cervix, one on each side, pressing the cervix inward as far as possible. Then move one finger on top and the other beneath the cervix, continuing to press inward, while pressing down with the abdominal fingers. If the uterus is in the midposition (Figure 8-13), it may not be possible to palpate the fundus with the abdominal hand. Confirm the location of the uterus as midline, regardless of its anterior, midposition, or posterior position. Also palpate the uterus for size, contour, and consistency. It should

feel smooth, firm, round, and flat. It should be mobile in the anterior–posterior plane. This examination should not cause pain, although a sensation of pressure is common.

9. Continue the bimanual examination by palpating the ovaries and surrounding area, called the adnexa. This term refers to the areas that are lateral to the uterus, which are taken up by the broad ligaments, and the structures located there. Again, notify the patient that during this part of the examination it is normal to feel pressure or a strange sensation of movement, but that they should state if there is any pain. Move the abdominal hand to the right-lower quadrant. The fingers inside the vagina remain facing upward. Now place both fingers in the right-lateral fornix. Press deeply inward and upward toward the abdominal hand. At the same time, with the abdominal hand, sweep the flat surface of the fingers deeply inward and obliquely down toward the pubis. Palpate the entire area in this manner, repeating this sweeping movement; at the same time, the fingers inside the vagina press upward, inward, and slide downward (**Figure 8-14**). This maneuver is then repeated on the left side.
10. Often normal ovaries are difficult to palpate because they are small, sometimes positioned deep in the pelvis, or obscured by the presence of abdominal adipose tissue or tense abdominal muscles. They are about 3 by 2 by 1 cm, smooth, and firm. If the ovaries are palpable, this examination usually causes momentary moderate pain when the ovaries are located; warn patients that a rapid sharp pain is common before starting this part of the examination. Palpable ovaries in individuals who are postmenopausal are reason for concern and require follow-up. If the ovaries are not palpated after thorough palpation with one or two sweeps, the examination is normal in the absence of any clinical signs or symptoms; no further repetition, pressure, or palpation is required. Usually, no other adnexal structures are palpable.
11. After the adnexal examination is completed, gently remove the fingers from inside of the vagina; use continued downward pressure to avoid pressure on the urethral structures and pubic bone. Take off and discard the examination glove. If this is the conclusion of the pelvic examination (i.e., rectovaginal examination is not being performed), help the patient sit up. Give them a moment to adjust their position and become comfortable, then offer tissues to wipe excess secretions and lubricant. Leave the examining room to allow privacy and time to dress, letting the patient know a discussion about the examination and next steps will occur after they are dressed.

Rectovaginal Examination

Learning to perform a gentle rectal examination is an important skill for any clinician, though it should be utilized sparingly with clear indication and full consent from the individual. Especially in asymptomatic individuals, this examination is often eliminated as part of routine screening and health maintenance. Many clinicians omit this examination because the vaginal examination allows for sufficient palpation of internal organs and because digital rectal examination to collect a stool sample for fecal occult blood testing is an unacceptable screening strategy for colorectal cancer screening (though it may be used to rule out gastrointestinal sources of otherwise unexplained anemia). A rectal examination is perhaps most useful if the uterus is retroflexed or retroverted, since this part of the pelvic examination allows palpation to a depth of an additional 2.5 cm, facilitating a more complete evaluation of some pelvic structures (**Figure 8-15**). It is usually an uncomfortable examination for the patient, but skilled clinicians complete this examination with sensitivity, skill, and often this exam is very brief. For people who engage in anal sex, rectal swabs for chlamydia, gonorrhea, or trichomoniasis can be self-obtained or provider obtained and do not necessitate internal palpation as part of the sampling.

Consent for a rectal examination should be separate from the vaginal examination, and not presumed based on the patient's consent for pelvic examination. Many patients will never have experienced this type of examination, so be very clear about the level of penetration and pressure prior to doing the examination. Inform them that this may be uncomfortable and may also cause a sensation similar to that of having a bowel movement. Assure the patient that even though this sensation may be present, a bowel movement will not occur. If conducted after a vaginal

FIGURE 8-14 **Adnexal examination.**

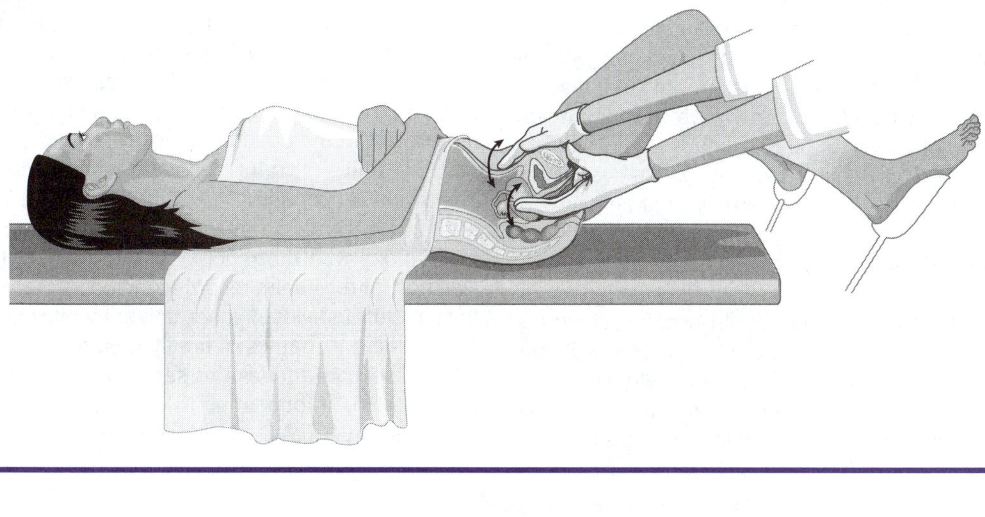

FIGURE 8-15 **Rectovaginal examination.**

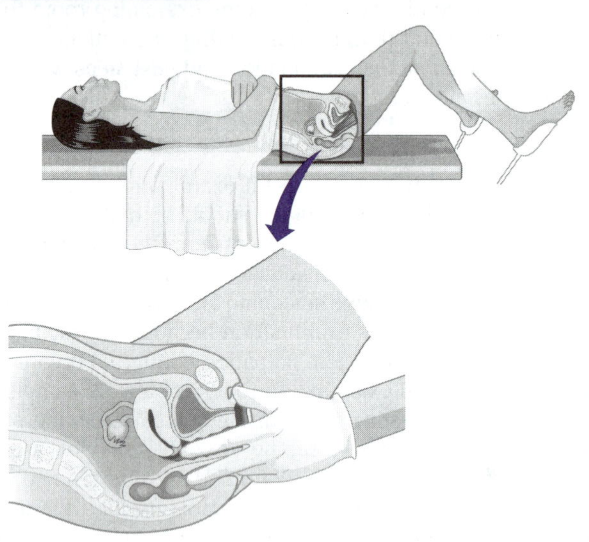

examination, before initiating the rectal examination, ask the patient's permission to begin this separate examination. Advise the patient that for ease in inserting the examining fingers, you will ask them to bear (push) down and at the same time will insert a finger inside their rectum. This should be explicitly discussed, as asking the patient to bear down and then inserting examining fingers with ease without their previous knowledge and consent is harmful. Alert them that once the examining finger is inserted, this examination will include rotating the finger and palpating internally, and the second part of the examination will include insertion of a separate finger into the vagina at the same time.

1. Put an examination glove on one hand, and lubricate the index and third fingertips with water-soluble gel. Place the third finger against the anus, ask the patient to bear down, and insert this finger into the rectum just past the sphincter. Palpate the anorectal junction and rotate the examining finger to sweep over the anterior and then the posterior rectum that can be reached above the sphincter. Note the sphincter tone, which should be moderate. The mucosal surfaces should feel smooth and uninterrupted.
2. Next, insert the index finger of the examining hand into the vagina until the posterior cervical fornix. Palpate the septum between the rectum and posterior vaginal wall for thickness. Ask the patient to bear down, which will bring the uterus about 1 cm closer to the examining finger. With the other hand, press firmly on the abdomen just above the pubis. The posterior surface of the uterus should be palpable, especially if it is retroverted. If the findings of the adnexal examination were questionable, repeat that examination as described previously.
3. Gently remove the examining fingers, inspect for secretions, and prepare a specimen for fecal occult blood testing if indicated. Remove and discard the gloves, and help the patient sit up. Give them a moment to adjust position and become comfortable, then offer tissues to wipe excess secretions and lubricant. Leave the examining room to allow privacy and time to dress, letting the patient know a discussion about the examination and next steps will occur after they are dressed.

CONCLUSION: SUMMING UP AND DOCUMENTING FINDINGS

It is important to take the time to review normal and abnormal findings from the examination. Describe expected findings as normal or healthy. If any abnormal findings occurred, they should be explained appropriately. The clinician should gauge how much detailed explanation, description, and thoughts on treatment, management, or follow-up should be presented based on the individual's desire for information, health literacy, and degree of severity of the finding. If the clinician is not sure of the implications of the finding, it is reasonable to say so, but also assure the patient that consultation with another health professional will be sought promptly and that a more complete explanation and plan will be forthcoming.

Encourage patients to voice their concerns, questions, and reactions to the examination. It is important not to presume that the patient "did great" or "everything went fine" just because the clinician did not note any verbal or nonverbal cues: trauma and trauma activation can look different for everyone. Ask how they are feeling to welcome both physical and emotional responses to the examination. Ask specifically if there is anything that can be modified during future examinations to improve comfort with any part of the examination, particularly the external and internal pelvic examinations. Attention to these issues demonstrates the clinician's commitment to understanding and responding to the individual. Discuss ways the patient may contact the provider after the examination with any recollected health history, new questions, or follow-up needs.

The final clinical responsibility in the history and physical examination is concise and accurate documentation of findings in the health record. Collaborating with the patient on what to chart and where, who can see charted information (parent/guardian, spouse, other clinicians), and being clear that all documentation becomes a legal record is part of the shared decision-making process. For example, documentation of pregnancy in the health record is not a neutral finding, as state and federal changes to abortion legislation may track patient pregnancy outcomes and the health record may be discoverable legal documentation (Tillman et al., 2023). It is helpful to document any modifications that were needed to ensure patient comfort during the examination, such as positioning, distraction techniques, or preferred language, so that future providers can do the same. Carry the empowerment that the provider brought to the clinical encounter through to the documentation. For example, avoid language such as "difficult," "noncompliant," or "nonadherent," which disempowers patient autonomy. Clinicians should balance clinically accurate documentation of the physical examination and recommendations with more personal information. Find space in the visit note or the health record to include social aspects, including the patient's individual goals, upcoming life plans such as school or celebrations, names of family members or relationships, and other aspects of the visit to serve as reminders of their unique character and a foundation to continue to build on the provider relationship with each subsequent visit.

References

Aaron, K. J., Griner, S., Footman, A., Boutwell, A., & Van Der Pol, B. (2023). Vaginal swab vs urine for detection of *Chlamydia trachomatis, Neisseria gonorrhoeae,* and *Trichomonas vaginalis:* A meta-analysis. *The Annals of Family Medicine, 21*(2), 172–179. https://doi.org/10.1370/afm.2942

AMA adopts new policy clarifying role of BMI as a measure in medicine. (2023, June 4). AMA Press Releases. https://www.ama-assn.org/press-center/press-releases/ama-adopts-new-policy-clarifying-role-bmi-measure-medicine

American Academy of Nursing. (2019). *Have you ever served in the military?* http://www.haveyoueverserved.com

American Academy of Pediatrics. (2021). *Equitable access to sexual and reproductive health care for all youth.*

American College of Obstetricians and Gynecologists. (2020). Sexual Misconduct. ACOG Committee Opinion No. 796. *Obstetrics & Gynecology, 135*(1), e43–e50. https://doi.org/10.1097/AOG.0000000000003608

American College of Obstetricians and Gynecologists. (2014). *reVITALize obstetric data definitions.* https://www.acog.org/About-ACOG/ACOG-Departments/Patien-Safety-and-Quality-Improvement/reVITALize-Obstetric-Data-Definitions

American College of Obstetricians and Gynecologists. (2018, reaffirmed 2024). The utility of and indications for routine pelvic examination (ACOG Committee Opinion No. 754). https://www.acog.org/clinical/clinical-guidance/committee-opinion/articles/2018/10/the-utility-of-and-indications-for-routine-pelvic-examination

American Psychiatric Association (Ed.). (2022). *Diagnostic and Statistical Manual of Mental Disorders: DSM-5-TR* (5th ed., text revision). American Psychiatric Association Publishing.

Association for Size Diversity and Health. (n.d.). *Health At Every Size® Principles.* https://asdah.org/haes/

Ballard, D. I., Mandhana, D. M., Tesfai, Y., Jacome, C. S., Johnson, S. B., Gionfriddo, M. R., Suarez, N. R. E., Perneth, S. A., Su, L., & Montori, V. M. (2024). Unhurried conversations in health care are more important than ever: Identifying key communication practices for careful and kind care. *Annals of Family Medicine, 22*(6), 533–538. https://doi.org/10.1370/afm.3177

Barbera, J. P., Cichon, B., Ankam, N., & Schwartz, B. I. (2024). Equitable care for patients with disabilities: Considerations for the gynecologic health care professional. *Obstetrics & Gynecology, 143*(4), 475–483. https://doi.org/10.1097/AOG.0000000000005493

Beauchamp, T., & Childress, J. (2019). Principles of biomedical ethics: Marking its fortieth anniversary. *American Journal of Bioethics, 19*(11), 9-12. https://doi.org/10.1080/15265161.2019.1665402. PMID: 31647760.

Bickley, L. S., Szilagyi, P. G., Hoffman, R. M., & Soriano, R. P. (2024). *Bates' guide to physical examination and history taking* (13th ed., revised reprint). Wolters Kluwer.

Campbell, L. R., Scalise, A. L., DiBenedictis, B. T., & Mahalingaiah, S. (2021). Menstrual cycle length and modern living: A review. *Current Opinion in Endocrinology, Diabetes & Obesity, 28*(6), 566–573. https://doi.org/10.1097/MED.0000000000000681

Centers for Disease Control and Prevention (CDC). (2024, April 2). *Lifesaving Naloxone.* Stop Overdose. https://www.cdc.gov/stop-overdose/caring/naloxone.html

Chor, J., Stulberg, D. B., & Tillman, S. (2019). Shared decision-making framework for pelvic examinations in asymptomatic, nonpregnant patients. *Obstetrics & Gynecology, 133*(4), 810–814.

Chung, R. J., Lee, J. B., Hackell, J. M., Alderman, E. M., COMMITTEE ON ADOLESCENCE, Alderman, E. M., Berlan, E. D., Chung, R. J., Colburn, M., Lee, J., Monge, M., Shafii, T., Grubb, L. K., Wallace, S. B., Amies, A.-M., Hua, L. L., Menon, S., Rahmandar, M. H., Vyver, E., ... Ferguson, E. (2024). Confidentiality in the care of adolescents: Policy statement. *Pediatrics, 153*(5), e2024066326. https://doi.org/10.1542/peds.2024-066326

Copen, C. E., Dittus, P. J., & Leichliter, J. S. (2016). Confidentiality concerns and sexual and reproductive health care among adolescents and young adults aged 15–25. *NCHS Data Brief, 2016*(266), 1–8.

Edelman, A., Boniface, E. R., Benhar, E., Han, L., Matteson, K. A., Favaro, C., Pearson, J. T., & Darney, B. G. (2022). Association between menstrual cycle length and coronavirus disease 2019 (COVID-19) vaccination: A U.S. cohort. *Obstetrics & Gynecology, 139*(4), 481–489. https://doi.org/10.1097/AOG.0000000000004695

Ellis, S. A., & Dalke, L. (2019). Midwifery care for transfeminine individuals. *Journal of Midwifery & Women's Health, 64*(3), 298-311. https://doi.org/10.1111/jmwh.12957. Epub 2019 Apr 8. PMID: 30957961.

Federative International Programme for Anatomical Terminology (FIPAT). (2019). *Terminologia anatomica* (2nd ed.). https://libraries.dal.ca/Fipat/ta2.html

Ferreyra, S., & Hughes, K. (1982). *Table manners: A guide to the pelvic examination for disabled women and health care providers.* Sex Education for Disabled People.

Guttmacher Institute. (2023, August 30). *Minors' access to contraceptive services.* State Laws and Policies. https://www.guttmacher.org/state-policy/explore/minors-access-contraceptive-services

Ilika, C. P., Eleje, G. U., Chiemeka, M. E., Ilika, F. N., Ikechebelu, J. I., Ilika, V. C., Ugwu, E. O., O for, I. J., Ogelle, O. M., Umeononihu, O. S., Mamah, J. E., Olisa, C. L., Ezeigwe, C. O., Nwankwo, M. E., Ofojebe, C. J., Okafor, C. C., Ekwebene, O. C., Nnabuchi, O. K., & Okafor, C. G. (2024). Effects of speculum lubrication on cervical smears for cervical cancer screening: A double blind randomized clinical trial. *PLOS ONE, 19*(5), e0292207. https://doi.org/10.1371/journal.pone.0292207

InterACT & Lambda Legal. (2018). *Providing ethical and compassionate health care to intersex patients: Intersex-affirming hospital policies.* https://www.lambdalegal.org/publications/intersex-affirming

Jarvis, C., & Eckhardt, A.L. (2024). *Physical examination & health assessment* (9th ed.). Elsevier.

Kim, G., Molina, U. S., & Saadi, A. (2019). Should immigration status information be included in a patient's health record? *AMA Journal of Ethics, 21*(1), 8–16.

King, D. W., Leskin, G. A., King, L. A., & Weathers, F. W. (1998). Confirmatory factor analysis of the clinician-administered PTSD scale: Evidence for the dimensionality of posttraumatic stress disorder. *Psychological Assessment, 10*(2), 90–96. https://doi.org/10.1037/1040-3590.10.2.90

LoGiudice, J. A., Tillman, S., & Sarguru, S. (2023). A midwifery perspective on trauma-informed care clinical recommendations. *Journal of Midwifery & Women's Health, 68*(2), 165–169. https://doi.org/10.1111/jmwh.13462

Madhu, C., Swift, S., Moloney-Geany, S., & Drake, M. J. (2018). How to use the Pelvic Organ Prolapse Quantification (POP-Q) system? *Neurourology and Urodynamics, 37*(S6). https://doi.org/10.1002/nau.23740

Magill, M., Martino, S., & Wampold, B. E. (2022). Goal setting and monitoring with alcohol and other drug use disorders: Principles and practices. *Journal of Substance Abuse Treatment, 132,* 108650. https://doi.org/10.1016/j.jsat.2021.108650

Marcell, A. V., Burstein, G. R., & American Academy of Pediatrics Committee on Adolescence. (2017). Sexual and reproductive health care services in the pediatric setting. *Pediatrics, 140*(5), e20172858.

Melms, L., Schaefer, J. R., Jerrentrup, A., & Mueller, T. (2021). A pilot study of patient satisfaction with a self-completed tablet-based digital questionnaire for collecting the patient's medical history in an emergency department. *BMC Health Services Research, 21*(1), 755. https://doi.org/10.1186/s12913-021-06748-y

O'Laughlin, D. J., Strelow, B., Fellows, N., Kelsey, E., Peters, S., Stevens, J., & Tweedy, J. (2021). Addressing anxiety and fear during the female pelvic examination. *Journal of Primary Care & Community Health, 12,* 2150132721992195. https://doi.org/10.1177/2150132721992195

Olson, S. M., Muñoz, E. G., Solis, E. C., & Bradford, H. M. (2024). Mitigating weight bias in the clinical setting: A new approach to care. *Journal of Midwifery & Women's Health, 69*(2), 180–190. https://doi.org/10.1111/jmwh.13578

Owens, L., Terrell, S., Low, L. K., Loder, C., Rhizal, D., Scheiman, L., & Seng, J. (2021). Universal precautions: The case for consistently trauma-informed reproductive healthcare. *American Journal of Obstetrics and Gynecology,* S0002937821008802. https://doi.org/10.1016/j.ajog.2021.08.012

Savoy, M., O'Gurek, D., & Brown-James, A. (2020). Sexual health history: Techniques and tips. *American Family Physician, 101*(5), 286–293.

Tillman, S. (2020). Consent in pelvic care. *Journal of Midwifery & Women's Health, 65*(6), 749–758. https://doi.org/10.1111/jmwh.13189

Tillman, S., Goodrum, B. A., Street, A. S., Premkumar, A., Ricardo, K. D., & Fleisher, J. (2023). Toward opt-in consent for pregnancy testing. *Journal of Midwifery & Women's Health, 68*(6), 705–709. https://doi.org/10.1111/jmwh.13597

U.S. Preventive Services Task Force, Barry, M. J., Nicholson, W. K., Silverstein, M., Chelmow, D., Coker, T. R., Davidson, K. W., Davis, E. M., Donahue, K. E., Jaén, C. R., Li, L., Ogedegbe, G., Pbert, L., Rao, G., Ruiz, J. M., Stevermer, J. J., Tsevat, J., Underwood, S. M., & Wong, J. B. (2023). Screening for depression and suicide risk in adults: U.S. Preventive Services Task Force recommendation statement. *JAMA, 329*(23), 2057. https://doi.org/10.1001/jama.2023.9297

U.S. Preventive Services Task Force, Bibbins-Domingo, K., Grossman, D. C., Curry, S. J., Barry, M. J., Davidson, K. W., Doubeni, C. A., Epling, J. W., Jr., Garcia, F. A., Kemper, A. R., Krist, A. H., Kurth, A. E., Landefeld, C. S., Mangione, C. M., Phillips, W. R., Phipps, M. G., Silverstein, M., Simon, M., Siu, A. L., & Tseng, C. W. (2017). Screening for gynecologic conditions with pelvic examination: U.S. Preventive Services Task Force recommendation statement. *JAMA, 317*(9), 947–953.

VanMeter, K. C., & Hubert, R. J. (2014). *Gould's pathophysiology for the health professions* (5th ed.). Saunders.

World Health Organization. (2018). *Female genital mutilation.* https://www.who.int/news-room/fact-sheets/detail/female-genital-mutilation

Yen, P. H., & Leasure, A. R. (2019). Use and effectiveness of the teach-back method in patient education and health outcomes. *Federal Practitioner: For the Health Care Professionals of the VA, DoD, and PHS, 36*(6), 284–289.

APPENDIX 8-A

Cervical Cytology Screening

The goal of this test is to obtain adequate cells from the cervical squamocolumnar junction for cytology screening. The squamocolumnar junction, or transformation zone, where the columnar endocervical epithelium and squamous ectocervical epithelium meet, is where most cervical cancers arise.

For many years, specimens were collected using a special wooden spatula (Ayer spatula), sometimes in conjunction with a cotton-tipped swab. The conventional method of preparing the sample for cytology is the Pap test, which entails applying the specimen to a glass slide. Limitations of this specimen collection and preparation method are well documented and include not obtaining sufficient endocervical cells for adequate laboratory cytologic evaluation; unavoidably leaving much of the cellular sample on the collection device when transferring the materials to the glass slide; and obscured detection of abnormal cells due to the presence of blood, mucus, air drying, or other artifacts on the slide. Newer specimen collection devices and liquid-based preparation methods have been developed to try to overcome these limitations and improve cervical cytology screening.

More recent specimen collection devices include endocervical brushes, a broom device that can simultaneously sample the ectocervix and endocervix, and extended-tip spatulas (**Figure 8A-1**). The use of cotton-tipped swabs is no longer recommended. Endocervical brushes plus spatulas, brooms, and extended-tip spatulas are all effective. Use the ectocervical device first when two devices are used (Massad et al., 2013).

Liquid-based methods for cervical cytology screening (ThinPrep, SurePath) allow for more complete removal of cellular material by rinsing the sampling devices in a liquid medium. Cells for cytologic examination are removed from the medium via a filtering process that minimizes the presence of obscuring artifacts. However, liquid-based methods are neither more sensitive nor more specific than the conventional Pap test for detecting cervical intraepithelial neoplasia (Arbyn et al., 2008; Siebers et al., 2009). An advantage of liquid-based cytology methods is that the sample can also be used to test for HPV deoxyribonucleic acid (DNA), chlamydia, gonorrhea, and trichomoniasis. This eliminates the need for a second visit for a cytologic abnormality that warrants HPV DNA testing. A disadvantage of liquid-based methods is their higher cost compared to the conventional glass slide cytology method. Additionally, liquid-based cytology is not considered diagnostic for trichomoniasis. If this test is positive for trichomoniasis, a nucleic acid amplification test (NAAT) should follow to confirm the presence of this infection (see **Appendix 8-B**). These considerations, and the failure of scientific evidence to establish clinically important differences, have led the USPSTF et al. (2018) to recommend that use of conventional cytology or liquid-based cervical cytology is acceptable. See Chapter 9 for cervical cancer and HPV screening recommendations.

FIGURE 8A-1 **Specimen collection devices for cervical cytology screening.**

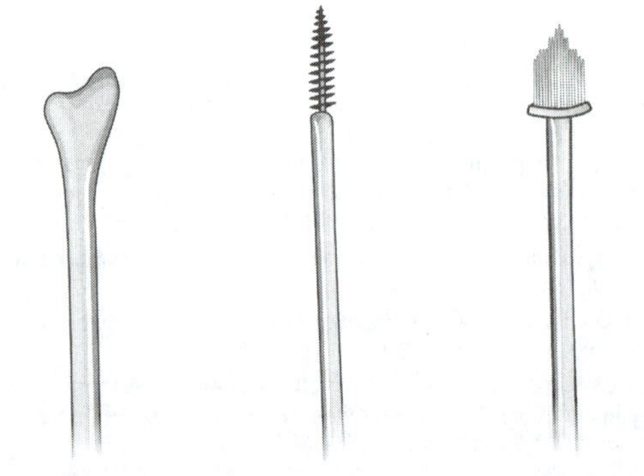

CONVENTIONAL METHOD FOR CERVICAL CYTOLOGY SCREENING

1. Assemble the necessary materials: a labeled container for one or two standard microscope slides, the slides, a spatula, an endocervical brush, and a canister of fixative.
2. Tell the patient that the Pap test will be performed, and they may feel slight pressure or discomfort, which is caused primarily from the contact of the sampling devices with the endocervix.
3. Visualize the cervix, using the speculum examination procedure described in this chapter.
4. Pick up the spatula, and insert the longer end into the cervical os. Press and rotate the spatula 360°, making sure it stays in direct contact with the inner surface of the cervical os (**Figure 8A-2**).

FIGURE 8A-2 **Obtaining cervical cells with a spatula.**

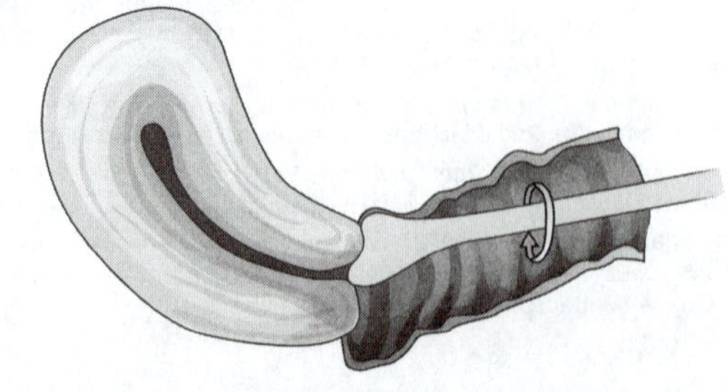

5. Pick up the glass slide, press the spatula flat against the surface, and smear the spatula across the slide (**Figure 8A-3**). Turn the spatula over, and spread the secretions from the second side of the spatula onto the slide. Discard the spatula. Some clinicians prefer to proceed to step 6 and place samples from the spatula and endocervical brush onto the slide after both specimens have been collected.
6. Insert the endocervical brush so that the bristles are fully in the cervical os, and rotate the brush 180° to 360°, which is one-half to one turn (**Figure 8A-4**).
7. Pick up the glass slide (or the second glass slide if using two); with firm pressure, roll the bristles of the endocervical brush across the slide surface (Figure 8A-3). If using one slide, recommendations vary as to whether to keep the spatula and endocervical brush samples separate (placing one on each half of the slide) or to place the endocervical brush sample over the spatula sample. Clinicians should consult their laboratory for the preferred preparation method. Discard the endocervical brush.
8. Promptly spray fixative onto the slide, holding the container about 12 inches away from the slide. Allow the sample to air dry for a few minutes before placing the slide in the transport container. Note that an assistant, if present, can hold the slides for the clinician and apply the fixative.
9. Continue the speculum examination, or prepare to collect additional specimens.

FIGURE **8A-3** **Preparation of the glass slide for cervical cytology screening.**

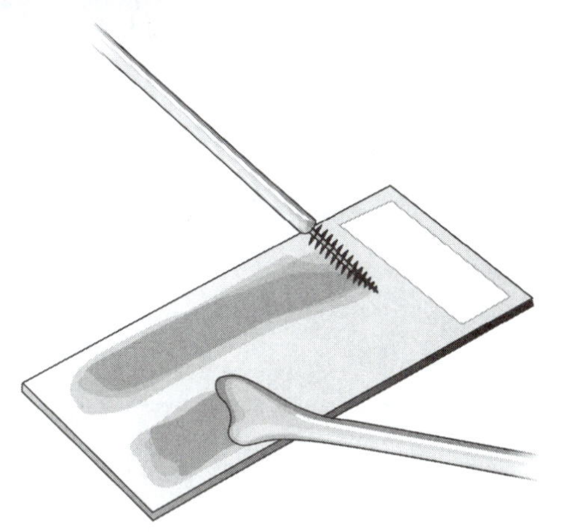

FIGURE **8A-4** **Obtaining cells with an endocervical brush.**

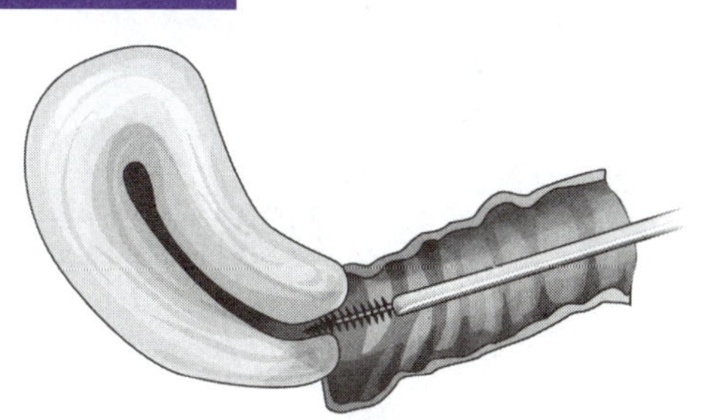

LIQUID-BASED METHODS FOR CERVICAL CYTOLOGY SCREENING

Specimen Collection with the Spatula and Endocervical Brush

1. Assemble the necessary materials: labeled vial of liquid medium, spatula, and endocervical brush. Take the lid off the vial.
2. Prepare the patient as described in step 2 for the conventional method.
3. Visualize the cervix as described in step 3 for the conventional method.
4. Collect a specimen with the spatula as described in step 4 for the conventional method.
5. Place the spatula into the vial and swirl vigorously 10 times to mix the specimen and the medium (**Figure 8A-5**). Remove and discard the spatula.
6. Collect the specimen with the endocervical brush as described in step 6 for the conventional method.
7. Place the endocervical brush into the vial and swirl vigorously 10 times to mix the specimen and the medium (Figure 8A-5). Discard the endocervical brush.
8. Screw the lid tightly and securely onto the vial.
9. Proceed as described in step 9 for the conventional method.

Specimen Collection with the Broom Device

1. Assemble the necessary materials: labeled vial of liquid medium and broom device. Take the lid off the vial.
2. Prepare the patient as described in step 2 for the conventional method.
3. Visualize the cervix as described in step 3 for the conventional method.

FIGURE **8A-5** **Placing cervical cell sample into liquid medium.**

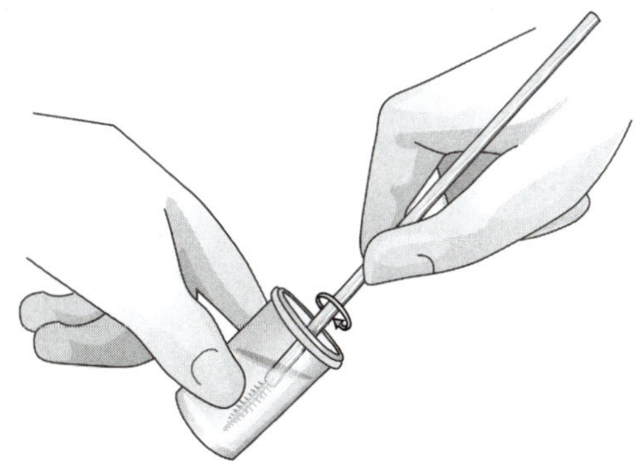

4. Insert the central bristles of the broom into the endocervical canal deep enough to allow the shorter bristles to fully contact the ectocervix (**Figure 8A-6**). Push gently and rotate the broom in a clockwise direction five times.
5. Place the broom into the vial and press firmly to the bottom of the vial so the bristles of the broom are forced apart. Swirl vigorously 10 times to mix the specimen and the medium (Figure 8A-5). Remove and discard the broom.
6. Screw the lid tightly and securely onto the vial.
7. Proceed as described in step 9 for the conventional method.

There is increasing research, evidence, and advocacy for patient self-collection for either HPV or cervical cytology. Please see Chapter 9 more for information about self-collection for these screening modalities.

FIGURE 8A-6 **Obtaining cervical cells with a broom device.**

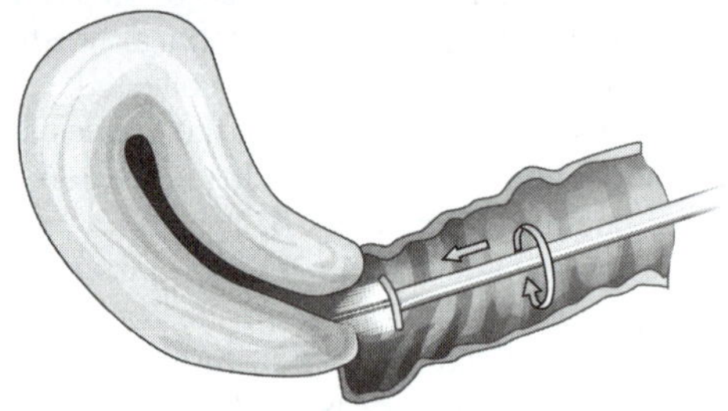

References

Arbyn, M., Bergeron, C., Klinkhamer, P., Martin-Hirsch, P., Siebers, A. G., & Bulten, J. (2008). Liquid compared with conventional cervical cytology: A systematic review and meta-analysis. *Obstetrics & Gynecology, 111*(1), 167–177.

Massad, L. S., Einstein, M. H., Huh, W. K., Katki, H. A., Kinney, W. K., Schirrman, M., Solomon, D., Wentzensen, N., & Lawson, H. W. (2013). 2012 updated consensus guidelines for the management of abnormal cervical cancer screening tests and cancer precursors. *Journal of Lower Genital Tract Disease, 17*(5), S1–S27.

Siebers, A. G., Klinkhamer, P. J., Grefte, J. M., Massuger, L. F., Vedder, J. E., Beijers-Broos, A., Bulten, J., & Arbyn, M. (2009). Comparison of liquid-based cytology with conventional cytology for detection of cervical cancer precursors: A randomized controlled trial. *Journal of the American Medical Association, 302*(16), 1757–1764.

U.S. Preventive Services Task Force, Curry, S. J., Krist, A. H., Owens, D. K., Barry, M. J., Caughey, A. B., Davidson, K. W., Doubeni, C. A., Epling, J. W., Jr., Kemper, A. R., Kubik, M., Landefeld, C. S., Mangione, C. M., Phipps, M. G., Silverstein, M., Simon, M. A., Tseng, C. W., & Wong, J. B. (2018). Screening for cervical cancer: U.S. Preventive Services Task Force recommendation statement. *JAMA, 320*(7), 676–686.

APPENDIX 8-B

Screening for *Chlamydia trachomatis, Neisseria gonorrhoeae,* and *Trichomonas vaginalis* Infections

NAAT is the recommended method for detecting gynecologic tract infections with *Chlamydia trachomatis*, *Neisseria gonorrhoeae*, and *Trichomonas vaginalis* (Centers for Disease Control and Prevention [CDC], 2014, 2015). *C. trachomatis*, *N. gonorrhoeae*, and *T. vaginalis* cultures should be reserved for specific indications, such as supporting research activities and monitoring resistance to treatment regimens. NAATs can be performed on vaginal swabs, endocervical swabs, rectal swabs, throat swabs, or urine specimens. Vaginal or rectal swabs, whether collected by the patient or the clinician, are the preferred sample type for *C. trachomatis* and *N. gonorrhoeae* NAATs over urine sampling. Endocervical swabs are acceptable if a pelvic examination is indicated. A urine specimen is also acceptable but may detect fewer infections when compared with vaginal and endocervical swabs (CDC, 2014). Vaginal swabs, endocervical swabs, and urine specimens are acceptable for *T. vaginalis* testing, and detection is similar among all three sample types (CDC, 2015). Several commercial NAAT products are available, including many that test for *C. trachomatis*, *N. gonorrhoeae*, and *T. vaginalis* from the same sample. Clinicians should follow the manufacturer's instructions when using these products.

To collect a vaginal or rectal swab specimen, the swab is inserted about 2 inches past the introitus or into the rectum and gently rotated for 10 to 30 seconds (**Figure 8B-1**). The swab should touch the walls of the vagina or rectum to absorb moisture. The swab is then withdrawn and placed into the transport medium. The sample may be self-collected by the patient or obtained by the clinician; self-obtained swabs are as accurate as, or more accurate than, clinician-obtained specimens (Lunny et al., 2015). A speculum or rectal examination is thus not required for this form of testing and should be considered only if other vaginal or cervical evaluation is needed beyond NAAT testing for these infections.

To collect an endocervical swab specimen, visualize the cervix using the speculum examination procedure. Remove all

FIGURE **8B-1** **Vaginal swab collection.**

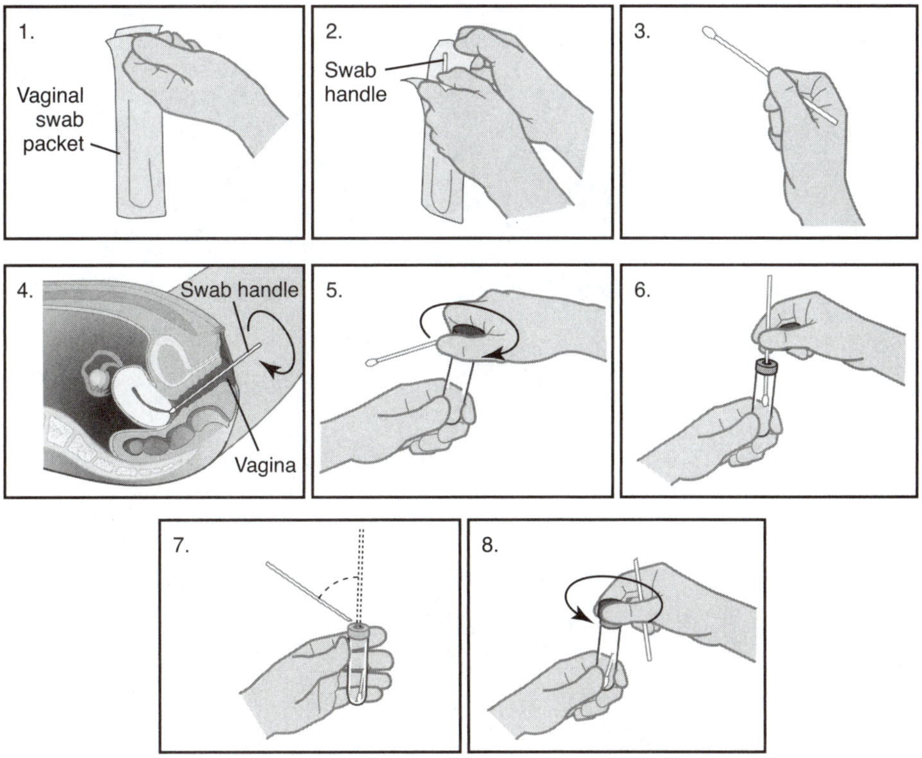

secretions and discharge from the cervix with a large swab. Insert the swab supplied by the manufacturer 1 to 2 cm into the cervical os, rotate it firmly at least twice against the walls of the canal, and allow it to remain in the os for the time recommended by the manufacturer. Withdraw the swab and place it into the transport medium. If the patient is engaging in oral and anal intercourse, the clinician or patient can self-swab similarly for these anatomical areas to complete STI screening.

References

Centers for Disease Control and Prevention. (2014). Recommendations for the laboratory-based detection of *Chlamydia trachomatis* and *Neisseria gonorrhoeae*—2014. *Morbidity and Mortality Weekly Report, 63*(RR02), 1–19. https://www.cdc.gov/mmwr/preview/mmwrhtml/rr6302a1.htm

Centers for Disease Control and Prevention. (2015). Sexually transmitted diseases treatment guidelines, 2015. *Morbidity and Mortality Weekly Report, 64*(3), 1–137.

Lunny, C., Taylor, D., Hoang, L., Wong, T., Gilbert, M., Lester, R., Krajden, M., & Ogilvie, G. (2015). Self-collected versus clinician-collected sampling for chlamydia and gonorrhea screening: A systematic review and meta-analysis. *PLOS ONE, 10*(7), e0132776.

APPENDIX 8-C

Preparing a Sample of Vaginal Secretions for Microscopic Examination

Vaginal secretions and exudates can be directly examined with a microscope to aid in the diagnosis of vaginal and sexually transmitted infections. See Chapters 21 and 22. Immediately after obtaining the vaginal secretions (whether by clinician collection or a patient's self-swab, as described in Appendix 8-B), mix one sample with normal saline solution; mix a second sample with a 10 percent solution of potassium hydroxide (KOH). *Candida albicans*, *T. vaginalis*, clue cells (epithelial cells with indistinct borders due to adherent bacteria) associated with bacterial vaginosis, and white blood cells can be seen in normal saline solution. Microscopy has poor sensitivity for *T. vaginalis* detection; NAAT testing is recommended if trichomoniasis is suspected (CDC, 2015). See Appendix 8-B and Chapter 21. Potassium hydroxide lyses trichomonads, white blood cells, and most bacteria, making visualization of *Candida* species easier. The presence of an amine or fishy odor with the addition of KOH to the vaginal secretions should be noted (whiff test) and is associated with, but not diagnostic for, bacterial vaginosis and trichomoniasis.

The CDC (2001) offers the following directions for collecting and preparing these specimens for microscopic examination:

1. Assemble the necessary materials: one or two standard glass microscope slides and cover slips, nonsterile cotton-tipped swabs, saline solution, and KOH solution. Some clinicians also use a small test tube.
2. Using a dropper or single-use blister pack of the solutions, place two to three large drops of saline on one slide and KOH on the second slide. Alternatives include the use of one slide (put drops of both solutions separately on it) or the test tube method (place drops of saline in a test tube and drops of KOH on a slide).
3. Obtain a specimen of vaginal discharge by either swabbing the vaginal walls and posterior fornix with a cotton-tipped swab or by sampling from the concave surfaces of the speculum blade after the speculum has been removed.
4. Mix the sample of the discharge with the drops of saline and KOH on the slides. Be sure to put the sample in the saline before the KOH, and keep the saline and KOH solutions separate. If using the test tube method, immerse the swab in the test tube, then use the swab to apply the premixed specimen onto a dry slide.
5. Cover each specimen with a glass cover slip. Avoid trapping air bubbles under the cover slip, which makes the microscopic examination more difficult. Put one edge of the cover slip into the mixed specimen, then lower the cover slip onto the specimen. Proceed as soon as possible to microscopic examination of the slide.

References

Centers for Disease Control and Prevention. (2001). *Program operations: Guidelines for STD prevention*. http://www.cdc.gov/std/program/medlab.pdf

Centers for Disease Control and Prevention. (2015). Sexually transmitted diseases treatment guidelines, 2015. *Morbidity and Mortality Weekly Report, 64*(3), 1–137.

APPENDIX 8-D

Anal Cytology Screening

Anal cytology screening is still an emerging and evolving field of study and clinical practice. Readers should cross-check for current recommendations. At the time of this writing, anal cytology screening is guided by risk thresholds which include age, sex of partners, HIV status, history of organ transplantation, history of vulvar precancer or cancer, history of cervical/vaginal HSIL or cancer, perianal warts, persistent HPV16, or autoimmune conditions (Stier et al., 2024).

The procedure to obtain anorectal cytology samples to screen for anal cancer proceeds as follows (University of California San Francisco Anal Neoplasia Clinic, Research and Education Center, 2025):

- Patients are asked not to douche or have an enema or insert anything into their anus for 24 hours prior to an anal cytology exam.
- Lubricants should not be used prior to obtaining a cytology sample because the lubricant may interfere with the processing and interpretation of the sample.
- We usually obtain the sample with the patient lying on their left side, but other positions are acceptable.
- The buttocks are retracted to visualize the anal opening and a Dacron or polyester tipped swab moistened in tap water is inserted for approximately 2 to 3 inches into the anus. The swab can be felt to pass through the internal sphincter so the sample is obtained from the junction of the anus and rectum, which is where most of the HPV-related lesions are found. This area is slightly above the region that corresponds anatomically to the dentate line.
- The swab is rotated 360 degrees with firm lateral pressure applied to the end of the swab, such that it is bowed slightly and then it is slowly withdrawn over a period of 15 to 30 seconds from the anus, continuing to rotate the swab in a circular fashion. The lateral pressure ensures that the mucosal surface, rather than rectal contents are sampled.
- The swab is either smeared directly onto a glass slide and fixed as a conventional Pap smear by placing it into alcohol, or the swab is placed in a preservative vial and vigorously agitated to disperse the cells for liquid-based cytology.
- Regardless of method used, the sample must be fixed quickly within 15 seconds in order to avoid drying artifact, which occurs easily and makes interpretation difficult.
- The slides are stained using the Papanicolau stain, hence the term "Pap smear," and then are examined by the pathologist.

References

American College of Obstetricians and Gynecologists. (2018, reaffirmed 2024). *The utility of and indications for routine pelvic examination* (ACOG Committee Opinion No. 754). https://www.acog.org/clinical/clinical-guidance/committee-opinion/articles/2018/10/the-utility-of-and-indications-for-routine-pelvic-examination

Beauchamp, T., & Childress, J. (2019). Principles of biomedical ethics: Marking its fortieth anniversary. *American Journal of Bioethics, 19*(11), 9-12. https://doi.org/10.1080/15265161.2019.1665402. PMID: 31647760.

Ellis, S. A., & Dalke, L. (2019). Midwifery care for transfeminine individuals. *Journal of Midwifery & Women's Health, 64*(3), 298-311. https://doi.org/10.1111/jmwh.12957. Epub 2019 Apr 8. PMID: 30957961.

Ferreyra, S., & Hughes, K. (1982). *Table manners: A guide to the pelvic examination for disabled women and health care providers.* Sex Education for Disabled People.

Stier, E. A., Clarke, M. A., Deshmukh, A. A., Wentzensen, N., Liu, Y., Poynten, I. M., Cavallari, E. N., Fink, V., Barroso, L. F., Clifford, G. M., Cuming, T., Goldstone, S. E., Hillman, R. J., Rosa-Cunha, I., La Rosa, L., Palefsky, J. M., Plotzker, R., Roberts, J. M., & Jay, N. (2024). International Anal Neoplasia Society's consensus guidelines for anal cancer screening. *International Journal of Cancer, 154*(10), 1694–1702. https://doi.org/10.1002/ijc.34850

University of California San Francisco Anal Neoplasia Clinic, Research and Education Center. (2025). *Obtaining a specimen for anal cytology.* https://ancre.ucsf.edu/obtaining-specimen-anal-cytology

CHAPTER 9

Periodic Screening and Health Maintenance

Paige Hardy

Taneesha Douglas

The editors acknowledge Kathryn Osborne who was the author of the previous edition of this chapter.

Primary preventive services refer to interventions aimed at preventing the onset of disease or injury before it occurs, whereas secondary preventive services are designed to detect disease or risk factors at an early stage, before symptoms develop, to facilitate timely treatment and reduce disease progression. The initial step in secondary prevention is assessment, which includes obtaining the patient's medical history, performing a physical examination, and evaluating data from laboratory tests. A comprehensive patient history is one of the most valuable screening tools available to the clinician. It affords the clinician an opportunity to receive detailed information about the patient and an opportunity to establish a therapeutic relationship with the patient. The patient's health history forms the basis for determining disease entities for which the patient is at risk and, therefore, requires further screening. A management plan is developed when risk factors are identified and should include measures that focus on reducing the short- and long-term consequences of any identified risks.

Cost containment continues to be critically important in today's healthcare environment, so it is imperative that clinicians make decisions about testing and treatment that are based on current evidence. It is the professional responsibility of every clinician to make healthcare delivery decisions that contain costs. As part of this responsibility, only tests and treatments with proven benefits should be used. Rather than conducting a battery of yearly, routine laboratory tests on every patient, the most effective approach to periodic screening is to individualize decisions about preventive health services by combining the best evidence with each patient's unique needs and circumstances (U.S. Preventive Services Task Force [USPSTF], n.d.).

In 1984, the U.S. Public Health Service gathered a panel of experts to examine the efficacy of preventive health services, including screening tests, counseling, immunizations, and chemoprevention. That panel—the U.S. Preventive Services Task Force (USPSTF)—remains active today and currently includes 16 experts from various private-sector specialty groups. The "task force works to improve the health of people nationwide by making evidence-based recommendations about clinical preventive services such as screenings, counseling services, and preventive medications" (USPSTF, n.d.). The initial findings of the USPSTF were published in 1989 as the *Guide to Clinical Preventive Services*. These findings were updated in 1996 and included the evaluation of more than 200 clinical services (USPSTF, 1996). Currently, the recommendations of the USPSTF are updated in an ongoing manner and published online for access by clinicians and the general public. As of 2024, the Task Force has recommendations on more than 88 topics. The USPSTF also provides the USPSTF Electronic Preventive Services Selector (the ePSS app), which can be downloaded to most mobile devices. Given that the work of the USPSTF is ongoing, and their recommendations are frequently updated, readers are advised to use ePSS or look for updates on the USPSTF website on a regular basis. (USPSTF, n.d.). The link to their website, the ePSS app, and additional resources for clinicians are listed in **Table 9-8** at the end of this chapter.

HEALTH MAINTENANCE: A NATIONAL PRIORITY

Passage of the Patient Protection and Affordable Care Act (ACA) in 2010 marked a change in U.S. national health policy relative to maintaining health through the delivery of preventive health services. The key objectives of the ACA were to expand Medicaid coverage to all individuals with incomes at or below 133% of the federal poverty level and to make lower-cost health insurance available for purchase (for those who do not qualify for Medicaid) on health insurance marketplaces, referred to as exchanges. However, a 2012 U.S. Supreme Court ruling allowed states to opt out of Medicaid expansion, leaving an estimated 1.9 million people in a "coverage gap" who are uninsured, as their income is too high for Medicaid but too low for ACA marketplace subsidies. If all states were to adopt Medicaid expansion, nearly 4.4 million people could become eligible for coverage (Kaiser Family Foundation, 2024a). Despite the 2012 ruling, millions of Americans continue to purchase lower-cost health insurance through the Health Insurance Marketplace.

Also included in the ACA are provisions that affect insurance coverage and reimbursement for health services. One such provision is that all individual and group insurance policies, whether sold on government-sponsored exchanges or privately, must include a predefined essential health benefits package. The essential health benefits package includes coverage for all preventive health services that receive an A or B rating from the USPSTF with no cost sharing (i.e., deductibles or copayments) for the individual (Kaiser Family Foundation, 2024b). However, a 2017 executive order issued by President Trump increased the availability of short-term health insurance policies that are not

TABLE 9-1 USPSTF Grade Definitions and Suggestions for Practice

Grade	Definition	Suggestions for Practice
A	The USPSTF recommends the service. There is high certainty that the net benefit is substantial.	Offer or provide this service.
B	The USPSTF recommends the service. There is high certainty that the net benefit is moderate or there is moderate certainty that the net benefit is moderate to substantial.	Offer or provide this service.
C	The USPSTF recommends selectively offering or providing this service to individual patients based on professional judgment and patient preferences. There is at least moderate certainty that the net benefit is small.	Offer or provide this service for selected patients depending on individual circumstances.
D	The USPSTF recommends against the service. There is moderate or high certainty that the service has no net benefit or that the harms outweigh the benefits.	Discourage the use of this service.
I statement	The USPSTF concludes that the current evidence is insufficient to assess the balance of benefits and harms of the service. Evidence is lacking, of poor quality, or conflicting, and the balance of benefits and harms cannot be determined.	Read the clinical considerations section of the USPSTF Recommendation Statement. If the service is offered, patients should understand the uncertainty about the balance of benefits and harms.

Reproduced from U.S. Preventive Services Task Force. (2024c). *Grade definitions*. https://www.uspreventiveservicestaskforce.org/uspstf/about-uspstf/methods-and-processes/grade-definitions

required to be ACA compliant and that usually exclude coverage of preventive health services (Kaiser Family Foundation, 2018). It is, therefore, incumbent upon all clinicians to remain aware of the various types of insurance coverage of the patients they serve, and the preventive services covered under qualified health plans, which are those that have received a grade of A or B from the USPSTF.

The intent of the USPSTF is to provide clinicians with a framework for decision making about the provision of preventive health services that is based on an extensive review of existing evidence for each preventive service. The current recommendation scheme assigns a letter grade to each recommendation that serves as a guide for informed and shared decision making. The grade that each service is assigned reflects the net benefit (benefits minus harms) and the quality of evidence upon which each recommendation is made (USPSTF, 2024c). The services designated as essential are those that the USPSTF recommends because there is a high (grade A) or moderate (grade B) degree of certainty that the net benefit from the service is substantial (grade A) or moderate to substantial (grade B). Services designated as grade C are those that the USPSTF has found to have such a small net benefit that they are not recommended for routine use in target populations, although grade C services may be justified for some patients (USPSTF, 2024c).

The USPSTF recommends against the use of grade D services—those for which there is a moderate or high degree of certainty that the service has no net benefit or that harms associated with the service outweigh the benefits. Services for which the USPSTF found insufficient evidence to recommend either for or against receive an I statement and no recommendation for use or nonuse. This designation indicates that the USPSTF could not assess the magnitude of benefits or harms with any degree of certainty (USPSTF, 2024c).

As shown in **Table 9-1**, the USPSTF updated its grade definitions in 2012 to reflect the periodic need to make screening decisions that are individualized based on patients' unique circumstances. **Table 9-2** explains the level of certainty relative to the net benefits of testing.

The screening recommendations of the USPSTF described here are intended for the general population of individuals who do not have signs or symptoms of disease or risk factors for specific disease entities. When no risk factors are found for a particular disease, a person is considered either not at increased risk for that disease or at average risk for the disease. However, people may experience changes in various aspects of their lives over time, and occasionally such changes are accompanied by developing risk factors. When that happens, there is a concomitant change in their risk status that is often accompanied by a need for additional screening. For example, a 30-year-old person who is not at increased risk for breast cancer experiences a change in risk status when they turn 40. The clinician must be aware of the various risk factors that may alter the risk status of individuals so that additional screening is obtained when needed.

This chapter focuses on the recommendations of the USPSTF that have received a grade of A or B, and it provides a brief summary of these evidence-based recommendations. The USPSTF recommendations and the guidelines developed by other professional groups are provided so that clinicians may compare and contrast them (**Table 9-3**). The USPSTF's published recommendations (USPSTF, 2024d), *Recommendations for Primary Care Practice,*

TABLE 9-2 Levels of Certainty Regarding Net Benefit

Level of Certainty[a]	Description
High	The available evidence usually includes consistent results from well-designed, well-conducted studies in representative primary care populations. These studies assess the effects of the preventive service on health outcomes. This conclusion is therefore unlikely to be strongly affected by the results of future studies.
Moderate	The available evidence is sufficient to determine the effects of the preventive service on health outcomes, but confidence in the estimate is constrained by such factors as: • The number, size, or quality of individual studies. • Inconsistency of findings across individual studies. • Limited generalizability of findings to routine primary care practice. • Lack of coherence in the chain of evidence. As more information becomes available, the magnitude or direction of the observed effect could change, and this change may be large enough to alter the conclusion.
Low	The available evidence is insufficient to assess effects on health outcomes. Evidence is insufficient because of: • The limited number or size of studies. • Important flaws in study design or methods. • Inconsistency of findings across individual studies. • Gaps in the chain of evidence. • Findings not generalizable to routine primary care practice. • Lack of information on important health outcomes. More information may allow estimation of effects on health outcomes.

Reproduced from U.S. Preventive Services Task Force. (2024c). *Grade definitions*. https://www.uspreventiveservicestaskforce.org/uspstf/about-uspstf/methods-and-processes/grade-definitions

[a]The USPSTF defines certainty as "likelihood that the USPSTF assessment of the net benefit of a preventive service is correct." The net benefit is defined as benefit minus harm of the preventive service as implemented in a general, primary care population. The USPSTF assigns a certainty level based on the nature of the overall evidence available to assess the net benefit of a preventive service.

which are available online, provide a more detailed description of the research underlying these recommendations and highlight the implications that the recommendations have for clinical practice. These published recommendations also provide detailed information for screening recommendations that have received a grade of C, D, or I; that is, screening tests that are not recommended for routine use or for which there is insufficient evidence to make a recommendation for or against their use. While the USPSTF uses binary gender language in its recommendations, clinicians should consider which guidelines may be appropriate for transgender and nonbinary individuals based on sex assigned at birth and individual risk factors.

Many of the current recommendations for routine screening are specific to people's sex assigned at birth. This is especially important when sex has been identified as a risk factor for the disease associated with the recommended screening. Therefore, binary gender terms are common in this literature and are used when necessary throughout this chapter. The authors and editors recognize that not all people assigned female at birth identify as female or women. The use of these terms is not meant to exclude people who do not identify as women and seek gynecologic care. Screening recommendations for individuals who are transgender or nonbinary may differ, especially with the use of gender-affirming treatments and procedures. The terminology in this chapter reflects screening recommendations based on risk factors, which often include one's biological sex; clinicians also need to consider anatomy and gender in individualizing patient care and screenings. Routine screening recommendations for people who are transgender, or nonbinary are evolving and are beyond the scope of this chapter. More detail on the care of patients who are transgender, or nonbinary can be found in Table 9-8 at the end of this chapter and in Chapter 11. Information about screening recommendations aimed at promoting sexual and reproductive health for people assigned male at birth is presented in Chapter 10.

GRADE A AND B SCREENING RECOMMENDATIONS

Alcohol Use

The current terminology for alcohol misuse is "unhealthy alcohol use." The reason for this change is that the USPSTF now combines risky drinking, alcohol misuse, hazardous drinking, and alcohol use disorder into "unhealthy alcohol use" to describe the spectrum of unhealthy drinking patterns.

The USPSTF (2018b) assigns a B recommendation to screening all adults age 18 and older (including pregnant

TABLE 9-3 Comparison of Screening Recommendations

	USPSTF	American College of Obstetricians and Gynecologists	American Cancer Society	Other Groups
Cervical cancer	Screen all women aged 21–65 years (grade A) using cervical cytology (Pap test) alone for women aged 21–29 years. Women aged 30–65 years may be screened every 3 years with Pap test alone, every 5 years with hrHPV testing alone, or every 5 years with hrHPV testing and Pap testing (co-testing). Recommends against screening women younger than age 21 (grade D). Recommends against screening women older than age 65 if they have had adequate prior screening and are otherwise not at risk for cervical cancer (grade D). Recommends against screening women who have had a total hysterectomy for benign disease (grade D).	The ACOG endorses the recommendations from the USPSTF In addition: These recommendations do not apply to individuals who are at high risk of the disease, such as those who have previously received a diagnosis of a high-grade precancerous cervical lesion or to individuals with in utero exposure to diethylstilbestrol (DES) or those with a compromised immune system (e.g., individuals with human immunodeficiency virus). Primary hrHPV testing every 5 years can be considered as an alternative to cytology-only screening in average-risk patients aged 25–29 years.	Start cervical cancer screening at age 25. Those aged 25–65 should have a primary HPV test every 5 years. If primary HPV testing is not available, screening may be done with either a co-test that combines an HPV test and Pap test every 5 years or a Pap test alone every 3 years. Those over age 65 who have had regular screening in the past 10 years with normal results and no history of CIN2 or more serious diagnosis within the past 25 years should stop cervical cancer screening. Once stopped, it should not be started again. People who have had a total hysterectomy (removal of the uterus and cervix) should stop screening (such as Pap tests and HPV tests), unless the hysterectomy was done as a treatment for cervical cancer or serious pre-cancer. People who have had a hysterectomy without removal of the cervix (called a **supra-cervical hysterectomy**) should continue cervical cancer screening according to the guidelines above.	The AAFP supports the recommendations of the USPSTF.

Breast cancer	Mammogram every 2 years for women aged 40–74 years (grade B). Insufficient evidence to recommend for or against screening after age 75 (I statement).	Offer CBE every 1–3 years for women aged 20–39 years and yearly for women age 40 and older. Annual or biennial mammogram for all women age 40 and older. Screening past age 75 should be done based on shared decision making with consideration of the woman's health status and life expectancy. Teaching BSE is not recommended. Breast self-awareness is recommended for women of all ages, and women should contact their healthcare provider regarding changes or concerns.	Offer all women aged 40–44 years the option to begin yearly mammogram screening. Yearly mammogram for all women aged 45–54 years. Mammogram every 1–2 years for all women starting at age 55 and continuing for as long as the woman is in good health and is expected to live 10 more years or longer. Women with certain risk factors may benefit from MRI screening in conjunction with mammogram. Recommend that women know how their breasts normally look and feel, and they should report any changes to their healthcare provider.	The AAFP supports the recommendations of the USPSTF.
Osteoporosis	Recommends routine screening for osteoporosis with bone density measurements for all women age 65 and older and screening younger women who are at increased risk (grade B). Although central DXA scan is used most often, peripheral DXA or QUS may be appropriate in some circumstances.	Concurs with the National Osteoporosis Foundation.		The AAFP supports the recommendations of the USPSTF. The National Osteoporosis Foundation recommends screening all women age 65 and older, and younger postmenopausal women who have had a fracture or who have one or more risk factors for osteoporosis, using DXA scan of the hip and spine.

(continues)

TABLE 9-3 Comparison of Screening Recommendations (*continued*)

	USPSTF	American College of Obstetricians and Gynecologists	American Cancer Society	Other Groups
Colorectal cancer	Screen all adults aged 50–75 years for colorectal cancer (grade A). Screening for colorectal cancer in adults aged 45 to 49 year (grade B). The risks and benefits of different screening tests vary. Because of limited available evidence, the USPSTF recommendation does not include serum tests, urine tests, or capsule endoscopy for colorectal cancer screening. Stool-based and direct visualization screening tests are recommended. The USPSTF recommends that clinicians selectively offer screening for colorectal cancer in adults aged 76 to 85 years. Evidence indicates that the net benefit of screening all persons in this age group is small. In determining whether this service is appropriate in individual cases, patients and clinicians should consider the patient's overall health, prior screening history, and preferences (grade C).	Recommends colorectal cancer screening beginning at age 45 for average-risk women. Preferred screening method: Colonscopy every 10 years. Other screening options: • CT colonography (virtual colonoscopy) every 5 years • Flexible sigmoidoscopy every 5 years • Fecal immunochemical test (FIT) annually • Guaiac-based fecal occult blood test (gFOBT) annually • Multi-targeted stool DNA test (mt-sDNA or Cologuard) every 3 years • Routine screening may be discontinued at age 75.	Starting at age 45, This can be done either with a stool-based test or with a visual exam. People who are in good health and with a life expectancy of more than 10 years should continue regular colorectal cancer screening through age 75. Recommendations for individuals aged 76–85 years, the decision to be screened should be based on a person's preferences, life expectancy, overall health, and prior screening history. Discontinue all screening after age 85.	The AAFP recommends screening for colorectal cancer in all adults starting at age 50 years and continuing until age 75 years. The AAFP recommends that clinicians selectively offer screening for colorectal cancer in adults aged 76 to 85 years The AAFP concludes that the evidence is insufficient to assess the benefits and harms for screening for colorectal cancer in adults aged 45 to 49 years.
Lung cancer	Screen all women aged 55–80 years with a 30-pack-year smoking history who have quit smoking within 15 years or who currently smoke. Screening should be done yearly with low-dose CT.		Yearly screening with low-dose CT for individuals who meet the following three criteria: • Age 55–74 years in good health • Currently smoke or quit smoking in the past 15 years • Have a 30-pack-year smoking history (1 pack per day for 30 years or 2 packs per day for 15 years)	

Ovarian cancer	Recommends against routine screening with tumor markers, ultrasound, or pelvic examination of asymptomatic women who are not at increased risk for ovarian cancer (grade D).	No techniques have proven to be effective in the routine screening of asymptomatic low-risk women for ovarian cancer. Clinicians should remain vigilant for signs and symptoms of disease. May recommend transvaginal ultrasound or CA 125 for certain women at high risk for ovarian cancer.	There are no recommended screening tests for ovarian cancer for women who do not have symptoms and are not at high risk of developing ovarian cancer. In studies of women at average risk of ovarian cancer, using TVUS and CA-125 for screening led to more testing and sometimes more surgeries, but did not lower the number of deaths caused by ovarian cancer.	The AAFP supports the recommendations of the USPSTF.
IPV	Screen all women of childbearing age for IPV.	Periodically screen all adolescents and women for IPV and reproductive and sexual coercion. Screen all pregnant women at the first prenatal visit and periodically during pregnancy and postpartum.		The AAFP supports the recommendations of the USPSTF.

Data from American Academy of Family Physicians. (n.d.). *Clinical preventive services recommendations. Cervical cancer.* https://www.aafp.org/family-physician/patient-care/clinical-recommendations/all-clinical-recommendations/cervical-cancer.html; American Academy of Family Physicians. (n.d.). *Colorectal cancer screening, Adults.* https://www.aafp.org/family-physician/patient-care/clinical-recommendations/all-clinical-recommendations/colorectal-cancer-adults.html; American Cancer Society. (n.d.). *Can ovarian cancer be found early?* American Cancer Society. Retirieved October 27, 2024 from https://www.cancer.org/cancer/types/ovarian-cancer/detection-diagnosis-staging/detection.html; American Cancer Society. (2024). *American Cancer Society guidelines for the prevention and early detection of cervical cancer.* https://www.cancer.org/cancer/types/cervical-cancer/detection-diagnosis-staging/cervical-cancer-screening-guidelines.html; American Cancer Society. (2024). American Cancer Society guideline for colorectal cancer screening. https://www.cancer.org/cancer/types/colon-rectal-cancer/detection-diagnosis-staging/acs-recommendations.html; American Cancer Society. *American Cancer Society Recommendations for the Early Detection* of Breast Cancer. https://www.cancer.org/cancer/types/breast-cancer/screening-tests-and-early-detection/american-cancer-society-recommendations-for-the-early-detection-of-breast-cancer.html; American College of Obstetricians and Gynecologists. (2017). *Breast Cancer Risk Assessment and Screening in Average-Risk Women.* https://www.acog.org/clinical/clinical-guidance/practice-bulletin/articles/2017/07/breast-cancer-risk-assessment-and-screening-in-average-risk-women; American College of Obstetricians and Gynecologists. (2012/2022). *Intimate Partner Violence.* https://www.acog.org/clinical/clinical-guidance/committee-opinion/articles/2012/02/intimate-partner-violence; American College of Obstetricians and Gynecologists. (2017). *The role of the Obstetrician–Gynecologist in the early detection of epithelial ovarian cancer in women at average risk.* American College of Obstetricians and Gynecologists. Retrieved October 27, 2024 from https://www.acog.org/clinical/clinical-guidance/committee-opinion/articles/2017/09/the-role-of-the-obstetriciangynecologist-in-the-early-detection-of-epithelial-ovarian-cancer-in-women-at-average-risk; American College of Obstetricians and Gynecologists. (n.d.). *Updated cervical cancer screening guidelines.* Retrieved October 1, 2024, from https://www.acog.org/clinical/clinical-guidance/practice-advisory/articles/2021/04/updated-cervical-cancer-screening-guidelines; National Osteoporosis Foundation. (n.d.). *Bone density exam/testing.* https://www.nof.org/patients/diagnosis-information/bone-density-examtesting/; Ray, J. & LaBundy, J. (2022). *Lower gastrointestinal tract disorders.* ACOG. https://www.acog.org/clinical/journals-and-publications/clinical-updates/2022/06/lower-gastrointestinal-tract-disorders and US Preventive Services Task Force. (2024). *Published recommendations.* Retrieved October 26, 2024, from https://www.uspreventiveservicestaskforce.org/uspstf/topic_search_results?topic_status=

Abbreviations: AAFP, American Academy of Family Physicians; BSE, breast self-examination; CA, cancer antigen; CBE, clinical breast examination; CT, computerized tomography; DXA, dual energy x-ray absorptiometry; HPV, human papillomavirus; hrHPV, high-risk HPV; IPV, *intimate partner violence*; QUS, quantitative ultrasound.

women) for unhealthy alcohol use; screening adolescents younger than age 18 has been assigned an I statement. Historically, research regarding the effects of alcohol on humans and animals has been conducted on males. Only recently has the research focus changed in an attempt to discover the effects of alcohol use on females. The findings of these studies have revealed that smaller quantities of alcohol can result in more severe damage to women (National Institute on Alcohol Abuse and Alcoholism [NIAAA], 2024c). According to a 2023 national survey on drug use and health, approximately 11.5 million women in the United States, ages 18 and older, are living with alcohol use disorder (AUD), a diagnosis outlined in the *Diagnostic and Statistical Manual of Mental Disorders,* Fifth Edition, Text Revision (DSM-5-TR) (NIAAA, 2024a). The DSM-5-TR categorizes AUD into three levels of severity: mild, moderate, and severe. Women who consume more than eight drinks per week or four drinks per day are considered at risk for developing AUD. This is considerably lower than the threshold for men (NIAAA, 2024b).

A variety of effective tools to screen for unhealthy alcohol use are available, and many of these can be found at the National Institute on Alcohol Abuse and Alcoholism website listed in Table 9-8 at the end of this chapter. To screen for unhealthy alcohol use, the USPSTF (2018b) recommends using either the Abbreviated AUDIT-C instrument or the Single Alcohol Screening Question (SASQ), in which patients are asked a single question about alcohol use: How many times in the past year have you had four or more drinks in a day? Both of these approaches have been found to have adequate sensitivity and specificity for detecting unhealthy alcohol use and can easily be applied in primary care settings (USPSTF, 2018b). Readers are advised that at the time of this writing, the USPSTF recommendation for unhealthy alcohol use was under review and is likely to change.

Cervical Cancer

The USPSTF assigns an A recommendation to screening all women aged 21 to 65 for cervical cancer (2024b). The recommended screening tests and screening intervals differ according to the age and existing risk factors of the individual. For women aged 21 to 29, the recommendation is to screen every 3 years using liquid-based or conventional cervical cytology alone, commonly called a Pap test. For individuals aged 30 to 65 years, the USPSTF (2024b) recommends that patients engage in shared decision making with their healthcare provider to select one of the following screening approaches that best meets their needs: (1) every 3 years with cervical cytology alone; (2) every 5 years with high-risk human papillomavirus (hrHPV) testing alone; or (3) every 5 years with hrHPV testing and cervical cytology (co-testing). The USPSTF found that the harms or potential harms outweigh the benefits and therefore recommends against (D recommendation) the following practices:

- Screening patients younger than age 21 years
- Screening patients older than age 65 years who have been screened adequately and who are not at increased risk for cervical cancer
- Screening patients who have had a hysterectomy with removal of the cervix and have no history of high-grade precancerous lesions (i.e., cervical intraepithelial neoplasia [CIN] grade 2 or 3) or cervical cancer (USPSTF, 2024b)

Chlamydia and Gonorrhea Infection

The USPSTF (2021a) assigns a B recommendation to screening all sexually active individuals including pregnant persons age 24 years and younger, and individuals including pregnant persons 25 years and older, who are at an increased risk for infection with chlamydia and gonorrhea. The recommendations are stratified by "men" and "women," although the net benefit estimates are driven by biological sex (i.e., male/female) rather than gender identity. The most significant risk factor for infection is age, with the highest infection rates in women occurring during ages 15 to 24 years. Additionally, women 25 years and older at increased risk of infection include those who have a new sex partner, more than one sex partner, a sex partner with concurrent partners, or a sex partner who has an STI; practice inconsistent external condom use when not in a mutually monogamous relationship; or have a previous or coexisting STI. Exchanging sex for money or drugs and history of incarceration also are associated with increased risk. In addition to individual risk factors, chlamydia and gonococcal infections are seen more frequently in particular communities. Clinicians should be aware of prevalence rates of infection in the communities where they practice (USPSTF, 2021a). The USPSTF recommends using nucleic acid amplification tests (NAATs) to diagnose chlamydia and gonorrhea infections, both of which can be tested using the same specimen. The U.S. Food and Drug Administration approves NAATs for use on urogenital and extragenital sites, including urine, endocervical, vaginal, male urethral, rectal, and pharyngeal specimens (USPSTF, 2021a).

Depression

The USPSTF assigns a B recommendation to screening all adults for depression, including patients who are pregnant or postpartum (USPSTF, 2023a). Screening for depression is an important aspect of women's health care because women are at higher risk for developing clinical depression than their male counterparts (National Institute of Mental Health, n.d.).

A variety of depression screening tools are available. The most commonly used are self-administered questionnaires that have been previously validated, such as versions of the Patient Health Questionnaire (PHQ), the Geriatric Depression Scale for older adults, and the Edinburgh Postnatal Depression Scale (EPDS) for postpartum and pregnant patients (USPSTF, 2023a). Perhaps the easiest tool to use in primary care settings is the PHQ-2, wherein a patient is asked about their ability to find pleasure in activities they usually enjoy and whether or not they have felt down, depressed, or hopeless. Patients with a positive screen should be further evaluated by clinicians who are skilled in the diagnosis and treatment of depressive disorders (USPSTF, 2023a). The USPSTF was unable to determine the optimal screening frequency but suggests that clinicians screen all adults who have not been previously screened and rescreen based on clinical judgment and the existence of risk factors for depression (USPSTF, 2023a).

The USPSTF recommends screening all adolescents aged 12–18 years for depression (USPSTF, 2022a). Validated tools include the Patient Health Questionnaire for Adolescents (PHQ-A) and adolescent-modified versions of the PHQ. The USPSTF has not established an optimal screening interval; instead, it advises repeat screening based on clinical judgment and risk factors. Because adolescents are infrequently seen for routine healthcare visits, opportunistic screening—performing a screen whenever an adolescent presents for care—is encouraged (USPSTF, 2022a).

Height and Weight

The USPSTF has made several counseling recommendations for women living in larger bodies, as discussed in Chapter 8. Body mass index (BMI) is the recommended method of identifying individuals at increased risk for morbidity and mortality related to body size. It is calculated by dividing a person's weight in kilograms by their height in meters squared. Overweight is defined as having a BMI in the range of 25 to 29.9. Anyone with a BMI of 30 or greater is classified as obese. BMI, however, has limitations as a health measurement. It does not differentiate between muscle and fat mass, nor does it account for variations in body composition, fat distribution, or metabolic health across different individuals and populations. Despite these limitations the USPSTF recommends its use as a screening tool, recognizing the clinician's judgment and additional assessment are necessary for a comprehensive evaluation of the individual's health risk.

The USPSTF provides B-grade recommendation that clinicians should offer referral for behavioral interventions to help with weight loss in adults who are obese. Most of the intensive behavioral weight loss interventions endorsed by the USPSTF last for 1 to 2 years, encourage self-monitoring of weight, and provide tools to support weight loss or weight loss maintenance (USPSTF, 2018c). All patients should be counseled on the importance of maintaining a healthy diet and regular exercise. Adults who adhere to national guidelines for a healthy diet and physical activity have lower cardiovascular morbidity and mortality than those who do not. All persons, regardless of their cardiovascular disease risk status, can gain health benefits from healthy eating behaviors and appropriate physical activity (USPSTF, 2020a). Readers are advised that at the time of this writing, updates are in progress for the USPSTF recommendation for healthy diet, physical activity, and weight loss.

Hypertension

The USPSTF assigns an A recommendation to screening for hypertension in adults 18 years and older without known hypertension; the routine screening of children and adolescents has been assigned an I statement. The recommended screening test for hypertension is a blood pressure measurement obtained in the healthcare provider's office using a sphygmomanometer (USPSTF, 2021c). The initial screening should be conducted after the patient has been seated and at rest for 5 minutes. The USPSTF also recommends confirming a diagnosis of hypertension with ambulatory blood pressure monitoring or blood pressure measurements taken in the patient's home prior to initiating treatment.

In addition to screening the general population, the USPSTF (2023b) assigns a B recommendation to screening all asymptomatic pregnant persons for hypertensive disorders. To achieve benefit from this screening, it is important to implement evidence-based management interventions for all persons with a positive screening result. A positive screening result for new-onset hypertension during pregnancy is defined as an elevated blood pressure reading (systolic blood pressure ≥140 mm Hg or diastolic blood pressure ≥90 mm Hg in the absence of chronic hypertension) measured twice at least 4 hours apart. A patient with multiple elevated blood pressure readings should have further diagnostic evaluation and clinical monitoring (USPSTF, 2023b).

Human Immunodeficiency Virus Infection

The USPSTF (2019c) assigns an A recommendation to screening all adolescents and adults, including pregnant people, aged 15 to 65 years for HIV; younger adolescents and older adults who are at increased risk for infection should also be screened. The USPSTF found insufficient evidence to recommend a screening interval, though the recommendation is to obtain a one-time screen for all patients aged 15 to 65 years to identify existing disease, with follow-up testing based on risk factors (USPSTF, 2019c). The recommended screening tests for HIV are those recommended by the Centers for Disease Control and Prevention (CDC), which include U.S. Food and Drug Administration-approved antigen/antibody immunoassays that are able to detect the HIV-1 p24 antigen and the HIV-1 and HIV-2 antibodies; reactive assays should be followed with supplemental testing to differentiate between HIV-1 and HIV-2 antibodies. When rapid HIV testing is used, conventional methods must be used to confirm initial positive findings (USPSTF, 2019c). At the time of writing, updates are in progress for USPSTF recommendations for HIV screening.

Intimate Partner Violence

The USPSTF assigns a B recommendation to screening all women of childbearing age (adolescents to women in their 40s) for intimate partner violence (USPSTF, 2018a). Several screening tools have high levels of sensitivity and specificity for identifying intimate partner violence, including the Extended-Hurt, Insult, Threaten, Scream (E-HITS); Humiliation, Afraid, Rape, Kick (HARK); Slapped, Threatened, and Throw (STaT); and the Partner Violence Screen (PVS) instruments. Each of these tools includes three to four questions and can be self-administered (USPSTF, 2018a).

According to the CDC (2024a), about 41% of women and 26% of men experienced contact sexual violence, physical violence, or stalking by an intimate partner during their lifetime and reported a related impact. Patients presenting with symptoms or injuries should receive detailed documentation of their injuries, medical treatment, counseling referrals, and a list of community resources that provide shelter and protection. See Chapter 15 for more information on IPV and Chapter 16 for more information on sexual assault.

Tobacco Use

The USPSTF gives an A recommendation for screening all adults for tobacco use. It advises individuals to quit using tobacco and encourages healthcare providers to offer behavioral interventions along with FDA-approved medications for cessation to nonpregnant adults who use tobacco. Additionally, the USPSTF recommends that clinicians inquire about tobacco use with all pregnant individuals, advise them to stop using tobacco, and provide behavioral interventions to those who use tobacco during pregnancy. A common approach to behavioral counseling involves the "5 As" framework. The five steps are: (1) ask about tobacco use; (2) advise on a quit attempt with clear, personalized messages; (3) assess the individual's willingness to quit; (4) assist with the quitting process; (5) arrange for follow-up and support (USPSTF, 2021f). Tobacco product use remains the leading cause of preventable disease and death in the United States. In 2022, 49.2 million (19.8%) or nearly 1 in 5 U.S. adults reported current tobacco product use (CDC, 2024b). Effective tobacco smoking cessation interventions for nonpregnant adults include behavioral counseling and pharmacotherapy, either individually or in combination. The behavioral counseling intervention type most often studied in pregnant persons who smoke was counseling. Scientific evidence demonstrates that patients who quit using tobacco are likely to realize substantial overall health benefits, regardless of the number of years of tobacco use, and that even brief interventions are effective at increasing quit rates (USPSTF, 2021f).

GRADE A AND B SCREENING RECOMMENDATIONS

The screening recommendations described thus far have applied primarily to all individuals, regardless of age. For several disease entities, however, age is a significant risk factor. Therefore, as people age, some additional screening recommendations apply.

Breast Cancer

The following recommendations apply to cisgender women, and anyone assigned female at birth (including transgender men and nonbinary individuals) who are 40 years or older and at average risk for breast cancer. Screening mammography every 2 years for those aged 40 to 74 years receives a B recommendation from the USPSTF (2024a). The task force found insufficient evidence to weigh the benefits or harms of screening mammograms in patients 75 years and older. It also found insufficient evidence to weigh the benefits and harms of supplemental screening for breast cancer using breast ultrasonography or magnetic resonance imaging (MRI) in patients identified to have dense breasts on an otherwise negative screening mammogram (USPSTF, 2024a). Both digital mammography and digital breast tomosynthesis (DBT, commonly referred to as "3D mammography") are effective screening methods for breast cancer (USPSTF, 2024a). Clinicians should be aware that while several health organizations issue guidelines for breast cancer screening and prevention, private insurance coverage of preventive services under the ACA is governed by recommendations from the USPSTF and the Health Resources and Services Administration (HRSA). Under these guidelines, private group and individual insurance plans and state Medicaid expansion programs must cover the following breast cancer screening and prevention services at no cost to the consumer: (1) screening mammography at least every 2 years and as frequently as once a year for those aged 40 to 74 with average risk for breast cancer; (2) genetic counseling and testing for mutation of the *BRCA1* and *BRCA2* genes in some individuals with a personal or family history of breast, ovarian, fallopian tube, or peritoneal cancer; (3) preventive medication for some individuals with elevated risk of breast cancer and at low risk for adverse medication effects (Kaiser Family Foundation, 2019). Following a review of the evidence, the USPSTF elected not to update their previous recommendations for breast self-examination and clinical breast examination. It is important for patients to remain cognizant of body changes and discuss their concerns with a healthcare provider. Refer to Chapter 17 for a more in-depth discussion of breast cancer.

Colorectal Cancer

The USPSTF (2021b) assigns a grade A to the recommendation that all adults aged 50 to 75 be screened for colorectal cancer. They assign a grade B for adults aged 45 to 49 to be screened for colorectal cancer. This recommendation is intended for patients at average risk for colorectal cancer. In this case, average risk is defined as having had no prior diagnosis of colorectal cancer, adenomatous polyps, or inflammatory bowel disease; no personal diagnosis or family history of known genetic disorders that predispose them to a high lifetime risk of colorectal cancer (such as Lynch syndrome or familial adenomatous polyposis).

Recommended screening tests, screening frequency, evidence of efficacy, and other considerations are listed in **Table 9-4**. Each of these options has advantages and disadvantages for the patient and the practice setting. Because of limited available evidence, the USPSTF recommendation does not include serum tests, urine tests, or capsule endoscopy for colorectal cancer screening. The USPSTF recognizes that maximizing the number of patients screened for colorectal cancer will have the greatest effect on reducing colorectal cancer deaths. Therefore, clinicians should discuss the risks and benefits, and the advantages and disadvantages, of each screening strategy and include patient preference in choosing the screening method that best fits the patient's needs. Clinicians providing health care for individuals who require screening should familiarize themselves with the risks, costs, and benefits of the various screening options. The USPSTF assigns a C grade to screening patients aged 76 to 85 years and recommends taking the patient's overall health and screening history into consideration when making decisions about screening for this age group (USPSTF, 2021b).

Hepatitis C Virus Infection

The USPSTF (2020c) recommends hepatitis C infection screening (grade B) for all adults aged 18 to 79 years. Pregnant adults should also be screened. HCV prevalence doubled in women aged 15 to 44 years from 2006 to 2014 (USPSTF, 2020c). Risk factors for hepatitis C infection include past or current intravenous or intranasal drug use, long-term hemodialysis, incarceration, being born to an infected mother, getting a tattoo at an unregulated establishment, and other exposure through percutaneous means. The most important risk factor for HCV infection is past or current injection drug use. In the United States, recent increases in HCV incidence have predominantly been among young persons who inject drugs. Clinicians may want to consider screening in adolescents younger than 18 years and in adults older than 79 years who are at high risk (USPSTF, 2020c). The recommended screening test is anti-HCV (hepatitis C virus) antibody testing and confirmation with polymerase chain reaction testing. Most adults need to be screened only once. Persons with continued risk for HCV infection should be screened periodically (USPSTF, 2020c).

Lipid Disorders

The USPSTF no longer assigns a stand-alone recommendation regarding routine screening for lipid disorders. However, they do provide recommendations for the use of statins to prevent cardiovascular disease in adults (USPSTF, 2022b). A detailed discussion regarding the use of this preventive medication is beyond the scope of this chapter. Readers should remain aware that the USPSTF recommends the use of moderate-dose statins (grade B)

TABLE 9-4 Characteristics of Colorectal Cancer Screening Strategies[a]

Screening Method[a]	Frequency[b]	Evidence of Efficacy	Other Considerations
Stool-Based Tests			
gFOBT	Every year	• Evidence from RCTs that gFOBT reduces colorectal cancer mortality • High-sensitivity versions (e.g., Hemoccult SENSA) have superior test performance characteristics than older tests (e.g., Hemoccult II) although there is still uncertainty about the precision of test sensitivity estimates. Given this uncertainty, it is unclear whether high-sensitivity gFOBT can detect as many cases of advanced adenomas and colorectal cancer as other stool-based tests	• Harms from screening with gFOBT arise from colonoscopy to follow up abnormal gFOBT results • Requires dietary restrictions and three stool samples • Requires good adherence over multiple rounds of testing • Does not require bowel preparation, anesthesia, or transportation to and from the screening examination (test is performed at home)
FIT	Every year	• Evidence from 1 large cohort study that screening with FIT reduces colorectal cancer mortality • Certain types of FIT have improved accuracy compared with gFOBT and HSgFOBT (20 μg hemoglobin per gram of feces threshold was used in the CISNET modeling)	• Harms from screening with FIT arise from colonoscopy to follow up abnormal FIT results • Can be done with a single stool sample • Requires good adherence over multiple rounds of testing • Does not require bowel preparation, anesthesia or sedation, or transportation to and from the screening examination (test is performed at home)
sDNA-FIT	Every 1 to 3 years	• Improved sensitivity compared with FIT per 1-time application of screening test • Specificity is lower than that of FIT, resulting in more false-positive results, more follow-up colonoscopies, and more associated adverse events per sDNA-FIT screening test compared with per FIT test • Modeling suggests that screening every 3 years does not provide a favorable (i.e., efficient) balance of benefits and harms compared with other stool-based screening options (i.e., annual FIT or sDNA-FIT every 1 or 2 years) • Insufficient evidence about appropriate longitudinal follow up of abnormal findings after a negative follow-up colonoscopy • No direct evidence evaluating the effect of sDNA-FIT on colorectal cancer mortality	• Harms from screening with sDNA-FIT arise from colonoscopy to follow up abnormal sDNA-FIT results • Can be done with a single stool sample but involves collecting an entire bowel movement • Requires good adherence over multiple rounds of testing • Does not require bowel preparation, anesthesia or sedation, or transportation to and from the screening examination (test is performed at home)
Direct Visualization Tests			
Colonoscopy[c]	Every 10 years	• Evidence from cohort studies that colonoscopy reduces colorectal cancer mortality • Harms from colonoscopy include bleeding and perforation, which both increase with age	• Screening and diagnostic follow-up of positive results can be performed during the same examination • Requires less frequent screening • Requires bowel preparation, anesthesia or sedation, and transportation to and from the screening examination

(continues)

TABLE 9-4 Characteristics of Colorectal Cancer Screening Strategies[a] *(continued)*

Screening Method[a]	Frequency[b]	Evidence of Efficacy	Other Considerations
CT colonography	Every 5 years	• Evidence available that CT colonography has reasonable accuracy to detect colorectal cancer and adenomas • No direct evidence evaluating effect of CT colonography on colorectal cancer mortality • Limited evidence about the potential benefits or harms of possible evaluation and treatment of incidental extracolonic findings, which are common. Extracolonic findings detected in 1.3% to 11.4% of exams; < 3% required medical or surgical treatment	• Additional harms from screening with CT colonography arise from colonoscopy to follow up abnormal CT colonography results • Requires bowel preparation • Does not require anesthesia or transportation to and from the screening examination
Flexible sigmoidoscopy	Every 5 years	• Evidence from RCTs that flexible sigmoidoscopy reduces colorectal cancer mortality • Risk of bleeding and perforation but less than risk with colonoscopy • Modeling suggests that it provides fewer life-years gained alone than when combined with FIT or in comparison to other strategies	• Additional harms may arise from colonoscopy to follow up abnormal flexible sigmoidoscopy results • Test availability has declined in the United States but may be available in some communities where colonoscopy is less available
Flexible sigmoidoscopy with FIT	Flexible sigmoidoscopy every 10 years plus FIT every year	• Evidence from RCTs that flexible sigmoidoscopy + FIT reduces colorectal cancer mortality • Modeling suggests combination testing provides similar benefits to those of colonoscopy, with fewer complications • Risk of bleeding and perforation from flexible sigmoidoscopy but less than risk with colonoscopy	• Additional potential harms from colonoscopy to follow up abnormal flexible sigmoidoscopy or FIT results • Flexible sigmoidoscopy availability has declined in the United States but may be available in some communities where colonoscopy is less available • Screening with FIT requires good adherence over multiple rounds of testing

Reproduced from U.S. Preventive Services Task Force. (2021b). *Colorectal cancer: Screening*. https://www.uspreventiveservicestaskforce.org/uspstf/recommendation/colorectal-cancer-screening#tab1

Abbreviations: CISNET, Cancer Intervention and Surveillance Modeling Network; CT, computed tomography FIT, fecal immunochemical test; gFOBT, guaiac fecal occult blood test; RCT, randomized clinical trial; sDNA-FIT, stool DNA test with fecal immunochemical test.

[a] To achieve the benefits of screening, abnormal results from stool-based tests, CT colonography, and flexible sigmoidoscopy should be followed up with colonoscopy.
[b] Applies to persons with negative findings (including hyperplastic polyps) and is not intended for persons in surveillance programs. Evidence of efficacy is not informative of screening frequency, with the exception of gFOBT and flexible sigmoidoscopy alone.
[c] As stated by the manufacturer.

to prevent cardiovascular mortality and events related to cardiovascular disease for all adults without a history of cardiovascular disease and who meet all of the following criteria:

- Age 40 to 75 years
- Have one or more risk factors for cardiovascular disease (including dyslipidemia)
- Have a calculated 10-year risk for a cardiovascular disease event of 10 percent or greater (USPSTF, 2022b)

Because the calculation of a 10-year risk for a cardiovascular event and the identification of dyslipidemia require universal lipid screening, it is necessary to screen all adults aged 40 to 75 years for dyslipidemia to identify those for whom preventive statin therapy is recommended (USPSTF, 2022b). This recommendation does not include a screening test or frequency of testing. However, the CDC recommends that asymptomatic adults without a personal or family history of cardiovascular disease or elevated cholesterol be screened every 4 to 6 years with serum measurements of total cholesterol, LDL, HDL, and triglycerides. Children should have an initial cholesterol test between the ages of 9 and 11, then again between 17–21 years (CDC, 2024c).

Osteoporosis

Screening women aged 65 and older for osteoporosis receives a B recommendation from the USPSTF (2018d). Screening younger postmenopausal individuals who are at increased risk for osteoporosis, as identified using a formal risk assessment tool, also receives a B recommendation. Factors associated with increased risk for the development of osteoporosis include low body weight (BMI less than 21), cigarette smoking, family history of osteoporosis or hip fracture, excessive alcohol intake, and white race. The USPSTF (2018d) recommends using previously validated tools, such as the Simple Calculated Osteoporosis Risk Estimation (SCORE) or the Fracture Risk Assessment (FRAX) instrument, to assess for increased osteoporosis risk in menopausal individuals younger than 65 years who have one or more risk factors for osteoporosis. The most commonly used test to screen for osteoporosis is dual-energy x-ray absorptiometry (DXA) of the hip and lumbar spine, although peripheral DXA and quantitative ultrasound may also be used (USPSTF, 2018d). The optimal frequency of screening has been minimally studied, but evidence suggests that repeat testing 4 to 8 years after the initial screen may be of little or no benefit (USPSTF, 2018d). Those in whom osteoporosis is identified should be counseled on the risks and benefits of various treatment options. Readers are advised that at the time of this writing, the USPSTF recommendation for osteoporosis screening was under review and is likely to change.

Screening Based on Risk

In addition to the previously discussed screening recommendations for generally healthy people across the life span, the USPSTF also provides guidance on screening based on specific risk factors. These recommendations take into account factors such as personal and family medical history, environmental exposures, and other conditions that may increase disease risk. It has also made recommendations for screening pregnant people. These recommendations are addressed in Chapters 32 and 33. The following sections outline USPSTF recommendations for individuals with risk factors that warrant modified screening approaches in primary care.

BRCA-Related Cancer

The USPSTF (2019a) has assigned a B recommendation to screening women for *BRCA*-related cancer risk, but only for those with a family history associated with an increased risk for *BRCA* gene mutations. It recommends against routine screening for *BRCA* risk and genetic counseling or testing for individuals without familial risk factors for *BRCA*-related cancer risk (grade D). The USPSTF recommends that those with one or more family members who have been diagnosed with a mutation on the *BRCA1* or *BRCA2* gene be offered a referral for genetic counseling and testing. All individuals with one or more family members who have been diagnosed with breast, ovarian, tubal, or peritoneal cancer should be screened for additional factors that may signal an increased risk for *BRCA* mutation. This screening can be done by primary healthcare providers using a previously validated family risk assessment tool, such as the Manchester Scoring System, the Referral Screening Tool (**Table 9-5**), the Ontario Family History Assessment tool, or the 7-Question Family History Screen (FHS-7) (**Table 9-6**). Each of these tools is designed to identify individuals who are at increased risk for *BRCA* mutations and who would therefore benefit from a referral for genetic counseling and, if indicated after counseling, genetic testing. Although it is appropriate for primary care providers to screen patients for *BRCA*-related cancer risk, those with a positive screen for increased *BRCA* mutation risk should be referred to a qualified healthcare provider for genetic counseling, additional screening, and, for some patients, testing for *BRCA* mutations (USPSTF, 2019a). Clinicians should remain aware of each patient's insurance coverage with an understanding that not all patients have health insurance and not all health insurance covers genetic counseling. Genetic counseling options and other resources are listed in Table 9-8 at the end of this chapter. Updates are currently in progress for BRCA-Related Cancers; readers should be advised the USPSTF recommendations may change. See Chapter 28 for a more in-depth discussion of gynecologic cancers.

TABLE 9-5 Referral Screening Tool

History of Breast or Ovarian Cancer in the Family? If Yes, Complete Checklist

Risk Factor	Breast Cancer at Age ≤ 50 Years	Ovarian Cancer at Any Age
Yourself		
Mother		
Sister		
Daughter		
Mother's side		
Grandmother		
Aunt		
Father's side		
Grandmother		
Aunt		
≥ 2 cases of breast cancer after age 50 years on same side of family		
Male breast cancer at any age in any relative		
Jewish ancestry		

Reproduced from U.S. Preventive Services Task Force. (2019a). *Final recommendation statement: BRCA-related cancer: Risk assessment, genetic counseling, and genetic testing.* https://www.uspreventiveservicestaskforce.org/uspstf/recommendation/brca-related-cancer-risk-assessment-genetic-counseling-and-genetic-testing#tab3

Referral if two or more checks in table.

Hepatitis B

The USPSTF (2020b) recommends screening all adolescents and adults at increased infection risk for hepatitis B virus (HBV) infection (grade B). Screening all pregnant people at the first prenatal visit receives an A recommendation (USPSTF, 2019b). Persons at increased risk for infection include those born in a country with high HBV prevalence rates, persons with parents from countries with high HBV prevalence rates who were not

TABLE 9-6 7-Question Family History Screen

No.	Questions
1	Did any of your first-degree relatives have breast or ovarian cancer?
2	Did any of your relatives have bilateral breast cancer?
3	Did any man in your family have breast cancer?
4	Did any woman in your family have breast and ovarian cancer?
5	Did any woman in your family have breast cancer before age 50 years?
6	Do you have two or more relatives with breast and/or ovarian cancer?
7	Do you have two or more relatives with breast and/or bowel cancer?

Reproduced from U.S. Preventive Services Task Force. (2019a). *Final recommendation statement: BRCA-related cancer: Risk assessment, genetic counseling, and genetic testing.* https://www.uspreventiveservicestaskforce.org/uspstf/recommendation/brca-related-cancer-risk-assessment-genetic-counseling-and-genetic-testing#tab5

One positive response initiates referral.

vaccinated as infants, and those who have never received HBV vaccine. Screening should also be considered for persons who are HIV positive, have household contacts or sexual partners of persons infected with HBV, have needle-sharing contacts, men who have sex with men, and those who use intravenous drugs. The CDC also recommends screening all adults age 18 or older at least once, persons with current or past hepatitis C virus infection, persons with sexually transmitted infections (STIs), and a history of STIs, or multiple sex partners. Persons incarcerated or formerly incarcerated in a jail, prison, or other detention setting; persons with a history of sexually transmitted infections or multiple sex partners; persons with elevated ALT or AST levels of unknown origin; those who are immunosuppressed and undergoing dialysis; and persons with a history of hepatitis C virus infection (CDC, 2023). The recommended screening test is the hepatitis B surface antigen (HBsAg), with confirmation of initially reactive tests. There was insufficient evidence to determine appropriate screening intervals for nonpregnant patients at continued risk for infection. Decisions regarding repeat testing should be made based on clinical judgment (USPSTF, 2020b).

Latent Tuberculosis

The USPSTF (2023c) recommends screening all individuals at increased risk for infection for latent tuberculosis (grade B). Populations with risk factors for latent tuberculosis infection include individuals who are former residents of countries with high prevalence rates and persons who live in, or have ever lived in, high-risk settings, such as homeless shelters, long-term care facilities, and correctional facilities. Prevalence patterns vary across the nation and globally; information about high-prevalence communities and facilities can be found at state or local health departments and the website of the World Health Organization. Individuals who are immunosuppressed or who have silicosis are also at greater risk for latent tuberculosis infection, though it is likely that regular screening is part of the ongoing care for these patients. Similarly, individuals who are in contact with persons who have tuberculosis, such as healthcare workers and personnel at correctional facilities, are at increased risk for latent tuberculosis infection, and it is likely that these persons are regularly screened as a matter of employment (USPSTF, 2023c). Clinicians may be called upon to conduct regular screening for any of these individuals. There are currently two screening tests available in the United States. The tuberculin skin test requires intradermal placement of purified protein derivative and a return to the clinic for interpretation of the patient's response 48 to 72 hours following placement. Interferon-gamma release assays require the collection of a venous blood sample that can be processed in a laboratory within 8 to 30 hours (USPSTF, 2023c). The optimal screening interval is unknown and should be determined based on individual risk factors (USPSTF, 2023c).

Lung Cancer

The USPSTF (2021d) recommends lung cancer screening for adults aged 50 to 80 years with a 20-pack-year (the equivalent of one pack per day for 20 years, or two packs per day for 10 years) smoking history who have either quit smoking within the past 15 years or who currently smoke (grade B). The recommended approach is yearly screening with low-dose computed tomography (CT). Screening should be discontinued 15 years after smoking cessation or with the development of a health problem that substantially limits life expectancy or the ability or willingness to have curative lung surgery (USPSTF, 2021d). Information regarding strategies to assist patients with smoking cessation can be found in Chapter 6.

Syphilis

The USPSTF (2022c) has assigned an A recommendation to screening all persons at increased risk and all pregnant people for syphilis infection. Those at increased risk for infection include those living with HIV, young adults, and those with a history of sex work, incarceration, or military service. In addition to individual risk factors, local prevalence rates for syphilis vary across the country. Clinicians should be aware of prevalence rates of infection in the communities where they practice (USPSTF, 2022c). Recommended screening tests include the Venereal Disease Research Laboratory (VDRL) and rapid plasmin reagin (RPR) test, followed by confirmation with treponemal antibody detection tests (FTA-ABS or TPPA). An alternative testing algorithm called the reverse sequence algorithm uses an automated treponemal test for the initial screening, followed by a nontreponemal test for reactive samples. Optimal screening intervals are not well established, though there is evidence that in persons living with HIV, screening every 3 months detects more syphilis infection than yearly screening (USPSTF, 2022c). Readers are advised that at the time of this writing, the USPSTF recommendation for syphilis infection screening in pregnant persons was under review and is likely to change.

Prediabetes and Type 2 Diabetes

It is estimated that more than 1 in 3 (97.6 million) U.S. adults have prediabetes, and 80% of them are unaware that they have this disease (CDC, 2024d). Prediabetes is a serious metabolic disorder that increases the risk for development of type 2 diabetes, heart disease, and stroke. When it is identified early, lifestyle changes can prevent or delay the progression from prediabetes to type 2 diabetes (CDC, 2024d). The USPSTF (2021e) assigns a B recommendation to screening all adults between the ages of 35 and 70 years who are overweight or obese (BMI greater than 25) for abnormal blood glucose as one component of a cardiovascular risk assessment; earlier screening may be considered for adults with additional risk factors for type 2 diabetes. It also recommends that all patients with abnormal blood glucose levels be offered or referred for effective preventive interventions (USPSTF, 2021e). Screening tests for prediabetes and type 2 diabetes include fasting plasma glucose, 2-hour post-load glucose tolerance test, and hemoglobin A1C. Normal and diagnostic thresholds for each of these are displayed in **Table 9-7**. The optimal screening interval is unclear, although the strongest evidence suggests that rescreening adults with normal blood glucose levels every 3 years is a reasonable approach (USPSTF, 2021e).

TABLE 9-7 Test Values for Normal Glucose Metabolism, IFG or OGTT, and Type 2 Diabetes

Test	Normal	Prediabetes	Type 2 Diabetes
Hemoglobin A1c level, %	< 5.7	5.7–6.4	≥ 6.5
Fasting plasma glucose level			
mmol/L	< 5.6	5.6–6.9	≥ 7.0
mg/dL		100–125	≥ 126
OGTT results (after 2 hours)			
mmol/L	7.8	7.77–11.04	≥ 11.1
mg/dL		140–199	≥ 200

Reproduced from U.S. Preventive Services Task Force. (2021c). *Final recommendation statement: Prediabetes and type 2 diabetes: Screening.* https://www.uspreventiveservicestaskforce.org/uspstf/recommendation/screening-for-prediabetes-and-type-2-diabetes. Abbreviations: OGTT, oral glucose tolerance test.

Abbreviations: OGTT, oral glucose tolerance test.

All positive test results should be confirmed with repeat testing.

TABLE 9-8 Resources for Clinicians

Resource	Description	Website
Guidelines for the Primary and Gender-Affirming Care of Transgender and Gender Nonbinary People	An excellent resource for clinicians providing care to transgender and nonbinary patients	https://transcare.ucsf.edu/guidelines
National Human Genome Research Institute	Provides links to online counseling support and advocacy groups and other resources for genetic counseling	https://www.genome.gov/For-Health-Professionals/Provider-Genomics-Education-Resources-advocacy-groups-online
National Institute on Alcohol Abuse and Alcoholism	Includes counseling interventions and validated tools used to screen for alcohol use disorder	https://www.niaaa.nih.gov/
U.S. Preventive Services Task Force (USPSTF)	A leading authority on health promotion and disease prevention	https://www.uspreventiveservicestaskforce.org/uspstf
USPSTF ePSS: Electronic Preventive Service Selector	App available for download to electronic devices; includes updated recommendations of the USPSTF	https://www.uspreventiveservicestaskforce.org/apps/
USPSTF published recommendations	Published recommendations of the USPSTF	https://www.uspreventiveservicestaskforce.org/uspstf/topic_search_results?topic_status=P

ADDITIONAL OBSERVATIONS

Changes in health policy, particularly changes in the laws that govern the insurance industry and reimbursement for various healthcare services, are likely to take place in the months and years ahead. Since the 2010 passage of the ACA, several attempts have been made to repeal the entire Act or portions of it, including provisions aimed at improving access to preventive health services. It is incumbent upon clinicians to remain cognizant of policy changes that influence the reimbursement of health services and to recognize that one component of patient advocacy is advocating for health policies that improve access to affordable health care.

The screening recommendations discussed in this chapter are intended for healthy, asymptomatic individuals unless otherwise specified. Healthcare providers are advised to remain alert for signs and symptoms or changes in health history that suggest the need for testing beyond the recommended screening described here. As noted earlier, the gynecologic history and physical examination provide excellent opportunities to gather important screening information about the patient. Answers to a few direct questions and close attention during the physical examination can give the clinician important information and should always be part of a routine patient encounter.

References

American Academy of Family Physicians. (n.d.). *Clinical preventive services recommendations. Cervical cancer.* https://www.aafp.org/family-physician/patient-care/clinical-recommendations/all-clinical-recommendations/cervical-cancer.html

American Academy of Family Physicians. (n.d.). *Colorectal cancer screening, Adults.* https://www.aafp.org/family-physician/patient-care/clinical-recommendations/all-clinical-recommendations/colorectal-cancer-adults.html.

American Cancer Society. (n.d.). *Can ovarian cancer be found early?* American Cancer Society. https://www.cancer.org/cancer/types/ovarian-cancer/detection-diagnosis-staging/detection.html

American Cancer Society. (2023). *American Cancer Society recommendations for the early detection of breast cancer.* https://www.cancer.org/cancer/types/breast-cancer/screening-tests-and-early-detection/american-cancer-society-recommendations-for-the-early-detection-of-breast-cancer.html

American Cancer Society. (2024). *American Cancer Society guidelines for the prevention and early detection of cervical cancer.* https://www.cancer.org/cancer/types/cervical-cancer/detection-diagnosis-staging/cervical-cancer-screening-guidelines.html

American College of Obstetricians and Gynecologists. (2017). *Breast cancer risk assessment and screening in average-risk women.* https://www.acog.org/clinical/clinical-guidance/practice-bulletin/articles/2017/07/breast-cancer-risk-assessment-and-screening-in-average-risk-women

American College of Obstetricians and Gynecologists. (2021). *Updated cervical cancer screening guidelines.* https://www.acog.org/clinical/clinical-guidance/practice-advisory/articles/2021/04/updated-cervical-cancer-screening-guidelines

American College of Obstetricians and Gynecologists. (2012/2022). *Intimate partner violence.* https://www.acog.org/clinical/clinical-guidance/committee-opinion/articles/2012/02/intimate-partner-violence

American College of Obstetricians and Gynecologists. (2017). *The role of the obstetrician–gynecologist in the early detection of epithelial ovarian cancer in women at average risk.* Retrieved October 27, 2024 from https://www.acog.org/clinical/clinical-guidance/committee-opinion/articles/2017/09/the-role-of-the-obstetriciangynecologist-in-the-early-detection-of-epithelial-ovarian-cancer-in-women-at-average-risk

Centers for Disease Control and Prevention. (2019). *Recommended adult immunization schedule for ages 19 years or older—United States, 2019.* https://www.cdc.gov/vaccines/schedules/downloads/adult/adult-combined-schedule.pdf

Centers for Disease Control and Prevention. (2023). *Screening and testing for hepatitis B virus infection: CDC recommendations.* https://www.cdc.gov/mmwr/volumes/72/rr/rr7201a1.htm?s_cid=rr7201a1_w

Centers for Disease Control and Prevention. (2024a). *About preventing intimate partner violence.* https://www.cdc.gov/intimate-partner-violence/about/index.html#:~:text=IPV%20is%20common.&text=Over%2061%20million%20women%20and,intimate%20partner%20in%20their%20lifetime.

Centers for Disease Control and Prevention. (2024b). *Current cigarette smoking among adults in the United States.* https://www.cdc.gov/tobacco/php/data-statistics/adult-data-cigarettes/index.html

Centers for Disease Control and Prevention. (2024c). National diabetes statistics report. https://www.cdc.gov/diabetes/php/data-research/index.html

Centers for Disease Control and Prevention. (2024d). *Prediabetes—Your chance to prevent type 2 diabetes.* https://www.cdc.gov/diabetes/prevention-type-2/prediabetes-prevent-type-2.html#cdc_generic_section_1-what-is-prediabetes

Centers for Disease Control and Prevention. (2024e). *Testing for cholesterol.* https://www.cdc.gov/cholesterol/testing/

Health Resources & Services Administration. (2019). *Women's preventive services guidelines.* U.S. Department of Health and Human Services. https://www.hrsa.gov/womens-guidelines-2016/index.html

Kaiser Family Foundation. (2018). *Understanding short-term limited duration health insurance.* https://www.kff.org/affordable-care-act/issue-brief/understanding-short-term-limited-duration-health-insurance/

Kaiser Family Foundation. (2019). *Coverage of breast cancer screening and prevention services.* https://www.kff.org/womens-health-policy/fact-sheet/coverage-of-breast-cancer-screening-and-prevention-services/

Kaiser Family Foundation (2024a). *How many uninsured are in the coverage gap and how many could be eligible if all states adopted the Medicaid expansion?* https://www.kff.org/medicaid/issue-brief/how-many-uninsured-are-in-the-coverage-gap-and-how-many-could-be-eligible-if-all-states-adopted-the-medicaid-expansion/

Kaiser Family Foundation (2024b). *Preventive services covered by private health plans under the Affordable Care Act.* https://www.kff.org/womens-health-policy/fact-sheet/preventive-services-covered-by-private-health-plans/

National Institute on Alcohol Abuse and Alcoholism. (2024a). *Alcohol use disorder (AUD) in the United States: Age groups and demographic characteristics.* https://www.niaaa.nih.gov/alcohols-effects-health/alcohol-topics/alcohol-facts-and-statistics/alcohol-use-disorder-aud-united-states-age-groups-and-demographic-characteristics#:~:text=According%20to%20the%202023%20NSDUH%2C%2028.1%20million%20adults%20ages%2018,AUD%20in%20the%20past%20year.&text=1%2C2-,This%20includes%3A,13.2%25%20in%20this%20age%20group)

National Institute on Alcohol Abuse and Alcoholism. (2024b). *Understanding alcohol use disorder.* https://www.niaaa.nih.gov/publications/brochures-and-fact-sheets/understanding-alcohol-use-disorder

National Institute on Alcohol Abuse and Alcoholism. (2024c). *Women and alcohol.* https://www.niaaa.nih.gov/publications/brochures-and-fact-sheets/women-and-alcohol

National Institute of Mental Health. (n.d.). *Women and mental health.* https://www.nimh.nih.gov/health/topics/women-and-mental-health/index.shtml

National Osteoporosis Foundation. (n.d.). *Bone density exam/testing.* https://www.nof.org/patients/diagnosis-information/bone-density-exam testing/

Ray, J., & LaBundy, J. (2022). *Lower gastrointestinal tract disorders.* ACOG. https://www.acog.org/clinical/journals-and-publications/clinical-updates/2022/06/lower-gastrointestinal-tract-disorders

U.S. Preventive Services Task Force. (n.d.). *About the USPSTF.* Retrieved October 27, 2024 from https://www.uspreventiveservicestaskforce.org/uspstf/about-uspstf

U.S. Preventive Services Task Force. (1996). *Guide to clinical preventive services* (2nd ed.). Williams & Wilkins.

U.S. Preventive Services Task Force. (2018a). *Final recommendation statement: Intimate partner violence, elder abuse, and abuse of vulnerable adults: Screening.* https://www.uspreventiveservicestaskforce.org/uspstf/recommendation/intimate-partner-violence-and-abuse-of-elderly-and-vulnerable-adults-screening

U.S. Preventive Services Task Force. (2018b). *Final recommendation statement: Unhealthy alcohol use in adolescents and adults: Screening and behavioral counseling interventions.* https://www.uspreventiveservicestaskforce.org/uspstf/recommendation/unhealthy-alcohol-use-in-adolescents-and-adults-screening-and-behavioral-counseling-interventions

U.S. Preventive Services Task Force. (2018c). *Final recommendation statement: Weight loss to prevent obesity-related morbidity and mortality in adults: Behavioral interventions.* https://www.uspreventiveservicestaskforce.org/uspstf/recommendation/obesity-in-adults-interventions

U.S. Preventive Services Task Force. (2018d). *Osteoporosis to prevent fractures: Screening.* https://www.uspreventiveservicestaskforce.org/uspstf/recommendation/osteoporosis-screening

U.S. Preventive Services Task Force. (2019a). *Final recommendation statement: BRCA-related cancer: Risk assessment, genetic counseling, and genetic testing.* https://www.uspreventiveservicestaskforce.org/uspstf/recommendation/brca-related-cancer-risk-assessment-genetic-counseling-and-genetic-testing

U.S. Preventive Services Task Force. (2019b). *Final recommendation statement: Hepatitis B virus infection in pregnant women: Screening.* https://www.uspreventiveservicestaskforce.org/uspstf/recommendation/hepatitis-b-virus-infection-in-pregnant-women-screening#fullrecommendationstart

U.S. Preventive Services Task Force. (2019c). *Final recommendation statement: Human immunodeficiency virus (HIV) infection: Screening.* https://www.uspreventiveservicestaskforce.org/uspstf/recommendation/human-immunodeficiency-virus-hiv-infection-screening

US Preventive Services Task Force. (2020a). *Healthy diet and physical activity for cardiovascular disease prevention in adults with cardiovascular risk factors: Behavioral counseling interventions.* https://www.uspreventiveservicestaskforce.org/uspstf/recommendation/healthy-diet-and-physical-activity-counseling-adults-with-high-risk-of-cvd

U.S. Preventive Services Task Force. (2020b). *Hepatitis B virus infection in adolescents and adults: Screening.* https://www.uspreventiveservicestaskforce.org/uspstf/recommendation/hepatitis-b-virus-infection-screening#fullrecommendationstart

U.S. Preventive Services Task Force. (2020c). *Hepatitis C: Screening.* https://www.uspreventiveservicestaskforce.org/uspstf/recommendation/hepatitis-c-screening.

U.S. Preventive Services Task Force. (2021a). *Chlamydia and gonorrhea: Screening.* https://www.uspreventiveservicestaskforce.org/uspstf/recommendation/chlamydia-and-gonorrhea-screening

U.S. Preventive Services Task Force. (2021b). *Colorectal cancer: Screening.* https://www.uspreventiveservicestaskforce.org/uspstf/recommendation/colorectal-cancer-screening#tab1

U.S. Preventive Services Task Force. (2021c). *Final recommendation statement: Hypertension in adults: Screening.* https://www.uspreventiveservicestaskforce.org/uspstf/recommendation/hypertension-in-adults-screening

U.S. Preventive Services Task Force. (2021d). *Final recommendation statement: Lung cancer: Screening.* https://www.uspreventiveservicestaskforce.org/uspstf/recommendation/lung-cancer-screening

U.S. Preventive Services Task Force. (2021e). *Final recommendation statement: Prediabetes and type 2 diabetes: Screening.* https://www.uspreventiveservicestaskforce.org/uspstf/recommendation/screening-for-prediabetes-and-type-2-diabetes

U.S. Preventive Services Task Force. (2021f). *Tobacco smoking cessation in adults, including pregnant women: Interventions.* https://www.uspreventiveservicestaskforce.org/uspstf/recommendation/tobacco-use-in-adults-and-pregnant-women-counseling-and-intervention

U.S. Preventive Services Task Force. (2022a). *Final recommendation statement: Depression and suicide risk in children and adolescents: Screening.* https://www.uspreventiveservicestaskforce.org/uspstf/index.php/recommendation/screening-depression-suicide-risk-children-adolescents

U.S. Preventive Services Task Force. (2022b). *Final recommendation statement: Statin use for the primary prevention of cardiovascular disease in adults: Preventive medication.* https://www.uspreventiveservicestaskforce.org/uspstf/recommendation/statin-use-in-adults-preventive-medication

U.S. Preventive Services Task Force. (2022c). *Final recommendation statement: Syphilis infection in nonpregnant adults and adolescents: Screening.* https://www.uspreventiveservicestaskforce.org/uspstf/recommendation/syphilis-infection-nonpregnant-adults-adolescents-screenin

U.S. Preventive Services Task Force. (2023a). *Depression and suicide risk in adults: Screening.* https://www.uspreventiveservicestaskforce.org/uspstf/index.php/recommendation/screening-depression-suicide-risk-adults

U.S. Preventive Services Task Force. (2023b). *Final recommendation statement: Hypertensive disorders of pregnancy: Screening.* https://www.uspreventiveservicestaskforce.org/uspstf/recommendation/hypertensive-disorders-pregnancy-screening

U.S. Preventive Services Task Force. (2023c). *Final recommendation statement: Latent tuberculosis infection in adults: Screening.* https://www.uspreventiveservicestaskforce.org/uspstf/recommendation/latent-tuberculosis-infection-screening

U.S. Preventive Services Task Force. (2024a). *Breast cancer: Screening.* https://www.uspreventiveservicestaskforce.org/uspstf/recommendation/breast-cancer-screening#bcei-recommendation-title-area.

U.S. Preventive Services Task Force. (2024b). *Final recommendation statement: Cervical cancer: Screening.* https://www.uspreventiveservicestaskforce.org/uspstf/recommendation/cervical-cancer-screening

U.S. Preventive Services Task Force. (2024c). *Grade definitions.* https://www.uspreventiveservicestaskforce.org/uspstf/about-uspstf/methods-and-processes/grade-definitions

U.S. Preventive Services Task Force. (2024d). *Published recommendations.* Retrieved October 26, 2024 from https://www.uspreventiveservicestaskforce.org/uspstf/topic_search_results?topic_status=P

CHAPTER 10

Male Sexual and Reproductive Health

Hanne S. Harbison

INTRODUCTION

Clinicians who provide gynecological health care have the opportunity to provide direct and indirect sexual and reproductive health (SRH) care for individuals assigned male at birth (AMAB) and/or who identify as male (Nurse Practitioners in Women's Health [NPWH], 2020). Indirect care includes providing partners with information on male SRH that they later share. Clinicians who practice in settings that care for male patients—for example, primary care practices, family planning clinics, sexually transmitted infection (STI) clinics, and infertility practices—may also provide direct male SRH care (NPWH, 2020).

This care is within the scope of clinicians who specialize primarily in gynecological health care. The *Women's Health Nurse Practitioner: Guidelines for Practice and Education* (NPWH, 2020) includes male SRH anatomy and physiology as well as the evaluation and management of common male SRH conditions, including contraception, infertility, STIs, and sexual dysfunction. The *Core Competencies for Basic Midwifery Practice* for STIs includes information on male partner evaluation, treatment, and referral (American College of Nurse-Midwives [ACNM], 2020). While the specific services offered may vary, all providers can positively affect male SRH. Caring for transgender and nonbinary individuals is also within the scope of midwifery practice (ACNM, 2021), and it is important to note that not all people AMAB identify as male or men, and not all people assigned female at birth (AFAB) identify as female or women. The terms *male*, *female*, *men* and *women* used in this chapter are reflective of the guidelines and research available and are not meant to exclude transgender and nonbinary people.

Clinicians must be familiar with colleagues in their community who provide male SRH care, such as urology specialists, so they have resources to contact for consultation, collaboration, and referral. This chapter provides a brief overview of essential content for clinicians who specialize in gynecologic care to provide SRH care for individuals AMAB and/or who identify as male.

REPRODUCTIVE ANATOMY

Male reproductive anatomy is made up of external and internal structures (see **Figure 10-1**). The external genitalia include the scrotum, testes, epididymis, and penis. These external structures produce and facilitate expulsion of sperm. The internal genitalia include the vas deferens, ejaculatory ducts, urethra, prostate, seminal vesicles, and bulbourethral (Cowper's) glands. These internal structures transport sperm from the testes to the urethral meatus.

Scrotum

The scrotum is a fibromuscular sac where the testes are suspended away from the body. The purpose of the scrotum is to maintain a temperature 1–2°C lower than the usual body temperature for normal spermatogenesis.

Testes

The testes have two functions: to produce sperm and to produce testosterone. Prenatally, the testes develop inside the abdomen, and at approximately 28 weeks' gestation they begin descending into the scrotum. At approximately 36 weeks' gestation they enter the inguinal canal. They migrate into the scrotal sac, where they are suspended by ducts, blood and lymph vessels, nerves, and the spermatic cord. After the descent is complete, the abdominal end of the inguinal canals close and disappear. The scrotal end of the canal tissue becomes the tunica vaginalis, which is the outer covering of the testes. If this closure does not occur completely or is weak, it may result in inguinal hernias.

The majority (80 percent) of the testicular volume is made up of seminiferous tubules. These are coiled ducts where sperm are produced. Surrounding the ducts is tissue containing blood and lymph vessels, fibroblast support cells, macrophages, mast cells, and Leydig cells. The Leydig cells comprise 1 to 5 percent of testicular volume and produce testosterone. After sperm are produced in the testes, they move to the epididymis where they mature.

Epididymis

The epididymis is a crescent-moon-shaped structure that rests on the posterior portion of each testicle. Each testicle has an adjacent epididymis. Each epididymis includes a single coiled duct that moves the sperm from the efferent ducts to the vas deferens. During the approximately 12 days of travel time through the epididymal ducts, the sperm receive nutrients and testosterone that allow them to mature. The sperm are then stored in the epididymal tail and vas deferens.

FIGURE 10-1 Midsagittal view of the male reproductive system.

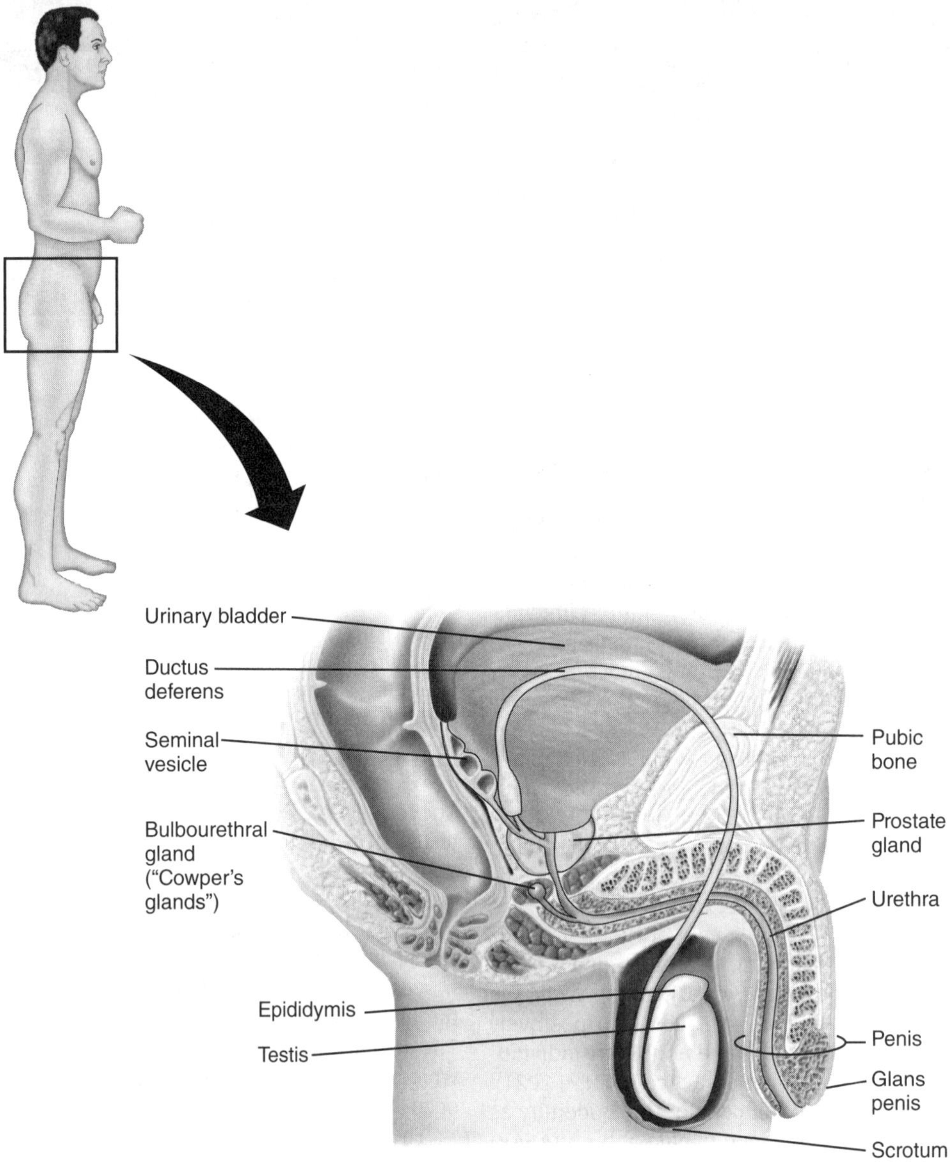

Vas Deferens, Ejaculatory Ducts, and Seminal Vesicles

The vas deferens are tubes that extend from the epididymis in the scrotum through the pelvis to the ejaculatory ducts. The vas deferens store and transport sperm into the urethra. The two seminal vesicles are composed of single coiled tubes, and they secrete the majority of seminal fluid. The seminal fluid has a role in coagulating semen, making it alkaline, and may potentiate capacitation of the sperm in the female reproductive tract.

Penis

The penis consists of the shaft and the glans. At birth, the glans is covered by the foreskin. If circumcision is performed, the foreskin is surgically removed. If the foreskin is left in place, the adhesions that connect it to the glans are gradually broken by erections in the first 3 years of life.

Penile tissue is made of three spongy cylinders: two paired corpus cavernosa and the corpus spongiosum. The corpus cavernosum are surrounded by the tunica albuginea, which provides protection and rigidity to erectile tissues. The urethra is surrounded by the corpus spongiosum. If it is not surrounded completely, the urethra may open on the ventral surface of the shaft (hypospadias) or on the dorsal surface (epispadias). Many infants who are born with hypospadias or epispadias will have these malformations surgically corrected.

The functions of the penis are to expel sperm and eliminate urine. The penis must be erect for sperm to be expelled. Erection is a complex process that will be briefly summarized here.

Stimulation of the penis triggers the release of neurotransmitters, which cause: (1) relaxation of the smooth muscles; (2) increased arterial dilation and blood flow; (3) trapping of blood in the corpus cavernosa; (4) compression of penile veins, which reduces blood outflow; (5) stretching of the tunica albuginea, which also compresses veins and decreases outflow; and (6) an increase in partial pressure of oxygen (PO_2) and intracavernous pressure, which lifts the penis to an erect state. The neurotransmitter primarily responsible for erection is nitric oxide. It leads to erection by increasing the production of cyclic guanosine monophosphate (cGMP), which relaxes the smooth muscles of the penis. The smooth muscles of the penis are contracted in a flaccid state and relaxed in an erect state.

Prostate

The prostate is a walnut-sized gland that weighs 20–30 grams in a young adult and is located between the bladder and the penis. Its primary function is to secrete fluid during ejaculation. The fluid has an alkaline pH that protects the sperm in a normally acidic pH of the vagina. The fluid also contains clotting enzymes and fibrinolysin that assist with sperm mobilization. The growth and functioning of the prostate are primarily controlled by testosterone. Within the prostate, testosterone is converted into its more active form, dihydrotestosterone (DHT).

REPRODUCTIVE PHYSIOLOGY

Hypothalamic–Pituitary–Gonadal Axis

The hypothalamic–pituitary–gonadal (HPG) axis regulates reproductive development and functioning in all people. In AMAB individuals, the HPG axis is responsible for testosterone and sperm production, phenotypic development during embryogenesis, and pubertal maturation (see **Figure 10-2**). The relevant hormone secreted by the hypothalamus is gonadotropin-releasing hormone (GnRH). Secretion is controlled by a pulse generator in the hypothalamus that releases GnRH approximately every 2 hours. GnRH is then transported directly to the anterior pituitary through the portal vascular system and neuronal pathways, rather than through systemic circulation.

From inside the anterior pituitary, GnRH stimulates the production and release of follicle-stimulating hormone (FSH) and luteinizing hormone (LH), which are both peptide hormones that attach to surface receptors on target cells. The target cells of LH in males are the Leydig cells in the testes. After it is attached to the Leydig cells, LH stimulates the conversion of cholesterol into testosterone and pregnenolone. The target cells of FSH in males are the Sertoli cells. FSH binds to the Sertoli cells and membranes within the testes, stimulating the growth of the seminiferous tubules. FSH is also responsible for initiating spermatogenesis during puberty and for maintaining spermatogenesis in adulthood.

The anterior pituitary also produces prolactin. It is hypothesized that prolactin plays several roles in AMAB individuals. It may increase LH receptors on Leydig cells, thus maintaining high levels of testosterone in the testes. Prolactin may affect libido and potentiate androgen effects on the accessory glands (seminal vesicles, prostate, and bulbourethral glands). An abnormally elevated prolactin level may suppress biosynthesis of testosterone.

Within the testes, the Leydig cells produce approximately 5 mg of testosterone per day. Testosterone is then metabolized into two compounds in the target tissues. The first is DHT via 5α-reductase. The second is estradiol through the action of aromatase. Testosterone and estradiol are both steroid hormones that are synthesized from cholesterol and are not stored, thus their levels are reflective of production rates. Testosterone is the primary hormone involved in the regulation of LH secretion. Testosterone also controls spermatogenesis and sexual differentiation in utero. DHT is primarily responsible for external development and sexual maturation during puberty. DHT acts on skeletal muscle tissue (increasing growth rate), bone marrow (increasing hemoglobin and hematocrit), skin (increasing and thickening sebaceous gland secretions), hair (making it coarse and thick and changing the distribution), and the musculature and cartilage of the larynx (resulting in voice changes). Estradiol is primarily responsible for regulating FSH secretion. Both testosterone and estradiol work through negative feedback to suppress GnRH secretion. Testosterone does this by binding to androgen receptors in the hypothalamus, while estradiol acts on the pituitary. The testes also produce the hormones inhibin and activin. Inhibin production is stimulated by FSH in the Sertoli cells, and it then inhibits FSH release from the pituitary through negative feedback. Activin stimulates FSH secretion.

With age there is a slow, progressive decline in testosterone and therefore sperm production. This decline starts at age 40 and continues at about 1% per year until death. The lower levels of testosterone lead to decreased responsiveness of the HPG axis. GnRH secretion is also decreased, and the pulses become less regular, leading to less effective stimulation of LH and FSH.

Spermatogenesis

The formation of sperm, called spermatogenesis, begins at puberty and continues throughout adult life. The process takes approximately 64 days and is controlled by intratesticular testosterone. The normal rate of sperm production is 1,200 sperm per second. Sperm production occurs within the seminiferous tubules, which are filled with Sertoli cells. The lumen between the Sertoli cells are lined with diploid male germ cells, called spermatogonia, that contain 46 chromosomes (23 pairs). The spermatogonia undergo mitotic division and produce two identical spermatogonium, each with 46 chromosomes. One of the spermatogonium remains a germ cell that is ready to divide again, while the other spermatogonium differentiates into a primary spermatocyte. The primary spermatocyte then divides via meiosis I and produces two daughter cells with 23 chromosomes called secondary spermatocytes. The two secondary spermatocytes undergo meiosis II and form four spermatids. The spermatids contain single copies of the 23 chromosomes, and they then differentiate into spermatozoa. The spermatozoa move via peristalsis of the seminiferous tubules into the rete testis, an area at the top of the testicle, and then into the epididymis where they complete maturation into sperm.

Sperm are made of three distinct sections: head, neck, and tail. The head contains DNA along with the acrosome, which is an organelle containing enzymes that can penetrate the outer layer of an egg during fertilization. The plasma membrane that covers the head also contains proteins that bind with the proteins in the zona pellucida of the egg. The axoneme complex in the proximal end of the tail is responsible for the sperm's motility.

FIGURE 10-2 **Hypothalamic–pituitary–gonadal axis.**

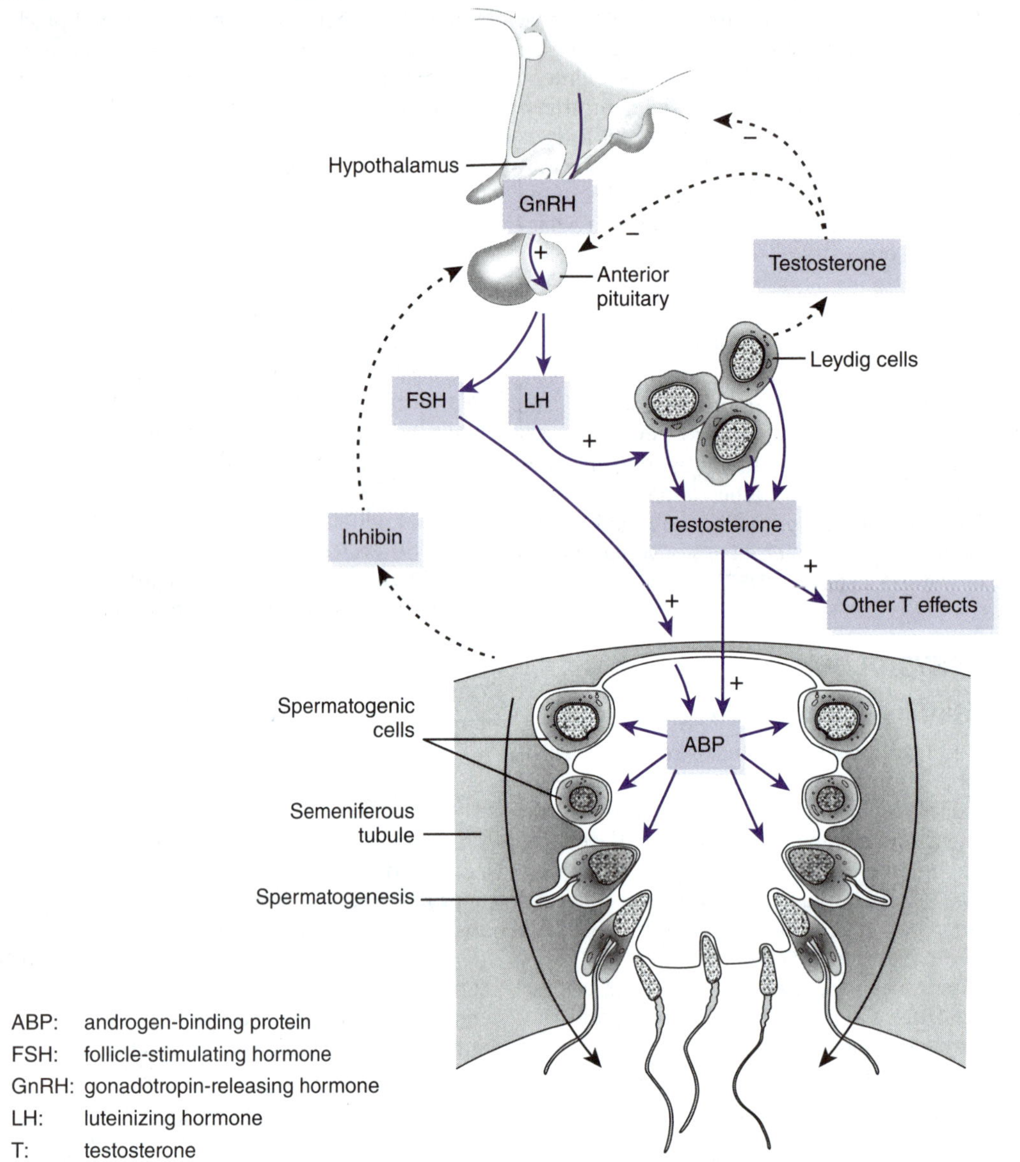

SEXUAL AND REPRODUCTIVE HEALTH ASSESSMENT

The U.S. Preconception Health and Healthcare Initiative (PCHHC) formed in 2004 as a public health partnership dedicated to improving preconception health for women. In 2015, the group added men as a focus for interventions (Anakwe et al., 2025; Verbiest et al., 2016). The PCHHC informed the "Providing Quality Family Planning Services: Recommendations of CDC and the U.S. Office of Population Affairs" report which includes recommendations for the services that should be offered to men at a family planning visit (Gavin et al., 2014; Gavin & Pazol, 2016; Gavin et al., 2017). A report by Marcell and the Male Training Center for Family Planning and Reproductive Health (2014), called *Preventive Male Sexual and Reproductive Health Care: Recommendations for Clinical Practice*, provides broader guidance for SRH services beyond the family planning setting. The report outlines the components of history taking, physical examination, laboratory tests, and counseling that should occur based on a comprehensive review of available literature and expert opinion and is an excellent resource for clinicians who provide male SRH care. The report contains detailed guidance and helpful checklists to implement the recommendations (Marcell & Male Training Center for Family Planning and Reproductive Health, 2014).

History

In addition to inquiries about medical and surgical history, medications, allergies, and immunizations—for example, human

TABLE 10-1 Six Ps of Sexual Health

Practices	Types of sex the patient engages in, including oral, vaginal, and/or anal sex
Partners	Number, sex, and concurrency of partners
Pregnancy prevention	What are the plans for contraception, if indicated
Protection from STIs	Condom use, including frequency of use and barriers to use
Past history of STIs	Personal and partner history of STI testing, diagnosis, and treatment
Pleasure/Problems/ Pride	Sexual satisfaction, functioning, concerns, and support for one's gender identity and sexual orientation

Data from Centers for Disease Control and Prevention. (n.d.). *A guide to taking a sexual history* [Publication No. 99-8445]. https://www.cdc.gov /std/treatment /sexualhistory.pdf

The National Coalition for Sexual Health. (2023). *Sexual health questions to ask all patients.* https://nationalcoalitionforsexualhealth.org/tools/for-healthcare -providers/Final-English-EssentialQuestions-updated-11.22.23.pdf

Abbreviation: STI, sexually transmitted infection.

papillomavirus (HPV) and hepatitis B—several history components specific to men's sexual health are recommended. The first is an assessment using the six Ps of sexual health approach described by the Centers for Disease Control and Prevention (CDC) and the National Coalition for Sexual Health (see **Table 10-1**). These questions provide a segue to the next two assessment areas: reproductive life planning and sexual functioning. Like standard pregnancy history questions for females, providers should ask males if they have ever caused a pregnancy, if they have tried and not been able to conceive with someone, and if they currently have children. Additionally, ask if they would like to have children, or more children, and if so, when. These questions will help guide discussions and/or referrals related to fertility and contraception. It is also essential to inquire about any concerns with sexual functioning. Although patients may be uncomfortable initiating this topic, sexual dysfunction can affect quality of life and may be symptomatic of other health problems, such as cardiovascular disease, depression, and diabetes. Include the following specific questions (Marcell & Male Training Center for Family Planning and Reproductive Health, 2014): Do you have trouble initiating or maintaining an erection? Do you experience premature or delayed ejaculation? Do you have pain with sexual activity? Are you concerned about loss of libido? Have you experienced priapism (erection lasting more than 4 hours)?

In their guidelines for preventive male SRH care, Marcell and the Male Training Center for Family Planning and Reproductive Health (2014) recommend including four additional areas of inquiry in the health history: intimate partner and sexual violence, alcohol and other drug use, tobacco use, and depression. Intimate partner violence can occur in any relationship regardless of the sex, gender, or gender identity of the individuals. In the United States, 33.6 percent of males experience rape, physical violence, or stalking by an intimate partner in their lifetime (Smith et al., 2018). Screening for intimate partner violence is discussed in Chapters 9 and 15. Alcohol use, tobacco use, and depression can affect SRH. Use of alcohol and other drugs can increase the probability that individuals engage in high-risk behaviors, including high-risk sexual behaviors that can lead to STI transmission and unintended pregnancy. Nicotine can impair reproductive function. Depression and some antidepressant medications can affect sexual function. Screening for alcohol use, tobacco use, and depression is addressed in Chapter 9.

Physical Examination

The physical examination will be directed, in part, by the reason for the patient's visit and any symptoms the patient reports during the history. Height, weight, body mass index, and blood pressure should be evaluated (Marcell & Male Training Center for Family Planning and Reproductive Health, 2014).

Although a genital examination is customarily performed during a male SRH visit, it is not required. Clinicians must consider whether a genital examination is warranted based on the reason for the visit and the patient's history; use a shared decision-making approach to make this determination. If a genital examination is performed, be attentive to the principles of trauma-informed care and the need for informed consent for the entire physical examination. Both are discussed in Chapters 5 and 8. Clinicians should also consider the potential need for a chaperone during male genital examinations. Any patient or provider who requests a chaperone should be accommodated, as noted in Chapter 8.

Oral Examination

It is important to examine the mouth because infections such as syphilis, HPV, herpes, and candidiasis can have oral manifestations. Inspect the lips, gums, tongue, and pharynx.

Genital Examination

The genital examination can be done with considerations for trauma-informed care for all individuals (see Chapter 7 for more information). The patient can be standing or supine on the examination table. The only examination components that should not be done supine are checking for hernias and varicocele. Examination of the genitalia begins with visual inspection. The provider should note the patient's development according to Tanner stages, assessing pubic hair distribution, scrotal skin, and the size of the testicles and penis. Next, palpate the groin bilaterally, checking for enlarged lymph nodes. While the patient is standing, have them cough or bear down and watch for any bulging, which can be evidence of a hernia.

The examination of the penis begins with inspection of the skin of the shaft, the prepuce (foreskin), and the glans. Note any rashes, lesions, ulcerations, erythema, or edema. The prepuce can be tight such that it cannot be retracted easily, which is referred to as phimosis. If the prepuce is retracted but cannot be returned to its original position due to edema, the patient may have paraphimosis, which is an emergent condition that requires prompt treatment. It is important to retract the prepuce on anyone that is not circumcised to examine the glans for condyloma, ulcers, discharge, and balanitis. Note the location of the urethral meatus, which should be at the tip of the penis. If the urethral meatus is not visible at the tip of the penis, check along the midline of the shaft for epispadias (urethral meatus located on the dorsal side of the penis) or hypospadias (urethral meatus located on the ventral side of the penis). If the provider has difficulty locating the meatus, it is helpful to ask the patient where their urine comes out. The examiner should next gently compress the meatus between the index finger and thumb and check for urethral discharge and erythema, as well as condyloma and ulcers that can occur inside the distal urethra. Although urethral discharge can be profuse, it may only be noted as a crust around the meatus or on the patient's underwear.

To examine the scrotum and testicles, start with inspecting the skin of the scrotal sac then lift the scrotum to examine the posterior surface. Next, palpate the scrotal contents, noting any swelling, tenderness, or masses. The testicles should be smooth, firm, mobile, and of equal size. Any painless nodule in the testicles is concerning for testicular cancer, and the patient should be referred for further evaluation. To palpate the epididymis, place the first two fingers on the posterior aspect of the scrotal sac and the thumb on the anterior aspect. Starting at the proximal end of the sac, the examiner moves their hands distally, applying gentle pressure to the vas deferens, then the epididymis, assessing for tenderness or masses.

Anal and Rectal Examination

The provider should perform a visual inspection of the anal area for any males that report rectal symptoms such as itching, lesions, and/or discharge. If the provider needs to examine the prostate, the patient can either be standing and leaning over the examination table or side-lying on the table. Inspect the anal area, looking for hemorrhoids, condyloma, and ulcerations. Next, using sufficient lubricant, insert a gloved index finger into the rectum as far as possible. Rotate the finger to the left, then the right, feeling for any masses. Then rotate the finger 180° to palpate the posterior prostate gland. Normally it should be smooth, nontender, and about the size of a walnut.

Additional Examinations to Consider

Depending on the patient's history, other body systems may be included in the physical examination. For example, the provider may need to conduct a neurological examination for a patient who reports erectile dysfunction, or a skin assessment for suspected syphilis or other skin condition. If a bladder or kidney infection is suspected, check for costovertebral angle tenderness. The genitourinary component of the examination can include the kidney, bladder, prostate, and genitalia. If there are any breast-related complaints, assess for gynecomastia, nipple discharge, and breast mass.

Laboratory Testing

The need for laboratory testing is guided by the patient's risk factors, history, and physical examination. Tests to consider include chlamydia, gonorrhea, trichomonas, syphilis, HIV, hepatitis B and C, and diabetes screening (U.S. Preventive Services Task Force, 2021; Marcell & Male Training Center for Family Planning and Reproductive Health, 2014).

SEXUALLY TRANSMITTED INFECTIONS

The incidence and prevalence of STIs vary depending on the infection. The causes of this discrepancy include health-seeking behavior differences, anatomical differences that increase or decrease susceptibility, sexual behavioral differences, and other factors. Women of reproductive age are more likely to interact with the healthcare system on a regular basis than men because of recommendations for annual examinations or their need for cervical cancer screening, contraception, or pregnancy-related care. The CDC recommendations for screening vary based on sexual behaviors, gender identity, and HIV status. The only infections for which there are routine screening recommendations in all males are HIV and hepatitis C (Workowski et al., 2021). For HIV, the recommendation is for screening one time between age 13–64, and for hepatitis C the recommendation is for a single screening over age 18. For all other STIs, screening is based on sexual behaviors and risk factors (Workowski et al., 2021). Sexual behavior influences an individual's risk for acquiring an STI. Risk factors include the number of partners, the infection status of partners, the infection prevalence within a sexual network, and the types of exposure (oral, genital, or rectal). The correct diagnosis and management of STIs is an essential component of SRH. Detailed information about STIs can be found in Chapter 22. This chapter includes STIs that are more common or only occur in males, with a focus on aspects that differ in males and females, such as incidence, clinical presentation, and diagnostic testing modalities (see **Table 10-2**). HPV is also included because of the availability of a vaccine for males.

TABLE 10-2 Aspects of Sexually Transmitted Infections That Differ Between Males and Females

Infection	Difference in Males
Chlamydia	Can cause urethritis and epididymitis More often symptomatic
Gonorrhea	More common More often symptomatic Can cause urethritis and epididymitis
Nongonococcal urethritis	Only occurs in males
Epididymitis	Only occurs in males
Syphilis	More common, particularly in men who have sex with men
HIV	More common, particularly in men who have sex with men

Chlamydia

Chlamydia is the most common reportable STI in the United States. In 2022, there were 1,649,716 cases of chlamydia reported, and of those, 602,851 cases were in males (CDC, 2022). Chlamydia infects columnar and transitional epithelial cells inside the urethra and rectum.

Chlamydia is asymptomatic in up to 50 percent of men who are infected (Mackern-Oberti et al., 2013). If a man has symptoms, they usually include dysuria; urinary frequency; clear, cloudy, or mucopurulent/mucoid urethral discharge; and urethral or meatal itching, tingling, or discomfort. In addition to urethritis, chlamydia can cause epididymitis, prostatitis, and proctitis.

TABLE 10-3 Treatment of Chlamydial Infections

Recommended Regimen	Alternative Regimens
Doxycycline 100 mg orally 2 times/ day for 7 days	Azithromycin 1 gm orally in a single dose **or** Levofloxacin 500 mg orally once daily for 7 days

Reproduced from Centers for Disease Control and Prevention. (2021). Sexually transmitted diseases treatment guidelines, 2021. *MMWR Recomm Rep*, *70*(4), 1–187.

Screening for chlamydia should include all sites where the person may have been exposed during sexual contact: oral, urethral, and/or rectal. A confirmatory diagnosis of chlamydia is made with a nucleic acid amplification test (NAAT). Although both urine and urethral specimens have high sensitivity (greater than 90 percent) and very high specificity (greater than 99 percent), first-catch urine testing is the preferred method in most settings because it is less invasive (U.S. Preventive Services Task Force, 2021; CDC, 2014). Because of high re-infection rates, people who test positive for chlamydia should be re-tested in 3 months (Workowski et al., 2021). Self-collected rectal swabs are also acceptable (Workowski et al., 2021). Treatment regimens for chlamydia can be found in **Table 10-3**.

Gonorrhea

Gonorrhea is the second most common reportable STI in the United States and is more common in males. In 2022, there were 648,056 cases of gonorrhea reported, and 60 percent of these occurred in males (CDC, 2022).

Although gonorrhea is most often asymptomatic in women, the majority of men will have mild or significant urethritis. Gonococcal urethritis is characterized by dysuria and often copious mucopurulent urethral discharge. There can also be swelling of the distal shaft and glans of the penis (a syndrome sometimes referred to as bull-headed clap). Like chlamydia, gonorrhea can cause epididymitis, prostatitis, orchitis, seminal vesiculitis, and infections of the Tyson and bulbourethral glands.

It is critical to test all sites of possible exposure to ensure accurate results because the prevalence of infection varies by anatomical site. In men who have sex with men, nationwide samples show urogenital gonorrhea positivity rates from 4.3 to 13.3 percent, rectal gonorrhea positivity rates from 7.6 to 18.1 percent, and pharyngeal gonorrhea positivity rates from 8.0 to 19.8 percent (CDC, 2019b). Gonorrhea can be diagnosed by a Gram stain of urethral secretions that has polymorphonuclear leukocytes and intracellular gram-negative diplococci, culture, or NAAT. The sensitivity of NAAT is superior to culture for *Neisseria gonorrhoeae* detection (Workowski et al., 2021). Treatment regimens for gonorrhea can be found in **Box 10-1**.

Nongonococcal Urethritis

Urethritis in males is a cluster of symptoms and signs associated with inflammation of the urethra from infectious or noninfectious causes. The symptoms and signs of urethritis include meatal pruritis, urethral discharge, and irritation and dysuria. Urethritis is classified as either gonococcal or nongonococcal. Approximately 5 to 20 percent of urethritis is caused by gonococcal infection (Bachmann et al., 2015). Nongonococcal urethritis (NGU) is a nonspecific diagnosis that has a number of causes. *Chlamydia trachomatis* is the most common cause of NGU and is responsible for 20 to 50 percent of cases. Other causative organisms include *Mycoplasma genitalium* (10 to 25 percent of cases), *Ureaplasma urealyticum* (5 to 10 percent), *Trichomonas vaginalis* (1 to 10 percent), adenovirus (2 to 4 percent), and herpes simplex virus (2 to 3 percent). Up to half the cases of NGU have no specific pathogen detected (Workowski et al., 2021).

Diagnostic criteria for urethritis can be found in **Box 10-2**. A diagnosis of NGU requires the differentiation of urethritis caused by gonorrhea from those not caused by gonorrhea. If the clinician observes urethral discharge or if the patient reports symptoms of urethritis, a urethral swab is collected for Gram stain and microscopic examination, if available. Individulas with urethritis should be tested for gonorrhea and chlamydia. *Mycoplasma* genitalium testing should be considered for patients with persistent or recurrent symptoms. In addition, consider *Trichomonas vaginalis* testing in areas or populations with high prevalence, an infected partner, and persistent or recurrent symptoms (Workowski et al., 2021).

BOX 10-1 Treatment of Uncomplicated Gonococcal Infections

Ceftriaxone 500 mg IM in a single dose

If cephalosporin allergy: Gentamicin 240 mg IM **plus** Azithromycin 2 gm PO in a single dose

If ceftriaxone is not available: Cefixime 800 mg PO in a single dose

Reproduced from Centers for Disease Control and Prevention. (2021). Sexually transmitted diseases treatment guidelines, 2021. *MMWR Recomm Rep, 70*(4), 1–187.

Abbreviations: IM, intramuscularly; PO, by mouth.

BOX 10-2 Diagnostic Criteria for Urethritis

In the setting of compatible symptoms, urethritis can be documented on the basis of any of the following signs or laboratory tests:

- Mucoid, mucopurulent, or purulent discharge on examination.
- Gram stain of urethral secretions demonstrating two or more white blood cells (WBCs) per oil immersion field.
- Positive leukocyte esterase test on first-void urine or microscopic examination of sediment from a spun first-void urine demonstrating 10 or more WBCs per high-power field.

Reproduced from Centers for Disease Control and Prevention. (2021). Sexually transmitted diseases treatment guidelines, 2021. *MMWR Recomm Rep, 70*(4), 1–187.

The CDC (2021) recommends oral treatment with doxycycline 100 mg twice daily for 7 days. If tests for CT, GC, and TV are all negative and the patient continues to have urethritis symptoms, NAAT testing for *Mycoplasma genitalium* is recommended. If resistance testing is available, it should be done. If the strain is macrolide sensitive, the treatment is doxycycline 100 mg twice daily for 7 days followed by Azithromycin 1 gm in a single dose, followed by Azithomycin 500 mg daily for 3 days. If the strain is macrolide resistant, the treatment is doxycycline 200 mg twice daily for 7 days followed by moxifloxacin 400 mg daily for 7 days. If no resistance testing is available, the treatment is doxycycline 100 mg twice daily for 7 days followed by moxifloxacin 400 mg daily for 7 days. Sex partners of individuals with NGU should be treated with the same regimen and should be tested for STIs. Counseling should include the importance of medication adherence, confirmation of diagnosis after NAAT test results, abstinence from sexual contact during treatment, and encouragement to return to the clinic if symptoms either do not resolve or return after treatment.

Epididymitis

Epididymitis is a syndrome unique to males. Inflammation of the epididymis can be either acute (lasting less than 6 weeks) or chronic (lasting 6 weeks or longer). The most common causes of acute epididymitis in sexually active males younger than 35 years are *Chlamydia trachomatis*, *Neisseria gonorrhoeae,* and *Mycoplasma genitalium*. Epididymitis can also be caused by enteric organisms such as *Escherichia coli*. In chronic epididymitis that is associated with an infectious agent, *Mycobacterium tuberculosis* is the most common cause. Other causes of both acute and chronic epididymitis include infection of the epididymis from bacteriuria due to bladder outlet obstruction (e.g., benign prostatic hyperplasia), trauma, cancer, or autoimmune diseases (Workowski et al., 2021).

The symptoms and signs of acute epididymitis are unilateral testicular pain and tenderness, hydrocele, and epididymal swelling. The examination should include palpation of the associated lymph nodes, epididymis, spermatic cord, and testicles. Additionally, the clinician needs to establish objective evidence of inflammation; there are three methods: (1) Gram stain of a urethral swab and the identification of two or more white blood cells (WBCs) per oil immersion field; (2) positive leukocyte esterase test on first-void urine; and (3) microscopic examination of sediment from centrifuged first-void urine that shows more than 10 WBCs per high-power field (Workowski et al., 2021). NAAT urine testing for *Chlamydia trachomatis* and *Neisseria gonorrhoeae* should also be performed. If a patient presents with sudden onset of severe unilateral pain and does not have other signs of infection, testicular torsion should be considered, and the patient should be immediately referred to a urologist or emergency department. Testicular torsion is a surgical emergency that needs to be addressed to prevent permanent damage to the testicle.

Treatment for epididymitis is initiated at the time of the visit; it is not recommended to defer treatment until laboratory results are available. Epididymitis treatment regimens are outlined in **Box 10-3**. Patients should be counseled regarding abstinence from sexual activity during treatment and the need for their partners to be tested and treated. They should also be advised to return for evaluation if they do not improve within 72 hours. Both chronic epididymitis and noninfectious acute cases should be managed by a urologist.

BOX 10-3 Epididymitis Treatment

Acute epididymitis most likely caused by sexually transmitted chlamydia and gonorrhea:

Ceftriaxone 500 mg IM in a single dose

plus

Doxycycline 100 mg orally twice/day for 10 days

Acute epididymitis most likely caused by sexually transmitted chlamydia and gonorrhea and enteric organisms (men who have insertive anal sex):

Ceftriaxone 500 mg IM in a single dose

plus

Levofloxacin 500 mg orally once/day for 10 days

Acute epididymitis most likely caused by enteric organisms:

Levofloxacin 500 mg orally once/day for 10 days

Reproduced from Centers for Disease Control and Prevention. (2021). Sexually transmitted diseases treatment guidelines, 2021. *MMWR Recomm Rep, 70*(4), 1–187.

Abbreviation: IM, intramuscularly.

Syphilis

Syphilis is another STI that is more common in males. Of the 59,016 primary and secondary syphilis infections reported in 2022 in the United States, 75 percent were in males (CDC, 2024). Despite occurring more commonly in males, the pathophysiology, diagnosis, presentation, and treatment of syphilis does not differ by sex. The populations at highest risk for syphilis include men who have sex with men, individuals who are HIV positive, and those who have a partner with syphilis. A summary of treatment regimens for syphilis in men who are HIV negative can be found in **Table 10-4**. More detailed treatment information about syphilis treatment, including treatment for men who are HIV positive, can be found in guidelines from the CDC (2021).

HPV

HPV is the most common STI in the United States. It is estimated to infect up to 80 percent of sexually active individuals at some point in their lives. Genital warts can be found on the penis, scrotum, lower abdomen, thighs, and in the perianal area. Genital warts are generally diagnosed based on visualization, but may need to be confirmed by biopsy if they appear atypical or do not respond to recommended treatments (CDC, 2021). They can be flat, papular or pedunculated, in clusters or dispersed, and be hyperpigmented compared to surrounding tissue. They are usually asymptomatic, but they can be painful or pruritic. There are both patient-applied and provider- applied treatment options. There is not sufficient data to say that any one treatment is superior to another, and they have varying side effects. The recommended approach to choosing a treatment is to use shared decision making while taking into consideration the number, location, and size of the warts as well as cost and convenience of treatment (CDC, 2021). Recommended treatment options can be found in **Table 10-5**. The full treatment guidelines are available from the CDC and see Chapter 22.

TABLE 10-4 Treatment of Syphilis for Men Who Are HIV Negative

Recommended	Alternatives if Allergic to Penicillin[a]
Primary, secondary, and early latent syphilis: Benzathine penicillin G 2.4 million units IM in a single dose Late latent syphilis, latent syphilis of unknown duration, and tertiary syphilis: Benzathine penicillin G 7.2 million units total, administered as three doses of 2.4 million units IM each at 1 week intervals	Primary, secondary, and early latent syphilis: Doxycycline 100 mg orally 2 times/day for 14 days **or** Tetracycline 500 mg orally 4 times/day for 14 days Late latent syphilis or latent syphilis of unknown duration: Doxycycline 100 mg orally 2 times/day for 28 days **or** Tetracycline 500 mg orally 4 times/day for 28 days Tertiary syphilis: Consult an infectious diseases specialist

Reproduced from Centers for Disease Control and Prevention. (2021). Sexually transmitted diseases treatment guidelines, 2021. *MMWR Recomm Rep, 70*(4), 1–187.

Abbreviation: IM, intramuscularly.

[a]There are limited data to support these regimens, so close follow-up is essential. Penicillin desensitization and treatment should be considered for persons with a penicillin allergy whose adherence to therapy or follow-up cannot be ensured.

TABLE 10-5 Treatment of Genital Warts

External anogenital warts	Patient-applied: Imiquimod 3.75% or 5% cream or Podofilox 0.5% solution or gel or Sinecatechins 15% ointment Provider-administered: Cryotherapy with liquid nitrogen or cryoprobe Surgical removal by tangential scissor excision, tangential shave excision, curettage, laser, or electrosurgery or Trichloroacetic acid (TCA) or bichloroacetic acid (BCA) 80%–90% solution
Urethral meatus warts	Cryotherapy with liquid nitrogen or Surgical removal
Intra-anal warts	Cryotherapy with liquid nitrogen or Surgical removal or Trichloroacetic acid (TCA) or bichloroacetic acid (BCA) 80%–90% solution *Management of intra-anal warts should include consultation with a colorectal specialist.*

Reproduced from Centers for Disease Control and Prevention. (2021). Sexually transmitted diseases treatment guidelines, 2021. *MMWR Recomm Rep, 70*(4), 1–187.

The 9-valent HPV vaccine (HPV9, Gardasil 9) is approved by the FDA for males aged 9 to 45 years for the prevention of genital warts, anal intraepithelial neoplasia, and anal cancer. Routine HPV vaccination is recommended for all children at age 11 or 12 years, but it can be started as early as age 9. Catch-up HPV vaccination is recommended for all persons who have not been adequately vaccinated through age 26. For adults aged 27 through 45 years who are not adequately vaccinated and most likely to benefit from vaccination, the CDC recommends shared decision making between the individual and their healthcare provider (Meites et al., 2019). HPV vaccination is not approved for use in adults older than 45 years.

SEXUAL DYSFUNCTION

Individuals can experience a number of different types of sexual dysfunction (see **Box 10-4**). These conditions can be lifelong (occurring from the first sexual encounter) or acquired (appearing later in life). The characteristic all sexual dysfunctions have in common is that they cause distress to the person experiencing them. Distress is required for a diagnosis of sexual dysfunction (McCabe et al., 2016). Sexual dysfunction can have a profound negative effect on an individual's well-being; thus, it is important to identify those who are experiencing these conditions and provide appropriate treatment. This section focuses on the two most common sexual dysfunction presentations in males: premature ejaculation and erectile dysfunction.

BOX 10-4 Sexual Dysfunctions in Men

Male hypoactive sexual desire disorder
Erectile dysfunction
Premature ejaculation
Delayed ejaculation
Retrograde ejaculation
Anejaculation
Anhedonic ejaculation
Hypohedonic ejaculation
Anorgasmia
Painful ejaculation or orgasm
Postorgasmic illness syndrome

Reproduced from McCabe, M. P., Sharlip, I. D., Atalla, E., Balon, R., Fisher, A. D., Laumann, E., Lee, S. W., Lewis, R., & Segraves, R. T. (2016). Definitions of sexual dysfunctions in women and men: A consensus statement from the Fourth International Consultation on Sexual Medicine 2015. *Journal of Sexual Medicine, 13*(2), 135–143.

Premature Ejaculation

Definition

Premature ejaculation (PE) can be lifelong (primary) or acquired (secondary). In 2014, the International Society for Sexual Medicine (ISSM) introduced an evidence-based definition of PE:

- Ejaculation which always or nearly always occurs prior to or within about 1 minute of vaginal penetration from the first sexual experience (lifelong PE), or a clinically significant reduction in latency time, often about 3 minutes or less (acquired PE).

AND

- Negative personal consequences, such as distress, bother, frustration, and/or the avoidance of sexual intimacy (Althof et al., 2014; Shindel et al., 2022).

Although this definition specifies vaginal penetration as a component of the definition, PE also occurs in men who have sex with men (Barbonetti et al., 2019; Shindel et al., 2022).

Prevalence

Using the ISSM definition, the prevalence of both lifelong and acquired PE is approximately 5% (Shindel et al., 2022). Additionally, as many as 50 percent of people with PE also have erectile dysfunction (El-Hamd et al., 2019).

Etiology

Ejaculation is a complex process that includes two phases: emission and expulsion. Emission is controlled by the autonomic nervous system, and expulsion is controlled by the somatic nervous system. The exact origin of PE is unknown, but a number of etiologies have been proposed and investigated. Etiologies of PE are typically divided into two categories: psychological factors, such as anxiety; and biogenic factors, such as 5-hydroxytryptamine receptor dysfunction (El-Hamd et al., 2019).

Diagnosis

The diagnosis of PE should be made using the ISSM definition. Patient and partner reports of the intravaginal ejaculatory latency time (IELT), which is the time between vaginal penetration and ejaculation, are well correlated with more objective stopwatch measures used in studies (Serefoglu et al., 2014). While IELT is the primary term in the literature, ejaculatory latency time is also applicable to nonvaginal penile sex (i.e., anal or oral). Two validated questionnaires can be helpful in PE diagnosis (Hatzichristou et al., 2016): the Premature Ejaculation Profile (PEP) (Patrick et al., 2009) and the Index of Premature Ejaculation (IPE) (Althof et al., 2006). A physical exam is recommended for lifelong PE. However, it is required for acquired PE in order to assess for other related issues such as erectile dysfunction, thyroid diseases, and prostatitis.

Management

A number of PE treatments are effective for increasing IELT (see **Box 10-5**). Other treatment outcomes, such as improving sexual satisfaction and ejaculation control, have not been evaluated consistently in PE research. Topical local anesthetics have been the mainstay of treatment for PE. More recently there have been multiple other medications that have shown effectiveness in treating it. The current American Urologic Association (AUA) Guidelines recommend daily SSRIs, and as needed topical anesthetics and clomipramine (Anafranil) (Shindel et al., 2022). There has also been recent evidence that an oxytocin receptor agonist (Cligosiban) is effective in treating lifelong PE (McMahon et al., 2019), but it is considered investigational. Pharmacologic and nonpharmacologic treatments can be used in combination for acquired PE, which can be more effective than using one alone. When assessing a patient's response to treatment, it is important to consider not only the time to ejaculation, but also if treatment is reducing the negative personal consequences of PE that are a component of the ISSM definition (Ciocanel et al., 2019).

BOX 10-5 Effective Treatments for Premature Ejaculation

Pharmacologic Treatments

Selective serotonin reuptake inhibitors:
Paroxetine
Citalopram
Sertraline
Fluoxetine
Dapoxetine
Oral and nasal clomipramine
Topical anesthetics:
Lidocaine/Prilocaine gel
Topical EMLA
Phosphodiesterase type 5 (PDE5) inhibitors (e.g., sildenafil)
Tramadol

Nonpharmacologic Treatments

Behavioral therapies
Acupuncture
Chinese medicine

Data from Ciocanel, O., Power, K., & Eriksen, A. (2019). Interventions to treat erectile dysfunction and premature ejaculation: An overview of systematic reviews. *Sexual Medicine, 7*(3), 251–269. https://doi.org/10.1016/j.esxm.2019.06.001

Note: These treatments have been evaluated in systematic reviews and found to be effective.

Erectile Dysfunction

Definition

Erectile dysfunction (ED) is defined as the "consistent or recurrent inability to attain and/or maintain penile erection sufficient for sexual satisfaction" (McCabe et al., 2016, p. 141).

Prevalence

The prevalence estimates for ED vary from study to study, but the trend of increasing prevalence with increasing age is consistent (Anderson et al., 2022). A recent study using data from the 2021 National Survey of Sexual Wellbeing found the prevalence of ED for people 18–24 was 17.9 percent; then it dropped slightly to 13.3 percent between 25–34, and 12.7 percent between 35–44. (Mark et al., 2024). The prevalence rises with age above age 45 with estimates of 25.3 percent between 45–54, 33.9 percent between 55–64, 48 percent between 65–74, and 52.2 percent for people over 75 (Mark et al., 2024). The increased prevalence of ED in older men reflects the fact that aging affects the vascular system, hormonal and neural function, and penile structure. In addition to age, the risk factors for ED include cigarette smoking, diabetes, cardiovascular disease, metabolic syndrome, genitourinary disease, and depression.

Etiology

A complex interplay between neurotransmitters, blood vessels, and musculature must occur for an erection. This process results in the arterial dilation and venous occlusion needed to achieve erection. Sexual stimulation triggers the release of neurotransmitters, and the primary neurotransmitter involved in erection is nitric oxide. Nitric oxide stimulates increased release of cyclic adenosine monophosphate (cAMP) and cyclic guanosine monophosphate (cGMP), which cause relaxation of the smooth muscles of the penis. This muscle relaxation is necessary to allow the penis to expand in volume and turgor, leading to the erect state. Simultaneously, the penile arteries dilate due to increased blood flow, and the blood is then trapped in the sinusoids. This leads to compression of the subtunical venous plexuses and reduces venous outflow. The tunica is also stretched, which occludes key veins and decreases venous outflow. The resulting increase in intracavernous pressure raises the penis from a flaccid to an erect state. The pressure can increase further with reflex contractions of the ischiocavernosus muscles during sexual stimulation.

The causes of ED are varied and often multifactorial. They can be anatomic, vasculogenic, neurogenic, endocrinologic, medication induced, or psychogenic (Burnett et al., 2018). The anatomic causes of ED include abnormality in structure or function of the vasculature, musculature, or nerves in the pelvis. There are multiple causes of vasculogenic ED. Any disease that leads to atherosclerosis or occlusion of veins or arteries (e.g., hypertension, hyperlipidemia, diabetes, or peripheral vascular disease) can contribute to ED. The association between cardiovascular disease and ED is sufficient that the presence of one should lead to screening for the other (Chaitoff et al., 2018; Burnett et al., 2018). Neurogenic ED results from dysfunction of the central nervous system or the nerves that innervate the penis. Neurologic conditions that can cause ED include stroke, Parkinson disease, Alzheimer disease, epilepsy, and trauma to the spinal cord from injury or surgery. Endocrinologic impotence is often related to hypogonadism, which can be the result of dysfunction of the HPG axis, hyperprolactinemia, hyperthyroidism, or hypothyroidism. Medications most commonly associated with ED include antiandrogens, antidepressants, and antihypertensives. Psychogenic (nonorganic) ED may be related to stress, anxiety, or depression. Psychogenic ED often has a sudden onset and is intermittent, while organic ED usually has a gradual onset and occurs consistently (Yafi et al., 2016).

Diagnosis

Patients often do not self-report ED to healthcare providers; thus, it is important to ask patients with risk factors if they have ED symptoms. Questions that are important to ask in the assessment include: the onset of symptoms, severity, how bothersome they are, if the problem is with attaining or maintaining an erection, contextual factors, presence or absence of nocturnal, morning or masturbation erections, and any previous therapies (Burnett et al., 2018). Complete guidelines for evaluation and treatment of ED are published by the American Urological Association (Burnett et al., 2018). Early intervention may prevent some of the symptoms from developing and subsequently decrease the psychologic and relational effects. The diagnosis and monitoring of response to treatment involves the use of patient-completed questionnaires. Two validated questionnaires are recommended: the International Index of Erectile Function (IIEF, Rosen et al., 1997) and the Male Sexual Health Questionnaire (MSHQ; Rosen et al., 2004).

Assessment and Management

Evaluation and treatment for ED should be done in consultation with a specialist. A patient who reports ED symptoms needs a complete health history, including sexual history, and physical examination. Laboratory tests are not required for ED diagnosis but are helpful in assessing for related conditions. Laboratory tests that could be considered include a lipid profile, fasting glucose, glycosylated hemoglobin (HgA1c), and serum total testosterone (Burnett et al., 2018). Due to the association of ED with cardiovascular disease, a concurrent assessment of cardiac risk should be performed using a standard tool such as the Framingham Risk Score.

Using a shared decision-making model that involves the patient and their partner(s) will allow the development of individualized goals and choice of treatment to reach those goals. There are a number of effective treatments for ED (see **Box 10-6**). The phosphodiesterase type 5 (PDE5) inhibitors (sildenafil, tadalafil, vardenafil, and avanafil) revolutionized the treatment of ED and are effective in improving sexual intercourse (Ciocanel et al., 2019). These medications increase the concentration of cGMP by blocking the enzyme that degrades it. It is important to note that PDE5 inhibitors augment an erection, but they do not initiate it. Their use must be closely monitored because there are potentially life-threatening interactions with nitrite-containing medications. If the cause of ED is anatomic, neurogenic, or endocrinologic, treatment of the underlying condition may be needed. There has been recent evidence that stem cell therapy improves neurogenic ED, but it is still considered investigational (Haahr et al., 2016; Burnett et al., 2018). There has also been recent evidence that hyperbaric oxygen therapy (HBOT) may improve vasculogenic ED (Saffati et al., 2023). For medication-induced ED, changing medications can be helpful when possible. Psychotherapy may be warranted for psychogenic ED.

CONTRACEPTION

There are four forms of male contraception: vasectomy, external condoms, coitus interruptus (withdrawal), and abstinence (avoiding vaginal contact with semen). Each of these methods is discussed in Chapter 13. This section focuses on vasectomy because it is the only one of these contraceptive methods that requires the involvement of a healthcare provider.

Vasectomy

Vasectomy is a highly effective and safe method for permanent contraception. It is more effective than female permanent contraception, with a 0.15 percent pregnancy rate in the first year after vasectomy compared to 0.5 percent for bilateral tubal ligation (Trussell et al., 2018). Complications after vasectomy are rare (up to 2 percent of procedures) and include hematoma, infection, and chronic scrotal pain (Yang et al., 2021). In the United States

BOX 10-6 Effective Treatments for Erectile Dysfunction

Pharmacologic Treatments

PDE5 inhibitors:
- Tadalafil
- Sildenafil
- Vardenafil
- Avanafil

Penile injection with papaverine and prostaglandin E1

Testosterone

Nonpharmacologic Treatments

Low-intensity shockwave therapy

Penile prosthesis implantation

Vacuum erection device

Hyperbaric oxygen therapy

Lifestyle interventions (diet, physical activity, and weight loss)

Psychological therapies (mixed evidence of improvement)

Data from Ciocanel, O., Power, K., & Eriksen, A. (2019). Interventions to treat erectile dysfunction and premature ejaculation: An overview of systematic reviews. *Sexual Medicine, 7*(3), 251–269. https://doi.org/10.1016/j.esxm.2019.06.001 and Wang, C. M., Wu, B. R., Xiang, P., Xiao, J., & Hu, X. C. (2023). Management of male erectile dysfunction: From the past to the future. *Front Endocrinol (Lausanne)*, 14, 1148834. https://doi.org/10.3389/fendo.2023.1148834

Note: These treatments have been evaluated in systematic reviews and found to be effective.

5–6 percent of males age 18–45 have had a vasectomy (Zhang & Eisenberg, 2022). There has been some evidence of an increase in vasectomy rates after the Supreme Court overturned *Roe v. Wade* (Bole et al., 2024).

Procedure

In contrast to tubal ligation, which must be performed in a surgical setting under general anesthesia, vasectomy is an outpatient procedure that can be performed with local anesthesia during an office visit. The procedure involves cutting and occluding the vas deferens bilaterally. This does not stop sperm production, but it prevents the sperm from entering the ejaculate. The preferred method is the no-scalpel technique. Compared to the conventional incisional method, the no-scalpel technique takes less time to perform, is less painful, results in fewer complications, and allows the patient to resume sexual activity sooner than other techniques (Yang et al., 2021). Patients are advised to avoid sexual activity for 1 week after the procedure so the surgical site can heal. Condoms or another method of contraception must be used for about 3 months after the procedure because azoospermia does not happen immediately. The American Urological Association recommends a semen analysis 8 to 16 weeks after the procedure; if azoospermia is not achieved, the semen analysis is repeated every 6 to 12 weeks until it shows azoospermia (Sharlip et al., 2012).

Counseling

The permanency of sterilization is an essential component of preprocedure counseling. Although it is possible to reverse a vasectomy, the potential to achieve a pregnancy can be affected. It is estimated that 28 to 40 percent of couples achieve pregnancy after vasectomy reversal (Yang et al., 2021). The effectiveness of reversal depends on the amount of vas tubing that was removed, the procedure used to occlude the cut tubes, and the amount of time that has passed since the original surgery. Patients should consider vasectomy only if they want permanent contraception. Other key points for preoperative counseling include the need for an additional contraceptive method until azoospermia is confirmed and the very small (1 to 2 percent) risk of procedure complications, such as hematoma, infection, and chronic scrotal pain. Additionally, patients should be advised that vasectomy does not protect against STIs or HIV.

TESTICULAR CANCER

Epidemiology

Testicular cancer is most often diagnosed in individuals aged 20 to 44 years old, with a mean age of 33 at diagnosis. It accounts for only 1 percent of all cancers in the United States (Giona, 2022). The majority (95 percent) of testicular cancers are germ cell tumors (Adra & Einhorn, 2017). The other 5 percent are caused by sex cord stromal tumors, lymphoid and hematopoietic tumors, tumors of the collecting ducts and rete testes, and tumors of the testicular adnexa. Approximately two thirds of patients with testicular cancer present with localized disease. The 5-year survival rate is 99 percent for localized disease and 75 percent for metastatic disease (American Society of Clinical Oncology, 2019).

Etiology

The etiology of testicular cancer has only been recently elucidated. Primordial germ cells (PGC) which transport genetic information, appear to undergo a malignant transformation in utero that leads to germ cell neoplasia in situ, which is then a precursor to germ cell tumors (GCT) (Chovanec & Cheng, 2022). Risk factors for testicular cancer include cryptorchidism (undescended testicle), personal or family history of testicular cancer, age, and intratubular germ cell neoplasia, as well as potential environmental exposures (Yazici et al., 2023). The primary modifiable risk factor is cryptorchidism. Those who have cryptorchidism are 4 to 6 times more likely to develop cancer in the affected testicle than those who do not have cryptorchidism; however, if cryptorchidism is surgically corrected before puberty, the relative risk is reduced to 2 to 3 times that of individuals who do not have cryptorchidism (Yazici et al., 2023).

Clinical Presentation

Most patients with testicular cancer present with a painless testicular mass. Some people will notice a heaviness or swelling in the affected testicle. Another common presentation is after a trauma to the testicles when the person notices the mass while doing a self-examination secondary to the injury. It is less common for someone to present with testicular pain or gynecomastia, which is caused by the tumor secreting beta human chorionic gonadotropin (Rovito et al., 2022; Baird et al., 2018). Pain can occur if the tumor is growing rapidly or has caused an intratesticular hemorrhage.

Assessment

Any testicular mass should be assumed to be cancer until proven otherwise. If a patient presents with a mass, or if a mass is found during an examination, the provider should do a thorough examination of both testicles. The examination should also include palpation for inguinal and supraclavicular lymphadenopathy, abdominal masses, and abdominal pain; inspection of the chest for gynecomastia; and auscultation of lung sounds to assess for metastatic disease (Baird et al., 2018). The differential diagnoses for testicular mass include epididymitis, orchitis, testicular torsion, and hematoma; less likely diagnoses include hernia, varicocele, or spermatocele. Testicular ultrasound is required for any suspicious mass.

Management

The initial treatment for all tumors is radical inguinal orchiectomy with removal of the testicle and spermatic cord to the level of the inguinal ring. The use of adjuvant chemotherapy is determined by the clinical staging. It is important to note that early detection and treatment are essential because these tumors have the potential for rapid growth, which can lead to increased morbidity and mortality. All patients should be offered sperm cryopreservation before treatment (Sineath & Mehta, 2019).

Testicular Self-Examination

Currently neither the U.S. Preventive Services Task Force (2010 nor the American Cancer Society (2019) recommend regular testicular self-examinations because they do not lead to earlier diagnosis or improved outcomes. For individuals with risk factors, it is expected that the provider will discuss the risks and potential benefits of self-examination with patients. Adolescent and young adult patients should be made aware of testicular cancer, including the signs and symptoms, and be advised to see a healthcare provider if they experience any problems or discover a mass.

CARE OF GAY AND BISEXUAL MEN AND AMAB TRANSFEMININE, TRANSGENDER, AND GENDER DIVERSE INDIVIDUALS

Health science literature and research often refers to sexual behaviors that people engage in, rather than how individuals identify, and terminology around sexuality is not universally agreed on (see Chapter 11). Data on health status and health-related behaviors for gay and bisexual men, transfeminine, transgender, and gender diverse individuals are limited and have been challenging to collect, in part because the terminology used to describe individuals is not standardized and is constantly changing (Morgan et al., 2020). This can present challenges for clinicians; however, care of these clients is not more complex than care for those who identify as heterosexual and/or cisgender. What is difficult is that health outcomes are directly influenced by lack of research, the quality of healthcare interactions, discrimination, stigma, lack of access to care, and a lack of providers trained in culturally responsive care.

A lack of access to quality, affordable, and appropriate care affects the health status of many gay and bisexual men, transfeminine, transgender, and gender diverse individuals. Compared to heterosexual men, they are twice as likely to delay or not receive health care due to cost (15 percent versus 33 percent) and fear of discrimination (8 percent versus 21 percent) (Caleb & Norris, 2025). They may also experience mistreatment in healthcare settings. For illustration, in a nationally representative U.S. survey about healthcare experiences, 26 percent of transgender respondents reported that providers used the wrong name or misgendered them. Additionally, 21 percent of transgender adults reported that their providers refused to document their gender dysphoria (Caleb & Norris, 2025).

To address these issues of inadequate care and discrimination, clinicians need to be trained in providing culturally responsive care to individuals of all sexual orientations and identities. Box 11-1 in Chapter 11 contains a number of resources for clinicians about providing culturally responsive care for LGBQT individuals. See Chapter 11 for a thorough discussion of care for lesbian, bisexual, and queer women and transgender and gender diverse individuals and Chapter 8 for more information on steps clinicians can take to create a care setting that is welcoming to people of all sexual orientations and gender identities.

CONCLUSION

This chapter has summarized the most common conditions clients AMAB will experience who are seeking sexual and reproductive-related health care. Some of these conditions can be managed independently by gynecologic providers, but many will need to be co-managed or referred to other specialists. It is important for gynecologic providers to be aware of these conditions so that they can best support and manage their AMAB clients.

References

Althof, S. E., McMahon, C. G., Waldinger, M. D., Serefoglu, E. C., Shindel, A. W., Adaikan, P. G., Becher, E., Dean, J., Giuliano, F., Hellstrom, W. J. G., Giraldi, A., Glina, S., Incrocci, L., Jannini, E., McCabe, M., Parish, S., Rowland, D., Segraves, R. T., Sharlip, I., & Torres, L. O. (2014). An update of the International Society of Sexual Medicine's guidelines for the diagnosis and treatment of premature ejaculation (PE). *Sexual Medicine, 2*(2), 60–90. https://doi.org/10.1002/sm2.28

Adra, N. & Einhorn, L. H. (2017). Salvage therapy for relapsed testicular cancer. *Oncotarget. 8*(41), 69200-69201. https://doi.org/10.18632/oncotarget.20573. PMID: 29050196; PMCID: PMC5642471.

Althof, S., Rosen, R., Symonds, T., Mundayat, R., May, K., & Abraham, L. (2006). Development and validation of a new questionnaire to assess sexual satisfaction, control, and distress associated with premature ejaculation. *Journal of Sexual Medicine, 3*(3), 465–475. https://doi.org/10.1111/j.1743-6109.2006.00239.x

American Cancer Society. (2019). *Can testicular cancer be found early?* https://www.cancer.org/cancer/testicular-cancer/detection-diagnosis-staging/detection.html

American College of Nurse-Midwives. (2020). *Core competencies for basic midwifery practice.*

American College of Nurse-Midwives. (2021). *Healthcare for transgender and gender non-binary people.*

American Society of Clinical Oncology. (2019). *Testicular cancer: Statistics.* https://www.cancer.net/cancer-types/testicular-cancer/statistics

Anakwe, A., Ortiz, K., Kotelchuck, M., & BeLue, R. (2025). Preconception health indicators among adult U.S. men: Race/ethnicity variations and temporal trends. *Andrology, 13*(1), 7–21. https://doi.org/10.1111/andr.13573

Anderson, D., Laforge, J., Ross, M. M., Vanlangendonck, R., Hasoon, J., Viswanath, O., Kaye, A. D., & Urits, I. (2022). Male sexual dysfunction. *Health Psychology Research, 10*(3), 37533. https://doi.org/10.52965/001c.37533.

Bachmann, L. H., Manhart, L. E., Martin, D. H., Seña, A. C., Dimitrakoff, J., Jensen, J. S., & Gaydos, C. A. (2015). Advances in the understanding and treatment of male urethritis [Suppl. 8]. *Clinical Infectious Diseases, 61*, S763–S769. https://doi.org/10.1093/cid/civ755

Baird, D. C., Meyers, G. J., & Hu, J. S. (2018). Testicular cancer: Diagnosis and treatment. *American Family Physician, 97*(4), 261–268.

Barbonetti, A., D'Andrea, S., Cavallo, F., Martorella, A., Francavilla, S., & Francavilla, F. (2019). Erectile dysfunction and premature ejaculation in homosexual and heterosexual men: A systematic review and meta-analysis of comparative studies. *Journal of Sexual Medicine, 16*(5), 624–632. https://doi.org/10.1016/j.jsxm.2019.02.014

Bole, R., Lundy, S. D., Pei, E., Bajic, P., Parekh, N., & Vij, S. C. (2024). Rising vasectomy volume following reversal of federal protections for abortion rights in the United States. *International Journal of Impotence Research, 36*, 265–268. https://doi.org/10.1038/s41443-023-00672-x

Burnett, A. L. (2016). Evaluation and management of erectile dysfunction. In A. J. Wein, L. R. Kavoussi, A. W. Partin, & C. A. Peters (Eds.), *Campbell-Walsh urology* (11th ed., pp. 643–668). Elsevier.

Burnett, A. L., Nehra, A., Breau, R. H., Culkin, D. J., Faraday, M. M., Hakim, L. S., Heidelbaugh, J., Khera, M., McVary, K. T., Miner, M. M., Nelson, C. J., Sadeghi-Nejad, H., Seftel, A. D., & Shindel, A. W. (2018). Erectile Dysfunction: AUA Guideline. *The Journal of Urology, 200*(3), 633–641. https://doi.org/10.1016/j.juro.2018.05.004

Caleb, S., & Norris, H. (2025). *The LGBTQI+ Community reported high rates of discrimination in 2024.* https://www.americanprogress.org/article/the-lgbtqi-community-reported-high-rates-of-discrimination-in-2024/

Celigoj, F. A., & Costabile, R. A. (2016). Surgery of the scrotum and seminal vesicles. In A. J. Wein, L. R. Kavoussi, A. W. Partin, & C. A. Peters (Eds.), *Campbell-Walsh urology* (11th ed., pp. 946–966). Elsevier.

Centers for Disease Control and Prevention. (n.d.). *A guide to taking a sexual history* [Publication No. 99-8445]. https://www.cdc.gov/std/treatment/sexualhistory.pdf

Centers for Disease Control and Prevention. (2014). Recommendations for the laboratory-based detection of *Chlamydia trachomatis* and *Neisseria gonorrhoeae*—2014. *Morbidity and Mortatlity Weekly Report, 63*(RR-02), 1–19.

Centers for Disease Control and Prevention. (2019a). *HIV and gay and bisexual men.* https://www.cdc.gov/hiv/group/msm/index.html

Centers for Disease Control and Prevention. (2019b). *Sexually transmitted disease surveillance 2018.* https://doi.org/10.15620/cdc.79370

Centers for Disease Control and Prevention. (2021). *U.S. Public Health Service: Preexposure prophylaxis for the prevention of HIV infection in the United States—2021 Update: A clinical practice guideline.* https://www.cdc.gov/hiv/pdf/risk/prep/cdc-hiv-prep-guidelines-2021.pdf

Centers for Disease Control and Prevention. (2024). *Estimated HIV incidence and prevalence in the United States, 2018–2022.* HIV Surveillance Supplemental Report 2024, *29*(1). https://www.cdc.gov/ hiv-data/nhss/estimated-hiv-incidence-and-prevalence.html

Chaitoff, A., Killeen, T. C., & Nielsen, C. (2018). Men's health 2018: BPH, prostate cancer, erectile dysfunction, supplements. *Cleveland Clinic Journal of Medicine, 85*(11), 871–880. https://doi.org/10.3949/ccjm.85a.18011

Chovanec, M., & Cheng, L. (2022). Advances in diagnosis and treatment of testicular cancer. *BMJ (Clinical research ed.), 379*, e070499. https://doi.org/10.1136/bmj-2022-070499

Ciocanel, O., Power, K., & Eriksen, A. (2019). Interventions to treat erectile dysfunction and premature ejaculation: An overview of systematic reviews. *Sexual Medicine, 7*(3), 251–269. https://doi.org/10.1016/j.esxm.2019.06.001

Dalby, J., & Stoner, B. P. (2022). Sexually Transmitted Infections: Updates From the 2021 CDC Guidelines. *American Family Physician, 105*(5), 514–520. https://www.aafp.org/pubs/afp/issues/2022/0500/p514.html

Do, D., Rodriguez, P. J., Gratzl, S., Cartwright, B. M. G., Baker, C., & Stucky, N. L. (2025). Trends in incidence of syphilis among US adults from January 2017 to October 2024. *American Journal of Preventive Medicine.* https://doi.org/10.1016/j.amepre.2025.03.008

El-Hamd, M. A., Saleh, R., & Majzoub, A. (2019). Premature ejaculation: An update on definition and pathophysiology. *Asian Journal of Andrology, 21*(5), 425–432. https://doi.org/10.4103/aja.aja_122_18

Gavin, L., Moskosky, S., Carter, M., Curtis, K., Glass, E., Godfrey, E., Marcell, A., Mautone-Smith, N., Pazol, K., Tepper, N., & Zapata, L. (2014). Providing quality family planning services: Recommendations of CDC and the US Office of Population Affairs. *Morbidity and Mortality Weekly Report Recommendations and Reports, 63*(RR04), 1–29.

Gavin, L., & Pazol, K. (2016). Update: Providing quality family planning services—recommendations from CDC and the US Office of Population Affairs, 2015. *Morbidity and Mortality Weekly Report, 65*(9), 231–234. https://doi.org/10.15585/mmwr.mm6509a3

Gavin, L., Pazol, K., & Ahrens, K. (2017). Update: Providing quality family planning services—recommendations from CDC and the U.S. Office of Population Affairs, 2017. *Morbidity and Mortality Weekly Report, 66*(50), 1383–1385. https://doi.org/10.15585/mmwr.mm6650a4

Giona, S. The epidemiology of testicular cancer. In: N. Barber, & A. Ali (Eds.). *Urologic cancers* [Internet]. Brisbane (AU): Exon Publications; 2022 Sep 12. Chapter 9. Available from: https://www.ncbi.nlm.nih.gov/books/NBK585983/ doi: 10.36255/exon-publications-urologic-cancers-epidemiology-testicular-cancer

Haahr, M. K., Jensen, C. H., Toyserkani, N. M., Andersen, D. C., Damkier, P., Sørensen, J. A., et al. (2016). Safety and potential effect of a single intracavernous injection of autologous adipose-derived regenerative cells in patients with erectile dysfunction following radical prostatectomy: An open-label phase I clinical trial. *EBioMedicine, 5*, 204–210. https://doi.org/10.1016/j.ebiom.2016.01.024

Hatzichristou, D., Kirana, P. S., Banner, L., Althof, S. E., Lonnee-Hoffmann, R. A., Dennerstein, L., & Rosen, R. C. (2016). Diagnosing sexual dysfunction in men and women: Sexual history taking and the role of symptom scales and questionnaires. *Journal of Sexual Medicine, 13*(8), 1166–1182. https://doi.org/10.1016/j.jsxm.2016.05.017

Mackern-Oberti, J. P., Motrich, R. D., Breser, M. L., Sánchez, L. R., Cuffini, C., & Rivero, V. E. (2013). *Chlamydia trachomatis* infection of the male genital tract: An update. *Journal of Reproductive Immunology, 100*(1), 37–53. https://doi.org/10.1016/j.jri.2013.05.002

Marcell, A. V., & Male Training Center for Family Planning and Reproductive Health. (2014). *Preventive male sexual and reproductive health care: Recommendations for clinical practice.* Male Training Center for Family Planning and Reproductive Health and Office of Population Affairs.

Mark, K. P., Arenella, K., Girard, A., Herbenick, D., Fu, J., & Coleman, E. (2024). Erectile dysfunction prevalence in the United States: Report from the 2021 National Survey of Sexual Wellbeing. *The Journal of Sexual Medicine, 21*(4), 296–303. https://doi.org/10.1093/jsxmed/qdae008

McCabe, M. P., Sharlip, I. D., Atalla, E., Balon, R., Fisher, A. D., Laumann, E., Lee, S. W., Lewis, R., & Segraves, R. T. (2016). Definitions of sexual dysfunctions in women and men: A consensus statement from the Fourth International Consultation on Sexual Medicine 2015. *Journal of Sexual Medicine, 13*(2), 135–143.

McCabe, M. P., Sharlip, I. D., Lewis, R., Atalla, E., Balon, R., Fisher, A. D., Laumann, E., Lee, S. W., & Segraves, R. T. (2016). Incidence and prevalence of sexual dysfunction in women and men: A consensus statement from the Fourth International Consultation on Sexual Medicine 2015. *Journal of Sexual Medicine, 13*(2), 144–152. https://doi.org/10.1016/j.jsxm.2015.12.034

McMahon, C., Althof, S., Rosen, R., Giuliano, F., Miner, M., Osterloh, I. H., Muirhead, G. J., & Harty, B. (2019). PEPIX Multi-Centre Study Group. The oxytocin antagonist cligosiban prolongs intravaginal ejaculatory latency and improves patient-reported outcomes in men with lifelong premature ejaculation: Results of a randomized, double-blind, placebo-controlled proof-of-concept trial (PEPIX). *Journal of Sexual Medicine, 16*(8), 1178–1187. https://doi.org/10.1016/j.jsxm.2019.05.016

Meites, E., Szilagyi, P. G., Chesson, H. W., Unger, E. R., Romero, J. R., & Markowitz, L. E. (2019). Human papillomavirus vaccination for adults: Updated recommendations of the Advisory Committee on Immunization Practices. *Morbidity and Mortality Weekly Report, 68*(32), 698–702. https://doi.org/10.15585/mmwr.mm6832a3

Morgan, R. E., Dragon, C., Daus, G., Holzberg, J., Kaplan, R., Menne, H., Smith, A. S., & Spiegelman, M. (2020, August). *Updates on terminology of sexual orientation and gender identity survey measures.* FCSM 20-03. Federal Committee on Statistical Methodology.

NIH Consensus Conference. (1993). Impotence. NIH Consensus Development Panel on impotence. *JAMA, 270*, 83–90.

Nurse Practitioners in Women's Health. (2020). *Women's health nurse practitioner: Guidelines for practice and education* (8th ed.). https://www.npwh.org/store/products/details/380

Papp, J. R. (2024). CDC laboratory recommendations for syphilis testing, United States, 2024. MMWR. *Recommendations and Reports, 73*(1). https://doi.org/10.15585/mmwr.rr7301a1

Patrick, D. L., Giuliano, F., Ho, K. F., Gagnon, D. D., McNulty, P., & Rothman, M. (2009). The Premature Ejaculation Profile: Validation of self-reported outcome measures for research and practice. *BJU International, 103*(3), 358–364. https://doi.org/10.1111/j.1464-410X.2008.08041.x

Rosen, R. C., Catania, J., Pollack, L., Althof, S., O'Leary, M., & Seftel, A. D. (2004). Male Sexual Health Questionnaire (MSHQ): Scale development and psychometric validation. *Urology, 64*(4), 777–782. https://doi.org/10.1016/j.urology.2004.04.056

Rosen, R. C., Riley, A., Wagner, G., Osterloh, I. H., Kirkpatrick, J., & Mishra, A. (1997). The international index of erectile function (IIEF): A multidimensional scale for assessment of erectile dysfunction. *Urology, 49*(6), 822–830. https://doi.org/10.1016/S0090-4295(97)00238-0

Rovito, M. J., Craycraft, M., Adams, W. B., Maresca, M., Saab, M. M., Cary, C., Gooljar, C., Martinez, S., & Abu Zanet, R. (2022). A cross-sectional analysis of testicular cancer symptom recognition and stage of diagnosis. *American Journal of Men's Health, 16*(3), 15579883221104900. https://doi.org/10.1177/15579883221104900

Saffati, G., Naeem, T., Guhan, M., Abello, A., Hinojosa-Gonzalez, D. E., Kaaki, B., Stocks, B. T., Lipshultz, L. I., & Khera, M. (2023). Hyperbaric oxygen therapy as a treatment for erectile dysfunction: A meta-analysis. *Sexual Medicine Reviews*, 12(1), 94–99. https://doi.org/10.1093/sxmrev/qead043.

Serefoglu, E. C., McMahon, C. G., Waldinger, M. D., Althof, S. E., Shindel, A., Adaikan, G., Becher, E. F., Dean, J., Giuliano, F., Hellstrom, W. J. G., Giraldi, A., Glina, S., Incrocci, L., Jannini, E., McCabe, M., Parish, S., Rowland, D., Segraves, R. T., Sharlip, I., & Torres, L. O. (2014). An evidence-based unified definition of lifelong and acquired premature ejaculation: Report of the second International Society for Sexual Medicine Ad Hoc Committee for the Definition of Premature Ejaculation. *Journal of Sexual Medicine, 2*(2), 41–59. https://doi.org/10.1111/jsm.12524

Sharlip, I. D., Belker, A. M., Honig, S., Labrecque, M., Marmar, J. L., Ross, L. S., Sandlow, J. I., & Sokal, D. C. (2015). *Vasectomy guideline 2015*. American Urological Association. https://doi.org/10.1016/j.juro.2012.09.080

Shindel, A.W., Althof, S. E., Carrier, S.,Chou, R., McMahon, C. G., Mulhall, J. P., Paduch, D. A., Pastuszak, A. W., Rowland, D., Tapscott, A. H., & Sharlip, I. D. (2022). Disorders of ejaculation: An AUA/SMSNA guideline. *Journal of Urology, 207*(3), 504–512. https://doi.org/10.1097/JU.0000000000002392.

Sineath, R. C., & Mehta, A. (2019). Preservation of fertility in testis cancer management. *Urologic Clinics of North America, 46*(3), 341–351. https://doi.org/10.1016/j.ucl.2019.04.010

Smith, S. G., Zhang, X., Basile, K. C., Merrick, M. T., Wang, J., Kresnow, M., & Chen, J. (2018). *The National Intimate Partner and Sexual Violence Survey: 2015 data brief—updated release*. National Center for Injury Prevention and Control, Centers for Disease Control and Prevention.

Trussell, J., Aiken, A. R. A., Micks, E., & Guthrie, K. A. (2018). Efficacy, safety, and personal considerations. In R. A. Hatcher, A. L. Nelson, J. Trussell, C. Cwiak, P. Cason, M. S. Policar, A. R. A. Aiken, J. Marrazzo, & D. Kowal (Eds.), *Contraceptive technology* (21st ed., pp. 95–128). Ayer Company Publishers.

U.S. Preventive Services Task Force. (2010). *Final evidence review: testicular cancer: Screening*. https://www.uspreventiveservicestaskforce.org/Page/Document/final-evidence-review96/testicular-cancer-screening

U.S. Preventive Services Task Force. (2021). Screening for Chlamydia and Gonorrhea: U.S. Preventive Services Task Force Recommendation Statement. *JAMA, 326*(10), 949–956.

Verbiest, S., McClain, E., & Woodward, S. (2016). Advancing preconception health in the United States: Strategies for change. *Upsala Journal of Medical Science, 121*(4), 222–226. https://doi.org/10.1080/03009734.2016.1204395.

Wang, C. M., Wu, B. R., Xiang, P., Xiao, J., & Hu, X. C. (2023). Management of male erectile dysfunction: From the past to the future. *Frontiers in Endocrinology (Lausanne), 27*(14), 1148834. https://doi.org/10.3389/fendo.2023.1148834.

Workowski, K. A., Bachmann, L. H., Chan, P. A., Johnston, C. M., Muzny, C. M., Park, I., Reno, H., Zenilman, J. M., & Bolan, G. A. (2021). Sexually transmitted infections treatment guidelines, 2021. *Morbidity and Mortality Weekly Report Recommendations and Reports, 70*(4), 1–192.

Yafi, F. A., Jenkins, L., Albersen, M., Corona, G., Isidori, A. M., Goldfarb, S., Maggi, M., Nelson, C. J., Parish, S., Salonia, A., Tan, R., Mulhall, J. P., & Hellstrom, W. J. G. (2016). Erectile dysfunction. *Nature Reviews Disease Primers, 2*(1), 16003. https://doi.org/10.1038/nrdp.2016.3

Yang, F., Li, J., Dong, L., Tan, K., Huang, X., Zhang, P., Liu, X., Chang, D., & Yu, X. (2021). Review of vasectomy complications and safety concerns. *The World Journal of Men's Health, 39*(3), 406–418. https://doi.org/10.5534/wjmh.200073

Yazici, S., Del Biondo, D., Napodano, G., Grillo, M., Calace, F. P., Prezioso, D., Crocetto, F., & Barone, B. (2023). Risk factors for testicular cancer: Environment, genes and infections—Is it all? *Medicina, 59*(4), 724. https://doi.org/10.3390/medicina59040724

Zhang, X., & Eisenberg, M. L. (2022). Vasectomy utilization in men aged 18–45 declined between 2002 and 2017: Results from the United States National Survey for Family Growth data. *Andrology, 10*, 137–142. https://doi.org/10.1111/andr.13093

CHAPTER 11

Gynecologic Health Care for Lesbian, Bisexual, and Queer Women and Transgender and Gender Diverse Individuals

Katie DePalma

The editors acknowledge Simon Adriane Ellis, who was author of the previous edition of this chapter.

INTRODUCTION

Health, and specifically gynecologic health, is experienced in the context of each person's life. It is experienced biologically, psychosocially, sexually, and spiritually by all people, including individuals of all sexual orientations and gender identities. However, numerous communities including lesbian, bisexual, and queer (LBQ) women and transgender and gender diverse (TGD) individuals, face inequitable barriers to respectful and informed gynecologic health care. It is important to recognize that care of LBQ women and TGD individuals is not inherently more complex than care for heterosexual or cisgender people, but health outcomes for this population are directly influenced by the quality of healthcare interactions and by minority stress. This chapter explores the special sexual and reproductive healthcare needs of LBQ women and TGD individuals through the frameworks of intersectional feminism and Reproductive Justice (SisterSong, n.d.) (see Chapter 2 for more information).

Throughout this chapter, we will refer to the broader lesbian, gay, bisexual, transgender/gender diverse, and queer community with the acronym LGBTQ+, with the "+" acknowledging other sexual orientation or gender identities as well as the everpresent evolution of language. As is discussed subsequently, gender and sexual orientation are separate contructs and can be associated with different healthcare needs or considerations. The more distinct groups will be referred to as TGD and LBQ when the umbrella term LGBTQ+ is not applicable or accurate.

GENDER AND SEXUAL MINORITIES IN THE UNITED STATES

In 2024, the U.S. population was estimated to be 340.1 million people, of which over 31 million people (almost 10% of the population) identified as lesbian, gay, bisexual, TGD, or queer (Jones, 2025; U.S. Census Bureau, 2024). This is a notable increase from 2014, when the estimate was only 3.7 percent of the population, and these numbers are expected to increase as the U.S. population ages. Due to an array of known and unknown factors, the percentage of each generation that identifies as LGBTQ+ is increasing significantly, with a dramatic comparison between Baby Boomers (3%) and Generation Z (23.1%) (Jones, 2025). Of these individuals, more identify themselves as women than as men (Newport, 2018). The LBQ and TGD communities represent a large and dynamic segment of the U.S. population with a wide range of gynecologic and other health needs. As this population grows, clinician competency must grow.

Support from Professional Organizations

Professional organizations in sexual and reproductive health have affirmed the importance of access to quality health care for women of all sexual orientations (American College of Nurse-Midwives, 2014, reaffirmed 2019; American College of Obstetricians and Gynecologists, 2012, reaffirmed 2024) and for TGD people (American College of Nurse-Midwives, 2012, revised 2021; American College of Obstetricians and Gynecologists, 2011, reaffirmed 2021; Nurse Practitioners in Women's Health, 2022). In fact, all major medical associations in the United States have declared gender-affirming care and surgery to be medically necessary for TGD individuals (Scheim et al., 2022).

LANGUAGE, CONCEPTS, AND CONSTRUCTS OF GENDER AND SEXUALITY

Clinicians may be intimidated or overwhelmed by perfectionist tendencies, trying to learn and use appropriate language, and by trying to unlearn socially engrained concepts of gender. Despite compassionate intentions, these feelings of being overwhelmed can present to patients as erasure, dismissal, or even disgust. Clinicians are encouraged to separate themselves from perfectionism and approach language and concepts with curiosity and respect, shifting power to patients to define themselves, and then following their leads.

Language and Definitions

There are no official definitions for "lesbian," "bisexual," "queer," "transgender," "nonbinary," or "gender diverse." Indeed, definitions and labels are constantly evolving and are often complex. For example, since the previous editions of this text, the term "gender nonconforming" was replaced by "nonbinary" which is now replaced by "gender diverse" in regards to general social preference. Some argue that narrowly defined categories are inherently problematic when it comes to sexual orientation and gender identity. FORGE, an organization that serves TGD people and their loved ones, articulates this as the "terms paradox"; terms are essentially meaningless in that there is no consensus on their definitions, yet they are crucial in that clinicians must ascertain the terms each person uses to define themselves and reflect them back when providing care (FORGE, 2012). The simplest way to think of this is that people are who they say they are, and clinicians should be respectful of this self-identification in the language they use when communicating with and about the people they serve. For purposes of clarity, this section outlines basic terms and concepts used in this chapter. **Table 11-1** summarizes these terms and concepts.

Concepts

It is important to emphasize that sexual orientation and gender identity are two separate concepts. Similarly, sex and gender are two separate concepts. Sex is a designation based on one's chromosomes and genitalia. While sex is often thought of as binary, consisting only of male or female, there are a substantial number of intersex people whose chromosomes or genitals fall somewhere in between these two designations. In this chapter, we will refer to sex based on assignment at birth: people assigned female at birth (AFAB), people assigned male at birth (AMAB), and intersex people.

Both sexual orientation and gender are dynamic and multifaceted. Sexual orientation describes the emotional, physical, and romantic attachments an individual has towards others

TABLE 11-1 Gender and Sexual Orientation Terminology

Term	Meaning
Agender	A person whose understanding of self is outside the concept of gender or does not align with a specific gender identity.
Asexual	A person who experiences little to no sexual attraction or desire for sexual activity. This does not mean a person does not engage in sexual activities.
Assigned female at birth (AFAB)	A person who was given the designation of female at birth based on the appearance of their genitals.
Assigned male at birth (AMAB)	A person who was given the designation of male at birth based on the appearance of their genitals.
Bisexual	A sexual orientation in which a person is attracted to people with both male and female gender identities.
Cisgender	Describes a person whose gender identity is in alignment with the sex they were assigned at birth. For example, a person who was assigned female at birth and identifies as a woman. Often shortened to "cis."
Gay	Frequently used as an umbrella term for all nonheterosexual people. Historically used to refer to a sexual orientation in which a person with a male gender identity is primarily attracted to other people with a male gender identity.
Gender	A social rather than biological construct that assigns specific roles, traits, and responsibilities to girls, women, boys, men, and gender diverse people. These characteristics vary among societies and cultures and also change over time.
Gender affirmation	Any process that strives to better align gender expression, social perception, or physical appearance with gender identity.
Gender binary	A social construct that recognizes only two mutually exclusive gender identities: male and female. In the United States, gender has historically been understood only through a binary construct; however, this is not in alignment with proven biologic variations of sex.
Gender diverse	An umbrella term describing a person whose gender identity is not limited to solely male or solely female.
Gender expression	The way in which a person outwardly expresses gender, which includes mannerisms, style of dress, behavior, and modifiable aspects of physical appearance.
Gender identity	A person's internal understanding of self in regard to gender. Gender identity may or may not be in alignment with one's sex or gender expression.
Gender nonconforming	Similar to nonbinary, this is an umbrella term describing a person whose gender identity is not limited to solely male or solely female.
Genderqueer	Similar to nonbinary, this is an umbrella term describing a person whose gender identity is not limited to solely male or solely female.

Term	Meaning
Intersex	A descriptor for individuals with variations of sex based on differences in chromosomes, anatomy, secondary sex traits, and/or hormones. Intersex is often used to describe sex chromosomes other than XX or XY or for genitals or gonads that do not appear male or female; however, many variations of intersex are not obvious at birth.
Lesbian	A sexual orientation in which a person with a female gender identity is primarily attracted to other people with a female gender identity.
Man	A person who identifies as male, regardless of sex assigned at birth.
Nonbinary	Describes a person whose gender identity is not limited to solely male or solely female. This umbrella term covers a diverse array of gender identities.
Pansexual	A sexual orientation in which a person is attracted to people of all gender identities, not limited to those with binary gender identities.
Queer	Umbrella term used to describe all nonheterosexual people. Historically it has been used as a derogatory slur by those outside of lesbian, gay, bisexual, and queer (LGBQ) and TGD communities; it is still experienced as derogatory by some community members. For other community members, "queer" is used as an empowering, reclaimed term that allows for discussion of sexual orientation outside of a binary construct of gender.
Sex	A construct that classifies people into separate categories based on their chromosomal makeup and the appearance of their genitals. One's natal sex is the sex that was assigned at the time of birth. Although sex is often thought of as binary, there is actually a great deal of human variation in regard to sex chromosomes.
Sexual orientation	A concept describing one's sexual attraction, identity, and behavior.
Trans feminine	Describes a person who was assigned male at birth and who identifies as female or on the feminine spectrum.
Transgender	Describes a person whose gender identity is not in alignment, in some way, with the sex assigned at birth. Transgender people can have binary or nonbinary gender identities. Often shortened to "trans."
Transgender man	A person who was assigned the female sex at birth and has a male gender identity. Transgender men may or may not pursue medical or surgical interventions to better align their physical appearance with their gender identity.
Transgender woman	A person who was assigned the male sex at birth and has a female gender identity. Transgender women may or may not pursue medical or surgical interventions to better align their physical appearance with their gender identity.
Trans masculine	Describes a person who was assigned female at birth and who identifies as male or on the masculine spectrum.
Two-spirit	Stemming from Indigenous North American cultures, this term refers to a person who possesses both a female and a male spirit. Two-spirit is considered a third gender and has a valued role in many Indigenous communities.
Woman	A person who identifies as female, regardless of sex assigned at birth.

Data from Human Rights Campaign. (2023, May 31). *Glossary of Terms*. Human Rights Campaign. https://www.hrc.org/resources/glossary-of-terms; Olson, S., & DePalma, K. (2024). Gender-affirming care. In J. Phillippi, & I. Kantrowitz Gordon (Eds.), *Varney's midwifery* (7th ed., pp. 532–534). Jones & Bartlett Learning.

(National LGBTQIA+ Health Education Center, 2024). Sexual attraction refers to whom, if anyone, a person desires sexually or fantasizes about, and it may be described as sexual preference or desire. Sexual identity refers to an individual's inner understanding of themselves regarding sexual orientation and the words they use to describe themselves as sexual beings. Sexual behavior refers to an individual's sexual partners and the sexual activities in which they engage. All people have all three components; in some people the three components are in alignment, while in other people they are different.

Lesbian has historically been used to refer to the sexual orientation of people assigned female at birth who are attracted to sexual partners who were also assigned female at birth; a better definition might be people with a female gender identity who are attracted to other people with a female gender identity. Individuals who identify as bisexual or pansexual are attracted to more than one gender identity. *Queer* is a reclaimed word that is used as an umbrella term to describe all people who are not heterosexual. The use of queer also allows people to describe their sexual orientation in an inclusive way that does not refer to a singular gender. Additionally, some people identify as asexual and experience little to no sexual attraction or desire for sexual activity.

Constructs

Gender

Gender is a social construct that assigns roles and attributes to people based on a society's or culture's beliefs about women, girls, men, boys, and gender diverse people. Like sexual orientation, gender identity has three components: sex assigned at birth, gender identity, and gender expression. *Sex assigned at birth* refers to the label that was placed on a person by the clinician attending their birth. *Gender identity* refers to one's understanding of themselves regarding their internal experience of gender. *Gender expression* refers to one's outward appearance or how they present to the world and includes things like dress, hair style, mannerisms, and other factors that communicate gender cues to others. In any given person, these components may be the same, or they may differ significantly. It is important to remember that a person's sexual orientation or appearance does not define that individual's gender identity, and vice versa.

Transgender is an umbrella term used to describe individuals whose gender identity is in some way different from their sex assigned at birth. Numerous terms describe this same concept; this chapter uses the term "transgender" for clarity. A transgender woman is a person who was assigned male at birth and has a female gender identity. A transgender man is a person who was assigned female at birth and has a male gender identity. These are examples of binary gender identities in which a person identifies as either male or female, but not both or neither. The term *cisgender* refers to someone whose gender identity matches the sex they were assigned at birth.

Genders Outside the Binary

In reality, a great number of people do not comfortably identify within this binary gender framework. Many people identify as somewhere between male and female, as both male and female, as alternately male or female, or as having no gender at all. A great number of terms are used to describe this relationship to the social construct of gender; for purposes of clarity, this chapter uses the term *gender diverse*. Because the terms *transgender woman* and *transgender man* are inherently binary, in this chapter the terms *trans feminine* and *trans masculine* will be used to refer to individuals who identify as more feminine or more masculine than the sex they were assigned at birth, rather than just those with a binary gender identity.

Affirmation of Gender

Gender affirmation refers to any process that strives to better align one's gender expression, social perception, or physical appearance with one's gender identity. Examples include seeking pharmacologic and/or surgical interventions to change secondary sex characteristics, wearing a particular style of clothing, and requesting the use of one's chosen name and pronoun in social interactions. Assumptions about desire for pharmacologic or surgical gender-affirming interventions can be problematic when caring for TGD patients, as they are often not aligned with an individual's goals and can diminish trust. A person's gender identity is valid regardless of whether they have pursued medical interventions. By leading with curiosity and respect, clinicians should base care plans on a patient's current anatomy and desired options for gender affirmation, if any.

Sexual Identity and Behavior

The fact that identity does not always mirror behavior can make the healthcare needs of LBQ women and TGD people complex to understand, despite care provision being quite straightforward. One cannot make assumptions about a patient's sexual behaviors based on identity alone. For example, there is well-established research showing that most lesbian-identified individuals have had male sex partners in their lifetime, including a significant number with recent male partners (CDC, 2021). Similarly, there is also data that shows a number of heterosexual-identified people have had recent same-sex partners (Mendelsohn et al., 2022). Like behavior, identity is fluid over time. Eighteen percent of 18- to 24-year-olds report at least one change in identity over a 5-year span, with cisgender women demonstrating greater fluidity in sexual identity than their male peers (Mittleman, 2023).

HISTORICAL AND SOCIOPOLITICAL INFLUENCES ON HEALTH

Minority Stress

Based on common logic and decades of research, we know that communities and individuals who are exposed to persistent increased stress related to societal discrimination experience more health disparities—Meyer (2003) describes this as *minority stress*. The specific groups and stressors vary by society, but the U.S. government is built upon inherently discriminatory structures, the effects of which are woven throughout current legislation, policy, and social power dynamics. In the United States, white cisgender heterosexual men are the most protected group, as they are intentionally written into foundational law. All other groups have varying degrees of disadvantage, arguably one of the most disadvantaged being Black and Indigenous transgender women. A broad and basic example of structural disadvantage woven into U.S. society is the lack of legal protection for over half of the U.S. population. Women were not mentioned in the protections of the U.S. constitution when it was written and it was not until 2025 that the executive branch acknowledged that the Equal Rights Amendment (ERA) is law. The U.S. government effectively ignored the ERA for almost a century, as it was created in 1923 and was ratified in 2020 and met legal criteria to become the 28th Amendment to the U.S. Constitution (Salas-Betsch & Kelly, 2024). At the time this chapter was written, we do not yet know the outcomes of how the ERA will inevitably be challenged in the courts.

In addition to sex, gender, and sexuality, clinicians must be aware of the intersectionality (Crenshaw, 1989) of other structurally oppressed identities and how that may influence health, as systems of oppression work synergistically in harming individuals with multiple marginalized identities. Examples of these identities include: any race or ethnicity that is not white and European, someone who is a migrant/immigrant/undocumented, someone who is poor or unhoused, religion other than Christianity, having a low level of education, one's degree of ability/disability, someone who is or has been incarcerated, using a language other than English, and having a larger body size. An individual's *allostatic load*, or cumulative chronic stress of personal life events, is inversely tied to physical and mental health (McEwan & Stellar, 1993; Guidi et al., 2020). Increased allostatic load or overload is associated with changes in biomarkers which increase the risk of conditions like cardiovascular disease, diabetes mellitus, preeclampsia, seizures, breast and ovarian cancers, periodontal disease, depression, and anxiety (Guidi, 2020). In addition to minority stress and allostatic load, the concept of *weathering* describes the impact of external stressors on health. Weathering is cumulative health effects of repeated exposure to structural exclusion, whether that be social, political, or economic (Geronimus, 2001). The concept of weathering is what explains that racism is what harms health, not race, or that transphobia is what harms health, not being transgender. While each framework is unique, it may be helpful to consider these concepts in sequence—systemic oppression and exclusion leads to allostatic overload, sustained allostatic overload leads to weathering and minority stress. Health care, and especially gynecologic care, of LBQ women and TGD individuals is complicated only by societal exclusion.

Historical Trauma

Historical trauma is the cumulative psychological harm experienced by a group of people, often over many generations, due to societal marginalization and violence (The Oxford Review, 2025). This type of trauma can persist for centuries and can affect the health of future community members, even those who did not directly experience specific events. Historical trauma of the LGBTQ+ community has differences from other communities based on race or religion because there is not a familial intergenerational component, though the trauma persists through communities. Unfortunately, violence inflicted on LGBTQ+ people persists in the United States and around the world. From blatant hate crimes on the individual level, to forced assimilation or rejection in communities, to political exclusion and attacks on a societal level, LGBTQ+ people have and continue to experience structural oppression. Consequently, those from outside the community should be cautioned against assumptions that social progress or isolated inclusive policies negate historical and ongoing trauma.

Social Determinants of Health

Adverse Childhood Events

Adult LBQ and TGD individuals report adverse childhood experiences at incredibly high rates. LBQ women reported childhood emotional abuse (72%), physical abuse (42%), sexual abuse (43%), and bullying (67%); transgender individuals reported childhood emotional abuse (75%), physical abuse (44%), sexual abuse (45%), and bullying (70%); and nonbinary individuals reported childhood emotional abuse (82%), physical abuse (40%), sexual abuse (41%), and bullying (53%) (Meyer et al., 2021).

Education and Economic Stability

In the United States, LGBTQ+ adults are unemployed at a rate that is twice the national level, and 68 percent of LGBTQ+ people report not making enough money to make ends meet (Meyer et al., 2021). In the LBQ and TGD populations, 48 percent of people live in low-income households with income lower than 200 percent of the national poverty level and 15 percent report recent housing instability (Meyer et al., 2021).

Violence and Harassment

In adulthood, 46% of LBQ women and 48% of TGD people report at least one instance of physical assault and half of LBQ women and 61% of TGD people have been threatened with violence (Meyer et al., 2021). Black and Latina trans women in the United States are affected by the highest rates of physical and sexual violence and homicide (Medina-Martinez et al., 2021). Trans feminine people of color are one of the most vulnerable groups and experience such high rates of violence due to a combination of hate crimes, intimate partner violence, lack of legal protections, lack of gun-control legislation, and anti-transgender laws in the United States (Everytown, 2024).

Resilience

There are many factors of resilience that can be considered social determinants of health. *Resilience* is a trait that all individuals possess and generally refers to the ability to adapt or recover in the face of adversity or threatening situations (Peel et al., 2022). In terms of health, having higher resilience can be protective against weathering and minority stress and therefore is associated with better health. Characteristics associated with resilience in the LGBTQ+ population are optimism, hope, emotional intelligence, transparency, low levels of internalized bias, and having social support (Peel et al., 2022). Social support is incredibly impactful and includes forms like family connectedness, social network size, safe environments, family and friend support, steady relationships, accepting work environments, and feelings of community connectedness (Peel at al., 2022). The LGBTQ+ community has been recognized for the ability to form deep interpersonal connectedness with friends; this is often referred to as *chosen family*. With many in the community having been rejected by their families of origin, chosen families can be deeply tied to resilience. Despite this, there is also harm that arises from within the community such as racism, ableism, transphobia, and the dismissal or erasure of nonbinary and bisexual identities. It is also important to recognize that while many groups with historical trauma are praised for their resilience, focusing on displays of resilience, instead of the reasons resilience is needed, only perpetuates societal harm by minimizing the role of the oppressor(s).

Barriers to Care

There are numerous barriers to accessing and receiving health care in the LBQ and TGD populations. While some barriers are related to socioeconomic disadvantages, most barriers stem from individuals associating healthcare environments and clinicians with a high likelihood of experiencing harm. This is highlighted in the TGD population, in which only about half (55.9%) of individuals have seen a clinician specifically for transgender-related care (Feldman et al., 2021) and 27% of individuals have been outright denied care (Scheim et al., 2022).

Financial Barriers

Barriers related to income and economic circumstances make health care less accessible in the LBQ and TGD populations. There are higher rates of poverty in TGD individuals as well as exclusion of gender-affirming care from many Medicaid programs (Scheim et al., 2022). Despite similar rates of insurance in the TGD population compared to the cisgender population (90.5% vs. 89.5%), more TGD individuals were likely to avoid care due to costs (Feldman et al., 2021). These costs can be associated with copays, deductibles, income lost from time off, and the fact that gender-affirming care may not be covered by insurance.

Clinician Knowledge and Attitude

Research has consistently revealed that a great number of healthcare clinicians and students have positive intentions regarding care of LGBTQ+ individuals, but that knowledge gaps are barriers to providing competent care (Gentile et al., 2020; Karpel et al., 2023; Stewart & O'Reilly, 2017). Cruciani et al. (2024) found that despite a majority of mental health clinicians having positive beliefs about the LGBTQ+ population, implicit bias remains prevalent and is tied to a lack of knowledge about the needs and culture of the group. The same study found that the clinicians' lack of understanding was often related to lack of awareness and apprehension and decreased confidence regarding language. It has also been studied that healthcare clinicians' self-efficacy improved after LGBTQ+ cultural competency training and that increased self-efficacy is significantly associated with clinicians' intentions (Rhoten et al., 2021). Though more research is needed, this information highlights the importance of increased education for clinicians, as awareness and knowledge can reduce implicit bias, allow for better access to care and health outcomes, and could even increase job satisfaction by increasing clinician confidence.

Healthcare Stereotype Threat

Healthcare stereotype threat is the fear of being judged or treated poorly due to a clinician's perception of harmful stereotypes about one's identity and this threat influences the health of LBQ and TGD individuals (Fingerhut et al., 2022; LeBlanc et al., 2024). Despite many clinicians having positive intentions, harms related to bias continue to limit access to safe health care for LBQ and TGD individuals—microaggressions and implicit bias remain common and even explicit bias persists in healthcare settings. Stereotypes that exist in U.S. society about LBQ and TGD people and clinicians are not immune to these generalized perceptions. Exposure to stereotypes and other threats to social identity can begin even before a patient meets a clinician—use of names and pronouns, institutional policies, ads and artwork in a waiting room, access to inclusive bathrooms, gendered gowns, options on forms and health records, and overhearing staff conversations can all be sources of exclusion for LBQ and TGD patients and can influence their comfort and safety in the visit. In both the LBQ (Ojeda-Leitner & Lewis, 2021) and TGD (LeBlanc et al., 2024) populations, healthcare stereotype threat is associated with not having a personal healthcare provider, more frequent poor mental and physical health days, and delaying in seeking care for health concerns. By effectively limiting access to health care and contributing to allostatic load, healthcare stereotype threat can worsen health outcomes and perpetuate health disparities.

Health Disparities

The research around LBQ and TGD health disparities has become more robust over the past decade. Very large national surveys (TransPop, Generations, and U.S. Transgender Survey) have shown the disparities in the TGD population to be consistent with disease due to minority stress (Feldman et al., 2021). As we will review, many of the health disparities affecting the LBQ and TGD populations can also be associated with lack of access to inclusive clinicians and avoidance or delay of care due to historical trauma and healthcare stereotype threat, in addition to minority stress.

Self-Rated Health

According to the TransPop and Generations surveys, about one in four LBQ and transgender people report poor or fair health, a rate that is higher (41%) in nonbinary individuals (Meyer et al., 2021). About half of LBQ women and TGD individuals report a debilitating health condition (45% and 53%, respectively) (Meyer et al., 2021). Additionally, nonbinary individuals experience more chronic health conditions than the rest of the trans community (Feldman et al., 2021).

Mental Health

The LBQ and TGD communities are impacted by higher likelihood of anxiety, depression, and severe mental distress (Scheim et al., 2022). The prevalence of symptoms consistent with serious mental illness is 32% in LBQ women, 39% in transgender individuals, and 51% in nonbinary individuals (Meyer et al., 2021). Lifetime suicidal ideation was reported in 77% of LBQ women and in 81% of TGD individuals while 32% and 42% reported past suicide attempts, respectively (Meyer et al., 2021). Additionally, sexual and gender minoritized people have higher rates of substance use (including tobacco and alcohol), substance use disorder, and polysubstance use when compared to the heterosexual population (Hughto et al., 2021; Lee et al., 2023, Medina-Martinez et al., 2021). In TGD individuals, family support, especially from parents, is associated with lower rates of severe mental health distress and suicide (Scheim, 2022).

Cardiovascular Health

Minority stress is well known to be associated with worse cardiovascular (CV) health outcomes and this is seen in gender and sexual minoritized communities. LBQ women experience higher rates of hypertension (HTN) and signs of disease appear about a decade earlier than in heterosexual women, many between the ages of 35 and 44 (Bonomo et al., 2024). LBQ and TGD individuals also have higher rates of stroke and dyslipidemia, and trans men have higher rates of myocardial infarction (Bonomo et al., 2024). It was previously concluded that trans feminine individuals on hormone therapy had higher rates of venous thromboembolism (VTE) and ischemic stroke; however, it is now known those results were due to a type of estrogen that is no longer used in hormone therapy and current research shows minimal increased risk of VTE or ischemic stroke (Bonomo et al., 2024).

Endocrine and Metabolic Health

Trans masculine individuals and LBQ women have a higher incidence of having larger body sizes and being exposed to weight discrimination is associated with poor health outcomes (Bonomo et al., 2024; Olson et al., 2024). Additionally, studies have shown that trans masculine individuals on hormone therapy have increased incidence of metabolic syndrome and its components of elevated systolic blood pressure, blood glucose, and triglycerides along with a decrease in HDL, whereas estrogen therapy in both trans and cis women was associated with decreased risk of metabolic syndrome (Hashemi et al., 2024). LGBTQ+ individuals also have higher rates of eating disorders and disordered eating than heterosexual and cisgender individuals (Parker & Harriger, 2020). The morbidity associated with weight bias and disordered eating is an important consideration for clinicians who provide care and education to LGBTQ+ patients.

Sexually Transmitted Infections

In AFAB individuals who have AFAB sex partners (often referred to as "women who have sex with women" or WSW in literature) have higher risk of acquiring or transmitting bacterial vaginosis (BV) (CDC, 2021). More studies are emerging that demonstrate sexual transmission of BV; this information is supported by the high rates of concordance between vaginal flora in monogamous

AFAB sex partners (Takemoto et al., 2019). This increased risk is related to less frequent use of barrier protection (like condoms or dental dams), having a partner with BV, having a new partner, sharing of sex accessories or enhancements, having receptive oral sex, having digital-oral or digital-anal sex (CDC, 2021).

In the TGD population, particularly trans feminine individuals, there are disproportionately high rates of HIV with a prevalence of 19% (Scheim et al., 2022). This disparity is likely further exacerbated by the effects of racism, as only 7% of trans feminine individuals living with HIV are white (Scheim et al., 2022).

Cancers

Higher rates of colon, liver, breast, ovarian, and cervical cancers are seen in LBQ women (Medina-Martinez et al., 2021). While data is very limited, LBQ and transgender individuals who are AFAB do have potential risk factors for some reproductive cancers including fewer pregnancies, less frequent use of combined oral contraceptive pills, higher rates of smoking, increased experience of healthcare discriminations, and potential discomfort or dysphoria with certain exams, leading to avoidance of cancer screening. LBQ women and TGD individuals who are AFAB and have not had mastectomy have a longer time from symptom onset to diagnosis of breast cancer and are three times more likely to experience recurrence than cisgender heterosexual women (Eckhert et al., 2023). It has also been found that the LBQ and TGD populations have higher rates of never having cervical cancer screening than cisgender and heterosexual populations, with the exception of Black trans men, who had higher rates of screening (Lin et al., 2024).

TGD individuals have higher incidence of viral and smoking-related cancers, likely related to social determinants of health and higher rates of tobacco and alcohol use (Cathcart-Rake et al., 2024). TGD individuals are generally under screened for cancer leading to later-stage diagnoses and earlier deaths, however trans feminine individuals on estrogen therapy appear to have lower rates of breast cancer (compared to cisgender women) and prostate cancer (compared to cisgender men) (Cathcart-Rake et al., 2025).

GENDER-AFFIRMING CARE

Gender-affirming care is best understood as care that allows for better congruence between one's gender presentation and gender identity. This type of care is not unique to TGD individuals, as a vast number of cisgender people have gender-affirming interventions. Examples include cisgender women who have breast augmentation or Brazilian butt lifts and cisgender men who have chest surgery for gynecomastia or who use exogenous testosterone to treat lower endogenous levels. However, gender-affirming interventions are not restricted, withheld, or politicized for cisgender people the way they are for TGD people. As mentioned at the start of this chapter, the fact that gender-affirming health care is medically necessary care for TGD individuals has been affirmed by all major medical associations in the United States (Scheim et al., 2022).

Social and Nonclinical Interventions for Gender Affirmation

There are many forms of gender-affirming interventions, including social interventions that require no assistance from clinicians. Social interventions include requesting others to use the name and pronouns that are aligned with one's gender identity, legally changing one's gender marker on identity documents, and making nonmedical changes to one's gender presentation through the use of dress, makeup, jewelry, prosthetics, and other resources.

Some nonmedical gender-affirming interventions do have potential health risks that clinicians should be aware of and discuss with their patients; these include the practices of binding and tucking. *Binding* refers to the practice of compressing the tissue of the chest to achieve a more masculine profile. The use of the term "chest" is an intentional alternative to the term "breast," and in this instance refers to the mammary glands located over the pectoral muscles. *Tucking* refers to the practice of tucking the external genitals to achieve a more feminine profile; this is achieved by placing the penis between the buttocks and moving the testes into the inguinal canals. Both binding and tucking can be associated with fewer instances of being misgendered and many trans people bind or tuck not only for affirmation, but for safety. Given that gender-affirming medical and surgical interventions are not desired by all TGD people and are not accessible to many, it is important to approach care through a lens of harm reduction.

Binding has been associated with improved mental health and reduced dysphoria in many trans masculine individuals but can also be associated with an array of negative health outcomes when not done in a safe manner. Health and safety issues are related to the technique used to bind and the amount of time spent with the chest compressed. Complications can include skin irritation, skin abrasions, skin infections, musculoskeletal pain, postural changes, shortness of breath, muscle wasting, restriction of activity, and rib fracture. To decrease the risk of complications, clinicians should encourage using a properly sized, commercially produced binder made of breathable fabric; limiting the amount of time spent binding per day; avoiding binding during sleep and exercise; and avoiding the use of products not specifically designed for binding, including adhesives of any kind, non-adhesive bandages or wraps, and plastic wrap. A very supportive sports bra can be worn as an alternative to a binder during exercise. Clinicians who avoid shaming patients who disclose binding practices and are knowledgeable regarding how to safely bind will be most equipped to reduce or avoid potential harm.

Tucking is a very common practice among trans feminine individuals, with about three-fourths of trans women reporting a history of tucking, most of whom report tucking every day and for over 8 hours a day (Malik et al., 2024). Common health problems related to tucking are itching (most common), rash, pain in testicles or penis, skin infection, problems urinating or ejaculating, and UTI. To decrease the risk of complications, clinicians should encourage using a properly sized pair of commercially produced compression underwear (often called a gaff); tucking only tight enough for a secure hold but not tight enough to cause pain; limiting the amount of time spent tucking per day; and avoiding the use of products not specifically designed for tucking, including adhesives of any kind. If adhesives must be used, patients should be counseled to use gentle medical tape and to use only medical-grade adhesive remover. Additionally, extensive tucking is associated with lower semen quality in regard to motile sperm count (de Nie et al., 2022). Clinician awareness of the potential implication of tucking is important when assessing patients' concerns and when counseling regarding safety or fertility preservation.

Clinical Interventions for Gender Affirmation

Gender-affirming hormone therapy (GAHT) involves the use of hormones and other medications to change one's secondary sex characteristics to better align with one's gender identity and to treat gender dysphoria. Of note, not everyone who identifies as TGD experiences dysphoria, and a better term in that case would be gender incongruence. A diagnosis of gender dysphoria, as defined by the DSM-5, is associated with clinically significant distress or impairment in social, occupation, or other important areas of functioning and at least six months of significant incongruence between an individual's experienced gender and assigned gender, evident via two or more of the following (American Psychiatric Association, 2013 & Hembree et al., 2017):

- the experienced gender is significantly incongruent with one's primary or secondary sex characteristics
- the desire to alter sex characteristics that are not congruent with experienced gender
- the desire for sex characteristics to be aligned with another gender
- the desire to be of a different gender than that assigned
- the desire to be treated as a different gender than that assigned
- the certitude that one's experienced and displayed emotions are that of another gender than their assigned gender (Data from Hembree, W. C., Cohen-Kettenis, P. T., Gooren, L., Hannema, S. E., Meyer, W. J., Murad, M. H., Rosenthal, S. M., Safer, J. D., Tangpricha, V., & T'Sjoen, G. G. (2017). Endocrine Treatment of Gender-Dysphoric/Gender-Incongruent Persons: An Endocrine Society Clinical Practice Guideline. *Endocrine Practice, 102*(11), 3869–3903. https://doi.org/10.1210/jc.2017-01658)

Hormones and medications are readily available and the provision of GAHT is routine primary care (Coleman et al., 2022) and thus within the scope of practice for advanced practice clinicians, including physician assistants, nurse practitioners, certified midwives, and certified nurse-midwives. Through increasing the number of clinicians who are confident in the management of GAHT, access to life-saving care can be expanded for TGD patients.

Management of gender-affirming hormones is about as complex as some contraceptive or menopause care. An important distinction, however, is that gender dysphoria is associated with high rates of suicidal ideation and there is no alternative to GAHT, and so some considerations or contraindications to hormone use in cisgender patients are not considered in the same way when used for gender affirmation. For example, tools such as the *US Medical Eligibility Criteria for Contraceptive Use* (US MEC) should not be used to guide decisions regarding the use of feminizing hormone therapy in trans feminine individuals. Instead, decisions should be made using a shared decision-making model and harm reduction approach. There are very few absolute contraindications to gender-affirming hormone therapy and, given the safe and straightforward nature of GAHT, multiple national and international professional organizations have created free toolkits for clinicians who provide GAHT. These toolkits provide easy-to-use care checklists for consent, typical regimens of medication dosing and indications, and initiation and follow-up management. See **Box 11-1** for some of these resources.

BOX 11-1 Gender-Affirming Professional Resources

Policy Guidance and Staff Training

The National LGBT Health Education Center, a program of the Fenway Institute. https://www.lgbtqiahealtheducation.org/

Glossary of Terms. The National LGBT Health Education Center. https://www.lgbtqiahealtheducation.org/glossary/en/

Sexual Orientation and Gender Identity (SO/GI) Collection Demonstration Videos. The National LGBT Health Education Center. https://www.lgbtqiahealtheducation.org/courses/so-gi-data-collection-training/

LGBTQIA+ Care Organizational Change Videos. The National LGBT Health Education Center. https://www.lgbtqiahealtheducation.org/courses/lgbtqia-affirming-care-demonstration-videos/

Trans 101. Cedar River Clinics. https://cedarriverclinics.org/transtoolkit/trans101/

Lyon-Martin's Intake Forms. TransLine. https://transline.zendesk.com/hc/en-us/articles/229380508-Lyon-Martin-s-Intake-Forms

Learning Resources and Continuing Education

Learning Resources. National LGBT Health Education Center. https://www.lgbtqiahealtheducation.org/

Clinical Care Modules and Cheat Sheets. Cedar River Clinics. https://cedarriverclinics.org/transtoolkit/clinicalcare/

Addressing the Healthcare Needs of Transgender and Non-Binary People. Cardea Services. https://cardea.matrixlms.com/visitor_catalog_class/show/1300264

Resources for LGBTQ+ Health Equity—For Patients. GLMA. https://www.glma.org/resources.php

Transgender and Gender Diverse Healthcare Protocols

(Pending revision in 2025) *Endocrine Treatment of Gender-Dysphoric/Gender-Incongruent Persons: An Endocrine Society Clinical Practice Guideline.* Hembree et al. (2017). https://www.endocrine.org/guidelines-and-clinical-practice/clinical-practice-guidelines/gender-dysphoria-gender-incongruence

(Pending revision in 2025) *Guidelines for the Primary and Gender-Affirming Care of Transgender and Gender Nonbinary People*; 2nd edition. UCSF Gender Affirming Health Program, Department of Family and Community Medicine, University of California San Francisco. Deutsch, M.B. (ED.). June 2016. Available at transcare.ucsf.edu/guidelines

Standards of Care for the Health of Transgender and Gender Diverse People, Version 8. World Professional Association for Transgender Health (WPATH). https://www.tandfonline.com/doi/pdf/10.1080/26895269.2022.2100644

Transgender Health Care Toolkit. Cedar River Clinics. http://www.cedarriverclinics.org/transtoolkit/
TransLine Hormone Therapy Prescriber Guidelines. TransLine. https://transline.zendesk.com/hc/en-us/articles/229373288-TransLine-Hormone-Therapy-Prescriber-Guidelines
Transgender Medical Consultation Service. TransLine. https://transline.zendesk.com/hc/en-us
Quick Guide: Gender Affirming Hormone Therapy by the Primary Care Provider. Johns Hopkins Medicine. https://www.hopkinsmedicine.org/-/media/center-for-transgender-health/documents/tgd-gaht-quick-guide.ashx

Healthcare Educators

Harvard Medical School's Sexual and Gender Minority Health Teaching Module Series. National LGBT Health Education Center. https://www.lgbtqiahealtheducation.org/collection/hms-sgm-health-teaching-module-series/

Research

Creating Welcoming and Affirming Clinical Studies for LGBTQIA+ Participants Toolkit. National LGBT Health Education Center. https://www.lgbtqiahealtheducation.org/collection/clinical-studies-toolkit/

For Patients and Families

Resources for LGBTQ+ Health Equity—For Patients. GLMA. https://www.glma.org/resources.php
Safer Sex for Trans Bodies. Whitman Walker Health and The Human Rights Campaign Foundation. https://www.hrc.org/resources/safer-sex-for-trans-bodies
Parents and Friends of Lesbians and Gays (PFLAG). https://pflag.org/
Patient Resources. Cedar River Clinics. https://cedarriverclinics.org/transtoolkit/patientresourcelinks/
Find LGBTQ+ friendly healthcare near you. GLMA. https://lgbtqhealthcaredirectory.org/

Gender-Affirming Hormone Management

After collecting a thorough history and establishing a diagnosis of gender dysphoria, the first step in GAHT management is to assess the patient's individual goals and desired outcomes. A question that can aid in this assessment might be, "What changes are you hoping to see?" Some patients have the goal of a binary gender presentation while others may prefer a nonbinary presentation and prefer a lower-dose protocol. Other important considerations are interest in gender-affirming surgeries (like mastectomy, breast augmentation, or "top surgery") or procedures (like hair removal or dermal fillers), fertility plans or goals, and contraceptive needs. Referrals to appropriate gender-affirming surgeons and fertility specialists should be made, as indicated.

After establishing goals and expectations, a full history and physical must be completed and documented. In this, clinicians are assessing any conditions or medication interactions that may be affected by gender-affirming medications. Conditions such as hypertension, diabetes, coronary artery disease, hyperlipidemia, obstructive sleep apnea, polycythemia, and risk for venous thromboembolism (VTE) should be addressed, as these conditions can be affected by testosterone or estrogen, whether endogenous or exogenous (Coleman et al., 2022). While these conditions do not preclude GAHT, they should be considered in the informed consent process. If an individual would not be further harmed by delaying GAHT, optimization of chronic health conditions would ideally be addressed before initiating hormones, though this is not mandatory. For example, a transgender woman in her 40s who smokes cigarettes will have an increased risk for VTE on estrogen therapy, and though not a contraindication, she should be fully informed of the risks and harm-reduction measures like smoking reduction or cessation should be discussed.

Next in the GAHT initiation process, clinicians should order baseline labs (CBC, CMP, estradiol, total testosterone, lipid profile, and hemoglobin A1c), assess capacity to give consent, complete the informed consent process, obtain informed consent, and provide prescriptions for GAHT. If no other referrals or consultations are warranted, this can be done on the same day. Of note, informed consent can be written or verbal and restrictive policies such as obtaining letters of support from mental health clinicians are antiquated and unnecessary, though clinicians must follow local legislation. If a patient prefers or requires further evaluation of current conditions or mental health support in the decision-making process, a follow-up visit should be planned before the decision to begin hormones is made. If a person desires to have biological offspring in the future or is uncertain, referral for a fertility preservation consultation should ideally, but not necessarily, occur before the initiation of hormones. There is scant evidence regarding the impact of GAHT on fertility, though modest evidence has shown successful fertility even after years of GAHT (Cheng et al., 2019).

For the ongoing management and maintenance of GAHT, clinicians should refer to the "Transgender and Gender Diverse Healthcare Protocols" section of Box 11-1. The protocols contain the most up-to-date evidence-based information set forth by professional organizations involved in gender-affirming health care and include information abouts specific drugs and dosing, titration, routine follow-up care timing, lab monitoring, and management of side effects. In general, the target testosterone and estrogen levels in GAHT maintenance are the typical testosterone and peak ovulatory estrogen levels in cisgender individuals, though individualized plans can vary.

Masculinizing Hormone Therapy

To achieve masculine sex characteristics and suppress estrogen, testosterone is used in masculinizing GAHT for AFAB individuals and can be administered parenterally by intramuscular (IM), subcutaneous (SQ) injection, transdermal gel, or patch. With brief education, injections can be self-administered (or administered by a support person) typically weekly and SQ routes have the benefit of smaller needles and less pain when compared to IM (Deutsch, 2016). For transdermal gel, it is important for clinicians to thoroughly educate patients on proper use which, for testosterone, involves daily application to the shoulder or upper arm, remaining dry for two hours, and avoiding contact of the gel with others, especially women, children, and pets, to avoid virilizing effects (Deutsch, 2016).

Complications or undesired side effects related to GAHT are not inherently reasons to discontinue therapy and they should be evaluated and treated as indicated. For example, in the case of polycythemia, peak testosterone level should be evaluated, pathology (such as obstructive sleep apnea) should be ruled out, and testosterone dosing and/or frequency should be adjusted as indicated. Additionally, therapeutic phlebotomy or blood donation may serve as a short-term treatment (Deutsch, 2016). See **Table 11-2** for typical effects of testosterone hormone therapy and associated risks. Absolute contraindications to gender-

TABLE 11-2 Expected Physical Changes, Time Course, and Risks Associated with GAHT

Effect	Onset	Time to Maximum Effect
Testosterone Regimen (Masculinizing)		
Acne/skin oiliness	1 – 6 months	1 – 2 years
Fat redistribution	1 – 6 months	2 – 5 years
Voice deepening	1 – 6 months	1 – 2 years
Cessation of menses	1 – 6 months	1 – 2 years
Clitoral enlargement	1 – 6 months	1 – 2 years
Vaginal atrophy	1 – 6 months	1 – 2 years
Facial and body hair growth	6 – 12 months	> 5 years
Hair loss (scalp)	6 – 12 months	> 5 years
Increased muscle mass	6 – 12 months	2 – 5 years
Risks associated with testosterone hormone therapy:		
Increased risk: Polycythemia, infertility, acne, alopecia, sleep apnea, weight gain, dyslipidemia	**Increased risk with the presence of additional risk factors:** Cardiovascular disease, diabetes mellitus	**No increased risk or inconclusive:** Low bone mass Breast, cervical, ovarian, or uterine cancers
Estrogen and Antiandrogen Regimen (Feminizing)		
Decreased spontaneous erections	1 – 3 months	3 – 6 months
Decreased sexual desire	1 – 3 months	Unknown
Softening of skin/decreased oiliness	3 – 6 months	Unknown
Decreased muscle mass	3 – 6 months	1 – 2 years
Breast growth	3 – 6 months	2 – 5 years
Decreased testicular volume	3 – 6 months	Variable
Decreased terminal hair growth	6 – 12 months	> 3 years
Increased hair on scalp	Variable	Variable
Decreased sperm production	Unknown	2 years
Voice changes	None	None
Risks associated with estrogen and anti-androgen hormone therapy:		
Increased risk: VTE, hyperkalemia (related to spironolactone), hypertriglyceridemia, weight gain	**Increased risk with the presence of additional risk factors:** Cardiovascular disease, cerebrovascular disease, meningioma (related to cyproterone), polyuria/dehydration (related to spironolactone), cholelithiasis, HTN, erectile dysfunction, diabetes mellitus, low bone mass/ osteoporosis, hyperprolactinemia	**No increased risk or inconclusive:** Breast and prostate cancer

Data from Coleman, E., Radix, A. E., Bouman, W. P., Brown, G. R., de Vries, A. L. C., Deutsch, M. B., Ettner, R., Fraser, L., Goodman, M., Green, J., Hancock, A. B., Johnson, T. W., Karasic, D. H., Knudson, G. A., Leibowitz, S. F., Meyer-Bahlburg, H. F. L., Monstrey, S. J., Motmans, J., Nahata, L., ... Arcelus, J. (2022). Standards of care for the health of transgender and gender diverse people, Version 8. *International Journal of Transgender Health, 23*(1), S1–S259. https://doi.org/10.1080/26895269.2022.2100644

affirming testosterone are not universally agreed upon but generally include active sex hormone-sensitive cancer (Deutsch, 2016), the inability to give informed consent, and pregnancy (due to potential virilization of the fetus).

Feminizing Hormone Therapy

Most feminizing GAHT protocols have a two-prong approach—the development of feminine sex characteristics via estrogen and the blockage of testosterone, most commonly via an antiandrogen. Estrogen in the form of estradiol can be administered by transdermal patch or gel, oral or sublingual tablet, or injection. Transdermal administration of estradiol is generally preferred when possible, as it is associated with quicker suppression of testosterone with lower dosing, bypasses the first-pass effect of the liver, and is associated with the lowest risk of VTE compared to other routes of administration (Cortez et al., 2024; Zucker et al., 2021). In fact, some studies showed no increased risk of VTE with transdermal estradiol (Deutsch, 2016).

Other forms of estrogen exist for the treatment of vasomotor symptoms of menopause in AFAB individuals, and while the management of menopause is similar to GAHT, those other forms have not been associated with therapeutic estrogen levels in trans feminine individuals. Additionally, ethinyl estradiol, the form of estrogen used in contraception, is associated with increased VTE risk and is no longer used in GAHT. Absolute contraindications to gender-affirming estrogen therapy are not universally agreed upon but generally include an active estrogen-sensitive cancer (Deutsch, 2016), the inability to give informed consent, and acute untreated VTE.

Most TGD individuals initiate gender-affirming hormones in adulthood after the development of secondary sex characteristics and some effects of pubertal testosterone are irreversible, such as voice deepening (Deutsch, 2016). To address potentially modifiable effects of testosterone, antiandrogens are commonly used along with estradiol in the most common feminizing GAHT protocols because these drugs can suppress endogenous testosterone, allow for a lower and safer dose of estradiol, and have modest feminizing effects on their own (Deutsch, 2016; Coleman et al., 2022). In the United States, spironolactone is the most commonly used antiandrogen medication and trans feminine individuals have the same risks as cisgender women, the most serious (though uncommon) being hyperkalemia (Deutsch, 2016). For patients with contraindications to spironolactone or who prefer a different medication, finasteride and dutasteride are other antiandrogen options (Deutsch, 2016).

Progesterone use in feminizing GAHT is not a component of standard protocols and is not supported by any strong evidence and, while it is unlikely to be harmful, concomitant use of estrogen and progesterone in GAHT is associated with a slightly greater VTE risk (Zucker et al., 2021; Deutsch, 2016). For patients who prefer to use progesterone as part of their GAHT, medroxyprogesterone acetate (Provera) is the most common form, and is anecdotally associated with positive increases in mood and libido as well as improved breast development in some individuals (Deutsch, 2016). In others, a negative effect on mood has been noted. Refer to Table 11-2 for typical effects of estrogen GAHT and antiandrogens and their associated risks.

As with testosterone GAHT, complications or side effects of estrogen GAHT should be addressed as indicated, but they do not necessitate the cessation of estrogen. An example of this is VTE while on estrogen. Management would include referral and temporary cessation of estrogen for the acute treatment of VTE, but transdermal estrogen may be later resumed, as there is no alternative to GAHT and management would be based on shared decision making and potentially include anticoagulation (Deutsch, 2016).

Surgical Affirmation of Gender

A wide variety of procedures are available for surgical gender affirmation, including procedures of the chest/breasts, genitals, body, face, head, and neck (see **Table 11-3**). Although many surgical procedures used in gender-affirming care are also used by cisgender patients for cosmetic appearance enhancement, when they are used for gender affirmation, they are both medically necessary and critical for the safety of TGD people. As such, these procedures should not be considered cosmetic. It is important for advanced practice clinicians to be aware of gender-affirming surgeries and procedures and their health implications in order to provide appropriate care post-procedure and to facilitate appropriate surgical referrals, as needed.

GYNECOLOGIC CARE

All trained reproductive health-care clinicians with an understanding of minority stress, trauma-informed care, and LBQ and TGD cultures have the capacity to provide evidence-based and affirming gynecologic care. As mentioned previously, LBQ and TGD individuals do not require inherently complicated care, as health and disease processes do not biologically differ from cisgender and heterosexual individuals. This section of the chapter will review special considerations for the care of LBQ and TGD individuals; however, please refer to Chapters 6, 8, 9, 12, 13, 19, 20, and 22 for more comprehensive information.

Health History and Organ Inventory

Care for any person should vary only due to specific risk factors and body parts an individual possesses—and, with the consent of the patient, it is the responsibility of the clinician to elicit that information. A trauma-informed approach to these conversations is necessary. This is especially true for LBQ and TGD patients given the harms associated with healthcare stereotype threat mentioned previously. Refer to **Box 11-2** for more information regarding creating safer spaces for conversations with LBQ and TGD patients. More information on trauma-informed care can be found in Chapter 5.

Organ Inventory

An assessment of what anatomy or organs a patient has should guide clinicians in making plans for care—this is especially true when providing gender-affirming or gynecologic care to TGD patients. Some refer to this assessment as making an *organ inventory* or *anatomical inventory* and this can be an effective way to be sure you are making evidence-based and comprehensive recommendations without becoming overwhelmed by concepts of sex, gender, and sexuality, especially if you are still building your confidence around these concepts. Two examples are:

1. Two patients report abnormal vaginal bleeding—one patient is a transgender woman, and the other is a cisgender woman with a history of a hysterectomy. A clinician would not recommend an endometrial biopsy for either, as neither patient's organ inventory has a uterus.

TABLE 11-3 Gender-Affirming Surgeries and Procedures

Facial Procedures
Brow contouring, hair transplant/hairline advancement, facelift following reconstruction of underlying skeletal structures, blepharoplasty (eyelid lift), cheek implants, chin reshaping, chondrolaryngoplasty (trachea shave)
Body Contouring
Liposuction, lipofilling, implants (pectoral, hip, gluteal, calf), monsplasty/mons reduction
Breast/Chest Procedures
Mastectomy with or without nipple-areola preservation, reconstruction/augmentation, liposuction
Genital Procedures
Phalloplasty (with or without scrotoplasty or prothesis): The use of flaps of tissue from donor sites to create a phallus and urethra via a series of three surgeries, typically. Donor sites include the radial forearm, anterolateral thigh, and abdomen. The new phallus may also include a penile implant to facilitate erection and insertive sex and has an average erect length of 14.1 cm. Compared to metoidioplasty, phalloplasty is associated with a larger phallus, greater potential for insertive sex, scarring at the donor site, and decreased erogenous sensation. *Metoidioplasty (with or without scrotoplasty or prosthesis):* A hormonally enlarged clitoris is released to create a phallus with an average erect length of 5.5 cm. Optional procedures that are often done simultaneously are urethral lengthening to the tip of the phallus and covered with adjacent skin, vaginectomy, and scrotoplasty. Compared with phalloplasty, metoidioplasty is associated with a less complex surgery (often one procedure), preserved erogenous sensation, a smaller phallus with limited ability for insertive sex. *Scrotoplasty:* Flaps of the labia majora are used to create a scrotum. Testicular implants may be placed during a subsequent procedure. *Vaginoplasty:* A vulva and vaginal canal are created using tissue from the penis, scrotum, and less commonly, the hip or abdomen. Typically, the urethra is shortened, the labia majora are created with scrotal skin, the labia minora created with penile skin, the citoris created from tissue from the glans, and the vaginal canal created with penile skin. This procedure requires frequent use of vaginal dilators for the first year to achieve desired vaginal size, followed by dilation 2–3 times a week for life for maintenance. *Vulvoplasty:* The same procedures as vaginoplasty to create the external genitalia only. No vagina, or a zero-depth vagina is created. *Orchiectomy:* Removal of one or both testicles. *Hysterectomy and/or salpingo-oophorectomy.*
Other Procedures
Hair removal (electrolysis, laser epilation), nipple or areolar tattoo, vocal cord shortening

Data from Coleman, E., Radix, A. E., Bouman, W. P., Brown, G. R., de Vries, A. L. C., Deutsch, M. B., Ettner, R., Fraser, L., Goodman, M., Green, J., Hancock, A. B., Johnson, T. W., Karasic, D. H., Knudson, G. A., Leibowitz, S. F., Meyer-Bahlburg, H. F. L., Monstrey, S. J., Motmans, J., Nahata, L., ... Arcelus, J. (2022). Standards of care for the health of transgender and gender diverse people, Version 8. *International Journal of Transgender Health, 23*(1), S1–S259. https://doi.org/10.1080/26895269.2022.2100644

2. A transgender man with no surgical history and a trans feminine patient with breast development on hormone therapy are both seen for well person care at 46 years old. Screening mammography would be recommended to both patients, as they both have mammary tissue. Be sure to refer to a trans-friendly radiology facility or, if not possible, inform the patients if that is not known about the facility.

While clinicians are not necessarily saying to patients "and now I'm recording an inventory of your organs," it is effectively the information gathered in a history and is what care should be based on. Incorporating the inventory into the electronic health record (EHR) is helpful for patients of any sex or gender (i.e., those with histories of appendectomy or hysterectomy) and can be an inclusive and effective way to address some health disparities in the TGD population (Grasso et al., 2021). Additional recommendations related to organ inventories in the EHR are tools to guide clinical decision making and population management tools (Grasso et al., 2021). An accurate organ inventory, health history, sexual health history, family history, and social history will guide clinicians to appropriate care and screening recommendations to discuss with patients.

Screening for Sexually Transmitted Infections

When assessing STI risk, sexual behavior—rather than sexual orientation or gender identity—is the most important factor. Sexual partners and sexual behaviors determine a person's risk for contracting and transmitting STIs. For example, a clinician may make assumptions about a cisgender lesbian's sexual practices without realizing that 53 to 97% of LBQ women have had AMAB sex partners (CDC, 2021). Clinicians must have knowledge about sexual practices and their associated risks and well as options for safer sex such as PrEP and appropriate barrier methods. Additionally, clinicians need to feel confident asking clarifying questions when needed, and approaching unfamiliar terms or

BOX 11-2 Trauma-Informed Suggestions for Gynecologic Care of LBQ and TGD Patients

- Have patients stay dressed and comfortably seated.
- Introduce yourself with your name and pronouns (and teach any other staff or students who interact with patients to do the same).
- Ask how the patient prefers to be addressed.
- Stay present and actively listen. Make eye contact, if appropriate.
- Give a disclaimer about the types of questions you will be asking and ask only questions that are relevant to the care you provide.
- It can be helpful to inform the patient that there are so many questions because you try not to make assumptions about anyone.
- Inform patients that if a question feels uncomfortable, they do not have to answer, or they may ask about the relevance of the question.
- Invite patients to have a support person present for the discussion, exam, or both.
- Ask about anything that the patient feels is important for you to know or do to make the visit feel safer for them.
- Remind patients that they are in control of the visit, and nothing should happen without their explicit consent and that consent can be withdrawn at any time.
- Use nonjudgmental language and ask clarifying questions as needed.
- Ask if there are alternatives to anatomical terms a patient prefers.
- Inform patients that after a conversation about their priorities and history, you will discuss recommendations for care and answer any questions. Only then will you proceed with any agreed-upon exams or procedures.
- When offering to have an additional staff member or chaperone present, inform patients of the reason and only invite that person in with the patient's consent.

practices with respectful curiosity to determine their relevance to care. Obtaining a thorough sexual health history will aid in determining an individual's STI risk and screening recommendations, regardless of gender or sexual orientation. More information on STIs can be found in Chapter 22.

Cancer Screening

It is widely agreed upon that if an individual has a body part that meets criteria for screening based on symptoms or risk factors, that person should be screened regardless of sexual orientation, gender identity, or gender-affirming hormone use (Coleman et al., 2022). For example, if a patient has a cervix, they should have cervical cancer screening per national guidelines, and the guidelines do not change based on medication use or sexual partners or practices.

For trans masculine individuals on GAHT, atrophy of genital tissue can begin early after initiating testosterone and can lead to pelvic exams that are painful and potentially emotionally distressing or dysphoric. Atrophic changes are associated with a 10-fold increase in unsatisfactory sampling of the cervix. Clinicians can improve the experience of pelvic care for trans men by using a small or pediatric speculum with a small amount of water-based lubricant. Additionally, vaginal estrogen for one to two weeks prior to an exam may decrease discomfort and increase the likelihood of adequate cervical sampling and this does not interfere with the gender-affirming effects of testosterone (Deutsch, 2016; Coleman et al., 2022). Clinicians may also use shared decision making to consider the option for high-risk HPV collection by the clinician or patient over cervical cytology screening.

Trans feminine individuals on GAHT experience growth of breast tissue, typically to Tanner stage 2 or 3, and should be screened for breast cancer according to the same guidelines for cisgender women. For trans masculine individuals who have undergone nipple and areolar-sparing mastectomy, a clinical chest exam of the peri areolar and subareolar areas should be done yearly or with any concerns (Deutsch, 2016; Coleman et al., 2022). More information on cancer screening recommendations can be found in Chapter 9.

Sexual Health

Sexual health is inextricably tied to overall health, and this fact is supported by decades of evidence and broad international professional endorsement (WHO, 2024). The American Sexual Health Association (ASHA) defines sexual health as:

> *the ability to embrace and enjoy our sexuality throughout our lives. It is an important part of our physical and emotional health. Being sexually healthy means: understanding that sexuality is a natural part of life and involves more than sexual behavior, recognizing and respecting the sexual rights we all share, having access to sexual health information, education, and care, making an effort to prevent unintended pregnancies and STIs and seek care and treatment when needed, being able to experience sexual pleasure, satisfaction, and intimacy when desired, and being able to communicate about sexual health with others including sexual partners and health care providers. (ASHA, 2025)*

This definition is in congruence with other health organizations and highlights the role of access to competent care in optimizing sexual health. Sexual health care, like other realms of care, should be based on the body parts an individual has and their practices, concerns, and goals. Care for LBQ and TGD populations only differs due to an increased emphasis on knowledgeable and inclusive clinicians. While clinicians should be empowered to ask respectful clarifying questions if they are unfamiliar with a term or practice, they are responsible for becoming educated regarding inclusive and comprehensive care without relying only on patients educating them. If a clinician lacks sex positivity, is unfamiliar with the spectrum of sexual practices, or makes assumptions based on stereotypes of queer or trans culture, it will be evident to the patient and is likely to perpetuate healthcare stereotype threat and close off communication.

In LBQ women and TGD individuals, if a clinician closes off communication, even unintentionally, there is an increased likelihood of patients feeling unsafe to discuss sexual health concerns due to fear of judgment. Consider the role of bias in the following scenario:

> *Shay is a lesbian-identified cisgender woman in her 30s who has not seen a clinician in the last 5 years. She is concerned because her libido has been low for the last 6 months despite a high level of attraction to her partner, who is also a cisgender woman. This concern brings Shay to schedule a gynecologic visit. During the visit, Shay explains her concern to the clinician. The clinician, who is open-minded but not educated on LBQ culture, is familiar with the stereotype that it is common and normal in lesbian relationships to have less sex. In an effort to be supportive and inclusive of Shay's identity, the clinician shares that low sex drive is common in long-term lesbian relationships and is not due to pathology, effectively dismissing Shay's concern.*

The clinician in this scenario was unintentionally negligent and may have missed significant health problems like depression or endocrine dysfunction and, because it was normalized, it could be years until Shay seeks care for this concern again. If she had received education on LBQ health, the clinician would have known that women who have sex with women have the highest frequency of orgasms, longer sexual encounters, and higher degrees of sexual intimacy and satisfaction than those who are heterosexual or have male partners (Dickman et al., 2024; Bondarchuk-Mclaughlin & Anderson, 2024) and that sexual satisfaction does not decline more than in heterosexual partnerships (Frederick et al., 2021). While all concerns of patients with any identity should be validated and explored, this brief interaction could lead to poor health outcomes, less trust, and even less access to future care.

In trans feminine individuals, assumptions about the role of external genitalia and sexual practices should be avoided, as many trans women do not experience dysphoria related to their genitals. For TGD individuals on estrogen therapy who experience the undesired loss of erectile function, pathology should be ruled out and treatment options such as sildenafil (Viagra) and tadalafil (Cialis) can be considered as well as reducing antiandrogenic agents (Deutsch, 2016). Similarly, trans masculine individuals on testosterone therapy should have any sexual concerns addressed according to their anatomy. For example, a concern for dyspareunia should be evaluated in the same way as for cisgender women. Pain or discomfort related to atrophic genital changes on testosterone can safely be treated with local estradiol cream (Estrace) without interfering with testosterone. More information on sexual health and alterations in sexual health can be found in Chapters 12 and 18, respectively.

Contraception

Contraceptive care is no different for LBQ or TGD patients and comprehensive information regarding this care can be found in Chapter 11.

In general, if someone is having the type of sex that can result in pregnancy and does not want a pregnancy, they should be offered contraception. For LBQ individuals, clinicians should remain aware that neither queer sexual orientation nor having a same-gender partner can rule out the potential for unintended pregnancy, as trans feminine partners can produce sperm, even if on estrogen hormone therapy.

Similarly, trans masculine individuals on testosterone therapy can conceive while on GAHT if they have a uterus and ovaries. Even with suppression of menses, ovulation may still occur. Studies have shown that up to a third of trans men on GAHT believe that testosterone is adequate contraception (Okano et al., 2022). Patients should be educated that gender-affirming hormones are not adequate contraception and additional protection is recommended to avoid unwanted pregnancy. While many trans masculine patients prefer to avoid estrogen, research shows that any form of hormonal contraception can be used in conjunction with testosterone and even estrogen-containing methods have been found not to interfere with GAHT effects (Okano et al., 2022). Contraceptive risks and benefits should be considered using the same guidelines as for cisgender women, such as the US Medical Eligibility Criteria for Contraceptive Use (US MEC).

Abortion Care

Individuals in the LBQ and TGD communities experience unwanted pregnancies and have abortions. Given what is known about healthcare stereotype threat and delayed access to care, it is also true that abortion care is difficult for these communities to access. Some TGD individuals who have had abortions have shared their experiences and provided recommendations to improve abortion care including inclusive intake forms (52% of respondents), staff use of gender-neutral language (48%), and enhanced privacy outside the clinic (24%) (Moseson et al., 2021).

Studies have shown that TGD individuals prioritize different factors than cisgender women when accessing abortion care. Medication abortion was chosen more frequently in TGD patients (61% of reported abortions) and the most common cited reasons for the choice of medication over procedural abortion was that it is less invasive and more private (Moseson et al., 2021). Clinicians can support LBQ and TGD individuals by increasing inclusive and respectful environments and practices and, in turn, increasing access to necessary health care. More information on abortion care can be found in Chapter 19.

Fertility Preservation and Family Building

Many LBQ and TGD adults would like to have biological children. For TGD individuals prior to and throughout transition, fertility preservation and other parenting options should be discussed and this support from clinicians is associated with positive patient experiences (Coleman et al., 2022). Please refer to Chapter 20 regarding further information on fertility, fertility preservation, and infertility.

Research is lacking regarding the long-term effect of testosterone GAHT on fertility; however, a number of trans masculine individuals return to baseline fertility after discontinuing testosterone (Deutsch, 2016). For trans masculine individuals on GAHT who plan to become pregnant, preconception care and counseling should be provided. In addition to routine care, counseling regarding GAHT management should be discussed, as testosterone is considered teratogenic to a developing embryo and is contraindicated in pregnancy. The optimal time to discontinue testosterone prior to pregnancy is unclear, and cessation can be associated with distress or dysphoria, so shared decision making should be used for an individualized approach. Generally, it is recommended that testosterone be discontinued prior to conception or cessation of contraception (Coleman et al., 2022).

There is also a lack of data regarding optimal time to resume testosterone in the postpartum period and this decision should also have an individualized approach. Some trans masculine individuals have goals to chest/breast feed and experienced lactation support has been a predictor of success (Coleman et al., 2022). Therapeutic testosterone is present in human milk and should be avoided during lactation due to a lack of data regarding infant safety; however, it can be resumed as soon as chest/breast feeding is discontinued (Coleman et al., 2022). Conversely, some trans masculine individuals may experience unwanted chest growth or lactation, even after chest contouring surgery, and should be supported in suppression and management of physical and emotional symptoms (Coleman et al., 2022). Trans feminine individuals may also wish to chest/breast feed and can be supported in doing so through lactation induction protocols, which is similar to lactation induction in cisgender nongestational parents (Coleman et al., 2022). Clients should be advised that the nutritional composition of milk from trans feminine individuals has not been studied and support around child feeding should be provided.

CONSIDERATIONS FOR SPECIFIC POPULATIONS

Adolescents

As previously mentioned, the number of LGBTQ+ individuals is steadily increasing with each younger generation, with over 23% of Generation Z identifying as a sexual or gender minority (Jones, 2025). As they access gynecologic care, approximately one in every four patients a clinician encounters will have LBQ and/or TGD identities. Suicide is the second-leading cause of death in 10- to 14-year-olds and the third-leading cause in 15- to 24-year-olds, with LGBTQ+ youth being four times more likely to attempt suicide than heterosexual cisgender youth (The Trevor Project, 2021). LGBTQ+ youth who had protective factors like supportive adults, safe spaces, and access to affirming care had significantly lower rates of suicide attempts (The Trevor Project, 2021).

As with adults, care for these populations is only complicated by the need for cultural competency and respect. Gynecologic care for LBQ and TGD youth does not differ from other identities and should include assessing safety, mental health, contraceptive and STI screening needs, sexual health and bodily autonomy, family planning services, appropriate referrals, comprehensive health education, and laying the groundwork for inclusive gynecologic care through adulthood.

For TGD youth, social affirmation and support from clinicians is protective in regard to health outcomes (Scheim et al., 2022). This can be as basic as using the correct pronouns and chosen name during care. As with adults, supportive families, specifically parents, safe environments, and community connectedness all increase resilience in TGD youth, so assessing their access to these and providing information for increased support should be an important component of care. In the setting of an unsupportive family, clinicians may be uniquely positioned to educate parents and provide resources for support, with the patient's permission. This affirmation and support is even more crucial in 2025 in the setting of hostile social and political threats aimed at TGD youth, their families, and their ability to access safe care.

Professional societies have documented support of gender affirmation for youth and have published guidelines and recommendations in the WPATH Standards of Care 8 (2022) and in the Endocrine Society's Clinical Practice Guidelines (2017). For TGD adolescents, delaying or blocking puberty decreases anxiety and depression and GAHT and surgical affirmation are associated with increased quality of life in this population (Scheim et al., 2022). This is most commonly done once Tanner stage 2 is reached via reversible gonadotropin-releasing agonists (GnRHa), often referred to as *puberty blockers*. This treatment pauses puberty and prevents the development of permanent secondary sex characteristics and allows for time for gender exploration, while also affirming the individual's identity (Lee & Rosenthal, 2023). While youth are often referred for gender-affirming hormone therapy once cognitive and emotional maturity allows for the ability to fully consent, reproductive health clinicians may be the first point of contact for patients and families asking questions and gathering information about gender-affirming options. Gender-affirming hormones for TGD youth have been strongly associated with improved mental health and a decrease in serious consideration of suicide (Lee & Rosenthal, 2023). Providing referrals to inclusive specialists may be an important aspect of care. For example, many adolescents have unclear parenting plans and clinicians should discuss fertility preservation with patients and families on an ongoing basis (Coleman et al., 2022) and provide referrals to trans-inclusive fertility specialists for more detailed discussion and planning.

For youth who are receiving care but not using GnRHa or GAHT, reproductive healthcare clinicians can offer supportive and affirming care in other ways. One example of this is offering options for cycle suppression via contraceptives in trans masculine youth after menarche who experience dysphoria related to menses. Another example is providing thorough education on the risks and benefits of binding or tucking and ensuring the safest method possible is used. Finally, clinicians are uniquely equipped to partner with local or national advocacy organizations and schools and engage in public education and policy shaping that supports and affirms TGD youth and their families.

Older Adults

The percentage of people over age 50 who are LGBTQ+ in the United States (3%) is drastically lower than younger generations (Jones, 2025). While social and political reasons account for some of this discordance, many in the younger generations recognize that access to many community elders was stripped away because of the structural neglect and violence of the AIDS epidemic. The older generation of LGBTQ+ people suffered the collective trauma of watching loved ones die from preventable deaths and yet continued to fight systems of oppression in the name of community. An impactful example of this is seen within the LGBTQ+ acronym. The history behind the order of the letters was to honor the "L" (lesbian community) who were some of the only individuals to actively support and advocate for HIV-positive gay men and trans women during the AIDS epidemic (APA, 2022). To this day, half of the U.S. population living with HIV is over 50 years old (Services and Advocacy for LGBTQ+ Elders (SAGE), 2021). This community has long needed to care for itself and with an aging population, it continues to bear the responsibility to advocate for and enact policies that support LGBTQ+ older people thriving.

The importance of supportive community, connectedness, and chosen family has been previously stressed in this chapter, and LGBTQ+ older people created a map for younger generations to maintain strong communities. Sadly, LGBTQ+ older people are twice as likely to live alone; four times less likely to have children; and more likely to experience poor health, poverty, and homelessness than cisgender heterosexual older people (SAGE, 2021). Health disparities in LGBTQ+ older people include higher rates of disability (41%), cardiovascular disease, healthcare stereotype threat (23%), higher rates of HIV and associated health problems, lack of inclusive long-term care facilities, high rates of loneliness and social isolation (53%), higher rates of tobacco and alcohol use, and higher rates of mental distress and suicidal ideation (SAGE, 2021).

Despite much structural adversity, LGBTQ+ older adults reported high rates of resilience in the landmark *The Aging and Health Report: Disparities and Resilience Among Lesbian, Gay, Bisexual, and Transgender Older Adults* (2011). The report showed high rates of resilience-promoting activities including feeling positive about community belonging (89%), engaging in regular wellness activities (91%), engaging in moderate physical activity (82%), and attending regular spiritual or religious activities (38%) (Fredriksen-Goldsen et al., 2011).

Clinicians should become knowledgeable regarding social and health disparities resilience factors impacting LGBTQ+ older adults and provide care that is culturally responsive to this. For example, assessing for social isolation at a routine gynecologic visit and responding with appropriate and inclusive resources could have more health benefits than a breast exam.

CONCLUSION

Lesbian, bisexual, and queer cisgender women and transgender and gender diverse individuals should have access to respectful and comprehensive gynecologic care that is based on their anatomy, practices, and personal goals. Most clinicians already have the clinical skills to provide this care because it is not inherently complicated by sexual or gender identities. Nearly all unique needs of these populations can be addressed by clinicians being educated on community history, current culture, health disparities, and barriers to safe care. With significant increases in the number of LBQ and TGD people in younger generations, ensuring cultural competency in health care has never been more important. As with care involving any disadvantaged identity, clinicians must remember that communities are not monoliths, and each patient is a unique person entrusting you not to harm them.

References

ACOG Committee on Health Care for Underserved Women (2012, reaffirmed 2024). ACOG Committee Opinion No. 525: Health care for lesbians and bisexual women. *Obstetrics and Gynecology, 119*(5), 1077–1080. https://doi.org/10.1097/AOG.0b013e3182564991

American College of Obstetricians and Gynecologists. (2011). Health care for transgender individuals. *Committee Opinion No. 512. Obstet Gynecol, 118*, 1454–1458.

American College of Nurse-Midwives. (2012, revised and reaffirmed 2021). *Position statement: Healthcare for transgender and gender non-binary people.*

American College of Nurse-Midwives. (2014, reaffirmed 2019). *Position statement: Health care for all families.*

American Psychological Association. (2022). *A guide to sexual orientation and gender diversity terms.* https://www.apa.org/ed/precollege/psychology-teacher-network/introductory-psychology/diversity-terms

American Sexual Health Association. (2025). *Understanding sexual health.* https://www.ashasexualhealth.org/sexual-health/

Bondarchuk-Mclaughlin, A., & Anderson, J. R. (2024). A systematic review on differences in sexual satisfaction of women as a function of sexual identity. *Psychology & Sexuality, 16*(1), 130–162. https://doi.org/10.1080/19419899.2024.2360998

Bonomo, J. A., Luo, K., & Ramallo, J. A. (2024). LGBTQ+ cardiovascular health equity: A brief review. *Frontiers in Cardiovascular Medicine, 11*, 1350603. https://doi.org/10.3389/fcvm.2024.1350603

Cathcart-Rake, E. J., Chan, A., Menendez, A., Markstrom, D., Schnitzlein, C., Chong, Y. W., & Dizon, D. S. (2025). Cancer care for transgender and gender-diverse people: Practical, literature-driven recommendations from the Multinational Association of Supportive Care in Cancer. *CA: A Cancer Journal for Clinicians, 75*(1), 68–81. https://doi.org/10.3322/caac.21872

Charlton, B. M., Reynolds, C. A., Tabaac, A. R., Godwin, E. G., Porsch, L. M., Agénor, M., Grimstad, F. W., & Katz-Wise, S. L. (2021). Unintended and teen pregnancy experiences of trans masculine people living in the United States. *International Journal of Transgender Health, 22*(1-2), 65–76. https://doi.org/10.1080/26895269.2020.1824692

Cheng, P. J., Pastuszak, A. W., Myers, J. B., Goodwin, I. A., & Hotaling, J. M. (2019). Fertility concerns of the transgender patient. *Translational Andrology and Urology, 8*(3), 209–218. https://doi.org/10.21037/tau.2019.05.09

Coleman, E., Radix, A. E., Bouman, W. P., Brown, G. R., de Vries, A. L. C., Deutsch, M. B., Ettner, R., Fraser, L., Goodman, M., Green, J., Hancock, A. B., Johnson, T. W., Karasic, D. H., Knudson, G. A., Leibowitz, S. F., Meyer-Bahlburg, H. F. L., Monstrey, S. J., Motmans, J., Nahata, L., . . . Arcelus, J. (2022). Standards of care for the health of transgender and gender diverse people, Version 8. *International Journal of Transgender Health, 23*(1), S1–S259. https://doi.org/10.1080/26895269.2022.2100644

Cortez, S., Moog, D., Lewis, C., Williams, K., Herrick, C. J., Fields, M. E., . . . & Baranski, T. (2024). Effectiveness and safety of different estradiol regimens in transgender females: A randomized controlled trial. *Journal of the Endocrine Society, 8*(8), bvae108.

Crenshaw, K. (1989). Demarginalizing the intersection of race and sex: A Black feminist critique of antidiscrimination doctrine, feminist theory and antiracist politics. *University of Chicago Legal Forum, 1989*(1), 139–167.

Cruciani, G., Quintigliano, M., Mezzalira, S., Scandurra, C., & Carone, N. (2025). Sexual and reproductive health practitioners' attitudes and knowledge regarding transgender, gender diverse, and non-binary patients: A mixed-method systematic review. *The Journal of Sexual Medicine, 22*(7), 1293–1295. https://doi.org/10.1093/jsxmed/qdaf115

Deutsch, M. B. (2016). *Guidelines for the primary and gender-affirming care of transgender and gender nonbinary people* (2nd ed.). UCSF Gender Affirming Health Program, Department of Family and Community Medicine, University of California San Francisco.

Dickman, K., Wetzel, G. M., & Sanchez, D. T. (2024). The role of partner gender: How sexual expectations shape the pursuit of an orgasm goal for heterosexual, lesbian, and bisexual women. *Social Psychological & Personality Science, 16*(5). https://doi.org/10.1177/19485506241235235

Eckhert, E., Lansinger, O., Ritter, V., Liu, M., Han, S., Schapira, L., John, E. M., Gomez, S., Sledge, G., & Kurian, A. W. (2023). Breast cancer diagnosis, treatment, and outcomes of patients from sex and gender minority groups. *JAMA Oncology, 9*(4), 473–480. https://doi.org/10.1001/jamaoncol.2022.7146

Everytown. (2024, February 13). *New Everytown data on transgender homicides reveals concentration in the South.* https://www.everytown.org/press/new-everytown-data-on-transgender-homicides-reveals-concentration-in-the-south/

Feldman J. L., Luhur W. E., Herman J. L., Poteat T., & Meyer I. H. (2021). Health and health care access in the US transgender population health (TransPop) survey. *Andrology, 9*(6), 1707–1718. https://doi.org/10.1111/andr.13052

Fingerhut, A. W., Martos, A. J., Choi, S. K., & Abdou, C. M. (2022). Healthcare stereotype threat and health outcomes among LGB individuals. *Annals of Behavioral Medicine: A Publication of the Society of Behavioral Medicine, 56*(6), 562–572. https://doi.org/10.1093/abm/kaab060

FORGE. (n.d.). *FORGE: Transgender aging, anti-violence, and empowerment.* https://forge-forward.org/

Frederick, D. A., Gillespie, B. J., Lever, J., Berardi, V., & Garcia, J. R. (2021). Debunking lesbian bed death: Using coarsened exact matching to compare sexual practices and satisfaction of lesbian and heterosexual women. *Archives of Sexual Behavior, 50*(8), 3601–3619. https://doi.org/10.1007/s10508-021-02096-4

Fredriksen-Goldsen, K. I., Kim, H.-J., Emlet, C. A., Muraco, A., Erosheva, E. A., Hoy-Ellis, C. P., Goldsen, J., Petry, H. (2011). *The aging and health report: disparities and resilience among lesbian, gay, bisexual, and transgender older adults—Key findings fact sheet.* Seattle: Institute for Multigenerational Health.

Gay and Lesbian Medical Association. (n.d.). *Resources—GLMA: Health Professionals advancing LGBTQ equality.* https://www.glma.org/resources.php

Gentile, D., Boselli, D., & MacNeill, E. (2020). Clinician's Experience and Self-Perceived Knowledge and Attitudes toward LGBTQ + Health Topics. *Teaching and Learning in Medicine, 33*(3), 292–303. https://doi.org/10.1080/10401334.2020.1852087

Geronimus, A. T. (2001). Understanding and eliminating racial inequalities in women's health in the United States: The role of the weathering conceptual framework. *Journal of the American Medical Women's Association (1972), 56*(4), 133–136, 149.

Grasso, C., Campbell, J., Yunkun, E., Todisco, D., Thompson, J., Gonzalez, A., Brewster, A., & Keuroghlian, A. S. (2021). Gender-affirming care without walls: Utilization of telehealth services by transgender and gender diverse people at a federally qualified health center. *Transgender Health*. https://doi.org/10.1089/trgh.2020.0155

Green, D. C., Parra, L. A., & Goldbach, J. T. (2022). Experiences of minority stress and access to health services among sexual minority people in the United States. *Health & Social Care in the Community*, 30, 1– 12. https://doi.org/10.1111/hsc.13883

Guidi, J., Lucente, M., Sonino, N., & Fava, G. A. (2020). allostatic load and its impact on health: A systematic review. *Psychotherapy and Psychosomatics, 90*(1), 11–27. https://doi.org/10.1159/000510696

Hashemi, L., Marijic Buljubasic, A., Budoff, M. J., Copeland, L. A., Jackson, N. J., Jasuja, G. K., Gornbein, J., & Reue, K. (2024). Gender-affirming hormone treatment and metabolic syndrome among transgender veterans. *JAMA Netw Open. 7*(7), e2419696. https://doi.org/10.1001/jamanetworkopen.2024.19696

Hembree, W. C., Cohen-Kettenis, P. T., Gooren, L., Hannema, S. E., Meyer, W. J., Murad, M. H., Rosenthal, S. M., Safer, J. D., Tangpricha, V., & T'Sjoen, G. G. (2017). Endocrine treatment of gender-dysphoric/gender-incongruent persons: An Endocrine Society clinical practice guideline. *The Journal of Clinical Endocrinology & Metabolism, 102*(11), 3869–3903. https://doi.org/10.1210/jc.2017-01658

Hughto, J. M. W., Quinn, E. K., Dunbar, M. S., Rose, A. J., Shireman, T. I., & Jasuja, G. K. (2021). Prevalence and co-occurrence of alcohol, nicotine, and other substance use disorder diagnoses among US transgender and cisgender adults. *JAMA Network Open, 4*(2), e2036512. https://doi.org/10.1001/jamanetworkopen.2020.36512

Human Rights Campaign. (2023, May 31). *Glossary of terms*. Human Rights Campaign. https://www.hrc.org/resources/glossary-of-terms

Jones, J. M. (2025). *LGBTQ+ identification in U.S. rises to 9.3%*. Gallup.com. https://news.gallup.com/poll/656708/lgbtq-identification-rises.aspx

Karpel, H. C., Sampson, A., Charifson, M., Fein, L. A., Murphy, D., Sutter, M., Tamargo, C. L., Quinn, G. P., & Schabath, M. B. (2023). Assessing medical students' attitudes and knowledge regarding LGBTQ health needs across the United States. *Journal of Primary Care & Community Health, 14*, 21501319231186729. https://doi.org/10.1177/21501319231186729

LeBlanc, M. E., Trinh, M. H., Zubizarreta, D., & Reisner, S. L. (2024). Healthcare stereotype threat, healthcare access, and health outcomes in a probability sample of U.S. transgender and gender diverse adults. *Preventive Medicine Reports, 42*, 102734. https://doi.org/10.1016/j.pmedr.2024.102734

Lee, J., Evans-Polce, R. J., Ahlquist, J., & Parker, M. A. (2023). Polysubstance use by sexual identity among U.S. adults, 2021. *Preventive Medicine, 177*, 107729. https://doi.org/10.1016/j.ypmed.2023.107729

Lee, J. Y., & Rosenthal, S. M. (2023). Gender-affirming care of transgender and gender-diverse youth: Current concepts. *Annual Review of Medicine, 74*, 107–116. https://doi.org/10.1146/annurev-med-043021-032007

Lin, E., Sleboda, P., Rimel, B. J., Chen, J. T., Hernandez, D. V., & Datta, G. D. (2024). Sexual orientation and gender identity inequities in cervical cancer screening by race and ethnicity. *Cancer Causes & Control: CCC, 35*(1), 133–151. https://doi.org/10.1007/s10552-023-01771-2

Malik, M., Cooney, E. E., Brevelle, J.-M., & Poteat, T. (2022). Tucking practices and attributed health effects in transfeminine individuals. *Transgender Health*. https://doi.org/10.1089/trgh.2022.0064

McEwan, B. & Stellar, E. (1993). Stress and the individual: Mechanisms leading to disease. *Archives of Internal Medicine (1960), 153*(18), 2093–2101. https://doi.org/10.1001/archinte.1993.00410180039004

Medina-Martínez, J., Saus-Ortega, C., María Montserrat Sánchez-Lorente, Sosa-Palanca, E., García-Martínez, P., & Mármol-López, M. I. (2021). Health inequities in LGBT people and nursing interventions to reduce them: A systematic review. *International Journal of Environmental Research and Public Health, 18*(22), 11801. https://doi.org/10.3390/ijerph182211801

Mendelsohn, D. M., Omoto, A. M., Tannenbaum, K., & Lamb, C. S. (2022). When sexual identity and sexual behaviors do not align: The prevalence of discordance and its physical and psychological health correlates. *Stigma and Health (Washington, D.C.), 7*(1), 70–79. https://doi.org/10.1037/sah0000338

Meyer I. H. (2003). Prejudice, social stress, and mental health in lesbian, gay, and bisexual populations: Conceptual issues and research evidence. *Psychological Bulletin, 129*(5), 674–697. https://doi.org/10.1037/0033-2909.129.5.674

Meyer, I. H., Wilson, B. D. M., & O'Neill, K. (2021). *LGBTQ people in the US: Select findings from the Generations and TransPop Studies*. Los Angeles, CA: The Williams Institute, UCLA School of Law.

Meyer, I. H., Wilson, B. D. M., Del Rosario, S., & O'Neill, K. (2021). *Identity, stress, and health of LGBTQ people in the US (data interactive)*. Los Angeles, CA: The Williams Institute, UCLA School of Law.

Mittleman, J. (2023). Sexual fluidity: Implications for population research. *Demography, 60*(4), 1257–1282. https://doi.org/10.1215/00703370-10898916

Moseson, H., Fix, L., Ragosta, S., Forsberg, H., Hastings, J., Stoeffler, A., . . . & Obedin-Maliver, J. (2021). Abortion experiences and preferences of transgender, nonbinary, and gender-expansive people in the United States. *American Journal of Obstetrics and Gynecology, 224*(4), 376-e1.

National LGBTQIA+ Health Education Center. (2024). *Glossary of terms*. https://www.lgbtqiahealtheducation.org/glossary/en/

Newport, F. (2018, May 22). *In U.S., estimate of LGBT population rises to 4.5%*. Gallup. https://news.gallup.com/poll/234863/estimate-lgbt-population-rises.aspx

Nie, I. de, Asseler, J., Meißner, A., Warem, I. A. C. V., Kostelijk, E. H., Heijer, M. den, Huirne, J., & Mello, N. M. van. (2021). A cohort study on factors impairing semen quality in transgender women. *American Journal of Obstetrics & Gynecology, 336*(3), (pp. p390.e1–390.e10). https://doi.org/10.1016/j.ajog.2021.10.020

Nokoff, N. J. (2022, January 19). DSM-5 criteria for gender dysphoria. www.ncbi.nlm.nih.gov. *National Library of Medicine*. https://www.ncbi.nlm.nih.gov/books/NBK577212/table/pediat_transgender.T.dsm5_criteria_for_g/

Nurse Practitioners in Women's Health. (2022). *Position statement: Healthcare for transgender and gender diverse individuals*.

Ojeda-Leitner, D., & Lewis, R. K. (2021). Assessing health-related stereotype threats and mental healthcare experiences among a LGBT sample. *Journal of Prevention & Intervention in the Community, 49*(3), 251–265.

Okano, S. H. P., Pellicciotta, G. G. M., & Braga, G. C. (2022). Contraceptive counseling for the transgender patient assigned female at birth. Aconselhamento contraceptivo para a pessoa transgênera designada mulher ao nascimento. *Revista brasileira de ginecologia e obstetricia: revista da Federacao Brasileira das Sociedades de Ginecologia e Obstetricia, 44*(9), 884–890. https://doi.org/10.1055/s-0042-1751063

Olson, S. M., Muñoz, E. G., Solis, E. C., & Bradford, H. M. (2024), Mitigating weight bias in the clinical setting: A new approach to care. *Journal of Midwifery & Women's Health, 69*, 180–190. https://doi.org/10.1111/jmwh.13578

The Oxford Review. (2025). *Historical trauma—Definition and explanation*. https://oxford-review.com/the-oxford-review-dei-diversity-equity-and-inclusion-dictionary/historical-trauma-definition-and-explanation/

Parker, L. L., & Harriger, J. A. (2020). Eating disorders and disordered eating behaviors in the LGBT population: A review of the literature. *Journal of Eating Disorders, 8*, 51. https://doi.org/10.1186/s40337-020-00327-y

Peel, E., Rivers, I., Tyler, A., Nodin, N., & Perez-Acevedo, C. (2022). Exploring LGBT resilience and moving beyond a deficit-model: findings from a qualitative study in England. *Psychology & Sexuality, 14*(1), 114–126. https://doi.org/10.1080/19419899.2022.2063754

Rhoten, B., Burkhalter, J. E., Joo, R., Mujawar, I., Bruner, D., Scout, N., & Margolies, L. (2021). Impact of an LGBTQ cultural competence training program for providers on knowledge, attitudes, self-efficacy, and intensions. *Journal of Homosexuality, 69*(6), 1030–1041. https://doi.org/10.1080/00918369.2021.1901505

SAGE. (2018, March 19). Home. *SAGE*. https://www.sageusa.org/

Salas-Betsch, I., & Kelly, K. (2024). *What comes next for the Equal Rights Amendment?* Center for American Progress. https://www.americanprogress.org/article/what-comes-next-for-the-equal-rights-amendment/

Scheim, A. I., Baker, K. E., Restar, A. J., & Sell, R. L. (2022). Health and health care among transgender adults in the United States. *Annual Review of Public Health, 43*(1), 503–523.

SisterSong. (n.d.). *About us: The herstory of reproductive justice (RJ)*. SisterSong. https://www.sistersong.net/about-x2

Stewart, K., & O'Reilly, P. (2017). Exploring the attitudes, knowledge and beliefs of nurses and midwives of the healthcare needs of the LGBTQ population: An integrative review. *Nurse Education Today, 53*, 67–77. https://doi.org/10.1016/j.nedt.2017.04.008

Takemoto, M. L. S., Menezes, M. de O., Polido, C. B. A., Santos, D. de S., Leonello, V. M., Magalhães, C. G., Cirelli, J. F., & Knobel, R. (2019). Prevalence of sexually transmitted infections and bacterial vaginosis among lesbian women: Systematic review and recommendations to improve care. *Cadernos de Saúde Pública, 35*(3). https://doi.org/10.1590/0102-311x00118118

The Trevor Project. (2021). *Facts about LGBTQ youth suicide*. https://www.thetrevorproject.org/resources/article/facts-about-lgbtq-youth-suicide/

U.S. Census Bureau. (2024). *New 2024 population estimates show nation's population grew by about 1% to 340.1 million since 2023*. https://www.census.gov/library/stories/2024/12/population-estimates.html

WHO. (2024). *Sexual health*. Who.int. https://www.who.int/health-topics/sexual-health#tab=tab_1

Zucker, R., Reisman, T., & Safer, J. D. (2021). Minimizing venous thromboembolism in feminizing hormone therapy: Applying lessons from cisgender women and previous data. *Endocrine Practice: Official Journal of the American College of Endocrinology and the American Association of Clinical Endocrinologists, 27*(6), 621–625. https://doi.org/10.1016/j.eprac.2021.03.010

CHAPTER 12

Sexuality and Sexual Health

Ella T. Heitzler
Kathryn Atkin
Mara Evans

Humans are inherently sexual beings, and sexual health is an essential component of health care. When sexual activity is voluntary, wanted, pleasurable, and noncoercive, it is healthy. Healthy sexual activity is associated with numerous health benefits, including improving cardiovascular health, affording protection from fatal coronary events, decreasing incidence of cancer and cancer-related mortality, decreasing levels of stress, slower cognitive decline in older individuals, and extending the life span (Cao et al., 2020; Gianotten, 2023; Wright et al., 2019). In women, increased frequency of orgasm has been shown to increase the pain threshold (Gianotten, 2023) and protect against mortality (Cao et al., 2020). Sexual well-being is positively associated with better sleep, immune function, mood, self-rated health, and life satisfaction, as well as increased happiness (Jackson et al., 2020; Gianotten, 2023; Gianotten et al., 2021). For people in intimate relationships, a higher initial level of sexual satisfaction enhances satisfaction with the relationship over time and greater sexual satisfaction may inhibit decline in satisfaction with the relationship over time (Quinn-Nilas, 2020). Sexual contact also stimulates oxytocin release, which is associated with wide-ranging health benefits (Ito et al., 2019).

Although sexual activity can deliver these benefits, sexual health is not often viewed as an essential component of health care and does not get addressed proactively by all clinicians (Zhang et al., 2020). People often have questions or concerns about their sexual health and function, and they may express these concerns to their clinicians. However, many patients believe the clinician should initiate the discussion about sexual health (Zhang et al., 2020). Clinicians care for people with a range of gender identities, sexual orientations, and relationship structures from a variety of socioeconomic, cultural, and religious backgrounds. Patients have the right to receive nonjudgmental, open, and direct communication, counseling, and therapy from clinicians regarding sexual health and concerns. Sexual concerns are addressed in more detail in Chapter 18. This chapter develops a solid knowledge base about the sexuality and sexual well-being of people assigned female at birth (AFAB) for use in clinical practice. Not all AFAB people identify as female or women; however, these terms are used occasionally in this chapter to be consistent with existing research literature. Use of these terms is not meant to exclude people who do not identify as women and seek gynecologic care. Information in this chapter is presented from a sex-positive perspective within a framework of patient-centered and trauma-informed care. The chapter aims to provide clinicians with tools to support patients in achieving the goals they establish for their sexual health and sexuality by delineating three cornerstones to sexual health: sexual self-knowledge, sexual agency, and control over pelvic muscles. Beginning with and interweaving definitions and a discussion of commonly used terminology, the chapter also addresses sexual practices, sexual desire, products to enhance sexual health, and assessment of sexual health. The chapter concludes with information about sexual health for specific populations and provides helpful resources for patients and clinicians (refer to **Appendix 12-A**).

DEFINITIONS OF KEY TERMS

Sexual Health

Increasingly, a plethora of terms are used to describe various aspects of human sexuality, sexual health, the sexual rights of individuals, and sexual orientation. **Box 12-1** contains definitions of sexual health from the World Health Organization and the American Sexual Health Association. In further recognition of the premise that sexual rights are essential to achieve sexual health, the World Association for Sexual Health issued the Declaration of Sexual Rights in 1999, which was subsequently revised in 2014 (World Association for Sexual Health, 2014).

For many people, sexual health is not something that is considered until its absence is noticed. In clinical situations, sexual health is frequently an undefined default state, devoid of any positive connotations, that describes the absence of infection, cancer, sexual violence, coercion, unintended pregnancy, or abnormal pregnancy. In contrast, when considered from a sex-positive framework, the definition of sexual health encompasses far more than a lack of negatives. A sex-positive working definition includes the appreciation that satisfying sexual activity stemming from sexual agency is healthy and contributes to overall well-being.

Sexual Pleasure

Per the World Association for Sexual Health, sexual pleasure can be defined as psychological and/or physical enjoyment and satisfaction that comes from solitary or shared erotic experiences. Erotic experiences may include: dreams, thoughts, feelings, or emotions (Ford et al., 2021). Sexual pleasure does not require achieving orgasm (Reis et al., 2021). When experienced in a self-determined, safe, private environment, sexual pleasure contributes to sexual

BOX 12-1 Definitions of Sexual Health

World Health Organization:

Sexual health is a state of physical, emotional, mental, and social well-being in relation to sexuality; it is not merely the absence of disease, dysfunction, or infirmity. Sexual health requires a positive and respectful approach to sexuality and sexual relationships, as well as the possibility of having pleasurable and safe sexual experiences, free of coercion, discrimination, and violence. For sexual health to be attained and maintained, the sexual rights of all persons must be respected, protected and fulfilled. (Reproduced from World Health Organization, 2006, p. 5)

American Sexual Health Association:

Sexual health is the ability to embrace and enjoy our sexuality throughout our lives. It is an important part of our physical and emotional health. Being sexually healthy means:

- Understanding that sexuality is a natural part of life and involves more than sexual behavior.
- Recognizing and respecting the sexual rights we all share.
- Having access to sexual health information, education, and care.
- Making an effort to prevent unintended pregnancies and STDs [sexually transmitted diseases] and seek care and treatment when needed.
- Being able to experience sexual pleasure, satisfaction, and intimacy when desired.
- Being able to communicate about sexual health with others including sexual partners and healthcare providers. (Reproduced from American Sexual Health Association, 2024, para. 4)

Reproduced from World Health Organization. (2006). *Defining sexual health: Report of a technical consultation on sexual health*, 28–31 January 2002, Geneva.

Reproduced from American Sexual Health Association. (2024). *Understanding sexual health*. http://www.ashasexualhealth.org/sexual-health/

health (Ford et al., 2021). Sexual experiences, arousability, body-esteem, age, sexual assertiveness, and sexual autonomy benefit a perons' sexual pleasure (Reis et al., 2021).

Sex, Gender, and Sexual Orientation

Sex is a designation based on chromosomes and genitalia. An individual's sex can be AFAB, assigned male at birth (AMAB), or intersex (i.e., chromosomes and genitalia fall between binary female and male designations). Gender is a social construct that assigns roles and attributes to people based on their sex assigned at birth. A person's gender identity, which is their understanding of their gender, may or may not match the sex they were assigned at birth. Gender identity and sexual orientation are distinct concepts (Bates et al., 2022), and individuals who fall outside of the cis-normative framework are often harmfully and erroneously stereotyped as being deviant or highly sexual beings (Howansky et al., 2021). Sexual orientation includes attraction, identity, and behavior—who a person desires sexually, how an individual identifies as a sexual being, and their sexual partners and activities. It is important to not make assumptions about an individual's sexual orientation based on their gender identity and vice versa. Gender and sexual orientation terms and concepts are discussed in detail in Chapter 11.

BOX 12-2 Sexual Violence of Women in the United States Reported in the 2016/2017 National Intimate Partner and Sexual Violence Survey

54.3 percent experienced contact sexual violence in their lifetime, with 4.7 percent experiencing this violence in the previous 12 months.

26.8 percent reported completed or attempted rape in their lifetime.

2.3 percent reported completed or attempted rape in the previous 12 months.

6.3 percent experienced attempted forced penetration.

23.6 percent experienced sexual coercion.

47.6 percent reported unwanted sexual contact in their lifetime.

Data from Basile, K. C., Smith, S. G., Kresnow, M., Khatiwada, S., & Leemis, R. W. (2022). *The National Intimate Partner and Sexual Violence Survey: 2016/2017 Report on Sexual Violence*. National Center for Injury Prevention and Control, Centers for Disease Control and Prevention.

Trauma-Informed Care

Trauma-informed care is a patient-centered framework that acknowledges that trauma from a variety of sources, including sexual violence, is common. Trauma-informed care assumes that an individual is more likely than not to have a history of trauma. Because it is statistically likely that a given patient has experienced trauma (refer to **Box 12-2**), it is best to provide care that is trauma informed with all patients. Trauma-informed care emphasizes physical, psychological, and emotional safety for both patients and providers. During interactions with patients, clinicians using a trauma-informed approach to care strive to help patients rebuild a sense of control and to not cause disempowerment. During a clinical encounter, a patient who has experienced trauma may display behaviors stemming from post-traumatic stress disorder (PTSD) that the clinician needs to recognize and respond to effectively. Signs of PTSD include shutting eyes, not responding, and complaining of tunnel vision or not being able to see clearly. Patients can be traumatized or retraumatized by well-meaning, but uninformed, providers. Chapter 5 provides more information about trauma-informed care, and Chapter 8 includes a trauma-informed approach to physical examination.

The American College of Obstetricians and Gynecologists (2019) reaffirmed in 2024 that in addition to practicing trauma-informed care in all patient interactions, clinicians should screen patients for a history of sexual violence/assault and nonconsensual sexual encounters. Experiencing sexual assault has numerous short- and long-term consequences, both physical and psychological. Unfortunately, screening does not regularly occur. When asked about sexual violence screening practices, only 40 percent of clinicians reported screening all of their pregnant cisgender patients, 21 percent reported screening nonpregnant cisgender patients, 39 percent reported screening all pregnant transgender patients, and 35 percent reported screening all nonpregnant transgender patients (Heitzler, 2024). Screening is key because only when a patient reports a history of sexual violence can clinicians further explore the ramifications the individual patient may be experiencing and offer services or resources to address sequelae.

SEXUAL PRACTICES AND BEHAVIORS

How individuals conceptualize and define sex varies widely. Clinicians need to be aware that the heteronormative lens that often equates sex with penile–vaginal intercourse represents a bias. Historically this bias is seen in the way sex is represented in research and clinical interventions, which does not accurately represent the conceptualizations of all individuals. For example, AFAB persons in same-sex relationships have reported defining sex much more broadly, conceptualizing the majority of intimate behaviors as sex, including partnered genital touching. Clinicians will build rapport by taking the lead from each patient as an individual when referring to definitions of what constitutes sex.

Sexuality involves a wide range of practices and behaviors, including fantasy, self-stimulation, noncoital pleasuring, erotic stimuli other than touch, the ability to identify what is wanted and pleasurable, enthusiastic consent, and communication about needs and desires. Sexual behaviors vary between and within individuals. In a study of their most recent sexual event, 83 percent of participants in the United States reported kissing, 69 percent cuddled, 67 percent used hands to stimulate genitals, 36 percent received oral sex, 40 percent gave oral sex, 23 percent rubbed genitals together, 13 percent used a sex toy, 3 percent had anal sex, and 81 percent had vaginal intercourse (Herbenick et al., 2023). Common sexual behaviors reported in another national U.S. survey included wearing sexy lingerie/underwear (75% of women, 26% of men), watching pornography (60% of women, 82% of men), reading erotic stories (57% of women and men), sending or receiving digital nude/seminude photos (54% of women, 65% of men), engaging in public sex (43% of women, 45% of men), and role playing (22% of women, 26% of men). Fewer participants reported engaging in threesomes (10% of women, 18% of men). The least common behaviors were going to BDSM parties (BDSM is an acronym that refers to some combination of bondage, discipline, dominance, submission, sadism, and masochism), participating in group sex and sex parties, and taking a sexuality class or workshop (less than 8%; Herbenick et al., 2017). These findings show that people engage in a wide variety of sexual practices.

Definitions of sexual practices may contain cultural and value-laden terms that are subject to different interpretations. Because it is not always easy to distinguish between aberrant and merely unconventional practices, clinicians must be aware of how they define normal and abnormal sexual practices. Is the sexual practice consensual? Does a particular behavior put the patient or their partner(s) at risk? If so, in what way, and is that risk one they understand and are willing to take? Is anyone else harmed by the behavior? Is the patient distressed by their behavior or interest? In general, unless the answer to one of these questions indicates the potential for coercion, unacceptable risk, or distress, clinicians must examine their own biases, avoid interacting judgmentally with a patient, and consider that what might otherwise be called a paraphilia (pejoratively labeled as sexual perversion or sexual deviation) is sexual arousal or sexual expression derived from atypical sources.

The *Diagnostic and Statistical Manual of Mental Disorders*, 5th ed., text revision (*DSM-5-TR*; American Psychiatric Association, 2022) distinguishes between atypical sexual interests (a paraphilia) and mental disorders involving these desires or behaviors. The diagnosis of a paraphilic disorder requires the individual to experience significant distress or functional impairment related to the paraphilia, or when the behaviors involve causing harm or functional impairment to oneself or others. Simply having an atypical sexual interest does not automatically require clinical care. These diagnostic criteria indicate that individuals who engage in consensual atypical sexual behavior should not be inappropriately labeled with a mental disorder (Reardon, 2025).

Sexual behaviors and practices that have been labeled as paraphilias in some cultures are considered normal in others (Moser, 2019). For example, at one time homosexuality was considered a paraphilia and given a medical diagnosis, and it is still considered as such in some societies. Another example of social stigma is BDSM. If a particular BDSM practice is nonconsensual, causes distress, or causes harm, it is listed in the *DSM-5* as a paraphilia. However, studies have found most adults have fantasies with BDSM themes and about half have engaged in BDSM at least one time. In fact, 8 to 70 percent of the general population include BDSM as part of their sexuality (De Neef et al., 2019). Nationally representative survey data also indicate sexual practices such as spanking (reported by more than 29%) and tying/being tied up (reported by more than 20%) are not uncommon (Herbenick et al., 2017). Literature suggests BDSM practitioners typically are highly educated, are less sexist and neurotic, have more confidence in their relationships, are more open to new experiences, and are more conscientious when compared to non-BDSM practitioners (De Neef et al., 2019).

Pornography

An important consideration is the impact of the widespread use of pornography may have on sexuality, sexual beliefs, and even body image. In a recent systematic review, Hoagland and Grubbs (2021) identified studies which indicated that in some situations, utilization of pornography is related to increased sexual functioning and satisfaction with sex, while in others pornography is related to less sexual satisfaction and functioning. More research is needed in this arena to clarify the relationship between pornography use and sexuality.

Celibacy, Monogamy, and Nonmonogamy

Celibacy involves the conscious choice to abstain from sexual activity, and it can be chosen within the context of a relationship or by those not currently in a relationship. Individuals may view this choice positively, as a means of giving their time and energy to other activities. Celibacy may also be chosen when one is between relationships or during a time when a partner is ill or away. Celibacy often refers to lack of sexual activity with another person; however, it is helpful to understand how a particular individual defines their own celibacy because, for example, masturbation is also sexual activity.

The term "monogamy" technically describes exclusive sexual and romantic love between two individuals (Kirton & McKeever,

2023), but may also be used to describe a relationship in which both partners are sexually or romantically (but not both) exclusive. The rules that determine which behaviors are and are not allowed within a monogamous relationship are unique to that dyad. Awareness of this nuance allows a clinician to avoid making mistaken assumptions about what monogamy means to an individual person's relationship. Infidelity within a relationship that is otherwise expected to be monogamous is termed "nonconsensual nonmonogamy."

Consensual nonmonogamy is an umbrella term for polyamory, swinging, or having an open relationship (Rosengren-Hovee, 2021). Consensual nonmonogamy is an intentional choice in which all parties know about and consent to the arrangement. This does not necessarily mean that all parties engage in sexual activity with one or more concurrent partners at all points in time; however, it does indicate that at least one person in the relationship is open to engage in interpersonal relationships that are not emotionally or sexually exclusive. At any given time, an individual in a consensual nonmonogamous relationship may or may not choose to engage in extradyadic sexual or emotional experiences. The perceived normalcy of monogamy, especially in Western cultures, is pervasive (Kirton & McKeever, 2023). This assumption is not evidence based and creates the potential for stigma in society and among clinicians. Clinicians often display bias, judgment, and lack of knowledge regarding diverse relationship structures (Campbell et al., 2023; Vaughan et al., 2019), and people in consensual nonmonogamous partnerships are often underserved as a result of that bias. In the course of providing clinical care, clinicians are familiar with the common concerns expressed by patients engaged in mutually monogamous relationships and may make an assumption that monogamy is the preferred structure or that extra dyadic pairings indicate infidelity. Consensual and nonconsensual nonmonogamous relationships are both often categorized by clinicians as including multiple partners or concurrent sexual partners, which may be considered problematic and defined as high-risk behavior. This may reflect provider bias given that people engaged in consensual nonmonogamous relationships have been shown to consistently employ safer and more protective sex practices than those who identify as monogamous and engage in infidelity (Gupta et al., 2023). It is imperative that clinicians examine their own bias and prepare themselves to interact constructively with patients engaged in relationship structures that are not familiar to them personally.

SEXUAL DESIRE

Possibly even more nuanced than gender and sexual behavior is sexual desire (often referred to a libido or sex drive), which has been defined as the motivation to engage in, or avoid, sexual acts. Biology may drive sexual species to engage in sex for reproduction; however, many other factors come into play that may motivate someone to engage in or avoid sexual activity (Gewirtz-Meydan et al., 2024). This motivation is molded by a continuum of biology, conditioning, psychology, culture, and society. Even having an orgasm during sexual debut impacts overall sexual desire in young adults (Peragine et al., 2022). Unfortunately, the concept of sexual desire is neither well defined nor well researched. While sexual desire has historically been considered mostly from the perspective of an individual, recent evidence implies sexual desire has both individual/solitary and dyadic components. Dyadic sexual desire includes interest in sexual acts with another person (or persons—whether their current partner or not), while solitary sexual desire includes interest in engaging in solo sexual behaviors like masturbation. This model also acknowledges the impact one's perception of their partner's sexual desire has on willingness to engage in sexual acts (Gewirtz-Meydan et al., 2024). Each person, clinician, and researcher defines desire in their own way. For some, the focus is on a physical sensation of wanting; for others, the key element is a sense of emotional craving; others experience a heightened subtle sense of excitement or arousal. Perhaps because of the elusive nature of desire or the fact that desire was thought to lie outside the realm of what can be measured with science, until recently sex researchers studied behavior rather than feelings, such as desire, that motivate behavior. William Masters and Virginia Johnson's research, which included filming research participants having sex, focused on sexual function (Masters & Johnson, 1966). Sexologists in the 1970s began examining what people desire, rather than their sexual behaviors. However, it was not until the late 1990s that full-scale research into sexual desire resumed when pharmaceutical companies began attempting to develop a female equivalent of sildenafil (Viagra), a medication to treat erectile dysfunction (Bueter & Jukola, 2020).

In the United States, the current interest in disorders of female sexual desire is relatively new. In 2015, the Food and Drug Administration approved the first pharmacological treatment for hypoactive sexual desire disorder in premenopausal women. Although many celebrate the approval as a significant win for women with hypoactive sexual desire disorder (HSDD), others criticize it as pharmaceutical medicalization or disease-mongering (Bueter & Jukola, 2020). A misconception that is central to the controversy is that one must experience desire to become aroused and engage in satisfying sex. Theories of the human sexual response cycle are presented later in the chapter (also refer to Chapter 18, Alterations in Sexual Function, for more information). An extremely valuable facet of these validated theories, supported by recent research, is that desire is very often responsive to stimuli or motivation for sexual contact, and one need not be aroused or actively desire sex to engage in fully satisfying sexual activity (Leavitt et al., 2019).

Sexual desire is shaped by a variety of factors, including familial and cultural rules. These forces mold how desire is perceived and experienced and what is considered acceptable versus taboo. Whether and what individuals desire sexually is also highly correlated with early conditioning. During early childhood, a person's sexual health is supported by maintaining autonomy and body integrity. During later childhood, avoiding sexual abuse, being supported in the right to choose relationships and sexual partners, and reproductive rights are key to developing sexual health. In adolescence and as a young adult, people need education and support to learn how to take responsibility for their own sexual health and rights (Sladden et al., 2021), as enjoyment at sexual debut likely has lasting impact on sexual desire (Peragine et al., 2022). Therefore, a person's self-perception and their presentation as a sexual being begin to form in early childhood, so gender-based social norms are also at play. Research continues to sharpen the understanding of the effects that early sexual experience can have on sexual desire later in life. While the body of evidence regarding human sexual conditioning is still developing, laboratory experiments with animals have shown that positive, pleasurable, satisfying early sexual experiences condition, through this positive feedback, preferences for partner characteristics and future sexual behaviors (Peragine et al., 2022; Quintana et al., 2019; Varas et al., 2024). In humans, research has shown that the neurotransmitters associated with arousal and potential pair bonding include noradrenaline, oxytocin, prolactin, dopamine, and opioids. During human orgasm, these neurotransmitters have been found to increase in the serum and the cerebrospinal fluid. This link between the experience of orgasm/sexual reward and the neurochemical mechanisms of pair bonding supports the idea that satisfying, pleasurable, and specifically orgasmic sexual experiences can condition an individual to desire particular sexual experiences with a particular partner who has particular traits (Coria-Avila et al., 2016).

Although conditioning impacts sexual desire preferences, humans show a tremendous capacity for erotic plasticity, sexual preferences and expression change across the life span, and many additional factors impact a person's sexual desire. For example, painful and unsatisfying sexual events can also impact a person's desire to participate in subsequent episodes, particularly if they have not communicated with their partner about the pain or stopped the activity that caused pain (Osterling et al., 2024). In addition, research shows that nonpenetrative sexual activity is often neglected as a source of creative sex play for women who are heterosexual, yet it may be less likely to cause pain and fear of recurrence. An individual's experience of their sexual identity, preferences, responses, and orientation is ever-changing. This allows an individual to rewrite the narrative of their sexual conditioning and increase their sexual agency. This plasticity can also cause shifts in an individual's perception of their sexual self that are unexpected, at which point they will benefit from validation and education to address those shifts and support them through these changes.

An individual's perception and interpretation of what they desire is shaped by their personal biology and psychosexual history and thus is influenced both positively and negatively by conditioning. For example, a person not adhering to sociocultural norms may have experienced trauma as a result. The alarming statistics shown in Box 12-2 on sexual violence underscore the possibility that for a patient presenting with sexual concerns, there is a statistically good chance that the issue may, at least in part, be related to sexual trauma. Clinicians addressing sexual concerns must consider the possibility that sexual trauma could be a contributing factor.

Trauma that impacts a person's sexuality may come from many sources. The majority of Americans (63.9% per one study and 83.2% per another) have experienced one or more adverse childhood experiences. Other sources of trauma, such as maltreatment or abuse, trafficking, or intimate partner violence also frequently occur. Additionally, trauma or retraumatization can be due to a past experience in interactions with the healthcare system—a seemingly routine pelvic examination; a potentially frightening or stigmatizing medical diagnosis; a painful procedure, such as an episiotomy, colposcopy, or biopsy; or difficult pregnancy or birth (ACOG, 2021). Perhaps most insidiously, implicit bias, lack of equity, and lack of inclusivity can harm individuals who are part of racial, ethnic, gender, or sexual minority communities or are members of other marginalized populations. Potentially traumatizing bias can be the result of clinic policies or due to the behavior of healthcare staff and clinicians. To prevent trauma and retraumatization during healthcare services, clinicians should consistently use a trauma-informed approach to care (refer to Chapter 5).

Trauma and conditioning based on past experiences, combined with sociocultural, religious, familial, and interpersonal perceptions of sexual desire, and the context within which those perceptions have developed, inform an individual person's concern about their own or their partner's sexual desire. Clinicians interact with people who have questions or concerns about their own or their partner's level of desire or perhaps about what they or their partner desire. Patients expressing concern about desire may benefit from clinician support in exploring how these factors may be influencing their concerns or limiting their own expression of desire. Refer to Chapter 18 for information on assessment and management of concerns about sexual desire.

SEXUAL SELF-KNOWLEDGE

Early experiences, combined with myriad socioeconomic and cultural factors, strongly impact a cornerstone to sexual health: self-knowledge. Sexual self-knowledge is being fluent in the language of one's own sexuality. It is the ability for a person to understand their own arousal and its physical manifestation and to recognize their own desire and preferences. With self-knowledge, if a person feels vaginal lubrication or engorgement, they can recognize it and, if appropriate, interpret those sensations as arousal. By the same token, when feeling an increase in lubrication due to sexual arousal, they would not ascribe the sensation to vaginal discharge or interpret engorgement as irritation or discomfort. Genital sexual arousal has measurable objective components that were observed by Masters and Johnson (1966), including swelling of the clitoral erectile tissue, production of lubricating secretions from the Bartholin glands, and other vaginal lubrication. Arousal also has subjective components, part of which is the subjective experience of each of these objective changes and the less easily measured range of emotions related to arousal. The matching of the objective signs—for example, measured engorgement and lubrication—with the subjective experience of arousal is called concordance. While concordance may occur, either aspect (subjective/emotional arousal or physiological arousal) can happen independently. The subjective experience of sexual arousal is not uniquely related to the experience of physiological response and is mediated by myriad additional cognitive and emotional mechanisms. Individuals may screen out their perception of physical sensations that are not consistent with what they deem appropriate or based on their sexual desires. These interpretations of physiologic responses are based on context and preferences. Information used to appraise one's state of sexual arousal is influenced by one's attitudes, beliefs, and values regarding sexuality and immediate contextual factors. For example, physiologic arousal in reaction to an unwanted stimulus may be filtered either consciously or unconsciously so that one may show physical manifestations of arousal, such as erection and orgasm, yet have no subjective experience of arousal. From a clinical perspective, providers need to foster trusting relationships with patients to facilitate full disclosure. Concordance is essentially a laboratory assessment; it is an interesting finding that may help people appreciate the importance of focusing on physical cues as sensations of arousal. Nevertheless, it is merely one small data point in the complex and critically important realm of sexual self-knowledge. Sexual self-knowledge encompasses layers upon layers of information that likely builds over the course of a person's life. As people progress through their lives, by attending to their own sexual interests and responses, they catalog all that they learn about what and who they find erotic, how they like to be touched, what is arousing, and what creates orgasm. Thus, while the popular media often stresses that sexual prime is associated with youth, lived experiences can bring both sexual self-knowledge and the capability of greater intimacy, potentially leading to greater sexual satisfaction than that experienced in younger years (Freihart et al., 2020).

Sexual Anatomy and Physiology

A person's understanding of their own sexual anatomy is an important precursor to sexual self-knowledge, the ability to gain sexual arousal and satisfaction, and communication of their needs and preferences to their partner(s).

The Clitoral Complex

All too often, information about even the most accessible portion of the clitoral complex may be incomplete or lacking altogether. Traditionally, many people's definition and understanding of the clitoris have been limited to what is merely the glans (head) and prepuce of the clitoris. In fact, anatomic, ultrasonographic, MRI, fMRI, and histologic studies are consistent in describing the components and characteristics of the variably named clitoris, clitoral complex, clitorourethrovaginal complex, or clitoral urethral complex. Whatever nomenclature is used, the clitoris is vast (refer to **Figure 12-1**) and incorporates the glans (head), shaft (body), crura (legs), clitoral (vestibular) bulbs, and neural plexus across much of the introitus and lower vagina (Mollaioli et al., 2021).

The G-Spot

There has been considerable controversy in the medical literature regarding the presence of a single anatomic G-spot, named after Ernst Gräfenberg, who published a report describing an erogenous zone in vaginas in the 1950s (Mollaioli et al., 2021). In the 1980s, the zone was further described by Ladas, Whipple, and Perry, who referred to it as a network of blood vessels, the female prostate (i.e. paraurethral glands and ducts), tissue around the bladder neck, and nerve endings (Mollaioli et al., 2021). Further, Addiego et al. (1981) describe a discrete, firm 1.5 to 2 cm area anterior to the urethra that, in one woman, enlarged by 50 percent with stimulation. However, a more recent study of 13 cadavers found that the components of the clitoral complex as described in the previous section and shown in Figure 12-1 were seen in all specimens, regardless of the age of the participant (Hoag et al., 2017). This is the largest anatomic study to date looking at the location of the putative G-spot. The dissections revealed the urethra deep to the epithelium of the anterior vagina and did not show any macroscopic structures other than the urethra and vaginal wall lining. Other than where the urethra abuts the clitoris distally, the researchers found no erectile or spongy tissue in the anterior vaginal wall. They concluded that the G-spot as a discrete anatomic entity, as has been described in the medical literature and discussed in the media, does not exist (Hoag et al., 2017). Rather, the clitorourethrovaginal complex (CUV), the area where the clitoris, urethra, vagina, and glands form an erogenous zone, may contribute to vaginally induced orgasm (Mollaioli et al., 2021). Stimulation to the anterior vaginal wall is pleasurable, arousing, and can facilitate orgasm in some women, which explains the enthusiasm for the concept of the original G-spot. However, the CUV, which includes the clitoris and the vaginal wall, provide an alternative explanation that indirect pressure and stimulation to clitoral structures underlying the vaginal wall anteriorly can cause the robust sexual response attributed to the putative G-spot.

FIGURE 12-1 **Clitoral complex.**

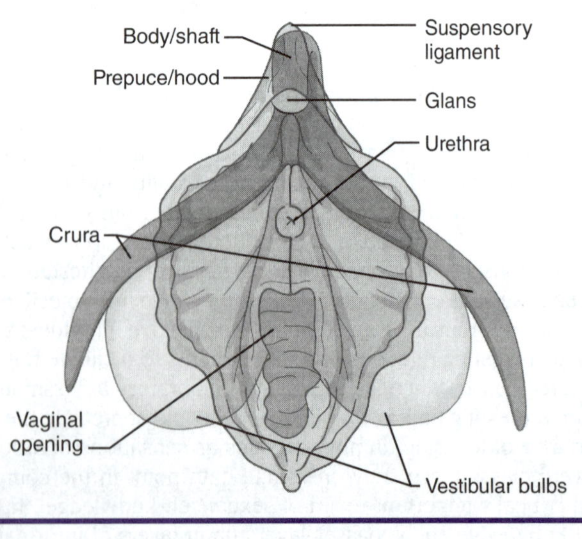

Courtesy of Phoebe S. Brown

Female Ejaculation and Squirting

Individuals with a CUV can emit four different fluids throughout arousal and orgasm: vaginal lubrication fluid (ultrafiltrated blood plasma from the vaginal wall), female ejaculate (thick whitish fluid produced by the paraurethral glands/female prostate which contains prostate-specific antigen), thin/dilute transparent urine (from the urinary bladder), and urine (via orgasmic incontinence) (Arias-Castillo et al., 2023; Pastor & Chmel, 2022). Therefore, individuals may ask clinicians if it is normal to experience involuntary fluid emission during sexual arousal or orgasm (also known as female ejaculation or squirting). In fact, 40 percent of adult women in a recent study reported having ever squirted (i.e., expelled fluid during sexual response), 60 percent found squirting to be pleasurable, and 20 percent reported always experiencing squirting and orgasm together (Hensel et al., 2024). However, it is important to get a sense of whether this is a welcome or a concerning experience. While it is likely that large amounts of fluid are the result of coital urinary incontinence, the amount reported can vary from less than 0.3 mL to more than 150 mL. Smaller amounts of fluid may reflect vaginal hyperlubrication or fluid produced by the greater vestibular glands (previously called Bartholin glands) or the paraurethral glands (previously referred to as the Skene glands). This scanty fluid is sometimes described as looking like watered-down or fat-free milk and may be reasonably described as ejaculate, in contrast to the large amounts of fluid seen with squirting or coital incontinence. Controlled laboratory studies during which emitted fluid was analyzed have shown emitted fluid has a varied biochemical makeup; female ejaculate contains PSA, glucose, and fructose, while fluid emitted during squirting includes uric acid/urea/creatinine, glucose, fructose, and may or may not include PSA (Pastor & Chmel, 2022).

Sexual Response

Sexual response involves both capacity (i.e., what someone is capable of experiencing) and activity (i.e., what the person actually experiences). Emotion and physiology are interwoven within the sexual response cycle. Traditionally, the Masters and Johnson (1966) model of sexual response, as adapted by Kaplan (1979), has been used to explain sexual response. Masters and Johnson began the modern movement toward an understanding of the sexual response cycle, and their description focuses on physiologic responses to stimuli. They identified two principal physiologic responses to sexual stimulation: vasocongestion and muscle tension. These responses are represented differently throughout the phases of the sexual response cycle. Later authorities incorporated both biologic and psychological components of sexual response (American Psychiatric Association, 2022; Kaplan, 1979).

The traditional female sexual response cycle, as described by Masters and Johnson and Kaplan, when modified to include the element of consent (Chalker, 1994), consists of four sequential phases: desire, excitement, orgasm, and resolution. The desire phase consists of sexual fantasy, thoughts, and awareness that sexual stimulation is wanted, albeit without the same degree of physiologic change that happens with arousal. Vasocongestion, muscle tension, and other physiologic changes build, peak and release, and then resolve during the excitement, orgasm, and resolution phases, respectively. During this cycle, progression occurs from a subjective sense of anticipation and pleasure to release and finally to relaxation.

In 2000, Basson described an alternative model of female sexual response that is circular rather than linear. Basson's original model was based on the theory that women are not motivated toward sexual activity by predominantly physical urges. In this model, women move from a sexually neutral state to seeking sexual stimuli when they sense either an opportunity to be sexual or a partner's need, or when they have an awareness of one or more of the potential benefits of sexual activity. Because sexual desire is a response rather than a spontaneous event—although a woman may experience what feels like spontaneous desire in the form of sexual dreams, thoughts, or fantasies—women are more likely to be at a baseline neutral state at the onset of a partnered sexual experience (Basson, 2000). Many sexually satisfied individuals do not experience spontaneous sexual desire (Basson et al., 2004). Rather, sexual arousal and responsive sexual desire may occur simultaneously after the decision to experience sexual stimulation. Basson et al. (2004) went on to endorse a composite model that reflects multiple reasons or incentives for sexual activity, including a sense of a sexual urge, which is beneficial but not essential, and the variable order and merging of responsive or triggered desire and subjective arousal. Thus, there are many variable reasons for sex, and the states of sexual desire and subjective arousal from meaningful sexual stimuli overlap. **Figure 12-2** is a diagram of the composite (circular and linear) model. This depiction allows for a sense of very early desire for sexual sensations, arousal, orgasm, or no sexual sensations at the onset of sexual engagement.

The relevance of the widely accepted current theoretical models of female sexual response based on Masters and Johnson, Kaplan, and Basson are an ongoing debate. A limitation of their work is that the studies were conducted via convenience sampling rather than random or population-based sampling (Quicke, 2023). To this end, Sand and Fisher explored a random sample of 580 female registered nurses aged 25 to 69 years old (Quicke, 2023). Participants were equally likely to endorse each of these different models of female sexual response as representing their own sexual experience. In addition to lending credibility to these models, this clearly points to the heterogeneity of sexual response. A more recent study by Ferenidou and colleagues surveyed 157 randomly selected female hospital employees and asked if their current sexual experiences were consistent with a linear model (merging the Masters and Johnson and Kaplan models) or with a circular model (based on Basson) (Quicke, 2023). Similar to the prior study, 70 percent of participants reported that their current sexual experiences were at times consistent with the linear model and at times with the circular model.

Interestingly, reports of having sex for insecurity reasons have been more consistently associated with the Basson model. Relationship contingency refers to deriving feelings of self-worth from romantic relationships. People of any sexual orientation who have relationship contingency are motivated to sustain relationships and increase intimacy, and they have been shown to be more likely to engage in sexual activity for these relational reasons. This can support sexual agency because having sex to improve intimacy is associated with autonomy and sexual satisfaction. Conversely, motivation to engage in sexual activities out of a desire to earn a partner's approval (i.e., duty sex) is associated with inhibition and sexual dissatisfaction (Metcalfe et al., 2024).

FIGURE 12-2 **Composite model of female sexual response.**[a]

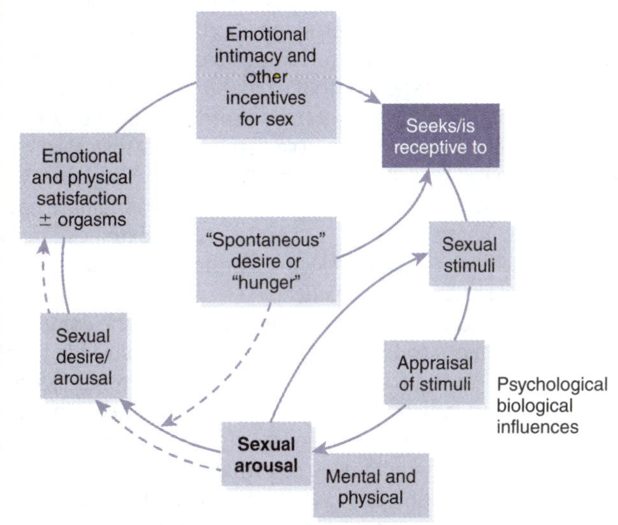

Reproduced from Basson R. (2001). Human sex-response cycles. *Journal of Sex & Marital Therapy, 27*(1), 33–43. https://doi.org/10.1080/00926230152035831

[a]This composite model of human sexual response reflects multiple incentives and overlapping phases of variable order. A sense of erotic desire may or may not be present initially: it can be triggered alongside sexual arousal resulting from attending to sexual stimuli. Sexual arousal comprises subjective (pleasure/excitement), and physical (genital and nongenital physical responses). Psychological and biological factors continuously modulate the brain's appraisal of the sexual stimuli (Brotto et al., 2016). The sexual and nonsexual outcomes influence present and future sexual motivation.

Another aspect of sexual response theory, the dual control model, was first introduced by Janssen and Bancroft of the Kinsey Institute (Bancroft et al., 2009; Janssen & Bancroft, 2007). The dual control model is based on research investigating neurotransmitters such as noradrenaline, dopamine, endocannabinoids, oxytocin, prolactin, serotonin, and opioids that impact sexual response. Each neurotransmitter creates and contributes to either sexual excitation or to a sexual inhibitory process. For example, dopamine stimulates the reward center and contributes to sexual excitation and responsiveness. Most serotonin pathways create sexual inhibition. This theory explains why medications that block serotonin and act on the dopamine pathway, such as flibanserin (Addyi), can increase sexual excitation (perceived as desire), while selective serotonin reuptake inhibitors can have negative sexual effects.

A central feature of the dual control model and the composite circular and linear model is the understanding that individuals vary greatly in their propensity for both sexual excitation and sexual inhibition. Much like the accelerator and brakes in a car, both processes occur simultaneously, and the resultant sexual response in a given individual is determined by the delicate balance between excitation and inhibition. Knowledge of individual variations in neurotransmitters and the continuous interplay between excitation and inhibition helps researchers and clinicians appreciate the wide variability seen in human sexuality. Validated instruments for measuring such propensities demonstrate similar variability in women and men.

SEXUAL AGENCY

Sexual agency is a cornerstone of sexual health though its definition has been somewhat of a subject of debate over the past several decades. Sexual agency is the concept that individuals have control over their own sexuality in a complex, multilayered, context-related and variable process (Vanwesenbeeck et al., 2021). Central to sexual agency is knowing what one likes sexually (sexual self-knowledge); being able to ask for it (sexual self-disclosure); the ability to say no (decline or rescind consent), maybe (explicitly limited consent), or yes (give enthusiastic consent); and the ability to initiate sexual interaction. Many other concepts discussed in this chapter contribute to sexual agency and sexual pleasure, or the lack of it, but simply put, the goal is for clinicians to support individuals in having control over all aspects of their sexuality (Reis et al., 2021).

The ability to ask for what one wants sexually, which is called sexual self-disclosure, is a crucial yet challenging aspect of sexual agency that relies on self-knowledge about sexual preferences to know which information about one's sexuality, anatomy, and preferences to communicate to a partner. A person's level of sexual self-disclosure is positively associated with their sexual satisfaction and sexual functioning (Sukhanova et al., 2022). Lower levels of body shame and higher levels of body appreciation are correlated with sexual self-disclosure, sexual assertiveness, and feelings of entitlement to sexual pleasure. There are many associated benefits of sexual agency, such as lower levels of sexual risk and greater levels of empowerment during sexual activity (Vanwesenbeeck et al., 2021).

Historically, there have been wide-ranging negative messages about female sexuality and stigmatizing representations of female bodies. These messages range from stereotyped images that teach women that their bodies are flawed or they are expected to have sex solely to please their partner (Carter et al., 2019), to extremes such as punishment by death for women who openly express their sexuality or are caught being sexual. Sexual guilt, negative body image, and sex-negative family attitudes and conditioning can negatively impact measures of sexual well-being, physiological satisfaction, psychological satisfaction, and one's ability to enjoy sex (Lamba et al., 2023; Reis et al., 2021). Feelings of body shame are pervasive and appear to be more common among women, individuals who have experienced sexual violence, and LGBTQ+ individuals (Saunders et al., 2024; Weaver et al., 2019).

Given the prevalence of sexual coercion and violence (refer to Box 12-2), clinicians often need to emphasize the skills an individual needs to be able to say no to unwanted sexual activity and to decline or withdraw consent. This means supporting an individual's ability to set limits on whether to engage in sexual activity, the type of sexual activity engaged in, and the timing of that activity. One example of limit setting is safer sex practices (e.g., condom use), which may require discussion between partners. Clinicians can assist individuals by providing interactive counseling conversations, active listening, and tools such as "condom comebacks" (refer to **Box 12-3**) to support an individual's sexual agency in the way they interact with their partners.

Consenting to wanted sex can be challenging in an environment where sexual activity may be stigmatized, regulated, or have unintended consequences. Even highly desired, pleasurable sex between consenting adults can result in transmission of STIs or undesired pregnancy. Developing sexual agency includes making increasingly conscious choices regarding one's own sexuality, sexual behavior, and sexual activity, including increasing the ability to initiate and consent to wanted sex.

A clinician can be a valuable resource by utilizing active listening skills and asking open-ended, focused questions designed to clarify negative conditioning about sex. In this way an individual can be assisted to sort out their own values about their sexuality and make conscious choices that are consistent with those values. Examples of these skills include paraphrasing: "So, I hear you saying that you feel like you have gotten some pretty strong negative impressions about masturbation from your mom. Do I have that right?" or, "It sounds like, on the one hand, you really enjoy it when your partner performs oral sex on you, and, on the other hand, you feel a bit embarrassed about it. Am I hearing that correctly?"

Sexual agency includes the ability to initiate sexual interaction or activity, either partnered or solo. This encompasses an individual's ability to initiate the type, timing, and range of sexual activity that they want. Traditionally, women have been at best considered passive partners in sexual encounters or at worst relegated to an assortment of sex-negative roles regarding sex (Farhane-Medina, et al., 2022). Given these constraining messages, it can be challenging for individuals to overcome familial, cultural, religious, or societal expectations to gain enough sexual agency to initiate sexual activity. In addition to these barriers, individuals who initiate sexual interaction run the risk of feeling disappointment or rejection because there is always the possibility that a partner might not be available or might not agree to engage in sex, or in the type of sex, that the individual is seeking. Individuals may experience, and therefore may be legitimately wary of, societal stigma, such as being termed promiscuous or a slut, in response to having taken an active role in initiating sex (Vanwesenbeeck et al., 2021).

BOX 12-3 Suggested Language for Individuals to Use in Conversations About Condoms

Comments for Individuals to Encourage Use of Barrier Methods

I can't wait to see you wearing nothing but a condom.

I feel sexier when I feel safe.

It's easier for me to relax and enjoy myself if I don't have to think about HIV or other STIs (or getting pregnant).

Comments from Partners About Barrier Methods with Suggested Responses

"It's not as comfortable (to have sex with a condom)."

- Riding without a seatbelt is more comfortable, too.
- If you're not comfortable using a condom, let's try something other than intercourse.

"Sex doesn't feel as good. I can't feel anything with a condom."

- Safe sex feels better!

"A condom spoils the mood. It ruins the moment. It's not spontaneous."

- (Putting the condom on together as part of foreplay.) I'll put it on for you or we can put it on together so the condom is part of the moment, it isn't interrupting it.
- The mood will come back.

"It takes too long (to put on a condom)."

- Let me help you put it on.
- We have all night!
- What's the rush?
- I'm not in a hurry.
- I like it when we take our time!

"Just this once . . . (let's have sex without a condom)."

- I don't ever have sex without a condom.
- So just this once I will have to say no.
- It only takes one time. Once is all it takes.
- The risk just isn't worth it to me.

"Don't you trust me?"

- I trust you not to put us at risk for infection.
- I trust you not to put us at risk for getting pregnant.
- I do trust you, but either of us could have an infection and not know about it.
- It's not a matter of trust.

Clinicians can help individuals gain sexual agency by supporting their efforts to initiate satisfying sexual encounters. This support can be accomplished by using active listening and paraphrasing, as described previously. Clinicians can also ask focused, open-ended questions designed to help an individual clarify what has worked well in terms of initiating sexual encounters in the past.

When proffering information or education about sexual health topics, an additional tool that a clinician can use is to sandwich the information between two questions, so the discussion remains centered on the individual rather than merely reciting advice. This process, which is called making an information sandwich, is helpful when a clinician has a piece of valuable information to share. For example, a clinician might say, "It sounds like you're saying that you feel like you are being pushy when you initiate sex with your partner. Are there any things you have tried in the past that let your partner know you would like to have sex but don't make you feel pushy?" Then, after the individual replies and the clinician paraphrases what was said, the clinician can offer a piece of information: "Sometimes people who are less interested in sexual interactions begin feeling interested when their partner frames sexual feedback in positive ways rather than as criticism." Then the clinician would follow this statement with another focused question like, "Have you noticed how you or your partner feels when sexual feedback is framed positively (I love it when you move really slowly) versus negatively (no, that's way too fast)?"

Given the importance of sexual self-disclosure, the benefit of framing information regarding preferences and giving positive feedback to a partner while minimizing critical feedback is important information for a clinician to share. Yet, at other times, saying "Don't do that!" to a partner is appropriate from a standpoint of safety and agency. Other important pieces of information that clinicians can sandwich between questions include descriptions of sexual anatomy (with visual aids); information about books, websites, videos, sexual lubricants, and sex toys; information about how to experience orgasm, including that orgasm generally requires clitoral stimulation and can be enhanced with cunnilingus (Rowland & Kolba, 2019; Curtis, 2023); condom comebacks for discussing condom use; and letting individuals know that spectatoring (mental distraction and self-judgment during sex) is a common barrier to sexual pleasure.

CONTROL OVER PELVIC MUSCLES

Another cornerstone of sexual health is awareness of, control over, and strength in the pelvic muscles—the ones that are under conscious control and are collectively referred to as the pelvic floor (more fully described in Chapter 7). There are many benefits to having control over the pelvic musculature. Pelvic floor control can decrease urinary incontinence and prevent pelvic organ prolapse. Control over the muscles distributed throughout the vagina and introitus can also aid sexual health and pleasure in multiple ways (Verbeek & Hayward, 2019). In the case of an individual who chooses to have penetration as part of sexual activity, the person can relax the muscles to facilitate various types of penetration. The individual can also relax the musculature to accommodate various positions. Tightening these muscles can help protect against deep dyspareunia if an individual experiences sensitivity deep in the pelvis or has pain with thrusting against the fundus due to a retroflexed uterus. The muscles surrounding the introitus and anus create a figure-eight shape that fully enshrouds and supports the clitoral complex, which explains how contracting these muscles can increase the physical stimulation to the clitoris (Bhat & Shastry, 2022; Omodei et al., 2019; Preda & Moreira, 2019; Tabatabaie et al., 2024).

A clinician can assess the pelvic musculature during any visit that includes a pelvic examination (Harm-Ernandes et al., 2021).

Most of the earliest data on the benefits of Kegel exercises utilized biofeedback machines for training women to identify and gain control of their pelvic muscles (Taylor & Henderson, 1986). During a biofeedback session, the patient relaxes and contracts the muscles in the pelvic floor, with the feedback helping the person to differentiate these muscles from the abdominal, thigh, and buttocks muscles. With time and feedback, the individual can learn to isolate the muscles that control the perianal region from the vaginal musculature. Biofeedback remains the gold standard for assessment and training the pelvic musculature. In many parts of the United States, there are physical therapists who specialize in sexual medicine and the pelvic floor. Clinicians should be familiar with those specialists in their area so they can provide timely, appropriate, high-quality referrals. An excellent source for referrals is the Academy of Pelvic Health Physical Therapy (APTA Pelvic Health). Their website (https://www.aptapelvichealth.org/ptlocator) allows users to search by geographic location and includes physical therapists specializing in a wide array of sexual and pelvic issues, including bladder or bowel incontinence, pelvic or genital pain, and concerns unique to pregnancy and the postpartum period.

If referral to a physical therapist or use of a biofeedback machine is not an option, a clinician can assess the strength of an individual's pelvic floor muscles and the person's current ability to identify and control those muscles during an office visit. The clinician begins by explaining the process, and if the individual agrees, the clinician places one or two fingers into the vagina, just as one would for a bimanual pelvic examination, and asks the person to grip the clinician's fingers with the vaginal muscles (Aljuraifani et al., 2019). The clinician can simultaneously grasp the individual's fingers in their own to reflect and transmit the information that the clinician gains during the examination. The clinician can note the baseline tone, control, and strength in the chart to compare these values with those obtained at future follow-up visits. Instruction on how to perform Kegel exercises should be given during the first visit. Refer to Chapter 23 for more information on Kegel exercises.

Kegel exercises can also be helpful for individuals who express concern about their ability to experience orgasm and who are interested in exploring ways to experience orgasm (Khosravi et al., 2022). To heighten awareness of sensual responses, an individual must allow time to explore these feelings and, to the greatest extent possible, banish the self-critic that might be hovering around. Distraction during sex with this spectatoring can easily interrupt focus and prevent orgasm. Often, distraction is worse with a partner, but even when an individual is alone masturbating, distraction due to spectatoring can prevent orgasm.

PRODUCTS TO ENHANCE SEXUAL HEALTH

Sexual Lubricants

The addition of exogenous lubrication to sexual activity has been credited with being as important to sex as communication. The use of sexual lubricants can facilitate wanted penetration, make good sex better, and allow penetration with larger things than might otherwise be accommodated, like multiple fingers or toys. For parts of the body that do not produce their own lubrication (the anus) or may no longer create enough lubrication (the postmenopausal vagina), the addition of exogenous lubrication can make contact or penetration pleasurable that would otherwise be painful or uncomfortable. The use of lubricants can be an important aspect of improving sexual health and well-being (Kennedy et al., 2021). With the World Health Organization prioritizing the promotion of sexual health as a key priority area, normalizing the use of lubricants for sexual pleasure, not only for treatment of vaginal dryness is key to helping to promote sexual well-being (Palacios et al., 2023).

In a systematic review that examined the use of lubricants for the promotion of sexual health and well-being, 21 studies were included that evaluated values and preferences related to use of lubrication, noting lubricant use is prevalent with 55 to 100 percent of participants in support of using lubricants. Water-based lubricants were generally preferred over oil-based or no use of lubricants and the reasons cited for using lubricants included a vast range of indications. Reasons identified included increased comfort, decreased dryness/pain/discomfort, increased pleasure for themselves and/or partner, partner's preference, improvement in orgasm, preference for sex to feel more wet, more fun, improved insertion, reduced risk of vulvovaginal or anal tearing, easier arousal, increased readiness for sex, decreased risk of condoms drying out or breaking and more enjoyable use of condoms (Kennedy et al., 2021).

The systematic review described above identified one study that suggested the use of lubricants increase sexual well-being but note a lack of recent data on lubricant use and its association with sexual pleasure and well-being. The authors concluded that lubricants play an important role in enhancing sexual pleasure, though further research is needed in this area (Kennedy et al., 2021).

Clinicians recommending sexual lubricants need to be familiar with data about the potential adverse effects of water-soluble lubricants, which can damage epithelial cells in the vagina, anus, and rectum, and can increase inflammatory markers in both the lower and upper genital tract (Wilkinson et al., 2019). It is well established that products containing nonoxynol-9 (N-9), an active ingredient in spermicides, can increase risk of HIV transmission (Van Damme et al., 2002), have detrimental effects on lactobacillus, disrupt the vaginal and rectal epithelial lining, and create sloughing that can cause epithelial ulceration (Stafford et al., 1998; Wilkinson et al., 2019). In addition, studies in vivo have seen an increase in inflammatory markers in both the lower and upper genital tract, which may increase susceptibility to other STIs including herpes simplex virus infection (Ayehunie et al., 2024).

Many water-based sexual lubricants not containing N-9 carry similar risks due to their high osmolality which can contribute to vaginal and anal epithelial disruption or damage (Palacios et al., 2023). Many of the products are made with high concentrations of glycerol, propylene glycol, polyquaternary compounds, or other ingredients that have 4 to 30 times higher osmolality than healthy vaginal fluid. The osmolality of healthy vaginal fluid is 370 plus or minus 40 mOsm/kg. In a 3-D model of human vaginal epithelium tissue, lubricants with osmolality greater than 4 times that of vaginal fluid (more than 1,500 mOsm/kg) markedly reduced epithelial barrier properties and showed damage in the tissue structure. Lubricants with osmolality greater than 1,500 mOsm/kg caused disruption in the parabasal and basal layers of cells and reduced barrier integrity. Guidance from the World Health Organization and United Nations Population Fund suggest water-based lubricants should not exceed 1,200 mOsm/kg and should have an acidic pH consistent with a health vaginal range (3.8–4.5) to ensure adequate vaginal lactobacillus production which has been shown to maintain vaginal health (Wilkinson et al., 2019). In an attempt to meet these specifications, several popular over-the-counter lubricants have been reformulated to meet the recommended osmolality and pH and a randomized trial by Palacios et al. (2023) demonstrated both safety and efficacy with these new reformulated products.

Household products such as cooking oils or lubricants may be preferred by some people but they can have a damaging effect on latex and therefore are not advised to be used with natural rubber latex condoms. These products include dairy butter, cooking oil, fish oil, palm or coconut oil, baby oil, mineral oil, suntan oil, burn ointment, hemorrhoid cream, petroleum jelly (Vaseline) and body/hand lotions. These products may have varying pH and osmolality so patients should be cautioned on their potential to impact vaginal flora if they are outside the recommended ranges provided by the World Health Organization (WHO, 2024).

Box 12-4 lists commercially available lubricants that have been tested and are shown to be toxic to epithelial cells or detrimental to lactobacillus in vitro and those that have been shown to be safe for rectal and vaginal epithelia. This is not an all encompassing list, but it includes lubricants that have been tested. As new data emerge, clinicians will have more practical information about which sexual lubricants to recommend. In the meantime, determining if the osmolality of a given lubricant is less than 1,200 mOsm/kg and has a pH of 3.8–4.5 is a good way to steer individuals toward choosing a safer product.

BOX 12-4 Sexual Lubricants

Nonirritating lubricants that are safe to use:

- Aloe Cadabra
- Female Condom 2 lubricant (silicone based)
- Good Clean Love
    - K-Y Natural Feeling Moisture Plus
- PRE
- Preseed
    - Queen V P.S. I Lube You
    - Reformulated K-Y Jelly
    - Reformulated K-Y Ultragel
- Restore
- Slippery Stuff
- Wet Platinum (silicone based)

Irritant lubricants that should be avoided:

- Astroglide
- EZ Jelly
- Boy Butter H20
- Elbow Grease
- ID Glide
- ID Glide (ultra long-lasting)
- K-Y Jelly
- K-Y personal lubricant
- K-Y Warming Jelly
- Replens

Data from Ayehunie, S., Landry, T., & Armento, A. (2024). Vaginal irritation testing-prospects of human organotypic vaginal tissue culture models. *In vitro cellular & developmental biology. Animal, 60*(6), 569–582. https://doi.org/10.1007/s11626-024-00907-1; Palacios, S., Hood, S., Abakah-Phillips, T., Savania, N., & Krychman, M. (2023). A randomized trial on the effectiveness and safety of 5 water-based personal lubricants. *The journal of sexual medicine, 20*(4), 498–506. https://doi.org/10.1093/jsxmed/qdad005; Wilkinson, E. M., Łaniewski, P., Herbst-Kralovetz, M. M., & Brotman, R. M. (2019). Personal and clinical vaginal lubricants: Impact on local vaginal microenvironment and implications for epithelial cell host response and barrier function. *The Journal of Infectious Diseases, 220*(12), 2009–2018. https://doi.org/10.1093/infdis/jiz412

Sexual Devices

Sexual devices, which may also be called sex toys, sex aids, and sexual enhancement products, can be valuable adjuncts to sexual health. Commonly used sexual devices include vibrators, penetrative devices (e.g., dildos, strap-ons), anal-specific devices (e.g., anal plugs), and air pulsation devices (Rubin et al., 2019). A wide variety of terms exist to describe this large set of products, but the most commonly accepted definition of sexual devices includes products that provide physical stimulation to the clitoris, vagina, rectum or other erogenous zone, with vibration, pulsation, pressure, or penetration (Dewitte & Reisman, 2021). Exploration with a vibrator or other sexual device can provide a pathway to experiencing or improving arousal and/or orgasm, whether an individual uses it for masturbation or with a partner. People can use sexual devices to experience wanted penetration without the need for a partner or exposure to STIs or pregnancy risk from penile–vaginal or penile–anal intercourse (Cervilla et al., 2024).

Despite the popularity of sexual devices, there is limited recent data on the use of sexual devices in the United States (Dewitte & Reisman, 2021). A nationally representative study by Herbenick et al. (2009) revealed 53 percent of women reported having used vibrators and another study conducted in Denmark, Norway, Sweden, Finland, France, and the United Kingdom revealed that more than half of the study respondents owned or previously owned a sex toy (Hald et al., 2024). Sexual devices have been around for centuries though only really became legitimate in the 1970s alongside the sexual revolution. Despite the increased legitimacy of sexual devices, in some circumstances they have remained somewhat controversial due to societal and cultural norms (Dewitte & Reisman, 2021; Hald et al., 2024). Additionally, some healthcare providers have reported feeling uncomfortable talking about devices or feel they are not well informed to provide guidance on what devices are available and how to initiate their use for improving sexual function (Dewitte & Reisman, 2021).

Some people believe that sexual devices are only intended for people who do not have a sexual partner or couples who are more adventurous, though people of all ages across the gender spectrum, single or coupled can benefit from sexual devices. By using devices solo, it can allow for individuals to identify what type of activities elicit sexual arousal and orgasm and therefore can help with allowing them to communicate their desires with a partner. Although sexual devices are beneficial for those not partnered, they appear to be used more commonly in partner play as they provide partnered people with the opportunity to shop for, choose, and explore ways to use the products together.

This can promote sexual communication and intimacy, including talk about fantasies and what they find erotic. Clinicians should validate and encourage use of sexual devices for both solo and partnered sexual activity by normalizing use (Dewitte & Reisman, 2021).

Individuals may express concern that they will become dependent on a sexual device. A clinician can use active listening skills to understand the full context of the concern that the person is expressing. For example, an individual may feel shame about the inability to orgasm with a partner, or perhaps the partner has expressed feelings of inadequacy. It can be helpful to know that after an individual's body has gained the ability to go from arousal to orgasm without a partner or with a sexual device, it becomes easier to reach orgasm consistently in other contexts and some sexual devices can be helpful for the treatment of certain sexual dysfunctions (Hald et al., 2024).

Vibrators are the most commonly used sexual device and are more often used externally providing direct clitoral stimulation, though individuals and partners gain benefit from using internally in increasing sexual pleasure. Factors to consider when selecting a vibrator include whether it is designed for external use or both external and internal use. Other considerations include shape; size (tiny bullet to large phallus shape); strength of vibration, including range of settings and speeds; power source (e.g., plug in to a power source, rechargeable, or disposable battery); volume (a consideration when living with or near others); and materials. Although there are insufficient data to guide evidence-based recommendations for safe use of sexual devices, there are known safety concerns about the chemical makeup of some of these products. The least allergenic and safest sexual devices are nonporous and are made from medical grade silicone, hypoallergenic metals, borosilicate glass or acrylonitrile butadiene styrene plastic (Rubin et al., 2019). One indication that a sexual device may be unsafe is if it has any detectable chemical or plastic smell, which is more common among less expensive products. This odor could suggest the item contains phthalates, which are chemicals used to make plastics more flexible and harder to break. Phthalates have been shown to adversely affect the reproductive systems of laboratory animals and more research is needed to fully understand their impact on human health (Sipe et al., 2023).

Patients often have questions about how to clean or disinfect sexual devices, though little research is available about the most effective way to clean and or disinfect sexual devices. It is important to note that cleaning generally refers to the removal of discharge and debris with soap and water where disinfection refers to a process that removes transmissible pathogens (Rubin et al., 2019). Clinicians should advise patients to wash devices after each use following the device manufacturer's instructions or consider disinfection or barrier methods to reduce infection risk associated with multi-partner use. STIs can be transmitted through sexual devices as research has demonstrated the persistence of HPV on porous and nonporous devices. For example, in a sample of women with positive vaginal human papillomavirus tests, the virus was detected on 70 to 90 percent of their vibrators immediately after use, on 40 percent immediately after cleaning, and on 0 to 2 percent 24 hours after cleaning (Anderson et al., 2014). Patients should be counseled to use disinfection or barrier methods between nonmonogamous partners or if diagnosed with an STI, bacterial vaginosis, or vulvovaginal candidiasis. They should also be informed that devices made with porous materials can be cleaned but they are not able to be disinfected and home disinfection methods have not been adequately studied to support one particular method (Rubin et al., 2019).

ASSESSMENT OF SEXUAL HEALTH

To provide excellent-quality sexual health care, clinicians should spend time exploring their own biases. While clinicians are not expected to have an exhaustive knowledge about all the specific details or the exact current nomenclature of the universal array of sexual practices their patients may choose, it is essential to not make assumptions about any aspect of an individual's sexuality and to take a sexual history nonjudgmentally with a genuine desire to understand. The standard for determining if a sexual practice, behavior, choice, or attitude is problematic is if it hurts the person, their partner(s), or someone else. If a patient's sexual choices are not comprehensible to the clinician, applying two fundamental principles—respect and genuine interest—will go a long way toward reaching the goal of maintaining rapport. Patient-centered, trauma-informed care means that even if the clinician "gets it wrong" (e.g., by misunderstanding what a client means about a specific practice), the patient will still feel safe and respected as the clinician prioritizes understanding their sexual situation. To "get it right," the clinician listens closely while a patient responds to focused, open-ended questions designed to clarify the patient's goals, risks, and priorities, which enable the clinician to offer appropriate services. Questions should be asked only if they are applicable to patient care, not out of curiosity.

When assessing sexual health, clinicians need to have a thorough anatomic understanding of genital anatomy, including the clitoris, and have visual aids available for patient education. In addition, part of taking and responding to a sexual history is knowing how medications (including contraceptives), medical diagnoses, and treatments affect sexual health. Gynecologic health clinicians do not need comprehensive knowledge of sex therapy or physical therapy techniques. They do need to know local physical therapists specializing in pelvic health and local sex therapists so they can make appropriate referrals. Online searchable directories are available for physical therapists specializing in pelvic health (https://www.aptapelvichealth.org/pt-locator) and sex therapists (www.aasect.org).

Although clinicians may not have the training, knowledge, skills, interest, and/or time to provide all potentially needed sexual health services, there are recommended frameworks that can help open a patient-centered conversation about sexual topics and provide the next steps. The most well-known and established of these is the PLISSIT model of addressing sexual function (Annon, 1976; refer to **Box 12-5**). This model includes four levels of intervention that move from basic to more complex: permission (P), limited information (LI), specific suggestions (SS), and intensive therapy (IT). The first level of the model, giving permission to discuss sexual health and raise sexual concerns, is applicable to all patients. The use of additional levels in the model will vary according to individual patients' needs and concerns, as well as the clinician's comfort, expertise, and time. Additionally, the ex-PLISSIT model developed by Taylor and Davis (2007) is an extension of the PLISSIT model with the goal to address the sexual well-being needs of individuals with an acquired disability or chronic illness and therefore is helpful to consider when providing care to patients with more complex

BOX 12-5 Using the PLISSIT Model in Sexual Health Care

- Permission: Give patients permission to discuss sexual health and raise sexual concerns.
- Limited Information: Give patients basic information about one or more sexual health topics, which may include patient handouts and lists of resources.
- Specific Suggestions: Make specific suggestions to address a patient's unique sexual health needs and concerns. This includes assessment and developing a plan, which may include one or more follow-up visits and/or referral to another clinician.
- Intensive Therapy: A minority of patients will require this level of intervention, which usually requires referral to a specialist.

Data from Annon, J. S. (1976). *Behavioral treatment of sexual problems: Brief therapy*. Harper & Row; Cicek Ozdemir, S., Dogan Gangal, A., & Senturk Erenel, A. (2024). The Effect of Sexual Counseling Based on PLISSIT and EX-PLISSIT Models on Sexual Function, Satisfaction, and Quality of Life: A Systematic Review and Meta-Analysis. *Archives of sexual behavior, 53*(9), 3485–3513. https://doi.org/10.1007/s10508-024-02898-2

needs (Cicek Ozdemir et al., 2024). Sexuality resources to share with patients, such as books and educational websites, can be found in Appendix 12-A.

History

It is essential for clinicians to assess their own biases when discussing sex and sexuality and monitor their own verbal and nonverbal responses as well as guarding against inadvertently displaying negative reactions, which are easily conveyed. People are sensitive to sexual criticism, so seeing a clinician have a visible reaction (e.g., negative facial expression) in response to one's sensitive disclosure can shame a patient and damage rapport (National Coalition for Sexual Health, 2022). Clinicians who are comfortable introducing topics of sexual health will establish a positive tone before beginning. Rapport and sufficient time for sensitive discussions are helpful before soliciting information that may be considered highly personal. In addition to ensuring privacy, take a sexual history in a place where the patient will be comfortable and interruptions can be minimized. Have the patient remain dressed and sit at eye level or above the interviewer. Such measures foster a sense of acceptance and respect by physically demonstrating an effort to not disempower the patient. Taking steps to mitigate against the power imbalance between the provider and the patient reduces possible feelings of intimidation and facilitates trust.

It is often best to begin with less threatening material, such as menstrual and pregnancy history, before moving to more sensitive topics such as a history of sexual violence and/or nonconsensual sexual encounters as well as current sexual practices. Closed-ended yes or no questions are appropriate for efficiently obtaining simple factual information like history of particular medical diagnoses. Often more information is obtained by asking open-ended questions focused on specific topic areas, such as how important pregnancy or STI prevention is to the patient. Allowing the sexual "story" to unfold in the way most comfortable to the storyteller yields more nuanced, detailed, and therefore more accurate information. How an individual interprets a question tells the clinician what aspect of the various potential answers are a priority. For example, asking, "Are you satisfied with the sex you're having?" will yield replies ranging from concerns about a partner's refusal to wear a condom, to excitement about a new partner, to a report of dyspareunia. As a clinician actively listens to the response to one open-ended question, they will hear within the reply the answer to several other sexual history questions. A clinician can redirect the discussion, when necessary, by utilizing paraphrasing rather than interrupting. For example, the clinician could say, "So I'm hearing you say you have been doing great with celibacy (the patient's words) until now and that you're thinking of becoming sexual with a new partner, so you'd like to look at your options for making sure your vagina will be okay because you've noticed that you are very dry. Do I have that right?" This allows the conversation to remain focused on the relevant issues and gives the patient an opportunity to further clarify their concerns.

Avoid using excessive medical terminology during an interview; both the clinician and the patient need to know the meanings of any terms used. Avoid euphemisms such as "slept with" or the broad term "sexually active" in favor of more specific terms like oral, vaginal, anal or other types of sex. Ask one question at a time, and allow enough time to answer. Statistical questions such as "How many times a week do you have sex?" are not helpful. Instead, ask the patient if they are satisfied with how frequently sex is occurring. Rather than asking whether a particular sexual experience has occurred (e.g., "Have you ever had sex without a condom?"), which tends to cause people to say no, it is better to ask how many times the experience has occurred. This technique suggests that the experience is normal. Techniques such as universalizing or prefacing questions by comments such as, "Many people," or "Other individuals I have talked with have said," may help a patient feel more comfortable when answering sensitive questions. In asking individuals to clarify the degree of satisfaction with their sex life, clinicians often get information about current sexual relationships so they can easily segue to asking about sexual communication, violence, consent, respect, and needs being met.

When taking a sexual history, it is important to inquire about behaviors, practices, and an individual's perception of their sexual experiences though it is equally important to obtain information about sexual orientation and gender identity (SO/GI). In terms of building rapport, it is helpful to hear how an individual defines and describes their own sexual orientation but the ultimate goal in obtaining this information is to improve the quality of care for all patients. The Institute of Medicine, the U.S. Department of Health and Human Services, as well as the Joint Commission all advocate for the routine collection of SO/GI data in clinical settings. The collection and reporting on SO/GI data in healthcare settings is essential to providing high-quality, patient-centered care to LGBTQ+ individuals, is an important part of efforts to better understand and address LGBTQ+ population health disparities, and allows opportunities to integrate the improvement of LGBTQ+ health into institutional and national quality improvement standards, policies, and practices (Streed et al., 2020). In addition to asking about and documenting

SO/GI, it is also important when taking a sexual history to ask questions about types of sexual activity, when and with whom they occurred, and how those experiences fit into the individual's goals for their sexual and reproductive life. For example, regardless of the patient's gender identity or sexual orientation, if they are having penile–vaginal intercourse, this could put them at risk for unwanted pregnancy. It is important for clinicians to understand that SO/GI does not correlate with what types of sex a person likes, and therefore clinicians should not make assumptions about what sexual acts their patients are engaging in based on their reported SO/GI.

An integral part of obtaining a sexual history includes asking questions that are designed to elicit risk for STIs, pregnancy, and intimate partner violence. For example, the CDC (n.d.) has established a set of sexual history questions (the five Ps) designed to address this aspect of sexual health. The five Ps is a list of possible relevant sexual history questions pertaining to partners, practices, protection from STIs, past history of STIs, and prevention of pregnancy. Refer to Chapter 22 for a complete list of the questions in the five Ps. In addition, the National Coalition for Sexual Health has expanded upon this approach of sexual history taking to include a sixth P that stands for "plus" and is meant to address sexual satisfaction, functioning, concerns and support for one's gender identify and sexual orientation (National Coalition for Sexual Health, 2022).

If an individual has already brought up sexual topics or concerns, the following introduction may not be necessary. If a clinician plans to bring up sensitive topics proactively, however, it may be helpful to prepare for the discussion. For example, a clinician can say, "I have a few questions about your sexual health and sexual practices. I understand that these questions are very personal, but they are important for your overall health." The clinician could add, "Just so you know, I ask these questions of all my adult patients, regardless of age, gender, or marital status. Like the rest of our visits, this information is kept in strict confidence" (CDC, n.d.). Alternatively, a clinician might take a neutral, straightforward approach: "At this point in the exam, I generally ask some questions regarding your sexual life. Will that be okay?" To ensure a productive sexual health conversation with patients so they can be assured the clinician is listening and able to assist, the clinician should employ some key techniques like asking direct questions in a professional and nonjudgemental manner. The term "partner" should be used when asking about the person's sexual relationships. After an individual has designated a word for their partner(s), such as "wife," "husband," or "boyfriend(s)," the clinician can then follow the lead and use the same term. Incorporating statements that highlight the commonality of the topics being discussed can help reassure patients that concerns about sexual health are widespread and normal, leading to a more open and comfortable conversation. This approach is called using ubiquity statements and it is meant to normalize sensitive discussions by emphasizing their prevalence. Stating "many individuals experience changes in their sexual health," can help patients feel less isolated in their experiences. If a patient seems reluctant to respond or answer a question, the clinician may consider rephrasing or explaining why the question is relevant and provide reassurance (National Coalition for Sexual Health, 2022).

Box 12-6 contains examples of open-ended questions of the type that clinicians can use in addition to the five Ps when taking a history focused on an individual's sexual life. In addition, much of the information gained from a complete health and gynecologic history pertains to sexual health. Refer to Chapter 7 for further information on history taking. Detailed assessment of risk for STIs can be found in Chapter 22. Assessment and management of sexual concerns is addressed in Chapter 18.

BOX 12-6 Examples of Sexual Health Assessment Questions

- Are you having sex of any kind with anyone?
- If no, have you ever had sex of any kind with another person?
- If yes, what kind of sex are you having (penis in vagina, oral, anal)? If the individual is having penile–vaginal sex, assess risk and desire for pregnancy.
- If the individual is in a relationship: How are things going for you with your sexual relationship?
- How do you feel about the sex you've been having?
- Are you satisfied with the quality of your sexual life? If not, what might make it better? or In what ways are you not satisfied?
- Is sex pleasurable for you?
- Do you masturbate?
- Do you use any form of lubrication during sex? or What kind of lubrication do you use during sex?
- Have you ever experienced an orgasm/climax? Have you experienced an orgasm with a partner? By yourself?
- What ways have you worked out to ask or show your partner what you like sexually?
- Do you feel comfortable initiating sex?
- How is it for you when your sexual partner initiates sex?
- Are there any sexual issues or concerns that you would like to discuss with me today?
- Sometimes people who (e.g., have just given birth, are diagnosed with cancer, are having chemotherapy, are dealing with fertility issues, have diabetes, have hypertension, have depression, are on this medication you are taking) have sexual issues. Have you experienced this?
- Many individuals around the time of menopause (or after menopause) have vaginal dryness or sometimes discomfort or even pain in their vaginal area. Have you experienced this?

Physical Examination and Diagnostic Testing

A physical examination and/or diagnostic tests may at times be indicated by history, the reason for seeking care (such as dyspareunia or symptoms of an STI), treatment goals, or need for referral. Physical examination and diagnostic testing to be considered in the evaluation of sexual concerns can be found in Chapter 18.

CONSIDERATIONS FOR SPECIFIC POPULATIONS

There are specific circumstances, such as certain medical conditions and medications, and particular times in a person's life when they could benefit from proactive questioning and support regarding their sexual life. Vulnerable times occur during all life stages: adolescence, sexual debut, pregnancy, postpartum, midlife, and older adulthood. Brief discussions of these considerations are included here to guide clinicians' treatment approaches. In addition, clinicians should be sensitive to the impacts that major life changes—such as changes in health, relationship, or financial status; or death of a loved one—can have on sexual health (Wickrama et al., 2022; Jones et al., 2024; Henning et al., 2023). Sexual concerns and dysfunction are addressed in Chapter 18.

Medical Factors

Medical diagnoses, chronic disease, or disabilities can significantly affect an individual's sexuality, often resulting in a diminished quality of life and higher rates of depression and anxiety (McGrath et al., 2021). In addition, some of the medications used to treat common medical conditions can have negative sexual effects (refer to Chapter 18). Because a given individual's response to a particular medication can vary, the clinician needs to ask a person about any effects they may be having. When doing so, it is better to avoid asking, "Are you doing well on this medication?" It is preferable to say something like, "Some people taking this medication report a change in their sexual response or sexual feelings. Now that I mention this, do you think you have noticed any differences?"

A clinician can be a valuable resource to a person who is taking a medication or who has a medical condition that may affect their sexuality. Similarly, clinicians can be immensely helpful in caring for people with cancer or surviving cancer, particularly those with breast or gynecologic cancers (Mangiardi-Veltin et al., 2023; Wilson et al., 2021); those who are recovering from surgery; and those struggling with fertility issues (Kelley & Kingsberg, 2024) by addressing possible sexual challenges, in addition to the health challenges.

The coronavirus (COVID-19) pandemic had a profound global impact, disrupting lives on health, financial, social and mental levels. Rates of sexual dysfunction increased while sexual activity decreased (Masoudi et al., 2022). Women, in particular, may have experienced greater disruption as they reporting decreases in arousal, increased pain, diminished orgasm, and lower satisfaction (Hessami et al., 2022).

Adolescents

Adolescence, which is generally defined as age 12 to 19 years, is a period of rapid physical change and potentially stressful psychosocial demands, including awareness of and changes in sexual feelings. It is also a time when sexual preferences are being formed, and early sexual experiences can contribute to preference conditioning. Adolescence marks a time for individuals to develop their sense of self, explore their sexual orientation, and affirm their gender identity (Long & Damle, 2024). Adolescents are influenced by their parents, peers, and society during this time and show a high interest in understanding the feelings and perceptions of the opposite sex (Bauer et al., 2020). Other factors which can influence one's sexual identity also include sexual knowledge, intimate relationship experiences, culture and religious exposures (Long & Damle, 2024). The adolescent period, marked by opportunities for self-discovery and sexual awareness, lays the foundation for behaviors essential to becoming a sexually healthy adult (Long & Damle, 2024) (refer to **Table 12-1**).

Adolescent sexual health researchers emphasize the primacy of supporting youth as they move through these developmental tasks (Kågesten & van Reeuwijk, 2021); however, most research and societal interest is focused instead on statistics about behavior. Familiarity with these statistics may be interesting but of minimal help to clinicians engaging with adolescents, except as reassurances that developing sexual self-concept and sexual agency results, in part, from sexual behavior and positively impacts future behavior (Maes et al., 2023). Although early sexual debut (often defined as before age 15) is associated with increased risk for adverse outcomes, such as STIs, substance use disorders, depression, and unwanted pregnancy (Fabersunne et al., 2024), it is important for clinicians to also understand that noncoercive, age-normative sexual experiences and romantic relationships during adolescence strongly predict positive parameters of physical, mental, emotional, and social health (Kågesten & van Reeuwijk, 2021).

When discussing sexual debut, it is important to consider terminology. The historical definition of virginity, which centers on vaginal-penile intercourse, excludes the experiences of LGBTQ+ individuals. A more nuanced, inclusive, and ambiguous understanding of virginity acknowledges the diverse ways youth define and experience sex. "Sexual debut" is a term that can be interpreted by the debutantes themselves, which is, after all, the meaning that clinicians seek when they ask a question about virginity.

Although sexual curiosity and self-exploration begins in infancy, during adolescence masturbation increases in frequency. Those who idenetify as males are more likely than females to masturbate. This discrepancy may be due to biology but also is rooted in social stigma. In a nationally representative sample of U.S. adolescents aged 14 to 17 years, 2018 data revealed that significantly fewer adolescents (39.5%) reported engaging in solo masturbation as compared to data from 2009 (56%) (Herbenick et al., 2021). Masturbation is an excellent way to learn about one's own sexual responses, genital anatomy, preferences, and orgasm. Solo sex also does not incur exposure to STIs or pregnancy. For young people who identify as female, masturbation is correlated with higher levels of self-awareness, body positivity, and satisfaction with relationships in the future (Long & Damle, 2024).

In recent years the percentage of adolescents reporting ever having sex has also decreased. Around 60 percent of U.S. adolescents have not had partnered sex (Abma & Martinez, 2023). The most common reason those identifying as female adolescents do not have partnered sex is that it is against their religion or morals (32.5%). The most common reason why those who identify as adolescent males say they do not have sex is that they have not found the right person yet (35.3%)(Abma & Martinez, 2023).

Partnered sexual activity includes a range of behaviors. While focusing on rates of penile–vaginal sex is a flawed, heteronormative, and incomplete measure, much research is devoted to it. For example, the lifetime prevalence of penile–vaginal sex increases with each year of age, and the timing varies little by gender (Abma & Martinez, 2023). Among a 2015–2019 sample of U.S. high school students, rates of condom use during last penile–vaginal intercourse were 49.7 percent for those who identified as females and 68.1 percent for individuals who identified as males (Abma & Martinez, 2023). Among young people aged 18 to 24 years who have had penile–vaginal sex, only 45.9 to 68.6 percent of individuals describe their first sexual experience as wanted

TABLE 12-1 Adolescent Behaviors to Support Healthy Sexuality

Appreciate one's own body.	Express one's sexuality while respecting the rights of others.
Practice masturbation to learn about personal responses, preferences, anatomy, and orgasm.	Discriminate between life-enhancing sexual behaviors and those that are harmful to self and/or others.
Understand everyone's right to pleasure and agency.	Use contraception effectively to avoid unintended pregnancy.
Seek further information about reproduction as needed.	Enjoy sexual feelings without necessarily acting on them.
Affirm that human development includes sexual development, which may or may not include reproduction or sexual experience.	Be supported to explore their sexual identity through self-discovery and sexual awareness.
Interact with all genders in respectful and appropriate ways.	Avoid contracting or transmitting a sexually transmitted disease.
Engage in sexual relationships that are consensual, non-exploitative, honest, pleasurable, and protected.	Act consistently with one's own values when dealing with an unintended pregnancy.
Seek early prenatal care.	Affirm one's own sexual orientation and respect the sexual orientation of others.
Develop and maintain meaningful relationships.	Know where to seek accurate information about sex and sexuality.
Make informed choices about family options and relationships.	Express love and intimacy in appropriate ways.
Demonstrate respect for people with different sexual values.	Exhibit skills that enhance personal relationships.
Express one's sexuality in ways that are congruent with one's values. Critically examine the world around them for biases based on gender, sexual orientation, culture, ethnicity, and race.	Assess the impact of family, cultural, media, and societal messages on one's thoughts, feelings, values, and behaviors related to sexuality. Exercise democratic responsibility to influence legislation dealing with sexual issues.
Explore age-normative sexual and romantic relationships.	Avoid behaviors that exhibit prejudice and bigotry.
Communicate effectively with family, peers, and romantic partners.	Reject stereotypes about the sexuality of different populations.
Enjoy and express one's sexuality throughout life.	Take responsibility for one's own behavior.

Reproduced from Sexuality Information and Education Council of the Unites States – SIECUS. Life Behaviors of a Sexually Healthy Adult. In Guidelines for Comprehensive Sexuality Education. 3rd edition.

(Abma & Martinez, 2023). This reflects the prevalence of sexual violence described earlier in this chapter and also points to a potentially remediable gap in adolescent sexual agency.

Oral sex rates have also decreased in recent years. Among U.S. 14- to 17-year-olds, 20.8 percent of individuals report receiving oral sex in 2009 whereas 2018 data reveal 9.9 percent of adolescents receiving oral sex (Herbenick et al., 2021). Adolescents may perceive oral sex as less risky considering chance of pregnancy, however oral sex carries STI risk for herpes, gonorrhea, chlamydia, syphilis and HIV (Moore-Petinak et al., 2022). This population may be vulnerable to STI transmission as only 7–10 percent of youths report using protection during oral sex (Moore-Petinak et al., 2022).

Anal sex is less common among adolescents. In the United States, 4.4 percent of adolescents report having ever had anal sex in 2009 versus 1.7 percent in 2018 (Herbenick et al., 2021). Anal sex is, however, more common in 18–49-year-olds where 17.8 percent of individuals report having had anal sex in the past year (Herbenick et al., 2021).

Data on sexual orientation and same-sex sexual behaviors for U.S. individuals reveal an increasing trend of those who identify as lesbian, gay, bisexual, or transgender (LGBT) (Flores and Conron, 2023). In a 2024 study, 9.3 percent of U.S. individuals identified as LGBT, this percentage increased among Gen Z individuals to 22.7 percent (Jones, 2025), although the majority of adolescents identify as heterosexual. Compared to older generations, it is more likely that younger Americans identify as something other than heterosexual. For Gen Z individuals in 2024, 59 percent identified as bisexual. (Jones, 2025). Chapter 11 discusses care for lesbian, bisexual, queer, transgender, and nonbinary adolescents.

Adolescents are planting the seeds for a life. Educators and sex education programs have an opportunity to address adolescent knowledge gaps in understanding sexual pleasure, desire, initiating and managing relationships, societal ideals, and the impact of pornography (Bauer et al., 2020). Clinicians frequently do not bring up sexual health or intimate relationship topics, and when these topics are discussed, it is brief (Lung et al., 2021).

Communication about sexual attractions, sexual orientation, and noncoital sexual behaviors may be the rarest, and discussion of contraception, however brief, appears to be more frequent (Lung et al., 2021). Communication about sexual behaviors, sexual agency, and protective behaviors is vital for the support of all adolescents and may be particularly lacking for LGBTQ+ adolescents or those with chronic illness or disabilities (Kågesten & van Reeuwijk, 2021). Clinicians can support adolescents with discussions about healthy relationships and education about anatomy, and by proactively addressing issues of pleasure and agency in addition to engaging them in discussions about protection from STIs, sexual violence, and undesired pregnancy. Clinicians have an opportunity to directly impact adolescent well-being through education and screening. As an example, though adolescents account for only 25 percent of the sexually active population, half of all newly contracted STI cases occur in adolescents (Long & Damle, 2024), and condom use has consistently declined since 2006 (Lindberg et al., 2021). By addressing these positive aspects of sexual health development, clinicians can also address other common adolescent health issues (Kågesten & van Reeuwijk 2021). Studies repeatedly indicate that higher levels of self-esteem, autonomy, sexual assertiveness, comfort, and openness are correlated with the ability to enact less risky behavior and an increased capacity for sexual satisfaction. Discussions with adolescents about sexual pleasure and tailored interventions have been shown to be effective strategies to improve STI and HIV prevention (de Vries et al., 2024). Adolescents will benefit from detailed information about sexual anatomy and function and diagrams of the clitoral complex. Clinicians should ensure that adolescents understand that the most likely route for most women or those AFAB to learn how to experience orgasm is with masturbation or a partner's hands or mouth rather than with penile–vaginal intercourse.

Pregnancy and Postpartum

Changes associated with pregnancy, the postpartum period, and lactation offer an opportunity to discuss sexuality and provide education for a childbearing couple's changing needs (Ollivier et al., 2020; Delgado-Perez et al., 2022; Grussu et al., 2021). Pregnant people may experience changes in sexual function with each trimester of pregnancy. During the first trimester, common symptoms, such as nausea and vomiting, breast tenderness, and fatigue, may impact interest in sex. It may be a time when a couple is feeling particularly close, being intimate, and enjoying nesting. Some individuals and some couples have anxiety about the pregnancy, which can impact their sexual activity. In the second trimester, pregnant persons often express heightened interest as they feel better. Even so, it is helpful if the clinician asks the person about feelings regarding their bodily changes, including increasing weight and body image as body acceptance is an important component of sexual health (Delgado-Perez et al., 2022). The third trimester can be associated with physical discomfort related to increasing size, especially when a person is near term. Fears about the effects of intercourse on pregnancy maintenance and harming the fetus may decrease sexual interest or pleasure at any time during pregnancy. As pregnancy progresses, sexual function declines. This is most apparent in the third trimester when a thickening of the muscle fibers within the vagina may decrease orgasmic response and vaginal vasocongestion may affect lubrication and dysparuenia (Grussu et al., 2021). A recent randomized controlled trial on the effect of pelvic floor muscle exercise on sexual functioning in the postpartum period found no improvement in sexual health or satisfaction for individuals who practice pelvic floor muscle exercises (Sobhgol et al., 2022).

There are surprisingly little data about sexual activity in the postpartum period. When examining the resumption of sexual activity during the postpartum period, research indicates that 50 percent or more of heterosexual couples had resumed penile–vaginal sex by 6–8 weeks postpartum with even more doing so by 6–12 months. However, the frequency of sexual activity during this time was reduced compared to prepregnancy levels (Grussu et al., 2021). Psychological and physical satisfaction during sex was lower both during pregnancy and after giving birth, relative to satisfaction before pregnancy (Grussu et al., 2021). Postpartum sexual concerns are common, distressing, and associated with decreased relationship well-being (Delgado-Perez et al., 2022). This is a time when clinicians have an opportunity to proactively ask about potential sexual issues to provide needed support, validation, and intervention, if appropriate.

During the postpartum period, there are immense emotional, psychological, relational, and physical changes and stressors with the potential to adversely impact sexuality (Grussu et al., 2021). Clinicians should remember that the postpartum period is a time of significant uncertainty and change. During this transition, sexuality—encompassing more than just physical factors—may vary greatly from person to person (Ollivier et al., 2020). Common challenges include loss of a sense of self; exhaustion; transitioning to roles and responsibilities of parenthood, which can be doubly stressful when considering the impact of family and sociocultural expectations about gender roles; new roles within the family; stress from competing priorities, such as work and other children; and new financial demands. Relationship dynamics in a couple change with the addition of a newborn to the family. These changes can herald some of the most precious moments in a couple's life together, yet they also have the potential for setting the couple up for alienation. For example, a partner may feel shut out of the chest/breastfeeding parent–infant dyad. Feelings of resentment or rejection detract from motivation to preserve or regain sexually satisfying interactions.

Postpartum stress for new parents has been shown to be negatively associated with sexual well-being, and more frequent positive sexual experiences predict lower perceptions of stress throughout this vulnerable period. Addressing sexual well-being with new parents may help postpartum women cope with stress and support relationship satisfaction (Rosen et al., 2021). A clinician can apply motivational interviewing techniques to help a person create potential solutions to sleep deprivation and prioritize time and space for intimacy. Clinicians can make suggestions to ease the pressures on new parents—perhaps a partner or family member will take an entire night with the newborn or be the one to get up to bring the newborn to the parent to chest/breastfeed to allow them more time for sleep.

Physical concerns include postpartum body changes that carry the potential to negatively impact self-image; discomfort or pain from birth trauma; and hormonal changes, such as lower estradiol and increased prolactin, that are associated with decreased desire and responsiveness to sex, vaginal dryness, and dyspareunia (Grussu et al., 2021; Rosen et al., 2021). Clinicians caring for individuals in the postpartum period can proactively ask open-ended, focused questions about these changes. Anticipatory guidance can help normalize the postpartum experience. For example, postpartum individuals may cope with dyspareunia, a common concern in the postpartum, by using lubricants, adopting new postures or avoiding painful postures during sex. For others sexuality takes on a different meaning in the postpartum and some individuals may desire intimacy in ways other than intercourse (Delgado-Perez et al., 2022).

Although vaginal dryness is more common among people who are chest/breastfeeding, it can occur in any postpartum person. Vaginal dryness may persist until ovulatory cycles resume. Those who are experiencing vaginal dryness can benefit from the use of lubricant to prevent dyspareunia (refer to the section on sexual lubricants for specific products to recommend and avoid). Nonpenetrative sexual activity may be less likely to cause pain until postpartum vaginal dryness resolves. Vaginal estrogen therapy may be beneficial for people who are breastfeeding (Smith et al., 2022).

Midlife

In midlife (40 to 65 years of age), a person's sexuality is as varied as people themselves. For those who have been having positive sexual experiences throughout their lives, with the cornerstones of sexual health in place, this time of life can be one of great sexual satisfaction because increased self-knowledge, sexual agency, and capacity for intimacy intertwine with the mastery they and their partner(s) may have developed (Barbee, 2022; Beerepoot et al., 2022). For some individuals, a decreased concern about avoiding pregnancy may increase sexual desire and lessen inhibitions. This may also be a time of relationship transition and changing family dynamics as children grow up and leave the household.

Alternatively, in a study following women aged 40 to 55 years old, sexual satisfaction decreased during the perimenopause years with vaginal dryness being a main factor (Cagnacci et al., 2020). In a study of individuals aged 40 to 64 years, 60.1 percent reported to be satisfied or very satisfied with their sex life. Similar findings were revealed among heterosexual individuals and those of sexual minorities. Those who were in better health physically and mentally, in a relationship, and had higher self-esteem were more likely to have greater sexual satisfaction (Buczak-Stec et al., 2023). Factors positively correlated with sexual satisfaction in menopause included regular physical activity, mental well-being, occurrence and frequency of orgasm before menopause, marital satisfaction, and emotional and social well-being (Shahrahmani et al., 2024).

During midlife, fluctuations and the eventual decrease in estrogen and androgen levels can affect the vulvar and vaginal mucosa (Cox et al., 2023). The term "genitourinary syndrome of menopause" (GSM) replaces the terms "vulvovaginal atrophy" and "atrophic vaginitis." The new term was created by a consensus panel because the prior nomenclature inadequately described the range of symptoms associated with physical changes of the vulva, vagina, and urinary tract. Many studies have shown the effectiveness in vaginal estrogen therapy in alleviating moderate to severe GSM symptoms (North American Menopause Society, 2020). Another effective way to maintain vaginal tissue pliability in perimenopause and after menopause is consistent sexual activity (North American Menopause Society, 2020). Other therapies for GSM are discussed in Chapters 14 and 21.

Older Adulthood

During older adulthood (after age 65), people continue to be sexual beings and enjoy sexual activity. There are strong associations between successful aging, fitness, and sexual satisfaction among older people in many countries (Beerepoot et al., 2022; Buczak-Stec et al., 2023; Henning et al., 2023). In a study considering satisfaction with their sex life, 45.6 percent of older individuals 65 years and older were satisfied or very satisfied (Buczak-Stec et al., 2023). The type of sexual activity people engage in often shifts with increasing age. This may mean taking adequate time for arousal and an increased emphasis and value placed on affection (Beerepoot et al., 2022). Allowing for change in what is sexually interesting is associated with sexual satisfaction. In later life, feelings of intimacy and closeness may arise from shared pleasures such as hobbies, cuddling, and kissing (Towler et al., 2023).

The transition from work to retirement can also significantly impact an individual's sexual satisfaction. Factors such as changes in free time, finances, responsibilities, self-perception, and marital dynamics all play a role. Research suggests that retirement can negatively affect both marital satisfaction and sexual satisfaction for men (Henning et al., 2023).The prevailing cultural view of older individuals as asexual beings has the potential to negatively affect sexual expression and activity, and it can become a self-fulfilling prophecy (Henning et al., 2023; Beerepoot et al., 2022). Further, the current cultural emphasis on youth, beauty, and thinness contributes to societal expectations about asexuality in older women. This time of life can continue the sexual satisfaction that occurred in midlife; the health benefits of sexual activity become increasingly evident. In addition to its cardiovascular benefits, sexual activity may also positively influence the immune system, enhance life enjoyment, reduce inflammation, decrease frailty, and improve personal perceptions of successful aging (Soysal & Smith, 2022). Sexual activity helps maintain the integrity of vulvar and vaginal tissues by supporting tissue pliability (North American Menopause Society, 2020). There is a clear link between sexual satisfaction and overall satisfaction with aging (Hajek & König, 2023).

Influences of Culture

A restrictive family upbringing or a belief that expressions of intimacy or sexuality are shameful or taboo may contribute to a person's inability to express themselves sexually. Religion also influences sexual attitudes, beliefs, and values and can exert a strong influence throughout a person's life (Shahrahmani et al., 2024). Some religious proscriptions may contribute to sexual concerns or problems. For example, a view that sexual intercourse is acceptable only for procreation may raise concerns when pleasurable sexual sensations are felt outside of a procreative context. Accepting or rejecting premarital sex, allowing or limiting contraception to prevent pregnancy, beliefs about monogamy, and condoning or rejecting LGBTQ+ people or nonheteronormative sex behaviors are examples of religious influences.

Society and culture are inextricably interwoven with sexuality and influence it as much as physiology and psychology. Society defines what sexual behavior is, identifies the norms for that behavior, and guides the behavior of individuals in a given culture. In part, people form their ideas of what is sexually appropriate and desirable from years of cultural scripting. These scripts can cause harm by interfering with healthy sexual functions and behaviors (Shahrahmani et al., 2024). The paradoxical and misogynistic notions that men who are sexually aggressive are viewed by society as favorable and that sexually aggressive women are condoned are examples of such cultural beliefs. In addition, sex role stereotypes often prescribe that genders also dictate who will initiate sexual activity and who will exercise sexual control.

Sexual myths are common in every culture and society, and they are a source of sexual misinformation. Often, they interfere with an experience of full sexual agency, reproducing traditional heteronormative gender norms. Myths surrounding sexuality and consent can cause significant harm by reinforcing stereotypes and attitudes that perpetuate rape culture and normalize sexual aggression. These misconceptions contribute to a societal environment where harmful behaviors are excused or overlooked, ultimately undermining efforts to promote healthy, respectful relationships (Reling et al., 2021). Other sexual myths are specific to older people, such as statements that older individuals are not interested in or capable of sexual expression, are physically unattractive, and are sexually undesirable.

A specific behavior may be defined as desirable by one cultural group and evil by another. Different views often exist regarding premarital, extramarital, and marital sex; appropriate sexual practices or positions; accepted foreplay activities; and duration of coitus. Clinicians need to be careful to avoid stigmatizing and making assumptions or judgments based on demographic, heteronormative, and cultural stereotypes.

CONCLUSION

Sexual health can contribute substantially to overall health throughout the life span. A trusted clinician who has a good rapport with a patient is in a unique position to support their safe progress toward sexual self-knowledge, sexual agency, and control over their pelvic musculature. It is essential for clinicians to provide care without judgment, using a patient-centered, trauma-informed approach, so that patients are comfortable discussing whatever questions and concerns they may have regarding their sexuality and can get accurate information, appropriate counseling, and relevant services. By fostering communication and, when needed, making appropriate referrals to other health professionals, clinicians can help each person enjoy their own version of sexuality.

References

Abma, J. C., & Martinez, G. M. (2023). Teenagers in the United States: Sexual activity, contraceptive use, and childbearing, 2015–2019. *National Health Statistics Reports, 196,* 1–23. https://dx.doi.org/10.15620/cdc:134957

Addiego, F., Belzer, E. G., Jr., Comolli, J., Moger, W., Perry, J. D., & Whipple, B. (1981). Female ejaculation: A case study. *Journal of Sex Research, 17*(1), 13–21. https://doi.org/10.1080/00224498109551094

Aljuraifani, R., Stafford, R. E., Hall, L. M., & Hodges, P. W. (2019). Activity of deep and superficial pelvic floor muscles in women in response to different verbal instructions: A preliminary investigation using a novel electromyography electrode. *Journal of Sexual Medicine, 16*(5), 673–679. https://doi.org/10.1016/j.jsxm.2019.02.008

Alvarez-Muelas, A., Sierra, J. C., Gomez-Berrocal, C., Arcos-Romero, A. I., Calvillo, C., & Granados, R. (2022). Study of sexual concordance in men and women with different typologies of adherence to the sexual double standard. *International Journal of Clinical and Health Psychology, 22*(2), 100297.

American College of Obstetricians and Gynecologists. (2019). ACOG committee opinion: Sexual assault. *Obstetrics & Gynecology, 133*(4), e296–e302.

American College of Obstetricians and Gynecologists. (2021). ACOG committee opinion: Caring for patients who have experienced trauma. *Obstetrics & Gynecology, 137*(4), e94–e99.

American Psychiatric Association. (2022). *Diagnostic and statistical manual of mental disorders* (5th ed., text revision).

American Sexual Health Association. (2024). *Understanding sexual health.* http://www.ashasexualhealth.org/sexual-health/

Anderson, T. A., Schick, V., Herbenick, D., Dodge, B., & Fortenberry, J. D. (2014). A study of human papillomavirus on vaginally inserted sex toys, before and after cleaning, among women who have sex with women and men. *Sexually Transmitted Infections, 90*(7), 529–531. https://doi.org/10.1136/sextrans-2014-051558

Annon, J. S. (1976). *Behavioral treatment of sexual problems: Brief therapy.* Harper & Row.

Arias-Castillo, L., Garcia, L, & Garcia-Perdomo, H. A. (2023). The complexity of female orgasm and ejaculation. *Archives of Gynecology and Obstetrics, 308,* 427–434. https://doi.org/10.1007/s00404-022-06810-y

Ayehunie, S., Landry, T., & Armento, A. (2024). Vaginal irritation testing—prospects of human organotypic vaginal tissue culture models. *In Vitro Cellular & Developmental Biology. Animal, 60*(6), 569–582. https://doi.org/10.1007/s11626-024-00907-1

Bancroft, J., Graham, C. A., Janssen, E., & Sanders, S. A. (2009). The dual control model: Current status and future directions. *Journal of Sex Research, 46*(2–3), 121–142. https://doi.org/10.1080/00224490902747222

Barbee, H. (2022). Harnessing progress: Gender, sexuality, and positive self-perceptions of aging in midlife. *Journal of Aging Studies, 61,* 101008. https://doi.org/10.1016/j.jaging.2022.101008

Basile, K. C., Smith, S. G., Kresnow, M., Khatiwada, S., & Leemis, R. Q. (2022). *The National Intimate Partner and Sexual Violence Survey: 2016/2017 Report on Sexual Violence.* Atlanta, GA: National Center for Injury Prevention and Control, Centers for Disease Control and Prevention.

Basson, R. (2000). The female sexual response: A different model. *Journal of Sex & Marital Therapy, 26*(1), 51–65. https://doi.org/10.1080/009262300278641

Basson, R. (2001). Human sex-response cycles. *Journal of Sex & Marital Therapy 27*(1), 33–43. https://doi.org/10.1080/00926230152035831

Basson, R., Leiblum, S., Brotto, L., Derogatis, L., Fourcroy, J., Fugl-Meyer, K., Graziottin, A., Heiman, J. R., Laan, E., Meston, C., Schover, L., van Lankveld, J., & Schultz, W. W. (2004). Revised definitions of women's sexual dysfunction. *Journal of Sexual Medicine,* 1, 40–48. https://doi.org/10.1111/j.1743-6109.2004.10107.x

Bates, N., Chin, M., & Becker, T. (2022). *Measuring sex, gender identity, and sexual orientation.* National Academies Press.

Bauer, M., Hammerli, S., & Leeners, B. (2020). Unmet needs in sex education—What adolescents aim to understand about sexuality of the other sex. *Journal of Adolescent Health, 67,* 245–252. https://doi.org/10.1016/j.jadohealth.2020.02.015

Beerepoot, S., Luesken, S. W. M., & Deeg, D. J. H. (2022). Enjoyment of sexuality and longevity in late midlife and older adults: The longitudinal ageing study Amsterdam. *Journal of Applied Gerontology, 41*(6), 1615–1624. https://doi.org/10.1177/07334648221078852

Beuter, A., & Jokola, S. (2020). Sex, drugs, and how to deal with criticism: The case of Flibanserin. In A. LaCase & B. Osimani (Eds.), *Uncertainty in pharmacology: Epistemology, methods, and decisions* (pp. 451–470). Springer.

Bhat, G. S., & Shastry, A. (2022). Sexually induced orgasm to improve postpartum pelvic floor muscle strength and sexual function in primiparous women after vaginal delivery: A prospective randomized two-arm study. *The Journal of Sexual Medicine, 19*(11), 1634–1643. https://doi.org/10.1016/j.jsxm.2022.08.189

Brotto, L., Atallah, S., Johnson-Agbakwu, C., Rosenbaum, T., Abdo, C., Byers, E. S., Graham, C., Nobre, P., & Wylie, K. (2016). Psychological and interpersonal dimensions of sexual function and dysfunction in women: An update. *Journal of Sexual Medicine, 13*(4), 538–571.

Buczak-Stec, E. W., Konig, H., & Hajek, A. (2023). Sexual satisfaction among sexual minority and heterosexual middle-aged and older adults. *Innovation in Aging, 7,* 1–11. https://doi.org/10.1093/geroni/igad010

Cagnacci, A., Venier, M., Xholli, A., Paglietti, C., & Caruso, S. (2020). Female sexuality and vaginal health across the menopausal age. *Menopause: The Journal of the North American Menopause Society, 27*(1), 14–19. https://doi.org/10.1097/GME.0000000000001427

Campbell, C., Scoats, R., & Wignall, L. (2023). "Oh! How modern! And . . . are you OK with that?": Consensually non-monogamous people's experiences when accessing sexual health care. *The Journal of Sex Research, 61*(9), 1377–1388. https://doi.org/10.1080/00224499.2023.2246464

Cao, C., Yang, L., Xu, T., Cavazos-Rehg, P., Liu, Q., McDermott, D., Veronese, N., Waldhoer, T., Ilie, P. C., Shariat, S. F., & Smith, L. (2020). Trends in sexual activity and associations with all-cause and cause-specific mortality among US adults. *The Journal of Sexual Medicine, 17,* 1903–1913. https://doi.org/10.1016/j.jsxm.2020.05.028

Carter, A., Ford, J. V., Luetke, M., Fu, T. J., Townes, A., Hensel, D. J., Dodge, B., & Herbenick, D. (2019). "Fulfilling his needs, not mine": Reasons for not talking about painful sex and associations with lack of pleasure in a nationally representative sample of women in the United States. *Journal of Sexual Medicine, 16*(12), 1953–1965. https://doi.org/10.1016/j.jsxm.2019.08.016

Centers for Disease Control and Prevention. (n.d.). *A guide to taking a sexual history.* http://www.cdc.gov/std/treatment/sexualhistory.pdf

Cervilla, O., Álvarez-Muelas, A., & Sierra, J. C. (2024). Relationship between solitary masturbation and sexual satisfaction: A systematic review. *Healthcare (Basel, Switzerland), 12*(2), 235. https://doi.org/10.3390/healthcare12020235

Chalker, R. (1994). Updating the model of female sexuality. *Sexuality Information and Education Council of the United States, 22,* 1–6.

Cicek Ozdemir, S., Dogan Gangal, A., & Senturk Erenel, A. (2024). The effect of sexual counseling based on PLISSIT and EX-PLISSIT models on sexual function, satisfaction, and quality of life: A systematic review and meta-analysis. *Archives of Sexual Behavior, 53*(9), 3485–3513. https://doi.org/10.1007/s10508-024-02898-2

Coria-Avila, G. A., Herrera-Covarrubias, D., Ismail, N., & Pfaus, J. G. (2016). The role of orgasm in the development and shaping of partner preferences. *Socioaffective Neuroscience & Psychology, 6*(1), 31815. https://doi.org/10.3402/snp.v6.31815

Cox, S., Nasseri, R., Rubin, R. S., & Santiago-Lastra, Y. (2023). Genitourinary syndrome of menopause. *Medical Clinics of North America, 107,* 357–369. https://doi.org/10.1016/j.mcna.2022.10.017

Curtis, L. (2023). Cunnilingus is very helpful in stimulating women to orgasm. *Archives of Gynecology and Obstetrics, 308*(6), 1899–1900. https://doi.org/10.1007/s00404-022-06839-z

Delgado-Pérez, E., Rodríguez-Costa, I., Vergara-Pérez, F., Blanco-Morales, M., & Torres-Lacomba, M. (2022). Recovering sexuality after childbirth. What strategies do women adopt? A qualitative study. *International Journal of Environmental Research and Public Health, 19,* 950. https://doi.org/10.3390/ijerph19020950

De Neef, N., Coppens, V., Huys, W., & Morrens, M. (2019). Bondage-discipline, dominance-submission and sadomasochism (BDSM) from an integrative biopsychosocial perspective: A systematic review. *Sexual Medicine, 7*(2), 129–144. https://doi.org/10.1016/j.esxm.2019.02.002

de Vries, A., den Daas, C., Willemstein, I. J. M., de Wit, J. B. F., & Heijne, J. C. M. (2024). Interventions promoting condom use among youth: A systematic review. *Journal of Adolescent Health, 74*(4), 644–656. https://doi.org/10.1016/j.jadohealth.2023.11.014

Dewitte, M., & Reisman, Y. (2021). Clinical use and implications of sexual devices and sexually explicit media. *Nature Reviews. Urology, 18*(6), 359–377. https://doi.org/10.1038/s41585-021-00456-2

Fabersunne, C. C., Milliren, C., Schuster, M. A., Elliott, M. N., Emery, S. T., Cuccaro, P. M., Davies, S. L., & Richmond, T. (2024). Sexual debut in early adolescence and individual, school, and neighborhood social capital. *Journal of Adolescent Health, 75,* 333–343. https://doi.org/10.1016/j.jadohealth.2024.04.007

Farhane-Medina, N. Z., Luque, B., Tabernero, C., & Castillo-Mayén, R. (2022). Factors associated with gender and sex differences in anxiety prevalence and comorbidity: A systematic review. *Science Progress, 105*(4), 368504221135469. https://doi.org/10.1177/00368504221135469

Flores, A., & Conron, K. (2023, December). *Adult LGBT Population.* Research that matters: Adult LGBT population in the United States; UCLA School of Law Williams Institute. https://williamsinstitute.law.ucla.edu/wp-content/uploads/LGBT-Adult-US-Pop-Dec-2023.pdf

Ford, J. V., Corona-Vargas, E., Cruz, M., Fortenberry, D., Kismodi, E., Philpott, A., Rubio-Aurioles, E., & Coleman, E. (2021). The World Association for Sexual Health's declaration on sexual pleasure: A technical guide. *International Journal of Sexual Health, 33*(4), 612–642. https://doi.org/10.1080/19317611.2021.2023718

Freihart, B. K., Sears. M. A., & Meston, C. M. (2020). Relational and interpersonal predictors of sexual satisfaction. *Current Sexual Health Reports, 12,* 136–142. https://doi.org/10.1007/s11930-020-00260-w

Gewirtz-Meydan, A., Sowan, W., Estlein, R., & Winstok, Z. (2024). Rights or obligations: The extent to which sexual desire and gender roles determine sexual intimacy in romantic relationships. *Journal of Sex & Marital Therapy, 50*(4), 482–497. https://doi.org/10.1080/0092623X.2024.2310693

Gianotten, W. L. (2023). The health benefits of sexual expression. In S. Geuens, A. P. Mivsek, & W. L. Gianotten (Eds.), *Midwifery and sexuality* (pp. 41–48). Springer.

Gianotten, W. L., Alley, J. C., & Diamond, L. M. (2021). The health benefits of sexual expression. *International Journal of Sexual Health, 33*(4), 478–493. https://doi.org/10.1080/19317611.2021.1966564

Grussu, P., Vincini, B., & Quatraro, R. M. (2021). Sexuality in the perinatal period: A systematic review of reviews and recommendations for practice. *Sexual and Reproductive Healthcare, 30,* 100668. https://doi.org/10.1016/j.srhc.2021.100668

Gupta, S., Tarantino, M., & Sanner, C. (2023). A scoping review of research on polyamory and consensual non-monogamy: Implications for a more inclusive family science. *Journal of Family Theory & Review, 16,* 151–190. https://doi.org/10.1111/jftr.12546

Hajek, A., & König, H. (2023). Sexual satisfaction and aging satisfaction among middle-aged and older adults. Evidence from a nationally representative study. *Archives of Gerontology and Geriatrics, 115,* 105102. https://doi.org/10.1016/j.archger.2023.105102

Hald, G. M., Pavan, S., & Øverup, C. S. (2024). Do sex toys make me satisfied? The use of sex toys in Denmark, Norway, Sweden, Finland, France, and the UK. *Journal of Sex Research,* 1–15. Advance online publication. https://doi.org/10.1080/00224499.2024.2304575

Harm-Ernandes, I., Boyle, V., Hartmann, D., Fitzgerald, C. M., Lowder, J. L., Kotarinos, R., & Whitcomb, E. (2021). Assessment of the pelvic floor and associated musculoskeletal system: Guide for medical practitioners. *Female Pelvic Medicine & Reconstructive Surgery, 27*(12), 711–718. https://doi.org/10.1097/SPV.0000000000001121

Heitzler, E. (2024, June 25–30). *Sexual violence screening practices of APRNs* [Poster presentation]. 2024 American Association of Nurse Practitioners Annual Conference, Nashville, TN.

Henning, G., Segel-Karpas, D., Bjork, M. P., Bjalkebring, P., & Berg, A. I. (2023). Retirement and sexual satisfaction. *The Gerontologist, 63*(2), 274–284. https://doi.org/10.1093/geront/gnac102

Hensel, D. J., von Hippel, C. D., Lapage, C. C., & Perkins, R. H. (2024). Vaginal squirting: Experiences, discoveries, and strategies in a U.S. probability sample of women ages 18–93. *The Journal of Sex Research, 61*(4), 529–539. https://doi.org/10.1080/00224499.2023.2243939

Herbenick, D., Bowling, J., Fu, T. J., Dodge, B., Guerra-Reyes, L., & Sanders, S. (2017). Sexual diversity in the United States: Results from a nationally representative probability sample of adult women and men. *PLoS One, 12*(7), e0181198. https://doi.org/10.1371/journal.pone.0181198

Herbenick, D., Fu, T., & Patterson, C. (2023). Sexual repertoire, duration of partnered sex, sexual pleasure, and orgasm: Findings for a U.S. nationally representative sample of adults. *Journal of Sex & Marital Therapy, 49*(4), 369–390. https://doi.org/10.1080/0092623X.2022.2126417

Herbenick, D., Reece, M., Sanders, S., Dodge, B., Ghassemi, A., & Fortenberry, J. D. (2009). Prevalence and characteristics of vibrator use by women in the United States: Results from a nationally representative study. *Journal of Sexual Medicine, 6*(7), 1857–1866. https://doi.org/10.1111/j.1743-6109.2009.01318.x

Herbenick, D., Rosenbergy, M., Golzarri-Arroyo, L, Fortenberry, J. D., & Fu, T. (2021). Changes in penile-vaginal intercourse frequency and sexual repertoire from 2009 to 2018: Findings from the National Survey of Sexual Health and Behavior. *Archives and Sexual Behavior, 51,* 1419–1433. https://doi.org/10.1007/s10508-021-02125-2

Hessami, K., Sayegh, N., Abdolmaleki, A. S., Bakht, S., Qaderi, S., Darabi, M., Shamsi, T., & Bagheri, F. (2022). Women's sexual function before and during COVID-19 pandemic: A systematic review and meta-analysis. *The Journal of Obstetrics and Gynaecology Research,* 48(9), 2285–2295. https://doi.org/10.1111/jog.15337

Hoag, N., Keast, J. R., & O'Connell, H. E. (2017). The "G-spot" is not a structure evident on macroscopic anatomic dissection of the vaginal wall. *Journal of Sexual Medicine, 14*(12), 1524–1532. https://doi.org/10.1016/j.jsxm.2017.10.071

Hoagland, K. C., & Grubbs, J. B. (2021). Pornography use and holistic sexual functioning: A systematic review of recent research. *Current Addiction Reports, 8,* 408–421. https://doi.org/10.1007/s40429-021-00378-4

Howansky, K., Wilton, L. S., Young, D. M., Abrams, S., & Clapham, R. (2021). (Trans) gender stereotypes and the self: Content and consequences of gender identity stereotypes. *Self and Identity, 20*(4), 478–495. https://doi.org/10.1080/15298868.2019.1617191

Ito, E., Shima, R., & Yoshioka, T. (2019). A novel role of oxytocin: Oxytocin induced well-being in humans. *Biophysics and Physicobiology, 16,* 132–139. https://doi.org/10.2142/biophysico.16.0_132

Jackson, S. E., Yang, L, Koyanagi, A., Stubbs, B., Veronese, N., & Smith, L. (2020). Declines in sexual activity and function predict incident health problems in older adults: Prospective findings from the English longitundinal study of ageing. *Archives of Sexual Behavior, 49,* 929–940. https://doi.org/10.1007/s10508-019-1443-4

Janssen, E., & Bancroft, J. (2007). The dual control model: The role of sexual inhibition and excitation in sexual arousal and behavior. In E. Janssen (Ed.), *The Kinsey Institute series. The psychophysiology of sex* (pp. 197–222). Indiana University Press.

Jones, J. (2025, February 20). *LGBTQ+ Identification in U.S. Rises to 9.3%.* Social & Policy Issues; Gallup. https://news.gallup.com/poll/656708/lgbtq-identification-rises.aspx

Jones, S., Albequerque, S., & Pascoal, P. M. (2024). Grief and sexual intimacy: Exploring therapists' views of bereaved clients. *International Journal of Sexual Health, 36*(3), 425–437. https://doi.org/10.1080/19317611.2024.2354815

Kågesten, A., & van Reeuwijk, M. (2021). Healthy sexuality development in adolescence: Proposing a competency-based framework to inform programmes and research. *Sexual and Reproductive Health Matters, 29*(1), 1–17.

Kaplan, H. (1979). *Disorders of sexual desire and other new concepts and techniques in sex therapy*. Brunner/Mazel.

Kelley, E. L., & Kingsberg, S. A. (2024). Sexuality and infertility. *Obstetrics and Gynecology Clinics of North America, 51*(2), 311–322. https://doi.org/10.1016/j.ogc.2024.02.005

Kennedy, C. E., Yeh, P. T., Li, J., Gonsalves, L., & Narasimhan, M. (2021). Lubricants for the promotion of sexual health and well-being: A systematic review. *Sexual and Reproductive Health Matters, 29*(3), 2044198. https://doi.org/10.1080/26410397.2022.2044198

Khosravi, A., Riazi, H., Simbar, M., & Montazeri, A. (2022). Effectiveness of Kegel exercise and lubricant gel for improving sexual function in menopausal women: A randomized trial. *European Journal of Obstetrics, Gynecology, and Reproductive Biology, 274*, 106–112. https://doi.org/10.1016/j.ejogrb.2022.05.022

Kirton, A., & McKeever, N. (2023). Trust, attachment, and monogamy. In D. Collins, I. V. Jovanovic, & M. Alfano (Eds.), *The moral psychology of trust* (pp. 295–312). Lexington Books.

Lamba, A., Mohajir, N., & Rahman, S. (2023). A review of the psychosocial factors that contribute to sexuality, female sexual dysfunction, and sexual pain among Muslim women. *Sexual Medicine Reviews, 11*(3), 156–173. https://doi.org/10.1093/sxmrev/qead019

Leavitt, C. E., Leonhardt, N. D., & Busby, D. M. (2019). Different ways to get there: Evidence of a variable female sexual response cycle. *Journal of Sex Research, 56*(7), 899–912. https://doi.org/10.1080/00224499.2019.1616278

Lindberg, L. D., Firestein, L., & Beavin, C. (2021). Trends in U.S. adolescent sexual behavior and contraceptive use, 2006-2019. *Contraception: X, 3*, 100064. https://doi.org/10.1016/j.conx.2021.100064

Long, J. R., & Damle, L. F. (2024). Adolescent sexuality. *Obstetrics and Gynecology Clinics of North America, 51*(2), 299–310. https://doi.org/10.1016/j.ogc.2024.02.004

Lung, S. L. M., Wincentak, J., Gan, C., Kingsnorth, S., Provvidenza, C., & McPherson, A. (2021). Are healthcare providers and young people talking about sexuality? A scoping review to characterize conversations and identify barriers. *Child: Care, Health, and Development, 47*(6), 744–757. https://doi.org/10.1111/cch.12892

Maes, C., Trekels, J., Impett, E., & Vandenbosch, L. (2023). The development of the Positive Sexuality in Adolescence Scale (PSAS). *The Journal of Sex Research, 60*, 45–61. https://doi.org/10.1080/00224499.2021.2011826

Mangiardi-Veltin, M., Hequet, D., Segura-Djezzar, C., Rouzier, R., & Bonneau, C. (2023). Sexuality after breast cancer, how to provide a global and contemporary approach. Bulletin du Cancer, *110*(1), 113–128. https://doi.org/10.1016/j.bulcan.2022.10.002

Masoudi, M., Maasoumi, R., & Bragazzi, N. L. (2022). Effects of the COVID-19 pandemic on sexual functioning and activity: A systematic review and meta-analysis. *BMC Public Health, 22*, 189. https://doi.org/10.1186/s12889-021-12390-4

Masters, W., & Johnson, V. (1966). *The human sexual response cycle*. Little, Brown.

McGrath, M., Low, M. A., Power, E., McCluskey, A., & Lever, S. (2021). Addressing sexuality among people living with chronic disease and disability: A systematic mixed methods review of knowledge, attitudes, and practices of health care professionals. *Archives of Physical Medicine and Rehabilitation, 102*, 999–1010. https://doi.org/10.1016/j.apmr.2020.09.379

Metcalfe, K. B., Kilimnik, C. D., & Meston, C. M. (2024). Predictors of duty sex frequency in women. *The Journal of Sexual Medicine*, 2024, 1–11. https://doi.org/10.1093/jsxmed/qdae137

Mollaioli, D., Sansone, A., Colonnello, E., Limoncin, E., Ciocca, G., Vignozzi, L., & Jannini, E. A. (2021). Do we still believe there is a G-spot? *Current Sexual Health Reports, 13*, 97–105. https://doi.org/10.1007/s11930-021-00311-w

Moore-Petinak, N., Strome, A., Waselewski, M., & Chang, T. (2022). Youths' knowledge and perceptions of health risks associated with unprotected oral sex. *Annals of Family Medicine, 20*, 72–76. https://doi.org/10.1370/afm.2761

Moser, C. (2019). DSM-5, paraphilias, and the paraphilic disorders: Confusion reigns. *Archives of Sexual Behavior, 48*(3), 681–689. https://doi.org/10.1007/s10508-018-1356-7

Nagoski, E. (2015). *Come as you are: The surprising new science that will transform your sex life*. Simon & Schuster.

Nagoski, E. (2024). *Come together: The science (and art!) of creating lasting sexual connections*. Ballantine Books.

National Coalition for Sexual Health. (2022). *Sexual health and your patients: A provider's guide*. https://www.nationalcoalitionforsexualhealth.org/tools/for-healthcare-providers/sexual-health-and-your-patients-a-providers-guide/

North American Menopause Society. (2020). *The 2020 genitourinary syndrome of menopause position statement of The North American Menopause Society. Menopause, 27*(9), 976–992. https://doi.org/10.1097/GME.0000000000001609

Ollivier, A. A., Aston, M. L., & Price, S. L. (2020). Exploring postpartum sexual health: A feminist poststructural analysis. *Health Care for Women International, 41*(10), 1081–1100. https://doi.org/10.1080/07399332.2019.1638923

Omodei, M. S., Marques Gomes Delmanto, L. R., Carvalho-Pessoa, E., Schmitt, E. B., Nahas, G. P., & Petri Nahas, E. A. (2019). Association between pelvic floor muscle strength and sexual function in postmenopausal women. *The Journal of Sexual Medicine, 16*(12), 1938–1946. https://doi.org/10.1016/j.jsxm.2019.09.014

Osterling, C., Harder, A., Borg, C., & de Jong, P. (2024). Factors involved in vulvar pain during sexual activity and persistence in sexual activity amidst pain [preprint]. https://doi.org/10.1101/2024.06.12.24308863

Palacios, S., Hood, S., Abakah-Phillips, T., Savania, N., & Krychman, M. (2023). A randomized trial on the effectiveness and safety of 5 water-based personal lubricants. *The Journal of Sexual Medicine, 20*(4), 498–506. https://doi.org/10.1093/jsxmed/qdad005

Pastor, Z., & Chmel, R. (2022). Female ejaculation and squirting as similar but completely different phenomena: A narrative review of current research. *Clinical Anatomy, 2022*, 1–10. https://doi.org/10.1002/ca.23879

Peragine, D. E., Skorska, M. N., Maxwell, J. A., Impett, E. A., & VanderLaan, D. P. (2022). A learning experience? Enjoyment at sexual debut and the gender gap in sexual desire among emerging adults. *The Journal of Sex Research, 59*(9), 1092–1109. https://doi.org/10.1080/00224499.2022.2027855

Preda, A., & Moreira, S. (2019). Incontinência urinária de esforço e disfunção sexual feminina: O papel da reabilitação do pavimento pélvico [Stress urinary incontinence and female sexual dysfunction: The role of pelvic floor rehabilitation]. *Acta Medica Portuguesa, 32*(11), 721–726. https://doi.org/10.20344/amp.12012

Quicke, D. L. J. (2023). *Female arousal and orgasm: Anatomy, physiology, behaviour and evolution*. Bentham Books.

Quinn-Nilas, C. (2020). Relationship and sexual satisfaction: A developmental perspective on bidirectionality. *Journal of Social and Personal Relationships, 37*(2), 624–646. https://doi.org/10.1177/0265407519876018

Quintana, G. R., Desbiens, S., Marceau, S., Kalantari, N., Bowden, J., & Pfaus, J. G. (2019). Conditioned partner preference in male and female rats for a somatosensory cue. *Behavioral Neuroscience, 133*(2), 188–197. https://doi.org/10.1037/bne0000300

Reardon, C. L. (2025, April 15). Paraphilic disorders: Background, etiology, epidemiology. *Medscape*. https://emedicine.medscape.com/article/291419-overview

Reis, J., de Oliveira, L., Oliveira, C., & Nobre, P. (2021). Psychosocial and behavioral aspects of women's sexual pleasure: A scoping review. *International Journal of Sexual Health: Official Journal of the World Association for Sexual Health, 33*(4), 494–515. https://doi.org/10.1080/19317611.2021.1910890

Reling, T. T., Becker, S., Drakeford, L., & Valaski, M. (2021). Exploring the influence of hookup culture on female and male rape myths. *Journal of Interpersonal Violence, 36*. https://doi.org/10.1177/0886260518801021

Rosen, N. O., Dawson, S. J., Leonhardt, N. D., Vannier, S. A., & Impett, E. A. (2021). Trajectories of sexual well-being among couples in the transition to parenthood. *Journal of Family Psychology, 35*(4), 523–533. https://doi.org/10.1037/fam0000689

Rosengren-Hovee, E. (2021). *The United States of monogamy* [Master's thesis; the University of North Carolina at Chapel Hill]. https://cdr.lib.unc.edu/concern/masters_papers/bz60d499f

Rowland, D. L., & Kolba, T. N. (2019). Relationship of specific sexual activities to orgasmic latency, pleasure, and difficulty during partnered sex. *Journal of Sexual Medicine, 16*(4), 559–568. https://doi.org/10.1016/j.jsxm.2019.02.002

Rubin, E. S., Deshpande, N. A., Vasquez, P. J., & Spadt, K. S. (2019). A clinical reference guide on sexual devices for obstetrician-gynecologists. *Obstetrics and Gynecology, 133*(6), 1259–1268. https://doi.org/10.1097/AOG.0000000000003262

Saunders, J. F., Nutter, S., Waugh, R., & Hayden, K. A. (2024). Testing body-related components of objectification theory: A meta-analysis of the relations between body shame, self-objectification, and body dissatisfaction. *Body Image, 50*, 101738. https://doi.org/10.1016/j.bodyim.2024.101738

Shahrahmani, N., Babezedeh, R., & Ebadi, A. (2024). Sexual satisfaction of postmenopausal women: An integrative review. *PLoS One, 19*(7), e0306207. https://doi.org/10.1371/journal.pone.0306207

Sipe, J. M., Amos, J. D., Swarthout, R. F., Turner, A., Wiesner, M. R., & Hendren, C. O. (2023). Bringing sex toys out of the dark: Exploring unmitigated risks. *Microplastics and Nanoplastics, 3*(1), 6. https://doi.org/10.1186/s43591-023-00054-6

Sladden, T., Philpott, A., Braeken, D, Castellanos-Usigli, A., Yadav, V., Christie, E., Gonsalves, L., & Mofokeng, T. (2021). Sexual health and wellbeing through the life course: Ensuring sexual health, rights and pleasure for all. *International Journal of Sexual Health, 33*(4), 565–571. https://doi.org/10.1080/19317611.2021.1991071

Smith, P. E., McLaughlin, E. M., Pandya, L. K., Hade, E. M., Lynch, C. D., & Hudson, C. O. (2022). A pilot randomized controlled trial of vaginal estrogen on postpartum atrophy, perineal pain, and sexual function. *International Urogynecology Journal, 33*, 3383–3390. https://doi.org/10.1007/s00192-022-05149-x

Sobhgol, S. S., Smith, C. A., Thomson, R., & Dahlen, H. G. (2022). The effect of antenatal pelvic floor muscle exercise on sexual function and labour and birth outcomes: A randomised controlled trial. *Women and Birth, 35*, e607–e614. https://doi.org/10.1016/j.wombi.2022.02.009

Soysal, P., & Smith, L. (2022). Sexual activity and successful aging. *European Geriatric Medicine, 13*, 1235–1238. https://doi.org/10.1007/s41999-022-00694-6

Stafford, M. K., Ward, H., Flanagan, A., Rosenstein, I. J., Taylor-Robinson, D., Smith, J. R., Weber, J., & Kitchen, V. S. (1998). Safety study of nonoxynol-9 as a vaginal microbicide: Evidence of adverse effects. *Journal of Acquired Immune Deficiency Syndromes and Human Retrovirology, 17*(4), 327–331. https://insights.ovid.com/crossref?an=00042560-199804010-00006

Streed, C. G., Jr, Grasso, C., Reisner, S. L., & Mayer, K. H. (2020). Sexual Orientation and Gender Identity Data Collection: Clinical and Public Health Importance. *American Journal of Public Health, 110*(7), 991–993. https://doi.org/10.2105/AJPH.2020.305722

Sukhanova, A., Pascoal, P. M., & Rosa, P. J. (2022). A behavioral approach to sexual function: Testing a moderation mediation model with expression of feelings, sexual self-disclosure and gender. *Journal of Sex & Marital Therapy, 48*(6), 607–627. https://doi.org/10.1080/0092623X.2022.2035867

Tabatabaie, N. S., Rasti Borujeni, F., Tavakol, Z., & Raeisi Shahraki, H. (2024). The effect of yoga and pelvic floor muscle exercise on sexual function and sexual self-esteem of reproductive-age women: A randomized clinical trial. *International Journal of Community-based Nursing and Midwifery, 12*(3), 188–198. https://doi.org/10.30476/IJCBNM.2024.101743.2441

Taylor, B., & Davis, S. (2007). The extended PLISSIT model for addressing the sexual wellbeing of individuals with an acquired disability or chronic illness. *Sexuality and Disability*, 25, 135–139. https://doi.org/10.1007/s11195-007-9044-x

Taylor, K., & Henderson, J. (1986). Effects of biofeedback and urinary stress incontinence in older women. *Journal of Gerontological Nursing, 12*(9), 25–30. https://doi.org/10.3928/0098-9134-19860901-08

The North American Menopause Society. (2020). The 2020 genitourinary syndrome of menopause position statement of The North American Menopause Society. *Menopause: The Journal of the North American Meonpause Society, 27*(9), 976–992. https://doi.org/10.1097/GME.0000000000001609

Towler, L. B., Graham, C. A., Bishop, F. L., & Hinchliff, S. (2023). Sex and relationships in later life: Older adults' experiences and perceptions of sexual changes. *The Journal of Sex Research, 60*(9), 1318–1331. https://doi.org/10.1080/00224499.2022.2093322

Van Damme, L., Ramjee, G., Alary, M., Vuylsteke, B., Chandeying, V., Rees, H., Sirivongrangson, P., Tshibaka, L. M., Ettiègne-Traoré, V., Uaheowitchai, C., Karim, S. S. A., Mâsse, B., Perriëns, J., & Laga, M. (2002). Effectiveness of COL-1492, a nonoxynol-9 vaginal gel, on HIV-1 transmission in female sex workers: A randomised controlled trial. *The Lancet, 360*(9338), 971–977. https://doi.org/10.1016/s0140-6736(02)11079-8

Vanwesenbeeck, I., Cense, M., van Reeuwijk, M., & Westeneng, J. (2021). Understanding sexual agency: Implications for sexual health programming. *Sexes, 4*, 378–396. https://doi.org/10.3390/sexes2040030

Varas, F. I., Saez-Rossel, V., Laborda, M. A., & Miguez, G. (2024). Sexual conditioning. In T. K. Shackelford (Ed.), *Encyclopedia of sexual psychology and behavior.* https://doi.org/10.1007/978-3-031-08956-5_131-1

Vaughan, M. D., Jones, P., Taylor, B. A., & Roush, J. (2019). Healthcare experiences and needs of consensually non-monogamous people: Results from a focus group study. *The Journal of Sexual Medicine, 16,* 42–51. https://doi.org/10.1016/j.jsxm.2018.11.006

Verbeek, M., & Hayward, L. (2019). Pelvic floor dysfunction and its effect on quality of sexual life. *Sexual Medicine Reviews, 7*(4), 559–564. https://doi.org/10.1016/j.sxmr.2019.05.007

Weaver, T. L., Elrod, N. M., & Kelton, K. (2019). Intimate partner violence and body shame: An examination of the associations between abuse components and body-focused processes. *Violence Against Women*, 1077801219873434. https://doi.org/10.1177/1077801219873434.

Wickrama, K., O'Neal, C. W., & Klopack, E. T. (2022). Midlife financial strain and later-life health and wellbeing of husbands and wives: Linking and moderating roles of couple intimacy trajectories. *Family Process, 61,* 1593–1609. https://doi.org/10.1111/famp.12749

Wilkinson, E. M., Łaniewski, P., Herbst-Kralovetz, M. M., & Brotman, R. M. (2019). Personal and clinical vaginal lubricants: Impact on local vaginal microenvironment and implications for epithelial cell host response and barrier function. *The Journal of Infectious Diseases, 220*(12), 2009–2018. https://doi.org/10.1093/infdis/jiz412

Wilson, C. M., McGuire, D. B., Rodgers, B. L., Elswick, R. K., & Temkin, S. M. (2021). Body image, sexuality, and sexual functioning in women with gynecologic cancer: An integrative review of the literature and implications for research. *Cancer Nursing, 44*(5), E252–E286. https://doi.org/10.1097/NCC.0000000000000818

World Association for Sexual Health. (2014). *Declaration of sexual rights.* https://worldsexualhealth.net/resources/declaration-of-sexual-rights/

World Health Organization. (2006). *Defining sexual health: Report of a technical consultation on sexual health, 28–31 January 2002, Geneva.*

World Health Organization. (2024, April 5). *WHO recommendations on self-care interventions: availability of lubricants during sexual activity.* https://www.who.int/publications/i/item/who-srh-23.4

Wright, H., Jenks, R. A., & Demeyere, N. (2019). Frequent Sexual Activity Predicts Specific Cognitive Abilities in Older Adults. *The journals of gerontology. Series B, Psychological Sciences and Social Sciences, 74*(1), 47–51. https://doi.org/10.1093/geronb/gbx065

Zhang, X., Sherman, L., & Foster, M. (2020). Patients' and providers' perspectives on sexual health discussion in the United States: A scoping review. *Patient Education and Counseling, 103*(11), 2205–2213. https://doi.org/10.1016/j.pec.2020.06.019

APPENDIX 12-A

Sexuality Resources for Patients and Providers

BOOKS

Comprehensive Information About Sex:

Joannides, P. (2021). *Guide to getting it on: Crush it in bed* (10th ed.). Goody Foot Press.

- This book uses informal language, quotations from interviewing a diverse demographic, and illustrations to provide accurate, approachable, and memorable information about sex and anatomy.

Rowland, K. (2020). *The pleasure gap: American women and the unfinished sexual revolution*. Seal Press.

- This book investigates the widespread sexual dissatisfaction among American women, revealing how cultural, psychological, and systemic factors contribute to a persistent disparity in sexual fulfillment. Drawing on interviews and research, she challenges outdated narratives and calls for a deeper understanding of desire, intimacy, and the right to pleasure.

Winston, S. (2010). *Women's anatomy of arousal: Secret maps to buried pleasure*. Mango Garden Press.

- A book with beautiful anatomy illustrations.

Desire:

Hall, K. (2004). *Reclaiming your sexual self: How you can bring desire back into your life*. John Wiley & Sons.

- This book explores sexual desire or lack thereof. A sex therapist discusses how to assert control over one's health and sexual life.

Nagoski, E. (2021). *Come as you are: Revised and updated: The surprising new science that will transform your sex life*. Simon & Schuster.

- This book presents science about desire in layperson's language with a focus on female sexuality.

Nagoski, E. (2024). *Come together: The science (and art!) of creating lasting sexual connections*. Ballantine Books.

Orgasm:

Cass, V. (2007). *The elusive orgasm: A woman's guide to why she can't and how she can orgasm*. Da Capo Press.

- A clinical psychologist who is also a sex therapist explores the causes of women's orgasm difficulties and how to remedy them. This book provides a full overview of women's sexual pleasure, covering sexual triggers, stages of arousal, the power of mind, and how women differ from men.

Mintz, L. (2017). *Becoming cliterate: Why orgasm equality matters—and how to get it*. HarperOne.

- This book addresses the persistent gap in sexual satisfaction between people of different genders, highlighting how cultural myths and inadequate sex education have contributed to the marginalization of pleasure for those assigned female at birth. Combining scientific research, personal narratives, and practical guidance, the book empowers individuals to advocate for their own pleasure and promotes a more inclusive, equitable approach to sexual well-being.

Disabilities and Sex:

Kaufman, M., Silverberg, C., & Odette, F. (2007). *The ultimate guide to sex and disability: For all of us who live with disabilities, chronic pain & illness*. Cleis Press.

- This book, written by a physician, a sex educator, and a disability activist, is the first complete sex guide for people who live with disabilities, pain, illness, or chronic conditions (although it is useful for anyone). This book provides readers with encouragement, support, and all the information they need to create a sex life that works for them.

Sexual Pleasure Techniques:

Kerner, I. (2010). *She comes first: The thinking man's guide to pleasuring a woman*. William Morrow, HarperCollins.

- This book provides a step-by-step guide to oral sex techniques.

Moon, A., & Diamond, K. (2018). *Girl sex 101*. Lunatic Ink.

- This book offers information about sex for women, and women lovers of all genders and identities, through playful and informative illustrations and voices.

Parenting and Children's Sexual Development:

Roffman, D. (2012). *Talk to me first: Everything you need to know to become your kids' "go to" person about sex*. Da Capo Press.

- This book is a teaching tool for parents in a time when children are exposed to sex and sexuality at an early age. It prepares parents to be the most credible and influential resource about sexuality in their children's lives.

Silverberg, C., & Smyth, F. (2015). *Sex is a funny word: A book about bodies, feelings, and YOU*. Seven Stories Press.

- This kid-friendly comic book is a resource about bodies, gender, and sexuality. It opens up conversations between young people and the adults in their lives.

Pregnancy and the Postpartum Period:

Young, M. (2016). *The ultimate guide to sex through pregnancy and motherhood: Passionate, practical advice for moms*. Cleis Press.

- The author uses her own personal experiences to discuss sex and sexuality throughout pregnancy and motherhood so that women are encouraged to embrace themselves, their feelings, and their desires.

WEBSITES AND ONLINE MEDIA FOR SEX EDUCATION

American Sexual Health Association: www.ashasexualhealth.org

I Wanna Know: Sexual Health for Teens and Young Adults: http://www.iwannaknow.org/

The Pleasure Project: www.thepleasureproject.org

Sex Smart Films: Promoting Sexual Literacy: www.sexsmartfilms.com

A Woman's Touch Sexuality Resource Center: www.sexualityresources.com

CHAPTER 13

Contraception

Amy Alspaugh

The editors acknowledge Rachel Newhouse, Patricia Aikins Murphy, Caroline M. Hewitt, and Cynthia Belew, who were coauthors of the previous edition of this chapter.

Contraceptive management is often a challenging undertaking, but providing family planning services offers clinicians the opportunity to empower people by helping them make choices that can truly alter their life courses. Of the more than 65 million individuals of reproductive age in the United States, three out of four have received at least one sexual or reproductive health service from a clinician, including 25 million individuals who sought services related to contraception (Frost et al., 2021).

The vast majority of U.S. individuals of reproductive age who use contraception choose nonpermanent methods (Frederiksen et al., 2024). Contraception can be highly effective at preventing pregnancy, depending on the type of contraception used. The majority of individuals using contraception (85%) are trying to prevent pregnancy, but 14 percent of contraception users are using a method solely for a noncontraceptive purpose, such as managing a health condition or for protection against sexually transmitted infections (Frederiksen et al., 2024).

When it comes to contraception, the challenge lies in helping each individual choose the method that best meets their needs and providing effective education so they can use the chosen method correctly and consistently. The importance of the healthcare clinician's role in guiding individuals to select the best option for their needs and in educating them on correct use cannot be overstated. Individuals of reproductive age have major knowledge gaps about contraceptive effectiveness, and they overestimate the effectiveness of pills, the patch, the vaginal ring, depot medroxyprogesterone acetate (DMPA), and condoms (Eisenberg et al., 2012; Kakaiya et al., 2017). Further, the majority of individuals incorrectly believe that using oral contraception is at least as hazardous to health as pregnancy (Kakaiya et al., 2017; Nelson et al., 2019). Misinformation about contraception is increasingly common, given the ease with which inaccurate information can spread across social media, in particular. Misinformation is not limited to patients (Swan et al., 2023), so it is critical that healthcare clinicians have up-to-date, accurate information about how contraceptive methods work and their adverse effects to assist individuals in making informed decisions.

Patient-centered contraception counseling that fully attends to the needs and priorities of the individual is one of the most important roles of a sexual and reproductive healthcare clinician (ACOG, 2022). Individuals report that they do not receive in-depth counseling on how to use their selected option. In addition, some feel pressured by their provider to select a certain method. There is continued reproductive coercion aimed mostly at individuals from minoritized backgrounds and those who are incarcerated (McCormick, 2021). Individuals have been pressured, and in some cases mandated by courts, to adopt long-acting methods of contraception (Gomez et al., 2014). Policies and counseling designed to steer individuals toward a particular method ignore the unique needs of the individual and undermine their autonomy. Family planning policies and encounters reflect racial inequality in the larger society. In particular, African American and Latina individuals report experiencing race-based discrimination when they seek family planning services (Mann et al., 2022; Manzer & Bell, 2021). Providers must make efforts to be aware of their own implicit biases and to stay informed about the social and political contexts of family planning to ensure that all individuals can choose freely from all contraceptive options, which is one aspect of Reproductive Justice (RJ). The growing RJ movement goes beyond the focus on access and individual choice to analysis of the social, economic, and structural constraints on an individual's reproductive decisions (Ross & Solinger, 2017). RJ is a critical framework from which to approach contraceptive care because RJ centers the needs, desires, and preferences of an individual as an expert in their own care needs, including, among other things, the ability to become pregnant and to choose not to become pregnant. Clinicians who provide care in a manner consistent with RJ will work to ensure that they provide unbiased, person-centered care that supports the bodily autonomy and individual agency of every person (Britton et al., 2020).

Discussing an individual's thoughts, feelings, and potential plan around growing a family is an important part of helping an individual find the best contraceptive method for them. Using one of many screening methods (**Table 13-1**), some version of reproductive life planning may assist the clinician to identify those who may need either contraception or preconception health care. These different approaches have their unique strengths and weaknesses. Across all approaches, it is essential to frame these questions as open-ended questions with no right or wrong answer. One Key Question is the shortest approach but may not create open dialogue for those who have more nuanced or complicated feelings about pregnancy and raising children (D. Allen et al., 2017). The PATH questions offer a person an opening to talk about degree of uncertainty regarding their goals and allows space for nuance and context on the relative importance

TABLE 13-1 Approaches for Reproductive Life Planning and Contraception Discussion

Approach	Questions
SINC[1]	Do you want to talk about contraception or pregnancy prevention during your visit today?
One Key Question[2]	Would you like to become pregnant in the next year?
Reproductive Life Plan[3]	1. Do you have any children now? 2. Do you want to have (more) children? 3. How many (more) children would you like to have and when?
PATH questions[4] • Pregnancy Attitudes • Timing • How important is prevention	1. Do you think you might like to have (more) children at some point? 2. If person is considering future parenthood: When do you think that might be? 3. How important is it to you to prevent pregnancy (until then)?

[1]Reproduced from The Regents of the University of California. What is SINC?. https://pcrhp.ucsf.edu/sinc
[2]Reproduced from Allen, D., Hunter, M. S., Wood, S., & Beeson, T. (2017). One Key Question®: First things first in reproductive health. *Maternal and Child Health Journal, 21*(3), 387–392. https://doi.org/10.1007/s10995-017-2283-2
[3]Reproduced from Callegari, L. S., Ma, E. W., & Schwarz, E. B. (2015). Preconception care and reproductive planning in primary care. *The Medical Clinics of North America, 99*(3), 663–682. https://doi.org/10.1016/j.mcna.2015.01.014
[4]Reproduced from Geist, C., Aiken, A. R., Sanders, J. N., Everett, B. G., Myers, K., Cason, P., Simmons, R. G., & Turok, D. K. (2019). Beyond intent: Exploring the association of contraceptive choice with questions about Pregnancy Attitudes, Timing and How important is pregnancy prevention (PATH) questions. *Contraception 99*(1), 22–26. https://doi.org/10.1016/j.contraception.2018.08.014

of contraceptive efficacy in their decision making (Geist et al., 2019). While none of these approaches are necessary, some of these questions may offer the opportunity to engage in dialogue with patients about their priorities and concerns. Simply asking "Would you like to talk about contraception or pregnancy prevention today" is also a patient-centered approach to guide your care (SINC, n.d.).

Many individuals report misconceptions about the risk of conception from unprotected sex and also the effectiveness and safety of contraceptive options (Manzer et al., 2023). Improved knowledge may encourage more consistent and effective contraceptive use. Specifically, overestimation of contraceptive risk and underestimation of health benefits are common and must be addressed. The small risks associated with contraception for most individuals are dwarfed by the health risks of pregnancy. In addition, the use of hormonal contraceptive methods may actually protect future fertility by decreasing the risk of endometriosis, ectopic pregnancy, pelvic inflammatory disease (PID), and abortion-related complications. Hormonal methods also decrease the risk of ovarian, endometrial, and colon cancer (Iversen et al., 2018; Wheeler et al., 2019). However, there is a growing movement away from hormonal contraception that clinicians may encounter in practice or share themselves. Evidence-based practice necessitates sharing what is known through scientific inquiry and identifying how this fits within the worldview, priorities, and perspectives of the individual. There is no perfect method for any person, but rather the method they want and are motivated to use.

The good news, however, is that more contraceptive options are available now than ever before. Contraceptive users today value more than efficacy from a method. They desire a method that is safe, convenient, and cost effective, and that has few side effects. How a method affects an individual's life—from side effects, such as daily spotting, to remembering to do something every day—may be a major determinant in consistency and continuation of use. In addition, knowledge about the noncontraceptive health benefits of some methods is increasing; this background enables individuals to make contraceptive choices that can have positive implications for their health. Most therapeutic uses of contraception are not approved by the U.S. Food and Drug Administration (FDA), although many are supported by evidence gathered through research studies. Clinicians frequently prescribe medications for conditions other than those for which they have FDA approval, and this off-label use is within the scope of prescriptive authority when sound rationale and evidence are used (U.S. Food and Drug Administration [FDA], 2018b).

Contraceptive counseling should never be guided by a clinician's bias about what is best for a particular person. Rather, the best method for any person is the one they want and are motivated to use. Clinicians should have information on all methods available and offer specific in-person information about methods the patient is medically eligible for and interested in. No clinician should make ethical, moral, or personal decisions about contraception for any patient that is outside of evidence-based medical eligibility criteria; instead, they should offer guidance while taking the patient's moral, ethical, and personal life choices into consideration. Clinicians should rely only on evidence-based contraindications to avoid unnecessarily restricting contraceptive options when determining whether the individual's history makes a particular method acceptable. The *U.S. Medical Eligibility Criteria for Contraceptive Use, 2024* from the Centers for Disease Control and Prevention (CDC) is the best evidence-based resource for determining whether a woman is a candidate for a particular method (A. Nguyen et al., 2024). In addition, evidence-based guidance on how to appropriately use contraceptive methods is available in the *U.S. Selected Practice Recommendations for Contraceptive Use, 2024* (Curtis et al., 2024). These two sources guide clinicians step by step through decision making in timing the initiation of contraception methods, side effect management, and presenting options that are safe for patients, depending on their personal history. These combined resources are available online from the CDC and in Contraception, a free mobile app created by the CDC. Clinicians cannot be expected to remember all the nuances to all of the different contraceptive methods, but they are responsible for having resources readily available to provide patients with a positive, evidence-based encounter.

A thorough knowledge of the available contraceptive methods, including their mechanisms of action, is imperative for providing contraceptive counseling that leads to a fully informed choice. Many pregnancy-capable people report wanting to share responsibility and decision making for contraceptive use with their partners, so their partners may need education as well (B. T. Nguyen & Jacobsohn, 2022; Rinehart et al., 2023). At times, they may need supportive counseling to negotiate contraceptive issues within their relationship.

In 2014, the CDC and the U.S. Department of Health and Human Services issued national quality standards for the provision of family planning services (Gavin et al., 2014). These recommendations, revised in 2024 (Romer et al., 2024), define which services should be offered in a family planning visit and give primary care providers the information they need to improve the quality of family planning services.

This chapter provides an overview of the various methods of contraception. Long acting hormonal contraception is described first, followed by permanent contraception. Hormonal methods, including short acting, emergency, and long acting contraception then bridge into non-hormonal methods, including physiologic and barrier methods. Data on efficacy and effectiveness, safety and side effects, noncontraceptive benefits, and the advantages and disadvantages of each method are presented. A full discussion of contraceptive counseling and management is beyond the scope of this chapter, but interested readers are referred to the recommended resources in **Appendix 13-A**.

CONTRACEPTIVE EFFICACY AND EFFECTIVENESS

The effectiveness of contraceptive methods is described in several ways. Efficacy, sometimes referred to as method failure or perfect use failure rates, is how well a method works inherently. Efficacy describes the likelihood that a pregnancy will occur even when the method is used consistently and exactly as prescribed. In most research studies, pregnancies that result from inconsistent or incorrect use are not included in method failure rates. Effectiveness, also termed typical use failure rates, is how well a method works in actual practice. Effectiveness describes all pregnancies that occur if a method is not used properly, such as in the case of inconsistent or incorrect use. The terms "efficacy" and "effectiveness" are often used interchangeably when discussing contraception, but in fact refer to different measures (Sundaram et al., 2017).

All contraceptive methods have inherent failure rates. Pregnancies may occur even with highly effective methods, such as sterilization (Schwarz et al., 2024). **Table 13-2** contains the effectiveness rates for contraceptive methods, and **Figure 13-1** is a visual summary of this information that is helpful to use with patients. Methods that are highly dependent on user consistency may have higher failure rates, but not all pregnancies occur as a result of user errors. Clinicians should never imply that pregnancies are the pregnant person's fault.

In addition to inherent method efficacy and consistent and correct use of a method, several other factors affect contraceptive failure rates. Most failures are concentrated in early usage. More fertile individuals will have experienced method failures sooner than those who are less fertile, and those who use contraception incorrectly or inconsistently will also get pregnant sooner than those with correct, consistent use. In addition, fertility in those who can get pregnant begins decreasing more rapidly at age 37 years; thus, any method used by younger individuals will have a higher failure rate than when the same method is used by older individuals (Sundaram et al., 2017). Other factors contributing to contraceptive success include the fertility of the partner, the motivation to avoid pregnancy (as opposed to simply wanting to space pregnancies), relationship status, and frequency of sexual intercourse (D'Souza et al., 2022).

LONG-ACTING REVERSIBLE CONTRACEPTION

Long-acting reversible contraception (LARC), which includes intrauterine devices (IUDs) and subdermal implants, refers to methods that prevent pregnancy for extended periods of time with no effort from the user. LARC removes the factors of user consistency and error from the contraceptive equation; therefore, its effectiveness is the highest of all contraceptive methods. LARC methods also have high satisfaction and continuation rates, compared with other methods (DeSisto et al., 2018; Ela et al., 2022). While there has recently been an effort to promote LARCs as the first choice method for every individual because of their superior efficacy (Brandi & Fuentes, 2020), this effort largely ignores the fact that individuals make contraceptive decisions based on a range of factors and effectiveness is only one among many reasons an individual may select a LARC. Further, there is a long history of reproductive coercion in the United States targeting low-income individuals and communities of color (Boydell & Smith, 2023). Low-income individuals of color have been forced and coerced into sterilization throughout the 20th century, often as a public health initiative in the vein of eugenics. There have been many attempts to legally force or entice individuals to use LARC as part of their criminal sentencing, and legislators proposed in the 1990s that low-income individuals should be financially incentivized to use Norplant levonorgestrel implants (Deparle, 1991; Hawkins, 2017). Providers may or may not intend to coerce their patients into using a specific method, LARC in particular, but all providers have a duty to ensure patients can make informed and autonomous choices in contraception, including the choice not to use a method or to use a less effective method (Holt et al., 2020; Littlejohn, 2021). Even though healthcare providers exhibit implicit racial and gender bias at the same levels as the general population, they have a higher responsibility to be aware of their own implicit biases and how they may contribute to disparities and coercion because of the unequal power between patient and clinician and the real ability to do harm (FitzGerald & Hurst, 2017). Further, provision of LARC methods that is rooted in justice, autonomy, and equity necessitates LARC removal that is free of provider barriers. Often, the same individuals who are targeted to receive LARCs experience greater barriers to removal (Amico et al., 2016; Fox et al., 2024; Howett et al., 2019), so ensuring removal is readily available, accessible, and affordable are key components to patient-centered LARC care.

Individuals of any age or parity can use LARC, including adolescents and those who are parous or nulliparous (Nguyen et al., 2024). The ease of use, high efficacy, and privacy provided by LARC methods are particularly relevant considerations for

TABLE 13-2 Contraceptive Method, Hormonal or Nonhormonal, Percentage of Individuals Experiencing an Pregnancy During the First Year of Typical Use and the First Year of Perfect Use of Contraception, and the Percentage Continuing Use at the End of the First Year, United States

	Hormone			% of Women Experiencing an Unintended Pregnancy Within the First Year of Use		% of Women Continuing
Method	**Estrogen**	**Progestin**	**Nonhormonal**	**Typical Use[1]**	**Perfect Use[2]**	**Use at One Year[3]**
No method[4]			x	85	85	
Spermicides[5]			x	21	16	42
Female condom[6]			x	21	5	41
Withdrawal			x	20	4	46
Diaphragm[7]			x	17	16	57
Sponge Parous Individuals			x	27	20	
Nulliparous Individuals			x	14	9	
Fertility awareness-based methods[8]			x	15		47
Ovulation method[8]			x	23	3	
TwoDay method[8]			x	14	4	
Standard Days method[8]			x	12	5	
Natural Cycles[8]			x	8	1	
Symptothermal method[8]			x	2	0.4	
Male condom[6]			x	13	2	43
Combined and progestin-only pills	x	x		7	0.3	67
Evra patch	x	x		7	0.3	67
NuvaRing	x	x		7	0.3	67
Depo-Provera		x		4	0.2	56
IUD ParaGard (copper T)			x	0.8	0.6	78
Skyla (13.5 mg LNG)		x		0.4	0.3	
Kyleena (19.5 mg LNG)		x		0.2	0.2	
Liletta (52 mg LNG)		x		0.1	0.1	
Mirena (52 mg LNG)		x		0.1	0.1	80
Nexplanon		x		0.1	0.1	89
Tubal occlusion			x	0.5	0.5	100
Vasectomy			x	0.15	0.1	100

Emergency Contraceptives: Use of emergency contraceptive pills or placement of a copper intrauterine contraceptive after unprotected intercourse substantially reduces the risk of pregnancy.

Lactational Amenorrhea Method: LAM is a highly effective, temporary method of contraception.[9]

Reproduced from Trussell, J., Aiken, A. R. A., Micks, E., & Guthrie, K. A. (2023). Efficacy, safety, and personal considerations. In Cason, P., Cwiak, C., Edelman, A., Kowal, D., Marrazzo, J. M., Nelson, A. L., Policar, M. (2023). *Contraceptive technology* (22nd ed.). Jones & Bartlett Learning. ISBN: 978-1284255034.

[1]Among *typical* couples who initiate use of a method (not necessarily for the first time), the percentage who experience an accidental pregnancy during the first year if they do not stop use for any reason other than pregnancy. Estimates of the probability of pregnancy during the first year of typical use for fertility awareness-based methods, withdrawal, the male condom, the pill, and Depo-Provera are taken from the 2006–2010 National Survey of Family Growth corrected for underreporting of abortion; see Trussell et al., 2018, for the derivation of estimates for the other methods.

[2]Among couples who initiate use of a method (not necessarily for the first time) and who use it *perfectly* (both consistently and correctly), the percentage who experience an accidental pregnancy during the first year if they do not stop use for any other reason. See Trussell et al., 2018, for the derivation of the estimate for each method.

[3]Among couples attempting to avoid pregnancy, the percentage who continue to use a method for 1 year.

[4]This estimate represents the percentage who would become pregnant within 1 year among women now relying on reversible methods of contraception if they abandoned contraception altogether. See Trussell et al., 2018.

[5]150 mg gel, 100 mg gel, 100 mg suppository, 100 mg film.

[6]Without spermicides.

[7]With spermicidal cream or jelly.

[8]About 80% of segments of fertility awareness-based method (FABM) use in the 2006–2010 National Survey of Family Growth (NSFG) were reported as calendar rhythm. Specific FABM methods are too uncommonly used in the United States to permit calculation of typical use failure rates for each using NSFG data; rates provided for individual methods are derived from clinical studies. The Ovulation and TwoDay methods are based on evaluation of cervical mucus. The Standard Days method avoids intercourse on cycle days 8 through 19. Natural Cycles is a fertility app that requires user input of basal body temperature (BBT) recordings and dates of menstruation and optional luteinizing hormone (LH) urinary test results. The Symptothermal method is a double-check method based on evaluation of cervical mucus to determine the first fertile day and evaluation of cervical mucus and temperature to determine the last fertile day.

[9]However, to maintain effective protection against pregnancy, another method of contraception must be used as soon as menstruation resumes, the frequency or duration of breastfeeds is reduced, bottle feeds are introduced, or the infant reaches 6 months of age.

FIGURE 13-1 Comparing typical effectiveness of contraceptive methods.

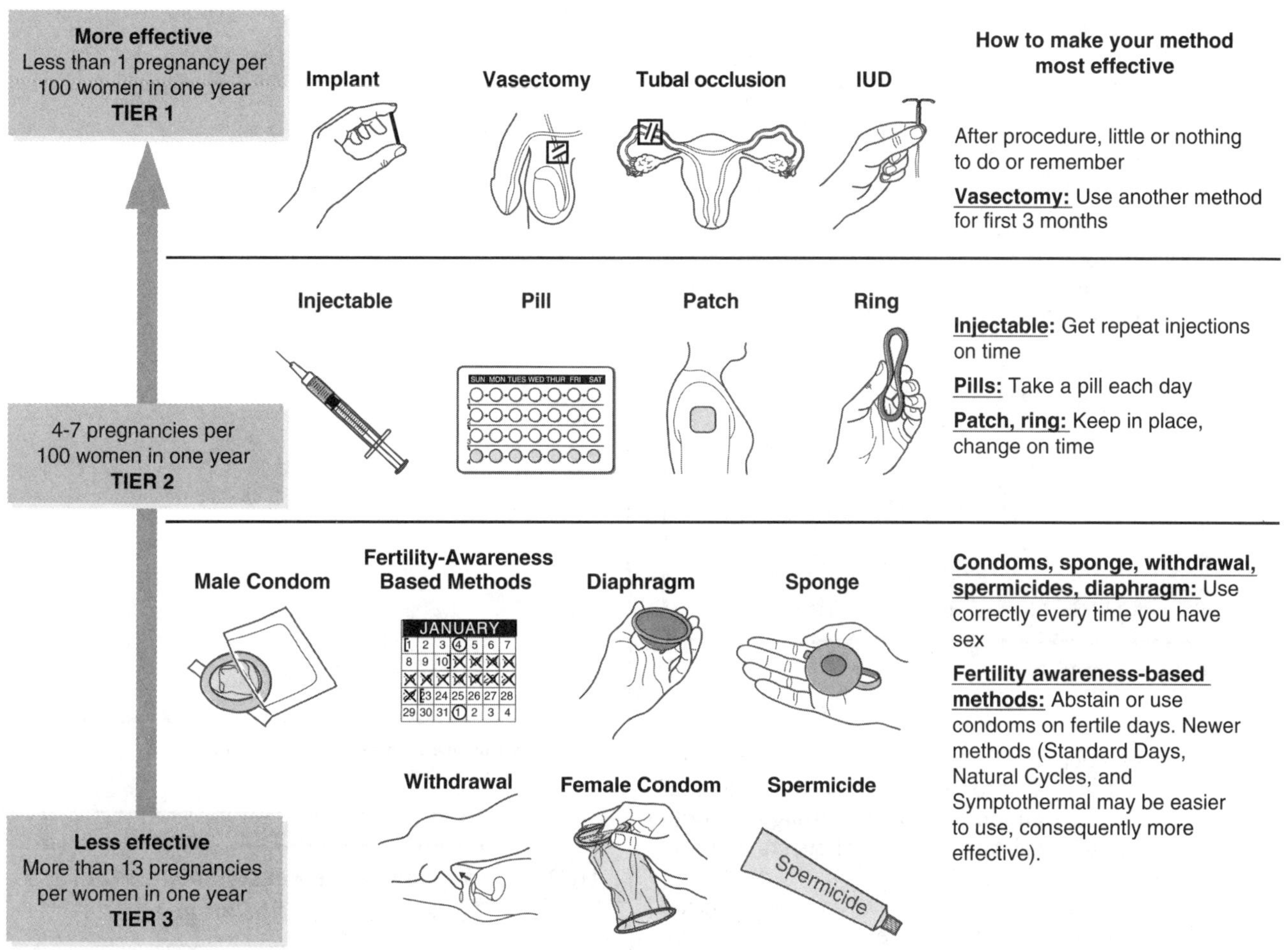

Reproduced from Trussell, J., Aiken, A. R. A., Micks, E., & Guthrie, K. A. (2023). Efficacy, safety, and personal considerations. In Cason, P., Cwiak, C., Edelman, A., Kowal, D., Marrazzo, J. M., Nelson, A. L., Policar, M. S. (2023). *Contraceptive technology* (22nd ed.). Jones & Bartlett Learning. ISBN: 978-1284255034.

adolescents or those who may want to keep their contraceptive method discrete. All LARCs can be inserted immediately postpartum, which may decrease patient-level barriers to use, but steps should be taken to ensure patient autonomy is centered (Moniz et al., 2017). Others barriers to use of LARC include provider inexperience with LARC methods and patient fears about safety (Moon & Smith, 2017). In addition, although LARC is more cost effective than most other methods over time, the high initial cost is a barrier to access.

Intrauterine Contraception

The use of medical devices placed in the uterus to prevent pregnancy dates back to the early 1900s. Although the infection risk with early devices was high, design improvements led to a variety of IUDs becoming available in the 1960s and 1970s (Tone, 2001). Popular devices were generally made of inert plastic, with single filament threads that protruded through the cervix into the vagina.

One prominent exception to this design was the Dalkon Shield, which was introduced in 1970. This device quickly became associated with a high risk of pelvic infection and infertility. It had a multifilament tail enclosed in a sheath; when the strings were cut, the protective sheath was compromised, and bacteria could ascend into the uterus inside the sheath (Nelson, 2000). Although other IUDs did not have the same design flaw, the adverse publicity and lawsuits associated with the Dalkon Shield tainted all IUDs, and these devices fell out of favor in the United States during the late 1970s.

Continued developments in design and scientific review of the risks and benefits associated with intrauterine contraception have led to a growing interest in this contraceptive method. IUDs are still underused due the high initial cost, lack of provider training in insertion, and misperceptions on the part of both healthcare providers and the public about safety (Yoost, 2014). There are five intrauterine contraceptives available in the United States, though others are used in other countries.

The copper IUD (T380A, Paragard) is a T-shaped device of polyethylene with copper wire wound around the stem and arms (**Figure 13-2**). A monofilament polyethylene thread is attached to a ball on the end of the stem (Alvarez et al., 1988).

FIGURE 13-2 Copper T380A intrauterine device (Paragard).

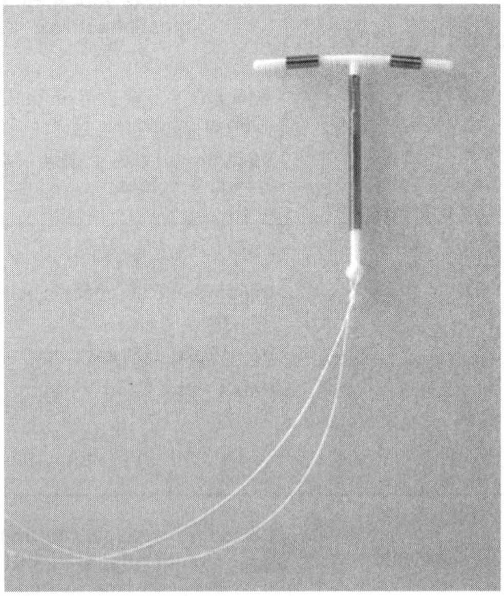

Reproduced from Teva Women's Health

FIGURE 13-3 Levonorgestrel intrauterine device.

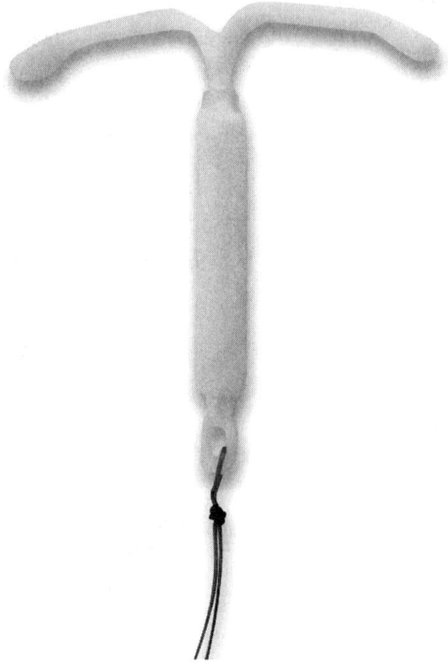

© Lalocracio/iStock/Getty Images Plus/Getty Images

The IUD releases copper ions that cause an inflammatory response; the ions are toxic for spermatozoa in the genital tract fluids, thus contraception is achieved through a sterile inflammatory response that has spermicidal effects (Ortiz & Croxatto, 2007).

Four IUDs containing levonorgestrel (LNG) are also available: Mirena, Liletta, Kyleena, and Skyla (Kaiser Family Foundation, 2020). These T-shaped IUDs feature a reservoir that releases LNG at varying doses; they contain no copper (**Figure 13-3**). After insertion, Mirena releases LNG at a rate of 20 mcg per day, Liletta at 18 to 19 mcg per day, Kyleena at 17.5 mcg per day, and Skyla at 14 mcg per day. Daily release rates decline over time as the device remains in place. The local delivery of progestin causes large changes in the amount and viscosity of cervical mucus, which serves to prevent sperm from entering the uterus (Natavio et al., 2013). Ovulation is suppressed in some individuals with these devices, particularly in the first year after its placement, but most cycles are ovulatory. The LNG IUDs have a monofilament thread. Skyla and Kyleena are the smallest devices and may be easier to insert for individuals with cervical stenosis or small uterine cavities; Liletta is available at a lower cost to public health clinics.

The copper IUD is approved for 10 years of use, but data suggests it may be effective for 12 years (Dethier et al., 2022). Mirena and Liletta, once approved for 5 years, have been recently updated to reflect data that shows they are effective for 8 years of use (Creinin et al., 2022; Jensen et al., 2022). Kyleena can be used for 5 years, and Skyla for 3 years (ACOG, 2018a).

Insertion of an IUD may occur at any time when it is reasonably certain an individual is not pregnant (**Box 13-1**) (Curtis et al., 2024). Insertion of a copper or LNG IUD can serve as emergency contraception (Salcedo et al., 2023). Postabortion, postplacental (within 10 minutes after expulsion of the placenta), and postpartum (at least 4 weeks postpartum) insertion may also be performed. The procedures for copper IUD and LNG IUD insertion differ and are beyond the scope of this chapter. The manufacturers provide insertion training for clinicians and can

BOX 13-1 How to Be Reasonably Certain a Patient Is Not Pregnant

They have no signs or symptoms of pregnancy AND any one of the following:

- is ≤ 7 days after the start of normal menses
- has not had sexual intercourse since the start of last normal menses
- has been correctly and consistently using a reliable method of contraception
- is ≤ 7 days after spontaneous or induced abortion
- is within 4 weeks postpartum
- is fully or nearly fully breastfeeding (exclusively breastfeeding or ≥ 85% of feeds are breastfeeds), amenorrheic, and < 6 months postpartum

Reproduced from Centers for Disease Control and Prevention. (2024). *How to be reasonably certain a woman is not pregnant.* https://www.cdc.gov/contraception/media/pdfs/2024/07/when-to-start-contraception-508.pdf

be contacted via their websites (http://www.paragard.com, http://www.mirena-us.com, http://www.skyla-us.com, https://www.kyleena-us.com, and http://www.liletta.com).

Effectiveness and Efficacy

Intrauterine contraception is extremely effective (Table 13-1). In a cohort of more than 58,000 IUD users, the pregnancy rate per 100 person-years was 0.06 for copper IUDs and 0.52 for LNG IUDs (Heinemann et al., 2015). Pregnancy may occur if partial or complete expulsion of the IUD occurs. The expulsion rate ranges from 2 to 10 percent, with most expulsions occurring in the first 3 months after insertion of the device. Although expulsion may be associated with cramping or bleeding, it may also go unnoticed. Individuals should be encouraged to check periodically for the strings to ensure the device is still in place.

Safety

Contemporary intrauterine contraceptives with monofilament threads are very safe for most individuals (A. Nguyen et al., 2024). Questions about their safety center on infection, future fertility, ectopic pregnancy, and risk of uterine perforation. A transient increase in infection rates occurs in the first 20 days after insertion, likely due to the insertion process or preexisting infection, with this risk reported to range from 1 to 10 cases per 1,000 individuals. The risk of infection returns to baseline thereafter. Antibiotic prophylaxis for insertion is not necessary (Curtis et al., 2024). The FDA has removed recommendations against the use of intrauterine contraceptives in individuals with more than one sexual partner. Sexually transmitted infection (STI) screening is not a requirement for IUD placement, but every individual for whom STI screening is recommended should be offered screening at the IUD insertion appointment (Curtis et al., 2024). If gonorrhea or chlamydia are detected, or if an individual with an IUD develops PID, the condition can be treated without removing the IUD. Please refer to the full *U.S. Selected Practice Recommendations for Contraceptive Use, 2024,* for more detailed information (Curtis et al., 2024).

Despite a common fear among patients, the use of an IUD does not appear to increase the rate of infertility (Hubacher et al., 2001). Actual rates of ectopic pregnancy among IUD users are up to tenfold lower than in nonusers, but if the method fails, the resulting pregnancies are more likely to be ectopic (Kopp-Kallner et al., 2022; Liu et al., 2024). Ectopic risk is slightly elevated but still well below baseline with a lower-dose hormonal IUD (e.g., 13.4 mg), so this may be an important consideration for an individual who has known risk factors for ectopic pregnancy (Elgemark et al., 2022).

Perforation of the uterus during insertion of an IUD occurs at a rate of 1.6 in 1,000 and is usually a benign event (Reed et al., 2022). The risk of perforation is higher in postpartum and breastfeeding individuals.

Previous concerns about the use of IUDs in nulliparous individuals, including adolescents, has largely been put to rest. Today, in fact, intrauterine contraception for adolescents should be as accessible as any other contraceptive option they may choose (Espey et al., 2019).

Side Effects

The most common side effects associated with a copper IUD are prolonged heavy bleeding and dysmenorrhea (X. Chen et al., 2018; Costescu et al., 2022). Menstrual blood loss can increase by as much as 50 percent with copper IUDs, as can the duration of menses. This initial heavy bleeding may improve over time (Sanders et al., 2018). Individuals switching from a hormonal method to the copper IUD may find this transition more concerning, as hormonal contraception has likely masked their normal menstrual pattern.

Unscheduled bleeding is common with LNG IUDs. As the duration of use increases, menstrual flow declines and amenorrhea often develops (X. Chen et al., 2018). Counseling prior to insertion of the device may help reduce anxiety about irregular bleeding. Individuals should be told that the bleeding does not represent hormonal fluctuations, but rather the shedding of the endometrial lining as an atrophic state is achieved. NSAIDs can be used to treat excessive bleeding with either type of IUD (Castillo et al., 2022).

Other side effects linked to LNG IUDs include lower abdominal pain, complexion changes and acne, back pain, breast tenderness, headaches, mood changes, and nausea, although all these effects decline with time, and they are noted in a minority of individuals (Adeyemi-Fowode & Bercaw-Pratt, 2019; Oliveira et al., 2024). In general, few hormonal side effects are observed with the low dose of progestin found in intrauterine contraceptives. As with other progestin-only methods, benign functional ovarian cysts are common, occurring in 8 to 12 percent of LNG IUD users. Most cysts are asymptomatic and resolve spontaneously (Nahum et al., 2015).

Noncontraceptive Benefits

LNG IUDs have many noncontraceptive benefits. Menstrual flow is reduced by as much as 90 percent (depending on which device is being used), and the Mirena device is FDA approved to treat heavy menstrual bleeding (Dean & Schwarz, 2018). The 52 mg LNG IUDs (Mirena, Liletta) can be used to treat idiopathic heavy or prolonged menstrual bleeding associated with adenomyomas and leiomyomas and are acceptable alternatives to endometrial ablation or hysterectomy (Dean & Schwarz, 2018). Reduced risks of endometrial cancer, ovarian, and cervical cancer are seen in IUD users (Cortessis et al., 2017; Wheeler et al., 2019). The progestin in LNG IUDs is sufficient to protect the endometrium as a component of hormone therapy. IUDs can be inserted during the late reproductive years and left in place through the transition to menopause.

Advantages and Disadvantages

Intrauterine contraception has the advantage of providing long-term contraception that is not coitus dependent and does not require adjustments to daily activities (such as remembering to take a pill every day). Contemporary intrauterine contraception options have effectiveness rates that are comparable to those of sterilization. Unlike permanent sterilization, however, intrauterine contraception offers the added advantage of being rapidly reversible, making this method ideal for those who desire long-term contraception but have not completed childbearing. IUDs are also discreet and private methods. Copper and LNG IUDs are effective contraceptive methods for individuals who have contraindications to estrogen-containing contraceptives. Reduced bleeding with the LNG IUDs can lead to substantial savings in the cost of sanitary products. Further, the IUD can be removed if the individual can feel their strings and is comfortable doing so, which decreases barriers to removal (Amico et al., 2020).

One of the biggest disadvantages of IUDs is their insertion process, which can cause cramping, pain, and anxiety at the time of placement. Pain associated with IUD insertions has, until recently, not been taken seriously which has perpetuated fear and mistrust among potential and current IUD users (R. H. Allen et al., 2025). Many systemic reviews have found conflicting evidence of effective pain management tools available for IUD insertions (Lopez et al., 2015; L. Nguyen et al., 2020), which has contributed to taking pain seriously. Local or pericervical lidocaine shows promise for addressing IUD insertion pain (Samy et al., 2019), and providers should remain attentive to pain and anxiety throughout IUD insertion.

There can be a high up-front cost for intrauterine contraception. Copper IUDs and LNG IUDs cost several hundred dollars, and a visit to a skilled clinician is needed for insertion. However, these are long-term contraceptives with no additional costs; thus, they are among the least expensive methods over time. Many clinicians require pre- or postinsertion visits to test for infections and follow-up, but this is not recommended for routine cases (Curtis et al., 2024). Requiring additional visits is not necessary or evidence based and serves as a barrier to individuals seeking LARC; same-day insertion should be the standard of care (Curtis et al., 2024; Holt et al., 2020).

Progestin Implant

A subdermal progestin implant is among the most effective methods of contraception. The single-rod etonogestrel implant (Nexplanon), available in the United States, is 40 mm long and 2 mm in diameter and contains 68 mg of etonogestrel that is released slowly over 3 years (**Figure 13-4**). Etonogestrel is the active metabolite of desogestrel. Nexplanon works by continuously releasing etonogestrel to suppress ovulation (Rocca et al., 2021). Clinicians need to be trained on the appropriate placement and skilled removal of the implant. Removing the etonogestrel implant is reportedly easier than was the case with previously used multiple-rod systems for several reasons: it is a single rod, slightly larger than the multiple-rod systems, and it is made of ethylene vinyl acetate, which is less flexible than the Silastic that was used to make older rods. It has a small amount of barium sulfate in order to make it visible on X-ray (Rocca et al., 2021).

FIGURE 13-4 **Single-rod etonogestrel implant (Nexplanon).**

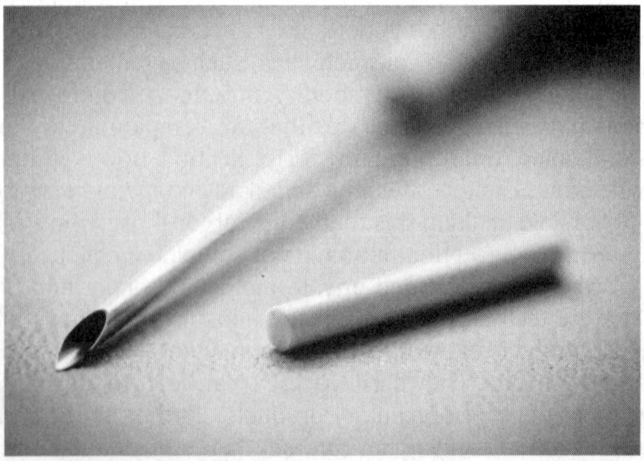

The implant can be inserted any time a clinician is reasonably certain the patient is not pregnant (see Box 13-1). After removal of the implant, etonogestrel levels are undetectable in most individuals within 1 week, and ovulation generally returns within 6 weeks, meaning this method has one of the quickest return to ovulation of any hormonal method (Girum & Wasie, 2018).

Efficacy and Effectiveness

The failure rates for the progestin implant are listed in Table 13-1. Its high rate of effectiveness is related to the intrinsic efficacy of the product and the fact that after it is inserted, there is very little possibility for user error.

Safety and Side Effects

Based on worldwide data, the progestin implant appears to be as safe as other progestin-only methods and is associated with similar side effects, such as irregular bleeding and amenorrhea (Rocca et al., 2021). Unscheduled bleeding is more common and persistent in implant users than in LNG IUD users and is the most common reason for discontinuation (Milliren et al., 2023; Peterson et al., 2019). Other side effects of the progestin implant include bruising and irritation at the insertion site, headache, acne, breast tenderness, and transient ovarian cysts (Rocca et al., 2021). In most studies, the implant has not been shown to cause weight gain (Zwayne et al., 2024), but a recent study showed weight gain patterns similar to DMPA among adolescents and young adults using the implant (Wernick et al., 2024).

Noncontraceptive Benefits

The progestin implant can decrease dysmenorrhea and endometriosis symptoms (Rocca et al., 2021). Further, the implant is a very discrete method that may be appealing for individuals who wish to keep their contraceptive use private for various reasons.

Advantages and Disadvantages

Advantages of the subdermal progestin implant include the presence of highly effective contraception following a single insertion procedure. This contraceptive effect is immediately reversible upon removal of the device. The implant is discreet but palpable, providing reassurance to the woman that it is in place and has not migrated. The major disadvantage and primary reason for discontinuation of use is irregular bleeding (Milliren et al., 2023). Patients should be proactively counseled to anticipate this side effect, and management such as use of NSAIDs for 5 to 7 days or daily use of panty liners should be discussed to reduce the negative effects of irregular bleeding (Curtis et al., 2024). Ulipristal acetate (UPA, 15 mg for 7 days) and tamoxifen (10 mg) have been shown to reduce irregular bleeding and improve satisfaction among implant users (Edelman et al., 2020; Zigler et al., 2018).

PERMANENT CONTRACEPTION

Permanent contraception, or sterilization, is one of the most prevalent contraceptive methods in the United States. People choose sterilization when they are sure they do not want any children or any more children. Among reproductive age individuals in the United States, 3 in 10 (31%) rely on a permanent method of contraception, either tubal occlusion or vasectomy (Frederiksen et al., 2024). Roughly 2 in 10 (21%) of reproductive age individuals reply on tubal occlusion, while 10 percent rely on vasectomy.

The popularity of permanent contraception, especially vasectomy, has been steadily increasing, including a notable rise in younger individuals, since the loss of federal protections for abortion (Bole et al., 2024). Although tubal occlusions and hysterectomies are much more frequent than vasectomies, vasectomies are more effective, safer, and less expensive (Yang et al., 2021). This is an important fact to consider when counseling patients and their partners who are interested in permanent sterilization.

Tubal Occlusion

Tubal occlusion, often referred to as tubal sterilization or female sterilization, involves permanently blocking the fallopian tubes, which prevents sperm from ascending the reproductive tract and thereby meeting and fertilizing an ovum released from the ovary. Tubal occlusion can be performed postpartum, postabortion, or as an "interval" procedure unrelated to pregnancy. In the United States, few tubal occlusion procedures are performed in conjunction with abortion; approximately half are done postpartum, and half are interval procedures. The surgical approaches employed include laparoscopy, mini-laparotomy, transcervical or hysteroscopic methods, and procedures concurrent with a cesarean birth (Marchand et al., 2022).

There are a variety of methods for occluding the fallopian tubes, including unipolar or bipolar electrocoagulation; mechanical occlusion using clips, rings, or bands; and ligation or salpingectomy, using one of several techniques. Procedures other than transcervical methods are generally effective immediately.

The only FDA-approved transcervical sterilization method (Essure) stopped being sold or distributed in the United States at the end of 2018. Essure was voluntarily taken off the market by Bayer after many reports of adverse events and a significant decrease in sales (U.S. FDA, 2018c). Essure was performed via hysteroscopy and could be done in an office setting. Essure involved placement of microinserts of metal and fibers into the fallopian tubes. After placement, tissue grows into the insert or matrix, effectively blocking the tubes. A hysterosalpingogram was performed 3 months after the procedure to confirm tubal occlusion, and individuals had to continue using reliable contraception until sterilization effectiveness was confirmed with hysterosalpingogram (Zite & Borrero, 2011). Despite Essure being taking off the market, it is important for clinicians to understand the method because thousands of individuals in the United States still have Essure as their method of contraception. It is not necessary to discontinue Essure if the patient already had it placed and is not experiencing related issues. For current information on the side effects, management, and status of Essure as a contraceptive method, clinicians should consult the FDA's *Essure Permanent Birth Control* webpage (U.S. FDA, 2022).

Efficacy and Effectiveness

Tubal sterilization is a highly effective contraceptive method (Table 13-1). Although the overall failure rate is low, failures do occur and are more frequent in individuals who are younger at the time of sterilization (Stuart & Ramesh, 2018). Failure rates are similar to those of other highly effective, long-term contraceptive methods, such as the progestin implant and intrauterine contraception.

Safety and Side Effects

Sterilization is a very effective method of contraception, but when pregnancy does occur after tubal sterilization, the risk of ectopic pregnancy is high. In the largest study of sterilization, one third of all post-sterilization pregnancies were ectopic (Peterson et al., 1997). An Australian study estimated the rates of ectopic pregnancy after tubal sterilization to be between 2.4 and 2.9 per 1,000 procedures. The rate was 3.5 times higher in individuals who were sterilized before the age of 28 years than among those sterilized after age 33 years (Malacova et al., 2014). Although studies often refer to sterilization generally, laparoscopic sterilization has higher rates of postsurgical ectopic pregnancy than hysteroscopic sterilization. Failed hysteroscopic sterilizations are more likely than laparoscopic sterilizations to result in live birth (Brandi et al., 2018).

Other risks are related to the surgical procedures used and include infection, hemorrhage, anesthesia complications, and surgical trauma or injury. The likelihood of these complications is very low, with such events occurring in fewer than 1 percent of all procedures (Stuart & Ramesh, 2018).

A "post-tubal ligation syndrome" has been described, which typically includes increased dysmenorrhea and abnormalities in the menstrual cycle. Some authorities believe such symptoms are more likely related to discontinuing hormonal contraceptives, or simply getting older and entering perimenopause. Studies show conflicting results as to whether menstrual patterns differ between those who have and have not had a tubal occlusion (Sadatmahalleh et al., 2016; Verma et al., 2023), so this topic requires more extensive research.

Noncontraceptive Benefits

There is a decreased risk of ovarian cancer following tubal sterilization via salpingectomy (Zadabedini Masouleh et al., 2023).

Advantages and Disadvantages

Tubal occlusion is a highly effective permanent method of contraception and is well suited to those who do not desire future fertility. The Patient Protection and Affordable Care Act (ACA) requires private insurance to cover tubal sterilization, but not vasectomy. States that have adopted Medicaid expansion cover female sterilization, and most states within this group cover male sterilization (Guttmacher Institute, 2024). However, some states have not expanded Medicaid and retain the authority to determine coverage for sterilization within their state (Kaiser Family Foundation, 2018). Additional barriers to access include requirements for a waiting period after signing a consent and minimum age requirements. Because contraception is one of the most common reasons reproductive-aged individuals seek health care, it is important to counsel those who are contemplating or undergoing sterilization about the continued need for preventive health services, such as cancer screening.

Sterilization regret is not uncommon, occurring for roughly 10 percent of those who undergo sterilization (Danvers & Evans, 2022; Siemons et al., 2022). Younger individuals tend to experience more regret, with regret decreasing with advancing age. Informed consent, including the availability, expense, and effectiveness of sterilization reversibility, is an important part of patient education.

Vasectomy

Vasectomy, also referred to as male sterilization, cuts or blocks both the right and left vas deferens, which are the small tubes that carry sperm from the testes to become part of the seminal fluid. Three techniques are used for occlusion of the vas deferens:

vasectomy, vassal occlusion, and vassal injection. Vasectomy is the most common technique (Velez et al., 2021).

Sperm account for only 5 percent of the semen that is produced by the prostate and other glands; thus, there is a minimal decrease in the amount of seminal fluid following male sterilization. Vasectomies have no effect on sex drive, hormone production, or sexual function.

Vasectomy includes two approaches, and both can be performed in an outpatient setting. The conventional vasectomy requires one midline or two lateral incisions in the scrotum. The vas is lifted out through the incision and occluded using one of a variety of methods, such as ligation, cautery, excision of a segment of the vas, or application of clips. The opening is then sutured. With the no-scalpel method, the skin of the scrotum is pierced, and the vas is exposed and blocked through an opening so small that it does not require stitches. A systematic review showed that the no-scalpel approach resulted in less bleeding, hematoma, infection, and pain, and a shorter operation time, than the traditional incision technique, with no difference in effectiveness (Cook et al., 2014).

Vasectomy is not immediately effective. Sperm are continually produced and transported through the reproductive tract, so some sperm will continue to be present distal to the site of the vasectomy. Generally, it takes between 15 and 20 ejaculations to clear all sperm from the reproductive tract. An analysis of semen should be done 8 to 16 weeks after vasectomy to ensure the procedure was successful. Until success has been confirmed with semen analysis, individuals should use additional contraceptive protection or abstain from sexual intercourse (Curtis et al., 2024).

Efficacy and Effectiveness

A systematic review estimated the failure rate of vasectomy to be less than 1 percent, which is similar to the rate associated with tubal occlusion (Sharlip et al., 2012) (Table 13-1).

Safety and Side Effects

Most individuals will experience some degree of postoperative discomfort; infection and scrotal hematoma occur on rare occasions (Yang et al., 2021). Some experience chronic testicular pain after vasectomy, but only a small percentage (3% or fewer) report pain that negatively affects their life or causes them to regret having had the procedure. Antisperm antibodies are more common among individuals who have had vasectomies than the general population, although this condition does not appear to be associated with any adverse health consequences. Studies on the relationship between vasectomy and prostate cancer differ in their findings (Baboudjian et al., 2022; Cheng et al., 2021; Xu et al., 2021). Likely, there is only a small increase in prostate cancer risk with vasectomy, a fact that will be especially important to discuss with those at elevated risk for prostate cancer (Minhaj Siddiqui et al., 2021).

Noncontraceptive Benefits

No benefits other than contraception have been demonstrated to date for vasectomy.

Advantages and Disadvantages

Vasectomy is a simple procedure that is less complicated and less costly than tubal occlusion for those wishing permanent contraception. Unlike tubal occlusion, 80 percent of vasectomies occur in an office under local anesthesia (Velez et al., 2021). As is true with tubal sterilization, regret may occur with naturally or with certain unanticipated life changes at roughly the same frequency as with tubal ligation. Vasectomies are more easily and successfully reversed than tubal occlusion, with success rates ranging from 65% to 90% (Dubin et al., 2021). Vasectomy does not prevent STIs.

HORMONAL METHODS

The FDA's approval of combined oral contraceptives (COCs) in 1960 marked a revolutionary change in reproductive rights and responsibilities for women and pregnancy-capable people. For the first time, individuals had access to a nearly 100 percent effective form of contraception that did not require the participation of a partner and was independent of the act of coitus. Contraceptive pills are some of the best-studied and most widely used medications available today; they remain the most popular form of reversible contraception in the United States (Guttmacher Institute, 2021).

Two types of hormonal contraceptives are available: those that contain progestin (progestin only) and those that contain progestin and estrogen (combined). Progestin, the synthetic version of the endogenous hormone progesterone, is highly effective alone as a contraceptive, but it may cause irregular bleeding. The addition of estrogen to progestin in combined methods results in more predictable bleeding patterns due to stabilization of the endometrium. Estrogen as a single agent for contraception requires doses that may cause unacceptable risks of serious side effects, such as thromboembolic events and endometrial hyperplasia. The synergistic activity of estrogen and progestin makes it possible to combine these hormones in lower doses to produce successful contraception than would be possible using either hormone alone (Bastianelli et al., 2018).

Combined contraceptive methods currently available in the United States include COCs, the patch, and the vaginal ring. Progestin methods include progestin-only pills (POPs), DMPA injections, subdermal implants, and LNG IUDs. The implant and IUDs are discussed in the section on LARC.

Both progestin and estrogen inhibit the hypothalamic–pituitary–ovarian axis and subsequent steroidogenesis. Progestins have several contraceptive effects, including preventing the luteinizing hormone (LH) surge and thereby inhibiting ovulation; thickening the cervical mucus, which inhibits sperm penetration and transport; changing the motility of the fallopian tubes so the transport of sperm or ova is impaired; and causing the endometrium to become atrophic, although it is unknown whether these changes are sufficient to prevent implantation in the rare event that fertilization occurs. Estrogen suppresses the production of follicle-stimulating hormone (FSH), thereby preventing the selection and emergence of a dominant follicle.

The primary mechanism of action of all hormonal contraceptive methods, with the exception of POPs and LNG IUDs, is preventing ovulation (refer to **Appendix 13-B**). Other contraceptive effects of progestin represent secondary mechanisms to prevent pregnancy if ovulation occurs. Many individuals who use contraception have fears about how long it will take to return to fertility after discontinuing their method. A systematic review demonstrated that within a year of discontinuing a contraceptive that inhibits ovulation, 80 percent of those attempting to conceive will become pregnant (Yland et al., 2020). POPs and LNG IUDs do not consistently inhibit ovulation; therefore, return to fertility is expected upon cessation of either method. The primary mechanism of action for both methods is thickening the cervical mucus; LNG IUDs also inhibit sperm from fertilizing an ovum.

In the past, a barrier to contraception use has been the requirement for a pelvic examination prior to initiation of hormonal methods. This is not necessary, and pelvic examination should not be a requirement for those seeking contraception, except for IUDs. Researchers have demonstrated that provision of oral contraceptives without a mandatory pelvic examination does not place individuals at higher risk of cervical cancer (Curtis et al., 2024).

None of the hormonal methods provide STI protection. For this reason, it is important to stress the concomitant use of barrier methods for those who are at risk of exposure to STIs.

Many popular myths exist regarding the health risks of hormonal methods, and the healthcare provider must be proactive in educating patients about both the safety and noncontraceptive benefits of these methods. Future fertility may be preserved through the decreased risk of PID and ectopic pregnancy associated with the use of hormonal methods (Schrager et al., 2020). Other benefits of hormonal methods include a decreased risk of several cancers (colon, ovarian, and endometrial) and a decreased risk of serious disease such as endometriosis, adenomyosis, rheumatoid arthritis, and asthma (Grandi et al., 2019; Nwaru et al., 2021; Salliot et al., 2022). Protection against ovarian and uterine cancer may persist as long as 28 years after discontinuation of these methods (Coelingh Bennink et al., 2024).

The relationship between hormonal contraception and breast cancer is subject to ongoing debate. Several recent meta-analyses identified an increased risk of breast cancer in specific subgroups of hormonal contraception users (Fitzpatrick et al., 2023; Kanadys et al., 2021; Satish et al., 2023; Torres-de la Roche et al., 2023). However, it is yet to be determined if the risk is elevated only in the short term or if the risk remains several decades after COC use (Fitzpatrick et al., 2023). An increased risk of cervical cancer is seen in long-term COC users (Bovo et al., 2023; Cortessis et al., 2017), though this association disappears when controlling for HPV status (Anastasiou et al., 2022). There is also an elevated risk for a rare, benign liver tumor, a hepatocellular adenoma, among those with a history of oral contraception use (Oldhafer et al., 2020).

During the first few postpartum weeks, the risk of venous thromboembolism (VTE; deep vein thromboses and pulmonary emboli) is greatly elevated; consequently, estrogen-containing contraceptives are contraindicated during this time. Progestin-only methods, including IUDs and implants, may be initiated immediately postpartum.

Combined Hormonal Methods

Early formulations of COCs contained unnecessarily high doses of hormones: 80 to 100 mcg of either ethinyl estradiol or mestranol and 1 to 5 mg of progestins. Since the 1970s, the trend has been toward lower-dose formulations that are equally effective, safer, and have a better side-effect profile. In addition to improving COC formulations, alternative delivery systems for combined contraception have been developed that allow individuals to avoid a daily dosing schedule. These alternative delivery systems include the combined contraceptive patch and the vaginal ring. This section begins by providing information about COCs, which is then followed by a discussion of the patch and the vaginal ring.

Combined Oral Contraceptives

Since the milestone introduction of COCs in the United States in 1960, many formulations of COCs have been developed. Each is unique while its patent protection remains in force. After the patent expires, however, generic formulations tend to outnumber the brand-name products, so the same formulation may have several names. COCs are classified as monophasic or multiphasic (biphasic, triphasic, or quadriphasic), depending on whether the dosage of hormones is constant or varies. There is no evidence that either monophasic or multiphasic formulations are a superior choice.

Most of the COCs available today contain 10 to 35 mcg of ethinyl estradiol, although a few COCs contain 50 mcg of ethinyl estradiol or mestranol, the methyl ether of ethinyl estradiol. Approximately 30 percent of mestranol is lost when it is converted to ethinyl estradiol; thus a 50 mcg mestranol pill is bioequivalent to a 35 mcg ethinyl estradiol pill. Estradiol valerate is found in the new quadriphasic COC.

COCs also contain one of several different progestins. The progestins are often referred to as belonging to the first, second, or third generation. With the exception of drospirenone, all progestins in COCs available in the United States are derived from C-19 androgens. These derivatives are classified into two categories: (1) the estranes, or chemical derivatives of norethindrone (norethindrone, norethindrone acetate, and ethynodiol diacetate); and (2) the gonanes, or chemical derivatives of norgestrel (norgestrel, its active isomer LNG, desogestrel, and norgestimate). Members of these categories differ in terms of both their bioavailability and their half-life. Caution should be exercised when comparing the potency or purported androgenicity of the various types of progestins by category. Rather, formulations should be judged on the clinical response of the individual.

Drospirenone, the only non-testosterone-derived progestin, is an analog of the diuretic spironolactone. Drospirenone has a mild potassium-sparing diuretic effect, necessitating that potassium levels be checked during the first cycle in individuals using angiotensin-converting enzyme (ACE) inhibitors, chronic daily NSAIDs, angiotensin-II receptor antagonists, potassium-sparing diuretics, heparin, or aldosterone antagonists. Those with conditions that predispose them to hyperkalemia should not use COCs containing drospirenone.

The initial choice of a particular COC should be made with the goal of providing the individual with safe, effective contraception. All low-dose (less than 50 mcg) COCs meet this requirement, so it is reasonable to provide a individual with whatever formulation is most cost effective, or whatever pill they request by name.

Instructions contained in the pill package insert include options for a Sunday start, a first day of menstrual cycle start, or any time within the first 5 days of one's cycle. All these options are based on the principle that as long as COCs are begun within the first 5 days of menses, there is contraceptive protection in the first cycle. The Sunday start has been the traditional approach in the United States because COC packages often reflect that regimen, and the withdrawal bleed does not usually occur on the weekend, which many may find preferable. The advantage of starting pills within the first 5 days of the menstrual cycle is that no backup contraceptive method is required during the first cycle. Individuals are advised to use additional contraception, such as condoms, with regimens having other starting points for the first 7 days of use.

An increasingly popular alternative approach is to utilize a "quick start" by beginning the pill any time in the menstrual cycle with additional contraception for the first 7 days. Instructions are given to take a pregnancy test in 2 to 4 weeks if unprotected sex occurred during the cycle. This practice has been shown to increase continuation rates for COCs initially and is not associated with an increased incidence of adverse bleeding patterns (Curtis et al., 2024). If the individual has had unprotected sex since their last cycle, emergency contraception may be offered at the same time if applicable. Further, the individual should be counseled that early pregnancy is possible at this time but will not be harmed by initiating a combined contraceptive method (Romer et al., 2024).

With the traditional cyclic schedule, users take 21 to 24 days of active COCs, followed by 4 to 7 days of inactive pills or no pills. During the hormone-free interval, bleeding from the withdrawal of estrogen and progestin occurs. This is technically a withdrawal bleed, rather than menses, and is based primarily on convention rather than science. Because it is not a real menses, the withdrawal bleed is usually lighter and shorter that an individual's usual menses. Extended (omitting the hormone-free interval for two or more cycles) and continuous (omitting the hormone-free interval indefinitely) COC regimens are popular, both for health indications and convenience. Monophasic pills are generally preferred for this use.

Efficacy and Effectiveness COCs require the individual's daily adherence to the dosing schedule, which can be compromised by many factors, resulting in a gap between efficacy and effectiveness (Table 13-1). Based on U.S. data related to pill use, it appears that approximately 7 percent of individuals will become pregnant unintentionally due to incorrect pill use (Sundaram et al., 2017). Common reasons for COC failure include not starting a new pack on time, missing pills, taking a break from the pill, and discontinuing the pill in response to expected side effects. The counseling and education provided by the clinician are critical to the ultimate success of the individual in avoiding pregnancy.

The most important pills to take in each cycle are the first and last active COCs, which ensure that the hormone-free interval does not exceed 7 days. During the hormone-free interval, pituitary stimulation of the ovaries by FSH is likely to resume, and follicular development may begin. Immature follicles stimulated during the hormone-free phase generally regress after the hormonal pills are resumed, and 7 consecutive days of pill use have been shown to be sufficient in suppressing any follicular function. Hormone-free intervals of less than 7 days have become increasingly standard (A. Nguyen et al., 2024). Patient instructions must stress the importance of starting a new pack on time and not taking more than 7 days off from the active pills. If an individual does extend the hormone-free interval beyond 7 days, they should be instructed to abstain from intercourse or use additional contraception until seven consecutive pills have been taken.

Missing a pill dose is almost universal among individuals who choose COCs for contraception. Missing a random pill now and then is unlikely to lead to a method failure, but unfortunately, this may lead to complacency regarding the importance of daily adherence to the schedule because individuals come to believe that inconsistent pill use is adequate. The probability of pill failure increases with repeated missed pills. This issue is complicated by the fact that instructions for those who miss a pill can be confusing. Current recommendations for late or missed pills can be found in **Figure 13-5**.

Many individuals believe that temporarily discontinuing, or taking a break from, COCs is beneficial. Ask open-ended questions to better understand the underlying fear or concern related to this belief. It is important to convey to individuals that the hormones found in the pill do not accumulate in the body, and the occurrence of a withdrawal bleed indicates that the endometrium is responding to the absence of hormones. There are no differences in the long-term fertility of those who use the pill intermittently and those who use the pill for many years.

Many of those who begin taking oral contraceptives discontinue their use before the end of 1 year; the most commonly reported reasons for discontinuation are side effects and difficulty obtaining contraception (Simmons et al., 2019). A misunderstanding about the management of side effects may compound this dissatisfaction. Clear information about the side effects commonly encountered during the first three cycles of pill use should be given. Whenever an individual begins a new COC, they should be encouraged to contact the clinician prior to discontinuing the pills if they experience unwanted side effects. In such a case, a different pill may be substituted without interrupting effective contraception.

A number of medications can modify the effectiveness of COCs. Pharmacologic mechanisms that alter medication metabolism include induction of liver enzymes, alterations in sex hormone-binding globulin, and medications that alter the first-pass effect in the gut. Medications that can reduce the effectiveness of COCs include one type of antiretroviral therapy (fosamprenavir), rifampin, and some anticonvulsants (e.g., carbamazepine, phenytoin, barbiturates, primidone, topiramate, oxcarbazepine, lamotrigine) (A. Nguyen et al., 2024). Despite popular cultural myths, antibiotics do not decrease the effectiveness of COCs, with the exception of rifampin. Those taking rifampin should use an alternative form of contraception in addition to COCs (A. Nguyen et al., 2024).

Safety and Side Effects COCs are among the most extensively studied medications available and are known to be extremely safe for healthy individuals. Many of the side effects associated with COCs are bothersome but not dangerous; however, serious complications are possible and are the basis of contraindications to COC use. These contraindications may be related to the direct effects of the hormonal ingredient, as in breast cancer, or they may result from hormonal effects on other systems, as in thromboembolism. The *U.S. Medical Eligibility Criteria for Contraceptive Use, 2024* provides an evidence-based guide to the contraindications to COC use (A. Nguyen et al., 2024). One must always weigh the risks of pregnancy in relation to the risks associated with contraceptive use.

All COCs increase the risk of VTE. The level of this risk appears to be related to the dose of estrogen and is greatest for those with clotting disorders, such as factor V Leiden, or a family history of thrombosis. Often, complications with pill use are the first time an individual discovers they have a clotting disorder. The various progestin components may contribute to the risk of VTE to a differing degree. Two different systematic reviews have found that combined hormonal pills using levonorgesterel as the progestin are less likely to cause venous thrombosis than those that utilize cyproterone acetate, desogestrel, drospirenone, or

FIGURE 13-5 **Recommended actions after late or missed COCs.**

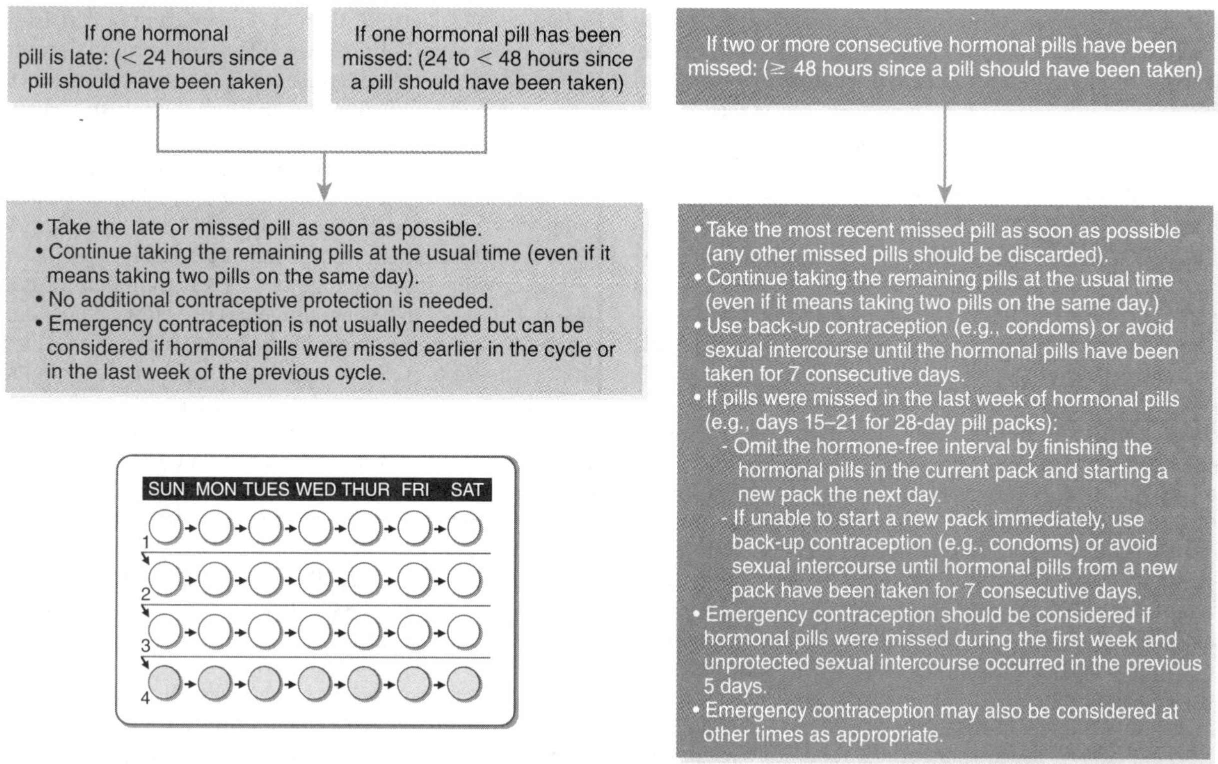

Reproduced from Curtis, K. M., Nguyen, A. T., Tepper, N. K., Zapata, L. B., Snyder, E. M., Hatfield-Timajchy, K., Kortsmit, K., Cohen, M. A., Whiteman, M. K., & Contributors (2024). U.S. selected practice recommendations for contraceptive use, 2024. *MMWR. Recommendations and reports: Morbidity and mortality weekly report. Recommendations and reports, 73*(3), 1–77. https://doi.org/10.15585/mmwr.rr7303a1

gestodene (de Bastos et al., 2014; Dragoman et al., 2018). The type of estrogen may also play a role in risk, with some studies suggesting a 33 percent reduction in VTE risk for E2-containing COCs compared to ethinylestradiol (Douxfils et al., 2024). COCs containing less than 50 mcg of estrogen do not appear to increase the risk of arterial thrombosis (myocardial infarction or stroke) in healthy nonsmoking individuals, including those older than 40 years. COCs may increase blood pressure in some individuals through an increase in plasma angiotensin. Because hypertension is a cofactor in the development of cardiovascular disease, blood pressure should be monitored in COC users (Curtis et al., 2024).

Metabolic effects of COCs may include development of benign hepatocellular adenomas, although this side effect is very rare with low-dose pills (Oldhafer et al., 2020). There does not appear to be an association between these benign tumors and the development of liver cancer. Low-dose COCs appear to create negligible changes in insulin levels or glucose levels and have no effect on the development of diabetes. Most comparisons of combination contraceptives have shown no significant difference in weight gain in pill users versus nonusers in large studies (Zwayne et al., 2024).

History of COC use, regardless of duration, does not affect breast cancer risk. There seems to be a small, time-dependent increased risk of breast cancer in users of combined oral contraceptives, with the highest risk occurring within 2 years of use. This elevated risk seems to disappear by the age of 55 (Karlsson et al., 2021). There may also be an elevated risk for cervical cancers among COC users, but newer research which looks at when the HPV infection was acquired, as opposed to when cervical cancer was diagnosed, finds no relationship between COC use and cervical cancer (Anastasiou et al., 2022).

Sexual dysfunction and changes in libido have been noted among COC users related to decrease in freely available testosterone among COC users. Sexual function changes that may occur among a minority of users includes general sexual response, desire, lubrication, orgasm, and relationship satisfaction. While these might not happen to many users, these changes can be very concerning when they do occur (Krapf & Goldstein, 2024). As part of evaluating any sexual concerns related to contraception, the clinician should do a thorough evaluation of other contributing factors, including pelvic floor dysfunction, relationship issues, and whether the use of vaginal lubricants and moisturizers would increase sexual function (Casado-Espada et al., 2019). Chapter 12 discusses assessment of sexual health and Chapter 18 addresses evaluation and management of alterations in sexual function. Depression and other mental health conditions, although rare, may be experienced but a small subset of COC users. Data suggests adolescent users may be especially at risk for reasons not fully understood (Kraft et al., 2024). Other side effects specific to estrogen include nausea, cervical ectopy and leukorrhea, telangiectasis, chloasma (darkening of sun-exposed skin), growth of breast tissue (ductal tissue or fat deposition), increased cholesterol content within the bile (which can lead to gallstones), benign hepatocellular adenomas, and changes in the clotting cascade. Effects specific to the androgenic impact of progestins include increased appetite and subsequent weight gain, mood changes and depression, fatigue, complexion changes, changes in carbohydrate metabolism, increased LDL and decreased HDL cholesterol, decreased libido, and pruritus. Effects that can be either estrogen or progestin related include headaches, hypertension, and breast tenderness. Many of the side effects that individuals associate with COCs occur either during the seven hormone-free days or appear to be associated with the demise of follicles recruited during the hormone-free interval (Noachtar et al., 2023). In some cases, a trial of extended or continuous use may be recommended to improve the symptoms that individuals experience at predictable times in their pill cycles.

Noncontraceptive Benefits The noncontraceptive benefits of COCs are numerous and often underappreciated (Coelingh Bennink et al., 2024; Schrager et al., 2020). Modern formulations of COCs have shown a 21–40 percent reduction in ovarian cancer with short- and long-term use (Iversen et al., 2018; Schrager et al., 2020). This reduction in risk persists for up to 25 years after pill use has stopped (Iversen et al., 2018). Likewise, COC use reduces the risk of endometrial cancer by approximately 34 percent. This risk reduction is greatest in individuals with additional risk factors for endometrial cancer, such as tobacco use and obesity (Karlsson et al., 2021). Individuals on COCs also experience lower rates of PID requiring hospitalization, fewer ectopic pregnancies, and lower incidence of endometriosis. These conditions are the most common causes of infertility; thus, the pill helps preserve fertility—not by conservation of ovulation, but rather through prevention of subfertility causes. Other well-documented noncontraceptive benefits of the pill include menstrual-related effects (discussed in the next paragraph), improvement in acne and hirsutism, and reduced incidence of benign breast conditions. Older studies demonstrated a reduced risk of developing functional ovarian cysts while individuals were on COCs, but this effect is less profound with the lower doses of hormones in currently used COCs (Maguire & Westhoff, 2011).

In addition to being effective contraceptive methods, COCs have many other therapeutic uses. For example, they regulate menstrual cycles and are useful in the management of abnormal bleeding patterns. While taking COCs, individuals experience lighter periods (withdrawal bleeds) that may treat or improve anemia. COCs can also be an effective treatment for mittelschmerz, dysmenorrhea, endometriosis, premenstrual symptoms, and the vasomotor symptoms of perimenopause (Schrager et al., 2020). Those who experience catamenial conditions—those that rise and fall in synchronicity with the menstrual cycle, such as menstrual migraines—may also find that COCs improve those conditions. Decreasing the number of withdrawal bleeding episodes per year via extended or continuous-use COCs may further diminish these problems.

Advantages and Disadvantages COC use is unrelated to coitus. Most individuals in the United States are familiar with the instructions for COC use, and this method is widely available in pharmacies and clinics. Confidence in the product is high because it has been on the market for more than 50 years and has been continually researched. Additionally, more than 30 different formulations of COCs are available, allowing for individualization based on response to the products. While it may be biologically plausible, there is not sufficient or consistent evidence demonstrating negative effects of hormonal contraception on breastfeeding (Bryant et al., 2019). The risk of VTE is increased in the immediate postpartum period, and as such the *U.S. Medical Eligibility Criteria for Contraceptive Use, 2024* classifies COC use in breastfeeding individuals who have no other risk factors for VTE in category 4 up to 21 days postpartum, in category 3 from 21 to 29 days postpartum, and in category 2 from 30 days postpartum on (A. Nguyen et al., 2024).

The obvious disadvantage of COCs is the need for daily pill taking. Patients can be encouraged to use apps or calendars that remind them to take their pills daily to reduce the incidence of late or missed pills. Some apps, such as Spot On from Planned Parenthood, provide reminders for all types of contraception in addition to evidence-based instructions on what to do in case of late or missed pills. Clinicians should connect patients to resources that increase consistent use. The ongoing cost of COCs can be problematic, although under the ACA, all private insurance companies and states with Medicaid expansion must cover at least one form of COCs. Particularly for young people, lack of privacy may also be an issue. Finally, some will find various side effects of COCs unacceptable.

Combined Contraceptive Patch and Vaginal Ring

The contraceptive patch (Xulane) and vaginal ring (NuvaRing, Annovera) share many similarities with COCs, yet they have some distinct differences. The patch and ring utilize delivery systems that allow for simpler dosing than daily pill taking. Both methods avoid the first-pass metabolism of COCs, allowing for lower-dose administration and potentially avoiding interactions with other medications.

The patch releases 20 mcg per day of ethinyl estradiol and 150 mcg per day of the progestin norelgestromin, the active metabolite of norgestimate. These active ingredients are rapidly absorbed and reach therapeutic serum concentrations within 24 to 48 hours. The thin beige patch, which is 1.5 inches square (approximately the size of a matchbook), is applied by the individual and is worn for 1 week at a time. The patch is changed weekly on the same day of the week for 3 weeks, then no patch is worn for 1 week to allow for a withdrawal bleed. As with COCs, no more than 7 days should pass between removal of the last patch and the beginning of the next patch cycle. The patch can be worn on the buttocks, upper arm, abdomen, and anywhere on the upper torso except the breasts (**Figure 13-6**).

The NuvaRing vaginal ring is colorless and flexible, with an outer diameter of about 2 inches (**Figure 13-7**). It releases 15 mcg per day of ethinyl estradiol and 120 mcg per day of the progestin etonogestrel, the active metabolite of desogestrel. The Annovera ring is white and flexible, 2.25 inches in diameter. It releases 13 mcg of ethinyl estradiol and 150 mcg of segesterone acetate a day. The active ingredients of each ring rapidly diffuse across the mucous membrane of the vagina and reach a steady state in the serum. The ring is left in place in the vagina for 21 days and then removed for 1 week, allowing for a withdrawal bleed. The ring provides a steady delivery of hormones, which leads to a very low serum concentration—approximately half of the serum concentration found with a 35 mcg COC.

FIGURE 13-6 **Locations for contraceptive patch placement: upper arm, upper torso (except breasts), abdomen, or buttocks.**

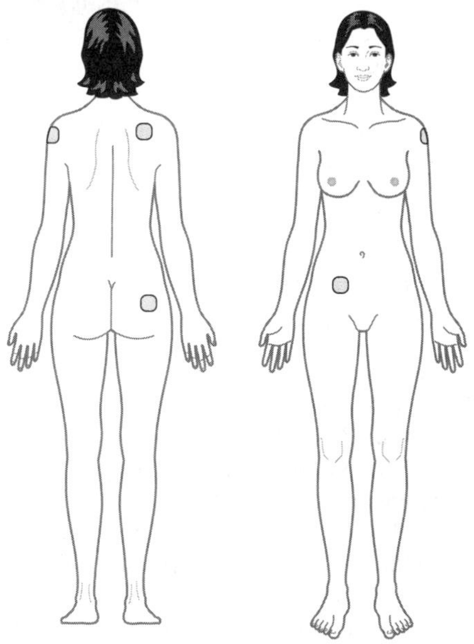

FIGURE 13-7 **Combined contraceptive ring.**

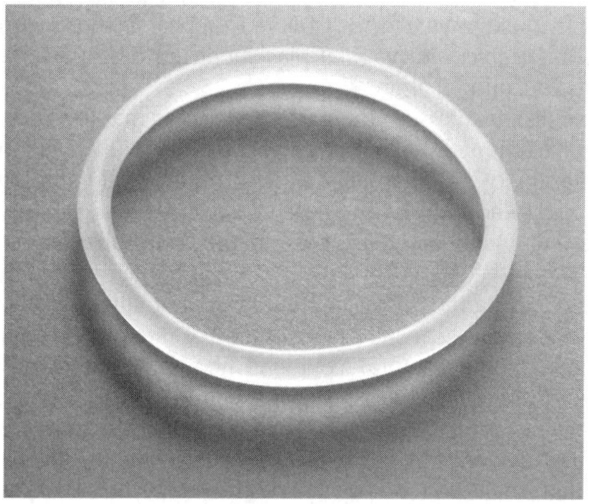

Efficacy and Effectiveness The patch and the vaginal ring have the same theoretical efficacy and typical use failure rates as COCs (Table 13-1). There is less opportunity for user error with the patch and ring because they do not need to be remembered daily. Each patch continues to emit hormones at therapeutic levels for at least 9 days after the second patch is applied (Nanda & Burke, 2018). The hormones emitted by the ring remain at therapeutic levels after 3 weeks; therefore, there is some margin of error if the product is not changed on time. As with COCs, extended use (omitting the patch- or ring-free week for two or more cycles) and continuous use (omitting the patch- or ring-free week indefinitely) of the patch and ring is common (Curtis et al., 2024).

The patch is effective only if it is completely attached to the skin; even partial detachment necessitates replacement. The exact placement of the ring in the vagina is not critical to its efficacy. Some studies have suggested increased failure rates of the patch in individuals who weigh more than 198 pounds or have a BMI > 30 kg/m^2. While this evidence is limited, clinicians should counsel patients on this possibility for decreased efficacy. Further, there may be an increased risk of venous thromboembolism (VTE) in individuals with a BMI > 30 kg/m^2 (Zwayne et al., 2024).

Safety and Side Effects *The U.S. Medical Eligibility Criteria for Contraceptive Use, 2024* currently specifies the same criteria for COCs, the patch, and the ring, except in individuals who have undergone malabsorptive bariatric surgery procedures who can safely use the patch and ring (Curtis, Tepper, et al., 2016). While it is theoretically possible that the nonoral delivery systems may result in different safety and side-effect profiles, no evidence has been published to support large differences in adverse effects or safety to date. Clinicians are cautioned to not presume that the patch and ring are safer than COCs. An individual who is not a candidate for COCs should not be given the patch or ring, either.

The patch has been associated with heightened concern about an increased risk of VTE. Studies have produced conflicting results on this topic (de Bastos et al., 2014). While hormone levels with the patch are typically higher than those with COCs, the clinical implications of these pharmacokinetic findings are unclear and do not necessarily indicate any increased risk of serious side effects. An FDA advisory committee concluded that the benefits of the patch (e.g., pregnancy prevention) outweigh the risk of VTE (U.S. FDA, 2015), with the exception of those with a BMI >30 (Zwayne et al., 2024).

In general, the side effects of the patch and the vaginal ring are very similar to those of COCs, such as breakthrough bleeding and nausea. In addition, the patch and ring have some unique side effects related to their delivery systems. In studies of the patch, approximately 20 percent of participating individuals experienced some skin irritation at the site of application, but fewer than 3 percent discontinued use for this reason (Lopez et al., 2013). The ring may be felt during intercourse, although this is not commonly cited as a reason for discontinuation. Although there is no increase in cervical cytologic changes with the vaginal ring, an increased incidence of vaginitis and leukorrhea has been noted (Lopez et al., 2013).

Noncontraceptive Benefits It is theoretically plausible that the noncontraceptive benefits of COCs may be realized with the patch and ring as well because these methods affect the hypothalamic–pituitary–ovarian axis in the same way as COCs; however, epidemiologic studies to support this theory are lacking. Caution must be exercised in attributing the same long-term benefits of COCs to the patch and ring in the absence of published evidence of this effect.

Advantages and Disadvantages The intrinsic advantage of the patch and ring is the avoidance of daily dosing, which may lead to greater effectiveness. A specific advantage of the vaginal ring is the lack of visible evidence of its use, which may appeal to some, particularly adolescents, who want to keep their contraceptive use private. The patch may appeal to those who are not comfortable with vaginal placement but desire a nondaily method of contraception.

One disadvantage of the patch and ring is that few formulations of each method are currently available. The development of a variety of products may allow for individual variations in response to hormones, and patch color choices may appeal to some individuals as well. These methods are also associated with ongoing costs. A final disadvantage of the patch and ring is that both methods still contain large amounts of active ingredients upon disposal. The presence of these chemicals has prompted environmental concerns about the effect of high doses of estrogen and progestin seeping into the water supply. In the future, a recommendation may be issued to place the used devices into a biohazard waste container instead of landfills.

Progestin-Only Methods

Progestin-only contraceptives are used continuously; there is no hormone-free interval, as occurs with combined methods. These contraceptive methods have minimal effects on coagulation factors, blood pressure, or lipid levels and are generally considered safer for individuals who have contraindications to estrogen, such as cardiovascular risk factors, migraine with aura, or a history of VTE. In spite of this belief, the product labeling for some progestin-only products mimics the labeling for products containing estrogen. The evidence-based *U.S. Medical Eligibility Criteria for Contraceptive Use, 2024* should be used, instead of product labels, to identify appropriate candidates for progestin-only contraception (A. Nguyen et al., 2024).

Progestin-only contraceptives do not provide the same cycle control as methods containing estrogen, and unscheduled bleeding is common with all progestin-only methods. Depending on the method, unscheduled bleeding occurs most frequently during the first 6 months of use, with a substantial number of users becoming amenorrheic by 12 months of use (ACOG, 2022). Overall blood loss decreases over time, making progestin-only methods protective against iron-deficiency anemia. With appropriate counseling, many individuals see amenorrhea as a benefit of these methods.

All progestin-only methods are likely to improve menstrual symptoms, including dysmenorrhea, menorrhagia, premenstrual syndrome, and anemia (Schrager et al., 2020). The thickening of cervical mucus seen with progestin methods is protective against PID.

Progestin-only contraceptives include progestin-only pills, injections, implants, and LNG IUDs. Implants and LNG IUDs are covered in the section on LARC.

Progestin-Only Pills

POPs, or mini-pills, that are available in the United States contain 0.35 mg of norethindrone. Each pill contains active ingredients; there is no hormone-free interval, as occurs with COCs. POPs must be taken not only daily, but also at the same time each day.

Efficacy and Effectiveness A recent analysis of studies found that progestin-only pills are more effective with typical use than traditionally thought, with an effective rate of around 98 percent (Zuniga et al., 2023). POPs do not suppress ovulation as reliably as COCs, but rather rely primarily on the contraceptive effect of thickened cervical mucus. The onset of cervical mucus thickening occurs 2 to 4 hours after a POP is taken and persists for 22 hours after each dose. For this reason, if intercourse generally occurs in the morning or evening, the POP should be taken at midday (Hatcher et al., 2019). If an individual ovulates while taking a POP, taking the pill as little as 3 hours late may allow the cervical mucus to return to its fertile state and render the contraceptive effect temporarily void. If taking a pill more than 3 hours later, the individual should take the missed pill as soon as possible, continue taking the pack even if this means taking two pills in one day, and using a back-up method until pills have been taken correctly, on time, for two consecutive days (Curtis et al., 2024). Despite this, studies suggest this method is used effectively by most who use it (Zuniga et al., 2023).

Safety and Side Effects POPs have the fewest contraindications of all hormonal methods. Contraindications to POP use can be found in the *U.S. Medical Eligibility Criteria for Contraceptive Use, 2024* (A. Nguyen et al., 2024) and include bariatric surgery via malabsorptive procedures, current or prior breast cancer, hepatocellular carcinoma, some anticonvulsants, and rifampin. Unscheduled bleeding and spotting are the side effects most commonly associated with POPs. Decreased effectiveness of POPs is possible when these agents are used in combination with rifampin or rifabutin (A. Nguyen et al., 2024).

Noncontraceptive Benefits Noncontraceptive benefits are described in the introduction to the "Progestin-Only Methods" section. The reductions in ovarian and endometrial cancer rates seen with COCs have not been reported with POPs.

Advantages and Disadvantages Each package of POPs contains one type of pill (vs. two or more types in a package of COCs), so there may be less confusion about which pill is to be taken. POPs are a safe method for most individuals who cannot take estrogen for medical reasons. Similarly, those who are sensitive to even low-estrogen pills, as manifested by nausea, breast tenderness, or hypertension, but who still want an oral contraceptive, may do well on POPs. All contraceptive steroids, including POPs, could impair lactation in theory; however, POPs are generally considered safe during breastfeeding (Stanton & Blumenthal, 2019). The contraceptive effect ends immediately upon discontinuation of POPs. Unlike all other hormonal contraception, POPs have recently become available over the counter, without a prescription. The pill increases access to an effective method of contraception that is widely safe to use (Hawkins, 2024).

Disadvantages of POPs, other than the side effects previously mentioned, include the need for careful adherence to the dosing schedule. Utilizing an alarm or watch that beeps daily at the same time may enhance compliance.

Progestin Injection

The DMPA injection (Depo-Provera, or Depo) has been approved as a method of contraception since 1995, although clinical trials with this agent were conducted in the 1960s and 1970s, and the medication was used for the treatment of endometriosis and as an off-label contraceptive prior to FDA approval. DMPA is a synthetic progestogen and a member of the pregnane family, but it differs from the estrane and gonane progestins found in oral contraceptives. DMPA is a powerful inhibitor of the hypothalamic–pituitary axis at the level of the hypothalamus.

DMPA is given as either a 150 mg intramuscular injection or a 104 mg subcutaneous injection that can be self-administered. Either injection is given every 11–13 weeks (average every 12 weeks). Intramuscular DMPA must be provided by a trained healthcare professional, which requires that the individual make regular visits for injections. Self-administration of the subcutaneous formulation is feasible and increases this method's convenience for those who find it difficult to get to a clinician's office. The subcutaneous formulation provides a dose that is 30 percent lower and a reduction in peak blood levels by 50 percent; however, it is more expensive because is it provided in a proprietary delivery system. Lower doses may reduce the metabolic side effects of weight gain and glucose intolerance, but currently no data supports this. Ovulatory suppression with this method often lasts longer than 13 weeks; however, because the contraceptive effect expires at this point in a minority of individuals, everyone is instructed to return for repeat doses at 13-week intervals (Curtis et al., 2024).

Although prescribing information advises that the first DMPA injection should be given during the first 5 days of the menses or postpartum (if not breastfeeding), the evidence-based *U.S. Selected Practice Recommendations for Contraceptive Use, 2024* advises that DMPA can be initiated any time, including immediately postpartum or postabortion (Curtis et al., 2024). If the individual or clinician is unsure whether or not they are pregnant, they should be reassured that DMPA has not been shown to harm an existing pregnancy (Curtis et al., 2024). Advise the individual to take a highly sensitive pregnancy test 2 to 4 weeks after the first injection because amenorrhea related to pregnancy may be interpreted as a normal effect of the method. Those who are given DMPA outside the previously mentioned ideal parameters for initiation of the method (off cycle) should be instructed to use a barrier method for the first 7 days while the serum levels are reaching adequate concentrations. The same instructions apply to individuals who are late for their injections. If an individual has engaged in unprotected intercourse in the previous 5 days, they should also be offered emergency contraception.

Efficacy and Effectiveness The failure rates for DMPA are listed in Table 13-1. The differences between theoretical efficacy and typical use probably reflect the pattern of individuals not returning on time for subsequent injections.

Safety and Side Effects Like other progestin-only methods, DMPA is safer than combination products overall and can be used by individuals who are not candidates for estrogen contraceptives. *The U.S. Medical Eligibility Criteria for Contraceptive Use, 2024* provides a complete list of contraindications and precautions regarding DMPA use (A. Nguyen et al., 2024).

In 2004, the following warning was added to the DMPA label:

> *Women who use Depo-Provera Contraceptive Injection may lose significant bone mineral density. Bone loss is greater with increasing duration of use and may not be completely reversible. It is unknown if use of Depo-Provera Contraceptive Injection during adolescence or early adulthood, a critical period of bone accretion, will reduce peak bone mass and increase the risk for osteoporotic fracture in later life. Depo-Provera Contraceptive Injection should not be used as a long-term birth control method (i.e., longer than 2 years) unless other birth control methods are considered inadequate.* (Information from Depo-Provera [Medroxyprogesterone Acetate Injectable Suspension])

Experts have called for removal of the FDA warning, citing abundant evidence that the effects of DMPA on bone density are considerably less than originally believed (ACOG Committee Opinion, 2004). While bone mineral density does decrease during DMPA use, a review of the literature determined that this decline in bone mineral density reverses after DMPA discontinuation (ACOG, 2014). This pattern is similar to the bone mineral density changes seen in individuals who breastfeed. Changes in bone mineral density are an intermediate outcome, but the truly important clinical outcome is fracture risk. In a retrospective study of more than 300,000 individuals using DMPA, COCs, or an LNG IUD, fracture risk was not increased in those who had used DMPA in the past, but there was a slight increased fracture risk in individuals currently using DMPA, compared to the other methods (Raine-Bennett et al., 2019).

ACOG does not recommend restricting DMPA initiation or duration based on concerns about bone mineral density. Likewise, the use of DMPA is not considered an indication for bone mineral density screening or initiation of medications to prevent osteoporosis, such as estrogen, bisphosphonates, or selective estrogen receptor modulators (ACOG, 2014). All individuals, regardless of contraceptive method, should be counseled about osteoporosis prevention, including weight bearing exercise and adequate intake of calcium and vitamin D via diet and/or supplements (Muñoz et al., 2020).

Uncertainty continues to exist regarding the impact of DMPA use on the risk of HIV transmission and progression, although a recent large, randomized controlled trial in four countries in Africa found no elevated risk of acquiring HIV among DMPA users, as well as LNG IUD and copper IUD users (Morrison et al., 2020). While the *U.S. Medical Eligibility Criteria, 2024* does not restrict the use of DMPA for those at risk of HIV exposure, as with all hormonal contraceptive methods, individuals should be aware that hormonal contraception does not protect against HIV or any other sexually transmitted infection (A. Nguyen et al., 2024).

Although there has been some past concern about the effect of DMPA on the development of diabetes, the *U.S. Medical Eligibility Criteria for Contraceptive Use, 2024* asserts that DMPA has little effect on short- or long-term diabetes control for insulin-dependent or non-insulin-dependent diabetes (A. Nguyen et al., 2024). However, DMPA is considered category 3 among individuals who have diabetes with nephropathy, retinopathy, neuropathy, other vascular disease, or diabetes $>$ 20 years in duration (A. Nguyen et al., 2024).

As with all progestin-only methods, side effects associated with DMPA include changes in bleeding patterns, with breakthrough bleeding and spotting occurring in the majority of individuals in the first 6 months of use. After 24 months of use, approximately 68–71 percent of individuals will have become amenorrheic (ACOG, 2022). With appropriate counseling, many see amenorrhea as a benefit of DMPA.

Weight gain is more clearly associated with DMPA than other methods, but even here the relationship is nuanced. Some studies show an associated between DMPA and weight gain, especially among those with a BMI > 30 (Zwayne et al., 2024). Other studies show no weight gain. Further, the vast majority of adolescents will experience no weight gain but 10 percent may gain excessive weight on DMPA (>10% of baseline body weight). Early weight gain may be an indication of consistent or excessive weight gain, so a baseline weight is essential with this method (Zwayne et al., 2024). Other side effects reported in a small minority of individuals on DMPA include nervousness, headache, decreased libido, and breast discomfort.

Noncontraceptive Benefits Noncontraceptive benefits of DMPA include a reduction in the number of seizures in individuals with epilepsy and seizure disorders (Humphrey et al., 2021). Unlike most other hormonal contraception, the effectiveness of DMPA is not decreased with the concomitant use of most anticonvulsant medications, making it ideal for individuals with seizure disorders who do not want to become pregnant (A. Nguyen et al., 2024). DMPA is also associated with a reduction in sickle cell crises in individuals with sickle cell disease (de Abood et al., 1997).

As is the case with all hormonal contraceptive options, individuals experience less menstrual bleeding and less dysmenorrhea with DMPA. Ectopic pregnancy, PID, and endometriosis are decreased in DMPA users—outcomes that are protective of future fertility.

Advantages and Disadvantages The advantages of DMPA include its high degree of efficacy, long-term nature, and noninterference with coitus. For those who want to keep their contraceptive choice private, there is no visible evidence of DMPA use. DMPA has long been used to achieve amenorrhea in individuals with mental or physical disabilities who have difficulty managing their menses.

The long-term nature of DMPA may be considered a disadvantage because the contraceptive effect may not cease immediately upon discontinuation. The time to return of ovulation varies widely, ranging from 15 to 49 weeks after the last injection (Curtis et al., 2024). DMPA requires that intramuscular injections be provided by a trained healthcare professional, so the individual must attend regular visits for injections. The subcutaneous formulation might improve continuation among those who find it difficult to get to a clinician's office. However, there remains the possibility of allergic reaction to either the progestin or the vehicle used for injection, or vagal reactions to the injection itself. Like all hormonal methods, DMPA does not provide any protection from STIs.

EMERGENCY CONTRACEPTION

Sperm can live for up to 5 days in the reproductive tract of pregnancy-capable people, and pregnancy can occur with intercourse 5 days prior to ovulation. The highest risk of pregnancy is in the 48 hours immediately preceding ovulation (Wilcox et al., 2000). However, due to the uncertainty of ovulation timing, emergency contraception is offered if unprotected intercourse occurs at any time in the menstrual cycle.

The Yuzpe, levonorgestrel (LNG), and Ulipristal acetate (UPA) emergency contraceptive pill (ECP) regimens, and the LNG and copper IUDs, may be used within 72 to 120 hours of unprotected intercourse. The Yuzpe and LNG methods have a dramatic decline in their effectiveness with time and should be used as soon as possible after unprotected intercourse. These two methods are ideally taken within 72 hours of unprotected intercourse, but they appear to have efficacy up to 120 hours after intercourse (Piaggio et al., 2011).

The Yuzpe regimen consists of combined ECPs that must contain at least 100 mcg of ethinyl estradiol and 0.50 mg of LNG, repeated in 12 hours. A dedicated combined ECP product is not available in the United States, but numerous COCs can be used as combined ECPs. COCs containing norgestrel are preferable to those with norethindrone because failure rates are slightly higher with norethindrone (Hatcher et al., 2019). Because the high dose of ethinyl estradiol causes unpleasant side effects and other ECP options are available, this regimen has largely fallen out of favor.

The most widely available over-the-counter emergency contraception is LNG ECPs, which usually contain a 1.5 mg single dose (Plan B One-Step and Next Choice One Dose). Previously, LNG ECPs were available over the counter only for those age 17 and older, and those age 16 and younger needed a prescription, but the age restrictions have now been lifted. There are no age or point-of-sale restrictions on buying 1.5 mg of LNG ECPs over the counter (American Society for Emergency Contraception, 2018). LNG ECPs are more effective than the Yuzpe regimen and have fewer side effects.

UPA, a selective progesterone receptor modulator provided as a single 30 mg dose, is the most effective oral emergency contraception method. The effectiveness of this medication does not decline within the 120-hour window after unprotected intercourse, as is the case for LNG and combined ECPs (Salcedo et al., 2023). UPA is available only by prescription and can be more difficult to find, so it is recommended to call a pharmacy first to verify if they carry UPA.

The copper and LNG IUDs are by far the most effective emergency contraception method, with a pregnancy rate of approximately 1 in 1,000 cases in which it is used for this purpose (Turok et al., 2021). They can be inserted as long as 5 days after unprotected intercourse. These methods are rarely utilized as emergency contraception in the United States partially due to the difficulty of coordinating the patient and clinic schedules in the 120-hour window of time. Evidence suggests that some individuals will choose the IUDs over ECPs if it is offered as an option, particularly if same-day insertion is available (Kohn & Nucatola, 2016).

Efficacy and Effectiveness

Factors influencing the risk of pregnancy when UPA or LNG is used for emergency contraception include body weight, the day of the cycle, and further intercourse during the same menstrual cycle after use of emergency contraception (ACOG, 2015).

Body weight has no impact on efficacy rates for the copper and LNG IUDs. Body weight does, however, impact the efficacy of the ECP pills, with the LNG ECPs in particular being much more sensitive to weight. Risk of failure when using LNG ECPs among individuals who are overweight is 1.5 times greater and among individuals with a BMI greater than 30 it is 3 to 8 times greater when compared to non-overweight users (Salcedo et al., 2023). Doubling the dose of LNG ECPs does not appear to decrease rates of follicular rupture. With UPA, overweight individuals have the same risk of pregnancy as non-overweight individuals. Among obese individuals taking UPA, however, the risk of pregnancy is doubled compared to nonobese individuals (Salcedo et al., 2023). Thus, UPA is a better ECP for overweight and obese individuals wishing to avoid pregnancy via a one-time pill. The copper and LNG IUD has the advantage of being highly effective in overweight and obese individuals and providing ongoing contraception. Despite the decreased efficacy of ECP pills, rates of pregnancy among overweight individuals taking ECPs was still quite low, 2.03 percent (Festin et al., 2017). It is essential to provide education and offer ECP, regardless of an individual's body weight or other characteristics, using person-centered, unbiased language.

LNG and UPA inhibit ovulation in 96 percent and 100 percent of cycles, respectively, when used prior to the onset of the LH surge (Brache et al., 2013). However, if given after the onset of the LH surge, these medications inhibit ovulation in 14 percent and 79 percent of cycles, respectively (Glasier, 2013). LNG is no more effective than placebo when used in the critical 5 days preceding ovulation. The risk of pregnancy with UPA use is half that seen with LNG (Glasier, 2014).

Both LNG and UPA delay ovulation. If individuals have repeated acts of unprotected intercourse after using ECPs, they are at a fourfold increased risk of pregnancy, compared with those who do not have further intercourse within the same cycle. If an individual has had repeated unprotected sex, including sex that has occurred more than 5 days prior, there is a potential presence of a preimplantation fertilized ovum. This possibility carries no risk for the individuals who wants to use LNG or UPA ECP, as no risks to the embryo or pregnant person have been identified (Salcedo et al., 2023). However, placing an IUD during this time carries the risk of miscarriage, preterm delivery, and septic abortion, which should be discussed with any individual considering an IUD as EC who has had unprotected sex more than 5 days ago during their current cycle (Salcedo et al., 2023).

Safety and Side Effects

The usual contraindications and precautions for ongoing COC and POP use do not apply to ECPs, but the usual contraindications and precautions to IUD use do apply when using this method for emergency contraception (Curtis et al., 2024). Neither the IUD nor oral emergency contraception methods cause abortion (Salcedo et al., 2023). Repeated doses of LNG and UPA ECP in the same cycle have not been associated with serious adverse effects.

Combined ECPs frequently cause nausea and vomiting, which can be reduced by giving an antiemetic, such as promethazine, prior to treatment. Spotting, changes in the next menses, headache, breast tenderness, and mood changes can also occur. These same side effects are sometimes noted with LNG ECPs but are much less frequent and less severe than those seen with combined ECPs (Salcedo et al., 2023). Headache, dysmenorrhea, nausea, and abdominal pain are the most frequently observed side effects with UPA (Salcedo et al., 2023). The copper and LNG IUD can cause the side effects discussed in the section on intrauterine contraception.

Advantages and Disadvantages

Emergency contraception is the only contraceptive method that can be used after intercourse. It is not an ideal method for ongoing method of contraception, however, and it provides no STI protection. Access to emergency contraception remains limited because only one method—LNG ECPs—is available without prescription. Clinicians can increase access to and timely use of emergency contraception by providing advance prescriptions to all individuals of reproductive age for UPA and/or recommending that patients purchase LNG ECPs in advance. Studies have shown that having ECPs at home increases the likelihood that they will be used when needed and does not promote sexual risk taking (Salcedo et al., 2023). Providing emergency contraception prescriptions over the phone as needed is another way to increase access.

NONHORMONAL METHODS

Nonhormonal contraceptive methods can be grouped into three general categories:

- Physiologic methods: Abstinence, coitus interruptus, lactational amenorrhea (breastfeeding), and fertility awareness-based method (FABM)
- Barrier methods: External condoms, vaginal barrier methods, and spermicides
- Permanent contraception (sterilization): Vasectomy and tubal occlusion

One additional contraceptive method that does not contain hormones—the copper IUD—is discussed in the section on intrauterine contraception. The physiologic and barrier nonhormonal contraceptive options, which are reversible, generally require motivated users, and most of these methods necessitate taking action with every act of sexual intercourse. In general, their efficacy is less than that of hormonal methods, but these options do not have systemic side effects. In addition, many barrier methods do not require clinician involvement. Nonhormonal methods may also be chosen because they fit within the individual's cultural beliefs. The permanent contraceptive options—tubal occlusion and vasectomy—are the only permanent forms of contraception and require certainty that future childbearing is not desired. Information about permanent contraception is presented in a separate section earlier in this chapter.

Physiologic Methods

Avoiding Vaginal Contact with Semen (Abstinence)

Abstinence has historically been centered around the moral and ethical concerns of sexual activity, not the scientific properties of the contraceptive method. People choose to abstain from all or certain types of sexual activity for many different reasons, and their choices should be respected. Abstinence can be important to a patient's faith or personal journey, and what abstinence means for each individual varies. Unfortunately, the varying definitions of abstinence could leave a patient at risk for pregnancy if they do not receive effective counseling (Society for Adolescent Health and Medicine, 2017). Many types of sexual engagement and arousal (e.g., kissing, petting, rubbing, same sex sexual activity) do not result in semen ejaculation near a vagina and thus effectively avoids pregnancy. However, ejaculation near the vaginal introitus without intercourse, which some may consider abstinence, can lead to pregnancy. This is why it is important to be explicit about asking what abstinence means to each patient who uses this method and educating them on how to avoid pregnancy. Clinicians should teach patients that the actual cause of contraception with abstinence is absence of semen near the vaginal introitus, not the absence of any sexual activity.

Efficacy and Effectiveness Avoiding vaginal contact with semen is 100 percent effective at preventing pregnancy. The effectiveness of this method for preventing STI transmission depends on what type of sexual contact the patient engages in. For example, individuals who avoid vaginal contact with semen but have oral sex are at risk for STI transmission.

Safety and Side Effects There are no safety considerations or side effects of this method.

Noncontraceptive Benefits There are no noncontraceptive benefits of abstinence.

Advantages and Disadvantages Avoiding vaginal contact with semen is readily available and completely effective. It can prevent certain STIs, including HIV infection via penile–vaginal transmission, but patients must be cautioned to avoid other sexual practices (e.g., oral sex and anal sex) that put them at risk for STIs (refer to Chapter 22).

Coitus Interruptus

Coitus interruptus, also known as withdrawal, is the removal of the penis from the vagina prior to ejaculation. Coitus interruptus prevents pregnancy by keeping sperm from entering the vagina. One in four individuals in a recent poll report using coitus interruptus in the past 12 months, and most will use this method at some point over the course of their lives (Frederiksen et al., 2024). Many who use coitus interruptus use it in rotation or combination with condoms and other more effective methods (Jones et al., 2014).

Efficacy and Effectiveness The theoretical efficacy of coitus interruptus is high, but the estimated typical failure rate is about 20 percent (Table 13-1). The long-held belief that pre-ejaculatory fluid contains sperm, which could theoretically cause pregnancy even if withdrawal were used correctly, has been subjected to small clinical studies with conflicting results (Killick et al., 2011; Patel et al., 2024).

Safety and Side Effects There are no contraindications to or side effects from using coitus interruptus.

Noncontraceptive Benefits There are no noncontraceptive benefits of coitus interruptus.

Advantages and Disadvantages Coitus interruptus is readily available, requires no supplies or cost, and is user controlled. Couples can use coitus interruptus intermittently when other methods are unavailable. Disadvantages include the need to use this method with every act of intercourse and the need to exert the self-discipline and control necessary to stop intercourse. Coitus interruptus does not prevent STI transmission because penile–vaginal contact occurs, and HIV and other STIs can be present in pre-ejaculatory fluid. Those who use coitus interruptus should be educated about emergency contraception as a backup method.

Lactational Amenorrhea Method

Infant suckling during breastfeeding increases maternal prolactin levels, which in turn inhibits ovulation; this is the physiologic basis of the lactational amenorrhea method (LAM) of contraception. Three conditions must be met for LAM to be effective: (1) exclusive or near-exclusive breastfeeding; (2) amenorrhea (no vaginal bleeding after 56 days postpartum); and (3) infant younger than 6 months (Van der Wijden & Manion, 2015). Breastfeeding education and support are beneficial for individuals using LAM.

Efficacy and Effectiveness Breastfeeding is an extremely effective method of contraception if the conditions for its use are met (Table 13-1). Failures typically occur when breastfeeding is nonexclusive or after the infant reaches 6 months of age. In these instances, the likelihood of ovulation increases, and the individuals may be unaware of the return to fertility.

Safety and Side Effects There are no contraindications to LAM, but breastfeeding is not recommended for individuals who are HIV positive in countries such as the United States where infant formula is accessible, or for individuals who are taking medications that could be harmful to the infant. The only side effects of LAM are those associated with breastfeeding, such as sore nipples and mastitis.

Noncontraceptive Benefits Individuals who breastfeed their infants have decreased risk of ovarian, endometrial, and breast cancers (Babic et al., 2020; Ma et al., 2018; Ye et al., 2024). Breastfeeding also has numerous benefits for infant, child, and lifelong health.

Advantages and Disadvantages LAM is readily available, free, and can be used immediately postpartum. The disadvantages of LAM are that it is available only to those who are breastfeeding, its duration of use is limited, and individuals may have difficulty sustaining the patterns of breastfeeding required to maintain contraceptive effectiveness. In addition, LAM does not provide protection from STIs.

Fertility Awareness-Based Methods (FABMs)

FABMs involve determining when an individual is most fertile during each month and using either abstinence or barrier contraception during that time to prevent pregnancy. The fertile window, or time when intercourse is most likely to result in pregnancy, occurs 5 days before plus the day of ovulation (Peragallo Urrutia et al., 2018). FABMs are also referred to as natural family planning and the rhythm method. Among individuals in the United States who use contraception, 13 percent use FABMs (Frederiksen et al., 2024).

The fertile window can be identified with calendar methods or by using signs and symptoms of ovulation. Calendar methods require counting the days in the menstrual cycle. For the calendar FABM, the individual records the length of 6 to 12 menstrual cycles and determines the longest and shortest cycles. They then use that information to identify the first (days in shortest cycle minus 18) and last (days in longest cycle minus 11) fertile days each month. The calculations must be updated with each cycle (Peragallo Urrutia et al., 2018). Because this method requires careful calculations that can be confusing, the Standard Days method was developed as a simpler calendar method. Individuals using the Standard Days method are advised to use abstinence or a barrier contraceptive on days 8 to 19 of the menstrual cycle. A color-coded set of beads called CycleBeads can be used in conjunction with the Standard Days method to help individuals keep track of their fertile window (http://www.cyclebeads.com). The Standard Days method is recommended for individuals whose cycles are 26 to 32 days in length (Peragallo Urrutia et al., 2018). There are also apps that can be used to track cycles for the FABM, including the Dot fertility app, which has been evaluated in a clinical trial (Jennings et al., 2019), and the Natural Cycles app, which has been permitted by the FDA to be marketed as a method of contraception (U.S. FDA, 2018a).

The postovulation method is another variation on the calendar method. With this method, the individual subtracts 14 days from her average cycle length to predict the day of ovulation. Abstinence or a barrier method is used during the first half of the cycle until the fourth morning after the predicted day of ovulation. This method requires the longest period of abstinence or use of additional contraception.

Signs and symptoms of ovulation include a rise in the basal body temperature and changes in cervical mucus. Using basal body temperature charting (refer to Chapter 20) in conjunction with the postovulation observations is beneficial, but predicting the fertile period with basal body temperature is difficult because ovulation occurs when the rise in temperature is observed, and it remains elevated for the rest of the cycle.

The Billings Ovulation Method assesses cervical mucus to determine the fertile window. Individuals check daily for the increased, clear, stretchy, slippery cervical secretions associated with ovulation. The fertile time lasts from the day when ovulatory cervical secretions are first observed until 4 days after they are last observed (Peragallo Urrutia et al., 2018).

The TwoDay method is a simplified version of the ovulation method. The woman checks daily for cervical secretions and is considered fertile any day that she has cervical secretions present or had them present the day before (Peragallo Urrutia et al., 2018).

The Symptothermal method involves observing multiple indicators of the fertile window; the most common combination is assessment of cervical mucus and daily basal body temperature charting. The cervical secretions can be used to identify the beginning of the fertile window, and the basal body temperature can be used to detect the end. Some individuals using the Symptothermal method also assess cervical position and signs of ovulation (e.g., mittelschmerz).

Home ovulation tests originally used for individuals with infertility can be used in conjunction with the calendar, ovulation, or Symptothermal methods to improve their effectiveness (Peragallo Urrutia et al., 2018).

The detailed information required for patient education about FABM is beyond the scope of this chapter. Readers are referred to the websites listed in **Box 13-2** for further information, including training courses for clinicians.

Efficacy and Effectiveness The theoretical efficacy of FABM varies according to the specific technique used (Table 13-1). The typical use failure rate reflects the difficulty of using these methods correctly and consistently. A systematic review concluded that the comparative efficacy of FABMs remains unknown (Peragallo Urrutia et al., 2018).

Researchers at the Institute for Reproductive Health demonstrated typical use effectiveness rates of 88 percent and 86 percent for the Standard Days method and the TwoDay method, respectively, and they have developed extensive resources for teaching these methods to providers, community health workers, and individuals (Institute for Reproductive Health, 2020). The Dot fertility app has a typical use effectiveness rate of 95 percent for individuals aged 18 to 39 years (Jennings et al., 2019).

Safety and Side Effects There are no health concerns with the use of FABM, but certain circumstances or conditions complicate their use. These factors include the postpartum period, breastfeeding, having an abortion immediately before use, recent menarche or perimenopause when cycles may be irregular, medications that alter the regularity of cycles or fertility signs, vaginal discharge, irregular vaginal bleeding, and conditions associated with elevated body temperature (Curtis et al., 2024). There are no side effects of FABM.

Noncontraceptive Benefits The principles of FABM can also be used to conceive when pregnancy is desired.

Advantages and Disadvantages Individuals may have to pay for FABM training or supplies (e.g., basal body thermometer, CycleBeads), but there is no ongoing cost unless a barrier contraceptive is used during the fertile window. These methods are user controlled and may be the only acceptable form of contraception for members of some religions and cultures. Further, some may appreciate how using fertility-awareness based methods increases their own bodily awareness (Ayala-Ramirez et al., 2023). Disadvantages include the need for detailed education, ongoing attention to identifying the fertile window, and abstaining from intercourse or using an additional contraceptive method several days each month. FABMs do not protect either partner from STIs, and users should be educated about emergency contraception. There is increasing concern about user privacy in the era of online, app-based fertility tracker apps, which has been exacerbated in our post-Roe health and legal landscape. For those with privacy concerns, the pregnancy app Euki has been designed with user privacy at the forefront (Stifani et al., 2023).

BOX 13-2 Websites for FABM Information

Billings Ovulation Method: http://www.boma-usa.org
Creighton Model FertilityCare System: http://www.creightonmodel.com
CycleBeads: http://cyclebeads.com
Dot fertility app: https://www.dottheapp.com
Marquette model: https://www.marquette.edu/nursing/institute-natural-family-planning/model.php
Natural Cycles app: http://naturalcycles.com
Symptothermal method (Couple to Couple League): http://ccli.org

Barrier Methods

All barrier methods must be applied at or near the time of intercourse, before any penile penetration, and ideally before any genital contact to avoid disruption in sex play. This requirement may be a problem for some couples due to the need to plan ahead, or for others who find the application of a barrier disruptive. Couples can be taught to apply or insert the barrier as part of their sex play. The coitus-dependent nature of barrier methods may be an advantage for couples who have infrequent intercourse.

Although these methods are less effective in preventing pregnancy than contemporary hormonal or intrauterine methods, interest in barrier contraception is on the rise again. This trend partly reflects the hormone-free aspects of barrier methods, but it largely indicates recognition of a barrier's potential role as dual protection against pregnancy and STIs, including HIV. The cervix is the point of entry for many sexually transmitted pathogens. Protecting the cervix via chemical or physical barriers is an expanding area of research in the prevention of STIs. Finally, barrier contraceptives can be used by most people because contraindications for their use are rare (Curtis et al., 2024).

External Condoms

The external condom, commonly called a male condom, is a thin sheath that is placed over the erect penis. It serves as a barrier to pregnancy by trapping seminal fluid and sperm and offers protection against STIs. In fact, early descriptions of condom use in the 1500s emphasized the condom's role in protection from syphilis and other diseases (Tone, 2001).

Latex condoms are manufactured and packaged with a rolled rim that is designed to be applied to the tip of the penis and then rolled down over the erect penis. It is important to note that there is a right side and a wrong side when the condom is rolled up; applying the condom with the wrong side out will prevent it from being placed properly and will potentially contaminate the outside of the condom with seminal fluid. Over the years, minor design changes to this rolled-rim construction have included enlarged tips to contain ejaculated fluid (**Figure 13-8**) and introduced various colors, sizes, flavors, and textured surfaces that are purported to enhance sexual pleasure. Some condoms add lubricants as well, including spermicidal lubricants. One-third of individuals report using a condom for contraception during the past year (Frederiksen et al., 2024).

Nonlatex condoms were developed in response to several concerns about latex. These condoms are made of polyurethane or a latex-like material called styrene ethylene butylene styrene. Nonlatex condoms are odorless, colorless, and nonallergenic. They transmit body heat better and have a looser fit, theoretically allowing more sensitivity. They can be used with any lubricant and do not usually deteriorate with the use of oil-based lubricants or under adverse storage conditions. Nonlatex condoms appear to have twice the odds of breakage or slippage during intercourse or withdrawal, compared to latex condoms (Festin, 2013). Many users prefer nonlatex over latex condoms; these preferences may translate into more consistent use. Consistent use and consumer familiarity with, and education about, nonlatex condoms may reduce the higher rates of breakage and slippage that have been reported in studies.

FIGURE **13-8** **External condoms: rolled-rim condom as packaged; unrolled condoms with rounded and extended tips.**

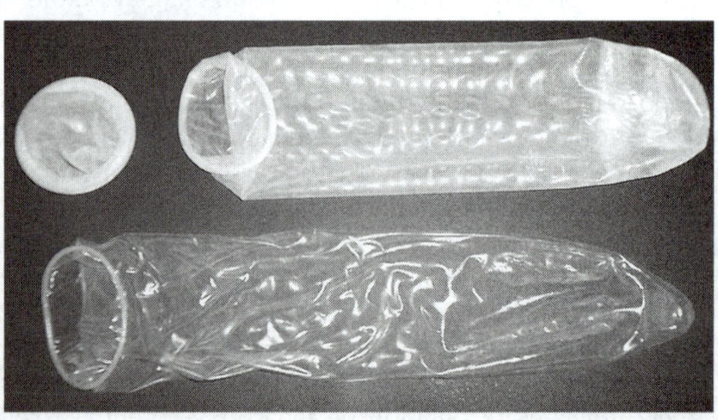

Efficacy and Effectiveness When used correctly and consistently, latex condoms are an effective form of contraception (Table 13-1). Condom failures are commonly related to breakage of the condom, slippage during intercourse, or while removing the condom. In general, pregnancy rates for nonlatex condoms are slightly higher than the corresponding rates for latex condoms, but it is within the range considered acceptable for barrier methods. As noted, nonlatex condoms have higher reported rates of breakage and slippage than latex condoms. It is unclear whether this difference is related to the product or to a lack of familiarity with the product.

Safety and Side Effects Latex condoms should not be used by persons with known latex allergies. Some individuals report genital irritation and discomfort from the use of condoms, an issue that may be related either to the condom or to concomitant lubricant use. Some condoms are lubricated with a spermicide—nonoxynol-9 (N-9)—that may produce genital irritation in some individuals (see the section on spermicides). One study of a polyurethane condom evaluated genital irritation across gender. Although no differences were observed among the men in each group, the female partners in the polyurethane group had significantly less genital pain, pruritus, and vaginal pain than their counterparts in the latex condom group (Steiner et al., 2003).

Noncontraceptive Benefits Condoms are routinely recommended for their noncontraceptive benefit of protection from STIs. Consistent use of latex condoms in sexually active HIV-serodiscordant couples reduces the incidence of HIV infection by more than 70 percent (Giannou et al., 2016). Condoms also offer statistically significant protection against gonorrhea, chlamydia, herpes simplex virus type 2, and syphilis, and they may protect individuals from trichomoniasis (Curtis et al., 2024). Although condoms do not appear to offer protection against HPV infection, their use is associated with higher rates of cervical intraepithelial neoplasia regression and cervical HPV infection clearance (Skorstengaard et al., 2019).

Advantages and Disadvantages Condoms have the advantage of being widely available on an over-the-counter basis, without the need for a clinician visit or prescription. Nonlatex condoms tend to be more expensive than their latex counterparts. The effectiveness of condoms is coitus dependent (**Table 13-3**). Correct use is critical to prevent breakage, slippage, and resultant unintended pregnancy. A potential disadvantage of using condoms as a contraceptive method is that they are male controlled. Individuals who are in relationships in which they cannot negotiate condom use with their partners need a method they can control.

Spermicides and Vaginal Gels

Spermicides are chemical barriers that are used either alone or in conjunction with a physical barrier (such as a condom, diaphragm, or sponge) to prevent pregnancy. The most common spermicides currently marketed in the United States contain N-9, which may be formulated as a gel, cream, foam, suppository, foaming tablet, or film. It is generally provided in 50–150 mg dosages. Other spermicidal compounds are available in other

TABLE 13-3 Advantages and Disadvantages of Barrier Methods[a]

Advantages	Disadvantages
Nonhormonal	Require planning
Do not require daily action	Require application at the time of intercourse and may be interruptive
Some are available without prescription	Breakage or slippage at time of intercourse may increase risk of unintended pregnancy
Some offer protection against STIs	

[a]All individuals relying on barrier or coitus-dependent methods should be aware of emergency contraception and be offered an advance prescription.

countries, such as octoxynol-9, benzalkonium chloride, and menfegol. Fewer than 0.2 percent of individuals report using spermicides as their primary method of contraception (Guttmacher Institute, 2021).

In 2020, the FDA approved Phexxi, a vaginal pH regulator. This gel does not kill sperm and is therefore not considered a spermicide. Rather, Phexxi alters vaginal Ph and reduces sperm motility, thus preventing ovulation (Coppola, 2021). It is made up of lactic acid (18 mg/g), citric acid (10 mg/g), and potassium bitartrate (4 mg/g) for 1.8%, 1%, and 0.4% strengths, respectively, in a preparation of 5 grams applied vaginally immediately before or within the hour of intercourse.

Efficacy and Effectiveness Studies comparing N-9 in various formulations (vaginal contraceptive film, foaming tablets, suppositories, and gels), each used without condoms or other physical barriers, showed pregnancy rates with typical use over 6 months in the 10 to 15 percent range, with some results as high as 28 percent (Table 13-1) (Raymond et al., 2004). These rates are higher than those for other barrier contraceptives. Formulations containing at least 100 mg of N-9 are associated with lower unintended pregnancy rates. Although the effectiveness of spermicides used as a sole agent is less than that of other contraceptive methods, spermicide use is more effective than using no method at all. Phase 3 clinical trials of Phexxi over a 7-cycle period showed a pregnancy rate of 13.7 percent (Coppola, 2021).

Safety and Side Effects N-9 is a surfactant, and surfactants can disrupt cell membranes. N-9 is an irritant to both animal and human tissue (Van Damme et al., 2002; Wilkinson et al., 2002). Frequent use is associated with increased reports of vaginal irritation. As an irritant, N-9 has the potential to disrupt or damage epithelial tissue in both the vagina and the rectum. The risk of this disruption increases with frequency of use and dose. Because intact tissue is the first defense against infection, use of N-9 could increase the risk of infection transmission by causing microabrasions in the epithelium. In addition, strong evidence indicates that N-9 does not reduce STIs among sex workers or individuals attending STI clinics. In fact, some research suggests that N-9 use can even increase the risk of HIV acquisition in high-risk individuals (Van Damme et al., 2002; Wilkinson et al., 2002).

Recommendations for the use of N-9 were developed in 2001 by a World Health Organization task force and reiterated in a 2006 report called *Sexual and Reproductive Health of Women Living with HIV/AIDS* (World Health Organization, 2020):

- N-9 should not be used for purposes of STI protection.
- N-9 should not be used by individuals who engage in multiple daily acts of intercourse.
- N-9 should not be used by individuals at high risk for HIV acquisition.
- N-9 should not be used rectally.
- Condoms should not be lubricated with N-9, but condoms lubricated with N-9 are more effective than not using condoms.

The *U.S. Medical Eligibility Criteria for Contraceptive Use, 2024* classifies spermicides as category 4 methods for individuals at high risk for HIV infection and as category 3 methods for individuals with HIV/AIDS. For those at low risk of HIV acquisition, however, N-9 products can be a valid contraceptive option (Curtis et al., 2024).

In individuals who use N-9 for contraception, the likelihood of developing specific genitourinary symptoms after 6 to 7 months of use is 13 to 17 percent for a yeast infection, 8 to 12 percent for bacterial vaginosis, 19 to 27 percent for vulvovaginal irritation, and 11 to 15 percent for urinary tract symptoms (but only 3 to 6 percent for culture-proven urinary tract infection). The likelihood of irritation and other genitourinary symptoms in the sexual partner ranges from 6 to 14 percent after 6 to 7 months of use. In the study that produced these findings, there was no comparison group to indicate whether these rates are higher than, lower than, or the same as the rates in the general population of sexually active individuals using contraception (Raymond et al., 2004). However, the reported rates are high enough to warrant counseling individuals to report symptoms so they can be evaluated, diagnosed, and properly treated.

Side effects with Phexxi were similar to those of a spermicide, but were much less prevalent, indicating that this may be a good alternative for individuals who have problems with the side effects of spermicide (Coppola, 2021).

Noncontraceptive Benefits Despite concerns about the potential for cervicovaginal epithelial disruption with N-9-based spermicides, vaginally applied chemical barriers remain appealing. This attraction stems largely from their potential to provide dual protection—they can be both spermicidal and microbicidal. Personally controlled, vaginally applied, lubricating microbicides offer great potential for protection against STIs, including HIV. Microbicide development and clinical trials are ongoing.

Advantages and Disadvantages Spermicides containing N-9 and Phexxi are widely available as over-the-counter products and do not require a prescription or clinician visit. Thus, they are readily accessible to individuals who need personally controlled, discreet, low-cost contraception. The effectiveness of spermicides is coitus dependent (Table 13-2). Disadvantages include low contraceptive effectiveness and the potential for symptoms of cervicovaginal irritation. As noted earlier, individuals who engage in multiple daily acts of intercourse or who are at high risk for STIs should avoid using spermicides containing N-9.

Diaphragms

The contraceptive diaphragm is a shallow dome-shaped cup that is inserted in the vagina to cover the cervix. Currently, less than 0.2 percent of individuals in the United States using contraception use the diaphragm (Guttmacher Institute, 2021). While older models had to be fitted with a bimanual exam and prescribed by a healthcare provider, the current model most widely used, Caya, does not require fitting by a healthcare provider (Curtis et al., 2024). All diaphragms require a prescription. Prior to insertion, about 4 ml (a teaspoon) of spermicide should be placed in the silicone membrane and spread around the rim. The diaphragm should be left in the vagina for at least 6 hours after intercourse, but no longer than 24 hours. A single diaphragm can be reused for up to 2 years.

Efficacy and Effectiveness The contraceptive efficacy of the diaphragm is similar to that of the external condom (Table 13-1). Traditional diaphragms are designed to be used in conjunction with a spermicide. The only study comparing differences in the contraceptive effectiveness of a traditional diaphragm depending on whether spermicide is used was underpowered and, therefore, could not reach firm conclusions (Bounds et al., 1995). The single-size diaphragm, Caya, has been shown to be as effective as a standard diaphragm when used with N-9 contraceptive gel (Schwartz et al., 2015).

During sexual excitement, the upper part of the vagina expands; thus, diaphragms and other devices that might be in contact with the vaginal walls during fitting may no longer provide a complete physical barrier to sperm migration during intercourse. Theoretically, an additional and important function of the diaphragm would be to maintain spermicide contact with the cervical os, thereby ensuring that sperm are trapped by the chemical barrier.

Safety and Side Effects The spermicide side effects discussed earlier in this chapter may also be experienced by diaphragm users. The *U.S. Medical Eligibility Criteria for Contraceptive Use, 2024* classifies the diaphragm as a category 3 or 4 method for individuals with HIV/AIDS or at high risk of HIV infection; this is solely due to concerns about the spermicide (Curtis et al., 2024).

The diaphragms available in the United States as of this writing are made of silicone and can be used by individuals with latex allergies. Water-based products (rather than those containing silicone) are recommended for individuals who wish to use a lubricant with silicone diaphragms. Irritation or even abrasions of the vaginal mucosa have been noted in those with improperly sized diaphragms or prolonged retention of the diaphragm in the vagina. Although no clear association with toxic shock syndrome has been demonstrated, diaphragms and other contraceptive barrier devices should not be left in the vagina for more than 24 hours, and their use during menses is discouraged.

Urinary tract infections are more common in diaphragm users than among individuals using hormonal contraceptives. Two factors may explain this phenomenon: (1) the rim of the diaphragm may exert pressure against the urethra, which might be perceived as frequency, dysuria, or incomplete bladder emptying, and may lead to infection; and (2) the spermicides used with the diaphragm can alter normal vaginal flora and may increase the likelihood of *Escherichia coli* bacteriuria (Hooton et al., 2000; Schreiber et al., 2006). However, risk of UTIs is slightly lower among Caya users (Lindh et al., 2021).

Noncontraceptive Benefits The diaphragm has possible or theoretical value in protecting the cervix from infection, but data demonstrating such a protective effect are not currently available. The only barrier methods known to reduce STIs are external and internal condoms.

Advantages and Disadvantages All available diaphragms require prescriptions. Diaphragms are user-controlled, nonhormonal contraceptive methods that are needed only at the time of intercourse (Table 13-2). One of the diaphragms currently available in the United States comes in multiple sizes with various diameters (**Figure 13-9**). This device must be fitted by a clinician, while the single-size diaphragm does not require clinician fitting (Schwartz et al., 2015).

As a result of the need for a clinician visit, diaphragms have a higher initiation cost than condoms, but they can be used for years with proper care. The only additional cost is the spermicide that must be used with the diaphragm. Diaphragms are washable and reusable. Proper use is important. Users should be counseled on the timing of insertion and removal, use of spermicide or other contraceptive gel, appropriate care of the device, and need for periodic reevaluation of the size.

Cervical Caps

Cervical caps are cuplike devices that cover the cervix. Smaller than diaphragms, they maintain their position over the cervix by suction, adhering to the cervix, or via a design that uses vaginal walls for support. The FemCap is the only cervical cap available in the United States.

The FemCap is made of silicone and has a design like an inverted sailor's cap (**Figure 13-10**). The dome covers the cervix, and the longer side of the brim fits into the back of the vagina. Three sizes are available, and selection is determined by pregnancy and birth history: the 22 cm FemCap is for individuals who have never been pregnant; the 26 cm FemCap is for individuals who have had a miscarriage, abortion, or cesarean birth; and the 30 cm FemCap is for individuals who have had a vaginal birth. The FemCap can be worn for as long as 48 hours, but, as with all vaginal devices, should not be used during menses. The device is designed to be used with a thin layer of spermicide around the outer brim. This method requires a prescription.

Efficacy and Effectiveness The FemCap was not as effective in preventing pregnancy as the traditional diaphragm in clinical

FIGURE 13-9 **Diaphragms.**

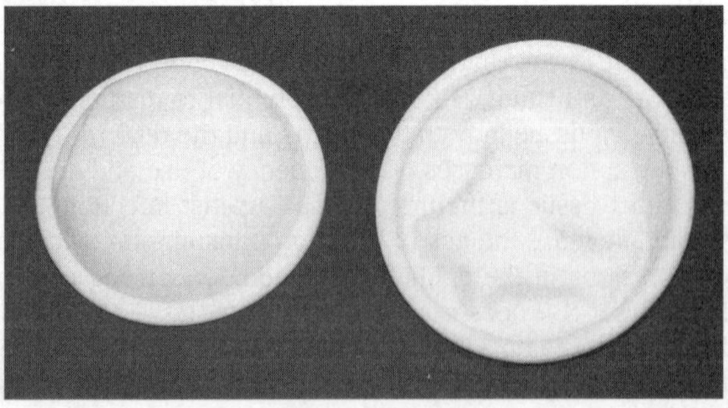

FIGURE 13-10 **The FemCap.**

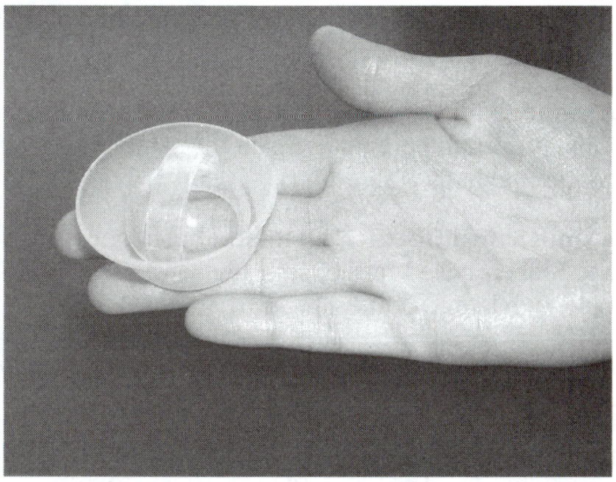

Courtesy of The Cervical Barrier Advancement Society and Ibis Reproductive Health.

FIGURE 13-11 **The Today sponge.**

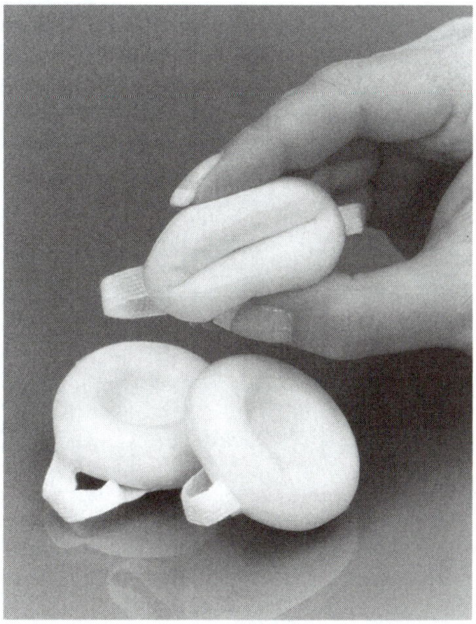

Courtesy of Mayer Laboratories, Inc.

studies; the extrapolated annual failure rates slightly exceed 20 percent (Lindh et al., 2021). Cervical caps may be less effective in individuals who have had children than in those who have not.

Safety and Side Effects In a randomized trial comparing FemCap to the traditional diaphragm, FemCap users had significantly fewer urinary tract infections (7.5%) than those in the diaphragm group (12.4%). In this same study, there were no differences in vaginitis, irritation, dysmenorrhea, or Pap test changes between the groups (Mauck et al., 1999).

Noncontraceptive Benefits The cervical cap has possible or theoretical value in protecting the cervix from infection, but there are no data to support this benefit. The only barrier methods known to reduce STIs are external and internal condoms.

Advantages and Disadvantages Cervical caps are coitus dependent (Table 13-2) and may be appropriate for individuals who do not want or cannot use hormonal contraception. The latex-free FemCap is appropriate for individuals who have, or whose partners have, latex allergies. In one study, individuals shared that they really appreciated how discreet the method was and felt their partner did not necessarily know they were using it during intercourse (Gollub et al., 2015). Insertion and removal of cervical caps may be complex for some; these individuals will need additional teaching and counseling to use this contraceptive method consistently and correctly. In a comparative study, more insertion and removal problems were noted with FemCap than with the traditional diaphragm (Lindh et al., 2021).

Caps require an initial cost for prescription, and purchase, but they should last for approximately 2 years with proper care. Ongoing costs include the purchase of spermicides. The FemCap website (http://www.femcap.com) provides detailed information about obtaining this device.

Vaginal Sponges

The Today sponge is a single-use, soft, absorbent polyurethane device that contains approximately 1,000 mg of N-9 spermicide; when moistened, the sponge gradually releases 125–150 mg of spermicide over 24 hours of use (**Figure 13-11**). Its primary contraceptive effectiveness derives from the gradual release of spermicide, but it also provides a physical barrier to the cervix and absorbs semen. The vaginal sponge can be used for multiple episodes of coitus over 24 hours without inserting more spermicide.

Efficacy and Effectiveness With typical use, pregnancy rates are somewhat higher among parous individuals who use contraceptive sponges than among individuals who use diaphragms, although rates for nulliparous individuals are similar (Table 13-1).

Safety and Side Effects Individuals who use the vaginal sponge tend to discontinue use at higher rates than individuals who use the diaphragm; more than 40 percent of those who used both methods stopped using the vaginal sponge in research studies. Allergic-type reactions such as dermatitis, erythema, irritation, and vaginal itching were more common with the sponge, although they occurred in only 4 percent of users (Kuyoh et al., 2003).

Noncontraceptive Benefits There are no data to suggest that the contraceptive sponge has value in protecting the cervix from infection; the only barrier methods known to reduce STIs are internal and external condoms.

Advantages and Disadvantages The sponge shares the advantages and disadvantages of other nonhormonal barrier, coitus-dependent methods (Table 13-2). It does not require a clinician visit or fitting and is available on an over-the-counter basis. Its single-use application may prove more expensive over time than methods that can be reused.

FIGURE 13-12 Internal condom.

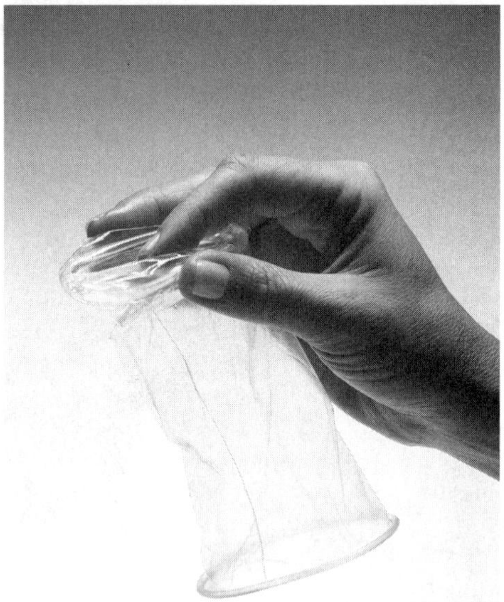

© Keith Brofsky/Photodisc/Getty Images

Internal Condom

The internal condom, previously called the female condom, is a barrier device designed to protect the cervix, vagina, and part of the vulva and perineum. It was developed as an alternative to external condoms to give pregnancy-capable individuals a nonprescription barrier contraceptive method that they could control and that would reduce their exposure to STIs.

The internal condom is a sheath made from a nitrile polymer, which is soft and smooth and quickly warms to body temperature (**Figure 13-12**). A small ring at the closed end of the sheath is inserted high in the vagina. A larger ring rests outside the vagina against the vulva and acts as a guide during penetration. This ring also maintains the sheath covering the full length of the vagina and prevents it from bunching up inside the vagina. The sheath is coated with a silicone-based nonspermicidal lubricant, and additional lubricant can be used as well.

The internal condom should not be used simultaneously with an external condom because this practice increases the risk of breakage. The internal condom should not be used with a diaphragm, cervical cap, or contraceptive vaginal ring because the inner ring of the internal condom fits into the same place by the cervix as those methods.

Efficacy and Effectiveness The effectiveness of the internal condom in preventing pregnancy is in the same range as that of other barrier methods (Table 13-1).

Safety and Side Effects The internal condom is made of a synthetic rubber, called nitrile, so it does not present problems for people with latex allergies.

Noncontraceptive Benefits The internal condom can protect against some STIs.

Advantages and Disadvantages The internal condom is a nonhormonal, personally controlled method that is available as an over-the-counter product. Internal condoms are less common, which means that more education is needed to support individuals who may want to use this method (B. A. Chen et al., 2019). However, internal condoms are an appealing option for many because they offer reproductive control that also provides protection against STIs (Fasehun et al., 2022).

Some find the internal condom difficult to insert, although this problem decreases with proper education (B. A. Chen et al., 2019). Although it is a user-controlled method, partner cooperation may still be necessary for consistent use; the partner's lack of acceptance is often cited as a reason for discontinuation. Internal condoms can be used only once and are more expensive than external condoms, so this method can be costly over time.

CONCLUSION

There are a plethora of options for individuals seeking contraception. There are short- and longer-term options, options that are permenant and reversible, and options that utilize homrones and options that do not. Individuals will likely use many of these methods over the course of their life, as sexual activity, preferences, and priorities change. There is not singular right method for any one person—the best method is the method they desire and can safely use. It is the provider's role to provide evidence-based education that is sensitive to the needs, priorities, and preferences of each individual. While this is not always a small task, person-centered, unbiased, evidence-based contraceptive education and counseling is critical to upholding patient autonomy and personal agency.

References

Adeyemi-Fowode, O. A., & Bercaw-Pratt, J. L. (2019). Intrauterine devices: Effective contraception with noncontraceptive benefits for adolescents. *Journal of Pediatric and Adolescent Gynecology, 32*(5S), S2–S6. https://doi.org/10.1016/j.jpag.2019.07.001

Ahrendt, H.-J., Nisand, I., Bastianelli, C., Gómez, M. A., Gemzell-Danielsson, K., Urdl, W., Karskov, B., Oeyen, L., Bitzer, J., Page, G., & Milsom, I. (2006). Efficacy, acceptability and tolerability of the combined contraceptive ring, NuvaRing, compared with an oral contraceptive containing 30 μg of ethinyl estradiol and 3 mg of drospirenone. *Contraception, 74*(6), 451–457. https://doi.org/10.1016/j.contraception.2006.07.004

Allen, D., Hunter, M. S., Wood, S., & Beeson, T. (2017). One Key Question(®): First Things First in Reproductive Health. *Maternal and Child Health Journal, 21*(3), 387–392. https://doi.org/10.1007/s10995-017-2283-2

Allen, R. H., Song, S., Weir, G. M., & White, K. O. (2025). "Stop gaslighting your patients": A quantitative and qualitative analysis of user experiences of IUDs on TikTok. *Journal of Pediatric and Adolescent Gynecology, 38*(4), 498–503. https://doi.org/10.1016/j.jpag.2025.02.003

Alvarez, F., Brache, V., Fernandez, E., Guerrero, B., Guiloff, E., Hess, R., Salvatierra, A. M., & Zacharias, S. (1988). New insights on the mode of action of intrauterine contraceptive devices in women. *Studies in Family Planning, 19*(5), 310.

https://www.jstor.org/stable/i307020?refreqid=excelsior%3Af1c746b07f36bf824c4a9591070d296d

American College of Obstetricians and Gynecologists. (2015). Practice Bulletin No. 152: Emergency Contraception. *Obstetrics and Gynecology, 126*(3), e1–e11. https://doi.org/10.1097/AOG.0000000000001047

American College of Obstetricians and Gynecologists. (2022). *Patient-Centered Contraceptive Counseling* (Committee Statement No. 1). American College of Obstetricians and Gynecologists. https://www.acog.org/clinical/clinical-guidance/committee-statement/articles/2022/02/patient-centered-contraceptive-counseling

American College of Obstetricians and Gynecologists (2004). *Depot Medroxyprogesterone Acetate and Bone Effects* (Committee Opinion No. 602). American College of Obstetricians and Gynecologists. https://www.acog.org/clinical/clinical-guidance/committee-opinion/articles/2014/06/depot-medroxyprogesterone-acetate-and-bone-effects

American College of Obstetricians and Gynecologists. (2014, reaffirmed 2019). Depot medroxyprogesterone acetate and bone effects. *Obstetrics & Gynecology, 123*, 1398–1402. https://www.acog.org/Clinical-Guidance-and-Publications/Committee-Opinions/Committee-on-Adolescent-Health-Care/Depot-Medroxyprogesterone-Acetate-and-Bone-Effects

American College of Obstetricians and Gynecologists. (2018a). ACOG committee Opinion No. 735: Adolescents and long-acting reversible contraception: Implants and intrauterine devices. *Obstetrics & Gynecology, 131*, e130–e139. https://www.acog.org/Clinical-Guidance-and-Publications/Committee-Opinions/Committee-on-Adolescent-Health-Care/Adolescents-and-Long-Acting-Reversible-Contraception

American College of Obstetricians and Gynecologists. (2018b). *Facts are important: Birth control does not cause abortion*. https://www.acog.org/advocacy/facts-are-important/hormonal-birth-control

American College of Obstetricians and Gynecologists (2022). General approaches to medical management of menstrual suppression: ACOG Clinical Consensus No. 3. *Obstetrics & Gynecology, 140*(3), 528–541. https://doi.org/10.1097/AOG.0000000000004899

American Society for Emergency Contraception. (2018). *Emergency contraception: A guide for pharmacies and retailers*. http://americansocietyforec.org/uploads/3/4/5/6/34568220/pharmacy_ec_access_overview.pdfAmico, J. R., Bennett, A. H., Karasz, A., & Gold, M. (2016). "She just told me to leave it": Women's experiences discussing early elective IUD removal. *Contraception, 94*(4), 357–361. https://doi.org/10.1016/j.contraception.2016.04.012

Amico, J. R., Stimmel, S., Hudson, S., & Gold, M. (2020). "$231 . . . to pull a string!!!" American IUD users' reasons for IUD self-removal: An analysis of internet forums. *Contraception, 101*(6), 393–398. https://doi.org/10.1016/j.contraception.2020.02.005

Anastasiou, E., McCarthy, K. J., Gollub, E. L., Ralph, L., van de Wijgert, J. H. H. M., & Jones, H. E. (2022). The relationship between hormonal contraception and cervical dysplasia/cancer controlling for human papillomavirus infection: A systematic review. *Contraception, 107*, 1–9. https://doi.org/10.1016/j.contraception.2021.10.018

Ayala-Ramirez, M., Grewe, M. E., Kaiser, J., Kennedy, E., Winn, M., & Urrutia, R. P. (2023). Understanding the perspective of women who use the Billings Ovulation Method®: A focus group study. *BMC Women's Health, 23*(1), 251. https://doi.org/10.1186/s12905-023-02398-w

Babic, A., Sasamoto, N., Rosner, B. A., Tworoger, S. S., Jordan, S. J., Risch, H. A., Harris, H. R., Rossing, M. A., Doherty, J. A., Fortner, R. T., Chang-Claude, J., Goodman, M. T., Thompson, P. J., Moysich, K. B., Ness, R. B., Kjaer, S. K., Jensen, A., Schildkraut, J. M., Titus, L. J., ... Terry, K. L. (2020). Association between breastfeeding and ovarian cancer risk. *JAMA Oncology, 6*(6), e200421. https://doi.org/10.1001/jamaoncol.2020.0421

Baboudjian, M., Rajwa, P., Barret, E., Beauval, J.-B., Brureau, L., Créhange, G., Dariane, C., Fiard, G., Fromont, G., Gauthé, M., Mathieu, R., Renard-Penna, R., Roubaud, G., Ruffion, A., Sargos, P., Rouprêt, M., & Ploussard, G. (2022). Vasectomy and risk of prostate cancer: A systematic review and meta-analysis. *European Urology Open Science, 41*, 35–44. https://doi.org/10.1016/j.euros.2022.04.012

Bastianelli, C., Farris, M., Rosato, E., Brosens, I., & Benagiano, G. (2018). Pharmacodynamics of combined estrogen-progestin oral contraceptives 3. Inhibition of ovulation. *Expert Review of Clinical Pharmacology, 11*(11), 1085–1098. https://doi.org/10.1080/17512433.2018.1536544

Bole, R., Lundy, S. D., Pei, E., Bajic, P., Parekh, N., & Vij, S. C. (2024). Rising vasectomy volume following reversal of federal protections for abortion rights in the United States. *International Journal of Impotence Research, 36*(3), 265–268. https://doi.org/10.1038/s41443-023-00672-x

Bounds, W., Guillebaud, J., Dominik, R., & Dalberth, B. T. (1995). The diaphragm with and without spermicide. A randomized, comparative efficacy trial. *Journal of Reproductive Medicine, 40*(11), 764–774. http://www.ncbi.nlm.nih.gov/pubmed/8592310

Bovo, A. C., Pedrão, P. G., Guimarães, Y. M., Godoy, L. R., Resende, J. C. P., Longatto-Filho, A., & Reis, R. D. (2023). Combined oral contraceptive use and the risk of cervical cancer: Literature review. *Revista Brasileira de Ginecologia e Obstetricia : Revista Da Federacao Brasileira Das Sociedades de Ginecologia e Obstetricia, 45*(12), e818–e824. https://doi.org/10.1055/s-0043-1776403

Boydell, V., & Smith, R. D. (2023). Hidden in plain sight: A systematic review of coercion and Long-Acting Reversible Contraceptive methods (LARC). *PLOS Global Public Health, 3*(8), e0002131. https://doi.org/10.1371/journal.pgph.0002131

Brache, V., Cochon, L., Deniaud, M., & Croxatto, H. B. (2013). Ulipristal acetate prevents ovulation more effectively than levonorgestrel: Analysis of pooled data from three randomized trials of emergency contraception regimens. *Contraception, 88*(5), 611–618. https://doi.org/10.1016/j.contraception.2013.05.010

Brandi, K., & Fuentes, L. (2020). The history of tiered-effectiveness contraceptive counseling and the importance of patient-centered family planning care. *American Journal of Obstetrics and Gynecology, 222*(4S), S873–S877. https://doi.org/10.1016/j.ajog.2019.11.1271

Brandi, K., Morgan, J. R., Paasche-Orlow, M. K., Perkins, R. B., & White, K. O. C. (2018). Obstetric outcomes after failed hysteroscopic and laparoscopic sterilization procedures. *Obstetrics and Gynecology, 131*(2), 253–261. https://doi.org/10.1097/AOG.0000000000002446

Britton, L. E., Alspaugh, A., Greene, M. Z., & McLemore, M. R. (2020). CE: An evidence-based update on contraception. *The American Journal of Nursing, 120*(2), 22–33. https://doi.org/10.1097/01.NAJ.0000654304.29632.a7

Bryant, A. G., Lyerly, A. D., DeVane-Johnson, S., Kistler, C. E., & Stuebe, A. M. (2019). Hormonal contraception, breastfeeding and bedside advocacy: The case for patient-centered care. *Contraception, 99*(2), 73–76. https://doi.org/10.1016/j.contraception.2018.10.011

Casado-Espada, N. M., de Alarcón, R., de la Iglesia-Larrad, J. I., Bote-Bonaechea, B., & Montejo, Á. L. (2019). Hormonal contraceptives, female sexual dysfunction, and managing strategies: A review. *Journal of Clinical Medicine, 8*(6), 908. https://doi.org/10.3390/jcm8060908

Castillo, K., Zambrano, K., Barba, D., Robayo, P., Sanon, S., Caicedo, A., & Jijon Chiriboga, A. J. (2022). Long-acting reversible contraceptives effects in abnormal uterine bleeding, a review of the physiology and management. *European Journal of Obstetrics, Gynecology, and Reproductive Biology, 270*, 231–238. https://doi.org/10.1016/j.ejogrb.2022.01.020

Chen, B. A., Blithe, D. L., Muraguri, G. R., Lance, A. A., Carr, B. R., Jensen, J. T., Kimble, T. D., Murthy, A. S., Schreiber, C. A., Thomas, M. A., Walsh, T. L., Westhoff, C., & Burke, A. E. (2019). Acceptability of the woman's condom in a phase III multicenter open-label study. *Contraception, 99*(6), 357–362. https://doi.org/10.1016/j.contraception.2019.02.006

Chen, X., Li, Q., Wang, X., Chen, J., Lv, W., Shi, B., Wang, H., Luo, J., & Li, J. (2018). Bleeding pattern difference between levonorgestrel intrauterine system and copper intrauterine devices inserted immediately post-abortion: A multicenter, prospective, observational cohort study in Chinese women. *Current Medical Research and Opinion, 34*(5), 873–880. https://doi.org/10.1080/03007995.2017.1421919

Cheng, S., Yang, B., Xu, L., Zheng, Q., Ding, G., & Li, G. (2021). Vasectomy and prostate cancer risk: A meta-analysis of prospective studies. *Carcinogenesis, 42*(1), 31–37. https://doi.org/10.1093/carcin/bgaa086

Coelingh Bennink, H. J. T., van Gennip, F. A. M., Gerrits, M. G. F., Egberts, J. F. M., Gemzell-Danielsson, K., & Kopp-Kallner, H. (2024). Health benefits of combined oral contraceptives—A narrative review. *The European Journal of Contraception & Reproductive Health Care: The Official Journal of the European Society of Contraception, 29*(2), 40–52. https://doi.org/10.1080/13625187.2024.2317295

Cook, L. A., Pun, A., Gallo, M. F., Lopez, L. M., & Van Vliet, H. A. A. M. (2014). Scalpel versus no-scalpel incision for vasectomy. *The Cochrane Database of Systematic Reviews, 2014*(3), CD004112. https://doi.org/10.1002/14651858.CD004112.pub4

Coppola, J. S. (2021). A new vaginal pH regulator for hormone-free, on-demand contraception. *Nursing for Women's Health, 25*(2), 152–155. https://doi.org/10.1016/j.nwh.2021.01.004

Cortessis, V. K., Barrett, M., Brown Wade, N., Enebish, T., Perrigo, J. L., Tobin, J., Zhong, C., Zink, J., Isiaka, V., Muderspach, L. I., Natavio, M., & McKean-Cowdin, R. (2017). Intrauterine device use and cervical cancer risk: A systematic review and meta-analysis. *Obstetrics and Gynecology, 130*(6), 1226–1236. https://doi.org/10.1097/AOG.0000000000002307

Costescu, D., Chawla, R., Hughes, R., Teal, S., & Merz, M. (2022). Discontinuation rates of intrauterine contraception due to unfavourable bleeding: A systematic review. *BMC Women's Health, 22*(1), 82. https://doi.org/10.1186/s12905-022-01657-6

Creinin, M. D., Schreiber, C. A., Turok, D. K., Cwiak, C., Chen, B. A., & Olariu, A. I. (2022). Levonorgestrel 52 mg intrauterine system efficacy and safety through 8 years of use. *American Journal of Obstetrics and Gynecology, 227*(6), 871.e1–871.e7. https://doi.org/10.1016/j.ajog.2022.05.022

Curtis, K. M., Nguyen, A. T., Tepper, N. K., Zapata, L. B., Snyder, E. M., Hatsfield-Timajchy, K., Kortsmit, K., Cohen, M., & Whiteman, M. K. (2024). U.S. selected practice recommendations for contraceptive use, 2024. *Morbidity and Mortality Weekly Report, 73*, 1–77. http://dx.doi.org/10.15585/mmwr.rr7303a1

Curtis, K. M., Tepper, N. K., Jatlaoui, T. C., Berry-Bibee, E., Horton, L. G., Zapata, L. B., Simmons, K. B., Pagano, H. P., Jamieson, D. J., & Whiteman, M. K. (2016). U.S. medical eligibility criteria for contraceptive use, 2016. *MMWR Recommendations and Reports, 65*(3), 1–104. https://doi.org/10.15585/mmwr.rr6503a1

Danvers, A. A., & Evans, T. A. (2022). Risk of sterilization regret and age: An analysis of the National Survey of Family Growth, 2015–2019. *Obstetrics and Gynecology, 139*(3), 433–439. https://doi.org/10.1097/AOG.0000000000004692

de Abood, M., de Castillo, Z., Guerrero, F., Espino, M., & Austin, K. L. (1997). Effect of Depo-Provera® or Microgynon® on the painful crises of sickle cell anemia patients. *Contraception, 56*(5), 313–316. https://doi.org/10.1016/S0010-7824(97)00156-X

Dean, G., & Schwarz, E. B. (2018). Intrauterine devices (IUDs). In R. A. Hatcher, A. L. Nelson, J. Trussell, C. Cwiak, P. Cason, M. S. Policar, A. R. A. Aiken, J. Marrazzo, & D. Kowal (Eds.), *Contraceptive technology* (21st ed., pp. 157–183). Ayer Company Publishers.

de Bastos, M., Stegeman, B. H., Rosendaal, F. R., Van Hylckama Vlieg, A., Helmerhorst, F. M., Stijnen, T., & Dekkers, O. M. (2014). Combined oral contraceptives: Venous thrombosis. *The Cochrane Database of Systematic Reviews, 3,* CD010813. https://doi.org/10.1002/14651858.CD010813.pub2

Deparle, J. (1991, May 12). The nation. As funds for welfare shrink, ideas flourish. *The New York Times*, p. 5.

DeSisto, C. L., Handler, A., Haider, S., Caskey, R., Peacock, N., Kottke, M., & Rankin, K. (2018). Women's informed choice and satisfaction with immediate postpartum long-acting reversible contraception in Georgia. *Contraception and Reproductive Medicine, 3,* 19. https://doi.org/10.1186/s40834-018-0073-x

Dethier, D., Qasba, N., & Kaneshiro, B. (2022). Society of Family Planning clinical recommendation: Extended use of long-acting reversible contraception. *Contraception, 113*, 13–18. https://doi.org/10.1016/j.contraception.2022.06.003

Douxfils, J., Raskin, L., Didembourg, M., Donis, N., Dogné, J.-M., Morimont, L., & Beaudart, C. (2024). Are natural estrogens used in contraception at lower risk of venous thromboembolism than synthetic ones? A systematic literature review and meta-analysis. *Frontiers in Endocrinology, 15*, 1428597. https://doi.org/10.3389/fendo.2024.1428597

Dragoman, M. V., Tepper, N. K., Fu, R., Curtis, K. M., Chou, R., & Gaffield, M. E. (2018). A systematic review and meta-analysis of venous thrombosis risk among users of combined oral contraception. *International Journal of Gynaecology and Obstetrics: The Official Organ of the International Federation of Gynaecology and Obstetrics, 141*(3), 287–294. https://doi.org/10.1002/ijgo.12455

D'Souza, P., Bailey, J. V., Stephenson, J., & Oliver, S. (2022). Factors influencing contraception choice and use globally: A synthesis of systematic reviews. *The European Journal of Contraception & Reproductive Health Care: The Official Journal of the European Society of Contraception*, *27*(5), 364–372. https://doi.org/10.1080/13625187.2022.2096215

Dubin, J. M., White, J., Ory, J., & Ramasamy, R. (2021). Vasectomy reversal vs. sperm retrieval with in vitro fertilization: A contemporary, comparative analysis. *Fertility and Sterility*, *115*(6), 1377–1383. https://doi.org/10.1016/j.fertnstert.2021.03.050

Edelman, A. B., Kaneshiro, B., Simmons, K. B., Hauschildt, J. L., Bond, K., Boniface, E. R., & Jensen, J. T. (2020). Treatment of unfavorable bleeding patterns in contraceptive implant users: A randomized controlled trial. *Obstetrics and Gynecology*, *136*(2), 323–332. https://doi.org/10.1097/AOG.0000000000003896

Eisenberg, D. L., Secura, G. M., Madden, T. E., Allsworth, J. E., Zhao, Q., & Peipert, J. F. (2012). Knowledge of contraceptive effectiveness. *American Journal of Obstetrics and Gynecology*, *206*(6), 479.e1–e9. https://doi.org/10.1016/j.ajog.2012.04.012

Ela, E. J., Broussard, K., Hansen, K., Burke, K. L., Thaxton, L., & Potter, J. E. (2022). Satisfaction, resignation, and dissatisfaction with long-acting reversible contraception among low-income postpartum Texans. *Women's Health Issues: Official Publication of the Jacobs Institute of Women's Health*, *32*(4), 334–342. https://doi.org/10.1016/j.whi.2022.02.006

Elgemark, K., Graner, S., McTaggart, J., Ramirez Löfström, J., Sörensen, D., Envall, N., & Kopp Kallner, H. (2022). The 13.5-mg, 19.5-mg, and 52-mg Levonorgestrel-releasing intrauterine systems and risk of ectopic pregnancy. *Obstetrics and Gynecology*, *140*(2), 227–233. https://doi.org/10.1097/AOG.0000000000004846

Espey, E., Yoder, K., & Hofler, L. (2019). Barriers and solutions to improve adolescent intrauterine device access. *Journal of Pediatric and Adolescent Gynecology*, *32*(5S), S7–S13. https://doi.org/10.1016/j.jpag.2019.03.010

Fasehun, L.-K., Lewinger, S., Fasehun, O., & Brooks, M. (2022). Barriers and facilitators to acceptability of the female condom in low- and middle-income countries: A systematic review. *Annals of Global Health*, *88*(1), 20. https://doi.org/10.5334/aogh.3612

Festin, M. R. (2013). Non-latex versus latex male condoms for contraception (2013). *The WHO Reproductive Health Library.* World Health Organization. https://extranet.who.int/rhl/topics/fertility-regulation/contraception/non-latex-versus-latex-male-condoms-contraception

Festin, M. P. R., Peregoudov, A., Seuc, A., Kiarie, J., & Temmerman, M. (2017). Effect of BMI and body weight on pregnancy rates with LNG as emergency contraception: Analysis of four WHO HRP studies. Contraception, 95(1), 50–54. https://doi.org/10.1016/j.contraception.2016.08.001

FitzGerald, C., & Hurst, S. (2017). Implicit bias in healthcare professionals: A systematic review. *BMC Medical Ethics, 18*(1), 19. https://doi.org/10.1186/S12910-017-0179-8

Fitzpatrick, D., Pirie, K., Reeves, G., Green, J., & Beral, V. (2023). Combined and progestagen-only hormonal contraceptives and breast cancer risk: A UK nested case-control study and meta-analysis. *PLoS Medicine*, *20*(3), e1004188. https://doi.org/10.1371/journal.pmed.1004188

Fox, K. R., Kameoka, A. M., Raidoo, S., Soon, R., Tschann, M., Fontanilla, T., & Kaneshiro, B. (2024). Patient barriers to discontinuing long-acting reversible contraception. *Maternal and Child Health Journal, 28*(2), 192–197. https://doi.org/10.1007/s10995-023-03878-z

Frederiksen, B., Diep, K., & Salganicoff, A. (2024, November 22). Contraceptive experiences, coverage, and preferences: Findings from the 2024 KFF Women's Health Survey. *KFF.* https://www.kff.org/womens-health-policy/issue-brief/contraceptive-experiences-coverage-and-preferences-findings-from-the-2024-kff-womens-health-survey/

Frost, J. J., Mueller, J., & Pleasure, Z. H. (2021). *Trends and differentials in receipt of sexual and reproductive health services in the United States: Services received and sources of care, 2006–2019.* https://doi.org/10.1363/2021.33017

Gavin, L., Moskosky, S., Carter, M., Curtis, K., Glass, E., Godfrey, E., Marcell, A., Mautone-Smith, N., Pazol, K., Tepper, N., & Zapata, L. (2014). Providing quality family planning services: Recommendations of CDC and the U.S. Office of Population Affairs. *Morbidity and Mortality Weekly Report, 63*(RR04), 1–29. https://www.cdc.gov/mmwr/preview/mmwrhtml/rr6304a1.htm

Geist, C., Aiken, A. R., Sanders, J. N., Everett, B. G., Myers, K., Cason, P., Simmons, R. G., & Turok, D. K. (2019). Beyond intent: Exploring the association of contraceptive choice with questions about Pregnancy Attitudes, Timing and How important is pregnancy prevention (PATH) questions. *Contraception*, *99*(1), 22–26. https://doi.org/10.1016/j.contraception.2018.08.014

Giannou, F. K., Tsiara, C. G., Nikolopoulos, G. K., Talias, M., Benetou, V., Kantzanou, M., Bonovas, S., & Hatzakis, A. (2016). Condom effectiveness in reducing heterosexual HIV transmission: A systematic review and meta-analysis of studies on HIV serodiscordant couples. *Expert Review of Pharmacoeconomics & Outcomes Research, 16*(4), 489–499. https://doi.org/10.1586/14737167.2016.1102635

Girum, T., & Wasie, A. (2018). Return of fertility after discontinuation of contraception: A systematic review and meta-analysis. *Contraception and Reproductive Medicine, 3*, 9. https://doi.org/10.1186/s40834-018-0064-y

Glasier, A. (2013). Emergency contraception: Clinical outcomes. *Contraception, 87*(3), 309–313. https://doi.org/10.1016/j.contraception.2012.08.027

Glasier, A. (2014). The rationale for use of ulipristal acetate as first line in emergency contraception: Biological and clinical evidence. *Gynecological Endocrinology, 30*(10), 688–690. https://doi.org/10.3109/09513590.2014.950645

Gollub, E. L., Cyrus, E., Dévieux, J. G., Jean-Gilles, M., Neptune, S., Pelletier, V., Michel, H., Sévère, M., & Pierre, L. (2015). "Men don't need to know everything": A field trial of a discreet, female-initiated, contraceptive barrier method (FemCap™) among Haitian-American women. *Culture, Health & Sexuality*, *17*(7), 842–858. https://doi.org/10.1080/13691058.2015.1005672

Gomez, A. M., Fuentes, L., & Allina, A. (2014). Women or LARC first? Reproductive autonomy and the promotion of long-acting reversible contraceptive methods. *Perspectives on Sexual and Reproductive Health, 46*(3), 171–175. https://doi.org/10.1363/46e1614

Grandi, G., Barra, F., Ferrero, S., Sileo, F. G., Bertucci, E., Napolitano, A., & Facchinetti, F. (2019). Hormonal contraception in women with endometriosis: A systematic review. *The European Journal of Contraception & Reproductive Health Care: The Official Journal of the European Society of Contraception*, *24*(1), 61–70. https://doi.org/10.1080/13625187.2018.1550576

Guttmacher Institute. (2021). *Contraceptive Use in the United States by Method.* Guttmacher Institute. https://www.guttmacher.org/fact-sheet/contraceptive-method-use-united-states

Guttmacher Institute (2024). *Insurance Coverage of Contraceptives.* https://www.guttmacher.org/state-policy/explore/insurance-coverage-contraceptives

Hatcher, R. A., Zieman, M., Lathrop, E., Haddad, L., & Allen, A. Z. (2019). *Managing contraception* (15th ed.). *Managing Contraception*.

Hawkins, D. (2017, July 28). Tennessee judge pulls offer to trade vasectomies, birth control implants for shorter jail sentences. *The Washington Post.* https://www.washingtonpost.com/news/morning-mix/wp/2017/07/28/tennessee-judge-under-fire-pulls-offer-to-trade-shorter-jail-sentences-for-vasectomies/

Hawkins, S. S. (2024). Approval of the first nonprescription oral contraceptive pill. *Journal of Obstetric, Gynecologic, and Neonatal Nursing: JOGNN*, *53*(5), 464–476. https://doi.org/10.1016/j.jogn.2024.08.001

Heinemann, K., Reed, S., Moehner, S., & Do Minh, T. (2015). Comparative contraceptive effectiveness of levonorgestrel-releasing and copper intrauterine devices: The European Active Surveillance Study for Intrauterine Devices. *Contraception, 91*(4), 280–283. https://doi.org/10.1016/j.contraception.2015.01.011

Holt, K., Reed, R., Crear-Perry, J., Scott, C., Wulf, S., & Dehlendorf, C. (2020). Beyond same-day long-acting reversible contraceptive access: A person-centered framework for advancing high-quality, equitable contraceptive care. *American Journal of Obstetrics and Gynecology*, *222*(4), S878.e1–S878.e6. https://doi.org/10.1016/j.ajog.2019.11.1279

Howett, R., Gertz, A. M., Kgaswanyane, T., Petro, G., Mokganya, L., Malima, S., Maotwe, T., Pleaner, M., & Morroni, C. (2019). Closing the gap: Ensuring access to and quality of contraceptive implant removal services is essential to rights-based contraceptive care. *African Journal of Reproductive Health*, *23*(4), 19–26. https://doi.org/10.29063/ajrh2019/v23i4.3

Hubacher, D., Lara-Ricalde, R., Taylor, D. J., Guerra-Infante, F., & Guzmán-Rodríguez, R. (2001). Use of copper intrauterine devices and the risk of tubal infertility among nulligravid women. *The New England Journal of Medicine*, *345*(8), 561–567. https://doi.org/10.1056/NEJMoa010438

Humphrey, K. N., Horn, P. S., Olshavsky, L., Reebals, L., & Standridge, S. M. (2021). Features of menstruation and menstruation management in individuals with Rett Syndrome. *Journal of Pediatric and Adolescent Gynecology*, *34*(2), 144–153. https://doi.org/10.1016/j.jpag.2020.11.002

Iversen, L., Fielding, S., Lidegaard, Ø., Mørch, L. S., Skovlund, C. W., & Hannaford, P. C. (2018). Association between contemporary hormonal contraception and ovarian cancer in women of reproductive age in Denmark: Prospective, nationwide cohort study. *BMJ (Clinical Research Ed.)*, *362*, k3609. https://doi.org/10.1136/bmj.k3609

Jennings, V., Haile, L. T., Simmons, R. G., Spieler, J., & Shattuck, D. (2019). Perfect- and typical-use effectiveness of the Dot fertility app over 13 cycles: Results from a prospective contraceptive effectiveness trial. *The European Journal of Contraception & Reproductive Health Care*, *24*(2), 148–153. https://doi.org/10.1080/13625187.2019.1581164

Jensen, J. T., Lukkari-Lax, E., Schulze, A., Wahdan, Y., Serrani, M., & Kroll, R. (2022). Contraceptive efficacy and safety of the 52-mg levonorgestrel intrauterine system for up to 8 years: Findings from the Mirena Extension Trial. *American Journal of Obstetrics and Gynecology*, *227*(6), 873.e1–873.e12. https://doi.org/10.1016/j.ajog.2022.09.007

Jones, R. K., Lindberg, L. D., & Higgins, J. A. (2014). Pull and pray or extra protection? Contraceptive strategies involving withdrawal among US adult women. *Contraception*, *90*(4), 416–421. https://doi.org/10.1016/j.contraception.2014.04.016

Kaiser Family Foundation. (2020, September 9). Intrauterine Devices (IUDs): Access for women in the U.S. *KFF*. https://www.kff.org/womens-health-policy/fact-sheet/intrauterine-devices-iuds-access-for-women-in-the-u-s/

Kaiser Family Foundation. (2018). *Sterilization as a family planning method*. https://www.kff.org/womens-health-policy/fact-sheet/sterilization-as-a-family-planning-method/

Kakaiya, R., Lopez, L. L., & Nelson, A. L. (2017). Women's perceptions of contraceptive efficacy and safety. *Contraception and Reproductive Medicine*, *2*, 19. https://doi.org/10.1186/s40834-017-0046-5

Kanadys, W., Barańska, A., Malm, M., Błaszczuk, A., Polz-Dacewicz, M., Janiszewska, M., & Jędrych, M. (2021). Use of oral contraceptives as a potential risk factor for breast cancer: A systematic review and meta-analysis of case-control studies up to 2010. *International Journal of Environmental Research and Public Health*, *18*(9). https://doi.org/10.3390/ijerph18094638

Karlsson, T., Johansson, T., Höglund, J., Ek, W. E., & Johansson, Å. (2021). Time-dependent effects of oral contraceptive use on breast, ovarian, and endometrial cancers. *Cancer Research*, *81*(4), 1153–1162. https://doi.org/10.1158/0008-5472.CAN-20-2476

Killick, S. R., Leary, C., Trussell, J., & Guthrie, K. A. (2011). Sperm content of pre-ejaculatory fluid. *Human Fertility*, *14*(1), 48–52. https://doi.org/10.3109/14647273.2010.520798

Kopp-Kallner, H., Linder, M., Cesta, C. E., Segovia Chacón, S., Kieler, H., & Graner, S. (2022). Method of hormonal contraception and protective effects against ectopic pregnancy. *Obstetrics and Gynecology*, *139*(5), 764–770. https://doi.org/10.1097/AOG.0000000000004726

Kraft, M. Z., Rojczyk, P., Weiss, T., Derntl, B., Kikinis, Z., Croy, I., & Heller, C. (2024). Symptoms of mental disorders and oral contraception use: A systematic review and meta-analysis. *Frontiers in Neuroendocrinology*, *72*, 101111. https://doi.org/10.1016/j.yfrne.2023.101111

Krapf, J. M., & Goldstein, A. T. (2024). Combined estrogen-progestin oral contraceptives and female sexuality: An updated review. *Sexual Medicine Reviews*, *12*(3), 307–320. https://doi.org/10.1093/sxmrev/qeae011

Kuyoh, M. A., Toroitich-Ruto, C., Grimes, D. A., Schulz, K. F., & Gallo, M. F. (2003). Sponge versus diaphragm for contraception: A Cochrane review. *Contraception*, *67*(1), 15–18. http://www.ncbi.nlm.nih.gov/pubmed/12521652

Lindh, I., Othman, J., Hansson, M., Ekelund, A.-C., Svanberg, T., & Strandell, A. (2021). New types of diaphragms and cervical caps versus older types of diaphragms and different gels for contraception: A systematic review. *BMJ Sexual & Reproductive Health*, *47*(3), e12. https://doi.org/10.1136/bmjsrh-2020-200632

Littlejohn, K. E. (2021). *Just get on the pill*. University of California Press. https://www.ucpress.edu/books/just-get-on-the-pill/paper

Liu, P., Meng, J., Xiong, Y., Wu, Y., Xiao, Y., & Gao, S. (2024). Contraception with levonorgestrel-releasing intrauterine system versus copper intrauterine device: A meta-analysis of randomized controlled trials. *EClinicalMedicine*, *78*, 102926. https://doi.org/10.1016/j.eclinm.2024.102926

Lopez, L. M., Bernholc, A., Zeng, Y., Allen, R. H., Bartz, D., O'Brien, P. A., & Hubacher, D. (2015). Interventions for pain with intrauterine device insertion. *The Cochrane Database of Systematic Reviews*, *2015*(7), CD007373. https://doi.org/10.1002/14651858.CD007373.pub3

Lopez, L. M., Grimes, D. A., Gallo, M. F., Stockton, L. L., & Schulz, K. F. (2013). Skin patch and vaginal ring versus combined oral contraceptives for contraception. *Cochrane Database of Systematic Reviews*. https://doi.org/10.1002/14651858.CD003552.pub4

Ma, X., Zhao, L.-G., Sun, J.-W., Yang, Y., Zheng, J.-L., Gao, J., & Xiang, Y.-B. (2018). Association between breastfeeding and risk of endometrial cancer: A meta-analysis of epidemiological studies. *European Journal of Cancer Prevention: The Official Journal of the European Cancer Prevention Organisation (ECP)*, *27*(2), 144–151. https://doi.org/10.1097/CEJ.0000000000000186

Maguire, K., & Westhoff, C. (2011). The state of hormonal contraception today: Established and emerging noncontraceptive health benefits [Suppl.]. *American Journal of Obstetrics and Gynecology*, *205*(4), S4–S8. https://doi.org/10.1016/j.ajog.2011.06.056

Malacova, E., Kemp, A., Hart, R., Jama-Alol, K., & Preen, D. B. (2014). Long-term risk of ectopic pregnancy varies by method of tubal sterilization: A whole-population study. *Fertility and Sterility*, *101*(3), 728–734. https://doi.org/10.1016/j.fertnstert.2013.11.127

Mann, E. S., Chen, A. M., & Johnson, C. L. (2022). Doctor knows best? Provider bias in the context of contraceptive counseling in the United States. *Contraception*, *110*, 66–70. https://doi.org/10.1016/j.contraception.2021.11.009

Manzer, J. L., & Bell, A. V. (2021). "We're a little biased": Medicine and the management of bias through the case of contraception. *Journal of Health and Social Behavior*, *62*(2), 120–135. https://doi.org/10.1177/00221465211003232

Manzer, J. L., Berndt, V. K., & Bell, A. V. (2023). Intersections between culture, contraception, knowledge and the body in the USA. *Culture, health & sexuality*, *25*(9), 1164–1179. https://doi.org/10.1080/13691058.2022.2141330

Marchand, G. J., Masoud, A. T., King, A. K., Brazil, G. M., Ulibarri, H. M., Parise, J. E., Arroyo, A. L., Coriell, C. L., Goetz, S. P., Moir, C. J., & Govindan, M. L. (2022). Salpingectomy, tubal ligation and hysteroscopic occlusion for sterilization. *Minerva Obstetrics and Gynecology*, *74*(5), 452–461. https://doi.org/10.23736/S2724-606X.22.05134-X

Mauck, C., Callahan, M., Weiner, D. H., & Dominik, R. (1999). A comparative study of the safety and efficacy of FemCap, a new vaginal barrier contraceptive, and the Ortho All-Flex diaphragm. *Contraception*, *60*(2), 71–80. https://doi.org/10.1016/S0010-7824(99)00068-2

McCormick, E. (2021, July 19). Survivors of California's forced sterilizations: 'It's like my life wasn't worth anything.' *The Guardian*. https://www.theguardian.com/us-news/2021/jul/19/california-forced-sterilization-prison-survivors-reparations

Milliren, C. E., DiVasta, A. D., Edwards, A. J., Maslyanskaya, S., Borzutzky, C., & Pitts, S. (2023). Contraceptive implant-associated bleeding in adolescent/young adult clinical practice: Associated factors, management, and rates of discontinuation. *The Journal of Adolescent Health : Official Publication of the Society for Adolescent Medicine*, *72*(4), 583–590. https://doi.org/10.1016/j.jadohealth.2022.11.007

Minhaj Siddiqui, M., Giovannucci, E. L., & Mucci, L. A. (2021). Can there be consensus on whether vasectomy is a prostate cancer risk factor? *Prostate Cancer and Prostatic Diseases*, *24*(4), 939–941. https://doi.org/10.1038/s41391-021-00400-w

Moniz, M. H., Spector-Bagdady, K., Heisler, M., & Harris, L. H. (2017). Inpatient postpartum long-acting reversible contraception: Care that promotes reproductive justice. *Obstetrics and Gynecology*, *130*(4), 783–787. https://doi.org/10.1097/AOG.0000000000002262

Moon, L. M., & Smith, K. M. (2017). Barriers to long acting contraception use in adolescents: A primary care provider survey. *Journal of Pediatric and Adolescent Gynecology*, *30*(2), 323–324. https://doi.org/10.1016/j.jpag.2017.03.120

Morrison, C. S., Hofmeyr, G. J., Thomas, K. K., Rees, H., Philip, N., Palanee-Phillips, T., Nanda, K., Nair, G., Onono, M., Mastro, T. D., Lind, M., Heffron, R., Edward, V., Deese, J., Beksinska, M., Beesham, I., Stringer, J. S. A., Baeten, J. M., & Ahmed, K. (2020). Effects of Depot Medroxyprogesterone Acetate, copper intrauterine devices, and levonorgestrel implants on early HIV disease progression. *AIDS Research and Human Retroviruses*, *36*(8), 632–640. https://doi.org/10.1089/AID.2020.0015

Muñoz, M., Robinson, K., & Shibli-Rahhal, A. (2020). Bone health and osteoporosis prevention and treatment. *Clinical Obstetrics and Gynecology*, *63*(4), 770–787. https://doi.org/10.1097/GRF.0000000000000572

Nanda, K., & Burke, A. E. (2018). Contraceptive patch and vaginal contraceptive ring. In R. A. Hatcher, A. L. Nelson, J. Trussell, C. Cwiak, P. Cason, M. S. Policar, A. R. A. Aiken, J. Marrazzo, & D. Kowal (Eds.), *Contraceptive technology* (21st ed., pp. 227–256). Ayer Company Publishers.

Nahum, G. G., Kaunitz, A. M., Rosen, K., Schmelter, T., & Lynen, R. (2015). Ovarian cysts: Presence and persistence with use of a 13.5 mg levonorgestrel-releasing intrauterine system. *Contraception*, *91*(5), 412–417. https://doi.org/10.1016/j.contraception.2015.01.021

Natavio, M. F., Taylor, D., Lewis, R. A., Blumenthal, P., Felix, J. C., Melamed, A., Gentzschein, E., Stanczyk, F. Z., & Mishell, D. R. J. (2013). Temporal changes in cervical mucus after insertion of the levonorgestrel-releasing intrauterine system. *Contraception*, *87*(4), 426–431. https://doi.org/10.1016/j.contraception.2012.09.034

Nelson, A. L. (2000). The intrauterine contraceptive device. *Obstetrics and Gynecology Clinics of North America*, *27*(4), 723–740. https://doi.org/10.1016/S0889-8545(05)70170-4

Nelson, A. L., Shabaik, S., Xandre, P., Kakaiya, R., Awaida, J., Mellon, M., Schiller, A., & Stohl, H. E. (2019). Perceptions of health risks associated with pregnancy compared to oral contraceptive use. *Contraception*, *100*(3), 193–195. https://doi.org/10.1016/j.contraception.2019.04.008

Nguyen, A., Curtis, K., Tepper, N., Kortsmit, K. M., Brittain, A. W., Snyder, E. M., Cohen, M. A., Zapata, L. B., & Whiteman, M. K. (2024). U.S. medical eligibility criteria for contraceptive use, 2024. *Morbidity and Mortality Weekly Report*, *RR-4*, 1–126. http://dx.doi.org/10.15585/mmwr.rr7304a1

Nguyen, B. T., & Jacobsohn, T. L. (2022). Post-abortion contraception, an opportunity for male partners and male contraception. *Contraception*, *115*, 69–74. https://doi.org/10.1016/j.contraception.2022.07.004

Nguyen, L., Lamarche, L., Lennox, R., Ramdyal, A., Patel, T., Black, M., & Mangin, D. (2020). Strategies to mitigate anxiety and pain in intrauterine device insertion: A systematic review. *Journal of Obstetrics and Gynaecology Canada: JOGC = Journal d'obstetrique et Gynecologie Du Canada: JOGC*, *42*(9), 1138–1146.e2. https://doi.org/10.1016/j.jogc.2019.09.014

Noachtar, I. A., Frokjaer, V. G., & Pletzer, B. (2023). Mental health symptoms in oral contraceptive users during short-term hormone withdrawal. *JAMA Network Open*, *6*(9), e2335957. https://doi.org/10.1001/jamanetworkopen.2023.35957

Nwaru, B. I., Tibble, H., Shah, S. A., Pillinger, R., McLean, S., Ryan, D. P., Critchley, H., Price, D. B., Hawrylowicz, C. M., Simpson, C. R., Soyiri, I. N., Appiagyei, F., & Sheikh, A. (2021). Hormonal contraception and the risk of severe asthma exacerbation: 17-year population-based cohort study. *Thorax*, *76*(2), 109–115. https://doi.org/10.1136/thoraxjnl-2020-215540

Oldhafer, K. J., Habbel, V., Horling, K., Makridis, G., & Wagner, K. C. (2020). Benign liver tumors. *Visceral Medicine*, *36*(4), 292–303. https://doi.org/10.1159/000509145

Oliveira, E. C. F. de, Senra, J. C., & Rocha, A. L. L. (2024). The impact of using the levonorgestrel-releasing intrauterine device on the incidence of acne in adolescents and young women. *The European Journal of Contraception & Reproductive Health Care: The Official Journal of the European Society of Contraception*, *29*(5), 233–238. https://doi.org/10.1080/13625187.2024.2379363

Ortiz, M. E., & Croxatto, H. B. (2007). Copper-T intrauterine device and levonorgestrel intrauterine system: Biological bases of their mechanism of action [Suppl.]. *Contraception*, *75*(6), S16–S30. https://doi.org/10.1016/j.contraception.2007.01.020

Patel, J., Nelson, A. L., & Nguyen, B. T. (2024). Low to non-existent sperm content of pre-ejaculate in perfect-use contraceptive withdrawal, a pilot study. *Contraception*, *140*, 110555. https://doi.org/10.1016/j.contraception.2024.110555

Peragallo Urrutia, R., Polis, C. B., Jensen, E. T., Greene, M. E., Kennedy, E., & Stanford, J. B. (2018). Effectiveness of fertility awareness-based methods for pregnancy prevention: A systematic review. *Obstetrics and Gynecology*, *132*(3), 591–604. https://doi.org/10.1097/AOG.0000000000002784

Peterson, A. M., Brown, A., Savage, A., & Dempsey, A. (2019). Prevalence of early discontinuation and associated factors among a retrospective cohort of etonogestrel contraceptive implant users. *The European Journal of Contraception & Reproductive Health Care: The Official Journal of the European Society of Contraception*, *24*(6), 475–479. https://doi.org/10.1080/13625187.2019.1666361

Peterson, H. B., Xia, Z., Hughes, J. M., Wilcox, L. S., Tylor, L. R., & Trussell, J., for the U.S. Collaborative Review of Sterilization Working Group. (1997). The risk of ectopic pregnancy after tubal sterilization. *The New England Journal of Medicine*, *336*, 762–767. https://doi.org/10.1056/NEJM199703133361104

Piaggio, G., Kapp, N., & von Hertzen, H. (2011). Effect on pregnancy rates of the delay in the administration of levonorgestrel for emergency contraception: A combined analysis of four WHO trials. *Contraception*, *84*(1), 35–39. https://doi.org/10.1016/j.contraception.2010.11.010

Raine-Bennett, T., Chandra, M., Armstrong, M. A., Alexeeff, S., & Lo, J. C. (2019). Depot medroxyprogesterone acetate, oral contraceptive, intrauterine device use, and fracture risk. *Obstetrics & Gynecology*, *134*(3), 581–589. https://doi.org/10.1097/AOG.0000000000003414

Raymond, E. G., Chen, P. L., & Luoto, J. (2004). Contraceptive effectiveness and safety of five nonoxynol-9 spermicides: A randomized trial. *Obstetrics & Gynecology*, *103*(3), 430–439. https://doi.org/10.1097/01.AOG.0000113620.18395.0b

Reed, S. D., Zhou, X., Ichikawa, L., Gatz, J. L., Peipert, J. F., Armstrong, M. A., Raine-Bennett, T., Getahun, D., Fassett, M. J., Postlethwaite, D. A., Shi, J. M., Asiimwe, A., Pisa, F., Schoendorf, J., Saltus, C. W., Anthony, M. S., Reed, S. D., Zhou, X., Ichikawa, L., . . . Anthony, M. S. (2022). Intrauterine device-related uterine perforation incidence and risk (APEX-IUD): A large multisite cohort study. *The Lancet*, *399*(10341), 2103–2112. https://doi.org/10.1016/S0140-6736(22)00015-0

Rinehart, D. J., Stowell, M., Barrett, K., Langland, K., Thomas-Gale, T., Al-Tayyib, A., & O'Connell, R. (2023). Exploring Family planning perspectives among men receiving medications for opioid use disorder: Implications for service development. *Journal of Addiction Medicine*, *17*(1), 21–27. https://doi.org/10.1097/ADM.0000000000001012

Rocca, M. L., Palumbo, A. R., Visconti, F., & Di Carlo, C. (2021). Safety and benefits of contraceptives implants: A systematic review. *Pharmaceuticals (Basel, Switzerland)*, *14*(6). https://doi.org/10.3390/ph14060548

Romer, S. E., Blum, J., Borrero, S., Crowley, J. M., Hart, J., Magee, M. M., Manzer, J. L., & Stern, L. (2024). providing quality family planning services in the United States: Recommendations of the U.S. Office of Population Affairs (Revised 2024). *American Journal of Preventive Medicine*, *67*(65), 541–586. https://doi.org/10.1016/j.amepre.2024.09.007

Ross, L. J., & Solinger, R. (2017). *Reproductive Justice*. University of California Press.

Sadatmahalleh, S. J., Ziaei, S., Kazemnejad, A., & Mohamadi, E. (2016). Menstrual pattern following tubal ligation: A historical cohort study. *International Journal of Fertility & Sterility*, *9*(4), 477–482. https://doi.org/10.22074/ijfs.2015.4605

Salcedo, J., Cleland, K., Bartz, D., & Thompson, I. (2023). Society of Family Planning Clinical Recommendation: Emergency contraception. *Contraception*, *121*, 109958. https://doi.org/10.1016/j.contraception.2023.109958

Salliot, C., Nguyen, Y., Gelot, A., Mariette, X., Boutron-Ruault, M.-C., & Seror, R. (2022). Lifetime female hormonal exposure and risk of rheumatoid arthritis in postmenopausal women: Results from the French E3N cohort. *Joint Bone Spine*, *89*(5), 105374. https://doi.org/10.1016/j.jbspin.2022.105374

Samy, A., Abbas, A. M., Mahmoud, M., Taher, A., Awad, M. H., El Husseiny, T., Hussein, M., Ramadan, M., Shalaby, M. A., El Sharkawy, M., Hatem, D., Alaa-El-Din Wali, A., Abd-El-Fatah, S. M., Hussein, A. H., & Haggag, H. (2019). Evaluating different pain lowering medications during intrauterine device insertion: A systematic review and network meta-analysis. *Fertility and Sterility*, *111*(3), 553-561.e4. https://doi.org/10.1016/j.fertnstert.2018.11.012

Sanders, J. N., Adkins, D. E., Kaur, S., Storck, K., Gawron, L. M., & Turok, D. K. (2018). Bleeding, cramping, and satisfaction among new copper IUD users: A prospective study. *PloS One*, *13*(11), e0199724. https://doi.org/10.1371/journal.pone.0199724

Satish, S., Moore, J. F., Littlefield, J. M., Bishop, I. J., & Rojas, K. E. (2023). Re-evaluating the association between hormonal contraception and breast cancer risk. *Breast Cancer (Dove Medical Press)*, *15*, 227–235. https://doi.org/10.2147/BCTT.S390664

Schrager, S., Larson, M., Carlson, J., Ledford, K., & Ehrenthal, D. B. (2020). Beyond birth control: Noncontraceptive benefits of hormonal methods and their key role in the general medical care of women. *Journal of Women's Health (2002)*, *29*(7), 937–943. https://doi.org/10.1089/jwh.2019.7731

Schreiber, C. A., Meyn, L. A., Creinin, M. D., Barnhart, K. T., & Hillier, S. L. (2006). Effects of long-term use of nonoxynol-9 on vaginal flora. *Obstetrics and Gynecology*, *107*(1), 136–143. https://doi.org/10.1097/01.AOG.0000189094.21099.4a

Schwarz, E. B., Chiang, A. Y., Lewis, C. A., Gariepy, A. M., & Reeves, M. F. (2024). Pregnancy after Tubal Sterilization in the United States, 2002 to 2015. *NEJM Evidence*, *3*(9), EVIDoa2400023. https://doi.org/10.1056/EVIDoa2400023

Schwartz, J., Weiner, D., Lai, J., Frezieres, R., Creinin, M., Archer, D., Bradley, L., Barnhart, K., Poindexter, A., Kilbourne-Brook, M., Callahan, M., & Mauck, C. (2015). Contraceptive efficacy, safety, fit, and acceptability of a single-size diaphragm developed with end-user input. *Obstetrics & Gynecology*, *125*(4), 895–903. https://doi.org/10.1097/AOG.0000000000000721

Sharlip, I. D., Belker, A. M., Honig, S., Labrecque, M., Marmar, J. L., Ross, L. S., Sandlow, J. I., & Sokal, D. C. (2012). Vasectomy: AUA guideline. *The Journal of Urology*, *188*(6), 2482–2491. https://doi.org/10.1016/J.JURO.2012.09.080

Siemons, S. E., Vleugels, M. P. H., van Balken, M. R., Braat, D. D. M., & Nieboer, T. E. (2022). Male or female sterilization—the decision making process: Counselling and regret. *Sexual & Reproductive Healthcare: Official Journal of the Swedish Association of Midwives*, *33*, 100767. https://doi.org/10.1016/j.srhc.2022.100767

Simmons, R. G., Sanders, J. N., Geist, C., Gawron, L., Myers, K., & Turok, D. K. (2019). Predictors of contraceptive switching and discontinuation within the first 6 months of use among Highly Effective Reversible Contraceptive Initiative Salt Lake study participants. *American Journal of Obstetrics and Gynecology*, *220*(4), 376.e1–376.e12. https://doi.org/10.1016/j.ajog.2018.12.022

SINC. (n.d.). *Person Centered Reproductive Health Program*. Retrieved November 27, 2024, from https://pcrhp.ucsf.edu/sinc

Skorstengaard, M., Suhr, J., & Lynge, E. (2019). Condom use to enhance regression of cervical intraepithelial neoplasia: Study protocol for a randomized controlled trial. *Trials*, *20*(1), 473. https://doi.org/10.1186/s13063-019-3564-4

Stanton, T. A., & Blumenthal, P. D. (2019). Postpartum hormonal contraception in breastfeeding women. *Current Opinion in Obstetrics & Gynecology*, *31*(6), 441–446. https://doi.org/10.1097/GCO.0000000000000571

Steiner, M. J., Dominik, R., Rountree, R. W., Nanda, K., & Dorflinger, L. J. (2003). Contraceptive effectiveness of a polyurethane condom and a latex condom: A randomized controlled trial. *Obstetrics & Gynecology*, *101*(3), 539–547. http://www.ncbi.nlm.nih.gov/pubmed/12636960

Stifani, B. M., Peters, M., French, K., & Gill, R. K. (2023). There's an app for it: A systematic review of mobile apps providing information about abortion using a revised MARS scale. *PLOS Digital Health*, *2*(7), e0000277. https://doi.org/10.1371/journal.pdig.0000277

Stuart, G. S., & Ramesh, S. S. (2018). Interval female sterilization. *Obstetrics and Gynecology*, *131*(1), 117–124. https://doi.org/10.1097/AOG.0000000000002376

Sundaram, A., Vaughan, B., Kost, K., Bankole, A., Finer, L., Singh, S., & Trussell, J. (2017). Contraceptive failure in the United States: Estimates from the 2006–2010 National Survey of Family Growth. *Perspectives on Sexual and Reproductive Health*, *49*(1), 7–16. https://doi.org/10.1363/psrh.12017

Swan, L. E. T., Cutler, A. S., Lands, M., Schmuhl, N. B., & Higgins, J. A. (2023). Physician beliefs about contraceptive methods as abortifacients. *American Journal of Obstetrics and Gynecology*, *228*(2), 237–239. https://doi.org/10.1016/j.ajog.2022.09.039

Tone, A. (2001). *Devices and desires: A history of contraceptives in America*. Hill and Wang. https://us.macmillan.com/books/9780809038169

Torres-de la Roche, L. A., Acevedo-Mesa, A., Lizarazo, I. L., Devassy, R., Becker, S., Krentel, H., & De Wilde, R. L. (2023). Hormonal contraception and the risk of breast cancer in women of reproductive age: A meta-analysis. *Cancers*, *15*(23), 5624. https://doi.org/10.3390/cancers15235624

Turok, D. K., Gero, A., Simmons, R. G., Kaiser, J. E., Stoddard, G. J., Sexsmith, C. D., Gawron, L. M., & Sanders, J. N. (2021). Levonorgestrel vs. copper intrauterine devices for emergency contraception. *The New England Journal of Medicine, 384*(4), 335–344. https://doi.org/10.1056/NEJMoa2022141

U.S. Food and Drug Administration. (2015). *Ortho Evra (norelgestromin/ethinyl estradiol) information.* https://www.fda.gov/drugs/postmarket-drug-safety-information-patients-and-providers/ortho-evra-norelgestrominethinyl-estradiol-information

U.S. Food and Drug Administration. (2018a). FDA allows marketing of first direct-to-consumer app for contraceptive use to prevent pregnancy. https://www.fda.gov/news-events/press-announcements/fda-allows-marketing-first-direct-consumer-app-contraceptive-use-prevent-pregnancy

U.S. Food and Drug Administration. (2018b). *Understanding Unapproved Use of Approved Drugs "Off Label."* https://www.fda.gov/patients/learn-about-expanded-access-and-other-treatment-options/understanding-unapproved-use-approved-drugs-label

U.S. Food and Drug Administration. (2018c). *Statement from FDA commissioner Scott Gottlieb, M.D., on manufacturer announcement to halt Essure sales in the U.S.; agency's continued commitment to postmarket review of Essure and keeping women informed* [Press release]. https://www.fda.gov/medical-devices/essure-permanent-birth-control/fda-activities-related-essure

U.S. Food and Drug Administration. (2022). *Essure permanent birth control.* https://www.fda.gov/medical-devices/implants-and-prosthetics/essure-permanent-birth-control#s1

Van Damme, L., Ramjee, G., Alary, M., Vuylsteke, B., Chandeying, V., Rees, H., Sirivongrangson, P., Tshibaka, L. M., Ettiègne-Traoré, V., Uaheowitchai, C., Karim, S. S. A., Mâsse, B., Perriëns, J., & Laga, M., on behalf of the COL-1492 Study Group. (2002). Effectiveness of COL-1492, a nonoxynol-9 vaginal gel, on HIV-1 transmission in female sex workers: A randomised controlled trial. *Lancet, 360*(9338), 971–977. https://doi.org/10.1016/S0140-6736(02)11079-8

Van der Wijden, C., & Manion, C. (2015). Lactational amenorrhoea method for family planning. *The Cochrane Database of Systematic Reviews, 2015*(10), CD001329. https://doi.org/10.1002/14651858.CD001329.pub2

Velez, D., Pagani, R., Mima, M., & Ohlander, S. (2021). Vasectomy: A guidelines-based approach to male surgical contraception. *Fertility and Sterility, 115*(6), 1365–1368. https://doi.org/10.1016/j.fertnstert.2021.03.045

Verma, P., Saxena, S., Gunjan, Hiremath, R. N., & Sinha, P. (2023). Comparative study on menstrual disorders in post-tubal ligated and non-ligated women. *Journal of Family Medicine and Primary Care, 12*(10), 2482–2487. https://doi.org/10.4103/jfmpc.jfmpc_880_23

Wernick, H. J., Abdel-Rasoul, M., Berlan, E. D., & Bonny, A. E. (2024). Body mass index changes among adolescents and young adults using the etonogestrel contraceptive implant. *Obstetrics and Gynecology, 144*(4), 553–561. https://doi.org/10.1097/AOG.0000000000005712

Wheeler, L. J., Desanto, K., Teal, S. B., Sheeder, J., & Guntupalli, S. R. (2019). Intrauterine device use and ovarian cancer risk: A systematic review and meta-analysis. *Obstetrics and Gynecology, 134*(4), 791–800. https://doi.org/10.1097/AOG.0000000000003463

Wilcox, A. J., Dunson, D., & Baird, D. D. (2000). The timing of the "fertile window" in the menstrual cycle: Day specific estimates from a prospective study. *British Medical Journal, 321*(7271), 1259–1262.

Wilkinson, D., Ramjee, G., Tholandi, M., & Rutherford, G. W. (2002). Nonoxynol-9 for preventing vaginal acquisition of HIV infection by women from men. *Cochrane Database of Systematic Reviews.* https://doi.org/10.1002/14651858.CD003936

World Health Organization. (2020). *World Health Organization/United Nations Population Fund prequalification programme guidance for contraceptive devices: Male latex condoms, female condoms and intrauterine devices (Annex 9).* In *WHO expert committee on specifications for pharmaceutical preparations: Fifty-fourth report* (WHO Technical Report Series, No. 1025). World Health Organization. https://apps.who.int/iris/handle/10665/332888

Xu, Y., Li, L., Yang, W., Zhang, K., Ma, K., Xie, H., Zhou, J., Cai, L., Gong, Y., Zhang, Z., & Gong, K. (2021). Association between vasectomy and risk of prostate cancer: A meta-analysis. *Prostate Cancer and Prostatic Diseases, 24*(4), 962–975. https://doi.org/10.1038/s41391-021-00368-7

Yang, F., Li, J., Dong, L., Tan, K., Huang, X., Zhang, P., Liu, X., Chang, D., & Yu, X. (2021). Review of vasectomy complications and safety concerns. *The World Journal of Men's Health, 39*(3), 406–418. https://doi.org/10.5534/wjmh.200073

Ye, D.-M., Bai, X., Xu, S., Qu, N., Zhao, N., Zheng, Y., Yu, T., & Wu, H. (2024). Association between breastfeeding, mammographic density, and breast cancer risk: A review. *International Breastfeeding Journal, 19*(1), 65. https://doi.org/10.1186/s13006-024-00672-7

Yland, J. J., Bresnick, K. A., Hatch, E. E., Wesselink, A. K., Mikkelsen, E. M., Rothman, K. J., Sørensen, H. T., Huybrechts, K. F., & Wise, L. A. (2020). Pregravid contraceptive use and fecundability: Prospective cohort study. *BMJ (Clinical Research Ed.), 371*, m3966. https://doi.org/10.1136/bmj.m3966

Yoost, J. (2014). Understanding benefits and addressing misperceptions and barriers to intrauterine device access among populations in the United States. *Patient Preference and Adherence, 2014*(8), 947–957. https://doi.org/10.2147/PPA.S45710

Zadabedini Masouleh, T., Etchegary, H., Hodgkinson, K., Wilson, B. J., & Dawson, L. (2023). Beyond sterilization: A comprehensive review on the safety and efficacy of opportunistic salpingectomy as a preventative strategy for ovarian cancer. *Current Oncology (Toronto, Ont.), 30*(12), 10152–10165. https://doi.org/10.3390/curroncol30120739

Zigler, R. E., Madden, T., Ashby, C., Wan, L., & McNicholas, C. (2018). Ulipristal acetate for unscheduled bleeding in etonogestrel implant users: A randomized controlled trial. *Obstetrics and Gynecology, 132*(4), 888–894. https://doi.org/10.1097/AOG.0000000000002810

Zite, N., & Borrero, S. (2011). Female sterilisation in the United States. *European Journal of Contraception and Reproductive Health Care, 16*(5), 336–340. https://doi.org/10.3109/13625187.2011.604451

Zuniga, C., Blanchard, K., Harper, C. C., Wollum, A., Key, K., & Henderson, J. T. (2023). Effectiveness and efficacy rates of progestin-only pills: A comprehensive literature review. *Contraception, 119*, 109925. https://doi.org/10.1016/j.contraception.2022.109925

Zwayne, N., Ebersole, A., Morse, J., & Lyman, E. (2024). Society of Family Planning Committee statement: Contraception and body weight. *Contraception*, 110725. https://doi.org/10.1016/j.contraception.2024.110725

APPENDIX 13-A

Recommended Resources

Books:

Hatcher, R. A., Nelson, A. L., Trussell, J., Cwiak, C., Cason, P., Policar, M., Edelman, A., Aiken, A., Marrazzo, J., & Kowal, D. (2021). *Contraceptive technology* (22nd ed.). Ayer Company Publishers, Inc.

Hatcher, R. A., Zieman, M., Lathrop, E., Haddad, L., & Allen, A. Z. (2019). *Managing contraception* (15th ed.). Managing Contraception.

Evidence-Based App for Clinicians:

CDC Contraception 2024 (includes the current *U.S. Medical Eligibility Criteria for Contraceptive Use* and *U.S. Selected Practice Resources for Contraceptive Use* from the CDC)

Evidence-Based Apps for Patients:

Dot Fertility and Period Tracker: https://www.dottheapp.com

Natural Cycles: https://www.naturalcycles.com/

Spot On Period Tracker: https://www.plannedparenthood.org/get-care/spot-on-period-tracker

Web Resources:

U.S. Medical Eligibility Criteria for Contraceptive Use, 2024: https://www.cdc.gov/reproductivehealth/contraception/mmwr/mec/summary.html

U.S. Selected Practice Recommendations for Contraceptive Use, 2024: https://www.cdc.gov/reproductivehealth/contraception/mmwr/spr/summary.html

APPENDIX 13-B

Primary Mechanisms of Action of Contraceptive Methods[a]

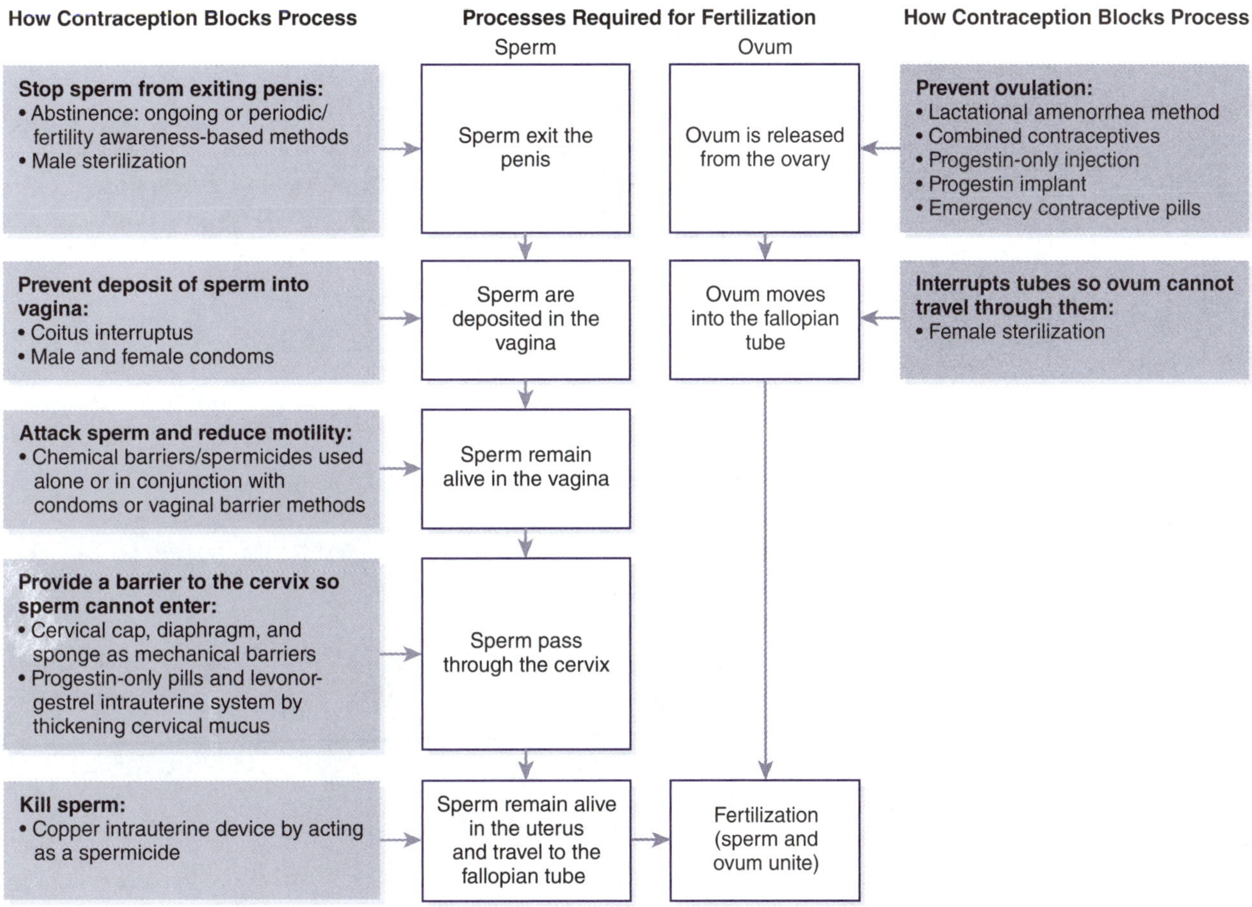

[a]Many methods have secondary mechanisms of action if the primary mechanism fails.

CHAPTER 14

Menopause

Ivy M. Alexander
Annette Jakubisin Konicki
Zahra A. Barandouzi
Christine Alexandra Bottone
Elizabeth Mayerson
Matthew Witkovic

The editors acknowledge Kathryn P. Atkin and Linda C. Andrist, who were co-authors of a previous edition of this chapter.

Menopause, defined by the North American Menopause Society as the final menstrual period and confirmed after 12 consecutive months of no menstrual bleeding, has emerged as a predominant health focus for many menopause-capable individuals (North American Menopause Society (NAMS), 2019). A major reason that menopause receives so much attention is the increasing number of people reaching midlife. Approximately 1.3 million individuals reach menopause each year in the United States, with the median age of natural menopause at 50–51 years (NAMS, 2019; Peacock et al., 2023). The baby boomer generation—people born between 1946 and 1964—is the largest middle-aged cohort ever recorded. With an estimated life expectancy of 80.2 years for menopause-capable individuals in the United States in 2022, many will live one-third of their lives after menopause (Centers for Disease Control and Prevention, 2024). We acknowledge that menopause affects women as well as other menopause-capable individuals who may not identify as women. We seek to promote inclusivity while addressing the diverse experiences of those navigating menopause. Throughout this chapter, a variety of terms are used, including menopause-capable individuals, individuals assigned female at birth (AFAB), people who menstruate or have menstruated, as well as woman/women especially when reviewing research and recommendations.

The historical emphasis on the end of reproduction ignores the myriad issues facing midlife menopause-capable individuals. Midlife brings with it many changes, such as children leaving home, illness or death of parents, and career changes. Transitions accompanying midlife include adjusting to the idea of mortality, adapting to changes in family relationships, becoming more authentic, and assessing and appreciating one's life experiences (Annual Meeting of The Menopause Society, 2023). During midlife, individuals continue to grow and develop psychologically. Increasingly, menopause is recognized as a life stage with potential for growth and development. The challenges experienced during this transition often serve as the basis for personal reflection and growth (Annual Meeting of The Menopause Society, 2023). Many individuals at midlife hold the perspective that they have processed the first half of their lives and are starting a new phase with a new lease on the second half of their lives. The transition to being postmenopausal reflects not only physical changes, but also may represent an empowering transformation to healthful self-focus.

THE MEDICALIZATION OF MENOPAUSE: A HISTORICAL PERSPECTIVE

The use of medication during perimenopause, the transition to postmenopause, and postmenopause has differed significantly over time. The view of menopause as a condition requiring medical treatment has foundations in the 19th century when the term "menopause" was first used by a French physician to describe a woman's post-reproductive years (Downham Moore, 2022; Kohn et al., 2019). Before this time, due to shorter life spans, little consideration was given to a person's post-reproductive life.

During the late 19th century, British physicians believed menopause was a form of insanity emanating from the uterus. Hysterectomy and institutionalization were common treatments, which were usually ineffective and likely harmful. Medications, such as opium and sedatives, and substances, such as lead, were also used with similar results (Downham Moore, 2022; Kohn et al., 2019). The discovery of reproductive endocrinology in the early 20th century led to the use of hormone therapy (HT) during menopause. The discovery of estrogen in the 1920s and progesterone in the 1930s were significant and largely responsible for the continued medicalization of menopause (Downham Moore, 2022; Kohn et al., 2019).

In 1942, conjugated equine estrogen (CEE) was used to produce Premarin and was recommended to "cure menopause" by preventing bothersome menopause-related symptoms, such as hot flashes, vaginal dryness, insomnia, and irritability, and to perpetuate youthfulness. Premarin was widely prescribed throughout the 1940s and 1950s. The sales of Premarin tripled from 1967 to 1975 after the 1966 publication of *Feminine Forever* written by American gynecologist Robert Wilson (Kohn et al., 2019; Wilson, 1966). This book, which was funded by a pharmaceutical company, described individuals after menopause as becoming "eunuchs" with withered breasts who begin a "living decay" (Wilson, 1966, p. 43). Estrogen was praised by Wilson as "one of the greatest biological revolutions in the history of civilization" (1966, p. 16) and was recommended for all individuals after menopause.

In 1975, researchers linked the use of estrogen to endometrial cancer (Cameron et al., 2024; El Khoudary et al., 2019; Kohn et al., 2019; Villa et al., 2024). By this time, Premarin was the fifth most popular drug in the United States. After the association between estrogen and endometrial cancer became widely known, the sales of Premarin dropped dramatically (Kohn et al., 2019).

During the late 1970s and early 1980s, continued research on menopause and menopause hormone therapy (HT, refer to **Table 14-1** for preferred terminology [NAMS, 2024]) demonstrated that adding progesterone to estrogen therapy for those with an intact uterus ameliorated the risk of endometrial cancer. Research during this time also found that HT decreased the risk of cardiovascular disease (CVD), bone fracture, and Alzheimer's disease (Kohn et al., 2019; Peacock et al., 2023). All-cause mortality in individuals taking HT also decreased. These findings, along with the established effectiveness of HT for symptomatic menopause, contributed to renewed increase in prescriptions for HT throughout the 1980s (Cameron et al., 2024; Villa et al., 2024).

Through the mid- and late 1980s, observational and case-controlled research results continued to show that HT prevented diseases associated with older age, such as osteoporosis and heart disease. Research results also demonstrated an increased risk of breast cancer related to HT use (Cameron et al., 2024; El Khoudary et al., 2019; Kohn et al., 2019; Peacock et al., 2023). These negative results were minimized because some of the results were contradictory. Some results showed an increased risk of breast cancer in individuals taking estrogen and progesterone therapy (EPT). Other results showed a decreased risk of breast cancer in those who took only estrogen therapy (ET). Still other studies demonstrated an increased risk of breast cancer with improved survival in individuals on HT (Cameron et al., 2024; Kohn et al., 2019; Peacock et al., 2023). Despite this, HT continued to be prescribed in increasing numbers due to the understanding that HT helped to reduce the risks of heart disease and the fact that the risk of death from CVD was higher than the risk of death from breast cancer. Until findings from the Women's Health Initiative (WHI) were released in 2002, many clinicians routinely recommended HT to most postmenopausal people, regardless of symptomatology (Cameron et al., 2024; El Khoudary et al., 2019; Villa et al., 2024).

TABLE 14-1 Preferred Terminology for Menopause Hormone Therapy

Term	Abbreviation and/or Explanation
Estrogen therapy	ET
Estrogen with progestogen therapy	EPT
Hormone therapy	HT; encompassing term including both ET and EPT
Progestogen	Encompassing term for progesterone and progestin

Data from North American Menopause Society (NAMS). (2024). Menopause glossary. https://www.menopause.org/for-individuals/menopause-glossary#E

Note: The North American Menopause Society (NAMS), now The Menopause Society (TMS), has urged clinicians, researchers, and the media to standardize terminology, which it considers essential for ensuring accurate communication. Note that the word "replacement" has been deleted from the terms "hormone replacement therapy" and "estrogen replacement therapy."

Results from the WHI, designed like a statin trial with the end point being outcomes on CVD, shifted the use of HT and ET to symptom management (Kohn et al., 2019; Peacock et al., 2023). The WHI findings for the HT arm upheld the known risks for breast cancer among those taking HT and identified risks for heart disease, stroke, and venous thromboembolism. Despite beneficial effects against osteoporosis-related fractures and colon cancer, the study had to be stopped early due to identification of cardiovascular, stroke, and venous thromboembolism risks among participants (Cameron et al., 2024; El Khoudary et al., 2019; Kohn et al., 2019; Peacock et al., 2023). Similarly, the ET arm was stopped early, in 2004, after a cumulative review of the data demonstrated an increased risk of stroke with no significant benefit for coronary artery disease (Cameron et al., 2024; El Khoudary et al., 2019; Kohn et al., 2019; Peacock et al., 2023).

The WHI findings were widely reported in the media, and the use of HT fell dramatically (Cameron et al., 2024; El Khoudary et al., 2019; Kohn et al., 2019; Peacock et al., 2023). Clinicians stopped recommending HT due to fear of breast cancer and doubtful cardiovascular benefit. Individuals with severe menopause-related symptoms had difficulty finding a healthcare provider who would prescribe HT, even if they were healthy and at low risk for breast cancer or CVD (Cameron et al., 2024; Downham Moore, 2022; Kohn et al., 2019; Peacock et al., 2023). The pendulum had swung from most peri- and most menopausal individuals receiving a recommendation to use and prescription for HT in the 1960s and 1970s, to most not receiving a prescription for HT by the early 2000s, regardless of menopause-related symptoms (Cameron et al., 2024; Downham Moore, 2022).

Fortunately, the research continued. Data from the WHI was still being examined, participants were followed over time, and new research studies were conducted. One of the criticisms of the initially reported WHI data was the finding that some associations were ignored, specifically the association of cardiovascular benefit with HT use among individuals younger than age 60 and reduced breast cancer overall in those taking ET in that arm of the WHI (Downham Moore, 2022). Continued examination of WHI data, along with ongoing research, has further clarified the indications for and risks associated with use of HT (Cameron et al., 2024; Canivenc-Lavier & Bennetau-Pelisser, 2023; Downham Moore, 2022; El Khoudary et al., 2019; Kohn et al., 2019). Additional research, conducted during the mid- to late 2000s and the following decade, focused on the timing of HT (e.g., what would the results be if HT were used in younger people who are just becoming postmenopausal?), length of use of HT, and further risk stratification (e.g., what might the differences be in women at low risk for breast cancer or CVD?) (Cameron et al., 2024; Villa et al., 2024). The compounds and formulations of HT were also examined (Canivenc-Lavier & Bennetau-Pelissero, 2023; Downham Moore, 2022). The estrogen used in the WHI was CEE; the progesterone used was medroxyprogesterone acetate (MPA) (Downham Moore, 2022; El Khoudary et al., 2019). This was seen as a limitation to the WHI, and later research evaluated the

BOX 14-1 NAMS 2022 Position Statement Recommendations for Menopause Hormone Therapy Use

- Hormone therapy (HT) is the most effective treatment for vasomotor and genitourinary symptoms of menopause. HT prevents bone loss and thus reduces fracture risk. The best risk-to-benefit ratio for HT use is among symptomatic women younger than age 60 or within 10 years of menopause onset, provided they have no contraindications to HT.
- Women older than age 60 or more than 10 years from becoming postmenopausal have more risk than benefit from HT because of higher absolute risks of coronary heart disease, stroke, venous thromboembolism, and dementia, which are more prevalent with age.
- Risks of HT differ depending on the type and formulation of HT used, the duration of HT use, the timing of HT related to either age or length of time since becoming postmenopausal, and whether progesterone is needed.
- Treatment with HT should be individualized with ongoing assessment of risk versus benefit. Generally, the lowest effective dose of HT should be used, and the duration of use should be based on need.
- Longer duration of HT may be safer for estrogen therapy regimens, compared to estrogen with progestogen regimens.
- HT may be continued for individuals older than 60 to 65 years based on the person's preference, quality of life, vasomotor symptoms, and need for osteoporosis prevention, keeping in mind the risk-to-benefit ratio and contraindications.
- Low-dose vaginal estrogen therapies may be used by postmenopausal women of any age for persistent genitourinary symptoms of menopause.
- Compounded bioidentical treatments present safety concerns due to lack of U.S. Food and Drug Administration (FDA) oversight and lack of standardization.

Data from North American Menopause Society. (2022). The 2022 hormone therapy position statement of the North American Menopause Society. *Menopause, 29*(7), 767–794. https://doi.org/10.1097/GME.0000000000002028

effects of various preparations of estrogen and progesterone. In 2022, NAMS published an evidence-based position statement on HT that included updates based on these most recent research findings (Cameron et al., 2024; NAMS, 2022; Peacock et al., 2023) (**Box 14-1**).

In summary, medical treatment for menopause-related symptoms has varied widely over time. HT, which did not exist before the 20th century, has been established as an effective treatment for menopause-related symptoms in postmenopausal individuals. However, knowledge of the risks and benefits of HT has continued to evolve. Although it is currently understood that becoming postmenopausal is a normal transition (Cameron et al., 2024; Downham Moore, 2022; NAMS, 2019, 2022), it is also understood that treating symptoms related to menopause as a healthcare issue of importance with available options for pharmacologic management, if so desired, is here to stay (Cameron et al., 2024; NAMS, 2022; Peacock et al., 2023).

NATURAL MENOPAUSE

Menopause occurs in response to normal physiologic changes in the hypothalamic–pituitary–ovarian axis. Refer to Chapter 7 for a detailed description of the menstrual cycle. During the perimenopausal period, which spans approximately 2 to 8 years prior to the last menstrual period, and for the 12 months of amenorrhea preceding menopause, fewer ovarian follicles develop in each menstrual cycle. Anovulation is common during this period because the follicles that do develop are less responsive to follicle-stimulating hormone (FSH), and the ovaries produce less estradiol, progesterone, and androgens. Thus, the usual negative feedback effect from elevated estrogen and progesterone levels on hypothalamic production of gonadotropin-releasing hormone (GnRH) is lost, and the anterior pituitary production of FSH and luteinizing hormone (LH) continues. Irregular menstrual cycles—characterized by longer or shorter cycles, heavier or lighter flow, periods of amenorrhea, and worsening or newly developing premenstrual symptoms—are common during this time. Eventually, ovarian follicle production stops, estrogen and progesterone levels remain low despite elevated FSH and LH levels, and menstruation ceases. The early postmenopausal period refers to the first 5 years following menopause when hormonal fluctuations often continue and rapid bone loss occurs, increasing the individual's risk for osteoporosis. The late postmenopausal period refers to 6 years after the final menstrual period through the remaining life span. This phase is marked by increasing genitourinary symptoms due to reduced estrogen levels and increased risks for CVD (NAMS, 2019; Sundheimer & Nathan, 2019).

An AFAB individual is born with approximately 1.2 million ovarian follicles. Throughout their life, fewer than 500 of these follicles are used during ovulation; most are lost through atresia until menopause, when approximately 1,000 follicles remain. The decline in follicles occurs at a constantly increasing rate, with a more rapid decline occurring with increasing age (NAMS, 2019; Sundheimer & Nathan, 2019).

Although it sounds like a smoothly functioning process, the transition to postmenopause is anything but smooth for many. Hormone levels can fluctuate wildly from day to day, causing many of the symptoms associated with perimenopause and the transition to postmenopause (**Box 14-2**). Hormone fluctuation is related to many factors, including the reduced number of responsive ovarian follicles, and does not correlate with symptoms. Due to these fluctuations, measuring hormones during this time does not provide meaningful clinical data to guide care and is not recommended (NAMS, 2019; Sundheimer & Nathan, 2019).

Contrary to popular belief, individuals continue to produce estrogen and androgens after menopause. Three types of estrogen exist:

- Estradiol (E_2), the most potent of the three, is the main estrogen produced during the reproductive years. It is present in low amounts in the postmenopausal years following peripheral conversion of androstenedione.

BOX 14-2 Symptoms Associated with Perimenopause and Postmenopause

- Acne
- Arthralgia
- Asthenia
- Decreased libido
- Decreased vaginal lubrication
- Depression
- Dizziness
- Dry eyes
- Dry/thinning hair
- Dyspareunia
- Dysuria
- Fatigue
- Forgetfulness
- Formication
- Headache
- Hirsutism/virilization
- Hot flashes/flushes
- Irregular menses/bleeding
- Irritability/mood disturbances
- Mastalgia
- Myalgia
- Nervousness/anxiety
- Night sweats
- Nocturia
- Odor
- Palpitations
- Paresthesia
- Poor concentration
- Recurrent cystitis
- Recurrent vaginitis
- Skin dryness/atrophy
- Sleep disturbances/insomnia
- Urinary frequency
- Urinary urgency
- Vaginal atrophy
- Vaginal/vulvar burning
- Vaginal/vulvar irritation
- Vaginal/vulvar pruritus

Data from North American Menopause Society. (2019). *Menopause practice: A clinician's guide* (6th ed.); Sundheimer, L. W., & Nathan, L. (2019). Menopause and postmenopause. In A. H. DeCherney, L. Nathan, N. Laufer, & A. S. Roman (Eds.), *Current diagnosis & treatment: Obstetrics & gynecology* (12th ed., pp. 989–1014). McGraw Hill.

- Estriol (E_3) is secreted by the placenta and synthesized from androgens produced by the fetus during pregnancy. It is present in nonpregnant individuals in small amounts as a byproduct of estradiol and estrone.
- Estrone (E_1), the weakest estrogen, is the primary estrogen present in children, men, and postmenopausal individuals. In the postmenopausal period, estrone is produced by adipose conversion of androstenedione secreted by the adrenals (95%) and, to a lesser extent, the ovaries (5%), and by metabolism of estradiol.

Postmenopausal ovaries no longer produce estrogen or functional follicles; however, the corticostromal and hilar cells of the stromal tissue are steroidogenic and produce significant levels of both androstenedione and testosterone for many years. Circulating levels of androstenedione in postmenopausal individuals are approximately half those of premenopausal individuals. Conversely, circulating levels of testosterone remain relatively constant in either premenopausal or postmenopausal individuals, partly due to the presence of high FSH and LH levels, which stimulate the ovarian stromal tissues to increase their testosterone production (NAMS, 2019; Sundheimer & Nathan, 2019).

The age at natural menopause ranges from 40 to 58 years, with a median age of 51–52 years (NAMS, 2019; Peacock et al., 2023). The age when menopause will occur is difficult to predict for an individual person, but it does correlate with the age when their mother or older sisters experienced menopause (Sundheimer & Nathan, 2019). Emerging data suggest that genetic factors may influence the age of menopause, and genome-wide association studies have had some success in revealing genetic determinants for menopause (Wang, et al., 2019).

A number of other factors that may affect the age at menopause have been studied. Cigarette smoking has consistently been found to correlate with age at menopause. Specifically, smokers are likely to experience menopause at a younger age than those who do not smoke (Zhu et al., 2018). Smokers are also at increased risk for early menopause, which is defined as menopause before age 45 (Whitcomb et al., 2018). Body size has been identified as a contributing factor to the age of menopause since body fat stores androstenedione and converts it to estrogen. Those with smaller bodies are at increased risk for early menopause, while those with larger bodies are likely to experience menopause later (Zhu et al., 2018). A higher level of education and history of oral contraceptive use are also associated with a later age at menopause (Gold et al., 2013). Multiple studies have examined race and ethnicity in relationship to individuals' experience of menopause (Chadha et al., 2016; Gold et al., 2013; Im et al., 2014; Solomon et al., 2016). Age at menopause appears to be related to health and socioeconomic factors (e.g., higher educational level, being employed, and better self-rated health status), rather than race and ethnicity.

MENOPAUSE FROM OTHER CAUSES

Menopause can also occur due to several other causes (Brent et al., 2023; NAMS, 2019). Induced menopause occurs following either surgical excision of both ovaries (bilateral oophorectomy) or ovarian function ablation caused by medication, chemotherapy, or radiation. Although menstruation and fertility cease immediately following surgical menopause, both may persist for several months after ablative treatments are given.

Primary ovarian insufficiency, previously referred to as premature ovarian failure or premature menopause, is a temporary or permanent loss of ovarian function leading to amenorrhea in those younger than 40 years. Primary ovarian insufficiency affects approximately 1 percent of AFAB reproductive age people, and can be related to a disease entity, or it can be medication induced or idiopathic (Brent et al., 2023; NAMS, 2019). It is often associated with other health problems, such as autoimmune and genetic disorders. Turner syndrome is the most common genetic disorder seen in those diagnosed with primary ovarian insufficiency, with most individuals with Turner syndrome reaching menopause by early adulthood (Viuff & Gravholt, 2022). Fragile x syndrome, Fanconi anemia, ataxia-telangiectasia, Bloom syndrome, Werner syndrome, and mumps infection have also been linked to primary ovarian insufficiency (Poteet et al., 2023).

Individuals who experience induced or premature menopause have early loss of fertility and often experience more severe symptoms. Not only does primary ovarian insufficiency affect quality of life, but it also increases the risk for developing CVD, osteoporosis, and cognitive impairment with aging. Untreated primary ovarian insufficiency also has been shown to decrease life expectancy and hormone therapy is recommended (Nash & Davies, 2024).

DIAGNOSING MENOPAUSE

Menopause is a retrospective diagnosis because it is based on the clinical absence of menses for 12 consecutive months. Serial FSH testing that revealed sustained levels greater than 40 mIU/mL was used in the past to determine menopause status. However, serum FSH testing is no longer required or recommended for determining menopause status because FSH levels can fluctuate, returning to normal, causing estrogen levels to rise unexpectedly high enough to trigger the LH surge needed for ovulation (NAMS, 2019; Peacock et al., 2023).

The Stages of Reproductive Aging Workshop (STRAW) created a staging system to standardize terminology when assessing reproductive aging in menopause-capable individuals. The initial workshop proposed stages of reproductive aging based on bleeding and FSH levels (Harlow et al., 2012). Ten years later, in 2011, the criteria were reevaluated by a multinational interprofessional team that incorporated newer data on FSH, anti-Müllerian hormone (AMH), antral follicle count, inhibin B, and postmenopausal changes in FSH and estradiol levels to create what is known as STRAW + 10 (Harlow et al., 2012; Harlow et al., 2023). Menstrual criteria do not apply to those with irregular cycles or those who have undergone hysterectomy or ablation. In these patients, endocrine markers are helpful (Harlow et al., 2023). For example, serum anti-Müllerian hormone (AMH) reflects the number of follicles remaining in the ovaries and a decline can indicate earlier menopause (Nelson et al., 2023). STRAW + 10 is the gold standard used to characterize reproductive aging. As shown in **Figure 14-1**, there are seven stages: five prior to and two after the final menstrual cycle with Stages -1 and -2 representing the transition to postmenopause and the onset of perimenopausal symptoms (Harlow et al., 2012; Harlow et al., 2023; Srivastava & Sreelatha, 2024).

AMH has been identified as a marker of ovarian reserve, although serum blood tests for AMH have been used primarily among those seeking fertility assessment. Research has identified that AMH may be helpful in identifying when an individual can expect to be postmenopausal; its level drops to an undetectable point approximately 5 years before menopause (Nelson et al., 2023). Limited data exist for the use of AMH testing outside of fertility assessment, and standardized assays using this test for prediction of menopause are lacking. Therefore, AMH testing to predict the time to menopause is not recommended; assessment of ovarian reserve with an AMH level is sometimes used in assessment of primary ovarian insufficiency (Nash & Davies, 2024).

Perimenopause refers to the time when individuals begin to experience cycle irregularities and other menopause-related symptoms, such as hot flashes and vaginal dryness, and it ends when the diagnosis of postmenopause is made after 12 months of amenorrhea. This period is often when people experience the most symptoms related to menopause, making this the most difficult period for many (Srivastava & Sreelatha, 2024). Because unexpected ovulation can occur in perimenopause, patients should be counseled accordingly, and can continue to use contraception if they desire. Refer to Chapter 13 for information about contraception. Perimenopausal individuals experience a high rate of unintended pregnancies; an estimated 75 percent of pregnancies in those older than age 40 are unplanned with an estimated 40 percent choosing to continue the pregnancy (Dalmijn et al., 2024).

Differential Diagnoses

Other health problems can mimic the symptoms of menopause and must also be considered when a person presents with perimenopause- and menopause-related symptoms (NAMS, 2019). These diagnoses may include diabetes, hypertension, arrhythmias, thyroid disorders (hypo- or hyperthyroid), anemia, depression, tumors, or carcinoma. A sample list of differential diagnoses is provided in **Table 14-2**. Medications, alcohol, or drug use can also cause many symptoms similar to those associated with perimenopause and menopause. For example, alcohol can cause warmth and flushing, which is like the experience of hot flashes. Complicating this is that some postmenopausal individuals are at increased risk for drinking alcohol, in particular binge drinking (Kronemyer, 2023).

Every patient presenting with suspected menopause-related symptoms must be carefully evaluated with a thorough history, physical examination, and selective laboratory testing (such as a complete blood count, fasting glucose, serum thyroid-stimulating hormone [TSH] level, and prolactin level) to accurately identify the cause of the symptoms. Often a person has several diagnoses to contend with at once, such as hypertension, diabetes, and postmenopause. Controlling diabetes and hypertension may also reduce menopause-related symptoms enough so they are no longer bothersome. It is important for the healthcare provider to keep in mind that many differential diagnoses for menopause-related symptoms may coexist with postmenopause.

PRESENTATION AND VARIATION OF THE MENOPAUSE EXPERIENCE

The experience of menopause is unique and personal. Some individuals have severe symptoms that disrupt all aspects of their lives, whereas others find menopause to be almost a nonevent and report no bothersome symptoms. Most symptoms that do occur are related to reduced levels of estrogen and progesterone.

FIGURE 14-1 **STRAW + 10 staging system for reproductive aging in individuals.**

Menarche (at stage −5) FMP(0) (at stage +1a)

Stage	**−5**	**−4**	**−3b**	**−3a**	**−2**	**−1**	**+1a**	**+1b**	**+1c**	**+2**
Terminology	**REPRODUCTIVE**				**MENOPAUSAL TRANSITION**		**POSTMENOPAUSE**			
	Early	Peak	Late		Early	Late	Early			Late
					Perimenopause					
Duration	variable				variable	1–3 years	2 years (1+1)		3–6 years	Remaining life span
PRINCIPAL CRITERIA										
Menstrual cycle	Variable to regular	Regular	Regular	Subtle changes in flow/ length	Variable length persistent ≥ 7 day difference in length of consecutive cycles	Interval of amenorrhea of ≥ 60 days				
SUPPORTIVE CRITERIA										
Endocrine										
FSH			Low	Variable	↑ Variable*	↑ ≥ 25 IU/L**	↑ Variable		Stabilizes	
AMH			Low	Low	Low	Low	Low		Very Low	
Inhibin B				Low	Low	Low	Low		Very Low	
Antral Follicle Count			Low	Low	Low	Low	Very Low		Very Low	
DESCRIPTIVE CHARACTERISTICS										
Symptoms						Vasomotor symptoms *Likely*	Vasomotor symptoms *Most Likely*			Increasing symptoms of urogenital atrophy

* Blood draw on cycle days 2–5 ↑ = elevated

** Approximate expected level based on assays using current international pituitary standard

Reproduced from Harlow, S. D., Gass, M., Hall, J. E., Lobo, R., Maki, P., Rebar, R. W., Sherman, S., Sluss, P. M., & de Villiers, T. J. (2012). Executive summary of the Stages of Reproductive Aging Workshop + 10: Addressing the unfinished agenda of staging reproductive aging. *The Journal of Clinical Endocrinology and Metabolism, 97*(4), 1159–1168. https://doi.org/10.1210/jc.2011-3362

Two types of estrogen receptors have been identified (alpha and beta); they are in the cognitive and vasomotor centers of the brain, as well as in the eyes, skin, heart, vascular system, gastrointestinal tract, breast tissue, urogenital tract, and bone. Progesterone receptors have been identified in the hypothalamus, pituitary, and vasomotor areas of the brain, as well as in the heart, vascular tissues, lung, breast, pancreas, gynecologic organs, and bones. As hormone levels rise and fall, related symptoms may develop. An individual's symptom experience may correlate with body size because adipose tissues store and convert androstenedione to estrogen. Additionally, individuals living in larger bodies are more likely to experience more frequent and severe hot flashes, poor quality of sleep, aches and joint pain, genitourinary symptoms, and reduced quality of life than individuals living in smaller bodies. (NAMS, 2019; Palacios et al., 2024).

Both the type (Box 14-2) and severity of menopause-related symptoms can vary. Symptoms usually begin in the perimenopausal period, then gradually increase in severity during the early postmenopausal period, reaching a peak in the first 2 years after the final menstrual period. The symptoms that individuals report most frequently are vasomotor in nature, including hot flashes, hot flushes, and sweats. Most symptomatic individuals will experience vasomotor symptoms on average for about 5 years after menopause, and approximately one-third of individuals will

TABLE 14-2 Examples of Differential Diagnoses with Symptoms Similar to Perimenopause- and Menopause-Related Symptoms

Diagnosis	Symptoms Similar to Perimenopause/Menopause
Anemia	Fatigue Cognitive changes (e.g., forgetfulness, short-term memory changes)
Anovulation	Amenorrhea
Arrhythmias	Fatigue Palpitations
Arthritis	Joint aches and pain
Depression	Fatigue Moodiness Anxiety Sleep disturbances, insomnia
Diabetes	Fatigue Hot flashes and heat intolerance
Hyperprolactinemia	Menstrual cycle changes
Hypertension	Headaches
Hyperthyroidism	Sleep disturbance, insomnia Nervousness, irritability Heat intolerance
Hypothyroidism	Fatigue Dry skin Cognitive problems (e.g., forgetfulness, short-term memory changes, poor recall)
Infections (viral illnesses, HIV, influenza, fever, tuberculosis, sexually transmitted infections)	Vasomotor symptoms (e.g., hot flushes, insomnia, palpitations, night sweats) Dyspareunia Cystitis symptoms (e.g., pelvic discomfort, increased urinary frequency, urinary urgency) Vaginitis (vaginal irritation, changes in vaginal discharge, dyspareunia)
Medication side effects	Hot flashes (can occur with some antihypertensives and lipid-lowering medications) Reduced libido and anorgasmia (can occur with some lipid-lowering medications and antidepressants)
Pregnancy Spontaneous abortion Uterine fibroids Uterine polyps Endometriosis Adenomyosis Ovarian cysts Ovarian tumors	Abnormal uterine bleeding Menstrual changes
Vulvar dystrophy	Vaginal atrophy Dyspareunia

experience these symptoms for 10 years or more after menopause (Freedman, 2014). Individuals whose vasomotor symptoms begin earlier in the transition to postmenopause are likely to have a longer total duration of symptoms and a longer persistence of symptoms after menopause. Black individuals have the longest duration of vasomotor symptoms, followed by Hispanic and white individuals; Chinese and Japanese individuals have the shortest duration (Avis et al., 2015). Race and ethnicity have shown not to be associated with severity of menopause depressive symptoms (Ji et al., 2021).

Hot flashes are experienced as an intense heat sensation and may or may not be followed by sweating, which can be profuse. They are characterized by a measurable increase in skin temperature and conductance, which is followed by a decrease in core body temperature. Hot flushes are like hot flashes and include a flushing over the face and upper chest, most likely due to peripheral vascular dilation. Vasomotor symptoms that occur during the night are termed night sweats. Hot flashes occur concurrently with a surge in LH levels. Although the relationship between LH secretion and body temperature change is poorly understood, the same mechanisms that trigger the hypothalamic event causing the temperature increase also stimulate GnRH secretion and cause LH elevation. Many individuals feel cold following a hot flash owing to the reduction in core temperature; this effect is exacerbated if sweating is also present. Postmenopausal individuals are more sensitive to core temperature changes because their thermoneutral zone—the range of internally recognized normal core body temperature—narrows (Freedman, 2014; Pérez-Medina-Carballo et al., 2023). Thus, when an individual's core temperature rises, they feel overly hot; when it falls, they feel overly chilled.

Sleep disruptions are also common, both during the menopause transition and in postmenopause. Some of these sleep changes are related to normal aging, such as reduced time in sleep stage 3 (early deep sleep) and sleep stage 4 (deep sleep and relaxation), more periods of brief arousal, and an overall decreased need for sleep. Hot flashes and sweats can further interrupt sleep (NAMS, 2019; Palacios et al., 2024). Poor sleep is associated with somatic, mood, and cognitive symptoms as well as performance deficits. Individuals experiencing poor sleep may demonstrate an inability to concentrate, lethargy, fatigue, difficulty performing tasks, and a lack of motivation. Additionally, poor sleep has been linked to some chronic illnesses, such as cardiac disease, diabetes, and depression (NAMS, 2019).

Urogenital changes from decreased estrogen lead to atrophy and affect all individuals not using estrogen replacement. Collectively identified as genitourinary syndrome of menopause (GSM), individuals may experience vaginal dryness and dyspareunia (Kagan & Rivera, 2018; NAMS, 2019, 2020, 2022). GSM can also predispose individuals to urinary tract infections. The risk of urinary incontinence increases with age; however, this condition is never considered normal. Refer to Chapter 23 for additional information on urinary incontinence. Low estrogen has been suggested as a factor contributing to the increased prevalence of urinary incontinence among postmenopausal individuals; however, decreases in serum estradiol levels have not been shown to cause or worsen symptoms of urinary incontinence among individuals who are transitioning to postmenopause (Li et al., 2024).

Many normal changes of aging can also affect sexual function, such as longer time to achieve vaginal lubrication and production of fewer vaginal secretions overall; reduced vaginal elasticity, pigment, rugation, and number of superficial epithelial cells, leading to increased petechiae and bleeding following minor trauma (including sexual activity); reduced lactobacilli populations, which increase pH and the risk of infection; and atrophy of adipose and collagen tissue in the vulva. Individuals may also experience lowered libido, lessened sexual activity, problems with their partner's sexual performance, or relationship problems that make them less interested in sex (NAMS, 2019, 2020, 2022). Whatever the causes of dyspareunia or sexual dysfunction may be, this subject is often difficult for individuals to broach with their clinicians. Thus, it is important for clinicians to ask individuals about sexual function and satisfaction and remain open to the fact that sexual expression can take many forms. Refer to Chapters 11, 12, and 18 for more information.

An individual's expectations for menopause may also affect their experience. These can range from no expectations to positive or negative expectations to uncertainty. Individuals with higher levels of perceived stress and negative attitudes toward menopause and aging are more likely to experience more severe symptoms. Similarly, an individual's response to menopause can affect the experience. Many people view menopause as a natural life transition and may not be interested in any treatment options besides lifestyle changes. Others see it as a disruption of their lives and a sign of aging that they want to minimize as much as possible. Many individuals identify menopause as a time for reflection and reevaluation of their lives and health (Johnston-Ataata et al., 2020).

MIDLIFE HEALTH ISSUES

Health risks change for individuals at midlife, partly due to the changed hormonal milieu and partly due to other normal aging processes. At this point in life, people are at increased risk for developing heart disease, osteoporosis, and diabetes. Weight management can also be a significant issue. Refer to Chapter 9 for a full discussion of routine health screening at midlife.

Changes in Body Size

Although individuals tend to associate increased weight with postmenopause, weight gain in midlife is primarily the result of lifestyle changes and aging processes and are related to a combination of both modifiable and nonmodifiable factors (Khandelwal, 2020). Regardless of racial background or body size, research shows that midlife individuals gain an average of 1.5 pounds each year during the fifth and sixth decade. This weight increase is partly due to the decrease in muscle mass that occurs with age and the associated decrease in resting metabolic rate (Ambikairajah, Tabatabaei-Jafari, & Cherbuin, 2019), and partly due to a decrease in activity that often accompanies midlife. Menopause-associated sleep disturbance, lack of estrogen, and mood disorders may also contribute to weight gain (NAMS, 2019). Maintaining one's weight through midlife usually requires a reduction in caloric intake and an increase in physical activity.

Not only does weight often increase at midlife, the tendency for central fat distribution is also heightened (Ambikairajah et al., 2019; Khandelwal, 2020). Premenopausal individuals typically have a gynoid (lower body) adipose tissue distribution that is primarily in the hips and thighs (pear-shaped body). As individuals age, however, adipose tissue is more in the android pattern, redistributing and accumulating at the waist (apple-shaped body). Abdominal adiposity and weight gain at midlife are significant issues. This can be associated with adverse metabolic outcomes, including dysglycemia, dyslipidemia, and hypertension, as well as increased risk of CVD, some cancers, and other serious health outcomes (Ambikairajah et al., 2019; Hales et al., 2020; Khandelwal, 2020).

Increased weight and central body changes may potentiate negative body image concerns for individuals. In addition, those who are overweight or obese have a greater frequency of vasomotor symptoms (Anderson et al., 2020). The 2014 joint clinical guidelines for interventions and counseling for individuals who are overweight and obese (the most current version of these guidelines) from the American Heart Association, the American College of Cardiology, and the Obesity Society are available to guide healthcare providers in identifying and treating individuals with overweight or obesity (Jensen et al., 2014). The American Heart Association also provides guidance for clinicians to counsel patients on dietary patterns (Volpp et al., 2023). When counseling patients, it is crucial for clinicians to remember that weight bias and stigma about weight gain can have a profound negative effect on individuals and their health. Counteracting these effects with patient-centered counseling strategies can reduce these negative experiences and build trust between the clinician and patient, providing further opportunities for a constructive clinician/patient relationship and health promotion (Puhl et al., 2021).

Cardiovascular Disease

Cardiovascular disease (CVD) is the number one cause of mortality for all people in the United States. CVD is an inclusive term that refers to conditions such as hypertension, valvular heart disease, and coronary heart disease, which lead to angina or myocardial infarction, stroke, arrhythmias, congestive heart failure, peripheral arterial disease, aortic disease, arterial and venous thrombosis, pulmonary embolism, and congenital heart defects. One in three menopause-capable individuals in the United States have some form of CVD, with more than 400,000 of them dying from CVD in the United States each year (Benjamin, et al., 2019). Due to advancements in prevention, diagnosis, and treatment, U.S. rates of CVD mortality have declined in recent years. Nevertheless, CVD is the most common cause of disability-adjusted life-years (a measure that considers both morbidity and mortality) among menopause-capable people the United States (Woodward, 2019). Notably, CVD disproportionately affects vulnerable populations, including those who have low socioeconomic status or whose race and ethnicity is non-white (Kandasamy & Anand, 2018).

The risk for CVD significantly increases after menopause. Menopause does not appear to solely increase CVD risk; chronologic aging also plays a role (El Khoudary & Thurston, 2018). Lipid changes in postmenopausal individuals include increases in total cholesterol, triglycerides, apolipoprotein B, and LDL cholesterol. HDL cholesterol levels may also change after menopause; however, the HDL cholesterol changes are not in a consistent direction, and their implications are less clear than other postmenopausal lipid changes (El Khoudary & Thurston, 2018). As menopause-capable individuals age, they experience a faster increase in left ventricular wall thickness and more age-related concentric remodeling than others. Postmenopausal individuals also have decreased elasticity in the vascular system and associated hypertension.

Prevention of risk factors and treatment of existing risk factors are key to reducing CVD-associated morbidity and mortality (Cho et al., 2020). Major risk factors for CVD include age, cigarette smoking, physical inactivity, family history of premature CVD, hypertension, dyslipidemia, obesity, and diabetes. Menopause-capable specific CVD risk factors include premature menopause and adverse pregnancy outcomes (APOs) (Arnett et al., 2019; Jowell et al., 2022; Søndergaard et al., 2020).

Type 2 Diabetes

The likelihood of developing type 2 diabetes increases with age and may be further increased by the biochemical, metabolic, and phenotypical changes associated with menopause (Lambrinoudaki et al., 2022). This disease disproportionately affects individuals of minority racial and ethnic groups, including Black, Native American, Latinx, Asian American, and Pacific Islander individuals. General risk factors for developing diabetes include overweight and obesity (BMI of 25 or greater), physical inactivity, history of gestational diabetes or polycystic ovary syndrome, family history of diabetes, age of 45 years or older, hypertension, dyslipidemia and obstructive sleep apnea–induced hypoxia (Ismail, Materwala, & Al Kaabi, 2021). In addition to significantly increasing the risk for CVD and cerebrovascular disease, diabetes increases the risk for developing infections, foot ulcers, peripheral vascular disease, peripheral neuropathy, nephropathy, and retinopathy (American Diabetes Association [ADA], 2024).

Individuals with impaired fasting glucose levels (100 to 125 mg/dL) or impaired glucose tolerance (2-hour post 75 gm glucose load of 140 to 199 mg/dL) are identified as having prediabetes. It is important to encourage lifestyle modifications, such as increasing activity levels, dietary changes, and weight loss, for those with prediabetes because such changes have been shown to delay or even prevent the onset of diabetes (ADA, 2024). The American Association of Clinical Endocrinologists recommends weight loss as the primary management goal for individuals with prediabetes through therapeutic lifestyle changes, medications, surgery, or a combination of these methods (Samson, et al., 2023). Insulin resistance is reduced with weight loss and can prevent progression to diabetes and improve lipids and blood pressure.

Managing diabetes can be more difficult for individuals after menopause. The effects of the hormonal changes of menopause on glucose homeostasis, insulin resistance, and insulin secretion are not completely understood (Samson et al., 2023). Decreased estrogen, relative increased androgenicity, weight gain, and changes in body composition may all contribute to the increased glucose levels identified during and after the transition to postmenopause (Slopien et al., 2018). The treatment goals for diabetes are to prevent complications and optimize quality of life (ADA, 2024). Lifestyle management includes weight management, healthy eating, physical activity and exercise, and smoking cessation (ADA, 2024). Most postmenopausal individuals with type 2 diabetes will need pharmacologic treatment (Paschou et al., 2019; Slopien et al., 2018). Metformin is the preferred first-line therapeutic option. Initiation of statin therapy in individuals older than age 40 with diabetes and controlling blood pressure are recommended to further reduce the risk of CVD and complications from diabetes (ADA, 2024).

Cancer

In 2024, the types of cancer most commonly causing mortality among menopause-capable individuals in the United States were estimated to be lung and bronchus (21%), followed by breast (15%), colon and rectum (8%), and pancreatic (8%) cancers. The types of cancer expected to be the most frequently diagnosed were breast cancer (30%), lung and bronchus (12%), colon and rectum (8%), and uterine (6%). Although mortality rates from cancer have decreased overall, death rates from uterine cancer have been increasing since mid-2000, particularly among Black, Hispanic, Asian American, and Pacific Islander individuals (National Cancer Institute, 2024). The risk of developing cancer, including breast and gynecologic cancers, increases with age, with approximately 88 percent of cancers being diagnosed in people 50 years or older (American Cancer Society, 2024). Any postmenopausal bleeding must be evaluated for potential endometrial or uterine cancer. Refer to Chapters 25 and 28 for more information. Additionally, Chapter 9 presents cancer screening recommendations, Chapter 17 provides information on breast cancer, and Chapter 28 addresses gynecologic cancers.

Osteoporosis

Osteoporosis is the most common bone disease in humans and is characterized by low bone mass, deterioration of bone tissue, and disruption of bone architecture resulting in reduced bone strength that increases the risk for fracture (LeBoff et al., 2022). Osteoporosis is the most common cause of morbidity among postmenopausal individuals, and osteoporotic fractures account for a large portion of morbidity and mortality among postmenopausal individuals, especially those older than 65 years (American College of Obstetricians and Gynecologists [ACOG], 2021, 2022; LeBoff et al., 2022). **Table 14-3** lists risk factors for osteoporosis.

Osteoporosis is categorized as primary, secondary, or idiopathic. Primary osteoporosis is associated with aging and affects menopause-capable individuals much more significantly than others. Adults achieve peak bone mass in their late 20s to mid-30s, after which time the rates of bone resorption and formation become relatively stable. Everyone requires estrogen for optimal bone health (ACOG, 2021, 2022; Anam & Insogna, 2021; LeBoff et al., 2022). As menopause-capable individuals age into their 30s and 40s, their bone resorption rate begins to exceed that of bone formation, resulting in a slow decline of bone mass. There is also a time-limited rapid bone loss triggered by menopause-associated estrogen deficiency. The rate of bone loss is most significant in the first year after menopause, between 1 and 5 percent, then slows to approximately 1 percent per year (Anam & Insogna, 2021; LeBoff et al., 2022).

Secondary osteoporosis occurs in response to medication (e.g., corticosteroids, anticonvulsants, or methotrexate) or disease processes (e.g., hyperthyroidism, chronic liver disease, or gastrointestinal diseases, such as malabsorption) that interfere with the normal process of bone formation and can affect people at any age (BHOG, 2022). Idiopathic osteoporosis is characterized by low bone density and fracture in young adults when no other cause is identified (NAMS, 2019).

Screening recommendations for osteoporosis can be found in Chapter 9. Bone mineral density (BMD) testing by dual energy x-ray absorptiometry (DXA) is a technique used to evaluate central

TABLE 14-3 Risk Factors for Osteoporosis

Potentially Modifiable Risk Factors	Nonmodifiable Risk Factors
Excessive thinness (BMI less than 21 kg/m^2) Hypogonadal states (e.g., anorexia, athletic amenorrhea, premature menopause, androgen insensitivity, hyperprolactinemia, Turner and Klinefelter syndromes) Nulliparity Lifestyle factors (e.g., cigarette smoking, excessive alcohol or caffeine intake, sedentary activity level, frequent falling, inadequate calcium or vitamin D intake) Medications (e.g., thyroid hormone, corticosteroids, anticonvulsants, aluminum-containing antacids, lithium, methotrexate, gonadotropin-releasing hormone, cholestyramine, heparin, warfarin, depot medroxyprogesterone acetate [Depo-Provera], premenopausal tamoxifen, selective serotonin reuptake inhibitors, proton pump inhibitors) Chronic diseases (e.g., endocrine disorders, gastrointestinal disorders, bone disorders, chronic liver disease, seizure disorders, prolonged immobility, eating disorders, chronic renal failure, frailty)	Advanced age Female gender Race (white and Asian individuals at greatest risk, followed by Hispanic and African American individuals) Personal history of fracture during adulthood Family history of osteoporosis First-degree relative with a history of fracture Genetic diseases (e.g., cystic fibrosis, Ehlers-Danlos syndrome, osteogenesis imperfecta, porphyria, Gaucher disease, hemochromatosis, Marfan syndrome, homocystinuria) Hematologic disorders (e.g., hemophilia, sickle cell, multiple myeloma, thalassemia, leukemia and lymphomas) Rheumatologic and autoimmune disease (e.g., systemic lupus erythematosus, rheumatoid arthritis, ankylosing spondylitis, thyroid disease)

Data from LeBoff, M. S., Greenspan, S. L., Insogna, K. L., Lewiecki, E. M., Saag, K. G., Singer, A. J., & Siris, E. S. (2022). The clinician's guide to prevention and treatment of osteoporosis. *Osteoporosis International, 33*(10), 2049–2102. https://doi.org/10.1007/s00198-021-05900-y

BMD at the spine and hip and is a vital component of the diagnosis and management of osteoporosis (Anam & Insogna, 2021; BHOG, 2022). Although DXA can also be used to evaluate wrist BMD, central testing is much more predictive of overall BMD and fracture risk. Quantitative computed tomography (CT) scan can be used to perform spine measurements and is particularly useful for testing individuals with arthritis because it is less likely to reflect osteocytes (Anam & Insogna, 2021; BHOG, 2022).

BMD results are reported as T-scores and Z-scores. The T-score identifies the number of standard deviations that the patient's BMD is greater or less than a young-adult, gender-matched norm. The Z-score is compared to the BMD of an age-, sex-, and ethnicity-matched referent population. Low bone mass (osteopenia) is present when the T-score is in the range of -1.0 to -2.5. Osteoporosis is present when the T-score is -2.5 or less. Severe or established osteoporosis is present when the T-score is -2.5 or less and low trauma fractures are present. T-scores are used in men older than age 50 and in postmenopausal individuals because they are the standard used to determine the risk for fractures. The International Society for Clinical Densitometry recommends using Z-scores instead of T-scores for premenopausal individuals, children, and others younger than 50 years, with Z-scores of -2.0 or less defined as "below the expected range for age" and those greater than -2.0 defined as "within the expected range for age." Z-scores are helpful for identifying individuals who should undergo an evaluation for secondary causes of osteoporosis (Anam & Insogna, 2021; LeBoff et al., 2022; Shuhart et al., 2024).

Individuals with osteoporosis are at increased risk for fracture. Although osteoporosis and low bone mass by themselves are painless and not functionally problematic, the risk for fracture puts a patient at significant risk. Following a hip fracture, there is an 8.4 to 36 percent increase in mortality and a 2.5-fold increased risk for a future fracture. Among survivors of such fractures, approximately 20 percent require long-term nursing home care, and only 40 percent fully regain their prefracture level of independence (Anam & Insogna, 2021; BHOG, 2022).

BOX 14-3 Strategies to Prevent Osteoporosis

- Adequate intake of calcium (1,200 mg/day in postmenopausal individuals)
- Adequate intake of vitamin D (800 to 1,000 international units [IU]/day for adults 50 years and older)
- Weight-bearing and resistance exercise
- Fall prevention
- Avoiding tobacco
- Moderating alcohol intake (fewer than two drinks per day for menopause-capable individuals)

Data from LeBoff, M. S., Greenspan, S. L., Insogna, K. L., Lewiecki, E. M., Saag, K. G., Singer, A. J., & Siris, E. S. (2022). The clinician's guide to prevention and treatment of osteoporosis. *Osteoporosis International, 33*(10), 2049–2102. https://doi.org/10.1007/s00198-021-05900-y

Patient Education for Preventing Bone Loss

Prevention is a key component of osteoporosis management. For perimenopausal and postmenopausal individuals, education should focus on prevention strategies (**Box 14-3**). Exercise is site specific and needs to be continued to maintain bone strength.

Management of Bone Loss

Medication management is recommended for patients with T-scores of -2.5 or less and for those with hip or vertebral fractures (LeBoff et al., 2022). For individuals with T-scores in the low bone mass range (-1.0 to -2.5), medication is recommended if they also have fractures or are at high risk for fracture (e.g., immobilized, taking glucocorticoids, or at high risk for falls).

For individuals with T-scores in the low bone mass range, use of the Fracture Risk Assessment Tool (FRAX®) is recommended to identify those who would realize a cost-effective benefit from initiating medication therapy (Kanis et al., 2017; Tosteson et al., 2008). Use of FRAX is reflected in many international guidelines. The U.S. adaptation is accessible online (https://www.bonehealthandosteoporosis.org/) and is applicable to those who have not previously been treated with medications. Information is entered for 11 different risk factors plus the hip raw BMD value (in g/cm^2) to calculate the 10-year probability for a hip fracture and the 10-year probability for any type of major osteoporotic fracture. If the hip fracture probability is equal to or greater than 3 percent, or if the risk for any major osteoporotic fracture is equal to or greater than 20 percent, medication therapy is recommended (LeBoff et al., 2022; Schini et al., 2024). FRAX results are often included in BMD reports.

The treatment decision must be weighed against the clinical presentation, the evaluation of potential secondary causes, and with the clinician recognizing the limitations of FRAX (Schini et al., 2024). The estimated fracture risk identified by adjusted FRAX provides an alert to the clinician that treatment may be useful. The intervention threshold—that is, the point at which treatment should be started for a specific individual—is determined mutually between the clinician and the patient. This threshold is different for each patient and is based on multiple factors, including the risks identified previously and the adjusted FRAX results (Anthamatten & Parish, 2019). Many of the variables considered in the FRAX instrument are dichotomous (e.g., yes/no) and do not capture variables that increase risk along a continuum (e.g., higher doses of corticosteroid increase risk for fracture). Additionally, the T-score used in the FRAX calculations is not the same as that obtained with DXA testing; however, when used in conjunction with the trabecular bone score, reflecting the mineral distribution in trabecular bone by giving an index of bone microarchitecture, increases the ability to predict fractures (Couraud et al., 2017).

Repeat BMD testing is an important component of evaluating the response to treatment and management of osteoporosis. Measurement is based on medical necessity, and the expected outcomes. It is recommended one year after treatment is initiated and if there has been a change in therapy. Once an effective threshold is reached, longer intervals of monitoring may be instituted (LeBoff et al., 2022). **Table 14-4** summarizes the available pharmacologic treatment options for osteoporosis in postmenopausal individuals. Combination therapy, initiated by an osteoporosis specialist, is also possible; usually a bisphosphonate (alendronate or risedronate) is combined with a drug from another class (e.g., estrogen or raloxifene).

TABLE 14-4 Pharmacologic Treatment Options for Postmenopausal Osteoporosis

Medication	FDA-Approved Indication	Considerations
Agents for Initial Therapy in Most Patients at High Risk for Fracture		
Alendronate (Fosamax) Alendronate plus vitamin D_3 (Fosamax Plus D or Binosto)	Prevention: 5 mg orally daily or 35 mg orally weekly Treatment: 10 mg orally daily Treatment: 70 mg orally weekly (70 mg dose also available with cholecalciferol/vitamin D_3 as Fosamax Plus D, 70 mg dose also available in an effervescent tablet as Binosto)	Use with caution if the patient has upper gastrointestinal disease, owing to its clinical association with dysphagia, esophagitis, and ulceration Contraindicated in individuals with hypocalcemia Take first thing in the morning on an empty stomach with an 8 oz glass of water; remain upright and take no other food or drink for at least 30 minutes Take 2 hours before antacids/calcium
Risedronate (Actonel, Atelvia)	Prevention or treatment: 5 mg orally daily, or 35 mg orally weekly, or 150 mg orally monthly	Same as alendronate
Zoledronic acid (Reclast)	Prevention: 5 mg intravenously once every 2 years Treatment: 5 mg intravenously once/year	Intravenous infusion is administered over a period of no less than 15 minutes Contraindicated in individuals with hypocalcemia
Denosumab (Prolia)	Treatment: 60 mg subcutaneously every 6 months	Reserved for use after failure of first-line agents Avoid in individuals with hypocalcemia

(*continues*)

TABLE 14-4 Pharmacologic Treatment Options for Postmenopausal Osteoporosis (*continued*)

Medication	FDA-Approved Indication	Considerations
Potential Agents for Initial Therapy in Patients Who Need Spine-Specific Therapy		
Ibandronate (Boniva)	Prevention or treatment: 150 mg orally once/month Treatment: 3 mg intravenously every 3 months	Same as alendronate for tablets but must remain upright and take no other food or drink for at least 60 minutes Intravenous injection is administered over a period of 15 to 30 seconds
Raloxifene (Evista)	Prevention or treatment: 60 mg orally daily	May cause hot flashes Not recommended if the patient is taking ET or EPT or has a history of venous thromboembolism
Agents for Patients Unable to Use Oral Therapy or at Exceptionally High Risk for Fracture		
Teriparatide (Forteo)	Treatment: 20 mcg subcutaneously daily	Reserved for use after failure of first-line agents in those with high fracture risk Safety and efficacy with more than 2 years of therapy not established
Abaloparatide (Tymlos)	Treatment: 80 mcg subcutaneously daily	Reserved for use after failure of first-line agents in those with high fracture risk Do not exceed 2 years of cumulative use of abaloparatide and parathyroid hormone analogs (e.g., teriparatide)
Romosozumab (Evenity)	Treatment: 120 mg subcutaneously monthly	Reserved for use after failure of first-line agents in those with high fracture risk Safety and efficacy with more than 1 year (12 months) of therapy not established
Denosumab (Prolia)	Treatment: 60 mg subcutaneously every 6 months	Reserved for use after failure of first-line agents Avoid in individuals with hypocalcemia
Zoledronic acid (Reclast)	Prevention: 5 mg intravenously once every 2 years Treatment: 5 mg intravenously once/year	Intravenous infusion is administered over a period of no less than 15 minutes Contraindicated in individuals with hypocalcemia
Other Agents Used in Managing Osteoporosis		
Calcitonin (Fortical, Miacalcin)	Treatment: 200 IU intranasal spray daily or 100 IU subcutaneous or intramuscular injection daily or every other day Use for 6 months or less	Not a first-line medication for osteoporosis Consider risk for malignancies prior to use Usually administered as nasal spray Has an analgesic effect on osteoporotic fractures Avoid in those allergic to calcitonin-salmon
Estrogen (e.g., Premarin, Ogen, Alora, Climara, Estrace, Menostar, Vivelle, Vivelle-Dot, Premphase,[a] Prempro,[a] femhrt,[a] Activella,[a] Prefest,[a] Climara Pro[a])	Prevention: Doses and routes vary[b]	Also effective in alleviating most symptoms of menopause Comes in pills or patches
Estrogen plus bazedoxifene (Duavee)		

Data from Camacho, P. M., Petak, S. M., Binkley, N., Diab, D. L., Eldeiry, L. S., Farooki, A., Harris, S. T., Hurley, D. L., Kelly, J., Lewiecki, E. M., Pessah-Pollack, R., McClung, M., Wimalawansa, S. J., & Watts, N. B. (2020). American Association of Clinical Endocrinologists/American College of Endocrinology clinical practice guidelines for the diagnosis and treatment of postmenopausal osteoporosis—2020 update. *Endocrine Practice, 26*, 1–46; Epocrates. (2024, July 24). Computerized pharmacology and prescribing reference [Mobile application software]. Retrieved from http://www.epocrates.com; LeBoff, M. S., Greenspan, S. L., Insogna, K. L., Lewiecki, E. M., Saag, K. G., Singer, A. J., & Siris, E. S. (2022). The clinician's guide to prevention and treatment of osteoporosis. *Osteoporosis international, 33*(10), 2049–2102; North American Menopause Society. (2019). *Menopause practice: A clinician's guide* (6th ed.).

Abbreviations: EPT, estrogen with progestogen therapy; ET, estrogen therapy.

Note: See prescribing reference for full information on doses, side effects, contraindications, and cautions.

[a]Also contains progestogen, which should be used in individuals with an intact uterus.

[b]Lowest effective dose should be used. The Food and Drug Administration (FDA) recommends considering nonestrogen osteoporotic agents when ET/EPT use is solely for the purpose of osteoporosis prevention.

Thyroid Disease

Thyroid disease is another health issue that must be considered at midlife. Thyroid disease affects menopause-capable individuals more often than others, and its incidence increases with age. Subclinical hypothyroidism is also more common as individuals age (Biondi & Cappola, 2022). Thyroid disorders can present with many of the same symptoms that occur during the transition to postmenopause, such as menstrual cycle changes or irregularities, disruption in sleep, fatigue, mood swings, heat intolerance, and palpitations (NAMS, 2019; Panda & Das, 2018). Although there is not a general consensus regarding who should be screened for thyroid disorders, the American Association of Clinical Endocrinologists recommends that screening should be considered in older patients, especially menopause-capable individuals, and the American Thyroid Association recommends that everyone older than 35 years be screened every 5 years (Panda & Das, 2018). NAMS (2019) recommends that clinicians maintain a high index of suspicion for thyroid disorders in midlife and postmenopausal individuals. Measurement of TSH is the initial step in assessing thyroid function (Panda & Das, 2018).

Depression

Despite the fact that most people progress through the transition to postmenopause without psychological symptoms, some individuals report symptoms of depression, anxiety, stress, or a decreased sense of well-being. There is an increased risk of depression during the transition to postmenopause, particularly among individuals with a history of depression, premenstrual syndrome, or postpartum depression (Maki et al., 2019). Risk factors that may contribute to depression include demographic factors (e.g., minority status, low income, low education, unmarried), psychological factors (e.g., trait anxiety, pessimism, rumination), social/environmental factors (e.g., lifetime adversity, trauma, current stressful situations, poor social support), health-related factors (e.g., smoking, physical activity, sleep disturbance, vasomotor symptoms. chronic pain, and comorbid medical conditions) (Bromberger & Epperson, 2018). The risk of clinical depression may also be increased around the transition to postmenopause; however, this has been the subject of less research than depressive symptoms. Routine screening for depression should be included when an individual presents with symptoms that appear to be related to the postmenopause transition, particularly in high-risk populations (Maki et al., 2019).

PATIENT EDUCATION FOR LIFESTYLE APPROACHES TO MANAGE MENOPAUSE-RELATED SYMPTOMS

Several lifestyle approaches have been demonstrated to reduce menopause-related symptoms, and many of these approaches also afford additional health benefits, such as reducing the risk for CVD, diabetes, and osteoporosis. Lifestyle approaches may encompass dietary changes, exercise, vitamins or supplements, vaginal lubricants and moisturizers, changes in clothing or environment, smoking cessation, stress management techniques, proper sleep hygiene, and activities to enhance cognitive function. Educating patients about lifestyle approaches is important as these nonpharmacological options may help manage symptoms and, in some cases, decrease or even obviate the need for pharmacological therapies.

Dietary Changes

Menopause-capable individuals are often advised to avoid certain foods or drinks which may be triggers for vasomotor symptoms (VMS). Examples of trigger foods can include alcohol, caffeine, spicy foods, and hot drinks. However, there are limited data to support a causative relationship between avoiding triggers and vasomotor symptom improvement (NAMS, 2019). Implementing a low-fat, vegan diet, with fruits, vegetables, whole grains, and legumes including a ½ cup of soybeans has been shown to reduce the frequency and severity for moderate to severe VMS (Barnard et al., 2021). Increased water intake is recommended because of the insensible loss of fluids through sweating among individuals who experience hot flashes. Despite limited data supporting the contention that consuming cool drinks improves menopause-related symptoms, water intake (especially cold water) appears to reduce symptoms such as skin dryness and may reduce the discomfort associated with hot flashes and sweating (NAMS, 2019). The usual water intake of six to eight glasses per day should be recommended. However, for menopause-capable individuals who experience urinary incontinence, water consumption may need to be restricted for social occasions when there is limited access to a bathroom.

Exercise

Levels of physical activity are not consistently linked to frequency of menopause-related symptoms (NAMS, 2019). Observational studies have reported fewer VMS in individuals who exercised regularly; however, several Cochrane reviews have found insufficient evidence to support exercise as a treatment for VMS, and in some individuals, exercise may trigger VMS (NAMS, 2019). Some evidence demonstrates that yoga and, to a lesser extent, aerobic exercise may be beneficial with less evidence to support resistance training (Money et al., 2024). Resistance training, walking, aerobic training, and self-directed programs such as cycling, swimming, and running, have been shown to improve quality-of-life scores in postmenopausal individuals (Berin et al., 2022; Nguyen et al., 2020). Even if exercise does not directly improve menopause-related symptoms, it improves general health, including a beneficial impact for cardiometabolic measures (Chrysant, 2020). The World Health Organization (WHO) recommends that individuals engage in a target range of 150–300 minutes per week of moderate-intensity exercise with multiple exercise types that provide bone health benefits (Bull et al., 2020).

Vitamins and Supplements

Selected vitamins and supplements may be useful in improving health; however, there is a lack of data demonstrating the effectiveness of vitamins and supplements for treating menopause-related VMS (NAMS, 2019). Oral vitamin E has been linked to improvements in nervousness, hot flashes, and insomnia. Vaginal vitamin E suppositories have shown improvements in genitourinary symptoms and sexual function (Feduniw et al., 2023). While there is a lack of high-quality studies in this area, vitamin E may offer a promising alternative or add-on treatment option. Omega 3 supplementation may help reduce VMS and improve sleep and depression symptoms (Iqbal et al., 2023). Additional randomized-controlled studies with larger sample sizes are needed to validate previous results.

The International Osteoporosis Foundation recommends that menopause-capable individuals age 50 and younger receive

1,000 mg of calcium from all sources daily, 1,200 mg are recommended at age 51 and older, 800–1,000 IU/day is the recommended intake for vitamin D with a target 25(OH)D blood level of 50 nmol/L for bone health at all ages (LeBoff et al., 2022).

Limited evidence supports the use of vitamins and supplements for the prevention of chronic diseases and all-cause mortality with the exception of a potential small benefit in decreasing cancer incidence with multi-vitamin use (O'Connor et al., 2022). Importantly, the potential for harm arises with excessive intake of some nutrients/supplements. Because of this, limiting dietary supplementation and instead encouraging midlife menopause-capable individuals to maintain a healthy diet is recommended. A diet consisting of complex carbohydrates, fruits and vegetables, proteins, adequate fiber, healthy fats, and low sodium can promote weight management, improve energy levels, and reduce the risk of developing type II diabetes, insulin resistance, CVD, and breast cancer (Erdélyi et al., 2023; Yuksel et al., 2021).

Vaginal Lubricants and Moisturizers

After menopause, about 45 percent of people will experience symptoms of vulvovaginal atrophy because of decreasing estrogen levels (Wasnik et al., 2023). Genitourinary syndrome of menopause (GSM) is the term now recommended to describe such symptoms, rather than vulvovaginal atrophy or atrophic vaginitis, as GSM encompasses the physiologic genitourinary tract changes and the variety of vulvovaginal (e.g., dryness, burning, irritation), sexual (e.g., inadequate lubrication, pain), and urinary (e.g., urgency, dysuria, urinary tract infections) symptoms associated with decreased estrogen levels (NAMS, 2020). GSM can have a significant effect on interpersonal relationships, daily activities, quality of life, and sexual function (NAMS, 2020). Additional information about GSM can be found in Chapter 21.

Individuals with mild symptoms of GSM often respond well to vaginal lubricants and moisturizers; these can be offered as an initial treatment option (NAMS, 2019, 2020). Vaginal lubricants can be used to relieve the friction and dyspareunia that results from vaginal dryness during intercourse. Several nonhormonal water-, silicone-, and oil-based lubricants and vaginal moisturizers are available as over-the-counter products (**Table 14-5**). Some vaginal lubricants contain capsaicin, which can cause significant burning for some individuals who have GSM; these lubricants should be avoided. Longer-acting vaginal moisturizers may be more appropriate for some individuals. These products are applied several times weekly, in addition to the use of a lubricant at the time of sexual activity. The moisturizers replenish and maintain moisture in the vaginal epithelial cells and provide longer relief while mimicking natural vaginal secretions. Moisturizers may be particularly beneficial for individuals who experience daily discomfort, and they can reduce symptoms of vaginitis by supporting a normal pH (NAMS, 2019, 2020). The therapy choice should be individualized, based on symptom severity, safety, effectiveness, and the individual's preference.

TABLE 14-5 Nonhormonal Vaginal Lubricants and Moisturizers

Lubricants	Moisturizers
Water based:	Feminease
Aloe Cadabra[a,b]	K-Y SILK-E
Astroglide	Luvena
Astroglide Gel Liquid	Me Again
Astroglide Liquid	Replens
Good Clean Love[a,b]	Silken Secret
Just Like Me	Sylk Natural
K-Y Jelly	Hyalo-gyn
Liquid Silk	
Pre-Seed[a,b]	
Slippery Stuff[a,b]	
Sliquid Organic[a,b]	
SYKL	
YES Personal Lubricant	
Silicone based:	
Astroglide X	
ID Millennium	
K-Y Intrigue	
Pink	
Pjur Eros (Bodyglide)[b]	
Uberlube	
Sliquid	
Oil based:	
Almond oil	
Coconut oil	
Elegance Women's Lubricants	
Olive oil	
Vitamin E oil	
YES OB	

Data from North American Menopause Society. (2019). *Menopause practice: A clinician's guide* (6th ed.); North American Menopause Society (2020). The North American Menopause Society position statement: The 2020 genitourinary syndrome of menopause position statement of The North American Menopause Society. *Menopause (New York, N.Y.)*, 27(9), 976–992. https://doi.org/10.1097/GME.0000000000001609; Shim, S., Park, K. M., Chung, Y. J., & Kim, M. R. (2021). Updates on therapeutic alternatives for genitourinary syndrome of menopause: Hormonal and non-hormonal managements. *Journal of Menopausal Medicine, 27*(1), 1–7. https://doi.org/10.6118/jmm.20034

Note: Lubricants are applied prior to or during sex. Moisturizers are applied on a regular basis (e.g., daily or two to three times/week).

[a]Osmolality less than 380 mOsm/kg, which is the maximum level recommended by the World Health Organization to minimize the risk of epithelial damage. Osmolality is only applicable to water-based lubricants; silicone- and oil-based lubricants do not have an osmolality value because they do not contain water.

[b]Propylene glycol-free. Propylene glycol can cause vaginal irritation for some individuals.

Lubricants are generally thought of as low-risk products; however, some individuals can be more susceptible to bacterial vaginosis when the pH and osmolarity of the lubricant are physiologically too different from the normal vaginal environment (Shim et al., 2021). Patients must be cautioned against using petroleum-jelly-based products (e.g., Vaseline), because these preparations can injure vaginal tissue, are not easily removed, and may increase the incidence of bacterial vaginosis (NAMS, 2019, 2020). Use of other products that contain additives such as fragrance, dye, spermicide, or flavors should also be discouraged because they often cause vaginitis or irritation. Douching is not effective for moisturizing and will remove normal flora, thereby increasing the risk for infection (NAMS, 2019, 2020). Because few tolerability studies are available for over-the-counter products, testing for 24 hours on a small skin area prior to intravaginal use is recommended. Studies have identified a correlation between cytotoxic and inflammatory vaginal epithelial cell changes with use of hyperosmolar vaginal lubricants (Ayehunie et al., 2018; Dezzutti et al., 2012; Wilkinson et al., 2019). Given that hyperosmolar products can also be irritating, low osmolality products without propylene glycol may be preferred (Riberio-Valadares et al., 2022). Natural oils, including olive, mineral, and coconut, provide a low-cost option for regular sexual activity and moisturizing (NAMS, 2019, 2020).

Clothing and Environment

Wearing layered clothes, breathable fabrics (e.g., cotton, linen), or moisture-wicking/cooling fabrics is recommended to reduce the discomfort associated with hot flashes and sweats. Avoiding turtlenecks, fabrics that do not allow circulation or absorb sweat (e.g., polyester, silk), and extra layers (e.g., slips, full-length stockings) is also recommended. Keeping the room temperature cool, opening a window and/or using a fan to circulate air, and using chilling towels and a chilling pillow can help reduce core body temperature and may be beneficial in reducing VMS related to menopause (NAMS, 2019).

Smoking Cessation

Smoking is associated with increased morbidity and mortality, especially related to CVD and cancers; increased rate of bone loss; and increased prevalence of VMS (Anderson et al., 2020; Nair et al., 2021; NAMS, 2022). Various pharmacologic and behavioral smoking cessation interventions are available. Ultimately, the best treatment is the one that is of greatest interest to a specific individual. The individual needs to be both interested in quitting and motivated to quit. The U.S. Preventive Services Task Force (USPSTF) recommends clinicians provide nonpregnant individuals who want to quit smoking with both pharmacotherapy, such as nicotine replacement therapy, and behavioral interventions. Combining the two intervention types is more effective than either alone (USPSTF, 2021).

Stress Management

Stress and anxiety have been associated with increases in the severity and frequency of hot flashes. Additionally, stress can negatively affect quality of life by causing sleep disturbances, decreasing libido, and aggravating medical conditions such as CVD (NAMS, 2019). At midlife, individuals may face multiple stressors, such as health changes for themselves or family members; financial concerns; loss of a parent; children leaving home; or relationship struggles with a partner, child, or parent.

Managing stress must be individualized because each person may find different tactics helpful. Individuals are encouraged to identify their own life stressors and find stress-relieving measures that work for them (NAMS, 2019). Some suggestions include regular exercise, meditation, relaxation techniques such as deep breathing or paced respiration, yoga, tai-chi, taking a lukewarm bath, reading, having a massage, seeking support from friends, or activities related to spirituality or religion. Many individuals find that yoga breathing—a variation of paced respiration—enhances relaxation and reduces hot flashes. Yoga breathing consists of a deep inhalation over a count of 5, holding the breath for a count of 7, and slowly exhaling over a count of 9. Systematic reviews and meta-analyses found that hypnosis, paced respiration, and cognitive behavioral therapy can significantly improve VMS. Yoga, relaxation, and mindfulness may also decrease hot flashes; however, additional research is necessary to confirm their benefit (Guo et al., 2019).

Sleep

Evaluating the cause of sleep disruptions is important for developing a management plan. If sleep disruption is related to hot flashes or other menopause-related symptoms, control of those symptoms will usually restore normal sleep patterns. Light blankets, cotton sleepwear or moisture-wicking pajamas, and a well-ventilated room are recommended for reducing nocturnal hot flashes. However, if sleep disruption is unrelated to hot flashes, such as sleep apnea, a more generalized approach is needed.

Developing good sleep hygiene is especially important for perimenopausal and postmenopausal individuals. Sleep hygiene refers to actions that cue the mind that it is time for sleep and allow the part of the brain that controls the body during sleep to take over. Developing regular routines prior to bedtime, such as brushing the teeth or changing into sleepwear, and doing something relaxing, such as paced respirations, progressive relaxation, guided imagery, taking a warm bath, reading a relaxing book, or drinking a warm beverage without caffeine, can help cue the mind that it is time to sleep. Similarly, activities that tend to stimulate the mind should be avoided just before bed, such as watching television, using electronic devices (e.g., smartphone, tablet, computer), reading a fast-paced or stimulating book, doing work, or exercise. Limiting blue-light exposure from electronic devices also helps reduce sleep disruptions. The bedroom should be reserved for sleep and sexual activities. This consideration is especially important for individuals who have difficulty falling asleep because doing work or watching television in bed can have a stimulating effect. Establishing regular times for sleep and waking is also important for developing good sleep patterns because this consistency will facilitate the development of normal daily routines.

Lifestyle changes that can help restore sleep patterns include avoiding caffeine, alcohol, and nicotine. The effects of caffeine can last as long as 20 hours in some individuals, so total elimination is preferable (NAMS, 2019). Although alcohol can have a sedative effect during the first half of the night, it may cause interruptions in the second half, including fragmented sleep and rebound awakening due to the effects of alcohol on the homeostatic regulation of sleep. Similarly, nicotine can prolong sleep onset and reduce overall sleep duration. Exercise can enhance sleep quality, reduce sleep latency, and increase the amount of time spent in deep sleep. However, timing of exercise is important because engaging in exercise close to bedtime will increase sleep latency (NAMS, 2019).

Sleep-restriction therapy can be considered to help reestablish a restorative sleep pattern. Use of relaxation techniques prior to bedtime may also benefit individuals with sleep difficulties. Additionally, acupuncture has been shown to improve sleep quality and quality of life among postmenopausal individuals with sleep disturbances (Zhao et al., 2023).

It is also important to educate individuals that they may require less sleep as they age. Although the amount of sleep required by adults is very individualized, and it is difficult to specify an exact amount of sleep that an individual may need, the National Sleep Foundation provides general guidelines. The recommended sleep duration is 7 to 9 hours from ages 26 to 64 years, and 7 to 8 hours for those 65 and older. However, it may be appropriate for some people who are 26 to 64 years to sleep 6 to 10 hours per night, and for those 65 and older to sleep 5 to 9 hours per night (Hirshkowitz et al., 2015).

Mental Function

Memory and cognitive function tend to decline with advancing age. During perimenopause, decreases in cognitive performance, such as deficits in attention, memory, and processing speed, commonly occur and appear to normalize in postmenopause (Conde et al., 2021). Although poor mental functioning is often associated with lack of sleep or high levels of stress, cognitive impairment can also be related to a myriad of medical problems. Thus, the first step in evaluating mental function is to complete a comprehensive assessment to identify potential causes of the cognitive deficit.

Some evidence suggests that individuals who engage in certain activities or lifestyle changes experience improved memory function and protection against dementia (NAMS, 2019). Maintaining an extensive social network and remaining physically active and mentally active by participating in activities that keep the mind engaged (e.g., intellectually stimulating work, puzzles, or other activities) can help maintain cognitive function. Increasing the intake of omega-3 fatty acids; not smoking; consuming alcohol only in moderation; and adapting lifestyle measures to reduce the risk for hypertension, diabetes, and high cholesterol have the added benefit of protecting against dementia and cognitive decline (NAMS, 2019).

PHARMACOLOGIC OPTIONS FOR MENOPAUSE-RELATED SYMPTOM MANAGEMENT

NAMS (2019, 2022), the International Menopause Society (Panay et al., 2024), and the revised Global Consensus on Menopausal Hormone Therapy (de Villiers et al., 2016) identify HT as the most effective therapy for menopause-related moderate to severe vasomotor symptoms. Individuals with mild vasomotor symptoms will often realize significant benefits from lifestyle changes alone or in combination with nonprescription remedies. Rather than defining severity of vasomotor symptoms by the number of hot flashes in a given day, most organizations now recognize severity based on level of bother, including sleep disturbance, and effect on quality of life for a menopause-capable individual (de Villiers et al., 2016; NAMS, 2019, 2022; Panay et al., 2024). In most people, hot flashes will eventually resolve over time without medication.

Systemic ET/EPT reduces hot flash severity and frequency significantly more than placebos (NAMS, 2019, 2022). Some antidepressant, antihypertensive, and anticonvulsant agents have also been shown to reduce vasomotor symptoms. **Table 14-6** lists HT products available in the United States. In their review of the efficacy of various preparations, the NAMS researchers concluded that there is no evidence to claim that one product is superior to another in terms of ability to provide symptom

TABLE 14-6 Oral and Transdermal Hormone Therapy Options*

Type	Product Name	Active Ingredient	Dosage
Estrogens, oral[a]	Estrace	17β-estradiol	0.5 mg, 1 mg, or 2 mg; 1 to 2 mg once daily
	Menest	Esterified estrogens	0.3 mg, 0.625 mg, 1.25 mg; once daily
	Premarin	CEE	0.3 mg, 0.45 mg, 0.625 mg, 0.9 mg, 1.25 mg; once daily
Estrogens, transdermal and topical preparations[a]	Minivelle, Vivelle-Dot, generic	17β-estradiol matrix patch	0.025 mg/d, 0.0375 mg/d, 0.05 mg/d, 0.075 mg/d, or 0.1 mg/d; one patch twice weekly (and 0.06 mg in generic only applied weekly)
	Climara	17β-estradiol matrix patch	0.025 mg/d, 0.0375 mg/d, 0.05 mg/d, 0.06 mg/d, 0.075 mg/d, or 0.1 mg/d; one patch once weekly
	Menostar[b]	17β-estradiol matrix patch	0.014 mg; apply once weekly
	EstroGel	17β-estradiol transdermal gel	0.75 mg/pump; one metered gel pump once daily applied from wrist to shoulder
	Elestrin	17β-estradiol transdermal gel	0.52 mg/pump; one to two metered pumps once daily applied to upper arm and shoulder
	Divigel	17β-estradiol transdermal gel	0.25 mg/packet, 0.5 mg/packet, 0.75 mg/packet, 1 mg/packet, or 1.25 mg/packet; one gel packet once daily applied to upper thigh
	Evamist	17β-estradiol transdermal spray	1.53 mg/spray; one to three sprays once daily applied to forearm
Estrogens, injection[a]	Delestrogen	Estradiol valerate	10 mg/mL, 20 mg/mL, or 40 mg/mL; 10 to 20 mg IM weekly

Type	Product Name	Active Ingredient	Dosage
Progestogens, oral	Provera, generic	MPA	2.5 mg, 5 mg, or 10 mg; continuously or on set cycle schedule
	Prometrium, generic	Micronized progesterone	100 mg or 200 mg; continuously or on set cycle schedule
	Generic[b]	Norethindrone	0.35 mg continuously or on set cycle schedule
	Aygestin[b]	Norethindrone acetate	5 mg continuously or on set cycle schedule
Combination estrogen–progestogen products, oral	Premphase	CEE (14 tabs), then CEE + MPA (14 tabs)	0.625 mg E once daily for 14 days, then 0.625 mg E + 5 mg P once daily for 14 days sequentially
	Prempro	CEE + MPA	0.3 mg E + 1.5 mg P, 0.45 mg E + 1.5 mg P, 0.625 mg E + 2.5 mg P, or 0.625 mg E + 5 mg P; once daily
	Jinteli	Ethinyl estradiol + norethindrone acetate	5 mcg E + 1 mg P once daily, continuously
	Generic	17β-estradiol + norethindrone acetate	2.5 mcg E + 0.5 mg P or 5 mcg E + 1 mg P; once daily
	Mimvey	17β-estradiol + norethindrone acetate	1 mg E + 0.5 mg P; once daily
	Angeliq	17β-estradiol + drospirenone	0.5 mg E + 0.25 mg D, 1 mg E + 0.5 mg D; once daily
	Activella	17β-estradiol + norethindrone acetate	0.5 mg E + 0.1 mg P or 1 mg E + 0.5 mg P; once daily
	Prefest	17β-estradiol (three tabs) then 17β-estradiol + norgestimate (three tabs)	1 mg E for 3 days, then 1 mg E + 0.09 mg P for 3 days; once daily sequentially
Combination estrogen–progestogen products, transdermal	Climara Pro	17β-estradiol + levonorgestrel	0.045 mg E + 0.015 mg P; once weekly
	CombiPatch	17β-estradiol + norethindrone acetate	0.05 mg E + 0.14 mg P or 0.05 mg E + 0.25 mg P; twice weekly
Combination estrogen–BZA product, oral	Duavee	CEE + BZA	0.45 mg E + 20 mg BZA; once daily
Combination estrogen–methyltestosterone[a]	Generic	Esterified estrogens + methyltestosterone	0.625 mg E + 1.25 mg MT or 1.25 mg E + 1.25 mg MT cycle 21 days on, 7 days off

Data from de Villiers, T. J., Hall, J. E., Pinkerton, J. V., Cerdas Pérez, S., Rees, M., Yang, C., & Pierroz, D. D. (2016). Revised global consensus statement on menopausal hormone therapy, *Climacteric, 19*(4), 313–315. https://doi.org/10.1080/13697137.2016.1196047; Epocrates. (2024, December 6). Computerized pharmacology and prescribing reference [Mobile application software]. Retrieved from http://www.epocrates.com; North American Menopause Society. (2019). *Menopause practice: A clinician's guide* (6th ed.); North American Menopause Society. (2022). North American Menopause Society. (2022). The North American Menopause Society position statement: The 2022 hormone therapy position statement of The North American Menopause Society. *Menopause: The Journal of The North American Menopause Society, 29*(7), 767–794. https://doi.org/10.1097/GME.0000000000002028; Panay, N., Ang, S. B., Cheshite, R., Goldstein, S. R., Maki, P., Nappi, R. E., & International Menopause Society Board. (2024). Menopause and HT in 2024: Addressing the key controversies—An International Menopause Society White Paper. *Climacteric 27*(5), 441–457. https://doi.org / 10.1080/13697137.2024.2394950.

Abbreviations: BZA, bazedoxifene; CEE, conjugated equine estrogens; d, day; D, drospirenone; E, estrogen; IM, intramuscularly; MPA, medroxyprogesterone acetate; MT, methyltestosterone; P, progestogen.

Note: See prescribing reference for full information on doses, side effects, contraindications, and cautions.

*Not comprehensive

[a]Consider adding progestogen if the individual's uterus is intact.

[b]Evidence-based use; not FDA approved for hormone therapy.

relief. **Table 14-7** lists nonhormonal prescription options and **Table 14-8** lists vaginal and intrauterine preparations available in the United States.

The only FDA-approved prescription therapy for treating hot flashes in individuals who are at high risk for, or who have been diagnosed with, breast cancer is paroxetine (Brisdelle). Other nonhormonal agents may also provide hot flash relief for those who have had breast cancer. Herbal alternatives to HT should be used with caution in individuals with contraindications to estrogen because many may have estrogen-like activity (Kenda et al., 2021).

TABLE 14-7 Nonhormonal Pharmacologic Options for Vasomotor Symptoms*

Drug	Dosage	Comments	Selected Side Effects	Selected Contraindications/ Cautions
Antidepressants: Selective Serotonin Reuptake Inhibitors (SSRIs) and Selective Norepinephrine Reuptake Inhibitors (SNRIs)				
Venlafaxine (Effexor XR)[a]	37.5 to 75 mg/day; up-titrate when starting therapy	Response is immediate	Nausea, vomiting, mouth dryness, decreased appetite	Concomitant use of MAO inhibitors; taper when discontinuing
Fluoxetine (Prozac)[a]	20 mg/day; up-titrate when starting therapy	Response is immediate	Asthenia, sweating, nausea, somnolence, anorgasmia, decreased libido	Concomitant use of MAO inhibitors or thioridazine; caution with warfarin; taper when discontinuing
Paroxetine (Paxil,[a] Brisdelle)	10 to 20 mg/day (Paxil); 7.5 mg at night (Brisdelle); 12.5 to 25 mg/day (extended release)	Response is immediate	Refer to fluoxetine; weight gain, blurred vision	Refer to fluoxetine; taper when discontinuing
Citalopram (Celexa)[a]	20 mg/day	Response is immediate	Abnormal bleeding/platelet function, glaucoma, seizure, somnolence, diaphoresis, insomnia	Ventricular arrhythmias, concomitant CNS depressant use, alcohol, hepatic impairment; taper when discontinuing
Desvenlafaxine extended release (Pristiq)[a]	50 mg/day	Response is immediate	Hyperlipidemia, anorgasmia, vomiting, tremor, proteinuria, anxiety	Concomitant CNS depressant use, alcohol, renal or hepatic impairment, bleeding risk, HTN; taper when discontinuing
Escitalopram (Lexapro)[a]	10 mg/day	Response is immediate	Abnormal bleeding/platelet function, seizure, headache, nausea, insomnia, fatigue, anorgasmia, reduced libido, constipation	Concomitant CNS depressant use, alcohol, hepatic impairment, recent myocardial infarction, congestive heart failure; taper when discontinuing
Anticonvulsants				
Gabapentin (Neurontin, Gralise)[a]	Initial dose 200 to 300 mg/day at bedtime, can increase to up to 300 mg three times/day at 3- to 4-day intervals		Somnolence, dizziness, ataxia, fatigue, weight gain	Avoid antacids within 2 hours of use; taper when discontinuing; adjusted dosing for creatinine clearance 30–60, avoid if <30
Antihypertensives				
Clonidine (Catapres)[a]	0.05 to 0.1 mg twice daily	Available as a patch, less effective than antidepressants or gabapentin	Dry mouth, drowsiness, dizziness, weakness, constipation, rash, myalgia, urticaria, insomnia, nausea, agitation, orthostatic hypotension, impotence, arrhythmias	Taper when discontinuing

Drug	Dosage	Comments	Selected Side Effects	Selected Contraindications/ Cautions
Methyldopa (Aldomet)[a] and belladonna, ergotamine, and phenobarbital (Bellergal)[a]		NAMS does not recommend due to limited efficacy data and potential for adverse effects		

Data from Azizi, M., Khani, S., Kamali, M., & Elyasi, F. (2022). The efficacy and safety of serotonin reuptake inhibitors and serotonin-norepinephrine reuptake inhibitors in the treatment of menopausal hot flashes: A systematic review of clinical trials. *IJMS 47*(3), 173–193. https://doi.org/10.30476/ijms.2020.87687.1817; de Villiers, T. J., Hall, J. E., Pinkerton, J. V., Cerdas Pérez, S., Rees, M., Yang, C., & Pierroz, D. D. (2016). Revised global consensus statement on menopausal hormone therapy, *Climacteric, 19*(4), 313–315. https://doi.org/10.1080/13697137.2016.1196047; Epocrates. (2024, December 6). Computerized pharmacology and prescribing reference [Mobile application software]. Retrieved from http://www.epocrates.com; North American Menopause Society. (2019). *Menopause practice: A clinician's guide* (6th ed.); North American Menopause Society. (2022). The North American Menopause Society position statement: The 2022 hormone therapy position statement of The North American Menopause Society. *Menopause: The Journal of The North American Menopause Society, 29*(7), 767–794. https://doi.org/10.1097/GME.0000000000002028; Panay, N., Ang, S. B., Cheshite, R., Goldstein, S. R., Maki, P., Nappi, R. E., & International Menopause Society Board. (2024). Menopause and HT in 2024: Addressing the key controversies—An International Menopause Society White Paper. *Climacteric 27*(5), 441–457. https://doi.org/10.1080/13697137.2024.2394950.

Abbreviations: CNS, central nervous system; HTN, hypertension; MAO, monoamine oxidase; NAMS, North American Menopause Society; XR, extended release.

Note: See prescribing reference for full information on doses, side effects, contraindications, and cautions.

*Not comprehensive

[a]Evidence-based use; not FDA approved for hormone therapy.

TABLE 14-8 Vaginal and Intrauterine Hormone Therapy Products*

Type	Product Name	Active Ingredient	Dose
Estrogen			
Vaginal hormone creams[a]	Estrace Vaginal	17β-estradiol	0.01% cream; 1 gm intravaginally one to three times/week
	Premarin	Conjugated equine estrogen (CEE)	0.625/gm; 0.5 to 2 gm intravaginally daily for 2 weeks, then taper gradually to lowest effective dose
Vaginal tablets[a]	Vagifem, Yuvafem	Estradiol hemihydrate	10 mcg; intravaginally once daily for 2 weeks then two times/week
Vaginal softgels[a]	Imvexxy	17β-estradiol	4 mcg or 10 mcg; intravaginally once daily for 2 weeks, then two times/week
Ring[a]	Estring	Micronized 17β-estradiol	7.5 mcg/24 hours, 2 mg/90 days; replace every 90 days
	Femring	Estradiol acetate	0.05 mg/day or 0.1 mg/day; replace every 3 months
Progestogen			
Gel	Crinone,[b] Prochieve[b]	Progesterone	4% gel (45 mg/applicator) every other day, give six doses; increase to 8% gel (90 mg/applicator) if no response
	Endometrin[b]	Micronized progesterone	100 mg insert
Intrauterine devices	Mirena[b]	Levonorgestrel	20 mcg daily, lasts for 5 years (52 mg over 5 years)
	Skyla[b]	Levonorgestrel	6 mcg/day (13.5 mg over 3 years)

Data from de Villiers, T. J., Hall, J. E., Pinkerton, J. V., Cerdas Pérez, S., Rees, M., Yang, C., & Pierroz, D. D. (2016). Revised global consensus statement on menopausal hormone therapy, *Climacteric, 19*(4), 313–315. https://doi.org/10.1080/13697137.2016.1196047; Epocrates. (2024, December 6). Computerized pharmacology and prescribing reference [Mobile application software]. Retrieved from http://www.epocrates.com; North American Menopause Society. (2019). *Menopause practice: A clinician's guide* (6th ed.); North American Menopause Society. (2022). The North American Menopause Society position statement: The 2022 hormone therapy position statement of The North American Menopause Society. *Menopause: The Journal of The North American Menopause Society, 29*(7), 767–794. https://doi.org/10.1097/GME.0000000000002028; Panay, N., Ang, S. B., Cheshite, R., Goldstein, S. R., Maki, P., Nappi, R. E., & International Menopause Society Board. (2024). Menopause and HT in 2024: Addressing the key controversies—An International Menopause Society White Paper. *Climacteric 27*(5), 441–457. https://doi.org/10.1080/13697137.2024.2394950.Note: See prescribing reference for full information on doses, side effects, contraindications, and cautions.

Note: See prescribing reference for full information on doses, side effects, contraindications, and cautions.

*Not comprehensive

[a]Consider adding progestogen if the individual's uterus is intact.

[b]Evidence-based use; not FDA approved for hormone therapy.

Therapy Considerations

Prior to prescribing HT, it is imperative that clinicians and their patients review any cautions or contraindications to hormone use (**Table 14-9**). The clinician must engage the individual in the decision-making process and weigh the risks, benefits, and scientific uncertainty with each patient to individualize their treatment options. The risk of breast cancer increases after 3 to 5 years of EPT (NAMS, 2019, 2022; Panay et al., 2024). As mentioned earlier, HT should not be used for protection against CVD or dementia. Use of HT within the first 10 years of menopause has not been shown to increase the risk for CVD (NAMS, 2019, 2022; Panay et al., 2024). Although some data indicate that beginning HT use in early postmenopause may have a cardioprotective effect, the only RCT that tested this hypothesis failed to find any such relationship (NAMS, 2019, 2022). Recent data do not support a decreased risk of dementia with HT use (NAMS, 2019, 2022).

Individuals considering using HT should have the recommended screening tests for health promotion and disease prevention in addition to a complete history and physical examination. Refer to Chapter 9 for screening recommendations. Special attention should be paid to any personal or family history of health problems that would contraindicate or increase personal health risks with ET or EPT use. If the individual is not at increased risk for HT, the clinician should explain the various protocols for administering HT: Et alone (for individuals without a uterus), EPT continuously or sequentially, estrogen with bazedoxifene, or local ET.

Hormone Therapy Protocols and Formulations

Estrogen Therapy

ET has been prescribed exclusively for individuals who have had a hysterectomy because the evidence (first reported in 1975) indicates that unopposed estrogen increases the risks for endometrial hyperplasia and cancer. Side effects of HT and strategies to manage them are listed in **Table 14-10**.

Estrogen–Progestogen Therapy

Combination estrogen and progestogen therapy can be taken either sequentially (S-EPT) or continuously (C-EPT). In the sequential regimen, an estrogen is taken daily with the addition of a progestogen in a cyclic fashion, usually on days 1 to 12 of the month. One side effect often noted with this therapy is that most people have a withdrawal bleed following the progestogen. To avoid this consequence, the continuous regimen was developed, in which the estrogen and progestogen are taken daily. Another option includes pulsed combination therapy, wherein the progestogen is taken for 2 days, followed by a day off, in a repeating pattern. The original idea was to reduce potential side effects from the progestogen; however, breakthrough bleeding is usually more problematic with this regimen. A less frequently used regimen is the cyclic regimen, in which estrogen is taken daily for the first 21 days of the cycle, then progestogen is added for days 12 to 21. A withdrawal bleed usually occurs between days 22 and 28, during which neither estrogen nor progestogen is taken. In addition, menopause-related symptoms usually rebound when the estrogen is not taken; therefore, few individuals opt for the cyclic regimen.

TABLE 14-9 Contraindications to Hormone Therapy and Adverse Effects

Selected Absolute Contraindications to Estrogen Use	Selected Adverse Effects of Estrogen Therapy
Known or suspected cancer of the breast	Uterine bleeding
Known or suspected estrogen-dependent neoplasia	Breast tenderness
History of uterine or ovarian cancer	Nausea
History of coronary heart disease or stroke	Abdominal bloating
History of biliary tract disorder	Fluid retention in extremities
Undiagnosed abnormal genital bleeding	Headache
History of or active thrombophlebitis or thromboembolic disorders	Dizziness
	Hair loss
Selected Absolute Contraindications to Progestogen Use	**Selected Adverse Effects of Progestogen Therapy**
Active thrombophlebitis or thromboembolic disorders	Mood changes
Liver dysfunction or disease	Possible increased uterine bleeding than if taking estrogen therapy alone
Known or suspected cancer of the breast	Breast tenderness, increased density
Undiagnosed abnormal vaginal bleeding	Lipid level changes
Pregnancy	Cancer (breast, hepatic, ovarian)
	Stroke, hypertension, myocardial infarction

Data from de Villiers, T. J., Hall, J. E., Pinkerton, J. V., Cerdas Pérez, S., Rees, M., Yang, C., & Pierroz, D. D. (2016). Revised global consensus statement on menopausal hormone therapy, *Climacteric, 19*(4), 313–315. https://doi.org/10.1080/13697137.2016.1196047; Epocrates. (2024, December 6). Computerized pharmacology and prescribing reference [Mobile application software]. Retrieved from http://www.epocrates.com; North American Menopause Society. (2019). *Menopause practice: A clinician's guide* (6th ed.); North American Menopause Society. (2022). The North American Menopause Society position statement: The 2022 hormone therapy position statement of The North American Menopause Society. *Menopause: The Journal of The North American Menopause Society, 29*(7), 767-794. https://doi.org/10.1097/GME.0000000000002028; Panay, N., Ang, S. B., Cheshite, R., Goldstein, S. R., Maki, P., Nappi, R. E., & International Menopause Society Board. (2024). Menopause and HT in 2024: Addressing the key controversies—An International Menopause Society White Paper. *Climacteric 27*(5), 441-457. https://doi.org/10.1080/13697137.2024.2394950.

TABLE 14-10 Management of Hormone Therapy Side Effects

Side Effect	Strategy
Fluid retention	Decrease salt intake; maintain adequate water intake; exercise; use an herbal diuretic or mild prescription diuretic
Bloating	Change to low-dose transdermal estrogen; lower the progestogen dose to a level that still protects the uterus; change the progestogen, or try micronized progesterone
Breast tenderness	Lower the estrogen dose; change the estrogen; decrease salt intake; change the progestogen; decrease caffeine and chocolate consumption
Headaches	Change to transdermal estrogen; lower the estrogen and/or progestogen dose; change to a C-EPT regimen; ensure adequate water intake; decrease salt, caffeine, and alcohol use
Mood changes	Lower the progestogen dose; change to a C-EPT regimen; ensure adequate water intake; restrict salt, caffeine, and alcohol consumption
Nausea	Take hormones with meals; change the estrogen; change to transdermal estrogen; lower the estrogen or progestogen dose

Data from Epocrates. (2024, December 6). Computerized pharmacology and prescribing reference [Mobile application software]. Retrieved from http://www.epocrates.com; North American Menopause Society. (2019). *Menopause practice: A clinician's guide* (6th ed.).

Abbreviation: C-EPT, continuous estrogen–progestogen therapy.

Estrogens

There are a variety of estrogen compounds: estrogens that are bioidentical and transformed into human estrogens, such as 17β-estradiol, estriol, and estrone; synthetic estrogen analogs, such as ethinyl estradiol; and nonhuman conjugated estrogens, such as CEE. CEE has been used in most clinical trials, including the WHI and the Heart and Estrogen/Progestin Replacement Study (HERS).

Estrogens differ in their target tissue response and dose equivalency. They can be administered either systemically or locally. Systemic preparations are available as oral tablets and transdermal patches, creams, sprays, and gels. Local preparations are available as creams, tablets, and rings. The vaginal ring releasing 0.5 mg or 0.1 mg per day of estradiol acetate over 3 months is the only local treatment that has proved effective in treating hot flashes (Epocrates, 2024, December 6; NAMS, 2019). Local treatment with estrogen theoretically avoids systemic absorption; however, in a seminal review of the studies on vaginal preparations, Crandall (2002) found that the ring has slightly more systemic absorption. Individuals who want to avoid systemic effects, such as breast cancer survivors, should probably use a different preparation until more evidence is available.

Progestogens

Progestogens are hormones that possess progestational properties. The most commonly prescribed progestogen was MPA, but others are being used with more regularity, such as micronized progesterone (which is bioidentical), norgestimate, and norethindrone acetate. Side effects of HT are listed in Table 14-10.

Estrogen–Bazedoxifene Therapy

Therapy combining CEE with bazedoxifene is taken daily and continuously. There may be some breakthrough bleeding early during therapy, but this tends to wane over time. This combination formulation is appropriate for individuals with an intact uterus. No progestogen is needed because the bazedoxifene protects against endometrial hypertrophy and malignancy.

Estrogen–Androgen Therapy

Therapy combining androgens and estrogens has been theorized to improve loss of libido in postmenopausal individuals; however, there is not enough scientific evidence from RCTs to say with certainty that testosterone plus estrogen is more effective than estrogen alone. Known side effects of androgens include alopecia, acne, deepening of the voice, and hirsutism. As of this writing, there are no menopausal androgen therapies approved by the FDA. Refer to Chapter 18 for additional information on use of androgen preparations and decreased sexual desire.

Natural Versus Bioidentical Hormones

Many individuals seek "natural hormones," believing they are safer and less likely to cause harmful side effects than pharmaceutically manufactured hormones (MacArthur et al., 2022; Thompson et al., 2017). The term "natural" refers to any product with principal components that originate from plant, animal, or mineral sources. Thus, this definition encompasses pharmaceutically manufactured hormones, which are derived from animal, plant, or mineral substances. Natural hormones are not necessarily identical to the hormones produced by an individual's body and must be processed to become molecularly identical to endogenous hormones (MacArthur et al., 2022; Thompson et al., 2017).

Frequently individuals requesting "natural hormones" are actually seeking bioidentical formulations (Endocrine Society, 2019; MacArthur et al., 2022; Thompson et al., 2017). Bioidentical hormones, which are identical in chemical and molecular structure to those made in the human body, are available through prescription from both conventional and compounding pharmacies. Bioidentical hormones do not have to be custom compounded. Several HT products that are FDA approved are bioidentical hormones. The bioidentical estrogens available in FDA-approved products are 17β-estradiol, estrone, estradiol acetate, and estradiol hemihydrate; bioidentical progesterone is available in micronized form (NAMS, 2019, 2022). Refer to Tables 14-6 and 14-8 for the names of FDA-approved products that contain these bioidentical hormones.

The term "bioidentical hormone therapy" was first used as marketing language for compounded products. Compounded bioidentical (cBHT) hormones are made in a compounding pharmacy and are not FDA approved. These formulations are often custom compounded for a specific individual, and customization may be based on salivary hormone testing. cBHT products may contain multiple hormones, including estrogen, progesterone, testosterone, and dehydroepiandrosterone (NAMS, 2019).

In 2018, the FDA partnered with the National Academy of Science, Engineering, and Medicine (NASEM) to assess cBHTs; they concluded that there is no evidence to support claims that cBHTs have fewer risks than FDA-approved HT products (Endocrine Society, 2019; NASEM, 2020). In fact, due to the lack of FDA approval and oversight for compounded products, custom-cBHTs do not have their safety, effectiveness, purity, potency, and quality verified (FDA, 2025; NASEM, 2020). Over 40 percent of individuals using HT in the United States use cBHT products, and most individuals are not aware that these products are not FDA approved (NAMS, 2019). Due to the widespread use of compounded products, the FDA has several initiatives to protect patients and improve the quality of compounded drugs. More information, including resources about compounding for clinicians and consumers, is available on the FDA website (https://www.fda.gov/drugs/guidance-compliance-regulatory-information/human-drug-compounding).

The International Menopause Society (Panay et al., 2024), Endocrine Society (2019), and Global Consensus Statement on Menopausal Hormone Therapy (de Villiers et al., 2016) advise against using compounded products for HT. NAMS (2019) and NASEM (2020) recommend cBHT be used only if there is a medical indication, such as an allergy or need for a dose or formulation that is not available in an FDA-approved product. Salivary testing to assess or monitor hormone levels is unreliable, is not supported by evidence, creates unnecessary expense, and should not be performed (Endocrine Society, 2019; NAMS, 2022; Panay et al., 2024).

Progesterone Creams

Several progesterone creams are available as over-the-counter products and from compounding pharmacies. FDA regulations are not currently enforced for these products, raising concerns about their purity and content like those with other cBHT products. Over-the-counter progesterone creams include products such as PhytoGest, Pro-Gest, and Endocreme; the stated progesterone content varies from less than 2 mg to 700 mg. These creams can also be prepared by compounding pharmacies.

Although some individuals taking systemic estrogens may want to use progesterone creams for endometrial protection to avoid systemic progesterone effects, no data supports this claimed protective effect. Some improvement has been seen in vasomotor symptoms among those using transdermal progesterone cream, compared with individuals serving as controls (British Menopause Society, 2021).

Plan of Care and Patient Education

NAMS (2019, 2022) and ACOG (2013, reaffirmed 2019) recommend initiating estrogen as ET and EPT at low doses, such as 0.3 mg CEE, 0.25 to 0.5 mg 17β-estradiol patch, or the equivalent. Studies have shown that these dosages provide adequate vasomotor relief. Progesterone doses in FDA approved combined EPT provide adequate endometrial protection (Stute et al., 2024). Using equivalent progesterone doses when using ET with added progesterone is advisable. Vasomotor symptoms usually begin to resolve 2 to 6 weeks after initiating HT. Transdermal estrogen has a lower risk for thrombotic activity and is recommended as a first-line treatment, especially for patients with chronic conditions such as hypertension and hyperlipidemia (ACOG, 2013, reaffirmed 2019; NAMS, 2019, 2022).

Patients should be offered anticipatory guidance about managing side effects if they occur. Research evidence has absolved HT from contributing to weight gain; however, fluid retention may make some people feel as if they are gaining weight. Table 14-10 lists possible side effects of HT and strategies to manage them.

Patients should return for a follow-up visit with the clinician in 6 to 8 weeks to evaluate their progress. If the initial dose of ET, EPT, or CEE combined with bazedoxifene does not provide adequate symptom relief, it can be increased, or a different combination can be tried. The decision to continue or discontinue HT should be revisited at least annually. On average, vasomotor symptoms last 7.4 years, but some individuals may experience them for 14 years or more (Avis et al., 2015). The duration of HT should be individualized based on the individual's symptoms and risk/benefit ratio (ACOG, 2013, reaffirmed 2019; de Villiers et al., 2016; NAMS, 2019, 2022; Panay et al., 2024). Decisions about extended use are complex due to a lack of adequate evidence about risks and benefits. Concerns include a potential increased risk of breast cancer with longer use and higher absolute risks for coronary heart disease, venous thromboembolism, and stroke in those who initiate HT at an age older than 60 years or more than 10 to 20 years from menopause onset (NAMS, 2019, 2022; Panay et al., 2024). Although the lowest dose for the shortest period of time has been the long-standing guiding principle for the duration of HT, NAMS notes that some individuals with more severe symptoms may need a higher dose and that individualizing care is key. When patients decide to discontinue therapy, they should be advised that there is approximately a 50 percent chance symptoms will recur. Rates of recurrence are similar whether HT is tapered or stopped abruptly (NAMS, 2019, 2022).

Several useful resources are available to assist with determining and evaluating an appropriate plan of care. The Menopause-specific Quality of Life (MENQOL) questionnaire can be used to identify an individual's most bothersome symptoms and more objectively track changes with treatment over time (https://download.lww.com/wolterskluwer_vitalstream_com/PermaLink/MENO/A/MENO_21_8_2013_10_30_BUSHMAKIN_MENO-D-13-00245_SDC1.pdf). Additionally, there are a number of mobile apps specific to menopause and osteoporosis management; for example, the MenoPro app by NAMS, the Well Woman Visit app by the Nurse Practitioners in Women's Health organization, the ACOG app, and the Food4Bones app by the Bone Health and Osteoporosis Foundation.

COMPLEMENTARY AND ALTERNATIVE MEDICINE OPTIONS FOR MENOPAUSE-RELATED SYMPTOM MANAGEMENT

The use of complementary and alternative medicine (CAM) is common in the United States, (Johnson et al., 2019). Approximately 51 percent of individuals use CAM to manage menopause-related symptoms at midlife (Johnson et al., 2019). More than half of individuals who use CAM for menopause symptom relief do not report this usage to their healthcare provider (Posadzki et al., 2013). Furthermore, the use of CAM to manage menopause-related symptoms is increasing (Peng et al., 2014). It is imperative for clinicians to ask patients about their use of CAM and to become knowledgeable about the CAM therapies that patients are using.

Herbals

Many individuals seek relief of menopause-related symptoms, especially vasomotor symptoms, by using herbal preparations. While future rigorous and well-designed studies are needed (Guo et al., 2019), there are promising results on the efficacy of herbal formulations in managing menopause-related symptoms (Portella et al., 2024). Because these products are generally identified as diet supplements, rather than as medications, they are not regulated by the FDA in the same way as prescription medications or other over-the-counter products. Federal regulations for these products do exist, but they are poorly enforced. This lax supervision raises questions about the purity, contents, and consistency from package to package or tablet to tablet. Various preparations of the same herbal product may contain different amounts of active ingredients (e.g., extract vs. tincture), and many products consist of mixtures of many different herbs in a single preparation, making dosing difficult. Furthermore, little is known regarding the interactions among various herbal products and prescription medications, over-the-counter medications or supplements, or other herbal products.

Despite these concerns, herbal products are widely used for menopause-related symptom relief (Portella et al., 2024). Several herbals are commonly included in combination products or in Chinese herb mixtures. **Table 14-11** provides information about some of these preparations.

TABLE 14-11 Herbals Commonly Used for Menopause-Related Symptom Relief

Product	Usual Dosage[a]	Purpose in Menopause	Comments
Black cohosh (*Cimicifuga racemosa*)	20 to 40 mg twice daily (proprietary standardized extract)	Vasomotor symptoms, insomnia, irritability, palpitations, headache	Multiple products and formulations available Evidence is conflicting regarding beneficial effect on menopause-related symptoms Safety for use longer than 6 months not established Can potentiate antihypertensives Wide variations in product ingredients, extraction processes, and purity Side effects rare, usually intestinal upset, headache, dizziness, hypotension, or painful extremities; inflammation of the lining of the stomach and intestines, nausea and vomiting, more common with higher doses Multiple case reports of liver failure, may be related to contaminants or use of a different cohosh species
Chaste tree berry (*Vitex agnus- castus*)	Dried fruit extract 3.2–40 mg by mouth daily for up to 6 months	Treatment of hot flashes Menstrual irregularity	More popular in Europe than in the United States; approved in Germany for PMS, mastalgia, and menopause symptoms Often found in combination products Evidence is conflicting regarding beneficial effect on menopause-related symptoms Side effects rare, usually nausea, vomiting, dry mouth, headache, dizziness, drowsiness, confusion, anxiety, intestinal upset
Dong quai (*Angelica sinensis*)	Two capsules 2 to 3 times/day; usually in combination products	Gynecologic conditions	Widely used in Asia No demonstrated benefit for menopause symptoms Often found in Chinese herb combination products (*Chinese Materia Medica* advises against giving it alone) A heating herb, can cause a red face, hot flashes, sweating, irritability, insomnia Contains coumarin derivatives; contraindicated in those taking anticoagulants Can cause photosensitivity, hypotension
Evening primrose oil (*Oenothera biennis*)	3 to 4 g daily in divided doses	Vasomotor symptoms such as hot flashes, mastalgia	Evidence is conflicting regarding beneficial effect on menopause-related symptoms Potentiates risk for seizure if taken by patients with seizure disorder, with phenothiazines, and with other medications that lower the seizure threshold Side effects include thrombosis, inflammation, immunosuppression, diarrhea, nausea, vomiting, bloating

(*continues*)

TABLE 14-11 Herbals Commonly Used for Menopause-Related Symptom Relief (*continued*)

Product	Usual Dosage[a]	Purpose in Menopause	Comments
Ginkgo (*Ginkgo biloba*)	40 to 80 mg of standardized extract 3 times daily	Treatment of memory impairment and attention disorders, memory changes	Insufficient research on safety and efficacy Memory changes often related to sleep disturbances, menopause-related sleep disturbances frequently related to vasomotor symptoms or other life stressors Side effects include mild gastrointestinal distress, headache, hypotension, allergic reactions, muscle spasms, arrhythmia, heart palpitations, dizziness, lowering of seizure threshold, increased bleeding after surgery; chronic use has been linked with subarachnoid hemorrhage, subdural hematoma, increased bleeding times
Ginseng (*Panax ginseng*)	200 mg to 3 grams by mouth daily for up to 12 weeks	General tonic Improved mood and concentration, treatment of fatigue, weakness, depression	Heavily adulterated Evidence is conflicting regarding beneficial effect on menopause-related symptoms Can cause uterine bleeding, mastalgia Contraindicated with breast cancer, monoamine oxidase inhibitors, stimulants, anticoagulants; may potentiate digoxin and others (multiple drug interactions) Side effects include rash (acne), nervousness, dizziness, insomnia, hypertension, headaches, low blood sugar, gastrointestinal problems
Kava (*Piper methysticum*)	150 to 300 mg of root extract daily in divided doses	Anxiety Insomnia Vasomotor symptoms	Systematic reviews indicate potentially effective for anxiety Banned in several countries due to hepatotoxicity; FDA recommends use only after consulting a provider; thus, it is not recommended Contraindicated with depression Side effects include gastrointestinal discomfort, impaired reflexes and motor function, weight loss, hepatotoxicity, rash
Licorice root (*Glycyrrhiza glabra*)	5 to 15 mg of root equivalent daily in divided doses; usually in combination products	Expectorant, anti-inflammatory, antiviral, antibacterial Menopause-related symptoms such as decreasing hot flashes	Found in many Chinese herb mixtures Contains flavonoids, coumarins, and terpenoids May relieve vasomotor symptoms Prolonged use can lead to high blood pressure, pseudo-hyperaldosteronism, heart problems, hypercortisolism, hypertension, hypokalemia, hypernatremia High doses can lead to primary aldosteronism, cardiac arrhythmias, cardiac arrest Contraindicated if the individual has hepatic or renal disease, diabetes, hypertension, arrhythmia, hypokalemia, hypertonus, pregnancy, or on diuretics
Passion flower (*Passiflora incarnata*)	Up to 800 mg daily of a dried alcoholic extract up to 8 weeks	Sleep disturbances, relief of hot flashes	Contains flavonoids Research shows mixed results in sleep improvement; may relieve vasomotor symptoms Menopausal sleep disturbances frequently related to vasomotor symptoms or other life stressors No side effects were reported with therapeutic doses

Product	Usual Dosage[a]	Purpose in Menopause	Comments
St. John's wort (*Hypericum perforatum*)	300 mg three times daily (standardized extract) for up to 12 weeks	Mild to moderate depression and anxiety Irritability Positive effects on vaginal dryness, libido, urinary tract problems, mental complications caused by menopause Vasomotor symptoms	Effective for treating depression Some data show efficacy in treating hot flashes Often combined with black cohosh for hot flashes Interferes with metabolism of many medications that are metabolized in the liver (e.g., estrogen, digoxin, theophylline); reduces INR levels; not to be used concomitantly with antidepressants, MAO inhibitors, immunosuppressants Side effects include gastrointestinal upset (minimized by taking with food), constipation, cramping, photosensitivity, rash, dry mouth, fatigue, dizziness, restlessness, insomnia, sensitivity to light
Valerian root (*Valeriana officinalis*)	300 to 600 mg daily aqueous extract 30 to 60 minutes before bed (insomnia); 150 to 300 mg aqueous extract each morning and 300 to 400 mg each evening (anxiety)	Treatment of hot flashes Insomnia Anxiety	Used for insomnia with intermittent dosing, for anxiety with chronic dosing Research showed improvement in sleep and depression/mood scales Some reports state there are no side effects, others identify mild side effects, including headache, uneasiness, excitability, arrhythmias, morning sedation, gastrointestinal upset, cardiac function disorders (with long-term use)
Wild yam (*Dioscorea villosa*)	It is possibly safe when used for up to 12 weeks	Menopause-related symptoms	Products claim that creams are converted to progesterone; however, the human body cannot convert topical or ingested wild yam into progesterone Research showed no benefit on menopause-related symptoms

Data from Guo, P.-P., Li, P., Zhang, X. H., Liu, N., Wang, J., Chen, D. D., Sun, W. J., & Zhang, W. (2019). Complementary and alternative medicine for natural and treatment-induced vasomotor symptoms: An overview of systematic reviews and meta-analyses. *Complementary Therapeutics for Clinical Practice, 36*,181–194. https://doi.org/10.1016/j.ctcp.2019.07.007; Hassen, G., Belete, G., Carrera, K. G., Iriowen, R. O., Araya, H., Alemu, T., Solomon, N., Bam, D. S., Nicola, S. M., Araya, M.E., Debele, T., Zouetr, M., & Jain, N. (2022). Clinical implications of herbal supplements in conventional medical practice: A US perspective. *Cureus, 14*(7), e26893. https://doi.org/10.7759/cureus.26893; North American Menopause Society. (2019). *Menopause practice: A clinician's guide* (6th ed.); WebMD. (2024). Vitamins & supplements. Available at: https://www.webmd.com/vitamins/index

Abbreviations: FDA, U.S. Food and Drug Administration; INR, international normalized ratio; MAO, monoamine oxidase; PMS, premenstrual syndrome.

Note: See prescribing reference for full information on doses, side effects, contraindications, and cautions.

[a]Dosages vary and differ according to form (e.g., tincture, liquid extract, drops, essential oil, standardized extract).

Phytoestrogens

Phytoestrogens are compounds derived from plants and are structurally like E_2. The most potent phytoestrogens are isoflavones, which are present in foods, such as soy (daidzein, genistein, and glycitein) and red clover (*Trifolium pratense*), and commercial preparations. Phytoestrogens can cause antiestrogenic effects by binding to estrogen receptors (Rietjens et al., 2017). They especially bind with beta receptors, which prompts some to classify isoflavones as selective estrogen receptor modulators (Guo et al., 2019).

Phytoestrogens have been extensively studied for vasomotor symptom management. Phytoestrogen use, including soy isoflavones (dietary, supplements, and extracts), red clover, and other phytoestrogens (genistein supplements, a phytoestrogen-rich diet, and topical wild yam cream) significantly reduced both hot flash frequency and vaginal dryness but not night sweats. Genistein and S-equol were found to provide significant improvement in hot flashes (Guo et al., 2019). Phytoestrogens, in low doses ($25\ mg/d \leq dose \leq 100\ mg/d$) and with long-term use, have also been found to reduce depression symptoms, particularly in postmenopausal individuals (Li et al., 2021). Soy isoflavones can improve quality of life (psychosexual, vasomotor, sexual, and physical scales) and may have beneficial effects on bone health. Soybeans and phytoestrogens have shown non-significant positive effects on vaginal atrophy (Saghafi et al., 2017). Studies evaluating the effects of phytoestrogens on cognitive function have been contradictory (Cui et al., 2019; Soni et al., 2014). Additionally, soy protein reduces circulating LDL and total cholesterol levels in adults (Blanko Mejia et al., 2019). NAMS has concluded that short-term use of soy isoflavones is effective for vasomotor symptoms, does not induce harmful effects on the endometrium or breast, and may be safe for breast cancer survivors (NAMS, 2019). Other classes of phytoestrogens include flavonoids, lignans, and coumestans. These phytoestrogens have much lower hormonal affinity and are generally not thought to be useful for menopause-related symptom management. They are found in some foods and food products and demonstrate some of the cardioprotective properties of isoflavones. Flavonoids are found in oils, spices, wine, tea, and some vegetables. Lignans are found in flaxseed oil, whole grains, and some fruits and vegetables. Coumestans are found in alfalfa sprouts, red beans, split peas, spinach, and some species of clover. Coumestan phytoestrogens can interfere with bleeding profiles and may interact with anticoagulants.

Acupuncture

Research findings evaluating acupuncture for the relief of menopause-related hot flashes have been contradictory. One concern is that many studies use sham acupuncture as the control, and sham acupuncture is thought to exert some effect (Kim et al., 2019). Manual acupuncture has been shown to be safer and more effective than hormone therapy for managing menopause-related symptoms and is recommended for treatment. However, the evidence supporting the effectiveness of other forms of acupuncture remains limited and inconclusive (He et al., 2021). Moreover, acupuncture may not significantly reduce the frequency of hot flashes but appears to produce hormonal changes like those of hormone therapy, such as increased E_2 and decreased FSH and LH. However, due to the low quality and limited number of trials reviewed, these findings are not conclusive. High-quality randomized controlled trials are needed to better establish the efficacy and mechanisms of acupuncture in this context (Liu et al., 2022).

CONCLUSION

Menopause is a key landmark in the lives of middle-aged menopause-capable individuals and women. This normal developmental stage gives people the opportunity to evaluate their health and risks for diseases of aging, and in turn institute lifestyle changes that can prevent disease and promote health. Although many individuals transition through perimenopause to postmenopause without incident, many also experience mild to severe vasomotor symptoms. Lifestyle modifications, pharmacologic therapies, and use of CAM can often decrease symptoms and improve an individual's quality of life. As the number of postmenopausal individuals increase, clinicians are in a prime position to counsel their patients about healthy aging.

References

Ambikairajah, A., Walsh, E., Tabatabaei-Jafari, H., & Cherbuin, N. (2019). Fat mass changes during menopause: A metaanalysis. *American Journal of Obstetrics & Gynecology, 221*(5):393–409e50, https://doi.org/10.1016/J.AJOG.2019.04.023

American Cancer Society. (2024). *Cancer facts and figures 2024*. https://www.cancer.org/content/dam/cancer-org/research/cancer-facts-and-statistics/annual-cancer-facts-and-figures/2024/2024-cancer-facts-and-figures-acs.pdf

American College of Obstetricians and Gynecologists. (2013, reaffirmed 2019). ACOG committee opinion no. 556: Postmenopausal estrogen therapy: Route of administration and risk of venous thromboembolism. *Obstetrics & Gynecology, 121*(4), 887–890. https://doi.org/10.1097/01.AOG.0000428645.90795.d9

American College of Obstetricians and Gynecologists. (2021, September). Clinical practice guidelines for osteoporosis prevention, screening, and diagnosis, ACOG clinical practice guideline no. 1. *Obstetrics & Gynecology 138*(3), 494–506. https://doi.org/10.1097/AOG.0000000000004514

American College of Obstetricians and Gynecologists. (2022). Management of postmenopausal osteoporosis: ACOG clinical practice guideline no. 2. *Obstetrics & Gynecology, 139*(4), 698–717. https://doi.org/10.1097/AOG.0000000000004730.

American Diabetes Association. (2024). Summary of revisions: Standards of care in diabetes—2024. *Diabetes Care, 47*(Suppl 1), S5–S10. https://doi.org/10.2337/dc24-SREV

Anam, A. K., & Insogna, K. (2021). Update on osteoporosis screening and management. *Medical Clinics, 105*(6), 1117–1134. https://doi.org/10.1016/j.mcna.2021.05.016

Anderson, D. J., Chung, H. F., Seib, C. A., Dobson, A. J., Kuh, D., Brunner, E. J., Crawford, S. L., Avis, N. E., Gold, E. B., Greendale, G. A., Mitchell, E. S., Woods, N. F., Yoshizawa, T., & Mishra, G. D. (2020). Obesity, smoking, and risk of vasomotor menopausal symptoms: A pooled analysis of eight cohort studies. *American Journal of Obstetrics and Gynecology, 222*(5), 478.e1–478.e17. https://doi.org/10.1016/j.ajog.2019.10.103

Annual Meeting of The Menopause Society. (2023, September 27–30). *Menopause, 30*, 1247–1305. https://doi.org/10.1097/GME.00000000000022882023

Anthamatten, A., & Parish, A. (2019). Clinical update on osteoporosis. *Journal of Midwifery & Women's Health, 64*(3), 265–275. https://doi.org/10.1111/jmwh.12954

Arnett, D. K., Blumenthal, R. S., Albert, M. A., Buroker, A. B., Goldberger, Z. D., Hahn, E. J., Himmelfarb, C. D., Khera, A., Lloyd-Jones, D., McEvoy, J. W., Michos, E. D., Miedma, M. D., Muñoz, D., Smith, S. C., Jr., Virani, S. S., Williams, K. A., Sr., Yeboah, J., & Ziaeian, B. (2019). 2019 ACC/AHA guideline on the primary prevention of cardiovascular disease: A report of the American College of Cardiology/American Heart Association Task Force on Clinical Practice Guidelines. *Circulation, 140*(11), e596–e646. https://doi.org/10.1161/CIR.0000000000000678

Avis, N. E., Crawford, S. L., Greendale, G., Bromberger, J. T., Everson-Rose, S. A., Gold, E. B., Hess, R., Joffe, H., Kravitz, H. M., Tepper, P. G., & Thurston, R. C. (2015). Duration of menopausal vasomotor symptoms over the menopause transition. *JAMA Internal Medicine, 175*(4), 531-539. https://doi.org/10.1001/jamainternmed.2014.8063

Ayehunie, S., Wang, Y.-Y., Landry, T., Bogojevic, S., & Cone, R.A., (2018). Hyperosmolal vaginal lubricants markedly reduce epithelial barrier properties in a three-dimensional vaginal epithelium model. *Toxicology Reports, 5*, 134-140. https://doi.org/10.1016/j.toxrep.2017.12.011

Azizi, M., Khani, S., Kamali, M., & Elyasi, F. (2022). The efficacy and safety of serotonin reuptake inhibitors and serotonin-norepinephrine reuptake inhibitors in the treatment of menopausal hot flashes: A systematic review of clinical trials. *IJMS 47*(3), 173–193. https://doi.org/10.30476/ijms.2020.87687.1817

Barnard, N. D., Kahleova, H., Holtz, D. N., Del Aguila, F., Neola, M., Crosby, L. M., & Holubkov, R. (2021). The Women's Study for the Alleviation of Vasomotor Symptoms (WAVS): A randomized, controlled trial of a plant-based diet and whole soybeans for postmenopausal women. *Menopause (New York, N.Y.), 28*(10), 1150–1156.

Benjamin, E. J., Muntner, P., Alonso, A., Bittencourt, M. S., Callaway, C. W., Carson, A. P., Chamberlain, A. M., Chang, A. R., Cheng, S., Das, S. R., Delling, F. N., Diousse, L., Elkind, M. S. V., Ferguson, J. F., Fornage, M., Jordan, L. C., Khan, S. S., Kissela, B. M., Knutson, K. L., . . . Virani, S. S. (2019). Heart disease and stroke statistics—2019 update: A report from the American Heart Association. *Circulation, 139*(10), e56–e528. https://doi.org/10.1161/CIR.0000000000000659

Berin, E., Hammar, M., Lindblom, H., Lindh-Åstrand, L., & Spetz Holm, A. C. (2022). Effects of resistance training on quality of life in postmenopausal women with vasomotor symptoms. *Climacteric: The Journal of the International Menopause Society, 25*(3), 264–270. https://doi.org/10.1080/13697137.2021.1941849

Biondi, B., & Cappola, A. R. (2022). Subclinical hypothyroidism in older individuals. *The Lancet Diabetes & Endocrinology, 10*(2), 129-141. https://doi.org/10.1016/S2213-8587(21)00285-0

Blanco Mejia, S., Messina, M., Li, S. S., Viguiliouk, E., Chiavaroli, L., Khan, T. A., Srichaikul, K., Mirrahimi, A., Sievenpiper, J. L., Kris-Etherton, P., Jenkins, D. J. A. (2019). A meta-analysis of 46 studies identified by the FDA demonstrates that soy protein decreases circulating LDL and total cholesterol concentrations in adults. *Journal of Nutrition 149*(6), 968-981. https://doi.org/10.1093/jn/nxz020

Brent, S., Christakis, M., & Shirreff, L. (2023). Primary ovarian insufficiency. *Canadian Medical Association Journal (CMAJ), 195*(28), E956–E956. https://doi.org/10.1503/cmaj.221712

British Menopause Society. (2021). *Tool for clinicians: Progestins and endometrial protection*. Available at: https://thebms.org.uk/wp-content/uploads/2021/10/14-BMS-TfC-Progestogens-and-endometrial-protection-01H.pdf

Bromberger, J. T., & Epperson, C. N. (2018). Depression during and after the perimenopause: Impact of hormones, genetics, and environmental determinants of disease. *Obstetrics and Gynecology Clinics of North America, 45*(4), 663–678. https://doi.org/10.1016/j.ogc.2018.07.007

Bull, F. C., Al-Ansari, S. S., Biddle, S., Borodulin, K., Buman, M. P., Cardon, G., Carty, C., Chaput, J. P., Chastin, S., Chou, R., Dempsey, P. C., DiPietro, L., Ekelund, U., Firth, J., Friedenreich, C. M., Garcia, L., Gichu, M., Jago, R., Katzmarzyk, P. T., Lambert, E., . . . Willumsen, J. F. (2020). World Health Organization 2020 guidelines on physical activity and sedentary behaviour. *British Journal of Sports Medicine, 54*(24), 1451–1462. https://doi.org/10.1136/bjsports-2020-102955

Camacho, P. M., Petak, S. M., Binkley, N., Diab, D. L., Eldeiry, L. S., Farooki, A., ... & Watts, N. B. (2020). American Association of Clinical Endocrinologists/American College of Endocrinology clinical practice guidelines for the diagnosis and treatment of postmenopausal osteoporosis—2020 update. *Endocrine Practice, 26*, 1–46.

Cameron, C. R., Cohen, S., Sewell, K., & Lee, M. (2024). The art of hormone replacement therapy (HRT) in menopause management. *Journal of Pharmacy Practice, 37*(3), 736–740. https://doi.org/10.1177/08971900231167925

Canivenc-Lavier, M. C., & Bennetau-Pelissero, C. (2023). Phytoestrogens and health effects. *Nutrients, 15*(2), Article 317. https://doi.org/10.3390/nu15020317

Centers for Disease Control and Prevention (CDC) National Center for Health Statistics. (2024, May 2). *Life expectancy*. https://www.cdc.gov/nchs/fastats/life-expectancy.htm

Chada, N., Chadha, V., Ross, S., & Sydora, B.C. (2016). Experience of menopause in aboriginal women: A systematic review. *Climacteric, 19*(1), 17-26. https://doi.org/10.3109/13697137.2015.1119112

Cho, L, Davis, M, Elgendy, I., Epps, K., Lindley, K. J., Mehta, P. K., Michos, E. D., Minissian, M., Pepine, C., Vaccarino, V., & Santos Volgman, A. (2020). Summary of updated recommendations for primary prevention of cardiovascular disease in women: JACC State-of-the-Art Review. *Journal of the American College of Cardiology, 75*(20), 2602–2618. https://doi.org/10.1016/j.jacc.2020.03.060

Chrysant, S. G. (2020). The cardiometabolic benefits of exercise in postmenopausal women. *Journal of Clinical Hypertension (Greenwich, Conn.), 22*(9), 1691–1693. https://doi.org/10.1111/jch.13968

Conde, D. M., Verdade, R. C., Valadares, A. L. R., Mella, L. F. B., Pedro, A. O., & Costa-Paiva, L. (2021). Menopause and cognitive impairment: A narrative review of current knowledge. *World Journal of Psychiatry, 11*(8), 412–428. https://doi.org/10.5498/wjp.v11.i8.412

Couraud, G., Souffir, C., Gaigneux, E., Kolta, S., Roux, C., & Briot, K. (2017) Adjusting FRAX® on TBS for identification of subjects at high risk of fractures. *Bone, 101*, 214–218.

Crandall, C. (2002). Vaginal estrogen preparations: A review of safety and efficacy for vaginal atrophy. *Journal of Women's Health, 11*(10), 857–877. https://doi.org/10.1089/154099902762203704

Cui, C., Birru, R. L., Snitz, B. E., Ihara, M., Kakuta, C., Lopresti, B. J., Aizenstein, H. J., Lopez, O. L., Mathis, C. A., Miyamoto, Y., Kuller, L. H., & Sekikawa, A. (2019). Effects of soy isoflavones on cognitive function: A systematic review and meta-analysis of randomized controlled trials. *Nutrition Reviews, 78*(2), 134–144. https://doi.org/10.1093/nutrit/nuz050

Dalmijn, E. W., Visse, M. A., & van Nistelrooij, I. (2024). Decision-making in case of an unintended pregnancy: An overview of what is known about this complex process. *Journal of Psychosomatic Obstetrics and Gynaecology, 45*(1), 2321461. https://doi.org/10.1080/0167482X.2024.2321461

de Villiers, T. J., Hall, J. E., Pinkerton, J. V., Cerdas Pérez, S., Rees, M., Yang, C., & Pierroz, D. D. (2016). Revised global consensus statement on menopausal hormone therapy. *Climacteric, 19*(4), 313–315. https://doi.org/10.1080/13697137.2016.1196047

Dezzutti, C.S., Brown, E.R., Moncla, B., Russo, J., Cost, M., Wang, L., Uranker, K., Ayudhya, R.P.K.N, Pryke, K., Pickett, J., LeBlanc, M.-A., & Rohan, L.C. (2012). Is wetter better? An evaluation of over-the-counter personal lubricants for safety and anti-HIV-1 activity. PloS One, 7(11), e48328. https://doi.org/10.1371/journal.pone.0048328

Downham Moore, A. M. (2022). *The French invention of menopause and the medicalisation of women's ageing: A history.* Oxford University Press. https://doi-org.ezproxy.lib.uconn.edu/10.1093/oso/9780192842916.001.0001

El Khoudary, S. R., Greendale, G., Crawford, S. L., Avis, N. E., Brooks, M. M., Thurston, R. C., Karvonen-Gutierrez, C., Waetjen, L. E., & Matthews, K. (2019). The menopause transition and women's health at midlife: A progress report from the Study of Women's Health Across the Nation (SWAN). *Menopause, 26*(10), 1213–1227. https://doi.org/10.1097/GME.0000000000001424

El Khoudary, S. R., & Thurston, R. C. (2018). Cardiovascular implications of the menopause transition: Endogenous sex hormones and vasomotor symptoms. *Obstetrics and Gynecology Clinics of North America, 45*(4), 641–661. https://doi.org/10.1016/j.ogc.2018.07.006

Endocrine Society (2006, reissued 2009, 2017, 2019). *Endocrine Society position statement: Compounded bioidentical hormone therapy*. Available at: https://www.endocrine.org/-/media/endocrine/files/advocacy/position-statement/position_statement_compound

Epocrates. (2024, December 6). *Computerized pharmacology and prescribing reference* [Mobile application software]. Retrieved from http://www.epocrates.com

Erdélyi, A., Pálfi, E., Tűű, L., Nas, K., Szűcs, Z., Török, M., Jakab, A., & Várbíró, S. (2023). the importance of nutrition in menopause and perimenopause—A review. *Nutrients, 16*(1), 27. https://doi.org/10.3390/nu16010027

Feduniw, S., Korczyńska, L., Górski, K., Zgliczyńska, M., Bączkowska, M., Byrczak, M., Kociuba, J., Ali, M., & Ciebiera, M. (2023). The effect of vitamin E supplementation in postmenopausal women—A Systematic Review. *Nutrients, 15*(1), 160. https://doi.org/10.3390/nu15010160

Freedman, R. R. (2014). Menopausal hot flashes: Mechanisms, endocrinology, treatment. *The Journal of Steroid Biochemistry and Molecular Biology, 142*, 115-120. https://doi.org/10.1016/s40695-015-0002-y

Gold, E. B., Crawford, S. L., Avis, N. E., Crandall, C. J., Matthews, K. A., Waetjen, L. E., Lee, J. S., Thurston, R., Vuga, M., & Harlow, S. D. (2013). Factors related to age at natural menopause: Longitudinal analyses from SWAN. *American Journal of Epidemiology, 178*(1), 70–83. https://doi.org/10.1093/aje/kws421

Guo, P.-P., Li, P., Zhang, X.-H., Liu, N., Wang, J., Chen, D.-D., Sun, W.-J., & Zhang, W. (2019). Complementary and alternative medicine for natural and treatment-induced vasomotor symptoms: An overview of systematic reviews and meta-analyses. *Complementary Therapies in Clinical Practice, 36*, 181–194. https://doi.org/10.1016/j.ctcp.2019.07.007

Hales, C. M., Carroll, M. D., Fryar, C. D., & Ogden, C. L. (2020). Prevalence of obesity and severe obesity among adults: United States, 2017–2018. *NCHS Data Brief, 360*, 1–8.

Harlow, S. D., Gass, M., Hall, J. E., Lobo, R., Maki, P., Rebar, R. W., Sherman, S., Sluss, P. M., & de Villiers, T. J. (2012). Executive summary of the Stages of Reproductive Aging Workshop + 10: Addressing the unfinished agenda of staging reproductive aging. *The Journal of Clinical Endocrinology and Metabolism, 97*(4), 1159–1168. https://doi.org/10.1210/jc.2011-3362

Harlow, S. D., Sievert, L. L., LaCroix, A. Z., Mishra, G. D., & Woods, N. F. (2023). Women's midlife health: The unfinished research agenda. *Women's Midlife Health, 9*(1), 1–7. https://doi.org/10.1186/s40695-023-00090-5

Hassen, G., Belete, G., Carrera, K. G., Iriowen, R. O., Araya, H., Alemu, T., Solomon, N., Bam, D. S., Nicola, S. M., Araya, M. E., Debele, T., Zouetr, M., & Jain, N. (2022). Clinical implications of herbal supplements in conventional medical practice: A US perspective. *Cureus, 14*(7), e26893. https://doi.org/10.7759/cureus.26893

He, Q. D., Zhong, Z. H., Liu, M. N., Tong, Z. Y., Wu, Q. B., & Chen, M. (2021). Efficacy and safety of acupuncture vs. hormone therapy for menopausal syndrome: A systematic review and meta-analysis. *American Journal of Chinese Medicine 49*(8), 1793–1812. https://doi.org/10.1142/S0192415X21500853.

Hirshkowitz, M., Whiton, K., Albert, S. M., Alessi, C., Bruni, O., DonCarlos, L., Herman, H. N., Katz, E. S., Kheirandish-Gozal, L., Neubauer, D. N., O'Donnell, A. E., Ohayon, M., Peever, J., Rawding, R., Sachdeva, R. C., Setters, B., Vitiello, M. V., Ware, J. C., & Adams Hillard, P. J. (2015). National Sleep Foundation's sleep time duration recommendations: Methodology and results summary. *Sleep Health, 1*(1), 40–43. https://doi.org/10.1016/j.sleh.2014.12.010

Im, E.O., Ko, Y., & Chee, W. (2014). Ethnic differences in the clusters of menopausal symptoms. Health Care for Women International, 35(5), 549-565. https://doi.org/10.1080/07399332.2013.815752

Iqbal, A. Z., Wu, S. K., Zailani, H., Chiu, W. C., Liu, W. C., Su, K. P., & Lee, S. D. (2023). Effects of omega-3 polyunsaturated fatty acids intake on vasomotor symptoms, sleep quality and depression in postmenopausal women: A systematic review. *Nutrients, 15*(19), 4231. https://doi.org/10.3390/nu15194231

Ismail, L., Materwala, H., & Al Kaabi, J. (2021). Association of risk factors with type 2 diabetes: A systematic review. *Computational and Structural Biotechnology Journal, 19*, 1759–1785.

Jensen, M. D., Ryan, D. H., Apovian, C. M., Ard, J. D., Comuzzie, A. G., Donato, K. A., Hu, F. B., Hubbard, V. S., Jakicic, J. M., Kushner, R. F., Loria, C. M., Millen, B. E., Nonas, C. A., Pi-Sunyer, X., Stevens, J., Stevens, V. J., Wadden, T. A., Wolfe, B. M., & Yanovski, S. Z. (2014). 2013 AHA/ACC/TOS guideline for the management of overweight and obesity in adults: A report of the American College of Cardiology/American Heart Association Task Force on Practice Guidelines and the Obesity Society [Suppl. 2]. *Circulation, 129*(25), S102–S138. https://doi.org/10.1161/01.cir.0000437739.71477.ee

Ji, X., Singleterry, S., Kulikova, A., Harrison, Y., Shivakumar, G., & Brown, E. S. (2021). Association of menopause symptoms with depressive symptom severity in a diverse community-based sample. *Maturitas, 143*, 78–80. https://doi.org/10.1016/j.maturitas.2020.09.009

Johnson, A., Roberts, L., & Elkins G. (2019). Complementary and alternative medicine for menopause. *Journal of Evidence Based Integrative Medicine 24*, 2515690X19829380. https://doi.org/10.1177/2515690X19829380. PMID: 30868921; PMCID:PMC6419242.

Johnson, P. J., Jou, J., Rockwood, T. H., & Upchurch, D. M. (2019). Perceived benefits of using complementary and alternative medicine by race/ethnicity among midlife and older adults in the United States. *Journal of Aging and Health, 31*(8), 1376–1397. https://doi.org/10.1177/0898264318780023

Johnston-Ataata, K., Flore, J., Kokanović, R., Hickey, M., Teede, H., Boyle, J. A., & Vincent, A. (2020). 'My relationships have changed because I've changed': Biographical disruption, personal relationships and the formation of an early menopausal subjectivity. *Sociology of Health & Illness, 42*(7), 1516–1531. https://doi.org/10.1111/1467-9566.13143

Jowell, A. R., Sarma, A. A., Gulati, M., Michos, E. D., Vaught, A. J., Natarajan, P., . . . & Honigberg, M. C. (2022). Interventions to mitigate risk of cardiovascular disease after adverse pregnancy outcomes: A review. *JAMA Cardiology,7*(3), 346–355.

Kagan, R., & Rivera, E. (2018). Restoring vaginal function in postmenopausal women with genitourinary syndrome of menopause. *Menopause, 25*(1), 106-108. https://doi.org/10.1097/GME.000000000000958

Kandasamy, S., & Anand, S. S. (2018). Cardiovascular disease among women from vulnerable populations: A review. *The Canadian Journal of Cardiology, 34*(4), 450–457. https://doi.org/10.1016/j.cjca.2018.01.017

Kanis, J. A., Harvey, N. C., Johansson, H., Oden, A., Leslie, W. D., & McCloskey, E. V. (2017). FRAX update. *Journal of Clinical Densitometry, 20*(3), 360–367.

Kenda, M., Glavač, Nagy, M., & Dolnec on behalf of OEMONOM. (2021). Herbal products used in menopause and for gynecological disorders. *Molecules 2021(26)*, 7421. https://doi.org/ 10.3390/molecules26247421. Available online: https://pmc.ncbi.nlm.nih.gov/articles/PMC8708702/pdf/molecules-26-07421.pdf

Khandelwal, S. (2020). Obesity in midlife: Lifestyle and dietary strategies. *Climacteric 23*(2), 140–147. https://doi.org/10.1080/13697137.2019.1660638

Kim, T.-H., Lee, M. S., Alraek, T., & Birch, S. (2019). Acupuncture in sham device controlled trials may not be as effective as acupuncture in the real world: A preliminary network meta-analysis of studies of acupuncture for hot flashes in menopausal women. *Acupuncture in Medicine: Journal of the British Medical Acupuncture Society, 38*(1), 37–44. https://doi.org/10.1136/acupmed-2018-011671

Kohn, G. E., Rodriguez, K. M., Hotaling, J., & Pastuszak, A. W. (2019). The history of estrogen therapy. *Sexual Medicine Reviews, 7*(3), 416–421. https://doi.org/10.1016/j.sxmr.2019.03.006

Kronemyer, B. (2023). Alcohol and menopause: A balancing act. *Contemporary Ob/Gyn, 68*(7), 26–27.

Lambrinoudaki, I., Paschou, S.A., Armeni, E., & Goulis, D. G. (2022). The interplay between diabetes mellitus and menopause: Clinical implications. *Nature Reviews Endocrinology, 18*(10), 608–622. https://doi.org/10.1038/s41574-022-00708-0

LeBoff, M. S., Greenspan, S. L., Insogna, K. L., Lewiecki, E. M., Saag, K. G., Singer, A. J., & Siris, E. S. (2022). The clinician's guide to prevention and treatment of osteoporosis. *Osteoporosis International, 33*(10), 2049–2102. https://doi.org/10.1007/s00198-021-05900-y

Li, J., Li, H., Yan, P., Guo, L., Li, J., Han, J., Qiu, J., & Yang, K. (2021). Efficacy and safety of phytoestrogens in the treatment of perimenopausal and postmenopausal depressive disorders: A systematic review and meta-analysis. *International Journal of Clinical Practice 75*(10), e14360. https://doi.org/10.1111/ijcp.14360. Epub 2021 Jun 3. PMID: 33987926.

Li, W., Wang, Z., Li, X., Luo, R., Huang, J., Liu, B., & Zhou, X. (2024). Associations between serum estrogen levels and urinary incontinence in women: A cross-sectional analysis of NHANES 2013 to 2016. *Urology (Ridgewood, N.J.), 188*, 63–69. https://doi.org/10.1016/j.urology.2024.04.029

Liu, C., Wang, Z., Guo, T., Zhuang, L., & Gao, X. (2022). Effect of acupuncture on menopausal hot flushes and serum hormone levels: A systematic review and meta-analysis. *Acupuncture Medicine 40*(4), 289–298. https://doi.org/10.1177/09645284211056655.

MacArthur, R. B., Mattison, D., & Parker, R. M. (2022). Compounded bioidentical hormone products, a path forward. *Journal of the American Pharmacists Association, 62*(1), 42–48. https://doi.org/10.1016/j.japh.2021.08.005

Maki, P. M., Kornstein, S. G., Joffe, H., Bromberger, J. T., Freeman, E. W., Athappilly, G., Bobo, W. V., Rubin, L. H., Koleva, H. K., Cohen, L. S., & Soares, C. N. (2019). Guidelines for the evaluation and treatment of perimenopausal depression: Summary and recommendations. *Journal of Women's Health (Larchmt), 28*(2), 117–134. https://doi.org/10.1089/jwh.2018.27099.mensocrec

Money, A., MacKenzie, A., Norman, G., Eost-Telling, C., Harris, D., McDermott, J., & Todd, C. (2024). The impact of physical activity and exercise interventions on symptoms for women experiencing menopause: Overview of reviews. *BMC Women's Health, 24*(1), 399. https://doi.org/10.1186/s12905-024-03243-4

Nair, A. R., Pillai, A. J., & Nair, N. (2021). Cardiovascular changes in menopause. *Current Cardiology Reviews, 17*(4), e230421187681. https://doi.org/10.2174/1573403X16666201106141811

Nash, Z., & Davies, M. (2024). Premature ovarian insufficiency. *BMJ (Clinical Eesearch Ed.), 384*, e077469. https://doi.org/10.1136/bmj-2023-077469

National Academies of Sciences, Engineering, and Medicine (NASEM). (2020). *The clinical utility of compounded bioidentical hormone therapy: A review of safety, effectiveness, and use.* Washington, DC: The National Academies Press.

National Cancer Institute. (2024). *Cancer stat facts: Common cancer sites.* Retrieved from https://seer.cancer.gov/statfacts/html/common.html

Nelson, S. M., Davis, S. R., Kalantaridou, S., Lumsden, M. A., Panay, N., & Anderson, R. A. (2023). Anti-Müllerian hormone for the diagnosis and prediction of menopause: A systematic review. *Human Reproduction Update, 29*(3), 327–346. https://doi.org/10.1093/humupd/dmac045

Nguyen, T. M., Do, T. T. T., Tran, T. N., & Kim, J. H. (2020). Exercise and quality of life in women with menopausal symptoms: A systematic review and meta-analysis of randomized controlled trials. *International Journal of Environmental Research and Public Health, 17*(19), 7049. https://doi.org/10.3390/ijerph17197049

North American Menopause Society. (2019). *Menopause practice: A clinician's guide* (6th ed.).

North American Menopause Society. (2020). The North American Menopause Society position statement: The 2020 genitourinary syndrome of menopause position statement of The North American Menopause Society. *Menopause (New York, N.Y.), 27*(9), 976–992. https://doi.org/10.1097/GME.0000000000001609

North American Menopause Society. (2022). The North American Menopause Society position statement: The 2022 hormone therapy position statement of The North American Menopause Society. *Menopause: The Journal of The North American Menopause Society, 29*(7), 767–794. https://doi.org/10.1097/GME.0000000000002028

North American Menopause Society. (2024). *Menopause glossary.* Retrieved August 1, 2024. https://www.menopause.org/for-women/menopause-glossary#E

O'Connor, E. A., Evans, C. V., Ivlev, I., Rushkin, M. C., Thomas, R. G., Martin, A., & Lin, J. S. (2022). Vitamin and mineral supplements for the primary prevention of cardiovascular disease and cancer: Updated evidence report and systematic review for the U.S. Preventive Services Task Force. *JAMA, 327*(23), 2334–2347. https://doi.org/10.1001/jama.2021.15650

Palacios, S., Chedraui, P., Sánchez-Borrego, R., Coronado, P., & Nappi, R. E. (2024). Obesity and menopause. *Gynecological Endocrinology, 40*(1), 2312885. https://doi.org/10.1080/09513590.2024.2312885

Panay, N., Ang, S. B., Cheshite, R., Goldstein, S. R., Maki, P., Nappi, R. E., & International Menopause Society Board (2024). Menopause and MHT in 2024: Addressing the key controversies—An International Menopause Society White Paper. *Climacteric, 27*(5), 441–457. https://doi.org/10.1080/13697137.2024.2394950.

Panda, S., & Das, A. (2018). Analyzing thyroid dysfunction in the climacteric. *Journal of Mid-life Health, 9*(3), 113–116. https://doi.org/10.4103/jmh.JMH_21_18

Paschou, S. A., Marina, L. V., Spartalis, E., Anagnostis, P., Alexandrou, A., Goulis, D. G., & Lambrinoudaki, I. (2019). Therapeutic strategies for type 2 diabetes mellitus in women after menopause. *Maturitas, 126*, 69–72. https://doi.org/10.1016/j.maturitas.2019.05.003

Peacock, K., Carlson, K., & Ketvertis, K. M. (2023, December 21). *Menopause.* StatPearls. https://www.ncbi.nlm.nih.gov/books/NBK507826/

Peng, W., Adams, J., Sibbritt, D. W., & Frawley, J. E. (2014). Critical review of complementary and alternative medicine use in menopause: Focus on prevalence, motivation, decision-making, and communication. *Menopause, 21*(5), 536–548. https://doi.org/10.1097/GME.0b013e3182a46a3e

Pérez-Medina-Carballo, R., Kosmadopoulos, A., Boudreau, P., Robert, M., Walker, C.-D., & Boivin, D. B. (2023). The circadian variation of sleep and alertness of postmenopausal women. *Sleep (New York, N.Y.), 46*(2), zsac272. https://doi.org/10.1093/sleep/zsac272

Portella, C. F. S., Silva, I. D. A., Simões, R. S., Ghelman, R., Baracat, E. C., Júnior, J. M. S., & Sorpreso, I. C. E. (2024). An overview of systematic reviews of medicinal plants and herbal formulations for the treatment of climacteric symptoms. *Journal of Herbal Medicine, 38*, 100863. https://doi.org/10.1016/j.hermed.2024.100863

Posadzki, P., Lee, M. S., Moon, T. W., Choi, T. Y., Park, T. Y., & Ernst, E. (2013). Prevalence of complementary and alternative medicine (CAM) use by menopausal women: A systematic review of surveys. *Maturitas, 75*(1), 34–43. https://doi.org/10.1016/j.maturitas.2013.02.005

Poteet, B., Ali, N., Bellcross, C., Sherman, S. L., Espinel, W., Hipp, H., & Allen, E. G. (2023). The diagnostic experience of women with fragile X-associated primary ovarian insufficiency (FXPOI). *Journal of Assisted Reproduction and Genetics, 40*(1), 179–190. https://doi.org/10.1007/s10815-022-02671-1

Puhl, R. M., Lessard, L. M., Himmelstein, M. S., & Foster, G. D. (2021). The roles of experienced and internalized weight stigma in healthcare experiences: Perspectives of adults engaged in weight management across six countries. *PloS One, 16*(6), e0251566. https://doi.org/10.1371/journal.pone.0251566

Riberio-Valadares, A. L., Kulak Junior, J., Paiva, L. H. S. D. C., Nasser, E. J., Silva, C. R. D., Nahas, E. A. P., Baccaro, L. F. C., Rodrigues, M. A. H., Albernaz, M. A., Wender, M. C. O., Mendes, M. C., Dardes, R. C. M., Strufaldi, R., Bocardo, R. C., & Pompei, L. M. (2022). Genitourinary Syndrome of Menopause. *Revista Brasileirade Ginecologia e Obstetricia: Revista da Federacao Brasileira das Sociedades de Ginecologia e Obstetricia, 44*(3), 319–324. https://doi.org/10.1055/s-0042-1748463

Rietjens, I. M. C. M., Louisse, J., & Beekmann, K. (2017). The potential health effects of dietary phytoestrogens. *British Journal of Pharmacology, 174*(11), 1263–1280. https://doi.org/10.1111/bph.13622

Saghafi, N., Ghazanfarpour, M., Sadeghi, R., Hosseini Najarkolaei, A., Ghaffarian Omid, M., Azad, A., Bakhtiyari, M., & Hosseini Najarkolaei, E. (2017). Effects of Phytoestrogens in Alleviating the Menopausal Symptoms: A Systematic Review and Meta-Analysis. *Iranian journal of pharmaceutical research: IJPR, 16*(Suppl), 99–111.

Samson, S. L., Vellanki, P., Blonde, L., Christofides, E. A., Galindo, R. J., Hirsch, I. B., Isaacs, S. D., Izuora, K. E., Low Wang, C. C., Twining, C. L., Umpierrez, G. E., & Valencia, W. M. (2023). American Association of Clinical Endocrinology Consensus Statement: Comprehensive Type 2 Diabetes Management Algorithm - 2023 Update. *Endocrine practice: official journal of the American College of Endocrinology and the American Association of Clinical Endocrinologists, 29*(5), 305–340. https://doi.org/10.1016/j.eprac.2023.02.001

Schini, M., Johansson, H., Harvey, N. C., Lorentzon, M., Kanis, J. A., & McCloskey, E. V. (2024). An overview of the use of the fracture risk assessment tool (FRAX) in osteoporosis. *Journal of Endocrinological Investigation, 47*(3), 501–511.

Shim, S., Park, K. M., Chung, Y. J., & Kim, M. R. (2021). Updates on therapeutic alternatives for genitourinary syndrome of menopause: Hormonal and non-hormonal managements. *Journal of Menopausal Medicine, 27*(1), 1–7. https://doi.org/10.6118/jmm.20034

Shuhart, C., Cheung, A., Gill, R., Gani, L., Goel, H., & Szalat, A. (2024). Executive Summary of the 2023 Adult Position Development Conference of the International Society for Clinical Densitometry: DXA reporting, follow-up BMD testing and trabecular bone score application and reporting. *Journal of Clinical Densitometry, 27*(1), 101435.

Slopien, R., Wender-Ozegowska, E., Rogowicz-Frontczak, A., Meczekalski, B., Zozulinska-Ziolkiewicz, D., Jaremek, J. D., Cano, A., Chedraui, P., Goulis, D. G., Lopes, P., Mishra, G., Mueck, A., Rees, M., Senturk, L. M., Simoncini, T., Stevenson, J. C., Stute, P., Tuomikoski, P., Paschou, S. A., Anagnostis, P., ... Lambrinoudaki, I. (2018). Menopause and diabetes: EMAS clinical guide. *Maturitas, 117*, 6–10. https://doi.org/10.1016/j.maturitas.2018.08.009

Solomon, D. H., Ruppert, K., Greendale, G. A., Lian, Y., Selzer, F., & Finkelstein, J. S. (2016). Medication use by race and ethnicity in women transitioning through the menopause: A study of women's health across the nation drug epidemiology study. *Journal of Women's Health, 25*(6), 599–605. https://doi.org/10.1089/jwh.2015.5338

Søndergaard, M. M., Hlatky, M. A., Stefanick, M. L., Vittinghoff, E., Nah, G., Allison, M., Gemmill, A., Van Horn, L., Park, K., Salmoirago-Blotcher, E., Sattari, M., Sealy-Jefferson, S., Shadyab, A. H., Valdiviezo, C., Manson, J. E., &Parikh, N. I. (2020). Association of Adverse Pregnancy Outcomes With Risk of Atherosclerotic Cardiovascular Disease in Postmenopausal Women. *JAMA cardiology, 5*(12), 1390–1398. https://doi.org/10.1001/jamacardio.2020.4097

Soni, M., Rahardjo, T. B. W., Soekardi, R., Sulistyowati, Y., Lestariningsih, Yesufu-Udechuku, A., Irsan, A., & Hogervorst, E. (2014). Phytoestrogens and cognitive function: A review. *Maturitas, 77*(3), 209–220. https://doi.org/10.1016/j.maturitas.2013.12.010

Srivastava, S., & Sreelatha, S. (2024). Perimenopause: Review article. *Journal of Gynecological & Obstetrical Research*, 1–3. https://doi.org/10.61440/JGOR.2024.v2.13

Stuenkel, C. A., Davis, S. R., Gompel, A., Lumsden, M. A., Murad, M. H., Pinkerton, J. V., & Santen, R. J. (2015). Treatment of symptoms of the menopause: An Endocrine Society clinical practice guideline. *The Journal of Clinical Endocrinology and Metabolism, 100*(11), 3975–4011. https://doi.org/10.1210/jc.2015-2236

Stute, P., Walker, L. J., Eicher, A., Pavicic, E., Kolokythas, A., Theis, S., von Gernler, M., von Wolff, M., & Vollrath, S. (2024). Progestogens for endometrial protection in combined menopause hormone therapy: A systematic review. *Best Practice & Research Clinical Endocrinology & Metabolism, 38*(2024), 101815. https://doi.org/10.1016/j.beem.2023.101815

Sundheimer, L. W., & Nathan, L. (2019). Menopause and postmenopause. In A. H. DeCherney, L. Nathan, N. Laufer, & A. S. Roman (Eds.), *Current diagnosis & treatment: Obstetrics & gynecology* (12th ed., pp. 989–1014). McGraw Hill.

Thompson, J. J., Ritenbaugh, C., & Nichter, M. (2017). Why women choose compounded bioidentical hormone therapy: Lessons from a qualitative study of menopausal decision-making. *BMC Women's Health, 17*(1), 97. https://doi.org/10.1186/s12905-017-0449-0

Tosteson, A. N., Melton, L. J., III, Dawson-Hughes, B., Baim, S., Favus, M. J., Khosla, S., Lindsay, R. L., & National Osteoporosis Foundation Guide Committee. (2008). Cost-effective osteoporosis treatment thresholds: The United States perspective. *Osteoporosis International, 19*(4), 437–447. https://doi.org/10.1007/s00198-007-0550-6

U.S. Food and Drug Administration (FDA). (2025). *Compounding and the FDA: Questions and answers*. https://www.fda.gov/drugs/human-drug-compounding/compounding-and-fda-questions-and-answers

U.S. Preventive Services Task Force. (2021). Interventions for Tobacco smoking cessation in adults, including pregnant persons: US Preventive ServicesTask Force recommendation statement. *JAMA, 325*(3), 265–279. https://doi.org/10.1001/jama.2020.25019

Villa, P., Bounous, V. E., Amar, I. D., Bernardini, F., Giorgi, M., Attianese, D., Ferrero, A., D'Oria, M., & Scambia, G. (2024). Hormone replacement therapy in post-menopause hormone-dependent gynecological cancer patients: A narrative review. *Journal of Clinical Medicine, 13*(5), Article 1443. https://doi.org/10.3390/jcm13051443

Viuff, M., & Gravholt, C. H. (2022). Turner syndrome and fertility. *Annales d'endocrinologie, 83*(4), 244–249. https://doi.org/10.1016/j.ando.2022.06.001

Volpp, K. G., Berkowitz, S. A., Sharma, S. V., Anderson, C. A. M., Brewer, L. C., Elkind, M. S. V., Gardner, C. D., Gervis, J. E., Harrington, R. A., Herrero, M., Lichtenstein, A. H., McClellan, M., Muse, J., Roberto, C. A., Zachariah, J. P. V., & American Heart Association (2023). Food Is Medicine: A Presidential Advisory From the American Heart Association. *Circulation, 148*(18), 1417–1439. https://doi.org/10.1161/CIR.0000000000001182

Wang, G., Lv, J., Qiu, X., & An, Y. (2019). Integrating genome-wide association and eQTLs studies identifies the genes associated with age at menarche and age at natural menopause. *PloS One, 14*(6), e0213953. https://doi.org/10.1371/journal.pone.0213953

Wasnik, V. B., Acharya, N., & Mohammad, S. (2023). Genitourinary Syndrome of Menopause: A narrative review focusing on its effects on the sexual health and quality of life of women. *Cureus, 15*(11), e48143. https://doi.org/10.7759/cureus.48143

WebMD. (2024). *Vitamins & supplements*. Available at: https://www.webmd.com/vitamins/index

Whitcomb, B. W., Purdue-Smithe, A. C., Szegda, K. L., Boutot, M. E., Hankinson, S. E., Manson, J. E., Rosner, B., Willett, W. C., Eliassen, A. H., & Bertone-Johnson, E. R. (2018). Cigarette smoking and risk of early natural menopause. *American Journal of Epidemiology, 187*(4), 696–704. https://doi.org/10.1093/aje/kwx292

Wilkinson, E. M., Laniewski, P., Herbst-Kravlovetz, M. M., & Brotman, R. M. (2019). Personal and clinical vaginal lubricants: Impact of local vaginal microenvironment and implications for epithelial cell host response and barrier function. *Journal of Infectious Disease, 2019*(220), 2009–2018.

Wilson, R. (1966). *Feminine forever*. Evans.

Woodward, M. (2019). Cardiovascular disease and the female disadvantage. *International Journal of Environmental Research and Public Health, 16*(7), 1165. https://doi.org/10.3390/ijerph16071165

Yuksel, N., Evaniuk, D., Huang, L., Malhotra, U., Blake, J., Wolfman, W., & Fortier, M. (2021). Guideline No. 422a: Menopause: Vasomotor symptoms, prescription therapeutic agents, complementary and alternative medicine, nutrition, and lifestyle. *Journal of Obstetrics and Gynaecology Canada: JOGC = Journal d'obstetrique et gynecologie du Canada: JOGC, 43*(10), 1188–1204.e1. https://doi.org/10.1016/j.jogc.2021.08.003

Zhao, F. Y., Zheng, Z., Fu, Q. Q., Conduit, R., Xu, H., Wang, H. R., Huang, Y. L., Jiang, T., Zhang, W. J., & Kennedy, G. A. (2023). Acupuncture for comorbid depression and insomnia in perimenopause: A feasibility patient-assessor-blinded, randomized, and sham-controlled clinical trial. *Frontiers in Public Health, 11*, 1120567. https://doi.org/10.3389/fpubh.2023.1120567

Zhu, D., Chung, H.-F., Pandeya, N., Dobson, A. J., Cade, J. E., Greenwood, D. C., Crawford, S. L., Avis, N. E., Gold, E. B., Mitchell, E. S., Woods, N. F., Anderson, D., Brown, D. E., & Mishra, G. D. (2018). Relationships between intensity, duration, cumulative dose, and timing of smoking with age at menopause: A pooled analysis of individual data from 17 observational studies. *PLoS Medicine, 15*(11), e1002704. https://doi.org/10.1371/journal.pmed.1002704

Zhu, D., Chung, H.-F., Pandeya, N., Dobson, A. J., Kuh, D., Crawford, S. L., Gold, E. B., Avis, N. E., Giles, G. G., Bruinsma, F., Adami, H.-O., Weiderpass, E., Greenwood, D. C., Cade, J. E., Mitchell, E. S., Woods, N. F., Brunner, E. J., Simonsen, M. K., & Mishra, G. D. (2018). Body mass index and age at natural menopause: An international pooled analysis of 11 prospective studies. *European Journal of Epidemiology, 33*(8), 699–710. https://doi.org/10.1007/s10654-018-0367-y

CHAPTER 15

Intimate Partner Violence

Abigail Howe-Heyman

The editors acknowledge Christina M. Boyland and Kelly A. Berishaj who were the authors of the previous edition of this chapter.

Content Warning: This chapter discusses sexual, emotional, and physical violence.

Intimate partner violence (IPV) is a serious global public health issue (World Health Organization, 2022) that may result in significant acute and chronic health consequences (Breiding et al., 2015). This chapter provides information on how clinicians may engage in both tertiary and secondary measures of IPV prevention. At the tertiary level, clinicians who have been properly trained and educated can provide high-quality, trauma-informed care and services that best meet the acute and chronic healthcare needs of patient–victims, leading to improved health and legal outcomes. At the secondary level, clinicians must be well versed in IPV screening and early identification of victims and perpetrators to intervene and prevent more severe health consequences associated with violence. Importantly, clinicians must also understand measures of primary violence prevention to stop abuse from ever occurring.

Since clinicians are instrumental in providing comprehensive, ongoing assessment and interventions for individuals who are experiencing IPV, it is crucial that they receive education about caring for victims of IPV and providing care from a trauma-informed approach. Part of this education is the understanding that sociocultural norms can have a significant influence on victims' ability to recognize, acknowledge, and report IPV. Stigma surrounding IPV disclosure, victimization, and divorce can prevent victims—especially those who identify as women—from disclosing IPV (Güler et al., 2023). Additionally, gender roles that dictate marital expectations and sexual norms can influence recognition and disclosure (Güler et al., 2023). Cultural concepts of preserving family honor and protecting children's well-being can also inhibit disclosure of IPV (Güler et al., 2023), and individuals who are immigrants may be afraid to report IPV because they fear deportation or persecution (ACOG, 2012).

DEFINITIONS

In keeping with the Centers for Disease Control and Prevention's (CDC) preferred terminology, a "victim" is the person who is the target of IPV, and a "perpetrator" is the person who inflicts the IPV.

IPV refers to "physical violence, sexual violence, stalking and psychological aggression (including coercive tactics) by a current or former intimate partner (i.e., spouse, boyfriend/girlfriend, dating partner, or ongoing sexual partner)" (Breiding et al., 2015, p. 11). An intimate partner can be further characterized as someone with whom a person has, or has had, a personal relationship; examples of these types of relationships include emotional connectedness, regular contact, ongoing physical contact and/or sexual behavior, identity as a couple, and/or familiarity and knowledge about each other's lives. Not all of these dynamics need be present to constitute a relationship. Further, the partner may or may not be someone that the victim lives with, and it can be a person of the same or different gender (Breiding et al., 2015).

TYPES OF INTIMATE PARTNER VIOLENCE

In 2015, the CDC's National Center for Injury Prevention and Control published uniform definitions for IPV and identified four main types: physical violence, sexual violence, stalking, and psychological aggression (Breiding et al., 2015). This remains the most current publication by the CDC and serves as the ongoing resource on IPV in the United States (U.S.). Thus, for the purposes of this chapter, the following definitions are used:

- Physical violence: The intentional use of physical force with the potential for causing death, disability, injury, or harm. Physical violence includes, but is not limited to, scratching; pushing; shoving; throwing; grabbing; biting; choking; shaking; hair pulling; slapping; punching; hitting; burning; using a weapon (gun, knife, or other object); and using restraints or one's body, size, or strength against another person. Physical violence also includes coercing other people to commit any of the above acts (Breiding et al., 2015, p. 11).
- Sexual violence: A sexual act that is committed or attempted by another person without freely given consent of the victim or against someone who is unable to consent or refuse. It includes forced or alcohol/drug-facilitated penetration of a victim; forced or alcohol/drug- facilitated incidents in which the victim was made to penetrate a perpetrator or someone else; nonphysically forced penetration that occurs after the victim is pressured verbally through intimidation or misuse of authority; intentional sexual touching; or noncontact acts of a sexual nature. Sexual violence can also occur when a perpetrator forces or coerces a victim to engage in sexual acts with a third party (Breiding et al., 2015, p. 11).
- Stalking: A pattern of repeated, unwanted attention and contact that causes fear or concern for one's own safety or

the safety of someone else (e.g., family member or close friend) (Breiding et al., 2015, p. 14).
- Psychological aggression: Use of verbal and nonverbal communication with the intent to harm another person mentally or emotionally and/or exert control over another person.

Psychological aggression is nonphysical acts of violence that may therefore not be perceived as aggression due to their covert and manipulative nature. This can include, but is not limited to, the following:

- Expressive aggression (e.g., name calling, humiliating, degrading, or acting angry in a way that seems dangerous).
- Coercive control (e.g., limiting access to transportation, money, friends, and family; excessive monitoring of a person's whereabouts and communications; monitoring or interfering with electronic communication, such as emails, instant messages, and social media, without permission; making threats to harm oneself; or making threats to harm a loved one or possession).
- Threat of physical or sexual violence (e.g., "I'll kill you"; "I'll beat you up if you don't have sex with me"; or brandishing a weapon), use of words, gestures, or weapons to communicate the intent to cause death, disability, injury, or physical harm; includes the use of words, gestures, or weapons to communicate the intent to compel a person to engage in sex acts or sexual contact when the person is either unwilling or unable to consent.
- Control of reproductive or sexual health (e.g., refusal to use birth control and coerced pregnancy terminations).
- Exploitation of victim's vulnerability (e.g., immigration status, disability, and undisclosed sexual orientation).
- Exploitation of perpetrator's vulnerability (e.g., perpetrator's use of real or perceived disability and immigration status to control a victim's choices or limit a victim's options); for example, telling a victim, "If you call the police, I could be deported."
- Gaslighting (i.e., mind games), such as presenting false information to the victim with the intent of making them doubt their own memory and perception (Breiding et al., 2015).

Reproductive and Sexual Coercion

Coercion is a common tactic used by abusers to gain power and control in IPV dynamics. In the National Intimate Partner and Sexual Violence Survey (NISVS), 39.7 percent of U.S. women reported some form of coercive control by an intimate partner (Smith et al., 2024). A specific form of coercive control is reproductive and sexual coercion. Sexual coercion is the use of behaviors and tactics with the intent to control and interfere with a partner's sexual decision making and/or coerce a partner to engage in sexual intercourse without using physical force (American College of Obstetricians and Gynecologists [ACOG], 2013, reaffirmed 2019). Sexual coercion is experienced by individuals across gender and sexual identities; over 1 in 5 lesbian women, nearly half of bisexual women, and over 1 in 5 heterosexual women in the United States have experienced sexual coercion in their lifetimes. More than 1 in 4 gay men, almost 3 in 10 bisexual men, and 1 in 10 heterosexual men report experiencing sexual coercion (Chen et al., 2023). The CDC does not include transgender people in their statistical reporting, and so there is not data that specifically addresses sexual coercion as a form of sexual violence in this population. A recent meta-analysis found that a median 25.0 percent of transgender people report experiencing sexual IPV in their lifetimes (Peitzmeier et al., 2020). Some tactics of sexual coercion include the repeated pressuring of a partner to have sex, threats to end the relationship if the victim will not have sex, pressuring sex without using contraception, and/or knowingly exposing a partner to sexually transmitted infections (STIs) (ACOG, 2013, reaffirmed 2019).

Abusers may interfere with contraception use to facilitate a pregnancy, including hiding, withholding, or damaging oral contraceptives; refusing to wear condoms, damaging condoms, or removing condoms during intercourse (stealthing); failing to withdraw when that is the agreed-upon contraceptive method; or removing other forms of contraceptives such as intrauterine devices, patches, or vaginal rings (ACOG, 2013, reaffirmed 2019). The abuser may further threaten harm or use violence against a partner to coerce them to become pregnant or to carry out a pregnancy. The abuser may also force the individual to terminate a pregnancy or inflict injuries with the intent to cause a miscarriage (ACOG, 2013, reaffirmed 2019). Although reproductive coercion can occur in the absence of physical violence, there is a strong association with reproductive coercion and IPV (Smith et al., 2024).

THEORIES OF INTIMATE PARTNER VIOLENCE

It can be difficult to understand why perpetrators inflict violence on their current or former romantic partners; theorists seek to explain this behavior from a variety of perspectives (Chester & DeWall, 2018). The General Aggression Model theorists focus on an individual's biological characteristics and situational factors that influence a perpetrator to become violent (Anderson & Bushman, 2002). Feminist theorists view IPV through a gendered lens (Basile et al., 2013). I^3 theorists focus on the circumstances that instigate an act of IPV, suggesting that the interplay of three processes—instigation, impellence, and inhibition—determine whether an intimate partner reacts with violence toward their partner (Finkel, 2014; Finkel et al., 2012). Others have identified specific biological, interpersonal, and intrapersonal qualities in an individual that increase the likelihood that they will perpetrate violence on a partner (Chester & DeWall, 2018). More recently, theorists have employed the ecological model to understand IPV, considering individual, relationship, community, and societal influences that contribute to violence in relationships (Tarzia, 2021). Considering IPV as a multifactorial phenomenon will help the clinician caring for victims and perpetrators to provide support without judgment.

Cycles of Intimate Partner Violence

IPV incidents fall along a continuum ranging from acts such as belittling and name calling with the intent to gain power and control, to the most severe form of abuse, intimate partner homicide. It is important for clinicians to understand the cycles of IPV to identify where the victim currently is in the cycle. This will help the clinician develop focused, individualized education and safety planning to best meet the patient's needs. Further, the victim may be more willing or able to accept information depending on where they are in the IPV cycle.

Walker (1980) was the first researcher to recognize that repetitive patterns or cycles can be discerned in abusive relationships, identifying three phases in the cycle of abuse. Later, the third

FIGURE 15-1 The four phases in the cycle of abuse.

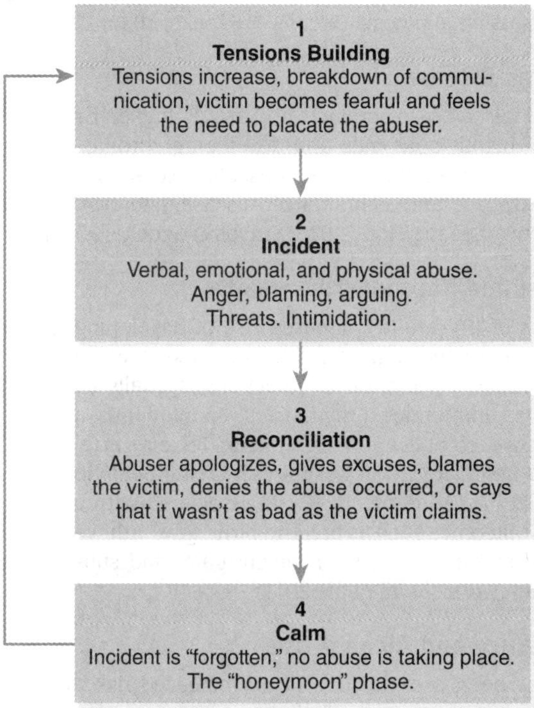

phase (reconciliation and calm) was separated into two different phases. Four phases are now identified in the cycle of abuse (refer to **Figure 15-1**):

1. Tension-building phase: This phase often includes verbal put-downs by the perpetrator, increased arguing, and, in some cases, the victim trying to appease the perpetrator.
2. Acute incident: This phase can include sexual assault, hitting, kicking, strangulation, and use of weapons.
3. Reconciliation phase: During this phase, the perpetrator will often repent for the abusive actions, will apologize, and may concede that the abuse occurred.
4. Calm or loving phase: During this phase, often referred to as the honeymoon phase, the perpetrator may apologize, promise it will never happen again, or deny the violence occurred. As time goes on, the calm phase may disappear altogether (Walker, 1980).

This theory continues to underpin contemporary understanding of IPV behaviors (Lutgendorf, 2019). An important aspect of the cycle of abuse theory is the acknowledgment that this cycle is not the same for everyone—some people may experience only some of the stages or none of the stages.

EPIDEMIOLOGY

Globally, 27 percent of individuals experience IPV in their lifetimes (Sardinha et al., 2022). In the United States, about 47 percent of women and 44 percent of men report that they have experienced some form of IPV during their lifetimes (Leemis et al., 2022). A median of 37.5 percent of transgender people report experiencing physical IPV during their lifetimes and 25.0 percent report experiencing sexual IPV during their lifetimes (Peitzmeier et al., 2020). When compared to cisgender people, transgender individuals are 1.7 times more likely to experience IPV (Peitzmeier et al., 2020). People who are victims of IPV have an increased risk for acute and chronic health consequences, including severe injury and/or death (Lutgendorf, 2019).

Physical violence—including being slapped, pushed, shoved, hit with a fist, kicked, slammed against something, choked, burned, or having a weapon used on them—is the most commonly experienced form IPV by both women (42.0%) and men (42.3%) (Leemis et al., 2022). Sexual violence, such as rape, sexual coercion, and unwanted sexual contact is reported by 19.6 percent of U.S. women and 7.6 percent of U.S. men (Leemis et al., 2022). More than 1 in 7 women and 1 in 20 men in the United States report being stalked by an intimate partner (Leemis et al., 2022). Almost half of women (49.4%) and men (45.1%) in the United States report psychological aggression by an intimate partner in their lifetime—this includes a partner demanding to know where they were and what they were doing, making decisions that should have been theirs to make, destroying something important to them, threatening to hurt themselves or kill themselves because they were upset, and trying to keep them from seeing or talking to family or friends (Leemis et al., 2022). Almost three-quarters of women in the United States report that they were first victims of IPV before age 25, including 27.1 percent who were first victimized before age 18 (Leemis et al., 2022). Among male victims, about two-thirds (62.1%) were first victimized by a partner before age 25, with 21.4 percent reporting IPV prior to the age of 18 (Leemis et al., 2022). Because the CDC does not include gender-diverse people in their reporting, there is limited national-level data to describe transgender and nonbinary people's specific experiences of IPV.

RISK FACTORS

IPV affects individuals of all backgrounds, but some circumstances can increase the risk of experiencing abuse. At the individual level, people who are marginalized by society, such as those who are younger aged, have intellectual disabilities, have limited education, or are facing mental illness or substance use disorder are at higher risk of IPV (Lutgendorf, 2019). Some relationship factors can also increase the risk of IPV, including short-term relationships, having other sexual partners, marital disagreements, and having a history of physical abuse as a child or witnessing IPV as a child (Lutgendorf, 2019). Residing in a community that has high levels of crime and unemployment, and a lack of social cohesion can also increase an individual's risk of experiencing IPV (Lutgendorf, 2019). Additionally, societal factors, such as gender inequality and cultural acceptance of IPV increase the risk of IPV (Lutgendorf, 2019).

THE EFFECTS OF INTIMATE PARTNER VIOLENCE

IPV directly affects a victim's physical and mental health; it can also have lasting financial, social, and family effects that ripple across generations. The impact also has repercussions for society as a whole. The estimated costs associated with IPV exceed \$3.6 trillion in lifetime expenses, \$2.1 trillion related to health care, \$1.3 trillion related to work and lost productivity, \$73 billion in criminal justice, and $62 billion in property loss and damage. In the United States, the estimated lifetime cost per woman who experiences IPV is $103,767 (Peterson et al., 2018).

Homicide and suicide of the IPV victim, perpetrator, or other individual, are the most serious outcomes of IPV. In the United States, nearly half of all female and one-tenth of male homicide victims are killed by intimate partners (AbiNader et al., 2023; Fridel & Fox, 2019). Among transgender and nonbinary homicide victims, 21 percent of homicides are perpetrated by intimate partners (Human Rights Foundation, 2021). Importantly, these IPV-related deaths are frequently tied to firearms, with more than 50 percent of IPV-related homicides caused by firearms (Tobin-Tyler, 2023). Identifying IPV and intervening prior to the escalation to fatal violence should be a key goal of clinicians (AbiNader et al., 2023).

Injuries

Although they do not always require medical intervention, approximately 35 percent of women victims and 21 percent of men victims will suffer an IPV-related injury. The injuries can range from minor (bruises and scratches), to moderate (cuts, major bruises, or black eyes), to serious injuries that require significant medical intervention (broken bones/teeth; knocked out after being hit, slammed against something, or strangled; head injury) (Leemis et al., 2022).

Mental Health

Victims of IPV are at 2.7 times higher risk of developing mental health disorders such as depression, anxiety, post-traumatic stress disorder (PTSD), and suicidal ideation and attempts than the general population (Kyle, 2023; World Health Organization, 2022). The risk of these mental health sequalae are increased in victims who have a prior history of mental health conditions, as well as in those experiencing more intense and recurrent violence (Stewart & Vigod, 2019).

Neurologic System

People who experience IPV often have long-term neurological consequences. Traumatic brain injury and hypoxia as sequelae of strangulation are the most common causes of neurologic injuries in victims of IPV (Haag et al., 2022), but symptoms may occur even in the absence of these injuries (Stubbs & Szoeke, 2022). Symptoms range from headache, dizziness, memory loss, blackouts, vision problems, hearing problems, and difficulty concentrating (Stubbs & Szoeke, 2022).

Cardiovascular System

Victims of IPV are more than two times as likely to have hypertension as those who do not experience IPV. IPV is also associated with greater rates of heart disease, chest pain, palpitations, and higher levels of inflammatory cardiovascular disease biomarkers (Stubbs & Szoeke, 2022).

Endocrine System

Experiencing IPV is associated with an increased risk of developing diabetes, likely because of high cortisol levels. Additionally, individuals who experience IPV are more likely than others to experience the adverse symptoms of menopause, such as night sweats, dyspareunia, and vaginal dryness (Stubbs & Szoeke, 2022).

Chronic Pain

Chronic pain is common in people who experience IPV, with 36.9 percent of victims reporting chronic pain (Leemis et al., 2022). IPV has been associated with body pain, pelvic pain, fibromyalgia, and temporomandibular joint disorder, as well as greater odds of using analgesia (Stubbs & Szoeke, 2022).

Chronic Disease

Individuals who experience IPV are at higher risk for poorer overall health outcomes and developing chronic disease such as gastrointestinal disorders, musculoskeletal conditions, respiratory disease and asthma, liver disease, and urinary and renal problems (Leemis et al., 2022; Stubbs & Szoeke, 2022).

Sexual and Reproductive Health

Victims of IPV are at increased risk of developing gynecologic problems. Gynecologic conditions related to IPV include pelvic pain, frequent urinary tract infections, sexually transmitted infections, unintended pregnancies, spontaneous abortion, and pregnancy complications (Clemente-Teixeira et al., 2022). IPV is also associated with sexual risk-taking behaviors (Chisholm et al., 2017). Additionally, IPV is associated with adverse pregnancy outcomes such as preterm birth, low birth weight, late and missed prenatal care, poor weight gain, and substance use in pregnancy (Chisholm et al., 2017).

Substance and Alcohol Use

IPV has been associated with an increased risk of abusing or becoming dependent on alcohol, smoking, intravenous drug use, needle sharing, and generalized substance use when compared to people who have not experienced IPV (Stubbs & Szoeke, 2022).

SCREENING FOR IPV

Establishing a Trauma-Informed Environment

When collecting the patient history, always document patient statements verbatim and in quotes. Do not try to modify language/terminology or try to paraphrase and summarize the history in your own words. If the patient uses slang that is not understood, the clinician should ask for clarification and document it in parenthesis. Always document "patient states" or "patient reports." Using terms such as "alleged" or "suspected" are not appropriate and can imply that the patient is not being an honest or accurate historian.

Screening for IPV is an important component of conducting a patient health history. Because of the statistical likelihood that a woman has or will face IPV at some point in her lifetime, the U.S. Preventive Services Task Force (USPSTF) recommends that clinicians routinely screen all pregnant and postpartum people and women of reproductive age for IPV (U.S. Preventative Services Task Force, 2025). USPSTF did not find evidence that screening for IPV in men or older women was valid or reliable and therefore is not currently recommended (U.S. Preventative Services Task Force, 2024) (a discussion of violence experienced by older adults is included at the end of this chapter). Despite this recommendation, it is estimated that only 2–50 percent of clinicians routinely screen for IPV (Alvarez et al., 2017; Burton & Carlyle, 2021).

When screening for violence, the clinician must cultivate an environment in which the victim feels safe and comfortable to disclose abuse. Lack of disclosure prevents the clinician from developing a plan of care that is appropriate to meet the patient's needs and may be a result of a deficit in the clinician's knowledge and skills in working with this highly vulnerable population. Victims may not disclose due to shame or fear of the repercussions for themselves and their families (Stewart & Vigod, 2019). It is important to inform the patient whether reporting the abuse is mandatory by law.

In addition to this, clinicians need to understand the importance of using appropriate screening tools and risk assessment instruments for their patient population. A recent systematic review by Garcia-Vergara et al. (2022) identified several assessment tools that are valid for use across cultures and primary languages. These instruments include: the Danger Assessment, the Danger Assessment for Immigrants, the Danger Assessment for Law Enforcement, the Danger Assessment-5, the Taiwan Intimate Partner Violence Danger Assessment, the Severe Intimate Partner Risk Predication Scale, the Lethality Screen, and the H-Scale (Garcia-Vergara et al., 2022). There should be no one except the clinician in the room during the screening process; this includes family, friends, and other staff members. The clinician should attempt to bar any interruption during the patient history to allow privacy in case the patient chooses to disclose. If the patient's partner has accompanied them to the exam, direct the partner to the waiting area during the examination. Do not ask but rather give a direct request so there is no option for the partner to remain in the room during the history or physical examination. This practice allows the patient to freely provide information to the clinician without fear of retribution from their partner.

If the patient brings their children to the office visit, it is imperative to ask that they wait outside during this portion of the exam. Screening for IPV in the presence of children raises a variety of safety concerns. Afterward, if the child talks to the perpetrator about the disclosure of IPV, the patient may be subjected to retaliation, such as further abuse or prohibiting further contact with the clinician. In addition, the child may be exposed to new information or be retraumatized by painful memories (Zink & Jacobson, 2003). Guidelines in the literature indicate that screening in front of children older than 3 years should be done only with prior permission from the parent, or only with general screening questions and sensitivity to the parent's nonverbal behaviors and comfort (Zink & Jacobson, 2003).

When screening the patient for violence and obtaining a health history, it is important for the clinician to be nonjudgmental and avoid victim-blaming statements or phrases, regardless of the circumstances surrounding the assault. The language the clinician uses can help foster a supportive, trusting relationship and disclosure of abuse. There are many reasons why a victim stays in an abusive relationship, and it is the clinician's job to support the patient in whatever decision they make about the relationship at this time. The victim may not be able to leave the relationship for physical, psychological, and/or socioeconomic reasons. If the victim grew up in a household where abuse was prevalent, they may view the abuse as normal and not recognize that healthy relationships are possible. They may rely on their partner for food, shelter, and transportation. They may have children in the home and no support system to help if they leave. They may be afraid that their partner will harm them, their children, family, or pets. Leaving a violent situation is often a process. According to the National Domestic Violence Hotline (2024), it takes a victim an average of seven times to leave their abuser before finally staying away.

A final consideration is to ensure that informed consent is part of the screening process. For the patient to answer screening questions in an informed manner, the clinician must educate the patient on what health information is protected by the federal privacy law, the Health Insurance Portability and Accountability Act (HIPAA), and what information the clinician may be mandated to report to law enforcement officials. In some states, clinicians are required to report all incidents of IPV to the police; in others, reporting is required only if a weapon, such as a gun or knife, was used. In many states, reporting is mandated to child welfare agencies if children are victims or witnesses of violence. Patients should be told this information before disclosure. In most states, the competent adult victim is the sole decision maker regarding whether they will file a police report (Stewart & Vigod, 2019). If the clinician is unsure about the duty to report, they should contact the local prosecutor's office to determine the requirements for mandated reporting. Clinicians can also obtain information about state IPV laws from their local law enforcement agency, prosecutor's office, or state attorney general's office. **Box 15-1** contains guidelines to facilitate a routine IPV assessment.

BOX 15-1 Guidelines to Facilitate a Routine IPV Assessment

1. Screen for IPV in a private and safe place with the patient alone (no children, partner, or family present).
2. If there is a language barrier, use a professional interpreter instead of family members.
3. Prior to administering a screening tool, it may be helpful to preface its use with a statement that generalizes violence in society and indicates that clinicians and many healthcare organizations support the routine screening of all patients for IPV.
4. Incorporate IPV screening into the routine medical history so all patients are screened routinely, regardless of whether abuse is suspected.
5. Develop and maintain relationships with community resources for people affected by IPV.
6. Keep printed take-home resources available, such as locations of shelters and hotline numbers.
7. Ensure that staff members receive training and regular updates about IPV.

With any yes answer on an IPV screen, a recommended interviewer response is, "Thank you for sharing. Can you give me an example? When was the last time?"

Data from American College of Obstetricians and Gynecologists. (2012, reaffirmed 2019). *Committee opinion no. 518: Intimate partner violence*. https://www.acog.org/-/media/Committee-Opinions/Committee-on-Health-Care-for-Underserved-Women/co518.pdf?dmc=1&ts =20160219T0918473135

Screening Tools

The USPSTF recommends that clinicians select from among four screening instruments to screen women for IPV: Humiliation, Afraid, Rape, Kick (HARK); Hurt, Insult, Threaten, Scream (HITS); Extended–Hurt, Insult, Threaten, Scream (E-HITS); Partner Violence Screen (PVS); and Woman Abuse Screening Tool (WAST) (USPSTF, 2025). (Refer to **Appendix 15-A**.)

HARK

HARK includes four questions that assess emotional and physical injury in the last year (Sohal et al., 2007). The tool was developed for use in the primary care setting and has a sensitivity of 81 percent and specificity of 95 percent. The questions have yes/no responses and should be administered by a healthcare professional (Andreu-Pejó et al., 2022).

HITS

HITS is a widely used tool for IPV screening that was first evaluated for use in the primary care setting. It is a four-item instrument with questions pertaining to how often one's partner has hurt (H), insulted (I), threatened (T), and/or screamed (S) at them. Each item is rated on a scale of 1 to 5 with a total of 10.5 or higher being a positive result (Sherin et al., 1998). With only four questions, it can be used for self-reporting or clinician administration. HITS is available in multiple languages. Additional versions of HITS have been developed; one that includes a question pertaining to sexual assault and a pediatric version (Andreu-Pejó et al., 2022). The sensitivity of the HITS is 30–88 percent, the specificity is 88–99 percent (Andreu-Pejó et al., 2022).

PVS

PVS is a three-item tool that was developed for use in the emergency department (Feldhaus et al., 1997). Three questions to ask: if the patient has experienced physical violence in the previous year and by whom, if the patient feels safe in their current relationship, and if there is a previous partner making the patient feel unsafe. A yes answer to any question indicates abuse. This survey should be administered by a professional. It has a sensitivity of 64.5–71.4 percent and specificity of 80.3–84.4 percent (Andreu-Pejó et al., 2022).

WAST

WAST includes eight items that assess physical and emotional IP, including the degree of tension and fear of the partner, the existence of emotional, physical, and sexual abuse (Brown et al., 1996). This instrument is used for patients to self-report and can be used in primary care settings. It has a sensitivity of 47–88 percent and specificity of 89–96 percent (Andreu-Pejó et al., 2022).

Responding to a Positive Screening Test

Immediate Response

Clinicians may feel unsure of how to respond and intervene after a victim discloses IPV. The first step is to thank the patient for sharing their experience with the clinician and reassure them that they do not deserve to be treated that way (Kyle, 2023; Paterno & Draughon, 2016). Next, the clinician should ask the victim if they want help and if so, offer assistance by sharing resources and developing a plan for safety. If the patient does not want help, a compassionate, nonjudgmental approach is important (Paterno & Draughon, 2016). With the patient's consent, the clinician should proceed with the following steps.

Additional Assessments

Before conducting any further assessments, the clinician should again remind the victim about any mandatory reporting requirements and limits on confidentiality. After obtaining consent, assessing for the timing of the violence will determine the capacity to refer the patient for a forensic exam, if they want to report the incident or collect evidence for possible future reporting. Victims should also be assessed for depression, substance use, lethality, intimate partner violence–related brain injury, strangulation injuries, and other physical injuries.

Danger Assessment The Danger Assessment (DA) is a valid and reliable instrument used to identify IPV victims who are at an increased risk of homicide (**Box 15-2**). The first portion of the DA should be completed in conjunction with a calendar. The victim is asked to mark the days on which abuse occurred and to rank the severity of the abuse. This method helps to recall events, raise awareness as to the severity, and reduce minimization of the abuse (Campbell et al., 2009). The second portion of the tool is a 20-item questionnaire pertaining to risk factors for intimate partner homicide. The DA takes approximately 20 minutes to complete. There are self-report scales that can be completed by the patient; however, it is recommended that the patient complete the tool along with a trained clinician, advocate, or law enforcement professional who can help score the tool and recommend appropriate resources based on the severity of the results (Campbell et al., 2009).

Screening for Intimate Partner Violence–Related Brain Injury

Victims of IPV should be screened for intimate partner violence–related brain injury (IPV-BI), particularly if the history includes numerous blows to the face, head, and neck; strangulation; or loss of consciousness or memory loss. Early detection and diagnosis can allow victims to obtain the appropriate care and rehabilitation to support their recovery from these injuries. There are many tools that can be used to screen for IPV-BI, though not one has been validated as a tool that consistently identifies brain injuries. Therefore, if a clinician obtains a positive IPV-BI screening test, the patient should be further evaluated before a diagnosis of brain injury is reached. The two most appropriate tools in the primary care setting are the HELPS-IPV and CHATS tools (Clarke et al., 2024).

The HELPS-IPV tool includes 20 questions and was developed specifically to screen for IPV-BI (Empire Justice Center, 2006). It is an adaptation of a tool that is used to screen a general population for traumatic brain injury (Picard et al., 1991).

The CHATS tool includes 12 yes/no questions and asks victims to select symptoms that they are experiencing from a list. This publicly available tool was developed by the Ohio Domestic Violence Network and can be easily accessed online (Ohio Domestic Violence Network: The Center on Partner-Inflicted Brain Injury, n.d.). Neither the HELPS-IPV nor CHATS screening instruments can be used to diagnose TBI, but affirmative responses suggest the need for further screening and assessment.

Strangulation Assessment

Strangulation is a form of asphyxia caused by the intentional application of external pressure to the victim's neck and throat. This pressure alters normal blood flow and/or breathing through

BOX 15-2 Danger Assessment

Several risk factors have been associated with increased risk of homicides (murders) of women and men in violent relationships. We cannot predict what will happen in your case, but we would like you to be aware of the danger of homicide in situations of abuse and for you to see how many of the risk factors apply to your situation.

Using the calendar, please mark the approximate dates during the past year when you were abused by your partner or ex-partner. Write on that date how bad the incident was according to the following scale:

1. Slapping, pushing; no injuries and/or lasting pain
2. Punching, kicking; bruises, cuts, and/or continuing pain
3. "Beating up"; severe contusions, burns, broken bones
4. Threat to use weapon; head injury, internal injury, permanent injury
5. Use of weapon; wounds from weapon

(If any of the descriptions for the higher number apply, use the higher number.)

Mark Yes or No for each of the following. ("He" refers to your husband, partner, ex-husband, ex-partner, or whoever is currently physically hurting you.)

____ 1. Has the physical violence increased in severity or frequency over the past year?
____ 2. Does he own a gun?
____ 3. Have you left him after living together during the past year?
3a. (If have never lived with him, check here: ____)
____ 4. Is he unemployed?
____ 5. Has he ever used a weapon against you or threatened you with a lethal weapon?
(If yes, was the weapon a gun?)
____ 6. Does he threaten to kill you?
____ 7. Has he avoided being arrested for domestic violence?
____ 8. Do you have a child that is not his?
____ 9. Has he ever forced you to have sex when you did not wish to do so?
____ 10. Does he ever try to choke you?
____ 11. Does he use illegal drugs? By drugs, I mean "uppers" or amphetamines, "meth," speed, angel dust, cocaine, "crack," street drugs or mixtures.
____ 12. Is he an alcoholic or problem drinker?
____ 13. Does he control most or all of your daily activities? For instance: does he tell you who you can be friends with, when you can see your family, how much money you can use, or when you can take the car? (If he tries, but you do not let him, check here: ____)
____ 14. Is he violently and constantly jealous of you? (For instance, does he say "If I can't have you, no one can.")
____ 15. Have you ever been beaten by him while you were pregnant? (If you have never been pregnant by him, check here: ____)
____ 16. Has he ever threatened or tried to commit suicide?
____ 17. Does he threaten to harm your children?
____ 18. Do you believe he is capable of killing you?
____ 19. Does he follow or spy on you, leave threatening notes or messages, destroy your property, or call you when you don't want him to?
____ 20. Have you ever threatened or tried to commit suicide?
____ Total "Yes" Answers

Thank you. Please talk to your nurse, advocate, or counselor about what the Danger Assessment means in terms of your situation.

Reproduced from Campbell, J. C. (2004). *Danger assessment*. http://www.dangerassessment.org; Campbell, J. C., Webster, D. W., & Glass, N. E. (2009). The danger assessment: Validation of a lethality risk assessment instrument for intimate partner femicide. *Journal of Interpersonal Violence, 24*, 653–674.

obstruction of the carotid arteries, jugular veins, and/or trachea, resulting in decreased oxygenation to the brain (Messing et al., 2022; Patch et al., 2023). Strangulation is a common and potentially lethal form of abuse. Death can result in as little as one minute if constant, consistent pressure is maintained on the neck (Training Institute on Strangulation Prevention, n.d.). Non-lethal strangulation can result in both acute and chronic sequelae. Traumatic injuries associated with strangulation include stroke, carotid artery dissection, brain injury, and miscarriage (Patch et al., 2023). Strangulation can also lead to long-term central nervous system injury such as loss of memory and problems with concentration (Patch et al., 2023).

Victims may use the term "choking" to describe being strangled. Healthcare providers, however, should not use the terms "choking" and "strangulation" interchangeably because they are separate concepts with different mechanisms of action (Brown, 2019; Stellpflug et al., 2022). Unlike strangulation, which is an intentional act committed by a perpetrator, choking occurs accidentally when the upper airway is obstructed by an external object, such as a piece of food. Choking can be corrected by utilizing the Heimlich maneuver and through removal of the offending object (Brown, 2019). Healthcare providers must use the medically and legally correct term when documenting the patient history.

Many victims who have been strangled will not seek care. One study found that as few as 5 percent of victims who had been strangled sought care within 48 hours (Strack et al., 2001). For those who do seek care, presenting symptoms may include throat pain, voice changes, or difficulty swallowing (Patch et al., 2023). When interviewing the patient, the clinician should ask about the modality of the strangulation—were one or two hands, a ligature, or a choke hold used; was the victim approached from the front or behind; and were they pinned against an object (Reckdenwald et al., 2022). Additional symptoms of strangulation that should be assessed include loss of consciousness, incontinence of bowel or bladder, loss of memory, breathing difficulties, nausea or vomiting, and headache. A greater number of symptoms should raise concerns about serious injury and all symptoms should be documented for forensic reporting (Reckdenwald et al., 2022). The healthcare provider should be alert to responses that signify the patient experienced oxygen deprivation in the brain, such as comments like "I saw stars," "I felt dizzy," "It felt like my head was going to explode," "I heard ringing in my ears," or "I don't remember."

Mental Health Assessment

Because of the high rates of mental health sequalae in victims of IPV, all victims should be screened for depression, anxiety, IPV, and suicidality (Salazar et al., 2023). Additionally, patients should be screened for substance use disorder (Paterno & Draughon, 2016). These assessments should be nonjudgmental and should be conducted for the purpose of identifying appropriate referrals and treatments.

SAFETY PLANNING

Regardless of whether the victim is ready to leave their relationship, all victims should be encouraged to develop a plan for safety. The clinician can encourage the patient to keep copies of vital documents (such as birth certificates, Social Security cards, and passports) and money hidden or at a trusted friend's house. The patient should also consider how to protect young children and how to obtain a restraining order or order of protection (Paterno & Draughon, 2016). Additional considerations include changing a routine, obtaining a new cell phone, and changing locks (Domestic Violence Crisis Center, n.d.).

Referrals

The clinician can offer referrals to a social worker, shelter, local support group, or legal services, based on availability. National resources such as the National Domestic Violence Hotline and the National Sexual Assault Hotline can be offered to all patients. If possible, the clinician should assist with reaching out to these resources while the patient is sitting with the clinician (Paterno & Draughon, 2016). Caution should be taken when providing written phone numbers or resources so that the patient's safety is protected.

DIAGNOSING INTIMATE PARTNER VIOLENCE IN THE ABSENCE OF A POSITIVE SCREENING TEST

Despite a thorough, trauma-informed screening, patients may not be ready or safely able to disclose abuse. Clinicians must be able to recognize other indicators of IPV in the absence of a positive screening test. Examples include a patient history that does not match the presenting injury, multiple injuries in various stages of healing, frequent walk-in or emergency department visits, a history of depression/anxiety disorders, and, importantly, multiple healthcare visits for vague somatic concerns (Chan & Sachs, 2023; Vicard-Olagne et al., 2022). The patient may not have access to identification or insurance cards, may not keep medical appoints or take prescribed medications, and may not follow directions about their care. Their partner may frequently be present in the healthcare system and appear controlling, do all the talking, and stay physically close to patient during the history or examination. The patient may appear fearful or quiet around the partner and defer all questions and decisions to the partner (Stewart et al., 2021).

Although it is never the clinician's role to force a disclosure, being aware that abuse may be occurring despite patient denial is important. The clinician needs to develop an appropriate plan of care that meets the patient's healthcare needs. Although the patient may not want to accept resources and referrals that address violence, the clinician can help by making sure the patient knows there are options should they want to leave the abusive relationship, and when they are ready, the clinician and the healthcare facility may be a safe place for the victim to go to seek help, support, and services.

PHYSICAL EXAMINATION

A thorough head-to-toe assessment should be conducted on clients suspected of being in an abusive relationship or who report being abused. The clinician must be able to perform a systematic physical examination that evaluates for the presence, severity, and timing of trauma or injury. Because most injuries affect the face, chest, breasts, and abdomen, special attention should be paid to these areas. If the victim reports sexual violence, a pelvic examination should also be included in the physical examination and should be conducted by a sexual assault examiner or clinician skilled in conducting a medical forensic examination. Refer to Chapter 16 for additional information on evidentiary examinations. As much as possible, the clinician should endeavor to make the physical examination minimally intrusive with the victim remaining in their clothing (Salazar et al., 2023).

Blunt Force Injuries

Bruise

A bruise is defined as internal bleeding of the skin from damage to the capillaries that is caused by impact with an edgeless object (Tirado & Mauricio, 2021). The term "bruise" can be used interchangeably with "contusion" or "ecchymosis." It is often helpful to use plain terminology that is easily understood. Using unnecessary medical jargon can be confusing when the patient is stressed or under duress and if there is potential for future legal proceedings. Each bruise should be documented separately. The patient's ability to heal and the color of the bruise is affected by many things, such as nutrition status, hemodynamic stability, age, environmental conditions, and medications; therefore, the stage of bruise healing is unpredictable and should never be included in the clinician's documentation (Tirado & Mauricio, 2021). A patterned bruise is limited to the capillaries of the contact area and will take a form consistent with the offending object. It is not a clinician's role to determine the offending object (Smock & Stack, 2021a). For example, if the injury looks consistent with a bite mark, do not document "bite mark"; rather, the documentation should state that an "oval" or "crescent-shaped" injury was noted.

Abrasion

An abrasion is the scraping away of a portion of skin or mucus membrane as a result of injury by mechanical means (Shrestha et al., 2024). Most often, abrasions are caused by friction and can include scratches, grazes, or bite marks. Additionally, abrasions may include trace evidence like dirt, gravel, or glass.

Laceration

A laceration can result from blunt force, crushing, tearing, ripping, shearing, overstretching, bending, or pulling apart that causes the skin to separate (Gosangi et al., 2021; Park et al., 2021). This injury has ragged and irregular margins that cause tissue bridging and often occurs over bony prominences. Trace material such as dirt, glass, or gravel may also be found. The terms "laceration" and "tear" can be used interchangeably. However, the term "cut" should never be interchanged with "laceration" because a cut is a penetrating injury, whereas a laceration is the result of a blunt force injury.

Petechiae

Petechiae are pinpoint nonraised, nonblanchable spots that are often red or purple. They are often the result of increased pressure, which causes capillary rupture that allows blood to seep into the tissue. Petechiae are often observed in soft tissue and mucous membranes.

Hematoma

A hematoma is swelling or a mass of blood (usually clotted) confined to an organ, tissue, or space that is caused by a break in a blood vessel caused by blunt force. A hematoma is not the same thing as a bruise.

Two areas of additional findings that the clinician should consider are erythema and point tenderness. Erythema is a superficial area of redness that can be caused by pressure or a blunt impact on the skin, such as pressure from being grabbed or held down or an impact to the area by a slap, punch, or kick. Point tenderness is a nonvisible area of soreness. When documenting point tenderness, measure the area of soreness from beginning to end and document the patient's amount of pain using an accepted pain scale.

Sharp Force Injuries

Sharp force injuries are produced by pointed objects or objects with sharp edges (Smock & Stack, 2021b). A few examples of objects that can cause sharp force injuries include knives, broken glass, ice picks, scissors, pens, screwdrivers, surgical instruments, barbed wire, or razor blades. Two types of sharp force injuries are incised wounds and stab wounds.

Incised Wounds

Incised wounds are longer than they are wide and are caused by a sharp instrument (Smock & Stack, 2021b). The term "cut" is interchangeable with "incision." The edges are smooth and clean without the presence of tissue bridging.

Stab Wounds

Stab wounds are puncture wounds that result from sharp or pointed objects forced inward by a thrust, movement, or fall (Smock & Stack, 2021b). Stab wounds are often deeper than they are long, which can increase the risk of internal bleeding and injury to vital organs.

Strangulation

The absence of external physical injuries should not be a consideration in whether the patient receives a medical evaluation for strangulation. In a landmark study by Strack et al. (2001), up to 85% of strangulation victims were found to have little to no obvious external visible injury. Physical exam should focus on airway, breathing, circulation, head/neck, neurological, skin and musculoskeletal assessments (Stellpflug et al., 2022). A comprehensive list of potential exam findings is presented in **Box 15-3**.

DOCUMENTATION

It is the responsibility of the clinician to accurately and thoroughly document in the medical record all findings from the patient assessment and evaluation. Inability to accurately identify and document a patient's injury can later lead to questioning of the accuracy and competence of the clinician and negatively impact outcomes during legal proceedings. Documentation of an injury should include a written narrative, a body diagram, and photo documentation.

Written Narrative

The written narrative is often the most significant portion of the patient record and may be the only document admissible in court. It is critical that the written narrative is accurate, fact based, and precise. It is important that each identified injury is separately documented. Documenting "multiple bruises" is inadequate and does not provide an accurate representation of injuries, nor does it pay respect to the suffering the patient endured. Documentation of each injury should include the anatomical location, type, measurement, and associated characteristics, such as color and pain. It is important to include any information the patient may report during injury documentation. For example, if documenting a small circular bruise on the patient's left arm and the patient says, "Oh, that's where he grabbed me," then record the following documentation: Left arm, 1 cm by 1 cm, circular, purple bruise. Patient states, "Oh, that's where he grabbed me."

Body Diagram

Body diagrams (**Figure 15-2**) provide an additional level of injury documentation that assists with visualization of where injuries occurred on the patient's body. The written narrative can be documented on the body diagram.

BOX 15-3 Signs and Symptoms of Strangulation (Stellpflug et al., 2022)

Airway/respiratory
- Hoarseness or stridor
- Cough
- Dyspnea
- Respiratory distress
- Hypoxia
- Hemoptysis
- Crackles or wheezes

Cardiovascular
- Cyanosis
- Arrhythmias
- Syncope
- Carotid bruit
- Neck swelling

Neurologic
- Altered mental status
- Seizures
- Stroke-like symptoms
- Urinary incontinence
- Loss of consciousness
- Headache

Dermatologic
- Ligature mark
- Neck or facial abrasions or lacerations
- Facial petechiae

Ophthalmologic
- Visual disturbances
- Conjunctival petechiae
- Hemorrhagic retinopathy

Gastrointestinal
- Swollen tongue
- Foreign body (blood, vomit, tissue) in oropharynx
- Pain with swallowing
- Difficulty swallowing
- Vomiting

Psychiatric
- Depression
- Post-traumatic stress

Data from Stellpflug, S. J., Weber, W., Dietrich, A., Springer, B., Polansky, R., Sachs, C., Hsu, A., McGuire, S., Gwinn, C., Strack, G., & Riviello, R. (2022). Approach considerations for the management of strangulation in the emergency department. *Journal of the American College of Emergency Physicians Open*, *3*(2), e12711. https://doi.org/10.1002/emp2.12711

Photo Documentation

Photo documentation is an additional tool used to help document an injury. It provides examiners with the ability to capture an injury at the time of occurrence because injuries change and heal over time. Photo documentation is a skill that requires education and training to ensure that the image is accurate and representative of the injury. Principles of medical forensic photography should be followed when photo documenting an injury. For discussion on the principles of medical forensic photography refer to Chapter 16.

FIGURE 15-2 Body diagram.

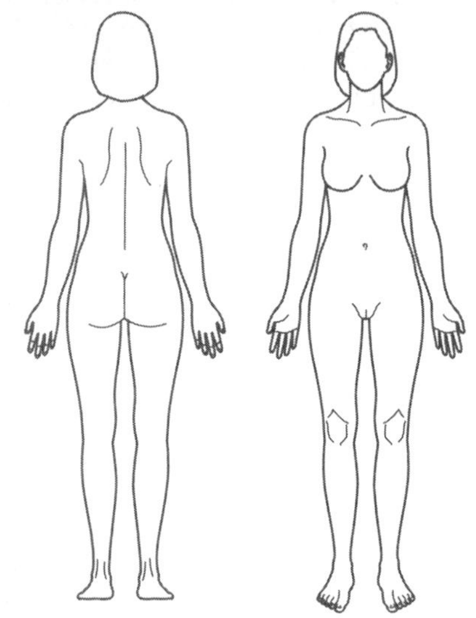

MANAGEMENT

Management of physical injuries will vary based on the type and severity of the injury. Life-threatening injuries should be addressed immediately with documentation deferred until after the patient is stable. Consider first if resuscitation, airway management, or hemorrhage control is needed (Salazar et al., 2023). Next, manage any life-threatening injuries and address vital-sign abnormalities (Salazar et al., 2023). When the patient is stable, further diagnosis and management should address the victim's physical and emotional well-being from a trauma-informed approach.

Diagnostic Testing

Laboratory testing or diagnostic imaging may be appropriate. Tests that may be ordered include a complete blood count (CBC), basic metabolic panel, liver enzymes, urinalysis, pregnancy test, hepatitis B and C, human immunodeficiency virus (HIV), syphilis, gonorrhea, and chlamydia (Salazar et al., 2023). Imaging may include computed tomography (CT) in the case of trauma to the head and brain, face, neck, spine, thorax, abdomen, or pelvis (Salazar et al., 2023). Plain radiography (x-ray) is appropriate for most bony injuries to the extremities or ribs or in the case of retained foreign bodies (Salazar et al., 2023). Ultrasound testing may be used to identify carotid artery injuries or to diagnose or assess a pregnancy (Salazar et al., 2023). Magnetic resonance imaging (MRI) is not used with regularity in assessing victims of IPV, except as a substitute for CTs in pregnant patients (Salazar et al., 2023).

Diagnostic testing should be ordered for patients who report strangulation and have symptoms that may indicate an injury. Laboratory testing is not indicated for the evaluation of strangulation injuries and should only be ordered based on the patient's clinical picture (Stellpflug et al., 2022). Imaging may be ordered to rule out life-threatening injuries such as laryngeal fracture or arterial dissection (Stellpflug et al., 2022). The gold standard imaging recommendation is a computerized tomography (CT) angiogram of the carotid and vertebral arteries.

Medical Management

Treatment should focus on managing physical injuries and psychiatric conditions. Some patients may need emergency evaluation by ophthalmology for eye injuries, vascular surgery for neck vessel injuries, neurology for brain injuries, or psychiatric evaluation for suicidality or other emergent psychiatric conditions (Salazar et al., 2023). Bite injuries should be treated empirically with antibiotics due to the high risk of infection. The first-line choice is a penicillin with a beta lactamase inhibitor (Salazar et al., 2023). A tetanus booster should be offered to anyone who has not had a vaccine in the past 10 years. For victims who have been sexually assaulted, postexposure prophylaxis and emergency contraception should be provided (refer to Chapter 16 for the detailed protocol).

If imaging is positive for a strangulation injury, a consult should be placed with neurology, neurosurgery, and potentially the trauma team (Stellpflug et al., 2022). A consult with an ears, nose, and throat specialist for dysphonia or dysphagia may be warranted. If the CT is negative, the clinician may consider keeping the patient under observation, based on the severity of signs and symptoms, or discharge the patient with education on home monitoring and when to return to the emergency department for an increase in symptoms (Stellpflug et al., 2022).

For patients experiencing acute anxiety or PTSD, pharmacologic and nonpharmacologic modalities can be offered. Nonpharmacologic options include meditation, relaxation techniques, and referral to behavioral or cognitive-behavioral therapy (Hameed et al., 2020; O'Doherty et al., 2023; Salazar et al., 2023). Low-dose oral benzodiazepines or antihistamines can be offered to manage acute mental health symptoms (Salazar et al., 2023). Referral to psychiatric providers may also be appropriate, based on the severity of symptoms.

CONSIDERATIONS FOR SPECIFIC POPULATIONS

Teen Dating Violence

Teen dating violence is a form of IPV that affects millions of adolescents in the United States (Centers for Disease Control and Prevention, 2024). Teen dating violence can occur in person or electronically through text messages and social media and may be in the form of physical violence, sexual violence, psychological aggression, or stalking (CDC, 2024). Many adolescents learn relationship norms through media, peers, their home environment, and other adults (CDC, 2024). Adolescents may consider behaviors such as name-calling, teasing, and jealousy as acceptable and even expect them as signs of a partner being interested or loving (CDC, 2024). The 2019 National Youth Risk Behavior Survey revealed that 1 in 12 teens report experiencing physical dating violence, and 1 in 12 also report experiencing sexual dating violence (Basile et al., 2020). Some teens are at higher risk of teen violence: female teens report higher rates of dating violence than male teens, and teens who identify as LGBTQ report higher rates of dating violence than those who identify as straight (Basile et al., 2020; Walls et al., 2019).

It is important to routinely screen adolescents for teen dating violence. Healthy and unhealthy relationship behaviors develop early and can have serious negative outcomes, including short-term or lifelong consequences. Adolescents who experience dating violence are more likely to experience IPV as adults; exhibit high-risk health behaviors, such as using tobacco, drugs, and alcohol; experience depression, anxiety, or post-traumatic stress disorder; exhibit antisocial behaviors such as lying, bullying, or hitting; plan or attempt suicide; or develop eating disorders (Centers for Disease Control and Prevention, 2024; Malherbe et al., 2023).

Education about teen dating violence should focus on healthy and unhealthy relationship behaviors and is most effective when initiated early (ACOG, 2018; Centers for Disease Control and Prevention, 2024). Clinicians should help adolescents define what healthy relationship behaviors look like and include a discussion on equality and partnership, honesty, respect, physical safety, sexual respectfulness, comfort, independence, and humor. Just as importantly, discussions on unhealthy behaviors, such as control, jealousy, dishonesty, physical or sexual violence, disrespect, intimidation, dependence, and hostility should also be held (ACOG, 2018).

CDC has developed evidence-based programs for communities to use to reduce teen dating violence. Dating Matters (also known as Strategies to Promote Healthy Teen Relationships) is a program that teaches 11- to 14-year-olds about healthy relationships and includes support and resources for parents, educators, and older adolescents. (https://vetoviolence.cdc.gov/apps/dating-matters-toolkit/content/youth-programs). The program has been found to reduce the incidence of teen dating violence and negative conflict resolution strategies among teens (Niolon et al., 2019).

The simple act of asking adolescents in a private and safe location about dating violence victimization and perpetration may be an important initial step toward effective intervention and prevention strategies. Questioning adolescents in a family planning clinic, emergency department, or pediatric setting about jealous or possessive partners could provide clues to the existence of dating violence. Because many adolescents accept physical and sexual aggression as normal in dating and partner relationships, clinicians can be invaluable in providing an alternative view by talking with them about types of behavior that are appropriate in a dating relationship. Early identification of teen dating violence in adolescents is critical because dating violence is often associated with IPV in adult life.

Pregnant People

Clinicians have long recognized that pregnancy can be a time in which pregnant individuals are at increased risk of IPV, either as a first-time victim or for an increase in severity. In the United States, approximately 6 percent of people who have recently given birth report experiencing IPV during pregnancy (D'Angelo et al., 2022). The effects of IPV in pregnancy can be severe, with an impact on the health of both the birthing person and the newborn. Pregnant people who experience IPV during pregnancy are at increased risk for depression; PTSD; high-risk behaviors, such as smoking and alcohol and substance use during pregnancy; late or missed prenatal care; and poor nutrition or inadequate weight gain during pregnancy (Agarwal et al., 2023).

In addition, pregnancy-associated homicide is a leading cause of pregnancy-related death. In 2018–2019, the pregnancy associated homicide rate was 3.62 deaths per 100,000 live births, exceeding the mortality rate of all other causes of death, such as hemorrhage, hypertension, or sepsis (Wallace et al., 2021). Firearms, assault by a sharp object, and strangulation are the causes of the majority of pregnancy-associated homicides (Wallace et al., 2021). Approximately half of pregnancy-related homicides occur during pregnancy and the other half occur in the first year postpartum (Wallace et al., 2021). Other causes of pregnancy-related death that may be associated with IPV are suicide and drug-related death. When taken as a whole, these three causes of death may account for as many as 40 percent of all pregnancy-associated deaths in the United States (Margerison et al., 2022).

IPV is also associated with adverse outcomes for the fetus, including preterm birth and low birth weight; small for gestational age; placental abruption; and fetal death (Agarwal et al., 2023). Children born to parents who experience IPV in pregnancy are also at higher risk of long-term sequalae such as developmental delays, behavioral health problems, and chronic health conditions (Agarwal et al., 2023).

Prenatal care provides a unique opportunity to build a trusting relationship with a provider. Pregnant people should be routinely screened for IPV at their initial prenatal appointment, at least once per trimester, during the postpartum period, and at yearly wellness visits (ACOG, 2012). Although pregnancy may offer a period of protection for some people who experience IPV in their relationships, patients should receive education that the abuse may resume, and they need to understand the implications abuse can have for both themselves and their children who are born into the abusive relationship. Even if the violence does not escalate, but simply continues at the previous rate, there are negative health effects associated with violence for both the pregnant person and their child.

Veterans

There is a growing awareness that a significant number of veterans experience IPV. Approximately 26 percent of veteran women and 24–37 percent of veteran men report experiencing IPV in the past year (Parr et al., 2021). When considering lifetime experiences of IPV, 58 percent of women veterans report having experienced IPV (Parr et al., 2021). Veterans are at risk for being both victims and perpetrators of IPV. The sequelae of IPV, such as PTSD and substance use, are also associated with combat experience, and these conditions may also lead to some veterans becoming perpetrators of IPV (Relyea et al., 2023). Thus, screening for the experience of IPV both as a victim and perpetrator is appropriate for this population and may help prevent escalating violence (Portnoy et al., 2023).

People with Disabilities

People with disabilities are at particular risk of IPV, as they may be reliant on an abusive partner. For women with disabilities, the risk of IPV is significantly higher than for women without disabilities (García-Cuéllar et al., 2023). It is important for clinicians to ask their patients who have disabilities if they are experiencing IPV. Also, many shelters are unprepared to make the needed accommodations for people with disabilities and are not trained or equipped to respond adequately (ACOG, 2012). Clinicians should identify shelters or community agencies that can support people with disabilities who are in abusive relationships.

Older Adults

Although IPV affects people of all ages, often the literature focuses on teens and people in their childbearing years, ignoring the unique problems of older adults who are experiencing IPV. The experience of IPV in older adults (often defined as adults over the age of 45) is frequently conflated with the concepts of elder abuse or family violence (McGarry et al., 2017; Ali & Rogers, 2023). However, violence in intimate partner relationships is also a concern that deserves attention from clinicians. Serious physical and emotional harm, and even death, may result from intimate partner violence at any age, but among older people, because of their physical vulnerability that increases with age, even low-severity violence can cause serious injury or death (Khurana & Loder, 2022; Yılmaz et al., 2023). Importantly, intimate partner violence can be experienced by all genders, and older men may be more likely to be victims of IPV than younger men (Durfee & Goodmark, 2021). Given the high rate of lifetime experience of IPV among transgender people, it is prudent to screen older transgender patients for IPV (Hillman, 2022). Because there is so little research into the experience of intimate partner violence among older adults, the USPSTF states that there is inadequate information to make screening recommendations for this population (U.S. Preventative Services Task Force, 2024).

Elder abuse and mistreatment may be viewed from an inadequate care perspective that obscures important issues. Some forms of elder abuse and mistreatment derive from inadequate care and are rooted in the dynamics of caregiving. Other forms of elder abuse and mistreatment, especially physical assaults, are family violence. Family violence involving older adults has been addressed by laws in all 50 states and the District of Columbia, requiring the reporting of elder or vulnerable person abuse (U.S. Department of Justice, n.d.). Clinicians are mandated by law to report a case if there is reasonable cause to suspect that an older adult patient has been the victim of abuse, neglect, or mistreatment. More than 1 in 10 adults who are 70 years of age or older (14.0%) have experienced some form of abuse in the past year, with 12.1 percent experiencing psychological abuse and 1.7 percent experiencing physical abuse (Rosay & Mulford, 2017). One in five victims (20.8%) were abused by both intimate and non-intimate partners (Rosay & Mulford, 2017). Accurate detection and assessment of elder patients who are subjected to abuse are critical duties of all clinicians, especially those in ambulatory care settings.

PREVENTING INTIMATE PARTNER VIOLENCE

IPV is a prevalent, serious, and preventable public health problem that affects people across genders, ages, cultures, and socioeconomic backgrounds, though racial/ethnic and sexual minority groups are disproportionately affected by IPV (Holditch Niolon et al., 2017). Prevention strategies for IPV include primary, secondary, and tertiary interventions. Primary prevention strategies to prevent IPV include teaching safe and healthy relationships, engaging influential adults and peers, disrupting the developmental pathways toward IPV, creating protective environments, strengthening economic supports for families, and supporting survivors to increase safety and lessen harms (Holditch Niolon et al., 2017). Clinicians may find these broad societal-level interventions to be aspirational, but providing trauma-informed care to individuals experiencing IPV can influence the safety, health, and well-being of the individual, their family, and generations that follow.

References

AbiNader, M. A., Graham, L. M., & Kafka, J. M. (2023). Examining intimate partner violence-related fatalities: Past lessons and future directions using U.S. national data. *Journal of Family Violence*, 1–12. https://doi.org/10.1007/s10896-022-00487-2

ACOG. (2012). ACOG Committee Opinion No. 518: Intimate partner violence. *Obstetrics and Gynecology*, *119*(2 Pt 1), 412–417. https://doi.org/10.1097/AOG.0b013e318249ff74

ACOG (2013). ACOG Committee Opinion No. 554: Reproductive and sexual coercion. *Obstetrics and Gynecology*, *121*(2 Pt 1), 411–415. https://doi.org/10.1097/01.AOG.0000426427.79586.3b

ACOG. (2018). ACOG Committee Opinion No. 758: Promoting Healthy Relationships in Adolescents. *Obstetrics and Gynecology*, *132*(5), e213–e220. https://doi.org/10.1097/aog.0000000000002945

Agarwal, S., Prasad, R., Mantri, S., Chandrakar, R., Gupta, S., Babhulkar, V., Srivastav, S., Jaiswal, A., & Wanjari, M. B. (2023). A comprehensive review of intimate partner violence during pregnancy and its adverse effects on maternal and fetal health. *Cureus*, *15*(5), e39262. https://doi.org/10.7759/cureus.39262

Ali, P., & Rogers, M. M. (Eds.). (2023). *Gender-based violence: A comprehensive guide*. Springer. https://doi.org/10.1007/978-3-031-05640-6

Alvarez, C., Fedock, G., Grace, K. T., & Campbell, J. (2017). Provider screening and counseling for intimate partner violence: A systematic review of practices and influencing factors. *Trauma, Violence & Abuse*, *18*(5), 479–495. https://doi.org/10.1177/1524838016637080

American College of Obstetricians and Gynecologists (ACOG) Committee opinion no. 554: Reproductive and sexual coercion. (2013). *Obstetrics and gynecology*, *121* (2 Pt 1), 411–415. https://doi.org/10.1097/01.AOG.0000426427.79586.3b

Anderson, C. A., & Bushman, B. J. (2002). Human aggression. *Annual Review of Psychology*, *53*, 27–51. https://doi.org/10.1146/annurev.psych.53.100901.135231

Andreu-Pejó, L., Valero-Chillerón, M. J., González-Chordá, V. M., Mena Tudela, D., & Cervera Gasch, A. (2022). Integrative review of the literature on screening for gender-based violence during pregnancy: Barriers, facilitators, and tools. *Nursing & Health Sciences*, *24*(3), 564–578. https://doi.org/10.1111/nhs.12967

Basile, K. C., Clayton, H. B., DeGue, S., Gilford, J. W., Vagi, K. J., Suarez, N. A., Zwald, M. L., & Lowry, R. (2020). Interpersonal violence victimization among high school students—Youth Risk Behavior Survey, United States, 2019. *Morbidity and Mortality Weekly Report Supplements*, *69*(1), 28–37. https://doi.org/10.15585/mmwr.su6901a4

Basile, K. C., Hall, J. E., & Walters, M. L. (2013). Expanding resource theory and feminist-informed theory to explain intimate partner violence perpetration by court-ordered men. *Violence Against Women*, *19*(7), 848–880. https://doi.org/10.1177/1077801213497105

Breiding, M. J., Basile, K. C., Smith, S. G., Black, M. C., & Mahendra, R. R. (2015). *Intimate partner violence surveillance: Uniform definitions and recommended data elements, version 2.0.* Retrieved from https://stacks.cdc.gov/view/cdc/31292?utm_source=chatgpt.com%2Fcdc_31292_DS1.pdf%2Fcdc_31292_DS1.pdf%2Fcdc_31292_DS1.pdf%2Fcdc_31292_DS1.pdf/cdc_31292_DS1.pdf

Brown, J. (2019). *Strangulation, domestic violence, and brain injury: An introduction to a complex topic*. https://biausa.org/public-affairs/media/strangulation-domestic-violence-and-brain-injury-an-introduction-to-a-complex-topic

Brown, J. B., Lent, B., Brett, P. J., Sas, G., & Pederson, L. L. (1996). Development of the Woman Abuse Screening Tool for use in family practice. *Family Medicine*, *28*(6), 422–428. https://pubmed.ncbi.nlm.nih.gov/8791071/

Burton, C. W., & Carlyle, K. E. (2021). Increasing screening for intimate partner violence and reproductive coercion: Understanding provider motivations. *Violence Against Women*, *27*(11), 1913–1929. https://doi.org/10.1177/1077801220969875

Campbell, J. C., Webster, D. W., & Glass, N. (2009). The danger assessment: Validation of a lethality risk assessment instrument for intimate partner femicide. *Journal of interpersonal violence*, *24*(4), 653–674. https://doi.org/10.1177/0886260508317180

Centers for Disease Control and Prevention. (2024). *About teen dating violence*. https://www.cdc.gov/intimate-partner-violence/about/about-teen-dating-violence.html

Chan, B., & Sachs, C. J. (2023). Intimate partner violence and sexual violence. *Emergency Medicine Clinics of North America*, *41*(2), 369–380. https://doi.org/10.1016/j.emc.2023.01.007

Chen, J., Khatiwada, S., Chen, M. S., Smith, S. G., Leemis, R. W., Friar, N. W., Basile, K. C., & Kresnow, M. (2023). *The National Intimate Partner and Sexual Violence Survey: 2016/2017 Report on Victimization by Sexual Identity*. Atlanta, GA.

Chester, D. S., & DeWall, C. N. (2018). The roots of intimate partner violence. *Current Opinion in Psychology*, *19*, 55–59. https://doi.org/10.1016/j.copsyc.2017.04.009

Chisholm, C. A., Bullock, L., & Ferguson, J. E. J., 2nd. (2017). Intimate partner violence and pregnancy: Epidemiology and impact. *American Journal of Obstetrics and Gynecology*, *217*(2), 141–144. https://doi.org/10.1016/j.ajog.2017.05.042

Clarke, A. D. A., Copas, C., Hannon, O., Padgett, C., Knight, J. M., Falkenberg, A., Varto, H., Mason, K., Wellington, C. L., van Donkelaar, P., Marks, J., Shultz, S. R., & Symons, G. F. (2024). Detecting a hidden pandemic: The current state and future direction of screening and assessment tools for intimate partner violence-related brain injury. *Neuroscience and Biobehavioral Reviews*, *167*, 105912. https://doi.org/10.1016/j.neubiorev.2024.105912

Clemente-Teixeira, M., Magalhães, T., Barrocas, J., Dinis-Oliveira, R. J., & Taveira-Gomes, T. (2022). Health outcomes in women victims of intimate partner violence: A 20-Year real-world study. *International Journal of Environmental Research and Public Health*, *19*(24), 17035. https://doi.org/10.3390/ijerph192417035

D'Angelo, D. V., Bombard, J. M., Lee, R. D., Kortsmit, K., Kapaya, M., & Fasula, A. (2022). Prevalence of experiencing physical, emotional, and sexual violence by a current intimate partner during pregnancy: Population-based estimates from the Pregnancy Risk Assessment Monitoring System. *Journal of Family Violence*, *38*(1), 117–126. https://doi.org/10.1007/s10896-022-00356-y

Domestic Violence Crisis Center. (n.d.). *Safety planning*. https://www.dvccct.org/is-this-abuse/safety-planning/

Durfee, A., & Goodmark, L. (2021). Gender, protection orders, and intimate partner violence in later life: A study of protective order filings in Arizona. *Journal of Interpersonal Violence*, *36*(21–22), 10479–10498. https://doi.org/10.1177/0886260519884688

Empire Justice Center. (2006). *Traumatic brain injury and domestic violence*. https://vawnet.org/sites/default/files/assets/files/2016-10/HELPSScreeningTool.pdf

Feldhaus, K. M., Koziol-McLain, J., Amsbury, H. L., Norton, I. M., Lowenstein, S. R., & Abbott, J. T. (1997). Accuracy of 3 brief screening questions for detecting partner violence in the emergency department. *JAMA*, *277*(17), 1357–1361.

Finkel, E. J. (2014). Chapter One—The I3 Model: Metatheory, theory, and evidence. In J. M. Olson & M. P. Zanna (Eds.), *Advances in Experimental Social Psychology* (Vol. 49, pp. 1–104). Academic Press. https://doi.org/10.1016/B978-0-12-800052-6.00001-9

Finkel, E. J., DeWall, C. N., Slotter, E. B., McNulty, J. K., Pond, R. S., Jr., & Atkins, D. C. (2012). Using I^3 theory to clarify when dispositional aggressiveness predicts intimate partner violence perpetration. *Journal of Personality and Social Psychology*, *102*(3), 533–549. https://doi.org/10.1037/a0025651

Fridel, E. E., & Fox, J. A. (2019). Gender differences in patterns and trends in US homicide, 1976–2017. *Violence and Gender*, *6*(1), 27–36.

García-Cuéllar, M. M., Pastor-Moreno, G., Ruiz-Pérez, I., & Henares-Montiel, J. (2023). The prevalence of intimate partner violence against women with disabilities: A systematic review of the literature. *Disability and Rehabilitation*, *45*(1), 1–8. https://doi.org/10.1080/09638288.2022.2025927

Garcia-Vergara, E., Almeda, N., Fernández-Navarro, F., & Becerra-Alonso, D. (2022). Risk assessment instruments for intimate partner femicide: A systematic review. *Frontiers in Psychology*, *13*, 896901. https://doi.org/10.3389/fpsyg.2022.896901

Gosangi, B., Lebovic, J., Park, H., Thomas, R., Gujrathi, R., Harris, M., Tornetta, P., & Khurana, B. (2021). Imaging patterns of lower extremity injuries in victims of intimate partner violence (IPV). *Emergency Radiology*, *28*(4), 751–759. https://doi.org/10.1007/s10140-021-01914-5

Güler, A., Lee, R. C., Rojas-Guyler, L., Lambert, J., & Smith, C. R. (2023). The influences of sociocultural norms on women's decision to disclose intimate partner violence: Integrative review. *Nursing Inquiry*, *30*(4), e12589. https://doi.org/10.1111/nin.12589

Haag, H. L., Jones, D., Joseph, T., & Colantonio, A. (2022). Battered and brain injured: Traumatic brain injury among women survivors of intimate partner violence—a scoping review. *Trauma, Violence & Abuse*, *23*(4), 1270–1287. https://doi.org/10.1177/1524838019850623

Hameed, M., O'Doherty, L., Gilchrist, G., Tirado-Muñoz, J., Taft, A., Chondros, P., Feder, G., Tan, M., & Hegarty, K. (2020). Psychological therapies for women who experience intimate partner violence. *Cochrane Database of Systematic Reviews*, *7*(7), Cd013017. https://doi.org/10.1002/14651858.CD013017.pub2

Hillman, J. (2022). Lifetime prevalence of intimate partner violence and health-related outcomes among transgender adults aged 50 and older. *Gerontologist*, *62*(2), 212–222. https://doi.org/10.1093/geront/gnab067

Holditch Niolon, P., Kearns, M., Dills, J., Rambo, K., Irving, S., Armstead, T. L., & Gilbert, L. (2017). *Intimate partner violence prevention: Resource for action*. Atlanta, GA.

Human Rights Foundation. (2021). *Dismantling a culture of violence: Understanding violence against transgender and non-binary peeople and ending the crisis*. https://reports.hrc.org/dismantling-a-culture-of-violence

Khurana, B., & Loder, R. T. (2022). Injury patterns and associated demographics of intimate partner violence in older adults presenting to U.S. emergency departments. *Journal of Interpersonal Violence*, *37*(17–18), Np16107–np16129. https://doi.org/10.1177/08862605211022060

Kyle, J. (2023). Intimate partner violence. *Medical Clinics of North America*, *107*(2), 385–395. https://doi.org/10.1016/j.mcna.2022.10.012

Leemis, R. W., Friar, N. W., Khatiwada, S., Chen, M. S., Kresnow, M., Smith, S. G., Caslin, S., & Basile, K. C. (2022). *The National Intimate Partner and Sexual Violence Survey: 2016/2017 Report on Intimate Partner Violence*. Atlanta, GA.

Lutgendorf, M. A. (2019). Intimate partner violence and women's health. *Obstetrics and Gynecology*, *134*(3), 470–480. https://doi.org/10.1097/aog.0000000000003326

Malherbe, I., Delhaye, M., Kornreich, C., & Kacenelenbogen, N. (2023). Teen dating violence and mental health: A review. *Psychiatria Danubina, 35*(Suppl 2), 155–159.

Margerison, C. E., Roberts, M. H., Gemmill, A., & Goldman-Mellor, S. (2022). Pregnancy-associated deaths due to drugs, suicide, and homicide in the United States, 2010–2019. *Obstetrics and Gynecology, 139*(2), 172–180. https://doi.org/10.1097/aog.0000000000004649

McGarry, J., Ali, P., & Hinchliff, S. (2017). Older women, intimate partner violence and mental health: A consideration of the particular issues for health and health-care practice. *Journal of Clinical Nursing, 26*(15–16), 2177–2191. https://doi.org/10.1111/jocn.13490

Messing, J. T., Campbell, J., AbiNader, M. A., & Bolyard, R. (2022). Accounting for multiple nonfatal strangulation in intimate partner violence risk assessment. *Journal of Interpersonal Violence, 37*(11–12), Np8430–np8453. https://doi.org/10.1177/0886260520975854

National Domestic Violence Hotline. (n.d.). *50 obstacles to leaving*. https://www.thehotline.org/resources/get-help-50-obstacles-to-leaving/

Niolon, P. H., Vivolo-Kantor, A. M., Tracy, A. J., Latzman, N. E., Little, T. D., DeGue, S., Lang, K. M., Estefan, L. F., Ghazarian, S. R., McIntosh, W. L. K., Taylor, B., Johnson, L. L., Kuoh, H., Burton, T., Fortson, B., Mumford, E. A., Nelson, S. C., Joseph, H., Valle, L. A., & Tharp, A. T. (2019). An RCT of Dating Matters: Effects on teen dating violence and relationship behaviors. *American Journal of Preventive Medicine, 57*(1), 13–23. https://doi.org/10.1016/j.amepre.2019.02.022

O'Doherty, L., Whelan, M., Carter, G. J., Brown, K., Tarzia, L., Hegarty, K., Feder, G., & Brown, S. J. (2023). Psychosocial interventions for survivors of rape and sexual assault experienced during adulthood. *Cochrane Database of Systematic Reviews, 10*(10), CD013456. https://doi.org/10.1002/14651858.CD013456.pub2

Ohio Domestic Violence Network: The Center on Partner-Inflicted Brain Injury. (n.d.). *Has your head been hurt? CHATS*. https://www.odvn.org/wp-content/uploads/2024/07/CHATS_May2024b.pdf

Park, C. W., Juliano, M. L., & Woodhall, D. (2021). Traumatic wounds. In K. J. Knoop, L. B. Stack, A. B. Storrow, & R. J. Thurman (Eds.), *The atlas of emergency medicine,* (5th ed.). McGraw Hill. https://accessmedicine.mhmedical.com/content.aspx?bookid=2969&sectionid=250461362

Parr, N. J., Young, S., Ward, R., & Mackey, K. (2021). VA Evidence-based synthesis program reports. In *Evidence brief: Prevalence of intimate partner violence/sexual assault among veterans*. Department of Veterans Affairs (U.S.).

Patch, M., Anderson, J. C., Alexander, K. A., Somoano, F. A., Kelen, G., Holbrook, D. S., & Campbell, J. C. (2023). Didn't put a label on it: Examining intimate partner strangulation within a diagnostic framework. *Journal of Advanced Nursing, 79*(4), 1575–1588. https://doi.org/10.1111/jan.15380

Paterno, M. T., & Draughon, J. E. (2016). Screening for intimate partner violence. *Journal of Midwifery and Women's Health, 61*(3), 370–375. https://doi.org/10.1111/jmwh.12443

Peitzmeier, S. M., Malik, M., Kattari, S. K., Marrow, E., Stephenson, R., Agénor, M., & Reisner, S. L. (2020). Intimate partner violence in transgender populations: Systematic review and meta-analysis of prevalence and correlates. *American Journal of Public Health, 110*(9), e1–e14. https://doi.org/10.2105/ajph.2020.305774

Peterson, C., Kearns, M. C., McIntosh, W. L., Estefan, L. F., Nicolaidis, C., McCollister, K. E., Gordon, A., & Florence, C. (2018). Lifetime economic burden of intimate partner violence among U.S. adults. *American Journal of Preventive Medicine, 55*(4), 433–444. https://doi.org/10.1016/j.amepre.2018.04.049

Picard, M., Scarisbrick, R., & Paluck, R. (1991). *HELPS Brain Injury Screening Tool*. Retrieved from https://abitoolkit.ca/assets/images/HELPS-tool.pdf

Portnoy, G. A., Relyea, M. R., Presseau, C., Orazietti, S. A., Bruce, L. E., Brandt, C. A., & Martino, S. (2023). Screening for intimate partner violence experience and use in the Veterans Health Administration. *JAMA Network Open, 6*(10), e2337685. https://doi.org/10.1001/jamanetworkopen.2023.37685

Reckdenwald, A., Powell, K. M., & Martins, T. A. W. (2022). Forensic documentation of non-fatal strangulation. *Journal of Forensic Sciences, 67*(2), 588–595. https://doi.org/10.1111/1556-4029.14958

Relyea, M. R., Presseau, C., Runels, T., Humbert, M. M., Martino, S., Brandt, C. A., Haskell, S. G., & Portnoy, G. A. (2023). Understanding veterans' intimate partner violence use and patterns of healthcare utilization. *Health Services Research, 58*(6), 1198–1208. https://doi.org/10.1111/1475-6773.14201

Rosay, A. B. P., & Mulford, C. F. P. (2017). Prevalence estimates and correlates of elder abuse in the United States: The National Intimate Partner and Sexual Violence Survey. *Journal of Elder Abuse & Neglect, 29*(1), 1–14. https://doi.org/10.1080/08946566.2016.1249817

Salazar, G. A., Palma, J. A., Box, M., & Brar, D. (2023). Evaluation and management of intimate partner violence in the emergency department. *Emergency Medicine Practice, 25*(Suppl 4), 1–37.

Sardinha, L., Maheu-Giroux, M., Stöckl, H., Meyer, S. R., & García-Moreno, C. (2022). Global, regional, and national prevalence estimates of physical or sexual, or both, intimate partner violence against women in 2018. *Lancet, 399*(10327), 803–813. https://doi.org/10.1016/s0140-6736(21)02664-7

Sherin, K. M., Sinacore, J. M., Li, X. Q., Zitter, R. E., & Shakil, A. (1998). HITS: A short domestic violence screening tool for use in a family practice setting. *Family Medicine, 30*(7), 508–512.

Shrestha, R., Krishan, K., Ishaq, H., & Kanchan, T. (2024). Abrasion. In *StatPearls*. StatPearls Publishing. Copyright © 2024, StatPearls Publishing LLC.

Smith, E. J., Bailey, B. A., & Cascio, A. (2024). Sexual coercion, intimate partner violence, and homicide: A scoping literature review. *Trauma, Violence & Abuse, 25*(1), 341–353. https://doi.org/10.1177/15248380221150474

Smock, W. S., & Stack, L. B. (2021a). pattern injuries of domestic violence, assault, and abuse. In K. J. Knoop, L. B. Stack, A. B. Storrow, & R. J. Thurman (Eds.), *The atlas of emergency medicine* (5th ed.). McGraw Hill. https://accessmedicine.mhmedical.com/content.aspx?bookid=2969&sectionid=250461273

Smock, W. S., & Stack, L. B. (2021b). Sharp-Force-Pattern Injuries. In K. J. Knoop, L. B. Stack, A. B. Storrow, & R. J. Thurman (Eds.), *The atlas of emergency medicine*, (5th ed.). McGraw Hill. https://accessmedicine.mhmedical.com/content.aspx?bookid=2969&sectionid=250461275

Sohal, H., Eldridge, S., & Feder, G. (2007). The sensitivity and specificity of four questions (HARK) to identify intimate partner violence: A diagnostic accuracy study in general practice. *BMC Family Practice, 8*, 49. https://doi.org/10.1186/1471-2296-8-49

Stellpflug, S. J., Weber, W., Dietrich, A., Springer, B., Polansky, R., Sachs, C., Hsu, A., McGuire, S., Gwinn, C., Strack, G., & Riviello, R. (2022). Approach considerations for the management of strangulation in the emergency department. *Journal of the American College of Emergency Physicians Open, 3*(2), e12711. https://doi.org/10.1002/emp2.12711

Stewart, D. E., MacMillan, H., & Kimber, M. (2021). Recognizing and responding to intimate partner violence: An update. *Canadian Journl of Psychiatry, 66*(1), 71–106. https://doi.org/10.1177/0706743720939676

Stewart, D. E., & Vigod, S. N. (2019). Update on mental health aspects of intimate partner violence. *Medical Clinics of North America, 103*(4), 735–749. https://doi.org/10.1016/j.mcna.2019.02.010

Strack, G. B., McClane, G. E., & Hawley, D. (2001). A review of 300 attempted strangulation cases. Part I: criminal legal issues. *Journal of Emergency Medicine, 21*(3), 303–309. https://doi.org/10.1016/s0736-4679(01)00399-7

Stubbs, A., & Szoeke, C. (2022). The effect of intimate partner violence on the physical health and health-related behaviors of women: A systematic review of the literature. *Trauma, Violence & Abuse, 23*(4), 1157–1172. https://doi.org/10.1177/1524838020985541

Tarzia, L. (2021). Toward an ecological understanding of intimate partner sexual violence. *Journal of Interpersonal Violence, 36*(23–24), 11704–11727. https://doi.org/10.1177/0886260519900298

Tirado, J., & Mauricio, D. (2021). Bruise dating using deep learning. *Journal of Forensic Sciences, 66*(1), 336–346. https://doi.org/10.1111/1556-4029.14578

Tobin-Tyler, E. (2023). Intimate partner violence, firearm injuries and homicides: A health justice approach to two intersecting public health crises. *Journal of Law, Medicine & Ethics, 51*(1), 64–76. https://doi.org/10.1017/jme.2023.41

Training Institute on Strangulation Prevention. (n.d.). *Strangulation in intimate partner violence: Fact sheet*. https://www.familyjusticecenter.org/wp-content/uploads/2017/11/Strangulation-in-Intimate-Partner-Violence-Fact-Sheet-2017-1.pdf

U.S. Department of Justice. (n.d.). *State elder abuse statutes*. https://www.justice.gov/elderjustice/elder-justice-statutes-0

U.S. Preventative Services Task Force. (2025). *Intimate partner violence and caregiver abuse of older or vulnerable adults: Screening*. https://www.uspreventiveservicestaskforce.org/uspstf/recommendation/intimate-partner-violence-and-abuse-of-elderly-and-vulnerable-adults-screening

Vicard-Olagne, M., Pereira, B., Rougé, L., Cabaillot, A., Vorilhon, P., Lazimi, G., & Laporte, C. (2022). Signs and symptoms of intimate partner violence in women attending primary care in Europe, North America and Australia: A systematic review and meta-analysis. *Family Practice, 39*(1), 190–199. https://doi.org/10.1093/fampra/cmab097

Walker, L. (1980). *The battered woman*. Harper & Row.

Wallace, M., Gillispie-Bell, V., Cruz, K., Davis, K., & Vilda, D. (2021). Homicide during pregnancy and the postpartum period in the United States, 2018–2019. *Obstetrics and Gynecology, 138*(5), 762–769. https://doi.org/10.1097/aog.0000000000004567

Walls, N. E., Atteberry-Ash, B., Kattari, S. K., Peitzmeier, S., Kattari, L., & Langenderfer-Magruder, L. (2019). Gender identity, sexual orientation, mental health, and bullying as predictors of partner violence in a representative sample of youth. *Journal of Adolescent Health, 64*(1), 86–92. https://doi.org/10.1016/j.jadohealth.2018.08.011

World Health Organization. (2022). *Intimate partner violence*. https://apps.who.int/violence-info/intimate-partner-violence/

Yılmaz, S., Gunay, E., Lee, D. H., Whiting, K., Silver, K., Koyuturk, M., & Karakurt, G. (2023). Adverse health correlates of intimate partner violence against older women: Mining electronic health records. *PLoS One, 18*(3), e0281863. https://doi.org/10.1371/journal.pone.0281863

Zink, T., Elder, N., & Jacobson, J. (2003). How children affect the mother/victim's process in intimate partner violence. *Archives of Pediatrics & Adolescent Medicine, 157*(6), 587–592. https://doi.org/10.1001/archpedi.157.6.587

APPENDIX 15-A

Screening Tools for IPV

HARK

HARK questions—one point is given for every yes answer.

H	HUMILIATION Within the last year, have you been humiliated or emotionally abused in other ways by your partner or ex-partner?
A	AFRAID Within the last year, have you been afraid of your partner or ex-partner?
R	RAPE Within the last year, have you been raped or forced to have any kind of sexual activity by your partner or ex-partner?
K	KICK Within the last year, have you been kicked, hit, slapped, or otherwise physically hurt by your partner or ex-partner?

A score of ≥ 1 is a positive screen.

Reproduced from Sohal, H., Eldridge, S., & Feder, G. (2007). The sensitivity and specificity of four questions (HARK) to identify intimate partner violence: A diagnostic accuracy study in general practice. *BMC Family Practice, 8,* 49. https://doi.org/10.1186/1471-2296-8-49

HITS (Hurt-Insult-Threaten-Scream) Domestic Violence Screening Tool

Please read each of the following activities and place a check mark in the box that best indicates the frequency with which your partner acts in the way depicted.

Date: ____________

Age: ____________

Sex: Male Female

Ethnicity: Caucasian __________ Hispanic __________ African American __________ Asian __________ Indian __________

How Often Does Your Partner?	Never	Rarely	Sometimes	Fairly Often	Frequently
1. Physically hurt you					
2. Insult or talk down to you					
3. Threaten you with harm					
4. Scream or curse at you					
	1	2	3	4	5
Total Score:					

Each item is scored from 1–5. Range between 4–20. A score greater than 10 signifies that you are at risk of domestic violence abuse, and should seek counseling or help from a domestic violence resource center such as the following:

The Family Place Hotline: 214.941.1991
Genesis Women's Shelter: 214.389.7700; Genesis Hotline– 214.946.HELP (4357)
Texas Council on Family Violence: 800.525.1978
National Domestic Violence Hotline: 1.800.799.SAFE (7233)

PVS—Partner Violence Screen

1. Have you been hit, kicked, punched, otherwise hurt by someone within the past year? If so, by whom?
2. Do you feel safe in your current relationship?
3. Is there a partner from a previous relationship who is making you feel unsafe now?

A score of ≥ 1 is a positive screen.

Reproduced from Feldhaus, K. M., Koziol-McLain, J., Amsbury, H. L., Norton, I. M., Lowenstein, S. R., & Abbott, J. T. (1997). Accuracy of 3 brief screening questions for detecting partner violence in the emergency department. *JAMA, 277*(17), 1357–1361.

WAST—Woman Abuse Screening Tool

These questions relate to the last 12 months.

1. In general, how would you describe your relationship?
   A. A lot of tension
   B. Some tension
   C. No tension
2. Do you and your partner work out arguments with . . .
   A. Great difficulty
   B. Some difficulty
   C. No difficulty
3. Do arguments ever result in you feeling put down or bad about yourself?
   A. Often
   B. Sometimes
   C. Never
4. Do arguments ever result in hitting, kicking, or pushing?
   A. Often
   B. Sometimes
   C. Never
5. Do you ever feel frightened by what your partner says or does?
   A. Often
   B. Sometimes
   C. Never
6. Has your partner ever abused you physically?
   A. Often
   B. Sometimes
   C. Never
7. Has your partner every abused you emotionally?
   A. Often
   B. Sometimes
   C. Never
8. Has your partner ever abused you physically?
   A. Often
   B. Sometimes
   C. Never

Scoring (range 0–16 points)
2 points per answer A
1 point per answer B
0 points per answer C

A score of 5 or higher indicates a positive screening test for IPV.

Source: Brown, JB, Lent, B, Brett, PJ, Sas, G, Pederson, LL. Development of the Woman Abuse Screening Tool for use in family practice. *Fam Med. 1996 Jun;28*(6):422-8.

CHAPTER 16

Sexual Assault and Human Trafficking

Lisa M. Hachey
Tamara Pavlik-Maus
Heather McCracken

The editors acknowledge Kelly A. Berishaj, who was the author of the previous edition of this chapter.

Trigger Warning: The following chapter addresses sensitive topics, including sexual assault and human trafficking. We acknowledge that these discussions can be triggering or emotionally difficult.

Sexual assault is a violent act committed for power and control. It often leads to both acute and chronic physical and psychological health consequences in victims and survivors (Basile et al., 2022) and is a significant global societal problem that can be prevented. Sexual assault and other forms of sexual violence, including human trafficking, are serious issues, and it is imperative that clinicians be properly educated to care for and treat all victims of sexual violence.

As with all encounters for health care, the individual's positionality, culture, values, and beliefs must be considered—this is especially important when caring for those who have experienced sexual violence. Certain populations require special consideration due to their heightened vulnerability compared to other survivor groups (U.S Department of Justice [DOJ], 2024). This includes individuals across various age groups, such as children, adolescents, and the older adults, who may face unique challenges in the aftermath of an assault. Additionally, the presence of physical or cognitive disabilities can significantly impact a survivor's ability to seek help and navigate the recovery process. Factors such as gender identity and sexual orientation also play a critical role in shaping the survivor's experience, as well as cultural issues that may influence perceptions of violence and the support available to survivors. Addressing these specific needs is essential to providing comprehensive care and support.

The age of the victim is important for many reasons. The very young and older adults may not have opportunities to report sexual violence if they are living with the perpetrator (U.S. Department of Justice Office on Violence Against Women [OVW], 2024). They may exhibit a sense of loyalty to the abuser if they rely on that person for food, shelter, and basic needs. Such victims may also be physically unable to leave the situation and find someone to whom they can report the sexual assault. This is important for all clinicians to consider, though the specific care of pediatric sexual assault patients is beyond the scope of this chapter. Children who are victims of sexual violence should receive care from clinicians who have additional specialty education and training in how to care for this vulnerable population.

Sexual assault of the elderly occurs more frequently in an institutional setting than in the home (Goldblatt et al., 2022). Elderly individuals are more likely to have bruising related to the effects of aging, decreased estrogen levels, and medication use (RAINN, n.d.). Furthermore, impairments in memory may prohibit accurate retelling of the assault, and physical decline can make the actual examination process more difficult (Goldblatt et al., 2022). Most states have mandatory reporting laws that apply to children and older victims of abuse.

People with developmental disabilities are almost three times as likely to experience violent victimization (46.2 per 1,000 age 12 or older), compared to those without disability (12.3 per 1,000) (DOJ, 2021b). Persons with cognitive disability suffer the highest incidence of violent victimization (DOJ, 2021b). In individuals with cognitive or developmental disability, there may be issues with obtaining informed consent to perform a forensic examination. It is best if the clinician is experienced in interviewing individuals with disabilities; alternatively, individuals with specialized interviewing skills may be called upon to obtain consent and assist with collection of the medical forensic history.

In persons with communication or physical disabilities, the clinician should ensure that the patient has access to adaptive devices. If the patient requests that caretakers or family members be present during the examination, it is crucial to minimize the influence of those individuals on the patient while relating the history of the assault. In the case of communication deficits, the use of an independent interpreter with no personal relationship to the patient may be required (OVW, 2024). Reporting the sexual abuse of disabled persons is mandated in every state.

Cultural values and beliefs vary greatly and may play a role in whether an individual reports sexual assault, and how they cope with the psychological and physical aftermath of the assault. Clinicians must be cognizant that these differences exist and adapt care to address the cultural needs of their patients during the provision of services.

For example, individuals of diverse racial or ethnic backgrounds may fear or distrust the healthcare system or worry about confidentiality and receiving fair, unbiased treatment (OVW, 2024). Immigrants, regardless of their legal status, may worry about the assault being reported to law enforcement and the impact that this would have on their presence in the country. If clinicians are aware of this, they can educate their patients on the process of applying for a U-visa, which allows immigrants who are victims of serious crime, including sexual assault, and who work with law enforcement to obtain temporary legal status to reside and work in the United States (U.S. Citizenship and Immigration Services, 2024).

In addition, in some cultures it is considered taboo to be touched or seen by opposite-sex clinicians. In such a case, it may be beneficial to have a same-sex clinician or someone of the same culture provide care for the individual. For some, the loss of virginity prior to marriage—even as a result of an assault—could lead to shunning by family or even prevention from marrying (OVW, 2024). Sexual assault in these instances may be a source of significant shame and embarrassment and could impact the individual's ability to seek care.

Individuals may also have the added barrier of limited English language proficiency. Any such difficulty in communicating may be exacerbated by the stress of the assault. It is important to make necessary accommodations for the individual's communication needs by offering a clinician who speaks the same language or utilizing interpreter services (OVW, 2024).

Although people of all genders and ages can be victims of sexual violence, this chapter focuses primarily on the care and treatment of adult and adolescent victims of sexual violence who were assigned female at birth (AFAB) and/or who identify as women or female, as well as transgender and nonbinary individuals, and the management of their healthcare needs related to the assault. The terms "women" and "female" are used in this chapter when discussing specific research findings and treatment modalities. Use of these terms is not meant to exclude those who do not identify as women and are seeking care because of sexual assault. The physical and psychological effects of sexual violence are presented in this chapter, along with information to assist clinicians in providing treatment according to the current standard of care. Throughout this chapter, the term "victim" is used when referring to a person who has recently been sexually assaulted, and the term "survivor" is used when an individual has begun to heal from the traumatic event. The term "patient" is used to describe and document the health care provided to a person who has been sexually assaulted. Resources for clinicians are provided in **Appendix 16-A**.

BOX 16-1 Types of Sexual Violence

- Completed or attempted forced penetration of a victim: Physical insertion of the penis into the vulva or anus, however slight; contact between the mouth and penis, vulva, or anus; or penetration of the anal or genital opening of another person by a hand, finger, or object.
- Completed or attempted forced acts in which a victim is made to penetrate a perpetrator or someone else: Includes when the victim was made to, or there was an attempt to make them, penetrate another without the victim's consent.
- Unwanted sexual contact: Intentional touching, either directly or through the clothing, of the genitalia, anus, groin, breast, inner thigh, or buttocks of any person without their consent. May also include making the victim touch the perpetrator.
- Noncontact unwanted sexual experiences: Does not involve physical contact. Includes unwanted exposure to sexual situations (voyeurism, exhibitionism, pornography), verbal or behavioral sexual harassment, threats of sexual violence, and taking/disseminating photographs of a sexual nature of another person.

Data from Basile, K. C., Smith, S. G., Breiding, M. J., Black, M. C., & Mahendra, R. R. (2014). *Sexual violence surveillance: Uniform definitions and recommended data elements, version 2.0*. National Center for Injury Prevention and Control, Centers for Disease Control and Prevention. http://www.cdc.gov/violenceprevention/pdf/sv_surveillance_definitionsl-2009-a.pdf

DEFINITIONS

"Sexual violence" is an umbrella term that refers to any sexual act, attempted or committed, against an individual who has not freely given consent (OVW, 2024). The types of sexual violence, listed in **Box 16-1**, include completed or attempted sex acts, unwanted sexual contact, and unwanted sexual experiences that do not include contact (Basile et al., 2014).

The term "sexual assault" refers to nonconsensual sex acts prohibited by federal, tribal, or state law (OVW, 2024). Rape is further defined as completed or attempted nonconsensual vaginal, anal, or oral penetration, no matter how slight, with any body part (penis, fingers, etc.) or object (Basile et al., 2022). The terms "sexual assault" and "rape" are often used interchangeably.

All acts of sexual violence involve a lack of freely given consent and include situations in which the person is unable to consent or refuse the sexual act (OVW, 2024). Inability to consent may occur as a result of alcohol or drug intoxication, whether the substances are consumed voluntarily or involuntarily. The individual could also be under the legal age of consent, have certain cognitive or physical disabilities, or be unconscious. Inability to refuse a sexual act refers to victims who are forced to comply under the threat of physical harm, psychological coercion, or the misuse of authority (Basile et al., 2022).

No clinical definition of sexual assault or rape has gained widespread acceptance. The lack of a consistent definition impedes the ability to accurately monitor the incidence of sexual violence and makes measuring risk and identifying preventive measures more difficult. It is important for clinicians to be familiar with their state's definitions of sexual violence and corresponding sexual assault laws to ensure they follow the practice and legal dictates in their jurisdiction (Basile et al., 2022).

EPIDEMIOLOGY

The 2016/2017 National Intimate Partner and Sexual Violence Survey (NISVS) Report on Sexual Violence by the Centers for Disease Control and Prevention (CDC) provide comprehensive data on the prevalence, demographic disparities, and long-term impacts of sexual violence in the United States (U.S.). Conducted between September 2016 and May 2017, the survey used a random-digit-dial method with landline and cell phones, targeting English- and Spanish-speaking adults aged 18 and older (Basile et al., 2022). With responses from 15,152 women and 12,419 men, the survey achieved national representativeness despite a 7.6 percent response rate, enhanced through follow-up efforts.

Key findings from the report highlight that sexual violence is widespread, with approximately 1 in 4 women (26.8%) and 1 in 26 men (3.8%) having experienced rape in their lifetimes, while about 1 in 2 women (47.6%) and 1 in 4 men (23.3%) reported unwanted sexual contact (Basile et al., 2022). The survey also categorizes sexual violence into types, including rape, sexual coercion, unwanted sexual contact, and sexual harassment, and reveals significant racial and ethnic disparities. For instance, lifetime prevalence rates are particularly high among non-Hispanic American Indian/Alaska Native and multiracial women, with nearly 48 percent of non-Hispanic multiracial women experiencing rape compared to 29 percent of non-Hispanic white women. Additionally, sexual violence often begins early, with most victims experiencing their first assault before age 25, which links early exposure to negative long-term health outcomes such as PTSD, chronic pain, and mental health challenges (Basile et al., 2022).

The 2016/2017 NISVS Report on Sexual Violence found most sexual violence perpetrators are predominantly male and known to their victims. Among female rape victims, 94 percent reported male perpetrators, with 56.1 percent identifying an acquaintance and 39.3 percent an intimate partner as the offender. Less than 20 percent of women reported a perpetrator who was a stranger. Male victims similarly reported a high incidence of male perpetrators, though cases of "being made to penetrate" more commonly involved female perpetrators. These patterns underscore the need for targeted prevention within trusted social networks to address the dynamics of known and gendered perpetrators in sexual violence cases (Basile et al., 2022).

According to the Bureau of Justice Statistics' *Criminal Victimization,* 2024 report, violent victimization remains substantially underreported in the United States. In 2024, the overall rate of violent victimization was 23.3 incidents per 1,000 persons age 12 or older, while only 11.2 of those victimizations per 1,000 were reported to law enforcement (Tapp & Coen, 2025). Because the Bureau of Justice Statistics (BJS) combines rape and sexual assault with other violent crimes, the reporting gap cannot be clearly quantified for sexual violence alone, which limits our ability to determine the actual prevalence or assess how effectively systems are responding. Stewart et al. (2024) note that many women choose not to report sexual violence because they expect to be disbelieved, fear being retraumatized by the process, or see little value in engaging with the system. Their findings suggest that non-reporting can be a deliberate and protective decision when weighed against ongoing structural and emotional barriers.

CLINICAL PRESENTATION AND CONCERNS FOLLOWING SEXUAL ASSAULT

In September 2023, ACEP reaffirmed its 2013 guidelines, *Evaluation and Management of the Sexually Assaulted or Sexually Abused Patient,* 2nd edition, underscoring their ongoing relevance. These guidelines outline medical evaluation, evidence collection, and psychological support, stressing coordinated community response, and serve as a resource for clinicians and support professionals. The U.S. Department of Justice, Office on Violence Against Women (OVW), incorporated the guidelines into its *National Protocol for Sexual Assault Medical Forensic Examinations* (3rd ed.; OVW, 2024).

After a sexual assault, deciding when or if to seek medical help is often complex and deeply personal. Some people may not feel ready for days, even weeks, before they are able to reach out for medical care (American College of Emergency Physicians [ACEP], 2013; ACEP, 2023; OVW, 2024). This delay can stem from powerful emotions like shame, self-blame, or fear of not being believed (Cuevas et al., 2018; Catton et al., 2023). Practical obstacles, such as lacking insurance, not having transportation, or concerns about retaliation can make it difficult to ask for support (DOJ, 2024). In nearly 80 percent of sexual assaults (DOJ, 2013a, revised 2016), the assailant is a current or former partner, friend, family member, or someone else they know. This familiarity can further complicate their decision to come forward (Basile et al., 2022).

Individuals seeking medical attention may prioritize testing and treatment for STIs, HIV, and pregnancy, along with addressing the physical and emotional effects of the assault (American College of Obstetricians and Gynecologists, 2019; Hassam et al., 2020). It is important for clinicians encountering survivors of sexual assault in the acute phase to understand both medical and legal requirements of care. It is recommended that these individuals be seen by a Sexual Assault Nurse Examiner (SANE) or Sexual Assault Forensic Examiner (SAFE) (OVW, 2024; ACOG, 2019), as they are specifically trained to document and preserve evidence for use in investigations and legal proceedings.

Acute Traumatic Injury

Immediately following sexual assault, the individual may present with a variety of general body injuries and/or injuries to the anogenital region. It is imperative to understand that although injury may be found, oftentimes a victim of sexual assault may present with no injuries at all. Further, a lack of injury should not be a factor that dissuades the clinician from treating a patient who has experienced sexual assault as a trauma victim.

Injuries from sexual assault can occur anywhere on the body, including the head, neck, oral cavity, torso, extremities, and anogenital region. Mild injuries may include abrasions, bruises, tenderness, or sore muscles and generally do not require clinical intervention. Moderate injuries often require intervention and include superficial tears or lacerations, bites, and chipped or broken teeth. Severe injuries that require extensive clinical intervention may include deep lacerations, broken bones, and traumatic brain injury (Basile et al., 2021). Injuries that are sustained during a sexual assault are generally categorized as mild, with moderate and severe injuries occurring only rarely (ACEP, 2013; McCormack et al., 2022). A mild categorization does not capture the profound psychological impact of the assault, which is often severe and can lead to numerous lifelong health-related consequences (Dworkin et al., 2017).

Several studies indicate that the incidence and detection of physical injuries after sexual assault vary based on examination timing, assault type, and assessment techniques. Based on the OVW (2024) guidelines, most survivors present for examination within 72 hours of the assault, with over half exhibiting general body injuries and nearly half showing anogenital injuries. Researchers noted survivors had general body injuries, with severity ranging from mild to severe, and noted that anogenital injuries were particularly common among individuals with no prior sexual intercourse or who experienced multiple forms of penetration (Hassam et al., 2020; Littleton et al., 2023).

Psychological Health

Behavioral responses to assault vary widely among individuals, making it essential for clinicians to understand that there is no single "normal" reaction to sexual assault. Some victims may present with evident signs of distress, such as crying, trembling, or expressions of anger. Conversely, other victims' reactions may be more composed and controlled, with minimal to no outward sign of distress (OVW, 2024).

Additionally, a person who has been sexually assaulted may have problems providing accurate details and recalling and recounting the assault secondary to the trauma of the event and the impairment that it has on brain functioning (Campbell, 2012; Laricchuita et al., 2023).

Dr. Rebecca Campbell, who is well recognized for her research on the neurobiology of trauma, has reported extensively about how the brain responds to a traumatic event such as a sexual assault. Her work identifies that the hormonal responses mediated by the hypothalamus, pituitary gland, and adrenal glands mount a fight, flight, or freeze response during the assault. In contrast, the hippocampus and amygdala play crucial roles in the processing, storing, and recollection of memories. If the information is emotionally charged, such as with an assault, it becomes much harder to encode that information into retrievable memories (Campbell, 2012; Laricchiuta et al., 2023).

Additionally, the hormones released during the stress response make recalling the details of the event even more difficult, which in turn further fragments the memories. Collectively, these effects explain why it is difficult for assault victims to recall the trauma in an orderly or organized manner. Their memory is disorganized and in pieces, and time may need to pass before they can recall the trauma, if they ever do. If alcohol was involved, there may have been no encoding of the memory, so there may be nothing left to retrieve (O'Callaghan & Ullman, 2024). Educating clinicians and members of the legal and criminal justice system about the effects of trauma on the brain and memory is crucial to help support individuals who have been victims of sexual assault as they attempt to navigate the criminal justice system and heal from the effects of their trauma.

Psychological symptoms may become more visible and severe in the weeks and months following the sexual assault. These responses can include fear, anger, anxiety, depression, substance use or abuse, and PTSD. Individuals who have been sexually assaulted are prone to more severe trauma responses when (1) the assault is completed rather than attempted, (2) the assailant is known to the person, (3) the individual experiences a freeze reaction or is restrained and unable to move during the assault, or (4) there is previous psychological trauma or a history of mental illness (Stewart et al., 2024).

The most significant factor influencing an individual's psychological health after experiencing sexual assault is the response from others, including clinicians, law enforcement, and support networks. Conversely, those who encounter victim-blaming, disbelief, lack of support, or even continued violence from any of these groups tend to experience more severe and lasting psychological impacts (SAMHSA, 2023).

EVALUATION OF THE SEXUAL ASSAULT PATIENT

Individuals who have been sexually assaulted are entitled to prompt, high-quality care to promote healing, minimize trauma, and increase the likelihood of recovering evidence from the assault (OVW, 2024). To coordinate these efforts effectively, a Sexual Assault Response Team (SART) can provide immediate interventions and services, including victim support, medical forensic care, and initiation of the criminal investigation (OVW, 2024). *A National Protocol for Sexual Assault Medical Forensic Examinations: Adults/Adolescents,* published by the VCW (2024), provides recommendations on the proper evaluation and management of individuals who have been sexually assaulted. This document provides a general overview of the forensic examination process; however, additional education and specialized training are recommended as best practice for optimal care and accuracy in evaluating sexual assault patients. Guided by trauma-informed care principles, the evaluation process centers on obtaining consent, gathering patient history, conducting a psychological assessment, performing a physical exam, obtaining detailed documentation, and diagnostic testing.

The Violence Against Women Act (VAWA) and the Sexual Assault Survivors' Bill of Rights (STOP) Act work together to strengthen legal protections and support systems for survivors of domestic violence and sexual assault. VAWA provides federal funding and resources improving law enforcement responses, victim services, and community-based prevention programs (OVW, 2024). The STOP Act stems from VAWA and establishes specific rights for survivors of sexual assault. This includes access to basic forensic examinations without requiring a police report and timely processing of evidence (OVW, 2024). These laws form the foundation for survivor advocacy and accountability within the legal system.

Forensic Examiners (SAFE)/(SANE) Referral

The OVW (2024) recommends clinicians serving as examiners of sexual assault victims have advanced knowledge and skill, as well as certification, in this specialty area of practice. When a clinician is not adequately trained to care for sexual assault victims, they should refer the patient to an available SAFE. These clinicians have completed the required didactic and clinical training to care for sexual assault patients. Often this role is assumed by a registered nurse, referred to as a SANE. The SANE performs all the components of the medical forensic examination, psychological and physical management of the patient, and relevant patient education. The International Association of Forensic Nurses (IAFN) provides educational guidelines and certification requirements for SANEs. For more information about the education, certification, and role of the SANE, refer to the IAFN website (http://www.iafn.org).

Communities should work to ensure that victims of recent sexual assault have access to healthcare professionals who are specially trained and clinically prepared to conduct medical forensic examinations. This complex, time-intensive care is significantly improved by specialized training, which promotes the delivery of consistent, high-quality care (OVW, 2024).

The medical forensic exam includes a complete patient history, a thorough physical examination with attention to trauma, a detailed anogenital examination as indicated by the patient history, and evidentiary collection. Clinicians treating individuals who have experienced sexual violence must be able to not only treat injuries and address health-related concerns, but also coordinate crisis intervention, collect evidence and maintain the appropriate chain of custody, follow jurisdictional reporting procedures, and testify in legal proceedings if necessary (ACEP, 2020; OVW, 2024).

Additionally, the clinician should ensure a safe and private setting is provided for the individual while waiting for the medical forensic examination, undergoing the examination, and participating in law enforcement reporting. The individual should be asked if they would like a victim services organization to be contacted so an advocate can be made available to offer crisis intervention, advocacy, and support to the patient before, during, and after the medical forensic examination (ACEP, 2013; OVW, 2024).

The clinician should also help the individual contact a support person, such as a family member or friend, if desired (ACEP, 2013; OVW, 2024). It is important that the clinician inform the individual and support person that information obtained during the examination may be used to prosecute a crime; thus, support persons could be subpoenaed to testify in court. It is important that persons who are present during the examination process do not participate in answering questions or influence the individual's answers in any way (OVW, 2024).

Consent

Prior to engaging in care of the sexual assault patient, the clinician must obtain two types of informed consent. The first is a general consent that signifies the individual has agreed to receive medical evaluation and treatment. The second form of consent grants the clinician permission to collect evidence and gives the individual the option to release the evidence to the appropriate law enforcement and criminal justice agencies if desired (OVW, 2024). The process of obtaining consent from the individual should follow agency policy, with consent generally obtained verbally, in writing, and in the presence of a witness.

In cases of reversible incapacitation (e.g., medication, drug, or alcohol ingestion and intoxication), the medical forensic examination should be deferred until the patient is legally able to consent. In cases when the patient is under the age of consent, is comatose, or is suffering from a permanent cognitive or developmental disability, consent should be obtained from the person legally responsible for making healthcare decisions for the patient as long as that person is not suspected of being the perpetrator (OVW, 2024). It is important for the clinician to follow state statutes regarding age of consent for medical forensic examinations and treatment for pregnancy and STIs because the age limit for consent in each situation varies by state.

Confidentiality and Reporting

Clinicians are required to maintain the privacy and confidentiality of patient health information as outlined in the federal privacy law, the Health Insurance Portability and Accountability Act (HIPAA), unless legally mandated to report to law enforcement officials. In some states, clinicians are required to report all incidents of sexual assault; in others, reporting is required only if a weapon, such as a gun or knife, was used during the crime. In other states, the competent adult victim is the sole decision maker regarding whether they will file a police report (OVW, 2024).

The careful balance between respecting patient confidentiality and fulfilling mandatory reporting obligations presents a complex challenge for clinicians in cases of sexual assault. Reporting requirements often hinge on the victim's age, the nature of their relationship to the alleged perpetrator, or the presence of any cognitive or physical vulnerabilities. Additionally, mandated reporting often extends to cases involving vulnerable adults, such as those who are older or who have disabilities, when there is suspicion or evidence of sexual assault (ACEP, 2013). Given the variation in state-specific requirements, clinicians are encouraged to consult local legal resources, such as the prosecutor's office or protective services, to clarify their reporting obligations.

When reporting is initiated, either at the patient's request or due to legal mandate, clinicians should explain the reporting procedure, maintaining transparency about the steps involved. Providing a private, quiet setting for the law enforcement interview helps preserve the patient's comfort and dignity, and clinicians should remain available to offer supportive presence throughout. Importantly, clinicians need to clarify that while healthcare settings uphold strict confidentiality, law enforcement is not held to the same standards; once health information is released, it can be shared with criminal justice entities involved in the prosecution (OVW, 2024). This delicate balance of maintaining patient trust while fulfilling legal duties underscores the importance of sensitive and informed communication in these cases.

It is essential for individuals to know they have the right to access medical care, including evaluation and treatment, even if they choose not to report the assault to law enforcement or engage with the criminal justice system. Additionally, they may receive this medical care without the obligation to undergo evidence collection (OVW, 2024). Importantly, they should be made aware that costs related to a medical forensic exam are covered through funds provided by each state's STOP Violence Against Women Formula Grant, regardless of their level of participation with law enforcement. Some individuals may need more time to consider their options before deciding to report, and they should be informed of the agency's policies on evidence storage, as well as how they can authorize the release of this material to law enforcement if they choose to do so later (OVW, 2024).

Post-Traumatic Stress Disorder

Individuals who are victims of sexual violence are at significant risk for developing PTSD, with studies showing that as many as one third to more than half of survivors are diagnosed with the disorder (Basile et al., 2022; APA, 2022). PTSD symptoms generally develop within 3 months of the trauma, though they may fluctuate over time. Approximately 50 percent of individuals with PTSD recover within 3 months, while others may experience symptoms for months or even years after the assault (APA, 2022). The diagnostic criteria for are defined by the American Psychiatric Association in the *DSM-5-TR*; refer to this source for complete criteria (APA, 2022). PTSD involves intrusive thoughts, avoidance, negative changes in mood and cognition, and heightened arousal, with a lifetime prevalence of 1 to 14 percent in the general population. Studies show that about 50 percent of female victims of sexual violence experience PTSD symptoms, with hyperarousal and re-experiencing symptoms playing key roles in the disorder's severity and progression, which impacts victims' treatment and recovery (Yang et al., 2023).

Sexual violence (SV) poses the highest risk for PTSD and deliberate self-harm (DSH), especially in women, who experience SV more frequently and engage in self-harm at higher rates than men (Brockdorf et al., 2023). SV-related PTSD symptoms are linked to self-harm, suggesting that survivors may engage in nonsuicidal self-harm to manage emotional distress caused by PTSD. Deliberate self-harm includes behaviors such as cutting, burning, and self-hitting, and is the strongest predictor of suicide attempts (Brockdorf et al., 2023). As many as 30 percent of female survivors who experience PTSD may turn to substances such as alcohol and drugs as coping mechanisms (Gong et al., 2019), and some may engage in self-harm behaviors (Cuevas et al., 2018). Younger survivors, particularly those from racial minority groups or who identify as bisexual, report higher rates of suicidal ideation. Furthermore, women who disclose their assault tend to report more trauma, increased drug use, and a higher incidence of suicide attempts. PTSD itself is a known risk factor for completed suicide (Cuevas et al., 2018). For these reasons, it is essential that clinicians assess suicide risk during the initial and all follow-up visits for victims of sexual assault.

Substance Abuse

The use of alcohol, marijuana, and other illicit drugs may be factors that increase a person's vulnerability to sexual assault because the effects of these substances prevent the person from being able to legally give consent (Gong et al., 2019). PTSD and substance use disorders (SUDs) frequently co-occur, with those who have PTSD being two to four times more likely to meet SUD criteria, particularly with substances like alcohol, nicotine, heroin, cocaine, and amphetamines. Nearly half (46.4%) of individuals with PTSD also have SUDs, and patients with both conditions experience higher symptom severity and poorer treatment outcomes than those with only one disorder (Gong et al., 2019).

In addition to this, sexual assault can lead to increased substance use and abuse in an attempt to cope with the trauma (Gong et al., 2019). The more severe the sexual trauma (e.g., completed rape), the more likely the person is to develop problematic substance use. Further, substance use may lead to an increase in risky sexual behavior, which in turn puts the person at risk for STIs and possible sexual dysfunction (Gong et al., 2019).

Sexual Dysfunction

Sexual dysfunction is a common and sometimes chronic problem after sexual assault—particularly loss of sexual desire and lack of ability to orgasm (Hassam et al., 2020; Littleton et al., 2023). Sexual dysfunction may also include an inability to become sexually aroused, slow arousal, pelvic pain associated with sexual activity, lack of sexual enjoyment, fear of sex, avoidance of sex, intrusive thoughts of the assault during sex, vaginismus, or abstinence (Hassam et al., 2020). Chapter 12 provides a thorough discussion of sexuality and the impact of stress on sexual functioning.

History

This section provides a general overview of the forensic examination process. However, additional education and specialized training are recommended as best practices to ensure accurate evaluations and optimal care for sexual assault patients. Using a trauma-informed approach, the clinician gathers comprehensive information related to the chief complaint, details of the assault, and the patient's general medical history (refer to Chapter 5). This history forms a foundation for guiding the physical examination, establishing medical and nursing diagnoses, and developing an appropriate care plan (OVW, 2024). It also assists in deciding whether forensic samples should be collected for potential analysis by a crime laboratory. It is essential that the clinician ensures the history is taken in the individual's primary language, especially for patients with limited English proficiency. Utilizing qualified interpreters can facilitate clear communication, allowing survivors to share their experiences and medical history accurately, which is crucial for effective treatment and care planning.

Although specific questions asked during the patient history may vary among agencies, **Box 16-2** provides an example of the type of information that should be requested from individuals who are being evaluated. Such information includes pertinent medical-surgical history, current medications, allergies, disabilities, immunizations, menstrual history, and recent consensual sexual contact (ACEP, 2013; OVW, 2024). Asking about gynecologic health and variances enables the clinician to distinguish between existing conditions and any trauma related to the assault. Furthermore, inquiry into recent consensual sexual contact is important for accurately interpreting DNA findings, allowing clinicians to differentiate expected DNA from forensic evidence associated with the assault.

It is essential to address questions specific to the sexual assault in a sensitive and supportive manner, and answers should be recorded in the patient's words. The intent of these inquiries is not to elicit a comprehensive narrative of the event but to gather pertinent information that will inform the physical examination, evidence collection, and treatment planning for the patient. Clinicians should prompt the patient to provide details regarding the time, date, and location of the assault (ACEP, 2013; OVW, 2024). The time and date are particularly critical, as they dictate the appropriate timing for certain medications and determine the admissibility of evidence based on jurisdictional guidelines (OVW, 2024). Identifying the location of the assault may also assist in tracing the origin of any debris present on the individual. Questions regarding post-assault activities, such as whether the individual showered, douched, used intravaginal products, consumed food or drink, smoked, brushed their teeth, changed clothes, or engaged in consensual intercourse, should also be asked to clarify the amount and type of evidence that may be found (ACEP, 2013; OVW, 2024).

The clinician should inquire about all orifices that may have been penetrated—such as the vagina, mouth, and anus—and the means of penetration (e.g., penis, finger, object). This information is vital for directing the examination and identifying potential evidentiary material (ACEP, 2013; OVW, 2024). Additionally, it is important to ask about drug or alcohol consumption immediately prior to the assault, as this can indicate whether the individual's ability to consent was compromised (ACEP, 2013; OVW, 2024). Specifically, clinicians should inquire about any loss of memory or consciousness, as this may signal a case of drug-facilitated rape. Prompt toxicology testing is crucial as detection of these substances is time-sensitive (OVW, 2024). Questions regarding the use of force or restraint during the assault are also critical, particularly if strangulation occurred. Strangulation is a particularly vicious act employed by perpetrators to exert control over their victims and is classified as a felonious assault in many jurisdictions. Patients with a history of strangulation should receive a thorough examination by a clinician who has received specialized training in this area. Refer to **Appendix 16-B** for signs and symptoms associated with strangulation cases.

Psychological Assessment

The clinician should assess the individual's psychological health throughout the examination. This part of the exam can be completed by asking about thoughts and feelings and by observing the patient's behavior. Each person copes differently with psychological trauma; thus, patients may present with a variety of behaviors, including anger, indifference, humor, emotional distress, or hostility (OVW, 2024). There is no normal response that is expected from someone who has been sexually assaulted. Psychological responses are dictated by previous experience

BOX 16-2 Information to Obtain During the Medical Forensic History

General Medical Questions

1. What is your relevant medical history that may impact the examination?
2. Have you experienced any recent injuries, surgeries, or diagnostic procedures in the anogenital area?
3. Are there any recent procedures that may have altered the appearance of your genitalia?
4. Do you have any medical conditions, such as clotting disorders, that we should be aware of?
5. Can you provide information about any allergies you may have?
6. What medications are you currently taking?
7. Do you have any acute or chronic health conditions we should consider?
8. If applicable, can you share your pregnancy history?
9. What is your immunization status?

Questions Regarding Recent Consensual Activity

1. Have you engaged in any recent consensual sexual activity? If so, can you specify the types (anal, vaginal, oral) and whether a condom was used?
2. Are there any recent consensual partners that we should be aware of in relation to any potential anogenital injuries?
3. Is there any additional information about recent contact that could help us understand the context of your injuries?
4. Have you noticed any trace amounts of bodily fluids that may be relevant to your case?
5. Would you like to discuss any specific concerns related to consensual partners in the context of your current situation?

Questions Concerning Post-Assault Activities

1. Can you describe any actions you took prior to the examination, such as urination, defecation, or bathing?
2. Did you wipe or clean your genital area or body before coming in for the examination?
3. Have you removed or inserted a tampon or any other item before the examination?
4. How much time has passed between the incident and your examination?
5. Is there anything else you did that might be relevant to the evidence we're collecting?

Questions Regarding the Offender Information and Location

1. Do you have any information about the number of suspected offenders involved in the incident?
2. If known, can you provide details about the gender of the suspected offenders?
3. Can you describe the location where the incident occurred (e.g., indoors, outdoors, in a vehicle, etc.)?
4. What were the physical surroundings of the assault (e.g., type of surface like carpet, dirt, grass)?
5. Are there any specific details about the location that might be relevant for evidence collection?
6. Is there any other information about the offenders or the location that you think might help guide the examination?

Questions Regarding Alcohol- or Drug-Facilitated Sexual Assault

1. Did you experience any memory loss or lapse of consciousness around the time of the incident?
2. Did you have any vomiting during or after the incident?
3. Were you given any food or drink by the suspected offender? If so, do you know what it was?
4. Did you voluntarily ingest any drugs or alcohol before or during the incident?
5. Would you consent to collecting toxicology samples to help with the investigation?
6. How much time has passed since the suspected ingestion of any substances?

Questions Regarding Sexual Assault

1. Was there penetration of genitalia? (e.g., vulva, hymen, and/or vagina of patient if applicable and however slight).
2. What was used for penetration? (e.g., finger, penis, or other object).
3. Was there penetration of the anal opening, however slight?
4. Was there oral contact with genitals (of patient by suspect(s) or of suspects by patient).
5. Was there contact with genitals (of patient by suspect(s) or of suspects by patient) or with the anus (of patient by suspect(s) or of suspects by patient).
6. Were any other non-genital act(s) involved such as licking, kissing, suction injury, strangulation, or biting?
7. During the assault, were other act(s) committed including use of objects for penetration and/or to injure, degrade, or humiliate in any way? Was there any use of restraints or taking of images or video by the offender(s)?
8. Did the assailant ejaculate and if so where (e.g., mouth, vagina, genitals, anus/rectum, body surface, on clothing, on bedding, or other)?
9. Was any contraception, including condom, or lubricants used?
10. Were any weapons involved?
11. Were there threats of or injury by hitting, grabbing, scratching, holding, pinching, biting, strangulation, burns (thermal and/or chemical), or involuntary ingestion of alcohol/drugs?
12. Is it possible the offenders were injured? (to know if evidence may be present on victim, for instance skin under the nails, or on suspect, such as scratches and bruises).

Data from U.S. Department of Justice. Office on Violence Against Women. (2024). *A national protocol for sexual assault medical forensic examinations: Adults/adolescents*, 3rd ed. https://www.justice.gov/ovw/media/1367191/dl?inline

and the presence of certain hormones in the body at the time of the assault and immediately following. Each person should be treated as an individual, with their response documented in the medical record. Further, it is important for the patient to be given as much control as possible throughout the examination, meaning that they have the right to decline any part of the evaluation, to take breaks as needed, and to have questions answered throughout the process (DOJ, 2024).

GENERAL PHYSICAL EXAMINATION

As previously discussed, the SANE/SAFE are trained to conduct the medical forensic examinations for sexual assault survivors. Their training ensures compassionate care and precise evidence collection. This chapter provides an overview of the key elements of the examination process. For detailed guidance on evidence-based procedures and examination standards, consult the *National Protocol for Sexual Assault Medical Forensic Examinations: Adults/Adolescents* (3rd ed.; OVW, 2024). Prior to beginning the examination, the individual's clothing and undergarments should be collected if they are the same items worn during the assault, with the individual being provided an examination gown. When removing their clothes, the individual should stand on a clean sheet or paper so that foreign material and debris that fall from them can be collected as evidence (ACEP, 2013; OVW, 2024). Each article of clothing should be packaged separately in a paper bag and marked with their name, date, time of collection, and name of the person collecting the evidence (ACEP, 2013).

The clinician should examine the individual's entire body, including their head, neck, oropharynx, extremities, and torso, looking for injury and foreign debris or biological fluids that could be collected as evidence (ACEP, 2013). All instances of acute injury should be documented on a body diagram (OVW, 2024) (refer to **Appendix 16-C**). Documentation should include the injury type, location, measurement, color, and if pain or tenderness is present.

Assessing the individual for signs, symptoms, and complications associated with strangulation, which has life-threatening consequences, should be included as part of the evaluation, particularly if the individual recounts that physical or mechanical force was applied to their face, neck, or upper chest. Individuals with a history of strangulation should receive a detailed examination with a clinician experienced in these types of injuries. Refer to Chapter 15 for detailed information on assessing the patient after strangulation.

Anogenital Examination

This section provides a general overview of a piece of the medical forensic examination process; however, additional education and specialized training are recommended as best practice for optimal care and accuracy in evaluating sexual assault patient injuries. Examination of the anogenital structures should align with the individual's history of the sexual assault (**Box 16-3** provides detailed steps for conducting the anogenital examination). For example, if the patient reports assault limited to the oral area, collection of genital specimens should be deferred. As with the entire evaluation process, the clinician should reconfirm verbal consent with the person prior to moving on to the anogenital examination because it may be psychologically traumatizing and physically painful, particularly if injury is present.

BOX 16-3 Steps of the Anogenital Examination

1. Visually inspect the perianal tissue for injury and the presence of foreign material.
2. Photograph the perianal tissue.
3. Collect evidentiary samples from the perianal tissue.
4. Palpate the perianal tissue for pain or tenderness.
5. Apply manual traction to the perianal tissue to examine perianal folds and the anal canal.
6. Photograph the anal canal if visualized.
7. Collect evidentiary samples from the anal canal.
8. Visually inspect the external genitalia (vulva) for injury and the presence of foreign material.
9. Photograph the external genitalia.
10. Collect evidentiary samples from the external genitalia.
11. Palpate the external genitalia for pain or tenderness.
12. Separate the labial folds to further examine external genital structures.
13. Apply manual traction to the labia minora to further examine external genital structures.
14. Apply toluidine blue dye (to external genital structures only) to assist with identification of external genital injury that is not visible by the unassisted eye.
15. With patient consent, complete a speculum examination to assess the internal genitalia (vaginal wall and cervix). Speculum examinations are completed on postpubescent females only.
16. Collect evidentiary samples from the internal genitalia.
17. Reinspect the external genitalia for injury that may have been caused by the speculum examination; document this finding if present.
18. Use a Foley catheter or other related technique to inspect the hymen for injury. The Foley technique is completed on postpubescent females only.

Perianal Tissue

If anogenital examination is indicated, the clinician should begin by visually inspecting the perianal area for signs of injury and foreign material. Evidentiary swabs should be collected prior to palpating the perianal tissue. The individual may be put in a knee–chest position while lying in a supine, prone, or side-lying position to assist with relaxation of the anal sphincter. Injury occurring to any part of the anogenital anatomy should be documented on a body diagram referencing the time on a clock, with 12:00 always being closest to the urethra. Further, documentation should include the injury: location, type, measurement, and other characteristics.

External Genitalia

Clinicians should examine the external genitalia and perineal area assessing for injury, foreign materials, and other findings in the following areas: abdomen, thighs, perineum, labia majora, labia minora, clitoral hood and surrounding area, periurethral tissue/urethral meatus, hymen, fossa navicularis, and posterior fourchette (OVW, 2024). Special attention should be paid to the posterior fourchette, as this is a common site for injury following sexual assault and consensual intercourse (OVW, 2024). Refer to Chapter 7 for discussion and illustrations of normal anatomy.

After the visual inspection of the external genitalia, photographs should be taken by the SANE if the individual provides consent. Evidentiary samples should then be collected, ensuring that the SANE clinician accurately documents the exact anatomical locations from which samples are obtained. Criminal sexual conduct laws can vary by state, and depending on the extent of the sexual assault (e.g., contact vs. penetration), different charges may apply. The location of DNA findings, such as on the hymen versus the labia majora, may influence the severity of criminal sexual conduct charges.

Internal Genitalia

If the individual consents, the vagina and cervix should also be assessed for injury or presence of foreign material by speculum examination. A small amount of water or saline may be used as lubrication to enhance patient comfort (DOJ, 2017); although some literature also supports the use of water-soluble non-spermicidal lubricant, additional research on whether or not this would interfere with evidence analysis is warranted with forensic examination.

Testosterone therapy can cause vaginal atrophy and decreased elasticity in trans-masculine individuals, which increases tissue fragility and the likelihood of tearing during an assault. Surgically constructed vaginas may also be more shallow, less flexible, and less lubricated, making them more susceptible to injury and subsequent risk of STI and HIV transmission. Genital injury may be particularly distressing for trans women when significant emotional or financial investment has been placed in the neovagina, and trans men may experience demasculinization or intensified dysphoria if forced vaginal penetration occurs (Oke, 2024). Vaginal swabs without speculum exam can be collected if the patient is unable to tolerate a speculum exam (DOJ, 2024).

Documentation

Thorough documentation by the clinician is crucial. The clinician may be responsible for documenting the results of the examination in both the patient's medical record and the evidence collection kit report. The medical record includes all information from the patient's admission, whereas the evidence collection kit report includes only the evidence collection consent form, a history of the assault, and information pertaining to evidence collection to assist the crime lab in analyzing samples. Only medical information that could affect evidentiary findings should be included in the kit report. If the sexual assault is reported to law enforcement, the evidence collection kit and report will be provided to the law enforcement agency and the state crime laboratory. The patient's medical record is not part of the evidence kit and should not be released to the referenced agencies unless required by law (OVW, 2024).

Diagnostic Testing

Sexually Transmitted Infections

Treating patients prophylactically is often preferable to performing STI testing unless the person presents with signs and symptoms consistent with an STI (CDC, 2021). Individuals evaluated soon after the sexual assault may not test positive for an STI as the infectious agent may not yet be present in sufficient quantities due to varying incubation times for each STI. Therefore, testing at this time would likely detect only pre-existing STIs and is often deferred in favor of prophylactic treatment with follow-up recommendations (CDC, 2021).

The CDC (2021) recommends that individuals being tested for STIs undergo nucleic acid amplification testing, which can detect the presence of *Chlamydia trachomatis* and *Neisseria gonorrhoeae*. These samples are collected from the site of penetration or attempted penetration. A urine sample or vaginal specimen can be used to test for *Trichomonas vaginalis*, and point-of-care (POC) testing or a vaginal wet mount is utilized for diagnosing bacterial vaginosis and candidiasis (CDC, 2021).

Based on the exposure risk, a baseline serum sample for HIV, hepatitis B virus (HBV), and syphilis may be indicated (CDC, 2021). For those individuals who have previously received the HBV vaccine, titers should be drawn to determine the immunization status. Those who receive initial STI testing should receive follow-up testing 2 weeks after the assault. Follow-up testing for HIV is recommended at 4 to 6 weeks and again at 3 months, and syphilis testing should occur at 6 weeks and again at 3 months (CDC, 2021).

Pregnancy

A baseline serum pregnancy test should be conducted with consent for any individual who can become pregnant, as the results may impact treatment options, including emergency contraception and antibiotics. Clinicians should not assume a person who has not menstruated in many months, for example because of testosterone therapy or perimenopause, cannot become pregnant. While the risk is low, it is still possible and should be ruled out (OVW, 2024).

Drug-Facilitated Sexual Assault

The use of alcohol or drugs compromises an individual's ability to consent to sexual activity, making it easier for a perpetrator to commit sexual assault. These substances inhibit a person's ability to resist and can prevent them from remembering the assault (DOJ, 2021a). Drug-facilitated sexual assault (DFSA), including alcohol-facilitated sexual assault, encompasses both voluntary and involuntary consumption of the substance used. A systematic review of literature on the topic by Anderson et al. (2017) found that (1) alcohol intoxication poses the greatest risk for DFSA; (2) lack of, or delayed reporting of DFSA to police or medical centers lead to an underestimation of the prevalence of DFSA; (3) there is poor conceptualization of DFSA and a need for systematic toxicological analysis exists; and (4) there is a greater need for systematic and detailed history taking from victims. A 2-year study published in 2017 by Richter et al. found that over half of the patients at an urban rape treatment center were victims of DFSA. Over the course of the study they also found that involuntary DFSA increased from one quarter to one third of the DFSA cases. Awareness of this risk is an important public health topic.

There are a variety of central nervous system (CNS) depressant drugs used to facilitate sexual assault, both prescription and over-the-counter, including benzodiazepines, antidepressants, muscle relaxants, antihistamines, sleep aids, hallucinogens, and opioids (Society of Forensic Toxicologists, n.d.). However, alcohol remains the biggest factor, particularly in combination with other drugs (Anderson et al., 2017; OVW, 2024). Toxicology is not routinely performed unless indicated by the patient's history and when DFSA is suspected. Testing for DFSA is recommended when an individual suspects they have been drugged and experiences symptoms such as loss of consciousness, drowsiness, fatigue, dizziness, memory loss, impaired motor skills, or severe intoxication. In some cases, the person may regain consciousness without remembering how they arrived at their current location. Voluntary drug and/or alcohol use should not diminish the perceived seriousness of the assault and should not alter or diminish the level of care provided to the victim. Coercion of substance use may be part of a power and control dynamic in an abusive relationship as well (OVW, 2024).

Drugs used to facilitate sexual assault are typically cleared from the body quickly; therefore, samples should be taken as soon as possible from the urine and blood as indicated (OVW, 2024). Most drugs clear more quickly from the bloodstream, so the first available urine sample is preferred as evidence. The drug is more concentrated and readily detected in the first sample. Clinicians should collect 100 mL of urine in a specimen cup with the preservative sodium fluoride and store refrigerated (OVW, 2024). While most drugs will be undetectable in the blood more than 24 hours after ingestion, blood may prove useful in a DFSA case if collected less than 24 hours after the incident. At least 12 milliliters of blood should be obtained in a gray-top test tube containing the preservative sodium fluoride and the anticoagulant potassium oxalate. The blood should be stored refrigerated. Toxicology samples are collected separately from the evidence collection kit because the samples may be tested in different laboratories. If not immediately tested, the toxicology samples should be refrigerated. Similar to the discussion about evidence collection, the chain of custody should be maintained for toxicology samples that may be related to a crime (OVW, 2024).

MANAGEMENT

A multidisciplinary approach is critical when addressing the needs of individuals who have experienced sexual assault. A Sexual Assault Response Team (SART) is useful to coordinate immediate interventions and services, including victim support, medical forensic care, and the initial criminal investigation (OVW, 2024).

It is important for clinicians to address physical and psychological health consequences; however, because sexual assault is a crime, the individual may also liaise with members of law enforcement, the legal system, and victim advocates (DOJ, 2017). A survivor-centered, trauma-informed approach by members of the team will help to achieve quality outcomes for the individual. A survivor-centered approach ensures the individual's needs are the top priority for all agencies involved. A trauma-informed approach recognizes that events such as sexual assault can be highly traumatic and result in poor outcomes for the survivor. Including survivor advocates as part of the team helps to ensure that a survivor-centered, trauma-informed process occurs (DOJ, 2017).

Advocacy Services

Survivor advocates should be involved early in the process to ensure that the individual's needs are being met and to help support them in dealing with the acute and chronic sequelae of sexual violence (DOJ, 2017). An advocate can serve as a support person, offer crisis intervention, provide information and referrals, and help ensure that the individual's rights and wishes are respected. Long-term resources, such as counseling, support groups, and legal advocacy, may also be offered (OVW, 2024).

Safety Planning

The clinician should assist the individual with contacting local law enforcement to file a report of the assault if they desire. The clinician may also partner with law enforcement officials and advocacy agencies to develop a plan to help ensure the individual's safety following sexual assault. Making sure the individual has a safe place to stay and a support system in place is important for both the physical and psychological health of the individual. If necessary, the advocacy services agency may be able to assist with finding emergency shelter or an alternative living arrangement if it is unsafe for the individual to return home. The agency may also be able to provide legal advocacy services, including assistance with obtaining a personal protection order and providing information and support while participating in legal proceedings (OVW, 2024).

Psychological Health

During the initial evaluation, the clinician must assess if the person's psychological health that is sufficient to determine a level of orientation, possible suicidal ideation, and need for referral for follow-up support, evaluation, or treatment. During this evaluation, visible signs of psychological distress may not be evident. The clinician should inform the patient that any type of psychological response is normal and that thoughts, feelings, and behavior may fluctuate or change over time (Dworkin et al., 2020).

A referral to a community-based agency that specializes in long-term management and care of the psychological needs of sexual assault victims should be offered. A watchful waiting approach may be implemented over several months in which the person engages in follow-up appointments with the referred agency. If during these appointments it is determined that the individual is suffering from alcohol or drug abuse, depression, psychotic symptoms, or suicidal ideation, or if they are self-harming or unable to participate in day-to-day activities, a referral to a qualified mental health clinician is recommended (Dworkin, 2020).

Pharmacological Management

STI Prevention

The most frequently diagnosed STIs among individuals who have been sexually assaulted are chlamydia, gonorrhea, trichomoniasis, and bacterial vaginosis (CDC, 2021). However, given the high incidence of these infections among sexually active individuals, establishing a direct link to the assault is not always feasible (CDC, 2021). Improperly treated and untreated chlamydia and gonorrhea infection can lead to pelvic inflammatory disease, ectopic pregnancy, and infertility in women; therefore, it is crucial for clinicians to consider prophylactic treatment following sexual assault. The CDC recommends empiric treatment for gonorrhea, chlamydia and trichomoniasis in females and gonorrhea and chlamydia for males at the time of visit, as follow-up visit compliance is low for survivors of sexual assault. Refer to **Box 16-4** for guidelines (CDC, 2021).

Patient education should emphasize the importance of avoiding sexual contact until the prescribed treatment regimen is completed. Patients should also be informed about signs and symptoms of STIs so they can seek evaluation and treatment if symptoms develop.

BOX 16-4 Prophylactic Antibiotic Therapy for STIs Post–Sexual Assault

Treatment for All Survivors:

- Chlamydia and Gonorrhea:
  - Single dose of ceftriaxone:
    - 500 mg intramuscularly for those < 150 kg
    - 1 g for those > 150 kg

PLUS:

- Females:
  - Doxycycline: 100 mg twice daily for 7 days orally
  - Metronidazole: 500 mg twice daily for 7 days orally (avoid if alcohol consumed within the past 24 hours)
- Males:
  - Doxycycline: 100 mg twice daily for 7 days orally

Counseling:

- Discuss benefits and side effects of medications.
- Consider alternative treatments for individuals with specific drug allergies (CDC, 2021).
- Emphasize the importance of refraining from sexual contact until the prescribed treatment regimen is completed.
- Educate on the signs and symptoms of STIs to ensure timely evaluation.

Data from Centers for Disease Control and Prevention. (2021, July 22). Sexually transmitted infections treatment guidelines, 2021: Sexual assault and abuse and STIs – Adolescents and adults. https://www.cdc.gov/std/treatment-guidelines/sexual-assault-adults.htm

BOX 16-5 Vaccination Recommendations Post–Sexual Assault

Hepatitis B (HBV) Vaccination:

- Administer the HBV vaccine at the time of the initial evaluation for those not previously vaccinated.
- Follow-up vaccinations:
  - 1–2 months after the first dose
  - 4–6 months after the first dose
- Hepatitis B immune globulin may be recommended for individuals not fully vaccinated post-assault if the assailant is known to be HbSAg + (CDC, 2021).

Human Papillomavirus (HPV) Vaccination:

- Offer HPV vaccination to individuals aged 9–26 who have not been fully vaccinated at the initial examination.
- Follow-up doses:
  - 1–2 months after the first dose
  - 6 months after the first dose
- For those under age 15, a two-dose schedule (0 and 6–12 months) is recommended (CDC, 2021).

Data from Centers for Disease Control and Prevention. (2021, July 22). Sexually transmitted infections treatment guidelines, 2021: Sexual assault and abuse and STIs – Adolescents and adults. https://www.cdc.gov/std/treatment-guidelines/sexual-assault-adults.htm

The CDC (2021) recommends administration of the HBV vaccine at the time of initial evaluation of an individual who has not been previously vaccinated, as postexposure vaccination can prevent infection (refer to **Box 16-5** for guidelines). Sexual assault survivors are also at risk for acquiring human papilloma virus (HPV). Those age 9–26 should be offered HPV vaccination at the time of the initial examination if they have not been previously vaccinated, or incompletely vaccinated as vaccine efficacy is high for HPV (CDC, 2021).

HIV Prevention

Transmission of HIV is also a concern in individuals who have been sexually assaulted. The risk of contracting HIV through receptive penile–vaginal intercourse is estimated at eight infections for every 10,000 exposures, or 0.08 percent (Centers for Disease Control and Prevention [CDC], 2021). Receptive penile–anal intercourse has a higher risk, estimated to be 138 infections for every 10,000 exposures, or 1.38 percent. Receptive penile–oral intercourse has a minuscule transmission risk, much lower than other forms of HIV transmission; nevertheless, it is not a zero risk (Patel et al., 2014). Sexual assault may potentially increase the likelihood of HIV transmission if the individual suffers trauma and bleeding. Other factors that increase transmission risk are the site of ejaculation, viral load in the ejaculate, and presence of genital lesions or current STIs in the survivor or assailant (CDC, 2021). Victims of sexual assault should be counseled on the importance of follow-up STI and HIV testing and adherence to prescribed treatment regimens to prevent these infections.

The clinician should consider several factors when deciding whether to recommend HIV nonoccupational postexposure prophylaxis (nPEP) to a person who has been sexually assaulted. Factors that increase the likelihood of HIV transmission include risk behaviors in the assailant (e.g., IV drug use, men who have sex with men) and high-risk characteristics of the assault (e.g., vaginal or anal penetration, ejaculation on mucous membranes, and exposure to blood) (CDC, 2021). An assault by multiple assailants or the presence of genital lesions or ulcers on the assailant or survivor also increases the possibility of transmission. It is important for the clinician to inform the individual of the known side effects of antiretroviral drugs and that close follow-up while taking the nPEP regimen is recommended. This information enables the patient to make an educated decision on whether they would like to begin nPEP therapy. The CDC algorithm for evaluation and treatment of possible nonoccupational HIV exposures can be a helpful decision-making tool. The National Clinician's Post Exposure Prophylaxis Hotline (PEP Line) (telephone: 888-448-4911) can also be helpful if a specialist is unavailable to assist (CDC, 2021).

If an individual chooses to begin nPEP, the regimen should be initiated as soon as possible. Effectiveness decreases with time and after 72 hours from the exposure, PEP is unlikely to be effective (CDC, 2016). A 28-day course of antiretroviral medications is generally prescribed. Currently, the preferred standard regimen includes the use of Truvada (combination of tenofovir 300 mg and emtricitabine 200 mg) once daily plus either raltegravir 400 mg twice daily or dolutegravir 50 mg once daily (CDC, 2016). The individual should be given a 3- to 7-day starter pack supply of medication with a prescription for the remaining amount or a prescription for the entire 28-day supply at the initial visit. This will allow the patient to start treatment immediately and improve compliance (CDC, 2024). The patient starting nPEP will need additional baseline lab testing, including serum creatinine, AST, and alanine aminotransferase at baseline as well as a follow up appointment with a PEP provider.

Pregnancy Prevention

Individuals who can get pregnant and are sexual assault survivors often fear the possibility of becoming pregnant. Unintended pregnancy following sexual assault is estimated to occur in 2 to 5 percent of cases. These statistics are similar to the risk of pregnancy from a one-time sexual encounter (OVW, 2024). Basile et al. (2018) estimated that nearly 2.9 million Americans have at some time in their life become pregnant as a result of rape. The National Intimate Partner and Sexual Violence Survey (Basile et al., 2022) found that 1 in 7 of the females who were raped became pregnant. All individuals who have been sexually assaulted should be informed of the risk of conception and the availability of emergency contraception. Both ACOG (2019) and IAFN (2022) recommend offering emergency contraception (EC) to all individuals of reproductive age who can become pregnant and are seen for sexual assault. If a clinician is not comfortable prescribing EC, another clinician must be provided to offer this standard of care. If one is unavailable, a plan should be in place for immediate referral or access to this time- sensitive care (OVW, 2024). A review of EC options and their mechanism of action, side effects and follow-up allows the patient to make an informed decision. This form of contraception can be quite effective if administered to an individual who seeks treatment immediately following sexual assault. It may be given within 72 to 120 hours of the assault depending on method, although its efficacy can decrease with time (OVW, 2024). If the individual vomits within 3 hours of receiving emergency contraception, it may be suggested that they take an additional dose of emergency contraception to ensure its efficacy (OVW, 2024).

One progestin-only emergency oral contraceptive option includes a single oral dose of 1.5 mg levonorgestrel (Plan B, Next Choice) or divided in two doses of 0.75 mg 12 hours apart and taken within 72 hours. Efficacy can be 81–90 percent but can be time dependent and may also decrease with a body mass index (BMI) over 25 (OVW, 2024). Ulipristal acetate (Ella) is a second-generation progestin-only emergency oral contraceptive with a 2.1 percent failure rate, and it can be taken up to 5 days after an assault. Research suggests that its efficacy may decrease in individuals with a BMI over 35. Both emergency contraceptive options work by inhibiting or delaying ovulation. While ongoing research continues, current data indicates that Ulipristal may be the more effective option for preventing pregnancy in individuals living in larger bodies. For more information on emergency contraception, please refer to Chapter 13 (OVW, 2024; Salcedo, 2023). This medication in combination with STI treatment my cause nausea and an antiemetic should be considered.

A second type of EC is available, and can provide not only emergency, but also ongoing contraception for up to 12 years. The copper intrauterine device (IUD) can be placed within 5 days (120 hours) of the assault and offers a 99 percent reduced risk of pregnancy. The copper IUD contains no hormones and primarily works by preventing sperm from reaching the egg. Research on the use of the levonorgestrel IUD for EC is continuing and is showing similar effectiveness rates when used within 5 days of intercourse (Salcedo et al., 2023).

An option not typically used due to significant nausea, the Yuzpe method is a combined estrogen–progestogen regimen of two tablets (0.05 mg ethinyl estradiol and 0.5 mg norgestrel or levonorgestrel) taken orally at the time of examination, with a repeat dose of two tablets given 12 hours later. An antiemetic agent may be offered with this option of emergency contraception (DOJ, 2024). More information on EC is available in Chapter 13.

Other Medications

Pain medication should be offered if indicated. The type of medication will depend on the severity of the individual's injury, but a nonsteroidal anti-inflammatory drug (NSAID) or acetaminophen is often sufficient for minor injury. The individual may be given an antiemetic agent because a common side effect of antibiotics, emergency contraceptives, and antiretrovirals is gastrointestinal distress. If the individual sustained an injury from a foreign object or a bite, a tetanus shot may also be recommended.

Patient Education

Prior to discharge, the individual should receive oral and written instructions regarding the care received during the examination. Both the oral and written instructions should be provided in their primary language if English is not their first language (OVW, 2024). Education should also emphasize the importance of medical follow-up and the availability of victim advocacy services. The clinician should inquire about safety concerns and, if necessary, facilitate referrals to appropriate agencies to assist with developing a safety plan for the individual.

FOLLOW-UP CARE

Follow-up care after a sexual assault is crucial for survivors, with medical assessments recommended within 1 to 2 weeks post-assault (CDC, 2021; OVW, 2024). During this follow-up, clinicians evaluate for sexually transmitted infections (STIs), complete necessary treatments, and ensure adherence to prescribed regimens. Effective communication regarding access to follow-up services is essential, particularly for those lacking a primary care provider or health insurance. Contacting survivors within 24 to 48 hours of the initial examination can enhance compliance with treatment plans (OVW, 2024).

Research indicates that survivors of sexual assault often experience significant, long-term health consequences. A study of 2,650 women diagnosed with sexual assault revealed they were four times more likely to have psychiatric disorders and eight times more likely to experience substance abuse issues compared to individuals who have not experienced sexual assault (Young-Wolff et al., 2018). Additionally, these individuals reported higher incidences of stress-related somatic conditions, gastrointestinal disorders, pain issues, and obesity. They also utilized psychiatric and obstetric-gynecological services more frequently. Nearly half of the survivors experienced mild injuries, with a substantial proportion facing ongoing health challenges (ACOG, 2019; Basile et al., 2021).

PREVENTION

The scope of sexual violence is vast, affecting nearly half of women and almost a third of men over the course of their lifetime

(Basile, 2022). This issue is frequently underreported and can have long-lasting effects on both physical and mental health. Effective prevention is crucial to addressing this national health crisis. In 1994, Congress passed the Violence Against Women Act to provide funding for prevention initiatives and support services for victims of violence (U.S. Congress, 1994/2022). Using this funding, the CDC established the Rape Prevention and Education (RPE) Program, to serve communities across the United States and its territories. The program utilizes a multilevel approach with strategies to prevent sexual violence, outlined in the Sexual Violence Prevention Resource for Action: A Compilation of the Best Available Evidence (Basile, 2016). This guide introduces the acronym STOP SV, which represents the following strategies (refer to **Box 16-6**). Each strategy is paired with specific interventions or programs to reinforce prevention efforts (Basile, 2022).

Integrating screening as a standard practice within these prevention initiatives can support early identification, intervention, and empowerment for individuals affected by sexual violence. ACOG recommends providers of women's healthcare screen all women for a history of sexual assault (ACOG, 2019). There are various tools available, such as the Two Question Screening Tool, that can quickly address history of IPV and sexual assault (McFarlane, 1995). If positive, responding in a way that acknowledges and validates the information without blame creates a safe environment for the survivor. The provider can then provide emotional support and resources to begin the healing process (refer to **Box 16-7**) (Hopkins & Kennedy, 2024).

Porat et al. (2024) reviewed community-based primary prevention efforts targeting sexual violence from 1985 to 2018 and found that most initiatives emphasize shifting beliefs and attitudes about sexual violence. Goals for prevention include both a decrease in perpetration and an increase in bystander involvement. The school-based curriculum program for adolescents and young adults, Safe Dates, developed by Vangie Foshee, began in 1996 to teach about relationship skills and dating violence. Follow-up data found a decrease in psychological, physical, and sexual dating violence perpetration and less physical dating violence victimization at all follow-up periods (Porat et al., 2024). Shifting Boundaries, also school based, focused on middle school students with classroom and building interventions (posters on dating violence, boundaries, and increased security). The Men's Program aimed to reduce perpetration by increasing empathy in undergraduate men on college campuses. The outcome surveys and focus groups conveyed that "participants reported increased awareness of sexual violence, improved understanding of consent, and greater belief in their ability to help victims of sexual violence" (Porat et al., 2024).

The review emphasized the *Bringing the Bystander* program, designed for undergraduate students, which emphasizes bystander intervention to prevent sexual violence. They discuss the role of community members in preventing sexual violence and help participants develop skills to safely intervene. Outcomes on follow-up survey are reported as "decreased rape myth acceptance, increased knowledge of sexual violence, increased prosocial bystander attitudes and feelings of self-efficacy, and increased self-reported bystander behaviors compared with the control group" (Porat et al., 2024). The most current prevention programs to decrease sexual violence have focused on changing beliefs, attitudes, norms, and bystander intervention. While such programs have shown success, the need for interventions specifically aimed at reducing the perpetration of violence are needed (Porat et al., 2024). As the CDC STOP SV guidelines point out, impacting public health will require a comprehensive approach that considers communities, schools, individual relationships, and broad social attitudes (Basile, 2022). A single program cannot resolve this issue; addressing the complexities of sexual violence requires collective efforts to transform social structures, belief systems, and behaviors both nationally and globally.

BOX 16-6 STOP Strategy Description

S – Promote social norms that protect against violence
T – Teach skills to prevent sexual violence
O – Provide opportunities to empower and support girls and women
P – Create protective environments
SV – Support victims

BOX 16-7 Two-Question Screening Tool

- "Have you ever been hit, slapped, kicked, or otherwise physically hurt by your partner?"
- "Have you ever been forced to have sexual activities?"

HUMAN TRAFFICKING

Background and Legal Framework

Human trafficking is a widespread and exploitative form of interpersonal violence with significant personal and public health consequences, disproportionately impacting women and young girls, who comprise approximately 80 percent of those exploited in the United States (Greenbaum et al., 2023). Often referred to as modern-day slavery, it is a pervasive global crisis that constitutes a severe violation of human rights, generating an estimated $150 to $300 billion annually, two-thirds of which comes from commercial sexual exploitation (U.S. Department of State, 2024; Walk Free, Global Slavery Index, 2023).

Defined by the Trafficking Victims Protection Act (TVPA) of 2020, human trafficking includes the recruitment, harboring, transportation, or obtaining of individuals through force, fraud, or coercion for involuntary servitude, peonage, debt bondage, or slavery (Walk Free, Global Slavery Index, 2023). This multibillion-dollar global enterprise affects significant numbers of people, including unaccompanied immigrant minors and individuals of the LGBTQ+ community, leading to a range of associated serious physical, emotional, and mental health issues (Baird & Connolly, 2023; Greenbaum, 2021). Victims are often invisible, and despite clinicians' perceptions, a substantial number of victims accessed healthcare services while being trafficked but were undetected (Walk Free, Global Slavery Index, 2023).

The United States categorizes both labor and sex trafficking as severe forms of trafficking in persons. The TVPA and its reauthorizations were established to provide comprehensive protections for victims and survivors of human trafficking and to strengthen the United States' response to combating trafficking crimes. Each reauthorization has progressively enhanced legal frameworks, expanded victim services, and increased collaboration between domestic and international entities (TBPA, 2000; Trafficking Victims Protection Reauthorization Act, 2003, 2005, 2008, 2013, 2017, 2018, 2024). Specifically, the TVPA defines:

- Labor trafficking as "the recruitment, harboring, transportation, provision, or obtaining of a person for labor or services, through the use of force, fraud, or coercion for the purposes of subjection to involuntary servitude, peonage, debt bondage, or slavery."
- Sex trafficking as "the recruitment, harboring, transportation, provision, obtaining, patronizing, or soliciting of a person for the purposes of a commercial sex act, in which the commercial sex act is induced by force, fraud, or coercion, or in which the person induced to perform such an act has not attained 18 years of age."

Under federal law, any commercial sex act involving a minor under 18 is automatically classified as child sex trafficking, as minors cannot legally consent to commercial sex, and proof of force, fraud, or coercion is not required. In contrast, cases involving adult victims must demonstrate elements such as force, fraud, coercion, or abuse of power to be legally considered trafficking (TVPA, 2000; U.S. Department of State, 2024). Defined as "any sex act on account of which anything of value is given to or received by any person," this legal framework ensures that minors engaged in such acts are protected as trafficking victims.

The strengthened anti-trafficking measures emphasize the prosecution of offenders, victim protection, and prevention of child trafficking. The Justice for Victims of Trafficking Act (JVTA) of 2015 further expanded protections by amending the Child Abuse Prevention and Treatment Act (CAPTA) to define "child abuse and neglect" as inclusive of "sex trafficking" and severe forms of trafficking affecting minors (Child Abuse Prevention and Treatment Act [CAPTA], 1988). While reporting laws vary, all U.S. states, the District of Columbia, and U.S. territories mandate reporting suspected child abuse and neglect to relevant authorities (Justice for Victims of Trafficking Act [JVTA], 2015; Rapoza, 2022).

The definitions in **Box 16-8** guide enforcement and victim support initiatives across U.S. jurisdictions, providing a legal framework to address and combat both forms of trafficking.

These definitions guide enforcement and victim-support initiatives across international and U.S. jurisdictions, providing a shared legal framework to identify and respond to human trafficking. The globally accepted Act–Means–Purpose (AMP) model was originally developed by the United Nations Office on Drugs and Crime (UNODC) to operationalize the definition established in the 2000 Palermo Protocol. The AMP framework was later formalized in UNODC's *Trafficking in Persons: Global Patterns* (2006) and the *Toolkit to Combat Trafficking in Persons* (2008), and is now widely used across U.S. federal agencies, including the U.S. Department of State. To meet the definition of trafficking, at least one element from each AMP category must be present (refer to **Box 16-9**) (United Nations, 2000; UNODC, 2006, 2008; U.S. Department of State, 2024).

BOX 16-8 Key Definitions of Trafficking Under U.S. Federal Law

- Minor Victims
  - Any commercial sex act involving a minor under 18 is classified as child sex trafficking.
  - Minors cannot legally consent to commercial sex, so no proof of force, fraud, or coercion is required (TVPA, 2000; U.S. Department of State, 2024).
- Adult Victims
  - Trafficking cases involving adults require evidence of force, fraud, or coercion for legal recognition (TVPA, 2000; U.S. Department of State, 2024).
- Commercial Sex Act
  - Defined as "any sex act on account of which anything of value is given to or received by any person," ensuring that minors involved in such acts are legally protected as trafficking victims (TVPA, 2000).
- Legislative Framework
  - The TVPA of 2000 established foundational protections and has been expanded over time.
  - The Justice for Victims of Trafficking Act (JVTA) of 2015 amended the Child Abuse Prevention and Treatment Act (CAPTA) to include "sex trafficking" as a form of child abuse and neglect (CAPTA, 1988).
- Mandated Reporting
  - All U.S. states, the District of Columbia, and U.S. territories require mandatory reporting of suspected child abuse and neglect, including trafficking (JVTA, 2015; Rapoza, 2022).

EPIDEMIOLOGY

Human trafficking is considered the fastest growing criminal activity worldwide with an estimated 40 to 50 million victims globally (Jain et al., 2022; Walk Free Foundation & International Organization for Migration, 2022). Current data from the International Labour Organization (ILO), Polaris Project, and the U.S. Department of State's Trafficking in Persons (TIP) Report (2024) underscore its massive scale. Vulnerable individuals are often trafficked or enslaved for various purposes that can overlap, including labor trafficking and sex trafficking, that continue from childhood into adulthood. The U.S. Department of State defines human trafficking broadly. In the United States, exploitation spans formal sectors such as construction and agriculture, informal work such as domestic and landscaping services, and commercial sex industries. Illegal commercial sex activities range from street-based work to tech-facilitated encounters, escort services, and more. Nail salons, massage parlors, and unregulated bodywork establishments may also serve as fronts for labor or sex trafficking (Baird & Connolly, 2023; Greenbaum et al., 2022; U.S. Department of State, 2024). For additional trafficking typologies refer to **Box 16-10**.

Adolescents of any nationality, legal status, gender, or age are vulnerable to multiple forms of trafficking, which can include sex

BOX 16-9 Elements of Human Trafficking—A-M-P Model

Act

- Recruitment, harboring, transportation, provision, obtaining, patronizing, or soliciting individuals.

Means

- Force: Use of physical restraint, monitoring, confinement, and physical harm (e.g., assault, beatings, burns).
- Fraud: False promises regarding employment, wages, working conditions, or relationships (e.g., love, marriage).
- Coercion:
  - Threats of harm to self or family.
  - Psychological abuse (e.g., captivity, isolation).
  - Confiscation of documents.
  - Blackmail using videos or photos.
  - Threats to report to authorities (e.g., immigration, law enforcement).

Purpose

- Exploitation through prostitution, pornography, sexual exploitation, or involuntary servitude, occurring in various locations, such as private homes, massage parlors, hotels, nail salons, online platforms, and other unregulated businesses may serve as "storefronts" for both labor and sex trafficking venues.

BOX 16-10 Trafficking Typologies

- Escort Services
- Illicit Massage, Health, and Beauty
- Outdoor Solicitation
- Residential
- Domestic Work
- Bars, Strip Clubs, and Cantinas
- Pornography
- Traveling Sales Crews
- Restaurants and Food Service
- Peddling and Begging
- Agriculture and Animal Husbandry
- Personal Sexual Servitude
- Health and Beauty Services
- Construction
- Hotels and Hospitality
- Landscaping
- Illicit Activities
- Arts and Entertainment
- Commercial Cleaning Services
- Factories and Manufacturing
- Remote Interactive Sexual Acts
- Carnivals
- Forestry and Logging
- Health Care
- Recreational Facilities

Reproduced from Polaris. *The typology of modern slavery*. https://polarisproject.org/the-typology-of-modern-slavery/

trafficking, stripping, online exploitation, performing in sexual venues, and the production of sexual abuse materials (Braun, 2024). Several factors contribute to adolescents becoming victims of trafficking. Due to their limited life experiences, need for acceptance, and underdeveloped impulse control, adolescents are particularly susceptible to manipulation, with many entering sex trafficking and exploitation between the ages of 11 and 17 (Greenbaum et al., 2023). Adolescents who have been abused (particularly sexually abused) or come from homes where abuse occurred are at higher risk. Other factors that place adolescents at high risk for becoming victims of sex trafficking include poverty, foster care, parental drug use, identification as LGBTQ+, and substance abuse (Wood, 2020). These factors make adolescents easier to recruit through the promise of money, a home, support, and being surrounded by people who care. Often the recruiter is someone the adolescent knows (Baird & Connolly, 2023; Polaris, 2023).

Global and U.S. Prevalence

Trafficking incidents are often facilitated by an organized network of recruitment, movement, and retention tactics designed to exploit vulnerable populations, including individuals experiencing economic hardship, discrimination, regional conflict, migration, homelessness, or gender-based violence. Violence, poverty, political instability, and environmental degradation have led to a surge of vulnerable populations in the Americas, including refugees and asylum seekers. In 2020, the region hosted 26 percent of the world's international migrants. Venezuela's crisis alone forced over 6 million citizens to flee by 2021 (Walk Free, Global Slavery Index, 2023). The Mexico–U.S. border remains the world's busiest migration route, with restrictive immigration policies through Central America pushing migrants toward the dangerous Darien Gap route—a treacherous 100-mile stretch of mountainous rainforest between Panama and Colombia. Migrants face extreme terrain, injury, wildlife threats, and risks of human trafficking or robbery by cabals or organized crime syndicates. Originally, many crossing the Darien Gap were from Haiti and Cuba, but more recently migrants from diverse regions are increasingly making this dangerous journey (Caitlyn Yates & Juan Pappier, 2023; Walk Free Foundation & International Organization for Migration, 2022).

The Polaris Project's U.S.-based National Human Trafficking Hotline highlights that annually, thousands of trafficking cases are reported across all 50 states, underscoring that human trafficking is not confined to any single region. In the United States, labor trafficking has also surged in specific sectors, especially with migrant and seasonal workers. Reports have highlighted increased labor trafficking among H-2A visa holders in agriculture, who often face abusive working conditions and are denied health services (Polaris, 2023). Globally and domestically, anti-trafficking organizations are seeing a yearly rise in reported cases, emphasizing the need for ongoing data collection and focused intervention efforts to address both forced labor and sexual exploitation across various industries. This data-driven approach can help shape stronger preventive measures, legal frameworks, and victim support systems to effectively combat trafficking.

Recruitment and Control

Traffickers use a combination of violence, coercion, and dependency to control victims, severely impacting their physical, reproductive, and mental health. Often victims lack freedom of movement or are closely monitored by traffickers. The high-risk conditions trafficked individuals face, including unsafe work environments and intentional harm, lead to accidental injuries and increased susceptibility to STIs, HIV, and unintended pregnancies. Dependency is further reinforced through financial manipulation, forced criminal acts, and deceptive recruitment tactics including false job offers. For minors, familial pressure plays a significant role. In 41 percent of child trafficking cases, family members often use psychological abuse and coercion to trap children into a trafficking situation (Barrick et al., 2024; Counter-Trafficking Data Collaborative [CTDC], 2024). Refer to **Figure 16-1**.

This control often involves complex psychological manipulation. Traffickers may initially build trust by meeting basic needs before introducing abuse and exploitation, creating strong trauma bonds that tie victims emotionally to their traffickers. This phenomenon, common among trafficking survivors, complicates interventions by reinforcing attachment to the trafficker as a survival mechanism. Additionally, trafficking risks heighten in environments marked by gang involvement, violence, and drug activity, requiring trauma-sensitive, nuanced approaches from healthcare providers to help survivors disengage safely (Wood, 2020).

While elements of interpersonal violence and sexual assault are present, human trafficking is characterized by a pattern of exploitative, complex, and repeated trauma, with each form of harm compounding the effects of the others. "Complex trauma" refers to the long-term effects of repeated exposure to multiple traumatic events, often occurring without the opportunity for recovery or healing between incidents. Victims of trafficking endure a cycle of manipulation, abuse, and coercion, which compounds the trauma experienced from interpersonal violence and sexual assault. Unlike isolated instances of harm, complex trauma creates deep psychological and emotional scars that hinder recovery, often making intervention and recovery more challenging (Chambers et al., 2024). Refer to **Figure 16-1**.

Clinical Presentation

Recognition and Red Flags

Traffickers often restrict victims' access to health care, leading to delays in receiving necessary care for acute injuries or illness and chronic disorders. As a result, victims frequently present with severe injuries or advanced illnesses. Traffickers enforce silence through threats, creating fear, stigma, and financial barriers that inhibit disclosure (Greenbaum, 2021). Fear of deportation, lack of funds, shame, criminal history, and concerns about judgment from healthcare providers further discourage victims from divulging information. Studies show between 28–88 percent of trafficking victims seek health care while being exploited, yet often go unnoticed by providing vague or inconsistent histories to avoid disclosure (Lawrence & Bauer, 2020; Stoklosa et al., 2015). Clinicians play a key role in identifying these individuals by noting clinical signs such as frequent reproductive health visits, STI or pregnancy tests, lack of identification, physical abuse, and apparent fear (Costa et al., 2019; Greenbaum et al., 2023; Hornor et al., 2023). Similar to those experiencing intimate partner violence, trafficking victims may present with vague symptoms inconsistent with their injuries. Indicators such as sexual trauma, tattoos, psychological effects, malnutrition, and lack of documentation suggest a need for sensitive screening (Barrick et al., 2024; Breiding et al., 2015; National Human Trafficking Training and Technical Assistance Center [NHTTAC], 2018; Richie-Zavaleta et al., 2021). Refer to **Box 16-11**.

Screening

The primary purpose of screening for human trafficking is to offer opportunities for intervention and access to resources while providing patient-centered, trauma-informed care. The PEARR Tool (Provide privacy, Educate, Ask, Respect, and Respond), developed by Dignity Health, HEAL Trafficking, and the Pacific Survivor Center, helps clinicians provide trauma-sensitive care to patients experiencing violence. The steps focus on providing privacy, educating patients about violence, asking open-ended questions, respecting patient autonomy, and responding with appropriate resources or referrals. This approach normalizes conversations about violence, fosters trust, and creates a safe place for patients to share their experiences (Dignity Health, 2019; Roe-Sepowitz et al., 2024). Refer to **Box 16-12** for HT screening questions.

Screening aims to:

- *Identify Red Flags:* Detect indicators of trafficking or coercion.
- *Prioritize Safety:* Ensure immediate and long-term safety for patients.
- *Empower Patients:* Provide education and resources to help patients make informed decisions about their health and safety.
- *Facilitate Referrals:* Connect patients to local services, advocacy organizations, and legal protections.
- *Promote Health Equity*: Address the disproportionate impact of HT on marginalized populations.

Health Implications and Trauma Responses

Exposure to severe, repetitive trauma often manifests in multifaceted physical, mental, and social health consequences. Physical health effects include injuries from violence, untreated infections, and the physical toll of labor in unsafe work or living conditions. In sexual exploitation cases, trafficking survivors are at high risk for STIs, including HIV/AIDS, unintended pregnancies, and reproductive health complications. Psychological trauma manifests as PTSD, depression, anxiety, suicide attempts, dissociation, and substance use disorders, all of which are exacerbated by the cumulative abuse and deprivation traffickers enforce to maintain control (Richie-Zavaleta et al., 2021). Refer to **Box 16-13** for a more detailed list.

Multidisciplinary Team Approach

Safety Planning and Referral

Safety planning is a critical component of managing care for trafficked individuals, who often return to exploitative situations

FIGURE 16-1 **Power and control wheel.**

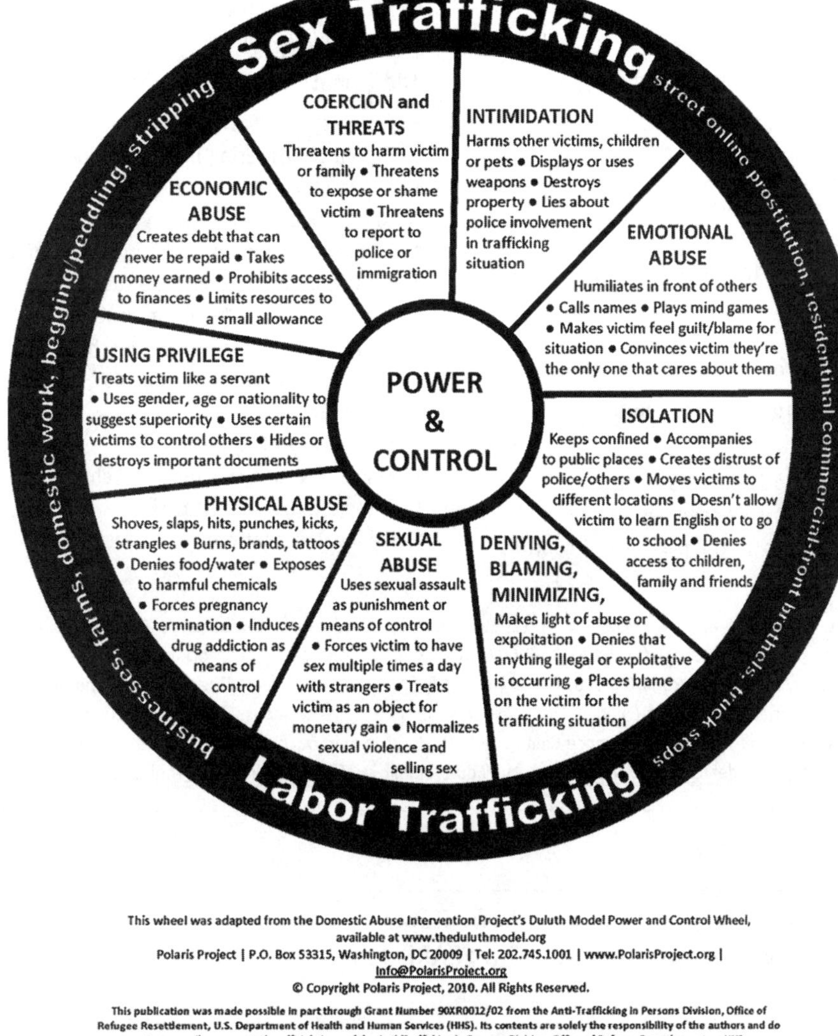
Sex Trafficking
street, online, prostitution, residential, commercial-front brothels, truck stops
Labor Trafficking
businesses, farms, domestic work, begging/peddling, stripping
COERCION and THREATS
Threatens to harm victim or family • Threatens to expose or shame victim • Threatens to report to police or immigration
INTIMIDATION
Harms other victims, children or pets • Displays or uses weapons • Destroys property • Lies about police involvement in trafficking situation
EMOTIONAL ABUSE
Humiliates in front of others • Calls names • Plays mind games • Makes victim feel guilt/blame for situation • Convinces victim they're the only one that cares about them
ISOLATION
Keeps confined • Accompanies to public places • Creates distrust of police/others • Moves victims to different locations • Doesn't allow victim to learn English or to go to school • Denies access to children, family and friends
DENYING, BLAMING, MINIMIZING,
Makes light of abuse or exploitation • Denies that anything illegal or exploitative is occurring • Places blame on the victim for the trafficking situation
SEXUAL ABUSE
Uses sexual assault as punishment or means of control • Forces victim to have sex multiple times a day with strangers • Treats victim as an object for monetary gain • Normalizes sexual violence and selling sex
PHYSICAL ABUSE
Shoves, slaps, hits, punches, kicks, strangles • Burns, brands, tattoos • Denies food/water • Exposes to harmful chemicals • Forces pregnancy termination • Induces drug addiction as means of control
USING PRIVILEGE
Treats victim like a servant • Uses gender, age or nationality to suggest superiority • Uses certain victims to control others • Hides or destroys important documents
ECONOMIC ABUSE
Creates debt that can never be repaid • Takes money earned • Prohibits access to finances • Limits resources to a small allowance
POWER & CONTROL
This wheel was adapted from the Domestic Abuse Intervention Project's Duluth Model Power and Control Wheel, available at www.theduluthmodel.org
Polaris Project | P.O. Box 53315, Washington, DC 20009 | Tel: 202.745.1001 | www.PolarisProject.org | Info@PolarisProject.org
© Copyright Polaris Project, 2010. All Rights Reserved.
This publication was made possible in part through Grant Number 90XR0012/02 from the Anti-Trafficking in Persons Division, Office of Refugee Resettlement, U.S. Department of Health and Human Services (HHS). Its contents are solely the responsibility of the authors and do not necessarily represent the official views of the Anti-Trafficking in Persons Division, Office of Refugee Resettlement, or HHS.

multiple times before permanently exiting. The clinician's role is to address the immediate healthcare needs and refer victims to a multidisciplinary team for comprehensive care coordination (Ruiz-Gonzalez et al., 2022). Early referral should involve a multidisciplinary team of social workers, case managers, and advocates to facilitate safety planning, which includes developing strategies to mitigate harm. Plans should be individualized, considering the patient's perception of their situation—whether they wish to remain, are in the process of leaving, or have already left. Risk assessment involves evaluating the patient's fear level and immediate and long-term safety needs. Indicators of escalating lethality, such as increased threats or violence, new threats of homicide or suicide, access to lethal weapons, or behaviors like strangulation, should be explored to address potential dangers. Providing discreet access to resources like the National Human Trafficking Hotline (1-888-373-7888) or Polaris text line ("BeFree" to 233733) ensures ongoing support while respecting patient autonomy (Costa et al., 2019; Greenbaum et al., 2023; Hachey & Phillippi, 2017).

Disposition and Follow-Up

The decision to admit a trafficked individual, refer for specialized services, or recommend outpatient follow-up should be determined by a clinically grounded, patient-centered approach. Admission may be necessary for medical reasons, such as ectopic pregnancy, PID, acute injuries, stabilization of chronic health conditions, substance abuse treatment, or psychological trauma. Outpatient follow-up can be recommended for patients whose immediate health and safety concerns are manageable without

BOX 16-11 Red Flags and Potential Indicators of Trafficking

Physical Indicators

- Delayed presentation to medical care
- Signs of physical, sexual, or dental trauma
- Evidence of physical violence, including torture
- Signs of neglect and malnourishment
- Substance use
- Multiple recurrent STIs
- Use of foreign objects to stop menstrual flow
- Multiple previous pregnancies
- Preventable work injuries due to lack of training or protective equipment
- Tattoos or other marks indicating ownership
- Evidence of untreated or ongoing medical conditions

Interpersonal Dynamics and Behavior Cues

- Accompanied by a controlling individual
- Companion insists on translating or refuses to leave
- Scripted, memorized, or restricted communication
- Companion answers questions for the patient and controls interaction
- Frequent glances to companion for approval
- Avoids eye contact with provider or companion
- Subordinate, hypervigilant, or fearful demeanor

Additional Behavioral Indicators

- Distrust of authority
- Difficulty answering basic questions (name, age, etc.)
- Apparent vs. reported age discrepancy or stated age older than appearance
- Inconsistent history and clinical presentation
- Possession of multiple fake IDs or hotel keys
- Inappropriate clothing for weather
- Truancy or absenteeism from school
- Lacks identification documents or documents taken by trafficker
- Excessive work hours
- Reluctance to speak on own behalf
- Possess large sums of cash
- Frequent relocation

Data from Costa, C. B., McCoy, K. T., Early, G. J., & Deckers, C. M. (2019). Evidence-based care of the human trafficking patient. *Nursing Clinics of North America, 54*(4), 569–584. https://doi.org/10.1016/j.cnur.2019.08.007; Greenbaum, J. (2021). Child labor and sex trafficking. *Pediatrics In Review, 42*(12), 639–654. https://doi.org/10.1542/pir.2020-001396; Hachey, L. M., & Phillippi, J. C. (2017). Identification and management of human trafficking victims in the emergency department. *Advanced Emergency Nursing Journal, 39*(1), 31–51. https://doi.org/10.1097/TME.0000000000000138; and National Human Trafficking Training and Technical Assistance Center. (2018). *Adult human trafficking screening tool and guide. Administration for children and families*. https://acf.gov/sites/default/files/documents/otip/adult_human_trafficking_screening_tool_and_guide.pdf

BOX 16-12 Human Trafficking Screening: The PEARR Tool

1. **Provide Privacy:**
   - Conduct discussions in secure, private spaces.
   - Ensure use of professional interpreters where language barriers exist.
2. **Educate:**
   - Normalize conversations about violence using brochures or safety cards with resources.
   - Frame the discussion broadly to reduce stigma and encourage disclosure.
3. **Ask:**
   - Engage in open-ended, nonjudgmental dialogue to assess for HT risk indicators.
   - Focus on safety and immediate needs without pressuring disclosure.
4. **Respect and Respond:**
   - Respect the patient's autonomy and decisions regarding disclosure and assistance.
   - If assistance is accepted, facilitate warm handoffs to advocates or community resources.
   - Provide discrete resources like hotline cards when a patient declines further help.
5. **Documentation and Follow-Up:**
   - Document concerns and actions taken while ensuring confidentiality.
   - Schedule follow-ups for continued rapport building and monitoring.

Screening Questions

General Safety and Well-Being

1. "Are you currently feeling safe where you live or work?"
2. "Do you have access to the things you need, such as food, clothing, or medical care?"

Indicators of Coercion or Control

3. "Is anyone preventing you from leaving your current situation?"
4. "Has anyone taken away your identification, money, or personal belongings?"

Work or Living Conditions

5. "Can you come and go as you please where you work or live?"
6. "Do you owe someone money or feel pressured to pay off a debt?"

Experience of Harm or Exploitation

7. "Has anyone ever threatened you or your loved ones if you didn't do what they asked?"
8. "Have you been forced or pressured to do something you didn't want to do, such as work or other activities?"

Approach to Asking Questions

- Be Trauma-Informed: Phrase questions gently, emphasizing patient safety and confidentiality.
- Normalize the Conversation: "I ask all my patients about their safety because we know violence and unsafe situations can affect health."
- Avoid Judgmental Language: Use neutral, supportive language to encourage honest responses.

Follow-Up Based on Responses

- If yes to any question, probe further with: "Would you like help finding resources or support?"
- If no or patient declines help, provide a hotline card discreetly.

Data from Roe-Sepowitz, D., Bracy, K., Gibbs, H., Stafford, R. L., Bernardin, B., & Stoklosa, H. (2024). PEARR tool training and implementation: Building awareness of violence and human trafficking in a hospital system. *Frontiers in Medicine, 11*, 1311584. https://doi.org/10.3389/fmed.2024.1311584

BOX 16-13 Trauma-Associated Medical and Mental Health Conditions

Category	Details
Psychological Trauma	• Normalizes sexual violence • Desensitization (repeated exposure to violence) • Intimidation • Disorientation (frequent relocations or isolation) • Coercion & manipulation • Shame • Frequent relocation • Induced dependence • Stigmatization • Depersonalization • Traumatic bonding • Self-inflicted injuries • Suicidal ideation and attempts • Cognitive impairment • Attachment disorder
Physical Trauma	• Physical abuse • Forced drug use • Deprivation (starvation, dehydration, sleep, sensory) • Sexual abuse • Torture/assault • Captivity • Debt bondage • Forced labor injuries • Restraint injuries (e.g., from handcuffs or ropes) • Exposure to unsanitary conditions
Mental Health Disorders	• Dissociative disorders • Depression • Addiction—psychological • Anxiety/fear • PTSD (hypervigilance and panic attacks) • Paranoia
Medical Conditions	• Malnutrition • Addiction—physical • Chronic infections (respiratory and urinary tract infections) • Untreated chronic illnesses (diabetes or hypertension) • Gastrointestinal issues (e.g., chronic abdominal pain, irritable bowel syndrome) • Neurological symptoms (headaches, dizziness) • Traumatic brain injury • Dental problems (broken teeth, extensive tooth decay, gum disease) • Musculoskeletal injuries (tissue trauma, fractures, contusions, sprains/strains) • Dermatological conditions (e.g., branding, burns, scars, rashes from poor hygiene or environmental conditions) • Reproductive health complications (menstrual irregularities, infertility, PID, STIs, pregnancy, abortions)

hospitalization. Follow-up appointments should prioritize continuity of care, addressing chronic illnesses, reproductive health, infectious diseases, and mental health conditions like PTSD, depression, and anxiety.

TRAUMA-INFORMED CARE: AN ESSENTIAL APPROACH

Healthcare organizations and clinicians need clear, multidisciplinary processes and procedures to facilitate effective responses when trafficking is suspected. These responses should prioritize the individual's urgent need for safety and management of the immediate presenting health issues. It is imperative that clinicians collaborate with local welfare and law enforcement agencies and establish policies and guidelines for the identification of adolescents who are at risk or are in a trafficking situation. Due to the hidden nature of this crime, raising awareness and increasing the education of clinicians to recognize signs of trafficking is essential (Gaitis, 2022; Jain et al., 2022).

The Substance Abuse and Mental Health Services Administration (SAMHSA) defines trauma as an experience that overwhelms an individual's capacity to cope and has lasting effects on their physical, mental, and emotional well-being. SAMHSA emphasizes the importance of trauma-informed care (TIC), which seeks to create environments that recognize the widespread impact of trauma, integrate knowledge about trauma into practice, and aims to avoid re-traumatization (SAMHSA, 2014; 2023). This approach involves understanding how trauma affects individuals and establishing services that support recovery in a compassionate, non-judgmental way. TIC is a critical framework in the management of trafficking survivors, emphasizing patient safety, empowerment, and collaboration (Dowdell & Speck, 2022). Refer to **Box 16-14**.

BOX 16-14 Key Principles of Trauma-Informed Care

- Safety and Trustworthiness: Creating a clinical environment where survivors feel secure encourages open communication.
- Empowerment: Allowing survivors to make decisions about their care fosters a sense of control and autonomy.
- Cultural Sensitivity: Recognizing cultural differences and providing access to interpreters ensures that patients can communicate effectively and feel respected.

SAMHSA's 2023 updated guidelines on trauma-informed care (TIC) emphasizes a structured, evidence-based approach for implementing trauma-sensitive practices. Building on its 2014 framework, the updates focus on creating environments that are physically, psychologically, and culturally safe while promoting systemic changes in organizational policies and culture (Dowdell & Speck, 2022; SAMHSA, 2023). This framework helps organizations recognize the pervasive effects of trauma and provide inclusive, resilience-building services that prioritize patient empowerment and community-specific needs.

Trafficking survivors with complex trauma require sensitive, trauma-informed approaches that prioritize safety, empowerment, and collaboration (SAMHSA, 2023). Within health care, TIC frameworks guide practitioners in addressing the unique needs of survivors, particularly those with experiences of sexual abuse, while preventing retraumatization and improving care accessibility (SAMHSA, 2023; Jain et al., 2022). Refer to Chapter 5.

Trauma Dynamics: Sexual Assault and Human Trafficking Distinction

While both sexual assault and human trafficking encompass severe traumatic events, they differ in scope, control dynamics, and varying degree of lasting impact on survivors. Sexual assault typically involves a single or repeated incident of unwanted sexual contact, which can lead to trauma responses such as PTSD, fear, and shame. Human trafficking involves prolonged, coercive control for the purpose of forced labor or sexual exploitation. The extended duration of trauma may trigger more complex trauma responses, such as dissociation, traumatic bonding, and psychological dependence on the trafficker. These responses can result in profound mental health issues and disruptions to a survivor's sense of identity. With a clear understanding of the distinctions in trauma impact, control dynamics, and legal frameworks, clinicians can better address the unique needs of survivors. This knowledge is essential for implementing interventions that promote recovery for both sexual assault and human trafficking survivors.

CONCLUSION

Sexual violence, including human trafficking and sexual assault, is a significant public health concern in the United States and globally. It is essential for survivors to understand their rights regarding medical evaluation and treatment. Survivors have the right to seek medical care without the obligation to report the assault to law enforcement, ensuring that their autonomy and choices are respected throughout the process. However, it is important to note that certain professionals may be mandated by law to report incidents of sexual assault, depending on the survivor's age and other factors, which can impact their decision making. It is vital that survivors are informed about the options available to them, including the importance of consent during the examination process and the significance of retaining the right to decide whether to engage with the legal system. Advocacy services can help survivors navigate these choices, providing resources that empower them to make informed decisions about their health and well-being.

Equally important is the recognition that healing and recovery are ongoing processes that require comprehensive support systems. Survivors should be connected to advocacy organizations that offer emotional support, counseling, and resources tailored to their unique needs. Prevention strategies aimed at educating communities about consent and healthy relationships are crucial in reducing the prevalence of sexual assault. Ultimately, fostering an environment that emphasizes respect, consent, and open dialogue about sexual violence is imperative for societal change. By prioritizing survivor-centered care, we can help individuals reclaim their autonomy, promote healing, and build resilience, ultimately contributing to a safer and more supportive community for all.

References

American College of Emergency Physicians. (2013). *Evaluation and management of the sexually assaulted or sexually abused patient* (2nd ed.). https://www.acep.org/globalassets/new-pdfs/sexual-assault-e-book.pdf.

American College of Emergency Physicians. (2023). *Evaluation and management of the sexually assaulted or sexually abused patient* (2nd ed.). https://www.acep.org/forensicmedicine/newsroom/fm-newsroom-articles/sept-20232/eval-and-management-of-SA

American College of Emergency Physicians. (2020). *Management of the patient with the complaint of sexual assault.* https://www.acep.org/patient-care/policy-statements/management-of-the-patient-with-the-complaint-of-sexual-assault/

American College of Obstetricians and Gynecologists (2019). ACOG COMMITTEE OPINION number 777 sexual assault. *Obstetrics and Gynecology, 133*(4), E296–E302. https://doi.org/10.1097/AOG.0000000000003178

American Psychiatric Association. (2022). *Diagnostic and statistical manual of mental disorders* (5th ed., text rev.). https://doi.org/10.1176/appi.books.9780890425787

Anderson, L. J., Flynn, A., & Pilgrim, J. L. (2017). A global epidemiological perspective on the toxicology of drug-facilitated sexual assault: A systematic review. *Journal of Forensic and Legal Medicine, 47,* 46–54. https://doi.org/10.1016/j.jflm.2017.02.005

Baird, K., & Connolly, J. (2023). Recruitment and entrapment pathways of minors into sex trafficking in Canada and the United States: A systematic review. *Trauma, Violence & Abuse, 24*(1), 189–202 https://doi-org.uc.idm.oclc.org/10.1177/15248380211025241

Barrick, K., Sharkey, T. C., Maass, K. L., Song, Y., & Martin, L. (2024). Expanding our understanding of traffickers and their operations: A review of the literature and path forward. *Trauma, Violence & Abuse, 25*(3), 2348–2362. https://doi.org/10.1177/15248380231210937

Basile, K., Smith, S., Kresnow M., Khatiwada S., & Leemis R. (2022). *The National Intimate Partner and Sexual Violence Survey: 2016/2017 Report on Sexual Violence.* National Center for Injury Prevention and Control, Centers for Disease Control and Prevention. https://www.cdc.gov/nisvs/documentation/nisvsReportonSexualViolence.pdf.

Basile, K., DeGue, S., Jones, K., Freire, K., Dills, J., Smith, S., & Raiford, J. (2016). *Sexual violence prevention resource for action: A compilation of the best available evidence.* Division of Violence Prevention National Center for Injury Prevention and Control, Centers for Disease Control and Prevention. https://www.cdc.gov/violence-prevention/media/pdf/resources-for-action/SV-Prevention-Resource_508.pdf

Basile, K. C., Smith, S. G., Breiding, M. J., Black, M. C., & Mahendra, R. R. (2014). *Sexual violence surveillance: Uniform definitions and recommended data elements, version 2.0.* National Center for Injury Prevention and Control, Centers for Disease Control and Prevention. https://stacks.cdc.gov/view/cdc/26326

Basile, K. C., Smith, S. G., Chen, J., & Zwald, M. (2021). Chronic diseases, health conditions, and other impacts associated with rape victimization of U.S. women. *Journal of Interpersonal Violence, 36*(23–24), NP12504–NP12520. https://doi.org/10.1177/0886260519900335

Basile, K. C., Smith, S. G., Liu, Y., Kresnow, M., Fasula, A. M., Gilbert, L., & Chen, J. (2018). Rape-related pregnancy and association with reproductive coercion in the U.S. *American Journal of Preventive Medicine, 55*(6), 770–776. https://doi.org/10.1016/j.amepre.2018.07.028

Braun, B. (2024). Human trafficking awareness in the emergency care setting: Joint position statement. *Journal of Forensic Nursing, 20*(3), E53–E56. https://doi.org/10.1097/JFN.0000000000000504

Breiding, M. J., Basile, K. C., Smith, S. G., Black, M. C., & Mahendra, R. R. (2015). *Intimate partner violence surveillance: Uniform definitions and recommended data elements, version 2.0.* National Center for Injury Prevention and Control, Centers for Disease Control and Prevention. https://stacks.cdc.gov/view/cdc/31292

Brockdorf, A. N., Gratz, K. L., Messman, T. L., & DiLillo, D. (2023). Trauma symptoms and deliberate self-harm among sexual violence survivors: Examining state emotion regulation and reactivity as dual mechanisms. *Psychology of Violence, 13*(1), 23–33. https://doi.org/10.1037/vio0000432

Campbell, R. (2012). *The neurobiology of sexual assault: Implications for law enforcement, prosecution, and victim advocacy* [Transcript]. National Institute of Justice. http://www.nij.gov/multimedia/presenter/presenter-campbell/pages/presenter-campbell-transcript.aspx

Catton, A. K. H., Dorahy, M. J., & Yogeeswaran, K. (2023). Disclosure of sexual victimization: Effects of invalidation and shame on re-disclosure. *Journal of Interpersonal Violence, 38*(13–14), 8332–8356. https://doi.org/10.1177/08862605231155122

Centers for Disease Control and Prevention. (2016). *Updated guidelines for antiretroviral postexposure prophylaxis after sexual, injection drug use, or other nonoccupational exposure to HIV—United States, 2016* (updated 2018). https://stacks.cdc.gov/view/cdc/38856

Centers for Disease Control and Prevention. (2019). *Sex trafficking.* https://www.cdc.gov/violenceprevention/sexualviolence/trafficking.html

Centers for Disease Control and Prevention. (2021). *Sexually transmitted infections treatment guidelines 2021: Sexual assault and abuse and STIs—Adolescents and Adults.* July 22, 2021. https://www.cdc.gov/std/treatment-guidelines/sexual-assault-adults.htm

Chambers, R., Gibson, M., Chaffin, S., Takagi, T., Nguyen, N., & Mears-Clark, T. (2024). Trauma-coerced attachment and complex PTSD: Informed care for survivors of human trafficking. *Journal of Human Trafficking, 10*(1), 41–50. https://doi.org/10.1080/23322705.2021.2012386

Child Abuse Prevention and Treatment Act of 1988, 42 U.S.C. § 5101 (1988).

Costa, C. B., McCoy, K. T., Early, G. J., & Deckers, C. M. (2019). Evidence-based care of the human trafficking patient. *Nursing Clinics of North America, 54*(4), 569–584. https://doi.org/10.1016/j.cnur.2019.08.007

Counter-Trafficking Data Collaborative. (2024). *Family members are involved in nearly half of child trafficking cases.* https://www.iom.int/sites/g/files/tmzbdl486/files/our_work/DMM/MAD/Counter-trafficking%20Data%20Brief%20081217.pdf

Cuevas, K. M., Balbo, J., Duval, K., & Beverly, E. A. (2018). Neurobiology of sexual assault and osteopathic considerations for trauma-informed care and practice. *Journal of Osteopathic Medicine, 118*(2), e2–e10. https://doi.org/10.7556/jaoa.2018.018

Dignity Health. (2019). *Human trafficking response program: Shared learnings manual.* https://www.dignityhealth.org/content/dam/dignity-health/pdfs/human-trafficking/dignity-health-htrp-sharedlearningsmanual-170512.pdf

Dowdell, E. B., & Speck, P. M. (2022). CE: Trauma-informed care in nursing practice. *AJN The American Journal of Nursing, 122*(4), 30–38.

Dworkin, E. R. (2020). Risk for mental disorders associated with sexual assault: A meta-analysis. *Trauma, Violence & Abuse, 21*(5), 1011–1028.

Dworkin, E. R., Menon, S. V., Bystrynski, J., & Allen, N. E. (2017). Sexual assault victimization and psychopathology: A review and meta-analysis. *Clinical Psychology Review, 56,* 65–81. https://doi.org/10.1016/j.cpr.2017.06.002

FORGE. (2024). *FORGE SAFE protocol: Trans-specific annotation* (2nd ed.). FORGE. https://evawintl.org/wp-content/uploads/SANE-protocol-trans-inclusive

Gaitis, K. K. (2022). Addressing the trauma of human trafficking victims in the UK. *Insights: A Series of Evidence Summaries,* 18. https://www.iriss. org. uk/resources/insights/addressing-trauma-human-trafficking-victims-uk

Goldblatt, H., Band-Winterstein, T., Lev, S., & Harel, D. (2022). "Who would sexually assault an 80-year-old woman?": Barriers to exploring and exposing sexual assault against women in late life. *Journal of Interpersonal Violence, 37*(5–6), 2751–2775. https://doi.org/10.1177/0886260520934440

Gong, A. T., Kamboj, S. K., & Curran, H. V. (2019). Post-traumatic stress disorder in victims of sexual assault with pre-assault substance consumption: A systematic review. *Frontiers in Psychiatry, 10,* 92. https://doi.org/10.3389/fpsyt.2019.00092

Greenbaum, J. (2021). Child labor and sex trafficking. *Pediatrics in Review, 42*(12), 639–654. https://doi.org/10.1542/pir.2020-001396

Greenbaum, J., Kaplan, D., Young, J., Council on Child Abuse and Neglect, Haney, S. B., Sirotnak, A. P., Asnes, A. G., Gavril, A. R., Gilmartin, A. B. H., Girardet, R. G., Heavilin, N. D., Laskey, A., Messner, S. A., Mohr, B. A., Nienow, S. M., Rosado, N., Forkey, H., Keefe, R., Keeshin, B., . . . Young, J. (2023). Exploitation, labor and sex trafficking of children and adolescents: Health care needs of patients. *Pediatrics, 151*(1), e2022060416. https://doi.org/10.1542/peds.2022-060416

Greenbaum, J., Sprang, G., Recknor, F., Harper, N. S., & Titchen, K. (2022). Labor trafficking of children and youth in the United States: A scoping review. *Child Abuse & Neglect, 131,* 105694. https://doi.org/10.1016/j.chiabu.2022.105694

Hachey, L. M., & Phillippi, J. C. (2017). Identification and management of human trafficking victims in the emergency department. *Advanced Emergency Nursing Journal, 39*(1), 31–51. https://doi.org/10.1097/TME.0000000000000138

Hassam, T., Kelso, E., Chowdary, P., Yisma, E., Mol, B. W., & Han, A. (2020). Sexual assault as a risk factor for gynaecological morbidity: An exploratory systematic review and meta-analysis. *European Journal of Obstetrics & Gynecology and Reproductive Biology, 255,* 222–230. https://doi.org/10.1016/j.ejogrb.2020.10.038

Hopkins, C., & Kennedy, E. (2024). Caring for survivors of sexual violence in primary care. *Women's Healthcare, 12*(1), 25–30. https://doi.org/10.51256/WHC022424

Hornor, G., Hollar, J., Landers, T., & Sherfield, J. (2023). Healthcare use and case characteristics of commercial sexual exploitation of children: Teen victims versus high-risk teens. *Journal of Forensic Nursing, 19*(3), 160–169. https://doi.org/10.1097/JFN.0000000000000402

IAFN reference for reference list – International Association of Forensic Nurses. (2022). *The use of emergency contraception after sexual assault.* https://www.forensicnurses.org/wp-content/uploads/2022/11/Final-2022-EC-Position-for-web.pdf

Jain, J., Bennett, M., Bailey, M. D., Liaou, D., Kaltiso, S.-A. O., Greenbaum, J., Williams, K., Gordon, M. R., Torres, M. I. M., Nguyen, P. T., Coverdale, J. H., Williams, V., Hari, C., Rodriguez, S., Salami, T., & Potter, J. E. (2022). Creating a collaborative trauma-informed interdisciplinary citywide victim services model focused on health care for survivors of human trafficking. *Public Health Reports, 137*(1_suppl), 30S–37S. https://doi.org/10.1177/00333549211059833

Justice for Victims of Trafficking Act of 2015, 34 U.S.C. § 20144 (2015).

Klein, L. B., Melnik, J., Curran, K., Luebke, J., Moore, K. M., Ruiz, A. M., Brown, C., Parker, D., Hernandez-White, I., & Walsh, K. (2024). Trauma- and violence-informed empowering care for sexual assault survivors. *Journal of Forensic Nursing, 20*(3), 166–173. https://doi.org/10.1097/JFN.0000000000000483

Laricchiuta, D., Panuccio, A., Picerni, E., Biondo, D., Genovesi, B., & Petrosini, L. (2023). The body keeps the score: The neurobiological profile of traumatized adolescents. *Neuroscience & Biobehavioral Reviews, 145,* 105033. https://doi.org/10.1016/j.neubiorev.2023.105033

Lawrence, M., & Bauer, P. (2020). Knowledge Base of nurses before and after a human trafficking continuing education course. *The Journal of Continuing Education in Nursing, 51*(7), 316–321. https://doi.org/10.3928/00220124-20200611-07

Littleton, H., Wright, L., Dodd, J. C., & Higgins, M. (2023). Gynecological health complaints among college women with sexual victimization histories: Examination of depression and anxiety as potential mediators. *Women's Health Issues, 33*(1), 105–112. https://doi.org/10.1016/j.whi.2022.06.001

McCormack, D., Subburamu, S., Guzman, G., Calderon, C., Darapaneni, R., Lis, R., Sima, N., Sperling, J., & Corbo, J. (2022). Traumatic injuries in sexual assault patients in the emergency department. *The Western Journal of Emergency Medicine, 23*(5), 672–677. https://doi.org/10.5811/westjem.2022.1.53994

McFarlane, J., Greenberg, L., Weltge, A., & Watson, M. (1995). Identification of abuse in emergency departments: Effectiveness of a two-question screening tool. *Journal of Emergency Nursing, 21*(5), 391–394. https://doi.org/10.1016/s0099-1767(05)80103-5

Munson, M. (2020). *Care, compassion and creativity: Trans survivors and forensic exams* [Webinar]. FORGE. https://forge-forward.org/event/forensic-exams-webinar-dec2020/

National Human Trafficking Training and Technical Assistance Center. (2018). *Adult human trafficking screening tool and guide.* Administration for Children and Families. https://nhttac.acf.hhs.gov/sites/default/files/2018-07/adult_human_trafficking_screening_tool_and_guide.pdfredflags

O'Callaghan, E., & Ullman, S. E. (2024). Are all substance-involved sexual assaults alike? A comparison of victim alcohol use, drug use, and combined substance use in sexual assaults. *Women & Criminal Justice, 34*(2), 88–106. https://doi.org/10.1080/08974454.2021.1914284

Oke, M.-J. (2024). Improving the forensic genital examination for trans and gender diverse sexual assault complainants: Three case reports. *International Journal of Legal Medicine, 138*(3), 899–909. https://doi.org/10.1007/s00414-023-03135-6

Patel, P., Borkowf, C. B., Brooks, J. T., Lasry, A., Lansky, A., & Mermin, J. (2014). Estimating per-act HIV transmission risk: A systematic review. *AIDS, 28*(10), 1509–1519. https://doi.org/10.1097/QAD.0000000000000298

Polaris. (2023). *National human trafficking hotline statistics.* https://polarisproject.org/wp-content/uploads/2020/07/Hotline-Trends-Report-2023.pdf

Polaris (2025). *The typology of human trafficking: Defining sex and labor trafficking in the United States.* https://polarisproject.org/the-typology-of-modern-slavery/

Porat, R., Gantman, A., Green, S. A., Pezzuto, J.-H., & Paluck, E. L. (2024). Preventing sexual violence: A behavioral problem without a behaviorally informed solution. *Psychological Science in the Public Interest, 25*(1), 4–29. https://doi.org/10.1177/15291006231221978

Rape, Abuse & Incest National Network (RAINN). (n.d.). *Elderly.* https://rainn.org/articles/elder-abuse

Rapoza, S. (2022). Sex trafficking: A literature review with implications for health care providers. *Advanced Emergency Nursing Journal, 44*(3), 248–261. https://doi.org/10.1097/TME.0000000000000419

Richie-Zavaleta, A. C., Villanueva, A. M., Homicile, L. M., & Urada, L. A. (2021). *Compassionate Care—Going the Extra Mile*: Sex trafficking survivors' recommendations for healthcare best practices. *Sexes, 2*(1), 26–49. https://doi.org/10.3390/sexes2010003

Richter, L. A., Fields, L., Bell, S., Heppner, J., Dodge, J., Boccellari, A., & Shumway, M. (2017). Characterizing drug-facilitated sexual assault subtypes and treatment engagement of victims at a hospital-based rape treatment center. *Journal of Interpersonal Violence, 32*(10), 1524–1542. https://doi.org/10.1177/0886260515589567

Roe-Sepowitz, D., Bracy, K., Gibbs, H., Stafford, R. L., Bernardin, B., & Stoklosa, H. (2024). PEARR tool training and implementation: Building awareness of violence and human trafficking in a hospital system. *Frontiers in Medicine, 11,* 1311584. https://doi.org/10.3389/fmed.2024.1311584

Ruiz-Gonzalez, C., Roman, P., Benayas-Perez, N., Rodriguez-Arrastia, M., Ropero-Padilla, C., Ruiz-Gonzalez, D., & Sanchez-Labraca, N. (2022). Midwives' experiences and perceptions in treating victims of sex trafficking: A qualitative study. *Journal of Advanced Nursing, 69, 78*(7), 2139–2149. https://doi.org/10.1111/jan.15165

Salcedo, J., Cleland, K., Bartz, D., & Thompson, I. (2023). Society of family planning clinical recommendation: Emergency contraception. *Contraception (Stoneham), 121,* 109958–109958. https://doi.org/10.1016/j.contraception.2023.109958

Society of Forensic Toxicologists. (n.d.). *Drug-facilitated sexual assault fact sheet.* (last visited November 2, 2024) https://www.soft-tox.org/assets/docs/DFSA_Fact_Sheet.pdf

Stewart, S., Willmott, D., Murphy, A., & Phillips, C. (2024). "I thought I'm better off just trying to put this behind me"—A contemporary approach to understanding why women decide not to report sexual violence. *The Journal of Forensic Psychiatry & Psychology, 35*(1), 85–101. https://doi.org/10.1080/14789949.2023.2292103

Stoklosa, H., Grace, A.M., & Littenberg, N. (2015). Medical education on human trafficking. *AMA Journal of Ethics, 17*(10), 914–921. https://doi.org/10.1001/journalofethics.2015.17.10.medu1-1510

Substance Abuse and Mental Health Services Administration. (2014). *SAMHSA's concept of trauma and guidance for a trauma-informed approach.* https://store.samhsa.gov/product/samhsas-concept-trauma-and-guidance-trauma-informed-approach/sma14-4884

Substance Abuse and Mental Health Services Administration. (2023). *Practical guide for implementing a trauma-informed approach.* SAMHSA. https://store.samhsa.gov/product/practical-guide-implementing-trauma-informed approach/pep23-06-05-005

Trafficking Victims Protection Act of 2000, Pub. L. No. 106-386, as amended through Pub. L. No. 118-42 (Mar. 9, 2024), 22 U.S.C. ch. 78. U.S. Government Publishing Office. https://www.govinfo.gov/app/details/COMPS-10421

Trafficking Victims Protection Reauthorization Act of 2003, Pub. L. No. 108-193, 117 Stat. 2875 (2003).

Trafficking Victims Protection Reauthorization Act of 2005, Pub. L. No. 109-164, 119 Stat. 3558 (2006).

Trafficking Victims Protection Reauthorization Act of 2008, Pub. L. No. 110-457, 122 Stat. 5044 (2008).

Trafficking Victims Protection Reauthorization Act of 2013, Pub. L. No. 113-4, 127 Stat. 54 (2013).

Trafficking Victims Protection Reauthorization Act of 2017, Pub. L. No. 115-393, 132 Stat. 5265 (2018).

Trafficking Victims Protection Reauthorization Act of 2018, Pub. L. No. 115-425, 132 Stat. 5472 (2019).

United Nations. (2000). *Protocol to prevent, suppress and punish trafficking in persons, especially women and children, supplementing the United Nations Convention against Transnational Organized Crime.* https://www.unodc.org/res/human-trafficking/2021protocol-tip_en.pdf

United Nations Office on Drugs and Crime. (2006). *Trafficking in persons: Global patterns* (pp. 50–51). United Nations.

United Nations Office on Drugs and Crime. (2008). *Toolkit to combat trafficking in persons* (pp. 12–13). United Nations.

U.S. Citizenship and Immigration Services. (2024). *Victims of criminal activity: U nonimmigrant status.* https://www.uscis.gov/humanitarian/victims-of-criminal-activity-u-nonimmigrant-status

U.S. Congress. (1994). Violence Against Women Act of 1994, Pub. L. No. 103–322, 108 Stat. 1902. Reauthorized 2022, Pub. L. No. 117–103.

U.S. Department of Justice. (2013, revised 2016). *Female victims of sexual violence, 1994–2010* [Special report]. http://www.bjs.gov/content/pub/pdf/fvsv9410.pdf

U.S. Department of Justice. (2017). *National best practices for sexual assault kits: A multidisciplinary approach.* https://www.ncjrs.gov/pdffiles1/nij/250384.pdf

U.S. Department of Justice. (2018). *Criminal victimization, 2017.* https://www.bjs.gov/content/pub/pdf/cv17.pdf

U.S. Department of Justice, Drug Enforcement Administration (2021a). *Drug-facilitated sexual assault.* https://www.dea.gov/sites/default/files/2018-07/DFSA_0.PDF

U.S. Department of Justice. (2021b). *Crime against persons with disabilities, 2009–2019—statistical tables.* https://bjs.ojp.gov/content/pub/pdf/capd0919st.pdf

U.S Department of Justice (2024). *Criminal victimization, 2023.* (NCJ 309335). https://bjs.ojp.gov/document/cv23.pdf

U.S. Department of Justice. Office on Violence Against Women. (2024). *A national protocol for sexual assault medical forensic examinations: Adults/adolescents* (3rd ed.). https://www.justice.gov/ovw/media/1367191/dl?inline

U.S. Department of State. (2024). *Trafficking in persons report: Office to Monitor and Combat Trafficking in Persons.* https://www.state.gov/reports/2024-trafficking-in-persons-report/

Victims of Trafficking and Violence Protection Act of 2000, Pub. L. No. 106-386, 114 Stat. 1464 (2000). https://www.govinfo.gov/content/pkg/PLAW-106publ386/pdf/PLAW-106publ386.pdf

Walk Free (2023). *Global slavery index.* (p. 173). Minderoo Foundation. https://cdn.walkfree.org/content/uploads/2023/05/17114737/Global-Slavery-Index-2023.pdf

Walk Free Foundation & International Organization for Migration (Eds.). (2022). *Global estimates of modern slavery: Forced labour and forced marriage*. International Labour Office.

Wood, L. C. N. (2020). Child modern slavery, trafficking and health: A practical review of factors contributing to children's vulnerability and the potential impacts of severe exploitation on health. *BMJ Paediatrics Open, 4*(1), e000327. https://doi.org/10.1136/bmjpo-2018-000327

Yang, S. B., Choi, S. S., Chang, H. Y., Kim, D., Lee, Y., & Lim, M. H. (2023). Central symptoms of post-traumatic stress disorder on adult victims of sexual violence: A network analysis. *Medicine, 102*(27), e34083. https://doi.org/10.1097/MD.0000000000034083

Yates, C., & Pappier, J. (2023, September 20). *How the treacherous Darien Gap became a migration crossroads of the Americas*. Migration Policy Institute. https://www.migrationpolicy.org/article/darien-gap-migration-crossroads-americas

Young-Wolff, K. C., Sarovar, V., Klebaner, D., Chi, F., & McCaw, B. (2018). Changes in psychiatric and medical conditions and health care utilization following a diagnosis of sexual assault: A retrospective cohort study. *Medical Care, 56*(8), 649–657.

APPENDIX 16-A

Clinician Resources

American College of Emergency Physicians (ACEP)
4950 W. Royal Lane
Irving, TX 75063-2524
1- 888-817-2237 (Phone or Text)
1-800-798-1822
1-972-580-2816 (Fax)
http://www.acep.org

AEquitas: The Prosecutors' Resource on Violence Against Women
High-quality guidance on sexual assault, trafficking, trauma-informed approaches, and legal considerations.
https://aequitasresource.org

Centers for Disease Control and Prevention (CDC)
1600 Clifton Rd. NE
Atlanta, GA 30333
1-800-CDC-INFO
http://www.cdc.gov
2021 Sexually Transmitted Infections Treatment Guidelines: https://www.cdc.gov/std/treatment-guidelines/default.htm

Division of Violence Prevention
National Center for Injury Prevention and Control
Centers for Disease Control and Prevention
Atlanta, Georgia
https://www.cdc.gov/violence-prevention/media/pdf/resources-for-action/SV-Prevention-Resource_508.pdf

End Violence Against Women International (EVAWI)
Training, best practices, and online modules tailored for multi-disciplinary professionals.
https://evawintl.org

FORGE
P.O. Box 1272
Milwaukee, WI 53201
(414) 559-2123
https://forge-forward.org/

HEAL Trafficking:
www.healtrafficking.org

International Association of Forensic Nurses (IAFN)
6755 Business Pkwy., Suite 303
Elkridge, MD 21075
1-410-626-7805
http://www.iafn.org

National Alliance to End Sexual Violence (NAESV)
655 15th Street NW, Suite 800
Washington, DC 20005
http://endsexualviolence.org

National Human Trafficking Resource Center and Hotline
(1-888-3737-888)
https://humantraffickinghotline.org

National Sexual Violence Resource Center (NSVRC)
2101 N Front Street, Governor's Plaza North, Building #2
Harrisburg, PA 17110
717-909-0715 (TTY)
1-877-739-3895
http://www.nsvrc.org

Polaris Project Website and Resource Center
Online Reporting, Education, and Resources
www.polarisproject.org

Office on Violence Against Women
U.S. Department of Justice
145 N Street NE
Washington, DC 20530
1-202-307-6026
https://www.justice.gov/ovw

Training Institute on Strangulation Prevention
A Program of Alliance for HOPE International
501 W. Broadway, Suite A #625
San Diego, CA 92101
1-888-511-3522
https://www.strangulationtraininginstitute.com/

RAINN
1220 L ST NW Suite 500
Washington, DC 20005
1-800-656-HOPE
http://www.rainn.org

APPENDIX 16-B

Signs and Symptoms of Strangulation

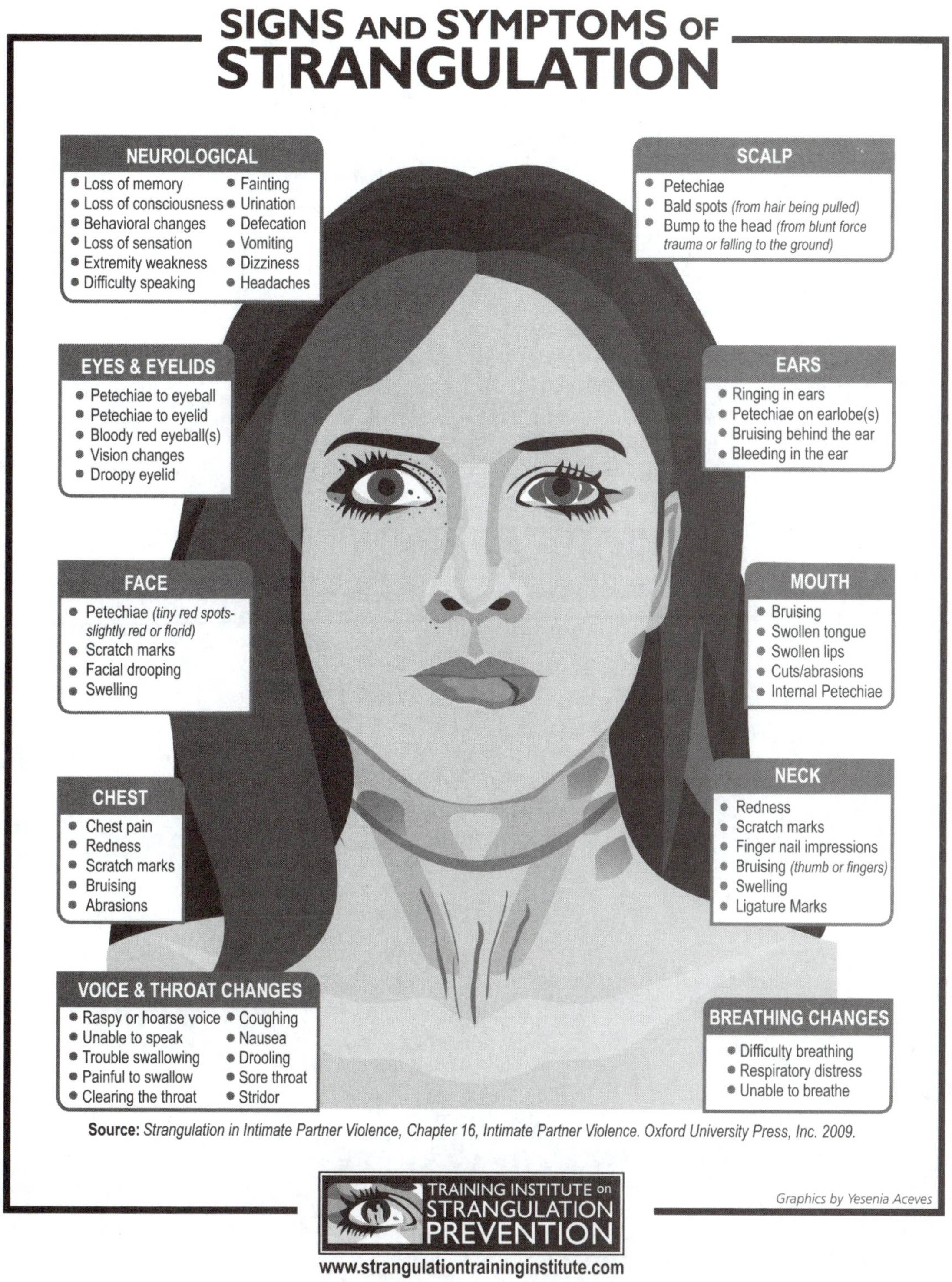

Reproduced from Training Institute on Strangulation Prevention. (2017). *Signs and symptoms of strangulation*. https://www.strangulationtraining institute.com/ Reprinted with permission of Phoebe S. Brown.

APPENDIX 16-C

Body Diagram

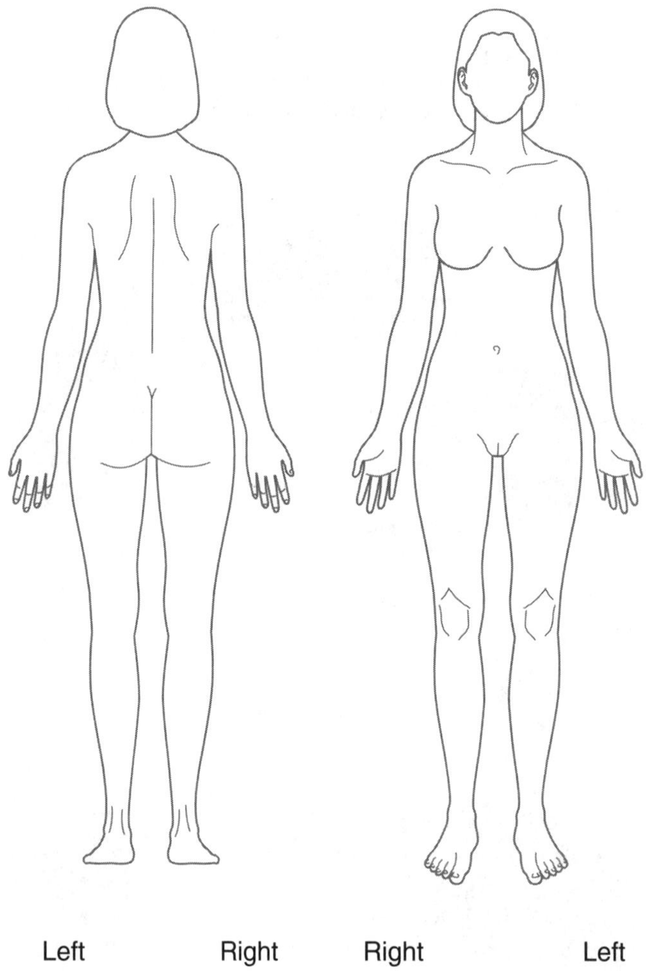

SECTION

3

Gynecologic Healthcare Management

CHAPTER 17

Breast Conditions

Bethany D. Sanders

The editors would like to acknowledge Kathryn J. Trotter, who was the author on a previous edition of this chapter.

For centuries, human breasts have garnered attention as a symbol of ideal beauty, a representation of one's gender identity, and a form of sustenance through lactation. Breasts have even been used as the model for champagne glasses (Epstein, 2025) yet at the same time, their exposure in some public spaces has been criminalized as "indecent" (Harbke & Lindemann, 2023). Depending upon the sociocultural context of the individual, breasts may be considered utilitarian, sexual, a burden, a source of fear, and may be subject to surgical alteration. As with most human features, breasts have basic similarities but unique variants, including different sizes, shapes, and asymmetries. Like any organ, the mammary gland deserves particular attention to symptomology, even if benign, and due diligence is required to verify any abnormalities or needed treatment. The clinician should be respectful, deliberate, and conscientious in the history, examination, and plan of care for breast concerns.

The presence of symptoms in the breasts that may be associated with pathology causes understandable concern for people. An individual may have an underlying fear, which may not be articulated or even conscious, that they have breast cancer. The meaning of their breasts to an individual will greatly influence how they react to having a breast condition. Providing adequate emotional support when a person presents with a breast condition is as important as ensuring accurate assessment, diagnosis, and management of the condition. The breast conditions that are the focus of this chapter are mastalgia, nipple discharge, benign breast masses, and breast cancer. Online resources for caring for individuals with breast conditions can be found in **Appendix 17-A**.

This chapter uses the term "breast" to refer to the mammary glands located over the pectoral muscles, and it uses the term "chest" to refer to the part of the body between the neck and the abdomen. The use of "breast" in this chapter is for clarity regarding the specific anatomy being discussed and is not meant to exclude people who do not use this term for their bodies.

MASTALGIA

Mastalgia, also called mastodynia or breast pain, is reported by approximately half of individuals presenting with breast concerns in the outpatient setting (Bui et al., 2024). The incidence of breast cancer in individuals presenting with breast pain is reported between 0–2.3 percent in radiological studies, although breast pain can be a significant source of anxiety (Holbrook, 2020). Mastalgia is classified as cyclic or noncyclic, depending on whether its presence is related to the menstrual cycle. Two-thirds of breast pain is cyclic (Li et al., 2021; Pleasant, 2022). Approximately 70 percent of individuals experience cyclic mastalgia, and breast pain may interfere with social, physical, and sexual activities (Fakhravar et al., 2021). Noncyclic mastalgia is less common, with approximately one-third of individuals reporting this symptom (Pleasant, 2022).

Etiology and Pathophysiology

Mild cyclic mastalgia is considered a normal physiologic condition caused by the hormonal changes of the menstrual cycle (Li et al., 2021). It is clearly linked to the reproductive cycle, with onset at menarche, monthly cycling, and cessation at menopause. Median age of individuals with cyclic mastalgia was reported to be 42 years old in one study (Arslan et al., 2016). Cyclic mastalgia occurs during the luteal phase of the menstrual cycle and lasts less than 5 days (Karimian et al., 2022). While the exact mechanism of cyclic mastalgia is not well understood, the effects of estrogen on stimulation of ductal cells, progesterone on stimulation of stromal cells, and prolactin on stimulation of ductal secretion of breast tissue are plausible contributors to cyclic mastalgia.

Mastalgia can also be caused by certain medications, including combined estrogen and progestin contraceptives (i.e., pills, NuvaRing, and OrthoEvra patch), estrogen-containing hormone therapy, selective serotonin reuptake inhibitors (SSRIs), haloperidol, amitriptyline, digoxin, methyldopa, cimetidine, spironolactone, oxymetholone, chlorpromazine, ketoconazole, and metronidazole (Sivarajah et al., 2020). In addition, mild mastalgia has been reported by less than 10 percent of individuals using a levonorgestrel intrauterine device (Teal et al., 2019).

Mastalgia is associated with a number of other conditions, including anxiety, depression, fatigue, panic disorder, eating disorders, posttraumatic stress disorder, alcohol use disorder, history of interpersonal violence, and irritable bowel syndrome (Sivarajah et al., 2020). Pain disorders such as fibromyalgia and chronic pelvic pain are frequent comorbidities with mastalgia (Sivarajah et al., 2020). Premenstrual syndrome (PMS) and premenstrual dysphoric disorders (PMDD) are conditions that, like cyclic mastalgia, occur during the luteal phase of the menstrual cycle. While mastalgia can occur as a symptom of PMS or PMDD, it is distinct in that there is not an emotional or affective component. The improvement in mastalgia that some individuals experience with SSRIs or hormonal contraceptives may be related to alleviation of the underlying neuroendocrine imbalance or hormone fluctuations triggering PMS or PMDD (Nappi et al., 2022).

Fibrocystic breast changes are common among people with mastalgia, although not all individuals with fibrocystic breast changes experience pain, and not all individuals with mastalgia have fibrocystic breast changes (Callé et al., 2023). Fibrocystic breast changes were originally called fibrocystic breast disease, but the associated constellation of symptoms has become increasingly recognized as common to many individuals; thus, these symptoms are no longer considered to constitute a disease. Such changes include tender, nodular, and swollen breast tissue.

Clinical Presentation

Three classifications are commonly used to distinguish the various types of breast pain: cyclic mastalgia, noncyclic mastalgia, and chest wall pain.

Cyclic mastalgia typically begins in the luteal phase of the menstrual cycle and subsides with menses. This pain is usually bilateral. It can be poorly localized but is most frequently associated with the outer quadrants, and it is described as soreness or aching. Individuals with large breasts, called macromastia, may be more likely to report breast pain than those without macromastia (Sivarajah et al., 2020).

In contrast, noncyclic mastalgia may be constant or intermittent and is unrelated to the menstrual cycle. Its incidence peaks at ages 40–50 (Bui et al., 2024). Noncyclic mastalgia is more likely to cause localized pain that is sharp or burning in nature. The left breast and right breast are equally likely to be affected when unilateral breast pain is reported (Ali & Faraj, 2023). Individuals with large, pendulous breasts may report shoulder grooving, neck pain, and back pain in addition to breast pain.

Chest wall pain is usually quite localized, becomes worse with movement, and is described as sharp or burning (Li et al., 2021). Extramammary causes of mastalgia are the least common type of mastalgia, affecting less than 5 percent of individuals in one clinical study (Ali & Faraj, 2023).

Assessment

History

The clinician must determine whether the mastalgia is cyclic or noncyclic, diffuse or focal, and must eliminate nonbreast causes of the discomfort, such as chest wall pain. When taking the history, ask the person about the timing (especially in relation to the menstrual cycle), frequency, location, nature, severity, and mitigating factors of the pain and its effects on their functioning. The use of an instrument, such as a visual analog scale or the Cardiff breast pain chart to rate pain may be helpful in evaluating mastalgia and monitoring the response to treatment (refer to **Figure 17-1**). Prospective evaluation of pain with a daily diary can be useful in differentiating cyclic and noncyclic mastalgia. In addition, the clinician should ask the individual about other breast symptoms, such as nipple discharge or breast mass, and whether there is a previous history of any type of breast disease or surgery.

Menstrual, pregnancy, lactation, and general medical histories are all necessary as part of a comprehensive assessment for mastalgia. Note current medications, including exogenous hormones. Although caffeine has not been definitively established as a causal factor, ask about the amount of caffeine intake in case a pattern exists. Caffeine contains the chemical methylxanthine, which causes dilation of blood vessels and overstimulation of breast cells and could theoretically result in mastalgia. However, the role of caffeine reduction in treatment of mastalgia is not supported by the literature (Bui et al., 2024).

Also obtain a family history, particularly regarding breast and ovarian cancer. A complete review of systems is helpful in eliminating nonbreast causes (refer to the discussion of differential diagnoses).

Physical Examination

Perform a comprehensive breast examination, including inspection and palpation of the breasts with the unclothed person in both the upright and supine positions, and evaluate the lymph nodes (refer to Chapter 8 for more details on conducting a physical exam). Assess for skin changes, nipple discharge, and breast masses. If the pain can be reproduced with examination, note its location. The chest wall structures should also be examined for nonbreast causes of pain.

FIGURE 17-1 The Cardiff breast pain chart.

This chart is to help you and your provider to see when your breast pain occurs. Record the amount of breast pain you experience each day by filling in the box as shown. For example, if you have severe breast pain on the fifth day of the month completely shade in the box under 5. For premenopausal individuals, note the first day that you start your period each month by writing the letter P in the box that corresponds to the date.

- severe pain • moderate pain • no pain

Month			1	2	3	4	5	6	7	8	9	10	11	12	13	14
15	16	17	18	19	20	21	22	23	24	25	26	27	28	29	30	31

Reproduced from Breast Cancer Now. Breast pain. https://breastcancernow.org/download-and-order-publications/breast-pain-bcc71

TABLE 17-1 Diagnostic Imaging Tests

Test	Source of Images	Best for Detecting	Limitations of Test
Mammogram	Radiographs (provide 2-D mammographic images)	Calcifications, masses, and architectural distortion	Cannot show if mass is solid or cystic; has lower sensitivity in individuals with dense breast tissue
Ultrasound	Sound waves	Differentiation of solid and cystic masses	Usually cannot show calcifications, not appropriate for screening
MRI	Magnetic fields, must be enhanced with gadolinium contrast	Tissue with increased blood flow, such as tumors; high sensitivity and negative predictive value	Expensive, limited to specific indications; high rate of false positive results (lack of specificity); specific protocols for implants
Tomosynthesis	Radiographs (provide 3-D digital images); use in conjunction with 2-D mammographic images	Architectural distortion, masses, and calcifications; increased cancer detection rates compared to conventional 2-D mammography	Slight increase in radiation exposure, compared with conventional mammogram (but often decreases repeat imaging, thus minimal glandular exposure)

Data from Bhushan, A., Gonsalves, A., & Menon, J. U. (2021). Current state of breast cancer diagnosis, treatment, and theranostics. *Pharmaceutics, 13*(5), 723; Bevers, T. B., Niell, B. L., Baker, J. L., Bennett, D. L., Bonaccio, E., Camp, M. S., Chikarmane, S., Conant, E. F., Eghtedari, M., Flanagan, M. R., Hawley, J., Helvie, M., Hodgkiss, L., Hoyt, T. L., Ivanovich, J., Jochelson, M. S., Kulkarni, S., Lancaster, R. B., Mauer, C., Maxwell, J., ... Stehman, K. (2023). NCCN Guidelines® Insights: Breast cancer screening and diagnosis, version 1.2023: featured updates to the NCCN guidelines. *Journal of the National Comprehensive Cancer Network: JNCCN, 21*(9), 900–909. https://doi.org/10.6004/jnccn.2023.0046.

Diagnostic Testing

Pregnancy testing should be performed, if indicated by the person's history, because tender breasts can be a sign of pregnancy. Diagnostic imaging is frequently used in the evaluation of breast conditions; however, it may not be necessary in cases of bilateral cyclical breast pain and may contribute to overuse of healthcare resources without increased detection of breast cancer (Bui et al., 2024). Information about imaging tests is provided in **Table 17-1**. If indicated by physical exam, a diagnostic mammogram with ultrasound can be performed for individuals older than 30 years; a targeted ultrasound alone is recommended for individuals younger than 30 years who have focal pain. For mastalgia without associated rash, mass, or nipple discharge, such diagnostic imaging is helpful only to rule out the unlikely diagnosis of cancer because there are no radiologic findings associated with diffuse mastalgia (Bui et al., 2024). However, with focal breast pain, radiologic tests may identify cysts or masses that correlate. The American College of Radiology regularly publishes evidence-based guidelines for appropriateness of breast imaging modalities for mastalgia (Holbrook et al., 2018). If a breast mass is discovered during the evaluation of mastalgia, it needs to be evaluated appropriately, as described later in this chapter.

Differential Diagnoses

Breast pain can originate from the breast with conditions such as pregnancy, mastitis, cysts, and abscess. Extramammary or nonbreast causes of pain are also important differential diagnoses. If the pain is reproducible with palpation of the chest wall, costochondritis or Tietze syndrome should be suspected (Pleasant, 2022). Costochondritis is characterized by inflammation of the costochondral or chondrosternal joints; the second through fifth costochondral junctions are most likely to be affected. Tietze syndrome is differentiated from costochondritis by the presence of swelling with or without erythema. Nonsteroidal anti-inflammatory drugs (NSAIDs) can be helpful in relieving the symptoms of both conditions. Individuals who bind their chest/breasts may experience mastalgia due to tissue compression (Sivarajah et al., 2020). In addition, breast pain may occur following injection of substances into the breast tissue for augmentation or following mastectomy (Sivarajah et al., 2020). Other potential etiologies of breast pain include medications (see the section on etiology), arthritis, mastitis, blunt trauma, pleuritis, cervical spondylitis, herpes zoster, cholecystitis, and myocardial ischemia (Bui et al., 2024).

Mastalgia is rarely the principal sign of a developing breast cancer, but the possibility of cancer increases when breast pain occurs postmenopausally in the absence of hormone therapy or is accompanied by skin changes or a palpable abnormality (Holbrook et al., 2019). Mastalgia related to breast cancer usually occurs in only one area of one breast and does not follow a cyclic pattern.

Management

After a clinician has ruled out malignancy and extramammary causes of mastalgia, attention turns to reassuring the individual that they do not have a serious illness and relieving their symptoms. In many cases, reassurance about benign breast findings will improve or relieve symptoms of mastalgia (Bui et al., 2024). In those with cyclical mastalgia, 20–30 percent will have spontaneous resolution within 3 months, compared to 50 percent in those with noncyclical mastalgia (Sivarajah et al., 2020). Nonpharmacologic, complementary, and alternative therapies may be successful in the treatment of mastalgia despite limited research to support their efficacy. Severe breast pain can be chronic and relapsing, and it may require pharmacologic treatment.

Nonpharmacologic Therapies

Reassurance is the first-line treatment for mastalgia and has been found to be effective for as many as 85 percent of individuals, with more success in those with mild or moderate symptoms than in those with severe mastalgia (Hafiz et al., 2018). Wearing a supportive and well-fitting bra is frequently recommended, especially for individuals with large, heavy breasts (Hafiz et al., 2018). One small study showed that a 6-week exercise regimen three times per week improved breast pain (Genc et al., 2017). Reductions in caffeine and dietary fat have shown limited effectiveness in diminishing breast pain; however, neither of these dietary recommendations is likely to be harmful. There is limited evidence that acupuncture at HT7 can be helpful (Shi et al., 2024). Despite a lack of data to support these treatment modalities, there is little risk of harm associated with massage therapy or yoga for alleviation of breast pain.

Pharmacologic Therapies

Reducing the dose or modifying the route of hormone therapy may be helpful in reducing breast pain in postmenopausal individuals. In individuals with mastalgia using hormonal contraception, trying a different contraceptive method or delivery system, such as changing from combined oral contraceptives to a nonoral combined method (i.e., NuvaRing or OrthoEvra patch), may sometimes prove helpful in reducing pain. Conversely, some individuals report an improvement in mastalgia with use of hormonal contraception, particularly combination oral contraception. The use of progesterone, either oral or topical, has not been found effective for treatment of mastalgia (Goyal & Mansel, 2016).

First-line pharmacologic therapy for breast pain is usually a topical nonsteroidal anti-inflammatory (NSAID). In particular, multiple studies have demonstrated the benefit of topical diclofenac sodium compared to placebos (Goyal & Mansel, 2016). Adverse effects with the use of topical NSAIDs can include elevated liver enzymes and photosensitivity. Limited evidence is available, however, to support the use of oral NSAIDs for improvement of mastalgia (Li et al., 2021).

Danazol, tamoxifen, and bromocriptine are additional pharmacologic therapies for mastalgia. However, all are associated with adverse side effects. Danazol is an antigonadotropin which suppresses luteinizing hormone and follicle-stimulating hormone. The U.S. Food and Drug Administration (FDA) has approved danazol for treatment of mastalgia; however, it is teratogenic and should not be used in individuals who may become pregnant (Li et al., 2021). Androgenic side effects are common with use of danazol and may include weight gain, menorrhagia, voice deepening, hair loss, acne, and muscle cramps. Side effects may be minimized by reducing the daily dose from 200 milligrams to 100 milligrams once improvement in mastalgia is appreciated (Goyal & Mansel, 2016). While tamoxifen, a selective estrogen receptor modulator, is not FDA approved for mastalgia, direct comparison between danazol and tamoxifen has demonstrated tamoxifen to have fewer side effects and therefore it is the preferred pharmacologic treatment (Li et al., 2021). Side effects include venous thrombosis, vasomotor symptoms, irregular menses, vaginal discharge, hair thinning, gastrointestinal disturbances, and weight gain (Goyal & Mansel, 2016; Li et al., 2021). Administration of 10 milligrams daily is associated with fewer side effects than 20 milligrams. As with danazol, tamoxifen is potentially harmful to fetal development and should not be used in individuals who may become pregnant. Bromocriptine, a dopamine agonist, is generally not recommended for treatment of mastalgia, as the side effects outweigh potential therapeutic benefits (Goyal & Mansel, 2016). Side effects include headaches, nausea, dizziness, increased libido, and compulsive gambling. Trigger point injections with lidocaine and steroids may also be effective treatment for mastalgia; however, studies are limited (Aphale et al., 2023).

Complementary and Alternative Therapies

Evening primrose oil, *Vitex agnus-castus, Nigella sativa,* chamomile, and flaxseed oil have all been suggested as herbal treatments for mastalgia but lack data from high-quality studies (Niazi et al., 2019). Supplementation with vitamins A, B_6, or E, or iodine or selenium, has not consistently demonstrated effectiveness in relieving mastalgia (ElSherif & Valente, 2022).

Surgical Therapies

Surgery is rarely indicated for the treatment of mastalgia and runs the risk of replacing a painful area with a painful scar. Potential surgical candidates include individuals with macromastia whose symptoms warrant reduction mammoplasty and those with refractory mastalgia who resort to mastectomy after nonsurgical options have proved unsuccessful in providing pain relief (El Maksoud et al., 2023; Hafiz et al., 2018). Mastectomy should be reserved for refractory cases and may not be curative (Hafiz et al., 2018). As with any surgery, the risks and benefits of this procedure must be considered.

Considerations for Specific Populations

Pregnant or Breast/Chestfeeding Individuals

Mastalgia is common during pregnancy and lactation. The pain in such cases is attributed to the proliferation of breast tissue and hormonal influences on that tissue. Mastitis is the most likely diagnosis when breast pain in a lactating person is accompanied by inflammation, erythema, chills, myalgia, and, in more advanced cases, fever. Mastitis is estimated to occur in up to 20 percent of breast/chestfeeding individuals (Louis-Jacques et al., 2023). Abscesses can also develop and should be suspected when mastitis is unresponsive to antibiotic therapy and the breast pain is worsening. Inflammatory breast cancer is also a consideration if an individual with suspected mastitis does not respond to antibiotic treatment (Hester et al., 2021). Refer to Chapter 34 for additional information about mastitis and abscess in persons who are breast/chestfeeding.

NIPPLE DISCHARGE

Nipple discharge is another breast symptom that often causes individuals to seek care; it is the third most common presenting symptom at breast clinics (Gulati et al., 2023). Approximately 3–5 percent of clinic visits for breast problems are related to nipple discharge (Stafford et al., 2021). The level of an individual's concern can range from minor embarrassment to fear and anxiety about underlying pathology. Nipple discharge can be classified as lactational, physiological, and pathological. Refer to **Color Plate 1** for an example of nipple discharge. Nipple discharge is usually the result of a benign process, but malignancy should always be considered in its evaluation as it is the presenting symptom in 5–12 percent of breast cancers (Patel et al., 2015).

Etiology, Pathophysiology, and Clinical Presentation

There are numerous etiologies of nipple discharge. Among the most common are pregnancy and lactation, galactorrhea, intraductal papilloma, mammary duct ectasia, and cancer. During pregnancy, individuals begin having bilateral milky discharge that can continue as long as 1 year after birth or the discontinuation of breast/chestfeeding. Clear nipple discharge during pregnancy, particularly in the third trimester, usually consists of colostrum which is yellow-clear and of a sticky consistency. Bloody nipple discharge during pregnancy or lactation can also occur as a result of the increased vascularity of the breasts and changes in the epithelium; however, evaluation is warranted (Mitchell & Johnson, 2022). Nipple discharge in individuals assigned male at birth should also be evaluated as its presence is associated with higher rates of breast cancer than nipple discharge in individuals assigned female at birth (Gulati et al., 2023).

Galactorrhea is physiological nipple discharge in an individual who has not been pregnant or lactated in the past 12 months. This type of discharge is usually bilateral and multiductal, and it may occur spontaneously or only with nipple or breast manipulation. The nipple discharge may range in color from white, green, brown, black, or yellow (Gulati et al., 2023). Galactorrhea is not caused by breast pathology (Stafford et al., 2021). Instead, it results from hyperprolactinemia, which may be caused by pituitary prolactin-secreting tumors, medications, hypothyroidism, stress, trauma, chronic renal failure, hypothalamic lesions, previous thoracotomy, and herpes zoster. Numerous medications can cause galactorrhea, including combined contraceptives containing estrogen and progestin, phenothiazines and other antipsychotics, tricyclic antidepressants, selective serotonin reuptake inhibitors (SSRIs), monoamine oxidase inhibitors (MAOIs), metoclopramide, domperidone, methadone, methyldopa, reserpine, verapamil, cimetidine, calcium-channel blockers, and amphetamines (Salzman et al., 2019). Most of these medications inhibit dopamine, which can lead to hyperprolactinemia. Hyperprolactinemia can also interfere with the normal menstrual cycle, resulting in anovulation, oligomenorrhea or amenorrhea, and infertility (Gupta et al., 2021). Marijuana use has also been implicated in nipple discharge (Breijyeh et al., 2021). Galactorrhea after breast augmentation surgery may occur (Sharma & Basu, 2021).

Pathological nipple discharge occurs spontaneously and is usually unilateral, uniductal, and serosanguinous or bloody (Gulati et al., 2023). Pathological nipple discharge is benign most of the time but requires further evaluation (Stafford et al., 2021). Intraductal papilloma and mammary duct ectasia are the most common causes of pathological nipple discharge. Intraductal papilloma typically occurs in individuals aged 35–50 years and results from proliferation of ductal epithelial cells in the duct. Mammary duct ectasia, in contrast, usually occurs in individuals ages 40–85 and results from dilation of the ducts with surrounding inflammation and fibrosis. Mammary duct ectasia can become chronic and lead to nipple inversion and skin retraction (Ni et al., 2023). Other risk factors for development of mammary duct ectasia include higher body mass index and history of lactation (Mohammed, 2021). Nipple discharge with mammary duct ectasia may be either unilateral or bilateral, multiductal, sticky, variable in color, and rarely occurs in individuals assigned male at birth (Ni et al., 2023). Mammary duct ectasia may also cause nipple discharge that is physiological in characteristics, rather than pathological (Gupta et al., 2021). Both intraductal papilloma and mammary duct ectasia may be accompanied by a palpable mass.

Although those with nipple discharge are often concerned that they have cancer, such pathology is the least likely etiology, but it must be considered carefully during assessment (Gulati et al., 2023). Cancer is more likely if the pathological nipple discharge is accompanied by a palpable mass or abnormal mammogram, or if the individual is older than age 50 (Stafford et al., 2021).

Assessment

History

Ask the person about the duration and color of their nipple discharge, whether it occurs spontaneously or only with manipulation of the nipple or breast, whether it is unilateral or bilateral, and whether it comes from one or more ducts on the nipple. Review the medications they are taking and determine whether any of them could cause galactorrhea. Note other breast symptoms such as mastalgia or breast mass and identify any history of any type of breast disease or surgery. Ask about symptoms of hypothyroidism (e.g., fatigue, weight gain, cold intolerance), hyperthyroidism (e.g., nervousness, weight loss despite increased appetite, heat intolerance), pituitary tumor (e.g., headaches, visual problems), and hyperprolactinemia (e.g., irregular menses, infertility, decreased libido) (Ghoreshi et al., 2022). Menstrual, pregnancy, lactation, general medical, and family histories should be obtained. Any family history of breast or ovarian cancer should be noted.

Physical Examination

Perform a comprehensive breast examination, including inspection and palpation with the person in both the upright and supine positions, and palpate the lymph nodes (refer to Chapter 8). If the nipple discharge can be reproduced, note the color, consistency, unilateral versus bilateral locations, and the number of ducts involved, using the clock method for documentation. Assess for skin changes, breast masses, and tenderness. Additional examination may be warranted based on the person's history, such as thyroid palpation if symptoms of a thyroid disorder are present or examination of the visual fields for individuals with galactorrhea who are not pregnant or breast/chestfeeding.

Diagnostic Testing

If the person has bilateral, milky discharge, perform a pregnancy test. If this test is negative, obtain a serum prolactin level and thyroid-stimulating hormone (TSH) measurement (Salzman et al., 2019). If hyperprolactinemia is present, imaging of the sella turcica with MRI should be performed to rule out a pituitary prolactin-secreting tumor (Vilar et al., 2019).

Evaluation of the person with nipple discharge depends on the presence or absence of a mass and the characteristics of the discharge. When a palpable mass is present, it should be evaluated as described later in this chapter. If the discharge is pathological in character, imaging recommendations are based on the person's age and biological sex (**Table 17-2**).

If the discharge is physiologic in character, the individual can be observed and advised to avoid nipple stimulation, with a follow-up examination occurring in 3 to 4 months. Avoiding nipple stimulation via compression is ideal. Breast imaging is not necessary for physiologic nipple discharge; however, persons should continue with routine breast cancer screening as discussed later in this chapter. Fecal occult testing for identification of blood in nipple discharge and cytology of the nipple discharge are no longer recommended (Gupta et al., 2021).

Additional diagnostic modalities that assist in ruling out malignancy include duct excision, ductoscopy, and ductography.

TABLE 17-2 Imaging Recommendations for Pathological Nipple Discharge

Age and Biological Sex	Initial Imaging	Additional Imaging
<30 years old		
Assigned female at birth	Breast ultrasound	Mammogram/digital breast tomosynthesis if indicated*
Assigned male at birth with or without history of estrogen therapy	Mammogram/digital breast tomosynthesis	Breast ultrasound if indicated*
30–39 years old		
Assigned female at birth	Breast ultrasound, mammogram, or digital breast tomosynthesis depending on individual and institutional preference	
Assigned male at birth without history of estrogen therapy	Breast ultrasound, mammogram, or digital breast tomosynthesis depending on individual and institutional preference	
Assigned male at birth with history of estrogen therapy	Mammogram/digital breast tomosynthesis	Concurrent breast ultrasound
>39 years old		
Assigned female at birth	Mammogram/digital breast tomosynthesis	Concurrent breast ultrasound
Assigned male at birth with or without history of estrogen therapy	Mammogram/digital breast tomosynthesis	Concurrent breast ultrasound

*Indications for additional imaging include elevated lifetime risk of breast cancer or suspicious findings on initial imaging.

Data from Expert Panel on Breast Imaging, Sanford, M. F., Slanetz, P. J., Lewin, A. A., Baskies, A. M., Bozzuto, L., Branton, S. A., Hayward, J. H., Le-Petross, H. T., Newell, M. S., Scheel, J. R., Sharpe, R. E., Jr, Ulaner, G. A., Weinstein, S. P., & Moy, L. (2022). ACR Appropriateness Criteria® Evaluation of Nipple Discharge: 2022 Update. *Journal of the American College of Radiology: JACR, 19*(11S), S304–S318. https://doi.org/10.1016/j.jacr.2022.09.020.

Excision of the affected duct or ducts allows for definitive evaluation, remains the gold standard, and may also be therapeutic; however, it may impair an individual's ability to breast/chest feed and peripheral lesions may not be able to be excised. Core needle biopsy is an alternative in some cases (Sanford et al., 2022). Core needle biopsy is preferred over fine needle biopsy due to its superior sensitivity and specificity (Sanford et al., 2022). Ductography is rarely used because it has low sensitivity, is technically difficult to perform, and may cause pain for the affected individual.

Differential Diagnoses

In addition to the conditions already described, sexual stimulation, infection or abscess, and Paget disease (described in the section on breast cancer later in this chapter) can cause nipple discharge.

Management

Pregnant people who express colostrum should be reassured that the discharge is benign and advised that avoiding nipple stimulation will generally lead to resolution of the discharge. Physiologic discharge has a similar management plan.

The treatment of galactorrhea unrelated to pregnancy or lactation depends on the etiology. Pituitary tumors may be treated surgically, with medications, or expectantly in certain circumstances (Tritos & Miller, 2023). Discontinuing a medication that causes galactorrhea or treating hypothyroidism if it is present may resolve the discharge. Bromocriptine and cabergoline can be used to treat galactorrhea, but symptoms often recur upon discontinuation of these medications; thus, long-term therapy is usually required.

Intraductal papillomas without atypia on core needle biopsy may be subject to active surveillance (Han et al., 2018). Palpable lesions or those with atypia should be excised (Hodorowicz-Zaniewska et al., 2019). Mammary duct ectasia can be managed expectantly with warm compresses (because it is associated with a benign process), or it can be surgically treated with removal of the subareolar duct system if symptoms are severe or recurrent (Pleasant, 2022).

If breast cancer is diagnosed, appropriate management should be initiated according to the disease stage, as is discussed in the breast cancer section later in this chapter.

BENIGN BREAST MASSES

A breast mass can be alarming for both the person and their clinician. Fortunately, most breast masses are benign; however, malignancy must always be considered in the evaluation of a breast mass. The likelihood of malignancy increases with age and risk factors for breast cancer, which are detailed in the breast cancer section later in this chapter.

Incidence, Etiology, and Clinical Presentation

The most common benign breast masses are fibroadenomas and cysts. Lipomas, fat necrosis, phyllodes tumors, hamartomas, and galactoceles may also be encountered.

Fibroadenomas, which are composed of both glandular (epithelial) and stromal (connective tissue) cells, are usually nontender, encapsulated, round, movable, and firm. Subtypes of fibroadenomas are defined by the histological features of the mass. They are the most common type of breast mass in reproductive age individuals, typically occurring in individuals between ages 15–35 (Ramala Jr. et al., 2023). Their incidence decreases with increasing age, and existing fibroadenomas tend to shrink after menopause. A single fibroadenoma is most typically seen, however multiple fibroadenomas can occur in some people. A proposed etiology for formation of these masses is the effect of estrogen on susceptible breast tissue.

Cysts are fluid-filled masses that are most commonly found in individuals aged 30–50 years (Pleasant, 2022). They are thought to result from ductal lobular obstruction due to dilation and proliferation of the breast ducts and acini. Breast cysts may be tender (Pleasant, 2022). Although many of these lesions can be dismissed as benign simple cysts requiring intervention only for symptomatic relief, complex cystic and solid masses require biopsy.

A lipoma is a benign fatty tumor that may occur anywhere in the body, but rarely in the breast tissue. It may be difficult for the clinician to palpate a lipoma due to the normal adiposity of the breasts (Okoye et al., 2022). Usually less than 5 centimeters in size, lipomas are generally slow growing, painless, well-circumscribed, mobile, and encapsulated (Busbaih et al., 2022). Lipomas typically occur in individuals ages 40–60.

Fat necrosis is a benign inflammatory process, usually the result of trauma to the breast, whether as a result of external force against the tissue (e.g., a seat belt in a motor vehicle accident) or subsequent to surgery, biopsy, infection, or radiation. It can occur in up to 25 percent of individuals following breast reconstruction due to lack of blood supply to the tissue flap (Lee et al., 2021).

Phyllodes tumors form from periductal stromal cells of the breast and present as a firm, palpable mass typically 4–5 centimeters in size. These typically large and fast-growing masses account for fewer than 1 percent of all breast neoplasms and most commonly occur in the upper outer quadrants of the breasts. Phyllodes tumors can be classified as benign, borderline, or malignant depending on the histological characteristics. The average age of an individual with a phyllode tumor is 45 years old (Lissidini et al., 2022).

Hamartomas are composed of glandular tissue, fat, and fibrous connective tissue; the average age at presentation for these masses is 45 years (Tazeoğlu et al., 2021). This breast mass is slow-growing and rare, accounting for less than 1 percent of breast lesions (Alran et al., 2022).

Galactoceles are milk-filled cysts that usually occur during or after lactation. They result from duct dilation and often have an inflammatory component (Peterson et al., 2023). Galactoceles may become infected or rupture spontaneously. Refer to **Color Plate 2** for an example of a breast mass.

Assessment

A person may present with a breast mass found on self-examination, or a mass may be discovered on clinical breast examination.

History

If the individual found the mass, determine when they first noticed it and any changes they have observed since that time. Ask about other breast symptoms, such as mastalgia or nipple discharge, and determine whether the individual has a history of any type of breast disease or surgery. Menstrual, pregnancy, lactation, and general medical histories should be taken. A family history of breast or ovarian cancer is particularly important, but to be thorough, all cancers in the family through a two-generation pedigree should be obtained.

Physical Examination

Perform a comprehensive breast examination, including inspection and palpation with the person in both the upright and supine positions, and evaluate the lymph nodes. If a mass is palpable, identify the size (in centimeters), the shape, and the consistency or texture. Determine whether the mass is discrete (well-delineated, distinct edges) or poorly differentiated, tender to palpation, and mobile or fixed. Assess for skin changes, nipple discharge, and lymphadenopathy. When documenting the location of a mass, draw a sketch of the breast with the site of the mass marked, or, more importantly, describe the position of the mass on the breast relative to a clock face, such as at 7 o'clock. Typical physical examination findings for benign breast masses are described in **Table 17-3**.

Diagnostic Testing

If the physical examination suggests a palpable area of concern, order an ultrasound if the individual is younger than age 30, and order a diagnostic mammogram with or without an ultrasound if they are 30 years or older. If the mass is suspicious for malignancy on physical examination and the person is at least 30 years of age, order a diagnostic mammogram and ultrasound (Gradishar et al., 2023). Ultrasound helps to distinguish a cystic mass from a solid mass, but it is not as accurate as tissue sampling. Mammography can be used to detect nonpalpable abnormalities if a person is of appropriate screening age or has a solid mass. Fibroadenomas appear as well-defined hyperechoic areas on ultrasound and rarely have calcified features on mammogram. Breast cysts appear as fluid-filled, round, well-demarcated lesions on imaging without wall thickening or internal septation. Lipomas may appear as a radiolucent nodule with a thin radiopaque capsule containing ring-shaped calcifications (Okoye et al., 2022). Fat necrosis typically appears as a calcified nodule lacking vascular supply on imaging (Lee et al., 2021). On mammogram, phyllode tumors appear as round or oval well-circumscribed dense masses (Lissidini et al., 2022). Hamartomas may have variable appearances on ultrasound due to different amounts of tissue types present in each mass; MRI may be useful to visualize the well-circumscribed dense smooth capsule (Tazeoğlu et al., 2021). Galactoceles appear as complex cysts without internal vasculature on ultrasound (Peterson et al., 2023).

Palpable breast masses may not be visible with diagnostic imaging tests, however, so these tests cannot rule out malignancy. Referral to a surgeon for further evaluation, such as biopsy or excision, is warranted.

Biopsy is required to definitively ascertain whether a mass is solid versus cystic and benign versus malignant. A fine-needle aspiration biopsy is a minimally invasive way to differentiate solid and cystic masses, and it provides for cytologic evaluation of a fairly superficial palpable mass. Fine-needle aspiration biopsy may also be therapeutic if the mass is filled with fluid. Tissue sample findings for benign breast masses are described

TABLE 17-3 Features of Benign Breast Masses

Type of Mass	Typical Physical Examination Findings	Tissue Sampling Findings
Fibroadenoma	Discrete, smooth, round or oval, nontender, mobile	Ductal epithelium, dense stroma, numerous elongated nuclei without fat
Cyst	Discrete, tender, mobile; size may fluctuate with menstrual cycle	Cyst fluid and inflammation
Lipoma	Discrete, soft, nontender, mobile	Fatty tissue
Fat necrosis	Ill defined, firm, nontender, nonmobile	Necrotic fat with inflammation
Phyllodes tumor	Discrete, firm, round, mobile, findings similar to a fibroadenoma but mass is usually larger	Stromal hypercellularity with glandular and ductal elements
Hamartoma	Discrete, nontender, mobile; may be nonpalpable with incidental diagnosis on imaging studies	Glandular tissue, fat, and fibrous connective tissue
Galactocele	Discrete, firm, sometimes tender	Fat globules

TABLE 17-4 Breast Tissue Sampling Procedures

Procedure	Description	Breast Target
Fine-needle aspiration biopsy	Tissue for cytologic evaluation aspirated with a small needle Differentiates solid and cystic masses	Palpable breast mass or thickening
Stereotactic-guided core-needle biopsy	Large-bore needle used to obtain cores of tissue for histologic examination Stereotactic mammography used for localization and targeting	Calcification seen on mammogram, masses or other abnormalities visible only by mammography (i.e., not visible with ultrasound)
Ultrasound-guided core-needle biopsy	Large-bore needle used to obtain cores of tissue for histologic examination Ultrasound used for localization and targeting	Solid or indeterminate lesion (most commonly a mass) seen on ultrasound
MRI-guided needle biopsy	MRI with intravenous contrast material used for localization and targeting	Lesions visible only with MRI
Needle-localized or seed-localized breast biopsy	Use of a wire (or radioactive seed) to localize an occult mammographic, sonographic, or MRI-detected abnormality prior to excisional biopsy	Mass or calcification seen on imaging in a location that cannot be effectively assessed with core biopsy
Excisional breast biopsy	Surgical procedure that requires a skin excision Mass is removed with a surrounding margin of normal-appearing tissue	Palpable breast mass, thickening or skin change; used for initial diagnosis only when needle biopsy is not feasible

in Table 17-3. If cytologic evaluation does not yield definitive findings, as may occur with atypical or complex fibroadenomas, a more invasive method of tissue sampling (**Table 17-4**) is required to rule out breast cancer or determine the type of tumor if the mass is benign (Gradishar et al., 2023; Ramala Jr. et al., 2023).

Differential Diagnoses

In addition to the types of breast masses already discussed, differential diagnoses for breast masses include fibrocystic changes, infection or abscess, and malignancy. Benign breast masses may also occur simultaneously in individuals with breast cancer. Individuals with fibrocystic breast tissue may present with a perceived mass, although these changes are typically associated with nodularity or thickening rather than formation of a discrete mass. Intradermal cysts, such as epidermal inclusion cysts and periareolar sebaceous cysts, occur in 3 to 5 percent of individuals assigned female at birth and are benign findings; however, they can cause discomfort when inflamed, especially if on the bra line (Yang et al., 2022). These cysts seem to be more prevalent in cigarette smokers and can be intermittently chronic.

Management

Management of benign breast masses depends on the type of mass. A fibroadenoma that has been definitively diagnosed by cytologic or histologic analysis does not need to be removed. Instead, it can be expectantly managed, and the person reassured that while fibroadenomas may change in size in response to hormone fluctuations, there is a very low risk of malignancy. Fibroadenomas usually decrease in size after menopause, and many resolve completely (Ramala Jr. et al., 2023). Some individuals may elect for removal of the fibroadenoma due to the size, discomfort, or cosmetic effects of the mass. Surgical removal is also indicated for fibroadenomas greater than 5 centimeters in size or if there are concerning features on imaging where further histological evaluation is necessary (Salati, 2021). Procedures for surgical removal include lumpectomy, excisional biopsy, cryoablation, radiofrequency ablation, and ultrasound-guided vacuum-assisted biopsy. Recurrence of the fibroadenoma after surgery may occur.

Management of cysts is based on symptoms, with these saclike structures sometimes requiring fine needle aspiration to treat large or painful cysts; however, cysts may recur (Pleasant, 2022). Asymptomatic simple cysts do not require intervention as the risk of malignancy is low. Complicated cysts will need biopsy of the debris to rule out atypia or malignancy.

Excision of a lipoma is not required if a breast mass is consistent with lipoma on clinical examination and tissue sampling and there are no suspicious findings at the site on mammography and ultrasound. Otherwise, excision should be performed. Some individuals may prefer excision for definitive pathology or due to distortion of the breast tissue caused by the lipoma. Subcutaneous deoxycholate injections and removal with liposuction are possible alternatives to surgical excision (Okoye et al., 2022). Fat necrosis typically resolves spontaneously, although resolution may take 2–3 years to occur (Lee et al., 2021).

Excisional biopsy is recommended for a biopsy-proven phyllodes tumor, and typically a wide margin of normal surrounding tissue is also removed due to the tendency for such masses to recur (Toussaint et al., 2021). Hamartomas may require excision for diagnosis but otherwise do not have to be removed and may be expectantly managed if no suspicious features are seen on imaging (Aminpour et al., 2022). Aspiration of a galactocele allows for diagnosis and appropriate treatment, however most galactoceles will resolve spontaneously after discontinuation of lactation (Peterson et al., 2023).

When benign breast masses are managed expectantly, the individual should be advised to report any new symptoms and encouraged to follow up with their clinician for examinations and diagnostic testing as recommended.

Considerations for Specific Populations

Adolescents

In approximately two-thirds of adolescents presenting with a breast mass, the diagnosis is a fibroadenoma. Ultrasound is the best diagnostic imaging test for this age group. Mammography is not indicated, and aspiration for diagnostic purposes can be avoided as there is risk of damaging still developing breast tissue (Salati, 2021). Observation of an asymptomatic fibroadenoma in an adolescent for 3–4 months prior to surgical intervention is recommended (Salati, 2021). Breast cancer in individuals younger than age 20 is very rare (Johnson et al., 2018).

Pregnant or Breast/Chestfeeding Individuals

Evaluation of palpable findings in pregnant and lactating persons is complicated by the complex breast parenchyma. Nevertheless, appropriate diagnostic imaging and breast tissue sampling should not be deferred. Ultrasound is generally preferred for imaging of breast lesions during pregnancy, although mammography with tomosynthesis may be appropriate in some cases. Use of MRI with contrast is contraindicated during pregnancy because of transplacental transfer of the radioactive agent and concern for fetal exposure; MRI without contrast is not sensitive for detection of breast lesions (Gradishar et al., 2023). Fibroadenomas may increase in size and become symptomatic during pregnancy and lactation in response to hormonal fluctuations (Ramala Jr. et al., 2023). Both ultrasound and mammography may be used during lactation and individuals should be advised to either feed or pump prior to imaging for their comfort (Gradishar et al., 2023).

Older Persons

The likelihood of malignancy increases with age. Among persons aged 55 years and older, 85 percent of breast masses are malignant. Masses in postmenopausal individuals are presumed to be malignant until proven otherwise (Jackson et al., 2022).

BREAST CANCER

Breast cancer is one of the most feared diseases, even though treatment of this condition has become increasingly successful in prolonging individuals' lives after diagnosis. From the Halsted radical mastectomy of the 1890s to breast-sparing surgery in conjunction with other treatment modalities, the management of breast cancer has changed dramatically over time. With increased public awareness and earlier detection, comprehensive treatment can be initiated promptly for this disease process. For the screening section below, content is specific to individuals assigned female at birth; given the rarity of breast cancers in individuals assigned male at birth and lack of data on transgender individuals, best practice for breast cancer screening remains unclear (Corso et al., 2023).

Incidence

After skin cancer, breast cancer is the most prevalent cancer diagnosed in the United States, with an incidence rate of more than 310,720 new invasive cases in 2024 (Giaquinto et al., 2024). One of every eight U.S. women (approximately 13%) will be diagnosed with breast cancer during their lifetime (Giaquinto et al., 2024). The risk increases gradually with age, with 84 percent of individuals diagnosed with breast cancer being over 50 years old. The median age at diagnosis is 62, but is seen at younger ages in Hispanic, Asian American, Pacific Islander, Black, American Indian, and Alaska Native populations. Breast cancer is the second-leading cause of cancer deaths in women after lung cancer (Siegel et al., 2024), but there are more than 4.1 million breast cancer survivors in the United States (Tonorezos et al., 2024).

Etiology

Two aspects of breast cancer are especially challenging: many of the risk factors are nonmodifiable, with only 20–30 percent of breast cancers being attributed to modifiable risk factors (Obeagu & Obeagu, 2024). In fact, fewer than 10 percent of those with breast cancer have an identified germ line mutation that puts them at known risk for this disease (American Cancer Society, 2021a). Known risk factors for developing breast cancer can be classified as nonmodifiable and modifiable, as listed in **Box 17-1**.

The discovery of the *BRCA1* and *BRCA2* genetic mutations was a monumental step in the understanding of breast cancer because mutations of these genes account for 5 to 10 percent of breast cancer cases (Force, 2019). In normal cells, these genes help prevent cancer by making proteins that keep the cells from growing abnormally. If a person inherits a mutated copy of either gene from a parent, they have a high risk of developing breast cancer during their lifetime with an autosomal dominant inheritance pattern. These mutations are also associated with an increased risk of developing ovarian, tubal, and peritoneal cancers. The estimated cumulative risk of breast cancer by age 70 was found to be 45 to 65 percent in women with a *BRCA* mutation (Force, 2019). Expanded panel testing is now available that can detect other genetic mutations in addition to *BRCA1* and *BRCA2*, which may also warrant management for increased risk. Given the growing knowledge base about genetic influences on the development of breast cancer, the genetic counselor has a significant role, working in collaboration with the healthcare team in the care of individuals with breast cancer as well as the identification of individuals with genetic mutations, which increase their cancer risk (Force, 2019).

BOX 17-1 Risk Factors for Breast Cancer

Nonmodifiable

- Individuals assigned female at birth
- Advancing age
- Personal history of invasive breast cancer, ductal carcinoma in situ, or lobular carcinoma in situ
- Family history of invasive breast cancer, ductal carcinoma in situ, or lobular carcinoma in situ, especially in first-degree relatives
- Inherited detrimental genetic mutations (primarily *BRCA1* and/or *BRCA2* although other genes have been identified as being related to development of breast cancer)
- Biopsy-confirmed proliferative breast lesions with atypia
- Dense breast tissue on mammogram
- High-dose radiation to chest, especially during puberty or young adulthood
- Menarche before age 12 years
- Menopause at age 55 years or older
- Personal history of endometrial or ovarian cancer

Modifiable

- Nulliparity
- First full-term pregnancy after age 30 years
- Never breast/chestfed a child
- Use of hormonal contraception
- Recent and long-term use of combined estrogen–progestogen hormone therapy after menopause
- Exposure to diethylstilbestrol during pregnancy for both mother and offspring
- Obesity
- Physical inactivity
- Consumption of alcoholic beverages
- Cigarette smoking

Data from American Cancer Society. (2022). *Breast cancer risk and prevention*. https://www.cancer.org/cancer/breast-cancer/risk-and-prevention.html

Other potential risk factors for premenopausal breast cancer include shift work, particularly at night (Hansen & Pedersen, 2024). Night shift work is classified as a probable breast carcinogen by the International Agency for Research on Cancer; however, further research is needed as it is currently unclear how the duration and frequency of night shift work affect an individual's cancer risk (Hansen & Pedersen, 2024). The relationship between cigarette smoking and breast cancer is not clearly elucidated, but evidence suggests that exposure increases the risk of premenopausal breast cancer (Daly et al., 2021). In addition, people who start smoking at a young age are at increased lifetime risk of breast cancer and the risk associated with smoking is compounded by the individual's alcohol intake (Daly et al., 2021). Due to hormonal manipulation, fertility treatments, such as ovulation-stimulating drugs, have been postulated to increase breast cancer risk, but there is no substantiated evidence (Barcroft et al., 2021). Furthermore, studies have yielded conflicting results about other lifestyle risk factors, such as diet, vitamin intake, and chemicals in the environment (Łukasiewicz et al., 2021). Research in this area is ongoing, with an emphasis on risk differences and tumor hormone receptor status.

Conversely, breast/chestfeeding has a slight protective factor against developing breast cancer. An individual's relative risk of breast cancer decreases by 4.3 percent for every 12 months of breast/chestfeeding (Stordal, 2023).

Physical activity decreases the risk of breast cancer, breast cancer recurrence, and death related to breast cancer. The reduction in risk increases as the amount of physical activity increases (Friedenreich et al., 2021). Maintaining a normal weight protects against breast cancer as well (Friedenreich et al., 2021).

The use of antiperspirants, a history of pregnancy termination, caffeine intake, microwaves, use of plastic serving ware and storage containers, cell phones, and bra usage are all disproven to contribute to an individual's risk of breast cancer development (American Cancer Society, 2021b; National Breast Cancer Foundation Inc., 2024).

Significant racial disparities in breast cancer exist. Black individuals have a higher risk of mortality from breast cancer compared to white individuals, while the highest rates of breast cancer diagnosis in the United States are in non-Hispanic white individuals (Jatoi et al., 2022). Hereditary factors alone do not explain these disparities, as evidenced by changing rates between racial and ethnic groups and types of breast cancer (Jatoi et al., 2022). Multiple factors contribute to these disparities, including healthcare access to screening and treatments, structural racism, and built environment.

Pathophysiology

Breast cancer develops when erratic cell growth and proliferation occur in the breast tissue. Which hormones are most critical in the development of breast cancer and why 60 to 70 percent of individuals who develop breast cancer have no identified risk factors remain unclear (National Breast Cancer

Foundation Inc., 2024). Although the discovery of pertinent genetic factors has clarified the predisposition toward developing breast cancer in some people, a significant amount of ongoing research is dedicated to further elucidating the development of this disease. In particular, by testing for biomarkers and tumor characteristics, personalized treatment plans have become the mainstay of breast cancer care.

Clinical Presentation and Types of Breast Cancer

Breast cancer may be detected by identification of a palpable lesion or by screening mammography. It is important to note that pain (or lack thereof) does not indicate the presence or the absence of breast cancer; nevertheless, pain is not usually a sign of breast cancer (Holbrook, 2020). Skin changes (e.g., nodules, dimpling, thickening) can also be the initial manifestation of breast cancer.

Most breast cancers are carcinomas, meaning the abnormal cells originate in epithelial cells of the breast (American Cancer Society, 2023b). Breast cancers that originate in the epithelial cells of glandular tissue, either ductal or lobular, are categorized as adenocarcinomas (American Cancer Society, 2023b). Refer to Chapter 7 for a discussion of breast anatomy and physiology. Breast cancers were historically categorized by histopathology; however, the heterogenous nature of breast cancers complicates this system. Thus, modern identification of breast cancer type relies on a combination of over 20 pathological, morphological, and molecular features (Rakha et al., 2023). One such morphological feature of importance is classification of breast cancer as either being in situ, meaning confined to the ductal or lobular tissue, or invasive, meaning abnormal cell growth extends outside of the ductal or lobular tissue.

Carcinoma In Situ

Ductal carcinoma in situ (DCIS), or intraductal carcinoma, is the earliest manifestation of breast cancer and involves abnormal cells that are confined to the ducts. This condition, which represents 20–25 percent of new breast cancer diagnoses in the United States (American Cancer Society, 2021c), is usually diagnosed in association with microcalcifications seen on mammography; it is rare to find a palpable mass in such cases (Grimm et al., 2022). DCIS is often referred to as a precancerous condition, although the likelihood of DCIS progressing to invasive cancer is unknown (Grimm et al., 2022). There may be a group of patients that may not require surgical excision and are candidates for an endocrine therapy agent such as tamoxifen (Grimm et al., 2022; Knowlton et al., 2022). The use of molecular testing may be helpful to determine likelihood of advance from DCIS to invasive carcinoma and guide treatment options while preventing overtreatment of low-risk tumors (Knowlton et al., 2022).

With lobular carcinoma in situ (LCIS), the abnormal cells are limited to the breast lobules. LCIS and atypical lobular hyperplasia are similar in that they are noninvasive lesions that differ from DCIS in that they do not progress to invasive cancer; thus, they are considered benign breast conditions. The term "lobular neoplasia" is often used to describe these conditions (American Cancer Society, 2023c). LCIS typically occurs in premenopausal individuals and is bilateral in about 20 percent of cases (Shaaban, 2021). A diagnosis of LCIS increases risk of future invasive breast carcinoma by 8 to 10 times; however, future cancers are as likely to be in the opposite breast as the previously diagnosed LCIS as in the same (American Cancer Society, 2023c; Shaaban, 2021).

Invasive Carcinomas

Invasive or infiltrating ductal carcinoma is the most common malignancy of the breast. Invasive ductal carcinoma usually presents as a discrete, solid mass, with malignant cells escaping the confines of the ducts and infiltrating the breast parenchyma. The most common sites of metastatic spread of such cancer are bones, liver, brain, and lungs (National Breast Cancer Foundation Inc., 2025).

Invasive or infiltrating lobular carcinoma is less common than ductal carcinoma (10–20% of all breast cancer). Individuals with invasive lobular carcinoma tend to be slightly older, with large tumor size, and more lymph node involvement at the time of diagnosis compared to individuals with invasive ductal carcinoma (Wilson et al., 2021). Invasive lobular carcinoma is more likely to be bilateral than invasive ductal carcinoma (Batra et al., 2023). The mass may be characterized only by thickening or induration, with margins that are diffuse and ill defined, both on physical examination and on mammogram. It is associated with a slow and unusual spread of metastases, including metastases to uterus, ovaries, gastrointestinal tract, and brain (National Breast Cancer Foundation Inc., 2025).

Paget Disease

Paget disease is a rare form of breast cancer (approximately 1% of all cases) that causes eczematous nipple changes and ulceration, itching, erythema, and nipple discharge that gradually extends into the areola. Over 90 percent of individuals with Paget disease will also have an underlying DCIS or invasive ductal carcinoma; however, fewer than 10 percent will have a palpable mass (Markarian & Holmes, 2022). Therefore, individuals with Paget disease who are demonstrating nipple change should be assumed to have underlying breast cancer and breast imaging should be obtained (Markarian & Holmes, 2022). Punch biopsy or full thickness excisional biopsy of the affected nipple and/or areola are the diagnostic tools for Paget disease.

Inflammatory Carcinoma

Inflammatory breast carcinoma is a rapidly progressive type of breast cancer, with more than half of all cases already demonstrating lymphovascular invasion at the time of diagnosis. Signs and symptoms of inflammatory breast carcinoma typically occur over a 6-month period (National Comprehensive Cancer Network, 2024). This type of carcinoma causes diffuse inflammatory changes of the breast skin with erythema, edema, warmth, skin thickening, and peau d'orange (fine dimpling that makes the breast skin appear similar to the skin of an orange). Thus, it can be mistaken for mastitis. Often there is not a distinct palpable mass.

Assessment

History

The initial history for an individual with a breast mass is the same as that described in the earlier section on benign breast masses. If the cancer is already diagnosed and classified as a T3 or T4 lesion (**Table 17-5**), the person should be asked about symptoms of metastases, such as bone pain, arthralgias, cough, jaundice, abdominal pain, headaches, visual disturbances, malaise, loss of appetite, unexplained weight loss, fever, and fatigue. Clinicians should remain vigilant for symptoms of metastasis in any individual with a history of breast cancer.

TABLE 17-5 TNM Classification of Breast Cancers

TNM Category	TNM Criteria
Primary Tumor (T)	
TX	Primary tumor cannot be assessed
T0	No evidence of primary tumor
Tis (DCIS) Tis (Paget disease)	DCIS Paget disease of the nipple *not* associated with invasive carcinoma and/or DCIS in the underlying breast parenchyma (Paget disease with a tumor is classified according to tumor size)
T1	Tumor 2 cm or smaller in greatest dimension (may be subdivided into T1mi, T1a, T1b, and T1c, depending on the exact size of the tumor)
T2	Tumor larger than 2 cm but not larger than 5 cm in greatest dimension
T3	Tumor larger than 5 cm in greatest dimension
T4	Tumor of any size with direct extension to the chest wall (T4a); ulceration and/or ipsilateral macroscopic satellite nodules and/or edema (including peau d'orange) of the skin (T4b); both T4a and T4b are present (T4c); inflammatory carcinoma (T4d)
Regional Lymph Nodes (N)	
NX	Regional lymph nodes cannot be assessed (e.g., previously removed)
N0	No regional lymph node metastases (by imaging or clinical exam)
N1 N1mi	Metastases in movable ipsilateral axillary node(s) Micrometastases (larger than 0.2 mm, but not larger than 2.0 mm)
N2	Metastases in ipsilateral axillary lymph nodes that are clinically fixed or matted (cN2a), or in clinically detected (by imaging studies or clinical examination) ipsilateral internal mammary nodes in the absence of clinically evident axillary lymph node metastases (cN2b)
N3	Metastases in ipsilateral infraclavicular lymph node(s) with or without axillary lymph node involvement (N3a), or in clinically detected (by imaging studies or clinical examination) apparent ipsilateral internal mammary lymph node(s) with clinically evident axillary lymph node metastasis (N3b), or metastases in ipsilateral clavicular lymph node(s) with or without axillary or internal mammary lymph node involvement (N3c)
Distant Metastases (M)	
M0	No clinical or radiographic evidence of distant metastases
M1	Distant detectable metastases detected by clinical or radiographic means (cM) and/or histologically proven metastases larger than 0.2 mm (pM)

Data from Gradishar, W. J., Moran, M. S., Abraham, J., Abramson, V., Aft, R., Agnese, D., Allison, K. H., Anderson, B., Bailey, J., Burstein, H. J., Chen, N., Chew, H., Dang, C., Elias, A. D., Giordano, S. H., Goetz, M. P., Jankowitz, R. C., Javid, S. H., Krishnamurthy, J., Leitch, A. M., ... Kumar, R. (2024). Breast Cancer, Version 3.2024, NCCN Clinical Practice Guidelines in Oncology. *Journal of the National Comprehensive Cancer Network: JNCCN, 22*(5), 331–357. https://doi.org/10.6004/jnccn.2024.0035.

Note: Clinicians may see two nomenclatures depending on the timing of classification. TNM is a dual system with a (pretreatment) clinical classification (cTNM or TNM) and a postsurgical histopathological classification (pTNM). This has important implications in recurrence and survival.

Physical Examination

The clinician should perform a comprehensive breast examination when breast cancer is suspected. Note any skin changes, palpable masses, and nipple discharge. A suspicious lesion is usually hard, is painless, and has irregular borders that may be immobile and fixed to the skin or surrounding breast tissue. Palpate for the axillary, cervical, and supraclavicular lymph nodes; enlargement of any of these nodes is suspicious. The lungs, abdomen, and neurologic system should also be examined to detect signs of metastasis. Refer to Chapter 8 for further information on breast examination.

Screening for Breast Cancer

Mammography was first introduced in the United States in 1930 in order to assess breast tumors prior to surgery (Nicosia et al., 2023). In the decades that followed, technological improvements led to the discovery that breast cancer could be detected by mammography before the progression to a palpable mass (Nicosia et al., 2023). A significant reduction in breast cancer mortality rates was found in the 1970s, which spurred the development of guidelines for screening mammograms (Nicosia et al., 2023).

Both the U.S. Preventive Task Force and the American Cancer Society issue recommendations for the age and frequency of screening mammograms; there are some differences between these recommendations as outlined in **Table 17-6** (American Cancer Society, 2023a; U.S. Preventive Services Task Force, 2024). Clinicians may want to engage individuals in frank conversations about risk factors, breast cancer-related anxiety, and preferences in order to determine which screening frequency to

TABLE 17-6 Recommendations for Breast Cancer Screening

Organization	Group	Recommendation
U.S. Preventive Task Force	Women ages 40–74	Screening mammogram every 2 years
	Women ages 75 and older	Insufficient evidence to evaluate benefits and harms of screening mammograms
	Women with dense breasts	Insufficient evidence to evaluate benefits and harms of supplemental screening with ultrasound or MRI
American Cancer Society	Women ages 40–44	Option for yearly screening mammogram
	Women ages 45–54	Screening mammogram yearly
	Women ages 55 and older	Screening mammogram every 1–2 years as long as general good health and life expectancy of at least 10 years
University of California San Francisco	Transgender individuals assigned male at birth ages 50 and with past or current hormone use of 5–10 years	Screening mammogram every 2 years
	Transgender individuals assigned female at birth who have not undergone mastectomy	Follow guidelines for cisgender women
	Transgender individuals assigned female at birth with history of mastectomy	Insufficient evidence for screening recommendation, technical limitations of mammography possible

Data from U.S. Preventive Task Force. (2024). *Breast cancer: Screening.* https://www.uspreventiveservicestaskforce.org/uspstf/recommendation/breast-cancer-screening

American Cancer Society. (2023). *American Cancer Society recommendations for early detection of breast cancer.* https://www.cancer.org/cancer/types/breast-cancer/screening-tests-and-early-detection/american-cancer-society-recommendations-for-the-early-detection-of-breast-cancer.html

UCSF Transgender Care. (2016a). *Screening for breast cancer in transgender women.* https://transcare.ucsf.edu/guidelines/breast-cancer-women

UCSF Transgender Care. (2016b). *Screening for breast cancer in transgender men.* https://transcare.ucsf.edu/guidelines/breast-cancer-men

follow. Guidelines specific to breast cancer screening for transgender individuals are also available (Table 17-6).

MRI is recommended for screening individuals at high risk for breast cancer (20% or greater lifetime risk), but evidence does not support the use of this modality for screening those at average risk (National Comprehensive Cancer Network, 2024). Thermography is not recommended for screening or diagnosis of breast cancer (National Comprehensive Cancer Network, 2024).

Diagnostic Testing

Diagnostic testing for breast cancer includes both imaging studies and tissue sampling. The diagnostic imaging tests most frequently used in the evaluation of breast cancers are mammography, ultrasound, and sometimes MRI (Table 17-2).

Mammography can identify breast cancers that are too small to palpate on physical examination, and it can detect both benign and malignant calcifications. Benign calcifications are typically characterized by their large, coarse, and scattered appearance. Malignant-appearing calcifications tend to be fainter, resembling grains of sand. With digital mammography and tomosynthesis, a wider range of tissue contrast can be seen; subtle contrast differences can be amplified with these technologies, and the images are immediately available. Mammography can also identify masses that ultrasound can then further characterize as solid or fluid filled. Solid masses require further intervention or follow-up, whereas simple fluid-filled cysts generally do not.

MRI is helpful in identifying occult breast cancer when there are axillary node metastases but no visible carcinoma on mammogram or ultrasound. This imaging technology can also assist with staging and therapy evaluation (National Comprehensive Cancer Network, 2025a). MRI should be used judiciously due to its expense and high false positive rate (lack of specificity); moreover, it may be unnecessary depending on findings of other imaging studies.

Breast tissue sampling procedures are described in Table 17-4.

Further Assessment When Breast Cancer Is Diagnosed

Several factors guide appropriate treatment options and serve as prognostic indicators when breast cancer is diagnosed. Malignancies are staged using the TNM system, which incorporates information on the size of tumor, lymph node involvement, and metastatic spread, and it now includes biologic factors (Table 17-5) (National Comprehensive Cancer Network, 2025a). Tumors are graded; grading indicates the tumor's extent of differentiation, or how closely the cells resemble normal tissue. A well-differentiated tumor has a more favorable prognosis than a poorly differentiated lesion (American Cancer Society, 2023b).

Advances in gene identification allow for identification of cancers based on expression of receptor types of the cancer cells—estrogen, progesterone, human epidermal growth factor receptor 2 (HER2). This system of classification guides treatment decisions and outcome prediction.

Approximately 70–75 percent of breast cancers have estrogen receptor expression (Orrantia-Borunda et al., 2022). Progesterone receptor expression is closely linked with estrogen receptors; therefore, it is rare for breast cancer to demonstrate high progesterone receptor expression in the absence of estrogen receptor expression (Orrantia-Borunda et al., 2022). More than 50 percent of breast cancers with high expression of estrogen receptors also have high progesterone receptor expression. Survival rates are higher in breast cancers with high expression of progesterone receptors (Orrantia-Borunda et al., 2022). There are four breast cancer molecular subtypes: luminal A, luminal B, human epidermal growth factor receptor 2 (HER2), and triple negative (Smolarz et al., 2022).

Luminal A breast cancer is defined as having high gene expression associated with estrogen receptors with or without progesterone receptors and low gene expression associated with proliferation and HER2 receptors (Smolarz et al., 2022). Individuals with this type of breast cancer are less likely to have relapse after treatment (Smolarz et al., 2022). This type of breast cancer generally has a good prognosis, and endocrine therapy may be appropriate treatment. Luminal B breast cancer also has high gene expression associated with estrogen receptors with or without progesterone receptors, but higher gene expression associated with proliferation. Luminal B subtype accounts for 10–20 percent of luminal breast cancers and is associated with poorer prognosis and higher rates of recurrence (Smolarz et al., 2022). Both chemotherapy and endocrine treatment may be appropriate for this subtype.

Breast cancers that are HER2 positive lack gene expression for estrogen and progesterone (Smolarz et al., 2022). This subtype accounts for 10–15 percent of all breast cancers and is generally fast growing and aggressive compared to luminal breast cancers (Smolarz et al., 2022). Treatment commonly includes chemotherapy specific to HER2 proteins and surgery.

Triple negative breast cancers lack receptors for estrogen, progesterone, and have no expression of the genes for HER2 receptors (Smolarz et al., 2022). Breast cancers with triple negative characteristics tend to occur in younger individuals and are associated with a poor prognosis due to high rates of relapse compared to other breast cancers. Triple negative breast cancers are often treated with chemotherapy although with limited efficacy, and research is ongoing to identify new therapies.

Other biomarkers in breast cancers, such as the radiosensitivity index and MRE11, vascular endothelial growth factor, androgen receptors, and proliferating cellular nuclear antigen, continue to be studied as a means to help predict individual recurrence risk and develop personalized treatment plans.

The status of the axillary lymph nodes is critical in determining treatment options for individuals with invasive breast cancer. For those who have early-stage tumors less than 5 cm in size and no palpable axillary lymph nodes, sentinel node biopsy provides necessary staging information without the associated morbidities of a full nodal dissection (e.g., lymphedema, immobility of the upper extremity, and accompanying diminished quality of life). With this technique, dye is injected into the region surrounding the tumor to identify the first nodes draining the breast. These one to six nodes that first drain the breast are termed the sentinel axillary nodes. The sentinel node or nodes that take up the tracer are removed (National Comprehensive Cancer Network, 2025a). If one or more sentinel nodes are positive, dissection of the Level I and II axillary lymph nodes is usually needed.

Additional tests are performed if there is evidence of advanced cancer (stage 3 or 4) to detect metastases. These tests routinely include a complete blood count, liver function tests, and a chest radiograph. Brain imaging, MRI, and a bone scan are not routinely done without symptoms, but abdominal and chest imaging (computed tomography [CT]) may be warranted if metastases are suspected (National Comprehensive Cancer Network, 2025a). A positron emission tomography (PET) scan may also be indicated when considering metastatic disease.

Differential Diagnoses

A palpable breast mass can be caused by any of the benign conditions discussed earlier in this chapter. Differential diagnoses for Paget disease include eczema, psoriasis, contact dermatitis, and, rarely, squamous cell carcinoma in situ arising in the skin (Bowen disease). Differential diagnoses for inflammatory carcinoma include breast abscess, infection, and mastitis. The presence of any of these conditions in a person who is not lactating is highly suspicious for malignancy.

Prevention

Two selective estrogen receptor modulators (SERMs), tamoxifen (Nolvadex) and raloxifene (Evista), and aromatase inhibitors, such as anastrazole (Arimidex) and exemestane (Aromasin), are used to prevent breast cancer in individuals who are at high risk for developing this disease; this indication is known as preventive therapy or chemoprevention (National Comprehensive Cancer Network, 2025b). To date, FDA approval for breast cancer prevention has been granted to only tamoxifen and raloxifene (National Cancer Institute, 2025). All these medications have potentially serious side effects. For example, SERMs are associated with thromboembolic events and endometrial cancer, and aromatase inhibitors have been linked to decreased bone mineral density, which can increase fracture risk (National Comprehensive Cancer Network, 2025b). Research supporting the use of particular agents continues, and the choice of agent should be made by the individual after consultation with a breast cancer expert and careful consideration of their individual factors and current evidence.

Individuals who are at very high risk for breast cancer due to genetic risk factors may elect to undergo prophylactic mastectomy, particularly after childbearing is complete. The benefits of risk reduction and decreased anxiety about the possibility of developing cancer must be weighed against the risks of the surgeries themselves. Given the complexity of risk assessment, discussions regarding risk reduction surgery should involve specialists (National Breast Cancer Foundation Inc., 2024).

Management

Suspected or diagnosed breast cancer requires collaborative care with breast cancer specialists, such as a surgeon or medical oncologist. Genetic specialists are now a more regular part of the team whose input may affect the final treatment plan. Reproductive planning may also be an important factor to consider. Primary treatment strategies for breast cancer include surgery, chemotherapy, radiation, hormone therapies, bisphosphonates, and monoclonal antibodies. A combination of these modalities is often used, and the specific therapies employed must be individualized based on a variety of clinicopathologic factors (e.g., cancer stage; age and menopausal status; ER, PR, and HER2 results; and genetic assays).

Breast-conserving surgery—lumpectomy or partial mastectomy—removes the cancer but not the breast itself. In addition to removal of breast tissue alone (total or simple mastectomy), mastectomy may include removal of the breast and Level I and II lymph nodes (modified radical mastectomy). Radical mastectomy, which includes removal of the breast, pectoralis major and minor muscles, and Level I to III lymph nodes, is no longer performed because it is associated with severe morbidities and does not offer any survival advantage over less radical surgery. Breast-conserving surgery may be performed instead of mastectomy depending on the characteristics of the breast cancer as well as individual risk factors. When mastectomy is performed, breast reconstruction is an option.

Chemotherapy may be administered after surgery (adjuvant therapy) or preoperatively (neoadjuvant therapy) to decrease the size of a large tumor prior to surgery. Use of chemotherapy agent is guided by the genetic and molecular results from tumor biopsy (National Comprehensive Cancer Network, 2025a).

Radiation therapy is used regularly following breast-sparing surgery and may also be administered after mastectomy. In addition, radiation is useful for treatment of locally advanced disease of the chest wall or breast, for palliation for bone pain from bone metastases, and to strengthen a region that contains bony disease that is at risk for pathologic fracture.

SERM, tamoxifen, and the aromatase inhibitors letrozole, exemestane, and anastrazole are the hormonal therapies used in breast cancer treatment when ER/PR receptors are positive. The duration of tamoxifen therapy varies, but may be up to 10 years (National Comprehensive Cancer Network, 2025a).

Ductal Carcinoma In Situ

Historically, DCIS was treated with mastectomy; however, more recently breast-conserving surgery is favored in the absence of widespread disease. Current options for DCIS treatment include breast-conserving surgery, with or without radiation, and, if individuals have large or high-grade tumors, total mastectomy. Tamoxifen therapy after surgery may be recommended, especially for those individuals who are ER positive. For postmenopausal individuals, tamoxifen or an aromatase inhibitor will be considered, with some advantage for the aromatase inhibitor therapy in people older than age 60 or for concerns of thromboembolism (National Comprehensive Cancer Network, 2025a). The most appropriate treatment strategy depends on patient characteristics, the extent of disease, and patient preferences.

Lobular Carcinoma In Situ

Optimal management of LCIS must balance the fact that this condition is a risk factor for cancer with the fact that it is not malignant per se. While management in the past has focused on surgical excision, current guidelines call for increased risk surveillance (National Comprehensive Cancer Network, 2024). Individuals 30 years old and older should undergo a yearly screening mammogram with tomosynthesis with consideration of yearly screening breast MRIs (National Comprehensive Cancer Network, 2024). Some individuals may elect for additional risk management strategies, including chemoprevention.

Invasive Breast Cancer

Treatment of invasive carcinoma depends on multiple factors, including the size and grade of the tumor, the involvement of lymph nodes, the presence of metastases, first-time diagnosis versus recurrent disease, and the results of ER/PR and HER2 testing. A combination of treatments, including surgery, chemotherapy, radiation, hormonal therapies, bisphosphonates (e.g., zoledronic acid [Reclast, Zometa] and pamidronate [Aredia]), and monoclonal antibodies may be used. FDA-approved monoclonal antibodies for use in treatment of invasive cancer include bevacizumab (Avastin), cetuximab (Erbitux), panitumumab (Vectibix), and trastuzumab (Herceptin). Poly (ADP-ribose) polymerase (PARP) inhibitors are offered to women with *BRCA* mutations and triple-negative breast cancer (i.e., no estrogen, progesterone, or HER2 receptors) (National Comprehensive Cancer Network, 2025a). When cancer has metastasized, the goal of treatment is control or palliative, rather than cure (National Comprehensive Cancer Network, 2025a).

Paget Disease

Suspicion for Paget disease should be high in any individual with nipple symptoms because diagnosis of this disease is often delayed. Breast-conserving surgery with complete excision of the nipple and areola to clear margins, followed by radiation, is recommended if the margins are negative. Mastectomy should be considered if the margins are positive or if the disease is multicentric or extends beyond the central portion of the breast. Tamoxifen therapy after surgery may be recommended, as with invasive breast carcinomas (National Comprehensive Cancer Network, 2025a).

Inflammatory Carcinoma

Individuals with signs and symptoms of inflammatory breast carcinoma may initially be treated with antibiotics because inflammatory carcinoma can be mistaken for mastitis. If a 7- to 10-day course of antibiotics does not result in complete resolution of symptoms, or if the cutaneous findings are highly suspicious, immediate mammography and referral for skin biopsy are indicated. Treatment of inflammatory carcinoma involves multiple modalities, including surgery, chemotherapy, radiation, hormonal therapy, aromatase inhibitors, and monoclonal antibodies (National Comprehensive Cancer Network, 2025a).

Emerging Evidence That May Change Practice

Recommendations regarding breast cancer screening, diagnostic techniques, and management are constantly evolving. As of March 2025, a search of clinicaltrials.gov identified more than 900 ongoing clinical trials related to breast cancer treatment alone. These trials will inevitably change clinical practice related to breast cancer, and clinicians must keep up to date about new developments. In addition, individuals at high risk for breast cancer, or those who already have breast cancer, should be encouraged to participate in clinical trials to help develop future treatment guidelines (National Comprehensive Cancer Network, 2025a).

Considerations for Specific Populations

Individuals with Dense Breast Tissue

As of September 2024, the Federal Drug Administration requires breast tissue density classification to be included in mammogram reports (Food and Drug Administration, 2023). This categorization is based on the imaging view and not the feel, shape, or size of the breast. According to the BI-RADS system, breast density is classified into four categories, from almost all fatty tissue to extremely dense tissue with very little fat: fatty tissue, scattered fibroglandular elements, heterogeneously dense tissue, or extremely dense tissue (Bodewes et al., 2022). Individuals who have dense breast tissue seem to have a slightly higher risk of breast cancer, compared to those with less dense breast tissue (Bodewes et al., 2022). It remains unclear why dense breast tissue is linked to breast cancer risk. Also, as breast density increases, mammography specificity decreases, and cancers can be missed. Adding tomosynthesis imaging to traditional 2-D mammogram has helped with breast cancer detection (National Comprehensive Cancer Network, 2024). No further imaging beyond mammography is recommended for individuals with dense breasts unless they have other factors that increase their risk of breast cancer (National Comprehensive Cancer Network, 2024).

Pregnant Individuals

The incidence of breast cancer in pregnancy is difficult to estimate; however, it is the most common cancer diagnosed during pregnancy. Breast cancer that is diagnosed either during pregnancy or within 1 year postpartum accounts for 0.2–2.6 percent of all breast cancers (Boere et al., 2022). The incidence of breast cancer in pregnant and postpartum persons is likely to increase with the trend toward delayed childbearing.

Diagnosis delays in this population are common because breast abnormalities can be difficult to detect in the presence of the normal breast changes that occur during pregnancy and lactation. Mammography, with appropriate abdominal shielding during pregnancy, and ultrasound can be used to evaluate a mass or other abnormality on clinical examination. Any palpable mass should be biopsied regardless of the imaging results.

Management of breast cancer during pregnancy must take into account the benefits and risks for both the individual and the fetus, and it can involve making complex decisions. Surgery—either mastectomy or lumpectomy—can be performed during pregnancy. Chemotherapy can be used during the second and third trimesters but requires close coordination between oncology and obstetric teams. Radiation is contraindicated during pregnancy (National Comprehensive Cancer Network, 2025a).

CONCLUSION

Breast concerns are frequently encountered by clinicians in the outpatient setting, in individuals of all ages. While many of these symptoms are ultimately benign, individuals often have anxiety or fear about the possibility of breast cancer. Navigating information about risk reduction and screening guidelines in an age of unfiltered information can be a balancing act that challenges both the individual and the clinician. The clinician's responsibility is to do their due diligence to thoroughly, and empathetically, evaluate the complaint and develop a patient-centered plan of care.

References

Ali, A. A., & Faraj, F. H. (2023). Clinicopathological profile of mastalgia in females: Incidence, types, and pathological correlations. A cross-sectional study. *Annals of Medicine and Surgery, 85*(10), 4764–4772.

Alran, L., Chamming's, F., Auriol-Leizagoyen, S., Velasco, V., Deleau, F., Brouste, V., Bonhomme, B., Ben Rejeb, H., Marty, M., & MacGrogan, G. (2022). Breast hamartoma: Reassessment of an under-recognised breast lesion. *Histopathology, 80*(2), 304–313.

The American Society of Breast Surgeons. (2016, 2018). *Concordance assessment of image-guided breast biopsies and management of borderline or high-risk lesions.* Retrieved January 22, 2025 from https://www.breastsurgeons.org/docs/statements/asbrs-ccs-concordance.pdf

American Cancer Society. (2021a). *Breast cancer risk factors you cannot change.* Retrieved April 15, 2025 from https://www.cancer.org/cancer/types/breast-cancer/risk-and-prevention/breast-cancer-risk-factors-you-cannot-change.html#:~:text=About%205%25%20to%2010%25%20of,passed%20on%20from%20a%20parent

American Cancer Society. (2021b). *Disproven or controversial breast cancer risk factors.* Retrieved February 12, 2025 from https://www.cancer.org/cancer/types/breast-cancer/risk-and-prevention/disproven-or-controversial-breast-cancer-risk-factors.html

American Cancer Society. (2021c). *Ductal carcinoma in situ: DCIS.* Retrieved March 2, 2025 from https://www.cancer.org/cancer/types/breast-cancer/about/types-of-breast-cancer/dcis.html

American Cancer Society. (2023a). *American Cancer Society recommendations for early detection of breast cancer.* Retrieved April 15, 2025 from https://www.cancer.org/cancer/types/breast-cancer/screening-tests-and-early-detection/american-cancer-society-recommendations-for-the-early-detection-of-breast-cancer.html

American Cancer Society. (2023b). *Your breast pathology report: Breast cancer.* Retrieved March 2, 2025 from https://www.cancer.org/cancer/diagnosis-staging/tests/biopsy-and-cytology-tests/understanding-your-pathology-report/breast-pathology/breast-cancer-pathology.html

American Cancer Society. (2023c). *Your breast pathology report: Lobular carcinoma in situ (LCIS).* Retrieved March 2, 2025 from https://www.cancer.org/cancer/diagnosis-staging/tests/biopsy-and-cytology-tests/understanding-your-pathology-report/breast-pathology/lobular-carcinoma-in-situ.html

Aminpour, N., Sogunro, O., Towfighi, P., Park, B. U., & Boisvert, M. (2022). Clinical management of myoid hamartomas of the breast: A case report and literature review. *Heliyon, 8*(11), e11723.

Aphale, R., Dhar, A., Kumar, S., Chintamani, Jatoi, I., Goyal, A., & Srivastava, A. (2023). ASOMA GUIDE for managing breast pain. *Indian Journal of Surgery, 85*(3), 702–712.

Arslan, M., Küçükerdem, H. S., Can, H., & Tarcan, E. (2016). Retrospective analysis of women with only mastalgia. *The Journal of Breast Health, 12*(4), 151.

Barcroft, J. F., Galazis, N., Jones, B. P., Getreu, N., Bracewell-Milnes, T., Grewal, K. J., Sorbi, F., Yazbek, J., Lathouras, K., & Smith, J. R. (2021). Fertility treatment and cancers—the eternal conundrum: A systematic review and meta-analysis. *Human Reproduction, 36*(4), 1093–1107.

Batra, H., Mouabbi, J. A., Ding, Q., Sahin, A. A., & Raso, M. G. (2023). Lobular carcinoma of the breast: A comprehensive review with translational insights. *Cancers, 15*(22), 5491.

Bodewes, F., Van Asselt, A., Dorrius, M., Greuter, M., & De Bock, G. (2022). Mammographic breast density and the risk of breast cancer: A systematic review and meta-analysis. *The Breast, 66*, 62–68.

Boere, I., Lok, C., Poortmans, P., Koppert, L., Painter, R., vd Heuvel-Eibrink, M. M., & Amant, F. (2022). Breast cancer during pregnancy: Epidemiology, phenotypes, presentation during pregnancy and therapeutic modalities. *Best Practice & Research Clinical Obstetrics & Gynaecology, 82*, 46–59.

Breijyeh, Z., Jubeh, B., Bufo, S. A., Karaman, R., & Scrano, L. (2021). Cannabis: A toxin-producing plant with potential therapeutic uses. *Toxins, 13*(2), 117.

Bui, A. H., Smith, G. J., Dyrstad, S. W., Robinson, K. A., Herman, C. R., Owusu-Brackett, N., & Fowler, A. M. (2024). An image-rich educational review of breast pain. *Journal of Breast Imaging*, wbae001.

Busbaih, Z., Saleh, A. A. A., AlMaghlouth, M. K., Albeladi, A. M., Alali, T., AlGhadeer, M. S., & Odeh, A. (2022). Giant breast lipoma: A case report. *Cureus, 14*(2), e22304.

Callé, C., Schmitt, F., Tse, G., & Tan, P.-H. (2023). Fibrocystic changes and cysts. In G. Tse, P.-H. Tan, & F. Scmitt (Eds.), *Fine needle aspiration cytology of the breast: Atlas of cyto-histologic correlates* (pp. 49-57). Springer.

Corso, G., Gandini, S., D'Ecclesiis, O., Mazza, M., Magnoni, F., Veronesi, P., Galimberti, V., & La Vecchia, C. (2023). Risk and incidence of breast cancer in transgender individuals: A systematic review and meta-analysis. *European Journal of Cancer Prevention, 32*(3), 207–214.

Daly, A. A., Rolph, R., Cutress, R. I., & Copson, E. R. (2021). A review of modifiable risk factors in young women for the prevention of breast cancer. *Breast Cancer (Dove Medical Press), 13,* 241–257.

El Maksoud, W. M. A., El-Amrawy, W. Z., & Sultan, M. H. (2023). Evaluation of therapeutic reduction mammoplasty for management of intractable mastalgia in female patients with large breasts. *The Egyptian Journal of Surgery, 42*(1), 346–354.

ElSherif, A., & Valente, S. A. (2022). Management of mastalgia. *Surgical Clinics, 102*(6), 929-946.

Epstein, B. S. (2025). *Champagne: A global history*. Reaktion Books.

Fakhravar, S., Bahrami, N., Qurbani, M., & Olfati, F. (2021). The effect of healthy lifestyle promotion intervention on quality of life in cyclic mastalgia via individual counseling: A randomized controlled clinical trial. *International Journal of Community Based Nursing and Midwifery, 9*(1), 55.

Food and Drug Administration. (2023). *Mammography Quality Standards Act. Federal Register,* https://www.federalregister.gov/documents/2023/03/10/2023-04550/mammography-quality-standards-act

Force, U. T. (2019). risk assessment, genetic counseling, and genetic testing for BRCA-related cancer: U.S. Preventive Services Task Force Recommendation Statement. *JAMA, 322*(7), 652–665. https://doi.org/10.1001/jama.2019.10987

Friedenreich, C. M., Ryder-Burbidge, C., & McNeil, J. (2021). Physical activity, obesity and sedentary behavior in cancer etiology: Epidemiologic evidence and biologic mechanisms. *Molecular Oncology, 15*(3), 790–800.

Genc, A., Celebi, M. M., Celik, S. U., Altman, E. D., Kocaay, A. F., Zergeroglu, A. M., Elhan, A. H., & Genc, V. (2017). The effects of exercise on mastalgia. Physician and Sportsmedicine, 45(1), 17-21. https://doi.org/10.1080/00913847.2017.1252702.

Ghoreshi, Z. a.-s., Akbari, H., Sharif-Zak, M., Arefinia, N., Abbasi-Jorjandi, M., & Asadikaram, G. (2022). Recent findings on hyperprolactinemia and its pathological implications: A literature review. *Journal of Investigative Medicine, 70*(7), 1443–1451.

Giaquinto, A. N., Sung, H., Newman, L. A., Freedman, R. A., Smith, R. A., Star, J., Jemal, A., & Siegel, R. L. (2024). Breast cancer statistics 2024. *CA: A Cancer Journal for Clinicians, 74*(6), 477–495.

Goyal, A., & Mansel, R. E. (2016). Mastalgia. In I. Jatoi & A. Roy (Eds.), *Management of Breast Diseases* (pp. 73–79).

Gradishar, W. J., Moran, M. S., Abraham, J., Abramson, V., Aft, R., Agnese, D., Allison, K. H., Anderson, B., Burstein, H. J., & Chew, H. (2023). NCCN Guidelines® Insights: breast cancer, version 4.2023: featured updates to the NCCN guidelines. *Journal of the National Comprehensive Cancer Network, 21*(6), 594–608.

Grimm, L. J., Rahbar, H., Abdelmalak, M., Hall, A. H., & Ryser, M. D. (2022). Ductal carcinoma in situ: State-of-the-art review. *Radiology, 302*(2), 246–255.

Gulati, M., Singla, V., Singh, T., Bal, A., & Irrinki, R. N. S. (2023). Nipple discharge: When is it worrisome? *Current Problems in Diagnostic Radiology, 52*(6), 560–569.

Gupta, D., Mendelson, E. B., & Karst, I. (2021). Nipple discharge: Current clinical and imaging evaluation. *American Journal of Roentgenology, 216*(2), 330–339.

Hafiz, S. P., Barnes, N. L., & Kirwan, C. C. (2018). Clinical management of idiopathic mastalgia: A systematic review. *Journal of Primary Healthcare, 10*(4), 312–323.

Han, S.-H., Kim, M., Chung, Y. R., La Yun, B., Jang, M., Kim, S. M., Kang, E., Kim, E.-K., & Park, S. Y. (2018). Benign intraductal papilloma without atypia on core needle biopsy has a low rate of upgrading to malignancy after excision. *Journal of Breast Cancer, 21*(1), 80.

Hansen, J., & Pedersen, J. E. (2024). Night shift work and breast cancer risk—2023 update of epidemiologic evidence. *Journal of the National Cancer Center, 5*(1), 94–103.

Harbke, C. R., & Lindemann, D. F. (2023). Objectification and reactions toward public female toplessness in the United States: Looking beyond legal approval. *Sexuality & Culture, 27*(1), 104–130.

Hester, R. H., Hortobagyi, G. N., & Lim, B. (2021). Inflammatory breast cancer: Early recognition and diagnosis is critical. *American Journal of Obstetrics and Gynecology, 225*(4), 392–396.

Hodorowicz-Zaniewska, D., Szpor, J., & Basta, P. (2019). Intraductal papilloma of the breast: Management. *Ginekologia Polska, 90*(2), 100–103.

Holbrook, A. I. (2020). Breast pain, a common grievance: Guidance to radiologists. *American Journal of Roentgenology, 214*(2), 259–264. https://doi.org/10.2214/ajr.19.21923

Holbrook, A. I., Moy, L., Akin, E. A., Baron, P., Didwania, A. D., Heller, S. L., Le-Petross, H. T., Lewin, A. A., Lourenco, A. P., & Mehta, T. S. (2018). ACR appropriateness criteria® breast pain. *Journal of the American College of Radiology, 15*(11), S276–S282.

Holbrook, A. I., Zhang, J., D'amico, K., Liu, Y., & Newell, M. S. (2019). The association of breast pain with malignancy. *Journal of Breast Imaging, 1*(3), 177–181.

Jackson, T., Carmichael, C., Lovett, K., Scott, M., Shakya, S., & Sotak, M. (2022). Approach to the patient with a palpable breast mass. *JAAPA, 35*(10), 22–28.

Jatoi, I., Sung, H., & Jemal, A. (2022). The emergence of the racial disparity in US breast-cancer mortality. *New England Journal of Medicine, 386*(25), 2349–2352.

Johnson, R. H., Anders, C. K., Litton, J. K., Ruddy, K. J., & Bleyer, A. (2018). Breast cancer in adolescents and young adults. *Pediatric Blood & Cancer, 65*(12), e27397.

Karimian, F., Akhavan, S., Marzoughi, A., Keramati, M. R., & Ashouri, M. (2022). Correlation between correction of menstrual irregularity and diminution of cyclic mastalgia. *Journal of Obstetrics, Gynecology and Cancer Research, 4*(4), 135–140.

Knowlton, C. A., Jimenez, R. B., & Moran, M. S. (2022). DCIS: risk assessment in the molecular era. *Seminars in Radiation Oncology, 32*(3), 189–197.

Lee, J., Park, H. Y., Kim, W. W., Lee, J. J., Keum, H. J., Yang, J. D., Lee, J. W., Lee, J. S., & Jung, J. H. (2021). Natural course of fat necrosis after breast reconstruction: A 10-year follow-up study. *BMC Cancer, 21,* 1–9.

Li, P., Simpson, A., & Dietz, J. (2021). Work-up and management of breast pain. *Annals of Breast Surgery, 5.*

Lissidini, G., Mulè, A., Santoro, A., Papa, G., Nicosia, L., Cassano, E., Ashoor, A. A., Veronesi, P., Pantanowitz, L., & Hornick, J. L. (2022). Malignant phyllodes tumor of the breast: A systematic review. *Pathologica, 114*(2), 111.

Louis-Jacques, A. F., Berwick, M., & Mitchell, K. B. (2023). Risk factors, symptoms, and treatment of lactational mastitis. *JAMA, 329*(7), 588–589.

Łukasiewicz, S., Czeczelewski, M., Forma, A., Baj, J., Sitarz, R., & Stanisławek, A. (2021). Breast cancer—epidemiology, risk factors, classification, prognostic markers, and current treatment strategies—An updated review. *Cancers, 13*(17), 4287.

Markarian, S., & Holmes, D. R. (2022). Mammary Paget's disease: An update. *Cancers, 14*(10), 2422.

Mitchell, K. B., & Johnson, H. M. (2022). Breast conditions in the breastfeeding mother. In *Breastfeeding* (pp. 572–593). Elsevier.

Mohammed, A. A. (2021). Mammary duct ectasia in adult females; risk factors for the disease, a case control study. *Annals of Medicine and Surgery, 62,* 140–144.

Nappi, R. E., Cucinella, L., Bosoni, D., Righi, A., Battista, F., Molinaro, P., Stincardini, G., Piccinino, M., Rossini, R., & Tiranini, L. (2022). Premenstrual syndrome and premenstrual dysphoric disorder as centrally based disorders. *Endocrines, 3*(1), 127–138.

National Breast Cancer Foundation Inc. (2024). *Risk factors.* Retrieved February 16, 2024 from https://www.nationalbreastcancer.org/breast-cancer-risk-factors/

National Breast Cancer Foundation Inc. (2025). *Metastatic breast cancer.* Retrieved March 2, 2025 from https://www.nationalbreastcancer.org/metastatic-breast-cancer/

National Cancer Institute. (2025). *Drugs approved for breast cancer.* https://www.cancer.gov/about-cancer/treatment/drugs/breast

National Comprehensive Cancer Network. (2024). *Breast cancer screening and diagnosis.* Retrieved March 2, 2025 from https://www.nccn.org/guidelines/guidelines-detail?category=2&id=1421

National Comprehensive Cancer Network. (2025a). *Breast cancer.* Retrieved March 2, 2025 from https://www.nccn.org/guidelines/guidelines-detail?category=1&id=1419

National Comprehensive Cancer Network. (2025b). *Breast cancer risk reduction.* Retrieved March 2, 2025 from https://www.nccn.org/guidelines/guidelines-detail?category=2&id=1420

Ni, Y., Tse, G., Tan, P.-H., & Schmitt, F. (2023). Inflammatory lesions of the breast. In G. Tse, P.-H. Tan, & F. Schmitt (Eds.), *Fine needle aspiration cytology of the breast: Atlas of cyto-histologic correlates* (pp. 43–48). Springer.

Niazi, A., Rahimi, V. B., Hatami, H., Shirazinia, R., Esmailzadeh-Dizaji, R., Askari, N., & Askari, V. R. (2019). Effective medicinal plants in the treatment of the cyclic mastalgia (breast pain): A review. *Journal of Pharmacopuncture, 22*(3), 131.

Nicosia, L., Gnocchi, G., Gorini, I., Venturini, M., Fontana, F., Pesapane, F., Abiuso, I., Bozzini, A. C., Pizzamiglio, M., & Latronico, A. (2023). History of mammography: Analysis of breast imaging diagnostic achievements over the last century. *Healthcare, 11*(11), 1596.

Obeagu, E. I., & Obeagu, G. U. (2024). Breast cancer: A review of risk factors and diagnosis. *Medicine, 103*(3), e36905.

Okoye, O. A., Obiesie, A. E., Azubuike, I. R., Ihekwoaba, E. C., & Anyanwu, S. N. (2022). Giant lipoma of the breast: Case report and review of literature. *Journal of the Nigerian Academy of Medicine, 1*(1), 31–33.

Orrantia-Borunda, E., Anchondo-Nuñez, P., Acuña-Aguilar, L. E., Gómez-Valles, F. O., & Ramírez-Valdespino, C. A. (2022). Subtypes of breast cancer. *Breast cancer [Internet].*

Patel, B. K., Falcon, S., & Drukteinis, J. (2015). Management of nipple discharge and the associated imaging findings. *The American Journal of Medicine, 128*(4), 353–360.

Peterson, M. S., Gegios, A. R., Elezaby, M. A., Salkowski, L. R., Woods, R. W., Narayan, A. K., Strigel, R. M., Roy, M., & Fowler, A. M. (2023). Breast imaging and intervention during pregnancy and lactation. *Radiographics, 43*(10), e230014.

Pleasant, V. (2022). Benign breast disease. *Clinical Obstetrics and Gynecology, 65*(3), 448–460.

Rakha, E. A., Tse, G. M., & Quinn, C. M. (2023). An update on the pathological classification of breast cancer. *Histopathology, 82*(1), 5–16.

Ramala Jr., S. R., Chandak, S., Chandak, M. S., & Annareddy, S. (2023). A comprehensive review of breast fibroadenoma: Correlating clinical and pathological findings. *Cureus, 15*(12), e49948.

Salati, S. A. (2021). Breast fibroadenomas: A review in the light of current literature. *Polish Journal of Surgery, 93*(1), 40–48.

Salzman, B., Collins, E., & Hersh, L. (2019). Common breast problems. *American Family Physician*, *99*(8), 505–514.

Sanford, M. F., Slanetz, P. J., Lewin, A. A., Baskies, A. M., Bozzuto, L., Branton, S. A., Hayward, J. H., Le-Petross, H. T., Newell, M. S., & Scheel, J. R. (2022). ACR Appropriateness Criteria® Evaluation of Nipple Discharge: 2022 Update. *Journal of the American College of Radiology*, *19*(11), S304–S318.

Shaaban, A. M. (2021). Why is LCIS important—Pathological review. *Current Breast Cancer Reports*, *13*, 132–140.

Sharma, S. C., & Basu, N. N. (2021). Galactorrhea/galactocele after breast augmentation: A systematic review. *Annals of Plastic Surgery*, *86*(1), 115–120.

Shi, H., Chen, H., Gao, S., Fang, J., Zhu, L., & Liu, Z. (2024). Acupuncture for cyclic and noncyclic breast pain in women: A systematic review and meta-analysis of randomized controlled trials. *European Journal of Integrative Medicine*, 102355.

Siegel, R. L., Giaquinto, A. N., & Jemal, A. (2024). Cancer statistics, 2024. *CA: A Cancer Journal for Clinicians*, *74*(1), 12–49.

Sivarajah, R., Welkie, J., Mack, J., Casas, R. S., Paulishak, M., & Chetlen, A. L. (2020). A review of breast pain: Causes, imaging recommendations, and treatment. *Journal of breast imaging*, *2*(2), 101–111. https://doi.org/10.1093/jbi/wbz082

Smolarz, B., Nowak, A. Z., & Romanowicz, H. (2022). Breast cancer—Epidemiology, classification, pathogenesis and treatment (review of literature). *Cancers*, *14* (10), 2569.

Stafford, A. P., Lucy, M., & Willey, S. C. (2021). Workup and treatment of nipple discharge—A practical review. *Annals of Breast Surgery*, *5*.

Stordal, B. (2023). Breastfeeding reduces the risk of breast cancer: A call for action in high-income countries with low rates of breastfeeding. *Cancer Medicine*, *12*(4), 4616–4625.

Tazeoğlu, D., Dağ, A., Arslan, B., & Berkeşoğlu, M. (2021). Breast hamartoma: Clinical, radiological, and histopathological evaluation. *European Journal of Breast Health*, *17*(4), 328.

Teal, S. B., Turok D. K., Chen, B. A., Kimble, T., Olariu, A. I., & Creinin, M. D. (2019). Five-year contraceptive efficacy and safety of a levonorgestrel 52-mg intrauterine system. *Obstetrics & Gynecology*, *133*(1), 63–70.

Tonorezos, E., Devasia, T., Mariotto, A. B., Mollica, M. A., Gallicchio, L., Green, P., Doose, M., Brick, R., Streck, B., & Reed, C. (2024). Prevalence of cancer survivors in the United States. *JNCI: Journal of the National Cancer Institute*, *116*(11), 1784–1790.

Toussaint, A., Piaget-Rossel, R., Stormacq, C., Mathevet, P., Lepigeon, K., & Taffe, P. (2021). Width of margins in phyllodes tumors of the breast: the controversy drags on?—A systematic review and meta-analysis. *Breast Cancer Research and Treatment*, *185*, 21–37.

Tritos, N. A., & Miller, K. K. (2023). Diagnosis and management of pituitary adenomas: A review. *JAMA*, *329*(16), 1386–1398.

U.S. Preventive Services Task Force. (2024). *Breast cancer: screening*. Retrieved April 15, 2025 from https://www.uspreventiveservicestaskforce.org/uspstf/recommendation/breast-cancer-screening

Vilar, L., Vilar, C. F., Lyra, R., & Freitas, M. d. C. (2019). Pitfalls in the diagnostic evaluation of hyperprolactinemia. *Neuroendocrinology*, *109*(1), 7–19.

Wilson, N., Ironside, A., Diana, A., & Oikonomidou, O. (2021). Lobular breast cancer: A review. *Frontiers in Oncology*, *10*, 591399.

Yang, S., Leng, Y., Chau, C., Ma, K., Fung, W., Chan, R., Yung, W., Leong, P., Li, O., & Wong, T. (2022). The ins and outs of male breast and anterior chest wall lesions from childhood to adulthood. *Clinical Radiology*, *77*(7), 503–513.

APPENDIX 17-A

Online Resources

American Cancer Society

The *American Cancer Society* provides resources for individuals with breast cancer and their caregivers, including plain language explanation of biopsy results. Patient handouts on understanding breast density and general breast cancer, links to clinical trial information, and general treatment information are available.

https://www.cancer.org/cancer/types/breast-cancer.html

National Cancer Institute's Breast Cancer

The *National Cancer Institute's Breast Cancer* page includes information about screening and testing, prevention, genetics, causes, treatment, clinical trials, cancer literature, research, and statistics. Materials for health professionals and patients are available.

Health Professional Version: https://www.cancer.gov/types /breast/hp

Patient Version: https://www.cancer.gov/types/breast

National Comprehensive Cancer Network

The *National Comprehensive Cancer Network* provides detailed evidence-based guidelines and algorithms for breast cancer screening, diagnosis, risk reduction, and treatment. Access to guidelines is available with registration for a free account.

https://www.nccn.org/guidelines/category_1

CHAPTER 18

Alterations in Sexual Function

Kathryn Atkin
Ella T. Heitzler
The editors would like to acknowledge Brooke M. Faught, who authored a previous edition of this chapter.

Over the past century, human sexuality evolved from a risqué topic to a more commonplace subject in media and among the general public. As a result, people seek clinician guidance more than ever on managing complications associated with healthy sexual functioning. Patient concerns about sexual health may reflect a normal variation of sexuality or simply indicate the need for patient education (e.g., inadequate knowledge about the sexual stimulation needed for arousal and/or orgasm). Distressing sexual concerns may also result from a medical or mental health condition, medication, or substance, or they may lead to an official diagnosis of sexual dysfunction.

This chapter is titled "Alterations in Sexual Function," because sexual function varies widely among people, and alterations in sexual function are not necessarily sexual dysfunction. A diagnosis of sexual dysfunction requires a component of distress. For example, a person who is unable to achieve orgasm, but is satisfied by their sexual relationship with their partner and not distressed by their lack of orgasm, is not considered to have a sexual dysfunction. Although not all sexual concerns are dysfunctional, this does not discount the right of patients and their clinicians to consider and implement safe and effective therapies, when appropriate, to improve sexual functioning. Every person should be considered as the unique individual that they are. Individualized care requires recognition that not all people assigned female at birth identify as female or women; however, these terms are often used in this chapter to align with current research and literature. Of note, the different sexual disorders discussed in this chapter utilize "female" in their names to facilitate effective use of this content in relation to the current evidence. Use of these terms is not meant to exclude people who do not identify as women and seek gynecologic care. Every person with sexual concerns should be evaluated from a holistic, unbiased, and nonjudgmental perspective and be provided with multimodal treatment options that may include an interdisciplinary healthcare team. This chapter focuses on women and those assigned female at birth. Content on alterations in sexual function for men and those assigned male at birth are in Chapter 10.

From a feminist perspective, it is important to appreciate the history of gender imbalance in treatment for sexual dysfunction. In 1998, the U.S. Food and Drug Administration (FDA) approved sildenafil (Viagra) for erectile dysfunction in men, which resulted in the expansion of disease-state awareness for male sexual dysfunction. In 1999, Laumann et al. published findings from the landmark National Health and Social Life Survey, which identified a larger proportion of women reporting sexual dysfunction than their male counterparts—43 versus 31 percent, respectively (Laumann et al., 1999). Yet, there were no FDA-approved medications for the libido, arousal, or orgasm domains of female sexual dysfunction until 2015, when flibanserin (Addyi) became the first medication to gain FDA approval for the indication of hypoactive sexual desire disorder in premenopausal women. At the time of flibanserin approval, nearly 30 FDA-approved medications already existed to directly or indirectly enhance sexual functioning of cisgender men. The issue is not whether a magic pill exists to cure a medical problem, but rather researcher, clinician, and government perception of gender equality in the development of treatments for sexual dysfunction. Although sexual health research focused on men immediately after sildenafil was approved by the FDA, women and those assigned female at birth now demand gender-specific research and treatment options for sexual dysfunction. A recent systematic review examined medicinal and nonmedicinal treatment options for the four domains of female sexual dysfunction: desire, arousal, orgasm, and sexual pain. This review found medications alone do not effectively treat female sexual dysfunction (Weinberger et al., 2019). These findings support the need for further high-quality research to identify effective treatment options for female sexual dysfunction.

This chapter begins with an overview of sexual response models and evolving definitions of female sexual dysfunction. This is followed by a description of the scope and etiology of sexual concerns in those assigned female at birth and a discussion of elements within the sexual health assessment. The remainder of the chapter focuses on the assessment and management of the three specific types of female sexual dysfunction: female sexual interest/arousal disorder, female orgasmic disorder, and genitopelvic pain/penetration disorder.

MODELS OF SEXUAL RESPONSE

Many models of sexual response have been proposed over the years. Alfred Kinsey (1953) was the original researcher of human sexuality, and he began his research in the 1950s. Approximately a decade later, Masters and Johnson (1966) published a linear model of sexual response that included a progressive occurrence of excitement, plateau, orgasm, and resolution. This model was believed to describe sexual response in both men and women. Another linear model proposed by Helen Singer Kaplan (1979) in the late 1970s was narrowed down to three phases: desire, arousal, and orgasm. In 2000, Dr. Rosemary Basson proposed a new model for female sexual response based on a changed perspective of female sexual dysfunction and desire disorders. Instead of the traditional model of excitement, desire, orgasm, and resolution, Basson (2000) describes many women as moving from a state of sexual neutrality to a state where they become motivated to seek stimuli that will cause sexual arousal. Orgasm is not always a necessary component to satisfying sexual encounters, according to Basson's model; other factors—such as emotional intimacy and relationship status—are of just as much importance as physiologic and biochemical changes. A diagram of Basson's model, as well as information about earlier sexual response models, can be found in Chapter 12.

DEFINITIONS OF FEMALE SEXUAL DYSFUNCTION

Various definitions of female sexual dysfunction have been proposed, and they remain inconsistent among different organizations and committees due to advancing research. To further complicate the situation, some organizations use the nomenclature of female sexual dysfunction, while others refer to female sexual disorder (Parish et al., 2021a). The *Diagnostic and Statistical Manual of Mental Disorders*, 5th ed. (*DSM-5*) in 2022 recognizes three categories of sexual disorder impacting those assigned female at birth: female sexual interest/arousal disorder, female orgasmic disorder, and genitopelvic pain/penetration disorder (American Psychiatric Association, 2022). These three *DSM-5* categories are used as the organizational structure for assessment and management of female sexual dysfunction in this chapter.

In 2016, the International Society for the Study of Women's Sexual Health (ISSWSH) published an article with suggested changes to the established sexual health nomenclature of the *DSM-5* (Parish et al., 2021a). The recommendations were generated by a consensus panel whose purpose was to unify terminology to improve interdisciplinary diagnosis and treatment of women with sexual dysfunction through use of consistent language. The definitions proposed by ISSWSH consensus panel include hypoactive sexual desire disorder, female genital arousal disorder, persistent genital arousal disorder, female orgasmic disorder, pleasure dissociative orgasm disorder, and female orgasmic illness syndrome.

Experts in sexual pain from three organizations—the International Society for the Study of Vulvovaginal Disease (ISSVD), ISSWSH, and the International Pelvic Pain Society (IPPS)—met in 2015 to develop revised terminology for persistent vulvar pain. The final consensus committee report includes two main categories of vulvar pain: vulvar pain caused by a specific disorder and vulvodynia (Parish et al., 2021a). In 2019, the ISSVD, ISSWSH and IPPS reconvened with a consensus panel to define the 11 descriptors of vulvodynia related to location (localized vs. generalized), provocation (provoked vs. spontaneous), onset (primary vs. secondary), and temporal pattern (persistent, constant, intermittent, immediate, or delayed) (Parish et al., 2021a). All three organizations suggest consideration of both the definition and description when diagnosing and treating vulvodynia.

Table 18-1 presents female sexual dysfunction terms and definitions in current use. Note that patient distress is a requirement for a diagnosis of sexual dysfunction. An important part of the evaluation of sexual concerns is determining whether the patient perceives the sexual dysfunction as distressing (American Psychiatric Association, 2022).

SCOPE OF THE PROBLEM

In the National Health and Social Life Survey, which was one of the first national U.S. surveys to address sexual concerns, 43 percent of women reported sexual dysfunction. Of the 1,486 women responding, 27–32 percent reported a lack of interest in

TABLE 18-1 Female Sexual Dysfunction Definitions

Type of Dysfunction	*Diagnostic and Statistical Manual of Mental Disorders*, 5th edition, text revision (APA, 2022).	International Society for the Study of Women's Sexual Health Consensus Panel; International Society for the Study of Vulvovaginal Disease (ISSVD), International Society for the Study of Women's Sexual Health (ISSWSH), and International Pelvic Pain Society Consensus Panel (IPPS) (as cited in Parish et al., 2021a)
Desire	Female sexual interest/arousal disorder	Hypoactive sexual desire disorder
Arousal	Female sexual interest/arousal disorder	Female cognitive arousal disorder Female genital arousal disorder Persistent genital arousal disorder
Orgasm	Female orgasmic disorder	Female orgasm disorders Female orgasmic illness syndrome
Sexual pain	Genitopelvic pain/penetration disorder	Vulvar pain caused by a specific disorder Vulvodynia

Data from American Psychiatric Association. (2022). *Diagnostic and statistical manual of mental disorders text revision* (5th ed.); Parish, S. J., Cottler-Casanova, S., Clayton, A. H., McCabe, M. P., Coleman, E., & Reed, G. M. (2021a). The evolution of the female sexual disorder/dysfunction definitions, nomenclature, and classifications: A review of DMS, ICSM, ISSWSH, and ICD. *Sex Med Rev, 9*, 36–56. https://doi.org/10.1016/j.sxmr.2020.05.001

sex, 22–28 percent were unable to achieve orgasm, 17–27 percent reported sex was not pleasurable, 18–27 percent described trouble lubricating, 8–21 percent experienced pain during sex, and 6–16 percent were anxious about performance, with the ranges reflecting variations among age groups (Laumann et al., 1999). A recent meta-analysis of 21 studies reported 50.75 percent of women of reproductive age have female sexual dysfunction (Alidost et al., 2021). The pooled prevalence of specific problems was 50.7 percent for low desire, 48.21 percent for low arousal, 37.6 percent for lubrication, 39.08 percent for pain, and 40.16 percent for orgasm difficulties (Alidost et al., 2021). Sexually related personal distress, as measured by the Female Sexual Distress Scale, was present in 50.2 percent of women of reproductive age; personal distress related to sex without dysfunction impacted 29.6 percent of women, while 20.6 percent reported at least one type of female sexual dysfunction (Zheng et al., 2020). A recent study indicated many transgender individuals assigned female at birth have low sexual pleasure scores; in fact, their arousal enjoyment, partner-related pleasure, and sexual self-efficacy scores were even lower than cisgender men or women (Gieles et al., 2023). Overall, published data indicate sexual concerns are common.

ETIOLOGY

Successful treatment of female sexual dysfunction requires an understanding of the etiology. Biologic, psychological, sociocultural, and interpersonal factors may all contribute. Etiologies may stem from numerous conditions and risk factors such as hormonal changes (decreased estrogen/androgens, diabetes, thyroid conditions), neurologic conditions (such as central and peripheral nervous system disorders), vascular conditions, infections, inflammatory conditions, iatrogenic causes (such as surgery, medications, or radiation), psychiatric diagnoses (anxiety and depression), and psychological factors (such as history of emotional/physical/sexual abuse, stress, relationship issues, or sociocultural factors) (Parish et al., 2019). The number and complexity of potential contributing factors highlights the importance of a comprehensive assessment and evaluation for those reporting sexual concerns.

GENERAL ASSESSMENT FOR SEXUAL CONCERNS

This section describes the general assessment of any patient presenting for care. Sexual health assessment and screening for sexual concerns is discussed in Chapters 8 and 12.Additional assessments specific to the different types of sexual dysfunction are detailed later in this chapter.

ISSWSH recommends all women be screened for sexual problems and concerns (Parish et al., 2019). When a patient screens positive for problems or concerns, a four-step model, proposed by ISSWSH, supports clinicians when (1) eliciting the patient's story, (2) reframing/naming the problem, (3) witnessing empathetically, and (4) either referring or assessing and providing treatment (Parish et al., 2019). Refer to **Box 18-1** for further detail. Overall, when assessing a patient for sexual dysfunction, it is necessary to determine whether the concerns have been lifelong (primary) or emerged more recently after a period of normal sexual function (secondary), and whether they are situational (specific to certain circumstances), or generalized (occur across all circumstances—masturbation, intercourse, manual stimulation, and so on). While proposing all clinicians screen using the four-step model, ISSWSH also provides advanced level competencies for clinicians who specialize in sexual health/medicine or have a strong interest in this area (Parish et al., 2019).

BOX 18-1 ISSWSH Process of Care for Identifying Sexual Concerns and Problems

- Begin by asking if they are sexually active:
  - If yes, ask what sexual concerns they have.
  - If no, ask if they have sexual concerns they would like to talk about or that have impacted their lack of sexual activity.
- When a concern or problem is detected, use the four-step model to engage the patient in discussion:
  - Step 1—Using patient-centered communication and open-ended questions, elicit the story of the problem and its impact on the patient (life, emotional well-being, and relationships).
  - Step 2—Name and (re)frame the sexual concern or problem, validating its importance.
  - Step 3—Witness the patient's story empathetically in an affirming way.
  - Step 4—Either refer to another clinician/specialist, or continue assessing and begin treatment as indicated.

Data from Parish, S. J., Hahn, S. R., Goldstein, S. W., Giraldi, A., Kingsberg, S. A., Larkin, L., Minkin, M. J., Brown, V., Christiansen, K., Hartzell-Crushanick, R., Kelly-Jones, A., Rullo, J., Sadovsky, R., & Faubion, S. S. (2019). The International Society for the Study of Women's Sexual Health process of care for the identification of sexual concerns and problems in women. *Mayo Clinic Proc, 94*(5), 842-856. https://doi.org/10.1016/j.mayocp.2019.01.009

Box 18-1 describes basic and core level assessment of sexual concerns. In addition, the Female Sexual Function Index (FSFI) can be helpful in assessment but should not replace a thorough sexual history. The FSFI questionnaire contains 19 items and is available online (http://www.fsfi-questionnaire.com). Other recommended screeners include the Brief Profile of Female Sexual Dysfunction and the Decreased Sexual Desire Screener (Parish et al., 2019).

History

Following a positive screen, the fourth step of ISSWSH's model includes either referring the patient or completing an assessment and providing treatment (Parish et al., 2019). Assessment of the patient with sexual concerns requires a comprehensive health history that includes physical and psychosocial history questions and assessment of their general and sexual health. Investigation of physical concerns should include surgeries, injuries, chronic illnesses, medications, and allergies. Reports of surgeries that could affect vascular or neurologic function of the genital tract and other erogenous areas, such as the breasts, indicate a need for further investigation. Past injuries to the pelvis, genital structures, spine, and even the brain can affect sexual response.

Chronic illnesses of relevance include, but are not limited to, thyroid disease, diabetes, hypertension/cardiovascular disease, certain cancers, chronic pain, prolactinoma, cognitive/psychiatric disorders, neurological disorders, neuromuscular disorders, and numerous gynecologic disorders (Parish et al., 2019). In addition, pregnancy history is important to review because pregnancy, birth, and lactation can pose unique challenges to sexual functioning. A review of medications is important as well because many drugs are known to cause or exacerbate sexual dysfunction (**Box 18-2**). For example, many mood-stabilizing medications, especially selective serotonin reuptake inhibitors (SSRIs), are known to contribute to sexual dysfunction (Parish et al., 2019); however, mental health conditions such as depression and anxiety are also risk factors for female sexual dysfunction.

The psychosocial history should include information about the individual's sexual orientation and their past and present partners and relationships. Never assume sexual orientation or monogamous relationship based on marital status, background, religious beliefs, or other sociodemographic factors. Some people may be uncomfortable answering sexual history questions in a face-to-face interview, so providing history forms for the patient to complete may yield more information about sensitive topics than verbally asking questions. Providing such forms prior to the appointment date allows the patient to answer intimate questions in the privacy of their own home.

Context and relationship stressors also need to be evaluated as a possible source of sexual dysfunction. For example, if a patient is or has experienced intimate partner violence, changing the time and location of sex is not an appropriate recommendation to help increase their sexual desire. In addition, using an intervention in such circumstances may lead to further deterioration of the individual's sexual health, and possibly even aggravate the violent episodes. It is not only important to utilize a trauma-informed approach (refer to Chapter 5 for further information), but also to conduct a thorough assessment. Ask the patient if they have a prior or present history of physical, emotional, or sexual abuse, or if they have ever been sexually assaulted. Assess for signs and symptoms of major depression and other mental health conditions, such as post-traumatic stress disorder and obsessive–compulsive disorder, as well as cognitive conditions that might affect memory and attention.

Partner sexual problems should be assessed, as partner dysfunction may adversely affect the patient's sexual health (Parish et al., 2019). Diet and exercise habits, life stressors, coping mechanisms, and body image can also be evaluated to rule out potential causes that are not medical in origin. It is important to inquire about the use of medications, alcohol, cigarettes, marijuana, and illegal drugs because these habits may be factors in sexual dysfunction. Additionally, the cultural and religious beliefs of the patient should be considered when evaluating and recommending treatment for sexual dysfunction. For example, if a patient is unable to achieve orgasm through intercourse, encouraging self-stimulation may not be an option if that practice conflicts with their religious or cultural beliefs.

Although many people presenting with issues related to their sexual health may have biologic etiologies, there is sometimes pressure to medicalize nonmedical symptoms in people seeking health care for sexual concerns. Individuals with sexual concerns may actually be experiencing normal variations of sexuality—a possibility that must be considered in the assessment. In this circumstance, referral to a sexuality educator or sex therapist can frequently prove beneficial. When evaluating a person who has a sexual concern, reviewing the normal sexual response may be all that is needed to reassure them that what they are experiencing is normal. The clinician may also need to evaluate the patient's understanding of normal sexual anatomy and function. One technique is to use a diagram to discuss genital anatomy and physiology. The sexual response cycle is often not well understood. For example, many people do not realize that the majority of people assigned female at birth cannot orgasm without direct or indirect stimulation of the glans clitoris. As a consequence, those who cannot achieve orgasm through penetrative intercourse often believe they have a problem. Discussing and describing sexual anatomy may give the patient enough information for them to understand and improve their sexual response.

BOX 18-2 Drugs Known to Cause or Exacerbate Female Sexual Dysfunction

- Anticonvulsants
- Antidepressants
- Antihistamines
- Antihypertensives and other cardiovascular agents
- Combined oral contraceptives
- Gonadotropin-releasing hormone (GnRH) agonists
- Hormonal agents
- Lipid-lowering agents
- Nonsteroidal anti-inflammatory drugs (NSAIDs)
- Opioid pain medications
- Psychotropic medications
- Substances including alcohol, amphetamines, cocaine, heroin, and marijuana

Data from Parish, S. J., Hahn, S. R., Goldstein, S. W., Giraldi, A., Kingsberg, S. A., Larkin, L., Minkin, M. J., Brown, V., Christiansen, K., Hartzell-Crushanick, R., Kelly-Jones, A., Rullo, J., Sadovsky, R., & Faubion, S. S. (2019). The International Society for the Study of Women's Sexual Health process of care for the identification of sexual concerns and problems in women. *Mayo Clinic Proc, 94*(5), 842-856. https://doi.org/10.1016/j.mayocp.2019.01.009

Physical Examination

The physical examination should specifically look for potential health conditions that could affect sexual function, such as undiagnosed diabetes or hypertension. Neurologic and vascular systems should be examined as well. If vulvar, vaginal, or pelvic pain is reported, a pelvic examination, including vulvovaginal examination, is important (Parish et al., 2019). Refer to Chapter 8 for pelvic examination techniques.

Diagnostic Testing

Laboratory testing is not usually required (Parish et al., 2019). Although a comprehensive battery of laboratory tests in every individual reporting sexual concerns is unnecessary, appropriate screening based on history and specific symptoms can facilitate individualized care. For example, may be appropriate based on symptoms or physical exam findings (Parish et al., 2019).

Testing for individuals presenting with sexual pain may include vaginal pH, sexually transmitted infection testing, and microscopy of vaginal secretions with normal saline and 10 percent potassium hydroxide (KOH) (Parish et al., 2019). Refer to Chapter 8 for microscopic examination techniques. In general, measurement of androgen levels, such as free and total testosterone, androstenedione, dihydrotestosterone, DHEA-S, and SHBG and albumin remains controversial. Assay methods vary in terms of their accuracy, precision, and reliability. A recent meta-analysis found total testosterone level was moderately associated with sexual desire and sexual function, but DHEA-S did not significantly impact desire (Maseroli & Vignozzi, 2022). Another meta-analysis, by Islam et al. (2019), found testosterone increased sexual function, desire, pleasure, arousal, responsiveness, self-image, and orgasm in postmenopausal women. However, off-label use of testosterone in premenopausal women remains questionable, as there is limited data which support their use. Therefore, there may be a benefit to evaluating serologic total testosterone levels in this population (Parish et al., 2021b).

Clinicians who obtain androgen levels must be well versed in the latest research on the topic so they can use this information appropriately. Additionally, there is the issue of how to manage a woman who is believed to have insufficient levels of endogenous testosterone. As of December 2024, there was no FDA-approved testosterone replacement product for women in the United States; however, testosterone products, including compounded testosterone, are widely recommended and used on an off-label basis (Parish et al., 2021b). This issue is discussed in more detail in the section on female sexual interest/arousal disorder.

Differential Diagnoses

The clinician should begin by categorizing the type of sexual dysfunction as sexual interest/arousal disorder, orgasmic disorder, or genitopelvic pain/penetration disorder (Table 18-1), keeping in mind that overlap among the types is frequent and common. Using the information obtained in the history, physical examination, and possibly laboratory testing, the clinician should then determine whether the source of the dysfunction is psychological, physiological, or a combination of the two. The remainder of this chapter presents specific assessment and management recommendations for each type of sexual dysfunction.

FURTHER ASSESSMENT AND MANAGEMENT OF SPECIFIC TYPES OF SEXUAL DYSFUNCTION

Female Sexual Interest/Arousal Disorder

Female sexual interest/arousal disorder (FSIAD) is the complete lack of, or significant reduction in, sexual interest or sexual arousal that is associated with three or more of the following six symptoms: (1) the absence or reduction of interest in sex; (2) an absence of or reduction in fantasies and erotic thoughts; (3) absent or decreased desire to initiate sexual encounters with their partner and usually unreceptiveness when the partner attempts to initiate such encounters; (4) absent or reduced sense of excitement/pleasure during sex; (5) absent or reduced response to sexual cues (e.g., verbal, visual); and (6) absent or reduced sensations in the genitals or elsewhere during sex. These symptoms must be distressing to the individual and must have persisted for a minimum of 6 months. The symptoms may be either lifelong or acquired after previously normal sexual function, and they may be either situational (occurring only in certain circumstances, such as penetrative intercourse) or generalized (occurring in all circumstances, such as penetrative intercourse, digital and manual stimulation, and masturbation). Severity may fall on a continuum from mild to moderate to severe distress over the symptoms. Lastly, there must be no other known mental health, physical, or substance-induced cause of the condition. It is important to recognize that gender diverse populations may not identify with or fit into the current sex and gender-based diagnostic categories described by the *Diagnostic and Statistical Manual of Mental Disorders*. Clinicians should understand that the symptoms and experiences that make up the diagnostic criteria for sexual dysfunctions are not dependent on the individual's gender or sex and diagnoses should be based on the individual's current reproductive anatomy and not necessarily their assigned sex at birth (American Psychiatric Association, 2022).

It must be emphasized that individuals presenting with female sexual interest/arousal disorder are distressed by their symptoms and are motivated to seek treatment. This is quite different from individuals with self-reported low sexual desire with no component of distress. There are a multitude of reasons an individual may experience low sexual desire without distress; for example, when they are not partnered, or more focused on other personal issues, or when their partner has health concerns that preclude the ability to be sexually active. Some individuals have low sexual desire for partnered sex although they enjoy self-stimulation. Masturbation is common and is considered a normal and healthy sexual behavior and in a study by Rowland et al. (2019), researchers identified that among women who were struggling to achieve orgasm, masturbation proved to be equally or more satisfying than partnered sex. Importantly, individuals who are asexual derive intimacy and pleasure from nonsexual activities and partnerships, and have varying levels of sexual attraction to others that range from a lack of sexual interest in anyone or anything to participation in some sexual activities. As with other sexual orientation identities, this may change over the course of a person's lifetime, and so screening for sexual concerns is still warranted. Notably, the defining feature for asexual individuals is that there is no distress associated with a lack of sexual interest, hence asexuality should not be classified as a sexual dysfunction. Refer to Chapter 11 for a further discussion of asexuality.

When evaluating patients with sexual interest/arousal disorders, it is important to understand that the diagnoses described by the *DSM-5* are appropriate in the context of the psychiatric compendium but there is concern that the combination of arousal and interest under one disorder has the potential to reduce diagnostic and treatment specificity, thereby impacting clinician judgment and patient care. Due to the fact that there is limited published data on the evaluation and treatment of FSIAD as a whole and that the evidence-based literature demonstrates that the desire and arousal should be considered as separate entities, the fourth International Consultation in Sexual Medicine (ICSM) as well as ISSWSH propose the use of the terms "hypoactive sexual desire dysfunction (HSDD)" and "female sexual arousal dysfunction (FSAD)" and recommends different assessment and management strategies (Parish et al., 2021a).

Assessment of Sexual Interest Disorder/Hypoactive Sexual Desire Disorder

Assessment of issues related to sexual interest should start with determining the duration of the concern and factors surrounding the symptoms. Has the individual always felt this way, or does their current state represent a change in their level of desire? It is important to look for any negative factors, either psychological or physical, that may affect desire. Does the person have a history of sexual abuse? Does the person have a partner? Does the partner have any sexual concerns? Are there conflicts about other issues in the person's relationship with their partner? Is the individual experiencing pain with intercourse? Other social factors that may influence desire include financial stress, small children who continue to require care at night, or work schedules that make it difficult for couples to find the time or energy to plan for sexual intimacy.

Frequency of sexual activity is another important factor to evaluate. Instead of experiencing a lack of sexual interest caused by a physical or psychological source, there may be a difference in expectations between the individual and their partner. There is a wide variation in the frequency, expectation, or desire to engage in sexual activity which can ultimately result in a discrepancy among partners in sexual desire. This is a common reason for couples to seek therapy, but this does not necessarily meet criteria for diagnosis of sexual interest/arousal disorder (Vowels & Mark, 2020). Among married individuals, there appears to be a positive correlation with sexual frequency and the quality and stability of the relationship as well as overall enjoyment with life (Lyons et al., 2024). It is important to inquire about whether the change in desire has resulted in a change in sexual frequency. Does the individual continue to have sex even when the encounters are unwanted? An individual who believes they do not have a choice about frequency of sex may first need to deal with issues of power and control in the relationship before it can be determined whether their sexual concern has a physical basis.

If an individual does not initiate sex, it is necessary to find out if they are willing to participate in and able to enjoy sex if the encounter is initiated by their partner. If so, the individual can be told that their pattern of response is normal for many individuals. Working with the individual, explore any changes that may have altered their satisfaction with their sexual relationship. Does the person experience orgasm with their partner? Although many anorgasmic people report satisfying sexual relationships, over time the lack of physical pleasure may decrease motivation to engage in sexual activity.

It is important to assess if individuals perceive that the negatives that may result from sex outweigh the positive rewards sex may yield. If an individual's need for intimacy is not being met during the sexual encounter because of either lack of time or fatigue, they may lose the motivation for future sexual encounters. Although the hormonal changes associated with menopause can affect desire, no longer having capacity for pregnancy may influence desire for sex after menopause or sterilization if pregnancy was a motivating factor. In addition, infertility and the associated testing, medications, interventions, and other therapies can medicalize sex and eliminate spontaneity. A systematic review and meta-analysis by Leeners et al. (2023), confirmed a diagnosis of infertility negatively impacts a couple's sexuality and increases the risk for sexual disorders.

Associated physical symptoms may also indicate that an individual's lack of interest may be the result of underlying illness. Fatigue may be related to thyroid dysfunction or sleep disorders. If the individual has a chronic medical condition, such as arthritis or back pain, it could contribute to making sex painful or uncomfortable. Sexual interest/arousal disorder may also be associated with thyroid disease, epilepsy, and renal disease. Screen the patient for use of medications (refer to Box 18-2) or a history of surgeries that could alter desire by changing hormone levels, particularly combined hormonal contraceptives, gonadotropin-releasing hormone (GnRH) agonists, antiestrogens, and hysterectomy or oophorectomy.

Menopause may be a time of decreased desire, which could be related to alterations in hormone levels and can subsequently lead to hot flashes, night sweats, fatigue, weight gain, vaginal dryness, and painful intercourse, though it is important to consider the cause may be multifactorial. Pelvic floor disorders such as urinary incontinence and pelvic organ prolapse are more common during menopause and appear to negatively impact sexual function (Stafne et al., 2024). The landmark PRESIDE study found the highest prevalence of distressing sexual arousal disorder occurs in the 45- to 64-year-old age range, with a greater decline in the 65 and older population (Shifren et al., 2008). This correlates with the decrease in estrogen production that occurs with menopause. Estrogen is known to play a critical role in sexual response and function and with the decline noted in menopause, a thinning and atrophy of the vaginal tissue can occur, potentially impacting sexual functioning (Lee et al., 2022). Since the PRESIDE study, multiple studies have found that sexual function worsens with menopause; however, there was no consensus as to which aspects of sexual function are most impacted, thus highlighting the importance of a holistic and comprehensive evaluation of sexual functioning in individuals regardless of their age (Christmas & Reed, 2024).

Testosterone plays an important role in sexual functioning and is produced both by the ovaries and the adrenal glands. Upon release into the bloodstream, testosterone binds to sex hormone-binding globulin (SHBG). When testosterone binds to androgen receptors, it has the ability to positively influence sexual function (Rojas-Zambrano & Rojas-Zambrano, 2024). Androgen levels can vary significantly from one individual to another though androgen production declines during menopause due to the age-related decline of ovarian and adrenal function. Additionally, the other two main factors that can decrease androgen levels are oophorectomy and oral estrogen therapy. Oophorectomy can result in a 50 percent loss of testosterone production, whereas oral estrogen therapy can increase SHBG, triggering a relative decrease in free testosterone levels (Uloko et al., 2022).

Androgen insufficiency can be diagnosed by history, exclusion of other causes of symptoms, and serum total testosterone measurement, although there is no established definitive total testosterone cutoff level that can be used to identify individuals with sexual dysfunction. Due to the limitations in testing previously described, SHBG and total testosterone should only be measured if the person is interested in initiating treatment for sexual arousal disorder with testosterone (Parish et al., 2021b).

Management of Sexual Interest Disorder/Hypoactive Sexual Desire Disorder

ISSWSH has a process of care for managing hypoactive sexual desire disorder that was developed by an international interdisciplinary committee of sexual medicine experts (Clayton et al., 2018). The process of care includes an algorithm for clinicians who are not experts in sexual medicine to address and manage hypoactive sexual desire disorder and provides a guideline for the treatment of both premenopausal and postmenopausal individuals with HSDD.

The appropriate treatment for decreased sexual interest in individuals depends on the etiology of this condition, but generally nonpharmacologic options are the preferred initial approach with an emphasis on optimizing health, well-being, education, and partner intimacy, and addressing modifiable risk factors. If relationship discord is affecting intimacy, the clinician should avoid suggesting a medical intervention and instead provide a referral to an appropriate therapist. Patients with undiagnosed or untreated physical or mental health conditions require applicable interventions to remedy the underlying illness. Consider changing any medications that may be affecting sexual desire (refer to Box 18-2). If decreased desire is related to pain with intercourse, the source of the pain should be diagnosed and treated. If sexual dysfunction already exists, be aware of how medical interventions may cause the sexual symptoms to increase in severity. For example, sexual dysfunction appears to increase by 50–70 percent among women with depression. At the same time, many antidepressants can lead to sexual side effects. SSRIs tend to carry the highest potential for sexual side effects, though serotonin-norepinephrine reuptake inhibitors (SNRIs), tricyclic antidepressants (TCAs), monoamine oxidase inhibitors (MAOIs), and first-generation antipsychotics can also increase sexual dysfunction (Pachano Pesantez & Clayton, 2021).

Individuals should be educated about normal alterations in desire that result from the aging process, longer duration of a relationship, and life changes such as those resulting from pregnancy, lactation, and menopause. For instance, even despite advances in health care to address sexual functioning in pregnancy, the overall quality of sexual functioning in pregnancy still declines among all domains of sexual function including desire, arousal, orgasm, and lubrication, resulting in decreased sexual activity over the course of pregnancy (García-Duarte et al., 2023). Additionally postpartum sexual dysfunction has been associated with multiple risk factors including depression, relationship stress, mode of delivery, amenorrhea, obesity, and hormonal changes. During lactation, prolactin levels are increased, and estrogen levels are decreased which can result in vaginal dryness and dyspareunia. Additionally, low sexual drive is associated with the release of oxytocin and lowering of androgens during lactation (Smetanina et al., 2023). Finally, sexual function often declines with advancing menopause status and distressing sexual concerns peak in the perimenopausal and early postmenopausal age group (ages 45 to 64), indicating another possible hormonal connection (Scavello et al., 2019).

Individual or couples counseling may help patients whose decreased desire is the result of life stressors or relationship problems. Some strategies to promote healthy sexuality among couples include planning time for intimacy, writing a to-do list of tasks that an individual may worry about during a sexual encounter and placing it outside the door prior to intimacy, and encouraging honest communication between partners (Vowels & Mark, 2020). In a systematic review by Sharifipour et al. (2024), cognitive behavioral therapy (CBT) was shown to help improve desire among reproductive-aged women presenting with sexual dysfunction. Additionally, a meta-analysis by Santos Silva et al. (2022) found sexual counseling programs to be an effective treatment approach among postmenopausal women presenting with sexual dysfunction. Mindfulness-based CBT also appeared to improve sexual desire and lead to positive results. Despite the benefits of counseling and CBT, treatment for HSDD appears to improve when utilizing a multifactorial approach that involves medication (Weinberger et al., 2019).

In August 2015, flibanserin (Addyi) was approved for use in the United States as the first-ever medication indicated for HSDD in premenopausal women. Flibanserin is a 5-HT_{1A} receptor agonist and 5-HT_2 receptor antagonist that has an approved dosing regimen of 100 mg to be taken orally once daily at bedtime, with expected improvement in satisfying sexual events within 8 weeks. Three randomized, double-blind, placebo-controlled trials demonstrated that flibanserin was effective for the treatment of HSDD when compared with placebo, noting an improvement in both desire and distress (Barakeh et al., 2024). Flibanserin has been shown to be safe when taken in combination with SSRIs or SNRIs and the most common side effects include dizziness, somnolence, nausea, fatigue, insomnia, and dry mouth. Nighttime dosing is recommended to avoid many of these potential side effects. Previously, alcohol consumption was contraindicated when taking flibanserin due to the possible risk for hypotension and syncope though recent data has demonstrated safety with concomitant use among healthy premenopausal women (Simon et al., 2020; Millheiser et al., 2019). As flibanserin is primarily metabolized by cytochrome P450 3A4 (CYP3A4), severe hypotension is a possible adverse reaction among individuals who are taking CYP3A4 inhibitor medications and therefore, reviewing all medications prior to initiating flibanserin is advised (Pachano Pesantez & Clayton, 2021). Although flibanserin is currently approved only for use in premenopausal women, published data support the safety and efficacy of this medication in postmenopausal women, though if no improvement is noted after 8 weeks, it would be prudent to discuss discontinuation of the medication (Simon et al., 2014; Pachano Pesantez & Clayton, 2021).

In May 2019, bremelanotide (Vyleesi), an injectable melanocortin receptor 4 agonist, became the second FDA-approved treatment for HSDD in premenopausal women. Bremelanotide 1.75 mg is delivered via a subcutaneous autoinjector on an as-needed basis in anticipation of sexual activity. Although the exact mechanism of action is unknown, bremelanotide is thought to increase excitation by enhancing dopamine and norepinephrine activity (Pachano Pesantez & Clayton, 2021). The RECONNECT study included two identical randomized, double-blind, placebo-controlled, phase 3 studies of bremelanotide for the treatment of HSDD in premenopausal women (Kingsberg et al., 2019). Compared with those taking a placebo, women taking bremelanotide had significantly increased scores on the desire domain of the FSFI at 6 months, indicating an increase in desire and reduction in distress based on the FSDS-Desire/Arousal/Orgasm (DAO) item 13 score. The most common side effects of bremelanotide include nausea (40%), flushing (20%), and headache (11%), although most respondents categorized symptoms as mild to moderate in severity (Kingsberg et al., 2019). A 1-year open-label extension of the RECONNECT study confirmed the safety of bremelanotide and demonstrated that women who continued the medication sustained improvement in their HSDD symptoms (Simon et al., 2019).

Individuals who have sexual side effects from SSRIs may find benefit in reducing the dose of the SSRI if their depression is mild but should be counseled appropriately regarding risk for relapse of depression symptoms. Additionally, providing patients with the option to switch to a different antidepressant with lower risk of sexual side effects could be a consideration and these medications include moclobemide, agomelatine, bupropion and reboxetine, mirtazapine, and possibly vortioxetine (Rothmore, 2020). Adding sustained-release bupropion SR (Wellbutrin) 300 mg once daily or buspirone (Buspar) 30 to 60 mg per day to the patient's regimen also has promising results, though close follow-up should occur to ensure the patient does not experience drug interactions (Barakeh et al., 2024). In addition, off-label use of bupropion SR (150 mg once daily for 1 week, then increase to 300 mg once daily) in individuals without a history of depression can improve desire and decrease distress and there is promising data that the addition of trazodone in combination with bupropion can improve HSDD symptoms in premenopausal women (Pyke & Clayton, 2019).

Transdermal estrogen therapy may be beneficial for an individual experiencing decreased desire after menopause, assuming hormone therapy is not contraindicated due to other health concerns, including the presence of one or more hormone receptive tumors, cardiovascular disease, and dementia (Clayton et al., 2018; Nappi et al., 2022). Additionally, evidence has demonstrated that testosterone can play a role in the treatment of HSDD, though until recently this has been an area of controversy. In 2021, ISSWSH published the Clinical Practice Guideline for the Use of Systemic Testosterone for HSDD which has helped to provide standards for the safe provision of testosterone to women with HSDD (Parish et al., 2021b). Yet as of December 2024, there were no androgen therapies approved by the FDA for use in people assigned female at birth; in contrast, the agency has approved oral, injectable, implantable, and transdermal androgen preparations for men. When the decision is made to initiate testosterone treatment for postmenopausal patients with HSDD, it is reasonable to prescribe an off-label male formulation at approximately one-tenth of the male dose if an approved female formulation is not available (Parish et al., 2021b).

Transdermal testosterone preparations are frequently used in symptomatic postmenopausal individuals, as they seem to provide the most physiological form of replacement therapy when administered as a patch, gel, cream, or spray. Prior to initiating therapy, clinicians should explain the off-label usage of testosterone for the treatment of HSDD and dosing should be aimed at maintaining testosterone concentrations in the physiologic premenopausal range (Parish et al., 2021b). In postmenopausal individuals receiving testosterone replacement for female sexual interest/arousal disorder, baseline serologic testing of total testosterone is suggested, with repeat testing at 3 to 6 weeks after treatment initiation. Patients on testosterone replacement should be monitored every 6 months for clinical effectiveness of treatment, and testosterone replacement should be discontinued if there is no perceived patient benefit at 6 months of use (Davis et al., 2019).

Known adverse effects from excessive androgen supplementation include hirsutism, acne, deepening of the voice, liver damage, hair loss, mood changes, and enlargement of the clitoris. Lowering of HDL cholesterol—that is, good cholesterol—levels can be avoided by using transdermal testosterone versus oral formulations (Davis et al., 2019). These potential risks must be discussed with the patient prior to prescribing androgen therapy and patients undergoing treatment should be assessed for signs of androgen excess with a plan to decrease the testosterone dose if symptoms are present (Parish et al., 2021b). To date, little evidence has been published to support the efficacy and safety of androgen supplementation in premenopausal women (Davis et al., 2019; Barakeh et al., 2024). Moreover, no causal relationship has been identified between exogenous testosterone use in women and cardiovascular disease and breast cancer (Davis et al., 2019; Lee et al., 2022).

Additional medications to treat hypoactive sexual desire disorder that remain in clinical development include a sublingual testosterone with sildenafil (Lybrido) (Bloemers et al., 2019), a sublingual testosterone with buspirone (Lybridos) (Gerritsen et al., 2020), as well as oral Dehydroepiandrosterone (DHEA) (Lee et al., 2022). Additionally, the use of tribulus terrestris, an herbal plant, in premenopausal individuals is thought to increase the levels of both free and bioavailable testosterone and is being considered as a treatment option for HSDD (Barakeh et al., 2024).

Assessment of Sexual Arousal Disorder

Patients should be asked whether they are experiencing vaginal lubrication or feelings of genital engorgement with sex play. It is important to determine whether the individual is having stimulation adequate to achieve arousal prior to their partner attempting penetrative intercourse and whether difficulty with arousal exists with all forms of sexual stimulation. Individuals with difficulties in achieving arousal should be assessed for physiologic conditions causing vascular or neurologic changes to the body. Diabetes, hypertension, and coronary artery disease can affect genital vasculature, for example. The patient should also be questioned about exercise or physical activities such as bicycle riding, horseback riding, and motorcycle riding where there is prolonged compression of the nerves and blood vessels leading to the genitals. Atrophic vaginitis and use of certain medications, particularly SSRIs, can also cause arousal disorders (ACOG, 2019). Other medications associated with arousal disorder include anticholinergics, antihistamines, monoamine oxidase inhibitors, tricyclic antidepressants, and antihypertensives. Smoking and alcohol use can also affect an individual's ability to achieve sexual arousal, which may provide a more enticing reason to stop smoking and limit alcohol use than simply citing the general health benefits from smoking cessation and limited alcohol use.

Although not included in the *DSM-5* criteria, the fourth ICSM and ISSWSH proposed subcategories of sexual arousal disorders to allow for greater specificity among the conditions. These subcategories include female cognitive arousal disorder (FCAD) which is characterized by the distressing difficulty or inability to attain or maintain adequate mental excitement associated with sexual activity and this is manifested by problems with feeling engaged, or mentally turned on or sexually aroused for a minimum of 6 months; female genital arousal disorder (FGAD), which is characterized by the distressing difficulty or inability to attain or maintain adequate genital response associated with sexual activity for a minimum of 6 months; and persistent genital arousal disorder (PGAD). PGAD is defined as the persistent or recurrent, unwanted or intrusive, distressing feelings of genital arousal or being on the verge of orgasm that is not associated with concomitant sexual interest, thoughts, or fantasies for a minimum of 6 months. It can be lifelong, acquired, generalized, or situational and associated with limited or no resolution or aggravated by sexual activity, aggravated by certain circumstances, leading to despair, emotional lability, catastrophizing, and or suicidality and present with inconsistent evidence of genital arousal on physical exam during symptoms (Parish et al., 2021a).

Management of Sexual Arousal Disorder

If arousal disorder is the result of inadequate stimulation of the clitoris, instructing the person on the use of artificial lubricants and clitoral stimulation may allow for adequate arousal to achieve orgasm. Vaginal moisturizers, lubricants, and topical arousal products may help increase stimulation, although caution should be urged given the potential for contact irritation. Many lubricants and arousal gels contain chemicals and vulvar irritants, such as glycerin, alcohol, and parabens, to which some people may be sensitive. Natural moisturizing products, such as coconut oil and emu oil, are often used as alternatives to traditional lubricants, although oil-based lubricants and moisturizers can affect condom integrity.

Arousal can also be impacted when individuals experience a decrease in estrogen levels due to menopause, ovarian removal, or with the use of hormonal contraceptives. When arousal appears impacted by estrogen deficiency, treatment with localized estrogen and/or testosterone therapy may be beneficial (refer to Chapter 14 for additional information on menopause) (Lee et al., 2022). Individuals who are breastfeeding may also benefit from localized estrogen therapy. Some vulvar skin conditions, such as lichen sclerosus and lichen planus, can result in scarring and clitoral phimosis, thereby decreasing clitoral sensitivity and increasing potential for irritation and pain (refer to Chapter 27). Vaginal Dehydroepiandrosterone (DHEA) has been shown to improve the symptoms of genitourinary syndrome of menopause (GSM)/dyspareunia by the estrogenic and androgenic actions that result with vaginal administration. This method could be considered for individuals experiencing dyspareunia related to menopause (Lee et al., 2022).

Sexual devices, which are also called sex toys and sex aids, can facilitate and enhance the sexual experience for individuals. Common sexual devices include vibrators, dildos, strap-on devices, anal plugs, and air pulsation devices (Rubin et al., 2019). Vibrators are commonly used to enhance genital arousal and increase the potential for orgasm. Such devices can be used for masturbation or with partnered sexual activity. If an individual does not have personal experience purchasing or using sexual devices, some counseling may be required to identify safe distributors and provide directions on proper use at home. For individuals who may be hesitant to consider sexual devices, normalizing their use can help them feel comfortable incorporating devices into their sexual practice. In some circumstances, referral to a sexuality educator or sex therapist can be helpful. There is an excellent clinical reference guide about sexual devices by Rubin et al. (2019). Refer to Chapter 12 for more information about vibrator use.

In 2000, the FDA cleared the Eros-CTD to treat sexual arousal and orgasmic disorders. Eros-CTD is a clitoral therapy device that fits over the clitoris and increases blood flow to the area by creating gentle suction. Further research is needed to determine the safety and efficacy of this device for the treatment of sexual arousal disorder (Lee et al., 2022). Many unapproved devices geared toward female sexual satisfaction are on the market and may prove to be beneficial during partnered sexual activity. Refer to Chapter 12 for more information about sexual devices.

Both cognitive behavioral therapy as well as mindfulness-based interventions have the potential to help individuals focus on the physical feelings of arousal and may enhance sexual arousal and improve sexual functioning. More research on this is needed to demonstrate the effectiveness of this approach (Lee et al., 2022).

Although not approved for use in women or people assigned female at birth, phosphodiesterase type 5 (PDE5) inhibitors, such as sildenafil have been shown to enhance genital blood flow and vaginal and clitoral vasocongestion and have been tested in clinical trials. Despite large scale placebo-controlled studies demonstrating oral sildenafil is well tolerated, it did not appear to perform better than placebo and at this time evidence does not support its use for treating women with sexual dysfunction (Lee et al., 2022). However, two randomized placebo-controlled studies have demonstrated that topically applied sildenafil cream appears to improve outcomes in women with sexual arousal disorder and was safe and well tolerated, suggesting a possible off-label treatment option (Thurman et al., 2024; Johnson et al., 2024).

Female Orgasmic Disorder

Female orgasmic disorder is present when there is a marked delay in, marked infrequency of, or absence of orgasm or reduced intensity of orgasm sensations lasting more than 6 months. To warrant this diagnosis, the anorgasmia cannot be related to other physical or mental health conditions or relational problems and must involve some degree of distress. Symptoms may have been present throughout the lifetime or they may be more recent, and they may be generalized to all types of sexual encounters or more situational encounters based on the type of stimulation. For example, many individuals require clitoral stimulation to reach orgasm but may be unable to orgasm during penetrative intercourse (situational), whereas other individuals cannot orgasm with any modality (generalized). In addition, some individuals who were previously orgasmic may not be able to orgasm after menopause with any mode of stimulation (secondary), whereas other individuals may have never been able to orgasm (primary). As the name states, this diagnosis is gender specific (American Psychiatric Association, 2022).

Assessment of Female Orgasmic Disorder

Assessment of orgasmic disorder begins with determining the duration and extent of the problem. Has the individual ever experienced an orgasm? If so, was the orgasm through self-stimulation or with a partner? Which sexual activities led to orgasm in the past? Inability to orgasm is often related to lack of sufficient stimulation. As noted previously, many people are unaware that most individuals need clitoral stimulation to reach orgasm. While not entirely visible when examining external vulvar structures, the clitoris is comprised of a substantial amount of erectile tissue analogous to the penis that extends deep into the pelvis. The clitoris can be stimulated both internally through the vagina and externally.

Other causes of orgasmic disorders may include history of trauma and physical or sexual abuse, particularly for individuals who have never had an orgasm; clitoral phimosis from vulvar skin disorders; chronic illness, such as diabetes, multiple sclerosis, chronic kidney disease, or fibromyalgia; pelvic disorders or surgery; use of medications, most notably SSRIs but also other antidepressants, antipsychotics, and mood stabilizers; alcohol, marijuana, and illegal drug use; relationship issues; partner sexual dysfunction; inadequate communication between partners; and cultural, religious, or familial beliefs or inhibitions. Inhibition of the orgasmic reflex may also occur for psychological reasons or as a response to genital pain (ACOG, 2019; Reiss et al., 2021; Parish et al., 2021a). Spectatoring, a concept proposed by

Masters and Johnson (1970), where individuals focus on their performance and/or the ability to please their partner by essentially viewing themself from the outside may lead to anxiety and inhibit arousal and the ability to orgasm because the focus is no longer on their own sensations.

It is also important to note that as part of the updated nomenclature provided by ISSWSH, female orgasmic illness syndrome is considered a separate classification and is characterized by peripheral or central aversion symptoms that may occur before, during, or after orgasm that can last for minutes, hours, or days after an orgasm. Peripheral symptoms may include diarrhea, constipation, abdominal pain, muscle aches, hot flashes, chills, diaphoresis, fatigue, and genital pain. Central symptoms may include confusion, disorientation, decreased verbal memory, insomnia, anxiety, depression, seizures, and headache. This syndrome has been associated with psychological, musculoskeletal, autoimmune, vascular, as well as peripheral and/or central neurologic pathophysiology (Parish et al., 2021a).

Management of Female Orgasmic Disorder

As part of the management process, it is critical to address any underlying cause of the orgasmic disorder. For example, consider referring individuals who have been subject to violence or abuse for counseling, and consider switching medications for individuals whose orgasmic disorder seems to be medication related.

There is no specific method for an individual to orgasm. For the individual who has never experienced orgasm, the clinician should begin by using a diagram to demonstrate genital anatomy to the person. During this education, it is important to explain to the individual that most people can orgasm only through direct or indirect stimulation of the clitoris. Individuals should be encouraged to try self-exploration of their genital area to determine which type of touching achieves the best response, if they are comfortable with this exercise. Practicing Kegel exercises allows the individual to control their muscular tension, which may decrease inhibition of the orgasmic response. For some individuals, the use of a vibrator will produce the required stimulation to orgasm.

Individuals who are uncomfortable with self-stimulation may be able to instruct their partner to provide direct clitoral stimulation either manually, with a vibrator, or with oral stimulation to lead to orgasm. Although individuals are able to orgasm with vaginal penetration, direct clitoral stimulation is more likely to lead to orgasm in the majority of individuals (Reed, 2022; Reis et al., 2021). Directed masturbation is one technique that involves mindfulness and cognitive behavioral techniques that involve genital stimulation with psychological tools to allow increased comfort with sexual feelings and stimulation by identifying challenges and attempting to reduce anxiety or spectatoring.

Despite being dated, *Becoming Orgasmic* (Heiman & Lopiccolo, 1988) is an excellent self-help guide for individuals who need more coaching to experience orgasm. Additional books recommended for individuals with orgasmic dysfunction can be found in **Box 18-3**. Cognitive behavioral therapy or sexual therapy may be useful for individuals with orgasmic disorder that does not resolve with self-help measures.

Pharmaceutical options for female orgasmic disorder are limited as there are no FDA-approved medications for arousal and orgasmic dysfunction in females. As mentioned previously in the discussion of female sexual interest/arousal disorder, off-label use of PDE5 inhibitors can prove beneficial to individuals battling anorgasmia related to insufficient arousal (Johnson et al., 2024). More research is needed on how to best treat female orgasmic disorder as there are currently limited options to clinicians as this time.

> **BOX 18-3 Recommended Books for Individuals with Orgasmic Dysfunction**
>
> *Becoming Cliterate: Why Orgasm Equality Matters—and How to Get It* by Laurie Mintz
>
> *Come As You Are: The Surprising New Science That Will Transform Your Sex Life* by Emily Nagoski
>
> *The Elusive Orgasm: A Woman's Guide to Why She Can't and How She Can Orgasm* by Vivienne Cass
>
> *She Comes First: The Thinking Man's Guide to Pleasuring a Woman* by Ian Kerner
>
> *Women's Anatomy of Arousal: Secret Maps to Buried Pleasure* by Sheri Winston
>
> *Your Blueprint for Pleasure: Discover the 5 Erotic Types to Awaken and Fulfill your Desire* by Jaiya

Genitopelvic Pain/Penetration Disorder

Genitopelvic pain/penetration disorder (GPPD) is present when an individual experiences one or more of the following: difficulty with vaginal penetration during sexual activity; vulvovaginal or pelvic pain during penetrative intercourse or attempted penetration; fear or anxiety about pain before, during, or after vaginal penetration; and the pelvic floor muscles tensing or tightening when vaginal penetration is attempted. To make this diagnosis, symptoms must be present for a minimum of 6 months, must cause significant distress, and cannot be better explained by another physical or mental condition (American Psychiatric Association, 2022). Even though ISSWSH has not published formal nomenclature for sexual pain, expert consensus broadens the GPPD category beyond difficulties with vaginal penetration to include pain with genital contact. The ICSM committee report on sexual dysfunction defines genital pain as any kind of genital or abdominal pain resulting from vulvodynia, chronic pelvic pain, or undiagnosed conditions. Vulvodynia refers to the general condition of idiopathic, chronic vulvar pain whereas dyspareunia indicates a common symptom of many genital pain conditions that includes but is not limited to pain during penetrative sexual activities (Parish et al., 2021a). In 2019, ISSWSH provided updated consensus guidelines on descriptors pertaining to vulvodynia. The 11 descriptors of vulvodynia were put into four groups: location (localized, generalized), provocation (provoked, spontaneous), onset (primary, secondary), and temporal pattern (persistent, constant, intermittent, immediate, delayed) (Bornstein et al., 2019).

Assessment of Genitopelvic Pain

In the evaluation of GPPD, it is important to determine the exact location and experience of the pain. Ask about the pain onset, duration, quality, and severity as well as any factors that cause the pain to improve or worsen. The timing of the pain in relation to the menstrual cycle should be assessed as well, especially if endometriosis is suspected. Determine whether painful sexual encounters occur with penetrative sexual activity only or with all internal and external stimulation. Ask if direct contact is required for pain or if arousal and orgasm result in pain independent from contact.

Causes of external pain may include vaginal infections, dermatologic disorders, atrophic vaginitis, trauma, allergy, and vulvodynia (persistent vulvar pain of at least 3 months duration without a clear identifiable cause). Vaginal infections to consider include vulvovaginal candidiasis, trichomoniasis, bacterial vaginosis, herpes simplex virus, and human papillomavirus (refer to Chapters 21 and 22). Dermatologic disorders that can cause pain with intercourse include lichen sclerosus, lichen planus, and lichen simplex chronicus (Hill & Taylor, 2021). Vulvar colposcopy and a punch biopsy may be indicated to properly diagnose any suspicious lesions or chronic skin conditions (refer to Chapter 27).

Individuals who are perimenopausal, postmenopausal, on long-term hormonal contraceptives, or lactating should be evaluated for atrophic changes to the vulvovaginal tissue (refer to Chapters 14 and 21). Genitourinary syndrome of menopause (GSM) is the term endorsed by ISSWSH and the North American Menopause Society to replace the terms vulvovaginal atrophy and atrophic vaginitis in premenopausal and postmenopausal individuals (NAMS, 2020; Parish et al., 2021a). GSM more appropriately describes the condition as a syndrome and acknowledges that it affects the entire urogenital tract. The use of certain medications, including tamoxifen, danazol, medroxyprogesterone acetate, and GnRH agonists, can result in GSM-like changes. Physical examination may demonstrate pale and dry vaginal walls with decreased rugae, vulvar fissures, petechiae, and loss of vulvar architecture. In addition, vaginal pH is typically greater than 5.0 in individuals with GSM (NAMS, 2020).

If the individual is using a latex barrier method for contraception, it is important to consider a latex allergy as the source of the pain. Although the condition is rare, some individuals are sensitive to human semen due to seminal fluid proteins. An individual with semen hypersensitivity can demonstrate localized vaginal symptoms after intercourse that include burning, vulvar pruritus, edema, and general discomfort and may also present with systemic symptoms of diffuse urticaria, angioedema, and malaise (Didziokaite et al., 2024). If the clinician suspects an individual has a seminal fluid allergy, and use of latex condoms does not alleviate symptoms, the person should be assessed for a concurrent latex allergy.

Individuals who report persistent vulvar pain or inability to achieve vaginal penetration secondary to pain should be evaluated for vulvodynia. Many of these individuals will describe experiencing pain while attempting to insert tampons prior to their first intercourse, but this condition can also develop in an individual with no previous vulvar pain. Individuals with chronic vulvar pain should also be assessed for mood disorders as there appears to be a correlation with anxiety and mood disorders with vulvodynia (Santangelo et al., 2023). Additionally, individuals should be screened for pain that began while on a combined oral contraceptive pill, allergic reactions, or chronic vaginal infections as well as signs of pelvic floor dysfunction like urinary urgency/frequency, incomplete bladder emptying, or constipation, which could be indicative of a hypertonic pelvic floor. To evaluate a person for vulvodynia, a detailed gynecologic examination of the vulvar anatomy should be performed using the cotton swab test to assess for pain. During this test, a cotton swab is used to palpate multiple different areas of the vulva. In patients with vulvodynia, they will often describe a sharp or burning sensation when certain areas of the vulva are lightly touched with the swab and if so, the pain is recorded on a numeric scale of 0–10 (Schlaeger et al., 2023). It is important for clinicians to understand that vulvodynia is generally the result of a multifactorial process and therefore obtaining a thorough history that helps to consider the 11 descriptors of vulvodynia described in **Box 18-4** will allow the clinician to work with the individual in helping to create a personalized treatment strategy (Santangelo et al., 2023).

An individual with vaginal pain or pain after vaginal intercourse should be evaluated for chronic vaginitis, atrophic vaginitis, and allergy. Trauma related to episiotomy or birth-related perineal lacerations may also be a source of sexual pain, with pressure during intercourse placed on the perineum or the outer third of the vagina. Deep pelvic pain or pain with thrusting may be caused by adenomyosis, endometriosis, pelvic adhesions, or adnexal pain (refer to Chapters 27 and 29). Nongynecologic etiologies (e.g., Crohn's disease, irritable bowel syndrome, painful bladder syndrome, and interstitial cystitis) can also cause deep pelvic pain (Hill & Taylor, 2021). Trying to reproduce the pain during pelvic examination may give an indication of the source of the pain, with attention to using a trauma-informed approach if this is attempted.

Management of Genitopelvic Pain

Treatment of GPDD depends on the etiology of the pain. Vaginal infections should be treated with appropriate antibiotic or antifungal medication. Dermatologic disorders of the genital area are often treated with topical corticosteroids (refer to Chapter 27). Clinicians should consider performing a vulvar biopsy to confirm the diagnosis before prescribing topical corticosteroids (Hill & Taylor, 2021).

A variety of vaginal estrogen preparations are available to treat perimenopausal and postmenopausal individuals with GSM (refer to Chapter 14). These products can also be used off label for short-term therapy in postpartum individuals with atrophic urogenital changes and in people with hypoestrogenic states due to various gynecologic conditions. Individuals who dislike the discharge associated with vaginal estrogen creams often prefer to use the vaginal tablets or ring.

Individuals who prefer to avoid hormonal medications or who are not candidates for vaginal estrogen can consider ospemifene, an FDA-approved, nonhormonal, selective estrogen receptor modulator (SERM). It is the only available product that is taken orally and approved for the treatment of vaginal dryness as well as moderate to severe dyspareunia. Prasterone, a nonhormonal vaginal insert used daily is approved for the treatment of moderate to severe dyspareunia in menopause and it utilizes the individual's own enzymatic pathway to convert the inactive steroid into estradiol and testosterone via intracellular metabolism (NAMS, 2020; Schlaeger et al., 2023). Fractional CO_2 vaginal laser treatments stimulate healthy collagen production and may improve symptoms of GSM, including vaginal dryness, itching, burning, and pain (NAMS, 2020). Additional studies support the potential use of fractional CO_2 laser therapy for postpartum perineal pain, vestibulodynia, and lichen sclerosus (Salgado et al., 2023; Filippini et al., 2019; Goldstein et al., 2023).

BOX 18-4 Vulvodynia Classification Chart

Descriptor	Definition	Notes
Location		
Localized	Pain involves a specific area of the vulva.	Pain is more likely to be provoked and typically affects the vestibule (Vestibulodynia) or clitoris (Clitorodynia).
Generalized	Pain involves the whole vulva.	Pain is more likely to be spontaneous and constant.
Provocation		
Provoked	Pain is triggered by physical contact.	May include sexual and nonsexual activities. For example, vaginal penetration, tight clothing, tampon insertion, cotton-tipped applicator pressure, fingertip pressure, prolonged sitting, etc.
Spontaneous	Pain occurs without any physical contact.	Pain arises without an identifiable trigger.
Onset		
Primary	Pain begins with the first instance of provoking contact.	Examples include pain during initial vaginal penetration from tampon insertion or intercourse.
Secondary	Pain develops after initially experiencing pain-free contact for a period of time.	Examples include pain with tampon insertion or intercourse after previously not experiencing pain.
Temporal Pattern		
Persistent	The pain lasts for at least 3 months.	The pain can be constant or intermittent.
Constant	Pain is always present.	Pain is continuous without relief/relapse in symptoms.
Intermittent	Pain occurs sporadically.	Pain is not always present and comes and goes at various times.
Immediate	Pain occurs with physical contact.	Pain is experienced during a provoking activity.
Delayed	Pain occurs after provoking physical contact.	Pain can develop minutes to hours following the provoking activity.

Data from American College of Obstetricians and Gynecologists. (2016, reaffirmed 2024). Persistent vulvar pain. ACOG committee opinion no. 673. *Obstetrics & Gynecology, 128*(3), p e78-e84, https://doi.org/10.1097/AOG.0000000000001645; Bornstein, J., Preti, M., Simon, J. A., As-Sanie, S., Stockdale, C. K., Stein, A., Parish, S. J., Radici, G., Vieira-Baptista, P., Pukall, C., Moyal-Barracco, M., Goldstein, A., & International Society for the Study of Vulvovaginal Disease (ISSVD), the International Society for the Study of Women's Sexual Health (ISSWSH), and the International Pelvic Pain Society (IPPS). (2019). Descriptors of vulvodynia: A multisocietal definition consensus (International Society for the Study of Vulvovaginal Disease, the International Society for the Study of Women Sexual Health, and the International Pelvic Pain Society). *Journal of Lower Genital Tract Disease, 23*(2), 161–163. https://doi.org/10.1097/LGT.0000000000000461; National Vulvodynia Association. (n.d.). *Definition and types of vulvodynia*. National Vulvodynia Association. Retrieved October 26, 2025 from https://www.nva.org/learnpatient/definition-and-types-of-vulvodynia/

Individuals with vulvodynia, including vestibulodynia, should wear cotton underwear and avoid common irritants to the vulvar area, such as glycerin-based lubricants, scented panty liners, and harsh soaps (Hill & Taylor, 2021). In addition, individuals with vulvar sensitivities should be encouraged to avoid self-treatment for perceived, undiagnosed infections. Multidisciplinary care can be particularly valuable for individuals with vulvodynia (Rains et al., 2024). Effective nonpharmacologic treatment modalities include pelvic floor physical therapy and cognitive behavioral therapy (Guillet et al., 2019; Morin et al., 2021). Likewise, acupuncture can be helpful for some individuals afflicted with vulvodynia (Schlager et al., 2022). Pharmacologic therapy options include topical lidocaine, oral antidepressants (e.g., tricyclics, SSRIs, SNRIs), and oral anticonvulsants (e.g., gabapentin, pregabalin); a variety of topical compounded therapies are used as well and include the off-label use of vaginal diazepam as well as vaginal hormonal methods (Santangelo et al., 2023). Botulinum toxin type A injections as well as low-molecular-weight-heparin have been considered as treatment options for vulvodynia (Schlager et al., 2022). Additionally, cannabis may play a role in pain management though further research is needed to understand the safety and efficacy of this approach (Barach et al., 2020). For individuals who do not obtain relief with nonpharmacologic, pharmacologic, or complementary and alternative therapies, surgical removal of the vestibule (modified vestibulectomy) can provide long-term pain relief (David & Bornstein, 2020). Due to the unknown etiology of vulvodynia, developing an effective treatment strategy for patients can present a challenge. There are many treatment options available; however, evidence is limited as to what the best course of action for treatment is. Working with patients collaboratively to obtain relief from symptoms is a place to start but clinicians need to advocate for further research to better understand the etiology of vulvodynia and rigorous controlled trials are needed to identify the most effective treatments for managing this complex condition (Schlager et al., 2022).

Treatment for pelvic pain with penetrative intercourse will depend on the source of the pain. Many individuals report feeling periodic sharp deep pain when their partner thrusts during intercourse or with use of penetrative sexual devices. This pain is often the result of the penis, fingers, or sex toys brushing against an ovary or the cervix. Teaching the individual to shift the position of their hips to change the angle of the uterus and ovaries may help to alleviate this type of pelvic pain. Individuals with pelvic infections, suspected or confirmed endometriosis, and vulvodynia should receive appropriate treatment to remedy these conditions. Pelvic floor physical therapy that includes dilators, EMG biofeedback, as well as TENS may also be beneficial in reducing pelvic pain by utilizing various modalities including stretching, massaging, dry needling, and deep diaphragmatic breathing techniques (Fernandez-Perez et al., 2023). A systematic review determined intravaginal, compounded diazepam vaginal suppositories can serve as an adjunctive treatment for high-tone pelvic floor dysfunction though more and larger studies are needed to confirm these potential effects (Stone et al., 2020). Additional information about treating pelvic pain can be found in Chapter 29.

REFERRAL TO THERAPISTS SPECIALIZING IN SEXUAL DYSFUNCTION

Clinicians who see individuals with sexual dysfunction should be aware of the counseling resources available in their communities. Circumstances that warrant referral to a therapist include, but are not limited to, long-standing dysfunction, multiple dysfunctions, history of sexual abuse, psychological disorder or acute psychological event, dysfunction with an unknown etiology, dysfunction that does not respond to therapy, poor relationship status, and negative portrayal of sex from parents as a child. The American Association of Sexuality Educators, Counselors and Therapists (AASECT) is a national organization that provides certification for sex therapists and sexuality counselors. Sex therapists are mental health professionals with specialized training in psychotherapy for sexual health and dysfunction. Sexuality counselors include individuals from a variety of professions who have advanced training in human sexuality. The AASECT website (https://www.aasect.org/) can help clinicians locate a certified sex therapist in their community.

In addition to mental health services, physical therapy should be considered for patients reporting sexual pain. APTA Pelvic Health, an academy of the American Physical Therapy Association (https://www.aptapelvichealth.org/ptlocator), can direct providers to local physical therapists who specialize in pelvic floor physical therapy.

CONCLUSION

Alterations in sexual function among women and those assigned female at birth are common, but fortunately knowledge and understanding of these conditions continue to grow. More research and clinician education are necessary to provide high-quality patient-centered care. In this, as in other evolving areas of health care, it is important for clinicians to stay up to date with new screening and treatment options.

References

Alidost, F., Pakzad, R., Dolatian, M., & Abdi, F. (2021). Sexual dysfunction among women of reproductive age: A systematic review and meta-analysis. *International Journal of Reproductive Biomedicine, 19*(5), 421–432. https://doi.org/10.18502/ijrm.v19i5.9251

American College of Obstetricians and Gynecologists. (2019). Female sexual dysfunction. ACOG practice bulletin no. 213. *Obstetrics & Gynecology, 134*(1), e1–e18.

American Psychiatric Association. (2022). *Diagnostic and statistical manual of mental disorders* (5th ed., text revision).

Barach, E., Slavin, M. N., & Earleywine, M. (2020). Cannabis and vulvodynia symptoms: A preliminary report. *Cannabis, 3*(2), 139–147. https://doi.org/10.26828/cannabis.2020.02.001

Barakeh, D., Mdaihly, H., & Karaoui, L. R. (2024). Pharmacotherapy of hypoactive sexual desire disorder in premenopausal women. *The Annals of Pharmacotherapy*, 10600280241253273. Advance online publication. https://doi.org/10.1177/10600280241253273

Basson, R. (2000). The female sexual response: A different model. *Journal of Sex and Marital Therapy, 26*, 51–65.

Bloemers, J., Gerritsen, J., van Rooij, K., de Leede, L., van der Geest, R., Frijlink, H. W., Koppeschaar, H. P. F., Olivier, B., & Tuiten, A. (2019). The effect of food on the pharmacokinetics of sildenafil after single administration of a sublingual testosterone and oral sildenafil combination tablet in healthy female subjects. *The Journal of Sexual Medicine, 16*(9), 1433–1443. https://doi.org/10.1016/j.jsxm.2019.06.015

Bornstein, J., Preti, M., Simon, J. A., As-Sanie, S., Stockdale, C. K., Stein, A., Parish, S. J., Radici, G., Vieira-Baptista, P., Pukall, C., Moyal-Barracco, M., Goldstein, A., & International Society for the Study of Vulvovaginal Disease (ISSVD), the International Society for the Study of Women's Sexual Health (ISSWSH), and the International Pelvic Pain Society (IPPS). (2019). Descriptors of vulvodynia: A multisocietal definition consensus (International Society for the Study of Vulvovaginal Disease, the International Society for the Study of Women Sexual Health, and the International Pelvic Pain Society). *Journal of Lower Genital Tract Disease, 23*(2), 161–163. https://doi.org/10.1097/LGT.0000000000000461

Christmas, M. M., & Reed, S. (2024). Sexual dysfunction after menopause: Guidelines for assessment and management. *Obstetrics and Gynecology Clinics of North America, 51*(2), 341–364. https://doi.org/10.1016/j.ogc.2024.02.007

Clayton, A. H., Goldstein, I., Kim, N. N., Althof, S. E., Faubion, S. S., Faught, B. M., Parish, S. L., Simon, J. A., Vignozzi, L., Christiansen, K., Davis, S. R., Freedman, M. A., Kingsberg, S. A., Kirana, P. S., Larkin, L., McCabe, M., & Sadovsky, R. (2018). The International Society for the Study of Women's Sexual Health process of care for management of hypoactive sexual desire disorder in women. *Mayo Clinic Proceedings, 93*(4), 467–487. https://doi.org/10.1016/j.mayocp.2017.11.002

David, A., & Bornstein, J. (2020). Evaluation of long-term surgical success and satisfaction of patients after vestibulectomy. *Journal of Lower Genital Tract Disease, 24*(4), 399–404. https://doi.org/10.1097/LGT.0000000000000552

Davis, S. R., Baber, R., Panay, N., Bitzer, J., Perez, S. C., Islam, R. M., Kaunitz, A. M., Kingsberg, S. A., Lambrinoudaki, I., Liu, J., Parish, S. J., Pinkerton, J., Rymer, J., Simon, J. A., Vignozzi, L., & Wierman, M. E. (2019). Global consensus position statement on the use of testosterone therapy for women. *The Journal of Clinical Endocrinology & Metabolism, 104*(10), 4660–4666.

Didziokaite, G., Kuznecovaite, A., Biliute, G., & Kvedariene, V. (2024). Case report: Human seminal plasma allergy diagnosis for a woman with unexplained infertility. *Frontiers in Medicine, 11*, 1403477. https://doi.org/10.3389/fmed.2024.1403477

Fernández-Pérez, P., Leirós-Rodríguez, R., Marqués-Sánchez, M. P., Martínez-Fernández, M. C., de Carvalho, F. O., & Maciel, L. Y. S. (2023). Effectiveness of physical therapy interventions in women with dyspareunia: A systematic review and meta-analysis. *BMC Women's Health, 23*(1), 387. https://doi.org/10.1186/s12905-023-02532-8

Filippini, M., Farinelli, M., Lopez, S., Ettore, C., Gulino, F. A., & Capriglione, S. (2019). Postpartum perineal pain: May the vaginal treatment with CO_2 laser play a key role in this challenging issue? *The Journal of Maternal-Fetal & Neonatal Medicine*. Advance online publication. https://doi.org/10.1080/14767058.2019.1628208

García-Duarte, S., Nievas-Soriano, B. J., Fischer-Suárez, N., Castro-Luna, G., Parrón-Carreño, T., & Aguilera-Manrique, G. (2023). Quality of sexuality during pregnancy: We must do something—Survey study. *International Journal of Environmental Research and Public Health, 20*(2), 965. https://doi.org/10.3390/ijerph20020965

Gerritsen, J., Bloemers, J., van Rooij, K., de Leede, L., van der Geest, R., Frijlink, H. W., Koppeschaar, H. P. F., Olivier, B., & Tuiten, A. (2020). The effect of food on the pharmacokinetics of buspirone after single administration of a sublingual testosterone and oral buspirone combination tablet in healthy female subjects. *Sexual Medicine, 8*(2), 186–194. https://doi.org/10.1016/j.esxm.2020.01.005

Gieles, N. C., van de Grift, T. C., Elaut, E., Heylens, G., Becker-Hebly, I., Nieder, T. O., Laan, E. T. M., & Kreukels, B. P. C. (2023). Pleasure please! Sexual pleasure and influencing factors in transgender persons: An ENIGI follow-up study. *International Journal of Transgender Health, 24*(2), 212–223. https://doi.org/10.1080/26895269.2022.2028693

Goldstein, S. W., Goldstein, I., Kim, N. N., Kellogg-Spadt, S., & Murina, F. (2023). Safety and efficacy of fractional CO_2 laser treatment to the vestibule: A randomized, double-blind, sham-controlled, prospective 3-site clinical study in women with vestibular pain. *The Journal of Sexual Medicine, 20*(6), 800–812. https://doi.org/10.1093/jsxmed/qdac053

Guillet, A. D., Cirino, N. H., Hart, K. D., & Leclair, C. M. (2019). Mindfulness-based group cognitive behavior therapy for provoked localized vulvodynia: A randomized controlled trial. *Journal of Lower Genital Tract Disease, 23*(2), 170–175. https://doi.org/10.1097/LGT.0000000000000456

Guz, S., Hecht, H. K., Kattari, S. K., Gross, E. B., & Ross, E. (2022). A scoping review of empirical sexuality research in social science literature. *Archives of Sexual Behavior, 51*(4), 2135–2145. https://doi.org/10.1007/s10508-022-02307-6

Heiman, J. R., & Lopiccolo, J. (1988). *Becoming orgasmic.* Simon & Schuster.

Hill, D. A., & Taylor, C. A. (2021). Dyspareunia in women. *American Family Physician, 103*(10), 597–604.

Islam, R. M., Bell, R. J., Green, S., Page, M. J., & Davis, S. R. (2019). Safety and efficacy of testosterone for women: A systematic review and meta-analysis of randomised controlled trial data. *The Lancet: Diabetes & Endocrinology, 7*(10), 754–766. https://doi.org/10.1016/S2213-8587(19)30189-5

Johnson, I., Thurman, A. R., Cornell, K. A., Hatheway, J., Dart, C., Brainard, C. P., Friend, D. R., & Goldstein, A. (2024). Preliminary efficacy of topical Sildenafil cream for the treatment of female sexual arousal disorder: A randomized controlled trial. *Obstetrics and Gynecology, 144*(2), 144–152. https://doi.org/10.1097/AOG.0000000000005648

Kaplan, H. (1979). *Disorders of sexual desire.* Brunner/Mazel.

Kingsberg, S. A., Clayton, A. H., Portman, D., Williams, L. A., Krop, J., Jordan, R., Lucas, J., & Simon, J. A. (2019). Bremelanotide for the treatment of hypoactive sexual desire disorder: Two randomized phase 3 trials. *Obstetrics & Gynecology, 134*(5), 899–908. https://doi.org/10.1097/AOG.0000000000003500

Kinsey, A. (1953). *Sexual behavior in the human female.* W. B. Saunders.

Laumann, E. O., Paik, A., & Rosen, R. C. (1999). Sexual dysfunction in the United States: Prevalence and predictors. *Journal of the American Medical Association, 281*(6), 537–544. https://www.ncbi.nlm.nih.gov/pubmed/10022110

Lee, J. H., Lee, J. E., Harsh, V., & Clayton, A. H. (2022). Pharmacotherapy for sexual dysfunction in women. *Current Psychiatry Reports, 24*(2), 99–109. https://doi.org/10.1007/s11920-022-01322-7

Leeners, B., Tschudin, S., Wischmann, T., & Kalaitzopoulos, D. R. (2023). Sexual dysfunction and disorders as a consequence of infertility: A systematic review and meta-analysis. *Human Reproduction Update, 29*(1), 95–125. https://doi.org/10.1093/humupd/dmac030

Lyons, H. A., Warner, D. F., & Orbuch, T. L. (2024). Sexual expression and subsequent marital quality among partnered older adults. *Archives of Sexual Behavior*, 10.1007/s10508-024-02956-9. Advance online publication. https://doi.org/10.1007/s10508-024-02956-9

Maseroli, E., & Vignozzi, L. (2022). Are endogenous androgens linked to female sexual function? A systemic review and meta-analysis. *The Journal of Sexual Medicine, 19*(4), 553–568. https://doi.org/10.1016/j.jsxm.2022.01.515

Masters, W., & Johnson, V. (1966). *Human sexual response.* Little, Brown.

Masters, W. & Johnson, V. (1970). *Human sexual inadequacy.* Little, Brown.

Millheiser, L., Clayton, A. H., Parish, S. J., Kingsberg, S. A., Kim, N. N., & Simon, J. A. (2019). Safety and tolerability of evening ethanol consumption and bedtime administration of flibanserin in healthy premenopausal female subjects. *Sexual Medicine, 7*(4), 418–424. https://doi.org/10.1016/j.esxm.2019.08.003

Morin, M., Dumoulin, C., Bergeron, S., Mayrand, M. H., Khalifé, S., Waddell, G., Dubois, M. F., & PVD Study Group (2021). Multimodal physical therapy versus topical lidocaine for provoked vestibulodynia: A multicenter, randomized trial. *American Journal of Obstetrics and Gynecology, 224*(2), 189.e1–189.e12. https://doi.org/10.1016/j.ajog.2020.08.038

Nappi, R. E., Tiranini, L., Martini, E., Bosoni, D., Righi, A., & Cucinella, L. (2022). Medical treatment of female sexual dysfunction. *The Urologic Clinics of North America, 49*(2), 299–307. https://doi.org/10.1016/j.ucl.2022.02.001

North American Menopause Society (NAMS) GSM Position Statement Editorial Panel. (2020). The 2020 genitourinary syndrome of menopause position statement of The North American Menopause Society. *Menopause, 27*(9), 976–992. https://doi.org/10.1097/GME.0000000000001609

Pachano Pesantez, G. S., & Clayton, A. H. (2021). Treatment of hypoactive sexual desire disorder among women: General considerations and pharmacological options. *Focus (American Psychiatric Publishing), 19*(1), 39–45. https://doi.org/10.1176/appi.focus.20200039

Parish, S. J., Cottler-Casanova, S., Clayton, A. H., McCabe, M. P., Coleman, E., & Reed, G. M. (2021a). The evolution of the female sexual disorder/dysfunction definitions, nomenclature, and classifications: A review of DSM, ICSM, ISSWSH, and ICD. *Sexual Medicine Reviews, 9*(1), 36–56. https://doi.org/10.1016/j.sxmr.2020.05.001

Parish, S. J., Hahn, S. R., Goldstein, S. W., Giraldi, A., Kingsberg, S. A., Larkin, L., Minkin, M. J., Brown, V., Christiansen, K., Hartzell-Cushanick, R., Kelly-Jones, A., Rullo, J., Sadovsky, R., & Faubion, S. S. (2019). The International Society for the Study of Women's Sexual Health process of care for the identification of sexual concerns and problems in women. *Mayo Clinic Proceedings, 94*(5), 842–856. https://doi.org/10.1016/j.mayocp.2019.01.009

Parish, S. J., Simon, J. A., Davis, S. R., Giraldi, A., Goldstein, I., Goldstein, S. W., Kim, N. N., Kingsberg, S. A., Morgentaler, A., Nappi, R. E., Park, K., Stuenkel, C. A., Traish, A. M., & Vignozzi, L. (2021b). International society for the study of women's sexual health clinical practice guideline for the use of systemic testosterone for hypoactive sexual desire disorder in women. *Journal of Women's Health (2002), 30*(4), 474–491. https://doi.org/10.1089/jwh.2021.29037

Pyke, R. E., & Clayton, A. H. (2019). Dose-finding study of Lorexys for hypoactive sexual desire disorder in premenopausal women. *The Journal of Sexual Medicine, 16*(12), 1885–1894. https://doi.org/10.1016/j.jsxm.2019.09.005

Rains, A., Bajzak, K., Miller, M. E., Swab, M., Logan, G. S., Jackman, V. A., & Gustafson, D. L. (2024). Multimodal and interdisciplinary interventions for the treatment of localized provoked vulvodynia: A scoping review of the literature from 2010 to 2023. *International Journal of Women's Health, 16*, 55–94. https://doi.org/10.2147/IJWH.S436222

Reed, M. A. (2022). Female sexual dysfunction. *Clinics in Plastic Surgery, 49*(4), 495–504. https://doi.org/10.1016/j.cps.2022.06.009

Reis, J., de Oliveira, L., de Oliveira, C., & Nobre, P. (2021). Psychosocial and behavioral aspects of women's sexual pleasure: A scoping review. *International Journal of Sexual Health: Official Journal of the World Association for Sexual Health, 33*(4), 494–515. https://doi.org/10.1080/19317611.2021.1910890

Rojas-Zambrano, J. G., & Rojas-Zambrano, A. R. (2024). Effects of testosterone hormone on the sexual aspect of postmenopausal women: A systematic review. *Cureus, 16*(8), e68046. https://doi.org/10.7759/cureus.68046

Rothmore J. (2020). Antidepressant-induced sexual dysfunction. *The Medical Journal of Australia, 212*(7), 329–334. https://doi.org/10.5694/mja2.50522

Rowland, D., Donarski, A., Graves, V., Caldwell, C., Hevesi, B., & Hevesi, K. (2019). The experience of orgasmic pleasure during partnered and masturbatory sex in women with and without orgasmic difficulty. *Journal of Sex & Marital Therapy, 45*(6), 550–561. https://doi.org/10.1080/0092623X.2019.1586021

Rubin, E. S., Deshpande, N. A., Vasquez, P. J., & Spadt, S. K. (2019). A clinical reference guide on sexual devices for obstetrician-gynecologists. *Obstetrics & Gynecology, 133*(6), 1259–1268.

Salgado, H. C., Drumond, D. G., Pannain, G. D., de Melo E Costa, L. G., Sampaio, F. S., & Leite, I. C. G. (2023). Randomized clinical trial with fractional CO_2 laser and Clobetasol in the treatment of vulvar lichen sclerosus: A clinic study of feasibility. *BMC Research Notes, 16*(1), 33. https://doi.org/10.1186/s13104-023-06300-7

Santangelo, G., Ruggiero, G., Murina, F., Di Donato, V., Perniola, G., Palaia, I., Fischetti, M., Casorelli, A., Giannini, A., Di Dio, C., Muzii, L., Benedetti Panici, P., & Bogani, G. (2023). Vulvodynia: A practical guide in treatment strategies. *International Journal of Gynaecology and Obstetrics: The Official Organ of the International Federation of Gynaecology and Obstetrics, 163*(2), 510–520. https://doi.org/10.1002/ijgo.14815

Santos Silva, I. M., Paula Pinto, M., & Gonçalves, D. (2022). Educational programs and sexual counselling for postmenopausal sexual dysfunction: A systematic review and meta-analysis. *The Journal of Sexual Medicine, 19*(1), 54–63. https://doi.org/10.1016/j.jsxm.2021.09.017

Scavello, I., Maseroli, E., Di Stasi, V., & Vignozzi, L. (2019). Sexual health in menopause. *Medicina (Kaunas, Lithuania), 55*(9), 559. https://doi.org/10.3390/medicina55090559

Schlaeger, J. M., Glayzer, J. E., Villegas-Downs, M., Li, H., Glayzer, E. J., He, Y., Takayama, M., Yajima, H., Takakura, N., Kobak, W. H., & McFarlin, B. L. (2023). Evaluation and treatment of vulvodynia: State of the science. *Journal of Midwifery & Women's Health, 68*(1), 9–34. https://doi.org/10.1111/jmwh.13456

Schlaeger, J. M., Suarez, M. L., Glayzer, J. E., Kobak, W. H., Meinel, M., Steffen, A. D., Burke, L. A., Pauls, H. A., Yao, Y., Takayama, M., Yajima, H., Kaptchuk, T. J., Takakura, N., Foster, D., & Wilkie, D. J. (2022). Protocol for double-blind RCT of acupuncture for vulvodynia. *Contemporary Clinical Trials Communications, 30*, 101029. https://doi.org/10.1016/j.conctc.2022.101029

Sharifipour, F., Qaderi, K., Peighambardoost, R., Zahedian, M., Azizi, F., & Faal Siahkal, S. (2024). Impact of cognitive behavior therapy on sexual dysfunction of women in reproductive age: A systematic review. *International Journal of Sexual Health: Official Journal of the World Association for Sexual Health, 36*(3), 287–301. https://doi.org/10.1080/19317611.2024.2360731

Shifren, J. L., Monz, B. U., Russo, P. A., Segreti, A., & Johannes, C. B. (2008). Sexual problems and distress in United States women: Prevalence and correlates. *Obstetrics & Gynecology, 112*(5), 970–978. https://doi.org/10.1097/AOG.0b013e3181898cdb

Simon, J., Kingsberg, S., Portman, D., Williams, L. A., Krop, J., Jordan, R., Lucas, J., & Clayton, A. H. (2019). Long-term safety and efficacy of bremelanotide for hypoactive sexual desire disorder. *Obstetrics & Gynecology, 134*(5), 909–917. https://doi.org/10.1097/AOG.0000000000003514

Simon, J. A., Clayton, A. H., Parish, S. J., Apfel, S. C., & Millheiser, L. (2020). Effects of alcohol administered with flibanserin in healthy premenopausal women: A randomized, double-blind, single-dose crossover study. *The Journal of Sexual Medicine, 17*(1), 83–93. https://doi.org/10.1016/j.jsxm.2019.10.004

Simon, J. A., Kingsberg, S. A., Shumel, B., Hanes, V., Garcia, M., Jr., & Sand, M. (2014). Efficacy and safety of flibanserin in postmenopausal women with hypoactive sexual desire disorder: Results of the SNOWDROP trial. *Menopause* (New York, N.Y.), *21*(6), 633–640. https://doi.org/10.1097/GME.0000000000000134

Smetanina, D., Awar, S. A., Khair, H., Alkaabi, M., Das, K. M., Ljubisavljevic, M., Statsenko, Y., & Zaręba, K. T. (2023). Risk of sexual dysfunctions in breastfeeding females: Protocol for a systematic review and meta-analysis. *BMJ Open, 13*(8), e074630. https://doi.org/10.1136/bmjopen-2023-074630

Stafne, S. N., Ulven, S. K. S., Prøsch-Bilden, T., & Saga, S. (2024). Pelvic floor disorders and impact on sexual function: A cross-sectional study among non-sexually active and sexually active women. *Sexual Medicine, 12*(2), qfae024. https://doi.org/10.1093/sexmed/qfae024

Stone, R. H., Abousaud, M., Abousaud, A., & Kobak, W. (2020). A systematic review of intravaginal diazepam for the treatment of pelvic floor hypertonic disorder. *Journal of Clinical Pharmacology, 60*(Suppl 2), S110–S120. https://doi.org/10.1002/jcph.1775

Thurman, A. R., Johnson, I., Cornell, K. A., Hatheway, J., Kim, N. N., Parish, S. J., Dart, C., Friend, D. R., & Goldstein, A. (2024). Safety of topical sildenafil cream, 3.6% in a randomized, placebo-controlled trial for the treatment of female sexual arousal disorder. *The Journal of Sexual Medicine, 21*(9), 793–799. https://doi.org/10.1093/jsxmed/qdae089

Uloko, M., Rahman, F., Puri, L. I., & Rubin, R. S. (2022). The clinical management of testosterone replacement therapy in postmenopausal women with hypoactive sexual desire disorder: A review. *International Journal of Impotence Research, 34*(7), 635–641. https://doi.org/10.1038/s41443-022-00613-0

Vowels, L. M., & Mark, K. P. (2020). Strategies for mitigating sexual desire discrepancy in relationships. *Archives of Sexual Behavior, 49*(3), 1017–1028. https://doi.org/10.1007/s10508-020-01640-y

Weinberger, J. M., Houman, J., Caron, A. T., & Anger, J. (2019). Female sexual dysfunction: A systematic review of outcomes across various treatment modalities. *Sexual Medicine Reviews, 7*(2), 223–250. https://doi.org/10.1016/j.sxmr.2017.12.004

Zheng, J., Skiba, M. A., Bell, R. J., Islam, R. M., & Davis, S. R. (2020). The prevalence of sexual dysfunctions and sexually related distress in young women: A cross-sectional survey. *Fertility and Sterility, 113*(2), 426–434. https://doi.org/10.1016/j.fertnstert.2019.09.027

CHAPTER 19

Pregnancy Diagnosis, Decision-Making Support, and Management of Abortion and Early Pregnancy Loss

Meghan Eagen-Torkko

Molly R. Altman

The editors acknowledge Katherine Simmonds, Frances E. Likis, and Julia Phillippi, who were authors of the previous edition of this chapter.

In the United States, approximately 6 million people become pregnant each year (Guttmacher, 2025a). Almost half of all pregnancies in the United States are unintended, unwanted, or mistimed (Bearak et al., 2022) and approximately 15–20 percent of clinically recognized pregnancies will spontaneously end (Quenby et al., 2021). At least one in four pregnancy-capable people in the United States will intentionally end a pregnancy in their lifetime (Jones & Jerman, 2022). While this number has been dropping for a number of years, prevalence has been increasing since the 2022 *Dobbs v. Jackson Women's Health* decision by the U.S. Supreme Court (Jones & Remez, 2024).

In the United States in particular, "abortion" is used in general discussion to refer to the intentional termination of a pregnancy in any trimester. However, "abortion" in health care refers to the ending of a pregnancy, from whatever cause, prior to 20 weeks from the last menstrual period. This complication in terminology has led to a situation in which management of intentional termination of pregnancy is seen as separate from that of spontaneous termination of pregnancy (i.e., early pregnancy loss, spontaneous abortion, miscarriage), and where people experiencing this management may not even realize that their care is clinically indistinguishable from intentional termination of pregnancy. Because of this, researchers recommend the use of "medication abortion" and "procedural abortion" to describe the mechanisms by which pregnancies may be completed, either intentionally or to resolve a spontaneous pregnancy loss, and that the word "abortion" be used to apply to all pregnancies that are terminated, whether intentionally or not (Upadhyay et al., 2023). This terminology is used throughout this chapter.

Clinicians who provide care to people of reproductive age are likely to encounter individuals who are pregnant as part of their clinical practice, in settings ranging from primary care to emergency departments to specialty sites. Pregnancy-related health care begins under a variety of circumstances. Some people visit a healthcare provider to confirm pregnancy or to receive education and support about their options. Others seek care only after deciding whether to continue or end a pregnancy. Individuals may also not realize they are pregnant until receiving a pregnancy diagnosis during a healthcare visit for another reason. After a person knows they are pregnant, they need to consider their options and decide whether to proceed with parenting, an abortion, or making an adoption plan. They may revisit this plan after obtaining fetal testing results or if their health or circumstances change. This chapter discusses the roles and responsibilities of clinicians in providing appropriate, safe, quality care to individuals across this pregnancy diagnosis, decision making, and management continuum.

CLINICAL AND ETHICAL COMPETENCE IN PREGNANCY-RELATED CARE

Historically, the concept of intention has been central to pregnancy discourse, including in previous editions of this chapter. More recently, there has been recognition of pregnancy intention as a population-level scientific construct that has limited applicability to individual-level patient care. Pregnancy intention does not necessarily predict a person's reaction to a pregnancy diagnosis or their decision about its resolution. For example, a person who did not intentionally become pregnant may be quite happy about the diagnosis and decide to continue the pregnancy and become a parent. In this chapter, we have shifted the focus from pregnancy intention preceding diagnosis to pregnancy diagnosis as a time of decision making that may require support and education from a clinician.

Providing any type of pregnancy-related care requires clinical competence and ethical conduct. Interprofessional core competencies for pregnancy-related care include (1) detecting pregnancy by using diagnostics appropriately; (2) providing patient-centered pregnancy options counseling that includes parenting, adoption, and abortion; (3) providing abortion screening, counseling, referrals, and aftercare; and (4) knowing relevant federal and state laws (Cappiello et al., 2016). Beyond these specific responsibilities, clinicians have an ethical duty to uphold patients' rights to autonomy and dignity in all stages of the process, from pregnancy diagnosis to resolution, across all potential outcomes.

Professional organizations have established ethical codes to guide health professionals in providing sound clinical care to patients, including when circumstances are morally complex. The American Nurses Association mandates that all nurses, including advanced practice registered nurses (APRNs), "practice with compassion and respect for the inherent dignity, worth, and uniqueness attributes of every person" (2025, Provision 1). This code applies to all clinical care, including those who present during the pregnancy discovery and resolution process.

The organizational statements in **Box 19-1** provide ethical and legal bases to ensure patient access to comprehensive reproductive health services, including pregnancy options counseling.

Professional Responsibilities

Providing care to individuals who are in the process of pregnancy diagnosis, decision making, or resolution includes allowing them to express their concerns, desires, and need for additional information in an environment that is free of judgment and stigma. Values clarification is a recommended practice for clinicians to explore the intersection of their personal beliefs and professional responsibilities to ensure patients' rights are upheld (Simmonds & Likis, 2011).

Although the clinical process to end a pregnancy, whether voluntary or spontaneous, is often the same, the experience of the pregnant person and those around them can be very different. Emotional and social responses to both spontaneous and intentional abortion can vary from deep grief to happiness, or any variation in between (Rocca et al., 2015; Lee et al., 2023). Because the emotional and social responses are so varied, it is important for clinicians caring for people who are pregnant or who have the potential for pregnancy to be comfortable supporting patients who may experience the full range of emotions related to their pregnancy and its end. Likewise, because abortion is a common experience, whether intended or spontaneous, familiarity with its management is important for all providers of sexual and reproductive health care, including within primary care settings.

Values Clarification

Values clarification is a technique that can be used to help individuals identify values, biases, and assumptions that may influence their actions. Values clarification related to pregnancy, abortion, adoption, and parenthood has been recommended for healthcare providers who provide clinical care to people of reproductive age as a strategy for avoiding or minimizing personal and professional conflicts. Several resources have been developed to support clinicians in this process (**Table 19-1**). Although most of these focus primarily on abortion, it is important for clinicians to also consider adoption and parenting because unexamined personal beliefs about any of these options can influence professional practice. Reproductive justice, defined as "the human right to maintain personal bodily autonomy, have children, not have children, and parent the children we have in safe and sustainable communities" (SisterSong, n.d.), may also be useful as a framework to introduce as part of the values clarification process. Although there is limited evidence that clinicians' engagement in pregnancy-related values clarification leads to improvements in patient outcomes or satisfaction with care, many reproductive-health-focused organizations and health professions educators encourage a process of self-reflection as essential for providing quality care.

While not all providers can or should provide medication and/or procedural abortion care, all providers need to be able to objectively discuss both intentional abortion and pregnancy loss with their patients and refer as needed. This is part of the American Nurses Association Code of Ethics (2025) and a requirement of all nurses (Eagen-Torkko & Levi, 2020). Clinicians who identify conflicts between their personal beliefs and professional responsibilities have an ethical duty to ensure patients will not be denied their right to respectful, unbiased care. This may require referring pregnant people to a colleague or a different practice setting that should not result in undue hardship, such as long-distance travel or delays in delivery of care. If patients are referred elsewhere, it is the referring clinician's responsibility to ensure the care includes factual, nondirective information about all available options. Crisis pregnancy centers—agencies known to provide biased counseling aimed at dissuading individuals from having abortions—are not acceptable referral sites for pregnancy decision-making support (Bryant & Swartz, 2018). Clinicians who cannot fulfill their duty to provide comprehensive, nondirective pregnancy options counseling are advised to not work in settings where such counseling is a frequent job responsibility (Higginbotham, 2002).

PREGNANCY DIAGNOSIS

A pregnancy test may be performed for diagnosis or to confirm previous testing. Urine pregnancy tests are inexpensive, noninvasive, reliable, and easy to perform in any setting where a urine sample can be appropriately obtained and handled. Pregnancy tests detect the presence of human chorionic gonadotropin (hCG), which is released from a fertilized egg (blastocyst) and then passes into the parental bloodstream and urine after implantation. Urine pregnancy tests provide a positive or negative finding, known as a qualitative result, within minutes. This type of test is usually positive by 14 days after fertilization or 4 weeks after the last menstrual period (LMP), which often corresponds to slightly before the first missed menses (Blackburn, 2017). A positive urine test, either at home or in the clinical setting, provides near certainty that a person is pregnant. False-positive results are unlikely in an otherwise healthy individual. A negative urine hCG test does not absolutely rule out the potential for pregnancy in the next few days if an individual has had vaginal contact with semen. Sperm can remain viable in the reproductive tract for 3 or more days, and a fertilized ovum floats within the reproductive tract for up to 7 days prior to implantation (Blackburn, 2017).

Blood serum pregnancy tests can detect hCG as early as 8 to 10 days after fertilization. The test can be ordered as either qualitative (positive or negative) or quantitative (numeric measure of the level of hCG). Serial quantitative hCG tests (also known as beta-hCG or BhCG, measuring the beta subunit of hCG) are useful for determining the viability of a pregnancy from implantation until 9 weeks' gestation, when hCG begins a physiologic decline (Landon et al., 2025). If there are concerns for ectopic pregnancy or nonviable pregnancy (e.g., abdominal or pelvic pain, bleeding, shoulder pain, syncope, history of ectopic pregnancy, or recurrent miscarriage), then following serial quantitative hCG levels can be helpful to identify the likelihood of a typically developing pregnancy prior to the ability to visualize the embryo

BOX 19-1 Statements of Professional Organizations

American Academy of Physician Associates

Reproductive decision making: Patients have a right to access the full range of reproductive healthcare services, including fertility treatments, contraception, sterilization, and abortion. Physician associates (PAs) have an ethical obligation to provide balanced and unbiased clinical information about reproductive health care.

When the PA's personal values conflict with providing full disclosure or providing certain services such as sterilization or abortion, the PA need not become involved in that aspect of the patient's care. By referring the patient to a qualified provider who is willing to discuss and facilitate all treatment options, the PA fulfills their ethical obligation to ensure the patient's access to all legal options. (Reproduced from American Academy of Physician Associates. (2024). Guidelines for ethical conduct for the physician associate profession.)

American College of Nurse-Midwives

The American College of Nurse-Midwives (ACNM) affirms the following:

- Procedural and medication abortion may be safely provided by trained midwives and other advanced practice clinicians (APCs).
- Midwives may provide medication and procedural abortion as part of their professional scope of practice. Professional scope refers to the role delineated by the profession itself, as opposed to legal scope, which refers specifically to the rapidly shifting legal and political regulations of a provider's role by the state.
- Both medication and procedural abortion pose low risks of post-abortion complications, such as infection or hemorrhage. Both options pose much lower risks than continuing a pregnancy and giving birth.
- Individuals have the human right to decide what is best for their health, bodies, lives, and families. ACNM opposes legislative, policy, or administrative efforts at the federal, state, and local levels to restrict or ban abortion as well as any efforts to render it less accessible.
- ACNM supports policy efforts that work to revise clinician scope of practice laws to include APCs as abortion providers, which will increase access to comprehensive reproductive health services.
- Telehealth abortion has been shown to be safe and effective. ACNM supports midwives in providing telehealth abortion care and opposes any legislative restrictions that limit the ability of midwives to provide these services.
- Self-managed abortion (SMA) is safe. SMA is abortion care that occurs outside of the established healthcare system, with no clinician contact. Midwives should be knowledgeable about the self-management process and supportive to those who choose this method. Midwives can and should support their clients utilizing SMA with pre- and post-abortion care services, such as ultrasounds and beta hCG testing. (Reproduced from American College of Nurse-Midwives, 2025, *Midwives as Abortion Providers Position Statement*)

American College of Obstetricians and Gynecologists

In its abortion policy, the American College of Obstetricians and Gynecologists (2022) recognizes that individual healthcare providers may hold personal beliefs about abortion but asserts that such beliefs should not compromise patient health, access to care, or informed consent in any way. Furthermore, the American College of Obstetricians and Gynecologists states that healthcare providers have an ethical obligation to provide pregnant people with accurate information about all options—including parenting, adoption, and abortion—that is free of personal bias so patients can make fully informed decisions. In addition, an American College of Obstetricians and Gynecologists (2014, reaffirmed 2025) Committee Opinion authored by the Committee on Health Care for Underserved Women endorses appropriately trained and credentialed advanced practice clinicians as providers of medication and first-trimester aspiration abortion services as a means to increase access to abortion.

National Association of Nurse Practitioners in Women's Health

The National Association of Nurse Practitioners in Women's Health's position statement on Access to Safe Abortion Care (2022) affirms that "abortion is an essential component of comprehensive reproductive healthcare." This statement also includes the assertion that the organization's leadership will ensure:

- Women's health nurse practitioners (WHNPs) and other advanced practice clinicians have access to continuing education programs and other resources for evidence-based information on abortion and on pregnancy options counseling.
- WHNP educational programs have access to evidence-based information on abortion and on pregnancy options counseling that can be incorporated into curricula.
- Collaborative engagement with other health professional organizations to advocate for access to abortion, as well as the full scope of reproductive healthcare, and policies that support initiatives to address inequities in all aspects of reproductive health.
- Research moves forward to promote best practices for access to high-quality abortion care. (Reproduced from National Association of Nurse Practitioners in Women's Health. (2022). Position statement.)

Data from American Academy of Physician Associates. (2024). *Guidelines for ethical conduct for the physician associate profession*; American College of Nurse-Midwives. (2023). Access to comprehensive sexual and reproductive health care services [Position statement]; Reproduced from American College of Obstetricians and Gynecologists. (2022). *Abortion policy* [Policy statement]; National Association of Nurse Practitioners in Women's Health. (2022). Position statement: Access to safe abortion care.

TABLE 19-1 Resources for Values Clarification

Title	Type of Resource	Where to Obtain the Resource
Abortion and Options Counseling: A Comprehensive Reference by Anne Baker (Hope Clinic for Women, 1995)	Book	Booksellers
The Abortion Option: A Values Clarification Guide for Health Professionals	Workbook	National Abortion Federation (https://prochoice.org/wp-content/uploads/abortion_option.pdf)
Values Clarification Workshop	Online workbook and activities guide	Reproductive Health Access Project (RHAP) (https://www.reproductiveaccess.org/resource/values-clarification-workshop/)

TABLE 19-2 Patient-Reported Pregnancy Indicators for Gestational Age Assessment

Patient-Reported Indicator	Assessment Modality	Estimated Gestational Age
Last normal menstrual period	Calculate days since first day of last menstrual period	From calculation
Probable date of conception	Calculate days since conception and add 2 weeks	From calculation
Pregnancy symptoms (e.g., breast/chest tenderness, nausea/vomiting)	Patient report	Typically appear no earlier than 6 weeks gestation
Fetal movement	Patient report	Typically appears no earlier than 16 weeks; most common 18–22 weeks

on ultrasound. Blood serum pregnancy tests are more expensive, and their results are not immediately available, so they are usually reserved for people with complications such as pain or bleeding. Because urine tests are so sensitive and rarely have false-positive results, a single positive urine pregnancy test is all that is needed to diagnose pregnancy.

Following diagnosis of pregnancy via positive hCG and/or other testing, patients may experience a wide range of responses, from disbelief or anger to joy. Shock is not an uncommon response, particularly for people who may have irregular menses or who may have believed pregnancy to be impossible. A bimanual exam may be useful to identify a range of gestational durations, but even experienced clinicians are often only able to estimate within a range of 2 weeks, which is often inadequate for planning future care, particularly for an unexpected pregnancy. Therefore, many clinicians will choose to defer an invasive exam in favor of an ultrasound. Duration of gestation can be established within 7 days with an early (first trimester) ultrasound; later ultrasounds are less reliable in establishing gestational duration (generally within 1–2 weeks in second trimester and 2–3 weeks in the third trimester), so early ultrasound in the case of uncertain last menstrual period (LMP) dates should be strongly considered. If LMP is known, Naegele's rule may be used to estimate the gestational duration. As with all pregnancies, multiple patient-reported indicators (pregnancy symptoms, probable date of conception, LMP if known) can be used to triangulate an estimated gestational duration in the meantime. **Table 19-2** provides the common patient-reported indicators used to help support gestational age assessment.

A major consideration of early pregnancy care is establishing location of pregnancy, and in this ultrasound can be very helpful. Ectopic pregnancies (those outside the uterus) cannot continue to term, and the recommendation is for intentional termination of ectopic pregnancies upon diagnosis. This is a life-threatening complication of pregnancy, and therefore its identification is paramount. Ectopic pregnancies can produce abnormally low levels of hCG, and some providers will repeat a BhCG test in 48–72 hours to ensure adequate rise in hCG levels (Blackburn, 2017). In a typically developing pregnancy, these are expected to double every 24–72 hours; failure to do so suggests either an abnormally located or abnormally developing pregnancy and needs further workup. Ectopic pregnancy is the primary concern of pregnancy location because it is potentially fatal, and can lead to infertility in those who survive, so prompt identification and treatment are essential. Once an intrauterine pregnancy is established on ultrasound, while heterotopic pregnancies (simultaneous intrauterine and ectopic pregnancies) exist, they are extremely rare and concern for ectopic all but vanishes.

Once hCG levels reach 4,000 mIU/mL (the "discriminant level"), a gestational sac and/or fetal cardiac motion should be detectable on transvaginal ultrasound (Park et al., 2023). Lack of either at this level or above suggests a "missed abortion" (a pregnancy that has ended but where the tissue remains in situ), a potential spontaneous abortion ("threatened abortion"), an ectopic pregnancy, and/or an incomplete abortion (in which case there would likely be tissue present in the uterus, though not necessarily identifiable morphology). If the last menstrual period and urine testing are used to establish pregnancy, the

TABLE 19-3 Interpretation of hCG Results

Key Event	hCG Finding	Implication
Positive serum or urine pregnancy test	15–25 mIU/mL (Park et al., 2023)	Probable sign of pregnancy
Gestational sac visible on US (discriminant level)	4,000 mIU/mL (Park et al., 2023)	Positive sign of pregnancy
Appropriate increase in hCG	Doubling every 48–96 hours (serum only)	Implies pregnancy is developing appropriately
Persistently elevated levels of hCG that continue to rise	At upper limit or beyond of reference range for an expected gestational age	Molar pregnancy, multiple gestations
Flat or declining serial hCG results	Failure to double appropriately, or any drop in the first trimester	Ectopic pregnancy, missed abortion, spontaneous abortion

TABLE 19-4 Types of Spontaneous Abortion (SAB)

Type	Definition	Symptoms	Prognosis
Threatened	Symptoms of SAB present Products of conception intact	Minimal vaginal bleeding Abdominal cramping Uterine size is equal to dates Cervical os is closed	Possible pregnancy loss
Inevitable	Symptoms of SAB increased in severity, to include cervical dilation Products of conception intact	Moderate vaginal bleeding Moderate to severe uterine cramping Uterine size is equal to dates Cervical os is dilated	Poor
Incomplete	Symptoms of SAB present, to include cervical dilation Partial products of conception expelled	Heavy vaginal bleeding Moderate to severe uterine cramping Uterine size is equal to dates Cervical os is dilated	Poor
Complete	Products of conception expelled in entirety following symptoms of SAB	Minimal vaginal bleeding Prior uterine cramping has subsided Uterus is prepregnancy size Cervical os is either closed or dilated	Pregnancy loss
Missed	Products of conception retained for up to 6 weeks following symptoms of SAB	Vaginal bleeding has occurred, subsided, and reoccurs No current uterine contractions, but there is a history of uterine cramping	Pregnancy loss
Recurrent	Three or more SABs occurring consecutively	Same as all previously listed types	Poor for maintaining future pregnancies without intervention; refer to assistive reproduction specialist

possibility of later conception and/or incorrect dating must be considered. In this case, repeating the ultrasound in 1–2 weeks is often reasonable; in the case of hCG > 4,000 mIU/mL there is no identifiable benefit as an intrauterine pregnancy, if present, should be visible (Park et al., 2023). However, there is also no clinical reason not to offer a repeat ultrasound to the patient if they desire. **Table 19-3** highlights how hCG results can be interpreted in early pregnancy.

Identification of Spontaneous Pregnancy Loss

Early pregnancy loss, defined as a spontaneous abortion in the first trimester, can be classified as (1) threatened abortion, (2) inevitable abortion, (3) incomplete abortion, (4) complete abortion, and (5) missed abortion. Each of these is included under spontaneous abortion, but the management and diagnosis of each varies. Refer to **Table 19-4** for definitions, symptoms, and prognosis for types of spontaneous abortion.

SAB can be diagnosed using a variety of assessments: (1) serial serum hCG; (2) auscultation or visualization of cardiac activity; (3) assessment of uterine size and expected findings for EGA; and (4) evaluation of cervical dilation and vaginal bleeding/passage of tissue, if any. Differential diagnoses include reproductive cancers, ectopic pregnancy, and hydatidiform mole. Once a nonviable pregnancy or pregnancy loss is identified, the patient has several options for management, most of which are discussed below. Both medication and procedural abortion are options in many cases, and the decision about which is preferred can be complex. While patients may feel an urge to make a decision quickly (or providers may), in a clinically stable patient a period of at least 2 weeks between diagnosis of a missed abortion and completion of that abortion is not associated with increased risks (Musik et al., 2021). Therefore, the provider has the opportunity to allow patients time for decision making in most cases. The exceptions are (1) infection, (2) significant blood loss leading to hemodynamic changes or significant anemia, and (3) life conditions that would make prompt ending of the pregnancy clinically preferable (lack of transportation or access to emergency care if needed, for example).

Ectopic Pregnancy

Ectopic pregnancy is the implantation of a fertilized ovum in locations other than the uterine cavity. The most common site of ectopic pregnancy is the fallopian tube (ACOG, 2018, reaffirmed 2025). It is the leading cause of first-trimester maternal mortality in the United States (Mullany et al., 2023). Ectopic pregnancies carry significant risk for pregnancy loss, tubal rupture, excessive blood loss, and future infertility due to tubal scarring. **Box 19-2** summarizes risk factors associated with ectopic pregnancy.

BOX 19-2 Risk Factors for Ectopic Pregnancy

- Previous ectopic pregnancy
- Any previous tubal surgery or tubal deformity
- History of ascending pelvic infection
- History of infertility
- Past or current use of intrauterine device[a]
- Assisted reproduction
- History of therapeutic abortion, especially with complications
- Age greater than 35 years (less significant risk factor)

Data from American College of Obstetricians and Gynecologists. (2018). ACOG Practice Bulletin No. 193: Tubal Ectopic Pregnancy. https://www.acog.org/clinical/clinical-guidance/practice-bulletin/articles/2018/03/tubal-ectopic-pregnancy

[a]Because use of an intrauterine device decreases the risk of pregnancy, the risk of ectopic pregnancy is lower; however, if pregnancy occurs with an intrauterine device in place, there is a higher risk that it is an ectopic pregnancy (ACOG, 2018, reaffirmed 2025).

Pelvic and abdominal pain and unexplained vaginal bleeding are the primary symptoms of ectopic pregnancy. The pain may be described as vague, sharp, diffuse, or unilateral. The person may have had a time of amenorrhea, and pregnancy may or may not already be diagnosed. A ruptured ectopic pregnancy is characterized by a sudden onset of vaginal bleeding and sharp, severe, unilateral abdominal pain. Following rupture, symptoms of significant blood loss and resulting shock may include hypotension, shoulder pain, and syncope.

Physical findings associated with ectopic pregnancy include cervical motion tenderness, a uterus that is not enlarged, adnexal mass, and adnexal tenderness. A transvaginal ultrasound evaluation is the minimum diagnostic evaluation of a suspected ectopic pregnancy, and it should be done by someone trained in obstetrical sonography. Often a serial hCG level is taken at the same time to confirm diagnosis. Management of an ectopic pregnancy should be by an obstetrician or maternal–fetal specialist. Differential diagnoses include appendicitis, pelvic inflammatory disease, bowel irritability or obstruction, cholecystitis, pyelonephritis, and ovarian torsion. However, all pregnancy-capable people who are sexually active and present with clinical signs and/or physical symptoms of ectopic pregnancy, such as abdominal pain and vaginal bleeding, should be screened for pregnancy regardless of whether they are using contraception (ACOG, 2018, reaffirmed 2025).

Management prior to a confirmed diagnosis includes close observation to avoid the medical emergency of tubal rupture. Early diagnosis also may facilitate the use of methotrexate to dissolve the products of conception and avoid tubal rupture. The presence of signs and symptoms of rupture requires prompt medical attention in an institution that is equipped with surgical capabilities. Close follow-up of the patient who experiences an ectopic pregnancy includes monitoring hCG levels, emotional support for unexpected pregnancy loss and for the possibly traumatic experience of medical emergency, and future fertility counseling.

Molar Pregnancy (Hydatidiform Mole)

Hydatidiform mole, also called molar pregnancy, is a form of gestational trophoblastic disease characterized by an abnormal proliferation of placental tissue that results in the development of a benign or malignant tumor. These abnormal growths appear as grapelike villi that fill the uterine cavity (**Figure 19-1**).

There are two types of molar pregnancies: partial, in which nonviable fetal tissue may be present; and complete, in which there is an absence of fetal tissue. In a partial molar pregnancy, the patient may present with symptoms of a missed SAB with uterine size as expected related to her last normal menstrual period. The typical presentation of a complete molar pregnancy is a uterine size greater than expected related to the last normal menstrual period and vaginal bleeding accompanied with passage of grapelike villi. Increased incidence of complications is associated with a complete molar pregnancy. The incidence of molar pregnancy is about 1 in 1,000 pregnancies and is more common in people of Southeast Asian origin. Other risk factors include age younger than 20 years or older than 40 years and history of molar pregnancy (Soper, 2021).

Symptoms of molar pregnancy can include dark or brown vaginal spotting; abdominal tenderness; unexpectedly severe and/or persistent nausea and vomiting (related to elevated

FIGURE 19-1 **Molar pregnancy.**

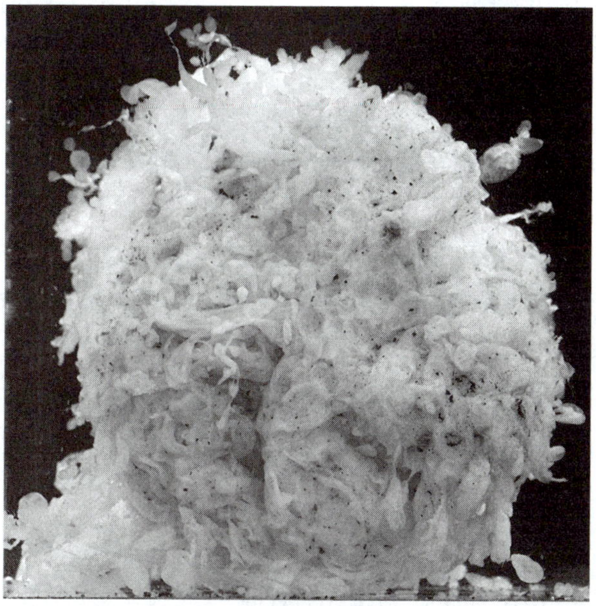

Courtesy of University of Cape Town Digital Pathology Collection.

levels of hCG compared to typical pregnancy); extreme fatigue; pelvic pain; coughing and shortness of breath; hemoptysis; and weight loss. Patients occasionally will pass clusters of villi from the vagina, which resemble tiny grapes, and fetal heart tones are not heard. Symptoms of preeclampsia may develop prior to 24 weeks. An ultrasound reveals a snowstorm pattern, lack of fetal parts, and lack of fetal movement. Levels of hCG will be consistently high and rising.

Management requires a referral to a maternal–fetal specialist. If a malignancy is diagnosed, a referral to an oncologist is necessary. Evacuation of the molar tissue may be accomplished pharmacologically or surgically. Follow-up care will include monitoring hCG levels to determine if the levels are decreasing, contraception, consultation with a maternal–fetal specialist, avoidance of pregnancy for 6 to 12 months, and emotional care (Soper, 2021).

NONDIRECTIVE PREGNANCY OPTIONS COUNSELING

The role of the clinician in pregnancy options counseling is well delineated. Many people, on discovering an unintended or mistimed pregnancy, will contact their usual provider to discuss pregnancy options. Others will opt to seek such care at a specialty clinic such as Planned Parenthood, often because of a fear of judgment by one's usual provider. Still others will seek this counseling later in a pregnancy, whether because of pregnancy complications, fetal testing, or changes in life circumstances. They may or may not bring a partner or others who are important to them, and it is important for the clinician not to make assumptions about the patient's intent, their feelings, or their relationship(s).

Options counseling is appropriate for patients who know they are pregnant and are undecided or unaware of all the options available to them, or who need more information to make their decision. Abortion counseling, in contrast, is appropriate for patients who have decided on abortion and are seeking emotional or educational support for their decision. While all clinicians are expected to be familiar with principles of nondirective counseling around issues of health care, it is challenging for some to provide such counseling around abortion care specifically. Therefore, clinicians who are aware that this presents a challenge for them are obligated to identify referral resources for nondirective options counseling and abortion counseling as needed, whether virtual or in their community.

Providing pregnancy options counseling is similar to options counseling for other healthcare decisions: The alternative courses of action are identified, the risks/benefits/alternatives of each are discussed, and the patient is supported in making their decision. However, unlike other healthcare decisions, pregnancy options are overwhelmingly between two relatively safe courses of action (abortion and continuing the pregnancy), and social, financial, emotional, family, and relational issues are more relevant to decisions (Recker et al., 2025). Therefore, key skills to develop for options counseling include (1) patient rapport, (2) listening (both active and passive), (3) reassurance of confidentiality, and (4) asking nondirective questions. These skills are all essential to health care more broadly, but if the clinician is uncertain of their facility with them, it is often helpful to observe a more experienced colleague or to seek additional training.

Although all people are individuals, a helpful stepwise process to use is:

1. Explore how the person feels about their pregnancy and the options available.
2. Explore their support system (for any decision) and assess any risks that exist (pregnancy sharply increases the risk of intimate partner violence [Roman-Galvez et al., 2021]).
3. Provide decision-making support (information, verbal support, nondirective questions) or establish a timeline for decision making. Since the Dobbs decision and the subsequent restriction or ban on abortion in many states, this step, as well as establishing an accurate duration of gestation, has become paramount as decisions will be affected by legal options available.
4. Provide or refer the pregnant person to the desired services. This last step is essential to completing options counseling.

These are also all appropriate to discussion of management of spontaneous abortion/early pregnancy loss, with the difference that "positive pregnancy test" is replaced with "diagnosis of nonviable pregnancy." In the case of a spontaneous abortion (early pregnancy loss), options can include management versus watchful waiting, and if intervention is chosen, on what timeline and within what parameters. In the case of a life-limiting fetal condition, the issue becomes more complex and is generally handled by a team, hopefully one with experience in perinatal hospice and genetic counseling, as well as maternal–fetal medicine. This kind of options counseling is beyond the scope of this text.

A comprehensive understanding of nondirective options counseling takes time and practice to develop. For newer providers, or for those who have not previously had many opportunities

TABLE 19-5 Examples of Language to Consider and to Avoid in Options Counseling

Recommended	Avoid

• How are you feeling about this pregnancy?
• Is there information that would be helpful to you in making your decision? What is it?
• How can I be most helpful to you in this decision?
• When you think about being pregnant, what are some of the feelings that come up? How about when you think about having an abortion? Parenting? Making an adoption plan?
• What values are important to you in making your decision?
	• Are you happy about the pregnancy?
	• Congratulations!
	  • You must be [so excited/upset/ etc.] . . .
	  • Your baby will be born on [EDD] . . .

for options counseling, there are a number of resources available through TEACH (Training in Early Abortion for Comprehensive Healthcare) at the University of California San Francisco, Nurses for Sexual and Reproductive Health (NSRH), and the Reproductive Health National Training Center (RHNTC, part of the Centers for Disease Control and Prevention), among others.

Exploration of Feelings

Rather than ask if the pregnancy was "intended," or "planned," consider asking how the patient feels about the test result or pregnancy. This is important regardless of where the patient first makes contact with the healthcare system; some people present for initial prenatal care and later opt for abortion, while others may make and cancel multiple appointments to terminate a pregnancy that they end up continuing. Delivering pregnancy test results is thus best done in a neutral, factual, but unmistakable way (e.g., "Your test was positive. This means that you are pregnant.") that then could be followed up with, for example, "How are you feeling about this?" Refer to **Table 19-5** for other example language to use.

It is very common for people to experience a variety of seemingly contradictory emotions, particularly immediately after learning of a pregnancy, and often the role of the clinician is to reflect back the patient's statements rather than to try to lead them to a decision. This can conflict with the time constraints of most clinics, and therefore many will schedule pregnancy test visits for extra time (although, of course, that does not help the surprise positive hCG in a patient scheduled for an IUD insert, for example).

Pregnancy options are really a two-step process: (1) whether or not to continue the pregnancy, and (2) whether, if continuing the pregnancy, to plan to parent. Rather than presenting three options ("abortion, adoption, or parenting?") as the question to answer, it can be helpful to the patient to take a stepwise approach and decide first if they want to continue the pregnancy, and if so, then tackle the question of parenting.

TABLE 19-6 Examples of Language to Use and Avoid When Identifying Support Systems and Risks

Suggested Questions	Avoid

• Who is important to you in your life? Can you discuss your decision with them?
• Does anyone know that you are or might be pregnant?
  • If someone knows, how did that person respond when they heard you are or might be pregnant?
  • If no one knows, how do you think other significant people in your life (e.g., partner, parents) might respond when they hear you are pregnant?
  • Is there anyone you could talk with about your pregnancy who you think would be supportive no matter what you decide to do?
	• Are your partner and/or parents going to support you?
	• It is important for you to tell your partner and/or parents about this.
	  • Dads often come around after they have some time.
	  • It will all work out in the end.

Identifying Support Systems and Risks

A helpful question to ask, if the pregnancy is not being diagnosed in this visit, can be, "Have you told anyone about the pregnancy/test results?" Another is, "Does anyone know you might be pregnant?" If the answer is no, following up on why that is (fear of judgment, fear of violence, no support system, etc.) will help to identify what support the person might need. If the patient says, "I can't tell anyone/I don't have anyone to tell," you might ask them if they have people in their life who have helped them through other hard things, or helped them make other decisions in the past. **Table 19-6** suggests language to use and avoid when assessing support systems and risks.

Assessing for intimate partner violence (IPV) and/or reproductive coercion are essential in any pregnancy, regardless of intended outcome. Sexual and reproductive coercion includes "explicit attempts to impregnate a partner against her will, control outcomes of a pregnancy, coerce a partner to have unprotected sex, and interfere with contraceptive methods" (American College of Obstetricians and Gynecologists, 2013, reaffirmed 2019). IPV can include emotional, financial, physical, or sexual violence or threats of violence (Centers for Disease Control and Prevention, 2024). Depending on the circumstances, including age, such disclosures may obligate breach of confidentiality and/or involvement of people besides the clinician. This may include referral to or consultation with other members of the healthcare team, community resources, and/or legal advisors. When the patient is a minor, reporting a pregnancy to Child Protective Services may be mandatory depending on the laws of the state. These limitations to confidentiality need to be made transparent to the patient prior to disclosure. More information on IPV is available in Chapter 15.

Supporting Decision Making or Setting Decisional Timeline

While some patients will immediately know their decision, many others, particularly those for whom the test results are a surprise, may need time to absorb the knowledge of their pregnancy. Likewise, people differ in their decisional speed, which can be affected by knowledge of pregnancy, familiarity with parenting, cognitive or developmental disability, religious or personal beliefs that may preclude abortion, and a host of other factors. The role of the clinician is to facilitate the individual process for this patient in this pregnancy, whether that includes sharing information (about fetal development, abortion care, fetal testing, support services available in the community, etc.) or assistance with setting a decisional timeline (making an appointment to review options in a week, for example). One way to proceed is to ask the patient whether they wish to discuss options immediately, not at all, or delay until a later time. This is a trauma-informed approach that allows the individual to identify which strategy will work best for them, while also ensuring that they have needed support and resources. **Table 19-7** reviews pregnancy options resources that may be helpful.

Another important component of pregnancy options counseling is ensuring that the individual is aware of the estimated gestational age of the pregnancy and any relevant clinical and legal implications. Postponing the decision about how to proceed can have important implications. In terms of abortion, an advancing gestation may preclude some methods (i.e., medication abortion), increase the cost, or eliminate the option altogether. For people who ultimately decide to continue a pregnancy, a delay in decision making may result in late initiation of prenatal care, which has been associated with poorer pregnancy outcomes and missed opportunities for early fetal risk assessment (Crequit et al., 2023).

MANAGEMENT AND/OR REFERRAL FOR CARE

Continuation of Pregnancy and Parenting

If the decision is made to continue the pregnancy, or if the patient is uncertain, they can be encouraged to initiate prenatal care and other recommendations for pregnancy (starting folic acid supplementation, avoiding potential teratogens, etc.). If the current clinician does not provide prenatal and/or birth care, the patient must be referred to one who does. For more information on promoting health in early pregnancy, refer to Chapter 32.

If the decision is made to parent, the clinician may refer the patient to early parenting supports as appropriate and available, such as public health nursing programs, early parenting support groups, and other similar services. Decisions about whether to parent or to make an adoption plan can occur anytime during pregnancy, and these decisions are not final until after birth.

TABLE 19-7 Patient Resources for Exploring Pregnancy Options

Title	Type	Where to Obtain the Resource	Description
All-Options Talkline	Telephone	1-888-493-0092	Peer-based counseling and support for people making decisions about a current pregnancy, as well as other pregnancy-related concerns (parenting, abortion, infertility, miscarriage). Free, confidential, nonjudgmental.
Are You Pregnant and Thinking About Adoption?	Fact sheet	Child Welfare Information Gateway (https://www.childwelfare.gov/pubPDFs/f_pregna.pdf)	Provides information about adoption, including community resources and considerations for fathers and relatives.
Pregnant? Need Help? Pregnancy Options Workbook	Web- and print-based workbook	PregnancyOptions.info (https://www.pregnancyoptions.info/pregnant.htm)	Features exercises for individuals undecided about what to do about a pregnancy and information on all three pregnancy options. Addresses topics such as decision making, getting support, male partners, fetal development, and spiritual and religious concerns.
Talking With Your Parent(s) About Your Pregnancy	Online resource	Abortion Care Network (https://www.abortioncarenetwork.org/exceptional-care/get-help/talking-with-your-parents-about-your-pregnancy/)	Resource created to assist young people explore their options and tell their parents about a pregnancy.
Unsure About Your Pregnancy? A Guide to Making the Right Decision for You	Brochure	National Abortion Federation (https://www.prochoice.org /pubs_research/publications/downloads/are_you_pregnant/pregnancy_guide_english.pdf)	Provides exercises for pregnant women who are undecided about their pregnancy. Website also provides links to information about all three options.

Clinicians should be familiar with some of the resources available in their area for both parenting and adoption, and they should offer these to patients as indicated. Some of the national resources are available in **Appendix 19-A**.

Continuation of Pregnancy and Adoption

Arrangements for adoption vary according to state law. Newborns may be placed for adoption through public or private agencies, independently with assistance from an adoption lawyer or facilitator, or formally or informally through kinship networks. Adoptions may be open or closed. Open adoptions vary in the degree of identifiable information and communication shared among the birth parents, child, and adoptive parents. In an open adoption, there may be ongoing contact between the families. Parents in a confidential or closed adoption do not know each other or have contact, but the adoptive parents are usually given relevant information about the birth parents, such as medical histories. Closed adoptions are much less common than in the past, and adopted individuals are required to have access to their birth records in many states (American College of Obstetricians and Gynecologists, 2012). The National Council for Adoption offers general information for pregnant women considering adoption on their website, and it advises people who are interested in this option to contact an agency in their area (refer to Appendix 19-A). Referring a person to a social worker or agency with expertise in adoption can be helpful because this is a complex and dynamic area in which accurate information may prove critical to the decision-making process. In the meantime, ensuring timely prenatal care access and support is crucial.

Abortion

As noted earlier in this chapter, "abortion" correctly refers to any pregnancy that does not end in a birth, whether that ending is spontaneous or intentional. Because the management of spontaneous pregnancy loss is essentially identical to an intentional abortion, the discussion of the clinical aspects of such management is shared with the discussion of the clinical aspects of intentional abortion. However, the emotions and decisions around each situation can be quite different, and the clinician should be sensitive to the needs of each individual patient in any case of pregnancy diagnosis or management.

CONTEXT FOR ABORTION IN THE UNITED STATES

In order to provide patient education and to assess the options available for a given patient, it is essential for any clinician caring for people of reproductive age to understand how intentional terminations of pregnancy are performed, the gestational ranges for each option, the risks and benefits of each, and the resources available in a given area. It is also important to understand the current legal status of abortion access, including management of ectopic pregnancy and spontaneous abortion/pregnancy loss in a given jurisdiction, and legal as well as physical safety for both the pregnant person and the provider. This is a more complicated landscape than even 5 years ago, and providers who are not extremely familiar with intentional termination of pregnancy regulations in their state are advised to update their knowledge regularly, using the resources in Appendix 19-A as a start. Patient education is a key component of clinical practice, but there are possibly no other areas of health care that are as legally and politically complex as that of abortion care.

Historical Context

While abortion has been a lightning rod of sorts for over a century and a half, for millennia it was largely both unregulated and not discussed (Reagan, 1995). Midwives and other community members managed "late" or "stuck" periods as they managed other aspects of sexual and reproductive health care, with herbal medicine and other traditional modalities, and while intentional termination of pregnancy may have been illegal in some places and times, those restrictions were often secondary to property concerns at a time when children were considered to be the property of their father and to have economic value to him. While the common King James version of the Bible does delineate punishment for causing a miscarriage, it is for causing one against the will of the pregnant person (Exodus 21:22-25). Even the Catholic Church, long considered at the forefront of anti-abortion work, did not consider abortion to be the moral equivalent of murder until 1869, almost 2,000 years after its initial founding (Castuera, 2017).

The changes in regulation for both contraception and abortion began in earnest in the Victorian Era, when a general opposition to sexuality and to participation by women in the larger society crashed against the burgeoning social changes of the Industrial Revolution, including increased immigration (Whittum & Rapkin, 2022). In the United States, banning abortion and contraception were also strategic ways to advance the agenda of the nascent physicians' professional movement—if midwives were associated with illegal acts like abortion, then not only could they be imprisoned, they would be perceived as illegitimate healthcare providers (Jenkins et al., 2023).

Abortion restrictions were not limited to the statehouse. The Comstock Act, named for then–Inspector General of the U.S. Postal Service Anthony Comstock, banned the use of the U.S. mail to distribute

> *[e]very article or thing designed, adapted, or intended for producing abortion, or for any indecent or immoral use; . . . and*
>
> *Every article, instrument, substance, drug, medicine, or thing which is advertised or described in a manner calculated to lead another to use or apply it for producing abortion, or for any indecent or immoral purpose; and*
>
> *Every written or printed card, letter, circular, book, pamphlet, advertisement, or notice of any kind giving information, directly or indirectly, where, or how, or from whom, or by what means any of such mentioned matters, articles, or things may be obtained or made, or where or by whom any act or operation of any kind for the procuring or producing of abortion will be done or performed, or how or by what means abortion may be produced, whether sealed or unsealed; and*
>
> *Every paper, writing, advertisement, or representation that any article, instrument, substance, drug, medicine, or thing may, or can, be used or applied for producing abortion, or for any indecent or immoral purpose . . . (18 U.S.C. § 1461, 1972)*

This essentially ended the ability of clinicians, even in less restrictive states, and activists to disseminate knowledge about safe abortion, which in turn led to an explosion in illegal unsafe abortion, often associated with organized crime (Reagan, 2023). Because of this lack of safety, by the year 1925, every state had banned intentional abortion. More liberal states allowed exceptions to save the life of the pregnant person, but that was often subject to review and consent of an "ethics board" of a hospital.

In response, clergy and others began civil disobedience to the intentional termination bans. One example is the Jane Collective, a group of Chicago laypeople who estimated that between 1969 and 1973 they provided almost 12,000 illegal but safe abortions (https://embryo.asu.edu/pages/jane-collective-1969-1973), at a cost one-tenth that of the going rate. Individual states liberalized their abortion laws as well, beginning with New York, Hawai'i, and Washington in 1970, but stopped short of overturning all restrictions (Whittum & Rapkin, 2022).

When the *Dobbs v Jackson Women's Health* Supreme Court decision (2022) overturned the *Roe v Wade* decision (1973), overnight it created a hodgepodge of abortion law in the United States, ranging from fully illegal to highly protected, with every variant in between. Increasing the complications are the shifts away from procedural abortion management for both intentional and spontaneous terminations of pregnancy and the delivery of this care via telehealth rather than in person following the 2023 decision by the Food and Drug Administration to allow remote abortion care (Jain et al., 2023). This shift reduces the reliance of any one state on its own regulations as long as delivery of the needed medications can occur (which requires the patient to seek telehealth services in a state where abortion is permitted and complete the visit there). However, the status remains rapidly shifting, and a national abortion ban remains possible.

FIRST-TRIMESTER ABORTION

Medication Abortion

As noted above, medication or pharmacologic abortion predates the modern healthcare system. However, the medications currently used in abortion both in the United States and globally are of relatively recent development, and the focus of this chapter is on mifepristone, methotrexate, and misoprostol as by far the most common and effective abortifacients currently available. While medications can be used for second- and third-trimester abortion, they rarely are in the United States, and this use has a somewhat increased risk of both hemorrhage and retained tissue (Kallner, 2023). Therefore, the focus will be on the use of medications in the first trimester of pregnancy, which is defined as up to 13 weeks from last normal menstrual period (LMP).

Mifepristone

Mifepristone, originally developed by French pharmaceutical company Roussel-Uclaf in 1980, is a synthetic progesterone antagonist (Spitz, 2010). It competitively binds to progesterone receptors in the uterus, blocking the ability of progesterone to inhibit uterine contractions and to maintain the endometrium, which effectively separates an early pregnancy from the endometrium (Mahajan & London, 1997). Used alone, mifepristone has a relatively high failure rate at pregnancy termination (approximately 10%) and has an unpredictable timing of action, which limits its utility as a monotherapy (Creinin et al., 2001). Therefore, it is almost always used in conjunction with misoprostol (refer to below), which decreases the failure rate to <1 percent (Ferguson & Scott, 2020).

TABLE 19-8 **2023 FDA REMS for Mifepristone**

Medication/ Procedure	2023 REMS
Mifepristone	200 mg PO (Day 0, at home or in office)
Misoprostol	800 mcg buccal or SL (Day 2, at home)
Visits	Telehealth acceptable
Restrictions	< 70d LMP, APC and physicians as prescribers

Mifepristone is an extremely safe medication, with few contraindications (refer to below); its most common side effect (besides vaginal bleeding, which is, of course, also its intended action) is nausea/vomiting (Sitruk-Ware, 2006). However, since its approval in 2000, it has been under increased FDA surveillance using the Risk Evaluation and Mitigation System (REMS), which requires registration of prescribers with the FDA and until 2023 prohibited dispensing mifepristone in a pharmacy (mandatory clinic dispensing). The REMS has failed to document significant risk using either the original FDA-approved protocol or the revised 2023 protocol (refer to **Table 19-8**).

Misoprostol

The second half of the standard medication abortion regimen used in the United States and other high-income countries is misoprostol, a synthetic prostaglandin analogue that attaches to receptors in smooth muscle to produce uterine contraction, among other effects (Krugh et al., 2024). Misoprostol is also widely used to manage missed abortion, incomplete abortion, postpartum hemorrhage, cervical ripening for labor induction, and treating gastric ulcers. Because of its cytokinetic action, fever lasting < 24 hours is common with misoprostol use for any indication and does not indicate infection. Diarrhea and nausea are also relatively common side effects, although somewhat dependent both on the dosage used and the route of administration (oral versus buccal, for example). Like mifepristone, misoprostol has few contraindications.

Misoprostol is widely used outside of the United States as a monotherapy in medication abortion, in part because of its extremely low cost and high efficacy compared to mifepristone alone. It is also used in some self-managed abortion, as it is readily available by mail and through informal sources. However, because mifepristone is currently available in the United States, and because efficacy is increased by using the two-medication regime, mifepristone + misoprostol is standard of care in the United States.

Methotrexate

Methotrexate is a folic acid antagonist that effectively blocks the ability of rapidly dividing cells to use folate. Without folate, the cells are unable to divide. Because of this mechanism of action, methotrexate is widely used in cancer treatment, as well as treatment of autoimmune disorders such as psoriatic arthritis, and ectopic pregnancy, and has been used for medication abortion in the United States. Because of its relatively high rate of side effects and the need to abstain from folic acid for several days prior to its use to maximize efficacy, it is rarely used in the United States for medication abortion, although that may change in the future depending on availability of mifepristone. While high doses of methotrexate have been used as a monotherapy, it is much less effective than a methotrexate-misoprostol regimen (Wiebe,1999).

Protocol, Considerations, and Follow-Up for Medication Abortion

Using the current FDA mifepristone + misoprostol regimen, there may be one, two, or no in-person visits. However, regardless of the number of visits, there are several factors to ensure safety when using medication abortion to end a pregnancy. First, ectopic pregnancy cannot be suspected, as none of the medications will effectively treat an ectopic pregnancy at the usual dosages (while methotrexate can be used to manage ectopic pregnancy, the dosage used is calculated differently and close evaluation before and after is required). Second, duration of pregnancy must be established. While the no-test protocol (National Abortion Federation [NAF], 2024) does not require ultrasound confirmation of gestational age, it does require certain knowledge of LMP. In the United States, mifepristone + misoprostol abortion can be used up to 70 days LMP (FDA, 2025), but is used off-label after these dates, as is misoprostol alone and oxytocin, as seen in "Later Abortion." Third, while there are relatively few contraindications to medication abortion using the standard protocols, the patient cannot, clearly, have any of them. Finally, there must be access to emergency care and adequate transportation if needed. While this need is very rare, identifying resources for it is a key part of safe abortion practice (NAF, 2024).

The no-test protocol is something of a misnomer, as a positive pregnancy test is part of the protocol. However, a home test, self-reported, is considered adequate, and the "no-test" refers to no clinical testing, including ultrasound. Instead, the clinician screens for symptoms of ectopic pregnancy (abdominal pain, particularly unilateral; syncope; shoulder pain; spotting), establishes a likely gestational age using LMP or known date of conception, screens for contraindications to medication abortion (presence of IUD; known contraindications; allergy to either medication; lack of access to emergency care if needed) and reviews the risks of opting out of clinical confirmation of gestational age. Thus, it is more accurately termed a test-optional protocol, and it can be completed safely via telehealth.

For the dual-medication protocol, 200 mg of mifepristone is taken orally on Day 1. Although access is limited, it is possible to send this prescription to a pharmacy for pickup; otherwise, it can be mailed or dispensed in clinic. During this first visit, whether telehealth or in person, the health history is reviewed, as are the LMP, any pregnancy symptoms, and any symptoms suggesting possible ectopic pregnancy. It is important to review with the patient that taking the first medication begins the abortion process, and despite claims by a few providers otherwise, it is not possible to "reverse" a medication abortion once begun (Stifani & Lavelanet, 2024).

The initial medication is followed 24–48 hours later by 800 mcg of misoprostol buccally (vs. orally). The majority (80% or more) of patients will end their pregnancy within 4 hours of misoprostol administration, so it is important for the patient to understand the range of normal for bleeding and pain, and for comfort measures to be readily available. The most common pattern of bleeding and pain is increasing cramping and bleeding, which peak with the passage of pregnancy tissue and should begin to resolve relatively quickly after that. Pain management can include nonpharmacologic measures (heating pad, massage, distraction, emotional support, etc.) as well as pharmacologic (NSAIDs, acetaminophen, and opioids). Bleeding should not exceed one pad/hour for more than 2 hours, and clots should not exceed the size of a lime. Most people are able to return to work or school the following day, but it is reasonable to support time off if needed.

If the pregnancy tissue does not pass within 4 hours, a second dose of misoprostol may be considered. Most providers encourage waiting 24 hours before repeating the dose, in order to minimize side effects, but it is not unsafe to repeat the dose sooner (WHO, 2022). Failure to have significant bleeding and cramping after two doses of misoprostol may indicate the need for evaluation, including ultrasound, but local abortion restrictions and other considerations should be included when planning care after two doses of misoprostol. The World Health Organization (WHO) considers repeated doses every 3 hours until completion of pregnancy termination to be acceptable practice (WHO, 2022), and with the rapidly shifting legal environment in the United States, seeking hospital care in the absence of hemorrhage or other urgent issues may be less desirable.

Follow-up after any abortion care includes ensuring needs for contraception, if any, are met. All methods except IUDs can be started on the same day as misoprostol administration; IUDs require completion of abortion prior to insertion of the IUD (NAF, 2024). However, while it is important to ensure that people have access to contraception if desired, abortion is not a consequence of failed contraception but rather a separate category of health care, and contraception may be neither needed nor desired by a given person. Ensuring access to contraception free from pressure or coercion to receive contraception is essential, given the history of reproductive coercion within health care.

While routine follow-up appointments may be offered, ultrasound to confirm completion of procedure is not required, and assessment of procedure completion is usually via history. Patient education prior to the abortion should include warning signs and symptoms of infection and retained tissue, as well as clear instructions on when to contact the provider versus seeking emergency care. This is particularly relevant for patients who may have traveled out of state or used telehealth to access abortion care due to local laws. It is important for both providers and patients to understand that medication abortion is overwhelmingly safe and effective, and that one of the major risks to it is legal risk in some jurisdictions.

Procedural Abortion

Procedural abortion, previously called "surgical abortion" (although it is not surgery) or generically referred to as a "D&C [dilation and curettage]" is one of the most common medical procedures performed in the United States (Kortsmit et al., 2023). In the first trimester, it has a safety profile better than that of tonsillectomy (Edmondson et al., 2022) and colonoscopy (Tomaszewski at al., 2021), but the narrative in the general population as well as politically has focused on its perceived danger. The most common risks to procedural abortion are similar to those of IUD placement (infection and perforation), and a landmark analysis of data in 2012 found that procedural abortion is approximately 12–14 times safer than continuing a pregnancy in the United States (Grimes & Raymond, 2012). The shift in terminology to "procedural abortion" is meant both to increase precision in language, and also to more accurately reflect the relative safety of abortion (Upadhyay et al., 2023).

Procedural abortion in the first trimester almost always refers to aspiration, which can be done with a mechanical suction similar to that used for airway maintenance, or with a manual vacuum aspirator (MVA), which is a handheld device similar to a large syringe with an extra valve added to avoid inadvertently injecting air into the uterus, which can be fatal. While dilation and curettage is taught routinely in OBGYN residency programs and is thus more familiar to many providers, risks of complication are higher with this procedure than with aspiration (Kakinuma et al., 2020) and it requires significant sedation and/or general anesthesia for patient tolerability. By contrast, aspiration procedures are routinely performed in stand-alone clinics or in offices, as well as in hospital settings, and the use of sedation or anesthesia is at the option of the patient.

Aspiration procedures (up until approximately 13–14 weeks) are a single-visit procedure. The duration of pregnancy is confirmed, with or without ultrasound, and a bimanual pelvic exam is used to identify uterine position and confirm size. Similar to an IUD placement, the provider inserts a speculum and uses a tenaculum or Allis clamp to provide traction to stabilize the uterus. It is standard to use a total of 10–20 mL 1–2% lidocaine, with or without bicarbonate as buffer, for a paracervical block. This is instilled into the lateral aspects of the cervical body at the cervicouterine junction. Injection site selection and pre-injection aspiration are essential to avoid inadvertent injection into the uterine arteries, which run approximately at 9 and 3 o'clock. The patient should be told to report any ringing in their ears, rapid heart rate, or numbness during the injection, as these may indicate lidocaine is being injected into the vessel. Instructions for performing a paracervical block are in **Appendix 19-B**.

The cervix is dilated using progressively larger cervical dilators, to a diameter that will accommodate the cannula for aspiration. The cannula selection is somewhat individual, but as a rule, the French measurement approximately equals the gestation in weeks LMP. Thus, an 8-week pregnancy would require an 8Fr cannula size. Cannulae are single-use and are available in rigid and flexible forms; the flexible cannulae are less likely to perforate the uterus but may not hold position adequately, particularly in larger sizes. The cannula is used with suction, whether mechanical or manual, to empty the uterus of tissue and blood. When the uterus is emptied, it will contract down and the walls will take on a characteristic "rough" feeling that has been compared to the front of the hard palate in the mouth.

The tissue should be examined prior to the end of the procedure, using water to separate the blood and the pregnancy tissue, and then floating the tissue above a light source to identify it. If inadequate tissue is seen, the uterus should be reaspirated and the new tissue examined to confirm procedure completion. Once completion is confirmed, an IUD may be inserted if desired. Routine ultrasound to confirm completion is not needed, assuming that adequate tissue is identified. A single dose of intraprocedural antibiotics is recommended for prophylaxis (Cheng et al., 2025).

Pain control during procedural abortion is similar in some ways to pain control for medication abortion. In both cases, nonpharmacologic methods like emotional support, hot pads, and other modalities are important to manage pain, and may be all that are needed. The role of abortion doula, similar to the role of birth doula, has started to emerge in some areas, and the limited research available suggests this support is helpful for some patients, and is recommended by most who experience it (Jefford et al., 2023). Pharmacologic pain options can include local anesthesia, narcotics, anxiolytics, oral or parenteral NSAIDs, sedation, and general anesthesia. With each step up the pain management scale, of course, risk also increases, and a discussion of this relative risk is important to have. However, it is also important for pain control decisions to be made as part of shared decision making with the patient, given their specific circumstances.

Aftercare for procedural abortion is similar to that of medication abortion. Most patients are able to leave the clinical facility shortly after their procedure, and do not have activity restrictions. Many patients return to work the next day, while others may prefer a day or two away from work or school. As with medication abortion, the concerning signs for procedural abortion are (1) flu-like illness, (2) fever >38C, (3) soaking >1 pad per hour for more than 1 hour, (4) passing clots larger than a lime, (5) increasing or severe pain, and (6) feeling very unwell or faint. All of these require evaluation, either in person or via telehealth, and part of pre-abortion counseling must be identifying the best process to access evaluation in a given area. Approximately 90 percent of counties have no abortion provider (Guttmacher, 2025a), and the distance that people travel to access abortion care has increased substantially in recent years (Rader et al., 2022), so finding an appropriate emergency care source in advance is essential.

As with medication abortion, contraception, if desired, can be started immediately after the procedure. While historically patients have been told to refrain from anything in the vagina for 2 weeks following a procedural abortion, there is little to no evidence to support this, and if pregnancy is desired, patients may start trying to conceive when they feel ready. If the procedural abortion was for a spontaneous abortion, patients may want to submit the pregnancy tissue for pathology and genetic testing. Some patients prefer not to know the sex of the fetus, for example, so this conversation should be had prior to any narcotics or sedation, with the knowledge that the pathology and genetic report will often be automatically released to the patient's chart, and they may not be able to avoid seeing it.

LATER ABORTION (>14 WEEKS LMP)

While later abortion is relatively rare (approximately 90 percent of intentional terminations and 98 percent of spontaneous abortions occur in the first trimester), it is increasing in frequency as people face more difficulty accessing intentional terminations promptly (Riley et al., 2024) and it carries more risks than early abortion (although still lower than carrying a pregnancy to term; Cheng et al., 2025). Therefore, it is important to understand the options and processes of second- and third-trimester abortion care, regardless of whether such care is provided. In particular, patients seeking intentional termination of pregnancy or care for pregnancy loss at later gestations have often had complicated journeys, whether because of fetal anomaly or difficulty accessing care, or for other reasons, and it is essential that staff and providers provide patient-centered and trauma-informed care.

Medication Abortion at Later Gestations

In the United States, medication abortion is not generally used in later gestations because of the availability and relatively lower risk of procedural abortions for these patients. The exception is when patients desire an induction abortion, in which labor is induced prior to viability and the fetus is delivered intact. This is most common for patients terminating a desired pregnancy, usually for fetal reasons. These abortions are very similar to any labor induction and usually start with misoprostol every 3–4 hours to ripen the cervix and, hopefully, induce contractions. Many providers will then switch to IV oxytocin (Pitocin) and offer parenteral or regional pain control when desired. While cervical change is often slow, delivery can be precipitous, and the provider should be alert for the possibility of retained tissues, particularly the placenta, and be ready to intervene if this occurs. In many circumstances, the patient can have photos taken of the fetus and bereavement care is often very helpful to their grieving process.

In some cases, induction abortions are used for intentional termination of pregnancy, particularly those in the third trimester. Although such abortions are rare, it is important to know that several states will provide this care if a patient needs it. The Guttmacher Institute (Guttmacher.org) keeps an updated list of abortion regulations by state and is a good resource to consult. This list is accessible here: https://states.guttmacher.org/policies.

Procedural Abortion in Later Gestations

Procedural abortion in later gestations share some similarities with earlier procedural abortion but have some changes that are specific to the larger fetal size, larger uterus, and need for greater dilation that are inherent in later abortion. The first consideration is cervical dilation, which is ideally done gradually to avoid the risk of weakening or lacerating the cervical musculature and potentially increasing the risk of preterm labor in future pregnancies. Because the fetal tissue is so much larger and because calcification of the fetal long bones begins at the end of the first trimester (Blackburn, 2017), significantly more dilation is required to safely remove the fetal and placental tissues in later gestations. This can be accomplished using sterilized compressed seaweed (laminaria japonica) or synthetic osmotic dilators (e.g., Dilapan) placed in the cervical os, which absorb moisture from the surrounding tissues and gradually stretch the cervical os.

For pregnancies prior to approximately 22 weeks LMP, 1 day of dilation may be adequate. For later gestations, the dilation may be done over 2 days to allow adequate time for cervical expansion. This can be quite uncomfortable, and also may result in spontaneous labor including delivery in itself, so patient education is essential prior to beginning the procedure. In addition, cervical preparation must be considered the start of the abortion procedure, because of the significant risk of infection and spontaneous labor if the abortion is not completed, and this should be part of the discussion with patients prior to starting the procedure.

For pregnancies greater than approximately 20 weeks LMP, most providers will provide intrafetal or intra-amniotic injections of lidocaine, digoxin, or potassium chloride to insure against a live delivery. While the best estimates of fetal neurological development place the capacity to experience pain at approximately 26–28 weeks LMP, many patients find it comforting that there is no chance of fetal pain after injection. The injection is done under ultrasound guidance using local anesthesia, usually on day 1 of the procedure.

The second stage of a later procedural abortion is the removal of fetal tissue using ring forceps and aspiration. As with earlier procedural terminations, completion of the procedure is verified with examination of the removed tissue. In later abortions it is also usual to use real-time ultrasound during the procedure to reduce the risk of perforation and retained products of conception (NAF, 2024). In particular, amnion and chorion are challenging to identify as complete through visual examination and can cause both subinvolution and infection.

As with earlier procedural terminations, contraception can be started immediately if desired. Some providers use a brief (<1 week) course of both antibiotics and uterotonics to reduce the risk of complications following the procedure, but neither are currently recommended in the postoperative period (NAF, 2024). IV or IM oxytocin (Pitocin) can be used in clinic to reduce the risk of hemorrhage from 18–24 weeks LMP (NAF, 2024), and periprocedural antibiotics are recommended (Cheng et al., 2025), usually beginning at the time of dilation. Patient teachings around bleeding parameters and signs of infection are the same as for earlier procedural abortions. **Table 19-9** compares these options.

Abortion can be performed as soon as pregnancy is detected, although some clinicians opt to wait until a gestational sac can be visualized on ultrasound or during postprocedure tissue examination, which is usually by 4 to 6 weeks' gestation. Aspiration abortion prior to 6 weeks' gestation has been shown to be safe and effective, particularly if protocols that guard against missed ectopic or continuing pregnancies are followed (Borchert et al., 2018; Planned Parenthood League of Massachusetts, 2019). Upper limits beyond which therapeutic abortion may be performed are based on legal (rather than medical) restrictions and vary from state to state. In recent years, an increase in legislative restrictions to abortion at the state level have been enacted in many parts of the country. Clinicians who provide care to the approximately 43 percent of women of reproductive age who live in states deemed hostile or very hostile to abortion rights may face new logistic and ethical challenges in helping patients access the services they desire (Nash, 2019).

A number of factors contribute to the decision about which abortion method will be used, including the gestational length of the pregnancy, patient preference, and provider training and availability. Nurse practitioners, nurse-midwives, and physician assistants can provide medication and/or procedural abortion in the large majority of the states that continue to have legal abortion (Guttmacher, 2025b; Jenkins et al., 2023). State-specific information about the current status of such laws and regulations and considerations for clinicians interested in offering abortion in their practice is available from Clinicians in Abortion Care/National Abortion Federation.

In addition to providing education and answering patients' questions about different abortion methods, clinicians who do

TABLE 19-9 Comparison of First-Trimester Abortion Options

Consideration	Early Aspiration Abortion	Medication Abortion
Invasive procedure	Yes	No, except if medication fails (less than 1–2%)
Anesthesia	If desired	Only if procedural intervention is needed and anesthesia is desired
Time to complete	Typically a few minutes; may be longer with advancing gestation	Typically 1 to 2 days from time of taking first medication (mifepristone); approximately 80 percent complete within 24 hours of taking misoprostol
Success rate	High, 99 percent	High, approximately 98–99 percent
Women's common perception of bleeding	Light	Moderate to heavy
Follow-up	Not required in most cases	Required to ensure completion of abortion
Number of visits to provider	One for procedure; may be more depending on state laws about required waiting period after counseling	Two (one to receive mifepristone and one for follow-up) unless provider follows protocols that allow for telemedicine prescribing and/or remote follow-up; may be more depending on state laws about required waiting period after counseling

not, or are not able to, provide abortion services must be able to relay pertinent information about specific referral sites, including the types of abortion available and gestational age limits, cost, type of insurance accepted; languages spoken; and likelihood of encountering protestors. State and institutional policies that can affect patients' abortion experiences—such as laws about pre- and postviability procedures, Medicaid, targeted regulation of providers, parental consent, state-mandated counseling, or waiting periods—should also be discussed. Resources for identifying abortion services in a particular state or region are listed in **Table 19-10**. Clinicians can also deepen their knowledge about local services by communicating directly with providers and staff from clinics and hospitals where abortions are performed, talking to colleagues, and asking patients about their abortion experiences.

The Abortion Care Network has developed a set of guidelines that both women and clinicians can use to find high-quality service delivery sites. The National Abortion Federation also has suggestions for determining if a clinic delivers safe, quality care (refer to Table 19-10). Given the illicit history of abortion in the United States prior to legalization and its continued illegality in many parts of the world, safety and quality are prominent concerns for many people that should be addressed as part of pregnancy options and abortion counseling.

Paying for Abortion

The majority of people in the United States pay out of pocket for their abortions, regardless of their insurance status (Jerman et al., 2016). A number of states restrict coverage of abortion under plans offered through insurance exchanges and for public employees; some also limit coverage of abortion by private insurers that are written in the state (Guttmacher Institute, 2019b). In 34 states and the District of Columbia, women who are Medicaid recipients are not covered for abortion because of the Hyde Amendment, which prohibits use of federal funds to pay for abortion services (Guttmacher Institute, 2025b). Given that the average cost of a first-trimester abortion in the United States is approximately $550 (Harned & Fuentes, 2023), this expense delays some people from obtaining services (Roberts et al., 2014). A number of independent state and national funds have been established to assist women seeking but unable to pay for an abortion. For information on these funds, refer to the National Network of Abortion Funds (https://abortionfunds.org/).

CONCLUSION

Abortion, whether spontaneous or intentional, is a common experience for many people. Management of pregnancy loss and intentional termination of pregnancy are not significantly different from a technical perspective but may require different kinds of support and resources for emotional responses afterwards. Access to safe abortion is identified as an essential health service by the World Health Organization and is considered within the scope of midwifery and nursing care by the relevant professional organizations. While nurses and midwives who opt not to participate in abortion care are protected by conscience clauses and other laws, they still are obligated under the ANA Code of Ethics (2024) and the ACNM Code of Ethics (2024) to refer patients as needed, and not to obstruct patient access to care. Because patient education and advocacy are key parts of nursing practice, it is essential for nurses to be adequately informed on abortion to appropriately educate and refer patients as needed.

TABLE 19-10 Resources for People Seeking Abortion Services

Organization	Where to Obtain the Resource	Description
Abortion Care Network	https://www.abortioncarenetwork.org/clinics/ Information on clinic locations can also be obtained by texting "hello" to 202-883-4620	List of independent abortion care providers who belong to the Abortion Care Network, organized by state
Abortion Clinics Online	http://abortionclinics.com	List of sites that offer abortion services, searchable by city and state
Bedsider	https://www.bedsider.org/where_to _get_it	Clinic locator that includes information on sites that provide abortion
Full Spectrum Doulas	http://www.fullspectrumdoulas.org	Information about doulas who provide abortion support
National Abortion Federation	1-877-257-0012	Provides referrals to quality abortion providers in the caller's area
	http://prochoice.org/think-youre-pregnant/find-a-provider	State-by-state map with information about state legislation that impacts abortion service delivery (e.g., waiting periods, mandated counseling) and contact information of National Abortion Federation member providers
	http://prochoice.org/think-youre-pregnant/i-want-an-abortion-what-should-i-expect	Includes questions to help determine if an abortion provider is safe
Planned Parenthood	1-800-230-PLAN (7526)	Helps the caller find the nearest Planned Parenthood health center
	https://www.plannedparenthood.org/health-center	Search for Planned Parenthood health centers by state or zip code
Radical Doula	http://radicaldoula.com	Includes profiles of doulas that provide full-spectrum care, including abortion support

References

18 U.S.C. § 1461 (1972). *Mailing obscene or crime-inciting matter.* https://uscode.house.gov/view.xhtml?req=granuleid:USC-prelim-title18-section1461&num=0&edition=prelim

AmericanAcademyofPhysician'sAssociates.(2021).*EthicalguidelinesforthePAprofession.* https://www.aapa.org/wp-content/uploads/2021/11/Guidelines-for-Ethical-Conduct-for-the-PA-Profession-7-1-21.pdf

American College of Nurse-Midwives. (2025). *Midwives as abortion providers position statement.* https://midwife.org/wp-content/uploads/2025/04/2025-ps_midwives-as-abortion-providers_amended.pdf

American College of Obstetricians and Gynecologists. (2012). ACOG committee opinion no. 528: Adoption. *Obstetrics & Gynecology, 119*(6), 1320[en dash]1324. https://doi.org/10.1097/AOG.0b013e31825af411. PMID: 22617617.

American College of Obstetricians and Gynecologists. (2013, reaffirmed 2019). ACOG committee opinion no. 554: Reproductive and sexual coercion. *Obstetrics & Gynecology, 121*(2), 411–415.

American College of Obstetricians and Gynecologists. (2014, reaffirmed 2025). *ACOG committee opinion no. 612: Abortion Training and Education.* https://www.acog.org/clinical/clinical-guidance/committee-opinion/articles/2014/11/abortion-training-and-education

American College of Obstetricians and Gynecologists. (2018, reaffirmed 2025). *ACOG Practice Bulletin No. 193: Tubal Ectopic Pregnancy.* https://www.acog.org/clinical/clinical-guidance/practice-bulletin/articles/2018/03/tubal-ectopic-pregnancy

American College of Obstetricians and Gynecologists. (2022). *Abortion policy: Statement of policy.* https://www.acog.org/clinical-information/policy-and-position-statements/statements-of-policy/2022/abortion-policy

American Nurses Association. (2025). Code of Ethics for Nurses with Interpretive Statements.

Bearak, J. M., Popinchalk, A., Beavin, C., Ganatra, B., Moller, A. B., Tunçalp, Ö., & Alkema, L. (2022). Country-specific estimates of unintended pregnancy and abortion incidence: A global comparative analysis of levels in 2015–2019. *BMJ Global Health, 7*(3), e007151.

Blackburn, S. T. (2017). *Maternal, fetal, & neonatal physiology: A clinical perspective.* Saunders.

Borchert, K., Wipf, H., Roeske, E., Clure, C., Traxler, S., & Boraas, C. (2018). Pregnancy of unknown location in abortion care: Management and outcomes. *Contraception, 97*(5), 463.

Bridwell, R. E., Long, B., Montrief, T., & Gottlieb, M. (2022). Post-abortion complications: A narrative review for emergency clinicians. *Western Journal of Emergency Medicine, 23*(6), 919.

Bryant, A. G., & Swartz, J. J. (2018). Why crisis pregnancy centers are legal but unethical. *AMA Journal of Ethics, 20*(3), 269–277.

Cappiello, J., Levi, A., & Nothnagle, M. (2016). Core competencies in sexual and reproductive health for the interprofessional primary care team. *Contraception, 93*(5), 438–445. https://doi.org/10.1016/j.contraception.2015.12.013

Castuera, I. (2017). A social history of Christian thought on abortion: Ambiguity vs. certainty in moral debate. *American Journal of Economics and Sociology, 76*(1), 121–227.

Centers for Disease Control and Prevention, U.S. Department of Health & Human Services. (2024). *About intimate partner violence.* https://www.cdc.gov/intimate-partner-violence/about/index.html.

Cheng, T., Kumar, N., Laursen, L., Achilles, S. L., & Reeves, M. F. (2025). Society of Family Planning Clinical Recommendation: Prevention of infection after abortion and pregnancy loss. *Contraception*, 110895.

Creinin, M. D., Schwartz, J. L., Pymar, H. C., & Fink, W. (2001). Efficacy of mifepristone followed on the same day by misoprostol for early termination of pregnancy: Report of a randomised trial. *British Journal of Obstetrics and Gynaecology, 108*(5), 469–473.

Crequit, S., Chatzistergiou, K., Bierry, G., Bouali, S., La Tour, A. D., Sghiouar, N., & Renevier, B. (2023). Association between social vulnerability profiles, prenatal care use and pregnancy outcomes. *BMC Pregnancy and Childbirth, 23*(1), 465.

Eagen-Torkko, M., & Levi, A. J. (2020). The ethical justification for conscience clauses in nurse-midwifery practice: Context, power, and a changing landscape. *Journal of Midwifery & Women's Health, 65*(6), 759–766.

Edmonson, M. B., Zhao, Q., Francis, D. O., Kelly, M. M., Sklansky, D. J., Shadman, K. A., & Coller, R. J. (2022). Association of patient characteristics with postoperative mortality in children undergoing tonsillectomy in 5 U.S. states. *JAMA, 327*(23), 2317–2325. https://doi.org/10.1001/jama.2022.8679

Ferguson, I., & Scott, H. (2020). Systematic review of the effectiveness, safety, and acceptability of mifepristone and misoprostol for medical abortion in low- and middle-income countries. *Journal of Obstetrics and Gynaecology Canada, 42*(12), 1532–1542.

Grimes, D. A., & Raymond, E. G. (2012). The comparative safety of legal induced abortion and childbirth in the United States. *Obstetrics & Gynecology, 119*(2 Part 1), 215–219.

Guttmacher Institute. (2025a). *Data center.* https://data.guttmacher.org/states/table?state=US&topics=58&dataset=data

Guttmacher Institute. (2025b). *State funding of abortion under Medicaid.* https://www.guttmacher.org/state-policy/explore/state-funding-abortion-under-medicaid

Harned, E., & Fuentes, L. (2023). *Abortion out of reach: The exacerbation of wealth disparities after* Dobbs v. Jackson Women's Health Organization. https://www.guttmacher.org/article/2023/01/abortion-out-reach-exacerbation-wealth-disparities-after-dobbs-v-jackson-womens

Higginbotham E. (2002). When your beliefs run counter to care. *RN, 65*(1), 69-72. PMID: 12465529.

Jain, D., Davies, M., Perritt, J., & Blasdell, J. (2023). The provision of medication abortion care via telehealth. *Women's Health Issues, 33*(4), 333–336.

Jefford, E., Marsden, J., & Ebert, L. (2023). The impact of abortion doulas on women and providers' outcomes: An integrative review of the evidence. *Sexual & Reproductive Healthcare, 37*, 100888.

Jenkins, J., Pitney, C., Nuzzo, M., & Eagen-Torkko, M. (2023). Midwifery and APRN scope of practice in abortion care in the early post-Roe era: Everything old is new again. *Journal of Midwifery & Women's Health, 68*(6), 734–743.

Jerman, J., Jones, R. K., & Onda, T. (2016). *Characteristics of US abortion patients in 2014 and changes since 2008.* https://www.guttmacher.org/report/characteristics-us-abortion-patients-2014?ref=popsugar.com&=___psv__p_49064103__t_w__r_www.popsugar.com%2Fhealth%2Fabortion-pill-advance-provision-49332675_

Jones, R. K., & Jerman, J. (2022). Population group abortion rates and lifetime incidence of abortion: United States, 2008–2014. *American Journal of Public Health, 112*(9), 1284–1296.

Kakinuma T., Kakinuma K., Sakamoto Y., Kawarai Y., Saito K., Ihara M., Matsuda Y., Sato I., Ohwada M., Yanagida K., Tanaka H., (2020). Safety and efficacy of manual vacuum suction compared with conventional dilatation and sharp curettage and electric vacuum aspiration in surgical treatment of miscarriage: A randomized controlled trial. *BMC Pregnancy Childbirth, 20*(1), 695. https://doi.org/10.1186/s12884-020-03362-4. PMID: 33198679; PMCID: PMC7667767.

Kallner, H. K. (2023). Medical abortion in the second trimester–an update. *Current Opinion in Obstetrics and Gynecology, 35*(6), 490–495.

Kortsmit, K., Nguyen, A. T., Mandel, M. G., Hollier, L. M., Ramer, S., Rodenhizer, J., & Whiteman, M. K. (2023). Abortion Surveillance - United States, 2021. *Morbidity and mortality weekly report. Surveillance summaries (Washington, D.C. : 2002), 72*(9), 1–29. https://doi.org/10.15585/mmwr.ss7209a1

Krugh, M., Patel, P., Maani, C. V. (2024). Misoprostol. *StatPearls.* Accessed at https://www.ncbi.nlm.nih.gov/books/NBK539873/

Landon, M. B., Galan, H. L., Jauniaux, E. R. M., Driscoll, D. A., Berghella, V., Grobman, W. A., Kilpatrick, S. J., & Cahill, A. G. (Eds.). (2025). *Gabbe's obstetrics: Normal and problem pregnancies* (9th ed.). Elsevier.

Lee, L., Ma, W., Davies, S., & Kammers, M. (2023). Toward optimal emotional care during the experience of miscarriage: An integrative review of the perspectives of women, partners, and health care providers. *Journal of Midwifery & Women's Health, 68*(1), 52–61.

Mahajan, D. K., & London, S. N. (1997). Mifepristone (RU486): A review. *Fertility and Sterility, 68*(6), 967–976.

Mullany, K., Minneci, M., Monjazeb, R., & C Coiado, O. (2023). Overview of ectopic pregnancy diagnosis, management, and innovation. *Women's health (London, England), 19*, 17455057231160349. https://doi.org/10.1177/17455057231160349

Musik, T., Grimm, J., Juhasz-Böss, I., & Bäz, E. (2021). Treatment options after a diagnosis of early miscarriage: Expectant, medical, and surgical. *Deutsches Ärzteblatt International, 118*(46), 789.

Nash, E. (2019). Abortion rights in peril—what clinicians need to know. *New England Journal of Medicine, 381*, 497–499. https://doi.org/10.1056/NEJMp1906972

National Abortion Federation (NAF). (2024). *Clinical policy guidelines for abortion care.* https://prochoice.org/wp-content/uploads/2024-CPGs-FINAL-1.pdf

National Association of Nurse Practitioners in Women's Health. (2022). *Position statement: Access to safe abortion care.* Accessed at https://www.npwomenshealthcare.com/position-statement-access-to-safe-abortion-care-2/#:~:text=The%20National%20Association%20of%20Nurse%20Practitioners%20in,it%20should%20be%20legal%2C%20safe%2C%20and%20accessible.&text=Current%20and%20potential%20state%20legislative%20restrictions%20target,services%20or%20counsel%20patients%20about%20such%20services

Park, K. E., Latack, K. R., Vestal, N. L., Ingles, S. A., Paulson, R. J., & Awadalla, M. S. (2023). Association of HCG Level with Ultrasound Visualization of the Gestational Sac in Early Viable Pregnancies. *Reproductive sciences (Thousand Oaks, Calif.), 30*(12), 3623–3628. https://doi.org/10.1007/s43032-023-01308-7

Planned Parenthood League of Massachusetts. (2019). *Medication abortion for pregnancy of unknown location (MAPUL)* (Clinicaltrials.gov identifier NCT04026789). https://clinicaltrials.gov/ct2/show/NCT04026789

Quenby, S., Gallos, I. D., Dhillon-Smith, R. K., Podesek, M., Stephenson, M. D., Fisher, J., Brosens, J. J., Brewin, J., Ramhorst, R., Lucas, E. S., McCoy, R. C., Anderson, R., Daher, S., Regan, L., Al-Memar, M., Bourne, T., MacIntyre, D. A., Rai, R., Christiansen, O. B., Sugiura-Ogasawara, M., ... Coomarasamy, A. (2021). Miscarriage matters: the epidemiological, physical, psychological, and economic costs of early pregnancy loss. *Lancet (London, England), 397*(10285), 1658–1667. https://doi.org/10.1016/S0140-6736(21)00682-6

Rader, B., Upadhyay, U. D., Sehgal, N. K. R., Reis, B. Y., Brownstein, J. S., & Hswen, Y. (2022). Estimated travel time and spatial access to abortion facilities in the US before and after the *Dobbs v Jackson Women's Health* decision. *JAMA, 328*(20), 2041–2047. https://doi.org/10.1001/jama.2022.20424

Reagan L. J. (1995). Linking midwives and abortion in the Progressive Era. *Bulletin of the History of Medicine, 69*(4), 569–598.

Reagan, L. J. (2023). From when abortion was a crime to abortion is a crime. *Bulletin of the History of Medicine, 97*(1), 11–21.

Recker, F., Kagan, K. O., & Maul, H. (2025). Advancing knowledge and public health: A scientific exploration of abortion safety. *Archives of Gynecology and Obstetrics*, 1–9.

Riley, T., Fiastro, A. E., Benson, L. S., Khattar, A., Prager, S., & Godfrey, E. M. (2024). Abortion provision and delays to care in a clinic network in Washington State after Dobbs. *JAMA Network Open, 7*(5), e2413847–e2413847.

Roberts, S. C., Gould, H., Kimport, K., Weitz, T. A., & Foster, D. G. (2014). Out-of-pocket costs and insurance coverage for abortion in the United States. *Women's Health Issues, 24*(2), e211-e218.

Rocca, C. H., Kimport, K., Roberts, S. C., Gould, H., Neuhaus, J., & Foster, D. G. (2015). Decision rightness and emotional responses to abortion in the United States: A longitudinal study. *PloS One, 10*(7), e0128832.

Román-Gálvez, R. M., Martín-Peláez, S., Fernández-Félix, B. M., Zamora, J., Khan, K. S., & Bueno-Cavanillas, A. (2021). Worldwide prevalence of intimate partner violence in pregnancy: A systematic review and meta-analysis. *Frontiers in Public Health, 9*, 738459.

Simmonds, K., & Likis, F. E. (2011). Caring for women with unintended pregnancies. *Journal of Obstetric, Gynecologic, and Neonatal Nursing, 40*(6), 794–807. https://doi.org/10.1111/j.1552-6909.2011.01293.x

SisterSong. (n.d.). *What is reproductive justice?* https://www.sistersong.net/reproductive-justice

Sitruk-Ware, R. (2006). Mifepristone and misoprostol sequential regimen side effects, complications and safety. *Contraception, 74*(1), 48–55.

Soper, John T. MD. (2021). Gestational trophoblastic disease: Current evaluation and management. *Obstetrics & Gynecology, 137*(2), 355-370. https://doi.org/ 10.1097/AOG.0000000000004240

Spitz, I. M. (2010). Mifepristone: Where do we come from and where are we going? Clinical development over a quarter of a century. *Contraception, 82*(5), 442–452.

Stifani, B. M., & Lavelanet, A. F. (2024). Reversal of medication abortion with progesterone: A systematic review. *BMJ Sexual & Reproductive Health, 50*(1), 43–52.

Tomaszewski, M., Sanders, D., Enns, R., Gentile, L., Cowie, S., Nash, C., Petrunia, D., Mullins, P., Hamm, J., Azari-Razm, N., Bykov, D., & Telford, J. (2021). Risks associated with colonoscopy in a population-based colon screening program: An observational cohort study. *CMAJ Open, 9*(4), E940–E947. https://doi.org/10.9778/cmajo.20200192

United States Food & Drug Administration (FDA). (2025), *Questions & answers on mifepristone for medical termination of pregnancy through ten weeks gestation.* https://www.fda.gov/drugs/postmarket-drug-safety-information-patients-and-providers/questions-and-answers-mifepristone-medical-termination-pregnancy-through-ten-weeks-gestation#GeneralInformation

Upadhyay, U. D., Coplon, L., & Atrio, J. M. (2023). Society of Family Planning Committee Statement: Abortion nomenclature. *Contraception, 126*, 110094.

Whittum, M., & Rapkin, R. (2022). History of abortion legislation in the United States. *Journal of Gynecologic Surgery, 38*(5), 320–323.

Wiebe, E. R. (1999). Comparing abortion induced with methotrexate and misoprostol to methotrexate alone. *Contraception, 59*(1), 7–10.

World Health Organization (WHO). (2022). *Abortion care guideline.* https://www.who.int/publications/i/item/9789240039483

APPENDIX 19-A

Resources on Reproductive Options, Legislation, and Policies

Abortion Care Network (http://www.abortioncarenetwork.org): Maintains a list of clinics that provide abortion across the United States.

All-Options (https://www.all-options.org): Resources and support for women seeking information and support for all pregnancy options.

Clinicians in Abortion Care (https://prochoice.org/health-care-professionals/ciac/about-ciac/): Membership organization representing certified nurse-midwives, nurse practitioners, physician assistants, and nurses working to increase access to comprehensive reproductive health care.

Global Abortion Policies Database (https://abortion-policies.srhr.org): Comprehensive information on abortion laws, policies, health standards, and guidelines for the World Health Organization and United Nations Member States.

Guttmacher Institute (http://www.guttmacher.org): Research and policy organization committed to advancing sexual and reproductive health and rights, including research and analysis for individual states (http://www.guttmacher.org/statecenter).

Kaiser Family Foundation (http://www.kff.org): Nonpartisan source of health facts and health policy analysis, including specifics regarding state policies and legislation (http://www.statehealthfacts.kff.org, click on "Women's Health").

National Abortion Federation (http://www.prochoice.org): Professional association of abortion providers that offers educational materials, information on relevant policies and legislation, an abortion provider locator, and a financial assistance program.

National Council for Adoption (http://adoptioncouncil.org/): Provides information for pregnant women considering adoption and resources for birth parents, adopted individuals, and adoptive families.

- General resources (https://www.adoptioncouncil.org/resources/general)
- Choosing adoption (https://www.adoptioncouncil.org/expectant-parents/about-adoption)
- Adoption agency search (http://www.adoptioncouncil.org/expectant-parents/find-an-agency/search)

National Network of Abortion Funds (http://www.fundabortionnow.org): Network of organizations across the United States that work to remove financial and logistical barriers to abortion access. Some funds help pay for abortions for women who need financial assistance.

APPENDIX 19-B

Instructions for Performing a Paracervical Block

1. **Review Contraindications**:
   - Allergy to lidocaine or local anesthetics
   - Current pregnancy (if not indicated)
   - Vaginal infection or bleeding disorder
2. **Gather Supplies:**
   - 20 mL of 1% lidocaine (or 10 mL of 2% lidocaine if 1% is unavailable)
   - 22g, 3.5 inch spinal needle or a 25g 1.5 inch needle with a needle extender
   - Syringe
   - Speculum
   - Tenaculum
   - Antiseptic solution and swabs
3. **Patient Preparation:**
   - Ensure informed consent.
   - Ask the patient to empty their bladder.
   - Perform a bimanual exam to assess uterine size and position.
   - Position the patient in lithotomy.

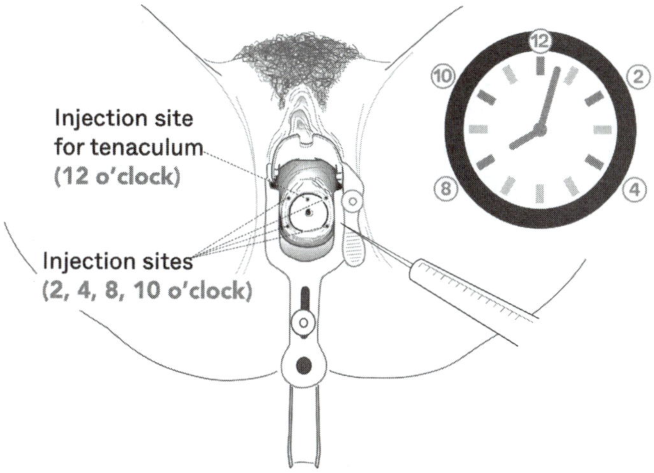

Reproduced from Ipas. (2023). Paracervical block technique. https://www.ipas.org/resource/paracervical-block-technique/

Procedure

1. **Antiseptic Prep:**
   - Insert the speculum.
   - Clean the cervix thoroughly with antiseptic-soaked swabs.
2. **Initial Lidocaine Injection:**
   - Inject **2 mL of lidocaine** superficially into the **anterior lip of the cervix at 12 o'clock**, where the tenaculum will be placed.
3. **Apply Tenaculum:**
   - Grasp the cervix at the 12 o'clock position with the tenaculum.
4. **Paracervical Block Injections:**
   - Inject the remaining lidocaine (approximately 18 mL) in **equal amounts** at the **cervicovaginal junction** at the following positions:
     - **2 o'clock**
     - **4 o'clock**
     - **8 o'clock**
     - **10 o'clock**
   - Alternatively, a **two-point technique** (4 and 8 o'clock) may be used for simpler procedures.
5. **Injection Technique Tips:**
   - Insert the needle **deeply (3 cm)** for more effective pain relief.
   - **Aspirate before injecting** to avoid intravascular administration.
   - Watch for signs of intravascular injection: metallic taste, dizziness, tinnitus, or bradycardia.

Post-Injection

- Wait **3–5 minutes** for anesthetic effect.
- Proceed with the gynecologic procedure.
- Monitor the patient for any adverse reactions.

Safety Notes

- **Maximum lidocaine dose**: 4.5 mg/kg or **200 mg total**
- Serious adverse events are **rare** but always monitor for bradycardia or systemic toxicity.
- Advanced practice providers (including nurse practitioners) trained in this technique show **comparable safety and efficacy** to physicians.

(Adapted from https://www.ipas.org/wp-content/uploads/2021/06/Paracervical-Block-Technique-PARABLK-E21.pdf)

CHAPTER 20

Fertility, Infertility, and Assisted Family Building

Signey Olson

The editors acknowledge Monica Moore, who was the author of the previous edition of this chapter.

INTRODUCTION

Fertility, or the biological ability to conceive a child, can hold personal meanings for many people and is often influenced by numerous biological and social factors. For some individuals, an intent to become a parent may begin in childhood or adolescence and can feel innate. For others, a desire to have children may occur later in life, gradually over time, or be triggered by specific circumstances. For yet others, a desire to parent may not occur at all. Each of these scenarios represents a normal response to the prospective idea of continuing the evolutionary cycle of reproduction.

The majority of cultures and communities around the world hold pronatalist views, in which there is a cultural perspective that promotes pregnancy, birth, and family building (Abramov et al., 2022). While cultural context can influence this process, the societal encouragement of procreation may feel like an expectation to some individuals and can add a complex emotional layer to the experience of those actively trying to conceive. Those intentionally opting not to pursue parenthood may also invoke cultural or societal judgments (Ashburn-Nardo, 2017). Definitions of femininity and womanhood have been socially constructed over time and are frequently interlaced with the ability to conceive and give birth (Kaźmierczak & Karasiewicz, 2019). Historically, infertility has been viewed as a problem specific to women, which is both physiologically inaccurate and does not acknowledge the diversity in gender of individuals wanting to become parents. This view is gradually changing due to clinical improvements in diagnosing various etiologies of infertility. These advancements have led to the recognition that sperm-related factors contribute to infertility just as frequently as factors related to a person's uterus and/or ovaries (Schlegel et al., 2021). Nevertheless, matters of reproduction, childbearing, and childrearing continue to be viewed societally as "women's issues."

In most instances, prospective parents often feel influenced by age, cultural norms, social support, the presence or absence of a romantic partner, and socioeconomic factors. Many individuals have grown up rehearsing to be parents, with some believing that their identities are dependent on childbearing. Individuals may come from cultural backgrounds in which pregnancy and parenthood hold a high social value and the community context supersedes the need for other factors to be present (WHO, 2024). For those actively hoping for pregnancy, discovering that they are unable to conceive can be both shocking and devastating. Infertility is a complex, multifactorial condition that generates a variety of meanings among those experiencing it and can significantly affect the physical, psychosocial, and economic aspects of a person's life (Shreffler et al., 2017). The process of seeking treatment for infertility as a patient, as well as the perspective of providing infertility treatment as a clinician can be an inherently humbling experience, as there are many aspects of human reproduction that remain unknown.

It is important not to conflate an individual's desire to parent with a desire for a biological child and/or a desire to become pregnant, as these are not synonymous. The concept and definition of family and parenthood are greatly influenced by the culture and society a person is raised in and lives in. This includes variation in the roles that individuals decide or prefer to take on, as parenthood is individually defined. Parental identity may not always equate to being a current caregiver for a child, as may be the case for individuals who have experienced pregnancy loss or the death of a child or parents who no longer have legal custody of their children (Weitz & Karlsson, 2021). Additionally, some people may not have contributed genetically to a pregnancy but hold a role as a parent in a child's life.

The logistical and psychological process of family building varies based on numerous individual factors. This chapter describes the incidence and causes of infertility, the assessment of individuals experiencing infertility, and treatments for infertility. The basic medical definition of infertility is discussed to be an age-dependent diagnosis based on the length of time individuals have been trying to conceive. For individuals under the age of 35, the diagnosis of infertility is given after the person has had regular, unprotected intercourse for 12 or more months without conception occurring. For individuals over the age of 35, infertility is an appropriate diagnosis after the person has been engaging in regular, unprotected intercourse for 6 months or more. However, this definition does not explicitly address physiological or social scenarios in which it is difficult or unlikely to meet this definition of infertility. Therefore, this chapter also reviews the concept that infertility may not always be related to physiological barriers, but rather may be related to the lack of gametes required to create a pregnancy and/or other societally influenced factors. The review of appropriate assessment and treatments for individual cases is discussed, including those who have already attempted conception and are experiencing a barrier, and those who are planning a pregnancy which requires some assistance. Additionally, the psychological effects of infertility can be vast and are explored later in this chapter. An overview of various options available beyond trying to conceive, including fostering, adoption, and child-free living is discussed, as are some of the potential ethical issues related to infertility.

The field of reproductive endocrinology and infertility (REI) care has greatly improved since the introduction in the United States of REI specialty fellowship for physicians in 1972 and the demand for REI services has continued to increase. However, this demand currently outpaces the availability of trained REI specialists. Currently, REI fellowships are a 3-year program following a 4-year OB/GYN residency and fewer than 50 fellowships are available in the United States (Feinberg & Rosenwaks, 2021). This leaves a significant gap in the number of patients who need access to REI services versus available REI clinics. Worldwide, it is estimated that an additional 12–13 million couples would be able to have children if fertility treatment services were accessible to them (Hariton et al., 2023). To address the increasing need for REI specialty care, expanded inclusion of advanced practice providers practicing to the full scope of their license is a beneficial approach in the provision of fertility care. These services may include routine gynecologic care and first trimester obstetric ultrasounds, saline sonograms, hysterosalpingograms, IUIs, endometrial biopsies, urgent evaluations for pain/bleeding, and new patient consultations. Additionally, continuity of care, protocol planning, and treatment management are appropriate within the advanced practice provider role.

Language

The etiologies, assessment, and management of infertility often relate to sex assigned at birth; therefore, available research in this field frequently uses gendered language meant to differentiate causes of infertility based on an individual's sex. However, given the spectrum of anatomy that individuals facing infertility possess, the use of clinical anatomy is prioritized throughout this chapter to enhance both inclusivity and clinical accuracy. The use of the terms assigned female at birth (AFAB) and assigned male at birth (AMAB) are used here to signify those who carry egg gametes and sperm gametes, respectively, with recognition that not all individuals with these designations at birth may have all expected reproductive organs. Social scenarios related to family building are vast and clinicians should also be sensitive to the fact that many individuals trying to conceive are prospective intentional single parents; thus, presumptive use of the term *partner* should be avoided in generalized discussions. It is also important for clinicians to recognize that pregnancy may occur through the blending of biology, both through that of romantic partners or platonic known donors. Polyamorous or genetically blended families may intentionally incorporate multiple individuals, either genetically or socially as co-parents or co-guardians.

When presenting or discussing the pathophysiology of infertility, attention should be given to avoid the use of terms that reflect negatively on patients. Clinicians should be mindful that individuals with infertility are often listening closely and may internalize subtle nuances in wording. For example, cervical mucus that is not receptive to sperm has sometimes been referred to as "hostile cervical mucus," and a cervix that prematurely dilates has sometimes been called an "incompetent cervix." Although this verbiage may be viewed as innocuous from a clinical perspective, this negative terminology can connote blame on the patient's part for the infertility, when in reality, the cause of infertility is largely out of their control. Clinicians should use alternative terms (e.g., short cervix or cervical insufficiency) that have a less negative implication to avoid exacerbating potential guilt and distress individuals may have about their infertility. Furthermore, commonly used clinical language regarding fertility includes comments such as noting a "successful pregnancy" or "unsuccessful cycle" and noting a person's "ability" to "achieve" a pregnancy. In relation to fertility treatment cycles, the phrases "a failed cycle" or "recurrent failure to implant" may also be used. While these words may seem accurate in conveying an outcome and may not always be inappropriate when discussing generalizations, they can also feel performance-oriented and may create the unintended illusion that infertility is something a person can control with enough effort. This can be most prominent when discussing individualized diagnosis and treatment with patients. Achievement-based language can also inappropriately project subjective values onto objective clinical findings or histories, such as infertility. Additionally, use of language that implies a person can control their fertility upholds the narrative of historical sexism on which modern gynecology was founded. Better alternatives include simply stating whether a treatment or attempt to conceive results in a pregnancy and/or the birth of a term infant such as, "this cycle unfortunately did not result in pregnancy" or "this cycle resulted in pregnancy and live birth." Additionally, stating that a "pregnancy occurred" (rather than "was achieved") or commenting that "a person did not become pregnant" are examples of ways to lessen the potential sting of effort-based language.

Reproductive Goals Counseling

Although routine assessment of pregnancy intention for all individuals with reproductive potential is recommended, clinicians cannot assume an individual's reproductive plan (American Society for Reproductive Medicine [ASRM] & American College of Obstetricians and Gynecologists [ACOG] Committee on Gynecologic Practice, 2024). Some clinicians have their own procreative biases and may hold an assumption that all individuals capable of pregnancy desire to be parents in the future. Many patients have life goals that do not include parenting. Additionally, the process of becoming pregnant may be intentional and planned for some people, but others may prefer a more passive approach to pregnancy. Thus, clinicians should understand that the act of making or discussing a reproductive plan may not feel beneficial to all patients and intentionality may be arbitrary to some individuals' reproductive paths.

A trauma-informed approach to care should be utilized in all aspects of reproductive health, including those pertaining to fertility and family building. More about trauma-informed care can be found in Chapter 5. It is most appropriate to ask patients, in a nonjudgmental manner, about their goals related to pregnancy and parenting with explicit recognition that not all individuals choose to pursue parenthood. Normalizing brief clinical discussions regarding fertility from a young age allows clinicians to provide evidence-based education and proactively dispel pregnancy or fertility misconceptions. Some patients may opt to avoid the use of contraception out of a fear of future infertility and the clinician may be able to explore whether younger-aged pregnancies are a reproductive goal the patient has (WHO, 2024). These discussions can be framed by reviewing that reproductive and sexual health and fertility are important components of overall health and may lend clues to other health considerations not directly linked to trying to conceive. Additionally, early education may decrease the number of patients who feel shocked or startled to learn about the influence of increasing age on fertility later in life. For younger patients, awareness of age-related fertility changes may allow for opportunities to explore proactive consideration of oocyte freezing, discussed later in this chapter. Importantly, conversations around fertility should always be characterized as theoretical unless the patient is actively hoping to conceive, using qualifying phrases such as "if you decide to conceive in the future . . ." or "should you decide to become pregnant later in life . . . ." The clinician should remain objective by demonstrating a neutral tone and refraining from disclosure of any personally held beliefs about the timing of pregnancy, particularly as it relates to older or younger age. Additionally, if a patient states they have no plans for pregnancy now or ever in the future, the clinician should not encourage the patient that they are likely to change their minds in the future, as this can be perceived as paternalistic and dismissive of the patient's current perspective.

A tool that has been developed to assist clinicians in directly identifying patients' pregnancy desires in a primary care setting is the One Key Question screening question, "Would you like to become pregnant in the next year?" (Allen et al., 2017). By utilizing this or a similar question during routine appointments, providers can discern the need for pre-pregnancy counseling, including information about fertility and infertility (ASRM & ACOG, 2024). A helpful framework for clinicians to utilize in these clinical conversations is Reproductive Justice (RJ), a term coined by Loretta Ross, a co-founder of SisterSong Women of Color Reproductive Justice Collective in 1994 (Ross & Solinger, 2017). RJ emphasizes that reproductive health decisions must be addressed within the context of external systemic oppression, understanding that these systems directly influence a person's ability to make autonomous reproductive choices for their body. This approach is relevant to a variety of reproductive health scenarios, including abortion care, LGBTQ+ affirming care, contraceptive access, and infertility, representing the reality that bodily autonomy is an essential foundation for all aspects of reproductive health (Tam, 2021; Barnes & Fledderjohann, 2020). More information on RJ can be found in Chapter 2.

SCOPE OF THE CONDITION

The global fertility rate can be calculated by the number of biological children born in the total population. Currently, the fertility rate worldwide is approximately 2.2 children per individual with gestational capacity with the United States having a slightly lower fertility rate of approximately 2 children per individual with gestational capacity, a significant decrease from historical rates (United Nations, 2024). The replacement level of global fertility is 2.1, which is expected to be the global rate in 2050. Rapid population decline and subsequent population aging occurs when sustained levels decrease to a level of 1.4 or fewer births per individual with gestational capacity (Fauser et al., 2024; Skakkebaek et al., 2019).

Some individuals who attempt to conceive find that pregnancy does not occur despite their efforts and a person's pregnancy history helps to categorize their infertility as primary or secondary. Primary infertility refers to a person of gestational capacity who has tried to conceive but has never been pregnant. Secondary infertility refers to a person who has previously given birth to one or more children who has either now been unable to become pregnant again or has been unable to carry a subsequent pregnancy to term. (Kolanska et al., 2022). The chance of an individual conceiving varies based on many separate factors. Monthly fecundability refers to the probability of pregnancy each month and is approximately 20 percent per cycle in couples with normal fertility (Practice Committee of the ASRM and the Practice Committee of the Society for Reproductive Endocrinology and Infertility, 2022; Taylor et al., 2020). Estimates of infertility in the United States vary slightly but are approximately 15 percent of individuals (Cox et al., 2022; Brannigan et al., 2024). However, less is known about individuals with infertility who do not seek testing or treatment.

Historically, infertility has been defined as the inability "to achieve a successful pregnancy after 12 months or more of regular unprotected intercourse" (Practice Committee of the ASRM, 2021c, p. 1255). In 2023, the American Society for Reproductive Medicine updated the medical definition of infertility:

> *"Infertility" is a disease, condition, or status characterized by any of the following:*
>
> - *"The inability to achieve a successful pregnancy based on a patient's medical, sexual, and reproductive history, age, physical findings, diagnostic testing, or any combination of those factors.*
> - *The need for medical intervention, including, but not limited to, the use of donor gametes or donor embryos in order to achieve a successful pregnancy either as an individual or with a partner.*
> - *In patients having regular, unprotected intercourse and without any known etiology for either partner suggestive of impaired reproductive ability, evaluation should be initiated at 12 months when the female partner is under 35 years of age and at 6 months when the female partner is 35 years of age or older."*
>
> *Nothing in this definition shall be used to deny or delay treatment to any individual, regardless of relationship status or sexual orientation." (Practice Committee of the ASRM, 2023)*

While this new definition does not fundamentally change the biologic parameters for medical infertility, the acknowledgment of the wide spectrum of family building factors is important, as many individuals do not have the type of sex that can result in pregnancy. Additionally, lesbian, gay, bisexual, transgender, nonbinary, and queer individuals experience increased disparities in the assessment and treatment of infertility (ACOG, 2024a; Ethics Committee of the ASRM, 2021b). Every person who desires biological and nonbiological parenthood should receive equitable care to pursue their family building goals in welcoming and affirming clinical environments. It is also important to note that intentional single parents and/or individuals who are not able to create a pregnancy with the combined anatomy and/or gametes of themselves and their partners may also meet the medical definition of infertility under certain circumstances. Because the definition of infertility relies on repeated sperm contact over a period of time, it is often unknown whether these individuals fall into the same category in terms of fecundity as their peers with regular sperm contact. This may lead some patients to feel surprised or defeated that low-intervention treatment such as vaginal, cervical, or intrauterine insemination does not quickly result in pregnancy.

Individuals may also construct their own definition of infertility which is influenced by the social context in which they live. For example, two individuals who have been trying to conceive for 3 months and have many friends who have recently become pregnant with no apparent difficulty may begin to see themselves as infertile even though they are not considered infertile according to the medical definition. Such a couple may become very anxious and request a referral to a fertility specialist but be advised to wait because they do not fit the medical definition of infertility. The clinician can validate the couple's concerns by taking a thorough history, acknowledging their fears, educating them on cycle tracking and expected chance of pregnancy, as well as scheduling a follow-up visit in 9 months. If they are pregnant, the visit can be canceled. If they are not pregnant, that visit is already scheduled, and their anxiety is not heightened by hearing that their clinician's first available visit is not for several weeks or months. Conversely, a clinician may advise nulligravid individuals over the age of 35 who are seeking routine gynecologic care that they should consider conceiving very soon because their childbearing years are almost over. While the clinician's intention may be to provide information about the age-related realities of fertility, this conversation can feel like unnecessary external pressure that assumes a desire to become pregnant and perpetuates a procreative bias, as described above.

Fertility and Age

The societal notion of a person's biological clock holds some aspects of physiologic reality, though it also holds much more individualized nuance that may be present in cultural narratives. It is generally believed that individuals born with ovaries are born with all the oocytes they will produce in their lifetime. This number varies individually but is likely near 1–2 million oocytes at birth and 300–500,000 at puberty. Peak fertility for an AFAB person is generally considered to be in their 20s to early 30s and typically begins a gradual decline around age 32, with a more rapid decline after age 37. By age 37, approximately 25,000 oocytes remain and by the time menopause commences at the average age of 51, only 1,000 oocytes remain (ACOG Committee on Gynecologic Practice and The Practice Committee of the ASRM, 2022). While these numbers are helpful estimates, individual fertility may not follow these exact parameters, and menopause may occur earlier or later than average. Additionally, the incidence of chronic conditions that may impair fertility (e.g., endometriosis, tubal blockage) increases with age, as does the incidence of spontaneous abortion related to chromosomal changes (ACOG Committee on Gynecologic Practice & The Practice Committee of the ASRM, 2022). Pregnancy risks and adverse neonatal outcomes are also known to be higher when individuals become pregnant at later ages. For AFAB individuals who are older than age 35, evaluation of fertility should be offered after 6 months of attempting pregnancy, instead of 1 year. While spontaneous pregnancy may take longer to occur with individuals > age 35, offering testing in this time-sensitive manner is advantageous in allowing individuals time to complete a comprehensive evaluation, which itself may take several months. Both the mean age at first birth and the birth rates of AFAB individuals aged 35 years and older continue to increase in the United States (CDC, 2024).

Sperm-related fertility is unique, in that individuals who produce sperm often remain fertile throughout their lives. Advanced paternal age (APA) refers to the age of the sperm-contributing individual and is generally considered to be age 40 and above, though there is little or no overall measurable decline in fertility rates before age 45 to 50. The children of APA individuals are believed to be at an increased risk of several health conditions, including neurodevelopmental disorders, congenital heart issues, other genetic disorders, as well as preterm birth and low birth weight. Stronger correlations were found between APA and increased incidence of psychiatric disorders and behavioral impairment for both the children and grandchildren of older fathers (Zweifel & Woodward, 2022). The effects of aging on sperm production and health are complex and influenced by declining testosterone levels, changes in testicular tissue and circulation, as well as age-related comorbidities. Pregnancy rates for the AFAB partners of sperm-producing individuals above age 50 are 23 to 38 percent lower than those for their counterparts who are younger than age 30; further, the time to conception is 5 times longer for sperm-producing individuals older than age 45, compared with sperm-producing individuals younger than age 25 (Taylor et al., 2020). Additionally, advanced paternal age is associated with an increased risk of spontaneous miscarriage in addition to infertility.

The prevalence of delayed biological parenthood is increasing for both those AMAB and AFAB due to a variety of individual considerations that make them want to have children at older ages. The contributing factors to this trend are multifactorial and likely represent a modern lifestyle shift, including increased pursuit of educational and career goals by reproductive-aged individuals and intentional or unintentional postponement of parenthood. With the increased use of technology to treat infertility, more options are available for individuals close to the end of their childbearing years. The growing use of preimplantation genetic screening and the availability of donor oocytes have enabled AFAB individuals in their mid-40s to 50s to conceive and carry a pregnancy to term. Although this flexibility provides more opportunities for AFAB individuals, it may also create more complex decisions for some patients regarding their priorities around use of their own biological gametes.

It is important for clinicians to carefully consider their language and tone when discussing age-related changes to fertility, as age is a nonmodifiable variable and can invoke a feeling of guilt or regret for some individuals who wish their life circumstances had led to attemptingconception at an earlier time in their life or who actively choose to delay childbearing in favor of other priorities (Adachi et al., 2020a, 2020b). Additionally, the intersection of sexism and gender norms can form a stark paradox where AFAB individuals are encouraged or expected to conceive and simultaneously shamed for prioritizing their reproductive goals. This same intersection can also apply to AFAB individuals who are either not in heterosexual relationships and/or not planning to conceive, in which the patriarchal value of expected fertility is not perceived to be upheld.

ETIOLOGY

Reproductive Anatomy and Physiology

An understanding of the anatomy and physiology of all variations of reproductive systems and the processes of fertilization and implantation is crucial to understanding the etiology of infertility. The discussion in this chapter is limited to an overview of fertilization and implantation. Reproductive anatomy and physiology are discussed in Chapter 7. While the anatomical term *fallopian tubes* may be better described as *uterine tubes,* as this more accurately refers to the location and function of these structures, as well as moves away from the use of anatomical terms that reference (prominently male) scientists and clinicians, the term *fallopian tubes* is still the most commonly used in the clinical setting and thus used in this chapter for functional clarity.

The processes of fertilization (also known as conception) and implantation involve several steps. During its journey through the reproductive tract, a sperm cell encounters obstacles at many different levels so that, in theory, the healthiest, most motile sperm arrive at the oocyte. This accounts for the large attrition rate seen from the millions of sperm that are deposited in the cervical canal to the hundreds that reach the fallopian tubes. Sperm must be produced and deposited in the vagina and then transported through the vagina, cervix, and fallopian tubes. Only motile sperm can pass through the cervical mucus and enter the uterus. This is the end of the journey for sperm with minimal motility and/or atypical morphology (i.e., head, neck, or tail differences that can be detrimental to sperm motility) because they are unable to proceed past this point. After they are in the uterus, the sperm are transformed by a process called capacitation, which changes their surface characteristics. Capacitation is essential to the sperm's ability to fertilize an ovum and enables the sperm to undergo the acrosome reaction, to bind to the zona pellucida, and to acquire hypermotility—all of which help to increase the sperm's ability to penetrate the ovum. The ovaries must produce a mature ovum (oocyte), which requires integrated functioning along the hypothalamic–pituitary–ovarian axis. The ovum is transported from the ovary into the fallopian tube, where it is fertilized by the sperm. The fertilized ovum then travels down the fallopian tube into the uterus. Implantation is the process by which the fertilized ovum attaches to the uterine wall and penetrates the uterine epithelium and the maternal circulatory system. Implantation can occur only if there is shedding of the zona pellucida, the protective membrane surrounding the oocyte, in a process called zona hatching.

Approximately 55 percent of infertility cases are due to at least one factor related to the gestational parent, and 35 percent of cases are due to primarily sperm-related factors (Taylor et al., 2020). In some cases where no apparent definable cause can be found, the diagnosis of unexplained infertility is then made. Of individuals experiencing unexplained infertility, approximately 30 percent meet the criteria for unexplained infertility after completing a fertility workup that does not identify a known cause of the infertility (Practice Committee of the ASRM, 2020a).

Causes of Infertility for Individuals with a Uterus and/or Ovaries

Alterations in the endocrine system resulting in ovulatory dysfunction make up the majority of fertility concerns for individuals with a uterus and ovaries (20 percent to 40 percent). Ovulatory dysfunction may involve either a total lack of ovulation or the occurrence of irregular ovulation. Anovulation is usually—but not always—evidenced by irregular menstrual bleeding patterns or amenorrhea. Numerous causes of ovulatory dysfunction are possible, stemming from any interruption of the hypothalamic–pituitary–ovarian axis. Etiologies of ovarian dysfunction include hyperandrogenic disorders, physiologic anovulation at either end of the reproductive spectrum, hyperprolactinemia, pituitary tumors, medication use, thyroid disorders, eating disorders, low body weight, possibly high body weight, and possibly stress. Further information about etiologies of anovulation can be found in Chapters 25 and 26.

Variations in genetics, sex characteristics, or chromosomes may also play a role as a cause of infertility. This includes individuals who have inherited genetic mutations in their DNA as well as those who are intersex with various combinations of sex traits and chromosomes (Poornima et al., 2020). The term *intersex* can be used to describe an individual whose internal and external body parts do not fall into those of male and female sex categories. This can include variation in hormones, gonads, sex chromosomes, and anatomical appearance. There are over 30 medically recognized variations of intersex traits and approximately 1.4 percent of the population is intersex, though many of these individuals may not know this about themselves unless they have undergone karyotype testing because some intersex traits are not outwardly visible. When patients or clinicians suspect an intersex variation may be present for the patient, a karyotype test should be run to determine if there is a variance in chromosomes such as Turner syndrome, which is characterized by a chromosomal result of 45X.

Fallopian tube and peritoneal disease and blockage make up approximately 30 to 40 percent of infertility cases in AFAB individuals, with pelvic inflammatory disease secondary to STIs such as gonorrhea and chlamydia being the primary cause. Please refer to Chapter 22 for more information about pelvic inflammatory disease. In some cases, the STI may have been asymptomatic and, therefore, gone unrecognized and untreated, resulting in tubal scarring; however, tubal scarring may result even when STIs are treated. Ectopic pregnancies are more likely to occur with tubal scarring due to destruction of the tubal cilia and/or distortion of the distal tube fimbriae. Other tubal factors that can impact fertility are stage III and IV endometriosis, which can cause severe adhesive disease, making oocyte and spermatozoa transport through the fallopian tubes very difficult; adhesions or blockage from uterine fibroids; hydrosalpinx; and blockage from a previous ectopic pregnancy or tubal surgery (Practice Committee of the ASRM, 2021d). Of note, IVF clinical pregnancy rates may be reduced by half in the presence of a hydrosalpinx due to the embryotoxic release of growth factor inhibitors (Harb et al., 2019). Racial disparities are significant in regard to tubal factor infertility, with studies showing Black women had higher rates compared to white women, likely due to increased rates of PID and STIs such as chlamydia and/or gonorrhea. This increased incidence continues to represent ongoing repercussions stemming from histories of reproductive violence experienced by enslaved individuals, mistrust of the healthcare system, and forced sterilizations (Gonullu et al., 2022).

Uterine pathology in the myometrium or endometrium is relatively rare as a cause of infertility, though other pelvic conditions to consider when assessing infertility include endometriosis of the pelvis, adenomyosis, Asherman syndrome, and other uterine pathology. Endometriosis is a complex inflammatory condition without a definitive etiology in which endometrial-like tissue is found attached to other organs, commonly near the uterus, ovaries, and peritoneal cavity. Paradoxically, endometriosis pain may not correlate with the extent of the disease process. For example, slight pain may be present with severe endometriosis, and severe pain may occur in conjunction with very minimal evidence of disease. This disease process can be elusive to diagnose and manage. Refer to Chapter 27 for further information about endometriosis.

Asherman syndrome is characterized by the formation of intrauterine adhesions, typically as a result of trauma to the uterine cavity (Dreisler & Kjer, 2019). These adhesions can be located within the uterus or inside the cervical canal, causing the cervix to become agglutinated. The lower uterine segment can have bands of adhesions crossing from the anterior endometrium to the posterior endometrium. Over time, and as white blood cells continually attack the adhesions, inflammation begins in the uterus, and these bands of adhesions become increasingly thicker. The functional layer of the uterus becomes unresponsive to hormonal stimulation, often resulting in a thin endometrial lining and potentially leading to amenorrhea, implantation concerns, or miscarriage. The most common causes of Asherman syndrome are uterine curettage postpartum to treat retained placenta or placenta increta, uterine curettage after incomplete spontaneous or medication abortion, myomectomy, and endometrial ablation (Dreisler & Kjer, 2019).

Other potential uterine causes of infertility include fibroids, endometrial polyps, and chronic endometritis. Cavity-distorting fibroids can be linked to infertility and they also may lower the success rates of assisted reproductive technology (ART) to treat infertility (Donnez et al., 2024; Don et al., 2023). Submucosal fibroids and large endometrial polyps that grow into the uterine cavity are the most likely to interfere with normal implantation and continuation of pregnancy. Subserosal fibroids are unlikely to interfere with fertility or pregnancy. Chronic endometritis appears to cause inhibition of embryo implantation during an in vitro fertilization (IVF) cycle if untreated (Li et al., 2020). Congenital anomalies of the uterus, such as a bicornuate uterus or septate uterus, are typically associated with pregnancy loss and complications but not infertility (Taylor et al., 2020). Additionally, the interaction between the immune system and pregnancy implantation is an area of ongoing research, including the effects of autoimmune disease on the uterine lining and overall fertility.

Causes of Infertility for Sperm-Producing Individuals

The perpetuation of the stereotype that infertility is typically due to a medical condition of an AFAB partner also results in the potential for sperm-producing partners to not consider themselves as a potential cause of the infertility. Some sperm-producing individuals may also have varying perspectives on how a diagnosis of infertility may intersect with their perception of their own masculinity (Pakpahan et al., 2023). However, in 20 percent of couples experiencing infertility, sperm-related concerns are found to be the sole cause of the inability to conceive. In another 30 to 40 percent of couples, a sperm-related concern contributes at least partially to infertility (Schlegel et al., 2021; ACOG, 2019). Sperm-related infertility can be divided into three main components: low or absent sperm production, sperm function concerns, or problems with sperm transport. Other causes of infertility for individuals assigned male at birth include idiopathic (40 to 50%), primary gonadal disorders (30 to 40%), disorders of sperm transport (10 to 20%), and hypothalamic–pituitary disorders (1 to 2%) (Taylor et al., 2020). Additionally, environmental factors such as increased air pollution appears to be associated with lowered semen quality (Margiana et al., 2025).

Sperm transport may be impaired by congenital absence of the vas deferens, which can be unilateral or bilateral, or by acquired obstruction of the vas deferens (e.g., infection, vasectomy).

Alteration in gonadal function can result from chromosomal disorders (e.g., Klinefelter syndrome, Y chromosome microdeletions), cryptorchidism (undescended testes), varicoceles, infections, medications, retrograde ejaculation, radiation, environmental exposures (such as industry chemicals, radiation, or heavy metals), and chronic illness such as celiac disease. Individuals with testes may experience infertility due to orchitis (testicular inflammation), which may occur secondary to viral infections, including gonorrhea and chlamydia (Taylor et al., 2020; Segal & Giudice, 2019). Symptoms of orchitis include high fever; unilateral, swollen, warm testicle; inflamed scrotum; and severe testicular pain. A varicocele is caused by a dilation of the pampiniform plexus of spermatic veins and occurs in 15 to 20 percent of postpubertal AMAB individuals. It is more common to diagnose a varicocele on the left than on the right because the left spermatic vein is longer and enters the left renal vein at a perpendicular angle (Taylor et al., 2020). A varicocele can range from minimal fullness to a bulge or large scrotal mass that, when palpated, feels like a "sack of worms." Although varicocele repair can improve semen parameters and sperm-related fertility, the effects are not immediate, and most improvement occurs 3 to 6 months after the procedure (Practice Committee of the ASRM, 2021b).

Thermoregulatory factors may negatively affect sperm production, although more research is needed to elucidate the details of these associations. The scrotal sac sits outside the body and is a protective mechanism against overheating. Increased temperature of the scrotum may represent an increased risk factor for infertility because it can alter sperm parameters and damage sperm membrane integrity (Hoang-Thi et al., 2022). Whether this is temporary or long-lasting is inconclusive and may be dependent on the frequency of certain activities. Thus, sperm-producing individuals who are trying to conceive a pregnancy should avoid the frequent use of hot tubs or saunas and avoid prolonged sitting in a vehicle.

Combined Causes

Other interactional causes of infertility include simultaneous factors from both the individual contributing the oocyte and the individual contributing the sperm. If an abnormal result is discovered in a workup for one individual, the clinician should still recommend continuing a comprehensive evaluation to determine whether multiple fertility barriers exist.

Unexplained Infertility

Unexplained infertility refers to scenarios of infertility in which no specific cause for the infertility can be identified using the existing methods of diagnosis. Unexplained infertility is a diagnosis of exclusion, meaning that all other possible causes of infertility must be ruled out. As scientific advances have enhanced clinicians' ability to identify an increasing number of causes of infertility, fewer people are being diagnosed with unexplained infertility. Having a known cause of their infertility may give individuals a sense of relief and a sense of what type of treatment is likely to be most effective. In contrast, a diagnosis of unexplained infertility can be especially distressing because individuals have no distinct etiology to treat that can improve their chance to conceive. This may lead to increased frustration, as well as financial strain if increased testing or treatment is pursued. In some cases, while the limitations of pretreatment testing may not be able to demonstrate an obvious cause of the infertility, data obtained through the process of fertility treatment may indicate where the problem lies.

Interestingly, a 2021 study conducted of couples whose fertility treatment cycles were postponed during the coronavirus disease 2019 (COVID-19) pandemic found that individuals who had previously been diagnosed with unexplained infertility and were scheduled to undergo in vitro fertilization treatment experienced an increased chance of conception during a 2-month period of national lockdown (Villani et al., 2021). Upon further exploration, the increased pregnancy rates were found to be associated with increased frequency of sexual intercourse, highlighting both infrequent intercourse as a possible cause of infertility and the importance of patient education regarding frequency of sperm contact.

Recurrent Pregnancy Loss

Approximately 15–25 percent of all pregnancies ultimately end in miscarriage and approximately 1–5 percent of individuals experience recurrent early pregnancy loss (RPL), which ASRM now defines as two or more losses of a clinical pregnancy (typically considered such after visibility on ultrasound) that occurs before 20 weeks' gestation (ASRM, 2021). Some patients and clinicians may also consider pregnancies that occur only via positive hCG with serum or urine testing (Genovese & McQueen, 2023). Previously, a diagnosis of RPL included only consecutive pregnancy losses, though it is now considered within criteria to include non-consecutive losses as well. The number of patients diagnosed with RPL appears to be on the rise, though this may be partially related to an increase of pregnancies identified in earlier gestation, as previously many individuals may not have had confirmed pregnancies prior to miscarriage. It is also likely to be associated with an increase in individuals conceiving at older ages, as the most common cause of pregnancy loss is fetal chromosomal aneuploidy, for which the risk increases with age.

The etiology of RPL is unknown in more than 50 percent of cases, often adding another complex layer to an emotionally challenging process. Some possible causes may include structural uterine anomalies in which implantation is difficult, chromosomal variations (sometimes due to age but not always), immunologic disorders, sperm dysfunction, infection, smoking, genetic disorders or genetic incompatibility between partners, untreated chronic medical conditions, and other yet to be determined reasons (Practice Committee of the ASRM, 2012; de Assis et al., 2024). When analyzing products of conception, chromosomal abnormalities were found less frequently for those with recurrent pregnancy loss compared to sporadic pregnancy loss. With increased number of pregnancy losses, the rate of chromosomal abnormalities continued to decrease (Lei et al., 2022). However, even after three or more pregnancy losses, an individual still has a 60–80 percent likelihood of going on to become pregnant and give birth to a full-term infant. Additionally, the field of reproductive immunology has emerged as a promising area of infertility treatment, particularly in regard to RPL. In addition to many of the other fertility evaluation tools in this chapter, the workup for RPL may include:

- Parental karyotypes
- Saline sonogram and/or hysteroscopy
- Antiphospholipid antibodies
- Endocrine evaluation
- Possibly endometrial sampling
- Sperm analysis or other sperm testing

Patients experiencing RPL often describe a deep sense of grief and varying degrees of self-blame and frustration. Research demonstrates that the grieving process after experiencing pregnancy loss is similar to the grief after the death of a close friend or family member. AFAB patients who have experienced recurrent pregnancy loss meet the diagnostic criteria for post-traumatic stress disorder (PTSD) and the associated trauma may have far-reaching implications after treatment has been stopped (Bindeman et al., 2025).

Stress and Trauma

There continues to be discourse surrounding the possibility of a link between increased stress and infertility. While it is clear that experiencing infertility can cause stress, the available research does not demonstrate that experiencing stress causes infertility. Patients experiencing infertility-related stress reported concerns of social isolation, stigma, sexual stress, financial strain, and feelings of identity loss (Woods et al., 2022). While some previous studies have shown that stress, anxiety, and depression may contribute to reduced chances of pregnancy with ART (Simionescu et al., 2021; Rooney & Domar, 2018; Dehkordi et al., 2025), this research is significantly limited by confounding variables regarding the timing of initiating treatment. However, the hypothesis that an underlying physiological stress response is a barrier to pregnancy continues to be perpetuated by both clinicians and the general public (Negris et al., 2021; Bakkensen et al., 2022). In their personal interactions, well-intentioned friends and family may recommend intended fertility-enhancing advice such as relaxation, decreased workloads, going on vacation, positive thinking, and other recommendations to "stop trying so hard." The efficacy of stress-reducing interventions on pregnancy outcomes are found to be anecdotal at best and these recommendations are inappropriate and dismissive of the efforts that individuals with infertility often go through (Bindeman et al., 2025). A more appropriate framing of stress in the clinical setting is discussing how evaluation of stress-reducing techniques may help to improve patients' quality of life while going through the emotional process of infertility and/or infertility treatment.

Research does suggest a possible link between individuals with increased adverse childhood experiences (ACE) scores and an increased likelihood of experiencing infertility and pregnancy loss, as well as numerous other chronic health conditions (Swift et al., 2024). These associations further confirm the need for a trauma-informed approach to fertility care to ensure patients do not experience additional harm.

ASSESSMENT OF INFERTILITY

Because a medical diagnosis of infertility is often not made until a person has attempted to conceive for 6–12 months, depending on their age, a fertility workup is often not initiated until this amount of time has elapsed. Infertility evaluation is recommended after 6 months for AFAB individuals age 35 and older and immediately recommended for AFAB individuals age 40 and older. However, earlier assessment is also recommended for individuals who have existing health conditions that have the potential to impair fertility (**Box 20-1**).

Assessment of fertility concerns for AFAB individuals who choose intentional single parenthood and lesbian, gay, bisexual, transgender, nonbinary, and queer individuals should be dependent on patient desire for fertility testing. Given the significant amount of time, money, and effort that goes into conception using donor gametes, it is reasonable to offer fertility testing for people who must utilize third-party reproduction to create a pregnancy.

Evaluation of infertility begins with a thorough history and physical examination. Clinicians who provide gynecologic care often perform limited assessment of AMAB partners (e.g., obtaining relevant history and ordering semen analysis) and then refer these patients to a urologist or other andrology specialist if additional evaluation is needed. Diagnostic tests for infertility are most useful and cost effective if they proceed sequentially in a logical order.

History

It is essential that the clinician initially obtain an accurate and detailed health history from the patient and partner(s) if applicable. This history will inform which diagnostic tests are recommended, how urgently these tests are performed, and how quickly the patient should return for a follow-up visit. In some cases, it may be helpful to gather a health history from partners separately in order to encourage the most complete evaluation. Given the large number of patients that clinicians must provide care for, however, obtaining a thorough infertility history in a timely manner while also providing compassionate care is a skill that is refined over time.

BOX 20-1 Indications for Immediate Infertility Evaluation

- History of irregular menses, oligomenorrhea, or amenorrhea of various etiologies
- Known or suspected uterine, tubal, or peritoneal disease
- Known or suspected stage 3 or 4 endometriosis
- Known or suspected sperm-related subfertility
- Other condition known to limit fertility

Data from American College of Obstetricians and Gynecologists Committee on Gynecologic Practice, & The Practice Committee of the American Society for Reproductive Medicine. (2014). Committee opinion No. 589: Female age-related fertility decline. Fertility and Sterility, 101(3), 633–634. https://www.ncbi.nlm.nih.gov/pubmed/24559617;

Practice Committee of the American Society for Reproductive Medicine. (2021c). Fertility evaluation of infertile women: A committee opinion. Fertility and Sterility, 116(5), 1255–1263. https://www.asrm.org/globalassets/_asrm/practice-guidance/practice-guidelines/pdf/fertility-evaluation-of-infertile-women-a-committee-opinion.pdf

The information to be gathered in history taking includes:

- Attempts and methods used to try to conceive (if any)
- Past and present medical history
- Pregnancy history
- Mental health
- Family health
- Genetic history
- Social information
- Sleep history, including sleep disorders (Lim et al., 2021)
- Occupational information
- Personal habits (including body movement, substance use, and nutrition)

Even if the patient is a previous patient of the clinician, their full history should still be reviewed in detail. The clinician should identify whether they have ever attempted to become pregnant before, as well as the duration of infertility if applicable, and any previous evaluation or treatment. The clinician should also ascertain whether a patient has previously used any type of contraception, and whether the potential for pregnancy has been present in the past, regardless of whether or not the individual was intentionally trying to become pregnant. For example, a patient may state that they have never tried to become pregnant, but did not use contraception and had regular unprotected intercourse with a previous sperm-producing partner for over a year without pregnancy occurring. This can also identify whether infertility might be temporarily related to contraception, such as the expected delayed return to fertility after discontinuation of the depot medroxyprogesterone acetate injection (Depo-Provera). The frequency of sperm contact, any sexual dysfunction, and history of STIs in either the patient or partner(s) as applicable are other important pieces of information to collect. A detailed gynecologic history, with particular attention to the menstrual and pregnancy histories and any previous surgeries or procedures, is crucial to the infertility evaluation. When obtaining the history of the patient's previous surgeries, make certain to identify the specific type of procedure (e.g., laparoscopic vs. open), the indication for the procedure, and any complications.

When asking about previous pregnancies, clarify whether the patient and/or partner if applicable have ever become pregnant together or with other partners. If so, obtain a pregnancy history, including whether the patient has had a dilation and curettage (D&C) or cesarean birth. Both of these surgical procedures can cause adhesion formation, which can potentially make it difficult for the oocyte to move through the fallopian tube or for the uterine lining to respond to hormonal fluctuations.

Note the occupation of the patient and/or partner if applicable, including exposure to environmental hazards, and substance use (Practice Committee of the ASRM, 2021c). Ask if the patient has had any abnormal Pap tests and, if so, what treatment they had because some cervical procedures can generate stenosis of the cervical os. Clinicians should also ask about a family history of congenital disorders, developmental delay, or reproductive problems. An important question in the infertility workup is asking AFAB patients the age that their mother and other maternal relatives experienced menopause. This question should also be asked to patients seeking routine gynecologic care and allows the clinician to screen for the likelihood of early menopause and identify appropriate candidates for fertility preservation earlier.

During the review of systems, ask the patient specifically about nipple discharge, hirsutism (some patients may utilize depilatory methods that can make it difficult for the clinician to ascertain the extent of hair growth on physical examination), pelvic and abdominal pain, and dyspareunia. Also ask about symptoms of thyroid disorders, such as fatigue, heat or cold intolerance, hair loss, and weight gain or loss (Practice Committee of the ASRM, 2021c).

When taking an infertility history for someone AMAB, ask about general health history, previous surgeries, current medications, and family genetic disorders that could interfere with conceiving. The reproductive history should include duration of infertility, frequency and timing of sex, and history of STIs. Ask if the patient has ever attempted to conceive with a previous partner. Note exposure to environmental or chemical toxins in the home or workplace and exposure to heat that could raise scrotal temperature. Ask whether the individual consumes alcohol, tobacco, herbal supplements, anabolic steroids, cannabis, amphetamines, cocaine, heroin, barbiturates, and other substances because the use of these can affect fertility (Practice Committee of the ASRM, 2021c; Practice Committee of the ASRM, 2024a). Lastly, assess for a history of any sleep disturbances or disorders, as there may be an association between sleep apnea and infertility for some patients (Lim et al., 2021).

Physical Examination

A complete physical examination of the patient, including a pelvic examination, is recommended (Practice Committee of the ASRM, 2021c). During the general examination, it is particularly important to note general vital signs including weight changes, blood pressure, and pulse; the presence of thyroid enlargement, nodules, or tenderness; acne, hirsutism, or androgenic alopecia that could indicate a hyperandrogenic disorder; and nipple discharge or visual changes that could indicate a pituitary mass. The pelvic examination should focus on identifying any variation of the genitalia, such as enlargement of the clitoris, tenderness, masses, and organ enlargement. Assess uterine size, shape, and mobility, and determine whether there is evidence of gynecologic infections or STIs. If infection is suspected, microscopic examination of vaginal secretions and urine chlamydia and gonorrhea testing should be performed (refer to Chapter 7). Most experts agree that a detailed reproductive history and semen analysis should be part of the initial evaluation of an AMAB partner, but there is no consensus on the indications for a complete physical examination. As a result, there are two approaches. One is to include a physical examination by an experienced clinician as part of the initial work-up (Barratt et al., 2017). For efficiency, many clinicians will refer the AMAB partner to a urologist or andrology specialist for a complete examination if there are abnormalities in either their reproductive history or semen analysis. A physical examination for an AMAB partner is also potentially indicated in couples with unexplained infertility (Practice Committee of the ASRM, 2021c).

Diagnostic Testing and Procedures

The basic diagnostic procedures that should be recommended in an initial evaluation include ovulation detection and obtaining a semen analysis from a partner or donor when applicable. More specific tests that may be warranted include serum hormone levels, ovarian reserve testing, lab work related to general health, sonohysterosalpingography, hysterosalpingography, transvaginal ultrasound, and hysteroscopy. Patient history should guide the clinician's decisions as to which testing is recommended and in which order so that time and money are not wasted. Evaluation generally proceeds from least invasive to most invasive testing. If an individual is ovulatory, it is preferable to organize the infertility evaluation according to the menstrual cycle. With this approach, many of the tests can be performed within the same month without hindering the patient's ability to conceive. It is also important to note that while laboratory testing, imaging, and surgical procedures can be valuable aspects of the fertility workup, there can be nuance and limitations to testing, as may be the case with unexplained infertility. Additionally, while some testing may help identify typical gamete characteristics associated with pregnancy, no testing currently exists to determine the inherent quality of oocytes or sperm.

Ovulation Detection

Basal Body Temperature An inexpensive, noninvasive method that can be used to detect ovulation is to monitor and record basal body temperature (BBT) each day upon awakening. If a person ovulates, the two phases of the reproductive hormonal cycle are characterized by consistently lower temperatures during the follicular phase and consistently higher temperatures during the luteal phase. Usually, a slight drop in temperature occurs just prior to ovulation, and a temperature increase of at least 0.4°F is expected after ovulation (**Figure 20-1**). A BBT thermometer, which is different from a fever thermometer, is calibrated in tenths of degrees, allowing for the detection of smaller changes in temperature. The individual should measure their temperature before rising from bed and before eating or drinking. The temperature can be obtained orally, vaginally, or rectally, but it should be taken the same way each time. Although fluctuations inevitably occur within each of the phases, plotting the temperatures on a graph demonstrates whether a biphasic pattern is present (Practice Committee of the ASRM, 2021c). The only caveat to BBT charting is that by the time a person's temperature has risen, they have already ovulated and might have missed their opportunity to conceive that month because contact with sperm should occur prior to ovulation. This information must be communicated effectively to the patient to avoid frustration that they have "wasted" a cycle. Recording the BBT is helpful because it can provide useful data for confirmation of ovulation and in predicting future timing of ovulation. Ideally, a patient's BBT should be recorded for at least three cycles because one menstrual cycle does not provide enough information.

Luteinizing Hormone (LH) Predictor Kits Although keeping a record of the patient's BBT may provide useful retrospective information, it can be cumbersome. An alternate and more accurate method of ovulation detection that provides real-time data is through the use of LH urine testing, often referred to as ovulation predictor kits, or OPKs, which patients can purchase over the counter and perform in their home. These may be in the form of LH paper strips, sticks, or digital tests. Individuals can either directly urinate onto the test or use a specimen collection cup to dip the test in their collected urine. Because the LH spike lasts about 24 hours, most individuals will receive a positive LH result for 1 day of their cycle and some individuals may receive a positive LH result for 2 days, depending on the timing of ovulation and testing. Reliability of urine LH testing varies, particularly for patients with polycystic ovary syndrome (PCOS) who can have

FIGURE 20-1 **Sample basal body temperature chart.**

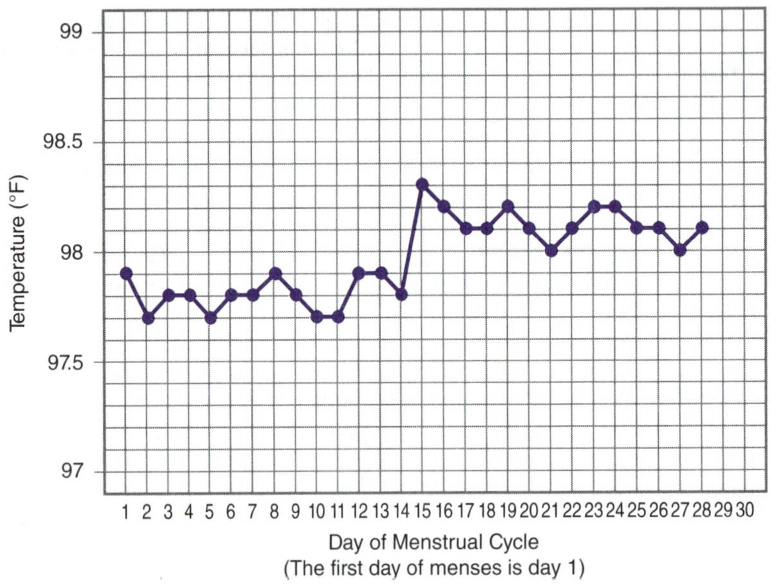

repeated false positive results due to excess LH stimulation. Because of this, many experts recommend that patients test daily until receiving a positive result and then test the following day as well, to determine if the LH surge has decreased and the result goes back to negative. An important teaching point for patients is that identification of an LH surge indicates that ovulation will likely occur within the next 24 to 36 hours, not at the exact time of the kit reading. For patients trying to time conception using an insemination procedure, the procedure should typically be scheduled the day following the positive LH result to optimize the motility of the sperm sample in relation to the timing of the oocyte release. Some patients may consider urine LH testing cost prohibitive if used for an extended period. However, ovulation predictor kits are often much less expensive and invasive than serial blood tests and ultrasounds to detect follicular maturation. As with BBT tracking, LH predictor kits should ideally be used for three cycles to obtain sufficient data regarding the likelihood of ovulatory cycles.

Serum Progesterone Measuring serum progesterone levels midway through the luteal phase (e.g., cycle day 21 of a 28-day cycle) can be helpful in confirming whether a person is ovulating, particularly if BBT charting or LH urine testing does not indicate a high likelihood of ovulation (Practice Committee of the ASRM, 2021c). If an individual with a menstrual cycle has a cycle that is greater than 28 days in length, this level should be drawn 1 week after ovulation occurs. For example, if a person has a 32-day cycle, ovulation likely takes place near day 18 and a progesterone level should be drawn on day 25. If a person has irregular menses, a random serum progesterone can indicate whether ovulation has spontaneously occurred in the recent past. A progesterone level greater than 3 ng/ml indicates the person has already ovulated; a serum progesterone level greater than 10 ng/ml is generally considered to be sufficient in supporting a pregnancy.

Semen Analysis

A basic semen analysis (BSA) is the primary assessment tool for AMAB individuals who produce sperm, as it can detect most sperm factor infertility and helps determine treatment options for sperm-related concerns, including intrauterine insemination (IUI), in vitro fertilization (IVF), and intracytoplasmic sperm injection (ICSI), discussed later in this chapter. In the past, a complete sperm evaluation often included at least two semen analyses, performed a month apart. Many experts now suggest performing one semen analysis and only repeating the analysis if an abnormal parameter is found, though normal fluctuations within the same individual can occur (Practice Committee of the ASRM & The Society for Male Reproduction and Urology, 2023). Differing results in separate semen samples most commonly occurs due to recent ejaculation, though they may also occur due to recent illness, laboratory analysis differences, smoking, medications, and failure of the patient to collect the entirety of the semen sample during collection. When applicable, it is important that semen analysis be performed early in the infertility evaluation so that sperm factor infertility can be diagnosed before an AFAB individual undergoes extensive diagnostic procedures. As discussed above, even when potential fertility barriers are identified in an AFAB individual, a sperm analysis should still be completed to determine whether the infertility is multifactorial. If potential variables influencing sperm analysis are modified, patients should wait at least 74 days before retesting, as this is the period of time required for sperm to fully develop (Punjani et al., 2021).

AMAB individuals should be provided with specific, standardized instructions before collecting a semen sample (Practice Committee of the ASRM & The Society for Male Reproduction and Urology, 2023). Semen can be collected by masturbation with ejaculation into a sterile container or by intercourse with ejaculation into a special collection condom that contains no toxins to sperm (if an individual is uncomfortable with masturbation).

Instructions should also include a defined period of abstinence 2 to 5 days prior to sample collection. Individuals with severe oligospermia should be instructed to adhere to a shorter duration of abstinence and may need to provide several sperm samples (Practice Committee of the ASRM & The Society for Male Reproduction and Urology, 2023). Although semen collection in the office or laboratory is preferred, some patients may prefer to collect their semen sample at home. In this case, no more than 1 hour should elapse between collection and microscopic examination of the semen sample, and the sample should be kept at room or body temperature during transport (Practice Committee of the ASRM & The Society for Male Reproduction and Urology, 2023). If an AMAB patient presents with a semen analysis that is older than 6 months, the semen analysis should be repeated because sperm parameters can change over time.

The World Health Organization (WHO) reference values are widely used to determine if a semen sample falls within normal ranges for semen volume and sperm concentration, motility, and morphology (Practice Committee of the ASRM, 2021b). The 2021 WHO reference values (**Table 20-1**) help to differentiate a semen sample as normal or atypical. It is important to appreciate that these values are reference ranges—they are *not* the minimum values needed for fertilization. Thus, an individual whose sperm parameters fall outside the ranges can be fertile, whereas an individual whose semen is within the ranges can experience infertility (Practice Committee of the ASRM, 2021b). If a patient's semen analysis indicates subfertility, the clinician should repeat the semen analysis a month from the first test prior to referring the patient to an andrology specialist.

Laboratory Testing

Utilization of serum lab testing is an essential aspect of an infertility evaluation and can help to identify some underlying fertility barriers which directly guide treatment options. Reproductive hormone tests will likely need to be repeated in order to assess the fluctuation of these levels across the various phases of the menstrual cycle. This can be helpful to explain to patients who may wonder why the same test needs to be drawn more than once (refer to **Table 20-2**). These may include general, primary care labs, as well as a more comprehensive endocrine workup.

TABLE 20-1 World Health Organization Reference Values for Semen Characteristics

Parameter	Reference Range
Ejaculate volume	1.3–1.5 mL
pH	7.2 or greater
Sperm concentration	$\geq 16 \times 10^6$ spermatozoa/mL
Total sperm number	≥ 39 ($\times 10^6$ spermatozoa/ejaculate)
Percentage motility	≥ 42%
Forward progression	≥ 30%
Normal morphology	≥ 4%
Sperm agglutination	Absent
Viscosity	2 cm or less thread after liquification

Data from World Health Organization. (2021). *WHO laboratory manual for the examination and processing of human semen* (6th ed.). https://www.who.int/publications/i/item/9789240030787

Ovarian Reserve Testing

Laboratory testing may also be performed to assess ovarian reserve, which is a term that refers to the quality and quantity of an AFAB individual's oocytes and their reproductive potential (Practice Committee of the ASRM, 2020b). Ovarian reserve gradually decreases with increasing age and may also be affected by other factors (refer to **Box 20-2**). Current methods of ovarian reserve testing assess the quantity of a person's remaining oocytes. This testing is intended to predict which patients may have poor outcomes in treatment cycles to guide their choice of infertility treatment options and predict the likelihood of successful treatment. Routine ovarian reserve testing in AFAB individuals who are attempting to conceive naturally is not recommended because its applicability in patients who are not undergoing treatment cycles has not been validated in the literature (Practice Committee of the ASRM, 2021c). However, some patients may request these labs and it is important that clinicians understand the nuance associated with the interpretation of these tests.

Serum anti-Müllerian hormone (AMH) has emerged as the most useful biochemical test of oocyte quantity (ovarian reserve). AMH is a hormone that is secreted by the granulosa cells that make up the tissue closest to the oocyte within small (up to 4 mm) ovarian follicles. As the quantity and hormonal sensitivity of primordial follicles declines with age, AMH levels gradually decline until they become undetectable by menopause. AMH testing is reliable and can be performed at any time in the menstrual cycle because levels remain relatively consistent within and between cycles. However, combined hormonal contraceptives may decrease AMH levels up to 50 percent in some individuals. Clinicians should therefore ensure patients have not been on these medications for the 3 months prior to drawing a serum AMH or the level may reflect an artificially lowered result. Additionally, while this test is often performed for patients inquiring about their fertility status, current guidelines do not recommend drawing AMH levels in patients without a diagnosis of infertility and who have not tried to conceive (ACOG, 2024c). Clinicians should counsel patients that the primary clinical use of AMH levels is to assess general ovarian reserve and establishing realistic expectations for ovarian response to gonadotropin medications used in IVF and/or oocyte cryopreservation cycles. Importantly, it cannot be utilized to predict person's current or future reproductive potential. Individuals under the age of 40 who are experiencing infertility and individuals under the age of 40 who are not experiencing infertility have been shown to have similar AMH levels (Hvidman et al., 2016). Therefore, obtaining an AMH levels may cause unwarranted anxiety without clinical benefit if found to be lower than average, as this test cannot predict future fertility or approximate timing of future menopause (Peate et al., 2025; Tehrani et al., 2022). Data shows that patients who receive evidence-based information about the limitations of AMH testing are less likely to desire having this test performed outside of a fertility clinic setting (Copp et al., 2024).

The antral follicle count (AFC) is the measurement of the number of follicles less than 10 mm in both ovaries during the early follicular phase using transvaginal ultrasound. Both the AMH level and antral follicle count appear to have high

TABLE 20-2 Reproductive Hormone Tests

Test	Indications	Source and Considerations
Progesterone (also known as P4)	Helpful in determining if ovulation has recently occurred, particularly if LH urine testing or BBT do not indicate ovulation	Produced only via the corpus luteum and will remain at levels of < 1.0 ng/mL in the follicular phase until ovulation has begun Levels of > 2 or 3 ng/mL typically indicate very recent ovulation, though these levels may also occur on the later end of the progesterone curve, immediately prior to menses Levels >10.0 ng/mL in the peak luteal phase are considered adequate to support a developing pregnancy
Follicle Stimulating Hormone (FSH)	Provides an assessment of ovarian reserve and increases over time as a person nears menopause Should be drawn in cases of amenorrhea and irregular menses	Produced in the pituitary gland and typically drawn on cycle days 2–5 for individuals with a 28-day cycle: levels < 10 mIU/mL in this early follicular phase indicate good ovarian function Some normal variation cycle to cycle and should always be drawn in conjunction with estradiol, as FSH has an inverse relationship with estradiol and will be suppressed by high estradiol
Luteinizing Hormone (LH)	May be helpful in a comprehensive workup for hyperandrogenism and/or possible polycystic ovarian syndrome (PCOS)	Produced in the pituitary gland and rarely drawn in relation to fertility, as the window of an LH surge is narrow If level is drawn on cycle days 2–5 for individuals with a 28-day cycle, results often range between 4–10 mIU/mL If level is incidentally drawn at the time of ovulation, results may indicate peak surges up to 50–100 mIU/mL
Estradiol (also called E2)	Provides supportive assessment of ovarian reserve in relation to FSH Should be drawn in cases of amenorrhea	Produced by ovarian follicles and typically drawn on cycle days 2–5 in a 28-day cycle: levels < 60 pg/mL are expected during this early follicular phase Levels typically not drawn mid-cycle unless going through fertility treatment. An individual mature follicle produces an average of 200 pg/mL of estradiol.
Anti-Müllerian Hormone (AMH)	Assessment of ovarian reserve	Produced by ovarian follicles and decreasing levels directly correlate to increasing age Should not be drawn while a person is taking combined hormonal contraception, as this may artificially suppress AMH levels up to 50% Levels ≥ 1.0 ng/mL indicate a high likelihood of the person having a positive response to gonadotropin medications used in IVF Typically, AMH will be elevated in those with PCOS, indicating a higher ovarian reserve, often levels are > 8 ng/mL

Data from Teede, H. J., Tay, C. T., Laven, J. J. E., Dokras, A., Moran, L. J., Piltonen, T. T., Costello, M. F., Boivin, J., Redman, L. M., Boyle, J. A., Norman, R. J., Mousa, A., & Joham, A. E. (2023). Recommendations from the 2023 international evidence-based guideline for the assessment and management of polycystic ovary syndrome. *The Journal of Clinical Endocrinology and Metabolism, 108*(10), 2447–2469. https://doi.org/10.1210/clinem/dgad463

Practice Committee of the American Society for Reproductive Medicine. (2024c). Current evaluation of amenorrhea: A committee opinion. *Fertility and Sterility, 122*(1), 52–60. https://www.asrm.org/globalassets/_asrm/practice-guidance/practice-guidelines/pdf/current_evaluation_of_amenorrhea.pdf

Practice Committee of the American Society for Reproductive Medicine. (2021c). Fertility evaluation of infertile women: A committee opinion. *Fertility and Sterility, 116*(5), 1255–1263. https://www.asrm.org/globalassets/_asrm/practice-guidance/practice-guidelines/pdf/fertility-evaluation-of-infertile-women-a-committee-opinion.pdf

Practice Committee of the American Society for Reproductive Medicine. (2020b). Testing and interpreting measures of ovarian reserve: A committee opinion. *Fertility and Sterility, 114*(6), 1151–1156. https://www.asrm.org/globalassets/_asrm/practice-guidance/practice-guidelines/pdf/testing_and_interpreting_measures_of_ovarian_reserve.pdf

Abbreviations: 17-OHP, 17-hydroxyprogesterone; FSH, follicle-stimulating hormone; LH, luteinizing hormone; TSH, thyroid-stimulating hormone.

[a]Signs of androgen excess include hirsutism, alopecia, acne, and virilization (clitoral hypertrophy, severe hirsutism, deepening of the voice, increased muscle mass, breast atrophy, and male pattern baldness).

specificity (78 to 92% and 73 to 100%, respectively) for screening for poor ovarian response to gonadotropin stimulation.

However, neither test has sufficient evidence as a screening test for failure to conceive (Practice Committee of the ASRM, 2020b). Other ways to measure ovarian reserve that are less commonly used, due to their lack of reliability and scheduling complexity, include obtaining serum FSH and estradiol levels on cycle day 2, 3, or 4 and/or performing a clomiphene citrate challenge test. Research has shown that a single FSH measurement is not predictive of ovarian reserve due to variations in FSH levels between and within cycles (Practice Committee of the ASRM, 2020b). The clomiphene citrate challenge test entails measuring serum FSH and estradiol levels on cycle day 3, administering clomiphene citrate (100 mg per day) from cycle days 5 to 9,

BOX 20-2 Risk Factors for Decreased or Diminished Ovarian Reserve

- Age greater than 35 years
- Family history of early menopause
- Minimal or absent response to gonadotropin medications
- Single ovary or history of previous ovarian surgery, chemotherapy, or pelvic radiation
- Unexplained infertility
- Autoimmune conditions

Data from Practice Committee of the American Society for Reproductive Medicine. (2021c). Fertility evaluation of infertile women: A committee opinion. *Fertility and Sterility, 116*(5), 1255–1263. https://www.asrm.org/globalassets/_asrm/practice-guidance/practice-guidelines/pdf/fertility-evaluation-of-infertile-women-a-committee-opinion.pdf

and repeating serum FSH and estradiol levels on cycle day 10. However, few clinicians use this test because it does not seem to have an advantage over existing simpler tests, such as AMH levels and antral follicle count which are less time intensive (Practice Committee of the ASRM, 2020b).

Additional Hormone Tests

Additional hormonal tests may be warranted if an individual has irregular menses, amenorrhea, galactorrhea, or signs of excess androgens. Hirsutism is the most frequent clinical manifestation of hyperandrogenism. After pregnancy is ruled out, additional tests may include prolactin, early follicular follicle-stimulating hormone (FSH), estradiol, free testosterone (direct by equilibrium dialysis or calculated from high-quality measurements of total testosterone and sex hormone-binding globulin), and 17-hydroxyprogesterone levels (drawn in the morning during the follicular phase) (Practice Committee of the ASRM, 2021c). Refer to Table 20-2 regarding indications for specific tests. Prolactin levels are generally of no value in AFAB individuals with infertility who are menstruating regularly unless galactorrhea, amenorrhea, or oligomenorrhea is present because elevated levels seem to not affect conception rates in this subgroup of patients (Practice Committee of the ASRM, 2021c). A repeatedly elevated serum prolactin level in the absence of lactation requires an MRI of the pituitary and sella turcica, with and without contrast, to rule out a pituitary neuroendocrine tumor, previously referred to as a pituitary adenoma or prolactinoma (Casar-Borota et al., 2025).

Additional Laboratory Testing

Other laboratory tests can be considered as indicated by the patient's history, refer to **Table 20-3** for a list of potential tests. In particular, thyroid testing and treatment may differ for those undergoing fertility evaluation or treatment in comparison to the general population, further explained below.

Thyroid Function Tests One of the tests that should be performed during the initial evaluation is a thyroid-stimulating hormone (TSH) level to detect thyroid dysfunction. Overt and subclinical (asymptomatic) hypothyroidism can have detrimental effects on reproductive, pregnancy, and fetal outcomes, so it is an important test to perform in reproductive-aged AFAB individuals. Current literature is unclear in terms of the optimal TSH level when attempting to conceive, though some data suggests an association between elevated TSH levels and unexplained infertility (Orouji Jokar et al., 2017). The most recent American Society for Reproductive Medicine (ASRM) guidelines advise that if the TSH level is found to be greater than 2.5 mIU/L but less than 4 mIU/L in patients experiencing infertility, the clinician should consider screening for thyroid antibodies and, if positive, levothyroxine treatment in this population may improve pregnancy outcomes (Practice Committee of the ASRM, 2024d). If thyroid antibodies are negative, the TSH level can be tested at regular intervals to ensure it does not exceed 4 mIU/L. If thyroid abnormalities are detected, they will need to be treated prior to the commencement of infertility treatment, or the infertility treatment may be less likely to result in pregnancy (Practice Committee of the ASRM, 2021c).

Sonohysterosalpingography and Hysterosalpingography

Sonohysterosalpingography is an inexpensive, minimally invasive test that uses transvaginal ultrasound to confirm the shape of the uterine cavity, measure the thickness of the endometrium, and assess the patency of the fallopian tubes. During a sonohysterosalpingogram (SHG), sterile saline is introduced into the uterine cavity via a catheter through the cervix to visualize the uterine cavity contour and detect uterine abnormalities such as polyps, submucosal fibroids, and septa. Two newer techniques, called HyCoSy (hysterosalpingo contrast sonography) and HyFoSy (hysterosalpingo foam sonography), entail slowly administering either foam or saline and air simultaneously (or alternating) with other contrast agents to create bubbles that can be visualized traveling through fallopian tubes, allowing the clinician to also assess tubal patency (Mandia et al., 2017; Devine et al., 2022).

Hysterosalpingography is a procedure in which radiopaque contrast is injected through a patient's cervix into their uterus. During a hysterosalpingogram (HSG), the transport of the contrast through the uterus and into the fallopian tubes is observed by radiograph. In a normal HSG, the contrast travels unobstructed; therefore, this test indicates whether the fallopian tubes are patent or if a structural abnormality is present in the uterus or tubes (Taylor et al., 2020). If there is concern that the patient has tubal pathology (e.g., history of an STI), doxycycline prophylaxis should be prescribed with 100 mg taken orally twice per day for 5 days, starting the day before the HSG. If hysterosalpingography cannot be obtained for financial or other reasons, chlamydia antibody testing can be performed as a screen for tubal blockage. If the chlamydia antibody test is negative, the likelihood of tubal pathology is less than 20 percent (Practice Committee of the ASRM, 2021c).

An SHG or HSG is ideally performed between cycle days 6 through 9 (of a 28-day cycle) and after menstruation ends to avoid interference from menstrual tissue and disruption of potential fertilization and implantation; however, these tests can be performed through cycle day 12. The SHG has better sensitivity and specificity for detecting anomalies of the uterine cavity than the HSG, and it allows the clinician to examine the ovaries via transvaginal ultrasound for abnormalities. In addition, the patient does not have to be exposed to the radiation hazards and risk of iodine allergy that occur with an HSG (Mandia et al., 2017). Both a HyCoSy and an HSG are excellent screening

TABLE 20-3 Additional Laboratory Tests Used in Infertility Evaluation

Test	Indications	Considerations
Thyroid-stimulating hormone (TSH) with free thyroxine (T_4)	Infertility, signs/symptoms of thyroid dysfunction	Consider subclinical hypothyroidism treatment
Prolactin	Irregular menses, amenorrhea, galactorrhea	Repeat serum prolactin if elevated on first draw, recommend pituitary MRI if both levels elevated Consider whether patient's medication history, breastfeeding, or incidental nipple stimulation may contribute to elevation of levels
Free testosterone (direct by equilibrium dialysis or calculated from high-quality measurements of total testosterone and sex hormone-binding globulin)	Irregular menses with signs of androgen excess[a]	
Morning, follicular phase 17-OHP	Irregular menses with signs of androgen excess[a]	Beneficial in ruling out congenital adrenal hyperplasia
Genetic karyotype	Certain variations in chromosomal composition can be linked to fertility concerns	Chromosomal variation is a normal part of human genetic makeup and should not inherently be considered pathologic
Vitamin D	Infertility, fatigue	Low vitamin D levels may be linked with decreased fertility
Hemoglobin A1c	Infertility, signs/symptoms of insulin resistance, family history of diabetes	Insulin resistance and diabetes may be linked with decreased fertility
Complete blood count	Infertility, fatigue	Anemia associated with decreased fertility
Genetic carrier screening	Preconception counseling	Should be offered to all individuals considering pregnancy before conception, including the sperm and oocyte contributors; provides opportunity for insight into their own genetic DNA and possible mutations Testing should never be required, as genetic screening may hold ethical implications for some individuals Due to the high number of mutations tested for, many individuals will screen positive for one or more mutations and patients should be referred to genetic counseling as needed, though many mutations may not have significant health implications Depending on the mutation, preimplantation genetic testing may be available with IVF
Chlamydia antibody testing	Screening for tubal blockage when hysterosalpingography cannot be obtained for financial or other reasons	

Data from Teede, H. J., Tay, C. T., Laven, J. J. E., Dokras, A., Moran, L. J., Piltonen, T. T., Costello, M. F., Boivin, J., Redman, L. M., Boyle, J. A., Norman, R. J., Mousa, A., & Joham, A. E. (2023). Recommendations from the 2023 international evidence-based guideline for the assessment and management of polycystic ovary syndrome. *The Journal of Clinical endocrinology and Metabolism, 108*(10), 2447–2469. https://doi.org/10.1210/clinem/dgad463

Practice Committee of the American Society for Reproductive Medicine. (2024c). Current evaluation of amenorrhea: A committee opinion. *Fertility and Sterility, 122*(1), 52–60. https://www.asrm.org/globalassets/_asrm/practice-guidance/practice-guidelines/pdf/current_evaluation_of_amenorrhea.pdf

Practice Committee of the American Society for Reproductive Medicine. (2021c). Fertility evaluation of infertile women: A committee opinion. *Fertility and Sterility, 116*(5), 1255–1263. https://www.asrm.org/globalassets/_asrm/practice-guidance/practice-guidelines/pdf/fertility-evaluation-of-infertile-women-a-committee-opinion.pdf

Practice Committee of the American Society for Reproductive Medicine. (2020b). Testing and interpreting measures of ovarian reserve: A committee opinion. *Fertility and Sterility, 114*(6), 1151–1156. https://www.asrm.org/globalassets/_asrm/practice-guidance/practice-guidelines/pdf/testing_and_interpreting_measures_of_ovarian_reserve.pdf

Abbreviations: 17-OHP, 17-hydroxyprogesterone; FSH, follicle-stimulating hormone; LH, luteinizing hormone; TSH, thyroid-stimulating hormone.

[a]Signs of androgen excess include hirsutism, alopecia, acne, and virilization (clitoral hypertrophy, severe hirsutism, deepening of the voice, increased muscle mass, breast atrophy, and male pattern baldness).

Abbreviations: CD, cycle day; DNA, deoxyribonucleic acid;; IVF, in vitro fertilization;; mIU, milli-international units; mL, milliter; ng, nanograms; pg, picogram; PCOS, polycystic ovarian syndrome tools for diagnosing tubal factor infertility, and one of these tests should be obtained prior to consideration of laparoscopy, which is the gold standard for diagnosing tubal occlusion but is an invasive procedure.

Transvaginal Ultrasound and Hysteroscopy

Transvaginal ultrasound can help identify uterine factors associated with infertility, such as fibroids and larger endometrial polyps. Transvaginal ultrasound can also detect the presence of endometriomas and polycystic-appearing ovaries, and it is used to obtain an antral follicle count when performed on day 2 to 4 of a menstrual cycle.

Hysteroscopy can be used for definitive diagnosis and treatment of intrauterine conditions causing infertility. This procedure allows the clinician to assess the uterine cavity and endometrium and detect and correct some uterine pathology, such as polyps, cavity-distorting fibroids, or intrauterine adhesions. A hysteroscopy is performed early in the follicular phase, typically from cycle days 7 through 11, and preferably after cessation of menses, for optimal visualization of the cavity (Wang et al., 2024).

Laparoscopy

The outside surfaces of the uterus, tubes, and ovaries can be observed via a laparoscope, which is inserted into the abdomen through the umbilicus. In this procedure, the pelvic organs are examined for any abnormalities, including structural alterations, endometriosis, or pelvic adhesions. Laparoscopy can be used not only for diagnosis of endometriosis, pelvic adhesions, and tubal pathology, but also for treatment of these by laser excision and salpingostomy or salpingectomy when necessary. Hysteroscopy may also be performed at the time of laparoscopy to evaluate the uterine cavity, such as in cases of suspected anatomic uterine defects (e.g., septum). Laparoscopy should be considered when advanced stage endometriosis, tubal occlusive disease, hydrosalpinx, or peritoneal factors are strongly suspected, but it is not recommended for routine evaluation without a specific indication (Ethics Committee of the ASRM, 2021d). Given that laparoscopy is an invasive diagnostic tool and other tests are available to assess tubal patency (i.e., HyCoSy and HSG), laparoscopy (with chromopertubation) is not used as a first-line assessment of tubal patency (Mandia et al., 2017).

Endometrial Biopsy

Endometrial biopsy should be used as an assessment only in patients strongly suspected to have endometrial pathology (e.g., cancer, chronic endometritis) (Ethics Committee of the ASRM, 2021d). Combining endometrial biopsy with a promising test called the endometrial receptivity assay, though, may more precisely time a patient's personal window of endometrial receptivity. An emerging body of research suggests that obtaining cells via endometrial biopsy and sending them to a laboratory that can identify specific genes involved in uterine receptivity might help determine a patient's specific window of implantation, as opposed to assuming that the window of implantation falls within the same 2-day window in all individuals (Ethics Committee of the ASRM, 2021d).

Endometrial Scratching

Also, a form of endometrial biopsy called an endometrial scratch, in which the endometrium is scraped as is done in a typical endometrial biopsy, may now be considered as part of the infertility treatment for individuals with a diagnosis of recurrent implantation failure (RIF) who do not conceive during ART despite having euploid embryos, satisfactory endometrial development, and good hormonal response. This scratch causes local injury to the endometrium so that substances involved in wound healing can be secreted because they are also important for the implantation process (van Hoogenhuijze et al., 2021; Vitagliano et al., 2019). Early studies found that patients who undergo endometrial scratching between day 7 of the previous cycle and day 7 of the embryo transfer cycle are slightly more likely to have a clinical and ongoing pregnancy in the following month, though there was no agreement on what degree and number of injuries (scratches) should be performed and when in the menstrual cycle this procedure should occur. Subsequent studies do not suggest a benefit and current guidelines do not support this procedure for patients (Mrosk et al., 2024).

Diagnostic Testing and Procedures That Are No Longer Recommended Routinely

Several diagnostic tests and procedures previously used in infertility assessment are no longer recommended during the initial infertility evaluation, though patients may inquire about them. These include the postcoital test, endometrial biopsy, and sperm penetration assay. Clinicians may occasionally encounter patients who have had these performed elsewhere; thus, it can be helpful to have some background knowledge regarding them.

A postcoital test was previously performed to determine if sperm cells continued to be present in a sample of cervical mucus obtained from the AFAB partner within a short period of time after having intercourse. However, this test is subjective and no longer recommended due to increased availability of treatments that can bypass potential cervical factors (e.g., IUI and IVF).

In the past, cells from endometrial biopsy were microscopically examined by a pathologist to assess the phase of the menstrual cycle and compare it to the self-reported day of the menstrual cycle by the patient. Endometrial biopsy was also considered the gold standard for the diagnosis of short luteal phase for many years. However, research has shown that it is not a valid diagnostic method and has a wide range of inter- and intrasubject variability; thus, it is no longer recommended for routine evaluation.

PREVENTION OF INFERTILITY

While the focus in infertility care has traditionally been on diagnosis and treatment, recently more attention has been paid to prevention. Many young adults, particularly young men, may not feel that fertility education is relevant to them and thus ongoing discussions regarding optimal ways to engage these populations in fertility education is warranted (Berthelsen et al., 2021). Young adults can be educated regarding ways to prevent STIs, such as barrier methods, which also have the added effect of offering some protection against future infertility, primarily a diagnosis of tubal infertility. Additionally, individuals can be taught to seek care early if they have symptoms or suspect they may have been exposed to infection. This can also reduce the chance of developing pelvic inflammatory disease (PID) and subsequent infertility. Paradoxically, certain contraceptive methods may protect future fertility by decreasing the risk of pelvic inflammatory disease and ectopic pregnancies. It is important for clinicians to address general health and lifestyle factors at preventive care visits, such as cigarette smoking, and alcohol and caffeine intake, not only for general health, but also because these are associated with reduced fertility (ACOG, 2024b). Oocyte freezing, discussed later in this chapter, is another potential method of infertility prevention, as the age of the oocyte is directly linked to the likelihood of pregnancy.

Federal or state government initiatives to reduce future infertility challenges may include the addition of fertility topics into sexuality education, expanded discussions on diagnosis and treatment of STIs, increased access to safe abortion care, postpartum care, and reducing environmental toxins. Additionally, expansion of ART coverage through both private and state Medicaid allows enhanced access to fertility services for individuals of various economic means (WHO, 2024).

MANAGEMENT OF INFERTILITY

Counseling patients considering fertility treatment on the predicted success rates of pregnancies and live birth is challenging given the number of individual factors that contribute to these outcomes (Sanders et al., 2021). Additionally, there are potential external barriers to accessing fertility treatment, including financial considerations, socioeconomic factors, geographical location, and availability of specialized and inclusive care. These barriers also contribute to the current body of research regarding fertility treatment outcomes.

Treatments for infertility are usually specific to an identified cause, though they may be empiric because a specific cause of infertility cannot be determined (unexplained infertility) or the medical criteria for infertility has not been met. Approaches to treatment recommendation in these instances raise nuanced issues about risks and benefits. Frequently, the least invasive and least costly option is recommended as first-line treatment. If that is unsuccessful, treatment then proceeds to more invasive and costly procedures. However, another appropriate approach is for the clinician to offer all available options up front with discussions regarding risks, benefits, costs, and the likelihood of success. This approach may be advantageous for patients who would prefer to start with the option most likely to be successful, even if it is more invasive or expensive. For example, although some individuals may choose less invasive treatments such as intrauterine insemination initially when there is no medical infertility or cause, others may opt to maximize their chances of pregnancy by proceeding immediately to more intensive treatments like in vitro fertilization (S. Olson, personal communication, November 13, 2019). Additionally, insurance coverage may play a significant role in the choice of treatment. Those with insurance coverage may be more likely to move on to more intensive treatments sooner, knowing that cost is not a significant barrier. However, for those without insurance coverage, it may still be preferable to choose IVF, with the understanding that it can be physiologically normal for it to take multiple cycles of insemination procedures for pregnancy to occur and those cycles may end up costing a similar amount when compared to one cycle of IVF. These nuances highlight the importance of the need for clinicians to take into account the physical and mental health, financial resources, and overall well-being of the patient and their partner(s), if applicable throughout the counseling and treatment process.

Nonpharmacologic Options

Patient Education

Education about when a person with a menstrual cycle is fertile is extremely important for individuals who are trying to conceive (Penzias et al., 2022). Individuals who have sperm contact every 1 to 2 days during this time have the highest pregnancy rates, but pregnancy rates are similar with sperm contact two to three times per week (Practice Committee of the ASRM and the Practice Committee of the Society for Reproductive Endocrinology and Infertility, 2022). Education about how to time intercourse or sperm contact with ovulation is all the information needed to improve conception rates for some patients.

Health-Promoting Behaviors

As discussed previously, the infertility evaluation is also an opportunity to discuss inclusion of health-promoting behaviors, including existing barriers to the integration of these behaviors. Some studies seem to suggest that individuals in larger bodies have decreased pregnancy rates and because of this, weight loss is frequently included as a recommendation for those facing fertility challenges (Hoek et al., 2022). However, research does not demonstrate weight loss as an effective intervention (Caldwell et al., 2024; Boyle et al., 2023). Body size is influenced by numerous factors, including genetics, epigenetics, psychological factors, endocrine function, social determinants of health, and exposure to weight stigma (Nutter et al., 2024). Many individuals who pursue intentional weight loss do so through the adoption of health-promoting behaviors such as increasing nutrient-dense foods that are high in fiber, limiting alcohol, increasing exercise, and cessation of smoking, all of which may individually improve overall health and/or fertility (Matheson, 2015). Thus, it is logistically unattainable to determine whether a decrease in weight is directly responsible for any improvement in health or fertility versus the positive cardiometabolic effects of these behaviors. Furthermore, pervasive cultural and medical perspectives continue to perpetuate the idea that weight is easily modifiable and possible to maintain long term, neither of which is demonstrated in research (Mauldin et al., 2022; Hall & Kahan, 2018). Screening for caloric restriction, disordered eating patterns, and overexercise are other essential components of fertility care, as these behaviors have the potential to damage the endocrine system and lead to reduced fertility. In addition, patients should be counseled that there is no safe level of alcohol use during pregnancy and caffeine consumption should be kept to less than 200 mg per day, though research does not exist to make these recommendations in the preconception period (ASRM & ACOG Committee on Gynecologic Practice, 2019).

Complementary and Alternative Therapies

In the United States, 26 to 96 percent of individuals seeking infertility treatment use complementary and alternative medicine (CAM), though only 20 percent of patients report use of these modalities to their clinicians. The decision to utilize CAM is likely influenced by cultural beliefs, length of time trying to conceive, geographical location, and level of education. Patients who have undergone multiple fertility treatments without becoming pregnant and those who experienced physiological or psychological difficulties with treatment are more likely to pursue CAM (Şahan et al., 2025; Sharifi et al., 2024). Additionally, the use of CAM has been closely focused on individuals with anovulation and PCOS-related fertility concerns. The most commonly used complementary and alternative treatments reported include vitamins and supplements, spiritual healing, herbal medicine, and acupuncture meditation (Sharifi et al., 2024).

The majority of research on the use of CAM to treat fertility yields conflicting results, however, among options of complementary and alternative therapies for infertility, several modalities demonstrated potential benefits:

- Herbal medicine and Traditional Chinese Medicine (TCM): Clinical pregnancy rates were increased, particularly for patients with anovulation and/or PCOS and those undergoing ART (Lee et al., 2021). TCM may improve fertility by reducing uterine inflammation, improving endometrial thickness, improving hormone levels, and improving follicular development (Feng et al., 2021).
- Coenzyme Q10 (CoQ10): A dosage of 30 mg CoQ10 daily for 3 months prior to fertility treatment resulted in significantly higher clinical pregnancy rates. Patients with diminished ovarian reserve also had higher clinical pregnancy rates after treatment, with an increased effect noted for younger individuals (Shang et al., 2024). Another study looking at ovarian aging showed patients under the age of 41 who had higher CoQ10 levels present in their follicular fluid were also found to have improved embryo quality and higher rates of pregnancy (Akarsu, 2017).
- Melatonin: A dosage of < 5 mg per day for at least 1 month may improve the quality of embryos in individuals of advanced age (Shang et al., 2024).
- Selenium, L-carnitine, Vitamin C, Vitamin E, Zinc, N-Acetyl-Cysteine: Supplements theorized to decrease oxidative stress may improve some aspects of semen parameters but data are lacking regarding pregnancy rates and numerous study limitations exist. Additionally, purity of supplements can vary significantly and more research is needed regarding sourcing and optimal therapeutic dosing (Lahimer et al., 2025; Dimitriadis et al., 2023).
- Psychotherapy: Improves psychological well-being but has mixed results regarding improvement of pregnancy rates.

Acupuncture

Acupuncture appears to improve anxiety levels in some patients but has mixed results regarding treatment of infertility and improvement of pregnancy rates (Bin et al., 2025; Quan et al., 2022; Lee et al., 2021). A 2022 systematic review showed that compared to control groups of nontreatment, both true and sham acupuncture (more superficially located acupuncture points not correlated with reproductive health) improved the live birth rate, biochemical pregnancy rate, clinical pregnancy rate, and implant rate for patients diagnosed with infertility. However, improved outcomes were not demonstrated in other categories such as the number of oocytes retrieved during IVF, improved embryo quality, or miscarriage rate. Because a significant increase in pregnancies occurred between nontreatment and both sham and true acupuncture, it is possible that a psychological or physiological placebo effect may explain these findings. Additionally, the timing of acupuncture treatment in relation to fertility treatment may impact results.

Pharmacologic Options

Progesterone Supplementation

A short duration of the luteal phase may also contribute to infertility. This condition is commonly referred to as luteal phase insufficiency, luteal phase deficiency, or inadequate luteal phase because it is associated with abnormally low levels of progesterone production by the corpus luteum. The term "luteal phase defect" is no longer used because it may reflect negatively upon individuals trying to conceive as previously explained. The luteal phase is important for sustaining the implantation of an embryo, and luteal phase insufficiency occurs when endogenous progesterone is not sufficient to maintain an adequate secretory endometrium, which is instrumental for the establishment of a healthy pregnancy. The corpus luteum must produce enough progesterone to support the endometrium until the placenta develops and takes over progesterone production. The luteal phase is considered short when fewer than 13 days elapse between the midcycle luteinizing hormone (LH) surge and the onset of menses (Taylor et al., 2020). Nevertheless, luteal phase insufficiency has not been proven as a cause of infertility, and its management in spontaneous or nonstimulated cycles is controversial, as noted later in this chapter (Practice Committee of the ASRM, 2021a).

With a typical luteal phase lasting 14 days, a shortened luteal phase is typically considered anything less than 10–11 days, though management of a short luteal phase is controversial. The Practice Committee of the ASRM (2021a) does not recommend treating luteal phase insufficiency in natural and unmedicated cycles. They do recommend treating conditions that could cause abnormal luteal function, such as hyperprolactinemia and thyroid disorders. Taylor et al. (2020) also do not recommend treating luteal phase insufficiency, noting that such therapy simply gets the patient's hopes up, delays menses if they are not pregnant, and increases stress. Nevertheless, some clinicians still treat luteal phase insufficiency with progesterone supplementation starting 2 to 3 days after a positive LH surge predictor kit, commonly due to the belief that there is a low risk of adverse effects.

Luteal phase support is a concern with ART due to suppression of endogenous LH release, which affects luteal function. Progesterone supplementation improves pregnancy outcomes in cycles with GnRH agonist or antagonist stimulation (Practice Committee of the ASRM, 2021a). Patients undergoing IVF usually begin progesterone supplementation from the time of egg retrieval until 8 to 10 weeks' gestation despite evidence that shorter durations of therapy have comparable live birth rates (Taylor et al., 2020).

The route of delivery for progesterone after an IVF cycle has also been cause for debate. Although progesterone intramuscular injection of 50 to 100 mg/1 cc in the gluteus maximus has been considered superior in its ability to quickly raise serum progesterone levels, it has some disadvantages. It generates lower endometrial progesterone levels than vaginal suppositories; the injections are difficult to self-administer because they must be injected into the gluteus maximus due to the progesterone being compounded in peanut, olive, or sesame oil; and the daily injections can be both painful and anxiety producing for patients. Providing an alternative to these injections has prompted researchers to evaluate the efficacy of vaginal progesterone delivery. Vaginal progesterone in the form of micronized progesterone suppositories (100 or 200 mg twice per day), gel (90 mg per day), or inserts (100 mg, 2 or 3 times per day) actually supports the endometrium more quickly than intramuscular injections. However, one systematic review and meta-analysis found intramuscular progesterone was associated with higher clinical pregnancy rates than vaginal progesterone (Mohammed et al., 2019). Oral progesterone is not recommended, as this route of administration is cleared from the body too rapidly.

Treatment of Subclinical Hypothyroidism

In contrast to overt hypothyroidism, management of subclinical hypothyroidism in AFAB individuals with infertility is controversial due to disagreement about the thresholds for diagnosis and conflicting findings regarding the association of subclinical hypothyroidism with infertility and the ability of treatment to improve outcomes. The ASRM defines subclinical hypothyroidism as a TSH level greater than the upper limit of normal (4 mIU/L for AFAB individuals who are not pregnant) with normal free T4 levels. There is some evidence that thyroid autoimmunity (as evidenced by the presence of thyroid antibodies) is associated with miscarriage and infertility. Levothyroxine treatment may improve pregnancy outcomes in these patients, especially if the TSH is greater than 2.5 mIU/L (Practice Committee of the ASRM, 2024e). **Table 20-4** summarizes the recent ASRM guidelines regarding management of subclinical hypothyroidism in patients with infertility.

Treatment of Sexual Dysfunction

For some individuals, sexual concerns such as erectile dysfunction (ED), ejaculatory anxiety, and lowered arousal can contribute negatively to both their sexual pleasure and ability to conceive through intercourse. When within their scope, clinicians should be knowledgeable about the use of ED medications such as sildenafil (Viagra) and tadalafil (Cialis) for patients, as they can be a straightforward treatment that addresses both fertility and sexual satisfaction. Patient education should also include counseling surrounding the use of alcohol, which is linked to erectile dysfunction, lower testosterone levels, and decreased sperm production. Additionally, for those undergoing fertility procedures, the precise timing in the menstrual cycle that is required for the production of a semen sample can lead to increased stress. A sperm-producing person may feel greater pressure to perform by producing semen on a schedule, and other patients may feel more anxious about having intercourse at planned times and abstaining at other times.

TABLE 20-4 Preconception Management of Subclinical Hypothyroidism in Patients with Infertility

Thyroid-Stimulating Hormone (TSH) Level	Management
Greater than 4 mIU/L	Treat with levothyroxine to maintain levels less than 2.5 mIU/L
2.5 to 4 mIU/L	Check thyroid antibodies If negative, monitor TSH and treat when greater than 4 mIU/L If positive, treat with levothyroxine to maintain levels less than 2.5 mIU/L

Data from Practice Committee of the American Society for Reproductive Medicine. (2024c). Subclinical hypothyroidism in the infertile female population: A guideline. *Fertility and Sterility, 121*(5), 765–781. https://www.asrm.org/globalassets/_asrm/practice-guidance/practice-guidelines/pdf/subclinical_hypothyroidism_in_the_infertile_female_population.pdf

Ovulation Induction

For individuals who experience irregular or absent ovulation, the utilization of ovulation induction medication can be an efficient way to address infertility. For AFAB individuals with anovulatory or unexplained infertility, the first-line medication for oral ovulation induction is most commonly clomiphene citrate (Clomid), though may include letrozole (Femara). These medications stimulate the HPO axis to grow one or more ovarian follicles that then ovulate and increase the chance of fertilization and implantation. These follicles may develop on one or both ovaries. Superovulation refers to the production of multiple follicles, as called a polyfollicular response. All mature follicles from both ovaries that are stimulated through the use of these medications will subsequently release with ovulation. The goal for patients with irregular or anovulation is to generate one or two mature follicles, though occasionally a higher response may occur. This response allows the person's menstrual cycle to be brought closer to the baseline of regular ovulation. For patients with unexplained infertility with regular cycles, clomiphene citrate should be used for superovulation to generate two to four mature follicles, which is more than the single follicle that typically ovulates per menstrual cycle. This increases the chance of fertilization and implantation by increasing the number of oocytes released, each with individual potential for pregnancy.

Appropriate monitoring of AFAB individuals using ovulation induction medications depends on the setting in which the patient is seen. The standard for patients being treated in a fertility clinic is to schedule a baseline appointment during cycle days 2–5 prior to starting medication. This visit typically includes serum bloodwork and a transvaginal or abdominal ultrasound to check for ovarian cysts, elevated estradiol, or other hormonal parameters that may interfere with the effectiveness of the medication (Garthwaite et al., 2020). If all tests look appropriate, the oral medication is started on cycle days 3, 4, or 5 and taken for 5 consecutive days. A second midcycle bloodwork and ultrasound appointment is then scheduled 5 days after the last pill to determine the ovarian response to the medication. Treatment decisions are made by evaluating same-day results of serum hormones coupled with the results of the ultrasound. If one or more follicles are mature and hormone levels are appropriate, a single dose of human chorionic gonadotropin (hCG) 250 mg (Ovidrel) is administered by the patient, which triggers the process of ovulation, and is followed by the subsequent scheduling of timed sperm contact, either through intercourse or insemination.

For individuals who do not have access to a fertility clinic, either due to geographical location or insurance limitations, it is acceptable for clinicians to prescribe ovulation induction medications without the above-described monitoring process (Lindheim et al., 2018). This approach is supported by the Reproductive Justice framework, which promotes bodily autonomy and the right to parent. In this case, alternative methods of ovulation detection may include BBT charting, monitoring of symptoms, and urine LH testing. However, without evaluation of hormone levels and visualization of ovarian response, it is not possible to know whether an individual had a positive response and how many mature follicles developed. Without this information, it can be difficult for clinicians to counsel on the risk of multiple gestation and for patients to fully undergo informed consent regarding this risk. Additionally, this approach may present challenges regarding efficacy related to dosage and timing of ovulation.

Clinicians must use ovulation induction methods judiciously and provide patients with education about these medications, including their risks and benefits, so they can make an informed decision about their use. Some studies in the 1990s found an association between the use of ovulation induction medications and ovarian cancer later in life. More recent studies have found that when confounding variables are controlled for, there is no evidence of an increased risk of ovarian or other cancers with fertility drug treatment (Practice Committee of the ASRM, 2024b). Consistent with most fertility therapies, pregnancy is most likely to occur in the first three to six cycles of ovulation induction medication use. Some clinicians recommend up to three cycles of ovulation induction medication for AFAB individuals with unexplained infertility and six cycles for AFAB individuals who are anovulatory. However, the number of recommended cycles varies and is dependent on multiple factors, including age, response to medications, and financial considerations, and it should be individualized for each patient.

Clomiphene Citrate

Clomiphene citrate, at an initial dose of 50 mg per day, works by binding to estrogen receptors in the hypothalamus, ovary, and endometrium, thereby blocking those receptors from detecting circulating endogenous estrogen. As a result, the hypothalamus perceives a hypoestrogenic state and increases its secretion of gonadotropin-releasing hormone (GnRH), which stimulates the pituitary to secrete FSH and LH. These hormones, in turn, stimulate the ovaries to produce a mature follicle in patients who do not ovulate regularly and multiple mature follicles in those who do ovulate regularly (Practice Committee of the ASRM, 2013). Each of these mature follicles then produces a peak amount of estrogen (estradiol); thus, more follicles will result in higher levels of estradiol.

Clomiphene citrate is taken orally once per day at the same time for 5 consecutive days. Patients are instructed to start clomiphene citrate on cycle day 3, 4, or 5 (prior to the formation of a dominant follicle) after the start of a spontaneous menses or menses induced with progestin withdrawal. The initial dose is typically 50 mg (Practice Committee of the ASRM, 2013). Ovulation usually occurs 14 days after the first dose, and it is common for ovulation to occur a couple of days later with clomiphene citrate use than it does in a person's natural cycle. The dose can be increased in increments of 50 mg if ovulation does not occur, up to a maximum dose of 250 mg, although most clinicians do not exceed a dose of 150 mg. Individuals with higher body weight may require higher doses than individuals with lower body weight (Practice Committee of the ASRM, 2013). The goal for clomiphene citrate therapy depends on whether a patient has preexisting regular or irregular menstrual cycles prior to medication. If an individual with a history of regular ovulation makes only one follicle while taking clomiphene citrate, it might be appropriate to consider an increased dose or different medication to increase the number of follicles produced and therefore increase the likelihood of pregnancy. However, if a patient produces more than four follicles while on medication, it is very important for the clinician to have an informed discussion with them about the increased chance of a multiple gestation pregnancy and associated potential risks. They may then choose to use a barrier contraception method or abstinence that month to prevent pregnancy altogether.

For patients who have existing irregular cycles, the ideal dosage is the one at which ovulation occurs. Commonly, individuals with irregular cycles produce only one follicle. This monofollicular response allows patients with irregular cycles to increase their chance of pregnancy similar to the baseline chances of monthly pregnancy for someone with regular cycles. If ovulation occurs at a specific dose, the patient should remain on that dose each month because an increased dose provides no advantage.

Clomiphene citrate should be used in conjunction with IUI; empiric treatment with clomiphene citrate with intercourse is no more effective than expectant management for unexplained infertility and, therefore, is discouraged (Practice Committee of the ASRM, 2013). The addition of insulin-sensitizing agents, such as metformin, to clomiphene or letrozole has been studied to determine whether there is a benefit in this combination. Results of these studies are limited by several variables and demonstrate a minimal to no increase in live births for patients with PCOS who have not responded to either medication by itself. Though, because research does not appear to show harm beyond gastrointestinal side effects, some clinicians may still opt to recommend these for certain patients (Kar & Maharana, 2023; Penzias et al., 2017). In general, metformin should be added only if the individual has a diagnosis of insulin resistance. Please refer to Chapter 26 for more information about PCOS.

Common side effects of clomiphene citrate are often due to its antiestrogenic actions and/or potential for a multifollicular response and include hot flashes, headaches, mood swings, thinning of the endometrium, ovarian enlargement, ovarian cysts, multiple gestation, and, less frequently, nausea and visual disturbances. Occasionally, patients may also report pelvic pain due to the formation of an ovarian cyst. In pregnancies that occur among AFAB individuals taking clomiphene citrate, 8 percent are multiple gestations. Almost all of those pregnancies (99% or more) are twin gestations; triplet and higher-order gestations are rare but possible (Bourdon et al., 2025).

A serum progesterone level is obtained around cycle day 21, or 5 to 7 days after a positive LH test or follicular ultrasound monitoring, to confirm that ovulation occurred. Close follow-up for ovarian enlargement is also warranted and, when available, should precede the administration of clomiphene citrate that month.

Clinicians should also know that clomiphene citrate can be used in the fertility setting to treat hypogonadism (low testosterone) in cisgender men, though in this context, the medication is most commonly prescribed by urologists and andrology specialists (Herzog et al., 2020).

Letrozole

The first-line medication for ovulation induction in patients who have PCOS is letrozole, after a landmark 2014 randomized controlled trial demonstrated it is more effective than clomiphene citrate for this subset of individuals (Legro et al., 2014; Reproductive Medicine Network+, the International Ovulation Induction, IPDMA Collaboration, Wang et al., 2019). Letrozole is also used as a second-line treatment for patients who do not become pregnant with clomiphene citrate. Unlike clomiphene citrate, it does not exert an antagonist effect on endometrial estrogen receptors. That and letrozole's short half-life (48 hours vs. about 14 days for clomiphene citrate) can avoid the unfavorable thinning effect that clomiphene citrate can have on the endometrium.

Letrozole is an aromatase inhibitor that decreases the amounts of estrogen produced by preventing the conversion of androgens to estrogens in the ovaries. Letrozole was first developed to suppress estrogen production in AFAB individuals with breast cancer, but it has been used on an off-label basis to induce ovulation. The decrease in estrogen production results in increased FSH secretion from the pituitary, which stimulates follicular development (Yang et al., 2021).

Like clomiphene citrate therapy, AFAB patients start taking letrozole on cycle day 3 and continue its use for 5 consecutive days. The initial dose can be 2.5 mg or 5 mg. If the patient does not ovulate, the dose can be titrated up to 7.5 mg. Patients should begin urine LH testing on cycle day 9 because they tend to ovulate sooner than in a natural cycle. Letrozole is not approved by the U.S. Food and Drug Administration (FDA) as an oral ovulation induction agent, but it is increasingly used in AFAB individuals who do not become pregnant with clomiphene citrate or who suffer from the adverse antiestrogenic effects of that medication. Due to its category X label, clinicians commonly begin with prescribing clomiphene citrate first for oral ovulation induction. As stated previously, the half-life of letrozole is 2 days, so by the time a person ovulates, the drug is completely out of their system and will not interfere with a developing oocyte. The most common side effects of letrozole are fatigue, hot flashes, and dizziness, due to the low levels of estradiol the medication causes (Yang et al., 2021).

Injectable Exogenous Gonadotropins

More potent ovulation induction medications such as injectable exogenous gonadotropins can be tried for AFAB patients who do not respond to clomiphene citrate or letrozole, though these are most commonly reserved for use in IVF. Often referred to as "stimulation medications" due to their effect on the ovaries, these medications are made up of recombinant or purified FSH (Follistim or Gonal-F) or human menopausal gonadotropins containing FSH and LH (Menopur). These medications work via bypassing the hypothalamus and pituitary to directly stimulate development of ovarian follicles. They are used in conjunction with hCG or a GnRH agonist, which is administered to induce the final stages of follicle maturation and subsequent oocyte release.

Due to their direct action on the ovaries, exogenous gonadotropins usually generate more mature follicles than oral medications and consequently increase the risk of ovarian hyperstimulation and multiple gestations. This risk can be mitigated by the use of low doses but is still present. When a multifollicular response is generated, it is impossible to control the number of oocytes that are fertilized and/or implanted and subsequently these treatment cycles may be canceled and patients recommended to abstain from sperm contact. The complexity and potential serious side effects of exogenous gonadotropins require careful treatment and extensive monitoring that is best performed by REI clinicians who are experienced in their use. Additionally, exogenous gonadotropins can be very expensive, which is a consideration for many people.

Insemination Procedures

Insemination procedures may be used to treat infertility or by individuals who wish to conceive but do not have a sperm-producing partner (e.g., AFAB individuals who are single or have AFAB partners). However, clinicians should counsel patients that insemination is not an appropriate treatment for all causes of infertility. Types of inseminations include vaginal insemination, intracervical insemination (ICI), and intrauterine insemination (IUI), though it is uncommon for vaginal insemination to be performed by clinicians and ICI is rarely the planned method of insemination. Many patients who opt for vaginal insemination will perform the insemination themselves. In most cases, only one vial of sperm is used per IUI, as repeated IUIs near ovulation have not demonstrated an increased chance of pregnancy (Khandavalli et al., 2020).

Medical or social indications for insemination may include:

- Use of donor sperm
- Use of frozen partner sperm (including when geographical challenges exist)
- A sperm-producing partner with a low sperm count
- Sexual or erectile dysfunction, dyspareunia
- HIV-serodiscordant couples (the process of washing sperm and intrauterine insemination have been demonstrated as excellent methods to minimize risk of seroconversion [Ethics Committee of the American Society for Reproductive Medicine, 2021c])
- Unexplained infertility
- Other scenarios in which insemination is the preferred method of sperm transport

Depending on the circumstances, sperm may be obtained from an intended parent, a known donor, or an anonymous donor. Timing of insemination must be precise and may be utilized during a patient's naturally occurring cycle or in conjunction with ovulation induction medications. For vaginal insemination, sperm for fresh sample insemination may be obtained by a sperm-producing partner or donor masturbating to collect semen in a sterile cup, which is loaded into a catheter and placed in the vagina.

For ICI and IUI, the semen is spun in a centrifuge to remove the seminal plasma, creating a more highly concentrated specimen of motile sperm that is then washed, combined with a sperm-friendly media, and inserted into the cervix or uterus. Clinicians must be aware that the use of unwashed sperm is contraindicated for IUI due to the presence of prostaglandins in semen, which can cause uterine cramping and mild to moderate inflammation.

When using donor sperm, FDA requirements mandate that the sperm donor have testing to rule out STIs prior to insemination. The sperm is usually frozen so the testing can be completed and results received as close to the time of sperm production as possible. Some clinics may require or recommend a quarantine time requirement, though this may be waived by the intended parent(s).

Although the sperm centrifuge procedure requires certain equipment and experience, performing the insemination is a simple procedure. A needleless syringe or other insemination device is used for vaginal insemination, most commonly performed by the patient themselves in the comfort of their own home. For ICI and IUI, the sperm are inserted into the cervix or uterus, respectively, via a flexible catheter attached to a syringe that contains the sperm. With intrauterine insemination, most patients experience symptoms such as mild to moderate uterine cramping. The training and supplies needed for insemination procedures are minimal; therefore, all reproductive healthcare clinicians—not just REI specialists—can easily provide these services and, in doing so, offer increased continuity of care for patients and their families.

Treatment for Tubal Blockage

Historically, tubal disease was treated surgically with fimbrioplasty or cannulation. However, poor pregnancy outcomes and poor tubal mucosal health postprocedure, coinciding with the availability of IVF, has made surgical tubal repair relatively obsolete in the United States. One exception is if a hydrosalpinx is present, surgical intervention may still be appropriate, as the fluid in the tubes can have detrimental effects on endometrial receptivity and embryo development even when the fallopian tubes are bypassed, such as with IVF (Practice Committee of the ASRM, 2021d). However, there are conflicting opinions about the standard of care for patients with infertility and hydrosalpinx (Van Voorhis et al., 2019). Ongoing patient education about transmission and prevention of STIs can be a powerful tool to prevent future infertility related to tubal blockages.

Treatment for Sperm-Related Infertility

Treatment for sperm factor infertility depends on the specific etiology. For example, certain hormonal conditions respond to medical therapy, and surgical repair of a varicocele can be beneficial. Some individuals who have previously had a vasectomy may choose to undergo a vasectomy reversal. Additionally, the use of testicular sperm aspiration (TESA) or percutaneous epididymal sperm aspiration (PESA) may be necessary in cases of azoospermia and utilizes surgical intervention to retrieve sperm instead of sperm collection using ejaculation (Gupta et al., 2023). Unfortunately, many causes of sperm-related infertility are either not identified or not amenable to treatment. In such cases, pregnancy can often still be achieved with other forms of ART such as intrauterine insemination (IUI) or in vitro fertilization (IVF).

Assisted Reproductive Technology (ART)

In Vitro Fertilization

The first IVF birth in the United States occurred in 1981, and today IVF is the most widely used ART procedure. More than 99 percent of the ART cycles in the United States are IVF (Centers for Disease Control and Prevention [CDC] et al., 2025). Currently, about 2 percent of live births are the result of IVF; thus, it is important for clinicians caring for pregnant individuals to understand the process of conception as it occurs via ART.

As of 2025, there are approximately 500 clinics in the United States that perform ART procedures. The Fertility Clinic Success Rate and Certification Act of 1992 requires these fertility clinics to report annual data to the CDC regarding the success rates for various procedures based on age. The Society for Assisted Reproductive Technology (SART) also maintains a comprehensive list of ART clinics, reports birth outcome data from clinics, and helps to develop industry standards. All U.S. clinics that perform ART must report procedural characteristics and outcomes to the Centers for Disease Control and Prevention, which publishes national and clinic-specific ART success rates (CDC, 2024).

Because IVF bypasses the fallopian tubes, it is commonly used in patients who have tubal blockage from structural conditions or secondary to pelvic infection or scar tissue. It is also used for patients who have not gotten pregnant with ovulation induction and IUI and when the etiology of infertility remains unknown. The likelihood that ART will be successful varies depending on a number of factors, most notably the age of the oocyte used. Younger individuals typically have higher AMH levels and thus a greater response to IVF medications. This results in a higher number of oocytes retrieved and available for fertilization, typically resulting in higher numbers of embryos per treatment cycle. For AFAB individuals in the United States using fresh embryos from their own oocytes, the percentage of ART cycles resulting in live births is 31 percent in AFAB patients younger than 35 years, 24 percent in patients aged 35 to 37 years, 15.5 percent in patients aged 38 to 40 years, 8 percent in patients aged 41 to 42 years, 3.2 percent in patients aged 43 to 44 years, and 1.6 percent in patients older than 44 years (CDC et al., 2024). Clinical conversations should balance reviewing realistic expectations for IVF outcomes (number of eggs retrieved and number of blastocysts) while also understanding the emotional complexity that may accompany age-related discussions.

In an IVF cycle, the ovaries are stimulated over the course of 10–14 days using injectable gonadotropin medication to produce multiple mature follicles. Throughout this time, the patient visits the fertility clinic every few days for pelvic ultrasound monitoring and hormonal bloodwork that must be obtained and interpreted the same day. The number of ovarian follicles that respond favorably and reach maturity through this process can vary significantly, depending greatly on the patient's age, AMH level, and dosage of medication used. For example, an average patient in their 20s may produce 15–30 follicles that reach maturity while an average patient in their 40s may produce 1–5 mature follicles. As the follicles develop, an injectable GnRH antagonist (ganirelix acetate or cetrorelix) is added in to prevent premature ovulation. Once the majority of follicles reach maturity, a single injection of hCG is administered, commonly referred to as a "trigger shot" due to its MOA of triggering the beginning of ovulation. The administration of the trigger shot must be precise and is typically administered exactly 36 hours prior to the egg retrieval, initiating the final maturation of the oocytes prior to ovulation. Before ovulation can then occur internally, the egg retrieval procedure is performed under sedation to extract the mature ova surgically. This procedure is typically performed by a specialized physician and involves aspiration collection of the fluid within each individual follicle. After all the follicles are aspirated, the embryologist will then microscopically analyze each extracted oocyte for visual characteristics to determine whether it is mature and able to be utilized, updating the clinical team regarding the total number of oocytes collected. Within approximately 4 hours of the egg retrieval, the oocytes are placed in a laboratory dish of gamete-friendly media and undergo fertilization. Sometimes the cause of infertility is the inability of the sperm to enter the ovum. Although a semen analysis measures sperm parameters, the ability of the sperm to fertilize an oocyte is just implied. Sperm abnormalities, then, are sometimes better understood in interaction with the ova, which is why an IVF cycle can be both diagnostic and therapeutic. The clinician can assess the fertilization capability of the sperm by noting the percentage of ova fertilized during that cycle. Fertilization takes place *in vitro* (external to the body), and can occur through two methods, conventional fertilization or intracytoplasmic sperm injection (ICSI).

Conventional In Vitro Fertilization Conventional fertilization can be used, in which sperm are simply placed in the same dish as one or more oocytes with the hopes of fertilization occurring without additional intervention. During laboratory conventional fertilization, the sperm first attaches to the external cells of the oocyte, beginning an acrosome reaction and enzyme release which allows it to penetrate the zona pellucida and result in fertilization.

Intracytoplasmic Sperm Injection (ICSI) Fertilization may also take place through a procedure called intracytoplasmic sperm injection (ICSI). During this procedure, the embryologist analyzes the sperm sample to choose individual sperm that have favorable characteristics and manually injects each oocyte with one sperm. This process bypasses the process of multiple sperm competing for entry through the oocyte's zona pellucida. ICSI has been utilized since 1990 and has been routinely used in repeat IVF cycles when previous fertilization results through the initial IVF cycle were low or absent (Practice Committees of the ASRM and the Society for Assisted Reproductive Technology, 2020). Historically this procedure was indicated when the male partner had a low sperm count or another form of sperm factor infertility, but it is increasingly being used with IVF procedures even when there is not a diagnosis of sperm factor infertility, such as in cases of preimplantation genetic screening or if fertilization was very poor or did not occur in an IVF cycle.

Embryonic Development Monitoring After the egg retrieval and initiation of fertilization, the embryologist evaluates the growing embryos on a daily basis, taking note of the expected versus actual embryonic development. Refer to Chapter 31 to review normal embryonic development. In some cases, embryos may develop slower than expected or undergo arrested development after several days of growth. Less frequently, there are no oocytes able to be fertilized and thus no embryos are created, likely indicative of a quality concern with either oocytes or sperm, or a compatibility concern.

Preimplantation Genetic Testing for Aneuploidy (PGT-A)
This is an optional genetic screening test performed in an IVF laboratory in which a sample of three to five cells are biopsied from an embryo at the blastocyst stage of development, typically on days 5, 6, or 7 after egg retrieval and fertilization occurs. Of note, the cells biopsied are taken from the trophectoderm of the embryo, which make up the outer layer of the blastocyst, and will eventually become the placenta. No biopsies are taken from the inner cell mass, which eventually forms the fetus. Results from PGT-A biopsies indicate whether an embryo is euploid (with the typical chromosomal make up of 46 chromosomes in 23 pairs) or carries aneuploidy (in which there is a gain or loss of one or more chromosomes) such as the case with Down syndrome and Turner syndrome (Greco et al., 2020). Additionally, an embryo may display mosaicism, in which the embryo displays more than two types of genetically different cells but still has the potential to result in a healthy infant without chromosomal variance. Several clinical questions arise from the use of this technology and potential results, including questions about genetic engineering (Yang et al., 2022). When counseling patients, it is important to note that these procedures do not in any way alter the existing DNA of the embryo but rather allow the intended parent(s) to prioritize the transfer of euploid embryos. For example, a patient with five embryos that have developed to the blastocyst stage may opt for PGT-A testing in order to know which embryo to transfer back first. Even for those paying out of pocket, the cost of PGT-A testing is often comparable to the cost of an embryo transfer. Thus, this testing may have a financial benefit in allowing fewer numbers of transfers to be needed before a pregnancy is achieved. A euploid embryo has approximately a 70 percent chance of resulting in pregnancy, seemingly independent of age. Untested embryos have an unknown potential for genetic alterations and hold closer to a 30–50 percent chance of pregnancy that is directly dependent on age. The sex of the embryo can also be predetermined, which is useful for sex-linked disorders, but it is controversial when sex selection is performed for nonmedical reasons (Ethics Committee of the ASRM, 2022). Some patients may also not want to know the sex of the embryo and care should be given not to accidentally reveal this. Current clinical guidance includes continuing to routinely offer typical prenatal genetic screening during the first trimester because PGT-A is not diagnostic and has the potential for false positives or negatives (Paulson, 2023).

Preimplantation Genetic Testing for Monogenic/Single Gene Disorders (PGT-M)
This optional screening test utilizes the same technique for embryo biopsy as PGT-A, but seeks to analyze single gene disorders when they are identified in personal or familial history. This evaluation allows individuals with known inherited disorders to select nonaffected euploid embryos for transfer, which can greatly increase the chance of implantation and reduce early pregnancy loss. A personalized test is created prior to the start of an IVF cycle, which is used to screen for individually selected gene variants. The use of this testing has increased due to heightened awareness, utilization of IVF, expanded insurance coverage, and improved identification of candidates with more broad use of expanded carrier screening in all settings. Interpretation and guidance regarding PGT-M results can be complex and should be done in conjunction with a genetics specialist. As with PGT-A, routine prenatal genetic screening tests should be offered, as PGT-M is not diagnostic (Ethics Committee of the ASRM, 2024b).

Embryo Transfer When one or more embryos have been identified for transfer back to the uterus for implantation, the embryo transfer procedure is scheduled. Embryos typically reach the blastocyst stage on day 5 after egg retrieval, though occasionally an embryo may be monitored until reaching the blastocyst stage around day 6 or 7. Historically, day 3 embryos prior to reaching the blastocyst stage were also transferred, though this is less common now, as blastocyst embryos are associated with higher rates of clinical pregnancies. The number of embryos transferred into a patient's uterus is based on a variety of factors, including age, perceived quality of embryos, previous success with infertility treatment, and whether or not this will be their only IVF cycle (Practice Committee of the ASRM & Practice Committee of the Society for Assisted Reproductive Technology, 2021e). For those undergoing PGT-A or PGT-M, no embryo transfer cycle is done in the days immediately following the egg retrieval in order to allow time for the genetic testing to occur. Once the genetic testing results are back, the embryo transfer is scheduled for the following cycle. Due to improving technology in cryopreservation techniques, the pregnancy rates for frozen embryo transfer cycles using the patient's own oocytes are actually higher than those for fresh embryo transfer cycles using the patient's own oocytes across all age groups (CDC et al., 2024).

Reciprocal IVF Reciprocal IVF is a specific type of IVF procedure in which a patient carries a pregnancy created with the oocyte of their partner—most commonly using donor sperm. While done for a variety of reasons, this process allows two partners to both be biologically involved—one contributing their genetics, and one as the gestational parent. This is different from the use of a gestational carrier, as both individuals involved in reciprocal IVF are intended parents. Though social circumstances and demographics frequently differ, the outcomes and live birth rates of reciprocal IVF cycles are similar to IVF cycles in which a donor oocyte is used (Aharon et al., 2020). Additionally, reciprocal IVF may be used for individuals in a polyamorous relationship who would like to involve three partners. In this case, a pregnancy may occur through combining an egg from one partner, sperm from another partner, with a third partner as the gestational parent.

Risks Associated with ART

Counseling patients on both short-term and long-term risks associated with IVF is an important aspect of informed consent. Some short-term risks of IVF include ovarian torsion, secondary to ovarian enlargement and heaviness from stimulation medication, which increases the chance of ovarian movement and subsequent torsion. Additionally, common and expected symptoms after an egg retrieval include abdominal discomfort such as bloating, cramping, and bruise-like tenderness, which typically dissipates within several days. Comfort measures after an egg retrieval procedure include prioritization of rest, hydration with plenty of fluids, OTC pain relief, heating packs, and consumption of high-sodium foods, which help in balancing the fluid shift that naturally occurs with this procedure.

Ovarian Hyperstimulation Syndrome A rare but potentially serious short-term complication associated with IVF includes ovarian hyperstimulation syndrome (OHSS). This condition results from the use of exogenous gonadotropins to stimulate the ovaries and specifically after the administration of the hCG trigger shot and subsequent egg retrieval. OHSS is most commonly seen in younger patients with higher AMH levels and in those with PCOS, as there are higher numbers of follicles and a stronger response to the medication is more common. Physiologically, OHSS involves ovarian enlargement secondary to IVF medication which causes increased capillary permeability and ovarian angiogenesis (increased formation of ovarian blood vessels), resulting in an intravascular fluid shift to the third space. This can result in signs and symptoms such as electrolyte imbalances, increased abdominal pressure and pain, nausea, vomiting, and ascites or edema. In rare cases, severe symptoms may require hospitalization and/or surgical intervention to carefully monitor and treat the potential risks of these fluid shifts. More recently, IVF treatment has expanded to include medication protocols aimed at minimizing the risk of OHSS (Practice Committee of the ASRM, 2024e).

Fetal Risks Though several potential adverse outcomes have been proposed with the use of IVF, ICSI, and embryo biopsy techniques like PGT-A/PGT-M, current research does not demonstrate an increased risk of fetal malformations or death secondary to these procedures nor support a causal relationship between these (Mao et al., 2024; Weiss, 2020).

Perinatal Risks Additionally, for individuals who became pregnant using IVF, there appears to be an increased association between postpartum hemorrhage and placental variation/anomalies, though it is unclear whether there is an identifiable cause of these complications (Kong et al., 2022; Tang et al., 2023). Some studies also demonstrate the possibility of increased pregnancy complications such as hypertensive disorders, preterm birth, and low birth weight (Mao et al., 2024). Though more research is needed, some research suggests that pregnancies created using oocytes from someone other than the gestational parent may have an increased risk of preeclampsia (Mascarenhas et al., 2021).

While some research does find an association between these conditions and the use of ART, it is unclear whether these technologies themselves directly cause these outcomes. Many experts believe this association may exist because individuals experiencing infertility sometimes have underlying conditions and genetic alterations, some of which may not be known or able to be identified with current technologies (Alteri et al., 2023). Through bypassing typical barriers in spontaneous conception, embryos with higher rates of anomalies may be more likely to result in pregnancy when IVF is utilized as compared to the same DNA when IVF is not utilized. This theory suggests that ART itself is less likely to be the cause of these associations and instead the underlying reason may be attributed to something that prevented pregnancy in the first place.

Multiple Gestation Risks Often contrary to public perception, the potential for a multiple gestation pregnancy is actually lower for IVF when compared to ovulation induction medication cycles (ACOG, 2020). This is because surgical egg retrieval and subsequent embryo transfer represent a more controlled procedure in which no oocytes are ovulating internally. Conversely, ovulation induction medications stimulate multiple follicles to mature and release multiple oocytes. Through shared decision-making, clinicians and patients can decide on an acceptable risk regarding the number of embryos to transfer (ASRM, 2021e). The risk of multiple gestation pregnancies is most effectively lowered by the use of single embryo transfers, which are done in 85.9 percent of cases and significantly decreases the chance of a multiple gestation pregnancy occurring and subsequent risks such as premature birth and low birth weight (ACOG, 2021; Penzias et al., 2021; Wang et al., 2019). When embryo quality is perceived to be lower or the patient is not planning to do more than one embryo transfer, these discussions may result in the decision to transfer back multiple embryos, which does increase the risk of a multiple gestation pregnancy (ASRM, 2021e).

Pregnancy After Fertility Treatment

Once an individual completes their embryo transfer or intrauterine insemination, a serum beta hCG test is drawn after a waiting period of 10–14 days, respectively. Often referred to as "the two-week wait," this time is often associated with significant anticipatory anxiety and questioning whether certain mild symptoms may be indicative of pregnancy. If a positive serum result occurs, it is typically then repeated two to three times to ensure the beta hCG level is rising appropriately. Once that has been established, an early pregnancy ultrasound is done to monitor the pregnancy development closely, often between 6 and 7 weeks. Because there is a higher incidence of ectopic pregnancies in those with fertility concerns, this close monitoring allows for quicker identification of these cases.

After a pregnancy has been initially documented, patients may feel anxious waiting for the next confirmation that the pregnancy is continuing to develop normally. Warning signs of miscarriage such as uterine cramping, vaginal bleeding, and fluctuation of breast tenderness are often forefront of these anxieties. Frequently identified incidentally during early first trimester ultrasound, subchorionic hemorrhages are approximately twice as likely for patients who have conceived through IVF and often cause episodic or ongoing vaginal bleeding. Importantly, subchorionic hemorrhage is not associated with miscarriage, a decreased rate of live birth, or preterm birth after IVF. Anticipatory guidance is a compassionate aspect of care and should be provided during this time.

Early ultrasounds may be repeated, depending on the individual circumstances and whether any signs or symptoms of potential miscarriage may be present. Most patients are transferred to their prenatal provider by approximately 8 weeks, gestation to continue care. Clinicians who care for prenatal patients who have conceived via fertility treatment should be sensitive to the challenging journey they may have been on. Some patients who have conceived via extensive treatment may prefer a more medicalized approach to pregnancy and seek frequent imaging or testing for reassurance of pregnancy and fetal health. Others may intentionally seek lower levels of prenatal intervention, when possible, to counter the previous, more intensive path of conception. Clinicians may be able to improve the psychological adjustment to pregnancy and maintenance of daily life by normalizing the diagnosis of infertility and conception through fertility treatment (Simionescu et al., 2021).

Fertility Preservation

Advances in the ART technologies used to treat infertility have created new opportunities for individuals to extend their reproductive windows and postpone some aspects of age-related fertility decline by cryopreserving genetic material such as oocytes, sperm, or embryos for potential future use. These gametes can remain cryogenically frozen indefinitely and age-related fertility changes are paused at the patient's age at the time of freezing (Walker et al., 2022). For example, an individual who freezes oocytes at age 30 but waits to conceive until age 38 will have an expected oocyte quality of a 30-year-old.

Initially this technology was used by patients facing disease- or treatment-related infertility, such those having chemotherapy and radiation for cancer or undergoing oophorectomy or orchiectomy for chemoprophylaxis (Lawson et al., 2017), but utilization has expanded to include other motivations (Baldwin et al., 2019). While once considered experimental, this label was removed in 2012 as a result of the greatly improved success rates since its initial use and the reassuring safety data related to infants born after oocyte cryopreservation (Ethics Committee of the ASRM, 2024c). This process is still frequently done for individuals who have been recently diagnosed with cancer and The Ethics Committee of the ASRM (2018) recommends that clinicians counsel patients about fertility preservation options and future reproduction prior to any gonadotoxic treatments or interventions that may affect fertility, such as chemotherapy. However, elective oocyte cryopreservation cycles have increased significantly within the past 10 years, likely a reflection of shifting social priorities as well as gradual increased coverage by some healthcare insurances (Walker et al., 2022). Interestingly, research shows that only 16–20 percent of individuals who freeze oocytes go on to utilize them in the process of getting pregnant. This low rate of utilization is theorized to be commonly due to spontaneous pregnancy occurring, thus eliminating the need to use the frozen oocytes, as well as other aspects of one's life such as career prioritization or difficulty finding a partner with whom to parent (Kakkar et al., 2023; Polyakov & Rozen, 2021).

While research does not indicate that prior use of gender-affirming hormones causes infertility if hormones are stopped, some transgender and nonbinary individuals may wish to consider cryopreservation of oocytes or sperm prior to pharmacologic and/or surgical gender-affirming interventions (Feil et al., 2023; Olson, 2025). Additionally, some research suggests that the baseline fertility for gender-diverse individuals may be lower than their cisgender peers prior to any initiation of hormones. Though not true for all individuals, multiple studies demonstrate that trans women are likely to have lower sperm count at baseline, prior to the initiation of gender-affirming hormones (de Nie et al., 2022; Marsh et al., 2019). Additionally, the frequency of tucking, discussed more in Chapter 11, in this population may further decrease semen parameters (Manafi et al., 2024). Additionally, some research suggests that trans men and gender diverse people AFAB may have higher rates of polycystic ovarian syndrome, which is associated with fertility challenges (Rangi et al., 2024; Gezer et al., 2022). However, clinicians should be aware that the utilization of gender-affirming testosterone does not cause PCOS (Pirtea et al., 2021).

This process can also allow individuals time to consider their readiness for parenthood and can be done for a variety of reasons beyond initiation of gonadotoxic medications such as not yet having a partner or wanting to accomplish specific life goals before having children. Increased education and awareness of age-related decline in fertility has led to interest in oocyte cryopreservation among individuals who want to delay childbearing due to a variety of life circumstances. Patients should be informed that their age at which the fertility preservation took place is strongly related to the chances of success because oocyte age determines pregnancy rate. In some cases, fertility preservation is done in order to screen for inherited genetic mutations. For these patients, it is often recommended to freeze more oocytes than average with the understanding that many oocytes are expected to carry the genetic mutation (Cermisoni et al., 2023).

Elective oocyte cryopreservation should be a discussion initiated by clinicians when appropriate for the clinical context, though not all reproductive healthcare providers provide this counseling. This may represent lack of clinician education or comfort with detailed discussions surrounding identification of appropriate candidates. Some potential barriers include clinicians underestimating the influence of age on egg quality and fertility, as well as an incomplete understanding of ART limitations and pregnancy outcomes (Chronopoulou et al., 2021). A simple recommendation that all clinicians can integrate is asking patients their mother's age at menopause, as this can help to identify individuals who may be at risk for premature ovarian insufficiency and thus may want to consider oocyte cryopreservation at an earlier age.

Cryopreservation has complex financial, ethical, and legal considerations. The research is unclear regarding the ideal age at which to undergo cryopreservation as well as the number of oocytes, sperm vials, and embryos to cryopreserve in order to have a high likelihood of a live birth, though most research suggests optimal timeframe is below 35–37 years of age (Ethics Committee of the ASRM, 2024c). Freezing oocytes at a younger age typically yields a higher quantity of oocytes which are also less likely to have age-related chromosomal changes. However, higher numbers of oocytes also may bring about logistical and ethical questions regarding storage of oocytes and costs associated, which can be prohibitively expensive and are frequently not covered by insurance (Plowden et al., 2025; Johnston et al., 2024). Individuals must also give instructions about what should be done with their cryopreserved spermatozoa, oocytes, or embryos if they die, divorce, or experience other life changes.

Third-Party Reproduction

Third-party reproduction refers to the biological and/or genetic involvement of one or more individuals who are not the intended parent(s) and do not plan to be involved in raising the child. This includes use of donor sperm, donor egg, donor embryo, and/or the use of a gestational carrier. Commonly, donor gametes are utilized by LGBTQ+ individuals but are also frequently utilized for heterosexual individuals as well. Meeting with a therapist who specializes in third-party reproduction is recommended for anyone using any form of donor gametes to discuss topics unique to this method of family building (Ethics Committee of the ASRM, 2024a). While some patients may view this recommendation as an additional barrier for those without all the gametes necessary to conceive, there are unique psychological considerations regarding the use of donor genetic material for intended parents as well as donor-conceived individuals.

Research demonstrates that donor-conceived individuals commonly desire and seek out additional information about the donor utilized in their conception (Casteels et al., 2024). Intended parents may feel conflicted about how and when to convey this information and some choose not to share it with their children. Best practices regarding parental disclosure of the use of donor genetics include early and frequent discussions with children who are donor conceived to ensure they are not surprised later in life to learn about their conception (Ethics Committee of the ASRM, 2019). Nondisclosure of the use of a donor has potential harms, including lack of knowledge of relevant medical history information and the psychological stress that people may experience when learning they are donor conceived. Conversely, early disclosure to donor-conceived children regarding their conception is associated with improved psychological well-being (Talbot et al., 2024; ESHRE Working Group on Reproductive Donation, 2022). These collective discussions may bring up nuanced perspectives on the value of genetic mirroring, kinship, and definition of family and parents of donor-conceived children should be prepared to provide support as needed (Martin, 2019).

The Donor Sibling Registry, linked later in this chapter, is a U.S. organization that serves donor-conceived people, egg donors, sperm donors, and embryo donors by providing connection, education, and resources related to the well-being of donor-conceived people. Additionally, an increase in the utilization of direct-to-consumer genetic testing may alter the timing or context in which individuals learn they were conceived with donor gametes. These tests may also inadvertently connect donor-conceived individuals to biological family members, including the donor who contributed to their conception (Darroch & Smith, 2021).

Donor Sperm

Intended parents may utilize donor sperm for a variety of reasons, including not being partnered to a sperm-producing individual or avoiding a genetically linked disorder. Donor sperm can be used for insemination procedures or with IVF. In the United States, donor sperm may be obtained from known or anonymous donors. Known donors are often a friend or acquaintance but may also be a sibling or relative of a patient's partner which allows a same-sex couple to combine some aspects of their individual genetics. Anonymous donors are found through various U.S. or international sperm cryobanks. Purchasing donor sperm can be expensive, with an average vial of frozen donor sperm costing approximately $1,000–$1,500 (Fairfax Cryobank, 2025; California Sperm Bank, 2025; Seattle Sperm Bank, 2025). Knowing that multiple treatment cycles are likely required to create a pregnancy, this cost can easily create a barrier. In the United States, anonymous donors can be further categorized into entirely anonymous donors and anonymous donors who are "open-ID," which allows children conceived with that sperm to obtain the contact information of the donor when the child reaches age 18.

Donor Egg

The use of an oocyte donor may be chosen when use of a patient's own oocytes has been unsuccessful, often due to diminished ovarian reserve and/or advancing age. As with donor sperm, intended parents may opt to use donor eggs to avoid a genetically linked disorder. Oocyte donors may be known to the intended parent(s), such as in the case of an oocyte donation from a friend or family member. Alternatively, intended parent(s) may utilize anonymous donor eggs. These donor oocytes are then fertilized in vitro with sperm, often from an AMAB partner (intended parent), and then transferred to an AFAB partner (embryo recipient and intended parent) for gestation.

Donor Embryo

A donor embryo refers to an instance in which the intended legal parent(s) do not contribute DNA to the creation of an embryo that they use to create a pregnancy. Sometimes an intended parent may carry the pregnancy and sometimes a gestational carrier is used. The decision to use a donor embryo may stem from various social or relationship scenarios, including two individuals who do not have the necessary biology to create a pregnancy or who have age-related fertility challenges. The contractual agreements are often facilitated by a fertility clinic, in which previous patients have opted to donate their remaining embryos after completion of their family building plans. As is the case with IVF, the potential for age-related complications is directly linked to the age of the person contributing the oocyte and to a slightly lesser degree, the age of the person contributing the sperm.

Gestational Carriers

A gestational carrier is a person with a uterus who carries a pregnancy for another person, couple, or family but does not contribute an oocyte and therefore is not biologically related to the child. Individuals who contract with the gestational carrier are referred to as the intended parent(s) and plan to be the social and legal parent(s) of the child. Utilizing a gestational carrier requires the use of ART, and the intended parent(s) may or may not be the source of the sperm and/or oocyte (Ethics Committee of the ASRM, 2023).

EVIDENCE FOR BEST PRACTICES RELATED TO INFERTILITY CARE

ASRM is an excellent resource for clinicians of all backgrounds to find continuing education resources regarding fertility evaluation and treatment options for infertility. Within the organization, an advanced practice provider group has been formed to continue the evolution of the role of these clinicians within the field of REI (Hariton et al., 2023). The Practice Committee of the ASRM regularly publishes updated national, evidence-based guidelines for infertility care (https://www.asrm.org/Guidelines). The guidelines are updated periodically and are considered the standard for delivery of ART care. Practices that offer ART are urged to follow the guidelines developed by the Practice Committee of the ASRM, Practice Committee of the Society for Assisted Reproductive Technology, and Practice Committee of the Society of Reproductive Biologists & Technologists. These guidelines address necessary personnel, the specialized training and experience required for personnel, ethical and experimental procedures, record keeping, and informed consent.

PSYCHOLOGICAL, FAMILY, RELATIONSHIP, AND SOCIAL ISSUES

This section presents some of the complex considerations related to infertility and its treatment. Infertility can have psychosocial effects on the individuals and couples involved and on their larger families. Being unable to become a parent due to infertility can be profoundly distressing for those experiencing it and extensive research suggests that there are many associated psychological concerns for those experiencing infertility. Individuals may grieve their deeply held expectations for what their life and/or family structure may look like. Common themes that individuals experiencing infertility report include feelings of loss of control, guilt, anger, grief, and isolation. These feelings may also lead to anxiety, depression, and in some cases, PTSD. It is important to note that these emotions should be considered a normal reaction to the experience of infertility rather than underlying psychological pathology (Bindeman et al., 2021). Commonly cited research demonstrates that patients with infertility experience a similar degree of emotional distress as patients diagnosed with cancer (Domar et al., 1993). For some individuals, the experience of infertility can become part of their identity and may feel all-consuming. Therefore, it is essential for clinicians to recognize the vast and unique pressures these patients with infertility may face outside of clinical interactions and understand that they can be an important source of emotional support and that the provision of fertility care involves far more than just physical treatment (Sharma & Shrivastava, 2022). Patients over the age of 42 who undergo IVF without the end result of a live birth may experience regret but also note that emotional support and insurance coverage contribute to the degree of regret they experience (Huang et al., 2021).

As stated earlier, individuals experience infertility within a socially pronatalist context and individuals may feel they are unable to contribute to their perceived societal expectations. Cisgender women in particular may view parenthood as a necessary way to confirm their gender identity and experience increased stress if unable to become pregnant (Grunberg et al., 2022). Infertility is also directly intertwined with family issues because it represents the inability to expand a family. Some people even view it as an inability to have a family, implying that two people in a couple are not a family by virtue of not having children and further emphasizing a societal bent toward pronatalism. Family and social gatherings can be extremely difficult for persons dealing with infertility because they may be directly confronted with their inability to conceive, especially if young children are present. Family issues may also extend to other people beyond the couple, such as the parents of people with infertility who are experiencing loss related to not being grandparents. Family members may pressure couples with infertility with comments such as, "Why are you taking so long to have a baby?," often not knowing about the individuals' attempts to conceive.

Deciding to Stop Treatment

Complicated psychological issues can come to the forefront surrounding a decision or inability to make a decision to stop infertility treatment. The introduction of new treatments and potential for robust fertility insurance coverage in some states may raise hopes and make it difficult to stop treatment for fear that there will be a feeling of not having done everything possible to conceive, which could then make it difficult to resolve infertility later. In this situation, the clinician should advise patients about their options, including the pros and cons of continuing treatment. Also, individuals should have financial discussions upfront and set mutually agreed-upon boundaries regarding the extent of treatment they will pursue and how much they will spend. Fertility treatments can be an enormous emotional and financial investment, depending on insurance coverage. While repeated treatments are ultimately likely to result in a live birth, the stress of infertility treatment itself may be the reason that individuals decide to cease ongoing treatment.

Psychological Interventions

Some evidence indicates that providing psychosocial interventions—particularly cognitive behavioral therapy and counseling—to patients being treated for infertility can be beneficial in terms of both decreasing psychological distress and improving clinical pregnancy rates (Talebi & Mirzaian, 2023; Jackson et al., 2025). Some infertility treatment centers now have a mental health professional on-site (Rooney & Domar, 2018), increasing the ease of access for patients. This type of specialist can be helpful not only for the patients, but also for clinicians and staff because caring for patients with infertility may be an emotionally charged experience. Clinicians must not become desensitized to the vulnerable nature of their work. Some data suggests that encouraging patients to maintain their normal routine as much as possible as a coping mechanism for the process of fertility treatment (Benyamini et al., 2017). The emotional, physical, financial, and societal pressures associated with infertility have the potential to cause relationship stress and while counseling may be helpful in mitigating some of the stress associated with fertility treatment, it cannot prevent all types of conflict that may arise and relationship separation may occur when individuals cannot reconcile their responses to these challenges. Of note, data shows that couples are less likely to divorce when state-mandated insurance coverage is accessible (Cintina & Wu, 2019).

Although there is a minimal amount of research on the experience of AMAB individuals during infertility treatments, some results show that these individuals reported feeling grief, inadequacy, stigmatization, and isolation—an important insight for clinicians who work with couples experiencing infertility (Wu et al., 2023).

Sexual Concerns

Individuals undergoing fertility treatment often report varying degrees of sexual concerns (Practice Committee of the ASRM &

Society for Male Reproduction and Urology, 2023). For some, this may be related to an increase in perceived pressure regarding the timing of sexual intercourse. Sometimes the act of having sex specifically for the purpose of becoming pregnant may lack the spontaneity of their previous sex life in which pleasure was prioritized. For others, they may feel as though their body is failing them in some way and engaging in activities with heightened emotions such as sex may feel too vulnerable (Okobi, 2021; Agarwal et al., 2022). Some patients also experience ongoing depression or anxiety related to their infertility, which may decrease their drive to have sex overall and/or result in other sexual dysfunction (Sater et al., 2022). When needed, these patients may also initiate the use of SSRI antidepressants, which may further contribute to a lowered libido.

Challenges of the Patient Experience

Seeking to understand the daily lived experience of patients going through fertility treatment can allow clinicians to cultivate compassion and empathy for the challenges their patients face. When patients are referred to a reproductive endocrinology and infertility specialist, they are typically seen for an initial intake appointment which results in an extensive plan for a fertility evaluation. This testing, detailed previously in this chapter, may be able to be completed within one menstrual cycle, but due to the time-sensitive nature of the tests and when the initial visit is scheduled within a person's menstrual cycle, this process can often take 2–3 months. Given that many patients have already been trying to conceive for some time prior to their first appointment, any delay in starting treatment may cause anxiety. Additionally, this testing may reveal new diagnoses or reasons for infertility, which may be emotionally difficult to process. During this time, if insurance is utilized, patients may learn if there are limitations to their coverage for procedures or medications, which may change their decision on which treatment to pursue. Prior to the start of treatment, large amounts of medications arrive by mail and understanding the purpose and timing of each medication in the protocol can feel overwhelming. For those who have not previously administered an injection, this prospect may also feel intimidating, especially given the high cost of medications. Once treatment is initiated, there are typically 5–10 early morning clinic appointments per menstrual cycle (depending on the type of treatment) to have blood drawn and vaginal ultrasounds performed. The frequency of visits can be challenging to integrate with a full-time job and/or other responsibilities and may require a medical note of necessity for work absences in some cases. This may create uncomfortable employment dynamics in which a supervisor becomes aware of a patient's infertility diagnosis. Sometimes these ultrasounds are done by their established clinician and other times it may be a rotation of different clinical staff. Additionally, the hormonal medications themselves may be associated with mood shifts for some patients. With each treatment monitoring visit, there can be heightened anxiety when anticipating a phone call that afternoon to discuss the results and next steps. In some cases, staff communication may not provide adequate compassion or detailed explanation of the process, leaving patients feeling frustrated. Difficulties related to communication access with the clinic staff and lack of clinical and logistical information have been included as some of the primary causes of patient stress. While these challenges are not the experience of every patient, the treatment process can feel vulnerable and emotionally demanding even when significant barriers are not encountered.

Fertility-Related Disparities

Accessing Treatment

Though The American Medical Association and The World Health Organization have clearly stated that access to infertility care is a basic human right, many factors contribute to the challenges that patients face accessing fertility treatment. Estimates vary in terms of social and geographical context, but the ASRM notes that only 38 percent of nulliparous American women with current fertility concerns have spoken to a clinician about their condition, and this often only entails receiving medical advice. (Ethics Committee of the ASRM, 2021d). Reasons for this are varied and may include financial constraints, geographic location, insurance limitations, perceived stigma, lack of education, age, lack of inclusive clinicians, and other factors. In relation to geographical location, research finds that patients who lived within a 9–10 mile radius were 21 percent more likely to pursue ART treatment and 68 percent more likely to pursue IUI treatment. The influence of geographic location was lessened with increased socioeconomic privilege (Lazzari et al., 2022). Significant fertility disparities also exist regarding body-based oppression, including racial, class, weight, and other identity-related factors that are unlikely to be explained solely by financial barriers (Komorowski & Jain, 2022). **Appendix 20-A** reviews organizations which may provide emotional support and/or financial assistance to patients experiencing infertility in various contexts.

Insurance Coverage

Insurance coverage and ability to afford treatments are often the largest contributing factors to whether fertility treatment is ultimately pursued. Some patients report feeling discouraged about the prospect of scheduling to see an infertility specialist, citing the perspective that fertility treatment may inherently be financially unattainable. While infertility is categorized as a disability under the American Disabilities Act, some people continue to believe that infertility is a choice, and treatment should be considered elective (Cummings, 2023). Private insurances in the United States vary widely in what types of testing and treatment they cover. As of 2025, 21 states require private insurance coverage of at least some infertility services (RESOLVE, 2025b). However, though there are several U.S. states in which Medicaid covers initial diagnostic fertility testing and limited, low-cost fertility medication, no U.S. state Medicaid program currently covers fertility treatment procedures such as IUI or IVF (RESOLVE, 2025a). For individuals using Medicaid with specific medical barriers to fertility such as fallopian tube blockage, use of ART procedures such as IVF may be the only way for them to conceive and thus create impenetrable barriers for these individuals. In caring for patients experiencing infertility who utilize Medicaid, clinicians must be aware of their own biases regarding family building, including potential beliefs about the number of children a person desires, partnership dynamics, financial resources, and use of contraception (Ethics Committee of the ASRM, 2021d). Additionally, clinicians who serve rural populations and/or communities that primarily utilize Medicaid should be familiar with basic infertility workups and initial lower intervention treatment options such as oral ovulation induction medications. While all patients deserve access to the standard ultrasound/serum hormone testing that ovulation induction medications should be used in conjunction with, informed consent and a harm reduction approach using the Reproductive Justice framework is appropriate in order to support patients' right to pursue parenthood.

Weight Bias

Higher body weights are often viewed as a potential barrier to conception, with some research citing lower rates of spontaneous pregnancy, higher rates of miscarriage, and lower rates of pregnancies after ART treatment for those in higher weight bodies (Nicoletti et al., 2022; Ward & McPhail, 2019). However, the effects of weight stigma, discrimination, and weight cycling are not accounted for in these statistics and are associated with numerous poor health outcomes, including internalized weight bias in which patients may self-ascribe negative traits to themselves (Nagpal et al., 2022). Some patients in larger bodies may be subject to harmful perspectives that individuals in higher weight bodies should not pursue pregnancy (Nagpal et al., 2022). Additionally, because weight-related discriminatory practices are common in health care and fertility care, many individuals living in larger bodies are often unable to access fertility care, even when they do have health insurance. The inability for these individuals to access fertility specialists is also likely to influence pregnancy outcomes. Furthermore, individuals with PCOS often have higher BMIs and access to fertility treatment is an essential component for those with PCOS and other anovulation challenges.

Fertility clinics commonly have a BMI threshold of 35–45 kg/m^2 for patients receiving care, with treatment being withheld unless they undergo a significant reduction in weight which can be unrealistic, harmful, and consume significant time, all of which may contribute negatively to conception chances (Kuyoro et al., 2022; Kelley et al., 2019). This commonplace policy is problematic for several reasons, including that BMI has been shown to be a poor representation of a person's health (Callahan, 2023). Additionally, because research has demonstrated that long-term reduction in weight is not possible for the majority of individuals and has a high potential to result in harmful weight cycling, its use as a motivator as a means of accessing fertility treatment is both ineffective and unethical (Kuyoro et al., 2022). Some patients who feel desperate to reach the BMI threshold may also pursue restrictive eating behaviors coupled with overexercise. Patients who are denied treatment on this basis may experience feelings of shame, guilt, and embarrassment, while often being told that their current weight would be likely to contribute to significant pregnancy risks. This paternalistic approach undermines a patient's ability to consent to their own threshold of accepted risk. Withholding fertility treatment, whether due to insurance or fertility clinic policies, on the basis of weight is unethical and has the potential to worsen distrust amongst individuals in larger bodies seeking to access necessary health care. Clinicians should be aware of their own biases and be well versed in strategies to reduce weight bias in their practice (Papini et al., 2025).

Racial Disparities

Fertility care contains multiple aspects of significant racial disparities, with Black, Indigenous, and other people of color (BIPOC) being less likely to be diagnosed with infertility, evaluated for fertility concerns, receive care with a fertility specialist, and pursue fertility treatment options (Merkison et al., 2023). Black patients are significantly less likely to receive fertility preservation counseling by oncologists compared with white patients (Swain et al., 2023). For those who do seek care, there is frequently a longer time period in which patients are trying to conceive prior to seeing a fertility specialist. One study demonstrated that Black and Hispanic women tried to conceive spontaneously for an additional 20 months longer before receiving care compared with white women, reporting concern for racial discrimination based on physical appearance and the potential for biased care which does not prioritize (Weiss & Marsh, 2023). Other studies of women of color report that some clinicians emphasize the use of contraception over planned conception, attempt to dissuade them from pregnancy, and display biased perceptions about hyperfertility, a harmful racial and ethnic stereotype that may persist in both clinical care and in some cultures (Merkison et al., 2023). Additionally, for those who seek treatment, there are lower rates of clinical pregnancies, higher rates of miscarriages, poor outcomes using IVF, increased pregnancy complications, and lower rates of live births (Huddleston et al., 2023; Ghidei et al., 2021). Several of the contributing factors to these poor outcomes are the effects of systemic racism as well as socioeconomic factors, including lower incomes and lower rates of health insurance that make it much less feasible to pursue fertility treatment options. These factors are likely due to a multitude of racially striated socioeconomic factors related to structural racism dating back to the transatlantic slave trade from West Africa to the Americas in the 16th to 19th centuries and the legacy of oppression. Additionally, the field of reproductive endocrinology and infertility care has a distinct lack of racial diversity and thus lower levels of cultural congruence, which may contribute to individuals opting to wait or to forgo care altogether (Merkison et al., 2023).

Many BIPOC individuals also have increased incidence of complex gynecologic conditions associated with fertility challenges, including uterine fibroids, endometriosis, adenomyosis, and gynecologic cancers (Katon et al., 2023). These chronic gynecologic conditions also have strong associations with the increased allostatic load, microaggressions, and weathering that intentionally marginalized individuals experience on a daily basis (Charifson et al., 2022). Little research has been done regarding the lived experiences of BIPOC individuals with infertility and further studies are needed to help determine ways to eliminate these disparities.

LGBTQ+ Fertility

For individuals without all the biological gametes necessary to create a pregnancy, there can be significant disparities. Some LGBTQ+ patients may encounter difficulties in accessing their insurance benefits even when fertility coverage is a stated benefit of the plan. This may be because of the differences that insurances and clinicians may have in defining infertility and coding fertility-related services. These challenges are one of the driving factors in ASRM's 2023 update of the medical definition of infertility. However, even when insurance plans will cover diagnostic testing and treatment, the vast majority of insurance companies do not cover the costs associated with donor sperm, donor egg, and donor embryos; thus, these costs are typically out of pocket, though they may sometimes be eligible for payment with a health savings account (HSA) or FSA (RESOLVE, 2025b).

This chapter reviewed fertility care that may be accessed by individuals of various sexual orientations and/or gender identities. When fertility evaluation and treatment are discussed in a gender-neutral way, with an emphasis on anatomy rather than gender, it allows this care to be imagined in an inclusive way by both patients and clinicians.

ETHICAL ISSUES

Patients and clinicians may face conflicting personal ethical considerations as well as societal narratives regarding the morality of their reproductive choices or circumstances. In addition to the disparities discussed above, the ethical issues within the fertility field can bring up uncomfortable questions that individuals and organizations may differ in opinion on. Some of these ethical questions occur as a result of the increasing use of technology and advancements in genetics; however, it is important to note that ethical issues existed prior to, and may be independent of, some of these advances in infertility treatment.

Cost

Historically, the field of infertility treatment has been a largely self-pay specialty and the majority of patients who access fertility services have higher incomes (Voigt et al., 2022). While more insurances are beginning to cover some aspects of treatment, most insurances do not fully cover the associated expenses. The high cost of infertility treatment raises the question of whether these therapies will continue to be limited to people with the financial means to afford them (Ethics Committee of the ASRM, 2021d; Plowden et al., 2025). These insurance coverage limitations, coupled with socioeconomic barriers, have the power to decide who is allowed to pursue parenthood and who is not, conveying a harmful social message of genetic worthiness. Demographics that are frequently denied functional access to fertility treatment include those with lower socioeconomic means, higher body weight individuals, and those on Medicaid.

Additional ethical concerns may stem from fertility clinics' operational and business structure. Some clinics may be consolidated or sold to private equity firms in an attempt to improve clinical efficacy, however this may inadvertently result in pressure for clinicians to recommend higher-cost treatments that have an increased likelihood of success (Saleh et al., 2023; Patrizio et al., 2022). Treatment option counseling should always be done in an objective manner by reviewing the available treatment plans and giving patients the ability to choose the one that aligns with their goals best.

Donor Gametes

Parties involved in various aspects of third-party assisted reproduction may include the oocyte donor, the sperm donor, the gestational carrier, and the intended parent(s). Sperm and egg cryobanks may be nonprofit or for-profit and have a number of policies and practices that may bring up ethical concerns. Healthcare professionals are often surprised to learn that there are no national legal requirements for cryobanks to follow and the cryobanks themselves set their own policies. The limits to the number of families a donor may donate to can vary significantly, as there is currently no process for ensuring these limits are followed and these numbers are based on parental self-reporting, which is not mandatory. The potential repercussions of this include whether pertinent and life-altering medical information may be missed without the ability to know about the existence of biological siblings and the ability to contact them and/or the donor themselves. The Donor Sibling Registry is a U.S.-based organization that offers resources and connection to donor-conceived individuals, their parents, and donors. Within the United States, it is not mandatory that anyone who conceives using donor gametes join this database; thus, incomplete data is a potential concern. Nevertheless, it is beneficial for facilitating knowledge of and communication with other parents of donor-conceived individuals and/or donor siblings. The U.S. Donor Conceived Council collects data from 20 U.S. sperm cryobanks that allows patients to compare some of these policies across multiple cryobanks. Tracked categories include whether there are (1) sperm donor psychological evaluation and counseling regarding potential consequences of donating; (2) limits to the number of families a donor may donate to; (3) operation of a sibling database or registry; (4) verification of donor information such as past and present medical information as well as contact information, genetic carrier screening, criminal history, educational background; (5) donor identity able to be released when the child turns 18 years old (U.S. Donor Conceived Council, 2023). Additionally, it has been documented that most cryobanks also primarily offer white sperm donors and a low number of donors who are Black, Indigenous, or other individuals of color, a practice which contributes to ongoing racial disparities within reproductive health settings. This lack of donors, which more accurately reflects specific racial, ethnic, and cultural characteristics, may lead some patients to seek donor sperm from an individual known to them (Tam et al., 2025; Karpman et al., 2018).

In regard to known oocyte or sperm donors, legal questions may arise regarding how the courts define the legal parent(s). This may be especially true in cases where a known sperm donor is used in the context of patients using self-vaginal insemination at home without medical documentation from a clinician that the known donor is not an intended parent.

Gestational Carriers and Surrogates

A genetic surrogate (sometimes called a traditional surrogate) is a person who carries a pregnancy that was conceived from their own oocyte but is not an intended parent. Although legal contracts put in place prior to pregnancy help to designate who the intended parent(s) are, not all states have laws to enforce this (Ethics Committee of the ASRM, 2023). In some cases, a genetic surrogate, who is connected to the pregnancy via both genetics and by carrying the pregnancy, may be granted parental rights. Because of these legal gray areas, genetic surrogacy is illegal in some states and is rare overall due to the ethical and legal complexity involved (Legal Professional Group of ASRM, 2024).

Gestational carriers, who carry a pregnancy that does not use their own DNA, have a separate set of potential ethical concerns. Motivation of gestational carriers has long been subject to speculation both from the public and those in the healthcare field, centering around concern for coercive for-profit practices at the expense of gestational carriers' health and well-being (Jacobson, 2022). Studies demonstrate that the majority of gestational carriers in the United States are white, married, lower- to middle-class individuals with some financial stability who have already given birth to their own children. Studies also report that most gestational carriers are satisfied with the experience of carrying a pregnancy for which they will not be parents. As with many other aspects of reproductive care, racial, ethnic, and socioeconomic disparities continue to persist worldwide regarding the use of gestational carriers (Jacobson, 2022).

Age

Possible ethical considerations may arise in relation to both younger and older ages of patients seeking treatment. Newer technologies have made it possible for some individuals to conceive at later ages. While sometimes this widens the reproductive window for some people, increased complications are seen in pregnancies of older individuals, including rates of preeclampsia, gestational diabetes, hypertension, and birth-related complications. Though it may not be an immediate consideration, children born to older parents are also more likely to experience psychological concerns related to early bereavement (Zweifel & Woodward, 2022).

In addition, some fertility clinics may have an age cutoff for accessing treatment services. Sometimes this cutoff may be specific to the use of the person's own oocytes versus the use of donor oocytes, given the lower likelihood of successful pregnancy outcomes when older oocytes are used. Given the potential for significant emotional implications associated with the use of donor gametes, this clinical discussion should focus on the option of donor oocytes rather than a recommendation. Conversely, while uncommon, there may be times in which a patient under the age of 18 seeks fertility services and clinicians may need to reflect on their personally held beliefs and bias toward younger-age family building. Additionally, clinicians should be aware of the signs of reproductive coercion and understand their state laws regarding reproductive access, taking into account whether the patient is legally emancipated.

Legal Concerns

Ongoing legislative changes and barriers to reproductive healthcare access may also be aimed at controlling the use of ART. Other legal decisions pertaining to abortion access, such as the 2022 *Dobbs v Jackson Women's Health Organization* and overturn of *Roe v Wade*, may not be intentionally focused on ART, but may be interpreted in ways that ultimately impact the provision of ART due to the many ways in which fertility and abortion care are intricately connected (ASRM Center for Policy and Leadership, 2022). Proposed or adopted personhood laws that seek to define conception as the beginning of life, may also apply to frozen embryos resulting from ART (Catchings, 2019). These laws would not only greatly influence the use of technologies involved in genetic testing and whether embryos could be disposed of but also have the potential to define what constitutes harm to an embryo. By defining embryos as people or potential people under the right circumstances, patients would not be able to discard any additional frozen embryos after completion of family building and be required to continue incurring the cost of cryopreservation storage or elect for an embryo transfer. In states in which abortion access is banned in cases of fetal anomaly, the use of PGT-A and PGT-M would likely change dramatically. Additionally, for laws seeking to hold individuals responsible for causing harm, potential legal questions arise regarding whether clinicians and/or companies could be held responsible for unforeseeable events such as the loss of electricity powering an embryo storage location.

Other medicolegal issues arise regarding the creation of frozen embryos and in what circumstances patients have the right to utilize these in the future. In cases where a couple subsequently divorces, there may be conflicting feelings regarding whether one parent is allowed to use an embryo made in their previous relationship and who the legal parents are. This may be directly related to age, as may be the case in which an AFAB individual is unable to use their own oocytes due to age but has previously frozen embryos at a younger age with a former partner and would like to use one of these embryos to create a pregnancy on their own or with a new partner.

Genetic Testing

Ethical concerns have also arisen in relation to the ability to perform preimplantation genetic screening and diagnosis with ART and under what circumstances this should be permitted. Questions regarding the degree to which genetic testing within fertility treatment options may intentionally or unintentionally enable discriminatory and ableist practices within medicine continue to be explored, particularly as it relates to preimplantation genetic diagnosis for nonlethal conditions. Some of the topics most connected include whether individuals should be allowed to use PGT-A solely for embryo sex selection in the absence of other chromosomal changes. For those with complicated genetic family histories, some patients may feel they have a duty to minimize or eliminate potential future transmission of genetic disorders to their children, though there are many ethical considerations regarding this (Yang et al., 2022). Historically, the transfer of affected or aneuploid embryos has previously not been an incorporated practice in many clinics, though this is changing.

Multiple Gestation Pregnancies

Another ethical dilemma can occur when several embryos are transferred into a patient's uterus and multiple embryos survive. This scenario may also occur with the use of a gestational carrier and many gestational carrier legal contracts specify an acceptable threshold of risk related to the number of embryos transferred. The presence of multiple embryos may create a high-risk situation for the person carrying a pregnancy as well as the embryos, and the individual may choose to reduce to one or two embryos to decrease this risk. Multifetal reduction may cause complex ethical and emotional issues to arise. Additionally, this procedure holds the risk of unintentionally disrupting the pregnancy and causing pregnancy loss to occur. Preventing high-order multiples by limiting the number of embryos transferred is advisable, and the majority of U.S.-based clinics are following these suggestions by performing elective single embryo transfer to individuals with a favorable prognosis, such as patients younger than age 35, gestational carriers, and individuals whose embryos were genetically tested prior to transfer, thus increasing the chance of successful implantation (Practice Committee of the ASRM & Practice Committee of the Society for Assisted Reproductive Technology, 2022).

These are just a few of the many ethical issues that arise in relation to infertility care and treatment. There are no simple answers to these conflicts, but they warrant consideration both from a societal perspective and on the level of caring for individual patients. The Ethics Committee of the ASRM regularly publishes reports that address ethical issues in infertility treatment (https://www.asrm.org/EthicsReports).

OTHER FAMILY BUILDING OPTIONS FOR INDIVIDUALS WITH INFERTILITY

Despite the array of infertility treatment, ART, and third-party reproduction options now available, some people will not be able to have children via any of these methods or choose to end treatment. Fostering, adoption, or child-free living may be options for individuals who are able to separate pregnancy from parenting, though it is important that in these conversations, children are not viewed as a commodity on the path to fulfillment of a person's desire to parent.

Fostering

Fostering refers to a commitment by an individual or couple to take care of a child or children when they cannot safely remain with their parent(s), without being the child's legal parent(s). Typically, this is for a limited amount of time and may include communication or interaction with the child's legal parent(s). Goals of fostering include reduction in rates of child maltreatment and reduced time awaiting permanent family care. Additionally, while not always possible, a critical goal of fostering is eventual reunification with the child or children's biological parent(s), who continue to maintain legal rights unless terminated by the court. In 2022, 30 percent of all children in foster care had parental rights terminated and thus were available for adoption (National Council for Adoption, 2024). In some cases, foster parents may eventually adopt the children in their care when reunification with the biological family is not possible. Only some of the individuals who consider adoption also consider fostering, which likely reflects the emotional challenges that accompany future potential reunification.

Adoption

Adoption is a legal process that intended adoptive parents undergo with the goal of providing a permanent home and family for a child or children. Prior to adoption being pursued, it is ethically necessary to attempt to keep children with their genetic family or community (Wulczyn, 2004). Those who wish to adopt may work with a public or private adoption agency, or they may work directly with an attorney and have an independent or private adoption. This process also typically involves amending the birth certificate of the adopted child to reflect the adoptive parent(s) names and the new legal name given by the adoptive parents if applicable.

Additionally, prospective parents may pursue either domestic or international adoption, depending on a variety of circumstances including ethnic or racial background, age of the adoptive child or children, and medical history of the adoptive child or children. Although adoption is considered by both people with and without infertility challenges, many individuals and couples ultimately do not take steps to pursue it, most likely due to the costs associated with adoption, the difficult application process, and other situational factors.

Women with infertility are four times more likely to consider adoption as compared to women without infertility. In some of these cases, adoption is viewed as a "backup plan" to biological parenthood, with patients waiting to initiate adoption only after extensive efforts pursuing fertility treatment (National Council for Adoption, 2024). However, experts caution that this perspective may hinder parental engagement in the adoption process and potentially convey to potential adoptive children a less committed approach to parenting if the child sees themselves as a secondary plan. Additionally, the higher rates of depression and anxiety associated with infertility may persist after stopping treatment and some prospective parents may inadvertently rush into the adoption process before taking the time to seek treatment. For individuals considering adoption after experiencing infertility, the emotional trauma of infertility, relationship stability, and potential mental health concerns should be addressed with an adoption professional and/or mental health professional prior to initiating the adoption process (National Council for Adoption, 2024).

Child-Free Living

Some individuals eventually decide to live their lives without children, either by choice or circumstance, which can be associated with internal or external stigma and judgment (Hintz & Brown, 2019; Nardo, 2017). People without children may sometimes be referred to as childless, but this term can connote a loss or absence and should be avoided unless preferred by the individual in reference. The term "child free" connotes that this state is a choice rather than something that occurred against their will. Granted, this situation was initially childlessness for those who hoped to conceive, but through the process of reconciling their loss, some people are able to come to a conclusion of their own volition to remain child free.

CONCLUSION

This chapter has reviewed pertinent clinical information regarding fertility, the diagnosis of infertility, and the process of individualized family building. Engaging patients in proactive discussions about their future fertility and parenthood goals at younger ages supports the hallmarks of reproductive justice and informed decision making. Primary care and general reproductive healthcare clinicians should be empowered to understand their scope of practice and provide fertility education and testing based on the physiological and social context of individual patient needs. Engaging in ongoing education on this topic also allows clinicians to better identify patients who may benefit from earlier interventions such as fertility cryopreservation in a timely manner. Above all, patient autonomy and a trauma-informed care approach should be prioritized in the fertility and infertility evaluation process to support the notion that there are many unique paths that can lead to the creation of a family.

References

Abramov, M., Shalom-Paz, E., & Benyamini, Y. (2022). Persevering in fertility treatments despite failures: Unrealistic optimism and the reality of a pronatalist culture. *International Journal of Behavioral Medicine, 29*(2), 209–219. https://doi.org/10.1007/s12529-021-10001-5

Adachi, T., Endo, M., & Ohashi, K. (2020a). Regret over the delay in childbearing decision negatively associates with life satisfaction among Japanese women and men seeking fertility treatment: A cross-sectional study. *BMC Public Health, 20*(1), 886. https://www.ncbi.nlm.nih.gov/pubmed/32513145. https://doi.org/10.1186/s12889-020-09025-5

Adachi, T., Endo, M., & Ohashi, K. (2020b). Uninformed decision-making and regret about delaying childbearing decisions: A cross-sectional study. *Nursing Open, 7*(5), 1489–1496. https://www.ncbi.nlm.nih.gov/pubmed/32802369 doi:10.1002/nop2.523

Agarwal, N., Bachmann, G., & Phillips, N. (2022). Impact of infertility on female sexual function. *Journal of Sexual Medicine, 19*(8), S31–S31. https://doi.org/10.1016/j.jsxm.2022.05.113

Aharon, D., Sekhon, L., Lee, J. A., et al. (2020). Perinatal outcomes in reciprocal vs. anonymous donor oocyte IVF cycles. *Fertility and Sterility, 114*(3), e271. https://doi.org/10.1016/j.fertnstert.2020.08.752 doi:10.1016/j.fertnstert.2020.08.752

Akarsu, S. Gode, F., Isik, A. Z., Dikmen, Z. G., & Tekindal, M. A. (2017). The association between coenzyme Q10 concentrations in follicular fluid with embryo morphokinetics and pregnancy rate in assisted reproductive techniques. *Journal of Assisted Reproduction and Genetics, 34*(5), 599–605. 10.1007/s10815-017-0882-x

Akpinar, F., Yilmaz, S., Karahanoglu, E., et al. (2019). Intimate partner violence in Turkey among women with female infertility. *Sexual and Relationship Therapy, 34*(1), 3–9. https://doi.org/10.1080/14681994.2017.1327711

Allen, D., Hunter, M. S., Wood, S., & Beeson, T. (2017). One key question®: First things first in reproductive health. *Maternal and Child Health Journal, 21*(3), 387–392. https://doi.org/10.1007/s10995-017-2283-2

Alteri, A., Cermisoni, G. C., Pozzoni, M., Gaeta, G., Cavoretto, P. I., & Viganò, P. (2023). Obstetric, neonatal, and child health outcomes following embryo biopsy for preimplantation genetic testing. *Human Reproduction Update, 29*(3), 291–306. https://doi.org/10.1093/humupd/dmad001

American College of Obstetricians and Gynecologists. (2018, reaffirmed 2024a). Marriage and family building equality for lesbian, gay, bisexual, transgender, queer, intersex, asexual, and gender nonconforming individuals [Committee Opinion No. 749]. *Obstetrics & Gynecology, 132*(2), e82–e86. https://doi.org/10.1097/AOG.0000000000002765

American College of Obstetricians and Gynecologists. (2018, reaffirmed 2024b). Committee opinion number 755: Well-woman visit. *Obstetrics and Gynecology, 132*(4), e181–e186. https://doi.org/10.1097/AOG.0000000000002897

American College of Obstetricians and Gynecologists. (2019, reaffirmed 2024c). *The use of Antimüllerian hormone in women not seeking fertility care. [Committee Opinion No. 773].* https://www.acog.org/clinical/clinical-guidance/committee-opinion/articles/2019/04/the-use-of-antimullerian-hormone-in-women-not-seeking-fertility-care

American College of Obstetricians and Gynecologists Committee on Gynecologic Practice and The Practice Committee of the American Society for Reproductive Medicine. (2014, reaffirmed 2022). Committee opinion 589: Female age-related fertility decline. *Fertility and Sterility, 101*(3), 633–634. https://www.ncbi.nlm.nih.gov/pubmed/24559617

American College of Obstetricians and Gynecologists. (2013, reaffirmed 2020). *Multifetal pregnancy reduction: ACOG committee opinion, number 719.* https://www.acog.org/clinical/clinical-guidance/committee-opinion/articles/2017/09/multifetal-pregnancy-reduction

American College of Obstetricians and Gynecologists. (2019). Infertility workup for the women's health specialist: ACOG committee opinion, number 781. *Obstetrics and Gynecology, 133(6),* e377–e384. https://doi.org/10.1097/AOG.0000000000003271

American College of Obstetricians and Gynecologists. (2021). Multifetal gestations: Twin, triplet, and higher-order multifetal pregnancies: ACOG practice bulletin, number 231.*Obstetrics and Gynecology, 137*(6), e145–e162. https://doi.org/10.1097/AOG.0000000000004397

American Society for Reproductive Medicine. (2021). *What is recurrent pregnancy loss (RPL)?* Reproductive Facts; American Society for Reproductive Medicine. https://www.reproductivefacts.org/globalassets/_rf/news-and-publications/bookletsfact-sheets/english-pdf/what_is_recurrent_pregnancy_loss_rpl_factsheet.pdf

American Society for Reproductive Medicine Center for Policy and Leadership. (2022). *State abortion trigger laws: Potential implications for reproductive medicine.* American Society for Reproductive Medicine. https://www.asrm.org/globalassets/_asrm/advocacy-and-policy/dobbs/state_abortion_laws_p2_oct_22.pdf

American Society for Reproductive Medicine & American College of Obstetricians and Gynecologists' Committee on Gynecologic Practice. (2019, reaffirmed 2024). Prepregnancy counseling: Committee opinion no. 762. *Fertility and Sterility, 111*(1), 32–42. https://doi .org/10.1016/j.fertnstert.2018.12.003

Ashburn-Nardo, L. (2017). Parenthood as a moral imperative? Moral outrage and the stigmatization of voluntarily childfree women and men. *Sex Roles, 76*(5), 393–401.

Awadalla, M. S., Bendikson, K. A., Ho, J. R., McGinnis, L. K., & Ahmady, A. (2021). A validated model for predicting live birth after embryo transfer. *Scientific Reports, 11*(1), 10800. https://www.ncbi.nlm.nih.gov/pubmed/34031492. https://doi.org/10.1038/s41598-021-90254-y

Bakkensen, J., Desai, K., Feinberg, E., & Lawson, A. (2022). Psychological stress and infertility: What do women in medicine believe? *Fertility and Sterility, 118,* e92–e93. 10.1016/j.fertnstert.2022.08.281

Baldwin, K., Culley, L., Hudson, N., & Mitchell, H. (2019). Running out of time: Exploring women's motivations for social egg freezing. *Journal of Psychosomatic Obstetrics and Gynaecology, 40*(2), 166–173. https://www.ncbi.nlm.nih.gov/pubmed/29648960 doi: 10.1080/0167482X.2018.1460352

Barnes, L., & Fledderjohann, J. (2020). Reproductive justice for the invisible infertile: A critical examination of reproductive surveillance and stratification. *Sociology Compass, 14*(2), e12745. https://doi.org/10.1111/soc4.12745

Barratt, C. L., Bjorndahl, L., De Jonge, C. J., Lamb, D. J., Osorio Martini, F., McLachlan, R. et al. (2017). The diagnosis of male infertility: An analysis of the evidence to support the development of global AHO guidance-challenges and future research opportunities. *Human Reproduction Update, 23*(6), 660-680.

Benyamini, Y., Gozlan, M., & Weissman, A. (2017). Normalization as a strategy for maintaining quality of life while coping with infertility in a pronatalist culture. *International Journal of Behavioral Medicine, 24*(6), 871–879.

Berthelsen, A. S. N., Gamby, A. L. N., Christensen, U., Schmidt, L., & Koert, E. (2021). How do young men want to receive information about fertility? Young men's attitudes towards a fertility campaign targeting men in Copenhagen, Denmark. *Human Reproduction Open, 2021*(3), hoab027. https://doi.org/10.1093/hropen/hoab027

Bin, C., Zhong, H., Zhang, S., Luo, Y., Su, J., Li, M., & Wei, S. (2025). Effects of acupuncture-related therapies on pregnancy outcomes among women undergoing in vitro fertilization and embryo transfer: A Bayesian network meta-analysis. *Journal of Assisted Reproduction and Genetics*, 1–14.

Bindeman, J. (2021). Psychological and medical perspectives on fertility care and sexual health, In K. Bergman & W. Petok (Eds.), *Psychological and medical perspectives on fertility care and sexual health.* Elsevier.

Bindeman, J., Abbasi, R., & Sacks, P. C. (2025). The mental health traumas of infertility: Impact and consequences. *Obstetrics and Gynecology Clinics of North America, 52*(1), 133–143. https://doi.org/10.1016/j.ogc.2024.10.005

Bourdon, M., Santulli, P., Beeker, N., Collier, M., Treluyer, J.-M., Tsatsaris, V., Pinson, P., & Chouchana, L. (2025). Impact of clomiphene citrate on multiple gestation births and perinatal outcomes: A nationwide cohort study. *Fertility and Sterility, 124*(2), 334–343. https://doi.org/10.1016/j.fertnstert.2025.04.005

Boyle, B. R., Ablett, A. D., Ochi, C., Hudson, J., Watson, L., Rauh, D., & Avenell, A. (2023). The effect of weight loss interventions for obesity on fertility and pregnancy outcomes: A systematic review and meta-analysis. *International Journal of Gynecology and Obstetrics, 161*(2), 335–342. https://doi.org/10.1002/ijgo.14597

Brannigan, R., Hermanson, L., Kaczmarek, J., Kim, S, Kirkby, E., & Tanrikut, C. (2024). Updates to male infertility: AUA/ASRM guideline. J Urol. https://www.auajournals.org/doi/10.1097/JU.0000000000004180

Caldwell, A. E., Gorczyca, A. M., Bradford, A. P., Nicklas, J. M., Montgomery, R. N., Smyth, H., Pretzel, S., Nguyen, T., DeSanto, K., Ernstrom, C., & Santoro, N. (2024). Effectiveness of preconception weight loss interventions on fertility in women: A systematic review and meta-analysis. *Fertility and Sterility, 122*(2), 326–340. https://doi.org/10.1016/j.fertnstert.2024.02.038

California Cryobank. *Sperm bank pricing—donor semen cost.* www.cryobank.com. https://www.cryobank.com/services/pricing/

Callahan, E. A. (Ed.). (2023). The science, strengths, and limitations of body mass index. In *Translating knowledge of foundational drivers of obesity into practice* (pp. 99–106). National Academies Press.

Casar-Borota, O., Burman, P., & Lopes, M. B. (2025). The 2022 WHO classification of tumors of the pituitary gland: An update on aggressive and metastatic pituitary neuroendocrine tumors. *Brain Pathology (Zurich, Switzerland), 35*(1), e13302. https://doi.org/10.1111/bpa.13302

Casteels, P., Nekkebroeck, J., & Tournaye, H. (2024). Perspectives on sperm donor anonymity: Insights from donor-conceived adults in Belgium. *Human Reproduction, 39*(9), 2021–2031. https://doi-org.proxy.library.georgetown.edu/10.1093/humrep/deae160

Casteels, P., Nekkebroeck, J., & Tournaye, H. (2024). Perspectives on sperm donor anonymity: insights from donor-conceived adults in Belgium. *Human Reproduction (Oxford), 39*(9), 2021–2031. https://doi.org/10.1093/humrep/deae160

Catchings, H. C. (2019). A "modern family" issue: Recategorizing embryos in the 21st century. *Louisiana Law Review, 80,* 1521.

Centers for Disease Control and Prevention, American Society for Reproductive Medicine, & Society for Assisted Reproductive Technology. (2025). *2022 assisted reproductive technology national summary report.* https://www.sartcorsonline.com/rptcsr_publicmultyear.aspx

Centers for Disease Control and Prevention. (2024a). *National health statistic reports: Infertility and impaired fecundity in women and men in the United States, 2015–2019.* https://www.cdc.gov/nchs/data/nhsr/nhsr202.pdf

Centers for Disease Control and Prevention. (2024b). *National ART surveillance system.* https://www.cdc.gov/art/php/nass/index.html#:~:text=Reporting%20requirements-,The%20Fertility%20Clinic%20Success%20Rate%20and%20Certification%20Act%20of%201992,these%20clinic%2Dspecific%20success%20rates

Charifson, M. A., Vieira, D., Shaw, J., Kehoe, S., & Quinn, G. P. (2022). Why are Black individuals disproportionately burdened with uterine fibroids and how are we examining this disparity? A systematic review. *F&S Reviews, 3*(4), 256–279. https://doi.org/10.1016/j.xfnr.2022.07.004

Chronopoulou, E., Raperport, C., Sfakianakis, A., Srivastava, G., & Homburg, R. (2021). Elective oocyte cryopreservation for age-related fertility decline. *Journal of Assisted Reproduction and Genetics, 38*(5), 1177–1186. https://doi.org/10.1007/s10815-021-02072-w

Cintina, I., & Wu, B. (2019). How do state infertility insurance mandates affect divorce? *Contemporary Economic Policy, 37*(3), 560–570. https://doi.org/10.1111/coep.12416

Cermisoni, G. C., Pisaturo, V., Vanni, V. S., Minetto, S., Pagliardini, L., Masciangelo, R., Candiani, M., Papaleo, E., & Alteri, A. (2023). Fertility preservation as an option for women with genetic disorders: Insights from a SWOT analysis on elective oocyte freezing and preimplantation genetic testing. *Life (Basel, Switzerland), 13*(7), 1483. https://doi.org/10.3390/life13071483

Copp, T., van Nieuwenhoven, T., McCaffery, K. J., Hammarberg, K., Cvejic, E., Doust, J., Lensen, S., Peate, M., Augustine, L., van der Mee, F., Mol, B. W., Lieberman, D., & Jansen, J. (2024). Women's interest, knowledge, and attitudes relating to anti-Mullerian hormone testing: A randomized controlled trial. *Human Reproduction (Oxford), 39*(9), 2010–2020. https://doi.org/10.1093/humrep/deae147

Cox, C. M., Thoma, M. E., Tchangalova, N., Mburu, G., Bornstein, M. J., Johnson, C. L., & Kiarie, J. (2022). Infertility prevalence and the methods of estimation from 1990 to 2021: A systematic review and meta-analysis. *Human Reproduction Open, 2022*(4), hoac051. https://doi.org/10.1093/hropen/hoac051

Cummings, J. (2023). Closing the reproductive divide: Expanding access to fertility services beyond the white nuclear family, *Law & Inequality, 253*, 41(2). https://doi.org/10.24926/25730037.686

Darroch, F., & Smith, I. (2021). Establishing identity: How direct-to-consumer genetic testing challenges the assumption of donor anonymity. *Family Court Review, 59*(1), 103–120. https://doi.org/10.1111/fcre.12553

de Assis, V., Giugni, C. S., & Ros, S. T. (2024). Evaluation of recurrent pregnancy loss. *Obstetrics and Gynecology, 143*(5), 645–659. https://doi.org/10.1097/AOG.0000000000005498

de Nie, I., Asseler, J., Meißner, A., Voorn-de Warem, I. A. C., Kostelijk, E. H., den Heijer, M., Huirne, J., & van Mello, N. M. (2022). A cohort study on factors impairing semen quality in transgender women. *American Journal of Obstetrics and Gynecology, 226*(3), 390.e1–390.e10. https://doi.org/10.1016/j.ajog.2021.10.020

Dehkordi, S. M., Khoshakhlagh, A. H., Yazdanirad, S., et al. (2025). The effect of job stress on fertility, its intention, and infertility treatment among the workers: A systematic review. *BMC Public Health, 25*, 542. https://doi.org/10.1186/s12889-025-21790-9

Devine, K., Dolitsky, S., Ludwin, I., & Ludwin, A. (2022). Modern assessment of the uterine cavity and fallopian tubes in the era of high-efficacy assisted reproductive technology. *Fertility and Sterility, 118*, 19–28. 10.1016/j.fertnstert.2022.05.020

Dimitriadis, F., Borgmann, H., Struck, J., Salem, J., & Kuru, T. (2023). Antioxidant supplementation on male fertility—A systematic review. *Antioxidants, 12*(4), 836. https://doi.org/10.3390/antiox12040836

Domar, A. D., Zuttermeister, P. C., & Friedman, R. (1993). The psychological impact of infertility: A comparison with patients with other medical conditions. *Journal of Psychosomatic Obstetrics and Gynaecology, 14*(Suppl), 45–52.

Don, E. E., Mijatovic, V., & Huirne, J. A. F. (2023). Infertility in patients with uterine fibroids: A debate about the hypothetical mechanisms. *Human Reproduction (Oxford), 38*(11), 2045–2054. https://doi.org/10.1093/humrep/dead194

Donnez, J., Taylor, H. S., Marcellin, L., & Dolmans, M.-M. (2024). Uterine fibroid–related infertility: Mechanisms and management. *Fertility and Sterility, 122*(1), 31–39. https://doi.org/10.1016/j.fertnstert.2024.02.049

Dreisler, E., & Kjer, J. J. (2019). Asherman's syndrome: Current perspectives on diagnosis and management. *International Journal of Women's Health, 11*, 191–198. https://doi.org/10.2147/IJWH.S165474

ESHRE Working Group on Reproductive Donation, Kirkman-Brown, J., Calhaz-Jorge, C., Dancet, E. A. F., Lundin, K., Martins, M., Tilleman, K., Thorn, P., Vermeulen, N., & Frith, L. (2022). Good practice recommendations for information provision for those involved in reproductive donation†. *Human Reproduction Open, 2022*(1), hoac001. https://doi.org/10.1093/hropen/hoac001

Ethics Committee of the American Society for Reproductive Medicine. (2018). Fertility preservation and reproduction in patients facing gonadotoxic therapies: An ethics committee opinion. *Fertility and Sterility, 110*(3), 380–386. https://doi.org/10.1016/j.fertnstert.2018.05.034

Ethics Committee of the American Society for Reproductive Medicine. (2019). Interests, obligations, and rights in gamete and embryo donation: An ethics committee opinion. *Fertility and Sterility, 111*(4), 664–670. https://www.asrm.org/practice-guidance/ethics-opinions/interests-obligations-and-rights-in-gamete-and-embryo-donation-an-ethics-committee-opinion-2019/

Ethics Committee of American Society for Reproductive Medicine. (2021a). Access to fertility treatment irrespective of marital status, sexual orientation, or gender identity: A committee opinion. *Fertility and Sterility, 116*(2), 326–330. https://www.asrm.org/globalassets/_asrm/practice guidance/ethics opinions/pdf/access-to-fertility-treatment-irrespective-of-marital-status-sexual-orientation-or-gender-identity.pdf

Ethics Committee of the American Society for Reproductive Medicine. (2021b). Access to fertility services by transgender and nonbinary persons: An ethics committee opinion. *Fertility and Sterility, 115*(4), 874–8. https://www.asrm.org/practice-guidance/ethics-opinions/access-to-fertility-services-by-transgender-and-nonbinary-persons-an-ethics-committee-opinion-2021/

Ethics Committee of the American Society for Reproductive Medicine. (2021c). Human immunodeficiency virus and infertility treatment: An ethics committee opinion. *Fertility and Sterility, 115*(4), 860 869. https://www.ncbi.nlm.nih.gov/pubmed/33832741 doi: 10.1016/j.fertnstert.2021.01.024

Ethics Committee of the American Society for Reproductive Medicine. (2021d). Disparities in access to effective treatment for infertility in the United States: An ethics committee opinion. *Fertility and Sterility, 116*(1), 54–63. https://doi.org/10.1016/j.fertnstert.2021.02.019

Ethics Committee of the American Society for Reproductive Medicine. (2022). Use of reproductive technology for sex selection for nonmedical reasons: An ethics committee opinion. *Fertility and Sterility, 117*(4), 720–725. https://www.asrm.org/globalassets/_asrm/practice-guidance/ethics-opinions/pdf/use_of_reproductive_technology_for_sex_selection.pdf

Ethics Committee of the American Society for Reproductive Medicine. (2023). Consideration of the gestational carrier: An ethics committee opinion. *Fertility and Sterility, 119*(4), 583–587. https://www.asrm.org/globalassets/_asrm/practice-guidance/ethics-opinions/pdf/consideration_of_the_gestational_carrier-pdfmembers.pdf

Ethics Committee of the American Society for Reproductive Medicine. (2024a). Gamete and embryo donation guidance. *Fertility and Sterility, 122*(5), 799–812. https://www.asrm.org/globalassets/_asrm/practice-guidance/practice-guidelines/pdf/gamete-and-embryo-donation-guidance-2024.pdf

Ethics Committee of the American Society for Reproductive Medicine. (2024b). Use of preimplantation genetic testing for monogenic adult-onset conditions. *Fertility and Sterility, 122*(4), 607–611. https://doi.org/10.1016/j.fertnstert.2024.05.165

Ethics Committee of the American Society for Reproductive Medicine. (2024c). Planned oocyte cryopreservation to preserve future reproductive potential: An ethics committee opinion. *Fertility and Sterility, 121*(4), 604–611. https://www.asrm.org/globalassets/_asrm/practice-guidance/ethics-opinions/pdf/planned_oocyte_cryopreservation.pdf

Fairfax Cryobank. *Fees*. https://fairfaxcryobank.com/fees

Families Rising. (2024). *Permanency planning/continuity of relationships*. https://wearefamiliesrising.org/positions-on-key-issues/permanency-planning/

Fauser, B. C. J. M., Adamson, G. D., Boivin, J., Chambers, G. M., de Geyter, C., Dyer, S., Inhorn, M. C., Schmidt, L., Serour, G. I., Tarlatzis, B., Zegers-Hochschild, F., & Contributors and members of the IFFS Demographics and Access to Care Review Board (2024). Declining global fertility rates and the implications for family planning and family building: An IFFS consensus document based on a narrative review of the literature. *Human Reproduction Update, 30*(2), 153–173. https://doi.org/10.1093/humupd/dmad028

Feil, K., Reiser, E., Braun, A. S., Böttcher, B., & Toth, B. (2023). Fertility, contraception, and fertility preservation in trans individuals. *Deutsches Ärzteblatt International, 120*(14), 243–250. https://doi.org/10.3238/arztebl.m2023.0026

Feinberg, E. C., & Rosenwaks, Z. (2021). Training the next generation of reproductive endocrinology and infertility subspecialists. *Fertility and Sterility, 115*(3), 567–568. https://doi.org/10.1016/j.fertnstert.2021.01.035

Feng, J., Wang, J., Zhang, Y., Zhang, Y., Jia, L., Zhang, D., Zhang, J., Han, Y., Luo, S., & Tamagno, G. (2021). the efficacy of complementary and alternative medicine in the treatment of female infertility. *Evidence-Based Complementary and Alternative Medicine: eCAM, 2021*, 6634309. https://doi.org/10.1155/2021/6634309

Garthwaite, H., Stewart, J., King, K., McGarry, K., & Wilkes, S. (2020). Ultrasound monitoring during first-cycle treatment with clomifene citrate: A national survey of compliance with NICE. *Human Fertility (Cambridge, England), 23*(3), 193–199. https://doi.org/10.1080/14647273.2018.1535201

Genovese, H. G., & McQueen, D. B. (2023). The prevalence of sporadic and recurrent pregnancy loss. *Fertility and Sterility, 120*(5), 934–936. https://doi.org/10.1016/j.fertnstert.2023.08.954

Gezer, E., Piro, B., Cantürk, Z., Çetinarslan, B., Sözen, M., Selek, A., Polat Işik, A., & Seal, L. J. (2022). The comparison of gender dysphoria, body image satisfaction and quality of life between treatment-naive transgender males with and without polycystic ovary syndrome. *Transgender Health, 7*(6), 514–520. https://doi.org/10.1089/trgh.2021.0061

Ghidei, L., Wiltshire, A., Raker, C., Ayyar, A., & Brayboy, L. M. (2021). Factors associated with disparate outcomes among Black women undergoing in vitro fertilization. *F&S Reports, 3*(2 Suppl), 14–21. https://doi.org/10.1016/j.xfre.2021.12.002

Gonullu, D. C., Huang, X. M., Robinson, L. G., Walker, C. A., Ayoola-Adeola, M., Jameson, R., Yim, D., & Awonuga, A. (2022). Tubal factor infertility and its impact on reproductive freedom of African American women. *American Journal of Obstetrics and Gynecology, 226*(3), 379–383. https://doi.org/10.1016/j.ajog.2021.06.002

Greco, E., Litwicka, K., Minasi, M. G., Cursio, E., Greco, P. F., & Barillari, P. (2020). Preimplantation genetic testing: Where we are today. *International Journal of Molecular Sciences, 21*(12), 4381. https://www.ncbi.nlm.nih.gov/pubmed/32575575. https://doi.org/10.3390/ijms21124381

Grunberg, P., Miner, S., & Zelkowitz, P. (2022). Infertility and perceived stress: The role of identity concern in treatment-seeking men and women. *Human Fertility (Cambridge, England), 25*(1), 117–127. https://doi.org/10.1080/14647273.2019.1709667

Gupta, S. N., Srinivas, B. V., & Pandey, D. (2023). 49: Does percutaneous epididymal sperm aspiration (PESA)-sperm attribute as the game changer in high-risk male factor fertility for intracytoplasmic sperm injection (ICSI)? *Fertility & Reproduction, 5*(4), 541–541. https://doi.org/10.1142/S2661318223742960

Hall, K. D., & Kahan, S. (2018). Maintenance of lost weight and long-term management of obesity. *Medical Clinics of North America, 102*(1), 183–197. https://doi.org/10.1016/j.mcna.2017.08.012

Harb, H., Al-Rshoud, F., Karunakaran, B., Gallos, I. D., & Coomarasamy, A. (2019). Hydrosalpinx and pregnancy loss: A systematic review and meta-analysis. *Reproductive Biomedicine Online, 38*(3), 427–441. https://doi.org/10.1016/j.rbmo.2018.12.020

Hariton, E., Alvero, R., Hill, M. J., Mersereau, J. E., Perman, S., Sable, D., Wang, F., Adamson, G. D., Coutifaris, C., Craig, L. B., Hosseinzadeh, P., Imudia, A. N., Johnstone, E. B., Lathi, R. B., Lin, P. C., Marsh, E. E., Munch, M., Richard-Davis, G., Roth, L. W., Schutt, A. K., . . . Devine, K. (2023). Meeting the demand for fertility services: The present and future of reproductive endocrinology and infertility in the United States. *Fertility and Sterility, 120*(4), 755–766. https://doi.org/10.1016/j.fertnstert.2023.08.019

Herzog, B. J., Nguyen, H. M. T., Soubra, A., & Hellstrom, W. J. G. (2020). Clomiphene citrate for male hypogonadism and infertility: An updated review. *Androgens, 1*(1), 62–69. https://doi.org/10.1089/andro.2020.0005

Hintz, E. A., & Brown, C. L. (2019). Childfree by choice: Stigma in medical consultations for voluntary sterilization. *Women's Reproductive Health, 6*(1), 62–75.

Hoang-Thi, A. P., Dang-Thi, A. T., Phan-Van, S., Nguyen-Ba, T., Truong-Thi, P. L., Le-Minh, T., Nguyen-Vu, Q. H., & Nguyen-Thanh, T. (2022). The impact of high ambient temperature on human sperm parameters: A meta-analysis. *Iranian Journal of Public Health, 51*(4), 710–723. https://doi.org/10.18502/ijph.v51i4.9232

Hoek, A., Wang, Z., van Oers, A. M., Groen, H., & Cantineau, A. E. P. (2022). Effects of preconception weight loss after lifestyle intervention on fertility outcomes and pregnancy complications. *Fertility and Sterility, 118*(3), 456–462. https://doi.org/10.1016/j.fertnstert.2022.07.020

Huang, D., Ransohoff, A., Boscardin, J., Jaswa, E., Cedars, M., & Huddleston, H. (2021). Patients' perceived level of counseling and emotional support, not number of cycles, strongly impacts decision regret after failed autologous IVF in women age 42 and over. *Fertility and Sterility, 116*(1), e8. https://doi.org/10.1016/j.fertnstert.2021.05.013 doi:10.1016/j.fertnstert.2021.05.013

Huddleston, A., Ray, K., Bacani, R., Staggs, J., Anderson, R. M., & Vassar, M. (2023). Inequities in medically assisted reproduction: A scoping review. *Reproductive Sciences (Thousand Oaks, Calif.), 30*(8), 2373–2396. https://doi.org/10.1007/s43032-023-01236-6

Hvidman, H. W., Bentzen, J. G., Thuesen, L. L., et al. (2016). Infertile women below the age of 40 have similar anti-Müllerian hormone levels and antral follicle count compared with women of the same age with no history of infertility. *Human Reproduction, 31*(5), 1034–1045. https://www.ncbi.nlm.nih.gov/pubmed/26965431. https://doi.org/10.1093/humrep/dew032

Jackson, P. L., Saunders, P., Mizzi, S., & Hallman, K. T. (2025). The efficacy of psychological interventions for infertile women: a systematic review and meta-analysis. *BMC Women's Health 25*, 506. https://doi.org/10.1186/s12905-025-04054-x

Jacobson, H. (2022). The ART clock: Temporal limits to assisted reproduction. *Reproductive Biomedicine & Society Online, 14,* 144–155. https://doi.org/10.1016/j.rbms.2021.10.004

Johnston, M., Fuscaldo, G., Sutton, E., Hunt, S., Zander-Fox, D., Rombauts, L., & Mills, C. (2024). Storage trends, usage and disposition outcomes following egg freezing. *Reproductive BioMedicine Online, 48*(4), Article 103728. https://doi.org/10.1016/j.rbmo.2023.103728

Kakkar, P., Geary, J., Stockburger, T., Kaffel, A., Kopeika, J., & El-Toukhy, T. (2023). Outcomes of social egg freezing: A cohort study and a comprehensive literature review. *Journal of Clinical Medicine, 12*(13), 4182. https://doi.org/10.3390/jcm12134182

Kar, S., & Maharana, L. (2023). Comparison of letrozole vs letrozole plus metformin as first line ovulation induction drug for infertile PCOS women. *Fertility & Reproduction, 5*(4), 587–587. https://doi.org/10.1142/S2661318223743266

Karpman, H. E., Ruppel, E. H., & Torres, M. (2018). "It wasn't feasible for us": Queer women of color navigating family formation. *Family Relations, 67*(1), 118–131. https://doi.org/10.1111/fare.12303

Katon, J. G., Plowden, T. C., & Marsh, E. E. (2023). Racial disparities in uterine fibroids and endometriosis: A systematic review and application of social, structural, and political context. *Fertility and Sterility, 119*(3), 355–363. https://doi.org/10.1016/j.fertnstert.2023.01.022

Kaźmierczak, M., & Karasiewicz, K. (2019). Making space for a new role—Gender differences in identity changes in couples transitioning to parenthood. *Journal of Gender Studies, 28*(3), 271–287. https://doi.org/10.1080/09589236.2018.1441015

Kelley, A. S., Badon, S. E., Lanham, M. S. M., Fisseha, S., & Moravek, M. B. (2019). Body mass index restrictions in fertility treatment: A national survey of OB/GYN subspecialists. *Journal of Assisted Reproduction and Genetics, 36*(6), 1117–1125. https://www.ncbi.nlm.nih.gov/pubmed/30963351 doi: 10.1007/s10815-019-01448-3.

Khandavalli, Y., Rai, S., & Lodha, R. S. (2020). Does increasing the number of inseminations per cycle increase the probability of conception? A randomized trial comparing single versus double intrauterine insemination. *International Journal of Reproduction, Contraception, Obstetrics and Gynecology, 9*(8), 3171–1378. https://doi.org/10.18203/2320-1770.ijrcog20203076

Klipstein, S., Azziz, R., Cameron, K., Collins, L., Coutifaris, C., Crockin, S., Daar, J., Davis, J., Farrell, R., Hammack-Aviran, C., Ginsburg, E., Katz-Jaffe, M., Kawwass, J., Racowsky, C., Rebar, R., Reindollar, R., Ryan, G., Samplaski, M., Schlegel, P., . . . Zweifel, J. (2021). Disparities in access to effective treatment for infertility in the United States: An ethics committee opinion. *Fertility and Sterility, 116*(1), 54–63. https://doi.org/10.1016/j.fertnstert.2021.02.019

Kolanska, K., Uddin, J., Dabi, Y., Mathieu d'Argent, E., Dupont, C., Selleret, L., Touboul, C., Antoine, J. M., Chabbert-Buffet, N., & Daraï, E. (2022). Secondary infertility with a history of vaginal childbirth: Ready to have another one?. *Journal of gynecology obstetrics and human reproduction, 51*(1), 102271. https://doi.org/10.1016/j.jogoh.2021.102271

Komorowski, A. S., & Jain, T. (2022). A review of disparities in access to infertility care and treatment outcomes among hispanic women. *Reproductive Biology and Endocrinology: RB&E, 20*(1), 1. https://www.ncbi.nlm.nih.gov/pubmed/34980166 doi:10.1186/s12958-021-00875-1

Kong, F., Fu, Y., Shi, H., Li, R., Zhao, Y., Wang, Y., & Qiao, J. (2022). Placental abnormalities and placenta-related complications following *in-vitro* fertilization: Based on national hospitalized data in China. *Frontiers in Endocrinology, 13*, 924070. https://doi.org/10.3389/fendo.2022.924070

Kuyoro, O., Brogan, C., & Goldman, R. H. (2022). Weight loss to meet bmi thresholds—Is this requirement worsening racial and ethnic disparities in assisted reproductive technology access? *Fertility and Sterility, 118*(4), e195–e196. https://doi.org/10.1016/j.fertnstert.2022.08.556

Lahimer, M., Capelle, S., Lefranc, E., Bosquet, D., Kazdar, N., Ledu, A., Agina, M., Cabry, R., & BenKhalifa, M. (2025). Micronutrient–antioxidant therapy and male fertility improvement during ART cycles. *Nutrients, 17*(2), 324. https://doi.org/10.3390/nu17020324

Lawson, A. K., McGuire, J. M., Noncent, E., Olivieri, J. F., Jr., Smith, K. N., & Marsh, E. E. (2017). Disparities in counseling female cancer patients for fertility preservation. *Journal of Women's Health (2002), 26*(8), 886–891. https://doi.org/10.1089/jwh.2016.5997

Lazzari, E., Baffour, B., & Chambers, G. M. (2022). Residential proximity to a fertility clinic is independently associated with likelihood of women having ART and IUI treatment. *Human Reproduction (Oxford, England), 37*(11), 2662–2671. https://doi.org/10.1093/humrep/deac205

Lee, J. W., Hyun, M. K., Kim, H. J. & Kim, D. (2021). Acupuncture and herbal medicine for female infertility: An overview of systematic reviews. *Integrative Medicine Research, 10*(3), 100694.

Legal Professional Group: A Professional Group of the American Society for Reproductive Medicine. (2024). *Surrogacy laws by state* [Review of *surrogacy laws by state*]. https://connect.asrm.org/lpg/resources/surrogacy-by-state?ssopc=1

Legro, R. S., Brzyski, R. G., Diamond, M. P., Coutifaris, C., Schlaff, W. D., Casson, P., Christman, G. M., Huang, H., Yan, Q., Alvero, R., Haisenleder, D. J., Barnhart, K. T., Bates, G. W., Usadi, R., Lucidi, S., Baker, V., Trussell, J. D., Krawetz, S. A., Snyder, P., . . . Zhang, H. (2014). Letrozole versus clomiphene for infertility in the polycystic ovary syndrome. *The New England Journal of Medicine, 371*(2), 119–129. https://doi.org/10.1056/NEJMoa1313517

Lei, D., Zhang, X.-Y., & Zheng, P.-S. (2022). Recurrent pregnancy loss: Fewer chromosomal abnormalities in products of conception? A meta-analysis. *Journal of Assisted Reproduction and Genetics, 39*(3), 559–572. https://doi.org/10.1007/s10815-022-02414-2

Li, Y., Yu, S., Huang, C., Lian, R., Chen, C., Liu, S., Li, L., Diao, L., Markert, U. R., & Zeng, Y. (2020). Evaluation of peripheral and uterine immune status of chronic endometritis in patients with recurrent reproductive failure. *Fertility and Sterility, 113*(1), 187–196.e1. https://doi.org/10.1016/j.fertnstert.2019.09.001

Lim, Z. W., Wang, I. D., Wang, P., Chung, C. H., Huang, S. S., Huang, C. C., Tsai, P. Y., Wu, G. J., Wu, K. H., & Chien, W. C. (2021). Obstructive sleep apnea increases risk of female infertility: A 14-year nationwide population-based study. *PloS one, 16*(12), e0260842. https://doi.org/10.1371/journal.pone.0260842

Lindheim, S. R., Glenn, T. L., Smith, M. C., & Gagneux, P. (2018). Ovulation induction for the general gynecologist. *Journal of Obstetrics and Gynaecology of India, 68*(4), 242–252. https://doi.org/10.1007/s13224-018-1130-8

Manafi, E., Belarmino, A. R., Mills, J. N., Eleswarapu, S. V., & Ng, G. Y. (2024). The impact of tucking on fertility among transgender women: A systematic review. *International Journal of Transgender Health*, 1–10. https://doi.org/10.1080/26895269.2024.2387643

Mandia, L., Personeni, C., Antonazzo, P., Angileri, S. A., Pinto, A., & Savasi, V. (2017). Ultrasound in infertility setting: Optimal strategy to evaluate the assessment of tubal patency. *BioMed Research International, 2017*, Article 3205895. https://doi.org/10.1155/2017/3205895

Mao, D., Xu, J., & Sun, L. (2024). Impact of trophectoderm biopsy for preimplantation genetic testing on obstetric and neonatal outcomes: A meta-analysis. *American Journal of Obstetrics and Gynecology, 230*(2), 199–212.e5. https://doi.org/10.1016/j.ajog.2023.08.010

Margiana, R., Odhar, H. A., Prasad, K., Oghenemaro, E. F., Rekha, M. M., Kumawat, R., Uthirapathy, S., Sharma, S., Kumar, M. R., & Nouri, M. (2025). Does outdoor air pollution cause poor semen quality? A systematic review and meta-analysis. *BMC Urology, 25*(1), Article 50. https://doi.org/10.1186/s12894-025-01728-4

Marsh, C., McCracken, M., Gray, M., Nangia, A., Gay, J., & Roby, K. F. (2019). Low total motile sperm in transgender women seeking hormone therapy. *Journal of Assisted Reproduction and Genetics, 36*(8), 1639–1648. https://doi.org/10.1007/s10815-019-01504-y

Martin, A. (2019). "Who do I look like?": Kinning and resemblance in the experience of French donor conceived adults. *Antropologia (Milano), 6*(2), 45–62. https://doi.org/10.14672/ada2019157845-62

Mascarenhas, S., Suff, N., & Shennan, A. (2021). Concurrent reciprocal IVF and risk of pre-eclampsia. *Journal of Obstetrics and Gynaecology: The Journal of the Institute of Obstetrics and Gynaecology, 2021,* 1–2. https://www.ncbi.nlm.nih.gov/pubmed/34907816. https://doi.org/10.1080/01443615.2021.1971177

Mauldin, K., May, M., & Clifford, D. (2022). The consequences of a weight-centric approach to healthcare: A case for a paradigm shift in how clinicians address body weight. *Nutrition in Clinical Practice, 37*(6), 1291–1306. https://doi.org/10.1002/ncp.10885

Merkison, J. M., Chada, A. R., Marsidi, A. M., Spencer, J. B. (2023). Racial and ethnic disparities in assisted reproductive technology: A systematic review. *Fertility and Sterility, 119*(3), 341–347. https://doi.org/10.1016/j.fertnstert.2023.01.023

Mohammed, A., Woad, K. J., Mann, G. E., Craigon, J., Raine-Fenning, N., & Robinson, R. S. (2019). Evaluation of progestogen supplementation for luteal phase support in fresh in vitro fertilization cycles. *Fertility and Sterility, 112*(3), 491–502e3. https://doi.org/10.1016/j.fertnstert.2019.04.021

Mrosk, P., Sandi-Monroy, N., Gagsteiger, F., Friedl, T. W. P., Hancke, K., & Bundschu, K. (2024). Endometrial scratching and intralipid treatment—No general recommendations. *Frontiers in Reproductive Health, 6,* Article 1505842. https://doi.org/10.3389/frph.2024.1505842

Nagpal, T. S., Salas, X. R., Vallis, M., Piccinini-Vallis, H., Alberga, A. S., Bell, R. C., da Silva, D. F., Davenport, M. H., Gaudet, L., Rodriguez, A. C. I., Liu, R. H., Myre, M., Nerenberg, K., Nutter, S., Russell-Mayhew, S., Souza, S. C. S., Vilhan, C., & Adamo, K. B. (2022). Exploring weight bias internalization in pregnancy. *BMC Pregnancy and Childbirth, 22*(1), 605–608. https://doi.org/10.1186/s12884-022-04940-4

National Council for Adoption. (2024). *A second choice but not second best: infertility, pregnancy loss, and adoption approval.* https://adoptioncouncil.org/publications/a-second-choice-but-not-second-best-infertility-pregnancy-loss-and-approval-to-adopt/

Negris, O., Lawson, A., Brown, D., Warren, C., Galic, I., Bozen, A., Swanson, A., & Jain, T. (2021). Emotional stress and reproduction: what do fertility patients believe? *Journal of Assisted Reproduction and Genetics, 38*(4), 877–887. https://doi.org/10.1007/s10815-021-02079-3

Nicoletti, A., Petersen, C. G., Massaro, F. C., Petersen, B., Vagnini, L., Ricci, J., Zamara, C., Oliani, A. H., Oliveira, J. B. A., Dieamant, F., & Franco, J. G. (2022). Female body mass index (BMI) influences pregnancy outcomes: An evaluation of 4349 IVF/ICSI cycles, *Human Reproduction, 37*(Suppl_1), deac105.063. https://doi.org/10.1093/humrep/deac105.063

Nutter, S., Eggerichs, L. A., Nagpal, T. S., Ramos Salas, X., Chin Chea, C., Saiful, S., Ralston, J., Barata-Cavalcanti, O., Batz, C., Baur, L. A., Birney, S., Bryant, S., Buse, K., Cardel, M. I., Chugh, A., Cuevas, A., Farmer, M., Ibrahim, A., Kataria, I., . . . Yusop, S. (2024). Changing the global obesity narrative to recognize and reduce weight stigma: A position statement from the World Obesity Federation. *Obesity Reviews, 25*(1), e13642. https://doi.org/10.1111/obr.13642

Okobi, O. E. (2021). A systemic review on the association between infertility and sexual dysfunction among women utilizing female sexual function index as a measuring tool. *Cureus, 13*(6), e16006. https://www.ncbi.nlm.nih.gov/pubmed/34336497 doi:10.7759/cureus.16006

Olson, S. (2025). *A person-centered approach to prescribing gender-affirming hormones, part one.* Presented at Virtual Clinician Course: Gender-Affirming Hormones, March 3, 2025.

Orouji Jokar, T., Fourman, L. T., Lee, H., Mentzinger, K., & Fazeli, P. K. (2018). Higher TSH levels within the normal range are associated with unexplained infertility. *Journal of Clinical Endocrinology and Metabolism, 103*(2), 632–639. https://www.ncbi.nlm.nih.gov/pubmed/29272395. https://doi.org/10.1210/jc.2017-02120.

Pakpahan, C., Ibrahim, R., William, W., Kandar, P. S., Darmadi, D., Khaerana, A. S. A., & Supardi, S. (2023). "Am I masculine?" A metasynthesis of qualitative studies on traditional masculinity on infertility. *F1000Research, 12,* 252. https://doi.org/10.12688/f1000research.131599.1

Papini, N. M., Nagpal, T. S., Whelan, A. R., Moore Simas, T. A., & Waring, M. E. (2025). Addressing weight stigma in perinatal care: Strategies for health care providers and organizations. *Women's Health Issues, 35*(1), 3–6. https://doi.org/10.1016/j.whi.2024.11.002

Patrizio, P., Albertini, D. F., Gleicher, N., & Caplan, A. (2022). The changing world of IVF: The pros and cons of new business models offering assisted reproductive technologies. *Journal of Assisted Reproduction and Genetics, 39*(2), 305–313. https://doi.org/10.1007/s10815-022-02399-y

Paulson, R. J. (2023). Is preimplantation genetic testing for aneuploidy (PGT-A) getting better? How can we know and how do we counsel our patients? *F&S Reports, 4*(4), 329–330. https://doi.org/10.1016/j.xfre.2023.11.002

Pearl, R. (1933). Factors in human fertility and their statistical evaluation. *The Lancet, 222*(5741), 607–611.

Peate, M., Copp, T., Lensen, S., Hammarberg, K., Simonis, M., Sandhu, S., Lieberman, D., & Vakkas, A. (2025). P-541 The psychosocial and behavioural consequences of anti-müllerian hormone (AMH) testing on women. *Human Reproduction (Oxford), 40*(Supplement_1). https://doi.org/10.1093/humrep/deaf097.847

Penzias, A., Azziz, R., Bendikson, K., Cedars, M. I., Falcone, T., Hansen, K., Hill, M., Jin-dal, S., Kalra, S., Mersereau, J., Reindollar, R., Shannon, C. N., Steiner, A., Tanrikut, C., Taylor, H., & Yauger, B. (2021). Guidance on the limits to the number of embryos to transfer: a committee opinion. *Fertility and Sterility, 116*(3), 651–654. https://doi.org/10.1016/j.fertnstert.2021.06.050

Penzias, A., Azziz, R., Bendikson, K., Falcone, T., Hansen, K., Hill, M., Jindal, S., Kalra, S., Mersereau, J., Reindollar, R., Shannon, C. N., Steiner, A., Tanrikut, C., Taylor, H., & Yauger, B. (2022). Optimizing natural fertility: A committee opinion. *Fertility and Sterility, 117*(1), 53–63. https://doi.org/10.1016/j.fertnstert.2021.10.007

Penzias, A., Bendikson, K., Butts, S., Coutifaris, C., Falcone, T., Fossum, G., Gitlin, S., Gracia, C., Hansen, K., La Barbera, A., Mersereau, J., Odem, R., Paulson, R., Pfeifer, S., Pisarska, M., Rebar, R., Reindollar, R., Rosen, M., Sandlow, J., & Vernon, M. (2017). Role of metformin for ovulation induction in infertile patients with polycystic ovary syndrome (PCOS): A guideline. *Fertility and Sterility, 108*(3), 426–441. https://doi.org/10.1016/j.fertnstert.2017.06.026

Pirtea, P., Ayoubi, J. M., Desmedt, S., & T'Sjoen, G. (2021). Ovarian, breast, and metabolic changes induced by androgen treatment in transgender men. *Fertility and Sterility, 116*(4), 936–942. https://doi.org/10.1016/j.fertnstert.2021.07.1206

Plowden, T. C., Whaley, N., & Christy, A. (2025). Infertility: Disparities and access to services: ACOG Committee Statement No. 14. *Obstetrics and Gynecology (New York. 1953), 145*(1), e51–e57. https://doi.org/10.1097/AOG.0000000000005769

Polyakov, A., & Rozen, G. (2021). Social egg freezing and donation: Waste not, want not. *Journal of Medical Ethics, 47*(12), e73–e73. https://doi.org/10.1136/medethics-2020-106607

Poornima, S., Daram, S., Devaki, R. K., & Qurratulain, H. (2020). Chromosomal abnormalities in couples with primary and secondary infertility: Genetic counseling for assisted reproductive techniques (ART). *Journal of Reproduction & Infertility, 21*(4), 269–274. https://www.ncbi.nlm.nih.gov/pubmed/33209743 doi:10.18502/jri.v21i4.4331

Power To Decide. *One key question.* https://powertodecide.org/one-key-question Updated 2025.

Practice Committee of the American Society for Reproductive Medicine. (2012). Evaluation and treatment of recurrent pregnancy loss: A committee opinion. *Fertility and Sterility, 98*(5), 1103–1111. https://www.asrm.org/globalassets/_asrm/practice-guidance/practice-guidelines/pdf/evaluation_and_treatment_of_recurrent_pregnancy_loss.pdf

Practice Committee of the American Society for Reproductive Medicine. (2013). Use of clomiphene citrate in infertile women: A committee opinion. *Fertility and Sterility, 100*(2), 341–348. https://doi.org/10.1016/j.fertnstert.2013.05.033

Practice Committee of the American Society for Reproductive Medicine. (2020a). Evidence-based treatments for couples with unexplained infertility: A guideline. *Fertility and Sterility, 113*(2), 305–322. https://www.asrm.org/globalassets/_asrm/practice-guidance/practice-guidelines/pdf/evidenece-based_treatments_for_couples_with_unexplained_infertility.pdf

Practice Committee of the American Society for Reproductive Medicine. (2020b). Testing and interpreting measures of ovarian reserve: A committee opinion. *Fertility and Sterility, 114*(6), 1151–1156. https://www.asrm.org/globalassets/_asrm/practice-guidance/practice-guidelines/pdf/testing_and_interpreting_measures_of_ovarian_reserve.pdf

Practice Committee of the American Society for Reproductive Medicine. (2021a). Diagnosis and treatment of luteal phase deficiency: A committee opinion. *Fertility and Sterility, 115*(6), 1416-1423. https://www.fertstert.org/article/S0015-0282(21)00128-X/fulltext

Practice Committee of the American Society for Reproductive Medicine. (2021b). Diagnosis and treatment of infertility in men: AUA/ASRM guideline part I. *Fertility and Sterility. 115(1),* 54–60. https://www.asrm.org/globalassets/_asrm/practice-guidance/practice-guidelines/pdf/diagnosis_and_treatment_of_infertility_in_men-aua-asrm_guideline_part_1.pdf

Practice Committee of the American Society for Reproductive Medicine. (2021c). Fertility evaluation of infertile women: A committee opinion. *Fertility and Sterility, 116*(5), 1255–1263. https://www.asrm.org/globalassets/_asrm/practice-guidance/practice-guidelines/pdf/fertility-evaluation-of-infertile-women-a-committee-opinion.pdf

Practice Committee of the American Society for Reproductive Medicine. (2021d). Role of tubal surgery in the era of assisted reproductive technology: A committee opinion. *Fertility and Sterility, 115*(5), 1143-1150. https://doi.org/10.1016/j.fertnstert.2021.01.051

Practice Committee of the American Society for Reproductive Medicine and the Practice Committee of the Society for Assisted Reproductive Technology. (2021e). Guidance on the limits to the number of embryos to transfer: A committee opinion. *Fertility and Sterility, 116(3),* 651–653. https://www.asrm.org/globalassets/_asrm

/practice-guidance/practice-guidelines/pdf/guidance_on_the_limits_to_the_number_of_embryos_to_transfer.pdf

Practice Committee of the American Society for Reproductive Medicine and the Practice Committee of the Society for Reproductive Endocrinology and Infertility. (2022). Optimizing natural fertility: A committee opinion. *Fertility and Sterility, 117*(1), 53–63. https://www.ncbi.nlm.nih.gov/pubmed/34815068. https://doi.org/10.1016/j.fertnstert.2021.10.007

Practice Committee of the American Society for Reproductive Endocrinology and Infertility, Quality Assurance Committee of the Society for Assisted Reproductive Technologies, and the Practice Committee of the American Society for Reproductive Medicine. (2022). Multiple gestation associated with infertility therapy: A committee opinion. *Fertility & Sterility, 117*(3), 498–511. https://doi.org/10.1016/j.fertnstert.2021.12.016

Practice Committee of the American Society for Reproductive Medicine. (2023). *Definition of infertility: A committee opinion*. American Society for Reproductive Medicine. https://www.asrm.org/globalassets/_asrm/practice-guidance/practice-guidelines/pdf/definition-of-infertility.pdf

Practice Committee of the American Society for Reproductive Medicine. (2024a). Tobacco or marijuana use and infertility: A committee opinion. *Fertility & Sterility, 121*(4), 589–602. https://doi.org/10.1016/j.fertnstert.2024.05.156

Practice Committee of the American Society of Reproductive Medicine. (2024b). Fertility drugs and cancer: A guideline. *Fertility and Sterility, 122*(3), 406–419. https://www.asrm.org/globalassets/_asrm/practice-guidance/practice-guidelines/pdf/fertility_drugs_and_cancer_2024.pdf

Practice Committee of the American Society for Reproductive Medicine. (2024c). Subclinical hypothyroidism in the infertile female population: A guideline. *Fertility and Sterility, 121*(5), 765–781. https://www.asrm.org/globalassets/_asrm/practice-guidance/practice-guidelines/pdf/subclinical_hypothyroidism_in_the_infertile_female_population.pdf

Practice Committee of the American Society for Reproductive Medicine. (2024e). Prevention of moderate and severe ovarian hyperstimulation syndrome: A guideline. *Fertility and Sterility, 121*(2), 230–244. https://www.asrm.org/globalassets/_asrm/practice-guidance/practice-guidelines/pdf/prevention-of-moderate-and-severe-ovarian-hyperstimulation-syndrome.pdf

Practice Committees of the American Society for Reproductive Medicine and the Society for Assisted Reproductive Technology. (2020). Intracytoplasmic sperm injection (ICSI) for non-male factor indications: A committee opinion. *Fertility and Sterility, 114*(2), 239–245. https://www.ncbi.nlm.nih.gov/pubmed/32654822 doi:10.1016/j.fertnstert.2020.05.032

Practice Committee of the American Society for Reproductive Medicine in Collaboration with the Society for Male Reproduction and Urology. (2023). Diagnostic evaluation of sexual dysfunction in the male partner in the setting of infertility: A committee opinion. *Fertility & Sterility, 120*(5), 967–971. https://www.asrm.org/globalassets/_asrm/practice-guidance/practice-guidelines/pdf/diagnostic_evaluation_of_sexual_dysfunction_in_the_male_partner.pdf

Punjani, N., Wald, G., Al-Hussein Alwamlh, O., Feliciano, M., Dudley, V., & Goldstein, M. (2021). Optimal timing for repeat semen analysis during male infertility evaluation. *F&S Reports, 2*(2), 172–175. https://doi.org/10.1016/j.xfre.2021.04.010

Quan, K., Yu, C., Wen, X., Lin, Q., Wang, N., & Ma, H. (2022). Acupuncture as treatment for female infertility: A systematic review and meta-analysis of randomized controlled trials. *Evidence-Based Complementary and Alternative Medicine, 2022*(1), 3595033.

Rangi, S. K., Rehmer, J., & Ferrando, C. A. (2024). Prevalence of polycystic ovarian syndrome in young and adolescent transmasculine patients presenting for gender-affirming care. *Journal of Pediatric & Adolescent Gynecology, 37*(1), 51–55. https://doi.org/10.1016/j.jpag.2023.09.003

Wang, R., Li, W., Bordewijk, E. M., Legro, R. S., Zhang, H., Wu, X., Gao, J., Morin-Papunen, L., Homburg, R., König, T. E., Moll, E., Kar, S., Huang, W., Johnson, N. P., Amer, S. A., Vegetti, W., Palomba, S., Falbo, A., Özmen, Ü., Nazik, H., ... International Ovulation Induction IPDMA Collaboration (2019). First-line ovulation induction for polycystic ovary syndrome: an individual participant data meta-analysis. *Human reproduction update, 25*(6), 717–732. https://doi.org/10.1093/humupd/dmz029

RESOLVE: The National Infertility Association. (2025a). *Coping with infertility tips*. https://resolve.org/get-help/helpful-advice/managing-infertility-stress/coping-techniques/

RESOLVE: The National Infertility Association. (2025b). *Insurance coverage by state* [Review of *insurance coverage by state*]. RESOLVE. https://resolve.org/learn/financial-resources/insurance-coverage/insurance-coverage-by-state/

Rooney, K. L., & Domar, A. D. (2018). The relationship between stress and infertility. *Dialogues in Clinical Neuroscience, 20*(1), 41–47.

Ross, L. J., & Solinger, R. (2017). *Reproductive justice*. University of California Press.

Şahan, Ö., Atilla, R., Höbek Akarsu, R., & Karakaş, S. (2025). Use of complementary and alternative medicine in infertility. *Alternative Therapies in Health and Medicine, 31*(3), 10–14.

Saleh, F. L., Adashi, E. Y., Sable, D. B., Kushnir, V. A., & Taylor, H. S. (2023). Changes to reproductive endocrinology and infertility practice, research, and training as investor mergers increase. *F&S Reports (Online), 4*(4), 332–336. https://doi.org/10.1016/j.xfre.2023.08.001

Sanders, K. D., Silvestri, G., Gordon, T., & Griffin, D. K. (2021). Analysis of IVF live birth outcomes with and without preimplantation genetic testing for aneuploidy (PGT-A): UK human fertilisation and embryology authority data collection 2016–2018. *Journal of Assisted Reproduction and Genetics, 38*(12), 3277–3285. https://www.ncbi.nlm.nih.gov/pubmed/34766235 doi:10.1007/s10815-021-02349-0

Sater, A. C., Miyague, A. H., Schuffner, A., Nisihara, R., & Teixeira, D. M. (2022). Impact of assisted reproduction treatment on sexual function of patients diagnosed with infertility. *Archives of Gynecology and Obstetrics, 305*(6), 1595–1604. https://www.ncbi.nlm.nih.gov/pubmed/35066622 . https://doi.org/10.1007/s00404-021-06367-2

Schlegel, P. N., Sigman, M., Collura, B., De Jonge, C. J., Eisenberg, M. L., Lamb, D. J., Mulhall, J. P., Niederberger, C., Sandlow, J. I., Sokol, R. Z., Spandorfer, S. D., Tanrikut, C., Treadwell, J. R., Oristaglio, J. T., & Zini, A. (2021). Diagnosis and treatment of infertility in men: AUA/ASRM guideline part I. *Fertility and sterility, 115*(1), 54–61. https://doi.org/10.1016/j.fertnstert.2020.11.015

Seattle Sperm Bank. *Prices*. https://www.seattlespermbank.com/services/prices/

Segal, T. R., & Giudice, L. C. (2019). Before the beginning: Environmental exposures and reproductive and obstetrical outcomes. *Fertility and Sterility, 112*(4), 613–621. https://www.ncbi.nlm.nih.gov/pubmed/31561863. https://doi.org/10.1016/j.fertnstert.2019.08.001

Shang, Y., Song, N., He, R., & Wu, M. (2024). Antioxidants and fertility in women with ovarian aging: A systematic review and meta-analysis. *Advances in Nutrition (Bethesda, Md.), 15*(8), Article 100273. https://doi.org/10.1016/j.advnut.2024.100273

Sharifi, F., Jamali, J., & Latifnejad Roudsari, R. (2024). The prevalence of complementary and alternative medicine use among infertile patients: A global systematic review and meta-analysis. *International Journal of Fertility & Sterility, 18*(4), 314–322. https://doi.org/10.22074/ijfs.2024.2005352.1482

Sharma, A., & Shrivastava, D. (2022). Psychological problems related to infertility. *Cureus, 14*(10), e30320. https://doi.org/10.7759/cureus.30320

Shreffler, K. M., Greil, A. L., & McQuillan, J. (2017). Responding to infertility: Lessons from a growing body of research and suggested guidelines for practice. *Family Relations, 66*(4), 644–658. https://doi.org/10.1111/fare.12281

Simionescu, G., Doroftei, B., Maftei, R., Obreja, B. E., Anton, E., Grab, D., Ilea, C., & Anton, C. (2021). The complex relationship between infertility and psychological distress (Review). *Experimental and Therapeutic Medicine, 21*(4), 306. https://doi.org/10.3892/etm.2021.9737

Skakkebaek, N. E., Jørgensen, N., Andersson, A.-M., Juul, A., Main, K. M., Jensen, T. K., & Toppari, J. (2019). Populations, decreasing fertility, and reproductive health. *The Lancet (British Edition), 393*(10180), 1500–1501. https://doi.org/10.1016/S0140-6736(19)30690-7

Swain, M., Miller, M., Cannella, C., & Daviskiba, S. (2023). Disparities in fertility preservation among patients diagnosed with female breast cancer. *Journal of Assisted Reproduction and Genetics, 40*(12), 2843–2849. https://doi.org/10.1007/s10815-023-02968-9

Swift, A., Berry, M., Fernandez-Pineda, M., & Haberstroh, A. (2024). An integrative review of adverse childhood experiences and reproductive traumas of infertility and pregnancy loss. *Journal of Midwifery & Women's Health, 69*(2), 258–278. https://doi.org/10.1111/jmwh.13585

Talbot, C., Hodson, N., Rose, J., & Bewley, S. (2024). Comparing the psychological outcomes of donor and non-donor conceived people: A systematic review. *BJOG: An International Journal of Obstetrics and Gynaecology, 131*(13), 1747–1759. https://doi.org/10.1111/1471-0528.17892

Talebi, F., & Mirzaian, B. (2023). The effect of cognitive-behavioral therapy on the infertility stress and marital burnout in infertile women. *Journal of Mazandaran University of Medical Sciences, 33*(226), 100–108. https://doaj.org/article/293e7d5f27bf4af79e7505900ae9187a

Tam, M. W. (2021). Queering reproductive access: Reproductive justice in assisted reproductive technologies. *Reproductive Health, 18*(1), 164. https://www.ncbi.nlm.nih.gov/pubmed/34340704. https://doi.org/10.1186/s12978-021-01214-8

Tam, M. W., Perez-Brumer, A., & Ross, L. E. (2025). Queer tax: Examining 2SLGBTQ+ Black, Indigenous, and People of Colour's experiences of accessing assisted reproductive technologies. *Social Science & Medicine (1982), 376*, Article 118053. https://doi.org/10.1016/j.socscimed.2025.118053

Tang, D., Cheng, Y., Feng, X., Li, X., & Coyte, P. C. (2023). The use of IVF/ICSI and risk of postpartum hemorrhage: A retrospective cohort study of 153,765 women in China. *Frontiers in Public Health, 11*, 1016457. https://doi.org/10.3389/fpubh.2023.1016457

Taylor, H. S., Pal, L., & Seli, E. (2020). *Speroff's clinical gynecologic endocrinology and infertility* (9th ed.). Wolters Kluwer.

Teede, H. J., Tay, C. T., Laven, J. J. E., Dokras, A., Moran, L. J., Piltonen, T. T., Costello, M. F., Boivin, J., Redman, L. M., Boyle, J. A., Norman, R. J., Mousa, A., & Joham, A. E. (2023). Recommendations from the 2023 International Evidence-Based Guideline for the Assessment and Management of Polycystic Ovary Syndrome. *The Journal of Clinical Endocrinology and Metabolism, 108(10)*, 2447–2469. https://doi.org/10.1210/clinem/dgad463

Tehrani, F. R., Firouzi, F., & Behboudi-Gandevani, S. (2022). Investigating the clinical utility of the anti-mullerian hormone testing for the prediction of age at menopause and assessment of functional ovarian reserve: A practical approach and recent updates. *Aging and Disease, 13*(2), 458–467. https://doi.org/10.14336/AD.2021.0825

United Nations Department of Economic and Social Affairs. (2025). *World fertility report.* https://www.developmentaid.org/api/frontend/cms/file/2025/08/undesa_pd_2025_wfr_2024_final.pdf

U.S. Donor Conceived Council. (2023). *2022 sperm bank data survey* [Review of *2022 sperm bank data survey*]. https://www.usdcc.org/wp-content/uploads/2023/04/Sperm-Bank-Survey_2022.pdf

van Hoogenhuijze, N. E., Mol, F., Laven, J. S. E., Groenewoud, E. R., Traas, M. A. F., Janssen, C. A. H., Teklenburg, G., de Bruin, J. P., van Oppenraaij, R. H. F., Maas, J. W. M., Moll, E., Fleischer, K., van Hooff, M. H. A., de Koning, C. H., Cantineau, A. E. P., Lambalk, C. B., Verberg, M., van Heusden, A. M., Manger, A. P., . . . Broekmans, F. J. M. (2021). Endometrial scratching in women with one failed IVF/ICSI cycle—outcomes of a randomised controlled trial (SCRaTCH). *Human Reproduction (Oxford), 36*(1), 87–98. https://doi.org/10.1093/humrep/deaa268

Van Voorhis, B. J., Mejia, R. B., Schlaff, W. D., & Hurst, B. S. (2019). Is removal of hydrosalpinges prior to in vitro fertilization the standard of care? *Fertility and Sterility, 111*(4), 652–656. https://doi.org/10.1016/j.fertnstert.2019.02.015

Villani, M. T., Morini, D., Spaggiari, G., Simoni, M., Aguzzoli, L., & Santi, D. (2021). Spontaneous pregnancies among infertile couples during assisted reproduction lockdown for COVID-19 pandemic. *Andrology (Oxford), 9*(4), 1038–1041. https://doi.org/10.1111/andr.12973

Vitagliano, A., Andrisani, A., Alviggi, C., Vitale, S. G., Sapia, F., Favilli, A., Martins, W. P., Raine-Ferring, N., Polanski, L., & Ambrosini, G. (2019). Endometrial scratching for infertile women undergoing a first embryo transfer: A systematic review and meta-analysis of published and unpublished data from randomized controlled trials. *Fertility and Sterility, 111*(4), 734–746.e2. https://doi.org/10.1016/j.fertnstert.2018.12.008

Voigt, P., Persily, J., Blakemore, J. K., Licciardi, F., Thakker, S., & Najari, B. (2022). Sociodemographic differences in utilization of fertility services among reproductive age women diagnosed with cancer in the USA. *Journal of Assisted Reproduction and Genetics, 39*(4), 963–972. https://doi.org/10.1007/s10815-022-02455-7

Walker, Z., Lanes, A., & Ginsburg, E. (2022). Oocyte cryopreservation review: Outcomes of medical oocyte cryopreservation and planned oocyte cryopreservation. *Reproductive Biology and Endocrinology: RB&E, 20*(1), 10. https://doi.org/10.1186/s12958-021-00884-0

Wang, R., Li, W., Bordewijk, E. M., Legro, R. S., Zhang, H., Wu, X., Gao, J., Morin-Papunen, L., Homburg, R., König, T. E., Moll, E., Kar, S., Huang, W., Johnson, N. P., Amer, S. A., Vegetti, W., Palomba, S., Falbo, A., Özmen, Ü., Nazik, H., . . . International Ovulation Induction IPDMA Collaboration (2019). First-line ovulation induction for polycystic ovary syndrome: an individual participant data meta-analysis. *Human Reproduction Update, 25*(6), 717–732. https://doi.org/10.1093/humupd/dmz029

Wang, Y., Tang, Z., Wang, C., Teng, X., & He, J. (2024). Whether hysteroscopy improves fertility outcomes in infertile women: A meta-analysis and systematic review. *Frontiers in Endocrinology, 15,* 1489783. https://doi.org/10.3389/fendo.2024.1489783

Ward, P., & McPhail, D. (2019). Fat shame and blame in reproductive care: Implications for ethical health care interactions. *Women's Reproductive Health, 6*(4), 225–241. https://doi.org/10.1080/23293691.2019.1653581

Weiss, M. S., & Marsh, E. E. (2023). Navigating unequal paths: Racial disparities in the infertility journey. *Obstetrics & Gynecology 142*(4), 940–947. https://doi.org/10.1097/AOG.0000000000005354

Weiss, R. (2020). Does preimplantation genetic testing increase the risk of adverse clinical outcomes? *The Science Journal of the Lander College of Arts and Sciences, 14*(1), 5–13. Retrieved from https://touroscholar.touro.edu/sjlcas/vol14/iss1/1

Weitz, Y. S., & Karlsson, M. (2021). Professional or authentic motherhood? Negotiations on the identity of the birth mother in the context of foster care. *Qualitative Social Work, 20*(3), 703–717. https://doi.org/10.1177/1473325020912815

Woods, B. M., Patrician, P. A., Fazeli, P. L., & Ladores, S. (2022). Infertility-related stress: A concept analysis. *Nursing Forum (Hillsdale), 57*(3), 437–445. https://doi.org/10.1111/nuf.12683

World Health Organization. (2021). *WHO laboratory manual for the examination and processing of human semen* (6th ed.). https://www.who.int/publications/i/item/9789240030787

World Health Organization. (2024). *Infertility.* https://www.who.int/news-room/fact-sheets/detail/infertility

Wu, W., La, J., Schubach, K. M., Lantsberg, D., & Katz, D. J. (2023). Psychological, social, and sexual challenges affecting men receiving male infertility treatment: A systematic review and implications for clinical care. *Asian Journal of Andrology, 25*(4), 448–453. https://doi.org/10.4103/aja202282

Wulczyn, F. (2004). Family reunification. *The Future of Children, 14*(1), 95–113. https://doi.org/10.2307/1602756

Yang, H., DeWan, A. T., Desai, M. M. ,et al. (2022). Preimplantation genetic testing for aneuploidy: Challenges in clinical practice. *Human Genomics, 16,* 69. https://doi.org/10.1186/s40246-022-00442-8

Yang, A. M., Cui, N., Sun, Y. F., & Hao, G. M. (2021). Letrozole for female infertility. *Frontiers in endocrinology, 12,* 676133. https://doi.org/10.3389/fendo.2021.676133

Zweifel, J. E., & Woodward, J. T. (2022). The risky business of advanced paternal age: Neurodevelopmental and psychosocial implications for children of older fathers. *Fertility and Sterility, 118*(6), 1013–1021. https://doi.org/10.1016/j.fertnstert.2022.10.029

APPENDIX 20-A

Patient Infertility Support and Resources

Organization	Description
AllPaths Family Building	Regional New England–based organization committed to providing support, education and advocacy to anyone facing complex family building challenges. Various free, virtual, peer-led support groups for a variety of demographics, including people experiencing pregnancy loss, pursuing IVF, military families, conceiving with donor genetics, LGBTQ+ individuals, and others. https://allpathsfb.org
American Society for Reproductive Medicine (ASRM), Mental Health Professional Group	A subsect group of mental health professionals who are involved with ASRM, whose mission is to address the mental health issues of patients experiencing infertility; to expand scientific and clinical knowledge of the field; and to educate and establish guidelines for mental health professionals practicing in assisted reproductive technology. Virtual and State-Specific Patient Support Groups: https://connect.asrm.org/mhpg/bookshelf/new-page2?ssopc=1
Baby Quest Foundation	National organization offering community support and financial assistance through fertility grants to those who cannot afford the high costs of procedures such as IVF (in vitro fertilization), gestational surrogacy, egg and sperm donation, egg freezing, and embryo donation. https://babyquestfoundation.org/
The Cade Foundation	National organization which provides information, support, and financial assistance to help needy infertile families overcome infertility. https://cadefoundation.org/
Donor Sibling Registry	National organization which assists individuals conceived as a result of sperm, egg, or embryo donation who are seeking to make mutually desired contact with others with whom they share genetic ties (available resources for donor siblings, donor offspring, parents of half-siblings, and biological parents). The DSR advocates for the right to honesty and transparency for donor-conceived people, promotes social acceptance and legal rights, and values the diversity of all families. https://donorsiblingregistry.com/
Expect Miracles Foundation	Expect Miracles Foundation's Surviving and Moving Forward (SAMFund) grants serve as a financial bridge to help young adult cancer survivors regain their financial footing toward their family building goals through family building grants twice a year. https://expectmiraclesfoundation.org/
Fat Positive Fertility	Online educational and support platform offering workshops, support groups, and resources for both patients and healthcare professionals. Run by fertility coach Nicola Salmon, author of *Fat and Fertile.* https://nicolasalmon.co.uk/
Fertility for Colored Girls	National organization which provides education, awareness, support and encouragement to African American women/couples and other women of color experiencing infertility https://www.fertilityforcoloredgirls.org/
Footsteps for Fertility Foundation	National organization created to raise awareness surrounding infertility, and provide grants for those who require fertility treatments such as IVF and IUI. https://footstepsforfertility.org/
InterNational Council on Infertility Information Dissemination (INCIID)	Largest infertility information and support organization in the United States which helps individuals and couples explore their family building options, provides education on the diagnosis, treatment, and prevention of infertility and pregnancy loss, and offers guidance to those considering adoption or child-free lifestyles. https://www.inciid.org/

Organization	Description
Jewish Fertility Foundation	National organization whose CEO and founder utilized IVF to conceive and provides financial assistance, educational awareness, and emotional support to Jewish families who have medical fertility challenges. https://jewishfertilityfoundation.org/
Journey to Parenthood	National organization which aims to help couples and individuals dealing with infertility achieve their dreams of becoming parents by providing financial and emotional support along their journey, as well as providing education and resources. https://journeytoparenthooddotorg.wpcomstaging.com/
LiveStrong Fertility	A subsect program of the LiveStrong Foundation which was created for those whose cancer diagnosis may affect their ability to create or add to their families; prospective patients must apply to determine eligibility. https://livestrong.org/how-we-help/livestrong-fertility/
Nest Egg Foundation	Organization which collaborates with medical and financial professionals, attorneys, and others who care about building families and aims to give an opportunity to those struggling with infertility via education and access to treatment. https://www.nesteggfoundation.org/
Operation Baby	National organization which provides education, advocacy, and financial assistance programs for active-duty and veteran couples diagnosed with medical infertility to help them achieve their dream of becoming parents through grants to offset costs associated with fertility treatments, surrogacy, and adoption. https://www.operationbaby.org/
Postpartum Support International, Fertility Challenges Support Group	This group is intended for those who have been actively trying to conceive for 6 months or longer or for any birthing person who needs medical intervention to achieve a successful pregnancy. It is led by PSI-trained facilitators (each with lived experience with primary and/or secondary fertility challenges). Struggling with fertility issues can be a lonely experience and this group helps provide an avenue for healing and hope. This group helps women and birthing people (gestational carriers) find support as they navigate the pain of fertility challenges. https://postpartum.net/group/fertility-challenges/
Rainbow Families	Washington, DC–based organization (with virtual events available nationally and internationally) which supports, educates, and connects LGBTQ+ families, parents, and prospective parents by offering a wide variety of education programs, support groups, opportunities to connect and more. https://rainbowfamilies.org/
Recurrent Pregnancy Loss Association	National organization created to support RPL patients and advance research towards understanding and eliminating recurrent pregnancy loss. https://rplassociation.org/
Return to Zero Hope	National online community of bereaved parents, families, and providers offering inclusive resources and holistic support for anyone whose life has been touched by loss, including infertility, secondary infertility, miscarriage, ending a wanted pregnancy, stillbirth, infant or toddler death, loss through surrogacy, or failed adoption. https://rtzhope.org/
RESOLVE: The National Infertility Association	National organization providing free support groups (including virtual and peer-led groups) for those experiencing fertility challenges, patient education, and advocacy. https://resolve.org/
Roaring Adventures	National organization which seeks to help first responders and active military personnel build and grow their families when facing infertility through education, support, and grants that help cover the expenses associated with adoption, medical treatment, gestational surrogacy, and other family building methods. https://www.roaringadventures.org/
Single Mothers by Choice	International organization for unpartnered individuals who purposefully decide to become mothers with the intention to parent by themselves. Local chapters and online community provide social support, resources, and discussion forums. https://www.singlemothersbychoice.org/

Organization	Description
Starfish Infertility Foundation	National organization committed to providing financial support for those struggling with infertility in the United States. https://www.starfishinfertilityfoundation.org
The Broken Brown Egg	Organization which provides resources and support for three major targets: Reproductive Justice and Health Equity, The Reproductive Health Careers Pipeline, Empowerment & Community. https://thebrokenbrownegg.org/
Worth the Wait	National organization whose mission is to empower young adult cancer survivors on their path to parenthood by providing financial support and educational resources for fertility treatments, adoption, and surrogacy while advocating for oncofertility within the healthcare system and beyond. https://worththewaitcharity.com/

CHAPTER 21

Gynecologic Infections

Kelly McBroom

The editors acknowledge Sharon M. Bond, who wrote the previous edition of this chapter.

Vulvovaginal health is a critical component for an individual's overall health, sexuality, self-perception, fertility, self-confidence, and ability to express intimacy. Vulvovaginal symptoms are among the most frequent reason patients seek care from a clinician. Recurrent urogenital infections have been found to have profound psychosocial impacts, with decreased scores on all aspects of quality of life for affected individuals (Thomas-White et al., 2023). Individuals perceive vulvovaginal symptoms, such as discharge, odor, pain, and itching, in unique ways. One person may be extremely uncomfortable with these symptoms, another may feel only minor distress, a third may be very anxious, and a fourth may be mildly concerned. Reactions depend on many factors, including their previous experiences or knowledge; concurrent or chronic medical conditions; societal, religious, and cultural beliefs; and the number and severity of symptoms (Murina, 2021; Thomas-White et al., 2023).

This chapter begins with an overview of promoting and maintaining vaginal health, the vaginal microbiome, vaginitis, vaginosis, and vulvovaginitis. The remaining sections address bacterial vaginosis (BV), vulvovaginal candidiasis (VVC), desquamative inflammatory vaginitis, atrophic vaginitis and genitourinary syndrome of menopause (GSM), toxic shock syndrome (TSS), greater vestibular gland duct cysts and abscesses (formerly known as the Bartolin gland), and infections related to genital piercing. Atrophic vaginitis and genital piercing are included in this chapter because they can be associated with an increased risk of genital infection. In addition, atrophic vaginitis can mimic the symptoms of some gynecologic infections and should be considered in the differential diagnosis of women with vulvovaginal symptoms. It is important to note that not all individuals with vulvovaginal symptoms identify as female or women. Gender-inclusive language is used throughout this chapter when possible, with the goal to include individuals across the gender spectrum and to recognize that clinicians whose scope of practice focuses on individuals assigned female at birth (AFAB) provide care not only for people who identify as women or female, but also for people who are transgender, gender expansive, and nonbinary.

PROMOTING AND MAINTAINING VAGINAL HEALTH

The vaginal environment is dynamic, unique, complex, and yet to be fully understood. Clinicians can help patients learn to protect the health of the vulva and vaginal environment by teaching them to adopt healthy personal behaviors, perform protective self-care activities, and recognize symptoms of vaginitis. The practices in **Table 21-1** can be helpful in maintaining vaginal health. Although not all the recommendations have been proven to prevent vulvovaginal infections in studies, they have been clinically observed as possibly helpful and are recommended by experts. Chapter 27 also discusses vulvar skin care.

Menstrual bleeding is a common human experience. Menstruators use an average of 10,000 menstrual products during their reproductive lives, including sanitary pads, tampons, pantiliners, wipes, douching solutions, and deodorant sprays and powders. These products have the potential to expose the user to endocrine disrupting chemicals (EDCs) through absorption by the vulvar and vaginal epithelium (Marroquin et al., 2024; Upson, 2022). Due to the high absorption efficiency, and permeability of the vaginal mucosa, this represents a significant exposure pathway. Despite known reproductive risks of EDC exposure including precocious puberty, endometriosis, female genital tumors and ovulation disorders, this issue has historically received little attention (Gao & Kannan, 2020).

Consumers and environmentalists have largely driven the recent research into chemical exposure in menstrual products, and this has been characterized in different countries across product types. A recent review of two dozen studies investigating chemical content in menstrual products demonstrated the widespread presence of EDCs including phthalates, dioxin, and volatile organic compounds (VOCs) (Kim, 2019). Three of these studies measured human biomarkers in whole blood concentrations of these chemicals in users, finding that the use of feminine powder increased ethylbenzene by 36 percent, and vaginal douching increased levels of 1.4 dichlorobenzene by 81 percent compared to non-users (Upson, 2022). In addition to EDCs, Singh et al. (2019) reported that tampon use over two menstrual cycles was associated with a 25 percent increase in mercury concentration due to bioaccumulation of toxic metals in the cotton plants that are a key constituent of tampons. Finally, Singh et al.'s BioCycle study suggests associations between tampon use and oxidative stress biomarkers (Singh et al., 2019).

In the single study examining products specifically from the United States, 24 EDCs were isolated in seven categories of feminine hygiene products collected in New York State (Gao & Kannan, 2020). While exposure to EDC and VOCs through menstrual products is clear, clinical implications are difficult to prove

TABLE 21-1 Promoting Vaginal Health

Area	Recommendations
Nutrition	• Eat a healthy diet that includes adequate servings of vegetables, fruits, and grains daily. • Limit intake of refined sugars, including soft drinks, fruit juices, and alcohol. • Eat unsweetened yogurt containing live, active cultures to add protective bacteria that may help control yeast. • Consider probiotic supplements or fermented foods to help balance the vaginal microenvironment.
General health	• Get adequate rest, with 7 to 8 hours of sleep per night. • Reduce and manage life stressors.
Hygiene	• Avoid douching, which can disturb the normal protective vaginal flora. • Avoid feminine sprays and hygiene products, scented soaps, bubble baths, and wet wipes. • Avoid unnecessary use of OTC (over-the-counter) vaginal creams, suppositories, and other treatments for vaginal symptoms, which are best evaluated by a healthcare provider. • Change pads, tampons, and menstrual cups frequently, using tampons and menstrual cups only during the menstrual cycle. • Avoid daily use of panty liners, which can prevent air flow to the vulva, trap moisture, and irritate vulvar skin. • Avoid vulvar shaving, waxing, and use of depilatories, which strip the vulva of protective hair, expose the skin to bacteria, and may lead to severe inflammatory reactions; unwanted vulvar hair can be clipped with scissors or a trimmer rather than shaved or waxed. • Clean diaphragms, cervical caps, and spermicide applicators after use. • Wipe front to back after urinating or defecating to avoid introducing anorectal bacteria to the vaginal and urethral area.
Sexual Expression	• Choose sex toys made of non-porous material which are easier to clean and disinfect. • Barrier use over sexual devices can reduce but not eliminate transmission of common viral and bacterial infections. • Avoid vaginal penetration following unprotected anal sex.
Clothing	• Wear cotton or silk undergarments, which are less likely to retain moisture than clothing made from synthetic fabrics. • Avoid extended use of tight-fitting or wet clothing near the genital area, such as bathing suits, jeans, yoga pants, and pantyhose; these items may increase the temperature near the vulva and encourage yeast growth.

Data from Holdcroft, A. M., Ireland, D. J., & Payne, M. S. (2023). The vaginal microbiome in health and disease—what role do common intimate hygiene practices play? *Microorganisms, 11*(2), 298. https://doi.org/10.3390/microorganisms11020298;

Marroquin, J., Kiomourtzoglou, M. A., Scranton, A., & Pollack, A. Z. (2024). Chemicals in menstrual products: A systematic review. *BJOG : An International Journal of Obstetrics and Gynaecology, 131*(5), 655–664. https://doi.org/10.1111/1471-0528.1766;

Mei, Z., & Li, D. (2022). The role of probiotics in vaginal health. *Frontiers in Cellular and Infection Microbiology, 12,* 963868. https://doi.org/10.3389/fcimb.2022.963868;

Rubin, E., Deshpande, N., Vasquez, P., & Kellogg Spadt, S. (2019). A clinical reference guide on sexual devices for obstetrician-gynecologists. *Obstetrics & Gynecology, 133*(6), 1259–1268. https://doi.org/10.1097/AOG.0000000000003262.

due to multiple confounders. More research is needed to describe transdermal and mucosal absorption rates, long-term biological and health risks to EDC exposure, dose dependent relationships, and descriptions of concurrent use of products for heavy menstruators (Gao & Kannan, 2020). While menstrual cups and underwear are increasing in market share, exposure has not been studied for these products.

THE VAGINAL MICROBIOME

The vaginal microbiome refers to a collection of microbial organisms that inhabit the human vagina, protect it, organize its environment, and respond to changes in hormonal levels, the menstrual cycle, pathogenic substances, medications, sexual activity, foreign bodies, contraceptive use, stress, and phase of life cycle. The vaginal microbiome, sometimes referred to as the vaginal ecosystem, plays a profound yet underappreciated role in the health of individuals, and together with the vaginal epithelium forms the primary defense against infection (Deka et al., 2021). The vagina is a lifelong passageway for menses, sperm, newborns, and an assortment of variable and unique secretions (Graziottin, 2024).

During reproductive years, vaginal secretions are normal and occur regularly. The numerous variations in the amount and characteristics of vaginal secretions are determined by physiology, timing in relation to the menstrual cycle, use of local or systemic medications, sexual practices, and pathology. Individuals who have adequate endogenous or exogenous estrogen will have vaginal secretions. The major source of these secretions is the cervical mucosa, although small amounts are also secreted by the Bartholin, sebaceous, sweat, and apocrine glands of the vulva. Unique combinations of organisms in the vagina are considered protective because they provide an initial line of defense against infection through production of lactic acid and hydrogen peroxide by *Lactobacillus* species.

Lactobacillus species are the dominant organisms in the vagina; they maintain the vaginal pH between 3.5 and 4.5. The presence of vaginal estrogen that accompanies the onset of puberty supports the growth of glycogen, which, in turn, nourishes growth of multiple *Lactobacillus* species. *Lactobacillus* metabolize glycogen to produce lactic acid, reducing the pH of the vaginal lumen, inhibiting growth of pathogenic organisms, and preventing colonization through the production of of bacteriocins and biosurfactants (Krakowsky et al., 2022). Some species of *Lactobacillus* also produce hydrogen peroxide, which in older studies was shown to exert antibacterial action against potentially harmful organisms. However, newer research is examining whether hydrogen peroxide has antimicrobial action or instead may merely represent the presence of a biomarker for *Lactobacillus* species (Tachedjian et al., 2018). It is primarily through the production of lactic acid and possibly hydrogen peroxide that *Lactobacillus* species exert their protective effects by inhibiting or directly eliminating pathogens. Conversely, the absence or depletion of *Lactobacillus* species is associated with impaired epithelial maturation, mucosal inflammation, decreased epithelial barrier function, and increased vulnerability to sexually transmitted infections (STIs) including HIV, infertility, and chronic vaginal conditions (Krakowsky et al., 2022). A vaginal environment lacking adequate *Lactobacillus* species has increased vaginal pH and facilitates growth of anaerobic organisms, such as *Gardnerella*, *Mobiluncus*, *Streptococcus*, *Ureaplasma*, *Corynebacterium*, *Escherichia coli*, and other opportunistic pathogens. Low prevalence of lactobacilli and subsequent dominance of anaerobic organisms may also be associated with an increased cervical cancer risk in patients infected with HPV (Rosario et al, 2023; Huang et al., 2024; Wu et al., 2021). However, some people with minimal lactobacilli populations appear to be healthy and do not report vaginal symptoms. Approximately 25 percent of individuals maintain a healthy vagina without lactobacilli either due to the presence of other, less familiar lactic-acid-producing organisms, such as *Megasphaera*, *Leptotrichia*, and *Staphylococcus* (Younes et al., 2018), or non-lactobacillary microbiota whose prevalence is based on the person's ethnicity (Buchta, 2018). Reasons for differences in the types of bacteria inhabiting the vagina are affected by a multitude of dynamic factors over a lifetime, and drivers that contribute to changes in the microbial community over time remain poorly understood (Gliniewicz et al., 2019).

Vaginal secretions provide physiologic lubrication and represent a response to the hormonal milieu. These secretions vary throughout the menstrual cycle and increase in amount around ovulation, during the premenstrual period, during pregnancy, and when sexual arousal occurs. Normal vaginal secretions are usually clear or cloudy and nonirritating in nature, although they may leave a yellow cast on clothing after drying. An increase in the amount of vaginal secretion is known as leukorrhea or physiologic discharge and is classically described as a thin or thick white discharge resulting from congestion of the vaginal mucosa and an increase in polymorphonuclear leukocytes (white blood cells) that are visible under microscopy (Graziottin, 2024). Leukorrhea may be seen under normal circumstances, such as pregnancy or menstruation, or in the presence of vaginal infection. Normal vaginal discharge is slightly slimy, nonirritating, and has a mild inoffensive odor. By comparison, the alkaline, shiny mucoid substance secreted by the cervix is more abundant than vaginal secretions and less viscous at ovulation. The amount of vaginal discharge is not, in itself, an indication of infection.

Life-Cycle Changes

A newborn assigned female at birth may have a mucous discharge for 1 to 10 days following birth as a result of in utero stimulation of the uterus and vagina by maternal estrogen. A similar mucoid discharge may be seen a few years before and after menarche as a result of increased estrogen production by the maturing ovaries. Pregnant individuals often report substantially increased mucus production, with a resulting profuse discharge, particularly during the last few weeks before childbirth.

Throughout the reproductive years, vaginal secretions and cervical mucus vary during the menstrual cycle. Typically, around day 9 of the menstrual cycle, rising levels of estradiol will increase the amount of cervical mucus, making it thin and watery to enable penetration of sperm immediately prior to ovulation. After ovulation occurs, progesterone secreted from the corpus luteum converts the cervical mucus into a thickened, tenacious barrier, impeding penetration by sperm by both its physical properties and immune functions.

Research has shown there are important differences in the bacterial communities and vaginal microbiomes among individuals that vary according to life stage, from newborn to menopause (Graziottin, 2024). Before menarche and following menopause estrogen levels are low; consequently, vaginal secretions are minimal. In premenarchal individuals, the vaginal epithelium is inactive and thin, the cells contain very little glycogen, lactobacilli are diminished or absent, and the vaginal pH is more alkaline, between 6 and 7. During this phase, multiple anaerobic organisms dominate the vaginal microbiome, primarily those found in the gut and respiratory tract (Itriyeva, 2020). Thus, the vulvovaginal environment in premenarchal females is particularly susceptible to irritation and infection, which can be introduced or exacerbated by practices such as inadequate or improper cleansing after urination or defecation, use of bubble baths and scented laundry detergents, and trauma from tight clothing. Consequently, most vulvovaginal symptoms in premenarchal patients result from infection related to hygiene or behavioral practices and can be treated with appropriate medications and education on proper cleansing and care of the genital area (Lanis et al., 2020). Any concerns regarding sexually transmitted infections should prompt an evaluation for abuse. (Refer to Chapter 22 for more information on STIs and Chapter 16 for sexual assault and trafficking.)

Among individuals in menopause, reduced levels of estrogen, as a result of diminished ovarian function, may lead to changes in the types of organisms found in the vaginal microbiome, compared with reproductive-age people. In 90 percent of patients of reproductive age, the vaginal environment is dominated by lactobacilli, whereas in menopause, anaerobic organisms dominate, most commonly *Gardnerella* species (Gliniewicz et al., 2019). Lower proportions of lactobacilli, decreased lactic acid production, and increased vaginal pH levels may impact anatomic and functional changes in the entire genitourinary tract (Gliniewicz et al., 2019). These physiologic changes affect up to

50 percent of menopausal patients not on menopausal hormone therapy, leading to reduced elasticity in the vaginal walls, diminished vaginal lubrication, increased risk of urinary symptoms (e.g., infection, nocturia, urgency), and dyspareunia. Estrogen therapy (systemic, local, with or without progestin) increases *Lactobacillus* species in the postmenopausal microbiome (Micks et al., 2024).

Transgender and gender diverse individuals may seek gender-affirming medical care, which might include testosterone therapy for transmasculine individuals, and vaginoplasty or the surgical creation of a neovagina for transfeminine patients (Birse et al, 2020; Moises da Silva et al., 2021). Gender-affirming hormone therapy has implications for the vaginal microbiome, and these environments are sparsely described in the literature, leaving practicing clinicians without guidelines for patient education and care (Krakowsky et al., 2022). Gender-affirming hormonal therapy is highly effective in the promotion of the development of secondary sex characteristics which are aligned with gender identity. In transmasculine individuals who are prescribed testosterone, there is a decrease in estrogen, which causes epithelial thinning, decreased levels of free glycogen in the mucosa, and a reduction in lactobacilli levels. The vaginal tissue of transmasculine patients demonstrates elevated levels of inflammation, edema, collagen fibrosis, and granulation tissue (Schardein et al., 2021). These individuals sometimes experience vaginal atrophy symptoms such as dryness, irritation, and dyspareunia that can have a negative impact on their quality of life and expression of intimacy. In these cases, topical estrogen therapy can be offered, but research is lacking on whether this is an effective treatment and results in increased lactobacilli, or whether this therapy might interfere with the desired masculinizing effects of testosterone (Krakowsky et al., 2022; Winston McPherson et al., 2019).

For transfeminine individuals, the primary surgical technique used to create a neovagina is penile inversion vaginoplasty. There are many variations on this technique with the desired outcome being concordant vulvar anatomy, and a moist vaginal canal with intact erogenous sensation. While both the female vaginal canal and the penile or sigmoid skin used to make the neovagina are composed of epithelial cells, penile skin lacks glycogen production, contains keratin and has a soft cornified outer layer. These characteristics suggest that a neovagina is not likely to support a *Lactobacillus*-dominated microbiota, which has implications for treatment of neovaginal complaints. Small studies on the microbiota of the neovagina demonstrate colonization with *Prevotella*, *Peptostreptococcus*, *Peptoniphilus*, and *Cornebacterium*, all of which are prevalent in testosterone-dominant vaginas, as well as the foreskin of the uncircumcised penis (Krakowsky et al., 2022; Winston McPherson et al., 2019). Interestingly, neovaginas constructed with sigmoid colon tissue are colonized by gut bacteria, suggesting that the neovaginal microbiome is dependent on the origin of the tissue used to create it. A recent systematic review examining the bacterial flora of the neovagina revealed a lack of both research and protocols for the role of oral probiotics, topical estrogen therapy of cleansing regimens to support neovaginal health (Stoehr et al., 2023).

There are many unanswered questions in the emerging field of transgender care. Data from TransPulse Canada suggest that nearly half of all individuals with neovaginas experienced gynecologic symptoms such as itching and malodorous discharge; and further, that traditional treatments were often ineffective, necessitating further research and the development of clinical guidelines for prevention and treatment of this community (Krakowsky et al., 2022).

Current research on the vaginal microbiome is complex and evolving. Reproductive health outcomes are closely affected by the health of the vaginal microbiome. Among pregnant people, researchers seek to establish interactions among the composition of the microbiome, vaginal secretions, and cervical length to develop point-of-care testing to assess patients at risk for premature birth, a leading cause of neonatal death globally (Witkin et al., 2019). Given its role in the health of reproductive-aged individuals globally, the vaginal microbiome is an important area of research by clinicians, microbiologists, and other scientists to further unlock its structure, function, and protective properties. Improved investment in resources, along with newer study models, sampling methods, and research designs, are needed to deepen understanding of vaginal and neovaginal health and potentially improve health globally (Anahtar et al., 2018). This research should include individuals from the transgender community as a step toward inclusive health care and the reduction of inequalities in care and access (American College of Obstetricians and Gynecologists' Committee on Gynecologic Practice and American College of Obstetricians and Gynecologists' Committee on Health Care for Underserved Women, 2021).

VAGINITIS, VAGINOSIS, AND VULVOVAGINITIS

Vaginitis is an inflammation of the vagina characterized by an increased vaginal discharge containing numerous white blood cells. Symptoms can include burning, irritation, dyspareunia, vulvovaginal itching, and a "fishy" vaginal odor. In contrast, vaginosis is not associated with an increase in white blood cells. Vaginitis and vaginosis occur when the vaginal environment is altered, either by microorganisms (**Table 21-2**) or by a disturbance allowing pathogens normally found in the vagina to proliferate. Vulvovaginitis, which is inflammation of the vulva and vagina, may be caused by vaginal infection or copious amounts of leukorrhea. In addition, chemical irritants, allergens, and foreign bodies may produce inflammatory reactions.

Vulvovaginal symptoms are common among patients with vaginas. Vaginal discharge was the most frequently reported symptom. BV, VVC, and trichomoniasis are the most common causes of abnormal vaginal discharge (AGOG Practice Bulletin 215, 2020). Refer to Chapter 22 for a discussion of trichomoniasis.

BACTERIAL VAGINOSIS

Incidence, Prevalence, and Scope

Bacterial vaginosis (BV) is the most common vaginal infection worldwide and is associated with a range of adverse public health issues, such as preterm birth, gynecologic postoperative infection, postpartum endometritis, and increased risk of STIs, HIV, and HPV infection (Muzny et al., 2022). African American and Hispanic populations are disproportionately affected, with BV prevalence among Black women at approximately 33.2 percent and Hispanic women at 30.7 percent while there is lower incidence among White (22.7%) and Asian (11.1%) populations. Recent research suggests that genetic ancestry might play an important role in risk (Murphy, 2024). BV recurrence rates are high, estimated at 80 percent

TABLE 21-2 Vaginal Symptoms and Findings

	Normal	Bacterial Vaginosis	Vulvovaginal Candidiasis	Desquamative Inflammatory Vaginitis
Vaginal pH	3.5 to 4.5	Greater than 4.5	Less than 4.5 (usually)	Greater than 4.5
Microscopy findings	Normal flora	With saline solution: Positive for clue cells, decreased lactobacilli	With KOH: Pseudohyphae with yeast buds	Abnormal flora, increase in inflammatory and parabasal cells, lactobacilli none or decreased
Discharge	White or clear Thin or mucoid	Thin, homogenous, grayish white, adherent	Thick or thin, white, curd-like (resembling cottage cheese), adherent	Purulent, yellow, profuse
Amine odor (KOH whiff test)	Absent	Present (fishy)	Absent	Absent
Vulvar pruritus	No	Mild, if present at all	Yes, swelling, excoriation, redness	Vulva mostly uninvolved, vaginal discomfort
Vaginal and/or vulvar skin changes	No	No	Erythema, edema, fissuring may occur with severe cases	Vaginal erythema may be present; petechiae or ecchymosis may be seen
Pelvic pain	No	No	No	No
Dysuria	No	Occasionally	Severe cases	Severe cases
Dyspareunia	No	Rarely	May or may not occur	Yes
Patient's primary concern	None or variable	May be asymptomatic; vaginal discharge, vaginal odor that is often worse after intercourse	Vaginal itching, burning, and/or discharge, or may be asymptomatic	Profuse discharge, rawness, burning, soreness, and sometimes severe dyspareunia

Data from Centers for Disease Control and Prevention. (2021). Sexually transmitted diseases treatment guidelines 2021. *Morbidity and Mortality Weekly Report, 70*(4), 1–187; Vaginitis in Nonpregnant Patients: ACOG Practice Bulletin, Number 215. (2020). *Obstetrics & Gynecology, 135*(1), e1–e17. https://doi.org/10.1097/AOG.0000000000003604

Abbreviation: KOH, potassium hydroxide.

at the 3-month mark following effective treatment with antibiotics (Coudray & Madhivanan, 2020; Plummer et al., 2023). The economic burden of BV within the United States is estimated at $4.8 billion (95% confidence interval [CI]: $3.7 to $6.1 billion), and the cost is approximately tripled if the costs of BV-associated preterm birth and individuals living with HIV are included (Muzny et al., 2022). Worldwide, approximately one-fourth of women in the general population meet the diagnostic criteria for BV (Peebles et al., 2019), with higher prevalence in the Middle East, North and Sub-Saharan Africa, and South Asia (Sousa et al., 2023).

Etiology and Pathophysiology

BV is not an infection per se but is caused by an imbalance in the normal microbiome. Normally, the vagina of reproductive-age and some postmenopausal patients is colonized with lactobacilli that produce hydrogen peroxide, lactic acid, and bacteriocins to maintain the pH of the vagina in an acidic range between 3.5 and 4.5. If the vaginal pH becomes more alkaline, an overgrowth of anaerobic and opportunistic organisms may occur. These anaerobes produce proteolytic enzymes which cause epithelial cell exfoliation and vaginal transudation, ultimately producing the characteristic symptoms of BV. Causative bacterial strains include *Gardnerella vaginalis*, *Prevotella* species, *Porphyromonas* species, *Bacteroides* species, *Peptostreptococcus* species, *Mycoplasma hominis*, and *Ureaplasma urealyticum*, as well as *Mobiluncus*, *Megasphaera*, *Sneathia*, and *Clostridiales* species (Plummer et al., 2023).

Although it is recognized that the vaginal environment of patients with BV undergoes a shift in vaginal flora which encourages overgrowth of anaerobic organisms, it remains unclear what events lead to these changes. Although BV is highly prevalent, 50 percent of people are reportedly asymptomatic (Coudray & Madhivanan, 2020). Researchers have investigated nutritional implications, socioeconomic factors, psychosocial stress, sexual activity, and behaviors (e.g., douching, use of pads, powders) to identify possible triggers for the development of BV. Some of these may be possible cofactors, but none have been found to be etiologic. The question of whether BV is sexually associated has surfaced repeatedly for decades, and the majority of epidemiologic studies support this hypothesis (Muzny et al., 2022; Plummer et al., 2020; Vodstrcil et al., 2021). A recent trial demonstrated that the addition of oral and topical antibiotic treatment for male partners reduced recurrence rates from 63 percent to 35 percent (Vodstrcil et al., 2025), suggesting that sexual transmission plays an important but not exclusive role in recurrence. Research also supports that copper IUDS may increase colonization by *G. vaginalis* and *A. vaginae*, leading to increased prevalence (Daniel et al., 2023).

An updated model of BV describes the pathogenesis of one key organism, *G. vaginalis*, and its capacity for development of a biofilm in the vagina resulting in a decrease of lactobacilli and subsequent increase in harmful anaerobic bacteria. Biofilms are communities of multiple types of bacteria that coalesce and embed within a cellular matrix, attaching themselves to the vaginal wall, effectively forming a scaffolding upon which bacteria attach. The subsequent desquamation of epithelial cells creates the "clue" cells which are diagnostic of BV. Bacterial biofilms are believed to develop in an effort to self-protect from environmental host defense mechanisms and challenges from antimicrobial drugs. A polymicrobial biofilm covering half or more of the vaginal epithelial surface is found in 90 percent of people with BV and 10 percent of those without BV (Plummer et al., 2023). Biofilms represent considerable concern among healthcare providers because their formation impedes antimicrobial activity, enhances the likelihood of antibacterial drug resistance, and provides a site where additional opportunistic pathogens may thrive, developing yet another source of infection. It is the process of biofilm development that likely affects high rates of recurrence and persistent BV symptoms despite appropriate therapy (Vodstrcil et al., 2021).

Clinical Presentation and Variations

Although BV is quite common, many individuals have no symptoms or concerns about vaginal discharge, irritation, or discomfort with intercourse. Some women report a fishy odor during urination or when removing undergarments. In the absence of symptoms, routine screening for BV is not recommended. When BV is present, the vulva is typically without erythema or edema; during speculum examination, a thin white or gray milky discharge may be seen coating the vaginal walls.

Assessment

History

A careful history may help distinguish BV from other causes of vaginitis if the patient is symptomatic. Individuals should be asked about duration and severity of symptoms and whether they have self-treated with OTC products. A complete history includes information about sexual behaviors and practices; use of tampons, sexual toys, douching, and menstrual hygiene products; and STI history and risk. Clinicians should elicit a menstrual and contraceptive history, including the use of condoms. The most common symptom reported by patients with BV is a malodorous discharge. The patient or their partner may notice a fishy odor after intercourse because semen releases vaginal amines. Reports of fishy odor, vaginal irritation, and increased thin vaginal discharge are considered the most significant findings. Some individuals also may experience mild irritation, vulvar pruritus, postcoital spotting, irregular bleeding episodes, vaginal burning after intercourse, and urinary discomfort. Previous occurrences of similar symptoms, diagnoses, and treatments should be investigated because recurrence is common (Plummer et al., 2023).

Physical Examination

The place to begin assessment of any vaginal concern is by thoroughly inspecting the vulva. Typically, there is no vulvar involvement specific to BV, although vaginal discharge is often present at the introitus. Following examination of the vulva, a speculum examination is performed to inspect the vaginal walls and cervix. When present, the vaginal discharge associated with BV is usually increased, thin, white or gray, and milky in appearance. The vaginal walls are usually pink or pale but not inflamed. The cervix may be smooth and pink, and it may or may not have notable discharge. A mucopurulent discharge or friability of the cervix suggests an infection other than BV or coinfection with an additional organism.

Diagnostic Testing

In symptomatic patients, diagnosis of BV can occur via clinical indicators (Amsel criteria), point-of-care testing (Nugent score), or molecular assays (Muzny et al., 2022); each diagnostic method has its strengths and limitations. A clinical diagnosis of BV can be reliably made using the classic Amsel criteria (Amsel et al., 1983; **Box 21-1**), in which three of four clinical indicators must be present for diagnosis, but this is limited by the microscopy skills of the practitioner and availability of a lab in a low-resource environment. Recent research suggests that the presence of two indicators offers similar specificity (Colonna & Steelman, 2023). The gold standard for BV diagnosis remains the Gram stain using the Nugent score. For the Nugent score, a vaginal smear is gram stained and the morphophytes present are counted and classified according to a semiquantitative scale. A score > 7 is diagnostic for BV. Due to the time-intensive nature of this exam, Gram staining is typically used in research protocols and is less commonly seen in office-based outpatient settings. Although

BOX 21-1 Criteria for Clinical Diagnosis of Bacterial Vaginosis

Clinical diagnosis of BV is based on the presence of three out of four of the following classic Amsel criteria:

- White, thin adherent vaginal discharge
- pH 4.5 or greater
- Positive whiff/KOH test
- Clue cells on microscopic examination (more than 20% of epithelial cells are clue cells)

Data from Amsel, R., Totten, P. A., Spiegel, C. A., Chen, K. C., Eschenbach, D., & Holmes, K. K. (1983). Nonspecific vaginitis: Diagnostic criteria and microbial and epidemiologic associations. *American Journal of Medicine, 74*(1), 14–22;

Abou Chacra, L., Fenollar, F., & Diop, K. (2022). Bacterial vaginosis: What do we currently know? *Frontiers in Cellular and Infection Microbiology, 11*, 672429. https://doi.org/10.3389/fcimb.2021.672429

Colonna, C., & Steelman, M. (2023). Amsel criteria. In *StatPearls*. StatPearls Publishing.

FIGURE 21-1 **Wet mount findings with bacterial vaginosis. A. No bacterial vaginosis: Presence of normal epithelial cells and *Lactobacillus*. B. Bacterial vaginosis: Clue cells and absence of *Lactobacillus*.**

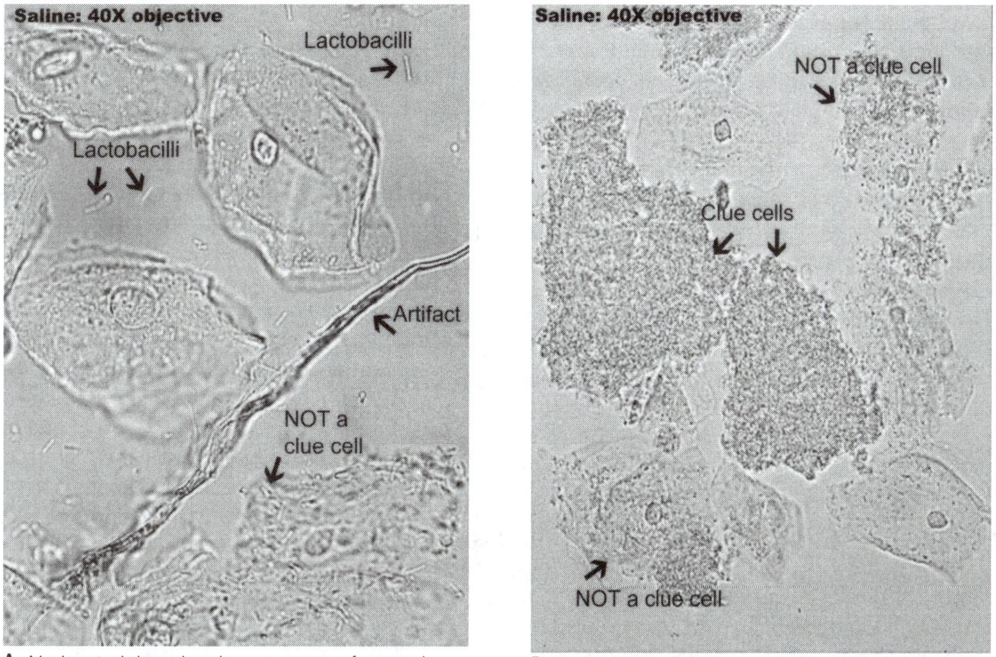

A No bacterial vaginosis: presence of normal epithelial cells and *Lactobacillus*.

B Bacterial vaginosis: clue cells and absence of *Lactobacillus*.

Reproduced from Washington State Department of Health STD/TB Program, Seattle STD/HIV Prevention Training Center, and Cindy Fennell, MS, MT, ASCP.

cytology reports may include comments such as "predominance of coccobacilli consistent with shift in vaginal flora," Pap testing is both nonspecific and not sensitive for diagnosing BV. Furthermore, vaginal cultures are not useful because BV is multibacterial in origin, and cultures are nonspecific. Although a wet mount and microscopy are important practices for outpatient settings, microscopy does have limitations with respect to accurate diagnosis in terms of sensitivity and specificity (Muzny et al., 2022; Sousa et al., 2023).

In order to perform a microscopic examination of vaginal secretions, a slide is prepared for wet mount examination using both 10 percent potassium hydroxide (KOH) and normal saline. The KOH solution is used to test for amine odor; amines are produced as a by-product of anaerobic metabolism. The fishy odor released when KOH is added to vaginal secretions on a slide or on the lip of the withdrawn speculum results in a positive KOH or whiff test. The presence of clue cells (vaginal epithelial cells coated with bacteria that obscure cell borders) in the sample with normal saline is a characteristic sign because this phenomenon is specific to BV (refer to **Figure 21-1**). In addition, a reduction in lactobacilli and typically very few white blood cells are noted. Increased numbers of white blood cells in addition to the presence of clue cells suggest concurrent vaginitis or a coinfection with trichomoniasis, chlamydia, or candidiasis. Clinicians often prefer microscopy for ease and cost, but data demonstrates that misdiagnoses are common either due to lack of microscopy skills or nonadherence to diagnostic criteria (Muzny et al., 2022).

Vaginal secretions can also be tested for pH. Nitrazine paper is sensitive enough to detect a pH of 4.5 or greater. Normal vaginal secretions have a pH in the range of 3.5 to 4.5. An elevated pH (4.5 or higher) is more commonly seen in the presence of BV, desquamative inflammatory vaginitis, or trichomoniasis. A sample for pH testing is best collected from the lateral walls of the vagina to ensure an accurate pH assessment; pH is more variable on the cervix, reflecting the current point in the patient's hormonal cycle. Although vaginal pH can be a useful adjunct test, it is nonspecific, and its results may be altered by the presence of blood in the vagina.

Given the time-intensive nature of the Nugent score, and the lack of sensitivity of the Amsel criteria (37–70%) emerging point-of-care testing (POCT) offers promise for improved diagnostics. The OSOM BV Blue Assay (Genzyme Diagnostics), is a dipstick test measuring sialidase levels, which are produced by *Gardnerella* and *Bacteriodes* species. Final results are available in 10 minutes and have high sensitivity (88–94%) and specificity (91–98%), as compared to Amsel which has much lower sensitivity (37–70%). A final POCT for settings lacking microscopy is the FemExam card (Cooper Surgical) which detects metabolic biproducts of *G. vaginalis* and measures vaginal pH (Muzny et al., 2022).

Due to the persistence of BV and the diagnostic and treatment challenges, molecular diagnostic assays have been developed to refine understanding. These tests are commonly done by direct DNA probe and nucleic acid amplification assays (NAAT), and can be run on self-collected vaginal swabs, and offer the advantage of improved sensitivity and specificity over the Amsel criteria or the Nugent score. Two examples are the Affirm VP assay (Becton Dickinson), and the DNA probe test by Quest Diagnostics. NAAT tests have the advantage of quantifying and describing BV-associated bacteria in addition to *G. vaginalis* and are typically used in research. Commercially available PCR assays include Labcorps NuSwab, Quest Diagnostics SureSwab, BD Max, Hologic Aptima BV, and MDL BV Panel (Muzny et al., 2022). Continued technological advances are needed to increase our understanding of the complexity of BV.

Differential Diagnoses

The differential diagnoses for BV include trichomoniasis, vulvovaginal candidiasis (VVC), presence of a foreign body, chemical vaginitis, contact vaginitis, desquamative inflammatory vaginitis, atrophic vaginitis, lactational vaginitis, chlamydia, gonorrhea, genital herpes, cervicitis, and normal physiologic discharge (Muzny, 2022). If vulvar itching is a symptom, clinicians should assess for and rule out vulvar dermatoses. Vulvar dermatoses are discussed in Chapter 27.

Prevention

Because the pathogenesis of BV is still not clearly understood, there are limited prevention strategies to recommend at this time. General health behaviors described earlier in this chapter may help prevent recurrent episodes of BV. Recent research into male-partner treatment to prevent the recurrence of BV demonstrated promising results. Monogamous couples in which the female partner received standard treatment and the male partner received both oral and topical antimicrobial treatment demonstrated 35 percent recurrence at 12 weeks versus 63 percent in the female treatment only group, a significant reduction (Vodstrcil et al., 2025). Estrogen increases the amount of glycogen in epithelial cells, favoring lactobacillus growth, which inhibits BV (Falconi-McCahill, 2019).

There is ongoing research into the use of probiotics for the prevention of BV (Mei, 2022). In a recent meta-analysis of 30 international studies (Jeng et al., 2020), probiotic intervention reduced the recurrence of vaginitis, improved the cure rate, and inhibited the growth of *Gardnerella sp*. In another meta-analysis of 18 studies (Liu & Yi, 2022), the combination of antibiotics and probiotics demonstrated a significant reduction in recurrence of BV compared with antibiotics alone. These studies focused primarily on *Lactobacillus acidophilus*, *Lactobacillis rhamnosus*, and *Lactobacillus crispatus*. Although this research is promising, this approach is still considered investigational and requires further study prior to incorporation into clinical guidelines (Sobel, 2024). For patients who are able to achieve remission following antibiotic administration, 600 mg of boric acid placed in the vagina nightly has been proven to be effective as a suppressive regimen (Surapaneni et al., 2021). Expert opinion holds that douching should be avoided.

Management

Pharmacologic Therapies

Table 21-3 outlines treatment guidelines for BV as recognized by the Centers for Disease Control and Prevention (CDC). The CDC recommends treatment for symptomatic patients. Vaginal metronidazole is not recommended for individuals with a known allergy to oral metronidazole; however, vaginal metronidazole can be used in people who do not tolerate oral metronidazole (CDC, 2021). Clindamycin cream is preferred in case of allergy or intolerance to metronidazole or tinidazole; however, patients should be advised that clindamycin may weaken latex condoms or contraceptive diaphragms. Treatment of sexual partners is not currently recommended in standing guidelines, but may become the standard of treatment due to the evidence of partner transmission discussed above. The CDC recommends all women with BV be tested for HIV and other STIs.

Complementary and Alternative Methods

CAM approaches to BV include nonconventional treatments and the use of phytomedicine to treat symptoms. Despite lack of definitive data, 65 percent report the use of alternative medicine to treat vaginitis (Falconi-McCahill, 2019), most commonly yogurt, garlic, tea tree oil, boric acid, and probiotics (refer to Table 21-4).

Researchers have explored the application of a variety of alternative measures, such as Ayurveda, homeopathy, mind–body intervention, traditional Chinese herbal compounds, phytotherapy, acupuncture, essential oils, vitamins, and diet therapies, for treatment of BV. Although the use of prebiotics and probiotics is promising and they have a generally acceptable safety profile, differences in study design, outcomes, types of species studied, method of administration, duration of use, targeted outcomes, and effectiveness have resulted in insufficient evidence for or against their use (Sobel & Mitchell, 2023). They continue to be aggressively marketed and may be reasonable treatment options for individuals who are uninsured, underinsured or have limited access to healthcare resources (Falconi-McCahill, 2019).

Essential oils of *Caledula officianalis*, *Hypericum perforatum* (St. John's Wort), *Berberris vulgaris* (Barberry root), and *Myrtus communis* (Myrtle) have been studied and compared to 0.75% metronidazole vaginal gel to treat and prevent recurrence of BV; all were found to be effective, but are not commercially available (Falconi-McCahill, 2019). Vitamins D and C have been investigated for the treatment of BV; both show statistically significant improvements in cure rates and decreased recurrence rates (Falconi-McCahill, 2019) and deserve further study. There are no studies supporting the use of douching to either treat or relieve BV symptoms (CDC, 2021), although it remains a common practice in the United States. Douching is associated with multiple reproductive health risks; therefore, this practice should be avoided, and the vagina should be cleansed using normal bathing and showering practices (Graziottin, 2024).

Referral

As many as 70 percent of individuals who experience an episode of BV report a recurrence within 3 to 6 months (Sobel, 2024). Indeed, recurrent BV remains a clinical enigma and a source of distress among affected patients and their healthcare providers. The CDC suggests treating patients with recurrent BV either by retreating with the original therapy or using a recommended therapy that differs from the original therapy. Those who experience multiple recurrences after initial treatment can use metronidazole gel intravaginally twice weekly for 4 to 6 months or monthly oral metronidazole with fluconazole (refer to Table 21-3). However, after suppressive therapy with vaginal metronidazole is discontinued, symptoms may recur. Individuals whose diagnosis is uncertain or who experience frequent recurrences that appear resistant to therapy can be referred to a healthcare provider who specializes in complex or recurring instances of

TABLE 21-3 Bacterial Vaginosis Treatment

Infection	Recommended Regimens	Alternative Regimens
BV	Metronidazole 500 mg orally twice/day for 7 days **or** Metronidazole gel 0.75%, one full applicator (5 g) intravaginally daily for 5 days **or** Clindamycin cream 2%, one full applicator (5 g) intravaginally at bedtime for 7 days **Pregnant women:** Metronidazole 500 mg orally twice/day for 7 days **or** Metronidazole 250 mg orally three times/day for 7 days **or** Clindamycin 300 mg orally twice/day for 7 days	Tinidazole 2 g orally once/day for 2 days **or** Tinidazole 1 g orally once/day for 5 days **or** Clindamycin 300 mg orally twice/day for 7 days **or** Clindamycin ovules 100 g intravaginally once at bedtime for 3 days **or** Secnidazole 2 g packet of granules sprinkled on applesauce, pudding, or yogurt and ingested within 30 minutes as a single dose[a] **Pregnant women:** None
Recurrent BV	*For patients who have not been treated with Clindamycin cream,* Clindamycin cream 2%, one full applicator (5 g) intravaginally at bedtime for 7 days **or** *Extended metronidazole regimen:* Oral metronidazole or tinidazole 500 mg daily for 7 days **or** Metronidazole gel 0.75% 5 g dose intravaginally once daily for 7 days **Followed by** Metronidazole gel 0.75% (5g) intravaginally twice weekly for 4–6 months prophylaxis	*Vaginal boric acid regimen:* Oral metronidazole or tinidazole 500 mg daily for 7 days **Then** Vaginal boric acid 600 mg intravaginally at night, to be continued for 21 days **and** Metronidazole gel 0.75% (5g) intravaginally twice weekly for 4–6 months
Investigational male-partner therapy	Metronidazole 400 mg tablets and 2% clindamycin cream applied to penile skin twice/day for 7 days	

Data from Vodstrcil, L. A., Plummer, E. L., Fairley, C. K., Hocking, J. S., Law, M. G., Petoumenos, K., Bateson, D., Murray, G. L., Donovan, B., Chow, E. P. F., Chen, M. Y., Kaldor, J., & Bradshaw, C. S. (2025). Male-partner treatment to prevent recurrence of bacterial vaginosis. *The New England Journal of Medicine, 392*(10), 947–957. https://doi.org/10.1056/NEJMoa2405404;

Centers for Disease Control and Prevention. (2021, July 19). *Bacterial vaginosis—STI treatment guidelines*. U.S. Department of Health and Human Services. https://www.cdc.gov/std/treatment-guidelines/bv.htm

vaginal symptoms or, in some cases, an infectious disease specialist. People with multiple, concurrent vaginal symptoms who also have chronic morbidities (e.g., those who have transplanted organs, diabetes, or forms of immune suppression) might also benefit from referral to a specialist for further evaluation. Individuals with HIV have a higher prevalence of BV and are more likely to have persistent infection, compared with those who do not have HIV (CDC, 2021); these patients may benefit from referral to an infectious disease specialist. Many academic medical centers offer specialty clinics to address chronic and recurring cases of vaginitis and vulvar syndromes.

The importance of completing the course of medication and avoiding alcohol both while taking metronidazole or tinidazole and after completing treatment (24 hours after treatment with metronidazole, 72 hours after treatment with tinidazole) must be emphasized. Inform patients that nitroimidazole antibiotics can cause a metallic taste, nausea, vomiting, and cramps even if they do not consume alcohol. There is no precaution statement from the manufacturer to avoid alcohol while using secnidazole. In addition, counsel patients to avoid intercourse until treatment is complete and to consistently use condoms. Advise patients to refrain from douching as a general practice and especially during treatment. Many individuals develop VVC symptoms following treatment with nitroimidazoles; therefore, providers often coprescribe an antifungal, such as one or two doses of fluconazole 3 to 5 days apart. Encourage patients to avoid self-diagnosis and self-treatment with OTC products because use of these products in the vagina may obscure microscopy findings, resulting in delayed diagnosis and additional costs to women who select an inappropriate product. Discuss what is currently known about BV, especially with women who have chronic recurring BV, to reassure them that long-term treatments, while not necessarily curative, can relieve symptoms and may reduce recurrence (Sobel, 2024).

TABLE 21-4 Alternative Measures for Managing Bacterial Vaginosis Symptoms

Intervention	Dosage	Administration	Use
Garlic clove	One peeled clove wrapped in cloth and dipped in olive oil, or capsule form	Overnight in vagina, change daily	BV
Boric acid powder	600 mg in gelatin capsule	Every day in vagina for 14 days (toxic if ingested orally)	BV
Cold milk, cottage cheese, yogurt	Compress or insert in vagina	Apply to affected area	Pruritus
Propolis (bee glue)	Vaginal cream or ovules	Topical; no dose given	BV
Probiotics	*Lactobacillus crispatus* IP174178	1 vaginal capsule for 14 days	BV
Probiotics	*Lactobacillus*: *L fermentum* 57A, *L plantarum* 57B, and *L gasseri* 57C	1 vaginal capsule for 7 days	BV
Probiotics	*Lactobacillus rhamnosus* GR-1 and *Lactobacillus reuteri* RC-14.	2 oral capsules twice daily for 6 weeks	BV

Data from Falconi-McCahill, A. (2019). Bacterial vaginosis: A clinical update with a focus on complementary and alternative therapies. *Journal of Midwifery & Women's Health.*, *64*(5), 578–591. https://doi.org/10.1111/jmwh.1301

Considerations for Specific Populations

Pregnant People

BV is associated with late miscarriage, chorioamnionitis, premature rupture of fetal membranes, preterm labor and birth, and postpartum endometritis (CDC, 2021). Despite these associations, there is no current recommendation to screen all asymptomatic pregnant patients for BV. In pregnant women at increased risk for preterm birth, the United States Preventative Services Task Force (USPSTF) concluded there is insufficient evidence for screening (I recommendation) (2020). Other women's health organizations have generally concurred. Although the CDC does not recommend routine screening for BV in high-risk asymptomatic women, their guidelines for BV management state symptomatic pregnant women should be treated (CDC, 2021). The American College of Obstetricians and Gynecologists (ACOG) finds that studies regarding screening pregnant women for BV are conflicting and thus show no clear benefit, but ACOG recommends treatment for symptomatic women during pregnancy, citing the same two studies referenced in the CDC guideline (American College of Obstetricians and Gynecologists [ACOG], 2006, reaffirmed 2019). In a recent prospective, multicenter RCT involving 6,671 pregnant individuals, there was no evidence found for a reduction in the rate of preterm birth or total costs with a PCR screen and treat strategy for asymptomatic pregnant patients (Bretelle et al., 2023).

Clinicians should treat symptomatic pregnant people who test positive for BV. Although treatment should reduce vaginal symptoms, it may or may not prevent adverse pregnancy outcomes. Patients with BV with a previous preterm delivery may benefit from screening and treatment, but there is insufficient data to recommend this routinely (Robinson, 2024). Clindamycin vaginal cream is not recommended in pregnancy because it is associated with low birth weight and neonatal infections in newborns whose mothers were treated with this medication (CDC, 2021); however, it is used in some Western European countries. Tinidazole is not recommended for use in pregnancy. Secnidazole is not recommended during pregnancy or breastfeeding. Guidelines for treatment can be found in Table 21-3.

Perimenopausal and Older Adults

Our understanding of BV in menopause is limited due to a lack of research on this population. In the postmenopausal state, characterized by decreased levels of endogenous estrogen production, there is a depletion of vaginal lactobacilli, and elevated vaginal pH, which result in a distinct microbiome very different from premenopausal patients. In addition, with lower levels of circulating estrogen, many patients experience vaginal dryness and irritation described as the genitourinary syndrome of menopause (GSM), which complicates BV diagnosis. As common current diagnostics (Amsel criteria and Nugent score) were validated on premenopausal subjects, there may be a role for BV molecular diagnostics such as NAATs and rRNA sequencing. Expert opinion suggests that treatment for vaginal symptoms in postmenopausal patients should begin with topical estrogen, and BV should be considered as a differential only if this is unsuccessful in alleviating symptoms (Van Gerwin et al., 2023).

Emerging Evidence

The most challenging aspect of clinical management of BV is the high rate of recurrence. This is thought to be largely due to the formation of the polymicrobial biofilm, but could also be due to antimicrobial resistance, reinfection, or colonization by nonsusceptible species, and is a fertile area of current research (Sousa, 2023). TOL-463 is a boric acid–based anti-infective with enhanced antibiofilm activity now in phase 2 trials, which has demonstrated to be safe and effective at reducing recurrence rates in combination with antimicrobials (Marrazo et al., 2019). Additionally, the potential of vaginal microbiome transplant for patients with intractable BV has been studied in very small investigational trials and shows promise but needs to be tested in RCTs with placebo (Sobel, 2024) prior to adoption.

VULVOVAGINAL CANDIDIASIS

Description

Vulvovaginitis is a general term for a collection of vulvar and vaginal symptoms, such as itching, burning, irritation, and sometimes dysuria or dyspareunia. VVC is a vulvovaginitis caused by *Candida* species, most commonly *C. albicans*. Species of the *Candida* genus can be found almost everywhere—in humans, animals, foods, nature, and hospitals. Most *Candida* species can be a component of the harmless, normal flora within an individual. However, in immunocompromised persons, *Candida* species can transform into opportunistic pathogens leading to systemic and overwhelming infections (Wychrij, 2025).

Incidence, Prevalence, and Scope

Worldwide, VVC is one of the most common infections of the lower genital tract. It is commonly referred to as a vaginal yeast infection. Approximately 75 percent of people with vaginas will experience at least one episode of VVC during their lifetime, and of these, about 40–45 percent will experience two or more episodes. Ten to twenty percent of patients will develop recurring VVC, described as four or more episodes in a year (CDC, 2021). VVC is further classified as uncomplicated VVC and complicated VVC, the later begin recurrent, severe, caused by a non-albicans species, or associated with other morbidities such as diabetes or immunocompromised conditions such as HIV, chemotherapy, or use of corticosteroids (CDC, 2021). Because *Candida* species are considered part of the normal flora of the genital tract and skin, they are not considered sexually transmitted pathogens although the same *Candida* species may be found among sexual partners.

Etiology and Pathophysiology

C. albicans is a normal inhabitant of the vagina and the most common cause of VVC. In many people, the presence of vaginal *Candida* causes no symptoms. *Candida* colonizes in or on other mucosal surfaces as well, such as the urinary, gastrointestinal, and respiratory tracts; on skin surfaces; and in the mouth. Although 90 percent or more of VVC episodes are believed to be caused by *C. albicans*, VVC can also be caused by non-*C. albicans* species, such as *Candida glabrata*, *Candida tropicalis*, *Candida parapsilosis*, and *Candida krusei*, although these types are less common causative species in the United States.

The development of VVC results from a change in the health of the vaginal environment (the host), leading to a change in the behavior of the *Candida*, shifting the organism from normal flora to pathogenic activity (CDC, 2021). Changes in health may lead to alterations in physiology, hormonal balance, and a diminished immune function. Common risk factors include diabetes mellitus, antibiotic use, increased estrogen levels, immunosuppression, and genetic factors. Possible risk factors with inconclusive causality include diet, COC use, intravaginal contraceptive devices and sexual behavior (Sobel & Mitchell, 2023; Wang et al., 2024).

Clinical Presentation and Variations

VVC can cause a spectrum of symptoms ranging from none at all to severe. *Candida* vulvovaginitis typically presents as a thickened, curd-like white discharge often visible at the introitus. The vulva and labia may be swollen and erythematous. Some individuals may report symptoms of vaginal irritation and dyspareunia but show no obvious external signs. Occasionally, clinicians may note evidence of VVC on examination, yet patients may be asymptomatic. During speculum examination, providers may notice erythematous vaginal walls with a white, adherent, clumpy discharge. In general, if VVC is the only diagnosis, there is usually no accompanying odor, although if additional types of vaginitis are also present, such as BV, there may be a noticeable amine odor. VVC and BV may occur concurrently. VVC is limited and localized to the genital tract and is not a systemic infection.

Assessment

History

The most common symptom of VVC is vulvar and possibly vaginal pruritus (Table 21-2). This itching may be mild or intense, interfere with rest and activities, and occur during or after intercourse. Some people report a feeling of dryness or dyspareunia. Others may experience painful urination because the urine flows over the vulva; this symptom usually occurs in individuals who have vulvar fissuring or excoriation resulting from scratching. Although no characteristic odor is associated with VVC, some people report a yeasty or musty smell. In addition to obtaining a thorough history of the patient's symptoms (their onset and course), it is valuable to identify predisposing host or behavioral risk factors (refer to **Figure 21-2**). Ask patients about the use of oral contraceptives, hormonal intrauterine device (IUD), contraceptive diaphragm, and recent use of antibiotics. What daily medications, including prescription, OTC, and herbal preparations, are used? Has the patient self-treated their current condition, and if so, how recently, what products were used, and were they effective? Have them describe routine bathing and hygiene practices, including use of feminine hygiene and laundering products, soaps, sprays, douches, and sex toys. Inquire about dietary practices, such as ingestion of highly sweetened beverages, soft drinks, and fruit juices. Are symptoms recurrent, and if so, how often? Behaviors such as wearing wet or damp clothing for prolonged periods of time after swimming or working out may increase moisture and facilitate growth of *Candida*.

Physical Examination

The physical examination begins with a thorough inspection of the vulva and vagina. Look for signs of redness, edema, or other possible causes of the patient's symptoms, such as contact or vulvar dermatitis. In the outpatient setting, a speculum examination and microscopic examination of vaginal secretions with saline and 10 percent KOH are performed. Most often the discharge is thick, white, and lumpy with the consistency of cottage cheese. Often the discharge is found in patches that adhere to the vaginal walls and labia. The labial folds and vagina are sometimes red and swollen or fissured and may exhibit excoriation. If vaginal discharge is extremely thick and copious, vaginal debridement with a cotton swab followed by application of vaginal antifungal medication may be useful. The cervix is not usually affected by the presence of vaginal and vulvar *Candida*, so although discharge may be present on the cervix, it does not typically cause cervicitis or bleeding that may been seen with other infections, such as trichomoniasis or chlamydia.

Diagnostic Testing

The presence of *Candida* in the vagina can be seen on routine wet mount preparation and, in the absence of symptoms, does not indicate infection because *Candida* species are part of the normal vaginal flora in 10-20 percent of patients. Although the characteristic spores and pseudohyphae may be seen on microscopy, these organisms may sometimes be confused with other cells and artifacts. Pseudohyphae are best seen with the addition of 10 percent KOH to the wet mount (**Figure 21-3**). During microscopy examination, check for other microorganisms, background material, and the presence of white blood cells. Vaginal pH is a

FIGURE 21-2 Host-related and behavioral risk factors for VVC.

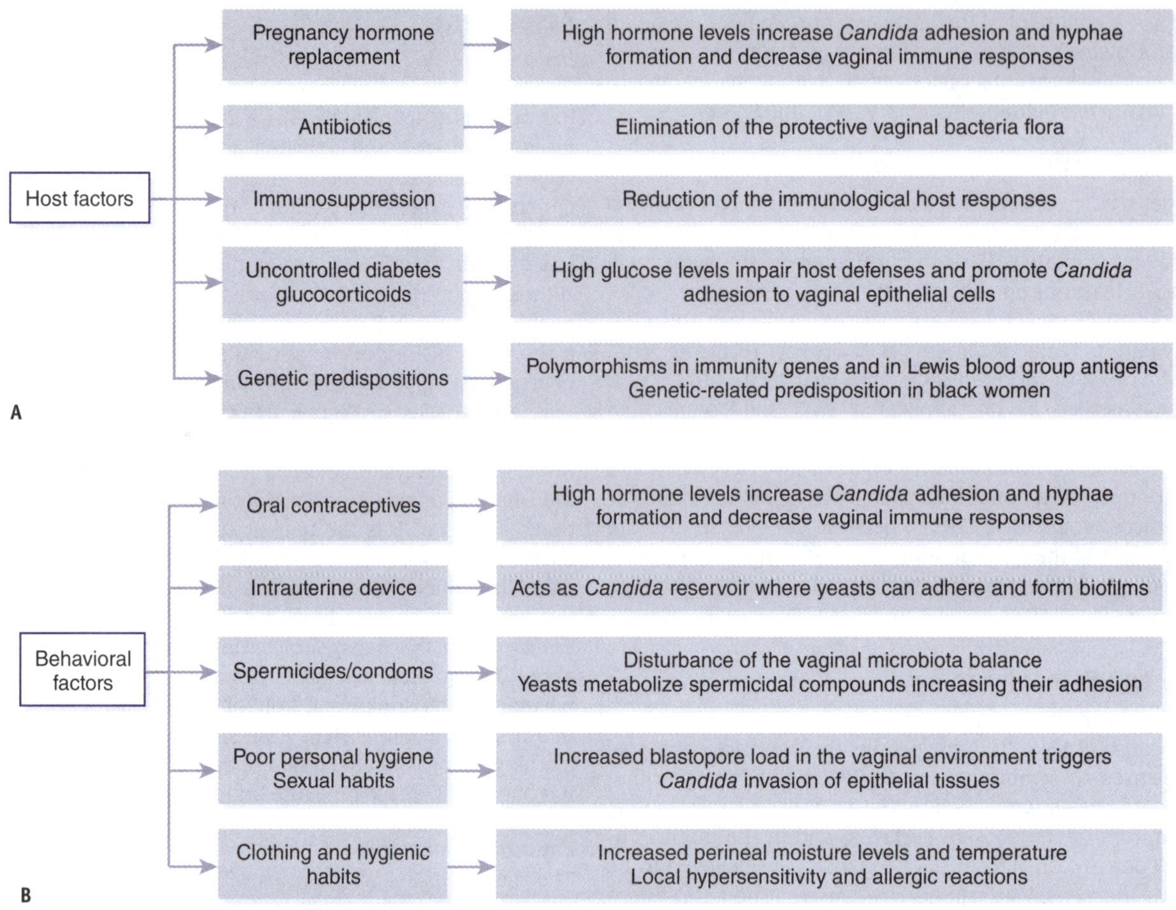

Reproduced from Gonçalves, B., Ferreira, C., Alves, C. T., Henriques, M., Azeredo, J., & Silva, S. (2016). Vulvovaginal candidiasis: Epidemiology, microbiology and risk factors. *Critical Reviews in Microbiology, 42*(6), 905–927. https://doi.org/10.3109/1040841X.2015.1091805

FIGURE 21-3 Wet mount findings with VVC.

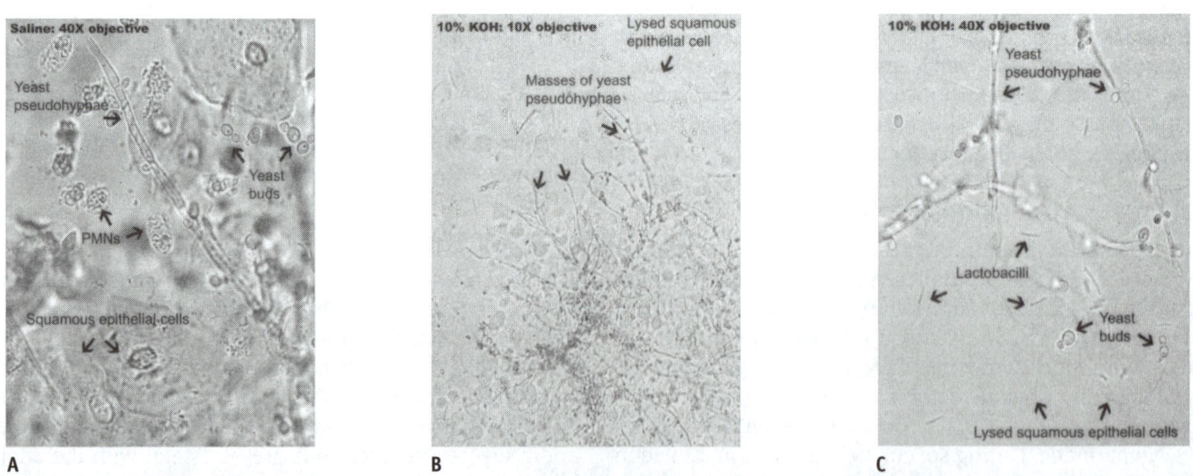

Reproduced from Washington State Department of Health STD/TB Program, Seattle STD/HIV Prevention Training Center, and Cindy Fennell, MS, MT, ASCP.
Abbreviation: PMNs, polymorphonuclear leukocytes/white blood cells.

useful, if not confirmatory, tool in assessing a range of vaginal irritations and can be tested using commonly available test strips. The normal vaginal pH in women with VVC ranges from 3.5 to 4.5. A normal vaginal pH is not sensitive enough to confirm a diagnosis of VVC because other similar symptoms will also present with a normal vaginal pH (e.g., contact dermatitis). However, if the pH is greater than 4.5, the clinician should suspect trichomoniasis, BV, atrophic vaginitis, or desquamative inflammatory vaginitis. Any blood in the vagina or cervical secretions will increase the pH.

In recurrent or resistant cases of VVC, vaginal cultures for *Candida* can confirm the diagnosis, identify less common species, and redirect treatment when candidiasis is suspected but the KOH wet smear is inconclusive (CDC, 2021). It is important to use a culture medium capable of identifying fungal organisms and to note this request on the laboratory form. Routine vaginal aerobic cultures will identify multiple types of normal vaginal flora and will not assist in the diagnosis of yeast species. The Gram stain method can also identify or confirm *Candida*, although it is infrequently used in the outpatient setting. Other modalities that are available but have fewer evidence-based studies supporting their efficacy include DNA probes and molecular testing methods. Yeast or fungal elements may be found incidentally on cervical cytology, but treatment is indicated only if the patient is having symptoms. *Candida* lives in the vagina as commensal, nonpathogenic organisms in many individuals, so these are often noted on cytology reports.

Differential Diagnosis

The differential diagnoses for VVC include BV, trichomoniasis, vulvar dermatitis (e.g., lichen sclerosus or lichen planus), chemical or irritant vaginitis, contact vaginitis, chlamydia, gonorrhea, genital herpes, atrophic vaginitis, desquamative inflammatory vaginitis, and normal physiologic discharge. Inadequate lubrication during coitus may also cause erythema and vulvar irritation. Clinicians should also consider candidiasis secondary to diabetes, pregnancy, HIV seropositivity, and infection with non-*C. albicans* species, such as *C. glabrata* or *C. tropicalis*.

Prevention

Candida organisms thrive in warm, damp environments, making the vagina an ideal location for its proliferation. Vaginal dysbiosis caused by the reduction of *Lactobacillus sp.* predisposes to VVC (Wang et al., 2024). However, when individuals increase their knowledge and understanding of presumed risk factors leading to VVC and manage them in their day-to-day lives, they can reduce their risk of VVC. Refer to the section on promoting and maintaining vaginal health at the beginning of this chapter.

Management

Given the wide availability of OTC therapies, many symptomatic individuals presume their symptoms are VVC related and choose to self-treat rather than see a healthcare provider. When self-treatment is ineffective and patients seek professional advice, accurate identification of the offending organisms is sometimes obscured by intravaginal OTC preparations. Only those who have been previously diagnosed with VVC and who are experiencing the same symptoms should attempt self-treatment with OTC medications. Any person whose symptoms persist or those who develop a recurrence of symptoms within 2 months of treatment should be evaluated by a clinician (CDC, 2021). Unnecessary or inappropriate use of OTC preparations is common and can lead to delays in treating other causes of vulvovaginitis.

VVC is classified as uncomplicated, complicated, or recurrent according to five features: clinical presentation, microbiology, host factors, response to therapy, and frequency of occurrence (CDC, 2021). After *Candida* is confirmed as the diagnosis, the clinician must then ascertain whether the infection is considered uncomplicated, complicated, or recurrent because this determination will guide appropriate treatment (refer to **Table 21-5**). Most individuals (80–90%) who have VVC will have uncomplicated disease. Those with complicated VVC will need special diagnostic testing and treatment regimens.

Nonpharmacologic

Individuals who have extensive irritation, swelling, and discomfort of the labia and vulva may find sitz baths helpful in decreasing inflammation and discomfort. Adding colloidal oatmeal to the bath may also decrease vulvar itching and inflammation.

Pharmacologic

A number of antifungal preparations are available for treatment of VVC (refer to **Table 21-6**), and no single brand is significantly more effective than another. Many effective topical azole drugs are available as OTC products; they have cure rates ranging

TABLE 21-5 Classification of Vulvovaginal Candidiasis

Uncomplicated VVC	Complicated VVC	Recurrent VVC (RVVC)
Sporadic or infrequent VVC **and** Mild to moderate VVC **and** Likely to be *C. albicans* **and** Immunocompetent people	RVVC **or** Severe VVC **or** Non-*C. albicans* candidiasis **or** People with diabetes, immunocompromising conditions (e.g., HIV infection), debilitation, or immunosuppressive therapy	Four or more episodes of culture-proven VVC in 1 year Pathogenesis of RVVC is poorly understood, and most individuals with RVVC have no apparent predisposing or underlying conditions Obtain vaginal cultures to confirm the clinical diagnosis and identify unusual species

Data from Centers for Disease Control and Prevention. (2021). Sexually transmitted diseases treatment guidelines 2021. MMWR. Recommendations and reports: Morbidity and mortality weekly report. *Recommendations and Reports, 70*(4), 1–187. https://doi.org/10.15585/mmwr.rr7004a1

TABLE 21-6 Vulvovaginal Candidiasis Treatment

Infection	Regimen
Uncomplicated VVC	**OTC intravaginal agents:** Clotrimazole 1% cream 5 g intravaginally for 7 to 14 days **or** Clotrimazole 2% cream 5 g intravaginally for 3 days **or** Miconazole 2% cream 5 g intravaginally for 7 days **or** Miconazole 4% cream 5 g intravaginally for 3 days **or** Miconazole 100 mg vaginal suppository, one suppository/day for 7 days **or** Miconazole 200 mg vaginal suppository, one suppository/day for 3 days **or** Miconazole 1,200 mg vaginal suppository, one suppository for 1 day **or** Tioconazole 6.5% ointment 5 g intravaginally in a single application **Prescription intravaginal agents:** Butoconazole 2% cream (single-dose bioadhesive product) 5 g intravaginally for a single application **or** Terconazole 0.4% cream 5 g intravaginally for 7 days **or** Terconazole 0.8% cream 5 g intravaginally for 3 days **or** Terconazole 80 mg vaginal suppository, one suppository for 3 days **Oral agent:** Fluconazole 150 mg oral tablet, one tablet in single dose **Pregnant women:** Topical azole therapy, applied for 7 days
Complicated VVC	**Recurrent VVC initial therapy:** Longer duration of initial therapy, such as topical azole for 7 to 14 days **or** Fluconazole 150 mg orally every third day for a total of 3 doses (days 1, 4, and 7) **or** Itraconazole 200 mg orally twice/day for 3 days **Recurrent VVC maintenance therapy:** Fluconazole 150 mg orally weekly for 6 months **or** Itraconazole 100 to 200 mg daily for 6 months **or** Miconazole 1,200 mg vaginal suppository, one suppository/week for 6 months **or** Intermittent use of topical treatments **Severe VVC:** Topical azole for 7 to 14 days **or** Fluconazole 150 mg in two sequential doses, second dose 72 hours after initial dose For severe vulvar symptoms, low-potency topical corticosteroid cream (clotrimazole–betamethasone or nystatin–triamcinolone) may be applied for 48 hours until antifungal medication begins its therapeutic effects **Non-*Candida albicans* VVC initial therapy:** Optimal treatment unknown; options include nonfluconazole azole drug (oral or topical) for 7 to 14 days **Recurrent non-*C. albicans* VVC:** Boric acid 600 mg in gelatin capsule vaginally once/day for 14 days (only when organism is culture-proven resistant to azoles) **HIV infection:** Should not differ from that of seronegative women

Data from Centers for Disease Control and Prevention. (2021).

from 80 to 90 percent among those who complete therapy (CDC, 2021), although there are increasing signs of resistance to azole therapies, even by *C. albicans* (Sobel, 2023). An alternative therapy to topical azoles for uncomplicated *Candida* is a single oral dose of fluconazole, 150 mg. For severe episodes of acute *Candida* vulvovaginitis, 150 mg of fluconazole may be prescribed and taken every 72 hours for two to three doses (CDC, 2021). In addition to the CDC-recommended therapies for recurrent VVC, 10 to 14 days of a topical therapy or oral fluconazole followed by fluconazole 150 mg weekly for 6 months shows high-quality evidence for efficacy.

Complicated VVC cases affect a relatively small number of people and are generally due to a recurrence of *C. albicans* or a non-*C. albicans* species, such as *C. parapsilosis*, *C. krusei*, or *C. glabrata*. Non-*C. albicans* yeast infections may not cause symptoms, so there is no need to treat asymptomatic women. When indicated, commonly prescribed azoles may not be effective against non-*C. albicans* species, posing some challenges in treatment. However, non-*C. albicans* infections generally respond favorably to azole medications but may require longer than the 1-to 3-day period of therapy recommended for uncomplicated VVC. The optimal treatment for non-*C. albicans* VVC is unknown. Oteseconazole, marketed as Vivjoa, was approved by the FDA in 2022 for recurrent VVC; however, availability and cost may impact accessibility (Vandecruys et al., 2023).

A recent comprehensive review reaffirmed the value of boric acid in the treatment of vaginitis conditions including both VVC and BV (Mitchell, 2024). The antibacterial, antifungal, antiseptic, and astringent properties of boric acid cause inhibition of growth in microbes and inhibit the formation of fungal and bacterial biofilm, demonstrating cure rates of 76 percent on average. The novel TOL-463, a combination of boric acid and ethylenediaminetetraacetic acid or boric acid/EDTA (et al., 2019) which was entering phase 2 clinical trials in 2022 holds great potential as a biofilm disruptor, demonstrating clinical cure rates of 81–92 percent in early trials with gel or vaginal insert. Compared with fluconazole for patients with *C. glabrata*, boric acid inserts were more effective, with an 81 percent cure rate compared to 60 percent with azole treatment (Müller et al., 2024).

Diabetes screening should be considered for those with recurrent infections and comorbidities, such as obesity or family history of diabetes. Testing for chlamydia, gonorrhea, and HIV is recommended if the history indicates the presence of risk factors for STIs. Refer to Chapter 22 for more information about STI risk factors and testing.

Complementary and Alternative Therapies

Although many patients will have successful treatment outcomes with antifungals, drug intolerance, treatment failure and recurrence, and antifungal resistant strains of *Candida* remain clinical challenges, and individuals may seek out more "natural" treatments. It is important to advise individuals that although complementary and alternative methods may be widely used, there is a lack of scientific study confirming safety and efficacy of most therapies (Cooke, 2022). Alternative and complementary therapies that are nonetheless widely used for VVC can be found in **Table 21-7**. Evidence-based complementary therapies currently under research include biotics (Wang et al., 2024), and plant-based remedies (Chauhan, et al., 2024), which while studied in animal models have not advanced to human trials.

Referral

People with evidence of systemic *Candida* should be referred to a specialist. Others who may benefit from referral to an infectious disease specialist include those with chronic, recurrent VVC who have comorbidities such as HIV or uncontrolled diabetes; those who have transplanted organs and are using immunosuppressant drugs or who have resistant non-*C. albicans* VVC; and those who are symptomatic and remain culture positive despite longer-term and/or maintenance therapy (CDC, 2021). Consider testing patients with recurrent, recalcitrant infection for diabetes, HIV, or other diseases that affect immune function, such as lupus, Crohn's disease, chronic fatigue syndrome, and others.

Emerging Evidence

VVC is an important public health problem whose etiology is not yet fully understood. Evolving research is revealing a new understanding of the pathogenesis of VVC, leading to a more complex set of circumstances working synchronously to facilitate infection. These etiologic factors involve host immune function, the composition of the vaginal microbiome, availability of estrogen, virulence of the specific organism, and changes in vaginal pH (Sobel, 2024; Wang et al., 2024). In a summary of two decades of work on prebiotics, probiotics, and postbiotics, especially in combination with traditional antifungals, Wang's work (2024) out of China notes multiple advantages, but calls for more definitive research, as well as for investigation of the potential of vaginal microbiome transfer as a promising area of inquiry. Four vaccines are mentioned in the literature with work dating back to 2012, but as of 2025 none have been approved (Wychrij et al., 2025). Ongoing studies of complementary and alternative methods of treatments are needed to verify safe and effective treatments for VVC.

Patient Education

It is essential for patients to complete the full course of prescribed antifungal treatment. If using intravaginal medication, instruct them to continue application during menstruation. Advise against tampon use during treatment because tampons will absorb the vaginal medication. If possible, individuals should avoid intercourse during treatment. If this is not feasible, use of a nonlatex condom during intercourse may decrease introduction of more organisms. However, it is important to advise people that vaginal creams and suppositories recommended for treatment of VVC are oil based, so they may weaken latex condoms and diaphragms.

Clinical observations and research have also suggested that wearing tight-fitting clothing and underwear and tights/leggings made of nonabsorbent materials creates an environment in which *Candida* can grow. Decreasing use of unnecessary antibiotics and reducing intake of refined sugars in the diet may diminish *Candida* colonization. Other studies continue to explore host genetic and microbiome factors, probiotic therapy, anti-*Candida* defense mechanisms, and genetic yeast factors that facilitate persistence of VVC. There is no evidence to treat the sexual partners of patients with recurrent VVC (Sobel, 2024).

The International Society for the Study of Vulvovaginal Disease has developed a mobile app, called Vulvovaginal Candidiasis, to assist with management of VVC. Available only for iOS devices, the application is targeted to clinicians but includes patient education materials.

TABLE 21-7 Alternative Measures for Managing Vulvovaginal Candidiasis

Intervention	Dosage	Administration	Use
Gentian violet	Few drops in water, 0.25–2%	Douche or local application	VVC
Vitamin C	500 mg 2 to 4 times/day	Orally	VVC
Acidophilus tablet	40 million to 1 billion units (1 tab) daily	Orally	VVC
Yogurt	One application to labia or in vagina	Hourly as needed	VVC
Garlic clove	One peeled clove wrapped in cloth and dipped in olive oil, or capsule form	Overnight in vagina, change daily	VVC
Boric acid powder	600 mg in gelatin capsule	Every day in vagina for 14 days (toxic if ingested orally)	VVC
Sassafras bark	Steep in warm water Compress	Wash affected area	VVC
Cold milk, cottage cheese, yogurt	Compress or insert in vagina	Apply to affected area	Pruritus
Tea tree oil	Soaked tampon or one suppository	One suppository daily	Vulvovaginal inflammation
Sodium bicarbonate (baking soda)	6 to 12 g/L of water 2 or 3 times/week 15 to 30 g/500 cc warm water	Use in bath 2 or 3 times/week Vaginal irrigation Reassess after 2 to 3 weeks	VVC
Propolis (bee glue)	Vaginal cream or ovules	Topical; no dose given	VVC
Povidone-iodine	Vaginal suppository	No dose given	VVC

Data from Felix, T. C., de Brito Röder, D. V. D., & dos Santos Pedroso, R. (2019). Alternative and complementary therapies for vulvovaginal candidiasis. *Folia Microbiologica, 64*(2);

Falconi-McCahill, A. (2019). Bacterial vaginosis: A clinical update with a focus on complementary and alternative therapies. *Journal of Midwifery & Women's Health, 64*(5), 578–591. https://doi.org/10.1111/jmwh.13013

Considerations for Specific Populations

Adolescent and Premenarchal Individuals

After menarche, adolescents may develop VVC for reasons and risk factors similar to those of reproductive-aged individuals. Although premenarchal patients often develop vulvovaginitis, inflammation is rarely caused by *Candida* unless inflamed skin has become secondarily infected. Most vulvovaginitis in the premenarchal age group originates as contact dermatitis because there is minimal to no estrogen in the vagina, resulting in a typically alkaline vaginal pH. Vulvovaginal inflammations in premenarchal patients that are not irritant dermatitis are usually bacterial in origin and caused by organisms such as *Haemophilus influenzae*, gastrointestinal pathogens, or pinworms, and should not be treated with OTC antifungal medications. Premenarchal individuals presenting with vaginal discharge need a thorough examination, a culture of the discharge, and appropriate treatment with antibiotics. In some cases, a foreign body may be responsible for odor and vaginitis. In any case, concern for sexual assault or molestation must be ruled out (ACOG, 2006, reaffirmed 2019).

Pregnant and Breastfeeding People

Pregnant people who suspect they have VVC should be counseled not to self-treat their symptoms, but instead to contact their healthcare provider. Currently, topical azoles are the only forms of treatment for VVC recommended for use by pregnant patients (CDC, 2021). Oral fluconazole is not recommended for use during pregnancy due to epidemiological links with congenital anomalies and spontaneous abortion in animal models. Until further studies are done, people are advised to avoid oral fluconazole during pregnancy. Fluconazole is found in breastmilk but is considered safe for use during breast and chestfeeding, especially for the treatment of breastfeeding individuals with *Candida* mastitis or whose infants have oral thrush (Drugs and Lactation Database, 2018).

Perimenopausal and Older Individuals

There are very few studies examining the prevalence and incidence of VVC during the climacteric. In perimenopause, VVC and colonization rates decline, but shift toward a more resistant non-albicans species (Willems et al., 2021). In general, following menopause, the occurrence of VVC declines considerably, except among individuals using hormone therapy due to the resulting increase in systemic estrogen. In a study comparing the incidence of VVC in postmenopausal individuals receiving HRT, culture-positive VVC was found in 49 percent versus 1 percent of those not on HRT, lending further support to disease models that find a relationship between hormone levels and occurrence of VVC (Denning et al., 2018). Symptoms commonly associated with VVC often mimic those of atrophic vaginitis (AV), creating the potential for misdiagnosis and ineffective treatment, which can further aggravate symptoms and impede effective diagnosis. Although VVC is not as common in the postmenopausal period as in reproductive years, it does occur and can be overlooked. More targeted epidemiological studies are needed to clarify the clinical implications in this demographic.

Global Variations

Denning et al. (2018) performed a systematic review examining the global burden of recurrent VVC to 2030, estimating that the population of women with RVVC each year will increase to almost 158 million, with largest increases seen in the Global South. This additional 20 million cases of RVVC in less resourced areas is exacerbated by imprecise diagnoses, incorrect empirical therapies, and the emergence of azole-resistant strains. In epidemiologic studies, there appear to be geographic differences with respect to etiologic species of *Candida* associated with VVC. For example, in older studies, researchers who examined the distribution of *Candida* worldwide found that species such as *C. glabrata*, *C. tropicalis*, and *C. parapsilosis* are more widespread and more commonly associated with VVC among countries in Asia and Africa, when compared with *C. albicans* as the dominant species associated with VVC in the United States. Higher-quality epidemiologic work is needed.

DESQUAMATIVE INFLAMMATORY VAGINITIS

Description

Desquamative inflammatory vaginitis (DIV) is a less well known and often overlooked vaginitis, which disproportionately impacts perimenopauseal and postmenopausal patients. DIV is characterized by a profuse, noninfectious vaginal discharge, accompanied by vaginal irritation, burning, and dyspareunia (Deka et al., 2021). DIV describes the occurrence of desquamation and inflammation, but its etiology is unknown. Expert consensus suggests that DIV is an inflammatory disorder with an immune component which includes a secondary disruption (Sobel, 2024). The predominant lactobacilli flora of the vagina are replaced with gram-positive coccobacilli, usually *E. coli*, leading to the old nomenclature of "aerobic vaginitis" (Sonthalia et al., 2020). The shift in vaginal flora is most likely a consequence of the inflammatory process and not the cause of it. The underlying mechanisms in understanding how or why the disruption of normal lactic-acid-producing bacteria occurs remains a conundrum, yet there is relatively little literature on the subject of DIV, compared with other types of vaginitis. DIV is a clinical syndrome based on nonspecific laboratory findings, signs, and symptoms (Deka et al., 2021; Mitchell et al., 2024). Often the diagnosis of DIV is one of exclusion that occurs only after more common conditions, such as trichomoniasis or severe atrophy, have been ruled out.

Incidence, Prevalence, and Scope

DIV is a less common vaginitis seen in pregnant, premenopausal, and postmenopausal patients. The true prevalence of DIV in the general population is difficult to determine because it is not commonly seen in general primary care and gynecologic health practices. However, in specialized vaginitis referral clinics, 8 percent of patients presenting with vaginitis were diagnosed with DIV, and tended to be older and in the perimenopause (Sobel, 2024). Although not well studied, DIV has been linked to premature birth, premature rupture of membranes, chorioamnionitis, and other adverse pregnancy outcomes (Zarmakoupi et al., 2024).

Etiology and Pathophysiology

The precise cause of DIV is uncertain, but signs and symptoms associated with DIV overlap with immune-related conditions, such as vaginal lichen planus. Similar to BV, DIV also appears to stem from a disruption of the normal vaginal microbiome. The vaginas of patients with DIV are colonized by bacteria such as *E. coli*, *Staphylococcus aureus*, group B streptococcus, and *Enterococcus faecalis*. Several etiologies have been proposed as playing a role in the development of DIV, yet they remain inconclusive. These etiologies include estrogen deficiency, bacterial infection, a specific type of gene known to be related to skin desquamation, and autoimmune or immune-induced conditions (Zarmakoupi et al., 2024). It is classified as primary or secondary, with primary being idiopathic, and secondary related to a drug interaction or other immune-mediated disorder (Sobel, 2024).

Clinical Presentation and Variation

When present, a typical manifestation of DIV is a profuse, purulent appearing, yellow discharge. It is generally homogeneous and without odor. The vagina is often erythematous, and erosions of the vaginal walls may be seen in severe instances. Patients report dyspareunia, vaginal/introital pain, and burning (Sobel, 2024). Symptoms may come and go, may last for some time, and may be severely or mildly symptomatic, suggesting a chronic or recurrent nature to the syndrome, necessitating long-term or maintenance therapy (Paavonen & Brunham, 2018; Reichman & Sobel, 2014). **Color Plate 3** compares features of normal vaginal flora, BV, and DIV.

Assessment

History

It is important to collect a detailed and thorough history, with an understanding of how long symptoms have persisted, whether they are recurrent or intermittent, and what treatments, both prescribed and self-administered, have been used. Inquire about menstrual and sexual history, recent gynecologic procedures, symptoms of urinary tract infection, and postpartum status. Ask patients about sexual behaviors and whether there is dyspareunia. Most people with DIV will have experienced vaginal symptoms for several months prior to a diagnosis being determined, and common symptoms are profuse vaginal discharge and dyspareunia (Deka et al., 2021).

Physical Examination

Assess the vulva for evidence of discharge, edema, erythema, and any other lesions. The vestibule is often erythematous. After the speculum is inserted, note the color, consistency, odor, and amount of vaginal discharge. Determine vaginal pH and assess whether testing for STIs may be indicated. Assess the vaginal walls for redness, ecchymotic rash, and focal or linear erosion. Colpitis macularis (strawberry cervix) or petechiae may be present, similar to inflammation seen with trichomoniasis infection. Examine the cervix for ectopy, bleeding, edema, and whether an IUD string is present (if relevant).

Diagnostic Testing

Because the exact cause of DIV has not been fully elucidated, methods for a precise diagnosis of DIV are also imprecise, and it is described as a diagnosis of exclusion (Deka et al., 2021). In the outpatient setting, microscopy and wet mount testing reveal findings consistent with inflammation, such as presence of immature squamous (parabasal) cells and large numbers of white blood cells, often greater than 100 per high-power field. Vaginal pH will be elevated over 4.5. Although pH testing provides useful information for assessment of several types of vaginitis, it is not sensitive for diagnosis and may be falsely elevated if red blood cells or cervical mucus are present. In sexually active patients *Neisseria gonorrhoeae, Chlamydia trachomatis,* and *Tricomonas vaginalis* must be excluded. Vaginal cultures are not recommended because cultures will identify multiple microbes in the vagina without being diagnostic.

Differential Diagnoses

The differential diagnoses for DIV include atrophic vaginitis, BV, VVC, trichomoniasis, presence of a foreign body, chemical vaginitis (e.g., from latex or spermicide), cervicitis, contact vaginitis, lactational vaginitis, chlamydia, gonorrhea, genital herpes, cervicitis, erosive lichen planus, pemphigus vulgaris, cicatricial pemphigoid, and normal physiologic discharge (Sobel, 2024). Common misdiagnoses include trichomoniasis and advanced atrophic vaginitis, but DIV does not respond to either a course of metronidazole or topical estrogen; thus, the clinician should be alerted to the possibility of DIV (Deka et al., 2021).

Prevention

Perhaps because there is no clear recognizable etiology to the development of DIV, there is limited, if any, literature on prevention. Although some studies suggest that certain probiotics may be useful in recolonizing and reacidifying the vagina to protect it from disease, the current state of the science is insufficient to develop guidelines or make recommendations for practice.

Management

Nonpharmacologic

There are no known nonpharmacologic therapies published for the treatment of DIV.

Pharmacologic

Evidence-based guidelines for the treatment of DIV have not been developed. Treatments presented here are recommendations from experts and published studies. Clindamycin cream is used for its anti-inflammatory activities. The topical glucocorticoid hydrocortisone can be also be used. Either clindamycin 2 percent cream or 300 to 500 mg of 10 percent hydrocortisone cream is inserted intravaginally each night at bedtime for 4–6 weeks. Alternately, topical clobetasol gel 0.05 percent 500 mg can be applied intravaginally for 1 week. Patients should then be reevaluated. Either clindamycin or hydrocortisone can be continued once or twice per week for 2–6 months as maintenance therapy. Clinicians may consider the addition of weekly oral fluconazole or local estrogen as therapy for associated conditions (Sobel, 2024). Eighty percent of patients respond to treatment within 3 weeks. Relapse is common, lending support to the perception of DIV as a chronic inflammatory process. Expert opinion suggests close follow-up monthly to ensure remission. Because DIV is often found to be chronic or recurrent, clinicians must recognize these signs and prepare to manage patients on maintenance or perhaps long-term suppressive therapy with periodic evaluation. For patients who do not respond to treatment, the immunosuppressant tacrolimus ointment can be applied to the vagina sparingly (Sobel, 2024).

Complementary and Alternative Therapies

There are no published recommendations regarding the treatment of DIV using complementary and alternative therapies.

Referral

Essential to formulating a diagnosis of DIV is the availability of office pH testing and skill in microscopy. A high-quality phase contrast microscope provides very clear images and can improve diagnostic accuracy of microscopy. Clinicians must have appropriate education and comfort in using microscopy to properly evaluate saline and KOH wet prep slides of the vaginal discharge. Refer to Chapter 8 for more information about microscopic examination of vaginal secretions. In addition to recognizing clue cells, yeast buds, and trichomonads, clinicians must also be able to identify parabasal cells, polymorphonuclear white blood cells, and background bacteria to put this information together with the clinical examination and the patient's history. DIV is often a diagnosis of exclusion; therefore, it is critical to rule out other causes of purulent vaginitis before consulting with or referring to a specialist.

Emerging Evidence

Scientists are studying factors that may predict both response to treatment and which individuals will require long-term therapy for management of symptoms. It is possible there are serologic biomarkers of autoimmune disease that could be found in individuals affected by DIV (Reichman & Sobel, 2020). Further research is needed to improve understanding of the vaginal microbiome, how to maintain colonization of protective bacteria, and how to improve host response to changes when they occur to protect the vagina and thus the reproductive health of all people worldwide.

Patient Education

After the diagnosis of DIV has been made and treatment begins, the majority of individuals experience significant improvement but not necessarily cure. Clinicians can talk with patients about the possibility of recurrence and chronicity of the syndrome, necessitating repeat office visits for reevaluation and perhaps incurring costs for long-term medications, particularly those requiring compounding and vaginal administration. Inform patients that DIV is not an STI and, based on current understanding, lifestyle, sexual practices, and behaviors do not cause DIV. Current literature does not describe a role for condoms in either prevention or symptom reduction, although safe sex practices are always important for protecting reproductive health. It is essential that patients complete all therapy as prescribed because this is key for decreasing symptoms.

ATROPHIC VAGINITIS AND GSM

Atrophic vaginitis (AV) is a symptomatic condition seen frequently among people experiencing decreased estrogen production as a result of perimenopause, postmenopausal status, premature ovarian failure, lactation, or another cause. AV may develop as a consequence of genitourinary syndrome of menopause (GSM), formerly known as vulvovaginal atrophy (VVA). GSM is a broader term that encompasses a range of vulvar, vaginal, and urinary tract symptoms and physical changes associated with estrogen deficiency. One rationale for the change in terminology from AV and VVA to GSM is to decrease stigma associated with terms such as atrophic and atrophy. Use of a less pejorative term, such as GSM, might help increase awareness and ease both patient's and clinicians' comfort levels in discussing this condition (Mili et al., 2021; North American Menopause Society [NAMS], 2020). Untreated GSM is a progressive condition that can significantly interfere with quality of life. AV is but one of a range of inflammatory, symptomatic syndromes resulting from GSM (NAMS, 2020).

Although AV is most frequently seen with GSM, it can occur as a distinct entity in individuals with decreased estrogen from any cause. Lactation and cancer treatments, such as surgical therapy and radiation, can also damage the vaginal epithelium, lead to vaginal stenosis, induce AV, and increase the risk of other vaginal infections. Medications and hypothalamic amenorrhea can also cause AV.

Incidence, Prevalence, and Scope

An estimated 27 to 84 percent of people in the menopausal transition have symptoms of GSM (NAMS, 2020). Many patients do not discuss these symptoms with their providers, often due to embarrassment, and they may not seek help to alleviate symptoms (Mili et al., 2021). For these reasons, GSM is frequently underdiagnosed. Among people who have been treated with chemotherapy or endocrine therapy for breast cancer, AV is believed to affect nearly 70 percent. As treatment for breast cancer advances, survivors are now living longer following treatment.

AV and other aspects of GSM have become significant quality of life issues for a growing population. In a systematic review of 27 studies, it was found that vaginal health is often not discussed by providers, awareness of treatment options is low, and the majority of patients who experience GSM are not satisfied with their treatment (Mili et al., 2021). Additionally, the high cost of menopausal therapies may make them cost prohibitive for patients, and lead clinicians to prescribe less effective treatments, resulting in undertreatment of symptoms (Bachmann & Pinkerton, 2024).

Etiology and Pathophysiology

During menopause, estradiol production decreases by 99 percent. In the vagina, the menopause transition is accompanied by decreased production of glycogen by vaginal epithelium and a decrease in lactic acid production by a diminishing number of lactobacilli, resulting in a lower vaginal pH, thus setting the stage for development of inflammation and overgrowth of abnormal cells. Diminished vaginal estrogen affects collagen, lubrication, and vascularity of the vaginal epithelium, predisposing people to vaginal irritation (Bachman & Pinkerton, 2024).

The physiology of lactational AV is similar to that of menopause-related AV; estrogen depletion is the primary etiology. The presence of estrogen increases the thickness and elasticity of the vaginal walls and promotes an acidic environment. In lactating individuals, high prolactin levels keep estrogen levels low, which can cause symptoms of vaginal dryness, vaginal discharge, and painful intercourse (Perelmuter et al., 2025). In a systematic review examining lactation-induced hormonal deficiency, a majority of patients reported AV, dryness, and sexual dysfunction (Perelmuter et al., 2025). Despite this finding, there is a lack of screening recommendations or treatment guidelines for postpartum visits (Perelmuter et al., 2024).

Pharmacologic therapies used as a component of breast cancer treatment—specifically aromatase inhibitors, such as anastrozole, letrozole, and exemestane—produce a symptomatic estrogen-deficiency state. Aromatase inhibitors prevent the conversion of androgens to estrogens, thereby causing vaginal dryness and dyspareunia (NAMS, 2020). Other conditions leading to a reduced estrogen state include surgical menopause (bilateral oophorectomy with or without removal of the uterus), use of medications such as gonadotropin-releasing hormone (GnRH) agonists used to treat endometriosis and uterine leiomyomata, and hypothalamic amenorrhea caused by excessive physical activity seen in athletes or among people with eating disorders such as anorexia (NAMS, 2020). In summary, a state of decreased estrogen, attributable to any cause, may result in AV.

Clinical Presentation and Variations

Up to 70 percent of individuals with AV may not report genital symptoms due to embarrassment or difficulty in speaking with clinicians about intimate concerns. Cultural or religious beliefs can contribute to this silence, and surveys of patients exploring menopausal experiences suggest that many people believe these symptoms are a normal part of the aging process (Bachman & Pinkerton, 2024). Those presenting with symptoms may be lactating, perimenopausal, menopausal, postmenopausal, or breast cancer survivors. In recognition of the prevalence of AV and GSM, their progressive nature, and the fact that patients often do not report symptoms of these conditions, it is incumbent on clinicians to ask people about their urogenital health during the course of routine physical examinations. Clinicians can assess premenopausal patients for contributing factors. Individuals with AV and GSM may report symptoms of vaginal dryness, burning, irritation, itching, discharge, odor, dysuria, urinary frequency, nocturia, and frequent urinary tract infections.

Assessment

History

Each gynecologic visit presents the clinician with an opportunity for conversation and education around sensitive topics. Due to the reticence of many patients to discuss intimate concerns, clinicians must be proactive in their approach. Common symptoms of AV include vaginal dryness and discomfort; decreased lubrication during sexual activity; dyspareunia; postcoital vaginal bleeding; decreased arousal, orgasm, or sexual desire; and urinary symptoms (Bachman & Pinkerton, 2024). People may have symptoms of AV whether or not they are sexually active. Premenopausal patients can also experience symptoms of AV. Systemic conditions such as breast and chestfeeding, postpartum estrogen deficiency, or use of certain medications can cause AV. Ask all patients about the use of GnRH agonist analogs (e.g., leuprolide), selective estrogen receptor modulators (SERMs; e.g., tamoxifen), aromatase inhibitors, danazol, and medroxyprogesterone. Also ascertain if they have experienced surgical menopause (i.e., removal of both ovaries) or another iatrogenic cause of estrogen deficiency, such as chemotherapy or radiation therapy. Transgender individuals taking testosterone commonly experience vaginal discomfort due to atrophy from testosterone-blocking estrogen production (Krakowsky et al., 2022; Winston McPherson et al., 2019).

Physical Examination

Vulvar examination may or may not reveal some degree of pelvic organ prolapse if the patient is postmenopausal. Tissues of the vulva may be thin, and a loss of subcutaneous fat may be noted. In severe cases of GSM, there may be no clear distinction between the labia minora and majora. The vaginal introitus may be stenotic. Speculum and bimanual examination may be painful and use of the smallest and most narrow speculum for the examination is recommended. The vagina may be shortened, and vaginal fornices may be flush with the surface of the cervix (Bachman & Pinkerton, 2024; NAMS, 2020). On examination, the vaginal epithelium is pale, with diminished rugae. Vaginal ulcerations may be present as a consequence of intercourse in an inadequately lubricated vagina. AV is characterized by scant vaginal secretions, elevated vaginal pH, and an increase in white blood cells. A yellow or light brown discharge may be noted. Petechiae may or may not be seen on the cervix. If performing a Pap test, the cervical os may be completely stenotic, and clinicians may be unable to insert either a cytobrush or broom collection device to obtain a sample.

Diagnostic Testing

The diagnosis of AV is often made based on elicited history and clinical findings. Although there are no specific diagnostic tests for this condition, some testing modalities can aid in diagnosis. Testing vaginal pH and calculating a vaginal maturation index (VMI) can be helpful. Vaginal pH is typically greater than 5.0. Clinicians can ask the cytology laboratory to perform vaginal maturation index testing.

On microscopy, white blood cells are often increased, while lactobacilli are diminished or absent. The background may contain multiple bacteria. The atrophic vagina is frequently repopulated with enteric organisms previously kept in check by the healthy, acidic vagina (NAMS, 2020). Parabasal cells with large nuclei are seen. Because they share similar clinical features and histories, it is possible for clinicians to misdiagnose AV and DIV. Both may present with similar patient histories, have similar appearances under microscopy, and are characterized by chronicity, challenging a clinician's diagnostic expertise. When uncertain about whether the diagnosis is AV or DIV, treat for AV first, then for DIV if the patient is still symptomatic (Mitchell et al., 2024).

Differential Diagnosis

The differential diagnoses for AV and GSM include bacterial vaginosis, vulvovaginal candidiasis, vulvar dermatitis, herpes lesions, vulvodynia, sexually transmitted infections, and normal physiologic discharge (Bachman & Pinkerton, 2024). Vulvovaginal dermatoses may be considered as differential diagnoses; these include lichen sclerosis, lichen planus, and lichen simplex chronicus, which are discussed in Chapter 27. Excluding precancerous or cancerous lesions of the internal or external genitalia should be included in the differential diagnoses because symptoms similar to AV may also arise in conjunction with cancer or extramammary Paget disease. If the diagnosis is unclear or if therapy has been ineffective, consider vaginal or vulvar biopsy.

Prevention

Prevention of AV secondary to menopause lies in recognizing that GSM is a chronic and recurring condition that significantly affects quality of life in many people, particularly following menopause. Therefore, prevention relies on clinicians' thorough review of health histories, identifying risk factors, and bringing the topic of GSM into the conversation of preventive health care. Preserving sexual function is a highly individual matter and may or may not be an important health concern. Sexual intercourse has been shown to enhance blood circulation to the vagina, while seminal fluid is rich with sexual steroids, prostaglandins, and essential fatty acids that help maintain strength and elasticity of vaginal tissues. Masturbation and use of sexual toys are also options for maintenance of vaginal health (NAMS, 2020). Currently, there are few, if any, data on the prevention of AV. Theoretically, it may be possible that regular use of low-dose vaginal estrogen may avert symptoms associated with AV (NAMS, 2020).

Management

Nonpharmacologic

The treatment for AV and GSM will depend on preference, severity of symptoms, effectiveness, and safety of treatments (NAMS, 2020). For many people, regular use of either a water-soluble or silicone-based lubricant will be adequate to maintain vaginal comfort during sexual intercourse (Mitchell et al., 2024). Lubricants and moisturizers are designed for short-term comfort; do not necessarily replace long-term therapies, such as estrogen, will not reverse physiologic changes associated with AV or GSM; and are generally more helpful for those having mild symptoms (Mitchell et al., 2024; Bachmann & Pinkerton, 2024). For some people, these short-term relief agents will be enough. A recent systematic review found vaginal moisturizers to be essentially equivalent to vaginal estrogen and recommend they be offered to those who wish to avoid hormonal therapies while affirming that vaginal lubricants do not offer long-term therapeutic effects (Casiano Evans et al., 2023).

There are differences between vaginal lubricants and vaginal moisturizers that are important for clinicians and patients to appreciate. The primary distinction is in their intended use and composition. Lubricants may be water-, silicone-, mineral-, or plant-based and are most useful for those whose primary concern is vaginal dryness during intercourse. Vaginal moisturizers are more likely to mimic vaginal secretions due to their rehydrating effect and adherence to the vaginal wall. Moisturizers are applied on a regular basis (usually twice per week) and are capable of lowering vaginal pH and exerting longer-lasting effects (2 to 3 days) than lubricants. Moisturizers and lubricants may also be useful for patients who are not sexually active but are experiencing uncomfortable day-to-day vaginal dryness (Bachman & Pinkerton, 2024). Lubricants and moisturizers can be safely used long term as needed for symptom relief. A topical application of 4 percent aqueous lidocaine may be applied topically to the vestibule as an adjunct to lubricants and moisturizers for women who are experiencing pain (Faubion et al., 2018). In addition to these products and pharmacologic treatments, individuals who have pelvic floor muscle dysfunction related to GSM may benefit from pelvic floor therapy, biofeedback, or referral to a sex therapist (Faubion et al., 2018). Refer to Chapters 12 and 14 for additional recommendations on the use of lubricants and moisturizers, including specific products to use or avoid.

Pharmacologic

A number of medications are used to treat AV and GSM, including vaginal estrogen, SERMs, and dehydroepiandrosterone (refer to **Table 21-8**).

Vaginal Estrogen Low-dose vaginal estrogen is the primary pharmacologic therapy for treatment of AV and can be used during lactation. Estrogen therapy promotes revascularization of

TABLE 21-8 Treatment Options for Atrophic Vaginitis and Genitourinary Syndrome of Menopause

Type	Product Name	Active Ingredient	Dose
Estrogen			
Vaginal cream	Estrace	17β-estradiol	0.5 to 2 g once/day for 2 weeks, then taper gradually to lowest effective dose, usually 0.5 to 1 g 1 to 3 times/week
	Premarin	Conjugated equine estrogens	0.5 to 2 g once/day for 2 weeks, then taper gradually to lowest effective dose, usually 0.5 to 1 g 1 to 3 times/week
Vaginal tablet	Vagifem, Yuvafem	Estradiol hemihydrate	10 mcg once/day for 2 weeks, then 10 mcg 2 times/week
Vaginal softgel	Imvexxy	17β-estradiol	4 mcg once/day for 2 weeks, then 4 mcg 2 times/week
Vaginal ring	Estring	Micronized 17β-estradiol	7.5 mcg/24 hours, replace every 90 days
	Femring[a]	Estradiol acetate	0.05 mg/day or 0.1 mg/day, replace every 3 months
SERM			
Oral tablet	Osphena	Ospemifene	60 mg once/day
Dehydroepiandrosterone (DHEA)			
Vaginal insert	Intrarosa	Prasterone (plant-derived version of endogenous DHEA)	6.5 mg once/day at bedtime

Data from The NAMS 2020 GSM Position Statement Editorial Panel. (2020). The 2020 genitourinary syndrome of menopause position statement of The North American Menopause Society. *Menopause (New York, N.Y.), 27*(9), 976–992. https://doi.org/10.1097/GME.0000000000001609

Danan, E. R., Sowerby, C., Ullman, K. E., Ensrud, K., Forte, M. L., Zerzan, N., Anthony, M., Kalinowski, C., Abdi, H. I., Friedman, J. K., Landsteiner, A., Greer, N., Nardos, R., Fok, C., Dahm, P., Butler, M., Wilt, T. J., & Diem, S. (2024). Hormonal treatments and vaginal moisturizers for genitourinary syndrome of menopause: A systematic review. *Annals of Internal Medicine, 177*(10), 1400–1414. https://doi.org/10.7326/ANNALS-24-00610

[a]This product provides systemic hormone levels to treat vasomotor symptoms in addition to GSM.

the vaginal epithelium and restores the normal pH of the vagina by increasing the number of lactobacilli. Estrogen improves the vaginal maturation index, improves epithelial integrity, and increases vaginal secretions. Estrogen, either topical or oral, can improve moderate or severe symptoms, and both preparations can be used at the same time (Danan et al., 2024). Low-dose vaginal estrogen can also lead to improvements in urinary symptoms of GSM, such as nocturia and urinary urgency and frequency, and decrease dyspareunia (NAMS, 2020). Vaginal preparations include creams, suppositories, rings, and ovules (refer to Table 21-6). Prescription vaginal estrogens are available as either estradiol or conjugated estrogen formulations. Although systemic or transdermal estrogen can be used for GSM, vaginal application is the preferred mode of delivery and is generally more effective than other routes when vaginal symptoms are the primary concern (NAMS, 2020). Multiple clinical trials and systematic reviews have confirmed the effectiveness of vaginal estrogen with respect to patients' subjective and objective outcome measures on symptoms of AV. Although the risk profile for vaginal estrogen is quite low, and vaginal administration produces hormone levels that are very low, compared with oral or other routes, patients using vaginal estrogen may experience VVC, breast pain, and vaginal bleeding.

An important concern regarding use of vaginal estrogen in individuals with a uterus is overgrowth and possible endometrial cancer as a result of unopposed estrogen use. Several studies have shown that low-dose vaginal estrogen therapy does not increase endometrial hyperplasia and can be safely used without a progestin after all other risk factors and benefits have been reviewed (NAMS, 2020). Because systemic absorption is limited by avoidance of first pass through the liver, an additional progestin is not needed if using only topical estrogen in patients with an intact uterus (NAMS, 2020). Currently there are insufficient data to recommend routine endometrial surveillance either by ultrasound or endometrial biopsy among asymptomatic women; any occurrence of vaginal bleeding requires appropriate investigation of the endometrium.

When selecting vaginal estrogen therapy with perimenopausal and postmenopausal patients, be sure to advise them that exclusive use of vaginal estrogen will not reduce hot flashes or reduce risk of osteoporosis; it will treat only AV and dyspareunia associated with GSM and may also reduce risk of frequent urinary tract infection, frequency, urgency, and nocturia not associated with infection (Bachman & Pinkerton, 2024). Many people are reluctant to initiate any hormonal therapy due to its associations with breast cancer and other safety concerns; however, vaginal estrogen therapy for AV and other symptoms of GSM is an underused therapy and likely safe for the majority of patients. Contraindications to the use of hormone therapy for treatment of AV include current breast cancer, history of estrogen-dependent cancer, active liver disease, history of pulmonary embolism or deep vein thrombosis, or known intolerance to any component of the hormonal preparation (Fait, 2019). A history of breast cancer is a relative contraindication to vaginal estrogen use, and although lifestyle modifications, lubricants, and moisturizers are preferred, use of low-dose vaginal estrogen treatment may be individualized for the patient in conjunction with their oncologist's review and oversight (Bachman & Pinkerton, 2024). Refer to Chapter 14 for additional information about menopause and estrogen therapy.

Selective Estrogen Receptor Modulators Ospemifene is a SERM with specific vaginal effects and is approved by the FDA for treatment of moderate to severe dyspareunia in postmenopausal people who are not candidates for vaginal estrogen. It is the only SERM approved specifically for breast cancer survivors. Originally developed to treat osteoporosis, ospemifene was approved by the FDA following multiple phase III trials for the treatment of dyspareunia resulting from GSM. The researchers found that treatment with ospemifene was highly effective compared with placebo, and no serious adverse events were reported (Palacios, 2020). Ospemifene improves vaginal maturation and pH, reduces the percentage of parabasal cells, and reduces most symptoms associated with dyspareunia caused by vaginal dryness. In addition, this therapy shows a protective effect on bone health, and improved lipid parameters. Finally, animal models suggest that ospemifene may inhibit tumor growth, exerting a mildly chemoprotective effect, a finding collaborated by a study demonstrating no difference in breast cancer incidence between survivors treated or untreated with the medication (Palacios, 2020).

Tamoxifen and raloxifene are SERMs used to reduce risk of breast cancer recurrence. However, in contrast to ospemifene, these drugs produce an estrogenic effect on the endometrium and exert antiestrogenic effects on the vaginal epithelium. Therefore, while their use in reducing breast cancer recurrence is well recognized, tamoxifen and raloxifene are not appropriate for treating vaginal symptoms associated with AV or dyspareunia of GSM. The use of tamoxifen and raloxifene is associated with endometrial hyperplasia and increased vaginal discharge (NAMS, 2020).

Dehydroepiandrosterone Intravaginal dehydroepiandrosterone (DHEA, Prasterone) has been shown in some studies to decrease pain with sexual activity in patients with moderate to severe dyspareunia. It reduces discomfort associated with GSM by decreasing parabasal cells, improving vaginal pH, and improving epithelial thickness, compared with placebo. It is produced as a vaginal suppository in a dose of 0.50 percent (6.5 mg) DHEA. Inserted nightly, it can metabolize to estrogen, exert a local action on the vaginal epithelium to improve maturation of cells (decrease immature, parabasal cells), and does not stimulate or thicken the endometrium or increase systemic circulation of sex hormones (Danan et al., 2024).

Compounded Bioidentical Hormones Many patients will seek out "compounded bioidentical menopausal hormone therapy" as these formulations are often advertised as more "natural," than synthetic hormone preparations. A recent ACOG position statement strongly discourages the use of these products when safer, effective, evidence-based and FDA-approved formulations are available, and calls on clinicians to provide comprehensive explanations about tailored therapy using effective communication and counseling (ACOG, 2023; Cuccu et al., 2024). Refer to Chapter 14 for more information.

Complementary and Alternative Therapies

About 47 percent of patients use complementary and alternative therapies (CAM) and/or supplements for vaginal symptoms associated with AV or GSM (Ullman et al., 2024). These include homeopathy, phytoestrogens, probiotics, vitamins, and mind-body practices. Recently, the Agency for Healthcare Research and Quality (AHRQ) and the Patient Centered Research Institute (PCORI) joined forces to complete a systematic review of CAM approaches supported by RCTs for the treatment of GSM. They included 57 clinical trials evaluating 39 unique CAM interventions. Overall, studies were small, short term, and conducted outside the United States. Outcome measures were nonstandardized, as were the herbal products tested, making comparison and synthesis impossible. Authors concluded that while research is in development, there continues to be a dearth of well-developed, adequately powered, placebo-controlled trials providing convincing evidence for translation into clinical practice (Ullman, 2024).

Referral

Individuals who do not respond to treatment or who have other poorly controlled comorbid conditions wielding a deleterious effect on quality of life can be referred to a gynecologic or menopausal specialist. Survivors of cancer, including breast and other cancers, who present with symptoms of GSM affecting quality of life may be cared for either by clinicians with appropriate training or in conjunction with an oncologist. Those whose general health or menopausal symptoms are beyond the clinician's ability and skills to manage over a long period of time can also be referred to a specialist.

Emerging Evidence

Fractional carbon dioxide vaginal laser therapy has emerged as a potentially promising treatment option for GSM, although it has not received wide support due to a lack of research on long-term effects. Vaginal lasers apply energy to the vaginal epithelium causing necrosis, which is thought to induce collagen remodeling, neovascularization, and elastin formation, resulting in improved vaginal elasticity and improvement in GSM symptoms (Salvatore et al., 2023). Vaginal energy devices (such as CO_2 lasers) have been licensed in Canada but are not approved by the FDA. In fact, the FDA issued a warning in 2018 about the safety risks associated with these procedures including scarring, dyspareunia, and recurring chronic pain, particularly if used for vaginal "rejuvenation" or other cosmetic indications (FDA, 2018). Two systematic reviews have been published, both demonstrating overall positive results for treatment of GSM. A systematic review and meta-analysis of 25 studies involving 1,152 patients examining both subjective and objective data showed significant statistical and clinical improvement in symptoms (dryness, itching, burning, dysuria, and dyspareunia) after this treatment, with notable improvement in patient sexual function indices (Filippini et al., 2022; Cuccu et al., 2024). The author noted that the review was limited by study heterogeneity, and the fact that included research was conducted in single centers without randomized controlled trials. A second meta-analysis with 542 participants had the same results. Three subsequent international RCTs with limited participants comparing laser treatment with sham therapy, estrogen cream, and hyaluronic acid demonstrated similar improvements in GSM symptomology, suggesting that this treatment might have a role as a nonhormonal therapeutic modality. Both the American College of Obstetricians and Gynecologists and the American Urogynecologic Society have consensus statements which hold that while energy-based treatments show promise, more research is needed prior to widespread adoption (Bachman & Pinkerton, 2024). The North American Menopause Society (NAMS) recommends that providers review all the available options that have established safety profiles, such as lubricants, moisturizers, vaginal estrogen, and other FDA-approved therapies (Pinkerton & Kingsberg, 2018).

Patient Education

It is important to make patients aware of the availability of treatment for GSM, which can occur not only in response to the menopause transition, but also in conjunction with other circumstances leading to an estrogen-deficient state. Clinicians can educate patients about changes that accompany the menopausal transition in addition to preservation of sexual health throughout the life cycle. It is important to discuss protecting sexual health while seeking to better understand individual needs. Regular, safe, painless sexual activity can help maintain vaginal health and delay AV symptoms by improving blood flow to the vagina and maintaining vaginal elasticity (Carlson & Nguyen, 2024). Sex steroids, prostaglandins, and essential fatty acids are components of seminal fluid and may be soothing to vaginal tissue if STIs are not a concern. For symptomatic, sexually abstinent individuals, masturbation, use of dilators, vibrators, and lubricants can promote stretching of vaginal tissue and minimize dryness symptoms. People using vaginal moisturizers are recommended to select those that are compatible with vaginal secretions and pH. The value of educating patients proactively about urogenital symptoms that may occur in response to a low-estrogen state has not been determined. Individuals using vaginal preparations should be informed that vaginal secretions may increase and, if using estrogen, they may be more likely to experience vaginal yeast symptoms.

Considerations for Specific Populations

Individuals With a History of Breast Cancer

Advances in treatment among people with breast cancer have resulted in improved survival rates and longer life spans with 5-year survival rates 91 percent and 99 percent for early-stage localized cancers (American Cancer Society, 2024). Sexual problems among this population are common due to the use of antiestrogen therapies and the onset of treatment-induced menopause. It is important to remember that younger survivors with AV may or may not be postmenopausal. First-line therapies include lifestyle modifications, such as smoking cessation, and nonhormonal options including the use of vaginal moisturizers and lubricants. However, for many, lifestyle modifications and nonhormonal therapies may not provide adequate relief of symptoms, and treatment must be guided by the type of breast cancer treatment a patient is receiving. A 2018 consensus recommendation from NAMS and the International Society for the Study of Women's Sexual Health (ISSWSH) concluded that there was insufficient data to confirm the safety of vaginal estrogen for this population. However, a recent large cohort study comprised of 49,237 breast cancer patients analyzing the time to breast cancer–specific mortality found that there was no increase in mortality in patients who used vaginal estrogen therapy compared to those who did not use HRT (McVicker et al., 2024). Similar findings were reported in a Danish observational cohort study with 8,461 patients; neither vaginal estrogen therapy nor menopausal hormone therapy increased risk of recurrence (Cold et al., 2022). For patients treated with selective estrogen receptor modulators (SERMs) such as tamoxifen, who have hormone-receptor negative disease, low dose vaginal estrogen or vaginal dehydroepiandostrerone (DHEA or Prasterone) are good second-line options (McVicker et al., 2024). For patients on aromatase inhibitors (AIs), designed to reduce serum estrogen levels, minimizing potential tumor exposure to serum estrogen, the evidence is less clear, and expert opinion generally does not endorse the use of DHEA or testosterone due to limited data on long-term safety, although small studies suggest that topical vaginal estrogen improves sexual function and VA without persistent serum elevations of estradiol (Melisko et al., 2017).

In summary, among survivors with estrogen-dependent cancer, use of vaginal estrogen should be individualized, best reserved for individuals unresponsive to nonhormonal methods, and reviewed in consultation with an oncologist (ACOG, 2016, reaffirmed 2018). In such cases, an informed discussion of risks and benefits is essential.

TOXIC SHOCK SYNDROME

Description

TSS is a rare, life-threatening, toxin-mediated infectious process with an acute onset characterized by fever, low blood pressure, a sunburn-like body rash, and end-organ damage (Berger et al, 2019; CDC 2024). TSS was first named in 1978 by two pediatricians and their colleagues who described a set of symptoms that included high fever, rash, headache, vomiting, and acute renal failure in young boys and girls ages 8 to 17 between 1975 and 1977 (Todd et al., 1978). Bacterial exotoxins induce lymphocyte activation, leading to rapid shock, multiorgan failure, and death. TSS can be menstrual or nonmenstrual in origin (Atchade et al., 2024). Although most commonly caused by *Staphlococcus aureus*, pregnant patients are often infected with *Streptococcus pyogenes*, with 91 percent of those infections reported in the postpartum period (Harris et al., 2023). A more fatal variant caused by *Clostridium sordellii* (Elkbuli et al., 2018) is sometimes found in the postpartum period and following termination of pregnancy. TSS is a medical emergency, requiring rapid recognition, immediate resuscitation, identification of toxin origin, and immediate antibiotic treatment (Atchade et al., 2024).

Incidence, Prevalence, and Scope

Staphylococcal TSS emerged into public awareness in 1980, when it became apparent that young menstruating women using highly absorbent tampons were at high risk for TSS infection. A decline in TSS infection occurred following public health messages regarding safe tampon use in conjunction with removal from the market of a highly absorbent tampon brand that contributed to risk. The incidence of TSS in the United States is estimated to be about 0.8 to 3.4 per 100,000; mortality rates range from 1.8 to 12 percent (Ross & Shoff, 2019). Clostridial TSS is relatively rare, with 16 gynecologic cases appearing in the world literature, and an 87.5 percent mortality rate (Elkbuli et al., 2018).

While menstrual TSS rates have decreased, tampon use remains a risk factor, and patients should be cautioned against the prolonged use of high absorbency tampons and leaving a single tampon in place for an extended period of time. TSS has also been reported in users of menstrual cups, diaphragms, vaginal contraceptive sponges, and cervical caps (Berger, 2019). In a systematic review and metanalysis on the leakage, safety and acceptability of the menstrual cup, Van Eijk et al. (2019) reported five cases of TSS among 3,319 participants. This is theoretically related to factors promoting the growth of *S. aureus*, such as the accumulation of blood providing a medium for bacterial growth.

Etiology and Pathophysiology

S. aureus was identified as the primary pathogenic agent for TSS, with *Streptococcus pyogenes* (group A streptococci) subsequently, but less frequently, implicated. Although there are similarities, there are important distinctions in TSS depending on the causative agent. TSS caused by *S. aureus* is generally secondary to a localized infection, whereas TSS caused by *S. pyogenes* is the consequence of an invasive infection. Both forms of TSS are now seen as separate entities with different case definitions (NNDSS, 2024). Moreover, staphylococcal TSS is further subdivided into menstrual and nonmenstrual illness. *S. aureus* is a common bacterium that is responsible for several diseases and conditions, including skin boils, acne, and some severe forms of food poisoning. Staphylococcal TSS may also occur in children. Some strains of *S. aureus* and *S. pyogenes* produce powerful toxins that result in massive immune cell activation and cytokine release, leading to shock and organ failure (Berger, 2019). A systematic review of 13 case reports of patients who developed TSS following insertion of IUDs suggests that this should be included in the differential if patients present with symptoms, although the evidence was low quality (Hutcherson et al., 2025).

Clinical Presentation

Streptococcal toxic shock syndrome typically presents generally with fever and chills, muscle aches and nausea and vomiting. Within 24–48 hours it causes hypotension, tachycardia, tachypnea, and early signs of organ failure (CDC, 2024).

Assessment

History

In addition to a careful history of the patient's symptoms, their onset, and the course of the infection, it is important for the clinician to identify other risk factors including recent use of tampons ore other vaginal devices, prior colonization or infection with TSS, and gram negative co-colonization (Berger, 2019). TSS can also be the causative factor in sudden deaths following surgery, syndromes with systemic inflammatory features, or any condition with acute local inflammation including a bacterial entry site, such as tattooing (Shreiner & Balikowski, 2025).

Physical Examination

Upon physical examination, dermatologic findings may differ depending on the stage of the illness. Early signs may include generalized erythematous and macular rash; generalized, nonpitting edema; and erythema of the palms and soles. After the acute phase, findings may include generalized maculopapular rash and desquamation of the fingers, palms, toes, and soles, followed by full thickness peeling. Alterations to the mucous membranes of the mouth (e.g., strawberry tongue), conjunctival erythema, and vaginal ulcerations may be present. Pelvic examination may reveal hyperemic vaginal mucosa and vulvar and vaginal tenderness (CDC, 2024).

Diagnostic Testing

There is no definitive test to diagnose TSS. The diagnosis is made on the basis of clinical manifestations meeting the 2011 CDC case definition (CDC, 2021) (refer to **Table 21-9**).

Differential Diagnosis

Numerous conditions can cause fever and/or rash. TSS should be considered in any person with unexplained fever and a rash during or immediately following menses or use of intravaginal menstrual products. Other conditions that should be included in the differential diagnoses include sepsis caused by other factors, drug reactions, coronavirus disease 2019 (COVID-19), Rocky Mountain spotted fever (RMSF), leptospirosis, Dengue fever, and Kawasaki disease (Chu, 2024).

Prevention

Prevention of TSS lies in education about early signs and symptoms of the illness so that medical care is sought as soon as possible. In addition, people can take steps to prevent its occurrence, such as using low-absorbency tampons, changing tampons frequently, alternating pad and tampon use, avoiding overnight use of tampons, not leaving a menstrual cup in place for more than 12 hours, and removing barrier contraception within 24 hours.

Management

TSS can constitute an acute, life-threatening emergency. Individuals with a suspected case of TSS need emergency evaluation and medical care. Clinicians in emergency department settings must have a high index of suspicion when young people present with symptoms of shock. It is essential that an infectious disease specialist be consulted as soon as possible. Mortality can be prevented with aggressive treatment (Harris et al., 2023). Patients with TSS require intensive medical care and aggressive intravenous fluid hydration. Soft tissue infections and necrotizing fasciitis require urgent management and surgical consultation. Sources of bacteria, such as menstrual tampons, menstrual cups, or wound packings, should be removed and cultured. Supportive care is a component of TSS management.

Pharmacologic

Treatment is based on the causative pathogen and differs for methicillin-susceptible *S. aureus* (MSSA), methicillin-resistant *S. aureus* (MRSA), or *Streptococcus*. Broad-spectrum antibiotics can be administered until cultures have returned and the spectrum of antibiotics can be reduced and appropriately determined. Initially, antibiotic coverage must include those effective against methicillin-resistant *S. aureus* (MRSA), given the prevalence of resistant strains. Clindamycin is often added to reduce toxin production, although it is rarely used alone because it is bacteriostatic and not bactericidal. Therapy should also cover gram-negative organisms. Penicillin is generally the preferred antibiotic for group A streptococci. Current recommendations are for 14 days of treatment. Vasopressors are used for patients in shock who are not improving on IV fluids alone. Intravenous immunoglobulin is believed to neutralize toxin activity. TSS patients are gravely ill and require intensive care unit management.

TABLE 21-9 CDC 2011 Case Definition for Toxic Shock Syndrome

Clinical Criteria	An illness with the following clinical manifestations:
	• Fever: temperature greater than or equal to 102.0°F (greater than or equal to 38.9°C)
	• Rash: diffuse macular erythroderma
	• Desquamation: 1–2 weeks after onset of rash
	• Hypotension: systolic blood pressure less than or equal to 90 mm Hg for adults or less than the fifth percentile by age for children younger than 16 years
	• Multisystem involvement (three or more of the following organ systems):
	  • Gastrointestinal: vomiting or diarrhea at onset of illness
	  • Muscular: severe myalgia or creatine phosphokinase level at least twice the upper limit of normal
	  • Mucous membranes: vaginal, oropharyngeal, or conjunctival hyperemia
	  • Renal: blood urea nitrogen or creatinine at least twice the upper limit of normal for laboratory or urinary sediment with pyuria (greater than or equal to 5 leukocytes per high-power field) in the absence of urinary tract infection
	  • Hepatic: total bilirubin, alanine aminotransferase enzyme, or asparate aminotransferase enzyme levels at least twice the upper limit of normal for laboratory
	  • Hematologic: platelets less than 100,000/mm^3
	  • Central nervous system: disorientation or alterations in consciousness without focal neurologic signs when fever and hypotension are absent

Laboratory Criteria for Diagnosis	Negative results on the following tests, if obtained: • Blood or cerebrospinal fluid cultures (blood culture may be positive for *Staphylococcus aureus*) • Negative serologies for Rocky Mountain spotted fever, leptospirosis, or measles
Case Classification	• Probable: a case that meets the laboratory criteria and in which four of the five clinical criteria described above are present • Confirmed: a case that meets the laboratory criteria and in which all five of the clinical criteria described above are present, including desquamation, unless the patient dies before desquamation occurs

Reproduced from Centers for Disease Control and Prevention. (n.d.). *Toxic shock syndrome (other than streptococcal) (TSS): 2011 case definition* (Reaffirmed 2021). https://wwwn.cdc.gov/nndss/conditions/toxic-shock-syndrome-other-than-streptococcal/case-definition/2011

Emerging Evidence

The role of intravenous immunoglobulin has been investigated for patients with staphylococcal TSS, but expert opinion does not support the use of this therapy unless the patient is unresponsive to other measures due to the potential for adverse effects. Similarly, there is some evidence that targeted decolonization of MRSA carriers who get TSS might offer some benefit (Chu, 2024).

Patient Education

Although TSS is rare, all people at risk for TSS should be educated about the signs and symptoms of this condition and steps to prevent its occurrence, such as using low-absorbency tampons, changing tampons frequently, alternating pad and tampon use, avoiding overnight use of tampons, not leaving a menstrual cup in place for more than 12 hours, and removing barrier contraception within 24 hours. Instruct patients who have had TSS not to use barrier contraceptive methods, tampons, or menstrual cups.

GREATER VESTIBULAR GLAND CYSTS AND ABSCESSES

Description

The greater vestibular glands (formerly Bartholin glands) are a pair of mucus-secreting, nonpalpable structures with duct openings within the posterolateral vulvar vestibule that provide a colorless, serous fluid to provide lubrication to the opening of the vagina. The greater vestibular glands are located at either base of the labia minora at approximately the 5 and 7 o'clock positions (Dole & Nypaver, 2019). The glands are small, about 5 mm wide, and are attached to a duct approximately 2.5 cm in length that opens into the vestibule at about the 4 and 8 o'clock positions. The purpose of the ducts is to transport fluid to the vestibule; however, obstruction or damage to the narrow ducts can result in blockage, leading to the development of a cystic mass or abscess (Dole & Nypaver, 2019). Obstruction may occur as a result of either nonspecific inflammation or trauma. Continued fluid secretion after obstruction results in cyst formation (Chen, 2024). Abscess formation occurs when the cystic fluid becomes infected. Development of a greater vestibular gland cyst does not always precede abscess formation, and the occurrence of an abscess is three times as common as a cyst (Chen, 2024). Composed of several types of tissue, the duct is primarily lined with squamous epithelium that transitions into the vulvar vestibule. Greater vestibular gland carcinoma and benign tumor formation are rare (Chen, 2024).

Incidence, Prevalence, and Scope

Approximately 2 percent of all reproductive-age individuals assigned female at birth will develop a greater vestibular gland cyst, and the incidence peaks at menopause (Chen, 2024). Most individuals with such a cyst are asymptomatic. However, greater vestibular duct cysts are a common reason for visits to the emergency department because they can come on suddenly, cause concern, can be associated with significant pain, and interfere with sexual activities. Progression of a cyst to abscess development usually occurs rapidly over 2 to 4 days, and most will spontaneously rupture within 3 to 4 days.

Etiology and Pathophysiology

Bartholin gland cysts and abscesses develop when the duct transporting fluid becomes blocked or is traumatized. Recent literature reports that approximately 2 percent of cases are caused by sexually transmitted organisms, but the majority are caused by opportunistic bacteria. In a prospective study including 224 patients, cystic aspirates contained 307 aerobic cultures and 118 anaerobic cultures with 78 isolates of *E coli*, 40 of *Staphylococcus spp.*, 32 of *Streptococcus spp.*, and 30 of *Bacteriodes spp.* (Chen, 2024).

Clinical Presentation

A vestibular gland mass may be present either as a cyst or an abscess. A cyst may be an incidental finding during a routine pelvic examination or by the individual, and it may be without symptoms. A vestibular gland cyst is shown in **Color Plate 4**. The cyst appears as a visible round or oval mass causing a crescent-shaped vestibular entrance. It is nontender but tense, and palpable swelling—usually unilateral and without erythema or inflammation—is apparent. A greater vestibular gland abscess is a very tender, edematous, fluctuant mass with erythema of the overlying skin. This is shown in **Color Plate 5**. When present, symptoms include varying amounts of pain or tenderness, difficulty sitting or walking, and dyspareunia. Labial edema and distortion are observable on the affected area. The affected area is rarely larger than 5 cm in size. An area of softening or pointing suggests an impending rupture. Extensive inflammation may cause systemic symptoms.

Assessment

History

Although the presence of a soft mass in the lower third of the vulva, usually unilateral, may seem like an obvious diagnosis, it is important to collect a thorough history and complete a careful examination. Ask about onset of symptoms, noting whether pain or noticeable discharge is present, if it is difficult to sit or walk, and presence of a fever. Ask if there is a history of Bartholin mass, vulvar surgery, or other related procedures. Assess for comorbidities, including diabetes, HIV, immune suppression, and pregnancy.

Physical Examination

It is important to palpate the mass to distinguish between a cyst and an abscess. Normally, greater vestibular glands are not palpable. Cysts are smaller (1–3 cm), typically soft, nontender and unilateral. A abscess is generally larger (3–6cm) and generally tender, warm, and fluctuant, often associated with erythema and edema in the surrounding tissue. There may be inguinal lymphadenopathy. Observe the immediate surrounding tissue to determine whether there is extension into the vaginal canal.

Diagnostic Testing

Although cultures are not necessary to initiate broad-spectrum antibiotic therapy for an enlarged gland or abscess, given the increasing prevalence of persons with immunocompromised health, cultures are recommended if the mass is draining to assess for MRSA (Chen, 2024). When cultures are collected, they are typically performed in the case of spontaneous drainage, at the time of incision and drainage (I&D), or if the abscess is aspirated when no incision is planned (Lazenby et al., 2019). Although rare, a biopsy is collected if there are findings that suggest malignancy, or if the patient is 40 years or older. Other pertinent findings requiring a biopsy include postmenopausal status, a mass with a solid component, a cyst or abscess that is fixed and not mobile, or a mass that persists despite treatment (Chen, 2024).

Differential Diagnoses

Differential diagnoses include Skene duct cyst, greater vestibular gland malignancy, vulvar malignancy, endometriosis, Gartner duct cyst, hematoma, hidradenitis suppurativa, abscess, neoplasm, STI, mesonephric cyst of the vagina, and epithelial inclusion cyst (Chen, 2024).

Prevention

To avoid greater vestibular gland cysts, advise patients to maintain good vaginal hygiene, avoid and seek treatment for STIs, and seek professional care when any vulvar mass or pain is noted during the course of routine self-care.

Management

Nonpharmacologic

The majority of vestibular duct cysts can be managed expectantly in the outpatient setting by healthcare providers. Small asymptomatic cysts (1 to 3 cm) do not require treatment and often rupture spontaneously. The fluid within the cyst is sterile, thus antibiotics are not indicated. Comfort measures include hygiene practices, nonprescription pain medications such as NSAIDs, and sitz baths. A follow-up office visit within a few days can determine resolution or abscess development.

Pharmacologic

Antibiotics are not routinely prescribed for greater vestibular gland abscesses, and expert opinion suggests a benefit for patients when the culture is positive for MRSA or patients are at high risk of MRSA colonization, if the abscess is recurrent, associated with systemic infection or in high-risk patients including those who are pregnant, immunocompromised, or have extensive cellulitis (Chen, 2024). When prescribed, antibiotic therapy should include coverage for staphylococcal species, including MRSA, and gram-negative organisms such as *E. coli* (Chen, 2024). Trimethoprim–sulfamethoxazole is the antibiotic of choice for first-line therapy, while amoxicillin–clavulanate, clindamycin, doxycycline, or cefixime are alternatives. Selection of a drug may be made based on culture sensitivities. When choosing clindamycin, providers must be aware of increasing resistance of clindamycin to community-acquired MRSA, and an infectious disease specialist may be consulted (Chen, 2019).

Surgical

Office-based treatment is indicated for a very symptomatic cyst or abscess. The aim of abscess treatment is to permit drainage of cyst contents and prevent reaccumulation of fluid. One management option is simple I&D, often performed in an office setting or in the emergency department. However, I&D is associated with a 13 percent rate of abscess recurrence (Chen, 2024), so most patients are managed with a Word catheter. A Word catheter is a device with a balloon tip that allows drainage and fistula formation to occur. This procedure can be done in an office setting. A Word catheter can be placed following a small incision using a local anesthetic. An incision is made just above the cyst, thereby creating a new duct. This process allows for continuous drainage and eventual healing over a period of 6 to 8 weeks. The use of a Word catheter is generally considered acceptable by most people, although depending on tolerance, an oral analgesic and local analgesic cream can be offered prior to instillation of lidocaine. A broad-spectrum antibiotic is prescribed following the procedure. Some find the presence of the Word catheter irritating or uncomfortable; sometimes the catheter will become dislodged prior to healing, thus increasing the risk of recurrence (Chen, 2019). Multiple resources detail precise steps and supplies needed to perform I&D with fistulization of a greater vestibular gland (Dole & Nypaver, 2019).

Marsupialization is a surgical procedure consisting of a wide excision of the mass and is reserved for recurrent abscesses. It is performed under spinal, epidural, or general anesthesia. A gynecologist or urologist performs marsupialization in the operating room. Marsupialization is generally done for individuals with large or recurrent Bartholin cysts or abscesses, those with systemic illness (e.g., advancing cellulitis), or older individuals. For those with latex allergy, marsupialization will be recommended over fistulization because the Word catheter stem is made from latex (Chen, 2019; Dole & Nypaver, 2019).

Excision of the greater vestibular gland is performed when other modalities have failed and definitive treatment is indicated, or when there is concern for Bartholin cancer (Chen, 2019). Another therapy involves an I&D procedure followed by an application of a silver nitrate stick (0.5 cm length) that is placed within the cyst cavity. The wound is covered with gauze, and the patient returns to the office within 2 days whereby the wound is cleaned of debris. This method is similarly effective compared to marsupialization (Chen, 2019).

Referral

Referral is indicated for marsupialization, recurrent cyst or abscess formation, and any solid mass, cyst, or abscess in people older than age 40 years to rule out neoplasm. An individual with signs or biopsy results showing possible cancer will be referred to a gynecologic oncologist. Pregnant people with Bartholin cysts or abscess may be referred to an obstetrician-gynecologist. Referral to an infectious disease specialist may be needed for those with systemic disease, those requiring intravenous therapy, or those needing hospitalization.

Patient Education

Although most individuals have no obvious risk factors for developing Bartholin cysts, some conditions may be seen more often among those who go on to develop abscesses. These include immunosuppression, such as HIV or diabetes. People of larger body size or inadequate vulvar hygiene may be predisposed to abscess development. Trauma to the vulva by shaving or waxing (thus breaking the protective skin barrier) or surgical procedures may also predispose people to abscess formation (Chen, 2019; Policar, 2017). Other than routine bathing and hygienic practices, avoidance of STIs, and seeking prompt evaluation for pain, there are no special steps that people need to take to avoid Bartholin gland cysts. A previous Bartholin gland cyst is a risk factor for recurrence (Chen, 2019).

Variations in Management for Specific Populations

Pregnant People

Characteristics of bacterial pathogens among pregnant and nonpregnant people are similar, and most will be treated using the same techniques. However, Bartholin cyst excision is not routinely performed during pregnancy or in the immediate postpartum period due to increased risk of bleeding (Chen, 2019). In a study comparing surgical treatment outcomes between pregnant and nonpregnant individuals, researchers found the incidence of Bartholin gland abscesses in pregnant individuals to be 0.13 percent. A history of Bartholin gland abscess was more common in pregnant than in nonpregnant patients (55% vs. 30.1%, $p < .05$). Although the rate of a positive culture was no different between the groups, *E. coli* was the most common pathogen found among both pregnant and nonpregnant people with Bartholin abscesses (Boujenah et al., 2017).

Older Individuals

Cancer of the Bartholin gland, although infrequent, is highest among people in their 60s and is approximately 0.1 to 5 percent of vulvar cancers and 0.001 percent of all female cancers (Chen, 2019). It usually occurs as a painless vulvar mass, adherent to underlying tissue. This accounts for a recommendation that patients aged 40 years and older have a biopsy when presenting with an enlarged Bartholin gland or cyst. Cyst drainage and biopsy, as opposed to gland excision, is recommended as an initial step in evaluation of older individuals because cancer of the Bartholin gland is rare (Chen, 2019).

INFECTIONS DUE TO GENITAL PIERCING

Description

The practice of body piercing has been around since ancient times and is described as the insertion of an ornament into a perforation made into the tissue for decorative, cultural, spiritual, or other reasons (Conte et al., 2023). Piercings in the genital area can be a form of sexual expression and possible sexual enhancement. The act of piercing the genitals can also be conceptualized as a ritual of reclaiming and redefining the body as a site of pleasure for survivors of violence or abuse (Association of Professional Piercers, 2024). Current literature primarily describes short-term complications that occur from a variety of medical and nursing perspectives. Practitioners should be aware of possible acute or chronic complications associated with genital piercings as well as effective treatment strategies and evidence-based aftercare.

Incidence, Prevalence, and Scope

Today, various forms of body art and piercing have become mainstream for a variety of reasons. Surveys suggest that 27–42 percent of adolescents and young adults (aged 13–29 years old) have body piercings at a site other than the earlobe (Desai & Breuner, 2023), although there is no data on the incidence of genital piercing specifically. Old research notes that fairly high proportion (13–18%) report removing their jewelry due to dissatisfaction or infection, although this has not been recently investigated (Desai, 2023). Conte and her colleagues (2023) performed a systematic review including a pooled analysis of 30,090 medical complications across 36,803 sites in 30,231 patients; of these complications, only 183 included the genitals. Seventy-four percent of the patients were female with a mean age of 27.8 years.

Etiology and Pathophysiology

Infections at piercing sites differ according to the general health of the individual, immune status, medications, body site that is pierced, skill of the person who performed the piercing, and level of aftercare by the patient. Tissue trauma and localized skin or cartilage infections are the most common complications of piercings, and *S. aureus* and *Pseudomonas aeruginosa* are the most frequent pathogens. Systemic infections following piercing are not common, although transmission of hepatitis B and C have been documented. A systematic review revealed case studies of endocarditis and meningitis, although these are rare. Other known systemic infections reported include tetanus, streptococcal septicemia, and staphylococcal and streptococcal toxic shock syndrome (Desai, 2024).

According to Conte et al. (2023), labial and clitoral genital piercings are prone to complication, with some estimates as high as 30–50 percent. Common issues include coital pain, loss of sensation, coital discomfort, and tearing or trauma to the genitals. The Association of Professional Piercers (APP) offers a different perspective, noting that the elastic and resilient characteristics of genital tissue cause these piercings to heal more quickly and with fewer complications than piercings at other sites. Female genital tissue specifically is designed to stretch during childbirth and heals rapidly from trauma. High levels of vascularity promote rapid healing, which diminishes risk of infection. Further, genital tissue is often covered by clothing, and rarely comes into contact with environmental pathogens (APP, 2024).

Noninfectious complications, such as metal allergies, bleeding, tissue trauma, and scarring have been observed (Conte et al., 2023). Other common complications of genital piercings include compromise of barrier contraceptive methods and keloid formation. Individuals with any increased vulnerability to infection (e.g., diabetes, HIV, use of steroid medications, anticoagulants) may be more likely to experience infection after a piercing procedure.

Clinical Presentation

Genital or intimate body piercings are typically performed on the breasts, nipples, clitoral hood, and labia majora and minora in females and on the glans penis and shaft in males. Clinicians may note genital piercings during the course of a routine physical examination. While most genital piercings will heal well, localized infections, bruising, inflammation, and skin reactions are possible. Little information exists on prevalence, but genitals are well vascularized and heal more quickly than other body piercing sites. Complications for genital piercings reported in the literature include prolonged priapism, recurrent condyloma acuminata, streptococcal toxic shock syndrome, allergic contact dermatitis, altered urinary flow, and compromised effectiveness of barrier contraception (Breuner, 2017).

Assessment

History

Patients may seek out either their primary care provider or their piercing professional for questions and concerns about genital piercings. It is important to take a thorough sexual history and a complete medical history to assess for chronic health problems, immune status, medications, and any past problems with piercings. Inquire about the patient's self-care of the pierced site. If the patient is experiencing problems with a piercing, ask if any topical treatments or OTC medications have been used. Clinicians can inquire about the credentials of individuals who performed the genital piercings and the patient's understanding of the piercer's qualifications, safety record, and licensure. Clinicians can familiarize themselves with techniques used for piercing and the types of body jewelry most commonly selected at genital sites, in addition to safe removal procedures when indicated.

Physical Examination

Female genital piercings include singular or multiple piercings of clitoral hood, inner and outer labia, and perineum (Desai, 2024). The location and type of body piercings, and the condition of the surrounding tissues, should be documented in the patient's health record in the event that injury or infection develops later. Inspect piercings and the surrounding area for redness, tenderness, itching, or skin changes, and ask the patient if they have any concerns.

Diagnostic Testing

Pathologic organisms most commonly associated with genital piercing infections include *E. coli*, *Klebsiella* species, *Proteus mirabilis*, *Enterococcus* species, and *Staphylococcus saprophyticus* (Conte et al., 2023). Infectious complications from piercing are typically local; systemic infections, although rare, can occur and require hospitalization and IV antibiotic therapy (Van Hoover et al., 2017). The Infectious Diseases Society of America (IDSA) has published a detailed set of guidelines that includes algorithms for diagnosis, management, and treatment of skin and soft tissue infections (Stevens et al., 2014, reaffirmed 2018). The guidelines include recommendations for management of superficial skin infections and those complicated by MRSA, and they assist clinicians in distinguishing infections that are mild, moderate, or severe.

Differential Diagnosis

Identifying the presence of infection and initiating early treatment with an appropriate regimen and follow-up care is essential. Furthermore, distinguishing systemic illness related to an infected genital piercing versus other causes of illness is key to successful treatment.

Prevention

Prevention of piercing-associated complications begins during a conversation with patients about potential health risks associated with genital piercings and informed decision making. An initial step is a review of preexisting health problems that may interfere with normal healing following a piercing (Lee et al., 2018). Individuals with cardiac conditions should avoid all piercings to reduce their risk of a rare but potentially serious endocarditis (Desai, 2024; APP, 2024). Those using anticoagulant medications, including aspirin or NSAIDs, have an increased risk of bleeding, so they should stop these medications at least 7 days prior to a piercing (Lee et al., 2018). Patients with allergies or diabetes, and those using steroid medications, are more likely to have poor healing. This is an important consideration prior to making a decision to have a piercing in a genital area.

Following a genital piercing, the most likely cause of infection and contamination is unprotected sexual contact. Body fluids and oral bacteria can contaminate any open wound, so all sexual contact during the healing phase must be fluid safe, either through the use of barriers such as condoms or dental dams, or by choosing abstinence. Additionally, manipulation and handling of the genital jewelry should be avoided during healing which generally takes 1–2 months (APP, 2024).

Stress to patients that their piercer should be a licensed or otherwise qualified individual who practices in accordance with state regulations in an environment that follows proper infection control procedures and uses sterile technique.

Management

Nonpharmacologic

It is recommended that patients who have had piercings be vigilant about aftercare of the site. Specific instructions from the piercing provider will likely include a minimum of twice daily cleansings with a mild soap solution or sterile saline wound wash (0.9% sodium chloride), and avoiding alcohol and hydrogen peroxide as these can delay healing. Patients should avoid touching the piercing site with unwashed hands, and should avoid swimming, saunas, and soaking the site in pools, hot tubs, or bathtubs for at least 2 weeks. Additionally, individuals should avoid shaving, waxing, or using commercial products in the genital area (APP, 2024).

Pharmacologic

Patients who have had piercings should avoid aspirin and NSAIDs to decrease risk of bleeding for at least 7 days following the procedure. Sites that show signs of infection, such as erythema, pus drainage, or cellulitis, should be cultured or referred for I&D in the event of an abcess. An appropriate antibiotic should be selected for coverage against *P. aeruginosa* (i.e., ciprofloxicin) and *S. aureus* (i.e., topical mucopiricin) based on culture results.

Referral

Patients should be referred to an infectious disease specialist when there is inadequate improvement with antibiotic use and wound care practices. If cultures do not identify an infectious organism, a tissue biopsy should be done.

Emerging Evidence

With increasing prevalence of piercings among all populations, clinicians need up-to-date, evidence-based practice guidelines to prevent and manage complications. Currently, there is limited published science in the field of genital piercing, and much of the current science is focused on identification and treatment of complications related to genital piercing. The Association of Piercing Professionals (2024) maintains a website with resources for healthcare providers, legislators, health inspectors and the general public. This resource features good information on safety, aftercare, regulations and legislation, and safe jewelry sourcing, and maintains a roster of licensed piercing professionals.

Patient Education

Providers are uniquely positioned to provide accurate health care information to all patients prior to decision making regarding genital piercings and body art (Desai & Breuner, 2023). Practitioners should familiarize themselves with types of genital piercing, genital jewelry, and how to remove it safely. Patients should be counseled to seek out licensed experienced practitioners in safe and sanitary environments which conform to state regulations as well as OSHA bloodborne pathogen standards. All tools must be sterile and needles must be single use. The piercing professional should use aseptic technique and practice trauma informed care maintaining the safety and comfort of the client, and should provide comprehensive aftercare instructions (APP, 2024; Desai, 2024).

Considerations for Specific Populations

Adolescents

Understanding and honoring the reasons why adolescents might pursue body art as a form of self-expression is critical for providers to provide compassionate, evidence-driven, nonjudgmental care to this population. Motivations for body modification are highly individual and can include decoration, expression of individuality, group affiliation, fashion, resistance, and sexual desire/gratification (Desai & Breuner, 2023). People seeking genital piercings report uniqueness (71%), sexual pleasure (77%), and self-expression (79%) as important factors in that decision (Kluger, 2020). Younger adolescents have different reasons for piercing in general than do college-age students, reporting aesthetics and fashion as the most common reasons for piercing, followed by feelings of transgression and curiosity (Conte et al., 2023). Adolescents younger than age 18 who are considering body piercing may need parental permission. Due to this limitation, some adolescents purchase over-the-counter piercing kits with unsterile components and low-quality jewelry which can lead to infection. Amateur piercers are at high risk of forgoing proper disinfection, and causing harm by improper anatomical placement which greatly increases risk of complications (APP, 2024). These patients should be given comprehensive information about the importance of seeking out piercing services from an experienced reputable professional in a clean and safe environment.

Pregnant and Breastfeeding Individuals

Patients should be discouraged from seeking out new genital piercings during pregnancy due to physiologic changes to the immune system, which have a negative impact on healing, and responsible piercing professionals will refuse to pierce pregnant individuals (APP, 2024). Current recommendations are to wait 3 months postpartum prior to considering a genital piercing, and 3 months following the cessation of breastmilk production to have a nipple piercing.

Genital piercing–related complications during pregnancy and labor have not been reported in the literature (Lee et al., 2018). It is recommended that genital jewelry should be removed prior to labor and birth due to the potential of labial swelling leading to tearing or injury to the infant during birth. Individuals who plan to have a cesarean birth may choose to leave genital piercings in place, but staff should take special care during procedures such as urinary catheter insertion to avoid urethral damage or infection. A general rule of thumb is that piercings should be removed if they are likely to interfere with a necessary procedure (i.e., intubation) or if the piercings become uncomfortable due to physiologic changes of pregnancy (Keltz Pomerantz, 2024).

CONCLUSION

Vulvovaginal health is a fundamental aspect of overall wellness, and has significant psychological, interpersonal, sexual, emotional, and economic impacts. This chapter has reviewed common vaginal dysbioses including bacterial vaginosis (BV), vulvovaginal candidiasis (VVC), desquamative inflammatory vaginitis, atrophic vaginitis, and genitourinary syndrome of menopause (GSM). In addition, it has provided an overview of more infectious conditions including toxic shock syndrome (TSS), greater vestibular gland duct cysts and abscesses, and complications related to genital piercing. While many of the infections considered in this chapter are age old, new understandings of the protective role of the vaginal microbiome and the relationships between vaginal dysbiosis and the formation of biofilms present reasons for optimism that these common infections may be addressed through further research. The vaginal microbiome in particular is an important area of research by clinicians, microbiologists, and other scientists to further unlock its structure, function, and protective properties. Improved investment in resources, along with newer study models, sampling methods, and research designs, are needed to deepen understanding of vaginal and neovaginal health and potentially improve health globally.

References

Abou Chacra, L., Fenollar, F., & Diop, K. (2022). Bacterial vaginosis: What do we currently know? *Frontiers in Cellular and Infection Microbiology, 11*, 672429. https://doi.org/10.3389/fcimb.2021.672429

American Cancer Society. (2024). *Survival rates for breast cancer.* Retrieved January 10, 2025 from https://www.cancer.org/cancer/types/breast-cancer/understanding-a-breast-cancer-diagnosis/breast-cancer-survival-rates.html

American College of Obstetricians and Gynecologists. (2006, reaffirmed 2019). ACOG clinical practice bulletin no. 72: Vaginitis. *Obstetrics & Gynecology, 107*(5), 1195–1206.

American College of Obstetricians and Gynecologists. (2016, reaffirmed 2018). ACOG committee opinion no. 659: The use of vaginal estrogen in women with a history of estrogen-dependent breast cancer. *Obstetrics & Gynecology, 127*, e93–e96.

American College of Obstetricians and Gynecologists. (2023). *Compounded bioidentical menopausal hormone therapy.* ACOG Clinical Consensus. Retrieved from https://www.acog.org/clinical/clinical-guidance/clinical-consensus/articles/2023/11/compounded-bioidentical-menopausal-hormone-therapy

American College of Obstetricians and Gynecologists' Committee on Gynecologic Practice and American College of Obstetricians and Gynecologists' Committee on Health Care for Underserved Women. (2021). Health care for transgender and gender diverse individuals: ACOG committee opinion, no. 823. *Obstetrics and Gynecology, 137*(3), e75–e88. https://doi.org/10.1097/AOG.0000000000004294

Amsel, R., Totten, P. A., Spiegel, C. A., Chen, K. C., Eschenbach, D., & Holmes, K. K. (1983). Nonspecific vaginitis: Diagnostic criteria and microbial and epidemiologic associations. *American Journal of Medicine, 74*(1), 14–22.

Anahtar, M. N., Gootenberg, D. B., Mitchell, C. M., & Kwon, D. S. (2018). Cervicovaginal microbiota and reproductive health: The virtue of simplicity. *Cell Host & Microbe, 23*(2), 159–168. https://doi.org/10.1016/j.chom.2018.01.013

Association of Professional Piercers. (2024). *Piercing FAQs.* https://safepiercing .org/safe_piercing_faq

Atchade, E., De Tymowski, C., Grall, N., Tanaka, S., & Montravers, P. (2024). Toxic shock syndrome: A literature review. *Antibiotics, 13*(1), 96. https://doi.org/10.3390/antibiotics13010096 cdc.gov+15researchgate.net+15pmc.ncbi.nlm.nih.gov+15

Bachman, G., & Pinkerton, J. V. (2024). Genitourinary syndrome of menopause (vulvovaginal atrophy): Clinical manifestations and diagnosis. *UpToDate.* Retrieved January 5, 2025, from https://www.uptodate/contents/genitourinary-syndrome-of-menopause-vulvovaginal-atrophy-clinical-manifestations-and-diagnosis

Berger, S., Kunerl, A., Wasmuth, S., Tierno, P., Wagner, K., & Brügger, J. (2019). Menstrual toxic shock syndrome: case report and systematic review of the literature. *The Lancet. Infectious diseases, 19*(9), e313–e321. https://doi.org/10.1016/S1473-3099(19)30041-6

Birse, K. D., Kratzer, K., Zuend, C. F., Mutch, S., Noël-Romas, L., Lamont, A., Abou, M., Jalil, E., Veloso, V., Grinsztejn, B., Friedman, R. K., Broliden, K., Bradley, F., Poliquin, V., Li, F., Yanavich, C., Burgener, A., & Aldrovandi, G. (2020). The neovaginal microbiome of transgender women post-gender reassignment surgery. *Microbiome, 8*(1), 61. https://doi.org/10.1186/s40168-020-00804-1

Boujenah, J., Le, S. N. V., Benbara, A., Bricou, A., Murtada, R., & Carbillon, L. (2017). Bartholin gland abscess during pregnancy: Report on 40 patients. *European Journal of Obstetrics, Gynecology, and Reproductive Biology, 212*, 65–68. https://doi.org/10.1016/j.ejogrb.2017.03.018

Bretelle, F., Loubière, S., Desbriere, R., Loundou, A., Blanc, J., Heckenroth, H., Schmitz, T., Benachi, A., Haddad, B., Mauviel, F., Danoy, X., Mares, P., Chenni, N., Ménard, J. P., Cocallemen, J. F., Slim, N., Sénat, M. V., Chauleur, C., Bohec, C., Kayem, G., . . . Groupe de Recherche en Obstetrique et Gynécologie (GROG) Investigators (2023). Effectiveness and costs of molecular screening and treatment for bacterial vaginosis to prevent preterm birth: The AuTop randomized clinical trial. *JAMA Pediatrics, 177*(9), 894–902. https://doi.org/10.1001/jamapediatrics.2023.2250

Breuner, C. C., Levine, D. A., & Committee on Adolescence (2017). Adolescent and young adult tattooing, piercing, and scarification. *Pediatrics, 140*(4), e20163494. https://doi-org.seattleu.idm.oclc.org/10.1542/peds.2017-1962

Brown, S. E., Tuddenham, S., Shardell, M. D., Klebanoff, M. A., Ghanem, K. G., & Brotman, R. M. (2023). Bacterial vaginosis and spontaneous clearance of chlamydia trachomatis in the Longitudinal Study of Vaginal Flora. *The Journal of Infectious Diseases, 228*(6), 783–791. https://doi.org/10.1093/infdis/jiad142

Buchta, V. (2018). Vaginal microbiome. Vaginální mikrobiom. *Ceska Gynekologie, 83*(5), 371–379.

Carlson, K., & Nguyen, H. (2024). Genitourinary syndrome of menopause. In *StatPearls.* StatPearls Publishing. Retrieved June 24, 2025, from https://www.ncbi.nlm.nih.gov/books/NBK559297/

Casiano Evans, E. A., Hobson, D. T. G., Aschkenazi, S. O., Alas, A. N., Balgobin, S., Balk, E. M., Dieter, A. A., Kanter, G., Orejuela, F. J., Sanses, T. V. D., & Rahn, D. D. (2023). Nonestrogen therapies for treatment of genitourinary syndrome of menopause: A systematic review. *Obstetrics & Gynecology, 142*(3), 555–570. https://doi.org/10.1097/AOG.0000000000005288

Centers for Disease Control and Prevention. (2021). Sexually transmitted infections treatment guidelines, 2021. *Morbidity and Mortality Weekly Reports Recommendation Reports, 70*(4), https://doi.org/10.15585/mmwr.rr7004a1

Centers for Disease Control and Prevention. (2024). *About streptococcal toxic shock syndrome.* National Center for Immunization and Respiratory Diseases. https://www.cdc.gov/group-a-strep/about/streptococcal-toxic-shock-syndrome.html

Centers for Disease Control and Prevention. (2021). *Toxic shock syndrome (other than streptococcal) (TSS): 2011 case definition* (Reaffirmed 2021). https://ndc.services.cdc.gov/case-definitions/toxic-shock-syndrome-2011/

Chauhan, V., Kumar, A., Tripathi, S., et al. (2024). An update on the pathogenesis and ethnopharmacological therapeutic approaches of vulvovaginal candidiasis. *Discover Public Health, 21*, 195. https://doi.org/10.1186/s12982-024-00274-y

Chen, K. T. (2019). Bartholin gland masses: Diagnosis and management. *UpToDate.* Retrieved March 4, 2020, from https://www.uptodate.com/contents/bartholin-gland-masses-diagnosis-

Cold, S., Cold, F., Jensen, M. B., Cronin-Fenton, D., Christiansen, P., & Ejlertsen, B. (2022). Systemic or vaginal hormone therapy after early breast cancer: A Danish observational cohort study. *Journal of the National Cancer Institute, 114*(10), 1347–1354. https://doi.org/10.1093/jnci/djac112

Colonna, C., & Steelman, M. (2023). Amsel criteria. In *StatPearls.* StatPearls Publishing.

Conte, S., Kamali, K., Muncey-Buckley, M., Abbas, K., Sabljic, T., & Mukovozov, I. M. (2023). Complications of body piercings: A systematic review. *Cutis, 112*(3), 139–145. https://doi.org/10.12788/cutis.0847

Cooke, G., Watson, C., Deckx, L., Pirotta, M., Smith, J., & van Driel, M. L. (2022). Treatment for recurrent vulvovaginal candidiasis (thrush). *The Cochrane*

Database of Systematic Reviews, 1(1), CD009151. https://doi.org/10.1002/14651858.CD009151.pub2

Coudray, M. S., & Madhivanan, P. (2020). Bacterial vaginosis—A brief synopsis of the literature. *European Journal of Obstetrics, Gynecology, and Reproductive Biology, 245*, 143–148. https://doi.org/10.1016/j.ejogrb.2019.12.035

Cuccu, I., Golia D'Augè, T., Firulli, I., De Angelis, E., Buzzaccarini, G., D'Oria, O., Besharat, A. R., Caserta, D., Bogani, G., Muzii, L., Di Donato, V., & Giannini, A. (2024). Update on genitourinary syndrome of menopause: A scoping review of a tailored treatment-based approach. *Life, 14*(11), Article 1504. https://doi.org/10.3390/life14111504

Danan, E. R., Sowerby, C., Ullman, K. E., Ensrud, K., Forte, M. L., Zerzan, N., Anthony, M., Kalinowski, C., Abdi, H. I., Friedman, J. K., Landsteiner, A., Greer, N., Nardos, R., Fok, C., Dahm, P., Butler, M., Wilt, T. J., & Diem, S. (2024). Hormonal treatments and vaginal moisturizers for genitourinary syndrome of menopause: A systematic review. *Annals of Internal Medicine, 177*(10), 1400–1414. https://doi.org/10.7326/ANNALS-24-00610

Daniel, A. L., Auerbach, S., Nazarenko, D., Agbemenu, K., & Lorenz, R. (2023). An integrative review of the relationship between intrauterine devices and bacterial vaginosis. *Nursing for Women's Health, 27*(2), 141–151. https://doi.org/10.1016/j.nwh.2023.01.007

Deka, N., Hassan, S., Seghal Kiran, G., & Selvin, J. (2021). Insights into the role of vaginal microbiome in women's health. *Journal of Basic Microbiology, 61*(12), 1071–1084. https://doi.org/10.1002/jobm.202100421

Denning, D. W., Kneale, M., Sobel, J. D., & Rautemaa-Richardson, R. (2018). Global burden of recurrent vulvovaginal candidiasis: A systematic review. *Lancet Infectious Diseases, 11*, e339–e347.

Desai, N., & Breuner, C. C. (2023). Tattoos and piercings in female adolescents and young adults. *Journal of Pediatric and Adolescent Gynecology, 36*(1), 14–17. https://doi.org/10.1016/j.jpag.2022.08.007

Dole, D. M., & Nypaver, C. (2019). Management of Bartholin duct cysts and gland abscesses. *Journal of Midwifery & Women's Health, 64*(3), 337–343.

Drugs and Lactation Database. (2018). Fluconazole. *National Library of Medicine*. https://www.ncbi.nlm.nih.gov/books/NBK501223/

Elkbuli, A., Diaz, B., Ehrhardt, J. D., Jr., Hai, S., Kaufman, S., McKenney, M., & Boneva, D. (2018). Survival from *Clostridium* toxic shock syndrome: Case report and review of the literature. *International Journal of Surgery Case Reports, 50*, 64–67. https://doi.org/10.1016/j.ijscr.2018.07.020

Fait T. (2019). Menopause hormone therapy: latest developments and clinical practice. *Drugs in context, 8*, 212551. https://doi.org/10.7573/dic.212551

Falconi-McCahill A. (2019). Bacterial vaginosis: A clinical update with a focus on complementary and alternative therapies. *Journal of Midwifery & Women's Health, 64*(5), 578–591. https://doi.org/10.1111/jmwh.13013

Faubion, S. S., Larkin, L. C., Stuenkel, C. A., Bachmann, G. A., Chism, L. A., Kagan, R., Kaunitz, A. M., Krychman, M. L., Parish, S. J., Partridge, A. H., Pinkerton, J. V., Rowen, T. S., Shapiro, M. C., Simon, J. A., Goldfarb, S. B., & Kingsberg, S. A. (2018). Management of genitourinary syndrome of menopause in women with or at high risk for breast cancer: Consensus recommendations from The North American Menopause Society and The International Society for the Study of Women's Sexual Health. *Menopause, 25*(6), 596–608. https://doi.org/10.1097/GME.0000000000001121

Felix, T. C., de Brito Röder, D. V. D., & Dos Santos Pedroso, R. (2019). Alternative and complementary therapies for vulvovaginal candidiasis. *Folia Microbiologica, 64*(2), 133–141. https://doi.org/10.1007/s12223-018-0652-x

Filippini, M., Porcari, I., Ruffolo, A. F., Casiraghi, A., Farinelli, M., Uccella, S., Franchi, M., Candiani, M., & Salvatore, S. (2022). CO2-laser therapy and genitourinary syndrome of menopause: A systematic review and meta-analysis. *The Journal of Sexual Medicine, 19*(3), 452–470. https://doi.org/10.1016/j.jsxm.2021.12.010

Gao, C. J., & Kannan, K. (2020). Phthalates, bisphenols, parabens, and triclocarban in feminine hygiene products from the United States and their implications for human exposure. *Environment International, 136*, 105465. https://doi.org/10.1016/j.envint.2020.105465

Gliniewicz, K., Schneider, G. M., Ridenhour, B. J., Williams, C. J., Song, Y., Farage, M. A., Miller, K., & Forney, L. J. (2019). Comparison of the vaginal microbiomes of premenopausal and postmenopausal women. *Frontiers in Microbiology, 14*(10), 193. https://doi.org/10.3389/fmicb.2019.00193

Gonçalves, B., Ferreira, C., Alves, C. T., Henriques, M., Azeredo, J., & Silva, S. (2016). Vulvovaginal candidiasis: Epidemiology, microbiology and risk factors. *Critical Reviews in Microbiology, 42*(6), 905–927. https://doi.org/10.3109/1040841X.2015.1091805

Graziottin A. (2024). Maintaining vulvar, vaginal and perineal health: Clinical considerations. *Women's Health (London, England), 20*, 17455057231223716. https://doi.org/10.1177/17455057231223716

Harris, K., Proctor, L. K., Shinar, S., Philippopoulos, E., Yudin, M. H., & Murphy, K. E. (2023). Outcomes and management of pregnancy and puerperal group A streptococcal infections: A systematic review. *Acta Obstetricia et Gynecologica Scandinavica, 102*(2), 138–157. https://doi.org/10.1111/aogs.14500

Hauth, J. C., Goldenberg, R. L., Andrews, W. W., DuBard, M. B., & Copper, R. L. (1995). Reduced incidence of preterm delivery with metronidazole and erythromycin in women with bacterial vaginosis. *New England Journal of Medicine, 333*(26), 1732–1736.

Holdcroft, A. M., Ireland, D. J., & Payne, M. S. (2023). The vaginal microbiome in health and disease—What role do common intimate hygiene practices play? *Microorganisms, 11*(2), 298. https://doi.org/10.3390/microorganisms11020298

Huang, R., Liu, Z., Sun, T., & Zhu, L. (2024). Cervicovaginal microbiome, high-risk HPV infection and cervical cancer: Mechanisms and therapeutic potential. *Microbiological Research*, 127857.

Hutcherson, T. C., Cieri-Hutcherson, N. E., Grosshans, M. A., Freemire, J., Meegan, E., Zu, V., & Tal, E. (2025). Systematic review of intrauterine contraceptive use and the development of toxic shock syndrome. *Journal of Pharmacy Practice*, 8971900241313402. Advance online publication. https://doi.org/10.1177/08971900241313402

Itriyeva K. (2020). Evaluation of vulvovaginitis in the adolescent patient. *Current Problems in Pediatric and Adolescent Health Care, 50*(7), 100836. https://doi.org/10.1016/j.cppeds.2020.100836

Jeng, H. S., Yan, T. R., & Chen, J. Y. (2020). Treating vaginitis with probiotics in non-pregnant females: A systematic review and meta-analysis. *Experimental and Therapeutic Medicine, 20*(4), 3749–3765. https://doi.org/10.3892/etm.2020.9090

Keltz Pomeranz, M. (2024). Maternal adaptations to pregnancy: Skin and related structures. *UpToDate.* Retrieved January 12, 2025, from https://www-uptodate-com/contents/maternal-adaptations-to-pregnancy-skin-and-related-structures

Kim, H. Y., Lee, J. D., Kim, J. Y., Bae, O. N., Choi, Y. K., Baek, E., Kang, S., Min, C., Seo, K., Choi, K., Lee, B. M., & Kim, K. B. (2019). Risk assessment of volatile organic compounds (VOCs) detected in sanitary pads. *Journal of Toxicology and Environmental Health, Part A, 82*(11), 678–695. https://doi.org/10.1080/15287394.2019.1642607

Kluger N. (2020). Manifestations cutanées et muqueuses des pratiques sexuelles [Cutaneous and mucosal manifestations of sexual practices]. *Annales de dermatologie et de venereologie, 147*(10), 629–636. https://doi.org/10.1016/j.annder.2020.04.022

Krakowsky, Y., Potter, E., Hallarn, J., Monari, B., Wilcox, H., Bauer, G., Ravel, J., & Prodger, J. L. (2022). The effect of gender-affirming medical care on the vaginal and neovaginal microbiomes of transgender and gender-diverse people. *Frontiers in Cellular and Infection Microbiology, 11*, 769950. https://doi.org/10.3389/fcimb.2021.769950

Lazenby, G. B., Thurman, A. R., & Soper, D. E. (2019). Vulvar abscess. *UpToDate*. Retrieved March 4, 2020, from https://www.uptodate.com/contents/vulvar-abscess

Lee, B., Vangipurim, R., Peterson, E., & Tyring, S. K. (2018). Complications associated with intimate body piercings. *Dermatology Online Journal, 24*(7), 1–8.

Liu, H. F., & Yi, N. (2022). A systematic review and meta-analysis on the efficacy of probiotics for bacterial vaginosis. *European review for medical and pharmacological sciences, 26*(1), 90–98. https://doi.org/10.26355/eurrev_202201_27752

Marrazzo, J. M., Dombrowski, J. C., Wierzbicki, M. R., Perlowski, C., Pontius, A., Dithmer, D., & Schwebke, J. (2019). Safety and efficacy of a novel vaginal anti-infective, TOL-463, in the treatment of bacterial vaginosis and vulvovaginal candidiasis: A randomized, single-blind, Phase 2, controlled trial. *Clinical Infectious Diseases: An Official Publication of the Infectious Diseases Society of America, 68*(5), 803–809. https://doi.org/10.1093/cid/ciy554

Marroquin, J., Kiomourtzoglou, M. A., Scranton, A., & Pollack, A. Z. (2024). Chemicals in menstrual products: A systematic review. *BJOG: An International Journal of Obstetrics and Gynaecology, 131*(5), 655–664. https://doi.org/10.1111/1471-0528.17668

McVicker, L., Labeit, A. M., Coupland, C. A. C., Hicks, B., Hughes, C., McMenamin, Ú., McIntosh, S. A., Murchie, P., & Cardwell, C. R. (2024). Vaginal estrogen therapy use and survival in females with breast cancer. *JAMA Oncology, 10*(1), 103–108. https://doi.org/10.1001/jamaoncol.2023.4508

Mei, Z., & Li, D. (2022). The role of probiotics in vaginal health. *Frontiers in Cellular and Infection Microbiology, 12*, 963868. https://doi.org/10.3389/fcimb.2022.963868

Melisko, M. E., Goldman, M. E., Hwang, J., De Luca, A., Fang, S., Esserman, L. J., Chien, A. J., Park, J. W., & Rugo, H. S. (2017). Vaginal testosterone cream vs estradiol vaginal ring for vaginal dryness or decreased libido in women receiving aromatase inhibitors for early-stage breast cancer: A randomized clinical trial. *JAMA Oncology, 3*(3), 313–319. https://doi.org/10.1001/jamaoncol.2016.3904

Micks, E., Reed, S. D., & Mitchell, C. (2024). The postmenopausal vaginal microbiome and genitourinary syndrome of menopause. *Clinical Obstetrics and Gynecology, 67*(1), 79–88. https://doi.org/10.1097/GRF.0000000000000832

Mili, N., Paschou, S. A., Armeni, A., Georgopoulos, N., Goulis, D. G., & Lambrinoudaki, I. (2021). Genitourinary syndrome of menopause: A systematic review on prevalence and treatment. *Menopause (New York, N.Y.), 28*(6), 706–716. https://doi-10.1097/GME.0000000000001752

Mitchell, C. M. (2024). Assessment and treatment of vaginitis. *Obstetrics and Gynecology, 144*(6), 765–781. https://doi.org/10.1097/AOG.0000000000005673

Mitchell, C. M., Reed, S. D., Diem, S. J., Manson, J. E., & Pinkerton, J. V. (2024). Genitourinary syndrome of menopause: Treatment. In R. B. Barbieri & UpToDate (Eds.),

UpToDate. Wolters Kluwer. Retrieved June 30, 2025, from https://www.uptodate.com/contents/genitourinary-syndrome-of-menopause-vulvovaginal-atrophy-treatment?csi=5d6fcf98-40b4-4469-8d37-7cae5f087897&source=contentShare

Moisés da Silva, G. V., Lobato, M. I. R., Silva, D. C., Schwarz, K., Fontanari, A. M. V., Costa, A. B., Tavares, P. M., Gorgen, A. R. H., Cabral, R. D., & Rosito, T. E. (2021). Male-to-Female Gender-Affirming Surgery: 20-Year Review of Technique and Surgical Results. *Frontiers in surgery, 8*, 639430. https://doi.org/10.3389/fsurg.2021.639430

Murina, P. F., Graziottin, A., Bagot, O., Panay, N., Thamkhantho, M., & Shaw, S. W. (2021). Real-world practices and attitudes towards intimate self-care: Results from an international women's survey. *Journal of Gynecology Obstetrics and Human Reproduction, 50*(10), 102192. https://doi.org/10.1016/j.jogoh.2021.102192

Murphy, K., Shi, Q., Hoover, D. R., Adimora, A. A., Alcaide, M. L., Brockmann, S., Daubert, E., Duggal, P., Merenstein, D., Dionne, J. A., Sheth, A. N., Keller, M. J., Herold, B. C., Anastos, K., & Aouizerat, B. (2024). Genetic predictors for bacterial vaginosis in women living with and at risk for HIV infection. *American Journal of Reproductive Immunology (New York, N.Y.: 1989), 91*(5), e13845. https://doi.org/10.1111/aji.13845

Muzny, C. A., Balkus, J., Mitchell, C., Sobel, J. D., Workowski, K., Marrazzo, J., & Schwebke, J. R. (2022). Diagnosis and management of bacterial vaginosis: Summary of evidence reviewed for the 2021 Centers for Disease Control and Prevention Sexually Transmitted Infections Treatment Guidelines. *Clinical Infectious Diseases: An Official Publication of the Infectious Diseases Society of America, 74*(Suppl_2), S144–S151. https://doi.org/10.1093/cid/ciac021

National Center for Complementary and Integrative Health. (2019). *Women's health and complementary approaches*. National Institutes of Health. https://nccih.nih.gov/health/womenshealth.htm

National Notifiable Disease Surveillance System. (2024). *Streptococcal toxic shock syndrome (STSS)* (streptococcus pyogenes). https://ndc.services.cdc.gov/conditions/streptococcal-toxic-shock-syndrome/ Retrieved January 10, 2025.

North American Menopause Society. (2020). The 2020 genitourinary syndrome of menopause position statement of The North American Menopause Society. *Menopause, 27*(9), 976–992. https://doi.org/10.1097/GME.0000000000001609

Owens, D. K., Davidson, K. W., Krist, A. H., Barry, M. J., Cabana, M., Caughey, A. B., . . . & U.S. Preventive Services Task Force. (2020). Screening for bacterial vaginosis in pregnant persons to prevent preterm delivery: US preventive services task force recommendation statement. *Jama, 323*(13), 1286–1292.

Paavonen, J., & Brunham, R. C. (2018). Bacterial vaginosis and desquamative inflammatory vaginitis. *New England Journal of Medicine, 379*(23), 2246–2254.

Palacios, S. (2020). Ospemifene for vulvar and vaginal atrophy: An overview. *Drugs in Context, 9*, 2020-3-2. https://doi.org/10.7573/dic.2020-3-2

Peebles, K., Velloza, J., Balkus, J. E., Scott McClelland, R., & Barnabas, R. V. (2019). High global burden and costs of bacterial vaginosis: A systematic review and meta-analysis. *Sexually Transmitted Diseases, 46*(5), 304–311. https://doi.org/10.1097/OLQ.0000000000000972

Perelmuter, S., Burns, R., Shearer, K., Grant, R., Soogoor, A., Jun, S., Meurer, J. A., Krapf, J., & Rubin, R. (2024). Genitourinary syndrome of lactation: A new perspective on postpartum and lactation-related genitourinary symptoms. *Sexual Medicine Reviews, 12*(3), 279–287. https://doi.org/10.1093/sxmrev/qeae034

Perelmuter, S., Stokes, C., Chapalamadugu, M., Drian, A., Zusman, G. L., Berdugo, J., Davide, M., Andy, C., Grant, R., Drew, T., Burns, R., Meurer, J., Shah, A., Contractor, S., Messafi, A., Thompson, A., Krapf, J., & Rubin, R. (2025). Postpartum and lactation-related genitourinary symptoms: A systematic review. *Obstetrics and Gynecology, 146*(1), 59–72. https://doi.org/10.1097/AOG.0000000000005940

Plummer, E. L., Sfameni, A. M., Vodstrcil, L. A., Danielewski, J. A., Murray, G. L., Fehler, G., Fairley, C. K., Garland, S. M., Chow, E. P. F., Hocking, J. S., & Bradshaw, C. S. (2023). Prevotella and gardnerella are associated with treatment failure following first-line antibiotics for bacterial vaginosis. *The Journal of Infectious Diseases, 228*(5), 646–656. https://doi.org/10.1093/infdis/jiad261

Plummer, E. L., Vodstrcil, L. A., Murray, G. L., Fairley, C. K., Danielewski, J. A., Garland, S. M., Chow, E. P. F., Bulach, D. M., Fethers, K. A., Hocking, J. S., & Bradshaw, C. S. (2020). Gardnerella vaginalis clade distribution is associated with behavioral practices and Nugent score in women who have sex with women. *The Journal of Infectious Diseases, 221*(3), 454–463. https://doi.org/10.1093/infdis/jiz474

Rademeyer, C., Farley, C. L., & Van Hoover, C. (2020). Health implications and counseling considerations for individuals with piercings and tattoos. *Nursing for Women's Health, 24*(3), 210–227. https://doi.org/10.1016/j.nwh.2020.03.006

Reichman, O., & Sobel, J. (2014). Desquamative inflammatory vaginitis. *Best practice & research. Clinical Obstetrics & Gynaecology, 28*(7), 1042–1050. https://doi.org/10.1016/j.bpobgyn.2014.07.003

Rosário, A., Sousa, A., Varandas, T., Marinho-Dias, J., Medeiros, R., Martins, G., Monteiro, P., & Sousa, H. (2023). Impact of cervicovaginal microbiome on the risk of cervical abnormalities development. *Journal of Medical Virology, 95*(5), e28762. https://doi.org/10.1002/jmv.28762

Ross, A., & Shoff, H. (2019). Toxic shock syndrome. *Stat Pearls*. https://www.ncbi.nlm.nih.gov/books/NBK459345/

Rubin, E., Deshpande, N., Vasquez, P., & Kellogg Spadt, S. (2019). A clinical reference guide on sexual devices for obstetrician-gynecologists. *Obstetrics & Gynecology, 133*(6), 1259–1268. https://doi.org/10.1097/AOG.0000000000003262

Salvatore, S., Ruffolo, A. F., Phillips, C., Athanasiou, S., Cardozo, L., Serati, M., & EUGA Working Group. (2023). Vaginal laser therapy for GSM/VVA: Where we stand now—A review by the EUGA Working Group on Laser. *Climacteric: The journal of the International Menopause Society, 26*(4), 336–352. https://doi.org/10.1080/13697137.2023.2225766

Schardein J. N., Li G., Zaccarini D. J., Caza T., Nikolavsky D. (2021). Histological evaluation of vaginal cavity remnants excised during neourethral stricture repair in transgender men. *Urology*. https://doi.org/10.1016/j.urology.2021.06.044

Schreiner, K., & Balikowski, M. (2025). Fatal toxic shock syndrome following tattooing. *Forensic Science, Medicine, and Pathology*, 10.1007/s12024-025-01068-7. Advance online publication. https://doi.org/10.1007/s12024-025-01068-7

Singh, J., Mumford, S. L., Pollack, A. Z., Schisterman, E. F., Weisskopf, M. G., Navas-Acien, A., & Kioumourtzoglou, M. A. (2019). Tampon use, environmental chemicals and oxidative stress in the BioCycle study. *Environmental health : a global access science source, 18*(1), 11. https://doi.org/10.1186/s12940-019-0452-z

Sobel, J. D. (2023). Resistance to fluconazole of candida albicans in vaginal isolates: A 10-year study in a clinical referral center. *Antimicrobial Agents and Chemotherapy, 67*(5), e0018123. https://doi.org/10.1128/aac.00181-23

Sobel, J. D. (2024). Bacterial vaginosis: Initial treatment. *UpToDate*. Retrieved January 6, 2025, https://www.uptodate.com/contents/bacterial-vaginosis-initial-treatment

Sobel, J. D. (2024). Bacterial vaginosis: Recurrent infection. *UpToDate*. Retrieved January 6, 2025, https://www-uptodate-com./contents/bacterial-vaginosis-recurrent-infection

Sobel, J. D., & Mitchell, C. (2023). Candida vulvovaginitis: Clinical manifestations and diagnosis. *UpToDate*. Retrieved June 25, 2025, https://www.uptodate.com/contents/candida-vulvovaginitis-clinical-manifestations-and-diagnosis

Sonthalia, S., Aggarwal, P., Das, S., Sharma, P., Sharma, R., & Singh, S. (2020). Aerobic vaginitis—An underdiagnosed cause of vaginal discharge—Narrative review. *International Journal of STD & AIDS, 31*(11), 1018–1027. https://doi.org/10.1177/0956462420913435

Sousa, L. G. V., Pereira, S. A., & Cerca, N. (2023). Fighting polymicrobial biofilms in bacterial vaginosis. *Microbial Biotechnology, 16*(7), 1423–1437. https://doi.org/10.1111/1751-7915.14261

Stevens, D. L., Bisno, A. L., Chambers, H. F., Dellinger, E. P., Goldstein, E. J. C., Gorbach, S. L., Hirschmann, J. V., Kaplan, S. L., Montoya, J. G., & Wade, J. C. (2014, reaffirmed 2018). Practice guidelines for the diagnosis and management of skin and soft tissue infections: A 2014 update by the Infectious Diseases Society of America. *Clinical Infectious Diseases, 59*(2), e10–e52. https://doi.org/10.1093/cid/ciu444

Stoehr, J. R., Moss, C., & Hamadian Jahromi, A. (2023). The microbiome of the neovagina: A systematic review and comparison of surgical techniques. *International Journal of Transgender Health, 25*(4), 623–633. https://doi.org/10.1080/26895269.2023.2237014

Surapaneni, S., Akins, R., & Sobel, J. D. (2021). Recurrent bacterial vaginosis: An unmet therapeutic challenge. Experience with a combination pharmacotherapy long-term suppressive regimen. *Sexually Transmitted Diseases, 48*(10), 761–765. https://doi.org/10.1097/OLQ.0000000000001420

Tachedjian, G., O'Hanlon, D. E., & Ravel, J. (2018). The implausible "in vivo" role of hydrogen peroxide as an antimicrobial factor produced by vaginal microbiota. *Microbiome, 6*(1), 29. https://doi.org/10.1186/s40168-018-0418-3

Thomas-White, K., Navarro, P., Wever, F., King, L., Dillard, L. R., & Krapf, J. (2023). Psychosocial impact of recurrent urogenital infections: A review. *Women's Health (London, England), 19*, 17455057231216537. https://doi.org/10.1177/17455057231216537

The North American Menopause Society (2020, September). The 2020 genitourinary syndrome of menopause position statement of The North American Menopause Society. *Menopause, 27*(9), 976–992. https://doi.org/10.1097/GME.0000000000001609

Todd, J., Fishaut, M., Kapral, F., & Welch, T. (1978). Toxic-shock syndrome associated with phage-group-I Staphylococci. *Lancet (London, England), 2*(8100), 1116–1118. https://doi.org/10.1016/s0140-6736(78)92274-2

Ullman, K. E., Diem, S., Forte, M. L., Ensrud, K., Sowerby, C., Zerzan, N., Anthony, M., Landsteiner, A., Greer, N., Butler, M., Wilt, T. J., & Danan, E. R. (2024). Complementary and alternative therapies for genitourinary syndrome of menopause: An evidence map. *Annals of Internal Medicine, 177*(10), 1389–1399. https://doi.org/10.7326/ANNALS-24-00603

Upson, K., Shearston, J. A. & Kioumourtzoglou, M. A. (2022). Menstrual products as a source of environmental chemical exposure: A review from the epidemiologic perspective. *Current Environmental Health Reports, 9*, 38–52. https://doi.org/10.1007/s40572-022-00331-1

U.S. Preventive Services Task Force. (2020). *Screening for bacterial vaginosis in pregnant adolescents and women to prevent preterm delivery: An updated systematic review for the US Preventive Services Task Force* (Evidence Synthesis No. 190). https://www.uspreventiveservicestaskforce.org/uspstf/draft-update-summary/bacterial-vaginosis-in-pregnant-adolescents-and-women-to-prevent-preterm-delivery-screening

Vaginitis in Nonpregnant Patients: ACOG Practice Bulletin, Number 215. (2020). *Obstetrics and gynecology* 2020, *135*, e1 Reaffirmed 2022.

Van Eijk, A. M., Zulaika, G., Lenchner, M., Sivakami, M., Nyothach, E., Unger, H., Laserson, K., & Phillips-Howard, P. A. (2019). Menstrual cup use, leakage, acceptability, safety, and availability: A systematic review and meta-analysis. *Lancet Public Health, 4*(8), e376–e393.

Van Gerwen, O. T., Smith, S. E., & Muzny, C. A. (2023). Bacterial vaginosis in postmenopausal women. *Current Infectious Disease Reports, 25*(1), 7–15. https://doi.org/10.1007/s11908-022-00794-1

Van Hoover, C., Rademayer, C.-A., & Farley, C. L. (2017). Body piercing: Motivations and implications for health. *Journal of Midwifery & Women's Health, 62*(5), 521–530. https://doi.org/10.1111/jmwh.12630

Vandecruys, P., Baldewijns, S., Sillen, M., Van Genechten, W., & Van Dijck, P. (2023). Oteseconazole: A long-awaited diversification of the antifungal arsenal to manage recurrent vulvovaginal candidiasis (RVVC). *Expert Review of Anti-infective Therapy, 21*(8), 799–812.

Vodstrcil, L. A., Plummer, E. L., Fairley, C. K., Hocking, J. S., Law, M. G., Petoumenos, K., . . . Bradshaw, C. S. (2025). Male-partner treatment to prevent recurrence of bacterial vaginosis. *New England Journal of Medicine, 392*(10), 947–957.

Vodstrcil, L. A., Muzny, C. A., Plummer, E. L., Sobel, J. D., & Bradshaw, C. S. (2021). Bacterial vaginosis: Drivers of recurrence and challenges and opportunities in partner treatment. *BMC Medicine, 19*(1), 194. https://doi.org/10.1186/s12916-021-02077-3

Walter, K. (2022). Premenopausal vaginitis. *JAMA, 327*(22), 2255–2255. https://doi.org/10.1001/jama.2022.9256

Wang, Y., Liu, Z., & Chen, T. (2024). Vaginal microbiota: Potential targets for vulvovaginal candidiasis infection. *Heliyon, 10*(5), e27239. https://doi.org/10.1016/j.heliyon.2024.e27239

Willems, H. M. E., Ahmed, S. S., Liu, J., Xu, Z., & Peters, B. M. (2020). Vulvovaginal candidiasis: A current understanding and burning questions. *Journal of fungi (Basel, Switzerland), 6*(1), 27. https://doi.org/10.3390/jof6010027

Winston McPherson, G., Long, T., Salipante, S. J., Rongitsch, J. A., Hoffman, N. G., Stephens, K., Penewit, K., & Greene, D. N. (2019). The vaginal microbiome of transgender men. *Clinical Chemistry, 65*(1), 199–207. https://doi.org/10.1373/clinchem.2018.293654

Witkin, S. S., Moron, A. F., Ridenhour, B. J., Minis, E., Hatanaka, A., Sarmento, S. G. P., Franca, M. S., Carvalho, F. H. C., Hamamoto, T. K., Mattar, R., Sabino, E., Linhares, I. M., Rudge, M. V. C., & Forney, L. J. (2019). Vaginal biomarkers that predict cervical length and dominant bacteria in the vaginal microbiomes of pregnant women. *mBio, 10*(5), e02242-19. https://doi.org/10.1128/mBio.02242-19

Wu, S., Ding, X., Kong, Y., Acharya, S., Wu, H., Huang, C., . . . Chen, H. (2021). The feature of cervical microbiota associated with the progression of cervical cancer among reproductive females. *Gynecologic Oncology, 163*(2), 348–357.

Wychrij, D. A., Chapman, T. I., Rayens, E., Rabacal, W., Willems, H. M. E., Oworae, K. O., Peters, B. M., & Norris, K. A. (2025). Protective efficacy of the pan-fungal vaccine NXT-2 against vulvovaginal candidiasis in a murine model. *NPJ Vaccines, 10*(1), 112. https://doi.org/10.1038/s41541-025-01171-4

Younes, J. A., Lievens, E., Hummelen, R., van der Westen, R., Reid, G., & Petrova, M. I. (2018). Women and their microbes: The unexpected friendship. *Trends in Microbiology, 26*(1), 16–32.

Zarmakoupi, P., Psarris, A., Karasmani, C., Antsaklis, P., Theodora, M., Syndos, M., Pampanos, A., Pappa, K. I., Domali, E., Thomakos, N., Akinosoglou, K., Tsiakalos, A., & Daskalakis, G. (2024). Cracking the code: Investigating the correlation between aerobic vaginitis and preterm labor. *Medicina (Kaunas, Lithuania), 60*(4), 648. https://doi.org/10.3390/medicina60040648

CHAPTER 22

Sexually Transmitted Infections

Heidi Collins Fantasia

INTRODUCTION

Sexually transmitted infections (STIs) are a major public health issue in the United States, with approximately 26 million new STIs occurring every year (Centers for Disease Control and Prevention [CDC], 2025). At any given time, approximately 20 percent, or one in five, individuals in the US have an STI. STIs cause significant disease burden, place heavy demands on healthcare services, and cost the U.S. healthcare system as much as $16 billion each year (CDC, 2025). As STI rates rise, so does the potential for antibiotic resistance to treat these infections (CDC, 2021). The term "sexually transmitted infection" does not refer to any one specific disease, but rather it refers to a pathogen that is able to cause infection via sexual contact (CDC, 2021). This term has replaced the older designation of sexually transmitted disease. Many infections never progress to diseases and the term STI helps reduce stigma associated with these infections (Lederer & Laing, 2017). STIs may be caused by a wide spectrum of bacteria, viruses, protozoa, and ectoparasites (organisms that live on the outside of the body, such as a louse). Common STIs are listed in **Table 22-1**.

Preventing, identifying, and managing STIs are essential components of reproductive and gynecologic health care. Clinicians can assume an important role in promoting a person's reproductive and sexual health by counseling about the risks of STIs, including HIV; encouraging sexual and other risk-reduction measures; and being familiar with assessment and management strategies related to STIs. Through screening, early detection, treatment, and education, clinicians can help individuals reduce their risk for STIs and improve their health.

This chapter begins with an overview of STI transmission, screening, and detection. Topics that need to be addressed when talking with a person who has been diagnosed with an STI are presented as well. The remaining sections address specific STIs, including HPV, genital herpes, chancroid, pediculosis pubis, trichomoniasis, chlamydia, gonorrhea, pelvic inflammatory disease (PID), syphilis, hepatitis B virus (HBV), hepatitis C virus (HCV), and HIV infection. The CDC "Sexually Transmitted Infections Treatment Guidelines" represents the standard of care for STI testing and treatment (CDC, 2021). These guidelines are updated periodically, and clinicians should always consult the most current version.

TRANSMISSION OF SEXUALLY TRANSMITTED INFECTIONS

The chance of contracting, transmitting, or having complications from STIs depends on multiple biologic, behavioral, social, and relationship risk factors (**Box 22-1**). That is, a myriad of microbiologic, hormonal, and immunologic factors influence individual susceptibility and transmission potential for STIs. These factors are partially influenced by a person's sexual practices and other health behaviors. Health behaviors, in turn, are influenced by socioeconomic factors and other social influences (Mollaei et al., 2023).

SEXUALLY TRANSMITTED INFECTION SCREENING AND DETECTION

Prompt diagnosis and treatment of STIs is important and individuals must know how to recognize the major signs and symptoms of all STIs and must be willing and able to obtain health care if they experience symptoms or have sexual contact with someone who has an STI. Clinicians have a responsibility to educate their patients regarding the signs and symptoms of STIs. This education may be provided at any visit, including when an individual comes in for their annual health examination or episodic care, seeks contraception, or obtains preconception or prenatal care.

Clinicians must also ensure that their patients know where and how to obtain care if they suspect they might have contracted an STI. Many local health departments have clinics specifically designed to treat STIs, with services often available for free or at a reduced cost.

Screening

All individuals who are sexually active should be screened for STIs regularly through history, physical examination, and laboratory studies based on risk factors. Information on screening in specific populations and age groups can always be found in the most current version of the CDC "Sexually Transmitted Infections Treatment Guidelines" (CDC, 2021). To identify individuals at increased risk, specific questions should be asked during the collection of a health history (**Box 22-2** and **Box 22-3**). The accuracy of risk assessment, however, depends on a person's

TABLE 22-1 Common Sexually Transmitted Infections

Infection	Causative Organism
Chancroid	*Haemophilus ducreyi*
Chlamydia	*Chlamydia trachomatis*
Genital herpes	Herpes simplex virus (HSV)
Genital warts	Human papilloma virus (HPV)
Gonorrhea	*Neisseria gonorrhoeae*
Hepatitis	Hepatitis B virus (HBV), hepatitis C virus (HCV)
HIV infection and AIDS	Human immunodeficiency virus (HIV)
Molluscum contagiosum	Molluscum contagiosum virus
Pubic lice	*Phthirus pubis*
Syphilis	*Treponema pallidum*
Trichomoniasis	*Trichomonas vaginalis*

BOX 22-1 Risk Factors for Sexually Transmitted Infections and HIV

- Previous or current sexually transmitted infection
- Sex with multiple or new partners
- Initiating sex at a young age
- Unprotected sex
- Sex with high-risk partners
- Sex with a partner who has HIV
- Sex in exchange for money or drugs
- Sex while intoxicated
- Recreational/illegal drug use
- Substance use disorder/alcohol use disorder
- Injection drug use
- Mental health conditions
- Age < 25 years
- Living in an area with high sexually transmitted infection/HIV prevalence
- Residing in a detention or correctional facility

Data from Centers for Disease Control and Prevention. (2021). Sexually transmitted infections treatment guidelines, 2021. *Morbidity and Mortality Weekly Report, 70*(4), 1–187; Mollaei, B., Ahmadi, K., & Yousefi, E. (2023). Risk and protective factors of high-risk sexual behaviors in young people: A systematic review. *International Journal of High Risk Behaviors and Addiction, 12*(1). https://doi.org/10.5812/ijhrba-131119

willingness to self-identify risk factors that may be seen as socially unacceptable or stigmatizing. Some individuals may not reveal such risk factors directly to clinicians, but they might be willing to do so if asked to fill out a questionnaire using questions similar to those given in the five Ps (Box 22-2). The five Ps—an instrument developed by the CDC—is one way to gather sexual history information in an organized and nonjudgmental way. Any person who has been diagnosed with an STI should also be screened for other STIs because comorbidity of such infections is high, and many STIs can be asymptomatic (CDC, 2021).

ASSESSMENT

The diagnosis of an STI is based on the integration of relevant history, physical examination, and laboratory data. A history that is accurate, comprehensive, and specific is essential for accurate diagnosis.

Generally, the history should be taken first, with the person dressed. Information should be collected in a nonjudgmental manner, avoiding assumptions about sexual preference. All partners should be referred to as "partners," rather than by sex or gender identification. It is helpful to begin with open-ended questions because they often elicit information that might otherwise be missed. These queries can be followed with symptom-specific questions and relevant history. Specific areas to address include the reason why the person has sought care and any symptoms they have noticed; a sexual history, including a description of the date and type of sexual activity; number of partners; whether they had contact with someone who recently had an STI; and all potential sites of infection (e.g., mouth, cervix, urethra, and rectum). Pertinent medical history includes anything that will influence the management plan, such as current medications, history of drug allergies, previously diagnosed chronic illnesses, and general health status. A menstrual and contraceptive history, including the date of the last menstrual period, must be obtained to determine if there is a possibility of pregnancy. When indicated, a systems review should be conducted that may assist in diagnosis of specific STIs. Any positive answers regarding symptoms should be followed up to elicit information about systemic and local onset, duration, and characteristics (Fantasia et al., 2025; Secor & Holland, 2024).

Before the physical examination is performed, the clinician should discuss the procedure to be followed so that patients have information on what the exam entails. Please refer to Chapter 5 on trauma-informed care for best practice recommendations. The physical examination begins with careful visualization of the external genitalia, including the perineum. Erythema, edema, distortions, lesions, trauma, and any other abnormalities are noted. Palpation can locate areas of tenderness. During the speculum examination, the vagina and cervix are inspected for edema, thinning, lesions, abnormal coloration, trauma, discharge, and bleeding. Thorough palpation of the inguinal area and pelvic organs through bimanual examination, milking of the urethra for discharge, and assessment of vaginal secretion odors is essential (Fantasia et al., 2025; Secor & Holland, 2024).

Appropriate laboratory studies will be suggested, in part, by the history and physical examination results. These tests include microscopic examination of vaginal secretions (wet mount testing for trichomoniasis, yeast, and bacterial vaginosis), chlamydia and gonorrhea testing, treponemal tests with reflex to Venereal Disease Research Laboratory (VDRL) or rapid plasma reagin (RPR) testing for syphilis, and a hepatitis B and C panel. When an

BOX 22-2 The Five Ps of Sexual Health

1. Partners
   - Are you currently having sex of any kind—oral, vaginal, anal—with anyone?
   - If no, have you ever had sex of any kind with another person?
   - In recent months, how many sex partners have you had?
   - What is/are the genders(s) of your sex partner(s)?
   - Do you or your partner(s) currently have other sex partners?
2. Practices
   - To understand your risks for sexually transmitted infections, I need to ask more specific questions about the kind of sex you have had recently. What kind of sexual contact do you have or have you had? What parts of your body are involved when you have sex?
   - Do you have genital sex, meaning "penis-in-vagina sex"?
   - Do you have anal sex, meaning "penis-in-rectum/anus sex"?
   - Do you have oral sex, meaning "mouth-on-penis/vagina/anus"?
   - Have you or any of your partners used drugs?
   - Have you exchanged sex for things you need (money, housing, drugs, etc.)?
3. Protection from STIs
   - Do you and your partner(s) discuss prevention of STIs?
   - If you use prevention tools, what methods do you use? (For example, male or female condoms, dental dams, etc.)
   - How often do you use these methods?
   - Have you received the human papilloma virus (HPV), hepatitis A, and hepatitis B shots?
   - Are you aware of pre-exposure prophylaxis or PrEP, a medicine that can prevent HIV? Have you ever used it or considered using it?
4. Past History of STIs
   - Have you ever been tested for STIs or HIV? Would you like to be tested?
   - Have you ever been diagnosed with an STI in the past? When? Did you get treatment?
   - Has your current partner or any former partners ever been diagnosed or treated for an STI? Were you tested for the same STI(s)? Do you know your partner(s)' HIV status?
5. Pregnancy Intention
   - Do you think you would like to have (more) children at some point?
   - When do you think that might be?
   - How important is it to you to prevent pregnancy (until then)?
   - Are you or your partner using contraception or practicing any form of birth control? Would you like to talk about ways to prevent pregnancy? Do you need any information on birth control?

Reproduced from Centers for Disease Control and Prevention. (2021). Sexually transmitted infections treatment guidelines, 2021. *Morbidity and Mortality Weekly Report, 70*(4), 1–187. https://www.cdc.gov/sti/hcp/clinical-guidance/taking-a-sexual-history.html

BOX 22-3 Gynecologic History Questions to Assess Risk of Sexually Transmitted Infections

Do you experience now or have you ever experienced the following:

- Frequent vaginal infections
- Unusual vaginal discharge or odor
- Vaginal itching, burning, sores, or warts
- STIs (ask about individual infections)
- Abdominal pain
- Pelvic inflammatory disease (PID)/infection of the uterus, tubes, or ovaries
- Sexual assault/rape
- Physical, emotional, or sexual abuse
- Abnormal Pap test
- Pain or bleeding with intercourse
- Severe menstrual cramps occurring at end of period
- Ectopic pregnancy

Data from Fantasia, H. C., Harris, A. L., & Fontenot, H. B. (2025). *Guidelines for nurse practitioners in gynecologic settings* (13th ed.). Springer; Secor, R. M., & Holland, A. C. (2024). *Advanced health assessment of women* (5th ed.). Springer.

STI is diagnosed, testing for other STIs is essential. The individual should be notified that HIV testing will be performed as part of screening unless they specifically decline it (see the section on HIV testing later in this chapter). Other laboratory tests, such as a complete blood count, urinalysis, and urine culture and sensitivity, should be obtained only if indicated. If the history or physical examination indicates possible pregnancy, a urine human chorionic gonadotropin (hCG) test should also be performed because treatment for STIs can differ in pregnant and nonpregnant persons and because certain antibiotics are contraindicated in pregnancy (CDC, 2021).

EDUCATION AND PREVENTION

Counseling is an essential part of caring for a person with an STI (**Box 22-4** and **Table 22-2**). A person with an STI will need support in seeking care at the earliest possible stage of symptoms. Counseling about STIs is essential for the following reasons:

- Preventing new infections or reinfection
- Increasing adherence to treatment and follow-up
- Providing support during treatment
- Assisting in discussions and disclosure with partners
- Increasing awareness of the serious potential consequences of untreated STIs

Effective treatment of STIs necessitates a careful, thorough explanation of the treatment regimen and follow-up procedures. Comprehensive and precise instructions about medications must be provided, both verbally and in writing. Side effects, benefits,

BOX 22-4 Patient Information About Sexually Transmitted Infections

The only certain way to prevent STIs is to avoid sexual contact with others. If you choose to be sexually active, there are things you can do to decrease your risk of developing an STI:

- Have sex with only one person who does not have sex with anyone else and who has no infections.
- Always use a condom or barrier and use it correctly, especially for higher-risk sexual activities such as anal and vaginal sex. Sex toys should be covered with a barrier and cleaned after use.
- Use clean needles if you inject drugs.
- Prevent and promptly treat other STIs to decrease your susceptibility to HIV infection and to lower your potential to spread infection if you are HIV positive.
- Wait to have sex until you feel you are emotionally and physically ready. The younger you are when you have sex for the first time, the more likely you are to get an STI. The risk of acquiring an STI also increases with the number of partners you have in your lifetime.

Anyone who is sexually active should do the following:

- Always use a condom or barrier unless you are having sex with only one person who does not have sex with anyone else and who has no infections.
- Have regular checkups for STIs even if you have no symptoms, and especially when having sex with a new partner.
- Learn the common symptoms of STIs. Seek health care immediately if any suspicious symptoms develop, even if they are mild.
- Avoid having sex during menstruation. Individuals with HIV are probably more infectious during menstruation.
- Use a condom for anal intercourse.
- Avoid douching. It removes some of the normal protective bacteria in the vagina and increases the risk of getting some STIs.

Anyone diagnosed with an STI should do the following:

- Be treated to reduce the risk of transmitting an STI to another person.
- Notify all recent and current sex partners and urge them to get tested and treated as soon as possible to reduce the risk of reinfection from an untreated partner.
- Follow the clinician's recommendations and complete the full course of medication prescribed. Have a follow-up test if necessary.
- Avoid all sexual activity while being treated.

Data from Centers for Disease Control and Prevention. (2021). Sexually transmitted infections treatment guidelines, 2021. *Morbidity and Mortality Weekly Report, 70*(4), 1–187; Fantasia, H. C., Harris, A. L., & Fontenot, H. B. (2025). *Guidelines for nurse practitioners in gynecologic settings* (13th ed.). Springer; Secor, R. M., & Holland, A. C. (2024). *Advanced health assessment of women* (5th ed.). Springer.

and risks of medications should be discussed. Unpleasant side effects or early relief of symptoms may sometimes discourage individuals from completing their medication course. All patients should be strongly urged to continue taking their medication until the full regimen is finished, regardless of whether their symptoms diminish or disappear a few days after they begin the therapeutic regimen. Stopping medication before the full course is completed can lead to treatment failure and contribute to medication resistance (CDC, 2021). Comfort measures that decrease symptoms such as pain, itching, or nausea should be suggested. Providing written information is a useful strategy because diagnosis of an STI is a time of high anxiety for many people, and they may not be able to hear or remember what they were told.

In general, individuals should refrain from sexual activity until all treatment is finished. After treatment, individuals should be urged to continue using condoms to prevent recurring infections. All individuals who have contracted an STI should be taught safer sex practices, if this education has not been provided already. Follow-up appointments should be made as needed (CDC, 2021; Fantasia et al., 2025).

In most situations involving STIs, sexual partners should be examined; thus, the patient is asked to identify and notify all partners who might have been exposed (partner notification). Individuals can notify their partners themselves or seek assistance through local health departments that can attempt to contact partners. More information on partner notification can be found in the CDC STI treatment guidelines (CDC, 2021). Expedited partner therapy (EPT) can also be utilized for treating sexual partners of individuals who have been diagnosed with gonorrhea or chlamydia. It is a harm reduction technique that extends treatment availability to those who are unable or unlikely to seek treatment in a timely manner (CDC, 2021). EPT involves providing medication or prescriptions to sexual partners, unless prohibited by law in the state of practice. More information can be found at https://www.cdc.gov/sti/hcp/clinical-guidance/expedited-partner-therapy.html.

REPORTING

Accurate identification and timely reporting of STIs are integral components of successful infection control efforts. Clinicians are required to report certain STIs to their state public health officials, who in turn report these infection rates to the CDC. Nationally notifiable STIs include chancroid, chlamydia, gonorrhea, HIV, and syphilis, and these are reportable diseases in all U.S. states (CDC, 2022). A full list of all nationally notifiable STIs can be found at the National Notifiable Diseases Surveillance System (NNDSS) website (https://www.cdc.gov/std/statistics/2022/nndss.htm#:~:text=Four%20STIs%20are%20nationally%20notifiable,gonorrhea%2C%20syphilis%2C%20and%20chancroid) (CDC, 2022). The requirements for reporting

TABLE 22-2 Sexual Risk Practices

Safest	Lower Risk	Possible Risk	High Risk
Behavior			
Abstinence from sexual activity Self-masturbation Mutual monogamy (both partners and no high-risk activities) Hugging, massage, or touching[a] Dry kissing Mutual masturbation Drug abstinence	Wet kissing Urine contact with intact skin Vaginal intercourse with condom Fellatio interruptus (penile–oral sex without ejaculation)	Cunnilingus (vaginal oral sex) Fellatio (penile-oral sex) Mutual masturbation with skin breaks Anal intercourse with condom	Unprotected anal intercourse Unprotected vaginal intercourse Unprotected oral–anal contact Fisting Multiple sexual partners Sharing uncleaned sex toys, douche equipment Sharing needles Vaginal intercourse after anal contact without new condom
Prevention			
Avoid all drug and sexual high-risk behaviors	Avoid exposure to potentially infected body fluids Consistently use condoms Do not share sex toys, needles, douching equipment	Use dental dam, female condom, or other barrier with cunnilingus Use condom with fellatio Avoid anal intercourse	If having anal penetration, use condom with intercourse, latex glove with digital/hand penetration Avoid oral–anal contact Consistent condom use for all acts of intercourse Avoid anal penetration Avoid exposure to potentially infected body fluids

Data from Alexander, I. M., Johnson-Mallard, V., Kostas-Polston, E., Cappiello, J., & Hubbard, H. S. (2023). *Women's health care in advanced practice nursing* (3rd ed.). Springer.
[a]Assumes no breaks in skin.

other STIs differ from state to state, and clinicians need to be aware of reporting laws in their practice area. Clinicians are legally responsible for reporting all cases of those infections identified as reportable. Additionally, individuals with STIs should be asked to identify and notify all partners who might have been exposed to the infection.

Confidentiality is a crucial issue for many patients. When an STI is reportable, the individual must be informed that their case will be reported and why. Failure to inform a person that their case will be reported is considered a serious breach of professional ethics. Additionally, individuals need to be aware that they may be contacted by a health department representative. They should be assured that the information reported to and collected by health authorities is maintained in strictest confidence. Reports are protected by individual state statute or regulation (CDC, 2021). Every effort, within the limits of the clinician's public health responsibilities, should be made to reassure patients that their confidentiality will be protected.

HUMAN PAPILLOMAVIRUS AND GENITAL WARTS

HPV infection is the most common STI in the United States and globally (CDC, 2024a). Its exact incidence is not known because clinicians are not required to report HPV cases. Nevertheless, as many as 13 million people in the United States are believed to become newly infected with HPV each year, and nearly all sexually active individuals who are unvaccinated will contract HPV at some point in their lives but may not be aware of the infection (CDC, 2021).

HPV comprises a group of double-stranded DNA viruses with more than 150 known serotypes, of which more than 40 can infect the genital tract, including the external genitalia, vagina, urethra, and anus (CDC, 2021). Most HPV infections are asymptomatic, subclinical, or unrecognized, and they clear spontaneously (CDC, 2021). HPV can cause genital warts, and persistent infection with high-risk, oncogenic strains, types 16 and 18, cause the majority of cervical, penile, vulvar, vaginal, anal, and oropharyngeal cancers. Most genital warts are caused by HPV types 6 and 11, which carry a low risk for progressing to invasive cancer.

Genital warts are most frequently seen around the vaginal introitus, under the foreskin, or on the shaft of the penis, but they can also occur on the cervix, vagina, urethra, perineum, scrotum, and anus/perianal area. Typically, the lesions present as small, soft papillary swellings occurring singularly or in clusters on the genital and anal–rectal region. This is shown in **Color Plate 6**. Growths can be flat, papular, or pedunculated (CDC, 2021). Warts are usually flesh colored in individuals who have light skin tones and darker on individuals with black or brown skin tones. Although they are usually painless and often asymptomatic, the lesions may sometimes be painful or pruritic, particularly when they are very large, inflamed, or ulcerated.

Assessment

An individual with HPV lesions may be asymptomatic or present with "bumps" in the genital area, including the vaginal introitus, vulva, labia, or anus. Symptoms such as vaginal discharge, itching, dyspareunia, and postcoital bleeding are possible, but less common (Fantasia et al., 2025; Secor & Holland, 2024). History of known exposure to the virus is important because of the potentially long latency period for HPV infection and the possibility of subclinical infections in men and women. Nevertheless, the lack of known exposure history cannot be used to exclude a diagnosis of HPV infection because viral transmission can occur between asymptomatic partners (CDC, 2021).

Physical inspection of the vulva, perineum, anus, vagina, and cervix is essential whenever HPV lesions are suspected or seen. Gloves should be changed between vaginal and rectal examinations to prevent the potential spread of vulvar or vaginal lesions to the anus (Fantasia et al., 2025). Because speculum examination of the vagina may block some lesions, it is important to rotate the speculum blades until all areas are visualized. When lesions are visible, the characteristic appearance previously described is considered diagnostic (CDC, 2021). In many instances, however, cervical lesions are not visible; moreover, some vaginal or vulvar lesions may be unobservable to the naked eye. Diagnosis is made by careful, thorough clinical examination of visible genital warts. Biopsy is often not necessary but can be considered if lesions are atypical, do not respond to treatment, or worsen during treatment (CDC, 2021). Perform testing for other STIs when genital warts are present.

Individuals with HPV lesions and genital warts should have cervical cancer screening according to national recommendations (CDC, 2021; ACOG, 2021). Guidelines regarding target ages and frequency of cervical cancer screening have and will continue to change as advances are made in science as well as increased population level rates of HPV vaccination. Updated Risk-Based Management Consensus Guidelines for Abnormal Cervical Cancer Screening Tests and Cancer Precursors (Perkins et al., 2020), published by the American Society for Colposcopy and Cervical Pathology (ASCCP), can be found at https://www.asccp.org/management-guidelines.

HPV DNA testing should be performed only in individuals aged 21 years and older with a Pap test result indicating atypical squamous cells of undetermined significance (ASC-US) or for individuals aged 30 years and older in conjunction with Pap testing for cervical cancer screening. HPV DNA testing is inappropriate in the following situations: for STI screening; in adolescents (age 20 and younger); for individuals with abnormal Pap test results other than ASC-US (e.g., atypical squamous cells cannot rule out a high-grade lesion [ASC-H], low-grade squamous intraepithelial lesion [LSIL], and high-grade squamous intraepithelial lesion [HSIL]); and as routine screening in individuals younger than age 30. People considering vaccination against HPV should not be tested for HPV prior to vaccination (CDC, 2021). The standard cervical cancer screening recommendations are presented in Chapter 9.

Although there are specific national guidelines for cervical cancer screening, there are no HPV-based algorithms for anal cancer screening. Data are insufficient to recommend routine anal cytology for cancer screening among the general population or subpopulations. A digital anal rectal examination may be considered for individuals with HIV or those who practice anal receptive intercourse. If anal cytology is done, there needs to be a mechanism to follow up on abnormal results, such as the availability of high-resolution anoscopy and biopsy. Shared decision making between the clinician and patient is necessary to guide screening options (CDC, 2021).

Differential Diagnoses

HPV lesions must be differentiated from molluscum contagiosum, condylomata lata, and carcinoma. Molluscum contagiosum lesions are half-domed, smooth, and flesh-colored to pearly white papules with depressed centers. Condylomata lata—a form of secondary syphilis—are generally flatter and wider than genital warts. Cancers to be ruled out include squamous cell carcinoma, carcinoma in situ, and malignant melanoma. HPV can also be confused with benign conditions such as skin tags and nevi (CDC, 2021; Fantasia et al., 2025). An extensive list of other differential diagnoses for vulvar lesions can be found in Chapter 27.

Prevention

The most clinically significant HPV types can now be prevented with vaccination. The bivalent vaccine (HPV2, Cervarix), the quadrivalent vaccine (HPV4, Gardasil), and the 9-valent vaccine (HPV9, Gardasil 9) all protect against HPV types 16 and 18, which cause the majority of cervical cancers. In addition, the quadrivalent and 9-valent vaccines protect against HPV types 6 and 11, which cause the majority of genital warts, and provide some protection against vulvar and vaginal cancers and precancers. The 9 valent HPV vaccine protects against another five strains of HPV (31, 33, 45, 52, and 58) that are responsible for additional cervical cancers (American College of Obstetricians and Gynecologists [ACOG], 2020; CDC, 2021). The 9-valent vaccine is the only HPV vaccine available in the United States, and practitioners outside the United States should confirm vaccine availability in their geographical area (ACOG, 2020; CDC, 2021).

Routine HPV vaccination is recommended for all youth aged 11 to 12 years. HPV vaccines can be given starting at age 9 and are also recommended for adolescents and individuals aged 13 to 26 years who were not vaccinated or did not complete the series earlier (CDC, 2021). In 2018, the FDA expanded the use of the 9-valent HPV vaccine to include individuals through the age of 45, which allows for increased vaccination beyond previous recommendations (U.S. Food and Drug Administration (FDA), 2018). In 2019, the Advisory Committee on Immunization Practices (ACIP) voted to recommend that all individuals routinely receive the HPV vaccine through age 26 (CDC, 2025b). For persons aged 27 to 45 years, the ACIP recommends shared decision making between the individual and their healthcare provider as to whether the HPV vaccine is beneficial (CDC, 2025a).

Ideally, vaccination should occur before an individual becomes sexually active and therefore has the potential for HPV exposure; nevertheless, previous sexual activity does not preclude receiving the HPV9 vaccine through age 45. Vaccination is recommended for individuals who have evidence of existing HPV infection, such as Pap test abnormalities or genital warts, to provide protection against HPV types that they have not yet acquired (CDC, 2021). Vaccination will not treat existing HPV infection, cervical cytologic abnormalities, or genital warts (ACOG, 2020; CDC, 2021).

The dosing schedule for 9-valent HPV vaccine is dependent on age. Prior to age 15, a two-dose schedule is followed in which an initial dose is given, and the second dose is given 6 to 12 months later (0, 6- to 12-month schedule) (CDC, 2025a). If vaccination is initiated after the 15th birthday, a three-dose schedule is followed, in which the second dose is given 1 to 2 months (and at least

4 weeks) after the first dose, and the third dose is given 6 months (and at least 12 weeks) after the second dose (0, 1–2, 6-month schedule). The series does not need to be restarted if the second and third doses are delayed, and the next vaccine can be given even if years have elapsed. The 9-valent HPV vaccine can be used to complete a vaccine series that was started with either the bivalent or quadrivalent formulations (CDC, 2019b). Revaccination with the 9-valent HPV vaccine is not recommended for individuals who previously completed vaccination with the bivalent or quadrivalent vaccines (ACOG, 2020). There is no recommendation for HPV testing prior to vaccination (ACOG, 2020; CDC, 2021).

The 9-valent HPV vaccine is not recommended during pregnancy, but it can be given during lactation (ACOG, 2020). Routine pregnancy testing prior to vaccination is not recommended. If an individual is found to be pregnant after the vaccine is given, the remaining vaccines in the series should be delayed until after they give birth, and the clinician should report the exposure to the vaccine manufacturer (Merck, 1-800-986-8999), but no intervention is needed (Merck, 2019). The 9-valent HPV vaccine is contraindicated for individuals with hypersensitivity to any vaccine component or an immediate hypersensitivity to yeast (CDC, 2019b). Syncope has been reported after administration of the 9-valent HPV vaccine, and therefore it is advisable to observe individuals for 15 minutes after each injection (Merck, 2019).

Management

The primary treatment goals for visible genital warts are removal or reduction of warts and relief of signs and symptoms, not eradication of the virus. If left untreated, genital warts may resolve, remain unchanged, or increase in size and number (CDC, 2021). Treatment of genital warts can be challenging. An individual often must make multiple office visits if clinician-administered regimens are used. Patient-applied treatments need to be repeated for months, and even with treatment, recurrence is common (CDC, 2021).

Treatment of genital warts should be guided by the individual's preferences, available resources, cost considerations, ability to return for multiple visits if needed, size and location of warts, and experience of the clinician. None of the treatments is superior to any of the others, and no one treatment is ideal for all people or all warts (CDC, 2021). Available treatments are outlined in **Table 22-3**. Any concurrent vaginal infections or STIs should also be treated along with the genital warts.

Patient Education

Individuals who are experiencing discomfort associated with genital warts may find that bathing with an oatmeal solution and drying the area with a hair dryer on a lower setting might provide some relief. Keeping the area clean and dry may also decrease discomfort. Cotton underwear and loose-fitting clothes that decrease friction and irritation may be helpful as well (Fantasia et al., 2025). Individuals should be advised to maintain a healthy lifestyle to aid the immune system and can also be counseled regarding diet, rest, stress reduction, and exercise. All people who smoke should be counseled in smoking-cessation techniques.

Counseling messages for individuals with HPV infection and genital warts are outlined in **Box 22-5**. The partners of those with genital warts should be evaluated and treated if lesions are present. Condoms or barriers should be used until both partners are lesion free and for as long as 9 months after the appearance of lesions because subclinical HPV may remain infectious (CDC, 2021). All sexually active individuals with multiple partners or a history of HPV should be encouraged to use latex condoms during intercourse to decrease HPV acquisition or transmission, although HPV transmission may still occur from areas not covered by a condom.

It also should be noted that the majority of HPV infections are vaccine preventable. Individuals have varying opinions regarding vaccines, which can be influenced by upbringing, religion, cultural norms, distrust of pharmaceutical companies, or concern regarding side effects and adverse reactions. Healthcare provider recommendation is the strongest predictor of vaccine acceptance. Clinicians should have clear and respectful conversations regarding vaccine hesitancy that provide evidence-based information but also address patient concerns.

Special Considerations

Adolescents

Ideally, individuals should be vaccinated in early adolescence, prior to the initiation of sexual activity. Vaccine effectiveness is increased when administered at younger ages. Cervical screening and HPV testing are not recommended for this age group.

Pregnant People

Although various options exist for treating genital warts, not all are safe during pregnancy. Specifically, podophyllin, sinecatechins, and imiquimod should be avoided in people who are pregnant. External genital warts can multiply during pregnancy

TABLE 22-3 Treatment of External Genital Warts

Patient-Applied Regimens	Clinician-Administered Regimens	Alternative Regimens
Podofilox 0.5% solution or gel **or** Imiquimod 3.75% or 5% cream **or** Sinecatechins 15% ointment	Cryotherapy with liquid nitrogen or cryoprobe, repeat applications every 1–2 weeks **or** Trichloroacetic acid or bichloracetic acid 80–90% **or** Surgical removal by tangential scissor excision, tangential shave excision, curettage, or electrosurgery	Intralesional interferon **or** Photodynamic therapy **or** Topical cidofovir **or** Podophyllin resin 10–25% in a compound tincture of benzoin[a]

Data from Centers for Disease Control and Prevention. (2021). *Sexually transmitted infections treatment guidelines, 2021.*

[a]Consider only if strict adherence to application guidelines is followed to avoid systemic toxicity.

BOX 22-5 Counseling Messages for Individuals With Human Papillomavirus and Genital Warts

The CDC recommends that the following key counseling points be conveyed to all persons with HPV:

- Genital HPV infection is very common and can be passed through vaginal, anal, or oral sexual contact.
- Most unvaccinated, sexually active adults will get HPV at some point in their lives, although most will never know it because HPV infection usually has no signs or symptoms.
- HPV infection usually clears spontaneously without causing health problems, but some infections progress to genital warts, precancerous conditions, and cancers. The types of HPV that cause genital warts are not the same as the types that can cause cancer.
- A diagnosis of HPV in one sex partner is not indicative of sexual infidelity in the other partner.
- Treatments are available for genital warts, but the actual virus cannot be eradicated.
- HPV does not affect fertility or the ability to carry a pregnancy to term.
- Correct and consistent condom use might lower the chances of giving or getting genital HPV, but condom use is not fully protective because HPV can infect areas that are not covered by a condom. The only way to definitively avoid giving and getting HPV is to abstain from sexual activity.
- Tests for HPV are available to screen for cervical cancer in certain individuals.
- One HPV vaccine is available in the United States; it protects against the HPV types that cause 70 to 85 percent of cancers and 90 percent of genital warts. The vaccine is most effective when all doses are administered before sexual contact.

The following key counseling points are for individuals diagnosed with genital warts and their partners:

- Genital warts are not life threatening. If they are not treated, genital warts might go away, stay the same, or increase in size or number. It is very unusual for genital warts to turn into cancer.
- It is difficult to determine how or when a person became infected with HPV. Genital warts can be transmitted even when no visible signs of warts are present and even after warts are treated.
- It is not known how long a person remains contagious after warts are treated or whether informing subsequent sexual partners about a history of genital warts is beneficial to their health.
- Genital warts commonly recur after treatment, especially in the first 3 months.
- People with external genital warts do not need more frequent Pap tests. Frequency of Pap tests for individuals with cervical HPV is determined based on the extent of HPV-related abnormality.
- STI screening for both sex partners is beneficial if one partner has genital warts.

Data from Centers for Disease Control and Prevention. (2021). Sexually transmitted infections treatment guidelines, 2021. *Morbidity and Mortality Weekly Report, 70*(4), 1–187.

and become friable. Unless the vaginal opening is obstructed by large warts, a cesarean birth is not warranted. The risk of HPV transmission to the neonate and subsequent development of respiratory papillomatosis is low, and the presence of small warts that do not block the vaginal opening does not preclude a vaginal birth (CDC, 2021).

Perimenopause

The perimenopause years occur during the fourth decade of life for many people. Individuals can receive the HPV9 vaccine through age 45 and knowing a patient's vaccine status is important information when considering management and treatment of HPV. Perimenopause does not preclude vaccination or change the cervical cancer screening interval.

Older People

Sexually active individuals of any age can become infected with HPV. The older a person is, the less likely they are to have been vaccinated against HPV. Clinicians should not make assumptions regarding disease and infection risk based solely on age and all individuals should be asked directly about sexual activity. Cervical cancer screening should be completed based on age, history, and national guidelines.

GENITAL HERPES

Genital herpes is a recurrent, incurable viral infection characterized by painful vesicular eruptions of the skin and mucosa of the genitals. Two types of HSV have been identified as causing genital herpes: HSV-1 and HSV-2. HSV-2 is usually transmitted sexually, whereas HSV-1 is transmitted either nonsexually or through oral–genital contact. Although HSV-1 is more commonly associated with gingivostomatitis and oral ulcers (fever blisters) and HSV-2 is more commonly associated with genital lesions, both types are not exclusively associated with those sites, and an increasing number of genital infections are being attributed to HSV-1 (CDC, 2021). HSV-2 infection significantly increases the risk of acquiring HIV, especially for women. HSV-1 infection does not appear to carry the same risk (CDC, 2021).

Genital herpes is one of the most common STIs in the United States, but its exact prevalence is unknown because HSV is not a reportable infection. It is the primary cause of genital ulcer disease in the United States. According to CDC surveillance data, the overall prevalence rate of genital HSV-2 among women is 15.9 percent, compared with 8.2 percent in men. Non-Hispanic individuals of African descent have the highest reported rates—approximately 34 percent, more than three times higher than the rates in white individuals (McQuillan et al., 2018). HSV prevalence also increases with a higher number of lifetime sex partners; seroprevalence has been reported as 5.4 percent in women with 1 lifetime sex partner, 18.8 percent in women with 2 to 4 lifetime partners, 21.8 percent in women with 5 to 9 lifetime partners, and 37.1 percent in women with 10 or more lifetime partners. Data are lacking on HSV prevalence among transgender and nonbinary individuals.

Although HSV rates are high, the majority of individuals who are positive for HSV-2 antibodies report that they have never had a clinician tell them they had genital herpes (CDC, 2021). Despite mild or unrecognized infections, the HSV virus can still be intermittently shed in the genital tract. As a result, most genital herpes infections are transmitted by individuals who do not know they have HSV or who do not have symptoms at the time of transmission (CDC, 2021).

An initial or primary genital herpes infection characteristically has both systemic and local symptoms and lasts approximately 3 weeks. Flu-like symptoms with fever, malaise, and myalgia first appear about a week after exposure, peak within 4 days, and subside over the next week. Multiple genital lesions develop at the site of infection and may be present anywhere in the anogenital area, including the vulva, perianal area, vagina, cervix, and penis. The lesions begin as small painful blisters or vesicles that become unroofed, leaving behind ulcerated lesions. This is shown in **Color Plate 7**. Individuals with a primary herpes infection often develop bilateral, tender inguinal lymphadenopathy; vulvar edema; vaginal discharge; and severe dysuria (Fantasia et al., 2025).

Ulcerative lesions last 4 to 15 days before crusting over, and new lesions may develop over a period of 10 days during the course of the infection. Cervicitis is also common with initial HSV-2 infections. The cervix may appear normal, or it may be friable, reddened, ulcerated, or necrotic if cervical lesions are present. A heavy watery to purulent vaginal discharge is possible. Extragenital lesions may be present because of autoinoculation. Urinary retention and dysuria may occur secondary to autonomic involvement of the sacral nerve root (Fantasia et al., 2025).

Individuals experiencing recurrent episodes of genital herpes typically develop only local symptoms that are less severe than those associated with the initial infection due to the initial immune response. Systemic symptoms are usually absent with recurrences, although the characteristic prodromal genital tingling is common. Recurrent lesions are unilateral, are less extensive than the original lesions, and usually last 7 to 10 days without prolonged viral shedding. Lesions begin as vesicles and progress rapidly to ulcers (Fantasia et al., 2025).

Assessment

Establishing a diagnosis of genital HSV can be challenging. Many individuals with HSV do not have overt and persistent symptoms. Thus, in making the diagnosis of genital herpes, a history of exposure to a person with HSV infection is important, although infection from an asymptomatic individual is common. A history of viral symptoms, such as malaise, headache, fever, or myalgia, could be suggestive of HSV infection. Local symptoms, such as vulvar pain, dysuria, itching, or burning at the site of infection, and painful genital lesions that heal spontaneously are very suggestive of HSV infection. The clinician should also ask about prior history of a primary infection, prodromal symptoms, vaginal discharge, dysuria, and dyspareunia.

During the physical examination, the clinician should assess for inguinal and generalized lymphadenopathy and elevated temperature. Carefully inspect the entire vulvar, perineal, vaginal, and cervical areas for vesicles, ulcers, or crusted areas. A speculum examination may be very difficult for the patient because of the extreme tenderness often associated with genital herpes. Genital lesions, especially those that are extremely tender, should be tested for HSV even if the appearance is not consistent with classic herpes lesions.

Although a diagnosis of HSV infection may be suspected from the patient's history and physical examination, it can be confirmed only by laboratory studies. Identification of HSV from nucleic acid amplification testing (NAAT) assay or by polymerase chain reaction (PCR) are the preferred tests for individuals who have genital ulcers or other mucocutaneous lesions. Viral culture is less sensitive than PCR, with the best culture yield found during a primary infection or if the specimen is taken during the vesicular stage of the infection—the sensitivity of a culture declines rapidly as lesions begin to heal. Both culture and PCR can be negative in a person with HSV infection because the virus is shed only intermittently (CDC, 2021).

Type-specific serologic tests are useful in confirming a clinical diagnosis given the frequency of false-negative HSV cultures, especially for individuals with healing lesions or recurrent infection. Antibodies are present within the first several weeks after infection and persist indefinitely. Clinicians should be certain to specifically request serologic type-specific glycoprotein G (IgG)-based assays. Serologic test options include laboratory-based assays and point-of-care tests using capillary blood or serum during a clinic visit. The sensitivity of these tests varies from 80 to 98 percent, and false-negative results can occur, especially in early-stage infection when antibodies are still developing. If there is a strong clinical suspicion of HSV in the presence of a negative result, testing can be repeated within a few months. The specificity of these assays is 96 percent or greater, and false-positive results can occur in individuals with a low likelihood of HSV infection.

Serologic screening for HSV is not recommended for the general population, but it should be considered for individuals who experience recurrent or atypical genital symptoms with negative HSV cultures, have a clinical diagnosis of genital herpes without laboratory confirmation, or have HIV. Testing should also be considered for asymptomatic partners of individuals with HSV infection (CDC, 2021). All patients with genital herpes should be tested for other STIs, including chlamydia, gonorrhea, syphilis, and HIV.

Differential Diagnoses

Differential diagnoses for HSV infection include syphilis, chancroid, lymphogranuloma venereum, and granuloma inguinale, as well as non-STI vulvar lesions such as those caused by Crohn's disease, Behcet syndrome, bacterial infection, trauma, or drug reaction (CDC, 2021; Fantasia et al., 2025; Roett, 2020).

Prevention

There is currently no vaccine available to prevent HSV infection, so changes in sexual behavior are the only way to protect against this infection. Safer sexual practices are detailed in Box 22-4 and Table 22-2. Although condoms provide some protection against HSV, they cover only a portion of the genital skin. Transmission of HSV via skin-to-skin contact, including oral–genital contact (oral sex), can still occur among partners, even in the absence of symptoms (CDC, 2021).

Management

Genital herpes is a chronic and recurring condition for which there is no known cure. However, HSV infection may produce few or no noticeable symptoms, especially if the infection is caused by HSV-1. Systemic antiviral drugs may partially control the symptoms and signs of HSV infections when used for primary or recurrent episodes, and they may completely control symptoms when used as daily suppressive therapy. These drugs do not cure the infection, however, nor do they alter the subsequent risk, frequency, or rate of recurrence after discontinuation. Three antiviral medications provide clinical benefits for genital herpes: acyclovir, valacyclovir, and famciclovir (**Table 22-4**). Topical antiviral therapy is not recommended due to its minimal benefits (CDC, 2021).

Systemic antiviral therapy should be given to all individuals experiencing their first genital herpes episode. Most people with a symptomatic first episode of genital HSV-2 infection will experience recurrent episodes of genital lesions; by comparison, recurrence is less common among individuals with genital HSV-1 infection. Lifelong intermittent, asymptomatic genital shedding occurs in people who have HSV-2 infection. Recurrent genital herpes can be treated with daily suppressive therapy, which decreases the frequency of recurrences and the risk of transmitting HSV; or episodic therapy may be implemented when lesions occur to help them heal more quickly. Episodic therapy should be started within 1 day of when the lesion begins or during the prodromal symptoms, if present. Individuals using episodic therapy should be provided with a prescription or medication in advance to facilitate immediate treatment of outbreaks. All individuals who have a history of HSV and desire suppressive therapy should be offered treatment if they do not have any contraindications to antiviral medications (CDC, 2021).

Oral analgesics, such as acetaminophen, aspirin, or ibuprofen, may be used to relieve pain and systemic symptoms associated with initial infections. Any topical agents should be used with caution because the mucous membranes affected by herpes are very sensitive. Ointments containing cortisone should be avoided. Occlusive ointments may prolong the course of infections.

Nonpharmacologic and complementary measures that may increase comfort for individuals when lesions are active include warm sitz baths; keeping lesions warm and dry by using a hair dryer set on cool or patting the area dry with a soft towel; wearing cotton underwear and loose clothing; applying cool witch hazel compresses followed by aloe vera gel or Burow's solution (Domeboro) to lesions daily as tolerated; and oatmeal baths. Topical application of vitamin E oil may reduce discomfort (Chang et al., 2023). However, these therapies are only for comfort and there is no evidence they increase healing time or decrease the severity of the outbreak (Fantasia et al., 2025; Roett, 2020).

Many complementary and alternative products are used for genital herpes, although no or only limited evidence supports the effectiveness of most of these products. The amino acid L-lysine has been used for active lesions and suppression. It is thought that L-lysine has an inhibitory effect on the amino acid L-arginine, which supports HSV infection. Minimizing consumption of the foods that contain arginine may help as well; these foods include coffee, grains, chicken, chocolate, corn, dairy products, meat, peanut butter, nuts, and seeds. Avoiding citrus foods may also be helpful (Chang et al., 2023).

TABLE 22-4 Treatment of Genital Herpes

Primary Infection[a]	Recurrent Infection	Suppressive Therapy
Acyclovir 400 mg orally 3 times/day for 7–10 days	Acyclovir 400 mg orally 3 times/day for 5 days*	Acyclovir 400 mg orally 2 times/day
or	**or**	**or**
Acyclovir 200 mg orally 5 times/day for 7–10 days*	Acyclovir 800 mg orally 2 times/day for 5 days	Famciclovir 250 mg orally 2 times/day
or	**or**	**or**
Famciclovir 250 mg orally 3 times/day for 7–10 days	Acyclovir 800 mg orally 3 times/day for 2 days	Valacyclovir 500 mg orally once/day **
or	**or**	**or**
Valacyclovir 1 gm orally 2 times/day for 7–10 days	Famciclovir 125 mg orally 2 times/day for 5 days	Valacyclovir 1 gm orally once/day
	or	
	Famciclovir 1 gm orally 2 times/day for 1 day	
	or	
	Famciclovir 500 mg orally once, followed by 250 mg 2 times/day for 2 days	
	or	
	Valacyclovir 500 mg orally 2 times/day for 3 days	
	or	
	Valacyclovir 1 gm orally once/day for 5 days	

Data from Centers for Disease Control and Prevention. (2021). Sexually transmitted infections treatment guidelines, 2021. *Morbidity and Mortality Weekly Report, 70*(4), 1–187.

[a]Treatment can be extended if healing is incomplete after 10 days of therapy.

*Effective but not recommended due to frequency of dosing.

** May be less effective than other valacyclovir or acyclovir dosing regimens in patients who have 10 or more episodes per year.

Vitamin and mineral supplementation has also been suggested for management of HSV and reduction of recurrent episodes. Specifically, vitamins B and C and the minerals zinc and calcium have been suggested as potentially helpful to prevent episodic HSV outbreaks (Chang et al., 2023). However, rigorous research in this area is lacking, and there is no established dose or evidence-based guidelines for vitamin and mineral supplementation.

Patient Education

Symptoms of HSV and whether the individual experiences recurrences depend on whether they have an infection with HSV-1 or HSV-2. Patients should be advised that viral shedding—and therefore transmission of HSV to a partner—is most likely with active lesions, but it can occur even while asymptomatic. Therefore, all current and future sex partners should be informed that the person has genital HSV infection. Individuals whose partners do not have HSV infection should refrain from sexual contact from the onset of the prodrome until the complete healing of lesions. During asymptomatic periods, condoms and suppressive therapy can be used to reduce the risk of transmission to partners who do not have HSV infection.

Special Considerations

Adolescents

Any sexually active individual or those who were previously sexually active can have a primary or recurrent HSV infection. Current recommendations for diagnosis or treatment do not differ based on age. Adolescents should be asked if they are sexually active and screened for STIs as indicated by their history and exam.

People Who Are Pregnant

Preventing neonatal herpes depends on preventing a primary infection during late pregnancy and avoiding exposure of the neonate to the HSV virus via shedding or exposure to active lesions during birth. Rates of HSV transmission to neonates are as high as 50 percent among pregnant people who first acquire HSV close to birth, but transmission rates are much lower in people with recurrent HSV or those who have a more remote history of primary infection (CDC, 2021). Individuals who have the capacity to become pregnant should be educated about the risk of neonatal HSV infection and be advised that if they become pregnant, they need to be certain to disclose their history of genital herpes to the clinicians providing their prenatal care and the care for their neonate (CDC, 2021). Individuals with a history of genital herpes can begin a suppressive regimen beginning no later than 36 weeks' gestation. Acyclovir 400 mg orally three times per day or valacyclovir 500 mg orally twice daily are recommended (CDC, 2021).

Individuals who have not had genital HSV should be counseled to abstain from vaginal intercourse and receptive oral sex if their partner is known or suspected to have oral or genital HSV. Individuals with a known history of HSV should be questioned during labor about active lesions or prodromal symptoms. Patients without lesions can give birth vaginally. Patients who have active lesions at the time of labor should have a cesarean birth to decrease the possibility of transmission to their neonate. Individuals with a history of HSV can take suppressive acyclovir during the third trimester to reduce the risk of an outbreak during labor and the subsequent need for cesarean birth (CDC, 2021).

Perimenopause and Older People

Any sexually active individual or those who were previously sexually active can have a primary or recurrent HSV infection. Current recommendations for diagnosis or treatment do not differ based on age. However, dose adjustments may be indicated. All three medications used to treat HSV—acyclovir, famciclovir, and valacyclovir—are excreted renally (Wilms et al., 2022). Although there are no recommendations for monitoring renal function prior to or during treatment, individuals with preexisting renal disease may require a dose reduction.

Individuals With HIV Infection

People who are immunocompromised, including those with HIV, can have prolonged or more severe episodes of HSV and HSV shedding is increased. HSV treatment guidelines for individuals with HIV are not different than for those without HIV, but treatment length may need to be extended for lesions to resolve. Additionally, intravenous antiviral treatment may be necessary for individuals with HIV and severe HSV (CDC, 2021).

CHANCROID

Chancroid is a bacterial infection of the genitourinary tract caused by the gram-negative bacteria *H. ducreyi*. Chancroid is uncommon in the United States and since 2016, less than five cases have been diagnosed each year (Gravett & Marrazzo, 2023). Globally, the highest number of cases are in Africa and lesser numbers in parts of Asia. Overall trends in chancroid are difficult to determine because the causative organism of chancroid is difficult to culture (Gravett & Marrazzo, 2023). Chancroid is a genital ulcer and therefore is a risk factor for HIV transmission. The incubation period for the infection, though not well established, usually ranges from 3 to 7 days (Gravett & Marrazzo, 2023).

Most individuals with chancroid present with a history of a painful macule on the external genitalia that rapidly changes to a pustule and then to an ulcerated lesion. This is shown in **Color Plate 8**. They may also develop enlarged unilateral or bilateral inguinal nodes known as buboes. After 1 to 2 weeks, the skin overlying the lymph node becomes erythematous, the center necroses, and the node becomes ulcerated (Gravett & Marrazzo, 2023). Autoinoculation from primary lesions is possible on opposing skin.

Assessment

A probable diagnosis of chancroid can be made when one or more painful genital ulcers are present; there is no evidence of syphilis (through dark-field examination of ulcer exudate or serologic testing at least 7 days after ulcer onset); the clinical presentation, ulcer appearance, and regional lymphadenopathy (if present) are typical for chancroid; and HSV testing of the exudate is negative (CDC, 2021). Because chancroid is more prevalent in certain geographic areas and less common in the United States, individuals should be asked about recent travel to or sexual activity with a partner from parts of Asia or Africa, where chancroid outbreaks are more common (CDC, 2021; Gravett & Marrazzo, 2023). Definitive diagnosis of chancroid is difficult because the organism can be identified only by culture on a special medium that is not used routinely; even when this technique is used, the sensitivity of the test is less than 80 percent (CDC, 2021). Testing for HIV and syphilis should be performed at the time of diagnosis and repeated in 3 months if initial testing was negative.

Differential Diagnoses

Differential diagnoses include syphilis, HSV, lymphogranuloma venereum, folliculitis, metastatic genital cancer (cervical, vagina, vulvar), and other vulvar lesions (Fantasia et al., 2025; Gravett & Marrazzo, 2023; Roett, 2020).

Prevention

There is no vaccine to prevent chancroid. General STI prevention strategies are detailed in Box 22-4 and Table 22-2.

Management

The recommended treatments for chancroid are azithromycin 1 gm orally in a single dose, ceftriaxone 250 mg intramuscularly (IM) in a single dose, ciprofloxacin 500 mg orally twice per day for 3 days, or erythromycin base 500 mg orally three times per day for 7 days (CDC, 2021). Individuals with comorbid HIV infection may require repeated or longer therapy (CDC, 2021).

Individuals should be reexamined 3 to 7 days after beginning therapy. If treatment is successful, symptomatic improvement should be apparent within 3 days of starting therapy. Objective clinical improvement should be noticeable on examination 7 days after treatment, although it may take more than 2 weeks for complete healing of large ulcers.

Patient Education

All partners who have had sexual contact with a person diagnosed with chancroid within 10 days preceding the onset of that individual's symptoms should be evaluated and treated, regardless of whether symptoms are present (CDC, 2021). Complete symptom resolution could take weeks, and permanent scarring is possible, even with successful treatment.

Overall, cases of chancroid are decreasing globally but are more prevalent in parts of Africa or Asia (Gravett & Marrazzo, 2023). Clinicians who suspect an individual may have chancroid should ask about sexual activity with a partner from a geographical area where chancroid is more common or if the person has engaged in commercial sex work with partners who may have traveled from these areas. Additionally, if a person is from an area of high susceptibility, the clinician can consider chancroid as a differential diagnosis. Chancroid has historically been linked to sexual networks, especially commercial sex work (Ogale et al., 2023). Clinicians should also consider the possibility of commercial sex trafficking if other findings from the history and physical are suspicious, such as unique tattoos, signs of trauma or violence, an older partner, homelessness or unstable housing, inconsistent health care, and history of STIs and/or unintended pregnancies (Fantasia, 2018).

Special Considerations

Infants, Children, and Adolescents

In the United States, sexual contact is the main route of transmission for chancroid. For infants and children in the United States, a diagnosis of genital ulcer disease from chancroid is highly suspicious for sexual abuse. Adolescents should always be asked about sexual activity when they present with symptoms that could indicate a sexually transmitted infection. However, nonsexual transmission of chancroid is more common in parts of African and Asia. Children who have recently immigrated to the United States or who have traveled to a country where chancroid is more common may not have contracted the infection through sexual contact. Careful history taking is critical in these situations.

Pregnant People

Although ciprofloxacin is generally considered safe during pregnancy, toxicity has been reported among infants who are breastfeeding. Consequently, one of the other antibiotics recommended for chancroid should be used in people who are pregnant or breastfeeding (CDC, 2021).

Perimenopause and Older People

There are no diagnostic or treatment considerations associated with perimenopause, menopause, or aging.

Individuals With HIV

Individuals who contract chancroid and also have HIV are more likely to experience a treatment failure and may require a longer duration of treatment (CDC, 2021). Additionally, ulcers may take a more prolonged time to heal.

PEDICULOSIS PUBIS

Pediculosis is a parasitic infection caused by any of three species of lice: *Pediculus humanus capitis* (head louse infecting the scalp), *Pediculus humanus corporis* (body or clothing louse infecting the trunk), and *Phthirus pubis* (pubic lice or "crabs"). *P. pubis* inhabits the genital area but may also be found in other hair-bearing areas of the body, including the axillae, chest, thighs, eyelashes, and head. An individual may be infected through sexual transmission or contact with infected clothing or bedding (Fantasia et al., 2025; Patel et al., 2021).

Assessment

Individuals with pediculosis usually present with pruritus caused by lice bites and deposition of saliva and fecal material into the skin. People may report seeing the lice or having a known exposure to a household member or sexual partner with head, body, or pubic lice (CDC, 2021). A history of shared clothing, bathing equipment, or bedding may also be given. Diagnosis is made by direct examination of the egg cases (nits) in the involved area. This is shown in **Color Plate 9**. Although the nits are usually visible to the naked eye, a hand lens and light can be helpful in identifying them. Black dots (excreta) may be visible on the surrounding skin and underclothing, and crusts or scabs may be seen in the pubic area. Individuals with pediculosis pubis should be tested for other STIs, including HIV, syphilis, chlamydia, and gonorrhea (CDC, 2021; Fantasia et al., 2025).

Differential Diagnoses

Differential diagnoses include anogenital eczema and pruritus, seborrheic dermatitis, pruritus vulvae, folliculitis, tinea cruris, and scabies (Fantasia et al., 2025). Other concomitant STIs should be ruled out as well (CDC, 2021).

Prevention

General STI prevention strategies are detailed in Box 22-4 and Table 22-2.

Management

Recommended treatments for pediculosis pubis include permethrin 1 percent cream rinse and pyrethrins with piperonyl butoxide. These medications are applied to the affected areas and washed off after 10 minutes. If symptoms do not resolve within a week and treatment failure is thought to be due to drug resistance, an alternative regimen consists of malathion 0.5 percent lotion applied for 8 to 12 hours and washed off. Oral ivermectin (250 mcg/kg) taken initially and repeated in 2 weeks is another alternative regimen, although this medication has limited ovicidal activity. Taking ivermectin with food increases this medication's bioavailability (CDC, 2021).

Patient Education

Advise individuals with pediculosis to wash all clothing, bed linens, and towels in hot water and to dry these items thoroughly on the hot cycle to destroy lice and nits. During treatment with topical agents, care should be taken to avoid contact with the eyes. Sexual partners within the past month should be evaluated and treated if necessary. Sexual contact should be avoided until the individual and their partners have been successfully treated and all linens and clothing have been decontaminated (CDC, 2021; Fantasia et al., 2025; Patel et al., 2021).

It is interesting to note that pubic hair removal has become a common practice among people globally, including in the United States. Cultural norms have shifted to suggest that pubic hair grooming is synonymous with sexual attractiveness and cleanliness, and removal has been associated with sexual activity, partner preferences, and healthcare examinations (Eltobgy et al., 2024). Some evidence suggests that pubic hair removal is associated with a decreased rate of pubic lice, but there is no current recommendation to educate clients to use this as a mechanism to reduce the risk of infection (CDC, 2021).

Special Considerations

Adolescents

There are no diagnostic or treatment considerations associated with adolescents. All adolescents should be asked about sexual activity and any symptoms of STIs.

Pregnant People

Individuals who are pregnant or lactating and have pubic lice should be treated. Permethrin or pyrethrins with piperonyl butoxide are recommended. Additionally, ivermectin is considered to be compatible with pregnancy and lactation and can be used as an additional or alternative treatment. In contrast, topical lindane has been shown to cause fetal harm and should not be used during pregnancy (CDC, 2021).

Perimenopause and Older People

There are no diagnostic or treatment considerations associated with perimenopause, menopause, or aging.

TRICHOMONIASIS

Trichomoniasis is caused by *T. vaginalis*, an anaerobic one-celled protozoan with characteristic flagella. This organism most commonly lives in the vagina in women and in the urethra in men. Many individuals are asymptomatic which facilitates transmission among sexual partners (Van Gerwen et al., 2023). Higher rates have been seen in specific populations of women, including those who are incarcerated and women who seek care at STI clinics (CDC, 2021). Trichomoniasis is sexually transmitted during vaginal–penile intercourse or vulva-to-vulva contact. Nonsexual transmission is possible but rare. Trichomoniasis is strongly associated with an increased risk of HIV transmission (CDC, 2021). Although trichomoniasis is often asymptomatic, individuals can experience a characteristically yellow to greenish, frothy, mucopurulent, copious, malodorous discharge. Inflammation of the vulva, vagina, or both may be present, and patients may have irritation, pruritus, dysuria, or dyspareunia. Typically, the discharge worsens during and after menstruation (CDC, 2021).

Assessment

In addition to the history of current symptoms, a careful sexual history, including information on last intercourse and last sexual contact, should be obtained from a patient with suspected trichomoniasis. Any history of similar symptoms in the past and treatment used should be noted. The clinician should determine whether the individual's partners were treated and whether there have been subsequent relations with new partners. Additional important information includes the last menstrual period, method of contraception, condom use, and use of other medications (Fantasia et al., 2025).

Inspect the external genitalia for excoriation, erythema, edema, ulceration, and lesions. On speculum examination, note the quantity, color, consistency, and any odor of the vaginal discharge. The cervix and vaginal walls may demonstrate characteristic tiny petechiae, often called "strawberry spots," especially after prolonged infection. This is shown in **Color Plate 10**. The cervix may bleed on contact. In severe infections, the vaginal walls, the cervix, and occasionally the vulva may be acutely inflamed. The pH of vaginal discharge is elevated (Fantasia et al., 2025; Van Gerwen et al., 2023).

Diagnosis has traditionally been made by point-of-care visualization of the typical one-celled flagellate trichomonads on microscopic examination of vaginal discharge (**Figure 22-1**). Although the specificity of this finding is 100 percent, this method has a sensitivity of approximately 51 to 65 percent. The slide must be viewed quickly (no longer than 20 minutes) to increase the chance of observing mobile trichomonads and ensure optimal results (Van Gerwen et al., 2023). Nonmotile trichomonads are more challenging to recognize. Microscopic examination of the wet mount may also reveal increased numbers of white blood cells, and a strong amine odor will be produced with the addition of potassium hydroxide to the specimen. Point-of-care tests that do not require microscopy are more commonly used and typically have higher sensitivity (more than 82%) and specificity (more than 95%) (CDC, 2021; Van Gerwen et al., 2023).

Culture is a sensitive and highly specific method of diagnosis, but it is no longer routinely performed because of the availability of nucleic acid amplification tests (NAATs). Culture should be performed when trichomoniasis is suspected but cannot be confirmed with microscopy or when NAAT is not available. Additionally, drug susceptibility testing to 5-nitroimidazole medications can be performed from the culture and this can be an important approach if a patient is experiencing persistent trichomoniasis infections despite adequate treatment (Van Gerwen et al., 2023). Although *T. vaginalis* may be an incidental finding on a Pap test, it is not considered diagnostic (even with liquid-based specimens), and confirmatory testing is still needed. All patients with trichomoniasis should be tested for other STIs, including chlamydia, gonorrhea, syphilis, and HIV (CDC, 2021).

FIGURE 22-1 **Wet mount findings with trichomoniasis.**

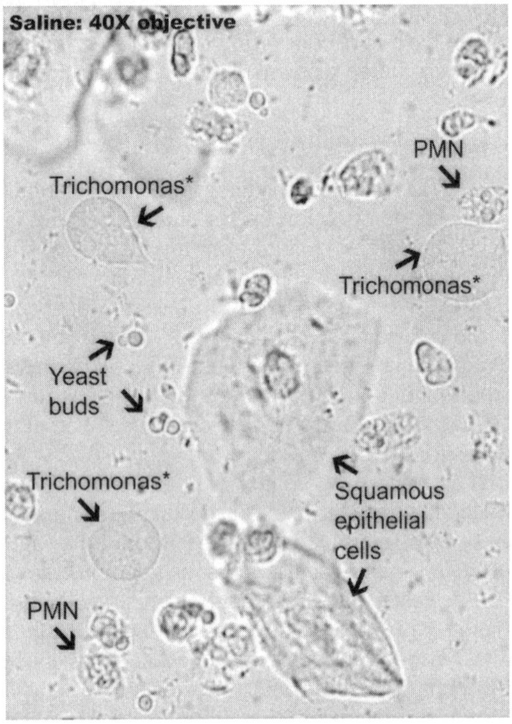

Reproduced from Washington State Department of Health STD/TB Program, Seattle STD/HIV Prevention Training Center, and Cindy Fennell, MS, MT, ASCP.

Note: Trichomonads must be motile for conclusive diagnosis.

Abbreviation: PMNs, polymorphonuclear leukocytes/white blood cells.

Differential Diagnoses

Differential diagnoses for trichomoniasis include other conditions that cause vaginal discharge, such as vulvovaginal candidiasis, bacterial vaginosis, chlamydia, and gonorrhea (Fantasia et al., 2025). Please refer to Chapter 21 for information about vulvovaginal candidiasis and bacterial vaginosis.

Prevention

General STI prevention strategies are detailed in Box 22-4 and Table 22-2.

Management

The nitroimidazoles are the only antimicrobial medications that are effective against *T. vaginalis*. The recommended treatment for trichomoniasis in women and people with vaginas is metronidazole 500 mg orally twice per day for 7 days. For men and people with penises, metronidazole 2 gm orally in a single dose is recommended. An alternate treatment regimen for people of any gender is tinidazole 2 gm orally in a single dose. Tinidazole is equivalent or superior to metronidazole in terms of cure and symptom resolution, and it has fewer gastrointestinal side effects, but it is more expensive than metronidazole. Topical metronidazole is less effective and not recommended (CDC, 2021).

Most recurrences of trichomoniasis are thought to be due to reinfection. If treatment failure occurs in a person after completing a course of metronidazole 500 mg orally twice daily for 7 days and they have been re-exposed to an untreated partner, a repeat course of the same regimen is recommended. If re-exposure has not occurred, then the person should be treated with either metronidazole or tinidazole 2 g once daily for 7 days. If infection persists, consultation with a specialist and testing for drug resistance is warranted (CDC, 2021).

Patient Education

Sex partners of individuals with trichomoniasis should also be treated, and all individuals should abstain from sex until both partners have been treated and are asymptomatic. Because rates of reinfection are high within the first 3 months after treatment, individuals should be evaluated within this time frame even if they and their partners have completed treatment (CDC, 2021). If it is not possible to retest someone at 3 months, they should be retested at the next healthcare appointment within a year from treatment.

Special Considerations

Adolescents

There are no diagnostic or treatment considerations associated with adolescents. All adolescents should be asked about sexual activity and any symptoms of STIs.

Pregnant People

Individuals who are pregnant and have trichomoniasis are at risk for pregnancy complications, including premature rupture of membranes, preterm labor and birth, and low-birth-weight infants (CDC, 2021). Metronidazole does cross the placenta but is not contraindicated in pregnancy and is considered to be low risk for the developing fetus. Pregnant individuals who are symptomatic should be tested and treated with metronidazole 500 mg orally twice daily for 7 days (CDC, 2021; Van Gerwen et al., 2023). Routine screening for asymptomatic individuals who are pregnant is not recommended.

Metronidazole is secreted in breast milk. With maternal oral metronidazole treatment, breastfed infants receive metronidazole in doses that are lower than those used to treat infections among infants. Although there is no evidence of adverse effects among infants exposed to metronidazole via breast milk, clinician judgment and shared decision making with parents is indicated as to whether to defer breastfeeding until maternal treatment with metronidazole is complete (CDC, 2021). There are limited data regarding tinidazole use during pregnancy but data from animal studies suggests there could be a moderate risk to the fetus. Therefore, tinidazole should be avoided during pregnancy and breastfeeding should be deferred for 72 hours after a single 2-g oral dose of tinidazole (CDC, 2021).

Perimenopause and Older People

There are no diagnostic or treatment considerations associated with perimenopause, menopause, or aging.

Individuals With HIV Infection

Women with HIV are at increased risk for infection with *T. vaginalis*. It is estimated that more than 50 percent of women and individuals assigned female at birth who have HIV may also be infected with *T. vaginalis* at some point in time, and this coinfection significantly increases their risk for PID, poor reproductive health, and possibly increased HIV transmission. Recommended screening for *T. vaginalis* among women and individuals assigned female at birth who have HIV includes screening upon entry to care and at least annually; more frequent screening can occur based on the individual's specific history and symptoms.

The recommended treatment for trichomoniasis in women with HIV infection is metronidazole 500 mg orally twice daily for 7 days (CDC, 2021).

CHLAMYDIA

Chlamydia, which is caused by the bacterium *C. trachomatis*, is the most commonly reported nationally notifiable infection in the United States and the most common bacterial STI. More than 1.6 million cases were reported to the CDC in 2022, with at least that many more estimated to have gone undetected (CDC, 2024a). Sexually active adolescents and women aged 15 to 24 years have nearly 3 times the prevalence of chlamydia compared to women aged 25 to 39 years, and women are infected twice as often as men. Risk factors for this infection include multiple sexual partners and not using barrier methods of contraception. The most serious complication of chlamydial infections for women is pelvic inflammatory disease (PID) (refer to the section on PID later in this chapter).

Chlamydial infections are usually asymptomatic and reported cases are often the result of asymptomatic screening. During the beginning of the COVID-19 pandemic, especially in 2020 and extending into 2021, many healthcare facilities limited in-person visits to patients with symptoms. Other clinics closed entirely or only provided visits via telehealth. Therefore, preventive visits where STI screening usually happens decreased. During 2020, the number of chlamydia cases decreased substantially, and this is likely a reflection of pandemic-related disruptions in health care, especially reproductive care (CDC, 2024).

Assessment

When assessing patients for chlamydia, in addition to obtaining information about risk factors, inquire about the presence of any symptoms while recognizing that chlamydia is usually asymptomatic. Individuals experiencing symptoms may report vaginal spotting or postcoital bleeding, mucoid or purulent cervical discharge, urinary frequency, dysuria, lower abdominal pain, or dyspareunia. Bleeding results from inflammation and erosion of the cervical columnar epithelium. Symptoms of chlamydia infection in women may mimic those of a urinary tract infection. In sexually active women who present with urinary symptoms only, it may be prudent to test a urine sample for chlamydia if urine is already being collected for dipstick analysis or culture (Fantasia et al., 2025).

Physical examination findings of abdominal guarding, referred pain, or rebound tenderness upon abdominal examination should raise the level of suspicion for PID. Cervical friability may be detected with the speculum examination. Discharge, if present, is characteristically mucopurulent. This is shown in **Color Plate 11**. During the bimanual examination, a patient may report cervical motion tenderness (pain with cervical movement), and the examiner may detect adnexal fullness and uterine tenderness. These findings are also suggestive of PID (Fantasia et al., 2025).

All sexually active people younger than age 25 should be screened for chlamydia annually (CDC, 2021). Individuals 25 years and older with risk factors (e.g., new or multiple partners, partner with an STI, partner who has other partners) should also be screened.

Chlamydia testing can be performed using urine or swab specimens from the endocervix or vagina. Screening procedures for chlamydial infection include NAATs, cell culture, direct immunofluorescence, enzyme immunoassay (EIA), and nucleic acid hybridization tests. NAATs are the preferred technique because they provide the highest sensitivity. Although they are less sensitive than urine or cervical/vaginal swabs, NAATs can also be used with liquid-based Pap tests. All patients with chlamydia should be tested for other STIs, including gonorrhea, syphilis, and HIV (CDC, 2021).

Differential Diagnoses

Differential diagnoses for chlamydia include gonorrhea, trichomoniasis, PID, appendicitis, and cystitis (Fantasia et al., 2025).

Prevention

General STI prevention strategies are detailed in Box 22-4 and Table 22-2. Postexposure prophylaxis (PEP) may be considered to prevent infection with chlamydia. Gay, bisexual, men who have sex with men, and transgender women who have a history of at least one bacterial STI (chlamydia, gonorrhea, syphilis) in the past 12 months should be counseled regarding the use of doxycycline PEP. Doxycycline 200 mg orally in a single dose is taken once within 72 hours of oral, vaginal, and/or anal sex. No more than 200 mg should be taken per 24 hours (Bachmann et al., 2024).

Although the pharmacokinetics of doxycycline indicate it is effective in both men and women, there is no current recommendation for the use of doxycycline PEP for cisgender women, cisgender men who have sex with women, transgender men, or nonbinary individuals. Clinicians should use clinical judgment and shared decision making with patients regarding use of doxycycline PEP in populations that fall outside of the CDC recommendations (Bachmann et al., 2024).

A prescription should be provided with enough refills to last until the next follow-up visit, which should be within 3–6 months, depending on individual patient characteristics.

Management

Recommendations for treatment of chlamydial infections are found in **Table 22-5**. Treatment of current and recent sexual partners is imperative. A test of cure to detect treatment failure (3 to 4 weeks after treatment) is not necessary unless a person is pregnant, has persistent symptoms, was unable to complete treatment, or may have been re-exposed or reinfected. A high prevalence of reinfection is observed among individuals who have had chlamydial infections in the preceding several months, usually from reinfection by an untreated partner. Clinicians should advise all individuals with chlamydia to be rescreened 3 months after treatment to assess for reinfection (CDC, 2021).

Treatment should be given as soon as possible after diagnosis because a delay may increase a person's chances of developing PID.

TABLE 22-5 Treatment of Chlamydial Infections

Recommended Regimens	Alternative Regimens
Doxycycline 100 mg orally 2 times/day for 7 days	Azithromycin 1 gm orally in a single dose **or** Levofloxacin 500 mg orally once/day for 7 days

Data from Centers for Disease Control and Prevention. (2021). Sexually transmitted infections treatment guidelines, 2021. *Morbidity and Mortality Weekly Report, 70*(4), 1–187.

Patient Education

All of the individual's sexual partners in the past 60 days should be referred for evaluation, testing, and presumptive treatment. If partners are unable or unwilling to be evaluated by a healthcare provider, expedited partner therapy should be considered if permitted by state law. Expedited partner therapy is the practice of treating sexual partners of individuals who have been diagnosed with chlamydia by providing medication, or prescriptions for medication, to the individual to provide to the partner. Examination of the partner is not necessary (CDC, 2021). All individuals should be advised to abstain from sex until their sexual partners are treated and to wait 7 days after single-dose treatment or until completion of a 7-day regimen before resuming sexual activity.

Special Considerations

Adolescents

Adolescents and individuals younger than age 25 have the highest rates of chlamydia. In 2022, nearly 58 percent of all cases of chlamydia were reported among persons aged 15–24 years (CDC, 2024; CDC, 2025). Screening and treating all sexually active adolescent and young adult women, even when asymptomatic, is essential to detect disease that can result in PID or tubal infertility (CDC, 2021). Clinicians should explain to adolescents why they are being screened for chlamydia even if they do not have symptoms or report high-risk sexual behavior.

People Who Are Pregnant

All people who are pregnant, younger than 25 years, and those who are at increased risk for chlamydia should be screened for chlamydia at their first prenatal visit and rescreened during the third trimester. Individuals aged 25 years and older should be screened based on risk factors (refer to the "Assessment" section), although many clinicians screen all pregnant individuals regardless of age. Asymptomatic screening in pregnancy may also be considered for individuals living in communities with high rates of documented chlamydia infections.

People who are pregnant and have been diagnosed with chlamydia should have a test of cure 3 to 4 weeks after the completion of treatment and again in 3 months to reduce the risk of neonatal transmission and infection. Chlamydia infection can cause conjunctivitis and pneumonia in neonates. Individuals who are pregnant should be treated with azithromycin 1 gm orally in a single dose. Doxycycline is known to discolor teeth and should be avoided in the second and third trimesters. An alternate treatment for chlamydia during pregnancy is amoxicillin 500 mg orally 3 times per day for 7 days (CDC, 2021).

Perimenopause and Older Adults

Chlamydia rates are lowest for individuals in the 45-54 and 55-64 age groups and very low for individuals aged 65 years and older (CDC, 2024; CDC, 2025). However, all sexually active individuals who have risk factors for chlamydia should be tested, regardless of age. Midlife individuals may have relationship changes leading to new sexual partners, such as divorce or the end of a long-term relationship. Due to biases associated with age and sexual activity, clinicians may erroneously assume older individuals are not sexually active. The postmenopausal decline in estrogen can cause mucosal vaginal tissue to become thinner and more susceptible to microabrasions that increase the risk of STI acquisition (Micks, 2024). Additionally, individuals who are not at risk for pregnancy because of age and postmenopausal status may not use condoms consistently. Clinicians should evaluate each person individually for STI risk factors and understand that genitourinary symptoms of menopause, such as dyspareunia, burning, discharge, and dysuria can be caused by STIs (Micks, 2024).

GONORRHEA

Gonorrhea, which is caused by the aerobic gram-negative diplococcus *N. gonorrhoeae*, is the second most common nationally notifiable STI in the United States, after chlamydia. In 2022, there were 648,056 cases of gonorrhea reported in the United States, although it is estimated that more than twice this number occur but are not diagnosed or reported (CDC, 2021; CDC, 2024; CDC, 2025). This is most likely because screening is not universal and many infections are asymptomatic, resulting in undiagnosed gonorrhea infections (Pollock et al., 2023). Currently, reported rates of infection are higher in men than in women, likely reflecting cases among men who have sex with men. Gonorrhea rates are highest in women who are aged 15 to 24 years (Kreisel et al., 2021b).

Gonorrhea is almost exclusively transmitted by sexual activity, primarily through genital-to-genital contact; however, it is also spread by oral-to-genital and anal-to-genital contact. Sites of infection can include the cervix, urethra, rectum, oropharynx, Skene glands, and Bartholin glands. In addition to age, other risk factors for this infection include early onset of sexual activity and multiple sexual partners.

The main complication of gonorrheal infections is PID. Women may also develop a pelvic abscess or Bartholin abscess. Disseminated gonococcal infection (DGI) is a rare complication of untreated gonorrhea. Symptoms of DGI can include bacteremia with chills, fever, skin lesions, acute septic arthritis, and possibly endocarditis and meningitis (CDC, 2021).

Assessment

Women and individuals assigned female at birth who have gonorrhea often remain asymptomatic and more than 80 percent may not have symptoms during the initial stages of infection (Fantasia et al., 2025; Tuddenham et al., 2022). When symptoms are present, they are often less specific than symptoms in men and those assigned male at birth. Women may report dyspareunia, a change in vaginal discharge, unilateral labial pain and swelling, or lower abdominal discomfort. Later in the course of infection, women may describe a history of purulent, irritating vaginal discharge or rectal pain and discharge. Menstrual irregularities may be the presenting symptom, with longer, more painful menses being noted or intermenstrual spotting and/or bleeding (Tuddenham et al., 2022). Women may also report chronic or acute lower abdominal pain. Unilateral labial pain and swelling may indicate Bartholin gland infection, whereas periurethral pain and swelling may indicate inflamed Skene glands. Dysuria, vague abdominal pain, or low backache may prompt women to seek care. Later symptoms may include fever (possibly high fever), nausea, and vomiting (Fantasia et al., 2025; Tuddenham et al., 2022). Refer to Chapter 21 for further information about Bartholin gland infection. In individuals assigned male at birth with urethral infection, dysuria and urethral discharge are often the presenting symptoms (Tuddenham et al., 2022).

Gonorrhea infections can also include the throat and rectum. The symptoms of gonococcal pharyngitis can include sore throat, pharyngeal erythema, exudate, and cervical lymphadenopathy. Rectal infections can result in anorectal pain, mucopurulent rectal discharge, bleeding, and tenesmus (Tuddenham et al., 2022). Rectal itching, fullness, and pressure are also commonly noted symptoms.

Physical examination is individualized based on the individual's presenting symptoms. The clinician should obtain vital signs and inspect the pharynx and oral cavity for erythema, edema, and lesions. In suspected pharyngeal infections, palpation for cervical lymphadenopathy is important. The abdomen should be palpated for masses, tenderness, and rebound tenderness. During the speculum examination, inspect the vaginal walls for discharge and redness, and examine the cervix for mucopurulent discharge, ectopy, and friability. This is shown in **Color Plate 12**. During the bimanual examination, observe for cervical motion tenderness, uterine tenderness, adnexal tenderness, and adnexal masses—all of these findings are associated with PID (Fantasia et al., 2025).

Annual screening for gonorrhea is recommended for all sexually active people younger than 25 years. Individuals who are 25 years or older should be screened annually based on risk factors such as inconsistent or absent condom use in nonmonogamous relationships, new or multiple partners, partner with an STI or other partners, and exchange of sex for drugs or money. Clinicians should also inquire about recent travel that included sexual partners outside the United States (CDC, 2021).

Gonorrhea testing can be performed by culture and NAATs. NAATs can be performed using urine or swab specimens from the endocervix or vagina. NAAT products vary, however, and clinicians must be certain that the test they are using is appropriate for the specimen type (CDC, 2021). Culture is also available for the detection of gonorrhea infection of the rectum and pharynx. People should be tested at all sites of possible exposure (Tuddenham et al., 2022). All patients with gonorrhea should be offered testing for other STIs, including chlamydia, syphilis, and HIV (CDC, 2021).

Differential Diagnoses

Differential diagnoses for gonorrhea include chlamydia, trichomoniasis, PID, appendicitis, and cystitis (Fantasia et al., 2025).

Prevention

General STI prevention strategies are detailed in Box 22-4 and Table 22-2. Postexposure prophylaxis (PEP) may be considered to prevent infection with gonorrhea. Gay, bisexual, men who have sex with men, and transgender women who have a history of at least one bacterial STI (chlamydia, gonorrhea, syphilis) in the past 12 months should be counseled regarding the use of doxycycline PEP. Doxycycline 200 mg orally in a single dose is taken once within 72 hours of oral, vaginal, and/or anal sex. No more than 200 mg should be taken per 24 hours (Bachmann et al., 2024).

Although the pharmacokinetics of doxycycline indicate it is effective in both men and women, there is no current recommendation for the use of doxycycline PEP for cisgender women, cisgender men who have sex with women, transgender men, or nonbinary individuals. Clinicians should use clinical judgment and shared decision making with patients regarding use of doxycycline PEP in populations that fall outside of the CDC recommendations (Bachmann et al., 2024).

A prescription should be provided with enough refills to last until the next follow-up visit, which should be within 3–6 months, depending on individual patient characteristics.

Management

Recommended therapies for gonorrhea are listed in **Box 22-6**. Treatment of current and recent sexual partners is imperative. Individuals who are treated for gonorrhea should be concomitantly treated for chlamydia if chlamydial infection has not been excluded. Quinolones are no longer used to treat gonorrhea because of the high prevalence of quinolone-resistant strains of the organism (CDC, 2021).

BOX 22-6 Treatment of Uncomplicated Gonococcal Infections of the Cervix, Urethra, and Rectum

Ceftriaxone 500 mg IM in a single dose for persons weighing < 150 kg*

If chlamydia has not been excluded, also treat with doxycycline 100 mg orally twice daily for 7 days

Alternate Regimens If Ceftriaxone Is Unavailable or a Documented Cephalosporin Allergy

Gentamicin 240 mg IM in a single dose

plus

Azithromycin 2 gm orally in a single dose

or

Cefixime 800 mg orally in a single dose**

Data from Information from Centers for Disease Control and Prevention. (2021). Sexually transmitted infections treatment guidelines, 2021. *Morbidity and Mortality Weekly Report, 70*(4), 1–187.

*For persons weighing > 150 kg, 1 gm of ceftriaxone should be given.

** If chlamydia has not been excluded, also treat with doxycycline 100 mg orally twice daily for 7 days.

A test of cure, typically performed 3 to 4 weeks after treatment, is not necessary for uncomplicated urethral or rectal infections. Individuals with pharyngeal gonorrhea should return within 7–14 days for testing with NAAT or culture (CDC, 2021). Decreased susceptibility of the infectious organism to cefixime has been reported, which has raised concerns about the potential for development of cephalosporin-resistant strains of *N. gonorrhoeae*. Additionally, cefixime has decreased efficacy against pharyngeal gonorrhea. Treatment with cefixime should be considered only if ceftriaxone is not available or if EPT is being used because a partner is unable to return to the clinician for treatment. It should not be prescribed based on the patient's preference for an oral medication instead of an injection or the patient not wanting to return to the office for treatment.

Clinicians must be vigilant for treatment failures (CDC, 2021). Individuals whose symptoms do not resolve after treatment should have a culture; any isolated gonococci should be tested for antimicrobial susceptibility. All individuals with gonorrhea should be retested 3 months after treatment due to the high rate of reinfection (CDC, 2021). If retesting at 3 months is not possible, individuals should be retested at the first appointment within 12 months.

Patient Education

If an individual has gonorrhea, all partners within the past 60 days or the last partner outside of that time period should be evaluated, tested and treated presumptively. Individuals and their partners should abstain from sexual activity for 7 days after single-dose injection treatment or oral therapy to avoid reinfection (CDC, 2021). The rationale for cotreatment of chlamydia should be explained. Safer sexual practices and strategies to prevent future infections need to be discussed in a nonjudgmental conversation.

Special Considerations

Adolescents

Gonorrhea rates are highest among individuals who are younger than 25 years old. All sexually active female adolescents younger than 25 years should be screened annually. There is currently no recommendation for annual screening for heterosexual males; however, males are involved in transmission. All adolescents should be asked about sexual activity and symptoms of STIs and screened appropriately.

People Who Are Pregnant

All people younger than age 25 who are pregnant should be screened for gonorrhea at their first prenatal visit. People aged 25 and older should be screened based on risk factors, although many clinicians screen all pregnant individuals. People who were diagnosed with gonorrhea in the first trimester and those who remain at high risk for gonorrhea throughout their pregnancies should be retested in the third trimester prior to birth to prevent maternal complications and neonatal infection. Gonorrhea can cause conjunctivitis in neonates. People who are pregnant should be treated with ceftriaxone 500 mg IM and azithromycin 2 gm orally as a single dose if chlamydia is present or has not been excluded. If a pregnant person is allergic to these medications, consultation with an infectious disease specialist is indicated (CDC, 2021).

Perimenopause and Older Adults

Gonorrhea rates are low for individuals in the 45–54 and 55–64 age groups and very low for individuals aged 65 years and older (CDC, 2024). However, all sexually active individuals who have risk factors for gonorrhea should be tested, regardless of age. Midlife individuals may also have relationship changes leading to new sexual partners, such as divorce or the end of a long-term relationship. Due to biases associated with age and sexual activity, clinicians may erroneously assume older individuals are not sexually active. The postmenopausal decline in estrogen can cause mucosal vaginal tissue to become thinner and more susceptible to micro abrasions that increase the risk of STI acquisition (Micks, 2024). Additionally, individuals who are not at risk for pregnancy because of age and postmenopausal status may not use condoms consistently. Clinicians should evaluate each person individually for STI risk factors and understand that genitourinary symptoms of menopause, such as dyspareunia, burning, discharge, and dysuria can be caused by STIs (Micks, 2024).

PELVIC INFLAMMATORY DISEASE (PID)

PID occurs in the upper genital tract and includes any combination of endometritis, salpingitis, tubo-ovarian abscess, and pelvic peritonitis (CDC, 2021). Each year approximately 1 million women in the United States will have an episode of acute PID (Yusuf & Trent, 2023). This estimate does not include women who have PID that is undiagnosed because it is asymptomatic or presents atypically. PID rates are the highest among individuals who are < age 25, often related to increased rates of gonorrhea and chlamydia (Yusuf & Trent, 2023).

Multiple organisms have been found to cause PID, and most cases are associated with infection by more than one organism. Common causative agents include *N. gonorrhoeae* and *C. trachomatis*. In addition to the pathogens that cause gonorrhea and chlamydia, a wide variety of anaerobic and aerobic microorganisms, including some found in the vaginal flora, are associated with PID (CDC, 2021), such as *Gardnerella vaginalis*, *Haemophilus influenzae*, and *Mycoplasma genitalium*. Bacterial vaginosis is common in individuals with PID and may facilitate the ascent of microorganisms into the upper genital tract, but it remains unclear whether treating bacterial vaginosis can reduce the incidence of PID (CDC, 2021).

Major health complications are associated with PID. Acute and chronic reproductive sequelae include tubo-ovarian abscess, ectopic pregnancy, infertility, chronic pelvic and abdominal pain, dyspareunia, and recurring PID (Yusuf & Trent, 2023).

As noted earlier, PID may be caused by a variety of infectious agents, and it encompasses a wide variety of pathologic processes; therefore, the infection can be acute, subacute, or chronic, and it may be associated with a wide range of symptoms. Diagnosis of PID is difficult because almost all of the most common signs and symptoms could accompany other urinary, gastrointestinal, or gynecologic tract problems. Accurate and prompt diagnosis is crucial to minimize long-term sequelae; thus, clinicians should maintain a high suspicion for PID and a low threshold for its diagnosis and treatment (CDC, 2021; Yusuf & Trent, 2023).

Assessment

When PID is suspected, the history taking must be comprehensive. Relevant history includes recent pelvic surgery, abortion, childbirth, dilation of the cervix, and insertion of an intrauterine device (IUD) within the past month. A thorough sexual risk history should be obtained, including the current or most recent sexual activity, number of partners, method of contraception, and use of condoms; this information will help the clinician identify possible increased risk for STI exposure (Fantasia et al., 2025; Yusuf & Trent, 2023).

The severity and extent of symptoms that individuals with PID experience vary widely. Historically, the abrupt onset of acute lower abdominal pain following menses has been considered the characteristic presenting symptom of PID. More recently, it has been recognized that symptoms of this infection can be very mild and nonspecific. Commonly reported symptoms include abdominal, pelvic, and low back pain; abnormal vaginal discharge; intermenstrual or postcoital bleeding; fever; nausea and vomiting; and urinary frequency (Yusuf & Trent, 2023). Individuals may report levels of pain ranging from minimal discomfort to dull, cramping, and intermittent pain to severe, persistent, and incapacitating pain. Pelvic pain is usually exacerbated by the Valsalva maneuver, intercourse, or movement. Rectal pain increases the suspicion for a pelvic abscess associated with PID (Yusuf & Trent, 2023). Symptoms of STIs among sexual partners also should be noted.

As part of the assessment for PID, the clinician should obtain vital signs and perform a complete physical examination. Although fever may be present, individuals with PID can be afebrile when they present for evaluation (Yusuf & Trent, 2023). Thus, absence of fever does not rule out PID. Physical examination may reveal adnexal tenderness, abdominal tenderness, uterine tenderness, and tenderness with cervical movement. Pelvic tenderness is usually bilateral. There may or may not be a palpable adnexal swelling or thickening. A pelvic mass suggests tubo-ovarian abscess (Fantasia et al., 2025; Yusuf & Trent, 2023).

A clinical diagnosis of PID is often made based on findings of pelvic organ tenderness and signs of lower genital tract infection, including mucopurulent cervicitis and cervical friability (Yusuf & Trent, 2023). There is no single laboratory test that can be used to detect upper genital tract infections. Instead, a pH test and wet mount of the vaginal secretions should be performed, along with tests for chlamydia and gonorrhea, although negative results do not rule out the presence of these infections in the upper genital tract. Other laboratory tests that are not needed for diagnosis but are recommended for individuals with clinically severe PID are a complete blood count (CBC) and erythrocyte sedimentation rate (ESR), which, if positive, increase the specificity of the PID diagnosis (Yusuf & Trent, 2023). All individuals with PID should be offered testing for syphilis and HIV as well. A pregnancy test will assist in identifying a potential ectopic pregnancy. Laboratory data are useful only when considered in conjunction with the history and physical examination findings. Pelvic ultrasound should be performed for individuals requiring hospitalization and those with a pelvic mass that was found on examination (Yusuf & Trent, 2023).

Clinical diagnosis of PID is imprecise; nevertheless, most diagnoses of PID are made clinically because laparoscopy and biopsy are too expensive and invasive to be practical screening tools. The CDC has established minimum criteria for beginning treatment of PID (**Box 22-7**) in recognition of the fact that delay in diagnosis and treatment of PID is associated with severe sequelae. In addition, a diagnosis of PID should be considered for an individual with any of the common symptoms of PID (CDC, 2021).

BOX 22-7 Diagnosing Pelvic Inflammatory Disease

Empiric treatment of PID should be initiated in sexually active young women and other women at risk for STIs if they are experiencing pelvic or lower abdominal pain, if no cause for the illness other than PID can be found, and if one or more of the following minimum criteria are present on pelvic examination:

- Cervical motion tenderness
- Uterine tenderness
- Adnexal tenderness

One or more of the following additional criteria can be used to enhance the specificity of the minimum criteria and support a diagnosis of PID:

- Oral temperature greater than 101°F (38.3°C)
- Abnormal cervical or vaginal mucopurulent discharge
- Presence of abundant numbers of white blood cells on saline microscopy of vaginal fluid
- Elevated erythrocyte sedimentation rate
- Elevated C-reactive protein level
- Laboratory documentation of cervical infection with *N. gonorrhoeae* or *C. trachomatis*

The most specific criteria for diagnosing PID include:

- Endometrial biopsy with histopathologic evidence of endometritis
- Transvaginal sonography or MRI techniques showing thickened, fluid-filled tubes with or without free pelvic fluid or tubo-ovarian complex, or Doppler studies suggesting pelvic infection (e.g., tubal hyperemia)
- Laparoscopic abnormalities consistent with PID

Data from Centers for Disease Control and Prevention. (2021). Sexually transmitted infections treatment guidelines, 2021. *Morbidity and Mortality Weekly Report, 70*(4), 1–187.

Differential Diagnoses

Symptoms of PID may mimic those associated with other conditions, such as ectopic pregnancy, endometriosis, ovarian cyst with torsion, pelvic adhesions, inflammatory bowel disease, and acute appendicitis (Fantasia et al., 2025).

Prevention

Perhaps the most important action a clinician can take to prevent PID is counseling. Primary prevention consists of education about avoiding STIs, whereas secondary prevention involves prompt treatment of lower genital tract infections to prevent ascension to the upper genital tract. Instructing patients in self-protective behaviors, such as practicing safer sex and using barrier contraceptive methods, is critical (refer to Box 22-4 and Table 22-2). Also important is the detection of asymptomatic gonorrheal and chlamydial infections through routine asymptomatic screening and screening of individuals with risk factors. Partner notification when an STI is diagnosed is essential to prevent reinfection (CDC, 2021; Yusuf & Trent, 2023).

Management

In the past, the majority of individuals with PID were hospitalized so that bed rest and parenteral therapy could be started. Today, most people with PID receive outpatient treatment, especially for mild PID, and do not experience any adverse reproductive outcomes (Fantasia et al., 2025). The decision of whether to hospitalize a patient should be based on each person's individual circumstances. To guide clinicians' decisions regarding hospitalization, the CDC (2021) has developed specific criteria for hospitalization, including the need to rule out surgical emergencies (e.g., appendicitis); pregnancy; no clinical response to oral antimicrobial therapy; inability to follow or tolerate an outpatient oral regimen; severe illness, nausea and vomiting, or high fever; and tubo-ovarian abscess.

Although treatment regimens vary with the infecting organism, broad-spectrum antibiotics are generally administered. Several antimicrobial regimens are effective, and no single therapeutic regimen appears to be superior to the others (**Table 22-6**). Substantial clinical improvement should occur within 72 hours of beginning treatment. Individuals who do not respond within this time frame should be reevaluated to confirm the diagnosis of PID; they may also need hospitalization (if being treated on an outpatient basis), additional testing, and surgical intervention. Individuals who do not respond to oral therapy and have a confirmed diagnosis of PID should be treated with an inpatient or outpatient parenteral regimen. Individuals on parenteral regimens can usually be transitioned to oral therapy 24 to 48 hours after they begin to show clinical improvement.

Patient Education

Health education is central to effective management of PID. Individuals should abstain from sexual activity until treatment has been completed, symptoms have resolved, and sexual partners have been adequately treated. Sexual partners within the past

TABLE 22-6 Treatment of Pelvic Inflammatory Disease

Parenteral Regimens	Oral/Intramuscular Regimens
Ceftriaxone 1 gm IV every 24 hours **plus** Doxycycline 100 mg orally or IV every 12 hours **plus** Metronidazole 500 mg orally or IV every 12 hours **or** Cefotetan 2 gm IV every 12 hours **plus** Doxycycline 100 mg orally or IV every 12 hours **or** Cefoxitin 2 gm IV every 6 hours **plus** Doxycycline 100 mg orally or IV every 12 hours **or** Clindamycin 900 mg IV every 8 hours **plus** Gentamicin loading dose IV or IM (2 mg/kg of body weight), followed by a maintenance dose (1.5 mg/kg) every 8 hours. Single-day dosing (3–5 mg/kg) may be substituted.	Ceftriaxone 500 mg IM in a single dose* **plus** Doxycycline 100 mg orally 2 times/day for 14 days **with** Metronidazole 500 mg orally 2 times/day for 14 days **or** Cefoxitin 2 gm IM in a single dose and probenecid 1 gm orally administered concurrently in a single dose **plus** Doxycycline 100 mg orally 2 times/day for 14 days with Metronidazole 500 mg orally 2 times/day for 14 days **or** Other parenteral third-generation cephalosporin (e.g., ceftizoxime or cefotaxime) **plus** Doxycycline 100 mg orally twice/day for 14 days with Metronidazole 500 mg orally twice/day for 14 days
Alternative parenteral regimen	
Ampicillin/sulbactam 3 gm IV every 6 hours **plus** Doxycycline 100 mg orally or IV every 12 hours **or** Clindamycin 900 mg IV every 8 hours **plus** Gentamicin loading dose IV or IM (2 mg/kg of body weight), followed by a maintenance dose (1.5 mg/kg) every 8 hours. Single-day dosing (3–5 mg/kg) may be substituted.	

*For individuals who weigh >150 kg, 1 gm of ceftriaxone should be given.

Data from Centers for Disease Control and Prevention. (2021). Sexually transmitted infections treatment guidelines, 2021. *Morbidity and Mortality Weekly Report, 70*(4), 1–187.

Abbreviation: IM, intramuscularly; IV, intravenously.

60 days preceding the onset of symptoms should be evaluated, tested, and treated presumptively for gonorrhea and chlamydia (CDC, 2021). Clinicians should explain to individuals the nature of their infection and encourage them to adhere to all therapy and prevention recommendations, emphasizing the necessity of taking all medication, even if their symptoms resolve before the course of therapy is completed. Any potential problems that would prevent a person from completing a course of treatment, such as lack of money for prescriptions or lack of transportation to return to a clinic for follow-up appointments, should be identified, and the importance of follow-up visits should be emphasized.

Special Considerations

Adolescents

Individuals who are < age 25 years are at high risk for chlamydia and gonorrhea. Approximately 50 percent of individuals who receive a diagnosis of acute PID are infected with either chlamydia or gonorrhea (CDC, 2021). All sexually active adolescents should be screened annually for asymptomatic chlamydia and gonorrhea and asked about behaviors that increase the risk of STIs. Prompt identification and treatment is important in the prevention of PID.

People Who Are Pregnant

People who are pregnant and have PID are at significant risk for maternal morbidity and preterm birth. They should be hospitalized and treated as inpatients with parenteral antibiotics. Consultation with an infectious disease specialist is warranted when a person has multiple antibiotic allergies (CDC, 2021).

Perimenopause and Older People

PID is most common in young people < 25 years of age and often not measured in national surveillance surveys beyond the age of 44 (Kreisel et al., 2021a). Although the risk of PID is lower among perimenopausal and older individuals, symptoms that are commonly associated with PID need to be investigated with the same approach used for younger people.

Individuals Using an Intrauterine Device

Many people use either copper-containing or levonorgestrel-releasing IUDs for contraception. An increased risk of PID is seen in the first 21 days after IUD insertion. If a person who is using either type of IUD is also diagnosed with PID, the device does not need to be removed immediately; indeed, it often does not need to be removed at all. Treatment should be initiated with a recommended antibiotic regimen. If no improvement is seen within 48 to 72 hours after beginning treatment, clinicians can consider removing the IUD (CDC, 2021). Please refer to Chapter 13 for more information about IUDs.

SYPHILIS

Syphilis is a systemic disease caused by *T. pallidum*, a motile spirochete. In 2022, more than 207,000 cases of syphilis, all stages and congenital syphilis, were reported in the United States (CDC, 2024). This represents the highest number of cases reported since 1950. Men who have sex with men continue to be disproportionately affected by syphilis and account for nearly half (45%) of all cases of syphilis among men. However, during 2021–2022, syphilis rates among women increased 19.2 percent which represents the increase in syphilis in the heterosexual population (CDC, 2024). The rise in syphilis rates among women contributes to the increase in rates of congenital syphilis (Amerson et al., 2022).

The increase in syphilis is related to complex and multifactorial issues that contribute to health inequities. Poverty and lack of health insurance reduce access to care; racism embedded into health care (either at the provider or system level) reduces screening and treatment; substance use, maternity care deserts, and inadequate federal funding for comprehensive STI prevention programs create an environment that supports the spread of syphilis (Fang et al., 2022).

Syphilis is a complex infection that can lead to serious systemic disease and even death when untreated. The infection can affect any tissue or organ in the body. Transmission is thought to occur by entry into the subcutaneous tissue through microscopic abrasions that can be created during oral, vaginal, or anal sex as well as sharing of sex toys (Bach & Heavey, 2021).

Syphilis is characterized by periods of active symptoms and periods of asymptomatic latency. It is divided into stages based on clinical findings, which helps guide treatment decisions (**Table 22-7**).

Primary syphilis is characterized by a primary lesion, or a chancre, which often begins as a painless papule at the site of inoculation and then erodes to form a nontender, shallow, indurated, clean ulcer that is several millimeters to a few centimeters in size. This is shown in **Color Plate 13A**. The chancre contains spirochetes and is most commonly found on the genitalia, although it may also occur on the cervix, perianal area, or mouth (Bach & Heavey, 2021; Fantasia et al., 2025).

Secondary syphilis is characterized by a widespread, symmetrical maculopapular rash on the palms of the hands and soles of the feet. This is shown in **Color Plate 13B**. Generalized lymphadenopathy is also present. The person may also experience fever, headache, and malaise. Condylomata lata (wartlike lesions) may develop on the vulva, perineum, or anus (Bach & Heavey, 2021; Fantasia et al., 2025).

If a person with syphilis is untreated, they enter a latent phase, which is asymptomatic for the majority of individuals. At this point, if the infection is still not treated, approximately one third of patients will develop tertiary syphilis. Cardiovascular (chest pain, cough), dermatologic (multiple nodules or ulcers), skeletal (arthritis, myalgia, myositis), and neurologic (headache, irritability, impaired balance, memory loss, tremor) symptoms can all develop in this stage. Dermatologic symptoms are shown in **Color Plate 13C**. Neurologic complications are not limited to tertiary syphilis; rather, a variety of syndromes (e.g., meningitis, meningovascular syphilis, general paresis, and tabes dorsalis) may span all stages of the disease (Bach & Heavey, 2021; Fang et al., 2022; Fantasia et al., 2025).

Assessment

Individuals with primary syphilis may be asymptomatic, or they may report an anogenital lesion that is typically raised, painless, and indurated. Most people with secondary syphilis (70%) will give a history of flu-like symptoms, including sore throat, malaise, headache, fever, myalgias, arthralgias, hoarseness, and anorexia. They may also report skin rashes on the trunk, extremities, palms, and soles that may be pruritic (Bach & Heavey, 2021; Fang et al., 2022; Fantasia et al., 2025). Some people experience alopecia and have a moth-eaten look or lose the lateral one-third of an eyebrow.

TABLE 22-7 Stages of Syphilis

	Primary	Secondary	Early Latent	Late Latent	Tertiary
Time after exposure	3–90 days (average 21)	4–10 weeks	1 year or less	More than 1 year	Years (usually 15–30)
Infectious routes	Sexual Vertical Chancre	Sexual Vertical	Sexual Vertical	Vertical	None
Clinical symptoms[a]	Chancre Regional lymphadenopathy	Chancre may still be present Skin lesions (papular rash of soles and palms, patchy alopecia, condylomata lata) Symptoms of systemic illness (fever, malaise, anorexia, weight loss, headache, myalgias) Lymphadenopathy	None	None	Cardiovascular syphilis (aortitis) Skin lesions (gumma)

Data from Centers for Disease Control and Prevention. (2021). Sexually transmitted infections treatment guidelines, 2021. *Morbidity and Mortality Weekly Report, 70*(4), 1–187; Fang, J., Partridge, E., Bautista, G. M., & Sankaran, D. (2022). Congenital syphilis epidemiology, prevention, and management in the United States: a 2022 update. *Cureus, 14*(12), e33009. https://doi.org/10.7759/cureus.33009

[a]In addition, neurosyphilis (central nervous system infection) can occur at any stage.

The physical assessment includes a general examination of the skin for alopecia, rash on the feet and palms, and condylomata lata. Additionally, the clinician should conduct a pharyngeal examination and inspect for enlarged inguinal nodes. Inspect the external genitalia for vulvar or perianal lesions and chancre at the point of inoculation. A speculum examination can assist in identifying lesions on the vaginal walls and cervix and for vaginal and cervical discharge. When history and clinical findings suggest the need, a neurologic examination may be performed as well (Fantasia et al., 2025).

Dark-field examination and direct fluorescent antibody for *T. pallidum* (DFA-TP) of lesion exudates or tissue will provide a definitive diagnosis of early syphilis, although these tests are not commercially available (CDC, 2021). The ability to confirm the diagnosis of syphilis depends on serology results obtained during the latency and late infection phases of the disease. Any test for antibodies may not be reactive in the presence of active infection because it takes time for the body's immune system to develop antibodies to any antigens. A presumptive diagnosis is possible with the use of two serologic tests: nontreponemal and treponemal.

Nontreponemal antibody tests, such as the VDRL and RPR, are used as screening tests and are relatively inexpensive, sensitive, moderately nonspecific, and fast. False-positive results can occur in patients with increased age, autoimmune disorders, malignancy, pregnancy, injection drug use, and recent vaccination (CDC, 2021). Sequential serologic tests should be obtained by using the same method (VDRL or RPR), preferably by the same laboratory. A high titer (more than 1:16) usually indicates active infection. A fourfold change in the titer (e.g., from 1:16 to 1:4 or from 1:8 to 1:32) is considered clinically significant. Treatment of syphilis usually causes a progressive decline in the pathogen's presence that may result in a negative VDRL or RPR, but low titers may persist. Rising titer (fourfold) or failure of titer to decrease fourfold within 6 to 12 months suggests reinfection or treatment failure (CDC, 2021).

The treponemal tests—the fluorescent treponemal antibody absorbed (FTA-ABS) test and the *T. pallidum* passive particle agglutination (TP-PA) assay—are used to confirm positive nontreponemal test results. Some clinical laboratories now also use a reverse screening protocol and are beginning to test samples with treponemal tests—a practice that may decrease the risk of false-positive results and identify individuals who have been previously treated for syphilis. Individuals with early primary or incubating syphilis may have negative test results.

Seroconversion usually takes place 6 to 8 weeks after exposure, so testing should be repeated in 1 to 2 months when a suspicious genital lesion exists. Treponemal antibody tests frequently stay positive for the remainder of the patient's life regardless of treatment or disease activity; therefore, treatment is monitored by VDRL or RPR titers. Tests for concomitant STIs, including HIV, should be offered as well (CDC, 2021).

No single test can confirm the diagnosis of neurosyphilis. Confirmation of this infection depends on a combination of tests, including cerebrospinal fluid (CSF) and reactive serologic tests in the presence of neurologic symptoms. Both a CSF-VDRL and CSF FTA-ABS can be performed, although routine CSF analysis in patients with primary or secondary syphilis is not recommended. Instead, testing of the CSF should be performed in specific situations; for example, in individuals with symptoms or signs of neurologic or ophthalmic disease, in individuals with persistent or recurring signs or symptoms, when titers increase fourfold, with high initial titers (1:32 or greater) that fail to decrease fourfold, in individuals with symptomatic late syphilis, and when evidence of active tertiary syphilis is found (CDC, 2021).

TABLE 22-8 Treatment of Syphilis for Individuals Who Are HIV Negative and Not Pregnant

Recommended	Alternatives If Penicillin Allergic[a]
Primary, secondary, and early latent syphilis: Benzathine penicillin G 2.4 million units IM in a single dose *Late latent syphilis, latent syphilis of unknown duration, and tertiary syphilis:* Benzathine penicillin G 7.2 million units total, administered as 3 doses of 2.4 million units IM each at 1-week intervals	*Primary, secondary, and early latent syphilis:* Doxycycline 100 mg orally 2 times/day for 14 days **or** Tetracycline 500 mg orally 4 times/day for 14 days *Late latent syphilis or latent syphilis of unknown duration:* Doxycycline 100 mg orally 2 times/day for 28 days **or** Tetracycline 500 mg orally 4 times/day for 28 days *Tertiary syphilis:* Consult an infectious diseases specialist

Data from Centers for Disease Control and Prevention. (2021). Sexually transmitted infections treatment guidelines, 2021. *Morbidity and Mortality Weekly Report, 70*(4), 1–187.

Abbreviation: IM, intramuscularly.

[a]There are limited data to support these regimens, so close follow-up is essential. Penicillin desensitization and treatment should be considered for persons with a penicillin allergy whose adherence to therapy or follow-up cannot be ensured.

Differential Diagnoses

Differential diagnoses include HSV, chancroid, scabies, HIV, genital warts, and drug eruptions or reactions (Fantasia et al., 2025).

Prevention

There is no vaccine for syphilis. General STI prevention strategies are detailed in Box 22-4 and Table 22-2. Postexposure prophylaxis (PEP) may be considered to prevent infection with syphilis. Gay, bisexual, men who have sex with men, and transgender women who have a history of at least one bacterial STI (chlamydia, gonorrhea, syphilis) in the past 12 months should be counseled regarding the use of doxycycline PEP. Doxycycline 200 mg orally in a single dose is taken once within 72 hours of oral, vaginal, and/or anal sex. No more than 200 mg should be taken per 24 hours (Bachmann et al., 2024).

Although the pharmacokinetics of doxycycline indicate it is effective in both men and women, there is no current recommendation for the use of doxycycline PEP for cisgender women, cisgender men who have sex with women, transgender men, or nonbinary individuals. Clinicians should use clinical judgment and shared decision making with patients regarding use of doxycycline PEP in populations that fall outside of the CDC recommendations (Bachmann et al., 2024).

A prescription should be provided with enough refills to last until the next follow-up visit, which should be within 3–6 months, depending on individual patient characteristics.

Management

Parenteral penicillin G is the preferred drug for treating individuals with all stages of syphilis (**Table 22-8**). It is the only proven therapy that has been widely used for individuals with neurosyphilis, congenital syphilis, and syphilis during pregnancy. Single-dose therapy is used to treat primary, secondary, and early latent syphilis. Individuals who have late latent, tertiary, or unknown-duration syphilis require weekly treatment for 3 weeks. Individuals with primary or secondary syphilis should have repeat clinical evaluation and serologic testing at 6 and 12 months after treatment. Individuals with latent or unknown-duration syphilis should have repeat clinical evaluation and serologic testing at 6, 12, and 24 months after treatment. Information on follow-up of individuals with tertiary syphilis is limited. Partner treatment is imperative, and management depends on the stage of the person's infection and the timing of the partner's exposure. Detailed recommendations can be found in the CDC treatment guidelines (CDC, 2021).

Patient Education

Significant education is necessary to improve adherence to treatment and monitoring and to reduce the risk of transmission to sexual partners. The primary treatment for syphilis involves parenteral administration of penicillin; therefore, individuals need to return to the office or clinic for the IM injection. This return visit, in addition to the other visits necessary for serologic monitoring, may present a hardship for some people. Any potential barriers to care and follow-up should be identified early and discussed.

Allergy history should be reviewed carefully. Even without a documented history of a penicillin allergy, such reactions are still possible. Individuals need to be aware that a Jarisch-Herxheimer reaction may occur. This sudden febrile episode typically happens within 24 hours of beginning treatment for syphilis. The fever is accompanied by other systemic symptoms, including myalgia and headache. Jarisch-Herxheimer reaction can be misinterpreted as a medication allergy. Treatment is supportive and includes antipyretics (CDC, 2021).

Partner notification when an individual has syphilis is essential. Transmission is most common during the first year of infection, especially when syphilitic lesions are present. State departments of public health can often assist with confidential partner notification. All sexual partners within 90 days preceding diagnosis of early, secondary, or early latent syphilis should be treated presumptively, even if serologic testing is negative. Partners outside the 90-day window should be tested and treated if positive. If serologic testing is not possible or partners are unable to complete follow-up, they should be treated presumptively.

Sexual contact should be avoided until the chancre has completely healed. Consistent condom use is important until follow-up serologic testing has demonstrated a response to treatment. The importance of HIV testing for patients and their partners should be stressed (CDC, 2021).

Special Considerations

Adolescents

There are no diagnostic or treatment considerations for adolescents who have syphilis. All sexually active adolescents should be asked about sexual activity and screened based on history and exam findings.

People Who Are Pregnant

All individuals should be screened for syphilis during their initial prenatal visit. Additional screening for people who live in geographic areas with high baseline rates of syphilis and for those who are at high risk for contracting the infection should be considered at 28 weeks' gestation and again at birth. People who have experienced an intrauterine fetal demise after 20 weeks' gestation should be tested for syphilis (CDC, 2021). Effective detection and prevention of congenital syphilis among neonates is dependent on early detection and treatment of pregnant individuals. For neonates with confirmed, probable, or possible congenital syphilis, penicillin in varying doses and formulations is the treatment in consultation with neonatology (CDC, 2021).

People who are pregnant, have been diagnosed with syphilis, and are allergic to penicillin should be desensitized and treated with penicillin. Although individuals should be treated with the penicillin regimen that corresponds to their disease stage, those with primary, secondary, or early latent infections can receive a second dose of benzathine penicillin 2.4 million units IM injection 1 week after the initial dose. Doxycycline and tetracycline are contraindicated in the second and third trimesters of pregnancy and do not prevent perinatal transmission of syphilis to the fetus. All people who are pregnant and have syphilis should receive care that is coordinated with infectious disease and obstetric specialists (CDC, 2021).

Perimenopause and Older People

Syphilis rates are often not measured in national surveillance surveys beyond the age of 44, although limited data indicate that rates are lower during the perimenopausal and postmenopausal years (CDC, 2024). However, the postmenopausal decline in estrogen can cause mucosal vaginal tissue to become thinner and more susceptible to micro abrasions that increase the risk of STI acquisition (Micks, 2024), especially if condoms are not used. Clinicians should evaluate each person individually for STI risk factors and screen for syphilis based on history and exam findings.

HEPATITIS B

Hepatitis B virus (HBV) is a blood-borne pathogen that is transmitted by percutaneous or mucosal exposure to infectious blood or body fluids (e.g., semen, saliva). In 2022, there were 2,126 cases of acute hepatitis B reported in the United States. After accounting for asymptomatic infections and underreporting, the CDC estimated that there were approximately 13,800 new infections in this country in 2022. The overall incidence (1.1/100,000) currently reported has declined significantly from the rate found in 1990 (8.5/100,000). The widespread use of HBV vaccination has contributed to this decline (CDC, 2021; CDC, 2024c).

Hepatitis B infection is caused by a large DNA virus and is associated with three antigens and their antibodies. Screening for active or chronic disease or disease immunity is based on testing for these antigens and their antibodies (**Table 22-9**). HBV is more infectious than HIV and HCV; HBV can survive outside the body for at least 7 days (CDC, 2021). HBV infection may be transmitted both parenterally and through intimate contact. In particular, hepatitis B surface antigen (HBsAg) has been found in blood, saliva, sweat, tears, wound exudate, vaginal secretions, and semen. Perinatal transmission does occur, but the fetus is not at risk of contracting the infection until making contact with contaminated blood at birth. HBV has also been transmitted by artificial insemination (CDC, 2021).

Factors that place a person at increased risk for HBV are those associated with STI risk in general (e.g., history of multiple sexual partners, multiple STIs, unprotected sex with a partner who has HBV), injection drug use, living in a household with one or more persons who have chronic HBV infection, and being born in or traveling to a country with a high incidence of HBV infection. With routine vaccination, occupational exposure to blood and body fluids (e.g., public safety workers exposed to

TABLE 22-9 Hepatitis B Serologic Tests

Name	Abbreviation	Purpose
Hepatitis B surface antigen	HBsAg	Indicates the patient has acute or chronic HBV infection and can transmit it to others
Hepatitis B surface antibody	Anti-HBs	Indicates the patient has immunity resulting from vaccination or previous infection
Total hepatitis B core antibody	Anti-HBc	Indicates the patient has previous or ongoing infection in an undefined time frame
Immunoglobulin M antibody to hepatitis B core antigen	IgM anti-HBc	Indicates the patient has had an acute infection within the past 6 months

Data from Centers for Disease Control and Prevention. (2024d). *Clinical testing and diagnosis for hepatitis B*. https://www.cdc.gov/hepatitis-b/hcp/diagnosis-testing/index.html

blood in the workplace, healthcare workers) occurs less commonly. Although HBV can be transmitted via blood transfusion, the incidence of such infections has decreased significantly since it became possible to test blood for the presence of HBsAg (CDC, 2021; CDC, 2024d).

HBV infection primarily affects the liver. It remains asymptomatic in as many as half of all individuals with the infection. When symptoms occur, they begin an average of 90 days after HBV exposure and usually last for several weeks. Symptoms of HBV infection include arthralgias, fatigue, anorexia, nausea, vomiting, fever, abdominal pain, clay-colored stools, dark urine, and jaundice. Approximately 5 percent of adults with HBV infection develop a chronic infection, and 15 to 25 percent of individuals with chronic HBV infection will die prematurely from liver cancer or cirrhosis (CDC, 2021; CDC, 2024c).

Assessment

Components of the history to be obtained when hepatitis B is suspected include symptoms of the infection and risk factors. Physical examination includes inspection of the skin for rashes, inspection of the skin and conjunctiva for jaundice, and palpation of the liver for enlargement and tenderness. Weight loss, fever, and general debilitation should be noted as well (CDC, 2024c).

Interpretation of test results for hepatitis B is complex (Table 22-9). Individuals who have negative HBsAg, anti-HBc, and anti-HBs tests are susceptible to infection, and vaccination should be considered. A person with a positive anti-HBs test with negative HBsAg and anti-HBc tests has immunity from vaccination. A person with a negative HBsAg test and positive anti-HBc and anti-HBs tests has immunity from previous infection that is now resolved. A person with acute hepatitis B infection will have positive HBsAg, anti-HBc, and IgM anti-HBc tests and a negative anti-HBs test. A person with chronic hepatitis B infection will have positive HBsAg and anti-HBc tests and negative IgM anti-HBc and anti-HBs tests. A person with a positive anti-HBc test and negative HBsAg and anti-HBs tests should be referred for further evaluation because this result has multiple interpretations, including resolved infection, false-positive anti-HBc, low-level chronic infection, and resolving acute infection (CDC, 2024b).

Individuals who have hepatitis B should be prepared to undergo repeat testing because HBV serologic markers may also be used to monitor the progression of the disease. Testing for other STIs, including HIV, should be performed as well.

Differential Diagnoses

Differential diagnoses include other forms of hepatitis (including hepatitis A and C as well as those caused by viruses, medications, and alcohol), biliary disease, and hemochromatosis (CDC, 2021; CDC, 2024b).

Prevention

Hepatitis B is a vaccine-preventable infection. All nonimmune individuals at risk of hepatitis B should be informed of the existence of a hepatitis B vaccine. Vaccination is recommended for all individuals who have had more than one sex partner within the past 6 months and anyone being evaluated or treated for an STI. In addition, the following individuals should be vaccinated: all children younger than 19 years; individuals who use injection drugs; residents and staff of facilities for developmentally disabled persons; individuals who have a sexual partner or household contact who is HBsAg positive; individuals with end-stage renal disease, chronic liver disease, or HIV; persons whose occupation exposes them to blood or body fluids; travelers to areas with high rates of HBV infection; and anyone who wants protection from HBV infection (CDC, 2021; Schillie et al., 2018). Multiple vaccinations are available, including one that protects against both the hepatitis B and hepatitis A viruses. Clinicians should consult current immunization schedules (https://www.cdc.gov/vaccines/hcp/imz-schedules/adult-age.html) and product information to determine the appropriate vaccine, dose, and frequency based on the patient's age; individual factors, such as immunocompromised status; and need to complete the vaccine series. The vaccine should be injected into the deltoid muscle.

Management

Individuals with a definite exposure to hepatitis B should be given hepatitis B immunoglobulin IM in a single dose as soon as possible, and preferably within 24 hours after exposure. There is no specific treatment for acute hepatitis B; recovery is usually spontaneous. For persons with chronic infections, several antiviral drugs are available; individuals can discuss treatment options for viral suppression with their healthcare providers (Schillie et al., 2018).

Patient Education

Education about preventing transmission of HBV to others is important. Individuals with chronic HBV should be referred to a specialist for management. Condom use with unvaccinated partners is important to prevent transmission. Other mechanisms to prevent transmission include covering cuts, not donating body fluids or organs, and not sharing household items that could be infected with blood. To avoid any further liver injury, individuals with HBV should avoid or limit alcohol consumption, refrain from taking any medications they have not discussed with their healthcare providers, and receive vaccinations for hepatitis A (CDC, 2021).

Individuals who are beginning the HBV vaccine series should be aware that completion of the series involves three injections that are typically administered over a 6-month period. Schedules and doses can vary slightly based on manufacturer guidelines (CDC, 2021). Most adults (90%) age 40 and younger achieve a protective antibody response after the third dose. Booster vaccination is not routinely recommended (Schillie et al., 2018). Individuals should be informed that reported side effects of vaccination are infrequent, with most involving pain at the injection site and mild fever. The HBV vaccine can be administered with other vaccines.

Special Considerations

Adolescents

Most adolescents in the United States are vaccinated for HBV because it is on the CDC immunization schedule. However, adolescents who were born outside of the United States or those who followed a modified or limited vaccine schedule may not have received all childhood vaccines. All sexually active adolescents should be asked about HBV vaccination status and offered the HBV vaccine if needed.

Pregnant People

All individuals who are pregnant should be tested for HBsAg at their initial prenatal visit, regardless of their previous vaccination status. Individuals who are pregnant, have not been vaccinated, and are at risk for acquiring the virus can be vaccinated during pregnancy. Pregnant people with HBV should be managed by infectious disease and obstetric specialists, and neonates whose mothers have HBV need to receive immunoprophylaxis after birth (CDC, 2021; Schillie et al., 2018).

Perimenopause and Older People

There are no specific recommendations for individuals who are peri- or postmenopausal and individuals in these age ranges can receive the HBV vaccine if not previously vaccinated. All individuals, regardless of age, should be assessed for HBV risk.

HEPATITIS C

HCV infection is the most common chronic blood-borne infection in the United States. An estimated 2.4 million individuals in the United States have chronic HCV, which is most prevalent in the 1945 to 1965 birth cohort. Although most transmission occurs via infected blood, sexual transmission can occur, especially in certain subgroups, including men who have sex with men, cocaine and intravenous drug users, and those who engage in group sex or traumatic sexual practices (CDC, 2021).

Hepatitis C is caused by a single-stranded RNA virus. Parenteral transmission is most common. Individuals at greatest risk for contracting the virus include current or former injection drug users, recipients of blood or solid-organ transplants prior to 1992, those who received clotting factor concentrate prior to 1987, and persons who have HIV (CDC, 2021). Approximately 15 to 25 percent of all individuals with an acute infection will clear the virus spontaneously and not develop chronic HCV, but the infection will become chronic in more than 75 percent of individuals. HCV infection is the leading cause of liver transplantation in the United States.

Assessment

Symptoms of acute HCV infection are often vague and nonspecific. Individuals may report fatigue, fever, abdominal pain, nausea, vomiting, anorexia, jaundice, dark urine, or clay-colored stool. The average time from exposure to emergence of symptoms is 4 to 12 weeks, but symptoms can occur as late as 24 weeks after exposure (CDC, 2021; CDC, 2023). Individuals should be asked about specific risk factors (described in the previous section) and sexual contact with a partner known to have HCV.

Decisions regarding testing for HCV are based on the history and physical examination findings. An algorithm for the recommended testing sequence for HCV (https://www.cdc.gov/hepatitis/hcv/pdfs/hcv_flow.pdf) and interpretation of HCV laboratory values (https://www.cdc.gov/hepatitis/hcv/pdfs/hcv_graph.pdf) can be found on the CDC website.

Differential Diagnoses

Differential diagnoses include other forms of hepatitis (including hepatitis A and B as well as those caused by viruses, medications, and alcohol), biliary disease, and hemochromatosis (CDC, 2021; CDC, 2023).

Prevention

Unlike hepatitis B, there is no vaccine for HCV. Prophylaxis with immune globulin is not effective in preventing infection after exposure (CDC, 2021). Prevention relies on avoiding contact with infected blood. Although the risk of transmission for this virus is smaller than that for HBV, HCV can be transmitted via sexual activity with a partner who has HCV, especially among individuals with HIV infection (CDC, 2021). In heterosexual, monogamous partners without HIV infection, sexual transmission to a discordant partner is rare (CDC, 2021).

Management

The goal of treatment is to reduce all-cause mortality and prevent or halt liver injury. Multiple medications can be used to treat HCV infection. The mainstay of treatment has been a combination of interferon and ribavirin with or without protease inhibitors, although there are newer medications with an improved side-effect profile. Members of this class of medications, called direct-acting antiviral agents, target viral enzymes and proteins throughout the viral life cycle and have a less complicated dosing regimen and higher tolerability. They include sofosbuvir and simeprevir and fixed-dose combination drugs. A full discussion of all treatment options is beyond the scope of this chapter but is available from the American Association for the Study of Liver Diseases and the Infectious Diseases Society of America (ASSLD) (2023).

Virologic cure is defined as the absence of HCV RNA 12 weeks after the completion of treatment. The optimal treatment regimen and timing of treatment are unclear, although the success rate for viral clearance appears to be higher when treatment begins in the acute phase of the infection. Treatment is recommended for all persons except those with a short life expectancy due to comorbid conditions. Coordination with a specialist in hepatitis management is advisable. Evaluation of chronic liver disease is imperative. Individuals who have HCV can receive vaccinations for hepatitis A and B if not already vaccinated (ASSLD, 2023; CDC, 2021).

Patient Education

Education about preventing transmission of HCV to others is important. Individuals with HCV should be referred to a specialist for management. To reduce the risk of transmitting this virus to others, people should be advised to not share personal household items (e.g., toothbrushes, razors) that may have blood on them. Any cuts or sores should be covered, and individuals with HCV should not donate blood, organs, or tissue. Sexual transmission is possible, although the risk is lower than with direct contact with infected blood. To protect partners, sexual activity in the presence of vaginal bleeding should be avoided. Condoms can be used with multiple partners or in the presence of coinfection with HIV. The benefit of condom use with low-risk, steady partners is uncertain. To avoid any further liver injury, people with HCV should avoid or limit alcohol consumption and refrain from taking any medications they have not discussed with their healthcare providers (CDC, 2021).

Rates of HCV infection are high among injection drug users. Counseling about the risks of continuing drug use is important, as is providing resources for substance abuse treatment. For individuals who are not ready or willing to discontinue drug use, the importance of using clean drug injection equipment and not sharing drug equipment with others should be stressed (CDC, 2021).

Special Considerations

Adolescents

HCV infection is poorly transmitted through sexual activity. However, all individuals should be assessed for their risk of HCV and prevention strategies should be discussed.

Pregnant People

Routine screening for HCV among all people who are pregnant is currently not recommended. Testing for HCV should be offered to pregnant people with known risk factors or for all pregnant individuals in settings where the prevalence of HCV is > 0.1 percent (CDC, 2021). The risk of perinatal transmission of the virus to the fetus varies, with the highest rates of transmission reported among pregnant individuals who have both HIV and HCV. Neonates whose mothers have HCV infection should be tested for this infection as well. HCV is not transmitted through breastmilk, but individuals with cracked and bleeding nipples should avoid this method of feeding until complete healing has taken place (CDC, 2021).

Perimenopause and Older People

There are no specific considerations for HCV among perimenopausal or postmenopausal individuals. Risk for HCV and testing should be based on individual history. All adults > age 18 should be screened for HCV at least once in their lifetime (CDC, 2021). In 1992, routine screening of donated blood and tissue began. Individuals who received a blood transfusion or solid organ transplantation prior to 1992 should have HCV testing documented.

Individuals With HIV

All individuals who are diagnosed with HIV should also be tested for HCV during their initial evaluation. If negative, people with HIV should be screened annually if they are at high risk for infection (e.g., high-risk sexual behavior, injection drug use, high prevalence of HCV in the community) (CDC, 2021).

HIV

In the early summer of 1981, the occurrence of several rare illnesses—such as *Pneumocystis carinii* (now called *Pneumocystis jiroveci*) pneumonia; *Mycobacterium* and *Mycobacterium intracellulare* infections; cryptosporidiosis; Kaposi sarcoma; and non-Hodgkin lymphoma—in a cluster of gay and bisexual men presented a medical mystery. It was subsequently solved by the identification of a single infectious agent that was destroying the immune system of persons who acquired it—the human immunodeficiency virus (CDC, 1981). Although the earliest identified victims of the HIV/AIDS epidemic were typically homosexual men, symptoms of the syndrome were identified in a woman within 2 months of the earliest reports of the infection in men. Within the first year of the epidemic, female partners of hemophiliacs with HIV, women using injection drugs, and female partners in heterosexual relationships in resource-poor countries, notably Haiti, were diagnosed with HIV/AIDS.

Deeply ingrained social and cultural forces that tend to devalue women, particularly women of color who are affected by poverty, perpetuated the tendency for HIV and AIDS to be considered a men's disease—more specifically, a disease of men who have sex with men. Additionally, the homophobia associated with HIV focused the attention on men who have sex with men as the sole population at risk for HIV. As a consequence, HIV/AIDS has historically been underdiagnosed in women. In 2022, nearly 7,000 women in the United States were diagnosed with HIV, which represented 18 percent of all new diagnoses (CDC, 2024d). The majority of new HIV diagnoses result from transmission from men who have sex with men (67%), heterosexual sexual contact (22%), and injection drug use (3%) (CDC, 2024d).

The Effect of HIV on the Immune System

The human immune system protects the body from invasion by a variety of microbes and tumor cells. The immune system is composed of two arms: humoral immunity, involved with antibody production; and cellular immunity, effected largely through T-helper lymphocytes (also known as CD4 cells). Central components of the cellular arm in the immune system are macrophages and CD4 cells.

HIV specifically targets CD4 cells, binding to the cell surface protein known as the CD4 receptor. The virus affects the cells in two ways: the absolute numbers of these cells are depleted, and the function of the remaining cells is impaired, resulting in a gradual loss of immune function. Progressive depletion of CD4 cells in peripheral blood occurs with advancing HIV infection, such that CD4 cell counts are used to estimate the cumulative immunologic damage caused by HIV. If its course is unimpeded, HIV can destroy as many as 1 billion CD4 cells per day. In addition to its aggressive destruction of the immune system, HIV is genetically highly variable and mutates with apparent ease (Ward et al., 2021).

HIV Transmission Issues Specific to Women and People Assigned Female at Birth

Several factors increase the risk for acquiring STIs, including HIV, among women and individuals assigned female at birth. In addition to the anatomically driven susceptibility of the female genitalia, the integrity of the tissues of the lower genital tract influences HIV transmission risk. Trauma during intercourse (including both vaginal and anal-receptive intercourse), STI-related inflammation or cervicitis, and an STI lesion (e.g., HSV ulcer or syphilitic chancre) may all increase susceptibility to HIV infection, as does any activity or condition that disrupts the tissues of the vagina. HIV can also be transmitted through receptive oral sex with ejaculation. Any condition that interrupts the integrity of oral tissues, including periodontal disease, increases the risk of HIV transmission in this manner (Adimora et al., 2021; Alexander et al., 2023).

Assessment

The CDC (2021) recommends that HIV screening be a routine part of clinical care for individuals aged 13 to 64 years in all health-care settings. All persons presenting for STI treatment should be screened for HIV at each visit where they have new symptoms. Individuals at high risk for HIV should be tested for the presence of the virus at least once per year. Individuals must be informed orally or in writing that HIV testing will be performed unless they decline (opt-out screening). Consent for HIV testing should be incorporated into the general consent for care. A separate consent form specific for HIV screening is neither required nor recommended (CDC, 2021).

All 50 states collect HIV surveillance data using confidential name-based reporting standards. Some states offer only confidential testing, whereas others also offer anonymous testing. State laws regarding HIV testing vary, and clinicians must be fully informed of regulations where they practice. Information about state HIV testing and reporting laws can be found on the CDC website (https://www.cdc.gov/hiv/policies/law/states/index.html).

HIV infection can be diagnosed by serologic tests that detect antibodies to HIV-1 and HIV-2 and by virologic tests that detect antigens to HIV or RNA. HIV screening is conducted with standard enzyme-linked immunosorbent assay (ELISA) or EIA tests that are sent to a laboratory, or with newer rapid HIV tests that can be performed at the point of care and yield results within minutes. If the screening test is reactive, then a more specific confirmatory test, such as the Western blot (WB) or an indirect immunofluorescence assay (IFA), is conducted. Although a negative antibody test usually indicates that a person does not have HIV, these tests cannot always detect an acute infection. A patient with a negative test who has known or suspected exposure to HIV should be retested at a time determined by history and possible exposure (CDC, 2021).

The CDC recommendations no longer require prevention counseling as part of a screening program. Nevertheless, such counseling is strongly encouraged for individuals who are seronegative for HIV but at increased risk for infection. Those who are at high risk for HIV or who have known or suspected exposure to the virus should also be counseled about the need for repeat testing (CDC, 2021).

A plan for treatment must be established, which includes prompt referral to a clinician with HIV expertise. Unless the individual is clearly immunocompromised and in need of immediate treatment for opportunistic infection, there is likely to be an interval between diagnosis and treatment decisions. The person can use this period to begin to adapt emotionally and psychologically to the diagnosis, make decisions about who must be told about the infection, and they can implement behaviors that are required to minimize the risk of transmitting the virus to others. Sensitive and nonjudgmental care at this time can help the individual make healthy accommodations in the face of the HIV diagnosis.

Differential Diagnoses

HIV infection is difficult to diagnose based on symptoms alone because signs of acute infection are often nonspecific, including fever, malaise, rash, myalgias, lymphadenopathy, sore throat, and headache (Fantasia et al., 2025). Other conditions that must be considered are upper respiratory infections, including influenza and tuberculosis, and viral infections, including mononucleosis. Immune disorders that place people at risk for opportunistic infections should also be considered (Fantasia et al., 2025).

Prevention

Preexposure Prophylaxis (PrEP)

Prevention of HIV can occur through different mechanisms, including behavioral change to reduce HIV exposure and pharmacologic intervention through the use of preexposure prophylaxis (PrEP) (CDC, 2021a). General guidelines to reduce the risk of all STIs, including HIV, can be found in Box 22-4 and Table 22-2.

A complete discussion of PrEP is beyond the scope of this chapter, but full guidelines for eligibility, medication use, and monitoring are available from the CDC (2021a). Briefly, PrEP is recommended as one preventive option for individuals who are HIV negative and use injection drugs, have sexual partners are known to have HIV, men who have sex with men, and all other individuals who are at substantial risk for contracting HIV (e.g., commercial sex workers, inconsistent or absent condom use, high number of sexual partners) (CDC, 2021a).

As of 2024, there are three PrEP formulations approved by the FDA for use in the United States:

1. Fixed-dose, oral combination of tenofovir disoproxil fumarate 300 mg and emtricitabine 200 mg taken daily. This is approved for use by all individuals.
2. Injectable cabotegravir 600 mg given IM. The initial two doses are given one month apart and then every 2 months thereafter. Oral cabotegravir may be given for 30 days prior to beginning injections to assess for tolerability to cabotegravir (CDC, 2021a). This can also be taken by all individuals.
3. Fixed-dose oral emtricitabine 200 mg and tenofovir alafenamide 25 mg. This is approved for men and transgender women.

Generally, individuals are clinically eligible for PrEP if the following conditions are met: (1) documented negative HIV test (antibody and antigen) in the week prior to starting PrEP; (2) no signs or symptoms of acute HIV infection; (3) estimated creatinine clearance > 60 mL/minute (for tenofovir/emtricitabine and > 30 mL/minute for emtricitabine/tenofovir alafenamide); (4) normal liver function (cabotegravir); and (5) not taking any medications that are contraindicated with their specific PrEP medication (CDC, 2021a). Different PrEP formulations have varied contraindications and warnings and clinicians should choose the formulation that is most appropriate for the individual.

Follow-up visits every 3 months are recommended for individuals taking PrEP to assess for HIV status and provide other services such as STI testing for those at high risk or to assess treatment services and needs for individuals who use injection drugs (CDC, 2021a). Renal function should be assessed every 6 months or at least yearly depending on the PrEP medication and patient medical history.

Prophylactic medication should be used in conjunction with risk-reduction services and behavior changes, including safer sex practices, to most effectively reduce HIV risk. Clinicians should expect the science to evolve in this area and new medications will be approved by the FDA. It is important to stay current with best practices for prescribing PrEP.

Management

Effective management and treatment of a person with HIV involves the use of antiretroviral therapy (ART) to improve health, decrease morbidity, prolong life, and reduce the risk of transmission to others (Adimora et al., 2021; Ward et al., 2021). More than 30 different antiretroviral medications are available; they belong to 8 classes: nucleoside reverse transcriptase inhibitors (NRTIs), nonnucleoside reverse transcriptase inhibitors (NNRTIs), protease inhibitors (PIs), fusion inhibitors (FIs), CCR5 antagonists, integrase strand transfer inhibitors (INSTIs), capsid inhibitors, and post-attachment inhibitors (National Institutes of Health, 2021).

Combination therapy with multiple ARTs is recommended (U.S. Department of Health and Human Services, 2024). Detailed treatment of HIV is beyond the scope of this chapter and is best provided by clinicians who are experienced in HIV management and infectious disease. Research activities directed toward development of new therapies and testing of different combinations of therapies can quickly change the state of the science. The AIDSinfo website (https://hivinfo.nih.gov/home-page) contains the most current recommendations for HIV/AIDS management and additional information can be found at https://clinicalinfo.hiv.gov/sites/default/files/guidelines/documents/adult-adolescent-arv/guidelines-adult-adolescent-arv.pdf.

Patient Education

In addition to clinical care, individuals with HIV need behavioral and psychosocial support and services. Comprehensive care is necessary to assist in coping with a disease that is associated with a high level of stigma (Adimora et al., 2021). HIV is a chronic condition that can be successfully managed and the importance of medication adherence, laboratory assessments, and follow-up care must be reviewed. Clinicians providing gynecologic care to individuals with HIV must be aware that the infection may necessitate adjustments to the usual standards of care, including STI screening, Pap test screening, and contraceptive choice (ACOG, 2016, reaffirmed 2019; CDC, 2021).

Special Considerations

Adolescents

In 2022, individuals between the ages of 13 and 24 accounted for 19 percent of all HIV diagnoses (CDC, 2024d). Sexually active adolescents should be evaluated for HIV risk factors and tested for HIV based on their history or symptoms. Sexually active adolescents who engage in behaviors that place them at a consistent, high risk of HIV exposure and acquisition and weigh at least 77 lbs are eligible for PrEP.

Pregnant People

All people who are pregnant should be tested for HIV at their initial prenatal visit, regardless of whether they were tested previously. Repeat testing at 36 weeks' gestation can be considered for individuals at high risk for HIV or for people who live in geographic areas where there is a high incidence of HIV among women (CDC, 2021). All individuals who are pregnant and have a new diagnosis of HIV during pregnancy should be educated about the benefits of ART and offered treatment. Without treatment, the rate of perinatal transmission of HIV to infants is approximately 30 percent, but it can decrease to 2 percent or less with specific interventions, including antiretroviral medication, planned cesarean birth, and avoidance of breastfeeding. All people who are pregnant and have HIV should be comanaged with obstetric specialists and HIV/infectious disease specialists. Updated guidelines on management of HIV in pregnancy can be found online (https://clinicalinfo.hiv.gov/en/guidelines) (AIDSinfo, n.d.).

Perimenopause and Older People

Rates of HIV are lower among older persons. Individuals aged 45–54 account for approximately 12 percent of infections. This rate drops to 8 percent among people aged 55–64 and 2 percent or less for individuals aged 65 and older (CDC, 2024d). However, all sexually active individuals who have risk factors for HIV should be tested, regardless of age. Due to biases associated with age and sexual activity, clinicians may erroneously assume older individuals are not sexually active. The postmenopausal decline in estrogen can cause mucosal vaginal tissue to become thinner and more susceptible to micro abrasions that increase the risk of STI acquisition, including HIV (Adimora et al., 2021; Micks, 2024). There are limited data on the use of PrEP among individuals who are aged 65 and older. Although no absolute contraindications exist, older adults may have higher rates of impaired hepatic and renal function. They are also more likely to experience comorbid health conditions which require medication treatment.

Additional Sexually Transmitted Infection Testing

All individuals who receive an initial diagnosis of HIV should be tested for other STIs and screened at least annually as part of comprehensive HIV care. Trichomoniasis is common among women who have HIV and therefore trichomoniasis screening should be done annually. Syphilis, chlamydia, and gonorrhea are also common and individuals should be screened for these infections. Cervical cancer screening should follow existing guidelines (CDC, 2021). Treatment of STIs for individuals diagnosed with HIV is addressed in the most current STI treatment guidelines (CDC, 2021).

CONCLUSION

STIs are among the most common health problems experienced in the United States and around the world. Women and people assigned female at birth experience a disproportionate amount of the burden associated with these illnesses, including complications of infertility, perinatal infections, poorer pregnancy outcomes, chronic pelvic pain, genital tract neoplasms, and potentially death. Additionally, these infections may interfere with an individual's lifestyle and cause considerable emotional and physical distress. Clinicians can help ameliorate the morbidity and mortality associated with STIs and other common infections by providing accurate, safe, sensitive, and supportive care.

Knowledge of STIs is constantly increasing and changing, with new and improved prevention, diagnostic, and treatment modalities being developed and reported on an ongoing basis. All clinicians have a responsibility to stay up to date on these developments by reviewing research, attending conferences, and being knowledgeable about recommendations and bulletins from the CDC. Furthermore, it is important that clinicians be aware of policies, recommendations, and guidelines in the state where they practice, which also may change frequently.

References

Adimora, A. A., Ramirez, C., Poteat, T., Archin, N. M., Averitt, D., Auerbach, J. D., Agwu, A. L., Currier, J., & Gandhi, M. (2021). HIV and women in the USA: What we know and where to go from here. *The Lancet, 397*(10279), 1107–1115. https://doi.org/10.1016/S0140-6736(21)00396-2

AIDSinfo. (n.d.). *Clinical guidelines.* U.S. Department of Health and Human Services. https://clinicalinfo.hiv.gov/en/guidelines

Alexander, I. M., Johnson-Mallard, V., Kostas-Polston, E., Cappiello, J., & Hubbard, H. S. (2023). *Women's health care in advanced practice nursing* (3rd ed.). Springer.

American Association for the Study of Liver Diseases and Infectious Diseases Society of America. (2023). *HCV guidance: Recommendations for testing, managing, and treating hepatitis C.* https://www.hcvguidelines.org/

American College of Obstetricians and Gynecologists. (2016, reaffirmed 2019). Gynecologic care for women and adolescents with human immunodeficiency virus: ACOG practice bulletin no. 167. *Obstetrics & Gynecology, 128*, e89–e110.

American College of Obstetricians and Gynecologists. (2020). Human papillomavirus vaccination: ACOG committee opinion no. 809. *Obstetrics & Gynecology 136*(2), e15–e21. https://doi.org/10.1097/AOG.0000000000004000

American College of Obstetricians and Gynecologists. (2021). *Updated cervical cancer screening guidelines.* https://www.acog.org/clinical/clinical-guidance/practice-advisory/articles/2021/04/updated-cervical-cancer-screening-guidelines

Amerson, E. H., Valladares, H. B. C., & Leslie, K. S. (2022). Resurgence of syphilis in the US—USPSTF reaffirms screening guidelines. *JAMA Dermatology, 158*(11), 1241–1243. https://doi.org/10.1001/jamadermatol.2022.3499

Bach, S., & Heavey, E. (2021). Resurgence of syphilis in the US. *The Nurse Practitioner, 46*(10), 28–35. https://doi.org/10.1097/01.NPR.0000790496.90015.74

Bachmann, L. H., Barbee, L. A., Chan, P., Reno, H., Workowski, K. A., Hoover, K., Mermin, J., & Mena, L. (2024). CDC clinical guidelines on the use of doxycycline postexposure prophylaxis for bacterial sexually transmitted infection prevention, United States, 2024. *Morbidity and Mortality Weekly Report, 73*(2), 1–8.

Centers for Disease Control and Prevention. (1981). *Pneumocystis* pneumonia—Los Angeles. *Mortality and Morbidity Weekly Review, 30*, 250–252.

Centers for Disease Control and Prevention. (2021). *Sexually transmitted infections treatment guidelines, 2021.* https://www.cdc.gov/std/treatment-guidelines/STI-Guidelines-2021.pdf

Centers for Disease Control and Prevention (2021a). *Preexposure prophylaxis for the prevention of HIV infection in the United States—2021 update: A clinical practice guideline.* https://www.cdc.gov/hiv/pdf/risk/prep/cdc-hiv-prep-guidelines-2021.pdf

Centers for Disease Control and Prevention. (2022). *National notifiable diseases surveillance system (NNDSS).* https://www.cdc.gov/nchs/hus/sources-definitions/nndss.htm

Centers for Disease Control and Prevention. (2023). *Clinical overview of hepatitis C.* https://www.cdc.gov/hepatitis-c/hcp/clinical-overview/index.html

Centers for Disease Control and Prevention. (2024). *Sexually transmitted infections prevalence, incidence, and cost estimates in the United States.* https://www.cdc.gov/sti/php/communication-resources/prevalence-incidence-and-cost-estimates.html

Centers for Disease Control and Prevention. (2024b). *Hepatitis B surveillance 2022.* https://www.cdc.gov/hepatitis/statistics/2022surveillance/hepatitis-b.htm

Centers for Disease Control and Prevention. (2024c). *Clinical testing and diagnosis for hepatitis B.* https://www.cdc.gov/hepatitis-b/hcp/diagnosis-testing/index.html

Centers for Disease Control and Prevention. (2024d). *HIV diagnoses, deaths, and prevalence.* https://www.cdc.gov/hiv-data/nhss/hiv-diagnoses-deaths-prevalence.html

Centers for Disease Control and Prevention. (2025). *Sexually transmitted infections surveillance, 2024 (provisional).* https://www.cdc.gov/sti-statistics/annual/index.html

Centers for Disease Control and Prevention. (2025a). *Advisory Committee on Immunization Practices (ACIP).* https://www.cdc.gov/acip/vaccine-recommendations/index.html

Chang, J. Y., Balch, C., Puccio, J., & Oh, H. S. (2023). A narrative review of alternative symptomatic treatments for herpes simplex virus. *Viruses, 15*(6), 1314. https://doi.org/10.3390/v15061314

Eltobgy, A., Aljabali, A., Farag, A., Elshorbgy, M., Hamed, M., Hamouda, E., Hamouda, H., Refaey, N., Kabeel, M., Amro, S., Abouheseba, T., & Tarek, M. (2024). Effects of pubic hair grooming on women's sexual health: a systematic review and meta-analysis. *BMC women's health, 24*(1), 171. https://doi.org/10.1186/s12905-024-02951-1

Fang, J., Partridge, E., Bautista, G. M., & Sankaran, D. (2022). Congenital syphilis epidemiology, prevention, and management in the United States: A 2022 update. *Cureus, 14*(12), e33009. https://doi.org/10.7759/cureus.33009

Fantasia, H. C. (2018). Examining the woman with anxiety, history of sexual violence, or intimate partner violence. In R. M. Secor & H. C. Fantasia (Eds.), *Fast facts about the gynecologic exam* (pp. 79–91). Springer.

Fantasia, H. C., Harris, A. L., & Fontenot, H. B. (2025). *Guidelines for nurse practitioners in gynecologic settings* (13th ed.). Springer.

Gravett, R. M., & Marrazzo, J. (2023). An ulcer by any other name: Non-herpes and non-syphilis ulcerative sexually transmitted infections. *Infectious Disease Clinics, 37*(2), 369–380. https://doi.org/10.1016/j.idc.2023.02.005

Kreisel, K. M., Llata, E., Haderxhanaj, L., Pearson, W. S., Tao, G., Wiesenfeld, H. C., & Torrone, E. A. (2021a). The burden of and trends in pelvic inflammatory disease in the United States, 2006–2016. *The Journal of Infectious Diseases, 224*(Supplement_2), S103–S112. https://doi.org/10.1093/infdis/jiaa771

Kreisel, K. M., Weston, E. J., Cyr, S. B. S., & Spicknall, I. H. (2021b). Estimates of the prevalence and incidence of chlamydia and gonorrhea among US men and women, 2018. *Sexually Transmitted Diseases, 48*(4), 222–231. https://doi.org/10.1097/OLQ.0000000000001382

Lederer, A. M., & Laing, E. E. (2017). What's in a name? Perceptions of the terms sexually transmitted disease and sexually transmitted infection among late adolescents. *Sexually Transmitted Diseases, 44*(11), 707–711. https://doi.org/10.1097/OLQ.0000000000000682

McQuillan, G., Kruszon-Moran, D., Flagg, E. W., & Paulose-Ram, R. (2018). Prevalence of herpes simplex virus type 1 and type 2 in persons aged 14–49: United States, 2015–2016. *NCHS Data Brief, 304*. Hyattsville, MD: National Center for Health Statistics. https://www.cdc.gov/nchs/data/databriefs/db304.pdf

Merck. (2019). *Highlights of prescribing information: Gardasil 9.* https://www.merck.com/product/usa/pi_circulars/g/gardasil_9/gardasil_9_pi.pdf

Micks, E. (2024). Sexually transmitted infections in midlife women. *Menopause, 31*(5), 430–432. https://doi.org/10.1097/GME.0000000000002345

Mollaei, B., Ahmadi, K., & Yousefi, E. (2023). Risk and protective factors of high-risk sexual behaviors in young people: A systematic review. *International Journal of High Risk Behaviors and Addiction, 12*(1), e131119. https://doi.org/10.5812/ijhrba-131119

National Institutes of Health. (2021). *What to start: Choosing an HIV treatment regimen.* https://hivinfo.nih.gov/understanding-hiv/fact-sheets/what-start-choosing-hiv-treatment-regimen

Ogale, Y. P., Ridpath, A. D., Torrone, E., Quilter, L. A., & Grey, J. A. (2023). A sore subject? An examination of national case-based chancroid surveillance. *Sexually Transmitted Diseases, 50*(8), 467–471. https://doi.org/10.1097/OLQ.0000000000001814

Patel, P. U., Tan, A., & Levell, N. J. (2021). A clinical review and history of pubic lice. *Clinical and Experimental Dermatology, 46*(7), 1181–1188. https://doi.org/10.1111/ced.14666

Perkins, R. B., Guido, R. S., Castle, P. E., Chelmow, D., Einstein, M. H., Garcia, F., . . . Schiffman, M. (2020). 2019 ASCCP risk-based management consensus guidelines for abnormal cervical cancer screening tests and cancer precursors. *Journal of Lower Genital Tract Disease, 24*(2), 102–131. https://doi.org/10.1097/LGT.0000000000000525

Pollock, E. D., Clay, P. A., Kreisel, K. M., & Spicknall, I. H. (2023). Estimated incidence and prevalence of gonorrhea in the United States, 2006–2019. *Sexually Transmitted Diseases, 50*(4), 188–195. https://doi.org/10.1097/OLQ.0000000000001763

Roett, M. A. (2020). Genital ulcers: Differential diagnosis and management. *American Family Physician, 101*(6), 355–361.

Schillie, S., Vellozzi, C., Reingold, A., Harris, A., Haber, P., Ward, J.W., & Nelson, A. P. (2018). Prevention of hepatitis B virus infection in the United States: Recommendations of the Advisory Committee on Immunization Practices. *Morbidity and Mortality Weekly Report, 67*(RR-1), 1–31. https://doi.org/10.15585/mmwr.rr6701a1

Secor, R. M., & Holland, A. C. (2024). *Advanced health assessment of women* (5th ed.). Springer.

Tuddenham, S., Hamill, M. M., & Ghanem, K. G. (2022). Diagnosis and treatment of sexually transmitted infections: A review. *Journal of the American Medical Association, 327*(2), 161–172. https://doi.org/10.1001/jama.2021.23487

U.S. Department of Health and Human Services. (2024). *Guidelines for the use of antiretroviral agents in adults and adolescents with HIV.* https://clinicalinfo.hiv.gov/sites/default/files/guidelines/documents/adult-adolescent-arv/guidelines-adult-adolescent-arv.pdf

U.S. Food and Drug Administration. (2018). Summary Basis for Regulatory Action, Gardasil 9. https://www.fda.gov/media/117054/download?attachment

Van Gerwen, O. T., Opsteen, S. A., Graves, K. J., & Muzny, C. A. (2023). Trichomoniasis. *Infectious Disease Clinics, 37*(2), 245–265. https://doi.org/10.1016/j.idc.2023.02.001

Ward, A. R., Mota, T. M., & Jones, R. B. (2021). Immunological approaches to HIV cure. *Seminars in Immunology,* 51, 101412. https://doi.org/10.1016/j.smim.2020.101412

Wilms, L., Weßollek, K., Peeters, T. B., & Yazdi, A. S. (2022). Infections with Herpes simplex and Varicella zoster virus. *JDDG: Journal der Deutschen Dermatologischen Gesellschaft, 20*(10), 1327–1351. https://doi.org/10.1111/ddg.14917

Yusuf, H., & Trent, M. (2023). Management of pelvic inflammatory disease in clinical practice. *Therapeutics and Clinical Risk Management, 19*, 183–192. https://doi.org/10.2147/TCRM.S350750

CHAPTER 23

Urinary Conditions

Jessica Wellette
Janell Senda

The editors acknowledge Mickey Gillmor-Kahn, Ying Sheng, and Janis M. Miller, who were authors in the previous editions of this chapter.

The focus of this chapter is the presentation, assessment, and treatment of urinary conditions, specifically urinary tract infections (UTIs), interstitial cystitis, overactive bladder, neurogenic bladder, and urinary incontinence (UI). This chapter mainly relates to people assigned female at birth (AFAB), independent of their gender identity. As genitourinary anatomy plays an important role in these conditions, the terms "female" or "woman" may occasionally be used throughout this chapter for consistency with the cited evidence. Use of these terms is not meant to exclude nonbinary and transgender individuals who seek gynecologic care.

URINARY TRACT INFECTIONS

Urinary tract infections (UTIs) are some of the most common complaints a clinician may encounter in a gynecologic or primary care setting. Although they can affect all populations, women and those assigned female at birth (AFAB) are at an increased risk of acquiring such infections and therefore proper identification and treatment of UTIs is an important skill for gynecologic providers. UTIs, especially when recurrent, can cause hospitalizations, multiple antibiotic courses, and can negatively affect a person's quality of life.

Scope of the Problem

On average, 1 in 3 individuals AFAB will have an uncomplicated UTI before 24 years of age and 50 percent will have at least one UTI in their lifetime (Aggarwal & Leslie, 2025; Cooper et al., 2022). Within one year of being diagnosed with a UTI, roughly 27–46 percent of patients will experience reinfection (Lala et al., 2023). About 15–25 percent of those patients will struggle with chronic or long-term UTIs (Cooper et al., 2022). The burden of this disease on people and society is great. Roughly 3.5 billion is spent every year in the United States treating UTIs (Aggarwal & Leslie, 2025).

The prevalence of bacteriuria increases with age. After menopause, most individuals have decreased lactobacilli in the vagina and a higher vaginal pH, which can lead to colonization with uropathogens (Kenneally et al., 2022). In long-term care settings, UTIs are one of the most common infections seen in AFAB patients. In elderly patients, one of the strongest risk factors for symptomatic UTIs is a previous history of UTIs. Other risk factors include cognitive decline, catheterization, bowel or bladder incontinence, functional disabilities, and dementia.

UTIs are the most common infection in pregnancy, affecting up to 15 percent of individuals. Anatomic and physiologic changes related to pregnancy place pregnant individuals at increased risk of UTIs, including pyelonephritis. Risk factors include young age, primiparity, diabetes, history of UTIs, anatomical abnormalities, malnutrition, and low socioeconomic status. Due to the increased risk of asymptomatic bacteriuria (ASB) developing into pyelonephritis, all pregnant patients should be screened for ASB early in their prenatal care or at least in the first or second trimester by clean catch urine. Most cases of pyelonephritis in pregnancy will occur in the second or third trimester. Pyelonephritis during pregnancy is associated with sepsis, acute respiratory distress syndrome (ARDS), disseminated intravascular coagulation (DIC), and anemia. Many clinicians choose to hospitalize pregnant patients with pyelonephritis, at least initially, to monitor for complications and ensure adequate treatment (Ansaldi & Martinze de Tejada Weber, 2023; Habak et al., 2024). Additional information on UTI in pregnancy can be found in Chapter 33.

Etiology

For a UTI to occur, a susceptible host and an active uropathogen is required. UTIs can be caused by many different bacteria and fungi, but the most common include *Escherichia coli*, followed by *Klebsiella pneumoniae*, *Enterococcus faecalis*, and *Proteus mirabilis*. Factors that can affect microbial colonization include urinary pH, oxygen tension, osmolarity, nutrient availability, potential adhesion sites, and immune interaction. The bladder epithelium must also be conducive to bacterial growth. Susceptibility may also include a genetic predisposition toward developing UTIs (Neugent et al., 2020).

The risk of developing a UTI for individuals assigned female at birth is mostly derived from their anatomy. The distance between the urethral meatus and the vaginal introitus and anus where most pathogens originate is shorter for individuals AFAB. Once a pathogen has entered the urethra, there is a relatively short distance to travel to the bladder, making infection more likely. Furthermore, the vaginal environment is moist, encouraging bacterial growth (Kenneally et al., 2022). **Box 23-1** lists additional risk factors for UTI.

BOX 23-1 Risk Factors for Urinary Tract Infection

- Female genital organs
- Previous UTI, including UTI in childhood
- Frequent or recent sexual activity
- Contraceptive diaphragm use
- Spermicide use
- Condom use
- Vaginal infections
- Anatomic abnormalities of the urinary tract
- Larger body size
- Diabetes
- Sickle cell trait or disease
- Urinary tract calculi
- History of UTI in first-degree relative
- Vaginal atrophy
- Incomplete bladder emptying
- Functional defects (overactive bladder and urinary incontinence)
- Rectocele, cystocele, urethrocele, or uterovaginal prolapse
- Catheter placement
- Surgery, especially if it involves the genitourinary tract and/or catheter placement
- Neurologic disorders or medical conditions requiring in-dwelling or repetitive bladder catheterization
- Increasing bacterial resistance to antibiotics

Data from CDCa. (2024, January 22). *Urinary tract infection basics.* cdc.gov/uti/about/index.html; NAFC. (2025). *Urinary tract infections in adults—symptoms, causes, and treatments.* nafc.org/urinary-tract-infection; Mititelu, M., Olteanu, G., Neacsu, S. M., Stoicescu, I., Dumitrescu, D. E., Gheorghe, E., Tarcea, M., Busnatu, S.S., Ionita-Mindrican, C.B., Tafuni, O., Belu, I., Popescu, A., Lupo, S., & Lup, C.E. (2024). Incidence of urinary tract infections and behavioral risk factors. *Nutrients, 16*(3), 446. https://doi.org/10.3390/nu16030446

Asymptomatic Bacteriuria

Research conducted through the Human Microbiome Project (HMP) has led the way in understanding the role of normal microbiota in health and disease. The urinary tract was previously thought to be a sterile environment. Urine samples containing any amount of bacteria were thought to be pathogenic or contaminated; however, research over the last decade has shown that the healthy urinary tract is a complex microbial community. The urobiome of those AFAB is commonly dominated by *Shigella, Lactobacillus, Enterococcus, Gardnerella, Prevotella, Sneathia, Escherichia,* and *Streptococcus*. When in balance, the presence of these microbes does not cause symptomatic illness. In fact, much like the vaginal environment, some of these microbes, like lactobacillus, are thought to aid the body in creating an environment unsuitable for some pathogens to thrive (Neugent et al., 2020; Kenneally et al., 2022). When out of balance, a pathogen will replicate in large numbers. However, not all overgrowth of bacteria (even types generally assumed to be pathogenic in nature), results in symptomatic illness.

TABLE 23-1 Types of Urinary Tract Infections

Infection	Definition	Signs and Symptoms
Asymptomatic bacteriuria	Bacteria present in the urine with no symptoms	None
Lower UTI/acute cystitis	Involves only the lower urinary tract: the bladder and urethra	Urinary frequency and urgency, dysuria, hematuria, suprapubic pain
Upper UTI/ pyelonephritis	Involves the upper urinary tract: one or both kidneys	Urinary frequency and urgency, dysuria, back pain, flank pain or tenderness, fever, chills, nausea, vomiting

Asymptomatic bacteriuria, by definition, does not cause the patient to experience any symptoms of urinary infection. ASB occurs in up to 5 percent of premenopausal patients, 2.8–8.6 percent of postmenopausal patients, and 1.9–9.5 percent of pregnant patients (Colgan et al., 2020). Many people will experience asymptomatic bacteriuria at some point. For some, it will be asymptomatic or may resolve on its own. For others, it may progress to symptomatic disease. It is not recommended to routinely screen for ASB in healthy nonpregnant patients (Colgan et al., 2020). Pregnant individuals are screened for asymptomatic bacteriuria during pregnancy to prevent serious sequala. Refer to Chapter 32 for screening during pregnancy.

Types of Urinary Tract Infections

Symptomatic UTIs can be divided into two general classifications: lower urinary tract infection, or cystitis, a relatively uncomplicated infection involving only the urinary bladder and urethra; and upper urinary tract infection, or pyelonephritis, an infection involving one or both kidneys (**Table 23-1**).

Acute Cystitis

Acute cystitis and UTI are terms that are often used interchangeably in the literature and in patient-clinician vernacular, despite acute cystitis being just one type of UTI. In acute cystitis, bacteria invade the lower urinary tract. Patients with acute cystitis typically present with lower urinary tract symptoms such as pyuria, urinary frequency, and two or more signs of lower abdominal discomfort (Mitrani-Gold et al., 2020). Uncomplicated cystitis occurs in healthy patients who are not pregnant, have no previous history of UTIs in the past 6 months (or two other UTIs in the past 12 months), immunocompetence, absence of urinary tract abnormalities, and have no signs of disease in the upper urinary tract. Cultures are not required for treatment in uncomplicated acute cystitis in otherwise healthy, nonpregnant patients, but should be considered if the patient is having persistent symptoms, treatment failure, or there is a need for bacterial identification (Lala et al., 2023). In the interest of decreasing antibiotic use, some investigators have studied treatment of lower UTIs with analgesics alone. However, studies have been inconclusive and at this time antibiotic treatment is still recommended (Barea et al., 2020).

Patients diagnosed with acute cystitis who are pregnant, have been treated for a UTI within the past 6 months (or two other UTIs in the past 12 months), are immunocompromised, or have a urinary tract abnormality are considered to have complicated cystitis and require culture and sensitivity (also called susceptibility) for definitive diagnosis and to verify the appropriate treatment. Clinically significant levels of bacteriuria on culture are 100,000 CFUs per mL. Immediate empiric treatment is still recommended for these patients. Treatment should not be delayed while awaiting culture and can later be tailored based on results if necessary.

Pyelonephritis

Pyelonephritis is a bacterial infection within the kidneys and renal pelvis which typically ascends from the urethra and bladder (Herness et al., 2020). Rarely, upper tract infection will arrive by descending through the bloodstream. Like acute cystitis, pyelonephritis is commonly the result of colonization with *E. coli*, accounting for 90 percent of cases (Herness et al., 2020). Pyelonephritis is most common in individuals AFAB between the ages of 15–29 years (Herness et al., 2020).

Like the other forms of UTI, pyelonephritis may be divided into uncomplicated and complicated infections. Uncomplicated pyelonephritis occurs in otherwise healthy patients with mild symptoms of upper tract infection and who are not pregnant or vomiting. Most of these infections can be treated on an outpatient basis if there are no other concerning complications and the patient can tolerate medications. Patients with severe symptoms, coexisting medical conditions, and/or a complex psychosocial situation may need hospitalization for treatment (Herness et al., 2020).

Symptoms of pyelonephritis typically include fever, chills, back pain, and costovertebral angle (CVA) tenderness. Other symptoms may include dysuria, urinary frequency and urgency, hematuria, tachycardia, nausea, vomiting, and diarrhea (Lala et al., 2023); however, in about 20 percent of cases, urinary symptoms can be absent (Herness et al., 2020). Pyelonephritis should be considered in any patient who presents with generalized symptoms and has a history of recent or recurrent UTIs. If left untreated, pyelonephritis may lead to sepsis, septic shock, and death (Herness et al., 2020).

Assessment

History Uncomplicated, nonrecurrent acute cystitis may be treated based on the patient's history alone; no laboratory testing is required. A report of new-onset dysuria, frequency, and urgency is adequate for diagnosis of simple acute cystitis. To rule out pyelonephritis, complicated or recurrent cystitis, a complete medical history should be taken, including questions outlined in **Box 23-2**. Significant back pain, nausea, vomiting, or generalized symptoms like fever or malaise should prompt pyelonephritis as a differential diagnosis. Preexisting conditions such as pregnancy, diabetes, immune insufficiency, history of recurrent infections, and abnormalities or alterations to urogenital anatomy would all be reasons to consider an acute cystitis as "complicated" and may indicate need for aggressive workup and treatment to prevent progression to pyelonephritis and or sepsis.

Older adults may not exhibit the typical symptoms of UTI such as urinary frequency and dysuria. Presenting complaints may differ and can include lethargy, generalized weakness, anorexia, new-onset urinary incontinence, or changes in mental status such as confusion or delirium (Lala et al., 2023; Rodriguez-Mañas, 2020). Older adults also have a higher incidence of nocturia and urgency at baseline as well as increased rates of asymptomatic bacteriuria (ASB); therefore, diagnosis can be difficult (Rodriguez-Mañas, 2020). Mental status changes in older patients with a UTI, especially those with preexisting dementia, are very common. However, the clinician must be cautious against assuming these changes are from bacteriuria alone and consider other potential causes of mental status change (Herness et al., 2020).

BOX 23-2 Questions to Identify Complicated Cystitis and Pyelonephritis

- Are you, or could you be pregnant?
- Have you had any fever or chills?
- Do you have any flank pain or back pain? Are you nauseated, or have you vomited?
- Have you ever had a urinary tract (bladder or kidney) infection? If so, when? How was it treated?
- Have you taken any medicines recently including: antibiotics, pain relievers, or other over-the-counter products?
- Do you have any other medical problems, including problems with the immune system, diabetes, or known urinary abnormalities?
- Do you self-catheterize or insert any products into the urethra?
- Have you ever had surgery on your urinary tract or genitals?
- Do you take any medications on a regular basis?
- Are you having any vaginal discharge or other vaginal problems? Are you concerned about sexually transmitted infections?

Physical Examination Physical examination of a patient with urinary symptoms is useful in ruling out worsening illness or other complications. Vital signs should be collected to assess for fever, tachycardia, or hypotension. Some patients with uncomplicated UTI may have suprapubic or abdominal tenderness which can be elicited on exam. Flank pain and tenderness in the presence of pyuria is highly suggestive for pyelonephritis (Herness et al., 2020). If the patient has clinical features consistent with other diagnoses such as vaginitis, pelvic inflammatory disease, or urinary incontinence, a pelvic exam should also be performed. A pelvic exam may also be useful in assessing for cystocele, vaginal atrophy, and pelvic organ prolapse, which could be the causative agent of recurrent UTIs (Aggarwal & Leslie, 2025).

Laboratory Testing In healthy, nonpregnant patients, routine laboratory screening for asymptomatic bacteriuria is not considered routine care (Hu & Pierre, 2019). The Women's Preventive Services Initiative is the only major organization that recommends annual screening in women (Hu, 2019). When a patient presents with urinary symptoms, the most common and cost-effective test for acute cystitis in the outpatient setting is point-of-care urinalysis (UA), also called a urine dipstick (Lala et al., 2023). This should be a clean-catch sample collected mid-stream after cleansing of the external genitalia to avoid contamination (Lala et al., 2023). Clinicians should closely evaluate for the presence of leukocyte esterase and nitrates as these are the most common indicators for acute cystitis (Bilsen et al., 2023; CDCa, 2024; Lala et al., 2023). The finding of nitrates on UA is the most reliable test for a UTI, having a sensitivity of 19–48 percent and specificity of 92–100 percent (Lala et al., 2023). Leukocyte esterase is also a useful indicator, but is not as reliable as nitrates (Lala et al., 2023). False positives can be caused by contamination or other vaginal infections, and false negatives can be caused by early infection, overly concentrated urine, and proteinuria (Lala et al., 2023). The co-occurring finding of nitrates and leukocyte esterase on UA has a positive predictive value of 85 percent (Lala et al., 2023). Hematuria may be present with acute cystitis or pyelonephritis but is not necessary for diagnosis. Hematuria can be either microscopic or gross (able to be observed without microscopy). Other causes of hematuria include nephrolithiasis, glomerulonephritis, polycystic kidney disease, renal or bladder malignancy, and various types of vascular, hematologic, or immune system disease (Willis & Tewelde, 2019). If a patient presents painless with hematuria, has a documented history of recurrent hematuria, or is at risk for bladder cancer (such as history of smoking), a referral to urology is appropriate.

Cultures for suspected uncomplicated UTI are not required but should be collected if the patient is having persistent symptoms, treatment failure, severe infection, is at high risk for antimicrobial resistance, or there is a determined need for bacterial identification (Aggarwal & Leslie, 2025; Lala et al., 2023). The American Urological Association (AUA) recommends obtaining a urine culture for each episode of acute cystitis in patients with recurrent UTIs (Aggarwal & Leslie, 2025). If there is any concern for pyelonephritis, cultures should be collected (Lala et al., 2023). Refer to **Box 23-3** for a list of appropriate and inappropriate reasons to obtain urine culture.

BOX 23-3 Urine Culture Stewardship

Urine Culture Indicated

- Complicated cystitis or suspected pyelonephritis
- Failed empiric therapy
- Dysuria, urgency, frequency, suprapubic pain or tenderness with flank pain, CVA tenderness, acute hematuria, or pelvic discomfort
- New onset or worsening sepsis with no identifiable cause
- Fever or altered mental status with evidence of another source
- Screening for asymptomatic bacteriuria in early pregnancy
- Pre-operative evaluation for urologic procedures

Urine Culture Not Indicated

- Simple acute cystitis in otherwise healthy persons (provider's discretion)
- Odorous, cloudy, or discolored urine in the absence of other localizing signs or symptoms
- Reflex urine cultures based on urinalysis results, such as pyuria, in the absence of other indications
- Urine culture to document response to therapy unless symptoms fail to resolve
- Screening for ASB in most people who are not pregnant
- Preoperative evaluations in most groups

Data from Centers for Disease Control and Prevention. (2024, March 13). *Urine culture stewardship in patient without indwelling urinary catheters*. https://www.cdc.gov/uti/hcp/clinical-guidance/culture-stewardship-without-catheter.html

Diagnostic Imaging Imaging is not typically required for acute cystitis but may aid in treatment if there is suspicion of other complications (Lala et al., 2023). Even recurrent UTIs do not routinely require cystoscopy or urological imaging (Aggarwal & Leslie, 2025). However, imaging should be considered for patients with a recurrent UTI in the presence of hematuria, or history of urolithiasis and relapsing infections (Aggarwal & Leslie, 2025). Preferred imaging includes ultrasonography or computed tomography (CT) scan of the abdomen and pelvis (Aggarwal & Leslie, 2025). Ultrasound can help detect hydronephrosis or abscess and CT can evaluate for nephrolithiasis, hydronephrosis, emphysematous changes, or abscess (Lala et al., 2023).

Differential Diagnoses

The differential diagnoses for dysuria, urinary urgency, and urinary frequency in AFAB individuals includes bacterial cystitis; pyelonephritis; interstitial cystitis/painful bladder syndrome (IC/PBS); vulvovaginal candidiasis; genitourinary syndrome of menopause; urethritis related to a sexually transmitted infection, gonorrhea or chlamydia; and normal physiologic changes of pregnancy (refer to Chapters 14, 21, and 22 for more information on these conditions). The differential diagnosis for a person presenting with pyelonephritis symptoms should also include nephrolithiasis. Usually, fever associated with pyelonephritis will resolve within 72 hours of treatment with appropriate antibiotics. Failure to resolve may indicate abscess, obstruction, or microbial resistance.

Management

Asymptomatic Bacteriuria

Although it is possible for asymptomatic bacteriuria to turn into an active, symptomatic infection, it is not currently recommended to treat asymptomatic bacteriuria in any population except pregnant people. Even in clinically significant colony counts (100,000 CFUs per mL), treatment is not recommended in any other population in the absence of urinary tract symptoms (Colgan et al., 2020).

Acute Cystitis

Acute uncomplicated UTIs can be managed in the outpatient setting. Telehealth is an option for patients who present with typical symptoms of acute cystitis (Aggarwal & Leslie, 2025). There is also evidence to support the safety of treating patients who self-diagnose acute cystitis and providing treatment without being seen in the clinical setting (Lala et al., 2023). The CDC recommends nitrofurantoin, trimethoprim/sulfamethoxazole (TMP-SMZ), and fosfomycin as appropriate first-line agents for treatment of acute cystitis in healthy nonpregnant, premenopausal individuals (CDC, 2024a). **Table 23-2** shows the treatment regimens for acute uncomplicated acute cystitis. A Cochrane Review found that the microbiological response (95% CI) was 0.766 for nitrofurantoin and 0.342 for placebo (Mitrani-Gold et al., 2020). Patients should see an improvement in their symptoms within 3 days of starting antibiotics (Lala et al., 2023). Ampicillin and amoxicillin should be avoided due

TABLE 23-2 Treatment Regimens for Acute Uncomplicated Cystitis

Drug	Dose and Duration	Common Adverse Effects	Comments*
Recommended Agents			
Nitrofurantoin monohydrate/macrocrystals	100 mg BID for 5–7 days	Nausea, headache	Resistance rare to date; may be useful for multidrug-resistant pathogens; cost varies; usually well tolerated; avoid if pyelonephritis is suspected due to poor tissue penetration and the patient's creatinine clearance is less than 45 mL/min.
Trimethoprim-sulfamethoxazole	160/800 mg BID for 3 days	Rash, urticaria, nausea, vomiting, hematologic signs	Excellent efficacy if local resistance < 20%; resistance prevalence is increasing; use with caution unless known susceptibility; inexpensive; extensive clinical experience; avoid during pregnancy, particularly first and third trimesters; avoid if estimated glomerular filtration rate (GFR) is less than 15 mL/min.
Fosfomycin trometamol	3 g single dose	Diarrhea, nausea, headache	Recommended as first-line therapy when other agents have failed or cannot be used. A single dose maintains therapeutic concentrations for 2–4 days and is comparable to a 7- to 10-day course with other agents. Can be used in conjunction with phenazopyridine for symptomatic relief.
Pivmecillinam	185 mg TID for 3–7 days	Carnitine deficiency: muscle aches, fatigue, hyperammonemia, weakness, cardiomyopathy, and confusion	Recommended when the risk for bacterial resistance is high; FDA approved in April 2024; very effective against *E. coli*. A dose reduction is recommended if the GFR is < 30 mL/min; it should not be used if the GFR is < 10 mL/min. Considered safe in first trimester of pregnancy.
Alternative Agents			
Amoxicillin-clavulanate	500/125 mg BID for 7 days	Antibiotic-associated diarrhea, *Clostridioides difficile* infection, drug-induced enterocolitis syndrome, drug-induced liver injury and hypersensitivity	Monitor renal, hepatic, and hematologic function if the patient is receiving prolonged therapy. If first dose, monitor for anaphylaxis. Do not prescribe if CrCl is < 30 mL/min or patient is on hemodialysis. Penicillin antibiotics are generally considered safe in pregnancy. Safe to use in breastfeeding but monitor infant for adverse effects.
Cephalexin	250 mg QID for 3–7 days	*Clostridiodes difficile* infection, hemolytic anemia and hypersensitivity reactions	Monitor renal, hepatic, and hematologic function with prolonged therapy. Monitor for anaphylaxis with first dose. Cephalosporins are considered safe in pregnancy. Give with caution in breastfeeding patients because it may cause diarrhea.
Fluoroquinolones	Dose varies by agent; 3-day regimen	Nausea, vomiting, diarrhea, headache, drowsiness, insomnia, tendon rupture, neuropathy	Risk may outweigh benefit for treatment of outpatient uncomplicated cystitis (FDA warning). Resistance prevalence increasing; cost varies; excellent efficacy; high collateral damage; better reserved for more serious conditions; avoid during pregnancy.

Abbreviations: FDA, U.S. Food and Drug Administration; BID, twice daily; TID, three times daily; QID, four times daily

Data from Lala, V., Leslie, S. W., & Minter, D. A. (2023). Acute cystis. In *StatPearls*. StatPearls Publishing; Aggarwal, N., & Leslie, S.W. (2025). Recurrent urinary tract infections. In *StatPearls*. StatPearls Publishing; Bono, M.J., & Leslie, S.W. (2025). Uncomplicated urinary tract infections. In *StatPearls*. StatPearls Publishing; UpToDate Inc. (2025). Amoxicillin and clavulante [Drug Information]. UpToDate Lexidrug. www-uptodate.com; UpToDate Inc. (2025). Cephalexin [Drug Information]. UpToDate Lexidrug. www-uptodate.com.

to high rates of resistance (Aggarwal & Leslie, 2025). Fluoroquinolones are contraindicated in pregnancy and should be avoided to minimize the development of quinolone resistance (Aggarwal & Leslie, 2025). It is also important to note that increased fluid intake alone will resolve about 20 percent of uncomplicated infections, so watchful waiting could be appropriate in an otherwise well patient with lack of severe symptoms (Lala et al., 2023). If antibiotic therapy is provided, allergies and length of treatment should be considered.

Complicated acute cystitis increases the risk of treatment failure or rapid progression related to patient demographics (pregnancy, age, catheterization, history of renal disease). Initial antibiotic selection is similar to uncomplicated acute cystitis while urine culture results are pending; treatment lengths are 10–14 days (Sabih & Leslie, 2024).

Patients with acute cystitis should respond to antibiotic therapy within 48 hours of initiation and should see a resolution of symptoms within 72 hours. If there is no improvement within 48 hours, then a repeat urine culture should be obtained along with urologic imaging to rule out other complications. Test of cure urinalysis or urine culture is not recommended with uncomplicated infection (Aggarwal & Leslie, 2025). If symptoms persist 72 hours after treatment, the clinician should consider a change in therapy or suspect an untreated source such as abscess or urolithiasis or a concurrent diagnosis like interstitial cystitis (Aggarwal & Leslie, 2025).

Acute cystitis can be extremely painful and cause significant disruption to a person's life. Phenazopyridine is an analgesic that can be used for symptomatic treatment of dysuria, burning, urgency, frequency, and pain associated with cystitis. The medication works by inhibiting nerve fibers in the bladder that respond to mechanical stimuli. Prescription phenazopyridine can be prescribed as 100–200 mg up to 3 times daily for 1–2 days. Over-the-counter phenazopyridine is available at a lower strength of 50–99.5 mg and can be taken up to 3 times a day. Phenazopyridine provides immediate relief while waiting for antibiotics to take effect. Patients should be reminded that the medication causes an orange discoloration of the urine so as not to be alarmed. Overall, the drug is very safe, but there are several adverse effects, including nausea, vomiting, diarrhea, headache, pruritus, ulceration, anaphylactoid-like reaction, methemoglobinemia, sulfhemoglobinemia, acute interstitial nephritis, discoloration of body fluids, aseptic meningitis, visual disturbances, renal or hepatic toxicity, jaundice, and renal calculi. Phenazopyridine can be safely taken with antibiotics. Phenazopyridine does cross the placenta and should only be used during pregnancy if indicated. The safety of phenazopyridine in breastfeeding is unknown and therefore use should be discouraged in breastfeeding patients (Eastham & Patel, 2023).

Treatment of pyelonephritis will depend on the severity of illness, likelihood of antibiotic resistance in the community, and patient history. As previously stated, uncomplicated pyelonephritis can be treated on an outpatient basis if the person is likely to be able to complete the treatment regimen and is able to return for follow-up. Suggest triaging people with pyelonephritis into one of three categories to determine the most appropriate location for treatment. Patients who are mildly ill may be managed completely at home. Those who are moderately ill, with or without vomiting, and can tolerate medications should be managed in the emergency department or an observation unit and can progress to outpatient care as symptoms start to resolve (Herness et al., 2020). Hospitalization is appropriate for severe illness, other conditions warranting increased surveillance, or if the individual is unable to manage an outpatient regimen. **Box 23-4** summarizes criteria for hospitalization.

BOX 23-4 Indications for Hospitalizing a Patient with Pyelonephritis

- Severe illness
- Pregnancy
- Immunocompromised
- Unstable or severe coexisting medical or psychosocial conditions
- Inability to tolerate oral treatment due to vomiting
- Inability to adhere to home therapy or return for follow-up due to age, living situation, or lack of social support
- Concurrent urinary tract obstruction

Data from Herness, J., Buttolph, A., & Hammer, N. C. (2020). Acute pyelonephritis in adults: Rapid evidence review. *American Family Physician, 102*(3), 173–180.

Antimicrobial selection should be individualized to the patient. The patient's clinical presentation and local resistance patterns should be taken into consideration when selecting an antibiotic. Ultimately, antimicrobial selection should be determined based on the results from urine culture. Fluoroquinolones and trimethoprim/sulfamethoxazole are supported as first-line oral therapies and considered Grade A evidence for uncomplicated acute pyelonephritis. However, microbial resistance to fluroquinolones and trimethoprim/sulfamethoxazole is increasing, making culture an imperative aspect of treatment. Nitrofurantoin and fosfomycin do not achieve adequate renal concentration and therefore should not be prescribed. Treatment options for pyelonephritis during pregnancy are limited due to lack of evidence. Options for outpatient treatment of pyelonephritis can be found in **Table 23-3**. After starting therapy, about 95 percent of patients will show improvement in symptoms within 48–72 hours. If there is no improvement, further workup should be completed and cultures should be repeated (Herness et al., 2020).

When to Refer

Patients with UTI symptoms or diagnosis sometimes require specialist care. **Box 23-5** presents indications for referral.

Patient Education

As personal hygiene plays a major factor in the prevention of UTIs, patient education is essential, especially in cases of recurrent disease. This includes voiding after intercourse and drinking plenty of fluids throughout the day. Patients may find using hygienic wipes instead of toilet paper to be beneficial. Patients should always wipe front to back and wash their hands before and after voiding. Patients should be encouraged to shower frequently and avoid taking baths. They should clean around the vagina with a soft, clean washcloth using gentle soaps without irritating ingredients such as fragrances or exfoliants. They should also avoid douching, vaginal sprays, or powders. Patients

TABLE 23-3 Outpatient Treatment Regimens for Pyelonephritis

Drug	Dose and Duration	Common Adverse Effects	Comments
Amoxicillin/ clavulanate	875/125 mg BID for 10–14 days	Antibiotic-associated diarrhea, clostridioides difficile infection, drug-induced enterocolitis syndrome, drug-induced liver injury and hypersensitivity.	Monitor renal, hepatic, and hematologic function if the patient is receiving prolonged therapy. If first dose, monitor for anaphylaxis. Do not prescribe if CrCl is < 30 mL/min or patient is on hemodialysis. Penicillin antibiotics are generally considered safe in pregnancy. Safe to use in breastfeeding but monitor infant for adverse effects.
Cefixime	400 mg once daily for 10–13 days	Abdominal pain, diarrhea, dyspepsia, flatulence, frequent bowel movements, loose stools, nausea, and vomiting.	Monitor renal and hepatic function with prolonged therapy. Monitor for anaphylaxis after first dose. No major birth defects or fetal maternal outcomes have been observed with cefixime. Risk with breastfeeding is unknown. Consider risks versus benefits.
Cefpodoxime	200 mg BID for 10–14 days	Headache, skin rash, diarrhea, nausea, abdominal pain, vomiting, and vaginal infection.	Monitor renal function. Monitor for anaphylaxis after first dose. Adverse effects were not observed in animal reproduction studies. Breastfeeding should be discontinued if used for treatment.
Cephalexin	500 mg BID for 7 days	Clostridioides difficile infection, hemolytic anemia, and hypersensitivity reactions.	Monitor renal, hepatic, and hematologic function with prolonged therapy. Monitor for anaphylaxis with first dose. Cephalosporins are considered safe in pregnancy. Give with caution in breastfeeding patients because it may cause diarrhea.
Ciprofloxacin	500 mg BID for 7 days	Aortic aneurysm/aortic dissection, arthropathy/arthralgia, CNS effects/ neuroexcitation, clostridioides difficile infection, glucose regulation/dysglycemia, hepatotoxicity, hypersensitivity, myasthenia gravis, peripheral neuropathy, phototoxicity/photoallergy, QT prolongation, tendinopathy/tendon rupture	With prolonged therapy monitor CBC, renal, and hepatic function. Monitor for signs and symptoms of mental status changes, tendinopathy, and peripheral neuropathy. Closely monitor blood sugar levels in diabetics. In pregnant and breastfeeding patients, alternative options should be considered.
Ciprofloxacin ER	1,000 mg once daily for 7 days	Aortic aneurysm/aortic dissection, arthropathy/arthralgia, CNS effects/ neuroexcitation, clostridioides difficile infection, glucose regulation/dysglycemia, hepatotoxicity, hypersensitivity, myasthenia gravis, peripheral neuropathy, phototoxicity/photoallergy, QT prolongation, tendinopathy/tendon rupture	With prolonged therapy monitor CBC, renal, and hepatic function. Monitor for signs and symptoms of mental status changes, tendinopathy and peripheral neuropathy. Closely monitor blood sugar levels in diabetics. In pregnant and breastfeeding patients, alternative options should be considered.

(*continues*)

TABLE 23-3 Outpatient Treatment Regimens for Pyelonephritis (*continued*)

Drug	Dose and Duration	Common Adverse Effects	Comments
Levofloxacin	750 mg once daily for 5 days	Aortic aneurysm/aortic dissection, arthropathy/arthralgia, CNS effects/ neuroexcitation, clostridioides difficile infection, glucose regulation, dysglycemia, hepatotoxicity, hypersensitivity, myasthenia gravis, peripheral neuropathy, phototoxicity/photoallergy, QT prolongation, tendinopathy/tendon rupture	Monitor renal, hepatic, and hematopoietic function with prolonged therapy. Monitor for altered mental status, signs and symptoms of tendinopathy and peripheral neuropathy. In diabetic patients, monitor blood glucose. Safe to give in pregnancy. Breastmilk should be discarded while taking this medication and for 2 days after last dose.
Trimethoprim/ Sulfamethoxazole	160 mg/800 mg BID for 14 days	Clostridioides difficile infection, liver injury, hematologic effects, hyperkalemia, hypoglycemia, hyponatremia, hypersensitivity, and kernicterus.	Monitor CBC, electrolytes, and renal function with prolonged therapy. Can be used in the first trimester when alternative antibiotics cannot be used. Relatively safe to use during breastfeeding. Alternative options should be considered if the infant is ill, jaundiced, premature, or if there is a risk for of bilirubin displacement or kernicterus.

Data from Herness, J., Buttolph, A., & Hammer, N.C. (2020). Acute pyelonephritis in adults: Rapid evidence review. *American Family Physician 102*(3), 173-180; UpToDate Inc. (2025). Amoxicillin and clavulanate [Drug Information]. UpToDate Lexidrug. www-uptodate.com; UpToDate Inc. (2025). Cephalexin [Drug Information]. UpToDate Lexidrug. www-uptodate.com; UpToDate Inc. (2025). Cefixime [Drug Information]. UpToDate Lexidrug. www-uptodate.com; UpToDate Inc. (2025). Cefpodoxime [Drug Information]. UpToDate Lexidrug. www-uptodate.com; UpToDate Inc. (2025). Ciprofloxacin [Drug Information]. UpToDate Lexidrug. www-uptodate.com; UpToDate Inc. (2025). Levofloxacin [Drug Information]. UpToDate Lexidrug. www-uptodate.com; UpToDate Inc. (2025). Trimethoprim-sulfamethoxazole [Drug Information]. UpToDate Lexidrug. www-uptodate.com

BOX 23-5 Indications for Referral to a Urologist or Gynecologist

- Suspected interstitial cystitis
- Resistant UTI after more than two failed treatment attempts
- More than three UTIs in 1 year
- Suspected kidney stones
- Complicated pyelonephritis

should be encouraged to complete their antibiotic regimens even if symptoms improve prior to completion. Patients should notify their provider if symptoms do not improve within 48 hours of taking antibiotics (Aggarwal & Leslie, 2025; CDC, 2024a; Lala et al., 2023).

Social and professional factors may limit an individual's ability to void at appropriate intervals, putting them at risk for developing a UTI. Certain professions, such as healthcare workers, teachers, military personnel, and factory workers, may work in settings where voiding on demand may be restricted or difficult. (Pierce et al., 2019a; Pierce et al., 2019b; Reynolds et al., 2019). Pierce et al. (2019b) specifically studied the voiding practices of nurses and midwives on the job and concluded that there was substantial room for improvement of voiding practices which could improve urinary symptoms in this population. Hectic work schedules and traveling can make voiding difficult. Limited access to restrooms or the fear that public restrooms are not clean enough can also be a barrier. This holding of one's urine can lead to lower urinary tract symptoms and urinary disorders (Jagtap et al., 2022). Education about the need for healthy bladder practices, including voiding when the urge is present, is important for all individuals. They should also be cautioned against the practice of limiting fluids to decrease the need to urinate (Kwok et al., 2022).

Prevention of Recurrent UTI

Many AFAB individuals develop recurrent or frequent UTIs. In fact, 20–30 percent of women who develop a UTI will have a recurrent UTI within 6 months (Cai, 2021). Older studies commonly define recurrent UTIs as two infections in the past 12 months and more recent studies define recurrent UTI as two infections within the past 6 months or three or more infections in 1 year (Aggarwal & Leslie, 2025; Jent et al., 2022). Risk factors include decreased fluid intake, delaying urination, dysfunctional voiding patterns, and wearing restrictive clothing (Cai, 2021).

Long-term prophylactic antibiotics is an option for patients with recurrent UTIs (Czajkowski et al., 2021). For asymptomatic patients, trimethoprim, trimethoprim/sulfamethoxazole, nitrofurantoin, cephalexin, and fosfomycin are available options (Czajkowski et al., 2021). Antibiotic prophylaxis can cause adverse events such as nausea, vaginal candidiasis, allergic reactions, and skin rashes. Other adverse events include drug toxicity, antimicrobial resistance, and alterations to the patient's microbiome. In 11 placebo-controlled trials, the risk of developing a UTI was 85 percent lower with prophylaxis treatment in comparison to placebo. For patients aged 65 years and greater, prophylactic antibiotics have been shown to be especially helpful if taken

BOX 23-6 Dosing Options for Urinary Tract Infection Antibiotic Prophylaxis

First-line antibiotic agents for recurrent UTI prophylaxis

- Nitrofurantoin 50–100 mg before bed (HS) daily
- Sulfamethoxazole and trimethoprim 40/200 mg HS daily
- Trimethoprim 100 mg HS daily

Second-line antibiotic agents for recurrent UTI prophylaxis

- Cephalexin 125 mg or 250 mg HS daily
- Cefaclor 250 mg HS daily
- Fosfomycin 3 gm every 10 days
- Norfloxacin 400 mg HS daily
- Pivmecillinam 185 mg daily

Reproduced from Aggarwal, N., & Leslie, S.W. (2025). Recurrent urinary tract infections. In *StatPearls*. StatPearls Publishing.

for more than 2 years (Czajkowski et al., 2021). Microbial resistance is a risk and has been noted more so with trimethoprim-sulfamethoxazole (Jent et al., 2022). Refer to **Box 23-6** for UTI prophylaxis regimens.

Intercourse increases the risk of UTI by up to 9 times (Cai, 2021). There may also be a link between spermicides and oral contraceptive use (Cai, 2021). Spermicide can increase the risk of *E. coli* periurethral colonization (Cai, 2021). Single-dose postcoital antibiotics may be helpful for people who find an association between sexual activity and UTIs. Individuals whose UTIs are unrelated to sexual activity can take a continuous low-dose antibiotic for 3 to 12 months (Anger et al., 2019).

Vaginal estrogen cream can be used to treat recurrent UTIs in postmenopausal women. As women age, estrogen depletion can affect lubrication, tissue elasticity, pH, and blood flow. There is also a decrease in lactobacillus which creates a more hospitable environment for bacterial growth (Rosenblum, 2020). Vaginal estrogen can help restore atrophic tissue and improve vaginal flora and pH (Kolman, 2019). The American Urological Association recommends that providers offer postmenopausal women vaginal estrogen for the treatment of recurrent UTIs (Aggarwal & Lesslie, 2025; Rosenblum, 2020). Vaginal estrogen is relatively safe with few side effects. Topical vaginal estrogen does not increase the risk of breast or gynecological cancers (Chambers et al., 2020; McVicker et al., 2024). However, collaborative discussion with the treating oncologist is encouraged before initiation.

Many patients now seek complementary and alternative measures prior to being prescribed medications. Clinicians should be knowledgeable and aware of alternative options for patients and be able to discuss safety and efficacy. Probiotics are an option for prophylactic treatment of recurrent UTIs. Probiotics act in the bladder by secreting bacteriocins and peptides which can inhibit bacterial growth. Probiotics generally have few side effects and are tolerated well. However, patients should be aware that cost and quality vary widely, so assistance in choosing an appropriate probiotic may be needed (Qasemi et al., 2023). Over-the-counter cranberry products such as juice, tablets, and powder have historically been used to prevent UTIs. Cranberries contain proanthocyanidins (PACs) which can decrease the ability of p-fimbriated *E. coli* to adhere to the urothelial cells within the bladder (Kolman, 2019). The recommended dose to prevent UTIs is 300 mL a day, which many people find difficult to consume (Kolman, 2019). A Cochrane Review found that cranberry products may help patients with frequent UTIs, children with UTIs, and patients who have had bladder interventions. However, the data from this study did not support the use of cranberry products to reduce the risk of UTIs in older people, pregnant individuals, or adults with neuromuscular dysfunction of the bladder and incomplete bladder emptying. The AUA guidelines support cranberry products; however, patients should be aware that effectiveness is variable, and alternative treatment options may be needed (Aggarwal & Leslie, 2025).

A recent systematic review found methenamine to be an effective and well-tolerated prophylactic antimicrobial agent. The combination of methenamine and vitamin C can be used to acidify the urine. Methenamine undergoes hydrolysis in the presence of urine, which results in the production of ammonia and formaldehyde. This causes antimicrobial activity by altering bacterial cells. Methenamine can be prescribed as 1 g by mouth twice a day or methenamine mandelate 1 g by mouth 4 times a day. Over-the-counter methenamine is available for UTI-related pain, but it is not as effective as the prescription. Patients with renal insufficiency, hepatic insufficiency, or severe dehydration should not take methenamine. It should not be taken with sulfonamides because it can cause urine to crystallize. High doses of methenamine (8 g daily for 3–4 weeks) have been associated with bladder irritation, painful and frequent urination, albuminuria, and hematuria (Aggarwal & Leslie, 2025; Li et al., 2024).

D-mannose is a sugar naturally found in various plants and fruits and commonly marketed as a supplement to reduce the risk of UTIs (Ala-Jaakola et al., 2022). It is thought to create a nonstick surface on the bladder wall as well as causative bacteria, therefore reducing the risk of UTI (Ala-Jaakola et al., 2022). D-mannose is relatively safe but can cause diarrhea and bloating (Ala-Jaakola et al., 2022). Prenatal studies in mice showed eye anomalies (Ala-Jaakola et al., 2022). For recurrent infections, it is recommended to take 500 mg twice daily. A Cochrane Review found that D-mannose played no role in the prevention of UTIs when compared to placebo and antibiotics (Cooper et al., 2022). This review did not support or refute the use of D-mannose as there are few recent RCTs that have shown any clinical benefit (Aggarwal & Leslie, 2025). Taking probiotics, D-mannose, and cranberry products for at least 6 months has been shown to reduce the rates of UTIs by 76 percent and drop antimicrobial use by 90 percent (Aggarwal & Leslie, 2025). Cost may be a barrier for some patients.

Immunizations for recurrent UTI prophylaxis appear promising. While not approved in the United States or Canada, there are several other countries already using vaccines such as Australia, United Kingdom, Sweden and Norway. The oral vaccine, MV140, has been shown to have good efficacy and minimal adverse effects in treating recurrent UTIs. The vaccine contains heat-inactivated strains of *E. coli, Klebsiella pneumoniae, Enterococcus faecalis*, and *Proteus vulgaris*. This induces antibody production and modifies the bladder's local immune response (Aggarwal & Leslie, 2025).

Traditional Chinese Medicine (TCM) has also been used for prevention of recurrent UTI. A systematic Cochrane review found that TCM was more effective than antibiotics when treating acute

UTIs and resulted in fewer recurrent episodes. There have been five published RCTs that showed TCM to be more efficacious than antimicrobial treatment. This is a promising option to prevent antimicrobial resistance or for patients who want to avoid antibiotics (van Wietmarschen et al., 2022). TCM should only be practiced under the supervision of an experienced practitioner.

URINARY INCONTINENCE

Urinary incontinence (UI) is the involuntary loss of urine that can be caused by several different conditions. The most common types of UI include stress urinary incontinence (SUI), urgency urinary incontinence (UUI), and mixed urinary incontinence (MUI) (refer to **Table 23-4**). For AFAB individuals, pelvic floor anatomy contributes to UI. This includes pliability of the pelvic floor, and a much shorter urethra located within (rather than outside) the pelvis.

UI can affect quality of life, self-esteem, body image, and sense of control. It can also be costly to patients and the healthcare system. In some resource-scarce areas of the world, a person may not be able to afford or find appropriate care, putting them at risk of isolation and depression. A holistic approach is crucial and should include assessment of urinary tract symptoms and other pelvic floor disorders. Patients should also be asked about social, psychological, community, emotional, and financial stressors. Referral should be considered to expedite diagnosis and treatment (Todhunter-Brown et al., 2022; Batmani et al., 2021).

Types of UI

The diagnosis of UI is typically broken down into three major categories—stress incontinence, urge incontinence, or mixed incontinence—as described in Table 23-4. Although these are the main categories of incontinence, others do exist in specific scenarios. Coital incontinence, postural incontinence, and nocturnal enuresis are all examples of other forms of incontinence. Neurogenic bladder (discussed later in the chapter) differs in that it is neither associated with stress or urgency but rather caused by overflow due to diminished sensation to urinate or the inability to control voiding at all (Atiemo & Stoffel, 2024).

TABLE 23-4 Types of UI

Type of Incontinence	Definition
Stress (urinary) incontinence	Involuntary leakage with effort or physical exertion, sneezing, or coughing
Urgency (urinary) incontinence	Involuntary loss of urine associated with urgency
Mixed (urinary) incontinence	Involuntary urine leakage associated with symptoms of both stress and urgency UI

Data from Denisenko, A. A., Clark, C. B., D'Amico, M., & Murphy, A. M. (2021). Evaluation and management of female urinary incontinence. *The Canadian Journal of Urology, 28*(S2), 27–32.

Scope of the Problem

UI is a common problem around the world and can significantly impact an individual's quality of life. UI is associated with an increased risk of anxiety, depression, isolation, sleep disturbances, and psychological distress. UI can also cause perineal rash, pressure ulcers, and UTIs (Todhunter-Brown et al., 2022). In older patients, UI can lead to falls resulting in fractures, which are the leading cause of death in people over 65 years of age (Batmani et al., 2021).

Most studies report the prevalence of UI in women between 25-45 percent, and this proportion increases with age (Milsom & Gyhagen, 2018). A meta-analysis (Batmani et al., 2021) found that 37.1 percent of older women and 77 percent of women living in nursing homes are affected by UI. Of patients who report UI, 49.8 percent reported SUI, 34.4 percent reported MUI, and 15.9 percent reported UUI. It is estimated that by 2050 almost 28.4 million AFAB people will have UI as compared to only 18 million in 2010 (Denisenko et al., 2021; Todhunter-Brown et al., 2022; Batmani et al., 2021).

Etiology and Pathophysiology

UI is defined as any occurrence or condition that elicits a moment of intravesical pressure that exceeds urethral pressure, resulting in involuntary urine loss. Continence is maintained as long as bladder pressure is less than urethral pressure. Both neurologic and structural abnormalities can contribute to the dysfunction of this system.

The bladder is a hollow muscular organ that can typically hold up to 600–650 mL of urine in people AFAB (Lavalle et al., 2023). The muscle of the bladder is called the detrusor. When the smooth muscle of the detrusor contracts, the low-pressure zone within the bladder is converted to a high-pressure zone, which is needed when an individual wishes to expel urine. Whenever an individual wishes to not expel urine, the detrusor is relaxed and the bladder serves as a low-pressure holding tank (Todhunter-Brown et al., 2022; Shermadou et al., 2023).

Dysfunction of the detrusor muscle can contribute to symptoms of UI (Rotem et al., 2024). Detrusor overactivity (DO) is a well-observed and discussed phenomenon contributing to urgency and urge incontinence. When the detrusor contracts unexpectedly (not during times of intentional micturition), the pressure can contribute to urine leakage. However, the exact mechanism for DO is not completely understood, and may be patient specific. The following three causes of DO have been hypothesized: (1) dysfunction of the musculature itself, as the detrusor is prone to fibrosis, inflammation, and decreased perfusion as it ages; (2) dysfunction of neurogenic mechanisms, including motor and sensory pathways; and (3) increased release of ATP from the urothelium during bladder filling, which can stimulate nerves associated with muscle activity (Rotem et al., 2024).

Conversely, detrusor underactivity (DUA), or the bladder's inability to contract adequately enough to empty the bladder, can cause chronic overfilling and retention of urine leading to situations where the bladder can overfill. When the building pressure surpasses the pressure of the urethra, overflow incontinence can occur. Similar to DO, DUA can be either from neurologic or muscular causes (Hartigan et al., 2019) (refer to section on neurogenic bladder later in this chapter). It should also be noted that this dynamic can occur when a person holds their urine regularly for long periods of time due to their profession or other reasons for infrequent micturition such as limited access to appropriate bathrooms. Alternatively, some people may experience bladder outflow obstruction (BOO), a condition where the urethra is blocked or kinked. A variety of conditions can mechanically cause BOO. In people AFAB, cystocele, or descent of the bladder due to weakened pelvic floor, is a common cause. Over time, emptying is chronically reduced resulting in eventual DUA (Makajeva et al., 2022; Hartigan et al., 2019).

The urethra is a high-pressure zone that is maintained by three distinct mechanisms: striated muscle contraction, the vascular plexus (a spongy, highly vascular submucosal layer which can control pressure via capillary engorgement), and the surrounding smooth muscle and connective tissues (Pipitone et al., 2021). The smooth muscle of the bladder extends longitudinally along the bladder to the most proximal 20 percent of the urethral length, including the internal urethral sphincter. The internal urethral sphincter is involuntarily controlled and keeps urine in the bladder. Striated circumferential muscle comprises most of the urethral length and is thickest at the midpoint of the urethra, where the external urethra sphincter is located. Because of the striated nature of the circumferential urethral muscle, it is under voluntary control, and in a healthy pelvic floor, volitional pelvic muscle contraction elicits increased urethral closure pressure (Todhunter-Brown et al., 2022). The urethra rests on the anterior vaginal wall, which is supported by the levator ani muscle. This muscle is commonly referred to as the pelvic floor or Kegel muscle and includes the pubovisceral muscle (also known as the pubococcygeus, iliococcygeus, and puborectal muscles) and its fibrous attachments. Upward-oriented forces of the levator ani form a resistive plate onto which the urethra is compressed when driven downward by increasing intra-abdominal pressure. This can occur with coughing, sneezing, and heavy lifting. The dynamic interrelationships among these factors are shown by the arrows in **Figure 23-1**. When an individual consciously contracts the pelvic floor muscles (i.e., striated urethral sphincteric muscle, levator ani muscle, and external anal sphincter), the urethra is closed, the bladder is lifted, and the anus is closed (Shermadou et al., 2023).

As the body ages, a decrease in urethral pressure is observed. One study showed that women between the ages of 61 and 65 had a 50 percent decrease in urethral pressure compared to women aged 36–40; the same study demonstrated a gradual reduction in functional urethral length after the age of 45. Several mechanisms are believed to contribute to this decreased pressure. A strong aging effect is observed with the striated circumferential urethral muscle. Muscle loss that naturally occurs with age is called sarcopenia. This causes atrophy of this muscle starting at its most superior point near the bladder neck and gradually extends down toward midurethra (Shermadou et al., 2023). The resultant low urethral pressure increases a person's risk of UI when the urine passively funnels into the upper portion of the urethra and is perceived as urgency. Smooth muscle density also decreases with age, as does the surrounding connective tissues. Some of this loss of muscle is believed to be caused by decreased innervation of these muscles over time. Finally, the incidence or likelihood of accruing another risk factor associated with UI (e.g., childbirth, hysterectomy, obesity, diabetes) increases as a patient ages (Pipitone et al., 2021). The levator ani muscle is a secondary control mechanism that operates through (1) its functional capacity to support the bladder and urethra from below and (2) its felt accessibility to a person for eliciting a volitional contraction that simultaneously prompts urethral striated muscle contraction. The pubovisceral portion of the levator ani muscle, however, is vulnerable to detachment from its origin at the pubic bone during childbirth (Lin et al., 2019).

Genetic Factors

Many studies have contributed to our knowledge that there is a genetic component to UI; however, the exact genes involved are unknown. Studies also point to environmental risk factors and epigenetics as contributing factors. Despite the findings that UI runs in families, the exact symptoms experienced by those family members may differ significantly, pointing to a genetic connection between subtypes of UI (Breinbjerg et al., 2023).

Pregnancy and Childbirth

Pregnancy, childbirth, and increased parity have long been associated with UI (Tähtinen et al., 2019; van Geelen at al., 2023). UI is commonly experienced during pregnancy due to increasing pressure of the enlarged uterus and fetal weight on the bladder, along with pregnancy-related hormonal changes including increased progesterone, increased relaxin, and decreased collagen levels. A systematic review and meta-analysis found that UI affects 9–75 percent of pregnancies and can impact people of every parity in any trimester. SUI is the most common type of UI reported, accounting for 63 percent of cases. Experiencing UI during pregnancy is a major risk factor for continuing to have SUI postpartum and later throughout life (Moossdorff-Steinhauser et al., 2021).

The prevalence and severity of UI are higher in women who have experienced vaginal childbirth versus those who have only had cesarean births (Tähtinen et al., 2019). It is estimated that 13–46 percent of people who give birth vaginally suffer some type of pelvic floor muscle injury during childbirth; the majority of these injuries is to the pubovisceral muscle (Vila Pouca et al., 2022), and as many as 66 percent of individuals with an additional demographic or obstetric risk factor for pubovisceral tear develop this condition (Sheng et al., 2019). The risk is greatest in people whose birthing experience includes use of forceps (Lin et al., 2019; Tähtinen et al., 2019). Varying degrees of pubovisceral muscle tears are possible, and many of them are chronic in nature. Regardless of severity, levator ani contraction force on attempt to contract is significantly reduced in individuals with pubovisceral tear, reducing the urethral closure pressure (Sheng et al., 2019).

Lifestyle Factors

Adequate water intake is crucial to urinary health; known benefits include prevention and treatment of a UTI and renal calculi (Perrier et al., 2021). However, it is also necessary that individuals provide themselves with adequate voiding to prevent overdistention of the bladder. Fluid intake habits—both amount and type of beverage—may contribute to UI. Some people inadvertently exacerbate or cause their UI by overconsumption of beverages without matching their void intervals to these higher intake amounts. Certain beverages, like citrus juices, caffeinated beverages, or those containing carbonation, have been found to be especially irritating to those with UI (Ha et al., 2025).

Smoking history is associated with UUI specifically, although the association in one study (Kawahara et al., 2020) was found

FIGURE 23-1 **Interrelationship of pelvic structures to achieve continence.**

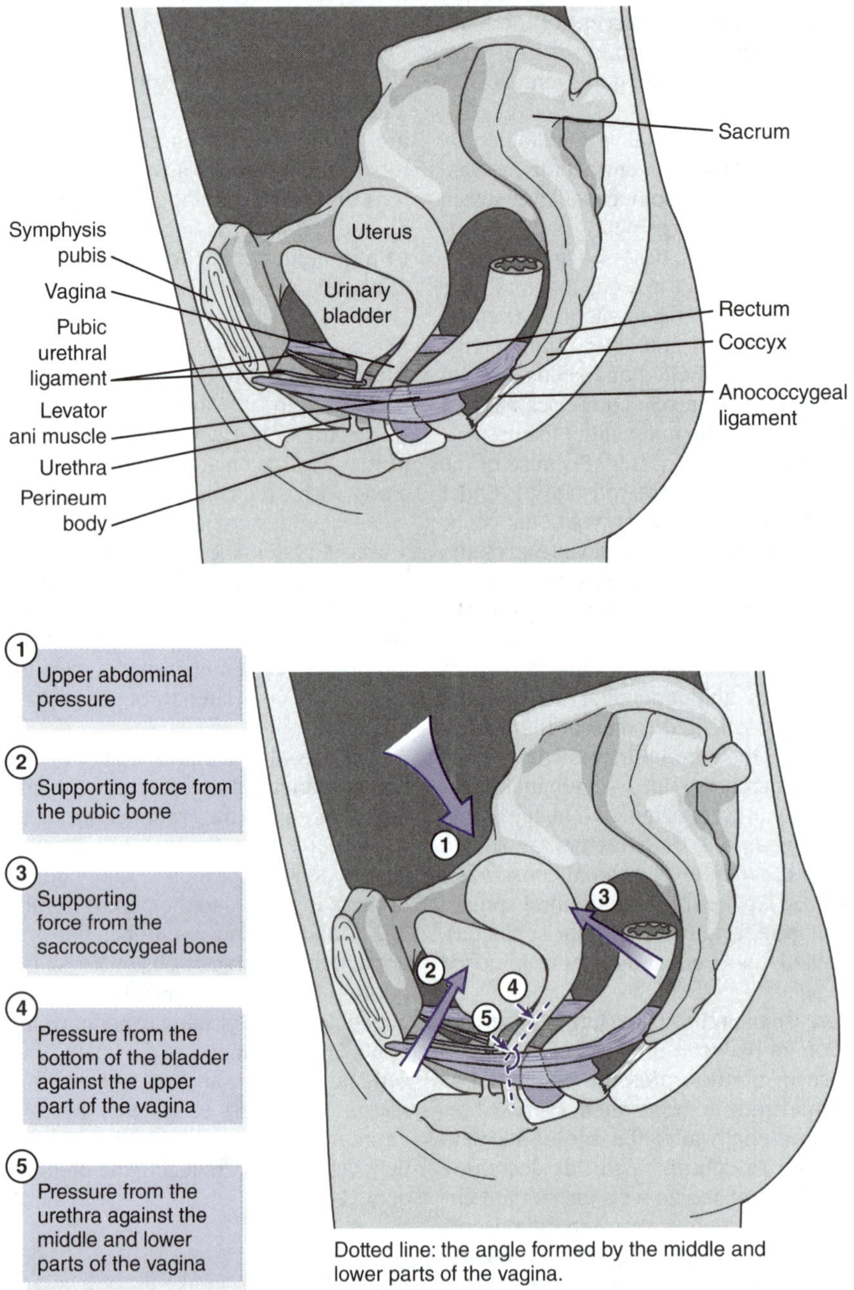

Abbreviations: AP, abdominal pressure; LA, levator ani; PB, pubic bone; US, urethral sphincter; V, vagina.
Data from Yang, X., Wang, X., Gao, Z., Li, L., Lin, H., Wang, H., Zhou, H., Tian, D., Zhang, Q., & Shen, J. (2022). The anatomical pathogenesis of stress urinary incontinence in women. *Medicina (Kaunas, Lithuania), 59*(1), 5. https://doi.org/10.3390/medicina59010005.

to be stronger in younger women and decrease with age as well as years since smoking cessation.

Having a larger body size has been identified as a predictor for the development of UI, with research showing that the longer an individual remains in a larger body, the greater their risk of developing UI (Batmani et al., 2021; Lamerton, 2021). Individuals with higher body mass indices also report more frequent episodes of UI, and having a larger body size after the age of 35 increases the likelihood of experiencing UI later in life. Research has shown that a 5–10 percent reduction in body weight can significantly reduce the frequency of UI episodes (Choi et al., 2022). When discussing this with clients, it is critical to recognize that individuals with larger bodies often face weight bias and stigma in healthcare settings, which can negatively impact their willingness to seek care and the quality of care they receive. Weight stigma can lead to internalized shame, avoidance of medical consultations, and delayed treatment for UI, exacerbating both physical symptoms and emotional distress (Gibbins et al., 2023). This stigma can also result in healthcare providers attributing UI solely to weight, potentially overlooking other contributing factors and reducing the likelihood of comprehensive, empathetic care (Dökmeci & Rizk, 2022). Addressing weight stigma is therefore essential not only for improving health outcomes but also for fostering a more inclusive and supportive healthcare environment for individuals affected by UI. Refer to **Box 23-7** for further risk factors for UI.

Urinary Incontinence Comorbidities

UI may sometimes be a symptom of broader system pathology. Coexisting diseases have been confirmed as precipitating risk factors that may independently or interdependently influence continence of urine. Such conditions include bacterial urinary tract infection, diabetes, neurologic disorders (e.g., multiple sclerosis, Parkinson disease, and cognitive impairment such as dementia or Alzheimer's disease), traumatic injury (e.g., spinal injury, pelvic trauma, and surgical trauma), heart disease and stroke, kidney disease, arthritis, back problems, visual impairments, constipation, and major depressive disorders (Johnson & Vaughan, 2019). In addition, many medications used for other conditions are associated with UI, such as diuretics, estrogen, benzodiazepines, tranquilizers, antidepressants, hypnotics, laxatives, and antibiotics (Lian et al., 2019; Handa et al., 2019; Johnson & Vaughan, 2019).

Urinary incontinence and disabilities are often associated; that is, UI is a significant cause of disabilities, and certain types of disabilities can either cause or exacerbate UI. Various types of UI can be secondary to other disease processes like stroke, mobility impairment, and dementia (Johnson & Vaughan, 2019). If the preexisting condition is neurologic in nature, the diagnosis of neurogenic bladder may be appropriate (refer to the section on neurogenic bladder). Depending on the degree of disability in a patient, caregiver involvement is often critical whether the patient resides at home or in a facility (Johnson & Vaughan, 2019). Patients may need assistance with timed or prompted voiding, physically accessing a restroom, or helping to avoid potential triggers. Although some medications may improve symptoms of UI for older and women with disabilities, a number of considerations must be taken into account before prescribing these agents. For patients who take multiple medications, drug interactions are difficult to avoid. Antimuscarinic agents can exacerbate cognitive impairment, especially in the frail elderly, and should be prescribed and dispensed with caution (Fontaine et al., 2021).

BOX 23-7 Risk Factors for Urinary Incontinence

- Age
- Race/ethnicity
- Larger body size
- Parity
- Smoking
- Diabetes
- Hysterectomy
- Vaginal delivery (especially forceps-assisted vaginal delivery)
- Menopause
- Education
- Hypertension
- Length of first and second stages of labor
- Urinary tract infections

Data from Denisenko, A. A., Clark, C. B., D'Amico, M., & Murphy, A. M. (2021). Evaluation and management of female urinary incontinence. *The Canadian Journal of Urology, 28*(S2), 27–32; Elders, A., Hagen, S., & McClurg, D. (2022). Conservative interventions for treating urinary incontinence in women: An overview of cochrane systematic reviews. *The Cochrane Database of Systematic Reviews, 9*(9), CD012337; Batmani, S., Jalali, R., Mohammadi, M., & Bokaee, S. (2021). Prevalence and factors related to urinary incontinence in older adults women worldwide: A comprehensive systematic review and meta-analysis of observational studies. *BMC Geriatrics, 21*(1), 212.

Clinical Presentation

Many people suffer from UI for years before discussing symptoms with their healthcare provider. Some individuals never seek treatment at all. Understanding health behaviors is complex; multiple variables contribute to a patient actively seeking medical help with a complaint. Personal belief that UI is a normal part of aging, fear that there is no cure or that the only cure is surgery, shame or embarrassment, fear of costs associated with treatment, the inconvenience of having to see a specialist, negative family support all may be barriers to a patient seeking help with their UI symptoms. Conversely, severity of symptoms, poor quality of life, and family/social support for seeking help are positive predictors of likelihood of seeking treatment (Rashidi et al., 2021).

Assessment

History

It is important to ascertain the full scope of UI in terms of its presence, frequency, duration, setting, severity, and impact on quality of life. The clinician should focus on the patient's experience and care priorities. Careful elucidation of the numerous underlying factors that can contribute to leakage, along with the individual's indication of which leakage situation is most important to address, can provide information to establish which of these more precise subcategories of UI is present and to determine treatment priorities.

The patient should be asked about previous testing and treatments; coexisting diseases that may be precipitating factors; medications; obstetric and physical impairment; social history, such as environmental issues and lifestyle including beverage intake patterns; any measures currently being used to contain the leakage; and the extent to which the individual is

TABLE 23-5 Medications and Substances That Can Affect UI

Effect	Medication or Substance
Decrease bladder contractility (retention and overflow UI)	Angiotensin-converting enzyme inhibitors (may also cause chronic cough) Antidepressants Antihistamines Antimuscarinics Antiparkinsonian agents Antipsychotics Beta-adrenergic agonists Calcium channel blockers Opioids Sedatives, hypnotics Skeletal muscle relaxants
Increase detrusor irritability or creatinine clearance (urge UI)	Alcohol Caffeine Diuretics
Increase urethral sphincter tone (retention and overflow UI)	Alpha-adrenergic agonists Amphetamines Tricyclic antidepressants
Decrease urethral sphincter tone (stress UI)	Alpha-adrenergic antagonists

Reprinted with permission from Jocelyn S. Hu, MD and Elyse Fiore Peirre, MD. Urinary Incontinence in Women: Evaluation and Management, Am Fam Physician 2019;100(6):339-348.

seeking or desiring treatment, from conservative to aggressive options (Denisenko et al., 2021). A list of common medications that can affect UI can be found in **Table 23-5.**

There are many screening tools to ascertain a patient's experience with UI. The 3 Incontinence Questions, the International Consultation on Incontinence Questionnaire Urinary Incontinence Short Form (ICIQ-UI), and the Revised Urinary Incontinence Scale (RUIS) are all examples of validated tools which can quickly and easily be used in an office setting (Hu & Pierre, 2019). A 3-day voiding diary is a valuable assessment tool for illuminating patterns that contribute to leakage in daily life such as drinking habits, voiding volumes, frequency of voids, daytime and nighttime urinary output, and episodes of incontinence (Denisenko et al., 2021). Many styles of bladder diaries are available; **Figure 23-2** provides one example. Regardless of the type of voiding diary used, four components are critical to record:

- Time of day and amount of voiding (provide a measurement hat for the toilet)
- Time of day when an episode of UI occurs
- A place to write a brief description of the UI episode and associated events
- Types and amounts of beverages consumed

Physical Examination and Diagnostic Testing

Assessing bladder capacity is done least invasively through a 3-day voiding diary. The largest void in the diary is an estimate of bladder capacity. The physical exam should include a pelvic exam which should assess for peri-urethral cysts, urethral hypermobility, and cystocele (Denisenko et al., 2021).

A clinical estimate of pubovisceral muscle tear can be made by palpatory assessment of the pubovisceral muscle body (Sheng et al., 2019). Palpatory assessment is performed using the index finger placed at the expected anatomical location of the middle pubovisceral muscle body as felt about 2 cm inside the vagina, with the finger curled to the right or left against the vaginal sidewall. The finger is lightly pressed against the vaginal sidewall and swept slightly up and down to palpate for fullness of the pubovisceral muscle body on one side, then on the other side, in an attempt to determine if the muscle body can be clearly felt (refer to **Figure 23-3**). Varying degrees of pubovisceral muscle tear can be definitively ascertained only by MRI (Sheng et al., 2019). However, palpation at the site of the pubovisceral muscle to assess for presence is a commonly used clinical approach and has been found to have high association with the risk of MRI-documented pubovisceral muscle tear (Sheng et al., 2019).

To determine whether the urethra is able to maintain a high margin of continence under the stress conditions of intra-abdominal pressure rise, a quantified standing stress test can be performed independently by the patient (Miller et al., 2021). This test is commonly referred to as the paper towel test. It is a quick, inexpensive, and noninvasive way to estimate the severity of stress-type leakage. The person does this test while standing with a comfortably full bladder; they cough very hard three times while holding a colored (blue or brown) trifold paper towel against their perineum. Urine loss onto the paper towel can be quantified; that is, visually measured as a wet area (**Figure 23-4**). One study showed that 38.9 percent of women who answered "no" on a questionnaire about UI did have some urine leakage on the paper towel test (Miller et al., 2021). Although a more definitive test for urethral sphincter deficiency is a urethral pressure profile, the equipment required to obtain such a profile is expensive and typically not readily accessible outside of specialty practices, and it is an invasive procedure.

It is important for the individual to validate the finding of stress-type leakage on the paper towel test as consistent with their experience of symptoms and the reason for seeking treatment. If the wet area on the paper towel corresponds to just a couple of drops of urine, this may not be the scenario that is troublesome to the patient at home. The clinician should ask, "Do you routinely cough this hard outside of the clinic setting, or undertake activities that would impose an equal level of pressure?" and "Is this the type of leakage that you experience and that you find bothersome?" If not, further assessment should be undertaken to determine the scenarios and additional causative factors that might account for the leakage that is considered bothersome.

During the visit, post-void residual (PVR) assessment and urinalysis (UA) should be collected to evaluate for UTI and hematuria (Denisenko et al., 2021). The PVR can be assessed through in-office catheterization; however, the use of US by means of a bladder scanner is much less invasive. Urine cultures are not necessary unless symptoms are suggestive of UTI. Typically, the type of UI can be diagnosed through history and physical exam.

FIGURE 23-2 **Voiding diary.**

Instructions:

Please record each time you drink fluids, you empty your bladder, you lose urine accidentally, and you perform pelvic muscle contractions for 3 consecutive days.

- "Time" columns: Be sure to write AM or PM.
- "Type" column: Write caffeinated or decaf for beverages such as coffee, tea, and cola. Other examples of beverage types include milk, juice, water, alcohol, milkshakes, etc.
- "Amount" column: Write one of the following numbers to indicate the amount of accidental urine loss:
  - 1 – leak a few drops
  - 2 – wet underpants, but not soak through
  - 3 – soak all the way through to outer clothes
  - 4 – possibly drip onto the floor
- "Urge" column: Write 'yes' if you had a sudden urge and couldn't get to the bathroom in time.
- "Activity" column: Please describe what you were doing when you accidentally lost urine (i.e., coughing, sneezing, laughing, reaching, jumping, lifting a heavy object, rising from chair, heard running water, etc.).

DATE BEGUN ___/___/___

Day 1

Awakening Time: __________ Bedtime: __________

Fluids I Drank Today:		
Time (AM/PM)	Type	Amount (oz/mL)

Urinated in Toilet:			
Time (AM/PM)	Time (AM/PM)	Time (AM/PM)	Time (AM/PM)

Accidental Leakage of Urine:			
Time (AM/PM)	Amount	Urge (Yes/No)	Activity

Urodynamic testing (UDS) is not necessary for most patients. However, in some patients with a history of anti-incontinence surgeries, mismatch between subjective and objective measures, significant voiding dysfunction, elevated PVR volume, MUI and a substantial urgency component, or neurogenic lower urinary tract dysfunction, UDS may be necessary. A filling cystometrogram can be performed. However, this procedure is invasive, uncomfortable, does not reflect a normal setting for the individual, and requires equipment that is typically not available in a nonspecialty clinical environment. Cystoscopy is an alternative

Courtesy of Dr. John DeLancey.

FIGURE 23-3 **Diagrammatic portrayal of index finger placement for palpatory assessment of the pubovisceral muscle body integrity.**

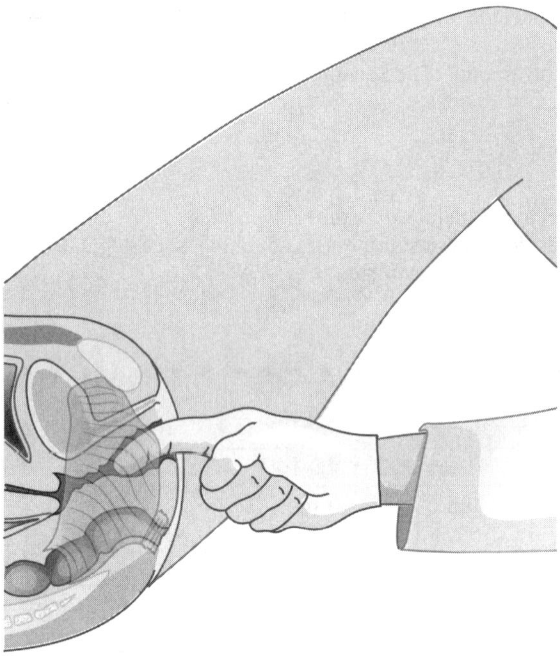

Courtesy of Dr. John DeLancey.

FIGURE 23-4 **Use of a paper towel to quantify volume of urine loss upon coughing.**

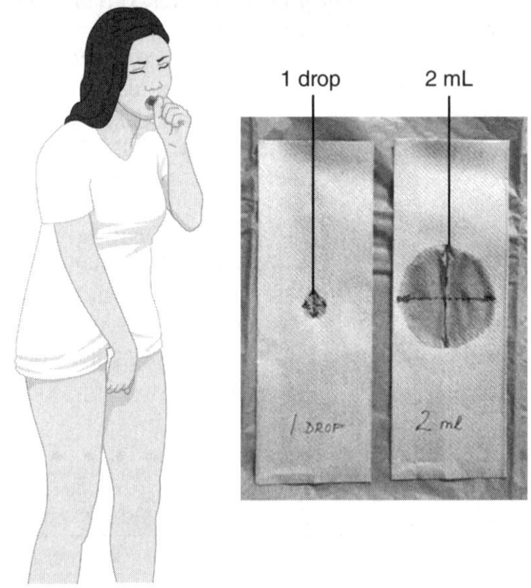

Data from Miller, J. M., Hood, M. M., Karvonen-Gutierrez, C. A., Richards-McCullough, K. C., & Harlow, S. D. (2021). Paper towel test as independently self-administered to quantify cough-related urine loss: Compliance and comparisons with survey-only data in SWAN. *Neurourology and Urodynamics, 40*(5), 1207–1216.

option for patients with concerns of lower urinary tract abnormalities (Denisenko et al., 2021).

Levator ani functional capacity to lift and stabilize the continence structures can be readily observed on a transperineal 2-D ultrasound. The test uses an external perineal probe and sagittal view of the bladder. This comfortable, simple assessment doubles as a quick and effective teaching aid in instructing a person on the pelvic muscle contraction technique. If ultrasound equipment is not available, the best clinical guess at functional loss (whether from pubovisceral muscle tear or genetic weakness) is obtained when a person continues to bear down or use the gluteal muscles when asked to contract their pelvic floor muscles. Specialty referral is appropriate to determine the cause in such a case.

Prevention

Prevention of UI may focus on a person addressing the following risk factors: obesity, pelvic floor dysfunction, excessive or ill-timed beverage intake, and treating underlying conditions which are risk factors for UI (like diabetes). Performing pelvic muscle exercises developing the Knack skill (discussed later in this chapter) encourages a strong pelvic floor which is important for prevention (Okeahialam et al., 2022). As a larger body size is one of the main risk factors for UI, encouraging healthy practices in body weight management would also be a strategy in prevention (Lamerton et al., 2021).

Management

Treatment for UI should be offered if the patient finds their symptoms distressing. Management of UI is aimed at reducing the factors that allow bladder pressure to exceed urethral pressure and generally follows a treatment pathway of less invasive to more invasive therapies. Nonpharmacologic treatments, such as lifestyle changes and strengthening of the pelvic floor should be considered first, followed by physical devices such as pessaries and medication management, and finally referral for a surgical consult if necessary (Okeahialam et al., 2022).

Nonpharmacologic Treatment

Patients often choose behavioral interventions as a first step for treatment of UI because these measures are less invasive and lower in risk than other treatments. Interventions related to beverage management and healthy toilet habits form the basis for initial treatment, but they depend on evaluation of a voiding diary. The diary can be both an assessment tool and an intervention. A person may not be fully aware of their own patterns and can find the self-monitoring experience to be illuminating. The diary also serves to monitor progress over time when a repeat diary is recorded later in treatment. Despite scant data to determine the mechanism by which specific ingredients produce UI, people who experience UI may benefit from reducing or eliminating beverages containing caffeine, artificial sweeteners, citrus juices, carbonation, and alcohol (Denisenko et al., 2021; Ha et al., 2025). This is especially beneficial for individuals with UUI (Denisenko et al., 2021).

BOX 23-8 Example of Bladder Training Protocol

1. Do not go out immediately in search of the bathroom
2. Inhibit the urination urge for at least 5 min
3. Sit down, if possible, relax the whole body and perform five consecutive contractions of the pelvic floor muscles associated with slow and deep breathing
4. Distract the mind by engaging in tasks that require mental but not physical effort (e.g., reading a topic of interest, making a phone call, making a to-do list, accessing a social network on an electronic device such as a smartphone or computer
5. Use self-affirmation: "I can do it; I can wait; I am in charge of my bladder."

Participants were instructed to progressively increase urination intervals during waking hours. Thus, after inhibiting the urge for 5 min, they were guided to progressively increase the intervals (15–20 min/week) until reaching 3–4 h between urinations.

Reproduced from Monteiro, S., Rocha, A. K., Valim, L., Silva, S. L. A. D., Riccetto, C., & Botelho, S. (2023). Bladder training compared to bladder training associated with pelvic floor muscle training for overactive bladder symptoms in women: A randomized clinical trial. *Neurourology and Urodynamics, 42*(8), 1802-1811.

Bladder training can help patients increase the interval between voiding and increase bladder capacity; it is especially recommended for people experiencing urge UI or overactive bladder (refer to the section in this chapter on overactive bladder) (Denisenko et al., 2021; Monteiro et al., 2023). A voiding diary should be evaluated prior to recommending bladder training so that baseline patterns can be established and the most appropriate adjustments identified.

Providing patients with a container that fits into their toilet for urine collection to monitor the color and amount of output is a valuable tool. This guideline helps monitor both void intervals and output.

There is no definitive protocol for bladder training. General principles include gradually holding one's urine for longer and longer periods of time, resulting in more consistent voiding patterns with less urgency, incontinence, and higher void volumes. One protocol for patients was offered by Monteiro et al. (2023) and is described in **Box 23-8**.

Conversely, the clinician may notice from a patient's voiding diary that they are voiding infrequently, having large volume voids, and are complaining of urgency or UUI, as would be the case in detrusor underactivity. In this case, the patient might benefit from working on voiding more frequently in a timed manner, such as every hour or every two hours until a normal voiding pattern is achieved.

Pelvic Floor Muscle Therapy

Pelvic muscle exercises, commonly known as Kegel exercises, constitute a repetitive pelvic floor muscle contraction regimen. The goal is to increase muscle mass and strength. Kegel exercises offer rehabilitation for people whose muscles are weakened, but they are not appropriate if the muscles are torn. Individuals who are unable to achieve a voluntary pelvic muscle contraction due to striated muscle loss or who have pelvic organ prolapse below the hymenal ring will probably be unable to effectively perform Kegel exercises due to mechanical misalignment from the latter problem.

Assessment of a person's ability to contract the levator ani muscle must be completed prior to recommending any pelvic muscle exercise for UI. Such exercises are likely to be ineffective (and frustrating) if a person is unable to voluntarily contract their levator ani muscle—as in the instance of a a pubovisceral muscle tear. It is important to ascertain that the individual is not bearing down (a potential indicator of pubovisceral muscle tear) during their attempt to contract the pelvic floor muscles (Okeahialam et al., 2022).

A practitioner can coach patients to perform Kegel exercises by instructing them to quickly engage the muscles as if they are attempting to prevent the flow of urine and prevent the passage of flatus (incorporating both the urethral striated muscle and the levator ani). This should be done without the patient tightening the muscles of the thighs or buttocks (Okeahialam et al., 2022).

The "Knack" is a pelvic muscle contraction strategically timed to a moment of expected loss of urine, whether from urge or stress-type triggers. Awareness of the triggers and learned Knack coordination skill allows a person to volitionally increase their margin of continence (urethral pressure higher than bladder pressure) at any moment of need during their day-to-day activities (Miller et al., 2020; Okeahialam et al., 2022). A more complete understanding of the Knack skill's applications can be viewed by people in an animated form on the Regents of the University of Michigan website (https://myconfident-bladder.com/), which portrays the intervention tested in Miller et al. (2020).

There is no consensus for exactly how patients should practice kegel exercises for the improvement of UI. **Figure 23-5** shows just one recommended regimen in which the patient should aim to practice 8–12 maximum strength pelvic floor contractions 3 times daily. Basic contractions are held for 1–2 seconds with 1–2 seconds of rest in between. Once the patient is skilled at engaging the necessary muscles, they can assess their baseline sustained contraction by attempting to hold the contraction for as long as possible (up to 10 seconds.) Rest between contractions should mirror the length of the contraction. For example, holding contractions for 6 seconds and resting for 6 seconds. Patients can work towards longer sustained contractions with practice. They can also work towards performing them in different positions and during varied activities. They can ultimately begin practicing the "Knack" with each incidence of coughing or sneezing (Okeahialam et al., 2022).

There are a variety of physical devices people AFAB can use to improve continence, the most common being continence pessaries (Denisenko et al., 2021). Continence pessaries are devices that are worn intravaginally and are designed to increase an individual's urethral pressure by supporting the anterior vaginal wall on which the urethra rests. Pessaries come in many forms (refer to **Figure 23-6**). Fitting may require a number of visits to find the correct size and type. Most providers start with a ring pessary due to their ease of insertion (Ma et al., 2020;

FIGURE 23-5 **Example of recommended regimen for Kegel exercises.**

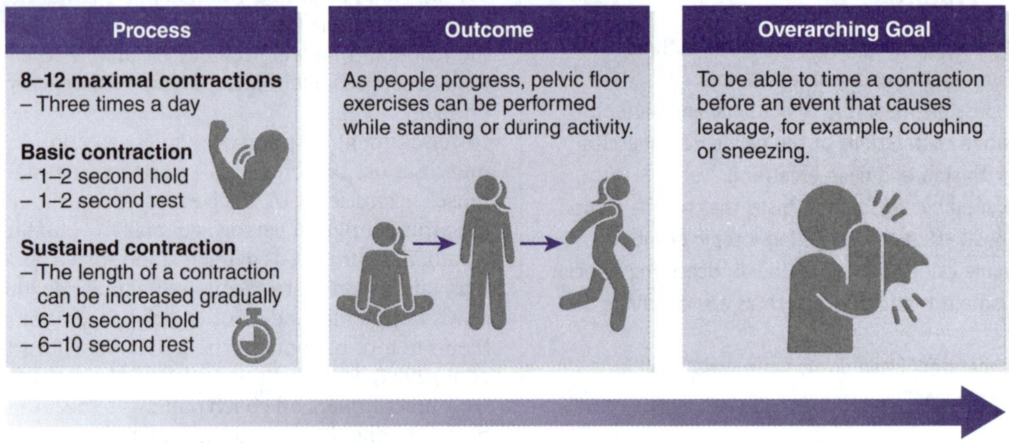

Data from Okeahialam, N.A, Oldfield, M, Stewart, E., Bonfield, C., Carboni, C. (2022). Pelvic floor muscle training: A practical guide. *British Medical Journal, 378,* e070186. https://doi.org/10.1136/bmj.e070186.

FIGURE 23-6 **Types of pessaries.**

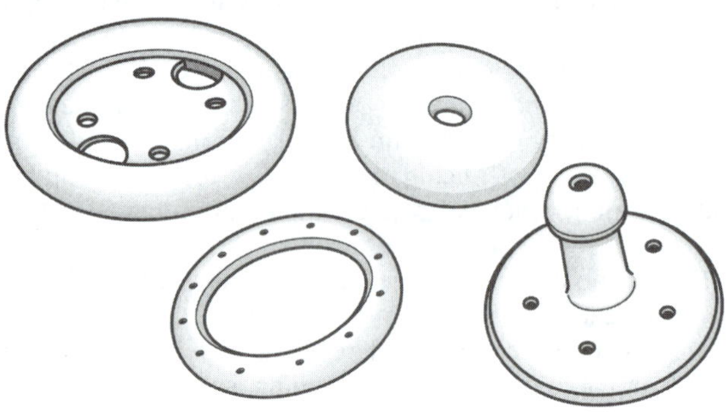

Xu et al., 2021). Once the pessary is in place, comfortable to the patient, and relieving symptoms adequately, it can stay in place for some time. In general, patients should remove their pessaries and wash them with soap and water (or return to the office to have this done for them) at least every 3 months (Trowbridge & Hoover, 2022). At least yearly, the provider should perform a speculum exam to check for vaginal erosion; if vaginal erosion occurs, the patient should stop using the pessary for at least 3 to 4 weeks. Vaginal estrogen cream can be prescribed to help heal the areas of erosion (Trowbridge & Hoover, 2022). A Cochrane Review found that when a continence pessary was used in conjunction with pelvic floor muscle training, there was greater improvement in symptoms (Todhunter-Brown et al., 2022).

Pharmacologic Treatment

Approved outpatient pharmacologic treatment for UI is limited to UUI; there are currently no medications approved for other types of UI (Trowbridge & Hoover, 2022). The major categories of medications include antimuscarinic (sometimes called anticholinergic) agents and β3-agonists. Antimuscarinic agents are considered first line for treatment of UUI. This includes oxybutynin (Ditropan) in various forms, including extended-release oral and patch products: tolterodine (Detrol), trospium (Santura), fesoterodine (Toviaz), darifenacin (Enablex), and solifenacin (Vesicare). These antimuscarinic drugs work by blocking the muscarinic receptors in the bladder which facilitate voiding by contracting the detrusor smooth muscle (Trowbridge & Hoover, 2022). Common side effects include dry mouth, dry/itchy eyes, constipation, blurred vision, palpitations, and impaired cognitive function in susceptible populations. Some drugs, like solifenacin and darifenacin, are urospecific, and therefore have less significant side effects (Fontaine et al., 2021). Extended-release formulations also have less side effects, especially dry mouth when compared to immediate release. Anticholinergics should not be prescribed to individuals with a previous sensitivity, narrow angle glaucoma, gastroparesis, or cognitive impairment. Recent studies have shown an increase in brain atrophy, dysfunction, and clinical decline (Fontaine et al., 2021; Trowbridge & Hoover, 2022).

β3-agonists target the storage phase by enhancing relaxation of the detrusor smooth muscle. β3-agonistsis have similar efficacy to anticholinergics but demonstrate a different side effect profile. For instance, mirabegron can cause headaches, nasopharyngitis, and elevated systolic blood pressure. Vibegron is the newest β3-agonist, and has fewer side effects but can cause an elevation in systolic blood pressure (Denisenko et al., 2021).

Tricyclic antidepressants (TCA), usually imipramine (Tofranil), and the selective serotonin and norepinephrine reuptake inhibitor (SSNRI) duloxetine (Cymbalta) have also been used on an off-label basis for urge-type UI but are not considered first-line pharmacologic agents for this indication (Trowbridge & Hoover, 2022).

Menopause can cause or exacerbate lower urinary tract symptoms including UI due to thinning of the vaginal and urethral tissues. Vaginal estrogen has been shown to be safe and effective in this population (Trowbridge & Hoover, 2022).

Surgical Treatment

If a patient suffers from UUI and conservative measures fail, they could be considered candidates for implantation of a sacral nerve stimulator or injection of botulinum toxin (Botox) into the bladder (Fontaine et al., 2021). Other forms of surgery are contraindicated for urge UI and can exacerbate urge symptoms that are related to detrusor instability.

A number of good surgical treatments for SUI are available when this condition is related to extrinsic sphincter deficiency or urethral hypermobility or both. Injection of bulking agents is used for urethral sphincter deficiency when SUI is primarily caused by poor urethral closure pressure and without hypermobility. There are two classes of bulking agents (solid microparticles in a liquid or gel carrier), and nonparticulate agents (homogenous gel). These medications are most commonly injected into the submucosa of the proximal urethra. Bulking agents are injected under local anesthesia by direct vision into the proximal urethra. This is an excellent option for patients who are not surgical candidates, or other agents failed. There is a high risk of treatment failure and multiple injections may be indicated to maintain symptom relief (Denisenko et al., 2021).

Surgical treatments for SUI also include several variations on surgical suspensions and slings. The aim of these procedures is to support and stabilize the urethra. Mid-urethral slings are generally considered the optimal technique (Chen et al., 2024; Denisenko et al., 2021; Kwon et al., 2021). The single incision sling is the least invasive of these procedures but offers a lower success rate than more invasive therapies. The tension-free vaginal tape sling procedure is also less invasive than other techniques and is typically performed on an outpatient basis. The tape can either be placed retropubically or through the obturator foramen (Chen et al., 2024). The retropubic approach is performed by inserting two needles through the retropubic space from the vagina to the abdomen or from the abdomen to the vagina. The success rate for this procedure is 51–81 percent. The transobturator approach was implemented in response to complications with the retropubic approach. During this procedure a sling is inserted into a horizontal plane underneath the middle of the urethra between the two obturator foramina. The success rate for this procedure is between 43–95 percent and patients have less urinary urgency, negative quality of life, and sexual dysfunction compared to the retropubic approach (Chen et al., 2024; Denisenko et al., 2021).

Adjustable slings are also available which enables the surgeon to make adjustments to the tension as needed (Kwon, et al., 2021). The autologous pubovaginal sling is another procedure that utilizes autologous fascia lata or rectus fascial tissue to recreate periurethral support. This is an excellent option for patients who had a previous mesh complication or failure, wish to avoid mesh, or are high-risk for poor wound healing. The success rate for this procedure is 85–92 percent (Chen et al., 2024; Denisenko et al., 2021).

More traditional surgeries, including urethral and bladder neck suspensions (Burch colposuspension, Stamey, Raz, and Gittes procedures) are also still performed (Kwon et al., 2021).

Complementary and Alternative Therapies

Many people use complementary and alternative therapies for UI, including biofeedback, acupuncture, yoga, Pilates, and tai chi. Data on the effectiveness of these interventions are scant at best.

Pelvic floor exercises have long been used and known to be effective for UI. More recently, some patients and therapists have been exploring the additional benefits of using additional modalities along with pelvic floor therapies including biofeedback, intravaginal electrostimulation, and weighted cones. Biofeedback uses an electronic machine to help people evaluate the effectiveness of their efforts, typically via a visual display. This adjunct therapy is used along with pelvic muscle exercise to facilitate skill development, particularly in the early stages of such treatment. Although studies demonstrate no statistically significant difference in reduction of urine leakage among groups undertaking pelvic muscle exercise with or without biofeedback, biofeedback may improve motivation in some (Alouini et al., 2022; Hagen et al., 2020; Todhunter-Brown et al., 2022). Similarly, other modalities to increase effectiveness of pelvic floor exercises have been studied including intravaginal electrostimulation and the use of weighted cones. These therapies do seem to show some clinical benefit, but it is inconclusive if they are any better than pelvic floor physical therapy alone (Stania et al., 2022; Burton et al., 2022). Therefore, these additions to pelvic floor training are not universally recommended but are still available for patients and clinicians who deem them appropriate. Acupuncture, including electro and laser acupuncture, has been investigated and found to have some clinical benefit for patients with UI (Kannon & Bello, 2023; Todhunter-Brown et al., 2022). Due to the vast differences in modalities and techniques used, more research should be done to further quantify the benefits. Acupuncture should always be performed by a skilled, licensed practitioner of Chinese medicine.

A meta-analysis conducted by Kannan et al. (2021) examined various mind–body techniques for the improvement of UI. tai chi, qigong, Pilates, yoga, and Paula exercises were included in the meta-analysis. Of these alternative modalities, only certain yoga poses showed a statistically significant improvement in symptoms. Even so, these studies were deemed low-quality evidence. Of note, no studies including AFAB individuals in the qigong and tai-chi intervention groups were identified. Given the relatively low cost and low risk of these interventions, improvement should be considered on a patient-by-patient basis and should not be discouraged if the patient reports improvement (Kannan et al., 2021).

When to Refer

Many individuals with UI will respond positively to behavioral instruction, pharmacologic treatments, or pessary use; some may be satisfied with education about UI, even if their symptoms persist. If management is ineffective, if it does not meet the individual's expectations for improvement, or if complicating factors are suspected, patients should be referred to a UI specialist or specialty clinic. If possible, referral to a urogynecologist or advanced practice nurse in urogynecology should be prioritized given these professionals' specialty training and practice. A listing of urogynecologists and continence nurse practitioners can be found on the American Urogynecologic Society website, Voices for PFD (n.d.) (http://www.voicesforpfd.org/p/cm/ld/fid=81).

Education about the various etiologies that underlie UI, and the full scope of treatment modalities is important in the evaluation of UI. Some people will choose an intervention because the results are more immediate and require less personal involvement;

others prefer to exhaust the full complement of behavioral approaches before considering pharmaceutical or surgical options. It is important to recognize UI as a nonspecific symptom of varying etiologies with different effects on individuals. Choice of treatment modalities must be made collaborating with the patient to determine their goals and the context of their symptom manifestation.

Patient Education

Educating patients regarding the basic anatomy and physiology of the urinary system can be helpful. Healthy bladder behaviors such as voiding patterns and fluid intake should be discussed. Most importantly, patients should be affirmed in their choice to seek care and that there are many potential treatment options, even if first line treatments do not work.

FUNCTIONAL DISORDERS OF THE URINARY TRACT

If lower urinary tract symptoms are present without any clear abnormality on genitourinary exam or urine studies, the clinician should consider the diagnosis of a functional urinary tract disorder such as overactive bladder (OAB), interstitial cystitis, which is sometimes called bladder pain syndrome (IC/BPS), or neurogenic bladder.

Interstitial Cystitis

Interstitial cystitis or bladder pain syndrome (IC/BPS) is a chronic condition hallmarked by urinary frequency and perceived bladder pain in the presence of a negative urine culture and no other defining pathology (Clemmens et al., 2022; Lim et al., 2024). If a patient's urinary symptoms last greater than 6 weeks, or a patient presents with multiple episodic complaints of a "urinary tract infection" for which the culture comes back negative, IC/BPS could be suspected once more serious pathology is considered and dismissed.

Scope

It has been estimated that 3.3 million AFAB individuals in the United States have been diagnosed with IC/BPS (Dobberfuhl, 2022). IC/BPS can be challenging to diagnose as many patients have no characteristic physical findings, and diagnosis is based on exclusion of other syndromes. This lack of physical evidence and reluctance of patients to discuss urinary symptoms for various reasons means this estimate likely does not capture the true number of those afflicted. Symptoms can significantly interfere with a patient's life; people diagnosed with IC/BPS report a lower quality of life with more pain, stress, sleep dysfunction, sexual dysfunction, and depression than their counterparts when matched for demographics (Hanno et al., 2022).

Pathophysiology

The etiology of IC/BPS is not yet fully understood and is likely multifactorial. The disease remains difficult to study due to the heterogenicity of symptoms and findings in those affected (Akiyama et al., 2020). Chronic inflammation is likely and has been attributed to many factors including immunological response, urothelial dysfunction, and urine cytotoxicity from either pharmaceuticals, bacteria, or changes in PH and osmolarity (Dobberfuhl, 2022; Lim et al., 2024). Notably, the glycosaminoglycan (GAG) layer of the endothelium is a thick mucus consistency comprised mainly of hyaluronic acid, chondroitin sulfate, heparin sulfate and keratin sulfate; it is the bladder's defense against toxins and irritants to the bladder wall, including urine (Ha & Xu, 2017; Sogutdelen & Citamak, 2022). It is likely that once an initial insult to this layer occurs and the urothelium is disrupted, afferent neurons in the bladder become upregulated and cause the central nervous system to dysregulate, resulting in an increased pain perception (Dobberfuhl, 2022).

It has been theorized that immune dysfunction plays a large role, and IC/BPS may in fact be an autoimmune disorder (Fallon et al., 2023; Dobberfuhl, 2022; Lim et al., 2024). Two distinct types of IC/BPS have been identified: IC/BPS with Hunner's Lesions (HIC) and IC/BPS without Hunner's Lesions (NHIC). A Hunner's Lesion (HL) is a small area of mucosal inflammation and ulceration found on cystoscopy (Clemens et al., 2022). Although both IC/BPS with and without HLs fall under the umbrella of IC/BPS, they are thought to have different pathophysiological etiologies. Urine, serum, and histological samples from these two groups of patients reveal distinct differences in the immunological cascade which occurs in patients with IC/BPS with and without HLs (Akiyama et al., 2020). Some experts argue for separation of the disorders for clearer diagnosis and treatment pathways (Akiyama et al., 2020; Fallon et al., 2023; Whitmore et al., 2019).

History

A thorough history should include a voiding/symptom journal, as well as the Interstitial Cystitis Symptoms Index (ICSI) or Interstitial Cystitis Problem Index (ICPI) (refer to **Figure 23-7**). Although neither of these tools are suggested to be used as diagnostic (Clemmens et al., 2022), they can be helpful in cataloging the relevant symptoms and can later be used as a symptom baseline when treatment follow-up occurs. High-frequency, low-volume voids and reports of painful urination or "bladder pain" in the absence of any other abnormal physical findings should suggest a diagnosis of IC/BPS (Clemmens et al., 2022). Although typically the complaint of pain is centered around the suprapubic and urethral area, patients can present with complaints of discomfort anywhere in the pelvis or external genitals and may describe this sensation in a variety of ways such as "pressure," or "burning" and may not use the word "pain." Patients may describe certain triggers, either dietary or activity based, that create a predictable pain response (Clemmens et al., 2022).

Urinary incontinence or gross hematuria are not typical patient complaints with IC/BPS and should warrant further investigation. The clinician should also consider risk factors for other diseases of the urinary system. For example, given the high rates of bladder cancer in smokers, a long smoking history should prompt the clinician to be more assertive in obtaining cystoscopy (Clemmens et al., 2022).

A sexual history is also relevant to see if a sexually transmitted infection (STI) such as gonorrhea, chlamydia, trichomoniasis, or even HSV should be included in the differential (refer to Chapter 22 for more information on STIs). There is research to suggest, as with most chronic pain syndromes, there is a link between IC and the patient's mental health. This is especially true in patients with a history of post-traumatic stress disorder and/or sexual trauma (Bendrick et al., 2022). Trauma-informed history taking is an essential skill for all clinicians (refer to Chapters 5 and 8 for more information on trauma-informed care).

Physical Exam

Relevant systems to examine include the gastrointestinal, neurological, psychological, and genitourinary systems, as well as a pelvic exam and assessment of the pelvic floor musculature

FIGURE 23-7 **Interstitial Cystitis Symptoms Index and the Interstitial Cystitis Problem Index.**

Interstitial Cystitis Symptoms Index (ICSI)	Interstitial Cystitis Problem Index (ICPI)
During the past month, how often have you felt the strong need to urinate with little or no warning? 0 __ Not at all 1 __ Less than 1 time in 5 2 __ Less than half the time 3 __ About half the time 4 __ More than half the time 5 __ Almost always	**During the past month, how much has each of the following been a problem for you?** **Frequent urination during the day.** 0 __ No problem 1 __ Very small problem 2 __ Small problem 3 __ Medium problem 4 __ Big problem
During the past month, have you had to urinate less than 2 hours after you finished urinating? 0 __ Not at all 1 __ Less than 1 time in 5 2 __ Less than half the time 3 __ About half the time 4 __ More than half the time 5 __ Almost always	**Getting up at night to urinate** 0 __ No problem 1 __ Very small problem 2 __ Small problem 3 __ Medium problem 4 __ Big problem
During the past month, how often did you most typically get up at night to urinate? 0 __ Not at all 1 __ Once per night 2 __ 2 times per night 3 __ 3 times per night 4 __ 4 times per night 5 __ 5 or more times per night	**Need to urinate with little warning** 0 __ No problem 1 __ Very small problem 2 __ Small problem 3 __ Medium problem 4 __ Big problem
During the past month, have you experienced pain or burning in your bladder? 0 __ Not at all 1 __ A few times 2 __ Fairly often 3 __ Usually 4 __ Almost always	**Burning, pain, discomfort, or pressure in your bladder** 0 __ No problem 1 __ Very small problem 2 __ Small problem 3 __ Medium problem 4 __ Big problem
Add the numerical values of the checked entries: ***TOTAL SCORE*** ________	*Add the numerical values of the checked entries:* ***TOTAL SCORE*** ________

Reproduced from Sirinian, E, Azevedo, K, Payne. C.K. (2005). Correlation between 2 interstitial cystitis symptom instruments. *Journal of Urology, 173,* 835–840.

(Lim et al., 2024). A post-void residual measurement, urinalysis, and urine culture should be obtained, along with tests for STIs if clinically relevant. The examiner should not find any abnormalities pointing toward other causes of pelvic pain, either in the physical exam or laboratory workup. Suprapubic or pelvic tenderness may or may not be elicited on exam (Lim et al., 2024).

Imaging

It is not necessary to obtain diagnostic imaging (such as CT or ultrasound) for a diagnosis of simple IC/BPS but it may be useful for ruling out other differentials or for identification of HLs (Clemens et al., 2022; Dobberfuhl, 2022; Whitmore et al., 2019). If diagnosis is in doubt, the patient is at high risk for bladder cancer, or there are findings suggestive of other pathology, imaging and cystoscopy (with or without biopsy) may be necessary.

Management

Patients need to be made aware that IC/BPS is a chronic condition that will likely require long-term and multimodal management. Initial management typically involves behavioral interventions such as bladder training, stress-management techniques, and avoidance of dietary triggers (Clemens et al., 2022; Lim et al., 2024). Given the high rate of PTSD and other psychological disorders in patients with IC/BPS, a referral for mental health services might be appropriate. Some patients with IC/BPS are found to have tight or tender musculature of the pelvic floor. In these patients, pelvic floor physical therapy has been shown to be effective but must be performed by a therapist specializing in pelvic floor disorders (Clemens et al., 2022). Cost and insurance coverage of physical therapy could be potential barriers and should be discussed with the patient.

Oral Medications

Pharmacologic management can involve a variety of medications used off-label, such as amitriptyline, cimetidine, cyclosporine A, methotrexate, azathioprine, and hydroxyzine. Currently, Pentosan polysulfate is currently the only drug on the market that is FDA approved for IC/BPS, but reports of efficacy are contradictory and it should be used with caution as it can cause long-term ocular complications (Clemens et al., 2022; Dobberfuhl, 2022; Lim et al., 2024). Cyclosporine A, azathioprine, and methotrexate are all immunosuppressants and should be used with extreme caution. Common dosing of these medications as well as relevant patient teaching can shown in **Table 23-6**.

Adjunct management for pain can include phenazopyridine, NSAIDS, gabapentin, or opioid pain medications as deemed appropriate by the provider. Opioid management is not typically required; however, in the event it is deemed necessary, patients should have a pain contract in place, be counseled regarding the addictive properties of opioids, and receive appropriate teaching on the use of naloxone (Clemens et al., 2022; Lim et al., 2024).

Monoclonal Antibodies

New research has found that certolizumab pegol, an anti-tumor necrosis factor alpha (anti TFA-*a)* can reduce symptoms of IC/BPS. Certolizumab pegol is approved for other autoimmune diseases, not specifically IC/BPS. However, studies show it can decrease bladder inflammation by interrupting mast-cell activation and therefore reduce symptoms of IC/BPS (Di et al., 2021).

Intravesical Instillations

A variety of therapies can be prepared and administered via an intravesical route. These types of medications are usually prescribed and administered by a urologist. They are typically done in the provider's office but can be administered at home if the patient has appropriate teaching and the ability to perform a self-catheterization. Many providers have their own "cocktail" which may involve two to four or more ingredients (Clemens et al., 2022; Jones et al., 2021). Intravesical therapies mostly fall into four categories: ingredients that help replace the GAG layer, analgesics, anti-inflammatories, anti-infectives, and compounds that aid the permeability of other ingredients. Some ingredients have more than one assumed mechanism of action and therefore could fit into multiple categories.

Dimethyl sulfoxide (DSMO) is the only drug approved for intravesical instillation for IC/BPS. Although its mechanism of action is not completely understood, it is believed to reduce inflammation by scavenging free radicals (Tomoe, 2023). Recent studies suggest it may only be effective in HIC. It should be used with caution with other agents as it can increase absorption of other substances, contributing to toxicity from other therapies (Clemens et al., 2022).

Intravesical lidocaine can be instilled for its analgesic effect. Alkalized lidocaine (AL) is typically more effective than non-alkalized lidocaine as it increases penetration into the epithelium and therefore is thought to improve efficacy; however, this can also increase the systemic absorption and chance of lidocaine toxicity (Clemens et al., 2022). Some providers use bupivacaine, a longer-acting lidocaine derivative (Lim et al., 2024).

Reinforcement of the GAG layer can be achieved via replacement of its main components—heparin, chondroitin sulfate, keratin sulfate, and hyaluronic acid. When studied as solo agents, none of these compounds have been shown to be of much benefit; however, when used in combination with one another, and/or AL, they can result in significant symptom relief for the patient (Ha & Xu, 2017).

TABLE 23-6 Oral Treatment Regimens for Interstitial Cystitis

Drug	Dose	Common Adverse Effects
Pentosan Polysulfate Sodium	100 mg PO TID	Nausea, diarrhea, headache, dyspepsia, abdominal pain, rash, edema. Maculopathy can occur (with long-term use). Recommend ophthalmic exam within 6 months of start and periodically.
Cyclosporine A	1.5–3 mg daily	Hypertension, dyslipidemia, edema, headache, paresthesia, hirsutism, hypertrichosis, renal toxicity, and susceptibility to infection.
Amitriptyline	Initiate 10 mg daily and titrate up to 50–100 mg daily as tolerated	Dry mouth, drowsiness, weight gain, dizziness, fatigue, constipation, orthostatic hypotension, QTc prolongation, and sexual dysfunction.
Cimetidine	300–400 mg BID	Dizziness, headache, and increased serum creatinine.
Hydroxyzine	25–75 mg as tolerated	Sedation, weakness, prolongation of QT interval, torsade de pointes, and acute generalized exanthematous pustulosis.
Methotrexate	7.5–12.5 mg weekly	Dizziness, alopecia, diarrhea, nausea, vomiting, thrombocytopenia, hepatotoxicity, severe bone marrow suppression, and aplastic anemia with concomitant NSAID use.
Azathioprine	50–100 mg daily	Malaise, nausea, vomiting, hepatotoxicity, and susceptibility to infection.

Data from Chen, P. Y., Lee, W. C., & Chuang, Y. C. (2021). Comparative safety review of current pharmacological treatments for interstitial cystitis/bladder pain syndrome. *Expert opinion on drug safety, 20*(9), 1049–1059. https://doi.org/10.1080/14740338.2021.1921733

Triamcinolone can be added for its anti-inflammatory properties and is especially useful in combination with DSMO. It is also recommended for patients in whom HLs have been identified (Lim et al., 2024).

Misoprostol can act as an anti-inflammatory and helps potentiate cyclosporine. While not currently a common treatment for IC/BPS, some studies have shown benefit (Lim et al., 2024).

Intravesical gentamycin has long been used to prevent urinary tract infections in patients who undergo frequent catheterization, especially when done in the home environment (Rutherford et al., 2024). No studies addressing its use in patients undergoing bladder installations for IC/BPS have been identified; however, its use can be seen in a variety of "cocktails" prescribed by urologists and is likely an appropriate addition (Lim et al., 2024).

Cystoscopy with short duration, low pressure hydrodistension is a technique used to rule out other pathology of the bladder and also allows the clinician to visualize HLs if present. Hydrodistension can also be therapeutic and has been shown to reduce clinical symptoms of IC/BPS (Clemens et al., 2022; Lim et al., 2024).

If HLs are observed during cystoscopy, the recommendation is for either immediate excision via fulguration with electrocautery, intra-lesion injections of triamcinolone, or both therapies in combination. This has been shown to improve symptoms significantly, although repeat treatments may be necessary in the future (Clemens et al., 2022). When these techniques are not successful, oral cyclosporine A may be considered. While this treatment has a high level of efficacy, it has significant side effects such as nephrotoxicity and immune suppression. For this reason, it should be used with extreme caution and only in patients with significant morbidity from their symptoms (Clemens et al., 2022; Dobberfuhl, 2022).

If the patient has failed pharmacotherapy (both oral and intravesical medications), then advanced therapeutic techniques may be necessary. Neuromodulation, typically via sacral nerve stimulation or posterior tibial nerve stimulation, has been effective in a number of patients; however, this technique is not approved by the FDA currently to treat pain, only for other LUTS such as frequency and urgency. Due to the constellation of symptoms typically present in IC/BPS, many patients could potentially meet criteria for neuromodulation, and many who have had it report improvement in the pain associated with IC/BPS. Even so, given the invasive nature of the therapy, it is only recommended after more conservative approaches have failed (Dobberfuhl, 2022; Padilla-Fernandez et al., 2022).

Botulism A detrusor (bladder wall) injections have been shown to decrease pain, inflammation, and the urge to frequently void. Urinary retention is a significant risk, so patients must be willing to self-catheterize. For this reason, although effective, botulism injections should only be considered in severe cases of IC/BPS where other therapies have failed. There is also a risk of urinary retention after botulinum toxin A bladder injections, which is why it is most useful in patients who can do intermittent self-catheterization if necessary (Clemens et al., 2022; Lim et al., 2024).

Surgery

If no other therapies have been effective and the patient is still having significant, quality-of-life affecting symptoms, a urologist might consider substitution cystoplasty or urinary diversion with or without cystectomy (Clemens et al., 2022; Dobberfuhl, 2022). This is, of course, a major surgery and should only be done by a specialist after significant counseling.

Referral

A urology or urogynecology referral should be considered if the diagnosis is unclear, cystoscopy (or other advanced therapy) is needed, or per patient preference. Referral is not typically warranted in cases of simple IC/BPS where treatment only includes lifestyle management and oral medications.

Overactive Bladder Syndrome

Although overactive bladder (OAB) shares significant symptom overlap with other urinary conditions, it is distinct as it is a nonstructural, non-infectious syndrome in which the patient experiences urinary urgency and frequency symptoms without chronic pain (which is indicative of IC/BPS) and may or may not result in urine leakage (which is consistent with UUI) (Dobberfuhl, 2022; Fontaine et al., 2021).

Scope

It is estimated that almost 30 million adults in America suffer from OAB (Dobberfuhl, 2022). The economic burden is estimated to be $26 billion annually (Fontaine et al., 2021). Patients describe their symptoms as very distressing and negatively impacting their lives (Torosis et al., 2023). Risk factors for OAB include obesity, advancing age, bladder outlet obstruction, and history of psychological stress or trauma (Torosis et al., 2023).

Pathophysiology

Like IC/PBS, the pathophysiology of OAB is unclear. Many etiologies have been suggested including: (1) dysfunction of the musculature of the pelvic floor; (2) central or peripheral neurogenic bladder dysfunction causing neurological hypersensitivity to stimuli; (3) bladder ischemia; and (4) excess ATP release from the bladder epithelium with bladder filling, creating chemical signaling informing the need to void (Chess-Williams & Sellers, 2023). Since UUI can sometimes be associated with OAB, it has been hypothesized for some time that UUI is a more severe form of OAB. In this classification, patients could be described as having OAB-dry or OAB-wet (UUI) subtypes. However, it is important to note that OAB patients without UI report their symptoms to be just as distressing as those with UI (Torosis et al., 2023). Furthermore, despite significant symptom overlap, OAB-dry patients describe symptoms that are more consistent with pelvic floor dysfunction and not consistent with UUI (such as feeling incomplete emptying, dribbling, or difficulty starting urination). For these reasons, it may be prudent to separate OAB and UUI as distinct but sometimes overlapping diagnoses.

History and Examination

As with other urinary conditions, the history should start with a review of a voiding/symptom diary. Urinary frequency and urgency with or without nocturia or urge incontinence could all indicate OAB (Fontaine et al., 2021). Some patients with OAB also complain of the feeling of incomplete voiding, difficulty starting stream of urine, and/or dribbling (Torosis et al., 2023). Pain should not be a predominant symptom. Physical examination and laboratory testing would be similar to other urinary conditions as the initial aim would be to rule out other pathology of the genitourinary system. Imaging and cystoscopy are generally not necessary (Fontaine et al., 2021). The diagnosis of OAB is generally made by symptomatology and exclusion of other etiologies.

TABLE 23-7 Oral Therapies for OAB

Drug	Dose	Uroselective?	Potential Adverse Events
Oxybutinin	5–15 mg PO once daily	No	Dry mouth, constipation
Oxybutinin	3.9 mg transdermal twice weekly	No	Dry mouth, constipation, redness at application site
Solifenacin	5–10 mg PO once daily	Yes	Dry mouth, constipation, blurred vision
Darifenacin	7.5–15 mg PO once daily	Yes	Dry mouth, constipation
Tolterodine	2 mg PO twice daily	No	Dry mouth, constipation, dry eyes
Trospium	20 mg PO twice daily	No	Dry mouth, constipation, abdominal pain
Fesoterdine	4–8 mg once daily	No	Dry mouth, constipation
Mirabegron	20–25 mg PO once daily	N/A	Hypertension

Reproduced from Fontaine, C., Papworth, E., Pascoe, J., & Hashim, H. (2021). Update on the management of overactive bladder. *Therapeutic Advances in Urology*, 13. https://doi.org/10.1177/17562872211039034

Treatments

Therapies can be consistent with others already mentioned for other urinary conditions. Bladder training, limiting fluid intake, avoidance of symptom triggers (including diuretics), and stress management are usually first steps in management (Fontaine et al., 2021).

If conservative management is not providing adequate symptom relief, there are multiple medications available, most of them being antimuscarinic agents (Fontaine et al., 2021). All of these agents can cross the blood–brain barrier and risk contributing to delirium and falls in older patients. Uroselective antimuscarinic agents have a slightly lower chance of systemic side effects and might therefore be safer in certain populations (Fontaine et al., 2021). Beta-agonists can also be used; although several beta-agonists are undergoing trials for OAB, mirabegron is the only one currently approved for this purpose (Fontaine et al., 2021). **Table 23-7** describes common therapies for OAB.

Referral

If conservative therapies fail, referral to a urologist is prudent for consideration of more advanced therapies. As with IC/BPS, intradetrusor injections of botulism a, sacral nerve stimulation, and posterior tibial nerve stimulation have all shown some promise in OAB for patients with significant symptoms who have failed lifestyle modification and pharmacologic therapy, but these therapies are not universally recommended (Fontaine et al., 2021).

Surgical options include augmentation cystoplasty, a technique where surgery is performed to increase the filling capacity of the bladder, and as a final resort, total urinary diversion; risks and benefits of any surgical procedure should be thoroughly reviewed with the performing surgeon (Fontaine et al., 2021).

Neurogenic Bladder

Patients may present with lower urinary tract symptoms stemming from underlying neurological disorders. The range of symptoms experienced will differ based on the underlying disease process (Atiemo & Stoffel, 2024).

Scope

Given the range of pathology that can contribute to neurogenic bladder and the range of symptoms, it is difficult to determine how many people are affected, and even harder to generalize their level of distress (Atiemo & Stoffel, 2024).

Pathophysiology

Any disease process which disrupts the neurological signaling between the brain and bladder can cause neurogenic bladder. The location of the breakdown in signaling will dictate what the resulting symptoms are. Etiologies stemming from the brain and subsacral spinal cord can result in a complete inability to control voiding. Pathology of the lower lumbar region and peripheral nerves result in a different presentation of symptoms, typically difficulty voiding, dribbling of urine, and incomplete emptying which can sometimes result in overflow incontinence. Some syndromes, like muscular sclerosis, can have both types of symptoms (Atiemo & Stoffel, 2024).

History and Examination

A patient may present with urinary symptoms or present for a neurologic complaint. Review of systems should probe the systems not included in the chief complaint and could include gastrointestinal, genitourinary, neurologic, and musculoskeletal systems as well as a brief psychological assessment. Depending on the disease state, the patient may complain of abrupt onset (stroke, spine injury) or gradual (cauda equina syndrome, MS) symptom onset. Any combination of acute and significant neurologic and urinary symptoms should prompt the provider to elevate the level of care, usually to the emergency department. Even some gradual onset disease processes can necessitate an emergency room visit, such as cauda equina syndrome. Examination should probe the same systems and also include lab studies screening for urinary abnormalities (urinalysis, PVR) as well as necessary screening tests for the suspected underlying disorder. **Table 23-8** describes the variety of symptoms, clinical presentation, and management options.

Treatment

Patients with NB can be characterized as low risk, unknown risk, and high risk. By "risk" in this context, we mean the chance of their condition resulting in further urologic complications like loss of renal function. This is separate from the prognosis of their causative disease process, which should be managed by

TABLE 23-8 Urinary Signs and Symptoms with Management Options of Common Neurologic Conditions

Neurologic Disease/Injury	Urodynamic Pattern	Clinical Presentation	Risk Stratification for Urologic Complications	Management Option
Supraportine: CVA, brain tumor, dementia	Synergic voiding, neurogenic detrusor overactivity, normal bladder compliance	Urinary incontinence	Low risk	Antimuscarinic/Beta-3 agonist Refer for urodynamic evaluation for persistent symptoms
Suprasacral: MS, spinal cord injury	Synergic/dyssynergic neurogenic detrusor overactivity, normal bladder compliance	Urinary incontinence, urinary retention, poor bladder compliance, and autonomic dysreflexia	Indeterminant/high risk	Refer for urodynamic evaluation with expectant management
Sacral/lower lumbar: Tethered cord, lumbar injury	Chronic nonrelaxing to fixed sphincter, detrusor areflexia, neurogenic detrusor overactivity, normal to reduced bladder compliance	Urine retention and recurrent UTI	Low risk	Intermittent catheterization, suprapubic catheter drainage
Diabetes	Detrusor areflexia, neurogenic detrusor overactivity, impaired bladder contractility, normal bladder compliance, and synergic voiding	Poor bladder sensation, urinary retention, and urinary incontinence	Low risk	Check PVR prior to expectant management

Reproduced from Atiemo, H. O., & Stoffel, J. T. (2024). A primer for primary care physicians managing neurogenic bladder patients. *The Urologic Clinics of North America, 51*(2), 305–311. https://doi.org/10.1016/j.ucl.2024.02.003

their neurology team. Management can include treating the underlying neurological disease (if possible), treating the urinary symptoms, or initiating self-catheterization if necessary. Often, neurogenic bladder requires careful coordination between the primary care provider, urology, and neurology.

Patient Education

The clinician should work closely with the patient to ensure that they understand the likely chronic nature of their symptoms and work to find toileting strategies that fit in with their daily lives. Support groups could be beneficial, especially if prognosis is poor.

CONCLUSION

Urinary conditions are common complaints encountered in clinical practice and result in significant burden to patients. Lower urinary tract symptoms can be acute or chronic in nature, and can be explained by a myriad of etiologies, including infectious, structural, neurological, and/or inflammatory. Differentiation of these distinct conditions, as well as appropriate history taking, examination, and treatment are essential skills for providers working in both primary care and gynecologic settings.

References

Aggarwal, N., & Leslie, S.W. (2025). Recurrent urinary tract infections. In *StatPearls*. StatPearls Publishing.

Akiyama, Y., Luo, Y., Hanno, P. M., Maeda, D., & Homma, Y. (2020). Interstitial cystitis/bladder pain syndrome: The evolving landscape, animal models and future perspectives. *International Journal of Urology: Official Journal of the Japanese Urological Association, 27*(6), 491–503. https://doi.org/10.1111/iju.14229

Ala-Jaakkola, R., Laitila, A., Ouwehand, A. C., & Lehtoranta, L. (2022). Role of D-mannose in urinary tract infections—A narrative review. *Nutrition Journal, 21*(1), 18. https://doi.org/10.1186/s12937-022-00769-x

Alouini, S., Memic, S., & Couillandre, A. (2022). Pelvic floor muscle training for urinary incontinence with or without biofeedback or electrostimulation in women: A systematic review. *International Journal of Environmental Research and Public Health, 19*(5), 2789. https://doi.org/10.3390/ijerph19052789

American Urogynecologic Society (Information for Women). (n.d.). http://www.augs.org or http://www.voicesforpfd.org

Anger, J., Lee, U., Ackerman, A. L., Chou, R., Chughtai, B., Clemens, J.Q., Hickling, D., Kapoor, A., Kenton, K.S., Kaufman, M., Rondanina, M.A., Stapleton, A., Stothers, L., Chai, T.C. (2019). Recurrent uncomplicated urinary tract infection in women: AUA/CUA/SUFU guideline. *The Journal of Urology, 202*, 282-289. https://doi.org/10.1097/JU.0000000000000296

Ansaldi, Y., & Martinez de Tejada Weber, B. (2023). Urinary tract infections in pregnancy. *Clinical Microbiology and Infection, 29*(10), 1249–1252. https://doi.org/10.1016/j.cmi.2022.08.015

Atiemo, H. O., & Stoffel, J. T. (2024). A primer for primary care physicians managing neurogenic bladder patients. *Urologic Clinics of North America, 51*(2), 305–311. https://doi.org/10.1016/j.ucl.2024.02.003. Epub 2024 Mar 12. PMID: 38609202

Barea, B. M., Veeratterapillay, R., & Harding, C. (2020). Nonantibiotic treatments for urinary cystitis: An update. *Current Opinion in Urology 30*(6), 845–852. https://doi.org/10.1097/MOU.0000000000000821

Batmani, S., Jalali, R., Mohammadi, M., & Bokaee, S. (2021). Prevalence and factors related to urinary incontinence in older adult women worldwide: A comprehensive systematic review and meta-analysis of observational studies. *BMC Geriatrics, 21*(1), 212. https://doi.org/10.1186/s12877-021-02135-8

Bendrick T. R., Sitenga G. L., Booth C., Sacco M. P., Erie C., Anderson D. J., Kaye A. D., & Urits, I. (2022). The implications of mental health and trauma in interstitial cystitis. *Health Psychology Research, 10*(4), 40321. https://doi.org/10.52965/001c.40321. PMID: 36425233; PMCID: PMC9680853.

Bilsen, M. P., Jongeneel, R. M. H., Schneeberger, C., Platteel, T. N., van Nieuwkoop, C., Mody, L., Caterino, J. M., Geerlings, S. E., Köves, B., Wagenlehner, F., Conroy, S. P., Visser, L. G., & Lambregts, M. M. C. (2023). Definitions of Urinary Tract Infection in Current Research: A Systematic Review. *Open forum infectious diseases, 10*(7), ofad332. https://doi.org/10.1093/ofid/ofad332

Bono, M. J., & Leslie, S. W. (2025). Uncomplicated urinary tract infections. In *StatPearls*. StatPearls Publishing.

Breinbjerg, A., Jørgensen, C. S., Borg, B., Rittig, S., Kamperis, K., & Christensen, J. H. (2023). The genetics of incontinence: A scoping review. *Clinical Genetics, 104*(1), 22–62.

Burton, C. S., Korsandi, S., & Enemchukwu, E. (2022). Current State of non-surgical devices for female stress urinary incontinence. *Current Urology Reports, 23*(9), 185–194. https://doi.org/10.1007/s11934-022-01104-x

Cai, T. (2021). Recurrent uncomplicated urinary tract infections: Definitions and risk factors. *GMS Infectious Diseases, 9,* Doc03. https://doi.org/10.3205/id000072

CDC. (2024a, January 22). *Urinary tract infection basics*. Cdc.gov/uti/about/index.html

CDC. (2024b, March 13). *Urine culture stewardship in patients without indwelling urinary catheters*. Cdc.gov/uti/hcp/clinical-guidance/culture-stewardship-without-catheter.htm

Chambers, L. M., Herrmann, A., Michener, C. M., Ferrando, C. A., & Ricci, S. (2020). Vaginal estrogen use for genitourinary symptoms in women with a history of uterine, cervical, or ovarian carcinoma. *International Journal of Gynecological Cancer: Official Journal of the International Gynecological Cancer Society, 30*(4), 515–524. https://doi.org/10.1136/ijgc-2019-001034

Chen, Y., Zhang, C., Yang, S., Chen, J., Peng, L., Chen, J., Shen, H., & Luo, D. (2024). Long-term outcomes of surgical interventions for stress urinary incontinence: A systematic review and network meta-analysis. *International Journal of Surgery (London, England), 110*(1), 520–528. https://doi.org/10.1097/JS9.0000000000000828

Chess-Williams, R., & Sellers, D. J. (2023). Pathophysiological mechanisms involved in overactive bladder/detrusor overactivity. *Current Bladder Dysfunction Reports, 18*(2), 79–88.

Choi, J. M., Jiang, J., Chang, J., Ziogas, A., Jiang, L., & Anton-Culver, H. (2022). Impact of lifetime obesity on urinary incontinence in the Women's Health Initiative. *The Journal of Urology, 207*(5), 1096–1104. https://doi.org/10.1097/JU.0000000000002380

Clemens, J. Q., Erickson, D. R., Varela, N. P., & Lai, H. H. (2022). Diagnosis and treatment of interstitial cystitis/bladder pain syndrome. *Journal of Urology, 208*(1), 34–42. https://doi.org/10.1097/ju.0000000000002756

Colgan, R., Jaffe, G. A., & Nicolle, L. E. (2020). Asymptomatic bacteriuria. *American Family Physician 102*(2), 99–104.

Cooper, T. E., Teng, C., Howell, M., Teixeira-Pinto, A., Jaure, A., & Wong, G. (2022). D-mannose for preventing and treating urinary tract infection. *Cochrane Database of Systematic Reviews 8*(8). https://doi.org/10.1002/14651858.CD013608.pub2

Czajkowski, K., Broś-Konopielko, M., & Teliga-Czajkowska, J. (2021). Urinary tract infection in women. *Menopause Review, 20*(1), 40–47. https://doi.org/10.5114/pm.2021.105382

Denisenko, A. A., Clark, C. B., D'Amico, M., & Murphy, A. M. (2021). Evaluation and management of female urinary incontinence. *The Canadian Journal of Urology, 28*(S2), 27–32.

Di, X. P., Luo, D. Y., Jin, X., Zhao, W. Y., Li, H., & Wang, K. J. (2021). Efficacy and safety comparison of pharmacotherapies for interstitial cystitis and bladder pain syndrome: A systematic review and Bayesian network meta-analysis. *International Urogynecology Journal, 32*, 1129–1141.

Dobberfuhl, A. D. (2022). Pathophysiology, assessment, and treatment of overactive bladder symptoms in patients with interstitial cystitis/bladder pain syndrome. *Neurourology and Urodynamics, 41*(8), 1958–1966. https://doi.org/10.1002/nau.2495

Dökmeci, F., & Rizk, D. E. E. (2022). *Insights into incontinence and the pelvic floor*. In Springer eBooks. https://doi.org/10.1007/978-3-030-94174-1

Eastham, J. H., & Patel, P. (2023). Phenazopyridine. In *StatPearls*. StatPearls Publishing.

Fallon, J., Tabansky Stern, I., Laurent, M., Birder, L., Moldwin, R. M., Stern, J. N. H. (2023). The immune system in interstitial cystitis/bladder pain syndrome and therapeutic agents, *Continence, 8*. 2772-9737, https://doi.org/10.1016/j.cont.2023.101057.

Fontaine, C., Papworth, E., Pascoe, J., & Hashim, H. (2021). Update on the management of overactive bladder. *Therapeutic Advances in Urology, 13*. https://doi.org/10.1177/17562872211039034

Gibbins, K. J., Abel, D. E., Carletti, A. A., Morrison, T., Sullivan, E. L., & Marshall, N. E. (2023). Weight bias in obstetrics. *Current Obstetrics and Gynecology Reports, 12*(1), 8–16. https://doi.org/10.1007/s13669-023-00348-9

Ha, B., Yanek, L. R., Harrington, B. J., Blomquist, J. L., Chen, C. C. G., Patterson, D., & Handa, V. L. (2025). Purported bladder irritant intake in women with urgency urinary incontinence. *Urogynecology, 31*(4), 352–360.

Ha, T., & Xu, J. H. (2017). Interstitial cystitis intravesical therapy. *Translational Andrology and Urology, 6*(S2). https://doi.org/10.21037/tau.2017.06.18

Habak, P. J., Carlson, K., & Griggs, Jr., R. P. (2024). Urinary tract infection in pregnancy. In *StatPearls*. StatPearls Publishing.

Hagen, S., Elders, A., Stratton, S., Sergenson, N., Bugge, C., Dean, S., Hay-Smith, J., Kilonzo, M., Dimitrova, M., Abdel-Fattah, M., Agur, W., Booth, J., Glazener, C., Guerrero, K., McDonald, A., Norrie, J., Williams, L. R., & McClurg, D. (2020). Effectiveness of pelvic floor muscle training with and without electromyographic biofeedback for urinary incontinence in women: Multicentre randomised controlled trial. *BMJ (Clinical research ed.), 371,* m3719. https://doi.org/10.1136/bmj.m3719

Handa, V. L., Roem, J., Blomquist, J. L., Dietz, H. P., & Muñoz, A. (2019). Pelvic organ prolapse as a function of levator ani avulsion, hiatus size, and strength. *American Journal of Obstetrics and Gynecology, 221*(1), 41.e1–41.e7. https://doi.org/10.1016/j.ajog.2019.03.004

Hanno P. M., Burks, D. A., Clemens, J. Q., Dmochowski, R. R., Erickson, D., FitzGerald, M. P., et al. (2011, updated in 2022). AUA Guideline for the diagnosis and treatment of interstitial cystitis/bladder pain syndrome. *Journal of Urology* https://www.auanet.org/documents/Guidelines/PDF/ICBPS%20Guideline.pdf

Hartigan, S. M., Reynolds, W. S., & Dmochowski, R. R. (2019). Detrusor underactivity in women: A current understanding. *Neurourology and Urodynamics, 38*(8), 2070–2076.

Herness, J., Buttolph, A., & Hammer, N. C. (2020). Acute pyelonephritis in adults: Rapid evidence review. *American Family Physician 102*(3), 173–180.

Hu, J. S., & Pierre, E. F. (2019). Urinary incontinence in women: Evaluation and management. *American Family Physician, 100*(6), 339–348.

Jagtap, S., Harikumar, S., Vinayagamoorthy, V., Mukhopadhyay, S., & Dongre, A. (2022). Comprehensive assessment of holding urine as a behavioral risk factor for UTI in women and reasons for delayed voiding. *BMC Infectious Diseases, 221*(1), 521. https://doi.org/10.1186/s12879-022-07501-4

Jent, P., Berger, J., Kuhn, A., Trautner, B. W., Atkinson, A., & Marschall, J. (2022). Antibiotics for Preventing Recurrent Urinary Tract Infection: Systematic Review and Meta-analysis. Open forum infectious diseases, 9(7), ofac327. https://doi.org/10.1093/ofid/ofac327

Johnson, T. M., 2nd, & Vaughan, C. P. (2019). Urological function and dysfunction in aging: Diagnosis and treatment. *Handbook of Clinical Neurology, 167*, 495–509. https://doi.org/10.1016/B978-0-12-804766-8.00027-3

Jones, P., Hjelle, K. M., Mohn, J., Gija Guðbrandsdottir, G., Roth, I., Asghar Chaudhry, A., Anne Kvåle Bergesen, A., & Beisland, C. (2021). Current status of intravesical therapies for bladder pain syndrome (BPS): A narrative review of emerging evidence. *Urology, 156,* e48–e57. ISSN 0090-4295. https://doi.org/10.1016/j.urology.2021.05.042.

Kannan, P., & Bello, U. M. (2023). Efficacy of various forms of acupuncture for the treatment of urinary incontinence in women: A systematic review and meta-analysis. *Explore (New York, N.Y.), 19*(1), 26–35. https://doi-org.10.1016/j.explore.2022.07.004

Kannan, P., Sy, S. L., & Boghra, S. (2021). Efficacy of mind-body therapies for the treatment of urinary incontinence in women: A systematic review and meta-analysis of randomized controlled trials. *Austin Journal of Women's Health, 8*(2), 1050.

Kawahara, T., Ito, H., Yao, M., & Uemura, H. (2020). Impact of smoking habit on overactive bladder symptoms and incontinence in women. *International Journal of Urology, 27*(12), 1078–1086.

Kenneally, C., Murphy, C. P., Sleator, R. D., & Culligan, E. P. (2022). The urinary microbiome and biological therapeutics: Novel therapies for urinary tract infections. *Microbiological Research, 259*, 127010. https://doi.org/10.1016/j.micres.2022.127010

Kolman, K. B. (2019). Cystitis and pyelonephritis: Diagnosis, treatment, and prevention. *Primary Care, 46*(2), 191–202. https://doi.org/10.1016/j.pop.2019.01.001

Kwok, M., McGeorge, S., Mayer-Coverdale, J., Graves, B., Paterson, D. L., Harris, P. N. A., Esler, R., Dowling, C., Britton, S., & Roberts, M. J. (2022). Guideline of guidelines: Management of recurrent urinary tract infections in women. *BJU International, 130* (Suppl 3), 11–22. https://doi.org/10.1111/bju.15756

Kwon, J., Kim, Y., & Kim, D. Y. (2021). Second-line surgical management after midurethral sling failure. *International Neurourology Journal, 25*(2), 111–118. https://doi.org/10.5213/inj.2040278.139

Lacy, M. E., Sidhu, N., & Miller, J. (2019). When does acute pyelonephritis require imaging? *Cleveland Clinic Journal of Medicine, 86*(8), 515–517. https://doi.org/10.3949/ccjm.86a.18096

Lala, V., Leslie, S. W., & Minter, D. A. (2023). Acute cystis. In *StatPearls*. StatPearls Publishing.

Lamerton, T. J., Mielke, G. I., & Brown, W. J. (2021). Urinary incontinence, body mass index, and physical activity in young women. *American Journal of Obstetrics and Gynecology, 225*(2), 164-e1.

Lavalle, L. L. F., Hermosa, P. C., Balanza, C. V., Cidre, M. J., Baños, J. L. G., Viegas, V., . . . & Guzmán, S. A. (2023). Bladder capacity in women with overactive bladder syndrome: A cross-sectional study. *Urology, 179,* 44–49.

Li, J. M., Cosler, L. E., Harausz, E. P., Myers, C. E., & Kufel, W. D. (2024). Methenamine for urinary tract infection prophylaxis: A systematic review. *Pharmacotherapy, 44*(2), 197–206. https://doi.org/10.1002/phar.2895

Lian, W. Q., Li, F. J., Huang, H. X., Zheng, Y. Q., & Chen, L. H. (2019). Constipation and risk of urinary incontinence in women: A meta-analysis. *International Urogynecology Journal, 30*, 1629–1634.

Lin, S., Atan, I. K., Dietz, H. P., Herbison, P., & Wilson, P. D. (2019). Delivery mode, levator avulson and obstetric anal sphincter injury: A cross sectional study 20 years after childbirth. *ANZJOG, 59*(4), 590, 596. https://doi.org/10.1111/ajo.12948

Lim Y., Leslie S. W., & O'Rourke S. (2024). Interstitial cystitis/bladder pain syndrome. In *StatPearls*. StatPearls Publishing. https://www.ncbi.nlm.nih.gov/books/NBK570588/

Ma, C., Xu, T., Kang, J., Zhang, Y., Ma, Y., Liang, S., & Zhu, L. (2020). Factors associated with pessary fitting in women with symptomatic pelvic organ prolapse: A large prospective cohort study. *Neurourology and Urodynamics, 39*(8), 2238–2245.

Makajeva, J., Watters, C., & Safioleas, P. (2022). Cystocele. In *StatPearls*. StatPearls Publishing.

McVicker, L., Labeit, A. M., Coupland, C. A. C., Hicks, B., Hughes, C., McMenamin, Ú., McIntosh, S. A., Murchie, P., & Cardwell, C. R. (2024). Vaginal estrogen therapy use and survival in females with breast cancer. *JAMA Oncology, 10*(1), 103–108. https://doi.org/10.1001/jamaoncol.2023.4508

Miller, J. M., Hawthorne, K. M., Park, L., Tolbert, M., Bies, K., Garcia, C., Misiunas, R., Newhouse, W., & Smith, A. R. (2020). Self-perceived improvement in bladder health after viewing a novel tutorial on Knack use: A randomized controlled trial pilot study. *Journal of Women's Health (Larchmt), 29*(10), 1319-1327. https://doi.org/10.1089/jwh.2018.7606

Miller, J. M., Hood, M. M., Karvonen-Gutierrez, C. A., Richards-McCullough, K. C., & Harlow, S. D. (2021). Paper towel test as independently self-administered to quantify cough-related urine loss: Compliance and comparisons with survey-only data in SWAN. *Neurourology and Urodynamics, 40*(5), 1207–1216.

Milsom, I., & Gyhagen, M. (2018). The prevalence of urinary incontinence. *Climacteric, 22*(3), 217–222. https://doi.org/10.1080/13697137.2018.1543263

Mititelu, M., Olteanu, G., Neacsu, S. M., Stoicescu, I., Dumitrescu, D. E., Gheorghe, E., Tarcea, M., Busnatu, S. S., Ionita-Mindrican, C. B., Tafuni, O., Belu, I., Popescu, A., Lupo, S., & Lup, C. E. (2024). Incidence of urinary tract infections and behavioral risk factors. *Nutrients, 16*(3), 446. https://doi.org/10.3390/nu16030446

Mitrani-Gold, F. S., Raychaudhuri, A., & Rao, S. (2020). Systematic review and meta-analysis to estimate the antibacterial treatment effect of nitrofurantoin for a non-inferiority trial in uncomplicated urinary tract infection. *Journal of Global Antimicrobial Resistance 22*, 68–77. https://doi.org/10.1016/j.jgar.2020.01.027

Monteiro, S., Rocha, A. K., Valim, L., Silva, S. L. A. D., Riccetto, C., & Botelho, S. (2023). Bladder training compared to bladder training associated with pelvic floor muscle training for overactive bladder symptoms in women: A randomized clinical trial. *Neurourology and Urodynamics, 42*(8), 1802–1811.

Moossdorff-Steinhauser, H. F. A., Berghmans, B. C. M., Spaanderman, M. E. A., & Bols, E. M. J. (2021). Prevalence, incidence and bothersomeness of urinary incontinence in pregnancy: A systematic review and meta-analysis. *International Urogynecology Journal, 32*(7), 1633–1652. https://doi.org/10.1007/s00192-020-04636-3

NAFC. (2025). *Urinary tract infections: causes, symptoms, and treatments*. nafc.org/urinary-tract-infection

Neugent, M. L., Hulyalkar, N. V., Nguyen, V. H., Zimmern, P .E., & De Nisco, N. J. (2020). Advances in understanding the human urinary microbiome and its potential role in urinary tract infection. *mBio, 11*(2). doi:10.1128/mBio.00218020

Okeahialam, N. A., Oldfield, M., Stewart, E., Bonfield, C., & Carboni, C. (2022). Pelvic floor muscle training: a practical guide. *bmj, 378*. doi:10.1136/bmj-2022-070186

Padilla-Fernández B., Hernández-Hernández D., & Castro-Díaz D.M. (2022). Current role of neuromodulation in bladder pain syndrome/interstitial cystitis. *Therapeutic Advances in Urology, 21*(14). https://doi.org/10.1177/17562872221135941

Perrier, E. T., Armstrong, L. E., Bottin, J. H., Clark, W. F., Dolci, A., Guelinckx, I., Iroz, A., Kavouras, S. A., Lang, F., Lieberman, H. R., Melander, O., Morin, C., Seksek, I., Stookey, J. D., Tack, I., Vanhaecke, T., Vecchio, M., & Péronnet, F. (2021). Hydration for health hypothesis: A narrative review of supporting evidence. *European Journal of Nutrition, 60*(3), 1167–1180. https://doi.org/10.1007/s00394-020-02296-z https://doi.org/10.1067/mob.2002.121089

Pierce, H., Perry, L., Gallagher, R., & Chiarelli, P. (2019a). Culture, teams, and organizations: A qualitative exploration of female nurses' and midwives' experiences of urinary symptoms at work. *Journal of Advanced Nursing, 75*(6), 1284–1295. https://doi.org/10.1111/jan.13951

Pierce, H. M., Perry, L., Gallagher, R., & Chiarelli, P. (2019b). Delaying voiding, limiting fluids, urinary symptoms, and work productivity: A survey of female nurses and midwives. *Journal of Advanced Nursing, 75*(11), 2579–2590. https://doi.org/10.1111/jan.14128

Pipitone, F., Sadeghi, Z., & DeLancey, J. O. (2021). Urethral function and failure: A review of current knowledge of urethral closure mechanisms, how they vary, and how they are affected by life events. *Neurourology and Urodynamics, 40*(8), 1869–1879.

Po-Yen Chen, Wei-Chia Lee, & Yao-Chi Chuang. (2021). Comparative safety review of current pharmacological treatments for interstitial cystitis/bladder pain syndrome. *Expert Opinion on Drug Safety, 20*(9), 1049–1059. https://doi.org/10.1080/14740338.2021.1921733

Qasemi, A., Lagzian, M., Rahimi, F., Khosravani Majd, F., & Bayat, Z. (2023). The power of probiotics to combat urinary tract infections: A comprehensive review. *Research in Biotechnology and Environmental Science, 2*(1), 1–11. https://doi.org/10.58803/RBES.2023.2.1.01

Rashidi, F., Hajian, S., Darvish, S., & Alavi Majd, H. (2021). Explaining factors affecting help-seeking behaviors in women with urinary incontinence: A qualitative study. *BMC Health Services Research, 21*, 1–10.

Reynolds, W. S., Kowalik, C., Delpe, S. D., Kaufman, M., Fowke, J. H., & Dmochowski, R. (2019). Toileting behaviors and bladder symptoms in women who limit restroom use at work: A cross-sectional study. *The Journal of Urology, 202*(5), 1008–1014.https://doi.org/10.1097/JU.0000000000000315https://doi.org/10.1007/s00192-015-2783-9

Rodriguez-Manas, L. (2020). Urinary tract infection in the elderly: A review of disease characteristics and current treatment options. *Drugs in Context, 9*, 2020-4-13. https://doi.org/10.7573/dic.2020-4-13

Rosenblum N. (2020). Update in female hormonal therapy: What the urologist should know. *Reviews in Urology, 22*(4), 182–185.

Rotem, R., Craven, S., Daykan, Y., Murphy, J., Galvin, D., & O'Reilly, B. A. (2024). Urodynamic insights: Exploring the relationship between detrusor overactivity and pelvic organ prolapse in women with urge incontinence. *Archives of Gynecology and Obstetrics, 309*(6), 2915–2920.

Rutherford, G., Tan, L. J., Aboumarzouk, O., de Souza, J., Khan, R., Somani, B., & Amer, T. (2024). Intravesical gentamicin treatment for recurrent urinary tract infections: A systematic review over the last two decades. *Journal of Clinical Urology, 17*(6), 536–544.

Sabih, A., & Leslie, S. W. (2024). Complicated urinary tract infections. In *StatPearls*. StatPearls Publishing.

Sheng, Y., Low, K. L., Liu, X., Ashton-Miller, J. A., & Miller, J. M. (2019). Association of index finger palpatory assessment of pubovisceral muscle body integrity with MRI-documented tear. *Neurourology & Urodynamics, 38*(4), 1120–1128. https://doi.org/10.1002/nau.23967

Sheng, Y., Liu, X., Low, L. K., Ashton-Miller, J. A., & Miller, J. M. (2020). Association of pubovisceral muscle tear with functional capacity of urethral closure: Evaluating maternal recovery from labor and delivery. *American Journal of Obstetrics and Gynecology, 222*(6), 598.e1–598.e7.

Shermadou, E. S., Rahman, S., & Leslie, S. W. (2023). Anatomy, abdomen and pelvis: bladder. In *StatPearls*. StatPearls Publishing.

Sogutdelen, E., & Citamak, B. (2022). Efficacy of intravesical cocktail therapy with or without dimethyl sulphoxide in interstitial cystitis. *Central European Journal of Urology, 75*(3), 299–304. https://doi.org/10.5173/ceju.2022.129

Stania, M., Niemiec, B., Kamieniarz, A., & Chmielewska, D. (2022). Intravaginal electrical stimulation as a monotherapy for female stress urinary incontinence: A systematic review and meta-analysis. *Complementary Therapies in Clinical Practice, 49*, 101624.

Tähtinen, R. M., Cartwright, R., Vernooij, R. W. M., Rortveit, G., Hunskaar, S., Guyatt, G. H., & Tikkinen, K. A. O. (2019). Long-term risks of stress and urgency urinary incontinence after different vaginal delivery modes. *American Journal of Gynecology, 220*(2), 181.e1–181.e8. https://doi.org/10.1016/j.ajog.2018.10.034

Todhunter-Brown, A., Hazelton, C., Campbell, P., Elders, A., Hagen, S., & McClurg, D. (2022). Conservative interventions for treating urinary incontinence in women: An overview of Cochrane systematic reviews. *The Cochrane Database of Systematic Reviews, 9*(9), CD012337. doi:10.1002/14651858.CD012337.pub2

Tomoe, H. (2023). Dimethyl sulfoxide: A review of pharmacology and clinical effect on interstitial cystitis/bladder pain syndrome. *Continence*, 8, 101058.

Torosis, M., Jackson, N., Nitti, V., & Ackerman, A. L. (2023). Overactive bladder patients with and without urgency incontinence: A spectrum of one condition or different phenotypes? *Urogynecology, 29*(1), 33–40.

Trowbridge, E. R., & Hoover, E. F. (2022). Evaluation and treatment of urinary incontinence in women. *Gastroenterology Clinics of North America, 51*(1), 157–175.

UpToDate Inc. (2025). Amoxicillin and clavulante [Drug Information]. *UpToDate Lexidrug*. Retrieved April 22, 2025, from www-uptodate.com.ckmproxy.vumc.org/contents/amoxicillin-druginformation?search=amoxicillin&source=panel_search_result&selectedTitle=1~150&usage_type=panel&kp_tab=drug_general&display_rank=1

UpToDate Inc. (2025). Cefixime [Drug Information]. *UpToDate Lexidrug*. Retrieved June 22, 2025, from www-uptodate.com.ckmproxy.vumc.org/contents/cefixime-drug-information?search=cefixime&source=panel_search_result&selectedTitle=1~31&usage_type=panel&kp_tab=drug_general&display_rank=1

UpToDate Inc. (2025). Cephalexin [Drug Information]. *UpToDate Lexidrug*. Retrieved June 22, 2025, from www-uptodate.com.ckmproxy.vumc.org/contents/cephalexin-drug-information?search=cephalexin&source=panel_search_result&selectedTitle=1~106&usage_type=panel&kp_tab=drug_general&display_rank=1

UpToDate Inc. (2025). Ciprofloxacin [Drug Information]. *UpToDate Lexidrug*. Retrieved June 22, 2025, from www-uptodate.com.ckmproxy.vumc.org/contents/ciprofloxacin-systemic-drug-information?source=auto_suggest&selectedTitle=1~4---3~4---ciprofl&search=ciprofloxacin%20systemic#F9611233

UpToDate Inc. (2025). Levofloxacin [Drug Information]. *UpToDate Lexidrug*. Retrieved June 22, 2025, from www-uptodate.com.ckmproxy.vumc.org/contents/levofloxacin-systemic-drug-information?source=auto_suggest&selectedTitle=1~2---3~4---levofl&search=levofloxacin%20systemic

UpToDate Inc. (2025). Trimethoprim-sulfamethoxazole [Drug Information]. *UpToDate Lexidrug*. Retrieved June 22, 2025,v from www-uptodate.com.ckmproxy.vumc.org/contents/trimethoprim-sulfamethoxazole-co-trimoxazole-drug-information?source=auto_suggest&selectedTitle=1~3---1~3---trimethoprim&search=trimethoprim%20sulfamethoxazole

van Geelen, H., & Sand, P. K. (2023). The female urethra: Urethral function throughout a woman's lifetime. *International Urogynecology Journal, 34*(6), 1175–1186. https://doi.org/10.1007/s00192-023-05469-6

Vila Pouca, M. C. P., Parente, M. P. L., Natal Jorge, R. M., DeLancey, J. O. L., & Ashton-Miller, J. A. (2022). Pelvic floor muscle injury during a difficult labor: Can tissue fatigue damage play a role? *International Urogynecology Journal, 33*(2), 211–220. https://doi.org/10.1007/s00192-021-05012-5

Whitmore, K. E., Fall, M., Sengiku, A., Tomoe, H., Logadottir, Y., & Kim, Y. H. (2019). Hunner lesion versus non-Hunner lesion interstitial cystitis/bladder pain syndrome. International *Journal of Urology, 6*(Suppl 1), 26–34. https://doi.org/10.1111/iju.13971

Willis, G. C., & Tewelde, S. Z. (2019). The approach to the patient with hematuria. *Emergency Medicine Clinics of North America, 37*(4), 755–769. https://doi.org/10.1016/j.emc.2019.07.011

Xu, H., Wu, W., Wang, X., & Xia, Z. (2021). A predictive model of choosing pessary type for women with symptomatic pelvic organ prolapse. *Menopause (New York, N.Y.), 28*(11), 1279–1286. https://doi.org/10.1097/GME.0000000000001849

CHAPTER 24

Menstrual Cycle Pain and Premenstrual Syndrome

Ruth E. Zielinski

Sarah Maguire

The editors acknowledge Kerri Durnell Schuiling, who was a coauthor of the previous edition of this chapter.

OVERVIEW

Much about menstruation and its accompanying symptoms remains taboo even today (Gopalan et al., 2024) with cultural stigma causing many menstruating people shame and reluctance to discuss discomforts (Åkerman et al., 2024). While the menstrual cycle is a normal physiologic process, normalizing the discomfort and pain that can accompany menstruation can lead to delays in healthcare seeking and stigma (Åkerman et al., 2024). Painful menses is often considered normal and natural even when it impacts quality of life (Ramos-Pichardo et al., 2020). People commonly assume the physical and emotional symptoms that often accompany menstruation are an expected part of their cycle and are to be endured in silence, even when those symptoms become disabling. Focusing on menstrual cycle disorders as a symptom or source of discomfort, rather than as a disease-oriented syndrome, provides a model for understanding this complex condition that includes biological, psychosocial, and sociocultural factors.

Most individuals with a uterus will experience some sort of functional cyclic pain or other related symptoms during the premenstrual and menstrual phases of their cycles (Mitsuhashi et al., 2022). Although cyclic changes (and often the accompanying discomforts) are a normative process, they can disrupt a person's sense of well-being. The menstrual cycle has three phases and is typically described in the context of a 28-day cycle, although the range of normal and other aspects often vary. Premenstrual symptoms may include psychological, physical, and behavioral changes—collectively termed premenstrual syndrome (PMS). Often, for the medical community to acknowledge menstrual pain and discomfort, variations must be identified as a disorder, thereby validating their existence and providing justification for research and formulation of treatment modalities. This chapter focuses on menstrual cycle pain and accompanying discomforts within a patient-centered, normalizing context. Refer to Chapter 7 for a comprehensive review of the menstrual cycle.

Not all people who are assigned female at birth and who experience menstrual cycle pain or premenstrual syndrome identify as female or women; however, these terms are used in this chapter when the literature cited included gender-specific study populations.

DYSMENORRHEA

Scope and Prevalence

Dysmenorrhea—defined as pain occurring with menstruation—is the most commonly reported gynecologic disorder (Ferries-Rowe et al., 2020). This definition does not accurately reflect the profound impact this condition has on people across all continents and cultures. Although a precise prevalence rate is difficult to determine due to varying definitions of dysmenorrhea, studies across the globe report prevalence rates as high as 83 percent (Amza et al., 2024). Among secondary and university age individuals, 71 percent reported painful periods with over 20 percent missing classes and 40 perent reporting a decrease in ability to concentrate and study due to menstrual discomforts (Armour et al., 2019). In addition to painful uterine cramping that begins with the start of menses, lasting from 8 to 72 hours, a myriad of additional symptoms may be experienced, including diarrhea, nausea, vomiting, diaphoresis, fatigue, headache, and sleep disorders (Baker & Lee, 2018). The effects of dysmenorrhea may impede a person's ability to work, attend school, exercise, and socialize (Li et al., 2024).

The significant impact on quality of life combined with the universal prevalence makes treating dysmenorrhea a global health priority (Amza et al., 2024). However, barriers—such as low rates of reporting symptoms to clinicians, lack of awareness about treatment options, and the absence of a clear method for categorizing symptom severity—lead to the belief that even disabling symptoms are a normal part of menstruation (Amza et al., 2024).

Dysmenorrhea is categorized as either primary or secondary. Primary dysmenorrhea is menstrual pain that is caused by myometrial contractions occurring in the absence of pelvic pathology and is associated with ovulatory cycles. Secondary dysmenorrhea is painful menses that is associated with underlying pelvic pathology, such as endometriosis or uterine fibroids (Rapkin et al., 2020; Taylor et al., 2020). Primary dysmenorrhea generally has its onset within 1 to 2 years of menarche (Rapkin et al., 2020). Individuals affected by dysmenorrhea report a significant impact on their ability to function in school because the pain is so debilitating it prevents them from attending classes and completing homework (Ezebialu et al., 2021). This can have far-reaching consequences for the educational success of those who suffer from this condition. Primary dysmenorrhea increases the risk for developing chronic pain conditions later in life, such as irritable bowel syndrome, interstitial cystitis, fibromyalgia, chronic headaches, and chronic low back pain (Oladosu et al., 2019; Li et al., 2020). In addition, the effects may exacerbate comorbid issues such as cystitis and irritable bowel syndrome (IBS) (Li et al., 2020).

The impact of the COVID-19 pandemic on reproductive health, both directly and indirectly, can be reflected in the reported effects on the menstrual cycle. Menstrual changes after COVID infection have been detailed in multiple studies; however, the symptoms (which included irregular or altered cycle lengths, heavier or lighter flow, amenorrhea, and increased clotting) varied widely between studies in both expression and frequency. The only finding consistently reported is increased pain with menses (Błażejewski & Witkos, 2023; Deogade et al., 2023; Sakurada et al., 2024). While the pathophysiologic action of the virus has yet to be completely identified, there are known inflammatory and immune effects which may explain the increased dysmenorrhea that people experience after infection (Deogade et al., 2023). Vaccination was also found to affect the menstrual cycle in populations globally with similar findings. Studies in Spain and Saudi Arabia both reported that more than 60 percent of participants reported menstrual cycle alterations after a first vaccine dose (Alshammari et al., 2024; Mínguez-Esteban et al., 2022). Similar to post-infection symptoms, participants described a range of changes, with heavy menstrual bleeding more common than amenorrhea or cycle irregularity. Dysmenorrhea, however, was the most consistent post-vaccine finding across studies (Alshammari et al., 2024; Contreras-Rendon et al., 2024; Farland et al., 2023; Matar et al., 2023; Payne et al., 2024; Smaardijk et al., 2024; Tandon et al., 2023; Trogstad et al., 2023). Although the vaccine was associated with menstrual cycle changes, clinicians can provide reassurance that the changes were temporary (Payne et al., 2024). An unexpected positive to the pandemic; university students who had experienced dysmenorrhea before the pandemic reported that they missed less school and felt more freedom to rest during their menstrual cycles due to the mandatory isolation (Ataş et al., 2023).

ETIOLOGY AND PATHOPHYSIOLOGY

Primary Dysmenorrhea

Primary dysmenorrhea is theorized to be caused by an excessive or imbalanced amount of prostanoids (particularly PGA2 and PGA2a), which are secreted by the endometrium during menstruation (Rapkin et al., 2020). Progesterone levels decrease in the late luteal phase, triggering the hormonal cascade that results in the sloughing of the endometrial lining and the release of prostaglandins, which then act on the uterine muscle, causing higher amplitude contractility and increased myometrial tone (Bernardi et al., 2017). One long-standing theory is that these strong, frequent uterine contractions cause hypoxia and potentially ischemia of the muscle, resulting in pain (Taylor et al., 2020). However, a recent study using ultrasound and MR imaging evaluated oxygenation throughout the menstrual cycle found that participants with dysmenorrhea had more tissue perfusion than the control group suggesting that the cause of menstrual pain may be more associated with uterine muscle inflammation (Cockrum et al., 2024). In addition to affecting the uterine muscle, prostaglandins, found in higher levels in individuals with dysmenorrhea, stimulate nociceptors throughout the body, resulting in increased pain signaling, and higher input of pain reports (Bernardi et al., 2017).

Secondary Dysmenorrhea

Secondary dysmenorrhea is caused by an underlying pathology, such as endometriosis (the most common cause), adenomyosis (the second most common cause), nonhormonal intrauterine devices, fibroids, and scarring from abdominal surgery or infection (Rapkin et al., 2020). The onset of secondary dysmenorrhea is typically 2 or more years after menarche, and it can usually be differentiated from primary dysmenorrhea through a detailed history, physical examination, and, if needed, pelvic imaging. The management of secondary dysmenorrhea is similar to that of primary dysmenorrhea; however, because the etiology has its roots in underlying pelvic pathology, finding the cause is imperative for treatment to be successful.

Clinical Presentation

The chief complaint for both primary and secondary dysmenorrhea is painful cramping with menses. Patients also report backache, pain that radiates into the thighs, nausea and vomiting, diarrhea, sweating, headaches, fatigue, and sleeping disorders (Ferries-Rowe et al., 2020). Symptoms occur during ovulatory cycles, beginning shortly before the onset of menses and persisting for 8 to 72 hours (Ferries-Rowe et al., 2020). Menstrual pain can lead to poorer sleep quality which can increase daytime sleepiness and impact quality of life (Ishikura et al., 2024). Among adolescents with dysmenorrhea, daytime sleepiness was correlated with increased suicide risk (Dong et al., 2023). Dysmenorrhea that does not improve with typical treatments and is accompanied by other symptoms, such as dyspareunia, heavy menstrual or postcoital bleeding, or infertility, should raise the clinician's suspicion for secondary dysmenorrhea (Ferries-Rowe et al., 2020).

Assessment History

Accurate diagnosis of dysmenorrhea requires a thorough history. While a family history of dysmenorrhea, especially those who experience early menarche, increases the risk of experiencing dysmenorrhea, whether this is related to genetics is unclear (Situmorang et al., 2024). Other factors that likely have a causative relationship with dysmenorrhea include a body mass index less than 20, menarche prior to age 12, longer menstrual intervals and duration of bleeding, irregular or heavy flow, history of sexual assault, and smoking (Taylor et al., 2020). A diet lower in protein and higher in simple carbohydrates has also been linked to dysmenorrhea (Güzeldere et al., 2024). Assessment of all potential factors during history collection improves the clinician's ability to develop individualized treatment plans. **Box 24-1** lists information that should be obtained at the gynecologic visit.

Physical Exam

A pelvic examination is unnecessary in an adolescent not at risk for sexually transmitted infections (STIs) who presents with classic primary dysmenorrhea symptoms. However, if during the history taking the clinician is unable to make a clear diagnosis of primary dysmenorrhea, a pelvic examination may become necessary. A pelvic examination is also warranted if there is a question of pelvic inflammatory disease, infection, adnexal cysts, endometriosis, adenomyosis, uterine fibroids, or a pelvic

BOX 24-1 History to Obtain at the Gynecologic Visit

Menstrual history:
- Age at menarche
- Family history of dysmenorrhea, endometriosis, or pelvic cancers
- Length of cycle, length of menses, estimated menstrual flow
- Presence of intermenstrual bleeding

Medical history:
- Any abdominal or pelvic surgeries
- Other chronic conditions (IBS, interstitial cystitis)
- History of mental illness (depression, anxiety)

Social history:
- Current tobacco use, diet, alcohol intake
- Amount and type of exercise
- Level of stress and methods for coping

Sexual and obstetric history:
- Age at first coitarche (first penetrative intercourse)
- Obstetric history, including route of delivery and complications
- Prior and current contraceptive use
- Pregnancy plans
- Sexual history, including number of partners and any dyspareunia
- History of sexually transmitted infections (STIs) and date of last testing
- History of sexual abuse or interpersonal trauma/violence

Dysmenorrhea symptom and treatment history:
- Description of symptoms, including onset, duration, and severity
- Treatments used, particularly response to NSAIDs
- Onset of dysmenorrhea symptoms in relation to menarche and menstrual cycle
- Impact on quality of life and activities of daily living

mass. Additionally, a rectal examination may be indicated if endometrial implants are suspected. Refer to Chapter 8 for steps in performing a pelvic examination.

Diagnostic Testing

Primary dysmenorrhea is a diagnosis made by a comprehensive history and physical examination that definitively rule out any other diagnosis. If the diagnosis cannot be confirmed by history and physical exam, or when the presentation is suspicious for secondary dysmenorrhea, imaging is indicated. Transvaginal and pelvic ultrasound are most useful when the suspected cause is structural, as in the case of fibroids or a congenital uterine anomaly (Taylor et al., 2020). It is important to remember that some differential diagnoses are not reliably identified by imaging, including endometriosis and interstitial cystitis, and may require referral.

BOX 24-2 Risk Factors for Dysmenorrhea

- Family history
- Age younger than 30 years
- Body mass index less than 20
- Smoking
- Early menarche (prior to age 12)
- Longer intermenstrual intervals and duration of bleeding
- Irregular or heavy flow
- History of sexual abuse
- Premenstrual molimina (symptoms)
- History of pelvic surgery

Data from Taylor, H. S., Pal, L., & Sell, E. (2020). *Speroff's clinical gynecologic endocrinology and infertility* (9th ed.). Wolters Kluwer.

Differential Diagnosis

Gynecologic conditions that should be considered in a differential diagnosis of secondary dysmenorrhea include endometriosis, endometrioma, adenomyosis, adnexal cysts, pelvic inflammatory disease, pregnancy (intrauterine or ectopic), and Müllerian malformations. Nongynecologic issues, such as musculoskeletal disorders, interstitial cystitis, and IBS, must also be ruled out (Taylor et al., 2020). The risk factors for dysmenorrhea are listed in **Box 24-2**.

Management

Although the best studied and most often recommended therapies currently are pharmacologic, there is some evidence for nonpharmacologic therapies as alternative or complementary approaches to relieving menstrual discomforts (Jo & Lee, 2018; Liu et al., 2022; Xu et al., 2020). Many online resources suggest the benefits of homeopathy or herbal medicine in relieving menstrual pain; however, rigorous, well-designed studies have not been undertaken recently (Liang et al., 2020). While evidence of efficacy is lacking, most complementary therapies can be used with minimal risk (Kim, 2020). Ideally, clinicians should provide evidence-based information to guide patients in choosing treatments that provide the best symptom relief.

Nonpharmacologic Treatment Options

Treatments that do not require medications can be utilized to decrease the symptoms of dysmenorrhea. These methods are referred to as alternative therapies when used alone, or as complementary therapies, when used in addition to pharmacologic interventions. A systematic review of 33 randomized controlled trials reported that there was a slight improvement in pain intensity with most of the treatments including exercise, herbs (fennel, ginger, or cinnamon), acupuncture, acupressure, aromatherapy, transcutaneous electrical nerve stimulation (TENS), topical heat, and yoga (Li et al., 2024). Most studies of alternative therapies for treatment of dysmenorrhea are limited by sample size and design rigor.

Heat The use of heat therapy to reduce menstrual pain has been studied and shows measurable improvement of symptoms (Jo & Lee, 2018). A systematic review of randomized clinical trials (RCTs) evaluating the benefit of nonpharmacologic treatments of dysmenorrhea found favorable outcomes when heat therapy was compared to placebo and analgesics (Jo & Lee, 2018). The use of heat, either as a solo treatment modality or as a complementary therapy to NSAIDs, often results in a significant amount of pain relief. Clinicians should advise patients that a temperature of approximately 104°F (40°C) is recommended. Heat may be applied as often as needed.

Lifestyle Changes Although the research is not robust, there is evidence that lifestyle modifications can improve dysmenorrhea symptoms. Avoiding smoking, limiting soda and sugary foods, and managing stress levels have all been shown to decrease reported pain levels (Biro & Bloemer, 2019). There is a considerable amount of evidence to support recommending physical activity to alleviate dysmenorrhea pain (Fuentes-Aparicio et al., 2023). High-intensity aerobic exercise for 30 minutes, three times per week, has been shown to be an effective intervention because it reduces prostaglandin production (Li et al., 2024).

Dietary Supplements There is a paucity of well-designed published studies about the efficacy of dietary supplements, such as vitamins and herbs. A study exploring the effect of vitamin E (200 IU daily) and omega-3 (300 mg daily) on dysmenorrhea pain found that each supplement was superior to placebo, with greater efficacy when administered together (Sadeghi et al., 2018). Omega 3 supplements may reduce menstrual pain and analgesic use, although no high-quality studies have been conducted (Snipe et al., 2024). Vitamin D supplementation may also provide improvement in reported pain when taken at a dose of at least 50,000 IU weekly (Chen et al., 2023). Associated symptoms such as sleep disturbances may also be addressed with nonpharmacologic options. A small study (N = 14) of participants with primary dysmenorrhea suggested that melatonin and meloxicam may improve sleep and decrease pain (Keshavarzi et al., 2018). One or more of these supplements in combination may be an option for patients who cannot or choose not to use pharmacologic methods for symptom relief. People who are interested in using herbal or homeopathic remedies should be referred to a knowledgeable herbalist or naturopathic clinician for the safest, most efficacious regimen.

Acupuncture, Aromatherapy, and Moxibustion Acupuncture, aromatherapy, and moxibustion treatments may improve dysmenorrhea symptoms and have minimal side effects (Li et al., 2024). A meta-analysis of 60 RCTs found that acupuncture was more effective than NSAIDs at reducing dysmenorrhea pain and related symptoms (Woo et al., 2018). However, as with most alternative therapies, more research is needed. Additionally, patients may find it challenging to find clinicians who are trained in acupuncture, aromatherapy, and moxibustion techniques because these treatment modalities are less commonly practiced in the United States and cost may be a deterrent for many individuals.

Pharmacologic Treatment Options

Non-Steroidal Anti-Inflammatory Drugs (NSAIDS) Currently, pharmacotherapy is the most common and most effective treatment for dysmenorrhea (Mardon et al., 2024). NSAIDs are considered the first-line pharmacologic choice for treatment of dysmenorrhea, although side effects, most often of a gastrointestinal nature, may occur (Tai & McAlindon, 2021). NSAIDs inhibit cyclooxygenase enzymes, thereby inhibiting the production of prostaglandins (Ferries-Rowe et al., 2020). This class of drugs carries some risk including bleeding, renal, heart, and liver disease (LaForge et al., 2023). Although aspirin is classified as an NSAID, it is less effective than others, such as ibuprofen (Nie et al., 2020), and even though acetaminophen has a weak impact on cyclooxygenase enzymes, it is not an NSAID and is not a first-line choice for treatment. Patients who use acetaminophen to treat their pain report fewer issues with indigestion but also less reduction in dysmenorrhea symptoms (Nie et al., 2020).

Clinical guidelines suggest initially recommending an NSAID for patients with dysmenorrhea (if there are no contraindications or drug sensitivities) and then assess pain and cycle control after 2 to 3 months (Ferries-Rowe et al., 2020). Counseling patients to begin treatment at the onset of menses or with associated symptoms typically results in requiring NSAIDs only for 2 to 3 days. Recommended therapeutic dosing is around the clock administration up to the daily maximum indicated by the manufacturer.

Combined Hormonal Contraceptives Although NSAIDs have consistently been reaffirmed as the first-line treatment, they fail to improve symptoms for approximately 18 percent of individuals with dysmenorrhea (Oladosu et al., 2019). Combined hormonal contraceptives are often used in the treatment of dysmenorrhea, particularly for those who also desire both cycle control and contraception. Combined hormonal contraceptives contain both estrogen and progestin and act to suppress ovulation and endometrial tissue growth, causing decreased prostaglandin production and menses volume, which results in lower intrauterine pressure and subsequent cramping (Francavilla et al., 2023). A continuous dosing regimen, in which the hormone-containing product is used for 84 days followed by a 4- to 7-day hormone-free period, decreases the frequency of menses and dysmenorrhea (Teal & Edelman, 2021; Schroll et al., 2023). Relief of symptoms occurs with both primary and secondary dysmenorrhea, particularly when a confirmed diagnosis of endometriosis has been made (Francavilla et al., 2023). Therefore, initiation of combined oral contraceptives for rapid relief of dysmenorrhea is recommended even before an investigation of possible causative pathology. However, it is important to know that long-term use of estrogen-containing products may exacerbate endometriosis, necessitating a change in treatment after further diagnostic testing (Chen et al., 2020).

Progestin Hormonal Methods Several routes of administration are available for progestin-only products, including oral pills, intradermal implants, intramuscular or subcutaneous injections, and intrauterine devices. Progesterone only contraceptive pills can be used to manage dysmenorrhea, specifically secondary dysmenorrhea caused by endometriosis (Koninckx et al., 2021). The benefit of oral progesterone is that it can decrease the amount of unpredictable bleeding compared with other progesterone methods; however, it must be taken daily which is challenging for many individuals (Teal & Edelman, 2021).

Progestin implants consist of a single etonogestrel-containing rod that is placed intradermally on the inner aspect of the upper arm. While the implant is currently labeled for 3 years of use, several studies have shown it to be effective contraception for 5 years (ACOG, 2024) although irregular bleeding may increase during the additional 2 years of use (Ali et al., 2017). As many as 81 percent of women report an improvement in dysmenorrhea symptoms with the use of progestin implants (ACOG, 2024; Ferrero et al., 2018). The implant's mechanism of action is primarily the suppression of ovulation, although the alteration of endometrial lining may also be a factor. Side effects include weight gain, acne, and menstrual bleeding changes that may present as amenorrhea or as frequent, infrequent, or prolonged bleeding, although only a small percentage of women choose to have the implant removed due to side effects (ACOG, 2024; Maceira et al., 2023).

Depot medroxyprogesterone acetate (Depo-Provera or DMPA) has been shown to decrease dysmenorrhea. It is administered by either intramuscular or subcutaneous injection every 90 days. As with the progestin implant, this method works by suppressing ovulation and decreasing endometrial tissue growth (ACOG, 2023). Amenorrhea is a commonly reported side effect. The use of DMPA has decreased since the U.S. Food and Drug Administration (FDA) issued a black box warning in 2004 due to the loss of bone mineral density with prolonged use. However, more current studies suggest that bone mineral density recovers after discontinuation (ACOG, 2023). Clinicians should provide detailed information to their patients about the risks and benefits of using DMPA and the FDA's black box warning so they can make informed decisions. DMPA should not be used for more than 2 years (ACOG, 2023). Additionally, it is suggested that adolescents be offered and counseled about other contraceptive options that have no effect on bone mineral density (ACOG, 2023).

There are several types of levonorgestrel- (progestin) releasing intrauterine devices (LNG-IUD) that are commonly used for contraception and management of heavy menstrual bleeding. They can be an effective option for treating dysmenorrhea due to endometriosis, adenomyosis, and leiomyomas (Teal & Edelman, 2021). Unlike progestin implants and injections, ovulation is not usually inhibited with an LNG-IUD. The beneficial effect in alleviating the pain of dysmenorrhea arises from the dramatic decrease in menstrual fluid volume and prostaglandin production. Counseling should include the impact on bleeding profile because irregular or prolonged bleeding during the first year occurs for over half of all users (ACOG, 2024; Lazorwitz et al., 2019). Conversely, amenorrhea is also common, with 20 percent of patients reporting one episode of amenorrhea lasting 90 days or more during the first year (Lazorwitz et al., 2019).

Surgical Intervention

Debilitating dysmenorrhea for which medical management is unsuccessful or contraindicated because of other medical conditions may warrant surgical intervention for alleviation of pain. The patient's desire for future childbearing influences the decision about the type of surgery. Options include a total hysterectomy or pelvic denervation, which spares the uterus and interrupts the transmission of sensation through the superior hypogastric plexus. In addition to complications inherent with any invasive abdominal or neurological procedure, neither option can deliver a guarantee of complete relief. Pelvic pain post-hysterectomy is a common occurrence (Sng et al., 2018) and a review of pelvic denervation procedures indicated success rates of approximately 85 percent in alleviating dysmenorrhea symptoms (Ramirez & Donnellan, 2017).

When to Refer

Although diagnosis and successful treatment of dysmenorrhea is often arrived at through primary care, there are situations when referral to a specialist is advisable. This is particularly true when secondary dysmenorrhea is suspected or when primary dysmenorrhea fails to respond to initial treatments, or when a diagnostic surgical procedure such as laparoscopy is indicated.

PREMENSTRUAL CYCLE SYNDROMES AND DYSPHORIC DISORDER: AN OVERVIEW

The physical and emotional symptoms often associated with the luteal (premenstrual) phase of the menstrual cycle include mastalgia, weight and appetite changes, emotional lability, and bloating. Symptoms typically begin the week prior to menses and resolve completely at the onset of bleeding. Although most people report premenstrual symptoms as mild and not interfering in their daily lives, a significant number experience significant, even disabling, effects (Liguori et al., 2023).

To provide validity to the symptoms people who menstruate experience, premenstrual syndrome (PMS) and premenstrual dysphoric disorder (PMDD) had to be identified, classified, and evidenced through scientific studies. Although the lack of understanding about menstrual disorders needed to be addressed in the clinical arena, these classifications led to the pathologizing of what many menstruating individuals have been experiencing throughout history. Recognized in the *International Classification of Diseases, 11th Revision* (*ICD-11*) manual developed by the World Health Organization (Harrison et al., 2021), PMS describes the cyclical recurrence of symptoms that impair a person's health, relationships, and occupational functioning. Unfortunately, even though PMS and PMDD are recognized by the scientific community, they may still be taboo subjects or derisively regarded. The term PMS is often used mockingly in Western culture; associated with irritability, mood swings, irrational behavior, and sometimes violence, with implications that people are incapable of rational thought during the premenstrual phase of their cycle. PMDD is a diagnostic label that applies to a much smaller number of menstruating people experiencing severe PMS with predominantly negative affective symptoms. Unfortunately, PMS/PMDD is often diagnosed based on symptoms that are actually part of other serious mental health conditions.

Global organizations such as the American Psychological Association, the American College of Obstetricians and Gynecologists, Royal College of Obstetricians and Gynaecologists, and the World Health Organization have not yet standardized global definitions of terms and diagnostic criteria. For continuity, this chapter will utilize the terminology that is commonly used in the United States.

Scope and Prevalence

Globally, premenstrual discomfort and mood changes are experienced by a large percentage of menstruating people across different cultures (Liu et al., 2024). Factors such as geographic location, marital status, education, and occupation appear to influence the prevalence and type of symptoms experienced and which symptoms are considered to be problematic

(Mitsuhashi et al., 2022). Although premenstrual disorders are recognized as a worldwide health concern, it is challenging to accurately determine the prevalence and severity of symptoms and their effect in global populations. This is due in large part to the historical lack of clear, internationally accepted definitions of terms and diagnostic criteria.

Prevalence studies of premenstrual symptoms report rates ranging from 12 to 92 percent with the large variance attributed to the lack of internationally recognized diagnostic criteria and under-reporting of not premenstrual symptoms. While many menstruating individuals experience premenstrual symptoms with ovulatory cycles, the diagnosis of premenstrual disorder, which encompasses both PMS and PMDD, is applied only when these symptoms are severe enough to cause impairment of daily activities and negatively impact quality of life (Öksüz & Guvenc, 2018). A frequently cited study details an incidence rate of 85 percent of women experiencing at least one symptom, with 20 to 25 percent reporting moderate to severe PMS, and 3 to 5 percent meeting criteria for PMDD (di Scalea & Pearlstein, 2019). Premenstrual disorders are conditions considered both acute and chronic, both having a significant impact on work, school attendance, social activities, and interpersonal relationships (Liu et al., 2024). The impact of the COVID-19 pandemic extended to prevalence of premenstrual disorders (Maher et al., 2022). Even individuals who were not infected with the COVID-19 virus experienced significant health impacts due to the situational isolation and stress. In a study conducted in the United Kingdom 64 percent of respondents reported worsening premenstrual symptoms and dysmenorrhea with associated increased anxiety and sleep disturbance as compared to pre-pandemic (Maher et al., 2022).

Etiology and Pathophysiology

The etiology of premenstrual disorder is not well defined (ACOG, 2023), but there are several theories to explain the symptoms and the cyclical timing of their occurrence. The most commonly accepted is that in some individuals premenstrual disorder symptoms occur when the hormonal fluctuation naturally occurring during the menstrual cycle adversely influences neurotransmitters (Tiranini & Nappi, 2022). This theory is supported by evidence that premenstrual disorder symptoms are not experienced during anovulatory cycles (such as during perimenopause or with use of ovulation-suppressing medication) unless those individuals receive add-back progesterone therapy (Tiranini & Nappi, 2022). Laboratory values for estrogen and progesterone levels are normal in individuals with PMS, leading to increased speculation that there is a neurobiologic vulnerability to the normal fluctuation of estrogen and progesterone (ACOG, 2023).

Progesterone and its main metabolite, allopregnanolone, peak during the luteal phase and decrease rapidly with menses, mirroring the timing of premenstrual disorder symptoms. Allopregnanolone is a powerful positive modulator of the $GABA_A$ receptor that, when activated, typically produces a sedative, anxiolytic effect. In individuals with premenstrual disorder, however, the response to allopregnanolone may be paradoxical, causing irritability, emotional lability, and depressed mood (Tiranini & Nappi, 2022). The medication dutasteride, a 5α-reductase inhibitor typically used to treat enlarged prostrate, blocks the conversion of progesterone into allopregnanolone. Preliminary studies indicate it may reduce mood symptoms associated with PMDD but it is not yet FDA approved for this use (Modzelewski et al., 2024).

Although the role played by serotonin is obscure, the efficacy of serotonin reuptake inhibitors (SSRIs) as a first-line therapy provides strong evidence of a relationship between serotonin and premenstrual disorders (di Scalea & Pearlstein, 2019). Evidence of the effect of gonadal hormones and neurotransmitters is supported by multiple studies; however, further research is needed to determine the pathophysiology of the atypical allopregnanolone response and the direction of the relationship. Whether the cause is abnormal levels of allopregnanolone (either above or below normal), an altered sensitivity to normal hormone production, inhibition of serotonin action, or another unidentified relationship between menstrual hormones and the brain is unclear (Tiranini & Nappi, 2022).

Neuroimaging of people with premenstrual disorders provides preliminary evidence that the hormonal fluctuations during the menstrual cycle lead to alterations in brain structure, plasticity, and function (Monteiro et al., 2024). In a current review of the literature, the authors conclude that the imaging methods used varied across studies and the findings were inconsistent, but that there did seem to be an association between higher levels of serotonin transporter binding potential in the midbrain during the luteal phase and depressive symptoms (Monteiro et al., 2024). Whether neuroimaging will eventually lead to consensus on the etiology of PMDD or how the findings may be helpful for the understanding and treatment of PMDD is unclear.

PMS, particularly mood changes, may result from a combination of stressors, a heightened stress response, lack of support, and a vulnerable period of biologic reactivity. There are many labels given to this set of stressors, including brain–gut neuroendocrine and decreased serotonin production syndromes (Shiha & Aziz, 2021). PMS has also been shown to be associated with several psychological conditions, such as overall reduced psychological well-being and mood disorders, including anxiety and depression (Yi et al., 2023). Both physical and psychological stressors are associated with increased PMS symptoms. Recent evidence suggests history of adverse childhood experiences (ACEs) of all types (sexual abuse, neglect, and violence) is associated with an increased risk for premenstrual disorder symptoms (Yang et al., 2022). The relationship between ACEs and premenstrual disorder is linear whereby the more ACEs a person experiences, the more likely they are to have more severe symptoms (Yang et al., 2022). Investigation into identifying risk factors for premenstrual disorders has often been inconclusive or yielded conflicting results. Two factors associated with increasing severity of premenstrual disorder symptoms are body mass index less than 18 and cigarette smoking (Mitsuhashi et al., 2022). While clinicians often tell patients to decrease caffeine and carbohydrate intake, these factors have not been shown to increase the likelihood or severity of premenstrual symptoms.

Assessment

Cyclic premenstrual pain and discomforts represent a cluster of symptoms that require the clinician and the patient to balance several seemingly dichotomous views: normative versus pathologic, one-dimensional versus multidimensional, acute versus chronic, and protocol versus individualized care. The conventional approach to assessment and diagnosis focuses on ruling out pathology. Data for assessment and diagnosis are obtained from the medical history, physical examination, and laboratory assessments. Finally, a list of differential diagnoses is identified. Although these are important steps, the goal for providing care related to the menstrual cycle and premenstrual experience is to explore what is normal and acceptable to the patient. A feminist approach to intervention focuses on patient-centered care, advocacy, health promotion, and self-care, integrated with the clinician's biomedical knowledge and skills. Listening to patients and helping them understand PMS and PMDD in the context of their life transitions, personal characteristics, and external stressors provides the support needed to make informed decisions for treatment.

Assumptions that underpin the assessment and therapeutic strategies for people experiencing premenstrual pain and discomforts include the following:

- Personal and social circumstances (for example, a supportive partner) have health effects that are as important as, if not more important than, the biologic changes of the menstrual cycle.
- Biologic changes should not be ignored but rather viewed in the context of biobehavioral relationships (for example, shifting levels of hormones).
- Many factors (for example, financial resources) can promote or prevent people from taking proactive steps in their healthcare decisions (Ussher & Perz, 2020).

Clinicians can have a significant influence on the health and well-being of patients with PMS and PMDD. Care of patients with these issues must be individualized and person-centered while also utilizing an evidence-based approach to assessing, diagnosing, and managing cyclic premenstrual pain and discomfort (Modzelewski et al., 2024). Although PMS and PMDD are separate diagnoses, their symptoms are similar (PMDD symptoms are typically more severe); therefore, the assessment approaches and therapeutic options may be similar (refer to **Table 24-1**).

History

A comprehensive evaluation of the patient's symptoms, as well as obstetric, gynecologic, and psychiatric history, are important to determine an accurate diagnosis. Assuring an accurate diagnosis of PMS or PMDD requires keeping a record of symptoms, severity, and timing of their onset and resolution in relationship to the menstrual cycle. The goal for assessment is to understand the individual's premenstrual experience and to help define and manage distressing symptoms and concomitant problems. Using an integrated approach to assess, diagnose, and treat premenstrual symptoms encourages the use of pharmacologic and nonpharmacologic treatment modalities. In addition, an integrated approach encourages individuals to participate in decision making and to take responsibility for aspects of the treatment regimens within their control, such as nutrition and exercise.

A prospective assessment of individual symptoms or symptom clusters—the recommended method—can be accomplished by the use of a calendar or symptom checklist that is kept for one or two consecutive cycles (Trépanier et al., 2023). This record provides evidence for patients when discussing symptoms with their clinician and can guide treatment options. Continued record keeping during treatment is also key to understanding the patient's individual response to pharmacologic and nonpharmacological remedies. Symptom monitoring essentially consists of educating individuals in self-diagnosis; it includes simply listing and rating feelings, symptoms, and behavioral changes and focusing on social and physical environmental factors. Patients can see symptom patterns that enable identification of the relationship between the symptoms and the circumstances of their lives that impact their menstrual cycle. Daily monitoring helps to determine the severity and pattern of symptoms as well as providing a basis for making and tracking healthy changes that lessen the intensity and impact of the symptoms.

An instrument for journaling symptoms that is commonly referenced in the literature is the Daily Record of Severity of Problems (DRSP) (Endicott et al., 2006). The DRSP is a prospective tool that the patient completes daily for two consecutive months prior to the clinician visit. It provides an accurate account of symptoms as they occur during the menstrual cycle and is a valid and reliable instrument that can be used to diagnose either PMS or PMDD (ACOG, 2023). A 2021 version is available for download from the International Association for Premenstrual Disorders website at https://iapmd.org/provider-resources. Alternatively there are smartphone apps which track symptoms that may be a preferred method for menstrual cycle tracking although there is evidence that people may be reluctant to pay for an app (Funnell et al., 2024).

Although prospective assessment is the recommended method for assessing symptom severity, distress, and pattern, retrospective assessment can be an initial first step in determining symptom distress (Henz et al., 2018). Retrospective tools, such as the Pre-Menstrual Symptoms Screening Tool (PSST) (Steiner et al., 2003), rely on recall of symptoms to provide a clinical picture. Recall is less accurate than reporting, but it may be preferred, particularly with adolescents who have difficulty adhering to daily recording. The PSST has been used and validated in a number of studies of premenstrual disorders globally (Pacitti et al., 2021). The PSST-A is a validated tool for screening with adolescents (Steiner et al., 2011). Retrospective symptom reports are likely to overestimate severity and do not provide data about symptom patterns; however, they can assist with diagnosis and ruling out other chronic illnesses. A retrospective assessment can include the following questions:

- In your own words, describe the pain and discomforts that are the most severe and distressing to you.
- What is the pattern of pain and discomforts during a typical menstrual cycle? How many days before, during, or after your period do you notice symptoms? Do the symptoms occur around ovulation?
- Does anything in particular—such as work stress, dietary influences, or exercise—worsen or alleviate your symptoms?

Determining Symptom Severity and Distress Patterns

It is important to delineate symptoms, their patterns, and ways they may be related to the menstrual cycle because premenstrual symptoms have no clearly defined cause. Some people may believe the symptoms they are experiencing are PMS but in actuality they have another condition, such as endometriosis, that worsened around the time of menstruation. In other instances, mood or behavior changes—which may have been heightened during the premenstrual phase—were attributed to PMS when, in fact, they were a result of external problems, such as work-related stress, relationship difficulties, problems with children, on-the-job harassment, violence, and other sources of anxiety, fear, and frustration.

Diagnostic Testing

There are no laboratory or imaging tests that can provide confirmation of a premenstrual disorder diagnosis. Although there is strong evidence that gonadal hormones play a role in expression

TABLE 24-1 Symptoms of PMS and PMDD

Symptoms	PMS	PMDD
Physical symptoms	Abdominal bloating and pain Mild weight gain from water retention Constipation, followed by diarrhea with the onset of the menses Headache Pelvic pain and cramping Fatigue Extremity edema Nausea/food cravings	Physical symptoms are same as PMS but typically more severe Abdominal bloating and pain Headache Pelvic pain and cramping Fatigue Extremity edema Nausea/food cravings
Psychological symptoms	Depression Anxiety Anger/irritability Insomnia Changes in libido Confusion, decrease in mental sharpness Social withdrawal Feelings of low self-esteem/poor self-image	Marked affective lability Marked irritability or anger or increased interpersonal conflicts Markedly depressed mood, feelings of hopelessness, or self-deprecating thoughts Marked anxiety, tension, feelings of being keyed up or on edge Decreased interest in usual activities Subjective sense of difficulty concentrating Lethargy Insomnia or hypersomnia Subjective sense of being overwhelmed or out of control
Diagnostic criteria	Symptoms begin up to 7 days prior to menses Remission of symptoms from cycle days 4 to 13 Symptoms are significant enough to impair activities of daily living Symptoms are charted during at least two cycles Symptoms are not due to another disorder (e.g., depression, anxiety, anemia, medication side effect, substance abuse disorder)	Include diagnostic criteria for PMS and significant distress or interference with work, school, social activities, or relationships with others APA *DSM-5* criteria for PMDD states one or more of the following affective symptoms must be present: • Emotional lability, increased sensitivity to perceived insult • Anger, irritability (most common) • Feeling hopeless, depressed mood, self-critical thoughts • Anxiousness, feeling of stress One or more of the following symptoms must be present for a total of five or more symptoms: • Poor concentration • Appetite changes, food cravings • Decreased interest in usual activities • Fatigue, diminished energy • Overwhelmed • Breast tenderness, bloating, weight gain, or aching joints and muscles • Hypersomnia or insomnia • (ACOG, 2023)

of premenstrual disorders, individuals with PMS and PMDD do not exhibit abnormal serum levels, compared with controls (Dilbaz & Aksan, 2021). Deeper insight into the etiology is necessary to identify precise testing for diagnosing premenstrual disorders. Currently, testing is used only to exclude differential diagnoses. Simple blood tests can identify conditions such as pregnancy, anemia, thyroid disorders, diabetes, or hypoglycemia. Ovarian hormone testing is unnecessary unless premature menopause (before age 40 years) is suspected.

Differential Diagnoses

The patterns and severity of symptoms are the best guide for determining whether a patient has PMS or PMDD and whether there is underlying etiology. Symptom-tracking charts and calendars, along with menstrual and health history data, provide essential clues for making a diagnosis. The defining characteristic of premenstrual disorder is timing—the cyclical onset of symptoms occurring after ovulation followed by a complete resolution by the end of menses. Without attention to timing, the presenting symptoms may suggest other conditions. Furthermore, the transition to menopause may be a vulnerable period when people experience the onset or a worsening of premenstrual disorder, especially mood disturbances and fatigue (Sander & Gordon, 2021).

Many medical and psychiatric conditions may be exacerbated in the premenstrual or menstrual phase of the cycle, leading an individual to believe that they must be experiencing PMS. For example, hypothyroidism, anemia, endometriosis, and physiologic ovarian cysts can mimic the signs and symptoms of PMS (Liguori et al., 2023). Other psychiatric disorders, such as substance abuse and eating disorders may worsen during the luteal phase of the menstrual cycle. Musculoskeletal pain syndromes, such as arthralgias, arthritis, and fibromyalgia, can cause symptoms that mimic those of premenstrual disorders (e.g., generalized pain, fatigue, sleep disturbances, or cognitive impairment) and may be misdiagnosed in people with moderate to severe premenstrual symptoms. Cyclic premenstrual pain that is severe and begins at midcycle or worsens before menstruation may indicate an underlying gynecologic condition, such as pelvic inflammatory disease, endometriosis, or chronic pelvic pain. In addition, migraine-type headaches appear to increase during the premenstrual and menstrual phases. Menstrual migraines tend to occur 1 to 3 days before menstruation begins or during the first day or two of menstruation when hormone levels drop considerably. Refer to Chapters 22, 27, and 29 for information about pelvic inflammatory disease, endometriosis, and chronic pelvic pain, respectively.

Premenstrual Disorders and Suicide Risk

Research has shown that people with PMS and PMDD are at greater risk for is a risk for suicidal ideation and attempts (Prasad et al., 2021). Patients with moderate to severe symptoms should be screened for suicide risk (Prasad et al., 2021).

Management: Setting Goals

Sometimes the process of assessment is therapeutic in itself—raising self-awareness and validating an individual's symptom experience. Setting goals and outcome criteria formalizes the plan of care and encourages participation in self-care. Goals should include both health-related outcomes and other outcomes, such as functional status and economic impact. Combination therapies, rather than single therapies, may be more beneficial (ACOG, 2023). Models of symptom management that combine self-care, social support, medical therapies, and psychosocial strategies applied to specific conditions have shown promising results (ACOG, 2023). Moreover, outcomes from symptom management programs suggest that when symptoms are comprehensively managed, people are more likely to remain in treatment and demonstrate improved outcomes (Liguori et al., 2023).

Health-Promoting Strategies

Regular physical activity has many health advantages and can significantly improve all aspects of PMS symptoms (Liguori et al., 2023). The type of exercise (e.g., walking, yoga) varies across studies as did the dosage so the optimal regimen is unclear and most likely varies widely from individual to individual. Clinicians should encourage regular physical activity tailored to the patient as an approach to improving overall health and potentially improving PMS symptoms rather than specify a certain exercise regimen. Strategies that generally promote overall health, such as eating a balanced diet, daily exercise, obtaining adequate sleep, and reducing stress, have long been promoted as actions that positively impact premenstrual symptoms. Although no particular diet has been shown to consistently offer relief from premenstrual disorders, clinicians often recommend decreasing refined sugar and simple carbohydrates, sodium, and dairy products (Modzelewski et al., 2024). Healthy, balanced diets that support overall health should be encouraged over a focus on specific dietary restrictions.

Nonpharmacologic Strategies

Quality studies are sparse for most nonpharmacologic interventions for premenstrual disorders despite growing public interest and an overwhelming volume of anecdotal information available on the internet. Although first-line recommendations continue to be pharmacologic, people who prefer or require nonpharmacologic interventions may benefit from these therapies.

Acupuncture/Acupressure

Studies of acupuncture as an intervention for alleviating PMS symptoms vary in the type of treatment administered, the number of sessions, and the treatment timing with the menstrual cycle (Carlini et al., 2022). A 2018 Cochrane Review found that symptom improvement has been reported in both physical and psychological PMS symptoms with acupuncture and acupressure (Armour et al., 2018). Although the lack of large RCTs limits the ability to robustly recommend acupuncture or acupressure, it remains an option with minimal side effects and minimal harm (ACOG, 2023).

Dietary and Herbal Supplements

Herbs that are most widely used in the treatment of PMS symptoms include *Vitex agnus-castus*, curcumin, cramp bark, and evening primrose oil; however, there is little evidence to document their safety or efficacy. These herbs are available without a prescription at many pharmacies and health food stores. Preliminary data indicate that curcumin (the compound responsible for turmeric's yellow hue) dietary supplements may be beneficial for the treatment of premenstrual disorders (Bahrami et al., 2021). In a small study of participants with premenstrual symptoms and dysmenorrhea, those in the treatment group (500 mg curcumin by capsule daily) had lower premenstrual symptoms than the control group and less pain although the difference did not reach statistical significance due to small sample size (Bahrami et al., 2021).

Native to the Mediterranean region and central Asia, *Vitex agnus-castus* (also known as chasteberry) is a shrub that produces small dark brown fruit that is processed into an extract or powder for ingestion. Although it has been used for centuries to treat menstrual irregularities and premenstrual disorders, and reports of side effects are rare, a systematic review of 14 studies found little evidence to support its efficacy in treatment of PMS (Verkaik et al., 2017). A more recent preliminary study suggested that *Vitex agnus-castus* along with vitamin B_6 and magnesium may decrease premenstrual physical symptoms as well as improve quality of life (Sureja et al., 2023). Additional information on the use of herbs and dietary supplements can be obtained by providers and patients from the National Center for Complementary and Integrative Health (https://nccih.nih.gov) or a textbook resource such as *Integrative Medicine*, 5th ed. (Rakel & Minichiello, 2022).

Because estrogen can lower calcium levels, supplemental calcium during the luteal phase of the menstrual cycle may be beneficial for premenstrual symptoms. A 2020 systematic review found sufficient evidence in 14 studies to support this, but noted that this conclusion was limited by small, non-RCT trials (Arab et al., 2020). While large studies of the effects on premenstrual disorders are lacking, calcium intake or supplementation at recommended levels (1,000–1,200 mg/day for supplementation not to exceed 2,500 mg/d total) is beneficial for overall health as well as bone health (ACOG, 2023).

Pharmacological Therapies

Selective Serotonin Reuptake Inhibitors (SSRIs) Typically, the first choice in pharmacologic treatment, especially for improvement of PMS and PMDD with predominantly emotional symptoms such as irritability, is selective serotonin reuptake inhibitors (SSRIs) (ACOG, 2023). A Cochrane Review of 34 RCTs comparing SSRIs to placebo suggests that SSRIs reduce symptoms in individuals with PMS and PMDD, compared to placebo (Jespersen et al., 2024). SSRIs were more effective when taken continuously versus only in the luteal phase of the menstrual cycle (Jespersen et al., 2024). Only three SSRIs—fluoxetine, sertraline, and paroxetine—have been approved by the FDA for treatment of PMDD, although essentially all SSRIs have been shown in RCTs to be efficacious in reducing PMS and PMDD symptoms (Reilly et al., 2023). Although the onset of SSRI therapeutic benefit when treating major depressive disorders can take several weeks, patients may report PMS and PMDD symptom improvement within a few days of starting SSRIs (Reilly et al., 2023). This may be because a different receptor site is involved with premenstrual disorders than with depressive disorders (Reilly et al., 2023).

Because of the relatively rapid onset of benefit from SSRIs, individuals can be treated with either continuous or intermittent therapy, which means taking the SSRI only during the second half of the menstrual cycle (**Box 24-3**). This type of dosing may decrease medication-related side effects and minimize exposure to pharmacotherapy but may decrease the efficacy of the treatment (Jespersen et al., 2024). Paroxetine is the only medication that should not be taken cyclically because it produces the most pronounced discontinuation effects.

Side effects associated with SSRIs may include gastrointestinal complaints, headaches, sleep disturbances, dizziness or drowsiness, unintended weight changes, and dry mouth (Jespersen et al., 2024). Some people have sexual side effects, such as decreased libido or difficulty achieving orgasm (Jespersen et al., 2024). Because side effects with SSRIs are dose dependent, trialing a lower dose or using the intermittent dosing regimen may reduce or resolve side effects. As when treating other conditions, the recommendation is to initially prescribe lower doses of SSRIs and increase after 1 to 2 months if indicated. Although improvement of symptoms was seen in low doses, some people experienced greater improvement with moderate doses (20 mg vs. 10 mg of escitalopram), particularly if intermittent or symptom-onset dosing is used (Reilly et al., 2023). SSRIs should be taken for at least two menstrual cycles to adequately assess their benefit or failure. Approximately 15 percent of people do not experience relief with these drugs after two cycles and may benefit from an increase in dosage, a switch to another SSRI, or initiation of an alternative therapy (ACOG, 2023).

BOX 24-3 Dosing Regimens of SSRIs for Treatment of PMS/PMDD

- Continuous: Daily dosing every day of the cycle; used for patients with concomitant mood disorder, difficulty adhering to nondaily dosing, or cycles that vary greatly in length
- Intermittent: Begin daily dosing of medication with ovulation and continue through the first 1 to 2 days of menses; used for patients with predictable cycles who prefer to avoid daily dosing, possibly due to side effects
- Semi-intermittent: Daily dosing with lower daily dose outside of luteal phase; used for patients who prefer or benefit from daily dosing and who want to minimize dose-dependent side effects
- Symptom-onset dosing: Begin daily dosing of medication with onset of symptoms and continue until the onset of menses; this is the most individually tailored regimen

Data from di Scalea, T. L., & Pearlstein, T. (2019). Premenstrual dysphoric disorder. *Medical Clinics of North America, 103*(4), 613–628. https://doi.org/10.1016/j.mcna.2019.02.007

Hormonal Contraception Combined oral contraceptives contain both estrogen and progesterone and have been widely used to treat symptoms of PMS and PMDD, although there is greater success in relieving physical symptoms, such as pain, than psychological symptoms, such as mood or anxiety. Combined hormonal contraception can be administered via pills, patch, or vaginal ring and are a preferred option for individuals who would like contraception in addition to premenstrual symptom management. Only combined oral contraceptives that contain the progesterone drospirenone in addition to ethinyl estradiol (DRSP-EE) are FDA approved to treat premenstrual disorders (National Library of Medicine, 2023). A 2023 Cochrane review of five RCTs examining only DRSP-EE COCs reported a reduction in overall PMS symptoms and improved ability to engage in social and work functions, but reinforced earlier findings of greater side effects such as breast pain, nausea, and intermenstrual bleeding (Ma & Song, 2023). There was also no difference noted between using combined oral contraceptives or placebo for reported premenstrual mood symptoms (Ma & Song, 2023). Despite only DRSP-EE formulations holding FDA approval for treatment of PMDD, a recent meta-analysis concluded that all combined oral contraceptives used in the studies improved PMS symptoms except mood (Ma & Song, 2023). The authors also noted that there was no significant difference between continuous and cyclic monthly dosing, despite earlier research suggesting that continuous dosing had greater efficacy (de Wit et al., 2021).

Additional Pharmacologic Approaches to Ovarian Suppression Other methods of ovarian suppression have been studied to determine their utility in treating PMDD. High doses of estrogen (100 to 200 mg/day via transdermal patches) demonstrated improvements in symptoms; however, due to the risks created by unopposed estrogen, progesterone must be added to the regimen, which can then cause a return of symptoms. Additionally, the evidence to support this recommendation is weak (Carlini et al., 2022). Progesterone-only regimens were reviewed and found to have no benefit on PMS symptoms (ACOG, 2023).

Gonadotropin-releasing hormone analogs are medications used to aggressively suppress ovulation and have been used for people who are unable to find symptom relief from other therapies. Although they are a powerful therapeutic tool, the menopause-like side effects can be significant and include vaginal dryness and atrophy, hot flashes, decreased libido, and insomnia. Add-back therapy may ameliorate some of the negative effects, but adding estrogen and progesterone may cause premenstrual

TABLE 24-2 Effectiveness of Various Therapies for Menstrual Cycle Pain, PMS, and PMDD

		Dysmenorrhea	PMS	PMDD
Lifestyle modification	Aerobic exercise	Effective	Effective	May be effective
	Yoga	May be effective	May be effective	No studies
	Decrease caffeine, sugar, or alcohol		May be effective	No studies
Dietary supplements	Calcium		May be effective	No studies
	B complex vitamins		May be effective	No studies
	Magnesium	May be effective		
	Fish oil	May be effective		
Herbal supplements	*V. agnus-castus* (chasteberry)		May be effective	May be effective
	Hypericum perforatum (St. John's wort)		May be effective	May be effective
Nonpharmacologic therapies	Cognitive behavioral therapy		May be effective	May be effective
	Bright light therapy		May be effective	May be effective
	Heat	Effective		
	TENS	May be effective		
	Acupuncture/massage	May be effective	May be effective	May be effective
Analgesics	Acetaminophen	May be effective		
	NSAIDs	Effective	May be effective	May be effective
Hormonal therapies	Combined estrogen/progesterone oral contraceptives	Effective	May be effective if drospirenone is the progesterone	May be effective if drospirenone is the progesterone
	Progesterone-only therapies	Effective	Not effective	Not effective
Other pharmacologic therapies	SSRIs, either continuous or cyclical		Effective	Effective
	Anxiolytics (short-term use only)			May be effective if anxiety is primary symptom

Abbreviation: TENS, transcutaneous electrical nerve stimulation.

symptoms to reoccur (Carlini et al., 2022). Surgical oophorectomy, an irreversible therapeutic option, should be considered only as a last resort (ACOG, 2023).

Table 24-2 lists the effectiveness of various therapies for menstrual cycle pain, PMS, and PMDD.

Considerations for Specific Populations

Although dysmenorrhea and PMS/PMDD may affect any person of reproductive age, clinicians must be sensitive to how they may affect specific populations uniquely.

Adolescents

Primary dysmenorrhea disproportionately affects younger individuals and symptoms are most pronounced in adolescents (Harley et al., 2024). Studies have also found that adolescents aged 13 to 19 years who have PMS/PMDD are at increased risk for depression and anxiety (Mann & Ts, 2023). Clinicians caring for young people should address menstruation, mood, and opportunities for education throughout the adolescent years. Although hormonal medications as a treatment may be beneficial for adolescents who also desire reliable contraception, there may be stigma or parental concern about its use. Additionally, the first-line treatment for premenstrual disorders, SSRIs, received an FDA black box warning in 2004 for use in adolescents due to concerns arising in 24 clinical trials about an increased rate of suicidal thoughts or attempts, although no deaths by suicide were reported by these studies. Therefore, while there is no contraindication to the use of SSRIs in adolescents, clinicians should use caution and close monitoring (ACOG, 2023).

People Who Are Pregnant

Two recent systematic reviews found overwhelming evidence that people with a history of PMS/PMDD are at greater risk for perinatal depression (Pereira et al., 2022), primarily postpartum (Cao et al., 2020). Although this is likely due to hormonal variations similar to those during the luteal phase of the menstrual cycle, the etiology remains unclear (Pataky & Ehlert, 2020). Cao et al. (2021) reported that participants who reported they "sometimes or often" had PMS were significantly more likely to develop postpartum depression, and recommended screening pregnant patients for a history of PMS to identify at-risk individuals.

Perimenopause and People Who Are Older

Although individuals typically experience relief of both dysmenorrhea and PMS/PMDD when the menstrual cycle ceases (Hantsoo et al., 2023), there is evidence that a history of PMDD is correlated with an increased likelihood of mood changes during perimenopause (Sander & Gordon, 2021). Individuals with a previous diagnosis of PMDD who are considering hormone replacement therapy for symptoms such as hot flashes should be counseled that the side effects of the added progesterone therapy (if needed for an intact uterus) may be very similar to PMDD symptoms (Sander & Gordon, 2021). More information regarding perimenopause and menopause is provided in Chapter 14.

CONCLUSION

Menstrual cycle disorders, including dysmenorrhea, PMS, and PMDD, are better understood now than they were in the past. More research, particularly related to lifestyle and nonpharmacologic options for treatment, is needed. Clinicians working collaboratively with their patients to ensure that their voice and opinions are heard and validated will result in the best outcomes. Integration of pharmacologic and complementary therapies is optimal to treat these conditions holistically and within the context of the patient's lived experience.

References

Åkerman, E., Wängborg, A., Persson, M., Sörensdotter, R., & Klingberg-Allvin, M. (2024). Navigating menstrual stigma and norms: A qualitative study on young people's menstrual experiences and strategies for improving menstrual health. *BMC Public Health, 24*, 1–14. https://doi.org/10.1186/s12889-024-20936-5

Ali, M., Akin, A., Bahamondes, L., Brache, V., Habib, N., Landoulsi, S., & Hubacher, D., (2017). For the WHO study group on subdermal contraceptive implants for women. Extended use up to 5 years of the etonogestrel-releasing subdermal contraceptive implant: Comparison to levonorgestrel-releasing subdermal implant. *Human Reproduction, 31*(11), 2491–2498. https://doi.org/10.1093/humrep/dew222

Alshammari, H., Alrabiah, A., Shaheen, S., Mazi, S., & Aljasser, R. (2024). Menstrual cycle changes after the COVID-19 vaccine: A cross-sectional study in Saudi Arabia. *Journal of Nature and Science of Medicine, 7*(3), Article 3. U-M Articles Search. https://doi.org/10.4103/jnsm.jnsm_169_22

American College of Obstetricians and Gynecologists' Committee on Clinical Consensus–Gynecology. (2022). General approaches to medical management of menstrual suppression: ACOG Clinical Consensus No. 3. *Obstetrics and Gynecology (New York, 1953), 140*(3), 528–541. https://doi.org/10.1097/AOG.0000000000004899.

American College of Obstetricians and Gynecologists. (2023). Management of premenstrual disorders: ACOG clinical practice guideline no. 7. *Obstetrics and Gynecology (New York, 1953), 142*(6). U-M Articles Search. https://doi.org/10.1097/AOG.0000000000005426

American College of Obstetricians and Gynecologists. (2023). *Depot medroxyprogesterone acetate and bone effects: Committee opinion no. 602.* https://www.acog.org/Clinical Guidance-and-Publications/Committee-Opinions/Committee-on-Adolescent-HealthCare/Depot-Medroxyprogesterone-Acetate -and-Bone-Effects

American College of Obstetricians and Gynecologists. (2024). Long-acting reversible contraception implants and intrauterine devices: Practice bulletin no. 186. *Obstetrics & Gynecology, 1*(30), e251–e269. https://www.acog.org/clinical/clinical-guidance/practice-bulletin/articles/2017/11/long-acting-reversible-contraception-implants-and-intrauterine-devices

Amza, M., Findeklee, S., Haj H., Sima, R., Poenaru, M., Popescu, M., & Pleş, L. (2024). Dysmenorrhea and its impact on patients' quality of life—A cross-sectional study. *Journal of Clinical Medicine, 13*(19), 5660. https://doi.org/10.3390/jcm13195660

Arab, A., Rafie, N., Askari, G., & Taghiabadi, M. (2020). Beneficial role of calcium in premenstrual syndrome: A systematic review of current literature. *International Journal of Preventive Medicine, 11*(1), 156. https://doi.org/10.4103/ijpvm.IJPVM_243_19

Armour, M., Ee, C. C., Hao, J., Wilson, T. M., Yao, S. S., & Smith, C. A. (2018). Acupuncture and acupressure for premenstrual syndrome. *Cochrane Database of Systematic Reviews.* https://doi.org/10.1002/14651858.CD005290.pub2

Armour, M., Parry, K., Manohar, N., Holmes, K., Ferfolja, T., Curry, C., MacMillan, F., & Smith, C. A. (2019). The prevalence and academic impact of dysmenorrhea in 21, 573 young women: A systematic review and meta-analysis. *Journal of Women's Health (2002), 28*(8), 1161–1171. https://doi.org/10.1089/jwh.2018.7615

Ataş, K., Poyraz IŞleyen, T., & Kaya Mutlu, E. (2023). The incidence of dysmenorrhea in university students during the COVID-19 pandemic and social isolation process: A cross-sectional study. *Turkiye Klinikleri Journal of Health Sciences, 8*(2), 284–291. https://doi.org/10.5336/healthsci.2022-93857

Bahrami, A., Zarban, A., Rezapour, H., Agha Amini Fashami, A., & Ferns, G. A. (2021). Effects of curcumin on menstrual pattern, premenstrual syndrome, and dysmenorrhea: A triple-blind, placebo-controlled clinical trial. *Phytotherapy Research: PTR, 35*(12), 6954–6962. https://doi.org/10.1002/ptr.7314

Baker, F. C., & Lee, K. A. (2018). Menstrual cycle effects on sleep. *Sleep Medicine Clinics, 13*(3), 283–294. https://doi.org/10.1016/j.jsmc.2018.04.002

Bernardi, M., Lazzeri, L., Perelli, F., Reis, F. M., & Petraglia, F. (2017). Dysmenorrhea and related disorders. *F1000Res*, 6, 1645. https://doi.org/10.12688/f1000research.11682.1

Biro, F. M., & Bloemer, N. L. (2019). Complementary medicine: Complementary and alternative health approaches in pediatric and adolescent gynecology. *Journal of Pediatric and Adolescent Gynecology, 32*(1), 3–6. https://doi.org/10.1016/j.jpag.2018.10.011

Błażejewski, G., & Witkos, J. (2023). The impact of COVID-19 on menstrual cycle in women. *Journal of Clinical Medicine, 12*(15), Article 15. U-M Articles Search. https://doi.org/10.3390/jcm12154991

Cao, S., Jones, M., Tooth, L., & Mishra, G. (2020). History of premenstrual syndrome and development of postpartum depression: A systematic review and meta-analysis. *Journal of Psychiatric Research, 121,* 82–90. https://doi.org/10.1016/j.jpsychires.2019.11.010

Cao, S., Jones, M., Tooth, L. & Mishra, G. (2021). Does premenstrual syndrome before pregnancy increase the risk of postpartum depression? Findings from the Australian Longitudinal Study on Women's Health. *Journal of Affective Disorders, 279,* 143–148. https://doi.org/10.1016/j.jad.2020.09.130.

Carlini, S. V., di Scalea, T. L., McNally, S. T., Lester, J., & Deligiannidis, K. M. (2022). Management of premenstrual dysphoric disorder: A scoping review. *International Journal of Women's Health, 14,* 1783–1801. https://doi.org/10.2147/IJWH.S297062

Chen, H., Malentacchi, F., Fambrini, M., Harrath, A. H., Huang, H., & Petraglia, F. (2020). Epigenetics of estrogen and progesterone receptors in endometriosis. *Reproductive Sciences (Thousand Oaks, Calif.), 27*(11), 1967–1974. https://doi.org/10.1007/s43032-020-00226-2

Chen, Y, Chiang, Y., Lin, Y., Huang, K., Chen, H., Hamdy, N., Huang, T., Chang, H., Shieh, T., Huang, Y. & Hsia, S. (2023). Effect of Vitamin D supplementation on primary dysmenorrhea: A systematic review and meta-analysis of randomized clinical trials. *Nutrients, 15*(13), Article 13. U-M Articles Search. https://doi.org/10.3390/nu15132830

Cockrum, R. H., Tu, F. F., Kierzkowska, O., Leloudas, N., Pottumarthi, P. V., & Hellman, K. M. (2024). Ultrasound and magnetic resonance imaging–based investigation of the role of perfusion and oxygen availability in menstrual pain. *American Journal of Obstetrics and Gynecology, 230*(5), 553.e1–553.e14. https://doi.org/10.1016/j.ajog.2024.01.018

Contreras-Rendon, A., Garcia Vences, E. E., & Olguin Ortega, A. A. (2024). The evaluation of menstrual alterations in Mexican women after vaccination against COVID-19. *Cureus, 16*(4), e58783. https://doi.org/10.7759/cureus.58783

Deogade, M. S., Tahlan, N., Anjum, S., Parwati, J. S., Bhati, D., Acharyya, A., & Nesari, T. M. (2023). Dysmenorrhea and heavy bleeding as complications in COVID-19-positive women: An observational study. *Journal of Family Medicine and Primary Care, 12*(9), 1849–1853. https://doi.org/10.4103/jfmpc.jfmpc_1988_22

de Wit, A. E., de Vries, Y. A., de Boer, M. K., Scheper, C., Fokkema, A., Janssen, C. A. H., Giltay, E. J., & Schoevers, R. A. (2021). Efficacy of combined oral contraceptives for depressive symptoms and overall symptomatology in premenstrual syndrome: Pairwise and network meta-analysis of randomized trials. *American Journal of Obstetrics and Gynecology, 225*(6), 624–633, https://doi.org/10.1016/j.ajog.2021.06.090

Dilbaz, B., & Aksan, A. (2021). Premenstrual syndrome, a common but underrated entity: Review of the clinical literature. *Journal of the Turkish German Gynecological Association, 22*(2), 139–148. https://doi.org/10.4274/jtgga.galenos.2021.2020.0133

di Scalea, T. L., & Pearlstein, T. (2019). Premenstrual dysphoric disorder. *Medical Clinics of North America, 103*(4), 613–628. https://doi.org/10.1016/j.mcna.2019.02.007

Dong, Q. Y., Yang, X. F., Liu, B. P., Zhang, Y. Y., Wan, L. P., & Jia, C. X. (2023). Menstrual pain mediated the association between daytime sleepiness and suicidal risk: A prospective study. *Journal of Affective Disorders, 328*, 238–244. https://doi.org/10.1016/j.jad.2023.02.041

Endicott, J., Nee, J., & Harrison, W. (2006). Daily record of severity of problems (DRSP): Reliability and validity. *Archives of Women's Mental Health, 9*(1), 43.

Ezebialu, I., Ezenyeaku, C., & Umeobika, J. (2021). Prevalence of dysmenorrhea and its contribution to school absenteeism among Nigerian undergraduate students. *Annals of Health Research (Onabanjo University Teaching Hospital), 7*(1), Article 1. U-M Articles Search. https://doi.org/10.30442/ahr.0701-07-116

Farland, L. V., Khan, S. M., Shilen, A., Heslin, K. M., Ishimwe, P., Allen, A. M., Herbst-Kralovetz, M. M., Mahnert, N. D., Pogreba-Brown, K., Ernst, K. C., & Jacobs, E. T. (2023). COVID-19 vaccination and changes in the menstrual cycle among vaccinated persons. *Fertility and Sterility, 119*(3), 392–400. https://doi.org/10.1016/j.fertnstert.2022.12.023

Ferrero, S., Evangelisti, G., & Barra, F. (2018). Current and emerging treatment options for endometriosis. *Expert Opinion on Pharmacotherapy, 19*(10), 1109–1125. https://doi.org/10.1080/14656566.2018.1494154

Ferries-Rowe, E., Corey., E., & Archer, J. (2020). Primary dysmenorrhea: Diagnosis and therapy. *Obstetrics and Gynecology (New York. 1953), 136*(5), 1047–1058. U-M Articles Search. https://doi.org/10.1097/AOG.0000000000004096

Francavilla, R., Petraroli, M., Messina, G., Stanyevic, B., Bellani, A. M., Esposito, S. M. R., & Street, M. E. (2023). Dysmenorrhea: Epidemiology, causes, and current state of the art for treatment. *Clinical and Experimental Obstetrics & Gynecology, 50*(12), 274–289. https://doi.org/10.31083/j.ceog5012274

Fuentes-Aparicio, L., C.-M., Ferran, Muñoz-Gómez, E., Mollà-Casanova, S., Aguilar-Rodríguez, M., Sempere-Rubio, N. (2023). Effects of therapeutic exercise in primary dysmenorrhea: An umbrella and mapping review. *Pain Medicine (Malden, Mass.), 24*(12), 1386–1395. https://doi.org/10.1093/pm/pnad104

Funnell, E. L., Martin-Key, N. A., Benacek, J., Spadaro, B., & Bahn, S. (2024). Preferences for and intention to use an app for premenstrual mental health symptoms using the Health Behaviour Model (HBM). *NPJ Women's Health, 2*(1), 1–10. https://doi.org/10.1038/s44294-024-00014-2

Gagnon, M. M., Moussaoui, D., Gordon, J. L., Alberts, N. M. & Grover, S. R. (2022). Dysmenorrhea across the lifespan: A biopsychosocial perspective to understanding the dysmenorrhea trajectory and association with comorbid pain experiences. *Pain (Amsterdam), 163*(11), 2069–2075. https://doi.org/10.1097/j.pain.0000000000002649.

Gopalan, S. S., Mann, C., & Rhodes, R. E. (2024). Impact of symptoms, experiences, and perceptions of the menstrual cycle on recreational physical activity of cyclically menstruating individuals: A systematic review. *Preventive Medicine, 184*, 107980. https://doi.org/10.1016/j.ypmed.2024.107980

Güzeldere, H. K. B., Efendioğlu, E. H., Mutlu, S., Esen, H. N., Karaca, G. N., & Çağırdar, B. (2024). The relationship between dietary habits and menstruation problems in women: A cross-sectional study. *BMC Women's Health, 24*(1), 397. https://doi.org/10.1186/s12905-024-03235-4

Harley, K. G., Watson, A., Robertson, S., Vitzthum, V. J., & Shea, A. (2024). Menstrual cycle characteristics of U.S. adolescents according to gynecologic age and age at menarche. *Journal of Pediatric & Adolescent Gynecology* 37(4), 419–425. https://doi.org/10.1016/j.jpag.2024.03.005

Harrison, J. E., Weber, S., Jakob, R., & Chute, C. G. (2021). ICD-11: An international classification of diseases for the twenty-first century. *BMC Medical Informatics and Decision Making, 21*(Suppl 6), 206. https://doi.org/10.1186/s12911-021-01534-6

Henz, A., Ferreira, C. F., Oderich, C. L., Gallon, C. W., Castro, J. R. S., Conzatti, M., Fleck, M. P. A., & Wender, M. C. O. (2018). Premenstrual syndrome diagnosis: A comparative study between the daily record of severity of problems (DRSP) and the premenstrual symptoms screening tool (PSST). Diagnóstico de síndrome pré-menstrual: um estudo comparativo entre o relato diário da gravidade dos problemas (DRSP) e o instrumento de rastreamento de sintomas pré-menstruais (PSST). *Revista brasileira de ginecologia e obstetricia: revista da Federacao Brasileira das Sociedades de Ginecologia e Obstetricia, 40*(1), 20–25. https://doi.org/10.1055/s-0037-1608672

Ishikura, I. A., da Silva Vallim, J. R., Fernandes, G. L., Moysés-Oliveira, M., Hachul, H., Tufik, S., & Andersen, M. L. (2024). Altered sleep and diurnal consequences in women with dysmenorrhea: Study from the EPISONO database. *Archives of Gynecology and Obstetrics, 310*(3), 1659–1667. https://doi.org/10.1007/s00404-024-07668-y

Jespersen, C., Lauritsen, M. P., Frokjaer, V. G., & Schroll, J. B. (2024). Selective serotonin reuptake inhibitors for premenstrual syndrome and premenstrual dysphoric disorder. *The Cochrane Database of Systematic Reviews, 8*(8), CD001396. https://doi.org/10.1002/14651858.CD001396.pub4

Jo, J., & Lee, S. H. (2018). Heat therapy for primary dysmenorrhea: A systematic review and meta-analysis of its effects on pain relief and quality of life. *Scientific Reports, 8*(1), 16252. https://doi.org/10.1038/s41598-018-34303-z

Keshavarzi, F., Mahmoudzadeh, F., Brand, S., Sadeghi Bahmani, D., Akbari, F., Khazaie, H., & Ghadami, M. R. (2018). Both melatonin and meloxicam improved sleep and pain with primary dysmenorrhea—Results from a double-blind cross-over intervention pilot study. *Archives of Women's Mental Health, 21*(6), 601–609. https://doi.org/10.1007/s00737-018-0838-x

Kim, S. D. (2020). Quality of safety reporting for complementary and alternative therapies for dysmenorrhea. *Complementary Therapies in Clinical Practice, 39*, 101160. https://doi.org/10.1016/j.ctcp.2020.101160

Koninckx, P. R., Fernandes, R., Ussia, A., Schindler, L., Wattiez, A., Al-Suwaidi, S., Amro, B., Al-Maamari, B., Hakim, Z., & Tahlak, M. (2021). Pathogenesis based diagnosis and treatment of endometriosis. *Frontiers in Endocrinology, 12*, 745548. https://doi.org/10.3389/fendo.2021.745548

LaForge, J. M., Urso, K., Day, J. M., Bourgeois, C. W., Ross, M. M., Ahmadzadeh, S., Shekoohi, S., Cornett, E. M., Kaye, A. M., & Kaye, A. D. (2023). Non-steroidal anti-inflammatory drugs: Clinical implications, renal impairment risks, and AKI. *Advances in Therapy, 40*(5), 2082–2096. https://doi.org/10.1007/s12325-023-02481-6

Lazorwitz, A., Aquilante, C., Dindinger, E., Harrison, M., Sheeder, J., & Teal, S. (2019). Relationship between etonogestrel concentrations and bleeding patterns in contraceptive implant users. *Obstetrics & Gynecology, 134*(4), 807–813. https://doi.org/10.1097/AOG.0000000000003452.

Li, X., Hao, X., Liu, J. H., & Huang, J. P. (2024). Efficacy of non-pharmacological interventions for primary dysmenorrhoea: A systematic review and Bayesian network meta-analysis. *BMJ Evidence-Based Medicine, 29*(3), 162–170. https://doi.org/10.1136/bmjebm-2023-112434

Liang, X., Wang, Q., Jiang, Z., Li, Z., Zhang, M., Yang, P., Wang, X., Wang, Y., Qin, Y., Li, T., Zhang, T., Wang, Y., Sun, J., Li, Y., Luo, H., & Li, L. (2020). Clinical research linking Traditional Chinese Medicine constitution types with diseases: A literature review of 1639 observational studies. *Journal of Traditional Chinese Medicine, Chung i tsa chih ying wen pan, 40*(4), 690–702. https://doi.org/10.19852/j.cnki.jtcm.2020.04.019

Liguori, F., Saraiello, E., & Calella, P. (2023). Premenstrual syndrome and premenstrual dysphoric disorder's impact on quality of life, and the role of physical activity. *Medicina (Kaunas, Lithuania), 59*(11), 2044. https://doi.org/10.3390/medicina59112044

Liisa Hantsoo, Jennifer L. Payne. (2023). Towards understanding the biology of premenstrual dysphoric disorder: From genes to GABA. *Neuroscience & Biobehavioral Reviews, 149* (105168), ISSN 0149-7634. https://doi.org/10.1016/j.neubiorev.2023.105168.

Liu, W., Wang, C. C., Lee, K. H., Ma, X., & Kang, T. L. (2022). Research methodology in acupuncture and moxibustion for managing primary dysmenorrhea: A scoping review. *Complementary Therapies in Medicine, 71*, 102874. https://doi.org/10.1016/j.ctim.2022.102874

Liu, X., Li, R., Wang, S., & Zhang, J. (2024). Global, regional, and national burden of premenstrual syndrome, 1990–2019: An analysis based on the Global Burden of Disease Study 2019. *Human Reproduction (Oxford, England), 39*(6), 1303–1315. https://doi.org/10.1093/humrep/deae081

Ma, S., & Song, S. J. (2023). Oral contraceptives containing drospirenone for premenstrual syndrome. *Cochrane Database of Systematic Reviews 2023, 6*(6), CD006586. https://doi.org/10.1002/14651858.CD006586.pub5

Maceira, D., Oizerovich, S., Perrotta, G., de León, R. G. P., Karolinski, A., Suarez, N., ... Chandra-Mouli, V. (2023). Acceptability and continuation of use of the subdermal contraceptive implant among adolescents and young women in Argentina: A retrospective cohort study. *Sexual and Reproductive Health Matters, 31*(1). https://doi.org/10.1080/26410397.2023.2189507

Maher, M., O' Keeffe, A., Phelan, N., Behan, L. A., Collier, S., Hevey, D., & Owens, L. (2022). Female reproductive health disturbance experienced during the COVID-19 pandemic correlates with mental health disturbance and sleep quality. *Frontiers in Endocrinology, 13*, 838886. https://doi.org/10.3389/fendo.2022.838886

Mann, P., & Ts, P. (2023). Premenstrual syndrome, anxiety, and depression among menstruating rural adolescent girls: A community-based cross-sectional study. *Cureus, 15*(12), e50385. https://doi.org/10.7759/cureus.50385

Mardon, A. K., Whitaker, L., Farooqi, T., Girling, J., Henry, C., Ee, C., Tewhaiti-Smith, J., & Armour, M. (2024). Investigational drugs for the treatment of dysmenorrhea. *Expert Opinion on Investigational Drugs, 33*(4), 347–357. https://doi.org/10.1080/13543784.2024.2326627

Matar, S. G., Nourelden, A. Z., Assar, A., Bahbah, E. I., Alfryjat, A. M., Hasabo, E. A., Matar, S. A., Bishtawi, S. N., Alhoubani, M., Yahia, A. B., Ragab, K. M., Salameh, L. M., Salameh, L. S. E., Zaazouee, M. S., Al-Kafarna, M., Elshanbary, A. A., Almadhoon, H. W., Bakdash, S. T., Adam, O. A. B., Malih, A. N., . . . Basheti, I. A. (2023). Effect of COVID-19 vaccine on menstrual experience among females in six Arab countries: A cross sectional study. *Influenza and Other Respiratory Viruses, 17*(1), e13088. https://doi.org/10.1111/irv.13088

Mínguez-Esteban, I., García-Ginés, P., Romero-Morales, C., Abuín-Porras, V., Navia, J. A., Alonso-Pérez, J. L., & de la Cueva-Reguera, M. (2022). Association between RNAm-Based COVID-19 vaccines and permanency of menstrual cycle alterations in Spanish women: A cross-sectional study. *Biology, 11*(11), 1579. https://doi.org/10.3390/biology11111579

Mitsuhashi, R., Sawai, A., Kiyohara, K., Shiraki, H., & Nakata, Y. (2022). Factors associated with the prevalence and severity of menstrual-related symptoms: A systematic review and meta-analysis. *International Journal of Environmental Research and Public Health, 20*(1), 569. https://doi.org/10.3390/ijerph20010569

Modzelewski, S., Oracz, A., Żukow, X., Iłendo, K., Sledzikowka, Z., & Waszkiewicz, N. (2024). Premenstrual syndrome: New insights into etiology and review of treatment methods. *Frontiers in Psychiatry, 15*, 1363875. https://doi.org/10.3389/fpsyt.2024.1363875

Monteiro, D. C., Ramos, C. da S., Alves, L. E. N. N., Cantilino, A., & Sougey, E. B. (2024). Functional and structural neuroimaging in premenstrual dysphoric disorder: A systematic review. *Journal of Psychiatric Research*, *175*, 205–210. https://doi.org/10.1016/j.jpsychires.2024.05.024

National Library of Medicine (2023). Drospirenone and ethinyl estradiol kit. *DailyMed*. https://dailymed.nlm.nih.gov/dailymed/drugInfo.cfm?setid=ea2fdcc3-f453-45f6-ae341bf3a2766eb7

Nie, W., Xu, P., Hao, C., Chen, Y., Yin, Y., & Wang, L. (2020). Efficacy and safety of over-the-counter analgesics for primary dysmenorrhea: A network meta-analysis. *Medicine*, *99*(19), e19881. https://doi.org/10.1097/MD.0000000000019881

Öksüz, E., & Guvenc, G. (2018). Relationship of premenstrual and menstrual symptoms to alexithymia among nursing students. *Perspectives in Psychiatric Care*, *54*(3), 391–397. https://doi.org/10.1111/ppc.12271

Oladosu, F. A., Hellman, K. M., Ham, P. J., Kochlefl, L. E., Datta, A., Garrison, E. F., Steiner, N. D., Roth, G. E., & Tu, F. F. (2019). Persistent autonomic dysfunction and bladder sensitivity in primary dysmenorrhea. *Scientific Reports*, *9*(1), 2194. https://doi.org/10.1038/s41598-019-38545-3

Pacitti, F., Iorio, C., Riccobono, G., Iannitelli, A., & Pompili, A. (2021). Assessment of premenstrual symptoms: Validation of the Italian version of the premenstrual symptoms screening tool. *Rivista di Psichiatria*, *56*(5), 246–253. https://doi.org/10.1708/3681.36672

Pataky, E. A., & Ehlert, U. (2020) Longitudinal assessment of symptoms of postpartum mood disorder in women with and without a history of depression. *Archives of Women's Mental Health, 23(3),* 391–99. https://doi.org/10.1007/s00737-019-00990-4

Payne, L. A., Wise, L. A., Wesselink, A. K., Wang, S., Missmer, S. A., & Edelman, A. (2024). Association between COVID-19 vaccination and menstruation: A state of the science review. *BMJ Sexual & Reproductive Health*, *50*(3), 212–225. https://doi.org/10.1136/bmjsrh-2024-202274

Pereira, D., Pessoa, A. R., Madiera, N., Macedo, A., & Pereira, A. T. (2022). Association between premenstrual dysphoric disorder and perinatal depression: A systematic review. *Archives of Women's Mental Health, 25,* 61–70. https://doi.org/10.1007/s00737-021-01177-6

Prasad, D., Wollenhaupt-Aguiar, B., Kidd, K. N., de Azevedo Cardoso, T., & Frey, B. N. (2021). Suicidal risk in women with premenstrual syndrome and premenstrual dysphoric disorder: A systematic review and meta-analysis. *Journal of Women's Health (2002)*, *30*(12), 1693–1707. https://doi.org/10.1089/jwh.2021.0185

Rakel, D. P., & Minichiello, V. (Eds.). (2022). *Integrative medicine.* Elsevier Health Sciences.

Ramirez, C., & Donnellan, N. (2017). Pelvic denervation procedures for dysmenorrhea. *Current Opinion in Obstetrics & Gynecology*, *29*(4), 225–230. https://doi.org/10.1097/GCO.0000000000000379

Ramos-Pichardo, J. D., Ortega-Galán, Á. M., Iglesias-López, M. T., Abreu-Sánchez, A., & Fernández-Martínez, E. (2020). Why do some Spanish nursing students with menstrual pain fail to consult healthcare professionals? *International Journal of Environmental Research and Public Health, 17*(21), 8173. https://doi.org/10.3390/ijerph17218173. PMID: 33167417; PMCID: PMC7663954

Rapkin, A. J., Lee, E., & Nathan, L. (2020). Pelvic pain and dysmenorrhea. In J. S. Berek (Ed.), *Berek & Novak's gynecology* (16th ed., pp. 251–278). Wolters Kluwer.

Reilly, T. J., Wallman, P., Clark, I., Knox, C.-L., Craig, M. C., & Taylor, D. (2023). Intermittent selective serotonin reuptake inhibitors for premenstrual syndromes: A systematic review and meta-analysis of randomised trials. *Journal of Psychopharmacology (Oxford, England)*, *37*(3), 261–267. https://doi.org/10.1177/02698811221099645

Sadeghi, N., Paknezhad, F., Rashidi Nooshabadi, M., Kavianpour, M., Jafari Rad, S., & Khadem Haghighian, H. (2018). Vitamin E and fish oil, separately or in combination, on treatmentof primary dysmenorrhea: A double-blind, randomized clinical trial. *Gynecological Endocrinology, 34*(9), 804–808. https://doi.org/10.1080/09513590.2018.1450377

Sakurada, Y., Matsuda, Y., Motohashi, K., Hasegawa, T., Otsuka, Y., Nakano, Y., Tokumasu, K., Yamamoto, K., Sunada, N., Honda, H., Hagiya, H., Ueda, K., & Otsuka, F. (2024). Clinical characteristics of female long COVID patients with menstrual symptoms: A retrospective study from a Japanese outpatient clinic. *Journal of Psychosomatic Obstetrics and Gynaecology*, *45*(1), 2305899. https://doi.org/10.1080/0167482X.2024.2305899

Sander, B., & Gordon, J. (2021). Premenstrual mood symptoms in the perimenopause. *Current Psychiatry Reports*, *23*(11), Article 11. U-M Articles Search. https://doi.org/10.1007/s11920-021-01285-1

Schrepf, A., Hellman, K. M., Bohnert, A. M., Williams, D. A., & Tu, F. F. (2023). Generalized sensory sensitivity is associated with comorbid pain symptoms: A replication study in women with dysmenorrhea. *Pain (Amsterdam), 164*(1), 142–48. https://doi.org/10.1097/j.pain.0000000000002676.

Schroll, J. B., Black, A. Y., Farquhar, C., & Chen, I. (2023). Combined oral contraceptive pill for primary dysmenorrhoea. *Cochrane Database of Systematic Reviews, 2023*(7). https://doi.org/10.1002/14651858.CD002120.pub4.

Shiha, M. G., & Aziz, I. (2021). Review article: Physical and psychological comorbidities associated with irritable bowel syndrome. *Alimentary Pharmacology & Therapeutics, 54 Suppl 1*, S12–S23. https://doi.org/10.1111/apt.16589

Situmorang, H., Sutanto, R. L., Tjoa, K., Rivaldo, R., & Adrian, M. (2024). Prevalence and risk factors of primary dysmenorrhoea among medical students: A cross-sectional survey in Indonesia. *BMJ Open*, *14*(10), e086052. https://doi.org/10.1136/bmjopen-2024-086052

Smaardijk, V. R., Jajou, R., Kant, A., & van Hunsel, F. P. A. M. (2024). Menstrual disorders following COVID-19 vaccination: A review using a systematic search. *Frontiers in Drug Safety and Regulation*, *4*. https://doi.org/10.3389/fdsfr.2024.1338466

Sng, B. L., Ching, Y. Y., Han, N.-L. R., Ithnin, F. B., Sultana, R., Assam, P. N., & Sia, A. T. H. (2018). Incidence and association factors for the development of chronic post-hysterectomy pain at 4- and 6-month follow-up: A prospective cohort study. *Journal of Pain Research*, *11*, 629–636. https://doi.org/10.2147/JPR.S149102

Snipe, R. M. J., Brelis, B., Kappas, C., Young, J. K., Eishold, L., Chui, J. M., Vatvani, M. D., Nigro, G. M. D., Hamilton, D. L., Convit, L., Carr, A., & Condo, D. (2024). Omega-3 long chain polyunsaturated fatty acids as a potential treatment for reducing dysmenorrhoea pain: Systematic literature review and meta-analysis. *Nutrition & dietetics: The Journal of the Dietitians Association of Australia*, *81*(1), 94–106. https://doi.org/10.1111/1747-0080.12835

Steiner, M., Macdougall, M., & Brown, E. (2003). The premenstrual symptoms screening tool (PST) for clinicians. *Archives of Women's Mental Health, 6*(3), 203–209. https://doi.org/10.1007/s00737-003-0018-4

Steiner, M., Peer, M., Palova, E., Freeman, E. W., Macdougall, M., & Soares, C. N. (2011). The premenstrual symptoms screening tool revised for adolescents (PSST-A): Prevalence of severe PMS and premenstrual dysphoric disorder in adolescents. *Archives of Women's Mental Health*, *14*(1), 77–81. https://doi.org/10.1007/s00737-010-0202-2

Sureja, V. P., Kheni, D. B., Dubey, V. P., Kansagra, J., Soni, Z. K., Bhatt, S. P., Mathuria, A., & Deshpande, S. S. (2023). Efficacy and tolerability evaluation of a nutraceutical composition containing vitex agnus-castus extract (EVX40™), pyridoxine, and magnesium in premenstrual syndrome: A real-world, interventional, comparative study. *Cureus*, *15*(8), e42832. https://doi.org/10.7759/cureus.42832

Tai, F. W. D., & McAlindon, M. E. (2021). Non-steroidal anti-inflammatory drugs and the gastrointestinal tract. *Clinical Medicine (London, England)*, *21*(2), 131–134. https://doi.org/10.7861/clinmed.2021-0039

Tandon, A., Kumar, N., Aggarwal, S., Anjana, Y., Sachdeva, M. P., Gupta, V., & Trilok-Kumar, G. (2023). Assessing menstrual changes among young Indian females post-SARS-CoV-2 vaccination. *Cureus*, *15*(12), e50025. https://doi.org/10.7759/cureus.50025

Taylor, H. S., Pal, L., & Sell, E. (2020). *Speroff's clinical gynecologic endocrinology and infertility* (9th ed.). Wolters Kluwer.

Teal, S., & Edelman, A. (2021). Contraception selection, effectiveness, and adverse effects: A review. *JAMA*, *326*(24), 2507–2518. https://doi.org/10.1001/jama.2021.21392

Tiranini, L., & Nappi, R. E. (2022). Recent advances in understanding/management of premenstrual dysphoric disorder/premenstrual syndrome. *Faculty Reviews*, *11*, 11. https://doi.org/10.12703/r/11-11

Trépanier, L. C. M., Lamoureux, É., Bjornson, S. E., Mackie, C., Alberts, N. M., & Gagnon, M. M. (2023). Smartphone apps for menstrual pain and symptom management: A scoping review. *Internet Interventions*, *31*, 100605. https://doi.org/10.1016/j.invent.2023.100605

Trogstad, L., Laake, I., Robertson, A. H., Mjaaland, S., Caspersen, I. H., Juvet, L. K., Magnus, P., Blix, K., & Feiring, B. (2023). Heavy bleeding and other menstrual disturbances in young women after COVID-19 vaccination. *Vaccine*, *41*(36), 5271–5282. https://doi.org/10.1016/j.vaccine.2023.06.088

Ussher, J. M., & Perz, J. (2020). Resisting the mantle of the monstrous feminine: Women's construction and experience of premenstrual embodiment. In C. Bobel, I. T. Winkler, B. Fahs, K. A. Hasson, E. A. Kissling, & T.-A. Roberts (Eds.), *The Palgrave handbook of critical menstruation studies*. Palgrave Macmillan. http://www.ncbi.nlm.nih.gov/books/NBK565639/

Verkaik, S., Kamperman, A. M., van Westrhenen, R., & Schulte, P. F. J. (2017). The treatment of premenstrual syndrome with preparations of *Vitex agnus castus*: A systematic review and meta-analysis. *American Journal of Obstetrics and Gynecology, 217*(2), 150-166. https://doi.org/10.1016/j.ajog.2017.02.028

Woo, H. L., Ji, H. R., Pak, Y. K., Lee, H., Heo, S. J., Lee, J. M., & Park, K. S. (2018). The efficacy and safety of acupuncture in women with primary dysmenorrhea. *Medicine, 97*(23), e11007. https://doi.org/10.1097/MD.0000000000011007

Xu, Y., Yang, Q., & Wang, X. (2020). Efficacy of herbal medicine (cinnamon/fennel/ginger) for primary dysmenorrhea: A systematic review and meta-analysis of randomized controlled trials. *The Journal of International Medical Research*, *48*(6), 300060520936179. https://doi.org/10.1177/0300060520936179

Yang, Q., Þórðardóttir, E. B., Hauksdóttir, A., Aspelund, T., Jakobsdóttir, J., Halldorsdottir, T., Tomasson, G., Rúnarsdóttir, H., Danielsdottir, H. B., Bertone-Johnson, E. R., Sjölander, A., Fang, F., Lu, D., & Valdimarsdóttir, U. A. (2022). Association between adverse childhood experiences and premenstrual disorders: A cross-sectional analysis of 11,973 women. *BMC Medicine*, *20*(1), 60. https://doi.org/10.1186/s12916-022-02275-7

Yi, S. J., Kim, M., & Park, I. (2023). Investigating influencing factors on premenstrual syndrome (PMS) among female college students. *BMC Women's Health*, *23*(1), 592. https://doi.org/10.1186/s12905-023-02752-y

CHAPTER 25

Normal and Abnormal Uterine Bleeding

Lee K. Roosevelt
Nora Drummond

The editors acknowledge Ruth Zielinski, who was a coauthor of the previous edition of this chapter.

INTRODUCTION

Abnormal uterine bleeding (AUB) is an all-encompassing term referring to any uterine bleeding that is irregular in amount, frequency, duration, or timing. It accounts for as many as one-third of all gynecologic visits (American College of Obstetrics & Gynecology, 2012, reaffirmed 2024). Although mortality from AUB is extremely uncommon, the significance of this condition lies in its effect on the physical, social, and emotional quality of life of the person experiencing the bleeding (Henry et al., 2020). People with menstrual-related problems are more likely to report anxiety, depression, insomnia, excessive sleepiness, and pain than people without menstrual-related problems (Behera et al., 2023; MacGregor et al., 2022; Wallace et al., 2022).

There are economic implications to AUB. People diagnosed with heavy menstrual bleeding (HMB) have significantly higher annual all-cause healthcare resource utilization and annual healthcare costs, compared to those who do not (Wang et al., 2022). These findings do not include intangible costs or productivity losses, such as time lost from work. Even by conservative estimates, AUB imposes a heavy economic burden.

People have identified that the impact of AUB on quality of life was not adequately addressed during clinical encounters, and clinicians' questions lack sufficient detail (Henry et al., 2020). Therefore, providing a thorough assessment of people with AUB is particularly important, sometimes necessitating multiple visits. However, it is also important to recognize that much of our knowledge and understanding of people's cyclicity is medicalized, socially constructed, or both. In some cases, "abnormal" bleeding represents a variation of normal, signifying the physiologic passage of a person's body into the next stage of development—for example, menarche or menopause. For this reason, it is vital to integrate the individual's unique lived experience into any conversations regarding menstrual cycle bleeding and to provide care that is focused on that individual's goals and preferences.

NORMAL UTERINE BLEEDING

Classifying what is meant by AUB necessitates a clear understanding of what is considered normal uterine bleeding. There is a wide variation of what constitutes normal uterine bleeding, and it is essential for healthcare providers to have a clear understanding of menstrual cycle and uterine bleeding physiology to assess what are normal versus potential interruptions of physiologic processes contributing to abnormal variations in uterine bleeding.

Normal uterine bleeding is regulated by two separate systems that work in concert with each other: the ovarian cycle and the uterine cycle. The ovarian cycle is responsible for the development and release of the oocyte in the ovary and follicular growth and maturation. The ovarian cycle consists of the follicular phase and the luteal phase. The uterine cycle involves the preparation of the inner lining of the endometrium for implantation of a fertilized ovum and shedding of the lining when implantation does not occur. The uterine cycle consists of the menstrual, proliferative, and secretory phases. The two cycles work concurrently and are tightly regulated by hormones released by the hypothalamus, pituitary gland, and ovary. A visual representation of the concurrent cycles is provided in **Figure 25-1**.

Normal uterine bleeding results from this functional hypothalamic–pituitary–ovarian axis (HPOA) and is a complex and remarkable sequence of hormonal events that leads to ovulation. If implantation does not occur, menses ensues. Normal menses varies widely in length, duration, and amount of flow, both among individuals and throughout an individual's reproductive life. Because the follicle, rather than the ovary, is responsible for estrogen and progesterone production, hormonal levels and hormonally mediated phenomena, such as volume of endometrium, can vary from month to month. Normal parameters are provided in **Table 25-1**. A key component of all sexual and reproductive health visits should be a thorough assessment of the menstrual cycle beginning with the question, "What does a normal menstrual cycle look like for you?" This open-ended, subjective question allows the person to describe their menstrual cycle and assign normalcy to the components that are not interfering with their quality of life or sense of health and wellness. Subsequent questioning may involve asking about length of time between cycles (the definition of day 1 is the first day of bleeding), duration of flow, and frequency with which they need to change pads or tampons, or empty their menstrual cup, to remain comfortable.

AUB NOMENCLATURE

AUB can occur as a normal physiologic event, such as perimenopausal changes in bleeding or ovulatory-induced changes related to puberty and adolescence. However, AUB can also signal potential pathology in need of attention, such as ectopic pregnancy or endometrial cancer. In 2007, FIGO

FIGURE 25-1 **Ovarian and uterine cycles.**

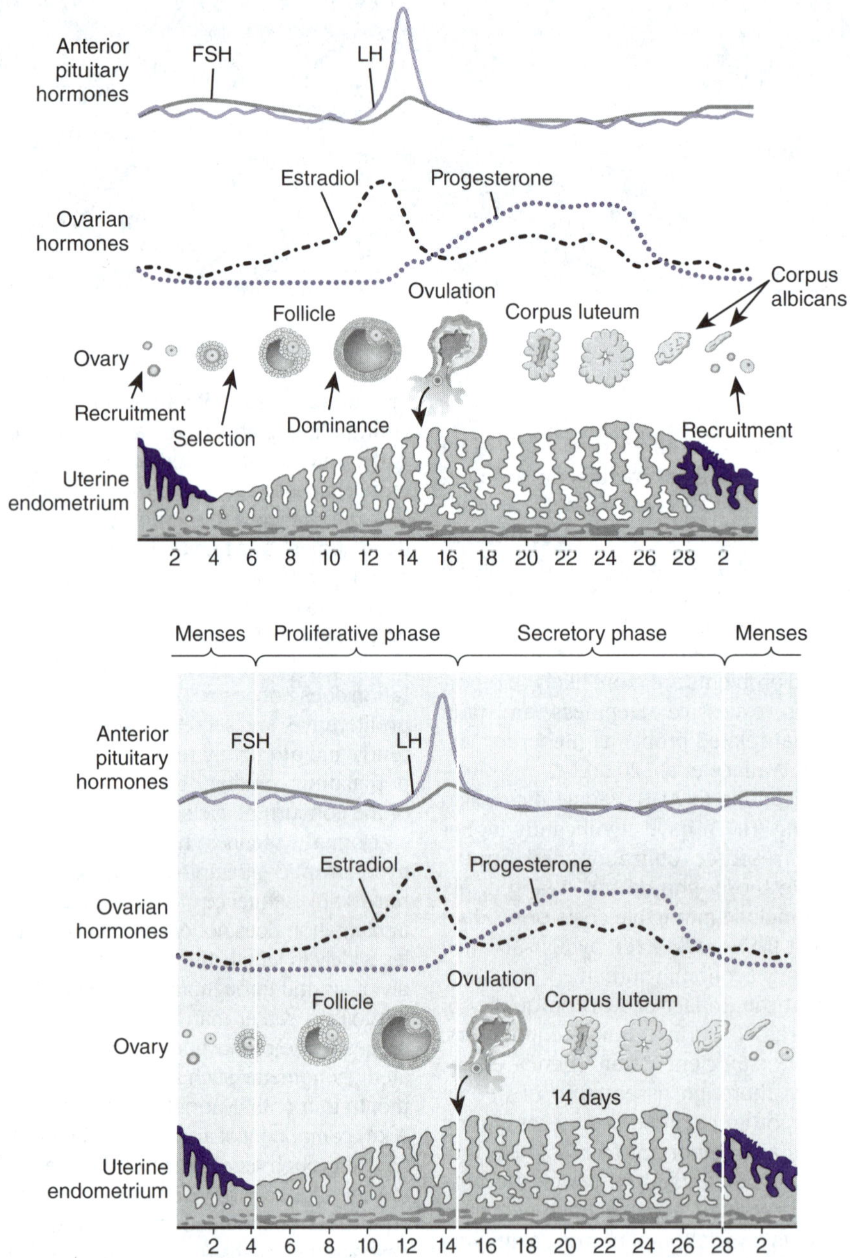

Reproduced from Nowak, R. A. (2018). Estrous and menstrual cycles. In *Encyclopedia of Reproduction: Volume 1-6,* Second Edition (Vol. 2, pp. 114–120). Elsevier. https://doi.org/10.1016/B978-0-12-801238-3.64631-7

revised the current standardized definitions in relation to AUB to ensure that healthcare providers speak the same language in research, diagnosis, and treatment. The system underwent additional modifications in 2009 and in 2018. The current system is referred to as PALM-COEIN. The acronym used to describe objective structural criteria (polyp, adenomyosis, leiomyoma, and malignancy and hyperplasia) is PALM, whereas the acronym COEIN describes categories that are unrelated to structural abnormalities (coagulopathy, ovulatory dysfunction, endometrial, iatrogenic, and not otherwise classified) (Munro et al., 2018). The components of PALM are generally discrete, structural entities that can be evaluated or measured visually using some combination of imaging techniques and histopathology; COEIN comprises entities that are

TABLE 25-1 Normal Uterine Bleeding

Parameter	Normal	Abnormal
Frequency	24 to 38 days	Absent (no bleeding)
		Infrequent (more than 38 days)
		Frequent (less than 24 days)
Duration	18–25 years old: 9 days or fewer 26–41 years old: 7 days or fewer 42–45 years old: 9 days or fewer	Prolonged (more than 8 days)
	Shortest to longest cycle variation 7 to 9 days or fewer	Shortest to longest cycle variation 8 to 10 days or more
Flow volume (patient determined)	Normal	Light
		Heavy

Data from Munro, M. G., Critchley, H. O. D., & Fraser, I. S. (2018). The two FIGO systems for normal and abnormal uterine bleeding symptoms and classification of causes of abnormal uterine bleeding in the reproductive years: 2018 revisions. *International Journal of Gynecology & Obstetrics, 143*(3), 393–408. https://doi.org/10.1002/ijgo.12666

not defined by imaging or histopathology and are considered nonstructural. By its nature, the not otherwise classified category includes a spectrum of potential entities that may or may not be measured or defined by histopathology or imaging techniques (Munro et al., 2018).

Another important distinction made by FIGO was the clear definition of what constitutes acute versus chronic AUB. These definitions remain unchanged since the 2018 update. Chronic nongestational AUB in the reproductive years is defined as bleeding from the uterus that is abnormal in duration, volume, frequency, and/or regularity and has been present for the majority of the preceding 6 months (Munro et al., 2018). Acute AUB is defined as an episode of heavy bleeding that is of sufficient quantity to require immediate intervention to minimize or prevent further blood loss. Although FIGO states that the subjective definition of "immediate intervention" should be made by clinicians (Munro et al., 2018), the authors of this chapter believe this should be a collaborative decision guided primarily by the person who is experiencing a bleeding episode that is disruptive enough for them to seek care.

In 2018, FIGO included a new section related to intermenstrual bleeding. Intermenstrual bleeding is described as bleeding between the cyclically regular onset of menses. Intermenstrual bleeding can be random or cyclic, which is predictable bleeding that may occur in the early, middle, or late part of the menstrual cycle (Munro et al., 2018).

SUBJECTIVE INFORMATION: THE EVALUATION

The Health History

The health history interview is a conversation with a purpose. The health history format provides an important framework for organizing the person's story into various categories pertinent to the person's present, past, and family history. The interviewing process that generates the person's story is fluid and requires empathy, effective communication, and relational skills to respond to patient cues, feelings, and concerns (Bickley, 2021).

Each symptom of AUB has attributes that must be classified, including context, associations, and chronology. In order to make an accurate diagnosis it is critical to understand the full context of the concern. Using a systematic approach—such as OLD CARTS (onset, location/radiation, duration, character, aggravating factors, relieving factors, timing, and severity) or OPQRST (onset, provocation/palliation, quality, region/radiation, severity, and time)—can be useful to address the essential attributes of bleeding concern, which are described in **Table 25-2**.

Identifying Other Causes of Vaginal Bleeding

In a patient with a concern of AUB, determining the location of the bleeding can be accomplished with a thorough and focused health history. People with AUB typically present with a concern about vaginal bleeding. However, there are many potential sources for genital tract bleeding, including the lower genital tract (vulva, vagina, or cervix), the urinary tract, or the gastrointestinal tract. A focused assessment includes questions that allow healthcare providers to begin to rule out bleeding from other locations (Kaunitz, 2019). The volume of bleeding gives some suggestion of the source of genital tract bleeding because heavy bleeding typically originates in the uterus, while spotting or light bleeding may originate from another genital tract site. If bleeding is consistently postcoital, that may suggest bleeding from the lower genital tract. If the person sees blood only after urination or a bowel movement, this may indicate a possible urinary or gastrointestinal tract concern, and further evaluation would be needed.

The Focused History

A detailed menstrual history is one of the most important components of the history-taking process for a person who presents

TABLE 25-2 Seven Attributes of a Symptom for AUB

Location	Where is the bleeding coming from? Does the person have pain? Where is the pain located? Where does it radiate to?
Quality	What is the pain like? What is the bleeding like? What is the pattern of bleeding like?
Quantity or severity	How severe is the bleeding? How concerning is the bleeding to the person? How often do they need to change their pad or tampon?
Timing	When did the bleeding start? How often does it occur? When does it occur in relation to the menstrual cycle? How long does the bleeding last?
Setting in which it occurs	Include environmental factors, personal activities, emotional reactions, or other significant life events, such as childbirth and initiation of contraception that may contribute to the AUB. Has the person experienced bleeding like this in the past? How long did it last?
Remitting or exacerbating factors	What makes it better? What makes it worse?
Associated manifestation	Has the person noticed anything else that accompanies it?

with AUB. The healthcare provider should determine the bleeding pattern by asking questions such as the following:

- When was the first day of your last menstrual period and several previous menstrual periods?
- How many days does the bleeding continue?
- How many days of full bleeding do you have, and how many days of light bleeding or spotting?
- Does bleeding occur between menstrual periods?
- How heavy is the bleeding? How often do you need to change your pad or tampon? Is it saturated when you change it? Does it wake you up from sleep, interfere with work activities, or cause you to soak through tampons or pads at a rapid rate?
- If the bleeding is irregular, how many bleeding episodes have there been in the past 6 to 12 months?
- What is the average time from the first day of one bleeding episode to the next?

Often, providing a calendar will help people answer questions more accurately. Their responses to these questions will help the healthcare provider begin to build a list of differential diagnoses that warrant further evaluation. Listening to the person is important for making an accurate diagnosis and allows the healthcare provider to find ways to provide them with needed support during the assessment.

In addition to a detailed menstrual history, it is essential to obtain a sexual history to determine the person's risk for pregnancy or sexually transmitted infections. If a person has any risk for pregnancy or is using contraception for menstrual control, it is necessary to obtain a thorough history of what method of contraception is being used, the duration of use, and if the method is being used as prescribed. Contraceptive history may reveal that their bleeding is mechanically caused by an intrauterine device (IUD) or is related to the use of hormonal contraception, such as oral contraceptives or injectable depot medroxyprogesterone acetate (Depo-Provera). In addition, inquire about hormone therapy in post- and perimenopausal people to rule out a history of taking unopposed estrogen. A detailed health history, including family and surgical history, provides information that may reveal underlying health conditions causing the abnormal bleeding.

It is important to include questions about lifestyle, such as drug and alcohol use, exercise patterns, nutrition, and social support systems. Obtain a complete medication history because glucocorticoids, tamoxifen, and anticoagulants may predispose people to AUB. Ask about use of over-the-counter and herbal medications—notably, the herb bromelain may increase the risk of bleeding. The answers to these questions will also provide necessary information on treatments people may have tried at home in an effort to balance hormones and control bleeding prior to seeking care from a healthcare provider.

Additionally, a thorough health history should include asking about symptoms of thyroid disorders (e.g., cold intolerance, fatigue, hyperactivity, weight gain or loss) and hormone-secreting tumors (e.g., hair loss, changes in breast size, hirsutism, headache, breast discharge). Findings in the health history may suggest the presence of a systemic disease; therefore, pay particular attention to signs and symptoms such as easy bruising, presence of petechiae, weight or appetite changes, and changes in elimination patterns. Given that bleeding and endocrine disorders can be inherited, it is important to look for familial patterns.

After completing the history and listening to the person's concerns, a healthcare provider is usually able to generate hypotheses as to what might be causing the AUB. A thorough review of systems should include assessment of all systems that support or refute these hypotheses. A thorough review of systems also avoids the trap of premature closure, or shutting down the person's story too quickly, which can lead to errors in diagnosis (Bickley, 2021).

THE OBJECTIVE EVALUATION

Physical Examination

A general physical examination should be performed to look for signs of systemic illness, such as fever, ecchymoses, enlarged thyroid gland, or evidence of hyperandrogenism (hirsutism, acne, clitoromegaly, or male pattern baldness). Similar to the review of systems, a thorough physical exam should include assessment of all body systems that support or refute the hypotheses of origins of the AUB. For example, acanthosis nigricans (darkening of the skin in folds and creases) may be seen in people with polycystic ovarian syndrome (PCOS). A breast examination should be done to assess for galactorrhea, a bilateral milky nipple discharge that could suggest the presence of hyperprolactinemia (Kaunitz, 2019). The amount of breast development is also an indicator of estrogen production or exposure to exogenous estrogen. Tanner staging is helpful when caring for adolescents because it can validate information from the history and may help determine the presence and length of ovulatory status. Observe for signs of anemia, such as pale skin tone and delayed capillary refill. Palpate the thyroid to identify enlargement or tumors related to hypothyroidism or hyperthyroidism. Vital signs, particularly the pulse rate, may also be helpful in diagnosing thyroid disorders. Refer to Chapter 3 for information about Tanner staging.

A pelvic examination is essential for a person of any age who is (or has been) sexually active or has abdominal pain, anemia, or bleeding that results in hemodynamic instability. A pelvic examination is most likely not necessary if the patient is an adolescent who is not sexually active, has recently begun menstruating, and has a normal hematocrit. A pelvic examination is helpful for identifying whether the genital anatomy is as expected, if the outflow tract is patent, and if estrogen depletion is present. As part of the pelvic examination, visually assess the external genitalia and the presence of pubic hair, which may indicate androgen production or exposure (Taylor et al., 2020). The absence of pubic hair does not always indicate an abnormality because pubic hair removal is relatively common (Caron, 2022). Visual inspection of the external genitalia may reveal clitoral hypertrophy and other signs of androgen excess. Observe for bruising, lacerations, lesions, or evidence of infection.

A speculum examination enables observation of the vagina and cervix for evidence of infection, trauma, or foreign objects. Cervical cultures to rule out infection and cervical cancer screening (if indicated) should be obtained at this time. When a pelvic examination is indicated for young, developmentally disabled clients who are not sexually active, or clients taking gender-affirming testosterone, a pediatric speculum should be considered; insert it with great care and gentleness using a trauma-informed approach (refer to Chapters 5 and 8). A pelvic examination in these instances may rarely need to be done under anesthesia if the person is too uncomfortable, either physically or emotionally. A bimanual examination provides the opportunity to assess for the presence of tumors, cervical polyps, ovarian cysts, uterine tenderness or enlargement, and adnexal pain or masses. If the bimanual examination is performed on a young adolescent, the clinician should use only one digit and, again, proceed with great care and gentleness.

Laboratory and Diagnostic Testing

Laboratory tests used to diagnose AUB can be invasive and expensive. Decisions regarding which tests to perform should be based on the differential diagnosis and directed by the information collected during the history and physical examination, including the person's age and reproductive status. General laboratory testing for AUB is summarized in **Table 25-3**.

TABLE 25-3 General Laboratory Testing for AUB

Test	Differential Diagnosis	Abnormal Results
Qualitative urine hCG	Pregnancy; threatened, missed, or incomplete spontaneous abortion	May be positive or negative
Quantitative serum hCG	Ectopic pregnancy or impending spontaneous abortion	Level lower than expected for gestational age, lack of significant increase in 48 hours and/or plateauing
CBC with platelets	Anemia	Hemoglobin less than 10 mg/dL
	Clotting abnormalities	Platelets less than 150,000 cells/mm^3
PT, aPTT, INR	von Willebrand disease, leukemia, prothrombin deficiency	PT greater than 13.5 seconds aPTT greater than 40 seconds INR greater than 1.1
Serum iron/ferritin	Iron-deficiency anemia secondary to bleeding	Serum ferritin levels less than 15 ng/mL
FSH	Amenorrhea due to menopause; premature ovarian failure	Levels greater than 30 mIU/mL, some texts cite 40 mIU/mL
Progesterone	Anovulatory	Levels less than 10 ng/mL
TSH	Hypothyroidism or hyperthyroidism	Levels less than 0.8 mU/L or greater than 4.0 mU/L
Pap test	Dysplasia; carcinoma	Atypical cells suggestive of dysplasia and/or carcinoma
Prolactin	Pituitary adenoma	Levels greater than 100 ng/mL
Cultures and/or microscopic examination of vaginal secretions	Vaginal infection (e.g., gonorrhea, chlamydia, trichomoniasis, vulvovaginal candidiasis)	Positive test or microscope

Abbreviations: aPTT, activated partial thromboplastin time; CBC, complete blood count; FSH, follicle-stimulating hormone; hCG, human chorionic gonadotropin; INR, international normalized ratio; PT, prothrombin time; TSH, thyroid-stimulating hormone.
Note: Refer to Chapter 21 regarding cultures and microscopic examination of vaginal secretions.

Differential Diagnosis and Laboratory Assessment of AUB

Additional tests should be ordered only for specific indications; for example, if the person describes heavy bleeding, is passing clots greater than 1 inch in diameter, and must change their pads or tampons frequently, particularly during the night, a serum ferritin test should be considered. **Table 25-4** includes laboratory tests that may be considered.

Although menstrual history alone is often sufficient to make the diagnosis of AUB, after organic, systemic, and iatrogenic causes are ruled out, other diagnostic tests may be required for definitive diagnosis of endometrial pathology. If a person is experiencing ovulatory dysfunction and is older than age 45, endometrial biopsy and pelvic sonography are recommended (American College of Obstetrics and Gynecology [ACOG], 2013a, reaffirmed 2025). If they are younger than age 45 and have a history of unopposed estrogen exposure, failed medical management, and persistent AUB, an endometrial biopsy should also be performed (ACOG, 2013a, reaffirmed 2025). The steps for performing an endometrial biopsy are provided in **Appendix 25-A**.

A convenient and reliable first-line diagnostic tool is transvaginal ultrasonography (abbreviated TVS for transvaginal scan). It is used for detecting polyps and submucosal fibroids, measuring endometrial thickness, evaluating pregnancy complications, and assessing ovarian masses (Keizer et al., 2018). In people who are premenopausal, TVS should be performed between days 4 and 6 of the menstrual cycle. In people who are postmenopausal (no longer cycling), TVS can reliably measure endometrial thickness and rule out endometrial carcinoma in people with a thin endometrium (defined as less than 5 mm). Endometrial thickness of 5 mm or greater on TVS in a postmenopausal person warrants further testing.

An endometrial evaluation in the form of a biopsy should be performed (preferably in the healthcare provider's office) for people aged 30 to 45 years with a negative β-hCG who have not responded to medical treatment, and it should be considered for those aged 19 to 29 years (ACOG, 2013a, reaffirmed 2025). For people aged 45 and older who present with suspected ovulatory dysfunction, an endometrial biopsy should be performed after ruling out pregnancy and prior to initiating medical management.

An endometrial biopsy is easily accomplished in the office setting and can be performed by clinicians who have the education and training required to carry out this test accurately and safely (American College of Nurse-Midwives, 2017). Endometrial biopsy can be useful in the diagnosis of both ovulatory and anovulatory AUB. It has a high overall accuracy in diagnosing endometrial cancer if an adequate specimen is obtained; however, this procedure can also miss endometrial cancer if less than 50 percent of the surface area of the endometrium is occupied by the cancer (ACOG, 2012, reaffirmed 2024). Essentially, a positive endometrial biopsy is more reliable than a negative one. Endometrial biopsy can also sometimes miss fibroids and polyps; thus, if these growths are suspected or need to be ruled out, imaging should be done. Most people can tolerate an endometrial biopsy in the clinic setting. Providing an anti-inflammatory medication, such as ibuprofen, 1 hour prior to the procedure can help alleviate cramping and discomfort experienced during the procedure. Some people may not be able to tolerate endometrial biopsy in the office setting, so a plan will be needed for more advanced sedation and anesthesia. When clinically feasible, TVS should be performed prior to endometrial biopsy

TABLE 25-4 Differential Diagnosis Laboratory Tests to Order

To Rule Out . . .	Laboratory Tests to Order
Endocrine causes of AUB	General laboratory tests plus prolactin, FSH, and LH levels (if premature ovarian failure is suspected)
Adrenal causes	General laboratory tests plus adrenal studies, testosterone levels
	Adjunct: CT scan of abdomen, cortisol levels
Hormone-producing tumor	General laboratory tests plus MRI, CT scan, cortisol levels
Structural abnormalities	General laboratory tests plus ultrasound
Infection	General laboratory tests plus gonorrhea and chlamydia tests and wet mount; consider need for WBC
Cervical or uterine pathology	General laboratory tests plus colposcopy with biopsy; endometrial biopsy; hysteroscopy
Amenorrhea	General laboratory tests plus FSH, LH, prolactin levels, TSH, T3, T4
Angiohemophilia (von Willebrand disease)	Ristocetin cofactor assay
Liver disease	Liver function tests
Renal disease	Renal function tests
Coagulation disorders other than angiohemophilia	PTT, PT, assessment of platelet function

Data from Taylor, H. S., Fritz, M. A., Pal, L., & Seli, E. (2020). *Speroff's clinical gynecologic endocrinology and infertility* (9th ed.). Wolters Kluwer.
Abbreviations: CT, computed tomography; FSH, follicle-stimulating hormone; LH, luteinizing hormone; PT, prothrombin time; PTT, partial thromboplastin time; T3, triiodothyronine; T4, thyroxine; TSH, thyroid-stimulating hormone; VWD, von Willebrand disease; WBC, white blood cell count.

because the endometrial lining may be disrupted by the endometrial biopsy, making ultrasound findings more difficult to interpret.

When an endometrial biopsy returns an insufficient tissue sample or cannot be performed, a hysteroscopic procedure would be performed. Hysteroscopy is considered the gold standard technique for diagnosis and managing AUB because it allows for direct visualization of the endometrial cavity and permits the healthcare provider to take directed biopsies (ACOG, 2012, reaffirmed 2024). MRI and computed tomography (CT) scan may be used to diagnose adnexal masses, adenomyosis, uterine fibroids, and pituitary adenomas. The costs of these technologies may be considered excessive if other types of evaluation methods would provide the same information (ACOG, 2012, reaffirmed 2024). However, MRI should be ordered if ovarian or endometrial cancer is suspected.

As mentioned previously, these diagnostic tests are generally not necessary for evaluation of a person with anovulatory AUB because often the menstrual history is sufficient for making a diagnosis. Nevertheless, an endometrial biopsy or hysteroscopy should always be included in the assessment of abnormal bleeding in people who are perimenopausal or postmenopausal. It should also be considered in individuals living in a larger body with long-term (3 or more years) unexplained abnormal bleeding, polycystic ovarian syndrome, diabetes, a family history of nonpolyposis colorectal cancer (Lynch syndrome) or any person whose endometrium has been exposed to unopposed estrogen (Tsakiridis et al., 2022).

DIFFERENTIAL DIAGNOSIS OF AUB

PALM: Structural Abnormalities

AUB can be caused by normal physiological processes, or it may be caused by life-threatening pathologies. A thorough and organized approach to diagnosis is necessary to prevent over-utilization of resources, unnecessary testing, delayed treatment, or missed or incorrect diagnosis. The PALM-COEIN schema allows the clinician to move through the differential diagnosis process in a systematic way to determine the most likely cause of AUB in a given patient. The PALM components focus on structural abnormalities; the COEIN components signify nonstructural causes of AUB.

AUB-P (Polyps)

Endocervical polyps are commonly occurring benign growths on the cervix. They are easily visualized with a speculum, appearing as smooth, deep to bright red growths that are fragile and bleed easily during examination. People with cervical polyps may present with a concern about vaginal bleeding. The bleeding associated with polyps often occurs during or after penetrative sexual intercourse. Endometrial polyps are usually benign growths of the endometrium consisting of connective, glandular, or muscular tissue; they are usually asymptomatic but are generally thought to contribute to AUB in some people. Within the FIGO classification system, polyps are classified as either present or not. The FIGO system does not indicate how many polyps must be present or how large they must be, although this information should be documented by the clinician and can be added as a subcategory. The FIGO Menstrual Disorders Committee is currently working on a subclassification system for polyps (Munro et al., 2018). Refer to Chapter 27 for more information on polyps.

AUB-A (Adenomyosis)

Adenomyosis is characterized by small areas of endometrial tissue within the myometrium. The principal symptoms are pain and heavy menstrual bleeding. The predominant predisposing factor for this condition is more than one pregnancy and history of miscarriage, curettage, endometrial resection, cesarean birth, or tamoxifen use (Abbott, 2017). The connection between adenomyosis and AUB is not well understood.

Definitive diagnosis of adenomyosis is made through histology. However, noninvasive ultrasonography and occasionally MRI can be used to detect the severity of the adenomyosis, which may include uterine enlargement (Abbott, 2017). Since the original publication of the FIGO system there have been advances in the diagnosis of adenomyosis. It has been demonstrated that 2-D TVS has similar sensitivity and specificity for the diagnosis of adenomyosis as MRI (Bazot & Daraï, 2018). With improvement in imaging technology, non-invasive diagnosis through ultrasonography or MRI is supported by the data (Abbott, 2017). Refer to Chapter 27 for more information on adenomyosis.

AUB-L (Leiomyoma)

Leiomyomas, commonly known as fibroids, are solid neoplasms composed of smooth muscle cells and fibroblasts (ACOG, 2021). Leiomyoma is a more accurate term than either fibroid or myoma for these benign tumors of the myometrium. Leiomyomas are the most common benign pelvic tumors in people and the leading indication for hysterectomy (ACOG, 2021). Many people who have leiomyomas have no symptoms and do not require treatment, although depending on their location within the uterus, they may contribute to AUB. Common symptoms include prolonged or heavy menstrual bleeding as well as pelvic pressure, urinary frequency, and constipation.

The prevalence of leiomyomas is 2–3 times higher among Black people compared with white people (ACOG, 2021). Black people typically develop leiomyomas at a younger age and are more likely to be anemic as a result of the leiomyoma. The difference in presentation is rooted in systemic racism and social determinants of health, and is not a result of biologic difference (Katon et al., 2023).

The primary classification system accounts for only the presence or absence of leiomyomas. Leiomyomas are further classified by a secondary category that labels their location within the uterus: submucosal and other. It is important to determine if the leiomyoma interferes with the endometrium (submucosal) because this type is more likely to cause AUB. The other category includes subserosal and intramural leiomyomas. The FIGO classification also has a Type 3 leiomyoma, which is not considered submucosal or other, but is classified in the other category. This type of leiomyoma contacts the endometrium and is 100 percent intramural (Munro et al., 2018). The sizes of leiomyomas are not included in the current classification system but could be considered with a tertiary classification system. This would further standardize the classifications of leiomyomas, thereby providing a reliable, accurate system for research studies and patient documentation. Refer to Chapter 27 for more information on leiomyoma.

AUB-M (Malignancy and Hyperplasia)

Malignancy and atypical hyperplasia are rare in people of reproductive age. However, these conditions must still be considered potential causes of AUB, particularly if a person is living in a larger body or has PCOS because of a well-documented increased risk of endometrial cancer (Johnson et al., 2023). People living in larger bodies have estimated odds ratios of 1.43 and 3.3, respectively, of developing endometrial cancer, compared with smaller people (ACOG, 2015, reaffirmed 2021). Furthermore, although Black people have a 30 percent decreased incidence of being diagnosed with endometrial cancer (compared to white people), they have a 2.5 times higher risk of death if they are diagnosed with endometrial cancer because of diagnosis at more advanced state of disease (ACOG, 2015, reaffirmed 2021). Similar to leiomyomas, this difference is rooted in systemic racism and social determinants of health, not an inherent biologic difference.

The most common symptoms of endometrial cancer are AUB and postmenopausal bleeding (ACOG, 2015, reaffirmed 2021). Therefore, malignancy must be ruled out in all people who are experiencing postmenopausal vaginal bleeding. Any person diagnosed with AUB-M will also have a subclassification of the malignancy using the World Health Organization or FIGO oncology staging systems. The PALM-COEIN AUB classification system is not meant to replace the oncology staging system. Refer to Chapter 28 for more information on malignancies and hyperplasia.

COEIN: Nonstructural Abnormalities

AUB-C (Coagulopathy)

The coagulopathy category encompasses a wide range of blood clotting disorders that can potentially cause AUB. Approximately 13 percent of people who present with AUB will have a blood clotting disorder, with angiohemophilia (von Willebrand disease) being one of the more commonly inherited bleeding disorders. Among young people with heavy bleeding, approximately 20 to 30 percent will have a diagnosis of angiohemophilia (ACOG, 2013b, reaffirmed 2021). People presenting with a concern for heavy menstrual bleeding who have a history of easy bruising and/or prolonged bleeding following dental work or surgery warrant further follow-up for angiohemophilia. The 2018 update to the FIGO system no longer includes AUB associated with pharmacologic agents that impair blood coagulation. Because it is iatrogenic in nature, this category of people with AUB is now included in AUB-I (Munro et al., 2018). The diagnosis of AUB-C is usually made by thoroughly reviewing the person's history and is confirmed by hematologic testing. Treatment includes consultation with a hematologist or other provider experienced in caring for coagulopathy disorders.

AUB-O (Ovulatory Dysfunction)

This category encompasses many different presentations of AUB, including amenorrhea and light or heavy menses that can occur in regular menstrual patterns or more or less frequently. Many cases of AUB-O stem from endocrinopathies including thyroid disorders, PCOS, excessive exercise, or extreme mental distress. Subcategories of AUB-O are defined as anovulatory uterine bleeding, amenorrhea (absence of bleeding), and ovulatory uterine bleeding.

Anovulatory Uterine Bleeding Anovulatory bleeding, in contrast to the typically regular, predictable bleeding experienced with ovulatory cycles, frequently leads to abnormal cycle intervals, excessively heavy bleeding, or lighter-than-normal bleeding. This type of bleeding tends to be heavy secondary to the high and sustained levels of unopposed estrogen that can result in endometrial hyperplasia. Endometrial hyperplasia, in turn, can result in episodes of amenorrhea, heavy menstrual bleeding, and intermenstrual bleeding. Anovulatory cycles, characterized by a lack of progesterone in the luteal phase, lead to an unstable, excessively vascular endometrium.

Table 25-5 identifies recognized physiologic and pathologic causes of anovulation.

Evidence from histologic and molecular studies suggests that anovulatory bleeding is the result of an increased density of abnormal vessels that have a fragile structure prone to focal rupture, which is then followed by the release of lysosomes (proteolytic enzymes) from surrounding epithelial and stromal cells and migratory leukocytes and macrophages (Taylor et al., 2020). This condition is generally caused by one of three hormonal imbalances: estrogen withdrawal, estrogen breakthrough, or progesterone breakthrough (ACOG, 2012, reaffirmed 2024).

Estrogen levels increase the thickness of the endometrium; thus, people with high sustained levels of estrogen tend to experience the heaviest menstrual bleeding. Estrogen breakthrough bleeding occurs as a result of the endometrium being stimulated by long-term, chronic, unopposed estrogen, such as that observed in people experiencing chronic anovulation. These people often include those who have PCOS, people with larger bodies, or those who are perimenopausal (Taylor et al., 2020). People with PCOS often experience estrogen breakthrough

TABLE 25-5 Physiologic and Pathologic Causes of Anovulation

Physiologic Causes
Pregnancy
Lactation
Adolescence
Perimenopause
Obesity
BMI less than 18
Excessive exercise
Pathologic Causes
Hyperandrogenic disorders (e.g., PCOS)
Hypothalamic dysfunction (secondary to anorexia nervosa)
Hyperprolactinemia
Iatrogenic (secondary to radiation therapy, chemotherapy, or medications)
Thyroid disorders
Primary pituitary disorders

Data from American College of Obstetricians and Gynecologists. (2013, reaffirmed 2022). ACOG practice bulletin no. 136: Management of abnormal uterine bleeding associated with ovulatory dysfunction. *Obstetrics & Gynecology, 122*(1), 176–185.

bleeding because of chronic anovulation (Taylor et al., 2020). Diseases or syndromes causing insulin resistance, such as PCOS, increase circulating levels of insulin, which in turn leads to an elevation in androgen production and concomitant anovulation (Azziz, 2018). The relationship between insulin and androgens is believed to be an underlying cause of PCOS (refer to Chapter 26).

Endocrine disorders may cause bleeding abnormalities; consequently, they should always be considered when evaluating a person with AUB. Although both thyroid disorders (hypothyroidism and hyperthyroidism) can result in a range of bleeding patterns, hypothyroidism is the more likely cause of amenorrhea, and hyperthyroidism more often results in heavy menstrual bleeding (Deshmukh et al., 2015). Pituitary disorders and some pituitary tumors may result in elevated levels of prolactin. Amenorrhea associated with elevated prolactin levels is due to prolactin inhibition of the pulsatile secretion of gonadotropin-releasing hormone (GnRH) (Taylor et al., 2020). Prolactin-secreting pituitary adenomas are the most common type of pituitary tumor (Taylor et al., 2020). Approximately one-third of people with elevated prolactin levels will also have galactorrhea. Nevertheless, some individuals (10%) have silent pituitary masses that are not endocrinologically active and have no adverse impact on health and well-being.

Progesterone breakthrough bleeding occurs when the ratio of progesterone to estrogen is elevated (ACOG, 2018, reaffirmed 2022). This type of AUB can occur in people using progestin-only pills or other forms of progestin-only contraception (Taylor et al., 2020). Heavy and/or irregular bleeding results from an imbalance in both the vasoconstricting and vasodilating properties of prostaglandins and platelet aggregation and inhibition (ACOG, 2012, reaffirmed 2024). The abnormal microvasculature is probably the cause of the abnormal bleeding that results from this phenomenon (Taylor et al., 2020).

The most common times for a person to experience irregular menstrual cycles are at the beginning and the end of their reproductive life cycle: postmenarche and perimenopause. The HPOA is most affected by the normal life-cycle transitions that occur during the first 2 years after menarche and 3 years prior to menopause (Taylor et al., 2020); thus, irregular bleeding during this time may be a reflection of normal functioning.

The least amount of variation in menses occurs during the childbearing years, which generally encompass ages 20 to 40, although most people will experience some variation from their established normal pattern from time to time. Even though bleeding patterns may fall within the range of normal, it is important to listen to the person's description prior to making a diagnosis because, for them, the bleeding may be abnormal and require some amount of reassurance, education, or follow-up.

Amenorrhea

The absence of menses, termed amenorrhea, is part of the spectrum of ovulatory disorders classified as AUB-O. The most common causes of amenorrhea are pregnancy, hypothalamic amenorrhea, and PCOS (ACOG, 2014b, reaffirmed 2021). According to Taylor et al., people meeting any of the following criteria should be evaluated for amenorrhea:

- No menses by age 14 in the absence of growth or development of secondary sexual characteristics
- No menses by age 16 regardless of the presence of normal growth and development of secondary sexual characteristics
- In people who have menstruated previously, no menses for an interval of time equivalent to a total of at least three previous cycles, or no menses over a 6-month period (2020, p. 343)

Amenorrhea can be categorized as either primary or secondary. Primary amenorrhea is the failure to begin menses by age 16. A number of disorders can be treated as soon as they are diagnosed, however, so any girl who has not reached menarche by age 15 or who has not had a menses within 3 years of thelarche should be evaluated (ACOG, 2014b, reaffirmed 2021). Secondary amenorrhea is defined as 3 months without a menses after menses has been established. The American Society for Reproductive Medicine recommends that any person experiencing 3 months of amenorrhea after the menses is established should be evaluated (ACOG, 2014b, reaffirmed 2021).

Nonpregnancy causes of amenorrhea include anatomic defects, ovarian failure, chronic anovulation, anterior pituitary disorders, and central nervous system disorders. Age is an important criterion in making the differential diagnosis of primary versus secondary amenorrhea, and it is relevant in determining the types of questions to ask when taking the health history. Primary amenorrhea in a young person may be indicative of HPOA disorder or anatomic factors, such as outflow tract obstruction. With primary amenorrhea, the physical examination should focus on identifying the maturation of secondary sex characteristics (e.g., Tanner staging for breast development and pubic hair pattern) and establishing outflow tract patency. The question of whether the person has had any bleeding from the vagina can assist in determining primary, secondary, and potential causes. Other important interview questions to consider relate to lifestyle patterns (e.g., exercise, medication, and drug use) and eating habits (e.g., possible eating disorders). A family history of anatomic or genetic abnormalities should be explored as well.

Normal menstrual function requires that four anatomic and structural components are in working order: uterus, ovary, pituitary, and hypothalamus. The clinician can then categorize the amenorrhea according to the site or level of disturbance (Taylor et al., 2020):

- Disorders of the genital outflow tract
- Disorders of the ovary
- Disorders of the anterior pituitary
- Disorders of the hypothalamus or central nervous system

Amenorrhea is often seen in people engaged in sports that focus on a lean body type or with strict weight standards. Relative Energy Deficiency in Sport (RED-S), formerly known as the Female Athletic Triad, is a syndrome marked by amenorrhea and often has characteristics of disordered eating and decreased bone mineral density (Kerns et al., 2022). Training for sport prior to menarche many even delay menarche for five months for each year of training. The pathophysiology of exercise-induced amenorrhea is complex and most likely due to the combination of low body fat and diminished secretion of GnRH. Lower GnRH levels result in fewer luteinizing hormone and follicle-stimulating hormone (FSH) pulses, which in turn decreases the amount of estrogen produced by the ovaries. The critical weight theory hypothesizes that some critical weight and amount of body fat exist that must be maintained for people to experience regular menstrual cycles (Taylor et al., 2020; Kerns et al., 2022).

Ovulatory AUB

Ovulatory dysfunction (AUB-O) includes a spectrum of disorders from amenorrhea to irregular heavy menstrual periods that are usually caused by an endocrinopathy such as PCOS (ACOG, 2012, reaffirmed 2024). Ovulatory AUB, one of the disorders of AUB-O, occurs significantly less often than abnormal bleeding due to anovulation; it is typically observed in the post-adolescent years and during the premenopausal years. Ovulatory abnormal bleeding tends to be cyclic and regular, although the bleeding patterns are often abnormal. The HPOA is intact, and the steroid hormone profile is normal in ovulatory AUB (ACOG, 2012, reaffirmed 2024).

Prolonged heavy menstrual bleeding is the pattern most frequently observed with ovulatory abnormal bleeding and is commonly associated with pelvic pathology such as uterine fibroids (leiomyomas), adenomyosis, or endometrial polyps (ACOG, 2021). Therefore, in people with ovulatory abnormal bleeding, an evaluation to rule out endometrial lesions and other pathology is indicated. Heavy menstrual bleeding is also frequently associated with bleeding dyscrasias, and as many as 20 percent of adolescents who present with heavy menstrual bleeding have a bleeding disorder (Taylor et al., 2020).

AUB-E (Endometrial)

Endometrial AUB usually occurs in a predictive and cyclical manner and includes heavy menstrual bleeding (Munro et al., 2018). AUB-E can also present with intermenstrual or prolonged bleeding patterns. All people of childbearing age who present with AUB should be considered pregnant until proven otherwise, and a urine or serum β-hCG must be included in the assessment. A thorough history and physical examination (including pelvic examination and cultures) will assist in ruling out infection as a cause of the abnormal bleeding. Although the role of infection is not discussed extensively in the current literature, *Chlamydia trachomatis* has been found to be associated with endometritis, which can produce intermenstrual bleeding as observed with this type of AUB. Thus, the clinician should discuss testing with the person as a means of possibly ruling this out as the causative factor (Munro et al., 2018). Other infections, such as gonorrhea, and endometritis may cause irregular spotting due to irritation and inflammation of the tissues of the cervix or endometrium.

The endometrium is a unique tissue that releases blood as a part of normal physiology. The etiology of AUB-E can involve a premature release of blood from the endometrium or disorders of local endometrial hemostasis. Platelets are involved in endometrial hemostasis very marginally at the time of menstruation. There can be a decrease of local endometrial vasoconstrictors (endothelin-1 and prostaglandin F_2), thereby causing vasodilation and heavy menstrual bleeding. Excessive amounts of plasminogen activator or decreased amounts of plasminogen activator inhibitor can also lead to heavy menstrual bleeding. The exact processes that happen during AUB-E are not well defined in the current literature. Consequently, there are no diagnostic tests that clinicians can use to confirm the presence of AUB-E; rather, it is a diagnosis of exclusion.

AUB-I (Iatrogenic)

Medications or devices that act on the endometrium or interfere with the ovulatory cycle can cause iatrogenic AUB. The Mirena, Skyla, Kyleena, Liletta, and Paragard intrauterine systems can also cause irregular spotting and bleeding after placement, although this phenomenon usually resolves within 3 to 6 months after placement. Other hormonal methods of contraception may also result in irregular or breakthrough bleeding. Medications that alter the serotonin reuptake process, such as antidepressants, can cause AUB-I related to a disturbance in the HPOA (Engler et al., 2024).

Some people with coagulopathy disorders take anticoagulant medications that could contribute to AUB. This category of bleeding was moved from AUB-C to AUB-I in the 2018 update to the FIGO system (Munro et al., 2018).

AUB-N (Not Otherwise Classified)

The AUB-N category may be used when possible causes of AUB other than those previously mentioned are being explored. For example, some people may experience AUB related to conditions such as arterial–venous malformations that do not fit into any of the other AUB categories (Munro et al., 2018). This category also leaves room for as-yet unidentified causes of AUB.

Special Considerations for Evaluating AUB

Trauma

Trauma to the genital tract can also cause AUB. Tampons can irritate the cervix and cause spotting. In addition, hymeneal tearing with tampon use or consensual penetrative intercourse can cause bleeding. People who have been sexually assaulted, particularly those who have not had sexual intercourse prior to the assault, may experience bleeding from lacerations and other injuries that affect the internal organs and genitals (ACOG, 2015, reaffirmed 2025).

Outflow Tract Causes of AUB

A properly functioning outflow tract (i.e., a patent uterus, cervix, and vagina) is a necessary component for normal menstrual flow. Anatomic abnormalities at any level of the outflow tract can interfere with normal menstrual flow and often result in amenorrhea. For example, uterine or cervical congenital structural abnormalities can cause obstruction and make menstrual flow impossible or abnormal. Rarely, segments of the Müllerian tube may fail to develop, resulting in abnormalities such as imperforate hymen, lack of a vaginal orifice, lapses in the continuity of the vaginal canal, or an absent uterus, cervix, uterine cavity, or endometrium. Obstruction of the vagina in the presence of a bulging, bluish-colored membrane indicates imperforate hymen. An obstructed bimanual examination warrants referral and follow-up for the possibility of either a vaginal septum or blind pouch. Obstruction of menses may lead to painful distention due to a menstrual blood collection, such as hematometra (blood in the uterus), hematocolpos (blood in the vagina), or hemoperitoneum (blood in the peritoneum). Affected people are genotypically and phenotypically normal females with functioning ovaries. Such abnormalities are uncommon except in people whose mothers were administered diethylstilbestrol (DES) during pregnancy, typically between the years 1938 and 1971. People with a history of multiple cervical procedures, such as dilation and curettage, or significant endometrial infections are at risk for scarring that may cause outflow tract AUB. If a person presents with amenorrhea with no history of infection or trauma and their pelvic examination and bimanual examination are normal, then an abnormality of the outflow tract is not likely.

MANAGEMENT OF AUB

Management goals for treating AUB are to (1) normalize the bleeding, (2) correct any anemia, (3) prevent cancer, and (4) restore quality of life. The clinician should always consider the person's choice of treatment when developing a plan of care. Concomitant therapy may be necessary to achieve these goals, particularly if the bleeding is severe and threatens hemodynamic stability. For example, a person who presents with severe bleeding from a raw and denuded endometrium may require high-dose estrogen to stop the bleeding. Estrogen therapy will provide rapid growth of a denuded endometrium. After the acute bleeding is under control, additional treatment options, such as oral contraceptives, use of the levonorgestrel intrauterine system, and progestin therapy (among others), are available for long-term treatment (ACOG, 2012, reaffirmed 2024). If testing reveals that the person is anemic because of the bleeding, iron therapy is recommended.

Age, desire for future fertility, and the person's preferences all need to be considered when determining treatment options for people with AUB. Treatment falls into two categories: treatment of acute bleeding, treatment of chronic bleeding, and treatment of amenorrhea. People who present with excessive heavy menstrual bleeding and who have a dangerously low hematocrit require physician consultation. All episodes of acute hemorrhagic bleeding should be managed by a physician in a hospital setting. Intravenous estrogen therapy is usually instituted in such cases. Following intravenous administration of estrogen, high-dose estrogen therapy should be continued orally, tapering to once daily when bleeding is under control and adding a progestogen such as medroxyprogesterone acetate (Taylor et al., 2020). This same treatment is effective for a person whose bleeding is acute but not yet considered an emergency.

Pharmacologic Management of Acute Non-Life-Threatening Heavy Menstrual Bleeding

A variety of pharmacologic choices are available for people with heavy menstrual bleeding, including combined oral contraceptives, progestogen-only therapy, and levonorgestrel-releasing IUDs. Medical therapies for heavy menstrual bleeding are shown in **Table 25-6**.

Estrogen Therapy

If a significantly denuded endometrium is suspected as the cause of heavy bleeding, then administration of high-dose estrogen usually will stop the bleeding and allow for further evaluation. Estrogen therapy stimulates rapid endometrial proliferation and resolves the bleeding from a denuded endometrium (Taylor et al., 2020). Concomitant use of antiemetics is indicated when high-dose estrogen is administered because of the nausea that often accompanies its use. The clinician needs to be mindful that estrogens—particularly high-dose estrogens—may precipitate thromboembolism and are therefore contraindicated in people with a history of thrombosis, other

TABLE 25-6 Medical Therapies for Heavy Menstrual Bleeding

Acute bleeding: Estrogen therapy[a]	• Replenish intravascular volume. • CEE 25 mg IV q 4 to 6 h as needed, then CEE 2.5 to 5.0 mg orally 4 times/day for 2 to 3 days, then add MPA 10 mg for 10 to 14 days (continue CEE). • COCs 2 to 3 times/day, then taper.
Acute bleeding: Progestin therapy	• Use only if endometrium is normal or increased in thickness. Treatment should continue for 3 weeks, decreasing to once/day after 7 to 10 days. • Medroxyprogesterone acetate 10 to 20 mg 2 times/day, or • Megestrol 20 to 40 mg 2 times/day, or • Norethindrone 5 mg 2 times/day.
Acute prolonged bleeding: Estrogen–progestin therapy	• Any monophasic COC beginning with one pill 3 times/day until bleeding stops, tapering to one pill daily. • Continue treatment for a minimum of 2 weeks.
Long-term/chronic management	• Cyclic MPA 10 mg/day for 10 to 14 days every 30 to 40 days. • Combined contraceptives (oral, patch, ring). • Oral micronized progesterone 300 mg for 10 to 14 days every 30 to 40 days. • Depo medroxyprogesterone acetate (Depo-Provera) 150 mg intramuscularly every 3 months. • LNG-IUS (Mirena, Skyla, Kyleena, or Liletta). • NSAIDs. • Tranexamic acid. • Drospirenone 4 mg/day.

Note: High doses of estrogen may precipitate a thrombotic event and therefore are contraindicated in people with a history of thrombosis or a family history of idiopathic venous thromboembolism. Also, warn the person using progestin therapy that withdrawal of progestin will result in heavy menses. In people who desire contraception, treatment with an estrogen–progestin contraceptive is a better choice (Taylor et al., 2020).

Abbreviations: CEE, conjugated equine estrogen; COC, combined oral contraceptive; LNG-IUS, levonorgestrel intrauterine system; MPA, medroxyprogesterone acetate; NSAIDS, nonsteroidal anti-inflammatory drugs.

[a]High-dose estrogen often causes nausea; therefore, concurrent treatment with an antiemetic is recommended.

coagulopathies, or family history of idiopathic venous thromboembolism. Conjugated equine estrogens (Premarin) 2.5 mg every 6 hours can be administered until the bleeding decreases or subsides, although therapy should not continue beyond 25 days. After estrogen therapy has been completed, a progesterone such as medroxyprogesterone acetate 10 mg should be administered for 10 days.

Combined Oral Contraceptives

For a person who is hemodynamically stable, a monophasic combined oral contraceptive administered 3 times daily should also result in the reduction of bleeding within 24 hours. The combined oral contraceptive is typically tapered to twice daily for 2 days, then one pill daily for 21 days of active pills followed by 7 days of placebo pills or no pills. An alternative to the 21/7 cycle is an extended regimen of 84 days of monophasic combined oral contraceptives followed by a 7-day pill-free interval. When the bleeding stops, 2.5 mg of conjugated equine estrogen (Premarin) can be administered daily, followed by the addition of 10 mg of medroxyprogesterone acetate (Provera) during the last 10 days of therapy to initiate withdrawal bleeding.

Progestogen Therapy

Progestogens can be used to treat chronic heavy bleeding that is due to anovulation. People with chronic heavy menstrual bleeding can be offered cyclic medroxyprogesterone acetate at doses of 10 mg per day for 10 to 14 days, with the therapy repeated every 30 to 40 days. Oral micronized progesterone (Prometrium) 200 mg should be taken at night because it can induce fatigue. Use Prometrium with caution in people with peanut allergies because peanut oil is used in the manufacturing process. **Box 25-1** describes progestogen therapy for chronic anovulation.

Progestogens are not as effective as estrogen in stopping acute bleeding, but they are effective for long-term treatment after the acute bleeding episode has been resolved. Additionally, progestogens may be the management regimen of choice if the person has contraindications to taking estrogen.

To induce normal bleeding, a progestogen is administered for 7 to 12 days each month. Withdrawal bleeding should occur within 2 to 7 days of discontinuing the progestogen. If bleeding fails to occur or if irregular bleeding persists, diagnostic reevaluation is necessary, and physician consultation is recommended. Do not use progestogen therapy if the person thinks they might be pregnant, even if their pregnancy test is negative.

If the person has no contraindications to their use, IUDs containing levonorgestrel are a particularly effective therapy for heavy menstrual bleeding caused by fibroids. People with fibroids are candidates for the LNG-IUS if the fibroid does not distort the uterine cavity and the uterus is less than 12 weeks' gestation in size.

Gonadotropin-Releasing Hormone Agonists

Gonadotropin-releasing hormone agonists (GnRHas), such as leuprolide acetate (Lupron), nafarelin acetate (Synarel), and goserelin acetate (Zoladex), may be used for a short period of time while a person is awaiting surgical treatment for heavy bleeding. Because GnRHas have many side effects related to estrogen deficiency, they are not considered for long-term treatment, unless they are combined with hormonal add-back therapy (Ali et al., 2022). GnRHa therapy is also quite expensive—another reason for using it only on a short-term basis. Nevertheless, these agents are very effective in stemming the bleeding with resultant amenorrhea. In the interim, the person's hemoglobin has time to rise, thereby optimizing surgical outcomes.

Nonhormonal Pharmacologic Management for Acute Heavy Menstrual Bleeding

NSAIDs (nonsteroidal anti-inflammatory drugs) are useful for ovulatory–idiopathic heavy menstrual bleeding. The heavier the bleeding, the better the effectiveness of NSAIDs, although their mechanism of action in curtailing heavy bleeding remains poorly understood. It is suspected that NSAIDs interfere with the transformation of arachidonic acid to cyclic endoperoxidases, thereby blocking the production of prostaglandins. Because they can also be an effective treatment for dysmenorrhea, NSAIDs may be a good option for people who have both heavy and painful menstrual bleeding. Optimally, an NSAID should be initiated 3 days prior to the start of menses, although some experts suggest waiting until the onset of menses to start treatment (Potter et al., 2021). All NSAIDs are contraindicated in people with ulcers or bronchospastic lung disease. **Box 25-2** identifies NSAIDs that are commonly used to manage heavy menstrual bleeding.

In 2009, tranexamic acid (Lysteda), an antifibrinolytic agent that reduces menstrual bleeding by 45 to 60 percent, was approved in the United States for the treatment of heavy bleeding (Taylor et al., 2020). This drug is particularly useful as a second-line option for people who cannot or do not wish to use hormonal options. It is also effective in managing the severe bleeding that accompanies angiohemophilia. Tranexamic acid treatment results in a significant reduction in blood loss, compared to placebo. A concern with use of this therapy is venous thromboembolism. Cases of venous and arterial thrombosis have been reported while using tranexamic acid, as have arterial and venous retinal occlusions (Tian et al., 2024). The use

BOX 25-1 Progestogen Therapy for Chronic Anovulation

- Medroxyprogesterone acetate (Provera) 10 mg for 10 days
- Norethindrone 5 mg twice per day for 10 days
- Oral micronized progesterone (Prometrium) 200 mg/day for 10 days
- Depo medroxyprogesterone acetate (Depo-Provera) 150 mg intramuscularly every 12 weeks
- Levonorgestrel-releasing intrauterine system (LNG-IUS)

BOX 25-2 NSAID Therapy for Heavy Menstrual Bleeding

- Mefenamic acid 500 mg 3 times per day (approved by the U.S. Food and Drug Administration)
- Ibuprofen 600 mg 3 times per day
- Naproxen sodium 550 mg loading dose, then 275 mg every 6 hours

of tranexamic acid is contraindicated in people with a history of, or who are at risk for, thrombosis. The prescribed dose is 1,300 mg taken 3 times per day for a maximum of 5 days per menstrual cycle. Side effects are rare but include nausea and leg cramps.

Surgical Management of Heavy Menstrual Bleeding

When medical therapy fails, surgical management options for heavy bleeding include dilation and curettage, endometrial ablation, uterine artery embolization, and hysterectomy. In the presence of a thin endometrium, medical therapy for excessive uterine bleeding is reasonable. The choice of surgical modality is based on a number of factors, including the person's initial response to medical management and their desire for future fertility (ACOG, 2021). Dilation and curettage is a temporary measure and not considered a long-term treatment for heavy menstrual bleeding.

Endometrial Ablation

Endometrial ablation was introduced in the 1990s as an alternative to hysterectomy. It is a less invasive procedure that results in destruction of the endometrium using heated fluid (either contained within a balloon or circulating freely within the uterine cavity), tissue freezing, microwave, or radiofrequency electricity (Leyland et al., 2024). Endometrial ablation should not be performed if a person desires to maintain their fertility. A potential issue with this therapeutic approach is that methods of screening for endometrial cancer after ablation, such as endometrial biopsy, may be challenging (Leyland et al., 2024). People at risk for endometrial cancer should be counseled prior to endometrial ablation about this potential risk. Ablation can be performed in the hospital or office setting and is usually performed with conscious sedation.

Uterine Artery Embolization

Uterine artery embolization (UAE) is an interventional procedure for people with AUB associated with leiomyomas who desire uterine preservation. Typically, uterine artery embolization is performed as an overnight hospital procedure by a radiologist. The objective is to occlude blood flow to the leiomyomas, shrinking them and decreasing their associated symptoms. Data are limited on the effects of UAE on fertility and future pregnancy and ovarian reserve. People considering a pregnancy after this procedure should be counseled that there may be a higher rate of miscarriage and pregnancy complications (ACOG, 2021). People should be counseled that they will have moderate to intense cramping and light vaginal bleeding for about a week after treatment. They should expect to see an improvement in menstrual bleeding approximately 2 to 3 months after the uterine artery embolization.

Hysterectomy

Each year, more than 600,000 people in the United States have a hysterectomy (Harvey et al., 2022). Advantages of hysterectomy have been reported, including improved quality of life, but postoperative morbidity, including postsurgical fatigue, weight change, and changes in sexual satisfaction, are widespread. People facing the decision to undergo hysterectomy, as with all surgeries, should be provided full information about the physical and emotional effects of the procedure and potential body image issues that may arise, including those related to perceptions of sexuality and femininity.

Alternative Treatments for Heavy Menstrual Bleeding

A systematic review of Traditional Chinese Medicine (TCM), compared to conventional Western medicine, was performed to determine the efficacy and safety of using Chinese herbal medicine for AUB. Four randomized clinical trials involving 452 women were reviewed. The conclusion was that all but one of the trials had methodological problems that rendered their findings unsuitable for use as evidence for practice. No adverse effects with the use of Chinese herbal medicine were identified, however, and findings in the satisfactory trial found that Chinese herbal medicine may be effective (Tu et al., 2009). In populations with ready access to TCM, many people chose it as a sole or adjunct therapy. In a study from Taiwan of 46,000 people diagnosed with AUB, 89.6 percent utilized TCM as part of their treatment plans (Lin et al., 2017). The use of TCM was associated with a reduced incidence of surgical management for abnormal uterine bleeding, regardless of comorbidities, childbirth status, or the use of common treatments such as TXA, progesterone, or NSAIDs (Lin et al., 2024). Formative research on animal models for several commonly utilized herbal formulations is ongoing but more research is needed to comprehensively describe clinical utility for available TCM preparations (K. Wang et al., 2020).

It is common for people in Iran to use purslane to treat symptoms of AUB. Purslane seeds are washed, dried, and ground into a powder, which can then be encapsulated. Purslane is said to exhibit estrogenic, anti-inflammatory, anti-proliferative, and analgesic effects and there are no known risks associated with purslane. There are a few very small studies which show some promise of improvement in the number of pads a person uses in a cycle, as well as self-reported quality of life measures (Khanam et al., 2021). Until further studies confirm this therapy's efficacy, people should be counseled that it may be beneficial but that studies are lacking.

In a randomized clinical trial in Iran, high school girls who were experiencing heavy menstrual bleeding were randomly allocated to receive a ginger or a placebo capsule. A dose of 250 mg of ginger in capsule form was administered 3 times per day starting from the first day of menstrual bleeding until the third day of menstrual bleeding. A significant decrease in menstrual bleeding was reported in the group receiving ginger, compared with the control participants (Kashefi et al., 2015).

Therapies such as green tea, vitamin D, and curcumin have been used for hundreds of years to treat AUB (Ciebiera et al., 2020). While there are limited studies to support their efficacy, the proposed biologic pathways for how these therapies may be useful is interesting and holds promise as potentially useful complementary therapies for people. There is a need for more human clinical trials involving these compounds before promoting widespread usage.

MANAGEMENT OF AMENORRHEA

For a person with amenorrhea, management depends on the determined cause of amenorrhea. Ovarian function abnormalities are the most common cause of amenorrhea, and estrogen production is the most reliable measure of ovarian function (Taylor et al., 2020). Tests to assess estrogen production include serum estradiol levels, progestogen challenge test, ultrasound measurement of endometrial thickness, and serum FSH concentration. A random serum estradiol level that is greater than 40 pg/mL indicates functioning ovaries. If the level is low, the person may be amenorrheic because of ovarian failure or hypothalamic amenorrhea.

A progesterone challenge test that produces withdrawal bleeding is indicative of functioning ovaries because bleeding will occur only if a sufficient amount of circulating estrogen is present. A progesterone challenge can be accomplished by administering micronized progesterone (Prometrium) 400 mg daily for 7 to 10 days or medroxyprogesterone acetate (Provera) 10 mg daily for 7 to 10 days. Withdrawal bleeding should occur within 7 to 10 days after the progesterone is discontinued if the level of endogenous estrogen is appropriate to produce a withdrawal bleed and the outflow tract is patent. If the person chooses to use micronized progesterone, it is suggested that they take this medication at bedtime because it can cause drowsiness in some people. If the response to the progesterone challenge is positive (withdrawal bleeding occurs), the person does not have galactorrhea, and their prolactin level is normal, the possibility of a pituitary tumor is effectively ruled out (Taylor et al., 2020). In this case, the diagnosis is anovulation, and the treatment is a progestogen for the first 10 days of each month or a combined contraceptive (pill, patch, or vaginal ring). The person should also be evaluated for PCOS. If the person does not have a positive progestogen challenge, then a physician consult is warranted for further evaluation and management options.

Serum FSH indirectly measures ovarian function, with lower levels of FSH indicating normally functioning ovaries. In contrast, an elevated result may indicate ovarian function disorder or disease and warrants further investigation. If the aforementioned tests reveal that the ovaries are producing estrogen and the FSH level is normal, the diagnosis is chronic anovulation (Taylor et al., 2020).

Thyroid disease and hyperprolactinemia are also common causes of anovulation, which can lead to amenorrhea. A TSH level can detect either hypothyroidism (TSH is elevated) or hyperthyroidism (TSH is low), both of which can cause amenorrhea. Menstrual cycles almost always return to normal after the thyroid level is normalized. Hyperprolactinemia is not always accompanied by galactorrhea (discharge from the nipples), but it can be diagnosed by obtaining a serum prolactin level in people with amenorrhea. Some medications, including antidepressants, opiates, calcium-channel blockers, and estrogens, can cause an elevated prolactin level; therefore, it is important to ask about medications when obtaining the health history. Hyperprolactinemia has many causes, but if it and the accompanying amenorrhea cannot be attributed to medication or another condition, then further evaluation to rule out pituitary tumors and hypothalamic mass lesions is necessary. A dopamine agonist is the treatment of choice for hyperprolactinemia (Taylor et al., 2020).

Table 25-7 lists the causes of primary and secondary amenorrhea.

All people with amenorrhea require management of this condition because if it is left untreated, hyperplasia and endometrial cancer can occur, regardless of the person's age. Typically, treatment consists of inducing menses using a progestogen, such as medroxyprogesterone acetate 5 to 10 mg daily for the first 12 to 14 days of the cycle. It is important for the person to know they are not protected against pregnancy during this treatment. If they do not have their menses, they should have a pregnancy test if they have engaged in intercourse during the treatment period. Oral contraceptive pills can also be used to induce a menstrual cycle.

Ovarian failure is diagnosed when low estrogen production is identified while the serum FSH is high. Premature ovarian failure can be due to many causes, including genetic conditions. For this reason, a karyotype test for all people younger than 30 years who have a diagnosis of ovarian failure is recommended. Ovarian failure may also be due to autoimmune diseases, particularly

TABLE 25-7 Causes of Primary and Secondary Amenorrhea

Primary Amenorrhea	Secondary Amenorrhea
Pregnancy	Pregnancy
Upper genital tract causes	Asherman syndrome
Müllerian agenesis (absence of uterus and vagina, normal secondary sex characteristics)	Cervical stenosis
Testicular feminization (absence of uterus, blind ending vaginal pouch, normal breast development, scant pubic and axillary hair)	Hormonal contraception
Lower genital tract causes	Hyperthyroidism/hypothyroidism
Labial agglutination	PCOS
Imperforate hymen	Pituitary tumor
Transverse vaginal septum	Premature ovarian failure
Hypergonadotropic hypogonadism	Menopause
FSH greater than 40 mIU/L Gonadal dysgenesis Ovarian enzyme disorder Resistant ovarian syndrome	Hypothalamic/central nervous system disorders (e.g., lifestyle stress, eating disorder, extreme athleticism)

Addison disease. Consequently, it is reasonable to test for antiadrenal antibodies in people who have premature ovarian failure (Taylor et al., 2020).

MRI assessment is suggested when there is no clear explanation for either hypogonadism or hyperprolactinemia. If no lesions are found, there is no need to perform further pituitary testing, and the diagnosis is functional hypothalamic amenorrhea (Taylor et al., 2020).

Functional hypothalamic amenorrhea is characterized by the absence of menses due to the suppression of HPOA in which no anatomic organic disease is identified (Pedreira et al., 2022). The typical picture of a person diagnosed with functional amenorrhea is an adolescent who is underweight, overexercises, and/or is experiencing a great deal of stress. In this setting, an energy deficit occurs, with a resultant negative impact on the HPOA. Treatment generally focuses on weight gain and exercise reduction, although psychological counseling may also be helpful. A goal of treatment is to offset the bone loss that occurs during the estrogen-deficient periods of time (Pedreira et al., 2022). The underlying pathophysiology of functional hypothalamic amenorrhea is not well understood, however, and more research about this condition is needed.

CONSIDERATIONS FOR SPECIFIC POPULATIONS

Adolescents

The American College of Obstetricians and Gynecologists Committee on Adolescent Health and the American Academy of Pediatrics encourage using the menstrual cycle as a vital sign because of the important information it provides about overall health (ACOG, 2015, reaffirmed 2025). First menses, termed menarche, has been stable at between 12–13 years old in well-nourished children in developed countries (ACOG, 2015, reaffirmed 2025).

Variations in nutritional status impact the maturation of the hypothalamus-pituitary-ovarian axis (HPOA) and individuals with higher BMIs may experience earlier menarche and those with lower BMIs may experience delays in menarche (Kabra & Fisher, 2022). Despite this variation, most adolescent people will experience menarche within 2–2.5 years of initial breast development (ACOG, 2015, reaffirmed 2021). The developing HPOA is also responsible for increased variability within and between menstrual cycles. HPOA immaturity may prevent estrogen from inducing luteinizing hormone release at midcycle, leading to follicular atresia and anovulatory cycles. Anovulatory cycles are common within the first 2 years following menarche, and cycle lengths between 21–45 days are normal. If anovulatory cycles persist beyond 2–3 years, other causes of anovulation should be considered including weight changes related to eating disorders, PCOS, thyroid disorders, diabetes mellitus, systemic lupus erythematous, kidney or liver disease. Adolescent people also experience greater variability in the day that menses occurs within their cycle than adults, resulting in less predictable ovulation and menses than adults (Kabra & Fisher, 2022).

Adolescents who present with heavy menstrual flow or long duration of menses at early in the reproductive years should be screened for coagulopathies. Coagulopathies account for between 20–53 percent of cases of heavy menstrual bleeding in adolescents compared to a 1–2 percent prevalence in adult patients (Kabra & Fisher, 2022). The most common coagulopathies causing heavy menstrual bleeding in adolescents are angiohemophilia followed by other platelet function disorders, thrombocytopenia, and clotting factor deficiencies (Kabra & Fisher, 2022).

Adolescents are more likely to present with nonstructural causes of abnormal uterine bleeding than structural causes (Kabra & Fisher, 2022). The most common endometrial cause of AUB in adolescents is endometritis associated with pelvic inflammatory disease (Kabra & Fisher, 2022). Contraceptive pills and devices are the most common cause of AUB in adolescents and comprehensive counseling on these effects should be discussed prior to initiation (Kabra & Fisher, 2022). It is important for clinicians to make no assumptions about an adolescent's sexual activity. It is essential to question adolescents about their sexual and gynecologic histories. Confidentiality is an important part of therapeutic interactions with all adolescents.

After a thorough history is obtained, decide if a pelvic examination is necessary. A pelvic examination should be done only if there is a specific indication for it, such as infection. Most adolescents with anovulatory bleeding can be treated with medication therapy (ACOG, 2015, reaffirmed 2025) and nutritional counseling. Teaching people who have significant anemia about consumption of a diet rich in iron and folic acid is important, and often a short course of iron supplementation is appropriate.

People with Disabilities

People with physical or mental disabilities and their caregivers may be particularly challenged by menstruation. It is important for the clinician to assess the level of knowledge the adolescent or adult has about their body and menstruation. Communication should be directed to the adolescent or adult, not to the caregiver (ACOG, 2019, reaffirmed 2024). It is important to ascertain if specific concerns need to be addressed. It is also important to use developmentally appropriate education to teach the person about hygiene, contraception, sexually transmitted infections, and abuse prevention (ACOG, 2019).

When the evaluation is complete, communicating with the person and their parents or caregiver is important. There may be a need to treat AUB, contraception may be desired, or menstrual suppression may be indicated (ACOG, 2022). If contraception is desired, the level of cognitive disability will help to determine which method might work best and to ensure that the individual is engaged in a consensual and safe relationships. Some contraceptives may not be suggested if the person is immobile (e.g., contraceptives that have venous thromboembolism risks associated with their use); therefore, the clinician should assess the risk–benefit profile prior to prescribing any option. If the family or caregiver is requesting a hysterectomy or sterilization procedure for the adolescent, it is important to find out the specific reason for the request and consider the ethical implications. Healthcare providers have an ethical obligation to educate people to the full extent of their cognitive abilities, maintain respect, maximize autonomy, and avoid ableist harm.

Perimenopause

The incidence of AUB increases as people approach menopause. The onset of anovulatory cycles represents a continuation of declining ovarian function. People should be educated early about health-promoting activities that can offset the risks associated with menopause, such as osteoporosis. They should be encouraged to exercise regularly and modify their diets to include foods rich in iron and calcium; in addition, if they smoke, they should be counseled about quitting (ACOG, 2014a, reaffirmed 2024).

Older People

One of the most important goals in the assessment of AUB is to rule out endometrial cancer, particularly in older people. Endometrial cancer is the most common gynecologic malignancy. It is the fourth most common cancer in people assigned female at birth in the United States after breast, lung, and colorectal cancers. The American Cancer Society recommends that all people experiencing menopause be informed of the risks and symptoms of endometrial cancer and be advised to seek evaluation if symptoms occur (American Cancer Society, 2020). Endometrial evaluation, including tissue sampling via endometrial biopsy, is recommended for all people 45 and older who present with AUB (ACOG, 2015, reaffirmed 2021).

Box 25-3 lists the risk factors for endometrial cancer. Notably, estrogen stimulation resulting in endometrial hyperplasia increases a person's risk for developing endometrial cancer. Symptoms of endometrial cancer include postmenopausal bleeding; thus, all uterine bleeding in a person who is postmenopausal should be considered cancer until proven otherwise.

BOX 25-3 Risk Factors for Endometrial Cancer

- Age 40 years or older
- Anovulation
- PCOS
- Family history of endometrial cancer
- New onset of heavy irregular bleeding, particularly after menopause
- Nulliparity
- Larger body size
- Unopposed estrogen stimulation of endometrium
- Tamoxifen therapy
- Infertility
- Type 2 diabetes

CONCLUSION

The clinical management of AUB is complex and requires the clinician to consider not only the physical etiology, but also the individual, emotional, and economic aspects of management. Age, history, and physical examination are reliable tools that suggest etiologic factors. It is essential to always rule out pregnancy first and to never assume the cause of the bleeding. Be thorough and consider all aspects of the PALM-COEIN classification system. If bleeding persists even in the face of negative or reassuring tests, reinitiate the investigation and consider consultation and referral. Order laboratory tests selectively, and always involve the person actively in the decision-making process and management plan.

References

Abbott, J. A. (2017). Adenomyosis and abnormal uterine bleeding (AUB-A)—Pathogenesis, diagnosis, and management. *Best Practice & Research. Clinical Obstetrics & Gynaecology, 40*, 68–81. https://doi.org/10.1016/j.bpobgyn.2016.09.006

Ali, M., Raslan, M., Ciebiera, M., Zaręba, K., & Al-Hendy, A. (2022). Current approaches to overcome the side effects of GnRH analogs in the treatment of patients with uterine fibroids. *Expert Opinion on Drug Safety, 21*(4), 477–486. https://doi.org/10.1080/14740338.2022.1989409

American Cancer Society. (2020, June 24). *Endometrial Cancer | Uterine Cancer*. https://www.cancer.org/cancer/types/endometrial-cancer.html

American College of Nurse-Midwives. (2017). Endometrial biopsy: American College of Nurse-Midwives. *Journal of Midwifery and Womens Health, 62*(4), 502–506. https://doi.org/doi: 10.1111/jmwh.12652. Epub 2017 Jul 18. PMID: 28719132.

American College of Obstetricians and Gynecologists. (2012, reaffirmed 2024). Practice Bulletin No. 128: Diagnosis of abnormal uterine bleeding in reproductive-aged women. https://www.acog.org/clinical/clinical-guidance/practice-bulletin/articles/2012/07/diagnosis-of-abnormal-uterine-bleeding-in-reproductive-aged-women

American College of Obstetricians and Gynecologists. (2013a, reaffirmed 2025). ACOG Practice Bulletin No. 136: Management of abnormal uterine bleeding associated with ovulatory dysfunction. https://www.acog.org/clinical/clinical-guidance/practice-bulletin/articles/2013/07/management-of-abnormal-uterine-bleeding-associated-with-ovulatory-dysfunction

American College of Obstetricians and Gynecologists. (2013b). Von Willebrand disease in women (ACOG Committee Opinion No. 580). *Obstetrics & Gynecology, 122*(6), 1368–1373.

American College of Obstetricians and Gynecologists. (2014a). Management of menopausal symptoms. Practice Bulletin No. 141. *Obstetrics & Gynecology, 123*, 202–216.

American College of Obstetricians and Gynecologists. (2014b). Primary Ovarian Insufficiency in Adolescents and Young Women. Committee Opinion No. 605. *Obstetrics & Gynecology, 124*(1), 193–197.

American College of Obstetricians and Gynecologists. (2015, reaffirmed 2025). Committee Opinion No 651: Menstruation in girls and adolescents: Using the menstrual cycle as a vital sign. *Obstetrics & Gynecology, 126*(6), e143–e146.

American College of Obstetricians and Gynecologists. (2018). ACOG Practice Bulletin No. 194: Polycystic Ovary Syndrome. *Obstetrics & Gynecology, 131*(6), e157–e171. https://doi.org/10.1097/AOG.0000000000002656

American College of Obstetricians and Gynecologists. (2019). Genetic syndromes and gynecologic implications in adolescents: ACOG Committee Opinion No. 768. *Obstetrics & Gynecology, 133*, e226-234.

American College of Obstetricians and Gynecologists. (2021). Committee on Practice Bulletins—Gynecology. Management of symptomatic uterine leiomyomas: ACOG practice bulletin, no. 228. *Obstetrics & Gynecology, 137*(6), e100–e115.

American College of Obstetricians and Gynecologists. (2022). General approaches to medical management of menstrual suppression: Clinical consensus no. 3. *Obstetrics & Gynecology, 140*, 528–541.

American College of Obstetricians and Gynecologists. (2015, reaffirmed 2021). Endometrial cancer: Practice bulletin no. 149. https://www.acog.org/clinical/clinical-guidance/practice-bulletin/articles/2015/04/endometrial-cancer

Azziz, R. (2018). Polycystic ovary syndrome. *Obstetrics & Gynecology, 132*(2), 321. https://doi.org/10.1097/AOG.0000000000002698

Bazot, M., & Daraï, E. (2018). Role of transvaginal sonography and magnetic resonance imaging in the diagnosis of uterine adenomyosis. *Fertility and Sterility, 109*(3), 389–397.

Behera, S., Gomanthi, B., & Behera, K. (2023). Sleep quality and depression among women with abnormal uterine bleeding (AUB). *International Journal of Nursing Education, 15*(2), 60–64.

Bickley, L. S. (2021). *Bates' Guide to Physical Examination and History Taking*. Wolters Kluwer.

Caron, S. L. (2022). To shave or not to shave: Exploring pubic hair removal among college students. *American Journal of Sexuality Education, 17*(2), 156–175. https://doi.org/10.1080/15546128.2021.2025182

Ciebiera, M., Ali, M., Prince, L., Jackson-Bey, T., Atabiekov, I., Zgliczyński, S., & Al-Hendy, A. (2020). The evolving role of natural compounds in the medical treatment of uterine fibroids. *Journal of Clinical Medicine, 9*(5), Article 5. https://doi.org/10.3390/jcm9051479

Deshmukh, P. Y., Boricha, B. G., & Pandey, A. (2015). The association of thyroid disorders with abnormal uterine bleeding. *Int J Reprod Contracept Obstet Gynecol, 4*(3), 701–708.

Engler, J., Filliter, C., Montastruc, F., Abenhaim, H., Rej, S., & Renoux, C. (2024). Risk of abnormal uterine bleeding associated with high-affinity compared with low-affinity serotonin and norepinephrine reuptake inhibitors. *Journal of Affective Disorders, 350*, 813–821. https://doi.org/10.1016/j.jad.2024.01.163

Harvey, S. V., Pfeiffer, R. M., Landy, R., Wentzensen, N., & Clarke, M. A. (2022). Trends and predictors of hysterectomy prevalence among women in the United States. *American Journal of Obstetrics and Gynecology, 227*(4), 611.e1-611.e12. https://doi.org/10.1016/j.ajog.2022.06.028

Henry, C., Jefferies, R., Ekeroma, A., & Filoche, S. (2020). Beyond the numbers—understanding women's experiences of accessing care for abnormal uterine bleeding (AUB): A qualitative study. *BMJ Open, 10*(11), e041853. https://doi.org/10.1136/bmjopen-2020-041853

Johnson, J.-E., Daley, D., Tarta, C., & Stanciu, P. I. (2023). Risk of endometrial cancer in patients with polycystic ovarian syndrome: A meta-analysis. *Oncology Letters, 25*(4), 1–9. https://doi.org/10.3892/ol.2023.13754

Kabra, R., & Fisher, M. (2022). Abnormal uterine bleeding in adolescents. *Current Problems in Pediatric and Adolescent Health Care, 52*(5), 101185. https://doi.org/10.1016/j.cppeds.2022.101185

Kashefi, F., Khajehei, M., Alavinia, M., Golmakani, E., & Asili, J. (2015). Effect of ginger (Zingiber officinale) on heavy menstrual bleeding: A placebo-controlled, randomized clinical trial. *Phytotherapy Research, 29*(1), 114–119. https://doi.org/10.1002/ptr.5235

Katon, J. G., Plowden, T. C., & Marsh, E. E. (2023). Racial disparities in uterine fibroids and endometriosis: A systematic review and application of social, structural, and political context. *Fertility and Sterility, 119*(3), 355–363. https://doi.org/10.1016/j.fertnstert.2023.01.022

Kaunitz, A. M. (2019). Abnormal uterine bleeding in reproductive-age women. *JAMA*. 321(21), 2126–2127. https://doi.org/10.1001/jama.2019.5248

Keizer, A. L., Nieuwenhuis, L. L., Twisk, J. W., Huirne, J. A., Hehenkamp, W. J., & Brölmann, H. A. (2018). Role of 3-dimensional sonography in the assessment of submucous fibroids: A pilot study. *Journal of Ultrasound in Medicine, 37*(1), 191-199.

Kerns, J., Itriyeva, K., & Fisher, M. (2022). Etiology and management of amenorrhea in adolescent and young adult women. *Current Problems in Pediatric and Adolescent Health Care, 52*(5), 101184. https://doi.org/10.1016/j.cppeds.2022.101184

Khanam, B., Begum, W., Tipo, F. A., & Naim, M. (2021). Effect of *Tukhme Khurfa* (purslane seeds) in abnormal uterine bleeding: A prospective study. *Advances in Integrative Medicine, 8*(3), 193–198. https://doi.org/10.1016/j.aimed.2020.03.001

Leyland, N., Laberge, P., Evans, D., Savard, E. G., & Rittenberg, D. (2024). Guideline No. 453: Endometrial Ablation in the Management of Abnormal Uterine Bleeding. *Journal of Obstetrics and Gynaecology Canada, 46*(9), 102641. https://doi.org/10.1016/j.jogc.2024.102641

Lin, Y.-R., Lin, W.-C., Wu, M.-Y., Lin, C.-L., Yang, S.-T., & Yen, H.-R. (2024). Complementary chinese herbal medicine treatment is associated with a reduction of surgical rate in patients with dysfunctional uterine bleeding: A propensity-score matched cohort study. *International Journal of Women's Health, 16*, 1361–1375. https://doi.org/10.2147/IJWH.S461730

Lin, Y.-R., Wu, M.-Y., Chiang, J.-H., Yen, H.-R., & Yang, S.-T. (2017). The utilization of traditional Chinese medicine in patients with dysfunctional uterine bleeding in Taiwan: A nationwide population-based study. *BMC Complementary and Alternative Medicine, 17*, 427. https://doi.org/10.1186/s12906-017-1939-1

MacGregor, R., Jain, V., Hillman, S., & Lumsden, M. A. (2022). Investigating abnormal uterine bleeding in reproductive aged women. *BMJ, 378*, e070906. https://doi.org/10.1136/bmj-2022-070906

Munro, M. G., Critchley, H. O. D., & Fraser, I. S. (2018). The two FIGO systems for normal and abnormal uterine bleeding symptoms and classification of causes of abnormal uterine bleeding in the reproductive years: 2018 revisions. *International Journal of Gynecology & Obstetrics, 143*(3), 393–408. https://doi.org/10.1002/ijgo.12666

Pedreira, C. C., Maya, J., & Misra, M. (2022). Functional hypothalamic amenorrhea: Impact on bone and neuropsychiatric outcomes. *Frontiers in Endocrinology, 13*, 953180. https://doi.org/10.3389/fendo.2022.953180

Potter, J., Sari, Z., & Lindblad, A. J. (2021). NSAIDs for heavy menstrual bleeding. *Canadian Family Physician, 67*(8), 598. https://doi.org/10.46747/cfp.6708598

Taylor, H. S., Fritz, M. A., Pal, L., & Seli, E. (2020). *Speroff's clinical gynecologic endocrinology and infertility* (9th ed.). Wolters Kluwer.

Tian, N., Sun, Y., Liu, Y., Jin, J., Chen, S., Han, H., Zhang, Y., & Li, Z. (2024). Safety assessment of tranexamic acid: Real-world adverse event analysis from the FAERS database. *Frontiers in Pharmacology, 15*, 1388138. https://doi.org/10.3389/fphar.2024.1388138

Tsakiridis, I., Giouleka, S., Koutsouki, G., Kostakis, N., Kalogiannidis, I., Kourtis, A., Athanasiadis, A., Goulis, D. G., & Dagklis, T. (2022). Investigation and management of abnormal uterine bleeding in reproductive-aged women: A descriptive review of national and international recommendations. *The European Journal of Contraception & Reproductive Health Care: The Official Journal of the European Society of Contraception, 27*(6), 504–517. https://doi.org/10.1080/13625187.2022.2112169

Tu, X., Huang, G., & Tan, S. (2009). Chinese herbal medicine for dysfunctional uterine bleeding: A meta-analysis. *Evidence-Based Complementary and Alternative Medicine: eCAM, 6*(1), 99–105. https://doi.org/10.1093/ecam/nem063

Wallace, K., Stewart, E. A., Wise, L. A., Nicholson, W. K., Parry, J. P., Zhang, S., Laughlin-Tommaso, S., Jacoby, V., Anchan, R. M., Diamond, M. P., Venable, S., Shiflett, A., Wegienka, G. R., Maxwell, G. L., Wojdyla, D., Myers, E. R., & Marsh, E. (2022). Anxiety, depression, and quality of life after procedural intervention for uterine fibroids. *Journal of Women's Health, 31*(3), 415–424. https://doi.org/10.1089/jwh.2020.8915

Wang, A., Wang, S., Owens, C. D., Vora, J. B., & Diamond, M. P. (2022). Health care costs and treatment patterns associated with uterine fibroids and heavy menstrual bleeding: A claims analysis. *Journal of Women's Health, 31*(6), 856–863. https://doi.org/10.1089/jwh.2020.8983

Wang, K., Gao, L., Zhang, Q., Zhang, Y., Yao, W., Zhang, M., Tang, Y., Ding, A., & Zhang, L. (2020). Revealing the mechanisms and the material basis of Rubia cordifolia L. on abnormal uterine bleeding with uniting simultaneous determination of four components and systematic pharmacology approach—Experimental validation. *Journal of Pharmaceutical and Biomedical Analysis, 189*, 113475. https://doi.org/10.1016/j.jpba.2020.113475

APPENDIX 25-A

Instructions for Performing an Endometrial Biopsy

Contraindications for endometrial biopsy:

- Viable intrauterine pregnancy
- Known or suspected cervical cancer
- Acute vaginal, cervical, or uterine infection
- Inability to visualize the cervical os
- Obstructing cervical mass or lesion

Before the procedure:

- Obtain a thorough history and pelvic exam and obtain TVS if indicated.
- Make certain there is a signed informed consent.
- Rule out pregnancy.
- Optional: Administer 600 to 800 mg ibuprofen or other NSAID 60 minutes prior to the procedure.

Supplies/equipment needed:

- Gloves, both sterile and nonsterile
- Appropriately sized vaginal speculum (Graves preferred)
- Cotton balls or large cotton swabs
- Antiseptic solution such as Betadine or Hibiclens
- Endometrial sampling device (at least two)
- Labeled formalin sample container
- Scissors
- Optional:
  - Local anesthetic, such as 2 percent lidocaine or 20 percent benzocaine gel
  - Tenaculum

Procedure:

1. Ask the patient to lie in the lithotomy position with their head elevated.
2. Perform a bimanual examination to determine uterine position and size.
3. Insert an appropriately sized speculum and ensure visualization of the cervix.
4. Cleanse the cervix with an antiseptic solution.
5. If a tenaculum is required (to align the uterus), place it on the anterior cervical lip and gently pull outward to straighten the cervical–uterine angle.
6. Open the needed equipment.
7. Don sterile gloves.
8. Insert the sampling device using moderate, steady pressure.
9. Advance to the uterine fundus and stop when resistance is felt.
10. Stabilize the sheath with the finger and thumb of one hand and pull the piston out as far as possible with the other hand to create suction.
11. Roll the sheath between the thumb and forefinger while simultaneously moving the sheath in and out of the fundus three or four times.
12. Do not bring the sheath outside the external cervical os until the sample is obtained because suction will be lost.
13. Withdraw the device when the lumen is as full of tissue as possible.
14. Cut the top of the distal tip with the scissors and plunge the contents into the formalin container.
15. Take a second sample using a new endometrial sampling device if the first sample appears insufficient.
16. Provide a pad or tampon in case of spotting after the procedure. Make sure the patient is fully recovered before leaving the room.

Note: Be sure to read sampling instructions on the endometrial sampling device you are using because there are slight differences in recommended techniques.

CHAPTER 26

Polycystic Ovarian Syndrome and Other Hyperandrogenic Disorders

Keely Robinson

The editors acknowledge Maureen Shannon, who was the author of the previous edition of this chapter.

Editor's Note: The literature on hyperandrogenic disorders, namely polycystic ovarian syndrome, is rapidly evolving as scientific understanding of hyperandrogenism continues to expand. It is important for readers of this chapter to be aware that at time of publication, though many studies exist, overall the evidence on this subject remains moderate to poor quality (Teede et al., 2023; Neven et al., 2024). There is much left to learn, and the editors are hopeful that the literature will continue to evolve in the coming years.

Hyperandrogenism is a complex endocrine disorder that can have systemic effects and cause distressing cosmetic changes. People assigned female at birth (AFAB) with hyperandrogenemia may have multifaceted concerns regarding their general health, fertility, appearance, and social acceptance. Given these broad implications, it is important for clinicians to approach people who have symptoms of hyperandrogenism with empathy and attentiveness. This chapter reviews the pathophysiology, clinical presentation, diagnostic evaluation, and therapy for hyperandrogenism, with a focus on the most common hyperandrogenic disorder, polycystic ovary syndrome (PCOS), including its systemic sequelae. It is important to note that not all AFAB people who have hyperandrogenic disorders identify as female or women. To ensure inclusive learning materials, we will use gender-neutral terms whenever possible throughout this chapter.

DESCRIPTION OF HYPERANDROGENIC DISORDERS

Scope of the Condition

Approximately 10 percent of AFAB people have clinical or biochemical evidence of excessive androgen production that results in various physical manifestations. Though PCOS is the most common, it is important to consider other possible diagnoses in the clinical and laboratory evaluation of the individual. Aside from PCOS, hyperandrogenism may be due to congenital adrenal hyperplasia, adrenal or ovarian tumors, ovarian hyperthecosis, gestational hyperandrogenism, and iatrogenic or idiopathic hyperandrogenism (Sharma et al., 2021; Esquivel-Zuniga et al., 2022). Because PCOS is the most common hyperandrogenic disorder, this chapter focuses primarily on PCOS.

PCOS has a prevalence rate of 6 to 20 percent of all AFAB people, depending on the diagnostic criteria used (Bahri Khomami & Teede, 2024; Siddiqui et al., 2022). In approximately 70 percent of individuals, the presenting clinical signs of PCOS reflect hyperandrogenism, including hirsutism, acne, androgenic alopecia, menstrual irregularity, and subfertility or infertility. People with PCOS also have an increased risk for adverse health outcomes, such as endometrial cancer, type 2 diabetes, cardiovascular disease, and metabolic syndrome (Lim et al., 2019; Rasquin et al., 2022; Bahri Khomami & Teede, 2024). In addition, people with PCOS may be at an increased risk of pregnancy complications if they conceive (Bahri Khomami & Teede, 2024). Consequently, they need to have regular, comprehensive, preventive health care and education to decrease their risk of developing the long-term sequelae associated with this syndrome.

Etiology

At the time of publication, investigations into the underlying mechanisms that contribute to the development of PCOS are ongoing, and the exact etiology remains unknown. Twin cohort studies have shown that in about 70 percent of cases, there may be a genetic component, and other studies hypothesize a combination of genetic predisposition together with environmental and epigenetic factors (Rasquin et al., 2022; Vatier et al., 2024). Many animal studies have shown that the mechanisms of PCOS may be driven by dysfunction in the hypothalamic–pituitary axis. Bioactive androgens, namely testosterone and dihydrotestosterone (DHT), bind to androgen receptors present in the brain, ovarian stroma, ovarian follicles, and corpus lutea while proandrogens, dehydroepiandrosterone (DHEA) and androstenedione, need to be converted into testosterone and DHT before they can bring about androgenic effects in the body. Mechanisms leading to the hyperandrogen state in PCOS along each of these pathways are being studied to better understand the underlying causes of PCOS (Walters et al., 2022).

In all AFAB people, the major circulating androgens are dehydroepiandrosterone sulfate (DHEA-S), DHEA, androstenedione, testosterone, and DHT. Testosterone is the most potent androgen. AFAB people normally produce amounts of testosterone in the range of 0.2 to 0.3 mg per day, 50 percent of which is derived from the peripheral conversion of androstenedione. The ovaries are the most common source of increased testosterone and androstenedione given the multiple sites of androgen receptors (Taylor et al., 2020; Walters et al., 2022).

The bioactivity and androgenicity of testosterone are determined by sex hormone-binding globulin (SHBG). Circulating testosterone is bound to SHBG, which is produced in the liver. It is normal for approximately 80 percent of circulating testosterone to be bound to SHBG, 19 percent to be loosely bound to albumin, and the remaining 1 percent to be left unbound. The unbound, free testosterone is mainly responsible for androgenicity, although the fraction associated with albumin makes some contribution to this condition (Taylor et al., 2020; Walters et al., 2022).

SHBG levels are increased by estrogen and thyroid hormone and suppressed by androgens and insulin. Therefore, in the presence of high levels of thyroid hormone or estrogen, more testosterone is bound, making less biologically available. If SHBG is suppressed or androgen production increases, the amount of free (unbound) testosterone will increase without necessarily increasing the total testosterone level, and the individual may develop symptoms of hyperandrogenism. Thus, because of the interplay among SHBG, insulin, thyroid hormone, estrogen, and androgen production, the total testosterone concentration may remain in the normal range, with symptoms reflecting only the decreased binding capacity of the SHBG and the increased percentage of unbound testosterone (Taylor et al., 2020).

Although testosterone is the major circulating androgen, DHT is the hormone responsible for the clinical expression of androgen stimulation in many androgen-sensitive tissues, such as the skin, pilosebaceous unit, and hair follicles. Conversion of testosterone to DHT is accomplished by 5α-reductase, an enzyme that is present in these target tissues. The sensitivity of the hair follicle to the effect of androgens is genetically predetermined and depends on the degree of 5α-reductase activity. In people who are genetically predisposed to excessive 5α-reductase activity, even normal levels of androgen can stimulate hair growth, leading to idiopathic hirsutism. Therefore, not all cases of hirsutism should be assumed to be related to hyperandrogenism or to PCOS as the mechanisms involved are multifactorial (Taylor et al., 2020).

In summary, the symptoms of hyperandrogenism include hirsutism, acne, alopecia, and, frequently, anovulation. These symptoms are caused by either an increase in androgen levels, a decrease in production of SHBG, or an increase in 5α-reductase activity in the skin and hair follicles. These changes result in the stimulation of the androgen-sensitive areas (Taylor et al., 2020). In preparing to diagnose and treat these symptoms, determining the source of the increased androgen production is the key to identifying and addressing the cause of hyperandrogenism.

Biochemical Features of Polycystic Ovary Syndrome

The pathogenesis of PCOS is complex and not completely understood, although many hormonal pathways have been identified as contributors to the syndrome. In addition, genetic, epigenetic, and environmental factors can influence the phenotypic variation in PCOS features, which can make diagnosis more challenging (Unfer et al., 2024). People with PCOS are predominantly anovulatory, and they typically maintain relatively steady levels of gonadotropins and sex steroids instead of experiencing the fluctuations in these levels characteristic of the normal menstrual cycle. Serum concentrations of luteinizing hormone (LH) are usually higher than those found in people who ovulate normally. The elevated LH levels are a result of increased pulse frequency and amplitude. People with PCOS have a relatively constant LH pulse frequency of approximately one pulse per hour, whereas people who are ovulatory experience cyclic variations in LH frequency. The increased LH pulse frequency is caused by increased gonadotropin-releasing hormone (GnRH) pulse frequency, which also causes follicle-stimulating hormone (FSH) levels to be at the low end of the normal range. FSH levels are also decreased because of the increased estrone levels resulting from peripheral conversion of increased androstenedione. People with PCOS generally exhibit an increased LH:FSH ratio (Taylor et al., 2020; Walters et al., 2022; Yang & Chen, 2024).

Most of the increased androgen production seen with PCOS occurs in the ovaries as a result of increased LH stimulation because increased LH pulse frequency stimulates ovarian theca cell production of androgens (Walters et al., 2022; Yang & Chen, 2024). People with PCOS may also have some increased androgen production in the adrenal glands. Additionally, insulin resistance, which results in compensatory hyperinsulinemia, is common in those with PCOS and can further contribute to hyperandrogenism. Increased insulin levels stimulate androgen production in the ovaries and suppress SHBG production in the liver. A cycle is created in which the elevated androgens and insulin suppress SHBG synthesis, resulting in an increase in free testosterone, which in turn exacerbates the insulin resistance (Taylor et al., 2020). In addition, the lower FSH levels found in people with PCOS impair follicle maturation and ovulation (Siddiqui et al., 2022; Walters et al., 2022).

CLINICAL PRESENTATION

Hirsutism

Hirsutism is defined as excessive terminal hair growth occurring in anatomic areas where the hair follicles are most androgen sensitive. Androgens cause transformation of fine, soft, unpigmented, vellus hair to coarse, dark, terminal hair in androgen-dependent areas of hair growth (Ilgan et al., 2019; Rasquin et al., 2022). Hirsutism is present in approximately 10 percent of the general AFAB population but is found in about 70 percent of people with PCOS. Common sites of involvement include the face and chin, upper lip, areolae, sternum, lower abdomen, lower back, inner thighs, and perineum. In addition, manifestations of hirsutism associated with PCOS develop over time and increase with larger body size, compared to the fairly rapid-onset hirsutism that is observed in association with neoplasms (Spritzer et al., 2022; Teede et al., 2023).

Hair follicle sensitivity to androgen stimulation is genetically determined, so not everyone's body will respond the same way with hair growth in the setting of exposure to increased androgens. The Ferriman-Gallwey scale is currently the only validated tool to assess for hirsutism (Ferriman & Gallwey, 1961; Hatch et al., 1981). It has, however, drawn criticism because the initial development of the tool was based on studies done on a largely homogenous population of white people. The Modified Ferriman-Gallwey scale is now most commonly used, accounting for variation in the diagnostic criteria based on race (Teede et al., 2023). This too has drawn criticism because it assumes that all people of a certain race have the same genetics, and it also does not account for people of mixed race backgrounds. This tool is the current standard of care for assessing the degree and extent of hirsutism, but clinicians should take care to be aware of these limitations when using the tool (Ilagan et al., 2019; Taylor et al., 2020). Refer to **Color Plate 29** for the scale.

Hirsutism as a symptom is not present in all people with PCOS as its causes are multifactorial. It depends on the genetic factors, how responsive the follicles are to androgens, interactions between circulating and local androgens, and other hormonal variables (Ilagan et al., 2019; Rasquin et al., 2022). The severity of hirsutism does not correlate with the severity of androgen excess, so those with significant biochemical hyperandrogenemia may present with only mild or no hirsutism (Spritzer et al., 2022).

Alopecia

In contrast to hirsutism, prolonged exposure to circulating androgens may paradoxically cause hair loss due to decreased density of androgen-sensitive scalp hair and reduced scalp coverage and volume. This process typically results in diffuse alopecia that includes hair loss at the vertex, crown, or a diffuse pattern with preservation of the frontal hairline, although bitemporal and frontal hair loss can be seen with more severe hyperandrogenemia (Carmina et al., 2019). A 2019 meta-analysis by Carmina et al. found that approximately 28 percent of people with PCOS have some form of alopecia, but it is rarely a presenting symptom.

Acne

Androgen stimulation of the pilosebaceous unit can cause enlargement of the sebaceous glands and increased secretion of sebum, leading to acne. Acne is a common finding in adolescents and usually regresses by the time affected individuals reach their mid-20s. In contrast, acne that persists beyond this time or presents when a person is in their mid-20s or 30s may be considered a sign of hyperandrogenemia, particularly if acne is accompanied by hirsutism or menstrual dysfunction or is resistant to treatment for these conditions. Acne is present in over 40 percent of people with PCOS (Ramezani Tehrani et al., 2021; Unfer et al., 2024).

Virilization

Virilization is characterized by clitoral hypertrophy, severe hirsutism, deepening of the voice, increased muscle mass, breast atrophy, and male-pattern baldness. This condition may indicate the presence of one of the less common causes of hyperandrogenism, such as adrenal or ovarian tumor, congenital adrenal hyperplasia, or hyperthecosis. It may also be associated with severe hyperinsulinemia. If the onset of virilization is sudden or the progression is rapid, this condition is particularly concerning for neoplasm (Bizuneh et al., 2025; Esquivel-Zuniga et al., 2022; Teede et al., 2023).

Menstrual Dysfunction and Infertility

People with hyperandrogenism may have various degrees of ovulatory dysfunction. Indeed, menstrual irregularity is a hallmark feature of PCOS. Infrequent menstrual cycles (cycle length greater than 38 days) is the most common presentation of overt menstrual dysfunction. People with PCOS may also present with amenorrhea (absence of menses). Those with amenorrhea may have significant endocrinopathies, including more severe hyperandrogenemia, increased serum LH and cortisol levels, and increased incidence of hyperinsulinemia (Yang & Chen, 2024). More rarely, people with PCOS may present with frequent cycles (cycle length less than 24 days). Bleeding is generally irregular and unpredictable and can be heavy as a result of continuous estrogenic stimulation of the endometrium and resultant endometrial hyperplasia. Typically, menstrual irregularity begins at menarche, but it can occur after regular cycles (Taylor et al., 2020).

Though menstrual cycle irregularities are most common in PCOS, regular menses do not rule out the possibility of oligo-anovulation. Subclinical menstrual dysfunction, in which people have regularly occurring menses but chronic anovulation, is common in individuals with PCOS (Jones & Sung, 2025).

Many people with hyperandrogenism experience infertility as a result of anovulation, although individuals with PCOS can ovulate intermittently. More than half of those with PCOS are fertile (i.e., they will become pregnant within 12 months of trying), although it may take them longer to conceive (Teede et al., 2023).

Polycystic Ovaries

Since Stein and Leventhal originally described the thickened, glistening, white, enlarged multicystic ovary in 1935, it has been clear that PCOS is associated with a classic ovarian morphology. In PCOS, polycystic ovaries are a result of chronic anovulation (Taylor et al., 2020). In 2023, a consensus group that included representatives from 71 countries developed international guidelines based on current evidence, which included recommendations for the use of ultrasound that take into account the life stage of the individual. Currently, ultrasound is not recommended for the diagnosis of PCOS within 8 years of menarche due to the high incidence of multifollicular ovaries in adolescents (Teede et al., 2019; Teede et al., 2023). The guidelines also note that there is a need to develop age-specific cutoff values for polycystic ovarian morphology (PCOM) criteria. The recommendation of the group is that when transvaginal ultrasonography is performed, updated equipment that has a frequency bandwidth of 8 MHz should be used. The threshold for the diagnosis of PCOM is 20 or more follicles and/or an ovarian volume of 10 ml or greater for either ovary (Teede et al., 2023).

Although the majority of people with PCOS have evidence of polycystic ovaries, the presence of this morphology is not required if other diagnostic criteria for the syndrome are met (Neven et al., 2024; Teede et al., 2023). Ultrasound can be a useful diagnostic tool for evaluation of presence of PCOM. The definition of polycystic ovaries does not apply to those who take combined oral contraceptives (COCs) because COCs modify ovarian morphology. In addition, people who do not meet the diagnostic criteria for PCOS can have polycystic-appearing ovaries on ultrasound (Neven et al., 2024).

Weight and PCOS

For PCOS and other endocrine disorders, changes in body size and composition are discussed in the literature. It is crucial, however, to be aware that body weight alone is not an appropriate measure for health and should always be considered together with other factors (Teede et al., 2023). Body mass index (BMI), though commonly used as a proxy for measuring health, is not a good measure for adiposity or health. Data show that BMI specifically is deeply rooted in racism and reinforces the harmful assumption that there is one ideal body type (Strings, 2023). There is a growing body of literature that provides data-driven evidence that weight-based counseling, counseling for weight loss, and weight shaming are overtly harmful and cause sequelae such as psychological distress, eating disorders, and substance use disorders (Fulton et al., 2023; Lessard & Puhl, 2021; Puhl et al., 2021; Teede et al., 2023). Though increased adiposity is a contributor to endocrine dysfunction in PCOS, take care to remember that weight alone is not an indicator of health; that BMI does not measure adiposity; and that counseling all people of certain body types to lose weight is harmful and does not improve health measures in the long term.

As adipose tissue plays an active role in the endocrine system, increased adiposity is associated with three alterations that interfere with normal ovulation:

- Increased peripheral aromatization of androgens, resulting in chronically elevated estrogen concentrations
- Decreased levels of hepatic SHBG, resulting in increased circulating concentrations of free estradiol and testosterone
- Insulin resistance, leading to a compensatory increase in insulin levels that stimulates androgen production in the ovarian stroma, resulting in high local androgen concentrations that impair follicular development (Taylor et al., 2020)

As a result, having increased adiposity may increase the likelihood of menstrual dysfunction and infertility (Taylor et al., 2020). People with PCOS with increased adipose tissue have been found to have worsened reproductive and metabolic outcomes, including increased testosterone and free androgen index, decreased SHBG, increased fasting glucose and fasting insulin, and a worsened lipid profile (Glueck & Goldenberg, 2019). People are also more likely to develop impaired glucose tolerance, type 2 diabetes, hypertension, dyslipidemias, and estrogen-dependent tumors than people with PCOS who are of normal or low weight (Glueck & Goldenberg, 2019). For these reasons, it is necessary to consider adiposity, rather than overall weight or BMI, in discussion of the pathogenesis of PCOS.

Insulin Resistance

Overall, approximately 50 to 70 percent of people with PCOS are insulin resistant, a condition that often results in compensatory hyperinsulinemia (American Diabetes Association, 2019; Glueck & Goldenberg, 2019). Hyperinsulinemia plays a pathogenic role in the etiology of PCOS by stimulating ovarian androgen production and decreasing serum SHBG concentrations. Increased adiposity further complicates the condition by increasing insulin resistance. Insulin resistance occurs in people with PCOS at any weight or size, but its frequency and magnitude are increased in people with PCOS who have more adipose tissue (Glueck & Goldenberg, 2019).

Dyslipidemia

Most individuals with PCOS (70%) have at least one lipid level that is borderline or high (Guo et al., 2022; Liu et al., 2019). Dyslipidemias commonly found in those with PCOS include decreased HDL cholesterol and increased triglycerides, LDL cholesterol, and non-HDL lipoproteins, reflecting more atherogenic apolipoprotein ratios. Additionally, prevalence of dyslipidemias is higher in individuals with PCOS regardless of weight or body size than in people without PCOS (Butler et al., 2023; Liu et al., 2019).

Metabolic Syndrome

Obesity, insulin resistance, and dyslipidemia are part of metabolic syndrome, which is a cluster of risk factors for cardiovascular disease and diabetes (Swarup et al., 2024; Teede et al., 2023). Criteria for diagnosing this condition are found in **Box 26-1**. People with PCOS have a threefold increase in the prevalence of metabolic syndrome, compared to those without PCOS (Lim et al., 2019). However, this risk appears to be modulated by the criteria used to diagnose PCOS, with higher associations reported in studies using the National Institutes of Health (NIH) criteria, compared to the Rotterdam or Androgen Excess and PCOS Society criteria (Cooney & Dokras, 2018). **Table 26-1** presents NIH, Rotterdam, and Androgen Excess and PCOS Society criteria for diagnosing PCOS.

BOX 26-1 Diagnostic Criteria for Metabolic Syndrome in AFAB People

Three or more of the following:

- Waist circumference of 88 cm (35 in.) or greater
- Triglycerides 150 mg/dL or greater, or drug treatment for elevated triglycerides
- HDL-C less than 50 mg/dL, or drug treatment for reduced HDL-C
- Systolic BP 130 m Hg or greater, and/or diastolic BP of 85 mm Hg or greater, or drug treatment for hypertension
- Fasting glucose 100 mg/dL or greater, or drug treatment for elevated glucose

Data from Swarup, S., Ahmed, I., Grigorova, Y., et al. Metabolic Syndrome. (2025). In *StatPearls*. StatPearls Publishing. https://www.ncbi.nlm.nih.gov/books/NBK459248/

Abbreviations: BP, blood pressure; HDL-C, high-density lipoprotein cholesterol.

TABLE 26-1 Diagnostic Criteria for Polycystic Ovary Syndrome

Source	Diagnostic Criteria
National Institute of Child Health and Human Development (Zawadzki & Dunaif, 1992)	• Clinical and/or biochemical hyperandrogenism • Menstrual dysfunction
Rotterdam PCOS Consensus Group (2004)	Exclusion of other etiologies and two out of three of the following: • Oligo- or anovulation • Clinical and/or biochemical signs of hyperandrogenism • Polycystic ovaries
Androgen Excess and Polycystic Ovary Syndrome Society (Azziz et al., 2009)	• Hyperandrogenism: Hirsutism and/or hyperandrogenemia • Ovarian dysfunction: Oligo-anovulation and/or polycystic ovaries • Exclusion of other androgen excess or related disorders

Cardiovascular Disease and Inflammatory Markers

Contradictory evidence exists regarding increased risk of cardiovascular events (e.g., myocardial infarction, stroke) in people with PCOS (Alalami et al., 2019; Cooney & Dokras, 2018).

However, emerging data show that individuals with PCOS have been documented to have an excess of numerous biochemical inflammatory and thrombotic markers of cardiovascular disease, including circulating cytokines and proarthrogenic factors, such as C-reactive protein, homocysteine, vascular endothelial growth factor, and plasminogen activator inhibitor-1. They also have a higher incidence of systemic inflammation associated with endothelial vascular dysfunction. This chronic inflammation can lead to higher incidence of conditions like coronary artery calcification. Previously, it was thought that increased adipose tissue led to increased inflammation, but a growing body of literature is showing that hyperandrogenemia may actually be the major contributing factor to this inflammation. Conclusive studies are ongoing at the time of publication of this chapter (Rudnicka et al., 2021; Wang et al., 2023).

Psychological Impact

The expression of hyperandrogenism (hirsutism, alopecia, and acne), the annoyance and unpredictability of irregular menstrual bleeding, and the potential experience of infertility can have significant negative impacts on an individual's psychological health and well-being. Additionally, the frequent occurrence of increased adiposity with hyperandrogenism can have a negative effect on self-esteem and self-image. Rates of depressive disorders, anxiety disorders, and binge eating are higher among those with PCOS than among those without the condition (Teede et al., 2023). PCOS may also be associated with decreased sexual satisfaction and lowered health-related quality of life; however, a meta-analysis of studies performed on this subject indicate that further research is necessary before conclusions can be drawn (Pastoor et al., 2024).

Cancer Risks

People with PCOS have been reported to have a threefold increased risk of developing endometrial cancer because of chronic unopposed estrogen stimulation of the endometrium (Ring et al., 2022; Shetty et al., 2023). Those who have more adipose tissue are thought to be at the greatest risk of developing endometrial cancer because the peripheral conversion of androgens to estrogen occurs in adipose tissue (Rotterdam ESHRE/ASRM-Sponsored PCOS Consensus Workshop Group [Rotterdam PCOS Consensus Group], 2004). Conclusive research into PCOS and risk for other gynecologic cancers is inconclusive at time of publication (Shetty et al., 2023).

ASSESSMENT

Individuals with hyperandrogenism can have a range of clinical manifestations and associated problems. Therefore, appropriate assessment, diagnosis, therapeutic management, and follow-up are essential.

History

A thorough history and physical examination will provide key information to the etiology of hyperandrogenism. During history taking, the clinician should ask about the individual's age at thelarche (onset of breast development), adrenarche (onset of pubic hair), and menarche, and the menstrual pattern since menarche. Obtain a complete pregnancy history, including time to conceive and history of miscarriages. Note the age of onset and progression of increased adiposity, hirsutism, seborrhea, acne, and alopecia, along with any treatments for these conditions and their success or failure. If alopecia is present, assess for other causes of hair loss, such as nutritional deficiencies, iron-deficiency anemia, thyroid dysfunction, recent surgery, rapid weight loss, or major illness (Carmina et al., 2019). Screen for symptoms of depression and anxiety as these conditions may be more common among those with PCOS than those without this condition (Pastoor et al., 2024; Teede et al., 2023).

PCOS is a diagnosis of exclusion, and clinicians must rule out other causes of the symptoms with which the individual is presenting. As discussed earlier in this chapter, other causes of hyperandrogenism symptoms include medication side effects, rare androgen-secreting tumors, thyroid dysfunction, diabetes, hyperprolactinemia, or Cushing syndrome (Rasquin et al., 2022; Teede et al., 2023).

A complete medication history is important to seek a possible pharmacologic cause of the symptoms. Medications that have been associated with hyperandrogenism include testosterone, anabolic steroids, danazol, certain progestins, glucocorticoids, and valproic acid (Hafsi & Kaur, 2023).

An important component of the history is determining whether the person has experienced rapid development of symptoms of hirsutism and any rapid progression to virilization over the course of several months. Ask the individual if they have experienced increased libido, increased muscle bulk, voice deepening, breast atrophy, or clitoromegaly. Although rare, these symptoms should raise the suspicion for an androgen-producing tumor (Taylor et al., 2020; Teede et al., 2023).

Considering other endocrine disorders that may present with symptoms similar to PCOS, assess the individual for signs and symptoms of thyroid dysfunction, diabetes, hyperprolactinemia, and Cushing syndrome. For thyroid dysfunction, symptoms include heat or cold intolerance, weight loss or gain, and constipation or increased stooling frequency. Assess for polydipsia, polyuria, and polyphagia as these can suggest glucose intolerance. For hyperprolactinemia or pituitary tumors, assess for presence of galactorrhea, visual disturbance, or headache. Though less common than thyroid or prolactin disorders, the clinician should also assess for Cushing syndrome, noting presence or absence of signs such as striae, mood changes, easy bruisability, or weight gain (Teede et al., 2023).

Additionally, the clinician should identify cardiovascular and metabolic risk factors, including cigarette smoking, history of hypertension, dyslipidemia, or diabetes. Ask about a family history of hirsutism, acne, infertility, diabetes, cardiovascular disease (especially first-degree relatives with premature cardiovascular disease occurring before age 55 in people assigned male at birth [AMAB] and before age 65 in AFAB people), dyslipidemia, or obesity (American College of Obstetricians and Gynecologists [ACOG], 2020).

Physical Examination

The physical examination should be geared toward establishing the degree of severity of hyperandrogenism and its related symptoms. In addition to assessing height and weight, measurement of the waist circumference is important in assessing the degree of adiposity in people with hyperandrogenism. Please refer to Chapter 8 for additional information about weight assessment. It is also important to measure blood pressure because abnormalities may indicate an increased risk for morbidity and mortality related to the metabolic syndrome (Teede et al. 2023).

Conduct a thorough skin examination, paying particular attention to the presence of hirsutism, acne, and alopecia. The pattern of body hair distribution and degree of hirsutism may be evaluated using a grading tool, such as the modified Ferriman–Gallwey scale. This is shown in **Color Plate 14**. When assessing for hirsutism, clinicians should ask the individual about possible self-treatment of hirsutism with hair removal as this can limit the efficacy of assessment (Teede et al., 2023).

Perform a thyroid examination and breast/chest examination to evaluate for thyroid conditions or evidence of galactorrhea. Observe for signs of Cushing syndrome, such as moon facies, dorsocervical fat pad (buffalo hump), and abdominal striae. Perform a complete pelvic examination, including evaluation of the clitoris for hypertrophy and bimanual examination to determine the size of the uterus and ovaries, as well as the presence of masses (ACOG, 2020).

Laboratory Testing

The laboratory assessments presented in this section are drawn mainly from the International Evidence-Based Guideline for the Assessment and Management of PCOS, a set of guidelines developed by experts from 71 countries, based on 52 systematic reviews of literature (Teede et al., 2023). A previous version of these guidelines was published in 2018, and the 2023 update has several key changes to assessment, including the addition of anti-Müllerian hormone (AMH), consideration of weight stigma and its sequelae in treatment of PCOS, and increased awareness of the need for accessible options for reproductive assistive technology for those seeking pregnancy (Teede et al., 2023).

For individuals not on hormonal contraception or hormone replacement therapy, all who have hyperandrogenism with ovulatory dysfunction should have prolactin; thyroid-stimulating hormone (TSH); 17-hydroxyprogesterone (17-OHP); and total and free testosterone tested (Teede et al., 2023). An AMH level is not required, especially if the individual already meets diagnostic criteria with anovulatory cycles and signs of hyperandrogenism. It can be used if the individual is an adult (not an adolescent) and ultrasound is not available to assess for PCOM. The level of AMH indicating PCOM is still being determined, but recent studies show that an AMH level above 5 ng/dL is strongly correlated with PCOM (Butt et al., 2022; Teede et al., 2023).

The prevalence of dyslipidemias in people with PCOS warrants baseline assessment of a fasting lipid profile (e.g., cholesterol, LDL cholesterol, HDL cholesterol, triglycerides). Glycemic status should be assessed at baseline by using a fasting glucose test, oral glucose tolerance test, or hemoglobin A1C (A1C), with the frequency of subsequent testing based on the results of the initial laboratory evaluation. A glucose tolerance test is the preferred method for this assessment as it is the most sensitive and specific, but it may not always be available. Testing for insulin resistance is not recommended due to the lack of accuracy (ACOG, 2020; Teede et al., 2023). People who have clinical signs of hyperandrogenism with regular menstrual cycles should be evaluated for ovulatory dysfunction by obtaining a serum progesterone level between days 20 and 24 of the menstrual cycle (Azziz, 2018; Bizuneh at al., 2025). If this luteal-phase progesterone level is less than 3 ng/mL, the cycle is considered oligo-anovulatory. Repeating the progesterone level during a second cycle can confirm the diagnosis of chronic oligo-anovulation and PCOS (Ranisalvjec et al., 2022).

The prolactin and TSH levels are used to exclude hyperprolactinemia and thyroid disorders as both can cause ovulatory dysfunction. Measurement of serum 17-OHP is performed to assess for nonclassical, or late-onset, congenital adrenal hyperplasia, which is characterized by excessive adrenal androgen production and can present very similarly to PCOS. The American College of Obstetricians and Gynecologists (2020) and International Evidence-based Guideline for the Assessment and Management of PCOS (Teede et al., 2023) recommend routine 17-OHP testing to rule out the aforementioned conditions when PCOS is suspected.

Routine measurement of androgen levels in people with clinical signs of hyperandrogenism has previously been considered somewhat controversial due to the variations in accuracy and sensitivity of testosterone assay methods. An individual may often have overt signs of hyperandrogenism with normal laboratory levels of androgens. The American College of Obstetricians and Gynecologists (2020) recommends routine free testosterone measurement either directly by equilibrium dialysis or calculated from high-quality measurements of total testosterone and SHBG. A recent systematic review demonstrated that total and free testosterone can be considered accurate if they are conducted with LC-MS/MS mass spectrometry laboratory methods and should be done routinely for assessment of hyperandrogenemia in PCOS (Bizuneh et al., 2025). Clinicians should remember, however, that due to the complexities of androgen conjugation, absence of hyperandrogenemia in the presence of overt signs of hyperandrogenism does not mean that hyperandrogenism is not present (Teede et al., 2023).

Testing for Cushing syndrome, which results from excess adrenal cortisol secretion, should be reserved for those with symptoms of this condition (ACOG, 2020; Taylor et al., 2020). Testing for Cushing syndrome consists of the overnight dexamethasone suppression test, requiring timed evening administration of oral dexamethasone followed by timed serum cortisol draw the following morning (Taylor et al., 2020).

Imaging Studies and Endometrial Biopsy

Pelvic ultrasonography can be used to assess for polycystic ovary morphology (PCOM) and identify endometrial hyperplasia in people who experience infrequent menses or are amenorrheic. Ultrasound, however, is not necessary for diagnosis of PCOS if the person presents with clinical signs of hyperandrogenism and anovulatory cycles (ACOG, 2020; Taylor et al., 2020; Teede et al., 2023). International guidelines recommend the use of transvaginal ultrasound with probes with a frequency of at least 8 MHz for optimal views of ovarian morphology (Teede et al., 2023). When this kind of ultrasound technology is used, a threshold of 20 or more follicles of 2 to 9 mm and/or an ovarian volume of 10 mL or more noted in either ovary is recommended for a diagnosis of PCOM. Clinicians should be aware that there is little standardization in training of radiologists for interpretation of ovarian follicles, so discussion of radiologic reports between clinician and interpreting radiologist may be necessary to arrive at an accurate interpretation of images (Teede et al., 2023).

An endometrial biopsy is recommended for any individual who has long-standing anovulation because of the risk for endometrial carcinoma. This risk is increased due to prolonged elevated estrogen seen with anovulation. If the individual is not using pharmacologic progesterone to balance this estrogen, they then have prolonged exposure to unopposed estrogen, increasing the risk for endometrial dysplasia and carcinoma. The decision to perform an endometrial biopsy should not be based on an individual's age because endometrial cancer can be encountered in young anovulatory individuals. It is the duration of exposure to unopposed estrogen that is critical, rather than the person's age (Shetty et al., 2023; Taylor et al., 2020). At time of publication, there were no standard guidelines for exactly when to perform endometrial biopsy for premenopausal people with PCOS with absent menses. Additionally, this decision is further complicated by the fact that there is not an agreed-upon radiologic definition for thickened endometrium in premenopausal people. A 2021 literature review demonstrated that endometrial pathologies were more frequently diagnosed with an endometrial thickness of greater than 1 centimeter, and 2023 international guidelines recommend endometrial biopsy in cases of persistent thickened endometrium (Giri et al., 2021; Teede et al., 2023). According to current ACOG guidelines, endometrial biopsy should always be performed for postmenopausal people with an endometrial thickness of greater than 4 millimeters (ACOG, 2018).

If a virilizing tumor is suspected but an adnexal mass is not palpable, transvaginal ultrasound of the ovaries is indicated. If no ovarian tumor is identified on ultrasound, adrenal CT imaging should be performed. Routine adrenal imaging should be avoided because it can lead to unnecessary evaluation of nonfunctioning adrenal masses (incidentalomas) (Taylor et al., 2020; Teede et al., 2023).

MAKING THE DIAGNOSIS OF POLYCYSTIC OVARY SYNDROME

As mentioned previously, the diagnosis of PCOS is one of exclusion (Bizuneh et al., 2025; Taylor et al., 2020; Teede et al., 2023). If history, physical examination, and laboratory testing rule out all other possible causes of hyperandrogenism, the most likely diagnosis is PCOS. It is important to remember that PCOS is a syndrome; thus, no single diagnostic criterion is sufficient for clinical diagnosis. Three sets of diagnostic criteria have been developed for PCOS (Table 27-1). Of these, the Rotterdam criteria and the Androgen Excess and PCOS Society criteria are the most widely applied, though the Rotterdam criteria continues to be most commonly utilized by clinicians (Azziz, 2018; Rasquin et al., 2022; Teede et al., 2023).

In addition to the diagnostic criteria, four specific phenotypes of PCOS have been identified (**Box 26-2**), and some evidence suggests that these subgroups differ biologically (Ganie et al., 2024). At a 2012 evidence-based methodology workshop on PCOS, the National Institutes of Health (NIH) endorsed the broad Rotterdam diagnostic criteria, which encompass the National Institute of Child Health and Human Development and Androgen Excess and PCOS Society criteria, and it recommended specifically identifying these phenotypes of PCOS in future research and data collection. Clinicians should be aware of which diagnostic criteria were used while reviewing research studies and should further clarify subgroups by phenotype in future studies (National Institutes of Health [NIH], 2012). At the time of publication, research into PCOS phenotypes and their clinical implications is ongoing (Barrea et al., 2021; Kiconco et al., 2021; Unfer et al., 2024).

BOX 26-2 Polycystic Ovary Syndrome Phenotypes

- Androgen excess + ovulatory dysfunction
- Androgen excess + polycystic ovarian morphology
- Ovulatory dysfunction + polycystic ovarian morphology
- Androgen excess + ovulatory dysfunction + polycystic ovarian morphology

Reproduced from National Institutes of Health. (2012). Evidence-based methodology workshop on polycystic ovary syndrome (PCOS). https://prevention.nih.gov/research-priorities/research-needs-and-gaps/pathways-prevention/evidence-based-methodology-workshop-polycystic-ovary-syndrome-pcos

DIFFERENTIAL DIAGNOSES

Differential diagnoses for hyperandrogenism include PCOS; congenital adrenal hyperplasia; hyperandrogenism, insulin resistance, and Acanthosis nigricans (HAIR-AN) syndrome; androgen-producing ovarian or adrenal tumors; idiopathic hirsutism; Cushing syndrome; thyroid disorders; androgenic medications; conditions associated with pregnancy; and hyperprolactinemia. The most likely of these is PCOS. Key points for differential diagnoses can be found in **Table 26-2**.

PREVENTION

PCOS cannot be prevented. Early detection and management are critical to appropriately manage metabolic and cardiovascular disease risk factors and cosmetic and psychological issues (ACOG, 2020; Teede et al., 2023).

MANAGEMENT

Management goals in people with PCOS are to treat current clinical manifestations and prevent or lessen the severity of long-term sequelae. Management should address any cosmetic manifestations of hyperandrogenism that the individual finds distressing and the psychological stress associated with PCOS.

Nonpharmacologic Management

Lifestyle Modification

All people with PCOS, regardless of their body size, would benefit from knowing the importance of a healthy diet and regular exercise in controlling symptoms of PCOS and preventing sequelae. Weight loss is recommended for people who are noted to have excess adipose tissue. Data support that reducing 5 percent or more of adipose weight decreases androgen levels and increases SHBG. Additional benefits can also include decreased hirsutism, resumption of ovulation, improved menstrual function, increased pregnancy rates, and reduced risk of miscarriage. As adipose tissue is an important part of the endocrine system, reducing adiposity can also improve fasting insulin, glucose, glucose tolerance, and lipid levels (Pfieffer, 2019; Taylor et al., 2020; Teede et al., 2023).

Clinicians should take care, however, in approaching this with patients and consider a weight-inclusive approach, supporting the individual's body image and mental health. The 2023 international PCOS guidelines include consideration for the harm that weight-loss approaches can do to an individual's body image and psyche. Assessing for an individual's current practices and goals for dietary and lifestyle changes and employing a

TABLE 26-2 Differential Diagnoses for Hyperandrogenism

Polycystic ovary syndrome (PCOS)	• Most common cause of hyperandrogenism, occurs in approximately 80% of AFAB people with androgen excess • Clinical and/or biochemical evidence of hyperandrogenism • Oligo-anovulation • Polycystic ovaries • Exclusion of other etiologies
Nonclassical congenital adrenal hyperplasia	• Occurs in approximately 2% of people with androgen excess • Clinically indistinguishable from PCOS • Elevated 17-hydroxyprogesterone (17-OHP), greater than 800 ng/dL
Hyperandrogenism, insulin resistance, and acanthosis nigrans (HAIR-AN) syndrome	• Occurs in approximately 4% of individuals with androgen excess • Severe hyperandrogenism, possible virilization • Acanthosis nigricans • Severe hyperinsulinemia/insulin resistance
Androgen-producing tumors (ovarian or adrenal)	• Rare • Acute, rapid course of virilizing symptoms • Testosterone usually elevated to more than 150 ng/dL in premenopausal people or more than 100 ng/dL in postmenopausal individuals • Palpable adnexal mass or mass on imaging of ovaries or adrenal glands
Idiopathic hirsutism	• Occurs in approximately 5% of individuals with androgen excess • Normal serum androgen levels • Normal ovulation by basal body temperature charting or luteal-phase progesterone measurements
Cushing syndrome	• Frequent referral diagnosis, one of the least common final diagnoses • Evidence of striae over abdomen, central weight distribution, muscle weakness, altered mood, easy bruisability • Failure of cortisol suppression after overnight dexamethasone suppression test
Thyroid disorders	• Palpable thyroid enlargement or mass • Suspect with presence of alopecia • Elevated thyroid-stimulating hormone
Androgenic medication use	• May be systemic or topical • Hirsutism is common
Pregnancy	• Rapid virilization occurs during pregnancy • Common causes: Pregnancy luteoma or theca-lutein cysts (hyperreactio luteinalis)
Hyperprolactinemia	• Galactorrhea • Elevated prolactin level

Data from Kanova, N., & Bicikova, M. (2011). Hyperandrogenic states in pregnancy. *Physiological Research, 60*, 243–252; Rotterdam ESHRE/ASRM-Sponsored PCOS Consensus Workshop Group. (2004). Evidence-based approach to cutaneous hyperandrogenism in women. *Journal of the American Academy of Dermatology, 73*, 672–690; Taylor, H. S., Pal, L., & Seli, E. (2020). *Speroff's clinical gynecologic endocrinology and infertility* (9th ed.). Wolters Kluwer; Teede, H. J., Tay, C. T., Laven, J. J. E., Dokras, A., Moran, L. J., Piltonen, T. T., Costello, M. F., Boivin, J., Redman, L. M., Boyle, J. A., Norman, R. J., Mousa, A., & Joham, A. E. (2023). Recommendations from the 2023 International Evidence-based Guideline for the Assessment and Management of Polycystic Ovary Syndrome. *The Journal of Clinical Endocrinology and Metabolism, 108*(10), 2447–2469. https://doi.org/10.1210/clinem/dgad463

harm-reduction, shared decision-making model of care is recommended (Teede et al., 2023). Simply instructing an individual to reduce calories and lose weight is harmful and should be avoided.

For individuals who identify dietary changes as a goal, clinicians should recommend an increase in consumption of fiber, whole grains, fruits, and vegetables. Specific macronutrient composition of the diet, such as high protein, low glycemic index, or very low carbohydrate consumption, has been studied, but there is not yet clear evidence to recommend any specific approach as being superior to the others (ACOG, 2020; Taylor et al., 2020; Teede et al., 2023).

If an individual identifies exercise as a goal area for lifestyle modification, the person should be advised to include at least 30 minutes of structured moderate intensity exercise per day and include muscle strengthening exercise on 2 nonconsecutive days per week (Teede et al., 2023). Exercise offers numerous health benefits even if weight loss does not occur. Evidence supporting the use of medications such as glucagon-like peptide-1 receptor agonists (GLP-1s) like liraglutide, semaglutide, and others like orlistat for people with PCOS remains limited, with a 2024 meta-analysis calling for further study (Goldberg et al., 2024). At the time of publication, current guidelines state that GLP-1s or orlistat can be considered for people with PCOS who desire weight reduction when lifestyle modifications are difficult to achieve or unsuccessful (Pfieffer, 2019; Teede et al., 2023). Structure and support for any weight management program are important, and the clinician must provide close follow-up, monitoring, and psychosocial support (Teede et al., 2023).

Mechanical Hair Removal

Contrary to popular belief, mechanically removing hair by shaving, plucking, waxing, or applying depilatory creams does not stimulate further hair growth. These methods may be used in conjunction with pharmacologic therapy to remove hair as needed. Electrolysis and photoepilation with laser or intense pulsed light (IPL) can be used for permanent hair reduction. Both strategies require several sessions of treatment and can cause pigment changes and scarring. The Endocrine Society recommends laser therapy over electrolysis because laser treatment is faster and less painful than electrolysis; however, electrolysis is less expensive than laser therapy (Martin et al., 2018; Pfieffer, 2019). Androgen-reducing medications may also be used.

Pharmacologic Management

This section focuses on pharmacologic treatment for individuals who are not trying to conceive. When selecting a medication, it is important to consider the specific treatment goals for the individual, such as improving clinical signs of hyperandrogenism (e.g., hirsutism, acne, and/or alopecia), regulating menstrual cycles, protecting the endometrium, and preventing long-term sequelae of PCOS. Most people have multiple treatment goals, and some individual medications (e.g., COCs and insulin-sensitizing agents) address more than one treatment goal.

Combined Oral Contraceptives (COCs)

COCs are recommended as a first-line pharmacologic treatment for people with PCOS (ACOG, 2020; Taylor et al., 2020; Teede et al., 2023). COCs treat hyperandrogenism by inhibiting LH secretion and subsequently LH-dependent ovarian androgen production, and by raising the concentration of SHBG, which binds free testosterone. As a result, COCs provide cosmetic relief of acne and hirsutism. These medications also regulate menstrual cycles and provide protection against endometrial cancer by interrupting the steady state of estrogen stimulation of the uterus and inducing a monthly withdrawal bleed (Azziz, 2018; Taylor et al., 2020; Teede et al., 2023).

A COC with a 20 to 35 mcg dose of ethinyl estradiol and a nonandrogenic progestin component is recommended. Formulations containing desogestrel, norgestimate, or drospirenone are commonly used because of their low androgenic effects (Barrionuevo et al., 2018; Teede et al., 2023).

The maximal effect of COCs on acne is usually observed within 2 months. In contrast, the maximal effect on hair growth may take as long as 9 to 12 months because of the length of the hair growth cycle. COCs as monotherapy may be insufficient to treat hirsutism (Barrionuevo et al., 2018; Teede et al., 2023). Nonoral combined contraceptives—the transdermal patch and the vaginal ring—are also likely to be beneficial for people with PCOS, but evidence on their use in this population is limited. People with PCOS can use transdermal or vaginal formulations of combined contraceptives instead of COCs if a nonoral method is preferable (Taylor et al., 2020). More detailed information about combined contraceptives can be found in Chapter 13.

Progestogens

People who have contraindications to or do not wish to take COCs can use progestogens to prevent endometrial hyperplasia and cancer. Individuals who need contraception can use the levonorgestrel-releasing intrauterine system, progestin-only pills, the depot medroxyprogesterone acetate injection, or the subdermal implant. People who do not need contraception can take a dose of 5 to 10 mg medroxyprogesterone acetate or 200 mg micronized progesterone daily for the first 14 days of each month. However, progestational therapy alone may not treat hirsutism (ACOG, 2020; Azziz, 2018; Taylor et al., 2020; Teede et al., 2023).

Research on progestin withdrawal therapy, sometimes called the "progestin challenge," for symptom treatment of PCOS is scant, but it can be a helpful tool for clinicians needing to distinguish between PCOS and functional hypothalamic amenorrhea (FHA). In this test, the clinician prescribes a daily dose of 10 mg oral medroxyprogesterone acetate for 5–10 days. Once the person stops using the progesterone, if they have a higher estrogen state as is seen with PCOS, they will have a withdrawal bleed. If they do not have a withdrawal bleed, then the clinician should assess further for FHA. This test is a diagnostic tool and not necessary if lab testing is available; it should not be confused with cyclic progestin therapy as mentioned above (Gordon et al., 2017; Shirin et al., 2021; Teede et al., 2023).

Antiandrogens

Antiandrogens are effective in the treatment of hirsutism, but they should always be used in combination with effective contraception in a person who is capable of pregnancy because of their potential for teratogenicity. Although COCs are generally used as a first-line treatment for hirsutism, in people whose hirsutism remains refractory after 6 months of COC use, the addition of an antiandrogen medication may be more effective than administration of either agent alone. Conversely, antiandrogens can be used as first-line therapy in those who do not want or need to take COCs. The antiandrogens include spironolactone, finasteride, and flutamide (Teede et al., 2023).

Spironolactone is the most commonly used medication effective in the treatment of hirsutism and androgenic alopecia. It works by inhibiting testosterone from binding to its receptors, thereby inhibiting its action. The usual dose is 50 to 100 mg daily, with the effects being dose dependent. It can take 6 months or longer to see the full clinical effect from this therapy. Side effects may include lightheadedness, dizziness, fatigue, diuresis, and increased risk of hyperkalemia. Spironolactone may also cause menstrual irregularity when used as monotherapy. Combination therapy with COCs reduces this side effect and improves clinical response (ACOG, 2020; Taylor et al., 2020; Teede et al., 2023).

Finasteride inhibits 5α-reductase activity, which blocks the conversion of testosterone to DHT in the skin. A dose of 5 mg per day is effective in decreasing hirsutism without engendering any adverse effects. This medication should be considered when COCs and spironolactone are ineffective for hirsutism. People who are treated with finasteride should be aware that this medication can increase risk for liver toxicity (ACOG, 2020; Teede et al., 2023).

Flutamide is a pure antiandrogen without progestogenic effects that has shown some benefit in treating hirsutism. Unfortunately, this medication is associated with hepatotoxicity that can cause liver failure and rarely, death (Alalami et al., 2019; Teede et al., 2023). For this reason, this medication is seldom used for people with PCOS.

Topical and oral minoxidil are being studied for treatment of androgen-related alopecia and are currently being used in clinical practice by some clinicians to treat PCOS-related alopecia. Topical minoxidil has been shown to have mixed efficacy, and oral minoxidil use has raised safety concerns due to its potency as a vasodilator. Overall, more studies are needed before any recommendations can be made about these medications in treatment of PCOS-related alopecia (Kaiser et al., 2023).

Insulin-Sensitizing Agents

Metformin is an oral antihyperglycemic agent whose primary mechanisms of action are inhibition of hepatic glucose production and increased peripheral insulin sensitivity. Metformin has been shown to increase ovulatory frequency and decrease androgen levels in those with PCOS, and it has minimal effect on weight. In people with PCOS and hyperinsulinemia, metformin decreases fasting insulin levels, blood pressure, and LDL cholesterol levels (ACOG, 2020; Attia et al., 2023; Teede et al., 2023).

Although metformin can treat some clinical manifestations of PCOS and has the potential to prevent or delay the onset of diabetes, routine therapy with this medication in all individuals with PCOS is not recommended. Metformin should be considered for individuals with impaired glucose tolerance, regardless of their weight or adiposity. This medication should not be given solely to treat hirsutism or promote weight loss as it has been shown to be ineffective for these purposes in treatment of PCOS. Metformin has also been used in infertility treatment for people with PCOS and can be used as a monotherapy and as an adjunct therapy for use with clomiphene citrate (Attia et al., 2023; Teede et al., 2023).

The usual dose of metformin is 1,000 mg to 2,500 mg per day, with the dose being started at 500 mg per day and gradually increased over 4 to 6 weeks. It is taken with meals to reduce this medication's gastrointestinal side effects. It is contraindicated in cases of impaired renal function, congestive heart failure, hepatic dysfunction, sepsis, or history of alcohol abuse. The most serious side effect of metformin is the development of lactic acidosis, although this is rare. Vitamin B_{12} deficiency can also occur. Gastrointestinal side effects, which are more common, include nausea, abdominal discomfort, diarrhea, and anorexia (Teede et al., 2023).

The thiazolidinediones, which are also known as glitazones, lower glucose levels by increasing the utilization of glucose by the skeletal muscles and decreasing hepatic glucose synthesis. Two related drugs, rosiglitazone and pioglitazone, have been investigated for use in PCOS, but due to limited to no efficacy and significant side effects like congestive heart failure, these medications are not recommended for treatment of PCOS (Melin et al., 2024).

Topical Preparations

Eflornithine HCl 13.9 percent (Vaniqa) is a topical cream approved for the treatment of facial hirsutism. This medication's primary mechanism of action is inhibition of the enzyme ornithine decarboxylase in human skin, which slows the rate of hair growth. It is not a depilatory, and hair growth returns after discontinuation of the cream, so it is recommended for use in conjunction laser hair removal (Rashid et al., 2022).

Ovulation Induction

Though this chapter is not discussing infertility as a diagnosis, for individuals seeking pregnancy, the infertility associated with PCOS can cause significant distress, and treatment of this condition should be managed, where possible, by the clinician treating other PCOS sequelae. Assessment of tubal patency prior to pharmacologic ovulation induction should be considered on a case-by-case basis and, where appropriate, letrozole is considered the first-line pharmacologic therapy for ovulation induction and can be considered for individuals with PCOS. Current guidelines also support the use of metformin in combination with clomiphene citrate (Teede et al., 2023). More information about infertility treatments is in Chapter 20.

Follow-Up

Patient education and comprehensive person-centered care are crucial to the successful management of PCOS and the reduction of negative long-term sequelae. Long-term follow-up with routine visits is appropriate to monitor response to treatment and development of complications. Screening for evidence of development of metabolic consequences must be undertaken at regular intervals. The clinician should assess the individual's blood pressure and any increase in adiposity at every visit (Pfieffer, 2019; Teede et al., 2023). If the baseline fasting lipid profile is normal, repeat this at usual intervals or sooner if the individual develops additional risk factors. If the baseline glucose tolerance test or A1C is normal, repeat this test following usual guidelines or sooner if the individual develops additional risk factors. Those with impaired glucose tolerance should undergo annual screening for diabetes (Teede et al., 2023).

Diabetes, hypertension, and dyslipidemia require prompt treatment (or referral for treatment) after diagnosis. Advise people that cigarette smoking and vaping further increases their risk for cardiovascular disease, and provide smoking cessation interventions for those who smoke or vape tobacco products.

Complementary and Alternative Therapies

Complementary therapies, such as acupuncture, reflexology, homeopathy, and herbal medicine, are increasingly available in the United States. Limited studies have been conducted to assess the efficacy of these modalities for PCOS, though some data are available. Jo et al. (2017) completed a systematic review of randomized controlled trials (RCTs) investigating the effect of acupuncture treatments on hormone levels and rates of ovulation and menstruation in those with PCOS, compared to people receiving traditional medications. There were statistically significant differences in ovulation rates and menstrual rates in those using acupuncture alone, as well as changes in some hormone levels (e.g., LH levels, LH/FSH ratios, fasting insulin levels) and pregnancy rates in individuals who received acupuncture in addition to metformin. A 2025 systematic review and meta-analysis built on these conclusions, showing that a combination of metformin with acupuncture, Chinese herbal medicine, and cupping had similarly favorable outcomes (Wu et al., 2025). Both systematic reviews, however, concluded that high-quality research was needed before any significant practice changes could be recommended (Jo et al., 2017; Wu et al., 2025).

Kwon et al. (2018) conducted a meta-analysis of RCTs and quasi-RCTs that compared the use of Chinese herbal medicine and moxibustion versus Western medicine for the treatment of PCOS. Compared to the Western medicine group, the people in the Chinese herbal medicine and moxibustion group had a significantly higher rate of pregnancy. Similarly, when Chinese herbal medicine and moxibustion were used as an adjunct to Western medicine, significantly higher pregnancy rates were observed.

A 2017 systematic review found that inositol supplementation may improve biochemical hyperandrogenism in people with PCOS as well as their ovulation and pregnancy rates, but the most recent international guidelines report that inositol should still be considered an experimental treatment with uncertain benefits (Arentz et al., 2017; Teede et al., 2023).

In short, as with other areas of PCOS research, higher-quality data are needed regarding complementary therapies. Current data show promising trends, however, and complementary therapies such as acupuncture can be considered in supporting individuals with PCOS.

When to Refer

Endocrinopathies

If diagnostic testing reveals that an individual has congenital adrenal hyperplasia, HAIR-AN syndrome, Cushing syndrome, hyperprolactinemia, or androgen-producing tumors, they should be referred to an endocrinologist. An endocrinology consultation should also be considered for individuals who are not responding to treatment for PCOS. Clinicians who are not experienced in the management of metabolic syndrome should seek appropriate consultation for treating people with PCOS who meet the criteria for metabolic syndrome.

Treatment of Infertility

Treatment of infertility in people with PCOS can be challenging and is beyond the scope of this chapter. Though access to reproductive assistance needs to be increased for people with PCOS, these individuals often require infertility care from a specialized clinician experienced in treating these conditions concomitantly. Information about infertility treatment can be found in Chapter 20.

CONSIDERATIONS FOR SPECIFIC POPULATIONS

Adolescents

Often, the symptoms of hyperandrogenism are not brought to the attention of the clinician until the person is in their late teens, early 20s, or even older. The most common causes of hyperandrogenism, however, usually become active in early adolescence. Premature adrenarche may be a consequence of hyperinsulinemia. These adolescents go on to develop clinical signs of hyperandrogenism and/or irregular menses, for which they often are treated symptomatically without undergoing a thorough assessment of the causes of symptoms. Menstrual irregularity is common soon after menarche but warrants investigation if it persists. The use of ultrasound to assist with the diagnosis of PCOS is not recommended in adolescents until they have had menstrual cycles for 8 years (Teede et al., 2023). This is because the normal morphology of the ovary during this time may demonstrate multiple follicles. Clinicians treating adolescents should consider hyperandrogenic conditions because early treatment may help ameliorate symptoms and prevent the development of adverse sequelae and psychological dysfunction (Taylor et al., 2020; Teede et al., 2023).

Pregnant Individuals

People with PCOS are at increased risk of several pregnancy complications including miscarriage, gestational diabetes, hypertensive disorders and preeclampsia, and preterm birth. Preconception assessment and intervention to support normal blood pressure, and glucose tolerance are recommended (Teede et al., 2023). People being treated for hyperandrogenism who become pregnant should be aware of the benefits and risks of any medications they are taking. Metformin use may be continued by some during pregnancy, but current data do not support its routine use. Some medications, such as finasteride, flutamide, and spironolactone, are contraindicated during pregnancy and should be discontinued immediately upon suspicion that the individual is pregnant (Teede et al., 2023).

Perimenopausal and Postmenopausal People

Individuals with PCOS often experience improved menstrual function with age, and evidence indicates that people with PCOS have prolonged reproductive function and increased ovarian reserve, compared to those who do not have PCOS. Age may improve other manifestations of PCOS, including ovarian morphology and serum testosterone levels (Cooney & Dokras, 2018). More studies need to be done regarding the general health of individuals with PCOS as they transition into menopause, but it is suspected that they have increased rates of higher weight, diabetes, and cardiovascular disease risk factors (Cooney & Dokras, 2018). Postmenopausal people who present with new-onset, severe, or worsening signs and symptoms of hyperandrogenism must be evaluated for androgen-secreting tumors and ovarian hyperthecosis (Teede et al., 2023).

CONCLUSION

PCOS is a complex, multifactorial disorder arising in the presence of various genetic and environmental factors. It affects the reproductive, endocrine, cardiovascular, dermatologic, and psychosocial health of a large number of individuals, but it is not well understood by clinicians or the public. Experts also recommend increased multidisciplinary awareness programs for clinicians and the public because the syndrome represents a major public health concern (NIH, 2012; Teede et al., 2023). Evidence shows that people with PCOS who are provided with detailed education regarding the syndrome, related health risks, and lifestyle changes and pharmacologic management strategies for symptoms report increased knowledge, motivation, and physical and psychological benefits, all of which benefit their long-term health. Clinicians should stay updated on changes in the literature and consider conversations and education about PCOS as essential to care for these individuals as making the diagnosis itself (Teede et al., 2023).

References

Alalami, H., Sathyapalan, T., & Atkin, S. L. (2019). Cardiovascular profile of pharmacological agents used for the management of polycystic ovary syndrome. *Therapeutic Advances in Endocrinology and Metabolism, 10*, 1–10. https://doi.org/10.1177%2F2042018818805674

American College of Obstetricians and Gynecologists. (2013). ACOG committee opinion no. 734: The role of transvaginal ultrasonography in evaluating the endometrium of women With postmenopausal bleeding. *Obstetrics and Gynecology, 131*(5), e124–e129. https://doi.org/10.1097/AOG.0000000000002631

American College of Obstetrics and Gynecology. (2020). ACOG practice bulletin No. 194: Polycystic ovary syndrome: Correction. *Obstetrics and Gynecology, 136*(3), 638. https://doi.org/10.1097/AOG.0000000000004069

American Diabetes Association. (2019). Classification and diagnosis of diabetes: Standards of medical care in diabetes—2019 [Suppl. 1]. *Diabetes Care, 42*, S13–S28. https://doi.org/10.2337/dc19-S002

Arentz, S., Smith, C. A., Abbott, J., & Bensoussan, A. (2017). Nutritional supplements and herbal medicines for women with polycystic ovary syndrome: A systematic review and meta-analysis. *BMC Complementary and Alternative Medicine, 17*, 1–24. https://doi.org/10.1186/s12906-017-2011-x

Attia, G. M., Almouteri, M. M., & Alnakhli, F. T. (2023). Role of metformin in polycystic ovary syndrome (PCOS)-related infertility. *Cureus, 15*(8), e44493. https://doi.org/10.7759/cureus.44493

Azziz, R. (2018). Polycystic ovary syndrome. *Obstetrics & Gynecology, 132*(2), 321–336. https://doi.org/10.1097/AOG.0000000000002698

Azziz, R., Carmina, E., Dewailly, D., Diamanti-Kandarakis, E., Escobar-Morreale, H. F., Futterweit, W., Janssen, O. E., Legro, R. S., Norman, R. J., Taylor, A. E., Witchel, S. F., & Task Force on the Phenotype of the Polycystic Ovary Syndrome of The Androgen Excess and PCOS Society. (2009). The Androgen Excess and PCOS Society criteria for the polycystic ovary syndrome: The complete task force report. *Fertility and Sterility, 91*(2), 456–488. https://doi.org/10.1016/j.fertnstert.2008.06.035

Bahri Khomami, M., & Teede, H. J. (2024). Addressing polycystic ovary syndrome in pregnancy care to improve outcomes. *JAMA Network Open, 7*(8), e2430549. https://doi.org/10.1001/jamanetworkopen.2024.30549

Barrea, L., Frias-Toral, E., Verde, L., Ceriani, F., Cucalón, G., Garcia-Velasquez, E., Moretti, D., Savastano, S., Colao, A., & Muscogiuri, G. (2021). PCOS and nutritional approaches: Differences between lean and obese phenotype. *Metabolism Open, 12*, 100123. https://doi.org/10.1016/j.metop.2021.100123

Barrionuevo, P., Nabhan, M., Altayar, O., Wang, Z., Erwin, P. J., Asi, N., Martin, K. A., & Murad, M. H. (2018). Treatment options for hirsutism: A systematic review and network meta-analysis. *The Journal of Clinical Endocrinology and Metabolism, 103*(4), 1258–1264. https://doi.org/10.1210/jc.2017-02052

Bizuneh, A. D., Joham, A. E., Teede, H., Mousa, A., Earnest, A., Hawley, J. M., Smith, L., Azziz, R., Arlt, W., & Tay, C. T. (2025). Evaluating the diagnostic accuracy of androgen measurement in polycystic ovary syndrome: A systematic review and diagnostic meta-analysis to inform evidence-based guidelines. *Human Reproduction Update, 31*(1), 48–63. https://doi.org/10.1093/humupd/dmae028

Butler, A. E., Moin, A. S. M., Reiner, Ž., Sathyapalan, T., Jamialahmadi, T., Sahebkar, A., & Atkin, S. L. (2023). HDL-associated proteins in subjects with polycystic ovary syndrome: A proteomic study. *Cells, 12*(6), 855. https://doi.org/10.3390/cells12060855

Butt, M. S., Saleem, J., Aiman, S., Zakar, R., Sadique, I., & Fischer, F. (2022). Serum anti-Müllerian hormone as a predictor of polycystic ovarian syndrome among women of reproductive age. *BMC Women's Health, 22*(1), 199. https://doi.org/10.1186/s12905-022-01782-2

Carmina, E., Azziz, R., Bergfeld, W., Escobar-Morreale, H. F., Futterweit, W., Huddleston, H., ... & Olsen, E. (2019). Female pattern hair loss and androgen excess: a report from the multidisciplinary androgen excess and PCOS committee. *The Journal of Clinical Endocrinology & Metabolism, 104*(7), 2875-2891.

Cooney, L. G., & Dokras, A. (2018). Beyond fertility: Polycystic ovary syndrome and long-term health. *Fertility & Sterility, 110*(5), 794–809. https://doi.org/10.1016/j.fertnstert.2018.08.021

Esquivel-Zuniga, M. R., Kirschner, C. K., McCartney, C. R., & Burt Solorzano, C. M. (2022). Non-PCOS hyperandrogenic disorders in adolescents. *Seminars in Reproductive Medicine, 40*(1-02), 42–52. https://doi.org/10.1055/s-0041-1742259

Ferriman, D., & Gallwey, J. D. (1961). Clinical assessment of body hair growth in women. *The Journal of Clinical Endocrinology & Metabolism, 21*(11), 1440–1447.

Fulton, M., Dadana, S., & Srinivasan, V. N. [Updated 2023 Oct 26]. Obesity, stigma, and discrimination. In *StatPearls*. StatPearls Publishing. https://www.ncbi.nlm.nih.gov/books/NBK554571/

Ganie, M. A., Chowdhury, S., Malhotra, N., Sahay, R., Bhattacharya, P. K., Agrawal, S., Jabbar, P. K., Suri, V., Rozati, R., Sreenivas, V., Baba, M. S., Wani, I. A., Rashid, H., Nair, A., Shukla, A., Arora, T., Kulkarni, B., & PCOS Study Group (2024). Prevalence, phenotypes, and comorbidities of polycystic ovary syndrome among Indian women. *JAMA Network Open, 7*(10), e2440583. https://doi.org/10.1001/jamanetworkopen.2024.40583

Giri, S. K., Nayak, B. L., & Mohapatra, J. (2021). Thickened endometrium: When to intervene? A clinical conundrum. *Journal of Obstetrics and Gynaecology of India, 71*(3), 216–225. https://doi.org/10.1007/s13224-020-01415-4

Glueck, C. J., & Goldenberg, N. (2019). Characteristics of obesity in polycystic ovary syndrome: Etiology, treatment, and genetics. *Metabolism Clinical and Experimental, 92*, 108–120.

Goldberg, A., Graca, S., Liu, J., Rao, V., Witchel, S. F., Pena, A., Li, R., Mousa, A., Tay, C. T., Pattuwage, L., Teede, H., Yildiz, B. O., & Ee, C. (2024). Anti-obesity pharmacological agents for polycystic ovary syndrome: A systematic review and meta-analysis to inform the 2023 international evidence-based guideline. *Obesity Reviews: An Official Journal of the International Association for the Study of Obesity, 25*(5), e13704. https://doi.org/10.1111/obr.13704

Gordon, C. M., Ackerman, K. E., Berga, S. L., Kaplan, J. R., Mastorakos, G., Misra, M., Murad, M. H., Santoro, N. F., & Warren, M. P. (2017). Functional hypothalamic amenorrhea: An Endocrine Society clinical practice guideline. *The Journal of Clinical Endocrinology and Metabolism, 102*(5), 1413–1439. https://doi.org/10.1210/jc.2017-00131

Guo, F., Gong, Z., Fernando, T., Zhang, L., Zhu, X., & Shi, Y. (2022). The lipid profiles in different characteristics of women with PCOS and the interaction between dyslipidemia and metabolic disorder states: A retrospective study in Chinese population. *Frontiers in endocrinology, 13*, 892125. https://doi.org/10.3389/fendo.2022.892125

Hafsi, W., & Kaur, J. (Updated 2023 May 3). Hirsutism. In *StatPearls*. StatPearls Publishing. https://www.ncbi.nlm.nih.gov/books/NBK470417/

Hatch, R., Rosenfield, R. L., Kim, M. H., & Tredway, D. (1981). Hirsutism: implications, etiology, and management. *American journal of obstetrics and gynecology, 140*(7), 815-830.

Ilagan, M. K. C. C., Paz-Pacheco, E., Totesora, D. Z., Clemente Chua, L. R., Jalique, J. R. K. (2019). The Modified Ferriman-Gallwey Score and hirsutism among Filipino women. *Endocrinology and Metabolism, 34*(4), 374–381.

Jo, J., Lee, Y. J., & Lee, H. (2017). Acupuncture for polycystic ovarian syndrome: a systematic review and meta-analysis. *Medicine, 96*(23), e7066.

Jones, K., & Sung, S. [Updated 2025 Mar 23]. Anovulatory bleeding. In *StatPearls*. StatPearls Publishing. https://www.ncbi.nlm.nih.gov/books/NBK549773/

Kaiser, M., Abdin, R., Gaumond, S. I., Issa, N. T., & Jimenez, J. J. (2023). Treatment of androgenetic alopecia: current guidance and unmet needs. *Clinical, cosmetic and investigational dermatology*, 1387-1406.

Kanova, N., & Bicikova, M. (2011). Hyperandrogenic states in pregnancy. *Physiological Research, 60*, 243–252.

Kiconco, S., Mousa, A., Azziz, R., Enticott, J., Suturina, L. V., Zhao, X., Gambineri, A., Tehrani, F. R., Yildiz, B. O., Kim, J. J., Teede, H. J., & Joham, A. E. (2021). PCOS phenotype in unselected populations study (P-PUP): Protocol for a systematic review and defining PCOS diagnostic features with pooled individual participant data. *Diagnostics (Basel, Switzerland), 11*(11), 1953. https://doi.org/10.3390/diagnostics11111953

Kwon, C.-Y., Lee, B., & Park, K. S. (2018). Oriental herbal medicine and moxibustion forpolycystic ovary syndrome: A meta-analysis. *Medicine, 97*(43), 12942. https://doi .org/10.1097/MD.0000000000012942

Lessard, L. M., & Puhl, R. M. (2021). Adolescents' exposure to and experiences of weight stigma during the COVID-19 pandemic. *Journal of Pediatric Psychology, 46*(8), 950–959. https://doi.org/10.1093/jpepsy/jsab071

Lim, S. S., Kakoly, N. S., Tan, J. W. J., Fitzgerald, M., Bahri Khomami, M., Joham, A. E., Cooray, S. D., Misso, M. L., Norman, R. J., Harrison, C. L., Ranasinha, S., Teede, H. J., & Moran, L. J. (2019). Metabolic syndrome in polycystic ovary syndrome: A systematic review, meta-analysis and meta-regression. *Obesity Reviews, 20*, 339–352. https://doi.org/10.1111/obr.12762

Liu, Q., Xie, Y. J., Qu, L. H., Zhang, M. X., & Mo, Z. C. (2019). Dyslipidemia involvement in the development of polycystic ovary syndrome. *Taiwanese Journal of Obstetrics & Gynecology, 58*(4), 447–453. https://doi.org/10.1016/j.tjog.2019.05.003

Martin, K. A., Anderson, R. R., Chang, J., Ehrmann, D. A., Lobo, R. A., Murad, M. H., Pugeat, M. M., & Rosenfield, R. L. (2018). Evaluation and treatment of hirsutism in premenopausal women: An Endocrine Society clinical practice guideline. *Journal of Clinical Endocrinology & Metabolism, 103*(4), 1233–1257. https://doi.org/10.1210/jc.2018-00241

Melin, J. M., Forslund, M., Alesi, S. J., Piltonen, T., Romualdi, D., Spritzer, P. M., Tay, C. T., Pena, A. S., Witchel, S. F., Mousa, A., & Teede, H. J. (2024). Effects of different insulin sensitisers in the management of polycystic ovary syndrome: A systematic review and meta-analysis. *Clinical Endocrinology, 100*(2), 149–163. https://doi.org/10.1111/cen.14983

National Institutes of Health. (2012). *Evidence-based methodology workshop on polycystic ovary syndrome (PCOS)*. https://prevention.nih.gov/research-priorities/research-needs-and-gaps/pathways-prevention/evidence-based-methodology-workshop-polycystic-ovary-syndrome-pcos

Neven, A. C. H., Forslund, M., Ranashinha, S., Mousa, A., Tay, C. T., Peña, A., Oberfield, S., Witchel, S., Teede, H., & Boyle, J. A. (2024). Prevalence and accurate diagnosis of polycystic ovary syndrome in adolescents across world regions: A systematic review and meta-analysis. *European Journal of Endocrinology, 191*(4), S15–S27. https://doi.org/10.1093/ejendo/lvae125

Pastoor, H., Mousa, A., Bolt, H., Bramer, W., Burgert, T. S., Dokras, A., Tay, C. T., Teede, H. J., & Laven, J. (2024). Sexual function in women with polycystic ovary syndrome: A systematic review and meta-analysis. *Human Reproduction Update, 30*(3), 323–340. https://doi.org/10.1093/humupd/dmad034

Pfieffer, M. L. (2019). Polycystic ovary syndrome: An update. *Nursing 2019, 49*(8), 34–40. https://doi.org/10.1097/01.NURSE.0000569748.65796.d1

Puhl, R. M., Lessard, L. M., Himmelstein, M. S., & Foster, G. D. (2021). The roles of experienced and internalized weight stigma in healthcare experiences: Perspectives of adults engaged in weight management across six countries. *PloS One, 16*(6), e0251566. https://doi.org/10.1371/journal.pone.0251566

Ramezani Tehrani, F., Behboudi-Gandevani, S., Bidhendi Yarandi, R., Saei Ghare Naz, M., & Carmina, E. (2021). Prevalence of acne vulgaris among women with polycystic ovary syndrome: A systemic review and meta-analysis. *Gynecological Endocrinology: The Official Journal of the International Society of Gynecological Endocrinology, 37*(5), 392–405. https://doi.org/10.1080/09513590.2020.1859474

Ranisavljevic, N., Huberlant, S., Montagut, M., Alonzo, P. M., Darné, B., Languille, S., Anahory, T., & Cédrin-Durnerin, I. (2022). Low luteal serum progesterone levels are associated with lower ongoing pregnancy and live birth rates in ART: Systematic review and meta-analyses. *Frontiers in Endocrinology, 13*, 892753. https://doi.org/10.3389/fendo.2022.892753

Rashid, R., Mir, S. A., Kareem, O., Ali, T., Ara, R., Malik, A., Amin, F., & Bader, G. N. (2022). Polycystic ovarian syndrome—Current pharmacotherapy and clinical implications. *Taiwanese Journal of Obstetrics & Gynecology, 61*(1), 40–50. https://doi.org/10.1016/j.tjog.2021.11.009

Rasquin, L. I., Anastasopoulou, C., & Mayrin, J. V. (2022) Polycystic ovarian disease. In *StatPearls*. StatPearls Publishing. https://www.ncbi.nlm.nih.gov/books/NBK459251/

Ring, K. L., Mills, A. M., & Modesitt, S. C. (2022). Endometrial hyperplasia. *Obstetrics and Gynecology, 140*(6), 1061–1075. https://doi.org/10.1097/AOG.0000000000004989

Rotterdam ESHRE/ASRM-Sponsored PCOS Consensus Workshop Group. (2004). Revised 2003 consensus on diagnostic criteria and long-term health risks related to polycystic ovary syndrome (PCOS). *Human Reproduction, 19*(1), 41–47.

Rudnicka, E., Suchta, K., Grymowicz, M., Calik-Ksepka, A., Smolarczyk, K., Duszewska, A. M., Smolarczyk, R., & Meczekalski, B. (2021). Chronic low grade inflammation in pathogenesis of PCOS. *International Journal of Molecular Sciences, 22*(7), 3789. https://doi.org/10.3390/ijms22073789

Sharma, A., & Welt, C. K. (2021). Practical approach to hyperandrogenism in women. *The Medical Clinics of North America, 5*(6), 1099–1116. https://doi.org/10.1016/j.mcna.2021.06.008. Epub 2021 Sep 8. PMID: 34688417; PMCID: PMC8548673.

Shetty, C., Rizvi, S. M. H. A., Sharaf, J., Williams, K. D., Tariq, M., Acharekar, M. V., Guerrero Saldivia, S. E., Unnikrishnan, S. N., Chavarria, Y. Y., Akindele, A. O., Jalkh, A. P. C., Eastmond, A. K., & Hamid, P. (2023). Risk of gynecological cancers in women with polycystic ovary syndrome and the pathophysiology of association. *Cureus, 15*(4), e37266. https://doi.org/10.7759/cureus.37266

Shirin, S., Murray, F., Goshtasebi, A., Kalidasan, D., & Prior, J. C. (2021). Cyclic progesterone therapy in androgenic polycystic ovary syndrome (PCOS)—A 6-month pilot study of a single woman's experience changes. *Medicina (Kaunas, Lithuania), 57*(10), 1024. https://doi.org/10.3390/medicina57101024

Siddiqui, S., Mateen, S., Ahmad, R., & Moin, S. (2022). A brief insight into the etiology, genetics, and immunology of polycystic ovarian syndrome (PCOS). *Journal of Assisted Reproduction and Genetics, 39*(11), 2439–2473. https://doi.org/10.1007/s10815-022-02625-7

Spritzer, P. M., Marchesan, L. B., Santos, B. R., & Fighera, T. M. (2022). Hirsutism, normal androgens and diagnosis of PCOS. *Diagnostics, 12*(8), 1922. https://doi.org/10.3390/diagnostics12081922. PMID: 36010272; PMCID: PMC9406611.

Strings, S. (2023). How the use of BMI fetishizes White embodiment and racializes fat phobia. *AMA J Ethics, 25*(7), E535–539. https://doi.org/10.1001/amajethics.2023.535

Swarup, S., Ahmed, I., Grigorova, Y., et al. [Updated 2024 Mar 7]. Metabolic syndrome. In *StatPearls*. StatPearls Publishing. https://www.ncbi.nlm.nih.gov/books/NBK459248/

Taylor, H. S., Pal, L., & Seli, E. (2020). *Speroff's clinical gynecologic endocrinology and infertility* (9th ed.). Wolters Kluwer.

Teede, H., Misso, M., Tassone, E. C., Dewailly, D., Ng, E. H., Azziz, R., Norman, R. J., Andersen, M., Franks, S., Hoeger, K., Hutchison, S., Oberfield, S., Shah, D., Hohmann, F., Ottey, S., Dabadghao, P., & Laven, J. S. E. (2019). Anti-Müllerian hormone in PCOS: A review informing international guidelines. *Trends in Endocrinology & Metabolism, 30*(7), 468–478. https://doi.org/10.1016/j.tem.2019.04.006

Teede, H. J., Tay, C. T., Laven, J. J. E., Dokras, A., Moran, L. J., Piltonen, T. T., Costello, M. F., Boivin, J., Redman, L. M., Boyle, J. A., Norman, R. J., Mousa, A., & Joham, A. E. (2023). Recommendations from the 2023 International Evidence-based Guideline for the Assessment and Management of Polycystic Ovary Syndrome. *The Journal of Clinical Endocrinology and Metabolism, 108*(10), 2447–2469. https://doi.org/10.1210/clinem/dgad463

Unfer, V., Kandaraki E., Pkhaladze, L., Roseff, S., Vazquez-Levin, M. H., Laganà A. S., Shiao-Yng, C., Yap-Garcia, M. I. M., Greene, N. D. E., Soulage, C. O., Bevilacqua, A., Benvenga, A. S., Barbaro, D., Pintaudi, B., Wdowiak, A., Aragona, C., Kamenov, Z., Appetecchia, M., Porcaro, G., Hernandez Marin, I., Facchinetti, F., Chiu, T., Pustotina, O., Papalou, O., Nordio, M., Cantelmi, T., Cavalli, P., Vucenik, I., D'Anna, R., Unfer, V. R., Dinicola, S., Salehpour, S., Stringaro, A., Montaninno Oliva, M., Tugushev, M., Prapas, N., Bizzarri, M., Espinola, M.S.B., Di Lorenzo, C., Ozay, A.C., & Nestler, J. (2024). When one size does not fit all: Reconsidering PCOS etiology, diagnosis, clinical subgroups, and subgroup-specific treatments. *Endocrine and Metabolic Science, 14*. https://doi.org/10.1016/j.endmts.2024.100159

Vatier, C., & Christin-Maitre, S. (2024). Epigenetic/circadian clocks and PCOS. *Human Reproduction (Oxford, England), 39*(6), 1167–1175. https://doi.org/10.1093/humrep/deae066

Walters, K. A., Moreno-Asso, A., Stepto, N. K., Pankhurst, M. W., Rodriguez Paris, V., & Rodgers, R. J. (2022). Key signalling pathways underlying the aetiology of polycystic ovary syndrome. *Journal of Endocrinology, 255*(1), R1–R26. Retrieved Apr 7, 2025, from https://doi.org/10.1530/JOE-22-0059

Wang, J., Yin, T., & Liu, S. (2023). Dysregulation of immune response in PCOS organ system. *Frontiers in immunology, 14*, 1169232. https://doi.org/10.3389/fimmu.2023.1169232

Wu, T., Liu, Y., Kong, F., Hu, J., Liu, Y., Yang, J., & Chen, J. (2025). Improvement of endocrine and metabolic conditions in patients with polycystic ovary syndrome through acupuncture and its combined therapies: A systematic review and meta-analysis. *Annals of Medicine, 57*(1), 2477295. https://doi.org/10.1080/07853890.2025.2477295

Yang, J., & Chen, C. (2024). Hormonal changes in PCOS. *The Journal of Endocrinology, 261*(1), e230342. https://doi.org/10.1530/JOE-23-0342

Zawadzki, J. K., & Dunaif, A. (1992). *Diagnostic criteria for polycystic ovary syndrome: Towards a rational approach*. Blackwell Scientific.

CHAPTER 27

Benign Gynecologic Conditions

Evelyn Addo-Wallace
Elizabeth Muñoz
Melicia Escobar
The editors acknowledge Katharine K. O'Dell and Eva M. Fried, who contributed to previous editions of this chapter.

This chapter addresses several benign gynecologic conditions that bring individuals to clinicians' offices seeking relief. Although they are not life-threatening, many benign gynecologic conditions can severely diminish quality of life for affected individuals. Labeling these conditions as benign refers to their lack of malignancy and not to their effects, which can be significant for individuals and their partners and families. The following conditions are discussed in this chapter:

- Conditions of the vulva
  - Skin cysts
    - Folliculitis, furuncles, carbuncles
    - Epidermoid and sebaceous cysts
    - Hidradenitis suppurativa
  - Dermatoses
    - Contact dermatitis
    - Lichen sclerosus
    - Lichen planus
    - Lichen simplex chronicus
    - Psoriasis
- Conditions of the uterus and cervix
  - Cervical and endometrial polyps
  - Uterine fibroids
  - Endometriosis
  - Adenomyosis
- Conditions of the adnexa
  - Ovarian cysts

Understanding of many of these conditions continues to evolve. Evidence suggests that several diagnoses–such as endometrial and cervical polyps, uterine fibroids, and endometriosis–are often associated and frequently occur together. It has been posited that this may be due to inflammatory or autoimmune pathways that these conditions have in common (Kolanska et al., 2020; van der Meijden et al., 2022). Some conditions, such as polyps and ovarian cysts, are easily treatable, while others, such as endometriosis and certain vulvar dermatoses, can be chronic or recurring. Clinicians can better care for patients when they have a solid understanding of these common gynecologic conditions.

Chronic and/or unpredictable conditions place a burden on individuals, their partners, families, and healthcare providers. The etiologies of these disorders are often poorly understood, and symptoms may be more bothersome than the physical findings suggest. Additionally, symptom severity can vary widely over time and among individuals with the same diagnoses, sometimes improving spontaneously without intervention. These factors make it challenging to establish an evidence base for optimal management using standardized clinical trials.

Because of this complexity, chronic gynecologic conditions can frustrate everyone involved and strain relationships between patients, their families, and their clinicians. At each healthcare visit, clinicians should actively listen, conduct a thorough assessment, and provide up-to-date, condition-specific information and management options. Individuals experiencing chronic or recurring gynecologic symptoms may also need support in setting realistic treatment goals, monitoring symptom changes, and adjusting management strategies over time.

Not all people assigned female at birth identify as female or women; however, these terms are used extensively in the literature. Use of these terms is not meant to exclude people who do not identify as women and seek care for the conditions discussed in this chapter. Seeking care for a body part that is incongruent with one's gender identity (e.g., a vulvar condition in a transmasculine person) may be particularly distressing. Clinicians should be cognizant of this and ask the person for their preferred language for referring to the body part in question.

CONDITIONS OF THE VULVA

Vulvar skin includes both keratinized and mucocutaneous surfaces. To help patients with vulvar skin changes, clinicians need a thorough understanding of this complex anatomy and basic history and physical examination skills. This section reviews two vulvar findings often seen in primary care: skin cysts and dermatoses. Please refer to Chapter 7 for information about the vulvar anatomy and Chapter 8 for history and physical examination skills. Refer to Chapters 21 and 22 for other conditions that affect the vulva and Chapter 18 for vulvar pain.

At least 20 percent of patients experience seriously bothersome vulvar discomfort, including itching, burning, pain, rashes, and lesions (Edwards et al., 2025). Some of these symptoms and signs are limited to the genital area, whereas others are manifestations of diffuse chronic diseases of the skin or mucous membranes. Differentiating among normal variations, benign disease, and malignancy is paramount. Optimal management planning is complicated because many vulvar skin conditions have similar appearances and symptoms, and a patient may have multiple conditions simultaneously.

Examples of the numerous differential diagnoses for vulvar skin conditions are presented in **Table 27-1**. A systematic approach to assessment should be used to avoid delay in identifying malignant changes and improve symptoms expediently. This section provides an overview of key points for evaluation and treatment needed to help individuals manage these benign conditions. Premalignant and malignant vulvar lesions are addressed in Chapter 28.

Assessment of Vulvar Skin Disorders

History

Ask patients about essential elements of their related health history, including onset and progression of symptoms; aggravating or alleviating factors, including any relationship to sexual activity; prior self- or prescribed treatments and their outcomes; and concomitant systemic changes, such as lymphadenopathy or skin, perianal, or oral mucosal disease. It is important to ask about all products used on the vulva and in the vagina, including what the patient uses to cleanse their vulva, personal care products (e.g., sprays, wipes), prescription and nonprescription medications, and douching (Mauskar et al., 2020). Increased risk of malignancy should be considered when patients report a prior history of high-risk human papillomavirus (HPV) or personal or close family history of skin malignancies, such as malignant melanoma. Personal or family history of systemic skin conditions, such as lupus, eczema, or psoriasis, may also guide diagnosis. Associated skin symptoms in sexual partners or close family members suggest a potential infectious process (Edwards et al., 2025; van der Meijden et al., 2022). Refer to Chapter 22 for information about sexually transmitted infections. Finally, assess for mental health status in the context of effects of reported symptoms including depression, anxiety, sexual discomfort, and suicidal ideation (Mauskar et al., 2020). Taking a holistic approach promotes trust upon which to build a comprehensive plan for management.

Physical Examination

While ensuring adequate visualization through patient positioning, conduct a thorough examination of the vulva beginning with the keratinized skin areas (e.g., inguinal folds, mons pubis, and labia majora) followed by the areas that are partially keratinized with modified mucous membranes (e.g., labia minora, clitoral

TABLE 27-1 Differential Diagnoses of Vulvar Skin Conditions

Erosions and Ulcers	Erythematous Papules and Plaques	Depigmentation
Aphthosis (oral–genital)	Basal cell carcinoma	Severe atrophy
Atrophic vaginitis	Candidiasis	Congenital hypopigmentation
Basal cell carcinoma	Condyloma acuminata (genital warts)	Halo nevus
Bechet syndrome	Contact dermatitis	Lichen sclerosus
Chancroid	Crohn's disease	Lichen simplex chronicus
Chemotherapy-induced reaction	Eczema	Tinea versicolor
Contact dermatitis	Erythema multiforme	Vitiligo
Herpes simplex	Folliculitis/epidermoid cysts	
Herpes zoster	Hemangiomas	
Impetigo	Hidradenitis suppurativa	
Melanoma	Intertrigo	
Stevens–Johnson syndrome	Lichen planus	
Syphilis	Lichen sclerosus	
Tuberculosis (genital)	Lichen simplex chronicus	
	Melanoma	
	Molluscum contagiosum	
	Nevi (moles)	
	Paget disease	
	Pemphigus/pemphigoid	
	Pityriasis versicolor	
	Psoriasis/inverse psoriasis	
	Scabies	
	Seborrheic dermatitis	
	Squamous cell carcinoma	
	Syphilis	
	Vulvar intraepithelial neoplasia	
	Vulvodynia/vestibulitis	

Data from Edwards, S. K., Lewis, F., Fernando, I., Haddon, L., & Grover, D. (2025). 2024 British Association for Sexual Health and HIV (BASHH) UK national guideline on the management of vulval conditions. *International Journal of STD & AIDS*, 9564624241311629. Advance online publication. https://doi.org/10.1177/09564624241311629; Fergus, K. B., Lee, A. W., Baradaran, N., Cohen, A. J., Stohr, B. A., Erickson, B. A., Mmonu, N. A., & Breyer, B. N. (2020). Pathophysiology, clinical manifestations, and treatment of lichen sclerosus: A systematic review. *Urology, 135*, 11–19. https://doi.org/10.1016/j.urology.2019.09.034; van der Meijden, W. I., Boffa, M. J., Ter Harmsel, B., Kirtschig, G., Lewis, F., Moyal-Barracco, M., Tiplica, G. S., & Sherrard, J. (2022). 2021 European guideline for the management of vulval conditions. *Journal of the European Academy of Dermatology and Venereology: JEADV, 36*(7), 952–972. https://doi.org/10.1111/jdv.18102

hood, and posterior fourchette). This distinction in types of epithelia can be helpful in making a diagnosis because some conditions tend toward specific areas of the vulva (Mauskar et al., 2020). Assessment of the patient's skin should go beyond the vulvar and perianal skin surfaces. Include palpation for systemic lymphadenopathy; careful inspection of the scalp, eyes, nasal mucosa, and oral mucosa; and examination of the abdominal, inguinal, and gluteal skin folds (Edwards et al., 2025). All surface inspection requires excellent lighting augmented by a magnifying glass or colposcope, if necessary. A speculum examination should be included to identify involvement of the vaginal mucosa. Invite the patient to localize their symptoms, pointing to areas of concern, to include in the documentation. Baseline and follow up photographic documentation may be included, with patient consent, in the medical record to monitor clinical progression or results of treatment (Mauskar et al., 2020).

Diagnostic Testing

Selective testing may aid diagnosis. For example, testing for concomitant infections may be helpful (e.g., tests for *Candida* or sexually transmitted infections, microscopy for scabies or vaginal pathogens). Microscopic examination of vaginal secretions should be considered in all patients with vulvovaginal symptoms (Mauskar et al., 2020). Please refer to Chapter 8 for more information about microscopic examination of vaginal secretions. Vulvar biopsy should be performed when the patient has any atypical, nonresponding, or otherwise concerning findings (American College of Obstetricians and Gynecologists [ACOG], 2021). A technique for vulvar punch biopsy is summarized in **Appendix 27-1**. Many vulvar skin conditions are correlated with autoimmune conditions. When clinical assessment suggests an autoimmune condition, tests may include thyroid evaluation and fasting blood sugar (Edwards et al., 2025; van der Meijden et al., 2022). Referral for allergy or patch testing may also be warranted.

Differential Diagnoses

A list of differential diagnoses for common vulvar lesions is provided in Table 27-1. Additionally, there are a wide variety of rare conditions affecting the vulva that are beyond the scope of this chapter. Unusual findings or inadequate response to standard treatment suggest the need for expedient referral to a dermatology specialist. It is also important to remember that concomitant skin conditions are common, and more than one therapy may be necessary. For example, lichen sclerosus (LS) can be present with incontinence-associated dermatitis and/or vulvovaginal candidiasis.

Prevention

There is scant to no evidence to support common genital skin care recommendations. For this reason, expert opinion continues to guide recommendations. **Box 27-1** summarizes the general advice for genital skin care that should be provided to patients with vulvar irritation (Edwards et al., 2025). Because sensitivities to products vary, each individual may need to experiment to find their optimal self-care regimen.

BOX 27-1 General Vulvar Skin Care Advice for Prevention and Management of Vulvar Irritation

- Avoid contact with irritants, which can include chronic irritative moisture (perspiration, incontinence, semen, antiseptics); feminine hygiene products; topical medications (anesthetics such as benzocaine, antifungals); soaps, shampoos, and bubble bath; and hair removal products.
- Hypoallergenic liquid body wash can be used to clean.
- Shower no more than once per day, rather than bathing; avoid excessive cleaning and drying. Use the hand (rather than a sponge or washcloth) for cleaning, avoid scrubbing, and pat gently dry.
- Remoisturize throughout the day with any nonperfumed, well-tolerated emollient; cold (refrigerated) moisturizers may help stop itching. Each person may need to perform their own skin test to find an emollient they can tolerate. Well-moisturized skin will feel less irritated and is better able to avoid infection.
- Avoid use of spermicides.
- Avoid tight-fitting clothing that can cause friction and perspiration buildup.
- Sleep without underwear.

Data from Edwards, S. K., Lewis, F., Fernando, I., Haddon, L., & Grover, D. (2025). 2024 British Association for Sexual Health and HIV (BASHH) UK national guideline on the management of vulval conditions. *International Journal of STD & AIDS*, 9564624241311629. Advance online publication. https://doi.org/10.1177/09564624241311629

Vulvar Skin Cysts

Cysts are closed cavities lined by epithelium and filled with fluid or semisolid material. They are common on the vulva. Many patients also have normal vulvar findings that can be confused with cystic pathology, so clinicians should be aware of these variations. Examples include vulvar papillomatosis (asymmetrical fingerlike projections around the vestibule or minora), Fordyce spots (prominent sebaceous glands), and angiokeratomas (benign blood vessel growths often seen on the labia majora) (Sally et al., 2021). Other common benign changes are reviewed in this section.

Folliculitis, Furuncles, and Carbuncles

Infected hair follicles on the vulvar skin are a common source of vulvar skin cysts. Small, scattered lesions, such as shaving folliculitis, are easily identified and will resolve with elimination of the precipitating factors in conjunction with warm compresses and/or application of topical antibacterial or antifungal agents if indicated by surrounding erythema. Larger infected cysts, such as vulvar furuncles and carbuncles, may require incision and drainage, culture, and/or systemic antibiotic treatment in patients with additional risks, such as immunosuppression, systemic signs of infection, or inadequate response to other treatments.

Epidermoid and Sebaceous Cysts

Epidermoid (keratin-filled) or similar sebaceous gland cysts can form on vulvar hair-bearing surfaces, with their prevalence increasing with aging. Patients often report concerns about these nodules and need reassurance of their benign nature (Sally et al., 2021). Both types of cysts are typically slow growing, rarely drain, often resolve spontaneously over weeks or months, and usually require no intervention. Patients should be advised to avoid any squeezing and manipulation of these cysts. If a patient reports serious discomfort due to size or site, surgical excision can be performed, remembering that new cysts are common.

Hidradenitis Suppurativa

Hidradenitis suppurativa is a chronic, relapsing inflammatory disorder of the hair follicles that can have a similar appearance to sebaceous cysts in its early stages. This can be observed in **Color Plate 15**. In individuals assigned female at birth, hidradenitis suppurativa is more likely to occur under the breasts and in the axillae and genital hair-bearing areas (Sabat et al., 2025). Unlike epidermoid cysts, hidradenitis suppurativa can be very painful, disfiguring, and odiferous, and it can have a profound negative effect on quality of life. As many as 4 percent of people in this group are affected, and the condition occurs most often during the reproductive years (Sabat et al., 2025). Optimal outcomes from treatment require early diagnosis and intervention, with appropriate referral as needed.

Hidradenitis suppurativa is posited to have genetic, hormonal, autoimmune, and epigenetic causes and is often seen in conjunction with Crohn's disease (Sabat et al., 2025). Plugged follicular units become distended with keratin and sebum and can rupture, resulting in inflammation, scarring, and formation of permanent draining sinus tracts. The inflammation is locally mediated, and removal of the contents will resolve individual lesions. Because the lesions are sterile, associated cellulitis and septicemia are rare.

In individuals assigned female at birth, androgen sensitivity plays a role in the expression of hidradenitis suppurativa. Symptoms are often limited to the reproductive years, may be premenstrually cyclic, and may be exacerbated by use of androgenic progestins (Sabat et al., 2025). Symptoms are also exacerbated by smoking, and an association has been noted with metabolic syndrome (Sabat et al., 2025). In contrast, this condition often improves temporarily during pregnancy and lactation, presumably due to estrogen dominance.

Early symptoms of hidradenitis suppurativa include deep-seated, painful nodules. They can become abscessed or draining sinuses, with bridging and scarring occurring over time (Sabat et al., 2025). Symptoms can be either chronic or recurring. Unlike furuncles, these lesions typically do not respond to antibiotic treatment and do tend to rupture and track subcutaneously, rather than coming to a head and discharging to the surface. For this reason, symptoms are exacerbated by squeezing, pinching, friction, and pressure, which promote rupture and inflammation of the underlying cyst.

In early disease, the differential diagnosis includes epidermoid cysts, folliculitis, and furuncles. Bartholin duct abscess and anogenital fistulae associated with Crohn's disease are included in the differential diagnosis for advanced disease (Sabat et al., 2025).

Due to a dearth of evidence, treatment strategies are based on expert opinion. Typically, they are multimodal, including behavioral, metabolic, medical, and surgical strategies (Sabat et al., 2025). Behavioral strategies center on avoidance of injury to the skin and limiting other exacerbating factors. Recommendations include gentle, friction-free local hygiene with a mild, soap-free cleansing bar; antiseptic cleansing, which may be helpful if the odor is bothersome; avoidance of pinching or squeezing; weight control; use of tampons rather than pads; avoidance of nicotine-related products, overheating, tight clothing, and excessive perspiration; zinc supplementation (e.g., zinc gluconate 90 mg/day); and comprehensive avoidance of dietary triggers, especially dairy (due to androgenic properties) and high-glycemic load products (Sabat et al., 2025).

Pharmacologic treatments include antibiotics for their anti-inflammatory effect and odor control, administered either topically (e.g., clindamycin 1 percent solution) or systemically (e.g., minocycline); antiandrogens such as drospirenone-containing oral contraceptives or finasteride 5 to 10 mg per day (the latter is used on an off-label basis with precautions due to teratogenicity); biologic therapies (e.g., tumor necrosis factor alpha antagonists), and adjunct immunosuppressives (e.g., high-dose, rapidly tapered prednisone for acute flares). These and other potential agents, including retinoids and phototherapy, may be more comprehensively available through a dermatologic referral. Biologicals, such as Adalimumab, are the newest type of medications used to treat hidradenitis suppurativa and are used in patients for whom other systemic medications have not proven effective or were not well tolerated. Because these medications are not recommended in patients with certain conditions, such as multiple sclerosis, it is important to complete a thorough medical history (Sabat et al., 2025). Surgical management options include unroofing of fluctuant lesions, both for early active nodules and branching severe lesions of advanced disease. Unroofing enhances drainage, resolution, and pain control, and it can be done by trained clinicians in primary care settings using only local anesthesia. It is typically accomplished by puncturing with sturdy surgical scissors held parallel to the skin surface or, for small lesions, punch biopsy (refer to Box 27-1). The need for more invasive surgical options may be reduced by early intervention. More invasive surgical options can be effective at limiting recurrence of symptoms but carry higher risk due to the prolonged healing time. If surgical treatment is performed, clients on biologicals should continue during the perioperative time to improve overall outcomes (Sabat et al., 2025).

Vulvar Dermatoses

Most dermatoses that affect either skin or mucous membranes can appear on the vulva. This section reviews general management of several vulvar dermatoses. Benign skin changes are differentiated from malignancy either clinically (by response to treatment) or by biopsy. Dermatoses, noninfectious by definition, generally involve an inflammatory reaction. They are often treated with high-potency topical corticosteroid preparations. Based on the severity of symptoms, steroid ointment may be selected based on the United States classification system ranking from superpotent (class I) to least potent (class VII) (**Table 27-2**). **Box 27-2** and **Box 27-3** provide general use considerations for patients and clinicians.

TABLE 27-2 Topical Corticosteroid Ointments by Class Used for Vulvar Dermatoses

Class	Potency	Medication	Strength
I	Super	Clobetasol propionate	0.05%
		Augmented betamethasone dipropionate	0.05%
		Diflorasone diacetate	0.05%
		Halobetasol propionate	0.05%
II	High	Amcinonide	0.1%
		Betamethasone dipropionate	0.05%
		Fluocinonide	0.05%
		Halcinonide	0.1%
III	Medium to High	Fluticasone propionate	0.005%
		Triamcinolone acetonide	0.5%
IV, V	Medium	Fluocinolone acetonide	0.025%
		Hydrocortisone butyrate	0.1%
		Hydrocortisone valerate	0.2%
		Mometasone furoate	0.1%
		Triamcinolone acetonide	0.025%, 0.1%
VI	Low	Alclometasone dipropionate	0.05%
		Desonide	0.05%
VII	Least	Hydrocortisone	1% and 2.5%

Data from Gabros, S., Nessel, T. A., & Zito, P. M. (2023). Topical corticosteroids. *StatPearls*. https://www.ncbi.nlm.nih.gov/sites/books/NBK537164/

BOX 27-2 Considerations for Advising Patients Using High-Potency Corticosteroid Products

- Surface application of a strong corticosteroid ointment can be a very safe, effective way to treat inflammation that causes genital skin irritation. Side effects related to misuse should be reviewed.
- Advise patients to apply the prescribed product to clean skin—a small, pea-sized amount in a very thin layer over only the affected area—and gently massage into skin until it disappears.
- Review signs and symptoms of an allergic response to the product, including rash, irritation, itching, or burning. Instruct patients to discontinue use and call their clinician if symptoms worsen during the first week of use. Use of ointments is recommended as they are usually better tolerated and stay on better than creams; creams generally have more additives.
- Advise against using the product on their face, near their eyes or mouth, or directly on acne, rosacea, or open sores without consulting their clinician.
- For daily use, nighttime application is best, with the treated skin uncovered (i.e., avoiding tight dressings or clothing).
- Encourage handwashing after each after application.
- The product should be kept away from children and pregnant or breastfeeding/chestfeeding individuals without clinician consultation.
- Overuse can result in over-absorption and high systemic steroid levels. Local effects include thinning, weakening, stretching, and changes in color of treated skin. Systemic effects include adrenal dysfunction, or Cushing syndrome, an adrenal gland disorder that includes symptoms such as rapid weight gain, generalized skin thinning, and new-onset depression. Additionally, the risk of altered glucose metabolism and diabetes increases.

Data from Mautz, T. T., Krapf, J. M., & Goldstein, A. T. (2022). Topical corticosteroids in the treatment of vulvar lichen sclerosus: A review of pharmacokinetics and recommended dosing frequencies. *Sexual medicine reviews, 10*(1), 42–52; Edwards, S. K., Lewis, F., Fernando, I., Haddon, L., & Grover, D. (2025). 2024 British Association for Sexual Health and HIV (BASHH) UK national guideline on the management of vulval conditions. *International Journal of STD & AIDS*, 9564624241311629. Advance online publication. https://doi.org/10.1177/09564624241311629.

Although treatments may be similar, expectations for response to treatment can be very different, making it especially important that clinicians are able to achieve an accurate diagnosis. This section addresses specific considerations for management of contact dermatitis, lichenoid disorders (sclerosus, planus, and simplex chronicus), and psoriasis. "Lichen" and "lichenoid" are dermatologic terms applied to inflammatory skin disorders that include flat, scaly patches with an appearance similar to plant lichen.

Vulvar dermatoses can result in both physical symptoms and psychological and relationship consequences. Individuals often suffer for years with symptoms and may present for care already feeling frustrated or hopeless. Body image, sexual function, and sleep can be deeply affected and should be evaluated and addressed. It is important to spend time reviewing realistic expectations for often long-term management and to explain that multiple dermatoses may be occurring concurrently and require multiple treatments. At the same time, the clinician should express a commitment to helping each patient obtain relief of symptoms and improvement in their quality of life. Centering patient autonomy in the treatment of vulvar dermatoses is crucial to promote effective corticosteroid use. Clinicians can reassure patients about drug safety, design treatment regimens that fit their lives, and take a nonjudgmental stance around adherence to the prescribed regimen (Rees et al., 2024). Patients with chronic dermatoses may also benefit from joining local or online support groups.

BOX 27-3 Guidelines for Prescribing Topical Corticosteroid Therapy

- Treat concomitant candidiasis (e.g., topical nystatin) because steroids can worsen candidal infection.
- Safety in pregnancy and breastfeeding has not been established; the smallest effective dose should be used if indicated.
- Ointments are typically preferred over creams, which are less adherent and more likely to contain potentially irritating additives.
- Potent or superpotent steroid therapy is often required for vulvar conditions because the modified mucous membranes of the vulva can be steroid resistant. Caution should be used when corticosteroids are applied to surrounding areas that are not steroid resistant (e.g., hair-bearing areas, perianal skin, and medial thighs) because atrophy can occur more easily in those areas.
- Taper protocols are typically used: corticosteroid (e.g., clobetasol propionate 0.05% ointment or similar agent) applied sparingly once nightly for 1 month, then tapered to every other day for 1 month, then twice weekly for 1 month.
- Carefully instruct the patient in use; a 30-gram tube should last 3 months.
- If symptoms recur with reduced frequency of application during tapering, use can be increased again to control symptoms.
- The patient should be reevaluated 3 months after initiating therapy; persistent or increased symptoms imply need for biopsy and/or referral. If the desired response is achieved, a low to medium potency may be sufficient for maintenance (typically 1 to 3 applications/week), or the patient may choose to stop treatment and restart when symptoms recur.
- Ongoing assessment for vulvar status should occur at least annually. Referral should be considered when symptoms are severe, involve the vagina, are unresponsive to therapy, or if management requires medications with which the clinician is unfamiliar.

Data from American College of Obstetricians and Gynecologists. (2020). Diagnosis and management of vulvar skin disorders: ACOG Practice Bulletin, Number 224. *Obstetrics and Gynecology, 136*(1), e1–e14; Edwards, S. K., Lewis, F., Fernando, I., Haddon, L., & Grover, D. (2025). 2024 British Association for Sexual Health and HIV (BASHH) UK national guideline on the management of vulval conditions. *International journal of STD & AIDS*, 9564624241311629. Advance online publication. https://doi.org/10.1177/09564624241311629; Mautz, T. T., Krapf, J. M., & Goldstein, A. T. (2022). Topical corticosteroids in the treatment of vulvar lichen sclerosus: A review of pharmacokinetics and recommended dosing frequencies. *Sexual Medicine Reviews, 10*(1), 42–52.

Contact Dermatitis

Irritant contact dermatitis and allergic contact dermatitis are often referred to collectively as contact dermatitis (ACOG, 2020). This can be observed in **Color Plate 16**. These two forms have distinguishing characteristics, which are summarized in **Table 27-3**. A detailed assessment will help in differentiating the various types and developing a plan for treatment and prevention. Individuals with either form of contact dermatitis should avoid provoking agents and use prescribed topical corticosteroids appropriately until symptoms resolve. Based on the severity of symptoms, a low- to very-high-potency steroid ointment can be selected, typically starting with use once or twice daily until the irritation has resolved.

Lichen Sclerosus

Table 27-4 compares benign lichenoid disorders. Lichen sclerosus (LS), one of the most common of these conditions, is a chronic mucocutaneous disorder that is characterized by inflammation, epithelial thinning and depigmentation, and dermal changes, which often include agglutination of the labia minora. It can be progressive or relapsing and remitting. Although it is most often genital, LS is occasionally identified in other body areas, including the trunk, neck, forearms, axillae, and under the breasts, often occurring on tissue that has undergone trauma (Edwards et al., 2025; Singh & Ghatage, 2020). LS was once thought to be primarily hormonally mediated because it is most often evident in individuals during adolescence and after menopause. Although affected individuals have been found to have variant hormone receptors, LS is now known to occur among all sexes at any age; it is likely predominantly an autoimmune disorder that manifests in genetically susceptible individuals (Fergus et al., 2020). Adolescents who develop LS prior to puberty are no longer thought to outgrow it, and they should be followed into adulthood for surveillance and maintenance therapy as needed. Early diagnosis and treatment can help prevent scarring and possibly prevent the change to malignancy (van der Meijden et al., 2022). Although events such as hormonal changes of menopause, infections, trauma, or persistent moisture from occlusive garments may act as precipitating factors, they are not causative. A small increased risk (3–6%) of vulvar cancer has been noted in individuals with LS (Fergus et al., 2020).

Patients presenting with LS can have a range of symptoms, from none to severely debilitating. Early symptoms may include dull, nonspecific vulvar irritation, whereas progressive disease often manifests with severe pruritus, burning, and associated dyspareunia. Perianal symptoms, including pruritus ani, painful defecation, and anal fissures, may also occur. Introital stenosis and loss of the structural architecture of the vulva occur with progressive disease. Phimosis of the labia minora over the clitoris can diminish sexual sensation and may result in a pseudocyst due to collection of keratin debris (ACOG, 2020). Introital stenosis may preclude sexual activity. Dribbling and dysuria may occur from fusion of the minora over the urethra, which may become completely obstructed.

On physical examination, patients with LS may have a range of genital skin findings, from maculopapular lesions, to coalescing plaques, to a classic, pale atrophic figure-eight depigmented formation surrounding the vulva and perianal area. This can be observed in **Color Plate 17**. The depigmented tissue has a "cigarette

TABLE 27-3 Differentiation of Contact Dermatitis

Factor	Irritant Contact Dermatitis	Allergic Contact Dermatitis
Etiology	Nonimmunologic	Hypersensitivity reaction to a preexisting allergen; other known systemic or skin allergies common
Common irritants	Perfumed soaps, feminine hygiene sprays and deodorants, bath bubbles and oils, colored or scented toilet paper, laundry detergents, sanitary napkins, tampons, condoms, spermicides, tight clothing, adult wipes, topical medications, and body fluids	Medications (e.g., anesthetics, antibiotics, antifungals, antiseptics, corticosteroids), douches, emollients, fragrances, nail polish, nickel, preservatives, rubber, sanitary napkins, spermicides
Symptom onset	Within 12 hours of exposure	Delayed (48 to 72 hours after exposure)
Symptoms	Burning, pruritus, pain	Similar to ICD
Signs	Acute: Erythema, edema, vesicles, ulcerations Chronic or subacute: Scale, excoriation	Similar to ICD
Management	Avoidance of provoking agent Cool packs or sitz baths, wet dressings with Burrow solution to decrease itching and burning Avoidance of scratching Topical corticosteroids until resolution of symptoms	Similar to ICD Severe cases: Oral corticosteroids and antihistamines may be warranted
Resolution	More rapid after elimination of irritants	Slower resolution after elimination of irritant(s)

Data from American College of Obstetricians and Gynecologists. (2020). Diagnosis and management of vulvar skin disorders: ACOG Practice Bulletin, Number 224. *Obstetrics and Gynecology, 136*(1), e1–e14.

Abbreviation: ICD, irritant contact dermatitis.

TABLE 27-4 Differentiation of Lichenoid Disorders of the Vulva

Factor	Lichen Sclerosus	Lichen Planus	Lichen Simplex Chronicus	Psoriasis
Etiology	Autoimmune, hereditary; hormone-receptor variant present Inflammatory, possibly oxidative stress	Autoimmune, hereditary, inflammatory condition	Local variant of atopic dermatitis; spontaneous onset or response to chronic friction/scratch, or psychological distress	Autoimmune, hereditary Triggers include infections, substance use, trauma to the skin
Incidence	Approximately 2%	Rare (less than 1%)	0.5%	Approximately 0.5–11.4%, 2–5% with genital lesions; most common autoimmune disorder
Age at onset	Bimodal age peak (prepuberty and early postmenopause); 20% of onset is in young adults	Most common in perimenopause and menopause	Most common in mid- to late adulthood	Any age; peak onset is adolescence to young adulthood
Distribution	Primarily affects genitalia; anal and perineal involvement common; extragenital and vaginal involvement are rare	Diverse; variant: oral, vulvar, and vaginal involvement	Vulva, particularly hair-growing areas, are most commonly affected, but can occur on any chronically irritated skin	Generally scattered (knees, elbows, scalp, nails, umbilicus, gluteal fold), but may be only vulvar

(*continues*)

TABLE 27-4 Differentiation of Lichenoid Disorders of the Vulva (*continued*)

Factor	Lichen Sclerosus	Lichen Planus	Lichen Simplex Chronicus	Psoriasis
Symptoms	Asymptomatic to severe itching, burning, dysuria, dyspareunia, apareunia, constipation; chronic or remitting	Asymptomatic to severe pain; vulvar itching, dysuria, dyspareunia; chronic or remitting	Severe itching; temporary relief by scratching or rubbing; excoriations are common because scratching offers relief	Asymptomatic or mild itch, burning, soreness; intermittent flares; common triggers: cold, dry climate, dry skin, stress; joint pain with related arthritis
Signs	Onset: Maculopapular coalescing plaques. Advanced: Ivory, "cigarette paper" skin; pale figure-of-eight around vulva and anus; fissures, ecchymosis, erosion, phimosis, and atrophy; agglutination may obscure clitoris, introitus, and/or urethra; lichenification if scratching; postinflammatory hyperpigmentation common	Type 1 (classic): Pruritic papular lesions of vulva, perineum, perianus; may have white reticulation/striae or hyperpigmentation after lesions have resolved in darker-skin Type 2 (hypertrophic): Rare; white hypertrophic, rough vulvar plaques, which may have ulcers Type 3 (erosive): Pain; erythematous erosions; serosanguinous discharge; white striae; friable, eroded vagina; adhesions, stenosis, with vaginal and/or clitoral obliteration possible; may have oral involvement	Onset: Mild erythema Advanced: Thickened patches, fissures, pallor, excoriations, hyperpigmentation; area may be denuded of pubic hair due to scratching	On vulva: Thin plaques, typically highly erythematous with scant scaling due to maceration; satellite lesions common Inverse psoriasis: Predominantly in skin folds
Malignant potential	Less than 6%	Rare	Not identified	Not identified
Differentiating factors	Symmetrical depigmentation in a figure-of-eight of pale, tissue-paper thin tissue around vulva and perianal area Loss of vulvar architecture with agglutination is common and supports the diagnosis	Vaginal (lesions and/or discharge) and/or oral involvement; can also affect scalp, skin, and nails Other diagnostic criteria: Well-demarcated erosions; white, hyperkeratotic borders; pain, burning, scarring, loss of genital architecture Association with other autoimmune disorders, including thyroid disease, is less common	Temporary relief with scratching; thickened keratinized skin; excoriations; lack of vaginal involvement; leathery quality to skin; vulvar architecture is typically intact	Family or personal history; thick, pale red to white scaly plaques outside the genital area; typically, thin, bright red, well-demarcated plaques without scaling on genitals; milder itch typical, excoriations uncommon

Factor	Lichen Sclerosus	Lichen Planus	Lichen Simplex Chronicus	Psoriasis
Management	Rule out other autoimmune disorders (thyroid, anemia, vitiligo, diabetes) Defer biopsy of symmetrical classic signs pending 3-month treatment trial First-line: clobetasol propionate or mometasone furoate steroid ointment tapered (e.g., daily for 1 month, every other day the next month, then twice weekly); daily use for 3 months is also an accepted treatment schedule Nonresponse warrants biopsy and/or referral Maintenance therapy after successful treatment is often needed (lowest effective dose, twice weekly, continuous or intermittent)	Swab excoriated lesions to rule out secondary infection Consider investigating for thyroid or other autoimmune diseases if suspected Type 1: May resolve spontaneously or may use emollient and medium-potency topical steroid Type 2: Superpotent topical steroid over 3 months or intralesional injection (triamcinolone) repeated in 6 to 8 weeks as needed Type 3: Superpotent topical steroid for 3 months; taper as symptoms improve, then maintenance (once or twice weekly); second-line includes tacrolimus, pimecrolimus, intralesional corticosteroid injection, oral prednisolone, antibiotics, or immunosuppressive (e.g., azathioprine, cyclosporine) Surgical repair of vaginal occlusion	Eliminate identifiable irritants Rule out secondary infection (e.g., yeast culture) Saline soaks to improve skin barrier function Topical xylocaine and oral antihistamine/anxiolytic (e.g., hydroxyzine) to break nighttime itch–scratch–itch cycle Nighttime sedative or antidepressant to control scratching (e.g., hydroxyzine or amitriptyline, respectively) Superpotent topical steroid ointment, tapered over 3 to 4 months until lichenification is totally resolved Intermittent application of ice (maximum 15 minutes) Cognitive behavioral therapy for concomitant mental illness	Biopsy seldom required for diagnosis Keep skin moist with emollients; careful exposure to sunlight may be helpful; topical medium followed by low-potency steroids Topical vitamin D analogues or coal tar preparations alone or in combination with steroids Systemic therapies include methotrexate, retinoids, cyclosporine, and biological agents (i.e., monoclonal antibodies)
Other considerations	Ongoing yearly vulvar examination warranted to identify early skin changes due to the small increased risk of vulvar cancer Advise patient to avoid sources of irritation	Specialist referral for erosive or vaginal disease because condition is highly debilitating Advise patient to seek urgent evaluation if concerning changes to texture or appearance are noted (e.g., lump, hardening, or ulceration) Early use of progressive vaginal dilators may improve and preserve vaginal integrity	Consider psychological component if resolution is atypical (e.g., obsessive–compulsive disorder) Avoid petroleum-based products	Referral and online support groups may be helpful for patients with extensive disease Systemic therapies should be avoided in pregnancy

Data from Edwards, S. K., Lewis, F., Fernando, I., Haddon, L., & Grover, D. (2025). 2024 British Association for Sexual Health and HIV (BASHH) UK national guideline on the management of vulval conditions. *International Journal of STD & AIDS*, 9564624241311629. Advance online publication. https://doi.org/10.1177/09564624241311629; van der Meijden, W. I., Boffa, M. J., Ter Harmsel, B., Kirtschig, G., Lewis, F., Moyal-Barracco, M., Tiplica, G. S., & Sherrard, J. (2022). 2021 European guideline for the management of vulval conditions. *Journal of the European Academy of Dermatology and Venereology : JEADV, 36*(7), 952–972. https://doi.org/10.1111/jdv.18102; American College of Obstetricians and Gynecologists. (2020). Diagnosis and management of vulvar skin disorders: ACOG Practice Bulletin, Number 224. *Obstetrics and Gynecology, 136*(1), e1-e14.

paper" appearance and is susceptible to fissuring, ecchymosis, and erosion with minimal trauma. The labia minora may agglutinate and fuse with the labia majora, and eventual phimosis may obscure the clitoris, urethra, and/or introitus. Irregular, patchy postinflammatory hyperpigmentation is often present, and biopsy may be needed to rule out malignant change (van der Meijden et al., 2022). Nongenital lesions on the neck, upper back, breasts, axillae, scalp, abdomen, or thighs are typically asymptomatic but may appear as pale, wrinkled papules or plaques (Singh & Ghatage, 2020). Some affected individuals may also have other autoimmune disorders, such as thyroid disease, vitiligo, or alopecia areata. Further, concurrent vaginal or vulvar infection is common, and patients should be tested for these at the time of diagnosis (van der Meijden et al., 2022).

In the presence of typical, symmetrical, lesions, biopsy is generally deferred pending a 12-week treatment trial (van der Meijden et al., 2022). Biopsy is often inconclusive in early-stage disease but is generally indicated for persistent areas of unusual pigmentation, hyperkeratosis, erosion, erythema, friability, focal atypical papules, or any time clinical diagnosis is uncertain. Additional evaluation could include thyroid testing due to the association of LS with other autoimmune diseases (refer to Table 27-1).

A condensed differential diagnosis for vulvar lesions is presented in Table 27-1. LS is most often confused with lichen planus (LP), lichen simplex chronicus (LSC), vitiligo, immunobullous disorders such as pemphigoid, and vulvar intraepithelial neoplasia.

Goals of treatment for LS include relief of symptoms, potential reversal of agglutination, prevention of further architectural distortion with loss of function, and prevention of potential malignant changes (ACOG, 2020). First-line treatment consists of superpotent topical corticosteroid ointment (refer to Table 27-3) twice daily until the skin texture normalizes, which usually takes about 4 months. Options for maintenance therapy, which has been shown to decrease the risk of vulvar squamous cell carcinoma, include a superpotent topical corticosteroid three times per week or a medium potency topical corticosteroid once daily (van der Meijden et al., 2022).

Patients with LS should be informed that this skin condition is chronic, and recurrence of symptoms is expected even after successful treatment. Recommendations for follow-up therapy vary. Some clinicians recommend maintenance corticosteroid application, whereas others recommend discontinuation of such therapy pending symptom recurrence (ACOG, 2020; van der Meijden et al., 2022).

Although evidence supporting this practice is limited, patients with LS may benefit from a yearly vulvar examination to provide for early detection of potential malignant skin changes and to detect any atrophy or irritation secondary to corticosteroid use (Edwards et al., 2025; van der Meijden et al., 2022). In addition, patients should be asked to contact the clinician if they notice interim changes in vulvar symptoms or appearance (van der Meijden et al., 2022). Referral to a sex therapist or counselor may also be indicated.

For patients with atypical findings, equivocal biopsy, or poorly controlled symptoms with appropriate topical corticosteroid treatment, referral to a specialist is warranted. Surgery is typically reserved for release of phimosis, introital stenosis, or excision of malignancy. Other experimental treatments include phototherapy, topical or systemic retinoids, and the topical calcineurin inhibitors pimecrolimus and tacrolimus (Edwards et al., 2025). Some especially thick plaques may require steroid injection into the lesion (van der Meijden et al., 2022). Use of experimental treatments, especially immunosuppressive agents, is done on an off-label basis and remains controversial because of the already small elevation in malignant potential attributed to LS.

Each patient should have education about chronicity and disease management to include hygiene measures and awareness of the appearance of their own vulva. The clinician should demonstrate where to apply the topical medication and the amount of product to be applied using a mirror. The clinician can also recommend a topical moisturizer to be applied on top of the ointment. Each patient should also be given information on sexual function to address comfort during sex (Smith et al., 2023). Additional information about sexual health and wellness can be found in Chapters 12.

Lichen Planus

Though fewer than 1 percent of all people assigned female at birth are affected by lichen planus (LP), it has the potential to be the most debilitating type of autoimmune-mediated, lichenoid inflammatory condition (Edwards et al., 2025). LP is typically identified on the vulva, scalp, skin, nails, and/or epithelial linings of the mouth and vagina (Edwards et al., 2025; van der Meijden et al., 2022). LS and LP can be very similar clinically and histologically, and some patients may not receive a differentiated diagnosis; however, involvement of the vaginal mucosa excludes LS (van der Meijden et al., 2022).

Clinical findings are used to differentiate three types of LP: type 1 (classical), type 2 (hypertrophic), and type 3 (erosive) (Edwards et al., 2025; van der Meijden et al., 2022). Further information is provided in Table 27-4. Type 3 (erosive) LP is the most likely to cause severe vulvovaginal symptoms. This can be observed in **Color Plate 18**. Its presentation can include severe genital pain with vaginal involvement, brightly erythematous erosions, white striae on erosion borders (Wickham striae), and serosanguinous discharge. Eroded vaginal epithelium can bleed easily with any penetration. Purulent-appearing discharge is common, and adhesion, stenosis, and obliteration of the vagina can occur. Excoriated lesions should be swabbed and tested for secondary infection (van der Meijden et al., 2022).

Some individuals have a variant of erosive LP called vulvovaginal–gingival syndrome, which involves similar highly erythematous, erosive, striated lesions on the gingivae, buccal mucosa, and tongue, as well as small papules or rough plaques. A second variant, inverse LP, results in erythematous papules and/or diffuse erythema without scale within moist skin folds (e.g., inguinal, axillary, gluteal, intramammary) (Edwards et al., 2025).

LP is typically treated with corticosteroids topically, intravaginally, intralesionally, and/or systemically, and patients can expect to experience a treatment response based on their type of LP (Table 27-4). Intractable cases may be treated with systemic immune modulators (Edwards et al., 2025). Erosive LP is most often managed by multidisciplinary specialists because it is the most painful, debilitating, and difficult-to-treat type. One treatment specific to erosive vaginal involvement is the use of vaginal dilators to help manage agglutination and stenosis and improve the patient's ability to resume or continue sexual penetration. For this treatment, the patient is taught to use progressively sized vaginal dilators, often in conjunction with intravaginal topical steroid ointment, holding the dilator in their vagina overnight with snug-fitting underwear. After the appropriate-size dilator is reached, they may need to continue its use at least weekly for maintenance of their vaginal patency. If labial or vaginal agglutination is bothersome, surgical intervention may be helpful after active inflammation is controlled (ACOG, 2020; Edwards et al., 2025). Patients should receive education about the frequency of recurrence and relapse.

Lichen Simplex Chronicus

Lichen simplex chronicus (LSC) (formerly called squamous hyperplasia, hyperplastic dystrophy, and leukoplakia) is a localized variant of atopic dermatitis (Edwards et al., 2025). LSC can arise spontaneously, often in individuals with other atopic conditions such as allergies or asthma, or it can be triggered by a vulvar disorder that causes pruritus. As they scratch, epidermal thickening and hyperproliferation of the cells (lichenification) occur. As the tissue thickens, blood flow is further compromised, and itching becomes increasingly intense as the itch–scratch–itch cycle progresses.

Presenting symptoms and signs of LSC typically facilitate the differentiation of this condition from LS and LP (Table 27-4). Affected individuals often report prior ineffective treatments for vague diagnoses, such as chronic yeast infections. Symptoms of itching can be continuous or recurrent, often for years, and typically are unique in that scratching or rubbing offer an intensely pleasurable temporary relief of the itch, especially at night.

Initial signs may include localized edema and erythema and mild exaggeration of the skin architecture. As the disease progresses, fissures, excoriation, epidermal thickening, and lichenified plaques will become visible. This can be observed in **Color Plate 19**. Hyperpigmentation or unusual whiteness of the tissue (from scale) may also be evident. A leathery texture to the skin may be observed or reported by the patients. Scratching in areas of hair growth is common, and pubic hair may be broken or eliminated by chronic scratching (ACOG, 2020; Edwards et al., 2025). Diagnosis can usually be made based on presentation, and biopsy is rarely necessary.

The goal of therapy is to break the itch–scratch–itch cycle and eliminate any secondary infections. Affected patients should be screened for infections, including sexually transmitted infections (due to increased susceptibility if excoriations are present), atrophic vaginitis, and desquamative inflammatory vaginitis (van der Meijden et al., 2022). If such an infection is identified, oral therapy should be considered to minimize potential vulvar irritation. For LSC itself, superpotent topical corticosteroid ointment (e.g., clobetasol propionate 0.05%) is the first-line treatment (Table 27-3, Box 27-3, and Box 27-4) (van der Meijden et al., 2022). Class 4 triamcinolone acetonide 0.1 percent can be used for daily maintenance therapy in cases of recurrence (van der Meijden et al., 2022). Long-term maintenance therapy is rarely indicated. Second-line treatments, such as tacrolimus or pimecrolimus, are typically reserved for specialist referral (Edwards et al., 2025).

Itching and scratching are often worse at night, and medications that provide sedation may be helpful in managing these nocturnal symptoms. Low-dose tricyclic antidepressants, such as amitriptyline or doxepin, may provide better and longer sedation than antihistamines (e.g., hydroxyzine, diphenhydramine) while also improving anxiety and depression, which are common associated symptoms in many patients with LSC (van der Meijden et al., 2022). Wearing gloves at night may also be helpful to interrupt the itch–scratch–itch cycle as can the use of topical, refrigerated petroleum jelly. Advise patients to minimize pubic hair grooming, consider replacing tampons and pads with a menstrual cup and/or reusable cloth pads, and keep their nails trimmed short. In the presence of anxiety, depression, or obsessive–compulsive disorder, cognitive behavioral therapy should be offered (Edwards et al., 2025; van der Meijden et al., 2022).

Psoriasis

Psoriasis is a chronic, immune-mediated disease for which there appears to be a genetic predisposition. Psoriasis is often seen in patients with other autoimmune or inflammatory disorders (including hidradenitis suppurativa) and can manifest in the skin and/or joints (psoriatic arthritis). Psoriasis can occur spontaneously or can be triggered by an immune insult, such as infection, smoking, excessive alcohol intake, physical trauma (e.g., tattoos or piercings), or medication (van der Meijden et al., 2022). Although the peak incidence of this disease is adolescence until age 30, it can develop at any age.

The most common form of psoriasis is characterized by well-demarcated, pale, erythematous papules or plaques covered with silvery white, often thick scale. These lesions are frequently found on the knees, elbows, scalp, and nails. Vulvar psoriasis can occur as an isolated manifestation or coexist with psoriasis on other body areas. Vulvar psoriasis is shown in **Color Plate 20**. On genital skin, which is typically moister, psoriasis-related plaques tend to be thinner and more intensely erythematous, with minimal scaling due to maceration. In severe cases, fissures may be noted (Edwards et al., 2025; van der Meijden et al., 2022). Inverse psoriasis is a variant that involves the development of red, well-demarcated plaques only in skin folds (e.g., natal, inguinal, gluteal). Satellite lesions are often present, and individuals with inverse psoriasis are often misdiagnosed and ineffectively treated for candidal intertrigo or incontinence-associated dermatitis.

Although vulvar psoriasis may be asymptomatic, symptoms may also include itching, burning, soreness, and fissuring of skin folds. Symptoms are typically less intense than with other lichenoid conditions. Many individuals report triggers of disease recurrence, including emotional stress; cold, dry weather with limited sunlight; and skin dryness. Affected skin may benefit from regular use of emollients and/or moisture barriers to improve skin moisture content. Avoidance of scented detergents and tight clothing may help prevent recurrent episodes. When flares occur, topical corticosteroids are the mainstay of therapy, but weak- to moderate-potency agents may be sufficient to control symptoms in many patients (Table 27-3, Box 27-3, and Box 27-4). Referral is indicated if vulvar psoriasis is unresponsive to corticosteroids. Follow-up of stable disease should occur every 1 to 3 months (van der Meijden et al., 2022).

Considerations for Specific Populations

Pregnant or Breastfeeding/Chestfeeding Individuals

Recommendations related to treatment in pregnancy and lactation may vary; however, limited amounts of topical low potency steroids are safe to use as directed in pregnancy and lactation (van der Meijden et al., 2022). Other second-line potential treatment agents, such as calcineurin inhibitors, antimetabolites including methotrexate, and retinoids, are contraindicated in pregnancy and/or lactation and may require avoidance of pregnancy for a period of time following treatment (van der Meijden et al., 2022). When topical steroids are not sufficiently effective in treating vulvar conditions, a pregnant person should be referred to a specialist (van der Meijden et al., 2022). Individuals who are breastfeeding/chestfeeding may experience a range of lactation-related genitourinary symptoms including atrophic vaginitis symptoms similar to those seen in menopause and may benefit from localized estrogen therapy and other nonpharmacologic treatments (Perelmuter et al., 2024). Refer to Chapter 21 for more information about assessment and treatment of atrophic vaginitis.

Postmenopause

In postmenopausal individuals, treatment of concomitant atrophic vaginitis with a topical estrogen product may play an important role in management. Refer to Chapters 14 and 21 for more information about atrophic vaginitis and genitourinary syndrome of menopause.

Influences of Culture

Ideas of genital health and beauty are socially constructed, highly influenced by societal factors (e.g., media, sexual health and wellness education) and even normative hetero-normative conceptions of how genitals should look and function (Mohammed et al., 2025). Patients presenting with bothersome genital skin symptoms may have strongly held and divergent beliefs about the importance of activities such as pubic hair removal, hygiene products, piercing, tattooing, cosmetic surgeries or genital cutting, and self-touch. Sexual partners may have difficulty understanding which skin conditions are infectious and which are not. Environmental factors, such as cold, dry weather, or heat and humidity, can aggravate many genital skin conditions. Continence care and basic hygiene can be very problematic in resource-scarce cultures, and highly effective steroid ointments may be unavailable or prohibitively expensive. Clinicians need to be sensitive and respectful of cultural norms while helping patients find safe, flexible, and nonirritating self-care routines to attain and maintain healthy genital skin.

CONDITIONS OF THE UTERUS AND CERVIX

Individuals with nonpregnancy-related concerns about their uterus and cervix often experience pain, bleeding, or worry about potential malignancy. This section explains how to evaluate and manage several common conditions that may cause these concerns, including cervical and endometrial polyps, uterine fibroids, and endometrial conditions such as endometriosis and adenomyosis. Chapter 7 discusses normal variations on physical examination, including cervical changes such as ectropion and Nabothian cysts. Chapters 21 and 28 cover infections and malignancies of the cervix and endometrium, respectively; Chapter 25 addresses the management of abnormal uterine bleeding.

Abnormal, irregular bleeding can cause significant social and sexual difficulties for individuals from cultures that have activity taboos related to menstrual bleeding. In addition, the lack of proven alternative therapies for treatment of uterine fibroids and the potential need for surgery may be problematic for those who prefer to avoid allopathic medicine. Fertility preservation may be of primary importance for individuals from some cultures and may warrant special consideration in treatment planning. All these concerns may also play a role in assessment and treatment planning for people with the benign conditions discussed in the remainder of this chapter, including polyps, uterine fibroids, endometriosis, adenomyosis, and ovarian cysts.

Polyps

Polyps grow from mucous membranes, and while their cause remains unknown, several factors have been postulated to contribute to their development. Increased estrogen stimulation, chronic inflammation, and vascular congestion have all been associated with polyp formation (Mansour & Chowdhury, 2023; Pegu et al., 2020). Although typically benign, polyps have malignant potential, making patient education essential as individuals consider their treatment options.

Cervical Polyps

Cervical polyps occur in approximately 2–5 percent of individuals with a cervix, but fewer than 1 percent of those polyps are malignant (Pegu et al., 2020). They can be single or multiple in number and are typically less than 3 cm in diameter, but they can be larger. Usually lobular or pear shaped, their stalk arises from the cervical canal and may be either short or long. Cervical polyps range in color from light pink to reddish purple if vascular congestion is present. This can be observed in **Color Plate 21**.

Cervical polyps are often asymptomatic and incidentally diagnosed on routine speculum examination. If symptoms occur, they typically include postcoital or intermenstrual bleeding. Differential diagnosis includes endometrial polyps, cervical carcinoma, and cervical leiomyomata, all of which also may protrude through the cervical os. Evaluation of the endometrium should be considered whenever a patient presents with irregular bleeding.

When cervical polyps are identified, patients will need to choose between observation and removal for histology (MacGregor et al., 2023). Up-to-date cervical cytology, HPV testing, and colposcopy are important aids to rule out high risk for dysplasia or malignancy. If the polyp is asymptomatic and the patient prefers the option of observation, they should be asked to report irregular or postcoital bleeding. If a person with cervical polyps experiences symptoms (e.g., irregular or postcoital bleeding, increased discharge) or has an atypical polyp (e.g., larger than 3 cm, necrotic, friable, irregular color), removal for histology is indicated (Pegu et al., 2020). Because polyps may indicate endometrial malignancy, some pathologists recommend that all cervical polyps be removed and sent for histology (Pegu et al., 2020). The patient should also be informed that if the polyp is removed, recurrence is not uncommon.

An experienced clinician can remove a simple cervical polyp in the office if the stalk insertion is clearly visible. To do this, the clinician gently grasps the polyp at the stalk with a ring forceps, applies clamped pressure for 3 to 5 minutes to achieve homeostasis, and then twists the forceps with gentle traction to remove the polyp. Because the vascular core of the polyp may sometimes bleed heavily during the procedure, a cautery option must be available. Cautery may also decrease the risk of recurrence. If the patient opts for removal, or if removal is indicated but the polyp base is not clearly identifiable, a transvaginal ultrasound can aid in differential diagnosis. In some cases, referral for operative hysteroscopy may be required for safe removal.

Endometrial Polyps

Endometrial polyps are similar to cervical polyps in that they are a hyperplastic overgrowth of the endometrial glandular and stromal cells with a vascular core. They can be single or multiple in number, and they may be asymptomatic or cause abnormal vaginal bleeding (Hurtado & Shetty, 2023). Endometrial polyps are typically smaller than 10 mm in size, and most polyps this size can be safely managed with observation (Nijkang et al., 2019).

Endometrial polyps most commonly affect individuals aged 30 to 50 years, but their prevalence does not appear to change after menopause. Because they are often asymptomatic, their incidence is unknown; estimates range from 7 to 50 percent of people with a uterus. Many people undergoing evaluation for infertility have endometrial polyps, but causation is not established. Factors such as age and polyp location may play a role (Nijkang et al., 2019; Vitale et al., 2021). Those with symptoms most often report abnormal bleeding (e.g., intermenstrual or postmenopausal). Malignant transformation appears to be uncommon, but endometrial polyps share similar risk factors with endometrial cancer, including increasing age, larger body habitus, hypertension, and use of selective estrogen receptor modulators that stimulate the endometrium (e.g., tamoxifen). Clinicians should have a heightened level of concern when unexpected bleeding occurs in individuals with these risk factors. Additionally, studies have identified a correlation between endometrial and colorectal polyps, such that the presence of one should alert the clinician to inquire about the other (Nijkang et al., 2019; Vitale et al., 2021).

Endometrial polyps are most commonly identified and evaluated using transvaginal ultrasound. In menstruating individuals, this imaging is optimally done around day 10 of the menstrual cycle to improve detection of polyps smaller than 10 mm (Nijkang et al., 2019; Vitale et al., 2021). Both color or power Doppler and contrast with or without 3-D imaging may improve visualization. If the findings are ambiguous, repeat imaging at a more optimal cycle time may be appropriate, or referral may be warranted. Saline infusion sonohysterogram is often used to facilitate visualization during ultrasound, and hysteroscopy (i.e., placement of a thin telescopic tube through the cervix and into the uterine canal) can be used for identification and biopsy. In perimenopausal and postmenopausal individuals, hysteroscopy and polypectomy are indicated (Giampaolino et al., 2020).

For asymptomatic endometrial polyps identified incidentally on ultrasound imaging in premenopausal individuals, conservative management, such as repeat imaging to establish stability, is an appropriate option (Nijkang et al., 2019; Vitale et al., 2021). Medications have a limited role in treating symptomatic polyps. Gonadotropin-releasing hormone (GnRH) agonists are sometimes used to shrink large polyps prior to hysteroscopic resection, but the cost-effectiveness of this therapy is not clear. The levonorgestrel intrauterine system (LNG-IUS) may help with resolution of endometrial polyps in those who report heavy menstrual bleeding (Vitale et al., 2021).

Specific Populations

Pregnant Individuals Cervical polyps may increase in size during pregnancy. The removal of cervical or endometrial polyps is contraindicated during pregnancy unless there is an urgent clinical indication. In such cases, a specialist should perform the procedure, or removal should be deferred until after delivery.

Postmenopause The risk of malignancy risk increases with age. Additionally, any vaginal bleeding in a postmenopausal individual warrants a comprehensive evaluation of the endometrium to rule out underlying pathology (Giampaolino et al., 2020).

Uterine Fibroids

Uterine fibroids, also known as myomas or leiomyomatas, are benign growths that arise from the smooth muscle of the uterus. They are classified based on their location within the uterine layers: subserosal fibroids arise on the external surface of the uterus; intramural or myometrial fibroids lie completely within the myometrium; and submucosal fibroids extend into the endometrium. This can be seen in **Figure 27-1**. Pedunculated fibroids, which grow on a stalk, are susceptible to torsion, necrosis, or prolapse through the cervical canal, where they can be confused with cervical polyps. Fibroids range in size from microscopic to large tumors weighing several pounds. Multiple fibroids are common, but solitary fibroids can also occur.

Incidence

Fibroids are highly prevalent, affecting up to 70 to 80 percent of individuals with a uterus by age 50. Approximately half of those with fibroids experience symptoms, including irregular bleeding and/or bowel and bladder pressure. Symptoms are most common in individuals in their 30s and 40s (Angioni et al., 2021). The etiology of fibroids remains poorly understood, though heredity and cumulative exposure to estrogen play roles in fibroid growth (Giuliani et al., 2020; Manyonda et al., 2020). Fibroids are the most common indication for hysterectomy in the United States.

Certain populations face a disproportionately higher burden of fibroids. Individuals of African descent, for example, have a great overall risk of developing fibroids, tend to have earlier onset, experience more severe symptoms, and a higher likelihood of requiring surgical intervention (Huang et al., 2023; Katon et al., 2023). This increased susceptibility may be linked to genetic and environmental factors, including protective adaptations against infections endemic to sub-Saharan Africa. Additionally, fibroid-related conditions such as alopecia, sarcoidosis, and keloids are more prevalent in this population, suggesting a potentially shared fibroproliferative pathway (Awonuga et al., 2022).

FIGURE 27-1 Uterine fibroids, classified by location.

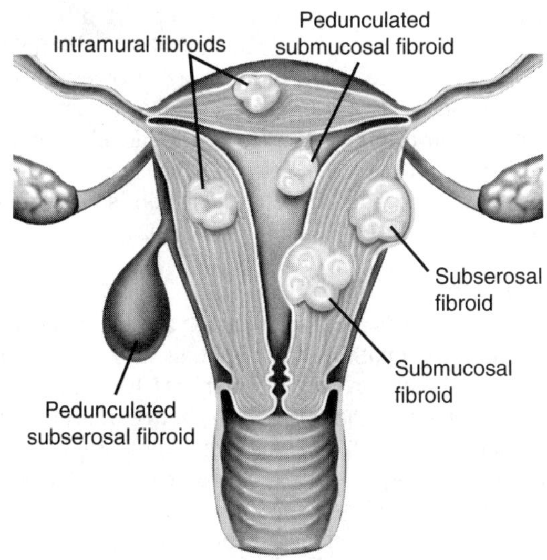

Disparities in fibroid outcomes persist even when access to care is equal, indicating the influence of cultural, socioeconomic, and genetic factors (Huang et al., 2023; Katon et al., 2023). Individuals of African descent report greater reductions in quality of life due to fibroids, often citing concerns such as heavy menstrual bleeding that leads to staining of clothes or bedding (Huang et al., 2023; Katon et al., 2023). They also experience longer delays in receiving an accurate diagnosis and are less likely to receive adequate information about treatment options (Martinez et al., 2024). Surgical management, including myomectomy and hysterectomy, is more common in people of African descent, potentially due to the earlier onset and increased severity of symptoms, as well as differences in treatment access and clinician recommendations (Huang et al., 2023).

The impact of fibroids can also be significant for people with physical or intellectual disabilities. Heavy menstrual bleeding associated with fibroids may pose unique challenges related to hygiene. In such cases, reducing or eliminating menstrual bleeding through medical management may be beneficial, whereas surgical sterilization is rarely appropriate (Wilbur et al., 2021).

Symptomatic fibroids are most common in the decade prior to menopause, in primiparous individuals, those living in larger bodies, and in persons of African descent; they are uncommon after menopause (Hurtado & Shetty, 2023). Although most people with fibroids do not have infertility or related pregnancy loss, fibroids can impede fertility, depending on their size and location (e.g., via blockage of sperm migration or of implantation due to the decreased blood supply and hypoestrogenic environment of the fibroids themselves) (Angioni et al., 2021; Donnez et al., 2024; Somigliana et al., 2021).

Etiology and Pathophysiology

The etiology of fibroids remains poorly understood (Guiliani et al., 2020; Manyonda et al., 2020). The extent of their expression in an individual's uterus appears to depend on a convergence of genetic, environmental, and lifestyle factors. They are known to arise from uterine smooth muscle (myometrium). The myometrial cells in fibroids are more similar to gravid rather than nongravid cells, suggesting they may be a manifestation of the type of myometrial stem cell stimulation and hyperproliferation normally seen in a pregnant uterus. Fibroids are composed of fibrotic tissue similar to that seen in keloids, suggesting a potential common etiology, which is supported by the more common occurrence of both keloids and fibroids in individuals of African ancestry (Awonuga et al., 2022). However, although keloid formation is always preceded by skin trauma, it is not clear that uterine trauma precedes fibroid development. Also, it is surprisingly unclear why fibroids, which result from highly hormone-sensitive cellular hyperproliferation, so rarely involve malignancy (less than 1%) (Giuliani et al., 2020).

Clinical Presentation

The majority of fibroids are asymptomatic and identified incidentally at ultrasound or pathology. Individuals who have symptoms typically report heavy or irregular menses, dysmenorrhea, pelvic pressure or pain, dyspareunia, or a change in urine or bowel control (Giuliani et al., 2020). Some individuals with fibroids may also have associated pregnancy-related problems, including infertility and pregnancy loss. When people report pain, it is often dull, crampy, and mild to moderate, but pain may become acute if torsion or necrosis occurs. Individuals with very enlarged fibroids may report an increase in abdominal girth and occasionally incorrectly assume they are pregnant. Fibroids (subserosal, intramural, or submucosal) can occasionally involve the cervix or protrude through the cervical canal and are visible or palpable as a mass on pelvic examination.

Assessment

Key factors in the health history of patients presenting with symptoms suggestive of uterine fibroids (e.g., abnormal uterine bleeding, pelvic pain or pressure) include a detailed menstrual and bleeding history and clear descriptors of related pain or pressure, helping to define any cyclic relationship. Those with symptoms should be asked about any difficulty achieving or maintaining pregnancy and any personal or family history of uterine fibroids.

Typically, fibroids are firm on palpation and nontender. Whether or not they are palpable will depend on their location and size. The uterus may be palpable abdominally if the fibroids are very large. On bimanual examination, the uterus may feel normal, smoothly enlarged, or irregular. Rectal examination may facilitate the identification of posterior fibroids. A pedunculated subserosal fibroid may be confused with a firm adnexal mass. Guarding or rebound tenderness can indicate irritation of the peritoneum related to torsion.

Definitive diagnosis of fibroids is usually made by ultrasound. In perimenopausal and postmenopausal individuals, endometrial cancer should be ruled out even if fibroids are identified because they may be concomitant conditions. Any person who reports frequent, heavy bleeding should have a hematocrit to evaluate the extent of blood loss.

Differential Diagnoses

Uterine fibroids are part of the differential diagnosis for abnormal uterine bleeding. Individuals can experience similar symptoms of pelvic pain and pressure with endometriosis and adenomyosis and with nonuterine conditions, such as ascites; disorders of the gastrointestinal tract (e.g., constipation, irritable bowel syndrome) or urinary tract (e.g., bladder diverticula, benign tumors); other gynecologic abnormalities (e.g., benign adnexal tumors); and neoplasia at any abdominal or pelvic location. Please refer to Chapter 25 for more information on abnormal uterine bleeding.

Management

No effective strategies for prevention or early intervention for fibroids have been identified, and conversion to malignancy is rare (Giuliani et al., 2020). Asymptomatic uterine fibroids are managed with observation. When fibroids become symptomatic, treatment options include medical therapies, surgery interventions (such as minimally invasive procedures or hysterectomy), uterine artery embolization, and MRI-guided high-frequency ultrasound therapy (MRgFUS) (Lebduska et al., 2023). Limited comparative outcomes data for these modalities exist, and few studies have included a representative number of individuals of African ancestry (Giuliani et al., 2020).

Generally, decisions about the timing and type of treatment are based on the number, size, and location of fibroids; the type and severity of symptoms; the individual's age and proximity to menopause; reproductive goals; and preferences regarding uterine preservation (Lebduska et al., 2023). No available medical treatments completely eliminate fibroids. An optimal treatment for symptomatic fibroids would effectively reduce fibroid size and symptoms over the long term while minimizing side effects and preserving fertility if desired. Current treatment options, summarized in **Table 27-5**, do not meet these criteria but instead aim to modify symptoms and/or temporarily shrink fibroids (Giuliani et al., 2020).

If an individual chiefly desires control of fibroid-related heavy bleeding, the use of oral progestogens, combination oral contraceptives, an LNG-IUS, or a short-term GnRH agonist may be sufficient. The LNG-IUS may improve dysmenorrhea as well, but it is contraindicated in fibroids that are submucosal, distort the uterine cavity, or are large (total uterine size greater than 12 cm). Chapter 13 contains additional information about the LNG-IUS.

Leuprolide, a GnRH agonist, is approved by the U.S. Food and Drug Administration (FDA) as a medical treatment to shrink fibroids temporarily (e.g., preoperatively or prior to attempting to become pregnant) and may temporarily control bleeding (refer to Table 27-5 and **Table 27-6**). Preoperative GnRH agonist treatment not only reduces fibroid volume (35 to 65% within 3 months of initiating treatment) but also increases systemic blood volume, thereby lowering the risks associated with surgery (Angioni et al., 2021; Lebduska et al., 2023). Major concerns for individuals using GnRH agonists include vasomotor symptoms and decreases in bone density, so only short-term treatment is approved. The effect of a GnRH agonist is temporary; fibroids will begin to regrow within months of discontinuation, and surgery or pregnancy attempts should ensue as soon as therapy is completed to maximize the benefits.

TABLE 27-5 Medical Treatment Options for Uterine Fibroids

Class	Target Symptoms	Considerations
Progestogens	May help control heavy bleeding	Reduce fibroid-associated endometrial hyperplasia LNG-IUS may improve dysmenorrhea but is contraindicated with submucosal fibroids or an irregularly shaped endometrial cavity No clear impact on fibroid size
Gonadotropin-releasing hormone agonist	Used to shrink fibroid prior to fertility treatment or surgery May control heavy bleeding	Approved only for short-term use (3 months) due to adverse-effect profile Fibroids can regrow quickly after treatment
Selective estrogen reuptake modulators	Shrink fibroid volume	Off-label use, limited data May increase cancer risk in other cells with extended use
Selective progesterone receptor modulators	May shrink fibroid volume, improve quality of life, and reduce bleeding	Off-label use
Aromatase inhibitors	May shrink fibroid volume	Off-label use, limited data, and high adverse-effect profile
Combined oral contraceptives	May improve periodic bleeding control and/or dysmenorrhea	No evidence that oral contraceptives either encourage or restrict growth of uterine fibroids; not contraindicated for individuals with fibroids
NSAIDs	May improve periodic bleeding control and/or dysmenorrhea	Rare but serious risks include gastrointestinal bleeding, acute renal failure, and congestive heart failure Data based on symptom improvement in individuals without fibroids Less effective than tranexamic acid, danazol, or LNG-IUS
Tranexamic acid	May improve bleeding	More expensive than some other treatment modalities
Iron supplements	May improve symptoms of iron deficiency anemia including fatigue, pica, headache secondary to heavy bleeding	Oral iron can cause constipation; IV iron can be expensive or inaccessible

Data from Donnez, J., Taylor, H. S., Marcellin, L., & Dolmans, M. M. (2024). Uterine fibroid-related infertility: mechanisms and management. *Fertility and Sterility, 122*(1), 31–39. https://doi.org/10.1016/j.fertnstert.2024.02.049; Giuliani, E., As-Sanie, S., & Marsh, E. E. (2020). Epidemiology and management of uterine fibroids. *International Journal of Gynecology & Obstetrics, 149*(1), 3–9. https://doi.org/10.1016/j.bpobgyn.2015.11.016; Lebduska, E., Beshear, D., & Spataro, B. M. (2023). Abnormal Uterine Bleeding. *The Medical Clinics of North America, 107*(2), 235–246. https://doi.org/10.1016/j.mcna.2022.10.014; Speciale, A. R., Ozpinar, K., Giani, M., Tureli, D., Fambrini, M., Vannuccini, S., & Petraglia, F. (2025). Selective progesterone receptor modulators for the treatment of dysmenorrhea: an update. *Expert Opinion on Pharmacotherapy, 26*(3), 257–264. https://doi.org/10.1080/14656566.2025.2451145

Abbreviation: LNG-IUS, levonorgestrel intrauterine system.

TABLE 27-6 **Gonadotropin-Releasing Hormone Agonists**

Product Names	Approved Indications	Route of Administration	Dosage
Leuprolide (Lupron)	Endometriosis and uterine fibroids	Intramuscular injection	3.75 mg monthly or 11.25 mg every 3 months
Nafarelin (Synarel)	Endometriosis	Nasal spray, 200 mcg per spray	400 to 800 mcg/day 400 mcg: One spray in one nostril in the morning, and one spray in the other nostril in the evening 800 mcg: One spray in each nostril twice/day
Goserelin (Zoladex)	Endometriosis	Subcutaneous injection in the upper abdomen	3.6 mg monthly

Data from Giuliani, E., As-Sanie, S., & Marsh, E. E. (2020). Epidemiology and management of uterine fibroids. *International Journal of Gynecology & Obstetrics, 149*(1), 3-9; Lebduska, E., Beshear, D., & Spataro, B. M. (2023). Abnormal uterine bleeding. *The Medical Clinics of North America, 107*(2), 235–246. https://doi.org/10.1016/j.mcna.2022.10.014; .

Note: These medications are contraindicated in pregnancy and must be used in conjunction with contraception. Refer to the specific prescribing reference for full information on doses, side effects, contraindications, and cautions.

Although surgery is rarely indicated for individuals with asymptomatic fibroids, they may choose surgical treatment if they have pedunculated fibroids due to the higher risk for torsion; related symptoms poorly controlled by medical treatments; or fibroids that obstruct other treatments (e.g., fertility or cancer interventions). Surgical options for the treatment of fibroids include myomectomy and hysterectomy (Lebduska et al., 2023). Hysterectomy is a definitive option for those who have severe symptoms, are distant from menopause, and have completed childbearing. Laparoscopically-assisted and transvaginal hysterectomies have been shown to reduce postoperative recovery time and infection risk. Nevertheless, open abdominal procedures continue to be performed for large fibroids, especially since the FDA issued warnings about power morcellation (debulking of large fibroids in situ to aid removal) carrying a risk of disseminating rare uterine sarcomas (ACOG, 2021; Sparic et al., 2022).

Myomectomy, in contrast, preserves the uterus and can be performed laparoscopically, abdominally, or hysteroscopically, depending on fibroid quantity, size, and location (Lebduska et al., 2023; Manyonda et al., 2020). Myomectomy does not prevent the growth of new lesions, and individuals choosing this option should be aware that they may require future procedures if symptomatic fibroids recur. Myomectomy can be performed in conjunction with a cesarean birth if indicated. In addition, myomectomy is not without risk both in terms of the surgery itself and the risk of uterine rupture and/or abnormal placentation in future pregnancies (Manyonda et al., 2020). Hysterectomy and myomectomy are both shown to improve quality of life, but there is little information about long-term satisfaction with either surgical option, and there is inadequate evidence to guide decision making based on characteristics of an individual fibroid. Therefore, the decision for type of surgery should be individualized based on the patient's desire and the surgeon's skill (Wallace et al., 2020).

Additional nonmedical, minimally invasive treatments are currently available or in development to resolve or decrease the size of fibroids through necrosis. These options include the FDA-approved procedures of uterine artery embolization (UAE) and MRgFUS, as well as cryomyolysis and temporary transvaginal occlusion of the uterine arteries (Lebduska et al., 2023). UAE is performed by interventional radiology and involves a guided injection of embolic particles to obstruct vascular supply of the fibroids. The limited evidence comparing UAE to surgery suggests that individuals who undergo UAE may be equally satisfied with their outcome, but up to 50 percent will require additional surgical treatment for fibroids within 5 years (Manyonda et al., 2020). Cryomyolysis involves the use of a probe to apply a cooling agent to necrose the fibroid and is not recommended for those who desire future fertility or who have concurrent diagnoses of endometriosis or adenomyosis along with their fibroids (Manyonda et al., 2020). Temporary transvaginal occlusion of uterine arteries is a technique used to treat fibroids by depriving them of blood supply. Pregnancy is not recommended after this procedure. Further, any nonsurgical treatment carries the risk of failing to identify a malignancy (Manyonda et al., 2020).

Although most uterine fibroids present as a chronic subacute condition, emergencies can occur. Torsion, which can cause acute, severe abdominal pain and necrosis, is a surgical emergency requiring immediate referral. Acute hemorrhage may also occur. Individuals with symptomatic fibroids who do not improve with medical management or are attempting pregnancy and meet the criteria for infertility should be referred for general gynecologic or specialist intervention.

Considerations for Specific Populations

Pregnant Individuals Research indicates that fibroids may affect pregnancy outcomes by distorting the uterine shape and affecting the function of the endometrium and myometrium (Michos et al., 2023). However, many individuals with fibroids have normal pregnancy outcomes. Given the increased risk of adverse pregnancy outcomes associated with fibroids, close observation is indicated. Potential complications include infertility, failed implantation, spontaneous abortion, preterm labor, placental abruption, malpresentation, cesarean birth, peripartum hysterectomy, and postpartum hemorrhage (Giuliani et al., 2020). Because many of these risks increase with advanced age, careful management is particularly important for those who are pregnant in their late 30s and 40s.

Perimenopause After menopause, the spontaneous decrease in hormone production typically results in reduction of fibroid size and symptom resolution. Exogenous hormone therapy after menopause is not contraindicated for individuals with fibroids if that treatment is otherwise warranted (Guiliani et al., 2020; Manyonda et al., 2020). For those who are perimenopausal or postmenopausal and present with enlarging fibroids, hysterectomy is indicated. Myomectomy, especially via power morcellation, is contraindicated in such individuals because the risk of occult cancers of the uterine corpus increases with aging (ACOG, 2021).

Endometriosis

Endometriosis is the presence of endometrial glands and stroma outside of the uterus. Outside of the uterus, endometrial implants have been identified in diverse sites, including the ovaries, anterior and posterior cul-de-sac, posterior broad ligaments, uterosacral ligaments, fallopian tubes, sigmoid colon, appendix, and round ligaments. Less commonly, histology has confirmed cases in other genital organs (e.g., vagina, vulva, cervix, perineum), the urinary tract, inguinal canals, elsewhere in the gastrointestinal tract, the respiratory system and diaphragm, the pericardium, surgical scars, and the umbilicus (Hirata et al., 2020). Individuals affected by endometriosis at any site may have cyclic or noncyclic pain that severely impairs their quality of life and also have increased risk for infertility and poor pregnancy outcomes.

Incidence

The true incidence of endometriosis is unknown, but it is thought to affect at least 10 percent of people assigned female at birth (Christ et al., 2021). This condition, which can be very burdensome, is present in more than 80 percent of those with chronic pelvic pain, 50 percent with infertility, and 50 percent of adolescents with dysmenorrhea (Beloshevski et al., 2024; Capezzuoli et al., 2022; Shim et al., 2024). Because many endometriosis studies are based on diagnoses confirmed by surgery, current understanding of incidence rates may underrepresent individuals from groups with less healthcare utilization.

Risk factors for endometriosis include genetic factors (sevenfold risk increase in people with symptomatic first-degree relatives), early menarche, short menstrual cycles, and active ovarian function (symptoms are uncommon in premenarche and after menopause) (Rahmioglu et al., 2023). Endometriosis is more common in white individuals than people of other races and ethnicities. In addition, a diagnosis of endometriosis is more likely associated with other pain syndromes (e.g., interstitial cystitis, fibromyalgia) and other autoimmune and atopic conditions (e.g., thyroid dysfunction, asthma), suggesting that this condition may involve both underlying alterations in immune surveillance and central sensitization (Beloshevski et al., 2024; Shim et al., 2024).

Etiology

An understanding of endometriosis etiology continues to evolve. Multiple mechanisms—hereditary, environmental, epigenetic, immunologic, mechanical, and hormonal—have been proposed to account for the ectopic distribution and activation of endometrial cells. These mechanisms (summarized in **Box 27-4**) may be responsible for the varied phenotypes of endometriosis, including asymptomatic lesions noted incidentally in unrelated surgeries; painful, deep endometriosis; and endometriomas (ovarian cysts containing endometrial tissue) (Nezhat et al., 2024). Studies suggest that microbleeding from endometriotic lesions may trigger a cascade of genetic and epigenetic insults that further increase inflammation and oxidative stress (Hirata et al., 2020; Signorile et al., 2022).

Molecular studies have provided additional insights. Individuals with endometriosis have been shown to have biochemically atypical endometrial cells, whether they are intrauterine or ectopic. Ectopic endometrial implants appear to function independently from the ovaries, producing their own endogenous estrogen de novo from cholesterol conversion, but lack progesterone receptors to balance this estrogen activity (Signorile et al., 2022). This progesterone resistance may play a more important role in disease progression and related infertility than estrogen dependence does (Cassani et al., 2024).

Clinical Presentation

Endometriosis can result in a wide range of often unpredictable symptoms, which may not correlate with the extent of visible implants and may obscure and delay diagnosis. On the one hand, endometrial implants may be seen incidentally during surgery

BOX 27-4 Proposed Mechanisms for the Development of Endometriosis

- Implantation of otherwise normal retrograde menstruation (observed as early as neonatally), which becomes activated in individuals with genetic or environmentally mediated susceptibility
- Spontaneous metaplasia of coelomic epithelium (the lining cells of body cavities) or mesenchymal stem cells
- Atypical differentiation of epithelial cells; triggers may include endogenous or exogenous biochemical or immunologic factors
- Mechanical spread, as during surgery (e.g., adenomyosis or the implants identified in abdominal surgical or episiotomy scars)
- Distant seeding of endometrial or stem cells via the lymphatic or circulatory system
- Dysregulation of organogenesis (especially of the uterine wall) in embryonic females (hereditary or environmentally mediated endocrine disruptors)
- Disruption of the junctional zone between the endometrium and myometrium

Chapron, C., Vannuccini, S., Santulli, P., Abrão, M. S., Carmona, F., Fraser, I. S., Gordts, S., Guo, S. W., Just, P. A., Noël, J. C., Pistofidis, G., Van den Bosch, T., & Petraglia, F. (2020). Diagnosing adenomyosis: an integrated clinical and imaging approach. *Human reproduction update, 26*(3), 392–411; Hirata, T., Koga, K., & Osuga, Y. (2020). Extra-pelvic endometriosis: A review. *Reproductive medicine and biology, 19*(4), 323–333; Signorile, P. G., Viceconte, R., & Baldi, A. (2022). New insights in pathogenesis of endometriosis. *Frontiers in medicine, 9*, 879015.

performed on asymptomatic patients. On the other hand, patients may present with severe to debilitating dysmenorrhea, dyspareunia, dyschezia, dysuria; or chronic or intermittent dull, throbbing, or sharp pelvic, abdominal or back pain; and they can experience associated infertility (Capezzuoli et al., 2022). Endometriomas may result in acute pain episodes (refer to the section on ovarian masses later in this chapter). Because of the diverse locations in which endometrial implants have been identified, extrapelvic endometriosis should be included in the differential diagnosis whenever patients report cyclic symptoms in any organ (Allaire et al., 2023).

Assessment

A detailed history should be obtained from any patient reporting chronic pelvic pain. The location and character of any dyspareunia should be assessed, along with menstrual cycle patterns, associated symptoms (e.g., dysmenorrhea, nausea and vomiting, diarrhea), fertility history, and family history of endometriosis. Discovery of the effects of this condition on quality of life and response to treatments may help with the differential diagnosis and facilitate a better understanding of the patient's attitude toward their symptoms. The clinician can also advise the patient to keep a diary of their symptoms, which may be of assistance in future care. Refer to Chapter 29 for more information about chronic pelvic pain.

Findings on physical examination may be limited or absent, but abdominal and pelvic examination, including a rectal examination, are indicated. When pelvic pain is present, it may be less traumatic to begin with a gentle single-digit vaginal examination to map the foci of pain, rather than with a speculum examination. Patients with endometriosis may exhibit condition-specific signs, such as pain or nodules at palpation of the posterior fornix or rectovaginal septum, tenderness or induration of the uterosacral ligaments, a tender non mobile uterus, and a tender enlarged adnexal mass (consistent with endometrioma). Palpation of the vaginal side walls and ancillary pelvic floor muscles may aid in differentiation of endometriosis from pelvic floor myalgias. Occasionally, endometrial implants are seen on the cervix or vaginal walls during speculum examination, appearing as nonblanching red or brownish/blackish areas or firm nodules. Asymptomatic lesions do not require treatment, although biopsy for histology is appropriate if the diagnosis is unclear.

There are no specific laboratory tests for endometriosis (Signorile et al., 2022). Biomarkers have been proposed, but reliable ones have not yet been identified. Patients with heavy or irregular bleeding may warrant endometrial biopsy and testing for anemia.

Transvaginal ultrasound is a relatively low-cost technology that can play a role in ruling out other diagnoses and that may identify endometriomas, adenomyosis, and, occasionally, deeply infiltrating endometriosis in the bladder, uterosacral ligaments, rectum, or rectovaginal septum. Transrectal ultrasound may identify bowel involvement and aid in surgical planning (Habib et al., 2020). MRI appears to add little to high-resolution ultrasound findings (Capezzuoli et al., 2022; Signorile et al., 2022).

Endometriosis can be diagnosed definitively only by histology and therefore requires surgical biopsy for confirmation. Diagnostic laparoscopy for staging is no longer recommended, however, because the extent of visible disease does not correlate well with symptoms or prognosis for future fertility (Capezzuoli et al., 2022).

Differential Diagnoses

Other gynecologic and nongynecologic causes of chronic pelvic pain include bladder pain syndromes, irritable bowel syndrome, pelvic floor muscle myalgias, and other gynecologic anatomic abnormalities (e.g., uterine fibroids, ovarian cysts, hydrosalpinx). Refer to Chapter 29 for a detailed discussion of pelvic pain.

Management

Individuals experiencing symptoms of endometriosis variants generally can choose among expectant management, medical therapies, and surgery. Goals of medical management include both symptom management and maintenance of desired fertility. Considerations relating to fertility are discussed in the next section, "Considerations for Specific Populations." Ovulation suppression is a primary target of medical therapy, with the goal to eliminate or reduce ectopic endometrial activity. Management of endometriosis can include GnRH agonists, danazol, progestins, and aromatase inhibitors (Allaire et al., 2023; Shim et al., 2024). Regardless, there continues to be significant variation in diagnosis and management across practice guidelines (Davenport et al., 2023). **Table 27-7** identifies several agents that have been shown to decrease patients' reported pain in randomized controlled trials, including combined estrogen and progestin contraceptives; progestins; GnRH agonists (e.g., goserelin, leuprorelin); and the synthetic androgenic hormone ethisterone (danazol) (Christ et al., 2021; Nezhat et al., 2024). There is insufficient evidence to compare the pain relief effectiveness of specific agents or specific regimens, either as initial treatment or for postsurgical maintenance. There is also insufficient evidence to support the use of acupuncture and other alternative or herbal treatments (ACOG, 2020; Christ et al., 2021). There is insufficient evidence to affirm that any medical treatments will improve the chances of successful pregnancy outcomes (ACOG, 2020; Capezzuoli et al., 2022; Christ et al., 2021). In addition, pain symptoms that do improve with such treatments may recur when medical therapy is discontinued. Additional medications directed at pain control, including neurotransmitter modulators and opioids, are used for chronic pelvic pain associated with endometriosis. They may improve a patient's quality of life if used judiciously but play no role in controlling the disease or preserving fertility.

Although surgery is required for definitive diagnosis of endometriosis, this modality is now reserved to treat people with debilitating symptoms and poor response or intolerance to medical therapy. Surgical options include laparoscopic conservative management (e.g., removal of endometrial implants, focal areas of adenomyosis, endometriomas, and distorting adhesions) and definitive surgery (e.g., complete hysterectomy with bilateral salpingo-oophorectomy).

Laparoscopic removal of implants and adhesions is effective for pain management and resolution of symptomatic endometriomas, although removal may decrease ovarian reserve (Christ et al., 2021). Excision is recommended over ablation to allow for histologic diagnosis. In addition, moderate-quality evidence supports a role for laparoscopic interventional surgery in increasing pregnancy and live birth rates for those with endometriosis and infertility. Following conservative surgery, endometriomas have a recurrence rate of approximately 30–50 percent. Therefore, for patients not seeking immediate pregnancy, medical suppression should be considered (Nezhat et al., 2024). Repeat procedures increase risks of postoperative adhesions and damage to ovarian reserve. Endometriomas larger than 4 cm are typically removed,

TABLE 27-7 Medical Treatments for Endometriosis

Category	Agents	Regimens	Adverse Effects	Considerations
Combined oral contraceptives	Pill, vaginal ring, transdermal patch	Cyclic or continuous (continuous may be more effective for pain management); no data to define optimal oral dosage	Minimal, compared to other agents (mood swings, low increased clot risk)	Long-term safety is well documented Inexpensive Limited data on pain management but appear comparable to other methods No data to support fertility preservation
Progestins	Oral (norethindrone, megestrol, or medroxyprogesterone acetate) Intramuscular injection (DMPA) Implant (etonogestrel rod) LNG-IUS	Continuous (implant or LNG-IUS), long-acting agents (injection every 3 months), or short-acting agents (daily oral) Medroxyprogesterone acetate and norethindrone acetate are FDA approved for endometriosis treatment	Irregular menstrual bleeding, breast tenderness, fluid retention, weight gain, and depression or mood instability	Pain reduction of typically 70–100% Decreased bone mineral density with long-term DMPA use LNG-IUS may be optimal for adenomyosis or postsurgical suppression due to low adverse effects
GnRHa	Depot injectable with quicker onset (leuprolide, goserelin) Nasal spray (nafarelin) Norethindrone acetate is FDA approved only as add-back therapy	Combine with add-back estrogen and/or progestogen, tibolone, bisphosphonates, or selective estrogen receptor modulators to limit bone loss and hot flashes	Hypoestrogenic symptoms (bone loss, vaginal atrophy, vasomotor symptoms)	Pain reduction as high as 100%, with 50% recurrence after discontinuation Decreases size of endometriomas Significantly more expensive than other treatments, with no evidence of superior outcomes Backup nonhormonal contraception is recommended Approval of an oral agent is pending; may decrease bone loss
Synthetic androgenic hormones	Ethisterone (danazol)	Oral daily	Hyperandrogenic and hypoestrogenic: Weight gain, muscle cramps, decreased breast size, acne, hirsutism, hot flashes, mood changes, depression, permanently lower voice	Pain relief similar to GnRHa but less well tolerated Concomitant use of effective contraception is imperative due to risks of virilization of female fetus
Aromatase inhibitors	Letrozole	Oral daily	Decreased bone density Vasomotor symptoms Pain Depression Cardiovascular effects	Pain control is similar to COC Must be combined with COC, progestin, or GnRHa to prevent ovarian hyperstimulation

Data from Allaire, C., Bedaiwy, M. A., & Yong, P. J. (2023). Diagnosis and management of endometriosis. *CMAJ: Canadian Medical Association journal = journal de l'Association medicale canadienne, 195*(10), E363–E371. https://doi.org/10.1503/cmaj.220637; Amro, B., Ramirez Aristondo, M. E., Alsuwaidi, S., Almaamari, B., Hakim, Z., Tahlak, M., Wattiez, A., & Koninckx, P. R. (2022). New Understanding of Diagnosis, Treatment and Prevention of Endometriosis. *International journal of environmental research and public health, 19*(11), 6725. https://doi.org/10.3390/ijerph19116725; Christ, J. P., Yu, O., Schulze-Rath, R., Grafton, J., Hansen, K., & Reed, S. D. (2021). Incidence, prevalence, and trends in endometriosis diagnosis: a United States population-based study from 2006 to 2015. *American journal of obstetrics and gynecology, 225*(5), 500.e1–500.e9. https://doi.org/10.1016/j.ajog.2021.06.067; Nezhat, F. R., Cathcart, A. M., Nezhat, C. H., & Nezhat, C. R. (2024). Pathophysiology and Clinical Implications of Ovarian Endometriomas. *Obstetrics and gynecology, 143*(6), 759–766. https://doi.org/10.1097/AOG.0000000000005587

Abbreviations: COC, combined oral contraceptive; DMPA, depot medroxyprogesterone acetate; FDA, U.S. Food and Drug Administration; GnRHa, gonadotropin-releasing hormone agonists; LNG-IUS, levonorgestrel intrauterine system.

even if asymptomatic, because they have been associated with ovarian cancers (Nezhat et al., 2024).

Individuals who have severe pain but wish to preserve their fertility and have not responded to other treatments may consider a presacral neurectomy (excision of the portion of the superior hypogastric plexus that provides sympathetic innervation to the uterus) (ACOG, 2020). This complex procedure is done infrequently but provides better long-term pain control, compared to laparoscopic procedures alone.

The definitive surgery for endometriosis is hysterectomy with salpingo-oophorectomy. Individuals may be most likely to choose hysterectomy if they do not desire a future pregnancy and have resistant symptoms that are severely impacting their quality of life. They should know that pain persists after definitive surgery in as many as 15 percent of people and may increase again over time in as many as 5 percent more (ACOG, 2020). Those who elect ovarian preservation benefit from bone preservation and positive cardiovascular effects but face a sixfold increase in the risk of persistent or recurrent symptoms (Nezhat et al., 2024). In contrast, the use of add-back estrogen after oophorectomy appears to have minimal effects on the risk of persistent or recurrent symptoms.

Endometrial ablation for superficial disease, UAE, and excision of localized disease may also be effective in selected situations. Aromatase inhibitors (AIs) may be able to suppress the endogenous estrogen production of ectopic endometrial implants (Amro et al., 2022; Kolanska et al., 2020; Signorile et al., 2022). Unfortunately, evidence of their effectiveness remains limited, the cost/benefit ratio is unclear, and the adverse effects of AIs can be severe, including loss of bone density, joint and muscle pain, hot flashes, mood swings, depression, cardiovascular disease, and genital atrophy. Consequently, AIs are typically reserved for severely affected patients and are used in combination with other medical therapies (Amro et al., 2022). In premenopausal women, AIs may induce ovulation and should be used with ovarian suppression (Kolanska et al., 2020).

Other potential agents under investigation for endometriosis management include statins, given that blocking cholesterol biosynthesis may inhibit bioconversion activity in implants (Qin et al., 2024); immunomodulators to modify immune surveillance for ectopic cells (Kolanska et al., 2020); angiogenesis inhibitors to limit implant proliferation (Chung & Han, 2022); synthetic steroids, which are used in other countries to treat endometriosis but are currently banned in the United States due to their risk of abuse as performance-enhancing drugs (de Souza Pinto et al., 2023); and valproic acid, which appears to reverse silencing of apoptotic genes that affect endometriosis (Psilopatis et al., 2023). Nonpharmaceutical agents under investigation include the antioxidant hormone melatonin (Li et al., 2022); certain isoflavones (e.g., pycnogenols), which may compete for and block estrogen receptors (Julio et al., 2024); and herbal agents with anticytokine and antioxidant properties (Julio et al., 2024). Further clinical trials are necessary to evaluate the therapeutic doses and effects of nonpharmaceutical agents on persons with endometriosis (Julio et al., 2024; Li et al., 2022).

Considerations for Specific Populations

Adolescents Endometriosis should be considered in the differential diagnosis of premenarcheal girls with chronic pelvic pain because cases of biopsy-confirmed symptomatic implants have been reported (Beloshevski et al., 2024; Capezzuoli et al., 2022; Shim et al., 2024; Signorile et al., 2022). Also, endometriosis is more common in girls with imperforate hymen or other obstructive Müllerian anomalies. First-line therapy for endometriosis in adolescents is menstrual suppression with a progestin-only or combined contraceptive. When effective, this should be continued until the patient desires pregnancy. NSAIDs should be the primary agent prescribed for pain relief in an adolescent with endometriosis. When symptoms persist despite medical management, surgical diagnosis should be considered. Endometriotic lesions may present differently in adolescents than in adults. Because of this difference in presentation, surgical diagnosis (when necessary) should be carried out by a gynecologic surgeon who is familiar with the appearance of endometrial implants in adolescents (Beloshevski et al., 2024; Capezzuoli et al., 2022).

When combined oral contraceptives (COCs) are recommended to young adolescents as the first-line treatment, some families may object, assuming this use may be a license to sexual activity. However, an open discussion with the adolescent and their family to review concerns, treatment safety profiles, and the expected potential benefits of endometriosis treatment (e.g., improved quality of life, prevention of central sensitization by good pain management, but no clear role in preventing infertility) may facilitate achievement of an optimal plan. Diagrams to demonstrate anatomy and physiology, along with handouts that can be reviewed at home, may be particularly helpful when caring for adolescents (Beloshevski et al., 2024; Capezzuoli et al., 2022; Shim et al., 2024).

Individuals With Infertility Despite the clear association between endometriosis and infertility, the mechanisms of this relationship remain unclear. Distortion of anatomy, inflammation, abnormal tubal transit, progesterone resistance, and implantation defects may all be involved (Kolanska et al., 2020). There is not universal agreement on the indications for surgical evaluation and therapy during infertility treatment. Age, duration of infertility, family history, pelvic pain, and stage of endometriosis should be taken into account when developing the management plan. For people with infertility and endometriosis, treatment may include expectant management after laparoscopy, superovulation (with gonadotropins) and intrauterine insemination, or in vitro fertilization. The use of GnRH agonists to suppress endometriotic activity for 3 to 6 months prior to in vitro fertilization may improve outcomes. Refer to Chapter 20 for more information about infertility.

Pregnant Individuals Although the etiology is unclear, individuals with endometriosis have increased risks when they do achieve pregnancy, including late miscarriage, preterm birth, fetal growth restriction, and antepartum hemorrhage (Kolanska et al., 2020). These outcomes may be related to progesterone resistance and/or the increased risk of subclinical atherosclerosis, a condition that is also associated with endometriosis.

Postmenopause Although symptoms of endometriosis typically resolve after menopause, some individuals may continue to experience issues. The persistence of symptoms may be due to estrogen produced by adipose tissue or the endometriotic lesions themselves (Amro et al., 2022). Individuals with endometriosis-associated infertility may have early-onset menopause. As many as 4 percent report ongoing symptoms after menopause, even in the absence of hormone therapy. Additionally, the use of hormone therapy or tamoxifen has been linked to recurrence of symptoms postmenopause. For symptomatic individuals with a history of endometriosis who request hormone therapy, use of combined estrogen and progestin or aromatase inhibitors have been suggested, but there is insufficient evidence to make a specific recommendation (Capezzuoli et al., 2022; Cassani et al., 2024; Christ et al., 2021). There is a small (less than 1%) but increased risk of endometriotic lesions becoming malignant after menopause, particularly on the ovaries. Therefore, obtaining tissue for histology is warranted for patients with persistent symptomatic endometriosis after menopause, particularly if there is vaginal bleeding or a mass (Cassani et al., 2024; Vitale et al., 2021).

Adenomyosis

Adenomyosis includes the presence of diffuse or localized (focal) endometrial cells within the myometrium. Focal adenomyosis is defined as a single nodule of endometrial tissue, while diffuse adenomyosis occurs when glands and stroma of endometrial tissue are found throughout the endometrium. Cystic adenomyosis is the term used to describe fluid-filled adenomyotic lesions. The presence of cystic lesions in adolescents and young adults up to age 30 is called juvenile cystic adenomyosis (Isaacson & Loring, 2020; Protopapas et al., 2020). It remains unclear whether adenomyosis is a variant of endometriosis or a unique condition. The two conditions are frequently associated, and adenomyosis is also commonly linked with the presence of endometrial polyps and uterine fibroids (Chapron et al., 2020; Isaacson & Loring, 2020; Moldassarina, 2023).

Incidence

Prevalence estimates range from 1 to 70 percent due to variability in definition and diagnostic criteria (Isaacson & Loring, 2020; Schrager et al., 2022). Up to 30 percent of people with adenomyosis are asymptomatic (Kho et al., 2021). Adenomyosis is most commonly diagnosed in the fourth and fifth decades of life, although this may be due to the increased frequency of hysterectomy at that time and subsequent histological examination of uterine tissue (Isaacson & Loring, 2020).

Proposed risk factors for adenomyosis include multiparity and history of uterine surgery, including dilation and curettage and cesarean birth. It is theorized that adenomyosis is due to disruption of myometrial integrity (Isaacson & Loring, 2020). Additionally, extended exposure to endogenous or exogenous estrogen is considered a risk factor due to the correlation of adenomyosis with early menarche, short menstrual cycles, COC use, and the observed phenomenon of disease regression after menopause (Isaacson & Loring, 2020).

Etiology and Pathophysiology

The etiology of adenomyosis is unknown. Some studies suggest a connection with high parity or uterine surgery that breaches the endometrial–myometrial junction, but other studies do not support this theory. Further, data collection is limited because definitive diagnosis of adenomyosis is made only by histologic examination following removal of myometrial tissue (Chapron et al., 2020; Donnez et al., 2024a; Stratopoulou et al., 2021). Other theories include a mechanism of tissue injury and repair in which endometrial tissue enters the myometrium and the possibility that the endometrial tissue grows in the myometrium during embryological development (Donnez et al., 2024a; Stratopoulou et al., 2021).

Clinical Presentation

The most common clinical presentation is patient report of dysmenorrhea, particularly dysmenorrhea that is severe and medication resistant, and abnormal uterine bleeding (Chapron et al., 2020; Isaacson & Loring, 2020). However, these symptoms are nonspecific for adenomyosis. Additional common symptoms include pelvic pain, dyspareunia, heavy cyclic menstrual bleeding, and infertility or subfertility (Chapron et al., 2020; Donnez et al., 20204a; Isaacson & Loring, 2020; Stratopoulou et al., 2021). One study also found adenomyosis to be associated with subjective reports of feeling swollen (Kho et al., 2021).

It is posited that adenomyosis contributes to abnormal uterine bleeding due to increased uterine mass, increased hormone production, and less effective uterine contractions (Kho et al., 2021). Although it is not clear that adenomyosis causes infertility, the two are frequently associated. As many as 25 percent of individuals undergoing fertility treatment are found to have adenomyosis (Moldassarina, 2023). It is theorized that adenomyosis contributes to infertility by impairing sperm transport, implantation, and placentation (Isaacson & Loring, 2020; Schrager et al., 2022).

Assessment

As with any pelvic pain condition, a detailed history, including menstrual history and associated symptoms, should be obtained. Refer to Chapter 29 for more about chronic pelvic pain. Physical examination signs may be absent or may include a diffusely enlarged uterus and or uterine tenderness (Isaacson & Loring, 2020). Additionally, clinicians should suspect adenomyosis when fibroids have been diagnosed but symptom severity is disproportionate to fibroid presence and also when dysmenorrhea is particularly severe or treatment resistant (Chapron et al., 2020; Kho et al., 2021). There is no laboratory test for adenomyosis. Although adenomyosis can be definitively diagnosed only by removal of myometrial tissue, junctional zone changes that are characteristic of adenomyosis can be seen with ultrasound or MRI (Schrager et al., 2022).

Differential Diagnoses

Because adenomyosis often presents along with endometriosis, endometrial polyps, uterine fibroids, and other uterine problems, it can be difficult to attribute symptom causality to any particular diagnosis (Donnez et al., 2024b). Further, disease severity as noted by ultrasound, MRI, or surgery and histology often does not correlate with symptom severity or future fertility (ACOG, 2010, reaffirmed 2018). Clinicians should also consider other gynecologic and nongynecologic causes of pelvic pain and abnormal uterine bleeding. Refer to Chapter 29 for a detailed discussion of pelvic pain.

Management

As with any condition, management is largely dependent on patient symptoms and goals. For patients who wish to preserve their uterus, the best-studied treatment for symptom management is the LNG-IUS, which can reduce pain and blood loss and, when used for 1 to 2 years, can result in a reduction in uterine size (Chapron et al., 2020; Schrager et al., 2022). Conversely, for those desiring a curative procedure who do not want to preserve their uterus, hysterectomy with or without ovarian preservation may be appropriate (Chapron et al., 2020). Individuals wishing to maintain fertility should be aware that uterine-conserving surgery may lead to adverse pregnancy outcomes, including risk of uterine rupture, and should be approached on a case-by-case basis (Donnez et al., 2024a; Gunther et al., 2022; Stratopoulou et al., 2021).

The use of GnRH analogs is often associated with reduced uterine volume, pain, and bleeding. However, there are no clear guidelines on the amount or duration of add-back therapy with this treatment (Schrager et al., 2022). Progestins have been shown to reduce pain and bleeding; combination contraceptives have been shown to reduce pain and bleeding and, if used continuously, can result in amenorrhea, but it appears these simply treat the symptoms rather than the adenomyosis itself. Further, NSAIDs demonstrate efficacy in reducing bleeding and pain, but there is no evidence that they help resolve the underlying condition (Moldassarina, 2023). There is no clear evidence to support the use of herbal medications, supplements, or other complementary therapies in the management of adenomyosis. However, patients may elect to manage symptoms with complementary modalities, such as acupuncture, that have been shown to address pain and discomfort in general.

Considerations for Specific Populations

Adolescents Cystic adenomyosis is more common in adolescents and individuals younger than age 30. Menstrual suppression with COCs and monitoring with ultrasound may be effective in differentiating these lesions from other types of cysts (Protopapas et al., 2020).

Individuals With Infertility For those wishing to preserve fertility and seeking fertility treatment, use of a GnRH analog prior to in vitro fertilization may be beneficial (Moldassarina, 2023).

CONDITIONS OF THE ADNEXA

Adnexal Masses

Although benign adnexal masses can arise in the fallopian tubes (e.g., hydrosalpinx, related to tubal occlusion from surgery or infection), the majority are ovarian. Ovarian masses can occur in any of the differentiated tissues of the ovary. Most adnexal masses are benign, but clinicians must remain vigilant to identify life-threatening conditions, such as malignancy and ectopic pregnancy. Refer to Chapters 28 and 33 for more information about malignancy and ectopic pregnancy. Even benign ovarian tumors can cause significant distress, including physical symptoms (e.g., pain, dyspareunia) and anxiety. Providing clear education on the causes, potential outcomes with and without treatment, impact on fertility, risk of recurrence, and its benign nature can help ease concerns and support follow-up care.

Incidence

The incidence of ovarian masses is unknown because it is likely that many are asymptomatic. They frequently appear as incidental findings on pelvic imaging. One in five individuals assigned female at birth develops at least one pelvic mass in their lifetime (Mobeen & Apostol, 2023). As expected, cystic masses were approximately twice as common in individuals who were actively menstruating, and most abnormal findings resolved spontaneously (Mobeen & Apostol, 2023).

Etiology and Pathophysiology

Common benign ovarian masses include functional (physiologic) ovarian cysts, mature cystic teratomas, serous or mucinous cystadenomas, and endometriomas (Mobeen & Apostol, 2023; Wolfman et al., 2020). Functional ovarian cysts are typically asymptomatic and resolve without intervention. Occasionally, they may rupture and produce the transient, acute pain of peritoneal irritation. In addition, an ovary enlarged by any type of cyst is more susceptible to torsion, with ovarian masses greater than or equal to 5 cm in diameter carrying an increased risk for surgical emergency (Wolfman et al., 2020).

Functional cysts include follicular, corpus luteal, and hemorrhagic cysts. Follicular cysts develop early in the menstrual cycle from unruptured follicles, are common, and are often asymptomatic. The pain that accompanies spontaneous follicular cyst rupture with ovulation is termed "mittelschmerz." If ovulation does not occur, the follicular cyst may continue to enlarge, with the already noted risks of symptomatic rupture or torsion (Limaiem & Mlika, 2023).

A corpus luteal cyst develops within the corpus luteum that forms in the ovary normally after ovulation. These cysts may persist into pregnancy and are also typically not symptomatic. Again, rupture-related pain is likely to be self-limiting, but severe pain may signal torsion (Limaiem & Mlika, 2023).

A hemorrhagic cyst can occur when a small vessel within any cyst lining erodes. The bleeding may be contained within the cyst or extrude into the peritoneal cavity and cause transient pain if rupture occurs. Although symptoms are typically self-limiting, heavy or continued bleeding may require emergent surgery.

Mature cystic teratomas, also called dermoid cysts, arise from the ovarian germ cell and are the most common ovarian tumors. They are filled with sebaceous material and often contain hair, bone, teeth, or other tissues from the germ layers. They can grow to be many centimeters in diameter, and ovarian torsion may occur.

Serous or mucinous cystadenomas arise from glandular tissue within the ovarian epithelium. They often persist but can be managed expectantly if they are small and have no concerning features. Mucinous cystadenomas can become very large, again increasing the risk of torsion.

Endometriomas, also known as chocolate cysts, are a form of endometriosis (refer to the previous section).

Clinical Presentation

The presentation of ovarian masses varies. They may be asymptomatic and identified as an incidental finding on imaging. When identified, the mass can range in size from less than a centimeter to basketball size and several pounds. Any size of ovarian mass may produce symptoms that typically include pressure, unilateral or bilateral pelvic pain, dyspareunia, irregular vaginal bleeding, and changes in bladder or bowel habits. Individuals may report diverse quality of discomfort, including dull, cramping pressure; sharp and intermittent stabbing; cyclic, bilateral, or abrupt and persistent pain; or any combination of these forms. Pain with abrupt onset often represents spilling of cystic fluid (serous and/or sanguineous) into the peritoneal cavity. Abrupt onset of severe pain may represent ovarian torsion, which occurs more commonly if the ovary is enlarged by a mass. When masses become large, abdominal girth can increase from the tumor and may be mistaken for pregnancy.

Assessment

Individuals with pelvic pain symptoms that suggest adnexal mass should be asked sufficient history questions to allow the clinician to quickly rule out the most morbid or life-threatening conditions, including ectopic pregnancy, appendicitis, ovarian torsion or infection, and malignancy. Key topics from the general health and gynecologic history include the specific characteristics of the symptoms the individual is experiencing; menstrual, sexual, and contraceptive history; any changes in vaginal bleeding or discharge; a pain scale; and a family history of risk factors, such as malignancy or endometriosis.

Taking the patient's vital signs will aid in ruling out infection, fever, and severe pain or shock. Systemic or atypical lymphadenopathy may suggest malignancy or infection. Unexplained weight gain or a disproportionate change in abdominal girth without weight gain may indicate large tumor growth.

Inspect, auscultate, and palpate the abdomen. Large masses may cause visible changes in the abdomen or may be palpable abdominally or on bimanual vaginal and rectal examination. Guarding or rebound tenderness can indicate peritoneal irritation.

Perform a complete pelvic examination, documenting the location, size, shape, texture, mobility, and tenderness of any palpable mass. Although pelvic and/or rectal examination are indicated, be aware that their sensitivity is limited, especially in individuals with higher body mass index (Ghosh & Rufford, 2023).

Pregnancy testing is essential in persons of reproductive age. Gonorrhea and chlamydia testing and complete blood count are warranted if a tubo-ovarian abscess is suspected. Although imaging is the first-line assessment for adnexal pathology, blood testing plays a role in multivariate index assays that have been developed in an attempt to predict malignant potential reliably and limit unnecessary intervention (Ghosh & Rufford, 2023). Tests appropriately ordered in primary care while specialist consultation is pending include cancer antigen 125 (CA-125), alpha fetoprotein, lactate dehydrogenase, and human chorionic gonadotropin (Lahoud et al., 2021). The CA-125 test is not reliable as a stand-alone modality for distinguishing benign and malignant masses, especially in premenopausal women, because the level of this protein is also elevated by endometriosis, fibroids, pelvic inflammatory disease, and other benign findings. In addition, no biomarkers have been demonstrated to be accurate for screening purposes because they can lead to unacceptably high rates of unnecessary intervention, without significant reduction in mortality.

Transvaginal ultrasound remains the first-line imaging modality for evaluation of ovarian masses (Ghosh & Rufford, 2023). Ultrasound will classify a mass as cystic, solid, or complex. Three-dimensional ultrasound may improve acuity, and color. Doppler ultrasound as an adjunct can assess measurement of blood flow in and around a mass. MRI and CT imaging are typically reserved for specific indications, such as determination of the origin of an associated non-ovarian pelvic mass (MRI) or evaluation for potential metastases (CT) (Ghosh & Rufford, 2023).

Differential Diagnoses

Table 27-8 offers an overview of the differential diagnoses for adnexal masses and some typical characteristics that may aid in achieving accurate diagnosis.

Management

Asymptomatic simple ovarian cysts less than 5 cm in diameter, including functional cysts and benign neoplasms, have a low probability of malignancy and can be followed with serial imaging (Ghosh & Rufford, 2023). There is little evidence-based guidance for timing of repeat ultrasounds, but they are generally obtained at 4- or 6-month intervals to establish stability. Many functional cysts will resolve within 3 months. Cysts that do not resolve in two to three menstrual cycles should be investigated further (Ghosh & Rufford, 2023; Mobeen & Apostol, 2023). Individuals who are receiving serial follow-up should be educated to report any increase in pain or other symptoms (e.g., bowel or bladder status). Although there is no evidence that they promote resolution of an existing cyst, combined hormonal contraceptives can be used to control repeated episodes of symptomatic functional cysts (Luo & Zhao, 2023).

Patients can be informed that complex and solid ovarian masses have been shown to resolve spontaneously in as many as 80 percent of cases (Ghosh & Rufford, 2023). However, these masses carry a higher risk of malignancy, and individuals should be referred to a reproductive health specialist or gynecologic oncologist for further evaluation (Ghosh & Rufford, 2023).

Teratomas and endometriomas can be managed expectantly when they are asymptomatic. When they resolve spontaneously, there does not seem to be an effect on future fertility. However, when they are excised, ovarian reserve appears to be affected. Surgery is indicated when these masses are particularly large, bothersome to the individual, or demonstrate increasing size on serial ultrasound (Ghosh & Rufford, 2023).

Considerations for Specific Populations

Adolescents Transabdominal ultrasound is a reasonable initial imaging modality in adolescents, including those who have not had vaginal intercourse. When premenarchal children or adolescents have an adnexal mass, they should be referred to a specialist, such as a gynecologic oncologist, due to the higher risk of malignancy in this age group (Triarico et al., 2020). Adolescents often develop functional cysts, including follicular and luteal cysts, due to the higher prevalence of anovulatory cycles in this age group. These cysts typically resolve spontaneously. If they are recurrently symptomatic, the adolescent may benefit from medical prevention, typically with combined hormonal contraceptives. In adolescents who also have irregular menses, hirsutism, or severe acne, polycystic ovary syndrome should be considered. Refer to Chapter 26 for additional information. Management of adnexal masses in adolescents should consider fertility preservation.

Pregnant Individuals With increased use of ultrasonography in pregnancy, adnexal masses are identified more frequently. These masses occur in 2 to 20 per 1,000 pregnancies, at a rate 2 to 20 times higher than in the age-matched general population (Cathcart et al., 2023). However, the majority resolve spontaneously, with approximately 70 percent regressing without intervention and only 2 percent found to be malignant (Cathcart et al., 2023). Approximately 75 percent of incidentally detected adnexal masses are simple cysts measuring less than 5.0 cm, of which 68–72 percent of those measuring 2.5-5.0 cm or exhibiting complex features resolve within 6 weeks postpartum (Cathcart et al., 2023). For cysts greater than 5 cm or those that persist, surgical intervention is warranted to mitigate the risk of ovarian torsion and assess for malignancy. The most common adnexal masses requiring surgical management during pregnancy include dermoid cysts (32%), endometriomas (15%), functional cysts (12%), serous cystadenomas (11%), and mucinous

TABLE 27-8 **Differential Diagnoses for Adnexal Masses**

Diagnosis	Distinguishing Typical Characteristics	Diagnostic Aids
Appendicitis, diverticular abscess	Gradual onset; fever, vomiting, unilateral pain	Complete blood count
Benign ovarian cysts (functional, cystadenoma)	Dull cramping pressure; sharp sudden pain with activity or on rupture—typically transient	Transvaginal ultrasound
Bladder diverticulum	Palpable mass, urinary symptoms	Imaging
Ectopic pregnancy	Symptoms vary and may include pelvic pain, vaginal bleeding, or missed menses	Pregnancy testing Transvaginal ultrasound
Endometrioma, endometritis	Dyspareunia, cyclic menstrual pain, pelvic tenderness	Transvaginal ultrasound
Hydrosalpinx/fallopian tube tumor	Pain, watery discharge	Transvaginal ultrasound
Malignancy	Symptoms may be vague, such as bloating, pelvic or abdominal pain, difficulty eating, early satiety, change in urine/bowels, increased abdominal size; individuals who have an adnexal mass prior to puberty or after menopause are at higher risk	Transvaginal ultrasound Blood assay/tumor markers (CA-125)
Mittelschmerz	Midcycle pain; temporary, predictable, may alternate sides	Typically none, possible transvaginal ultrasound
Ovarian torsion	Sudden onset pain, severe, often unilateral; associated nausea or vomiting	Complete blood count Transvaginal ultrasound
Pelvic inflammatory disease, tubo-ovarian abscess	Gradual onset; fever, vomiting, purulent discharge	Complete blood count Chlamydia and gonorrhea testing
Ruptured cyst (follicular or corpus luteum)	Sudden onset, after activity or intercourse, may exhibit unilateral pain	Hematocrit Transvaginal ultrasound if needed
Teratoma	Dull, cramping, persistent, noncyclic	Transvaginal ultrasound
Uterine fibroid	Predominantly menstrual symptoms: Cyclic pain, dysmenorrhea; menorrhagia	Transvaginal ultrasound

Data from Cathcart, A. M., Nezhat, F. R., Emerson, J., Pejovic, T., Nezhat, C. H., & Nezhat, C. R. (2023). Adnexal masses during pregnancy: diagnosis, treatment, and prognosis. *American journal of obstetrics and gynecology, 228*(6), 601–612. https://doi.org/10.1016/j.ajog.2022.11.1291; Ghosh, B., & Rufford, B. (2023). A practical approach to managing post-menopausal women with ovarian cysts. *Obstetrics, Gynaecology & Reproductive Medicine, 33*(6), 153-159; Mobeen, S., & Apostol, R. (2023). Ovarian Cyst. In *StatPearls*. StatPearls Publishing. https://www.ncbi.nlm.nih.gov/books/NBK560541/; Wolfman, W., Thurston, J., Yeung, G., & Glanc, P. (2020). Guideline No. 404: Initial Investigation and Management of Benign Ovarian Masses. *Journal of Obstetrics and Gynaecology Canada, 42*(8), 1040–1050.e1. https://doi.org/10.1016/j.jogc.2020.01.014

cystadenomas (8%) (Cathcart et al., 2023). Given the low risk of malignancy and acute complications, expectant management is appropriate unless there is rapid or atypical growth (Cathcart et al., 2023). Laparoscopic surgery is considered a safe option for managing ovarian cysts during pregnancy (Cagino et al., 2021; Cathcart et al., 2023). However, the tumor marker, CA-125, is physiologically elevated in pregnancy and should not be used in the evaluation of adnexal masses during this period (Cathcart et al., 2023; Ghosh & Rufford, 2023).

Postmenopause Postmenopausal individuals are at increased risk for ovarian cancer. Those with a personal or familial history of breast cancer or BRCA1 or BRCA2 mutation should be followed with particular diligence (Ghosh & Rufford, 2023). Benign functional cysts are rare in this age group. Any adnexal mass in a postmenopausal person should be considered highly suspicious for malignancy and thoroughly evaluated to include transvaginal ultrasound and CA-125. In postmenopause, ovarian cysts may present as acute abdominal pain (Ghosh & Rufford, 2023).

CONCLUSION

In conclusion, patient education and awareness are essential components in the management of benign gynecologic conditions. Although these conditions are not malignant, their impact on daily functioning, emotional well-being, and intimate relationships can be profound. Clinicians play a critical role in helping patients understand the nature of their symptoms, the range of treatment options available, and the importance of ongoing care. Empowering individuals with accurate information fosters shared decision making, reduces stigma, and enhances trust in the patient-clinician relationship—ultimately improving health outcomes and quality of life for those affected by these common, yet often misunderstood, conditions.

References

Allaire, C., Bedaiwy, M. A., & Yong, P. J. (2023). Diagnosis and management of endometriosis. *CMAJ: Canadian Medical Association Journal = Journal de l'Association Medicale Canadienne, 195*(10), E363–E371. https://doi.org/10.1503/cmaj.220637

American College of Obstetricians and Gynecologists' Committee on Practice Bulletins—Gynecology (2020). Diagnosis and management of vulvar skin disorders: ACOG practice bulletin, no. 224. *Obstetrics and Gynecology, 136*(1), e1–e14. https://doi.org/10.1097/AOG.0000000000003944

American College of Obstetricians and Gynecologists. (2021). Uterine morcellation for presumed leiomyomas. *Obstetrics and Gynecology, 137*, 552–553. https://doi.org/10.1097/AOG.0000000000004292

Amro, B., Ramirez Aristondo, M. E., Alsuwaidi, S., Almaamari, B., Hakim, Z., Tahlak, M., Wattiez, A., & Koninckx, P. R. (2022). New understanding of diagnosis, treatment and prevention of endometriosis. *International Journal of Environmental Research and Public Health, 19*(11), 6725. https://doi.org/10.3390/ijerph19116725

Angioni, S., D'Alterio, M. N., & Daniilidis, A. (2021). Highlights on medical treatment of uterine fibroids. *Current Pharmaceutical Design, 27*(36), 3821–3832. https://doi.org/10.2174/1381612826666210101152820

Awonuga, A. O., Chatzicharalampous, C., Thakur, M., Rambhatla, A., Qadri, F., Awonuga, M., Saed, G., & Diamond, M. P. (2022). Genetic and epidemiological similarities, and differences between postoperative intraperitoneal adhesion development and other benign fibro-proliferative disorders. *Reproductive Sciences, 29*(11), 3055–3077. https://doi.org/10.1007/s43032-021-00726-9

Beloshevski, B., Shimshy-Kramer, M., Yekutiel, M., Levinsohn-Tavor, O., Eisenberg, N., & Smorgick, N. (2024). Delayed diagnosis and treatment of adolescents and young women with suspected endometriosis. *Journal of Gynecology Obstetrics and Human Reproduction, 53*(3), 102737. https://doi.org/10.1016/j.jogoh.2024.102737

British Society for the Study of Vulvar Disease. (2023). Guidance on taking a vulval 'punch' biopsy. https://bssvd.org/wp-content/uploads/2023/08/TAKING-A-PUNCH-BIOPSY-OF-THE-VULVA-updated-26.3.23.pdf.

Cagino, K., Li, X., Thomas, C., Delgado, D., Christos, P., & Acholonu Jr., U. (2021). Surgical management of adnexal masses in pregnancy: A systematic review and meta-analysis. *Journal of Minimally Invasive Gynecology, 28*(6), 1171–1182.e2. https://doi.org/10.1016/j.jmig.2021.01.020

Capezzuoli, T., Rossi, M., La Torre, F., Vannuccini, S., & Petraglia, F. (2022). Hormonal drugs for the treatment of endometriosis. *Current Opinion in Pharmacology, 67*, 102311. https://doi.org/10.1016/j.coph.2022.102311

Cassani, C., Tedeschi, S., Cucinella, L., Morteo, V., Camnasio, C. A., Tiranini, L., Martini, E., & Nappi, R. E. (2024). Menopause and endometriosis. *Maturitas, 190*, 108129. https://doi.org/10.1016/j.maturitas.2024.108129

Cathcart, A. M., Nezhat, F. R., Emerson, J., Pejovic, T., Nezhat, C. H., & Nezhat, C. R. (2023). Adnexal masses during pregnancy: diagnosis, treatment, and prognosis. *American Journal of Obstetrics and Gynecology, 228*(6), 601–612. https://doi.org/10.1016/j.ajog.2022.11.1291

Chapron, C., Vannuccini, S., Santulli, P., Abrão, M. S., Carmona, F., Fraser, I. S., Gordts, S., Guo, S. W., Just, P. A., Noël, J. C., Pistofidis, G., Van den Bosch, T., & Petraglia, F. (2020). Diagnosing adenomyosis: an integrated clinical and imaging approach. *Human reproduction update, 26*(3), 392–411. https://doi.org/10.1093/humupd/dmz049

Christ, J. P., Yu, O., Schulze-Rath, R., Grafton, J., Hansen, K., & Reed, S. D. (2021). Incidence, prevalence, and trends in endometriosis diagnosis: A United States population-based study from 2006 to 2015. *American Journal of Obstetrics and Gynecology, 225*(5), 500.e1–500.e9. https://doi.org/10.1016/j.ajog.2021.06.067

Chung, M. S., & Han, S. J. (2022). Endometriosis-associated angiogenesis and anti-angiogenic therapy for endometriosis. *Frontiers in Global Women's Health, 3*, 856316. https://doi.org/10.3389/fgwh.2022.856316

Coutinho, L. M., Assis, W. A., Spagnuolo-Souza, A., & Reis, F. M. (2022). Uterine fibroids and pregnancy: How do they affect each other? *Reproductive Sciences (Thousand Oaks, Calif.), 29*(8), 2145–2151. https://doi.org/10.1007/s43032-021-00656-6

Chronic Pelvic Pain: ACOG Practice Bulletin, Number 218. (2020). *Obstetrics and gynecology, 135*(3), e98–e109. https://doi.org/10.1097/AOG.0000000000003716

Davenport, S., Smith, D., & Green, D. J. (2023). Barriers to a timely diagnosis of endometriosis: A qualitative systematic review. *Obstetrics & Gynecology, 142*(3), 571–583. https://doi.org/10.1097/AOG.0000000000005255

de Souza Pinto, L. P., Ferrari, G., Dos Santos, I. K., de Mello Roesler, C. R., & de Mello Gindri, I. (2023). Evaluation of safety and effectiveness of gestrinone in the treatment of endometriosis: a systematic review and meta-analysis. *Archives of Gynecology and Obstetrics, 307*(1), 21–37. https://doi.org/10.1007/s00404-022-06846-0

Donnez, J., Stratopoulou, C. A., & Dolmans, M. M. (2024a). Endometriosis and adenomyosis: Similarities and differences. *Best Practice & Research. Clinical Obstetrics & Gynaecology, 92*, 102432. https://doi.org/10.1016/j.bpobgyn.2023.102432

Donnez, J., Taylor, H. S., Marcellin, L., & Dolmans, M. M. (2024b). Uterine fibroid-related infertility: Mechanisms and management. *Fertility and Sterility, 122*(1), 31–39. https://doi.org/10.1016/j.fertnstert.2024.02.049

Edwards, S. K., Lewis, F., Fernando, I., Haddon, L., & Grover, D. (2025). 2024 British Association for Sexual Health and HIV (BASHH) UK national guideline on the management of vulval conditions. *International Journal of STD & AIDS*, 9564624241311629. Advance online publication. https://doi.org/10.1177/09564624241311629

Fergus, K. B., Lee, A. W., Baradaran, N., Cohen, A. J., Stohr, B. A., Erickson, B. A., Mmonu, N. A., & Breyer, B. N. (2020). Pathophysiology, clinical manifestations, and treatment of lichen sclerosus: A systematic review. *Urology, 135*, 11–19. https://doi.org/10.1016/j.urology.2019.09.034

Gabros S., Nessel, T.A., & Zito, P.M. (2023). Topical corticosteroids. In *StatPearls*. StatPearls Publishing. https://www-ncbi-nlm-nih-gov.proxy.library.georgetown.edu/books/NBK532940/

Ghosh, B., & Rufford, B. (2023). A practical approach to managing post-menopausal women with ovarian cysts. *Obstetrics, Gynaecology & Reproductive Medicine, 33*(6), 153–159.

Giampaolino, P., Della Corte, L., Di Filippo, C., Mercorio, A., Vitale, S. G., & Bifulco, G. (2020). Office hysteroscopy in the management of women with postmenopausal bleeding. *Climacteric, 23*(4), 369–375. https://doi.org/10.1080/13697137.2020.1754389

Giuliani, E., As-Sanie, S., & Marsh, E. E. (2020). Epidemiology and management of uterine fibroids. *International Journal of Gynaecology and Obstetrics: The Official Organ of the International Federation of Gynaecology and Obstetrics, 149*(1), 3–9. https://doi.org/10.1002/ijgo.13102

Günther, V., Allahqoli, L., Gitas, G., Maass, N., Tesch, K., Ackermann, J., Rosam, P., Mettler, L., von Otte, S., & Alkatout, I. (2022). Impact of adenomyosis on infertile patients—Therapy options and reproductive outcomes. *Biomedicines, 10*(12), 3245. https://doi.org/10.3390/biomedicines10123245

Habib, N., Centini, G., Lazzeri, L., Amoruso, N., El Khoury, L., Zupi, E., & Afors, K. (2020). Bowel endometriosis: Current perspectives on diagnosis and treatment. *International Journal of Women's Health, 12*, 35–47. https://doi.org/10.2147/IJWH.S190326

Hirata, T., Koga, K., & Osuga, Y. (2020). Extra-pelvic endometriosis: A review. *Reproductive Medicine and Biology, 19*(4), 323–333. https://doi.org/10.1002/rmb2.12340

Huang, D., Magaoay, B., Rosen, M. P., & Cedars, M. I. (2023). Presence of fibroids on transvaginal ultrasonography in a community-based, diverse cohort of 996 reproductive-age female participants. *JAMA Network Open, 6*(5), e2312701–e2312701.

Hurtado, S., & Shetty, M. K. (2023). Post-menopausal bleeding: Role of imaging. *Seminars in Ultrasound, CT and MRI, 44*(6), 519–527. https://doi.org/10.1053/j.sult.2023.10.003

Isaacson, K., & Loring, M. (2020). Symptoms of adenomyosis and overlapping diseases. *Seminars in Reproductive Medicine, 38*(2-03), 144–150. https://doi.org/10.1055/s-0040-1721795

Julio, T., Fenerich, B. A., Halpern, G., Carrera-Bastos, P., Schor, E., & Kopelman, A. (2024). The effects of oral nutritional supplements on endometriosis-related pain: A narrative review of clinical studies. *Journal of Gynecology Obstetrics and Human Reproduction*, 102830.

Katon, J. G., Plowden, T. C., & Marsh, E. E. (2023). Racial disparities in uterine fibroids and endometriosis: A systematic review and application of social, structural, and political context. *Fertility and Sterility, 119*(3), 355–363. https://doi.org/10.1016/j.fertnstert.2023.01.022

Kho, K. A., Chen, J. S., & Halvorson, L. M. (2021). Diagnosis, evaluation, and treatment of adenomyosis. *Jama, 326*(2), 177–178. https://doi.org/10.1001/jama.2020.26436

Kolanska, K., Alijotas-Reig, J., Cohen, J., Cheloufi, M., Selleret, L., d'Argent, E., Kayem, G., Valverde, E. E., Fain, O., Bornes, M., Darai, E., & Mekinian, A. (2020). Endometriosis with infertility: A comprehensive review on the role of immune deregulation and immunomodulation therapy. *American Journal of Reproductive Immunology, 85*(3), e13384. https://doi.org/10.1111/aji.13384

Lahoud, R., O'Shea, A., El-Mouhayyar, C., Atre, I., Eurboonyanun, K., & Harisinghani, M. (2021). Tumour markers and their utility in imaging of abdominal and pelvic malignancies. *Clinical Radiology, 76*(2), 99–107. https://doi.org/10.1016/j.crad.2020.07.033

Lebduska, E., Beshear, D., & Spataro, B. M. (2023). Abnormal Uterine Bleeding. *The Medical clinics of North America, 107*(2), 235–246. https://doi.org/10.1016/j.mcna.2022.10.014Li, Y., Hung, S. W., Zhang, R., Man, G. C., Zhang, T., Chung, J. P., Fang, L., & Wang, C. C. (2022). Melatonin in endometriosis: Mechanistic understanding and clinical insight. *Nutrients, 14*(19), 4087. https://doi.org/10.3390/nu14194087

Limaiem, F., & Mlika, M. (2023). Ovarian cystadenoma. In *StatPearls*. StatPearls Publishing. https://www.ncbi.nlm.nih.gov/books/NBK536950/

Luo, L., & Zhao, G. (2023). Analysis of the effectiveness of evidence-based management care combined with psychological care in ovarian cyst debulking. *Archives of Clinical Psychiatry, 50*(2).

MacGregor, B., Munro, M. G., & Lumsden, M. A. (2023). Therapeutic options for the management of abnormal uterine bleeding. *International Journal of Gynaecology and Obstetrics: The Official Organ of the International Federation of Gynaecology and Obstetrics, 162*(Suppl 2), 43–57. https://doi.org/10.1002/ijgo.14947

Mansour, T., & Chowdhury, Y. S. (2023). Endometrial polyp. In *StatPearls*. StatPearls Publishing. https://www.ncbi.nlm.nih.gov/books/NBK557824/

Manyonda, I., Belli, A. M., Lumsden, M. A., Moss, J., McKinnon, W., Middleton, L. J., Cheed, V., Wu, O., Sirkeci, F., Daniels, J. P., McPherson, K., & FEMME Collaborative Group (2020). Uterine-artery embolization or myomectomy for uterine fibroids. *The New England Journal of Medicine, 383*(5), 440–451. https://doi.org/10.1056/NEJMoa1914735

Martinez, C., Olig, E., Pachalla, S., & Findley, A. (2024). Racial disparities in medical management of uterine fibroids prior to myomectomy or hysterectomy. *Journal of Racial and Ethnic Health Disparities*, 10.1007/s40615-024-02048-3. Advance online publication. https://doi.org/10.1007/s40615-024-02048-3

Mauskar, M. M., Marathe, K., Venkatesan, A., Schlosser, B. J., & Edwards, L. (2020). Vulvar diseases: conditions in adults and children. *Journal of the American Academy of Dermatology, 82*(6), 1287-1298.

Mautz, T. T., Krapf, J. M., & Goldstein, A. T. (2022). Topical corticosteroids in the treatment of vulvar lichen sclerosus: A review of pharmacokinetics and recommended dosing frequencies. *Sexual Medicine Reviews, 10*(1), 42–52. https://doi.org/10.1016/j.sxmr.2021.03.006

Michos, G., Dagklis, T., Papanikolaou, E., Tsakiridis, I., Oikonomou, K., Mamopoulos, A. M., Kalogiannidis, I. A., & Athanasiadis, A. (2023). Uterine leiomyomas and infertility: A comparison of national and international guidelines. *Cureus*. https://doi.org/10.7759/cureus.50992

Mobeen, S., & Apostol, R. (2023). Ovarian cyst. In *StatPearls*. StatPearls Publishing. https://www.ncbi.nlm.nih.gov/books/NBK560541/

Mohammed, G. F., Al-Dhubaibi, M. S., AbdElneam, A. I., Bahaj, S. S., & Al-Dhubaibi, A. M. (2025). Exploring female genital self-image: A psychological and sociocultural perspective. *Sexual Medicine Reviews*, qeaf006. Advance online publication. https://doi.org/10.1093/sxmrev/qeaf006

Moldassarina R. S. (2023). Modern view on the diagnostics and treatment of adenomyosis. *Archives of Gynecology and Obstetrics, 308*(1), 171–181. https://doi.org/10.1007/s00404-023-06982-1

Nezhat, F. R., Cathcart, A. M., Nezhat, C. H., & Nezhat, C. R. (2024). Pathophysiology and Clinical implications of ovarian endometriomas. *Obstetrics and Gynecology, 143*(6), 759–766. https://doi.org/10.1097/AOG.0000000000005587

Nijkang, N. P., Anderson, L., Markham, R., & Manconi, F. (2019). Endometrial polyps: Pathogenesis, sequelae and treatment. *SAGE Open Medicine, 7*, 2050312119848247. https://doi.org/10.1177/2050312119848247

Pegu, B., Srinivas, B. H., Saranya, T. S., Murugesan, R., Priyadarshini Thippeswamy, S., & Gaur, B. P. S. (2020). Cervical polyp: Evaluating the need of routine surgical intervention and its correlation with cervical smear cytology and endometrial pathology: A retrospective study. *Obstetrics & Gynecology Science, 63*(6), 735–742. https://doi.org/10.5468/ogs.20177

Perelmuter, S., Burns, R., Shearer, K., Grant, R., Soogoor, A., Jun, S., Meurer, J. A., Krapf, J., & Rubin, R. (2024). Genitourinary syndrome of lactation: A new perspective on postpartum and lactation-related genitourinary symptoms. *Sexual Medicine Reviews, 12*(3), 279–287. https://doi.org/10.1093/sxmrev/qeae034

Psilopatis, I., Vrettou, K., Fleckenstein, F. N., & Theocharis, S. (2023). The impact of histone modifications in endometriosis highlights new therapeutic opportunities. *Cells, 12*(9), 1227. https://doi.org/10.3390/cells12091227

Protopapas, A., Grimbizis, G., Athanasiou, S., & Loutradis, D. (2020). Adenomyosis: Disease, uterine aging process leading to symptoms, or both?. *Facts, views & vision in ObGyn, 12*(2), 91–104. PMID: 32832923; PMCID: PMC7431194.

Qin, X., Wang, Q., Xu, D., Sun, Y., Xu, W., Wang, B., Yang, Z., & Hao, L. (2024). Atorvastatin exerts dual effects of lesion regression and ovarian protection in the prevention and treatment of endometriosis. *European Journal of Pharmacology, 964*, 176261. https://doi.org/10.1016/j.ejphar.2023.176261

Rahmioglu, N., Mortlock, S., Ghiasi, M., Møller, P. L., Stefansdottir, L., Galarneau, G., Turman, C., Danning, R., Law, M. H., Sapkota, Y., Christofidou, P., Skarp, S., Giri, A., Banasik, K., Krassowski, M., Lepamets, M., Marciniak, B., Nõukas, M., Perro, D., Sliz, E., ... Zondervan, K. T. (2023). The genetic basis of endometriosis and comorbidity with other pain and inflammatory conditions. *Nature genetics, 55*(3), 423–436. https://doi.org/10.1038/s41588-023-01323-z

Rees, S., Arnold, S., Kherlopian, A., & Fischer, G. (2024). Attitudes toward proactive topical corticosteroid use among women with vulval lichen sclerosus. *Journal of Lower Genital Tract Disease, 28*(2), 183–188. https://doi.org/10.1097/LGT.0000000000000791

Sabat, R., Alavi, A., Wolk, K., Wortsman, X., McGrath, B., Garg, A., & Szepietowski, J. C. (2025). Hidradenitis suppurativa. *Lancet (London, England), 405*(10476), 420–438. https://doi.org/10.1016/S0140-6736(24)02475-9

Sally, R., Shaw, K. S., & Pomeranz, M. K. (2021). Benign "lumps and bumps" of the vulva: A review. *International Journal of Women's Dermatology, 7*(4), 383–390. https://doi.org/10.1016/j.ijwd.2021.04.007.

Schrager, S., Yogendran, L., Marquez, C. M., & Sadowski, E. A. (2022). Adenomyosis: Diagnosis and Management. *American Family Physician, 105*(1), 33–38.

Shim, J. Y., Laufer, M. R., King, C. R., Lee, T. T. M., Einarsson, J. I., & Tyson, N. (2024). Evaluation and management of endometriosis in the adolescent. *Obstetrics and Gynecology, 143*(1), 44–51. https://doi.org/10.1097/AOG.0000000000005448

Signorile, P. G., Viceconte, R., & Baldi, A. (2022). New insights in pathogenesis of endometriosis. *Frontiers in Medicine, 9*, 879015. https://doi.org/10.3389/fmed.2022.879015

Singh, N., & Ghatage, P. (2020). Etiology, clinical features, and diagnosis of vulvar lichen sclerosus: A scoping review. *Obstetrics and Gynecology International, 2020*, 7480754. https://doi.org/10.1155/2020/7480754

Smith, A. B., Muhammad, N. I., Cigna, S. T., & Krapf, J. M. (2023). A systematic review of sexual health consequences among women with lichen sclerosus. *Sexual Medicine Reviews, 11*(1), 8–14.

Somigliana, E., Reschini, M., Bonanni, V., Busnelli, A., Li Piani, L., & Vercellini, P. (2021). Fibroids and natural fertility: A systematic review and meta-analysis. *Reproductive Biomedicine Online, 43*(1), 100–110. https://doi.org/10.1016/j.rbmo.2021.03.013

Sparić, R., Andjić, M., Babović, I., Nejković, L., Mitrović, M., Štulić, J., Pupovac, M., & Tinelli, A. (2022). Molecular Insights in Uterine Leiomyosarcoma: A Systematic Review. *International Journal of Molecular Sciences, 23*(17), 9728. https://doi.org/10.3390/ijms23179728

Speciale, A. R., Ozpinar, K., Giani, M., Tureli, D., Fambrini, M., Vannuccini, S., & Petraglia, F. (2025). Selective progesterone receptor modulators for the treatment of dysmenorrhea: An update. *Expert Opinion on Pharmacotherapy, 26*(3), 257–264. https://doi.org/10.1080/14656566.2025.2451145

Stratopoulou, C. A., Donnez, J., & Dolmans, M. M. (2021). Origin and pathogenic mechanisms of uterine adenomyosis: What is known so far. Reproductive Sciences (Thousand Oaks, Calif.), 28(8), 2087–2097. https://doi.org/10.1007/s43032-020-00361-w

Triarico, S., Capozza, M. A., Mastrangelo, S., Attinà, G., Maurizi, P., & Ruggiero, A. (2020). Gynecological cancer among adolescents and young adults (AYA). *Annals of Translational Medicine, 8*(6), 397. https://doi.org/10.21037/atm.2020.02.41

van der Meijden, W. I., Boffa, M. J., Ter Harmsel, B., Kirtschig, G., Lewis, F., Moyal-Barracco, M., Tiplica, G. S., & Sherrard, J. (2022). 2021 European guideline for the management of vulval conditions. *Journal of the European Academy of Dermatology and Venereology: JEADV, 36*(7), 952–972. https://doi.org/10.1111/jdv.18102

Vitale, S. G., Haimovich, S., Laganà, A. S., Alonso, L., Di Spiezio Sardo, A., Carugno, J., & From the Global Community of Hysteroscopy Guidelines Committee (2021). Endometrial polyps: An evidence-based diagnosis and management guide. *European Journal of Obstetrics, Gynecology, and Reproductive Biology, 260*, 70–77. https://doi.org/10.1016/j.ejogrb.2021.03.017

Wallace, K., Zhang, S., Thomas, L., Stewart, E. A., Nicholson, W. K., Wegienka, G. R., Wise, L. A., Laughlin-Tommaso, S. K., Diamond, M. P., Marsh, E. E., Jacoby, V. L., Anchan, R. M., Venable, S., Larry, G. M., Lytle, B., Wang, T., & Myers, E. R. (2020). Comparative effectiveness of hysterectomy versus myomectomy on one-year health-related quality of life in women with uterine fibroids. *Fertility and Sterility, 113*(3), 618–626. https://doi.org/10.1016/j.fertnstert.2019.10.028

Wilbur, J., Morrison, C., Iakavai, J., Shem, J., Poilapa, R., Bambery, L., Baker, S., Tanguay, J., Sheppard, P., Banks, L. M., & Mactaggart, I. (2021). "The weather is not good": Exploring the menstrual health experiences of menstruators with and without disabilities in Vanuatu. *The Lancet Regional Health. Western Pacific, 18*, 100325. https://doi.org/10.1016/j.lanwpc.2021.100325

Wolfman, W., Thurston, J., Yeung, G., & Glanc, P. (2020). Guideline no. 404: Initial investigation and management of benign ovarian masses. *Journal of Obstetrics and Gynaecology Canada, 42*(8), 1040–1050.e1. https://doi.org/10.1016/j.jogc.2020.01.014

APPENDIX 27-A

Technique for Vulvar Punch Biopsy

A successful biopsy provides a nondistorted specimen for optimal pathologic interpretation. Cutting or shaving with a scalpel blade or scissors may be used to obtain samples of raised or pedunculated lesions. For flat to slightly raised lesions, a 3 to 6 mm Keyes punch biopsy is often used as follows:

1. Explain the procedure to the patient and offer time for questions.
2. Identify the areas to be biopsied; typically, this includes either the entirety of a small lesion or the most suspicious areas of all larger lesions (e.g., atypically pigmented, raised, or irregularly contoured margins).
3. Cleanse the area with povidone–iodine or chlorhexidine.
4. To decrease the patient's discomfort from the local anesthetic injected into this sensitive area, consider initial superficial desensitization with ice or a topical anesthetic (e.g., 2.5% lidocaine with 2.5% prilocaine in a cream base left in place up to 60 minutes on keratinized skin or 20 minutes on mucous membranes; application on mucous membranes is an off-label use).
5. Lidocaine solution (1 to 2%) with epinephrine is commonly used as the injected local anesthetic, although epinephrine should be avoided near the clitoris. A tuberculin or 30-gauge needle is held bevel up, with the solution injected slowly to form a bleb under and just beyond the margins of the chosen biopsy sites. The clinician should wait approximately 3 minutes following lidocaine injection and confirm numbness with the patient before proceeding.
6. The punch biopsy is held directly perpendicular to the skin surface to avoid distortion and is rotated back and forth 180 degrees to just reach the subcutaneous adipose (full thickness); the sample should then be lifted with a tissue forceps, released with a small surgical scissors, and placed in preserving medium, such as formalin.
7. Specimen sites smaller than 4 mm typically do not require closure; any bleeding can be stopped with pressure (using a sterile gauze or swab) or application of aluminum chloride or silver nitrate. If a suture is used, removable silk may be more pliable and comfortable on sensitive surfaces than dissolvable suture (e.g., 4-0 chromic). Removable suture is typically removed in 5 to 14 days depending on the amount of stress on the site.
8. Review any hygiene precautions and expectations for discomfort, bleeding, and follow-up.

Data from British Society for the Study of Vulvar Disease. (2023). Guidance on taking a vulvar 'punch' biopsy. https://bssvd.org/wp-content/uploads/2023/08/TAKING-A-PUNCH-BIOPSY-OF-THE-VULVA-updated-26.3.23.pdf.

CHAPTER 28

Gynecologic Cancers

L'Oréal Kennedy

The editors would like to acknowledge Nancy Maas and Kristi Robinia the authors of Gynecologic Cancers for the 4th edition of Gynecologic Health Care.

Gynecologic cancers are serious, life-threatening diseases. Many symptoms of these diseases are vague and subtle, making early diagnosis, treatment, and successful recovery difficult. Not all people with gynecologic organs identify as female or women, and as such, nongendered terms will be used as much as possible throughout this chapter.

A humanistic approach that integrates patient-centered care with medical and sociopsychological perspectives serves to equalize the power imbalance between an individual and their clinician. Clinicians using this approach actively listen to their patients and assess them in the context of their lived experiences, culture, and socioeconomic class. Such clinicians are less likely to miss hearing a patient's vague symptoms that may be warnings of underlying disease and instead encourage them to provide more information that may be helpful in making an accurate diagnosis. Clinicians using a humanistic approach are cautious, thoughtful, and think critically, using the most recent evidence in assessing and formulating treatment for the disease. They provide their patients with information that is critical to informed consent and decision making. Sensitive clinicians who use good listening skills are the practitioners who have helped decrease the number of cancer deaths in people who were misdiagnosed when their voices were ignored.

Gynecologic cancers are defined as cancer of the uterus, cervix, ovary, vulva, and vagina. In 2023, there were approximately 114,810 new diagnoses of gynecologic cancers in the United States and 34,020 deaths resulting from these cancers (Siegel et al., 2023). Prevention and early recognition of health problems, such as gynecologic cancers, is the primary goal of clinicians who provide health care for people with gynecologic organs. For each person, genetic, behavioral, and environmental factors will influence their risk of developing a gynecologic malignancy.

VULVAR CANCERS

Description of Vulvar Cancer

Incidence and Prevalence

Vulvar cancer accounted for approximately 6 percent of all reproductive-organ cancers and 0.7 percent of all cancers in people with gynecologic organs in 2024 (American Cancer Society [ACS], 2025). The age-adjusted rate of new cases of vulvar cancer in 2024 was 2.6 per 100,000 (Surveillance, Epidemiology, and End Results Program [SEER], n.d.-a). The overall 5-year survival rate for a person with vulvar cancer is 86 percent if it is localized or considered stage 1 (National Comprehensive Cancer Network [NCCN], 2022; SEER, n.d.-a). Prognosis is significantly impacted by lymph node involvement (Jaeger et al., 2022). The overall 5-year survival rate for people with regional lymph node involvement is 47 percent, and this rate decreases to 22 percent when the cancer has metastasized to distant sites (Abu-Rustum et al., 2024; SEER, n.d.-a).

Carcinoma of the vulva is primarily a disease of postmenopausal individuals (Olawaiye et al., 2021). The average age of vulvar cancer diagnosis is 65 to 74 years, and the average age at death is 76 years. Between 2012–2021, the rate of vulvar cancer increased by 0.6 percent each year (SEER, n.d.-a). Vulvar cancers that occur at younger ages have increased in recent years, with a 38 percent increase in incidence under the age of 60, which may be related to infection with human papillomavirus (HPV) (Olawaiye et al., 2021). Older age is associated with a higher risk of mortality after controlling for competing risks such as age, stage, and radiation (Hafez et al., 2022).

Etiology and Pathophysiology

Vulvar squamous cell cancer accounts for greater than 80 percent of vulvar carcinomas. Rare types include basal cell carcinoma, adenocarcinoma related to extra-mammary Paget's disease, Bartholin gland carcinoma (squamous, adenocarcinoma, or transitional cell carcinoma), and sarcoma (Olawaiye et al., 2021). Research has shown that squamous cell vulvar carcinomas differ in terms of etiology, pathogenesis, and clinical significance (Dasgupta et al., 2020). In 2012, a consensus group co-sponsored by the College of American Pathologists and American Society for Colposcopy and Cervical Pathology recommended using "lower anogenital squamous terminology (LAST)" to describe low-grade (LSIL) and high-grade (HSIL) vulvar lesions in order to unify nomenclature (Gadkari et al., 2022). The World Health Organization (WHO) adopted these terms and retained the use of differentiated vulvar intraepithelial neoplasia (dVIN) in 2014 (Dasgupta et al., 2020). In 2015, the International Society for the Study of Vulvovaginal Disease Terminology of Vulvar Squamous Intraepithelial Lesions moved to divide these lesions into the following three categories, each correlating with the risk of progression to cancer over time (Olawaiye et al., 2021):

- Low-grade squamous intraepithelial lesion (LSIL) includes flat and exophytic condyloma (koilocytosis) as well as HPV lesions that are not associated with vulvar cancer and may resolve spontaneously without treatment (Gadkari et al., 2022).
- High-grade squamous intraepithelial lesions (HSIL), formerly termed usual type vulvar intraepithelial neoplasia (VIN), is related to HPV and tends to occur in individuals aged 40–44 years with a second peak incidence after age 55. These lesions can present as basaloid or warty, and greater than 80 percent contain HPV. Infection with HPV types 16 (77.2%), 33 (10.6%), 18 (2.6%) (Dasgupta et al., 2020), and 31 (2.8%) (Brusen Villadsen et al., 2021) carry the highest risk for progression of HSIL to squamous cell cancer of the vulva. Although the presence of vulvar HSIL confers an increased risk of vulvar cancer, most cases do not progress to squamous cell cancer. An estimated 9 to 16 percent of untreated HSIL develops into invasive disease compared to 3 percent of treated HSIL (Dasgupta et al., 2020).
- In vulvar intraepithelial neoplasia, differentiated type (dVIN), high-risk, abnormal squamous cells are present. This type of lesion has a higher rate of progression to squamous cell cancer and less than 2 percent are related to HPV infection (Olawaiye et al., 2021). It occurs most commonly in people in the sixth and eighth decades of life and is associated with chronic inflammatory dermatoses such as lichen sclerosus and lichen simplex chronicus (Wang et al., 2023). The lifetime risk of lichen sclerosus progressing to dVIN is 4–5 percent (Pouwer et al., 2020). Untreated dVIN resulting from lichen sclerosus has a median time of progression between 9 and 23 months. Lichen sclerosus is underdiagnosed and thus undertreated. Early diagnosis, prompt treatment, and close surveillance are imperative to decreasing the incidence of vulvar cancer in this subgroup (Kesic et al., 2022). Refer to Chapter 27 for more information about lichen sclerosus.

Risk factors for vulvar cancer are similar to those for cervical neoplasia related to acquisition of HPV and include early age at first intercourse, multiple sexual partners, and smoking (Hafez et al., 2022). Early sexual contact and infection with HPV provides more time for malignant transformation of HSIL to vulvar cancer. Infection with HIV is a risk factor due to its potential for immunosuppression, which can increase susceptibility to persistent HPV infections and, in turn, increases the risk of vulvar cancer. In addition, immunosuppression is linked to decreased ability of the immune system to limit cancer growth and spread (Bucchi et al., 2022). Increased age and inflammatory conditions of the vulva are risk factors more specific to dVIN (Wang et al., 2023).

Carcinogenesis of vulvar squamous cell cancer involves the transformation of either HSIL or dVIN precursor lesions to cancer. Approximately 80 percent of precancerous vulvar lesions are HPV positive whereas vulvar squamous cell carcinoma is predominantly HPV-independent, a discrepancy that remains unexplained (Brusen Villadsen et al., 2021). Both genetic and epigenetic changes are associated with the pathogenesis of vulvar cancer, and mutations are detected more often with increasing tumor stage. DNA mutations resulting in vulvar cancer are acquired, not hereditary, and develop over the course of a person's life; consequently, the risk for vulvar cancer is not inherited (Xing & Fadare, 2020).

Genetic research indicates that people with both HSIL- and dVIN-associated vulvar cancer have genetic mutations of the p53 tumor suppressor gene, which plays a key role in the carcinogenesis of many types of cancer (Xing & Fadare, 2020). The p53 protein normally stops proliferation of DNA-damaged cells. It senses DNA damage and initiates DNA repair; or, when the DNA damage cannot be repaired, the p53 protein triggers cell apoptosis, thereby preventing unregulated proliferation of mutated cells (ACS, 2022). Research indicates that mutation of the p53 gene is more prominent in the development of dVIN, and a p53 mutation may also be present in cases of lichen sclerosus (Xing & Fadare, 2020). The prognostic value of p53 mutations is unclear; however, vulvar cancers with p53 mutations are associated with significantly lower 5-year survival rates (Pouwer et al., 2020).

Clinical Presentation

Vulvar cancer is often asymptomatic. When signs and symptoms do occur, there is often a prolonged history of vulvar pruritus reported. Less common symptoms are vulvar bleeding and discharge. On physical examination, the most obvious sign is a visible lesion. The lesion may be a lump, ulcerated, warty, pigmented, painful, or pruritic (Olawaiye et al., 2021). Lesions may be single or multifocal; the color can vary from white to red, gray, blue, or brown; and affected skin may be raised or thickened (Kesic, Vieira-Baptista, & Stockdale, 2022). Two-thirds of squamous cell carcinomas occur on the labia majora and minora and may be multifocal, affecting the vagina, urethra, anus, and cervix. Advanced disease may present with a lump in the groin related to lymph node metastasis (ISSVD, 2023).

Malignant melanoma is the second most common neoplasm of the vulva, although it is very rare with an incidence of 0.1 per 100,000 (Olawaiye et al., 2021). These lesions may be located on the labia minora or clitoris and appear pigmented. The cutaneous melanoma "ABCDE" (asymmetry, border irregularity, color, diameter, and evolution [of size, shape, or color]) criteria should be employed and these patients urgently referred to a gynecologic oncologist for further evaluation (Falcicchio et al., 2022). Extramammary Paget disease is an adenocarcinoma of the vulva characterized by eczematoid or well-demarcated patchy erythematous plaques with a "strawberry and cream" appearance. Due to their likeness to eczema and dermatitis (rashes), these malignancies are underdiagnosed and usually discovered once they are locally advanced (Caruso et al., 2023). Rarely, adenocarcinoma involving the apocrine Bartholin glands can occur and originate either from intraepithelial lesion or invasion from a primary anorectal, urothelial, endocervical, or endometrial adenocarcinoma (Olawaiye et al., 2021).

Assessment

History and Physical Examination

Patients should see their clinicians at least yearly for a wellness exam, with pelvic examination being a shared decision with the clinician based on identified risks and benefits. This preventive visit provides an opportunity for therapeutic communication, which may help to identify risks for vulvar cancer that the patient may not recognize as needing follow-up (ACOG, 2018, reaffirmed 2024). Because HPV infection is a known risk factor for vulvar cancer, the clinician should ask about sexual activity and relationships, use of barrier protection, previous history or exposure to sexually transmitted infections (STIs), and HPV immunization status. Smoking status should be discussed related to its strong association to vulvar cancer. Additionally, clinicians need to ask about a history of lichen sclerosis, previous diagnosis of HSIL or dVIN of the vulva, Paget disease, malignant melanoma, or a recurrent or persistent Bartholin cyst because these conditions are associated with a risk of developing vulvar cancer (Olawaiye et al., 2021; Kesic et al., 2022).

Thorough patient education about when and how to perform a vulvar self-examination using a mirror may be helpful in early identification of vulvar lesions and is especially important for people with a previous history of vulvar cancer. Pap tests are no longer recommended for all people with gynecologic organs, and the Committee on Gynecologic Practice, Society of Gynecologic Oncology (2018) and American College of Obstetricians and Gynecologists (2018, reaffirmed 2024) recommends that pelvic examinations be performed as indicated by history or reported symptoms. Pelvic examination is an appropriate component of a comprehensive physical examination for any person with known risk factors for vulvar cancer or a person who reports symptoms suggestive of gynecologic malignancy (Committee on Gynecologic Practice, Society of Gynecologic Oncology, 2018; American College of Obstetricians and Gynecologists, 2018, reaffirmed 2024). Patients with a history of cervical or vaginal cancer and those with lichen sclerosis should be examined regularly, and all individuals reporting or found to have a vulvar lesion must be thoroughly evaluated to rule out malignancy (Olawaiye et al., 2021; Kesic et al., 2022). Refer to Chapter 9 regarding Pap tests.

Genital neoplasia is often multifocal. Thus, careful examination of the entire genitalia for lesions, including the vulva, vagina, cervix, perineum, perianal area, and anus, should be performed as part of the pelvic examination. Vulvar cancer that is not associated with HPV infection often presents as a single mass on the labia majora or minora. In HPV-positive vulvar cancer, lesions tend to be multifocal, with concurrent cervical neoplasia more common (Abu-Rustum et al., 2024). The femoral and inguinal lymph nodes should be palpated routinely during pelvic examination because vulvar squamous cell cancer most often spreads to these nodes, and lymph node metastasis is the single most prognostic indicator of survival in vulvar cancer (Abu-Rustum et al., 2024; Jaeger et al., 2022). In addition, examination of the urethra, bladder, and rectum may be appropriate to determine metastasis and spread (NCI, 2020a).

Diagnostic Testing

Diagnosis of vulvar cancer is made by identifying a lesion through visual inspection and then obtaining confirmation with a biopsy (Committee on Gynecologic Practice, Society of Gynecologic Oncology, 2016, reaffirmed 2019; Abu-Rustum et al., 2024; Olawaiye, Cuello, & Rogers, 2021). Biopsy should be done on any lesion where diagnosis cannot be made based on clinical presentation, lesions that do not respond to treatment, and any that have an atypical vascular appearance or are rapidly changing in size, border, or color (Committee on Gynecologic Practice, Society of Gynecologic Oncology, 2016, reaffirmed 2019). Vulvoscopy may assist in the diagnosis of vulvar cancer in people who have persistent pruritus or vulvar pain but do not present with specific lesions, and it may be helpful in defining the extent of disease (Committee on Gynecologic Practice, Society of Gynecologic Oncology, 2016, reaffirmed 2019; Olawaiye, Cuello, & Rogers, 2021). Additional diagnostic testing may include colposcopy of the cervix and vagina because of the association of vulvar cancer with other gynecologic neoplasia. A CT scan, MRI, or positron emission tomography (PET) scan of the pelvis and groin may be helpful in detecting any enlarged lymph nodes, urethral or bladder involvement, or erosion of underlying bony structures and may assist in staging the cancer (if detected) (Olawaiye et al., 2021). Laboratory workup may include complete blood count, liver and kidney function, cervical cytological testing, and HIV testing (Abu-Rustum et al., 2024).

Unfortunately, delays in the diagnosis of vulvar cancer are common and both patients and clinicians may contribute to the delay. Common causes of late-stage diagnosis of vulvar cancer include patients not seeking treatment when initial symptoms occur because symptoms are assumed to be due to normal aging or hesitancy in reporting them related to fear, shame, or embarrassment. Clinicians may not perform pelvic exams due to absence of genital bleeding, lack of appropriate resources in exam rooms, unavailability of a chaperone for the exam, and virtual appointments (Goodman, 2021). Experts recommend that a biopsy be performed of growing lesions, ulcers, bleeding lesions, discolored areas, indurated areas, and lesions either resistant or unresponsive to treatment (Kesic et al., 2022).

Differential Diagnoses

When establishing differential diagnoses for vulvar disorders, the clinician should consider basic vulvar changes, inflammatory conditions, and neoplasia (Gupta et al., 2024). The following are potential differential diagnoses to consider prior to making a diagnosis of vulvar cancer:

- Papillomatosis
- Vulvar psoriasis
- Bartholin gland cyst
- Lichen planus
- Lichen sclerosus
- Vulvar nevi, melanosis, or melanoma
- HPV infection with or without HSIL
- Paget disease
- Differentiated VIN
- Vulvar neoplasia

Prevention

Primary Prevention

The HPV vaccine has been shown to decrease the risk of vulvar HSIL and consequently vulvar cancer (Committee on Gynecologic Practice, Society of Gynecologic Oncology, 2016, reaffirmed 2019). Most cases of HPV-associated cancer in the United States are caused by the HPV genotypes 16 and 18 (CDC, 2024c). Immunization with the 9-valent HPV vaccine protects against genotypes 6, 11, 16, 18, 31, 33, 45, 52, and 58. The Centers for Disease Control and Prevention (2024a) and Society of Gynecologic Oncology (2021) recommend that the HPV vaccine routinely be given to all children aged 11 to 12 years and as young as 9 years old. Catch-up vaccination is recommended for all people up to

26 years old. Although sexually active people can receive the vaccine, it may be less effective in those who have already been exposed to HPV (Adjei Boayke et al., 2022). It is important for clinicians to provide education to their patients (or to their patients' parents or guardian, if patients are younger than the age of consent) about the benefits and risks of HPV vaccination and to encourage vaccination at office visits (Society of Gynecologic Oncology, 2021; CDC, 2024a).

Prevention of vulvar cancer should also focus on its other risk factors. Sexually active people should receive education on using barrier protection to limit their risk of exposure to HPV and HIV infection. Because cigarette smoking is strongly associated with the development of HPV-associated HSIL, smoking cessation should be encouraged (Committee on Gynecologic Practice, Society of Gynecologic Oncology, 2016, reaffirmed 2019).

Secondary and Tertiary Prevention

There are currently no specific screening recommendations for the prevention of vulvar cancer (Committee on Gynecologic Practice, Society of Gynecologic Oncology, 2016, reaffirmed 2019). Clinicians should emphasize the importance of vulvar self-examination and routine gynecologic visits to ensure prompt evaluation and treatment of all precancerous and cancerous lesions (Foundation on Women's Cancer, Society of Gynecologic Oncology, 2024). In addition, identification and treatment of vulvar dermatologic disorders, such as lichen sclerosis, may reduce the risk of dVIN and subsequent cancer (Committee on Gynecologic Practice, Society of Gynecologic Oncology, 2016, reaffirmed 2019; Kesic, Vieira-Baptista, & Stockdale, 2022).

Management

Biopsy for vulvar cancer may include the primary lesion and sentinel node biopsy in early-stage disease (NCI, 2020a; Nica et al., 2019) or removal and biopsy of the inguinal and femoral nodes, depending on primary tumor characteristics, imaging, and sentinel node results (NCCN, 2020; Nica et al., 2019). Lymph node metastasis in vulvar cancer is highly correlated with poorer prognosis, with a higher number of involved lymph nodes and involved lymph nodes in the groin and pelvis associated with decreased survival rates (NCCN, 2020; Nica et al., 2019; Jaeger et al., 2022). Staging for vulvar cancer utilizes two systems that describe characteristics of the primary tumor and the extent of cancer spread. The American Joint Committee on Cancer (AJCC) tumor–node–metastasis (TNM) system first classifies vulvar cancer growth by direct tumor extension to nearby organs, such as the vagina, urethra, or anus, then secondarily by local lymph node involvement, and finally by presence or absence of distant metastasis (American Joint Committee on Cancer, 2020). Categories include the following:

- The T category describes the primary tumor according to its size and location.
- The N category refers to the extent of cancer in the regional lymph nodes that drain fluid from the area of the tumor.
- The M category identifies whether the cancer has spread to distant areas in the body (e.g., from the vulva to the lungs) by vascular or lymphatic channels.

The AJCC's TNM categories correspond to staging of vulvar cancer by the International Federation of Gynecology and Obstetrics (FIGO). Vulvar cancer staging according to the FIGO guidelines is outlined in **Table 28-1**.

TABLE 28-1 2021 FIGO Staging for Carcinoma of the Vulva

FIGO Stage	Description
I	Tumor confined to the vulva
IA	Tumor size ≤ 2 cm and stromal invasion ≤ 1 mm[a]
IB	Tumor size > 2 cm or stromal invasion > 1 mm[a]
II	Tumor of any size with extension to lower one third of the urethra, lower one-third of the vagina, lower one-third of the anus with negative nodes
III	Tumor of any size with extension to upper part of adjacent perineal structures, or with any number of nonfixed, nonulcerated lymph node
IIIA	Tumor of any size with disease extension to upper two thirds of the urethra, upper two thirds of the vagina, bladder mucosa, rectal mucosa, or regional lymph node metastases ≤ 5 mm
IIIB	Regional[b] lymph node metastases > 5 mm
IIIC	Regional[b] lymph node metastases with extracapsular spread
IV	Tumor of any size fixed to bone, or fixed, ulcerated lymph node metastases, or distant metastases
IVA	Disease fixed to pelvic bone, or fixed or ulcerated regional[b] lymph node metastases
IVB	Distant metastases

Olawaiye, A. B., Cuello, M. A., & Rogers, L. J. (2021). Cancer of the vulva: 2021 update. *International journal of gynaecology and obstetrics: the official organ of the International Federation of Gynaecology and Obstetrics, 155 Suppl 1*(Suppl 1), 7–18. https://doi.org/10.1002/ijgo.13881

[a] Depth of invasion is measured from the basement membrane of the deepest, adjacent, dysplastic, tumor-free rete ridge (or nearest dysplastic rete peg) to the deepest point of invasion.

[b] Regional refers to inguinal and femoral lymph nodes.

Abbreviation: FIGO, International Federation of Gynecology and Obstetrics.

The majority of people with vulvar cancer are diagnosed with early-stage, localized disease (Abu-Rustum et al., 2024). Risks for lymph node metastasis include depth, thickness, amount of differentiation, and degree of extension of the primary tumor (NCI, 2020a; Abu-Rustum et al., 2024; Jaeger et al., 2022). Vulvar cancer lesions that are well differentiated tend to be minimally invasive, whereas poorly differentiated, anaplastic lesions are more likely to be deeply invasive (NCI, 2020a). Vulvar cancer spreads primarily through lymph nodes, starting in the superficial inguinal nodes, traveling to the deep inguinal nodes, into pelvic nodes, and then to iliac and paraaortic nodes (Chow et al., 2021). The incidence of lymph node involvement in vulvar cancer is approximately 30 percent (Weinberg & Gomez-Martinez,

2019; NCI, 2020a). Hematogenous spread to distant sites such as the lungs or bones occurs in approximately 4 percent of patients (NCI, 2020a; Chow et al., 2021).

Referral

Patients presenting with symptoms or questionable lesions need to be referred to a gynecologist or a gynecologic oncologist who has expertise in cancer surgery. Further referral should be considered for individuals with lesions on the clitoris or in the urethra to minimize impairment of urinary or sexual function (Committee on Gynecologic Practice, Society of Gynecologic Oncology, 2016, reaffirmed 2019). Treatment is recommended for all people with vulvar cancer and for those with either HSIL or dVIN precursor lesions (Committee on Gynecologic Practice, Society of Gynecologic Oncology, 2016, reaffirmed 2019). Management of vulvar neoplasia should be tailored to the individual and guided by a multidisciplinary cancer center team. Psychosexual counseling services should be offered throughout treatment for all people with preinvasive and invasive disease (Olawaiye et al., 2021).

Pharmacologic Treatment

When invasion is not a concern, HSIL can be treated with surgical excision, laser ablation, or medical therapy (Committee on Gynecologic Practice, Society of Gynecologic Oncology, 2016, reaffirmed 2019). Topical therapy with imiquimod 5 percent, which is an immune modulator, has been shown to effectively treat about half of people who have HSIL that has not progressed to invasive disease, with an average length of treatment being 16 weeks (Committee on Gynecologic Practice, Society of Gynecologic Oncology, 2016, reaffirmed 2019; NCI, 2020a). Follow-up is recommended for 2–3 years due to a 30–40 percent risk of recurrence (Olawaiye et al., 2021).

Laser Treatment

Laser excision is also an acceptable option for the treatment of vulvar HSIL when cancer is not suspected. It can be used for single or multifocal lesions, although the risk of recurrence may be higher than with surgical wide excision, particularly with multifocal disease (Committee on Gynecologic Practice, Society of Gynecologic Oncology, 2016, reaffirmed 2019; Boonlikit & Tangterdchanakit, 2024), and scarring in areas of treatment has been reported (NCI, 2020a). Regular follow-up is important because people treated for HSIL are considered to remain at risk for recurrent HSIL and vulvar cancer throughout their lifetime (Committee on Gynecologic Practice, Society of Gynecologic Oncology, 2016, reaffirmed 2019; NCI, 2020a; Gupta et al., 2024).

Surgical Treatment

Surgical resection is the standard treatment for patients with dVIN and vulvar cancer, regardless of the stage of the disease (Committee on Gynecologic Practice, Society of Gynecologic Oncology, 2016, reaffirmed 2019; Gupta et al., 2024). Localized wide excision involves removing the tumor and at least a 1 to 2 cm margin of normal tissue surrounding the tumor to limit recurrence (Abu-Rustum et al., 2024; Olawaiye, Cuello, & Rogers, 2021). Such surgery is the preferred intervention for patients with unifocal lesions and early-stage vulvar cancer (Olawaiye, Cuello, & Rogers, 2021). Radical vulvectomy may be required for FIGO stage 3 and 4A disease which indicates extension to nearby structures and/or lymph nodes (Chow et al., 2021). When radical vulvectomy is performed, reconstructive plastic surgery may lower the rate of wound dehiscence, vaginal introital stenosis, sexual dysfunction, and urinary problems postoperatively (Caretto et al., 2023).

Because groin invasion carries a much higher mortality risk, appropriate surgical lymph node management is the single most important factor in reducing mortality from vulvar cancer (Abu-Rustum et al., 2024; Olawaiye, Cuello, & Rogers, 2021; Jaeger et al., 2022). The utilization of the sentinel lymph node is increasing and thereby reducing the need for node dissection, a process which can result in significant morbidity. A sentinel lymph node is the first node in a chain and if it is negative, dissection of that chain is unnecessary (Olawaiye, Cuello, & Rogers, 2021). Sentinel lymph node excision may be considered for those with smaller, localized lesions (Abu-Rustum et al., 2024; Olawaiye, Cuello, & Rogers, 2021). Inguinal and femoral lymph node excision is recommended when sentinel lymph node biopsy is positive, when higher-grade vulvar tumors are present, or when diagnostic testing indicates cancer spread (Olawaiye, Cuello, & Rogers, 2021). Lymph node dissection is performed either unilaterally or bilaterally using separate incisions from the primary tumor to promote healing and limit surgical complications (Abu-Rustum et al., 2024; Olawaiye, Cuello, & Rogers, 2021).

Radiation therapy is considered for larger tumors, lymph node involvement, close margins (< 5 mm), and concurrently with chemotherapy (chemoradiation) as an alternative to surgery when the removal of all pelvic organs and structures (exenteration) such as the urethra, bladder, rectum, and anus would be necessary to obtain clear margins. Immunotherapy and chemotherapy can be used when rare histology or metastatic disease are present or in palliative care settings (Olawaiye, Cuello, & Rogers, 2021).

Emerging Evidence That May Change Management

Research into the genetic and molecular alterations that play a role in the carcinogenesis of vulvar cancer may lead to greater insight into the etiology of vulvar cancer, assist in the development of clinical trials, and could provide individuals with vulvar cancer alternative treatment options, including new targeted therapies (Sand et al., 2019; Olawaiye, Cuello, & Rogers, 2021). Although there are currently no targeted therapies approved for management of this disease, potential genetic and molecular targets for vulvar cancer have been identified, such as EGFR, PI3K, CDK2NA, and PTEN (Olawaiye, Cuello, & Rogers, 2021). Targeted therapy approaches are at the forefront of improving treatment and outcomes for all people who have gynecologic cancers.

Patient Education

Treatment side effects and their impact on a person's quality of life vary with the type of vulvar cancer treatment. Prior to treatment, people diagnosed with vulvar cancer require anticipatory education about the potential complications of any therapeutic option. Evaluation and discussion should then continue with each follow-up visit. Side effects from surgical treatment may include distortion of the anatomy and function which can negatively impact activities of daily living (Paez Lopez et al., 2024).

Complete inguinofemoral dissection is associated with a high risk of early complications including wound infection, wound breakdown, and lymphatic leakage, and late complications such as lower limb lymphedema, and erysipelas/lymphangitis (Caretto et al., 2023). Radiation can cause vaginal stenosis, urinary incontinence, and chronic bowel and bladder irritation (Proppe et al., 2024) whereas surgery can lead to sexual, anal and/or urinary dysfunction due to scarring, mutilation, and damage to nerves and blood vessels. Given that patients who undergo vulvar surgery and/or radiation may experience the aforementioned complications as well as sexual dysfunction and anxiety, depression, and low self-confidence, it is imperative that they work with mental health professionals during and after treatment (Malandrone et al., 2021).

Using a vaginal dilator 3 to 4 times a week or regular sexual intercourse can help to stretch vaginal tissues and are used to prevent vaginal stenosis. Dilator kits with hard plastic appliances of varying sizes are recommended. Patients should start by inserting the smallest dilator, gradually increasing the dilator diameter with the goal of full vaginal insertion of the largest size without discomfort (Memorial Sloan Kettering Cancer Center, 2024). If introital stenosis occurs, the clinician may need to use a pediatric speculum for vaginal visualization and insert only a single digit when palpating the vagina.

Some degree of sexual dysfunction is almost always present with definitive treatment of vulvar cancer. In particular, problems with arousal, orgasm, vaginal dryness, and sexual relationships are commonplace (Lagana et al., 2021; Memorial Sloan Kettering, 2024). Vaginal dryness may be helped by the use of vaginal lubricants which can be extremely helpful in relieving vaginal and vulvar symptoms, especially when an adequate amount and consistency of application is utilized (Memorial Sloan Kettering, 2024). Referral to a physical therapist who specializes in pelvic floor physical therapy may be considered. Physical therapy can reduce urinary symptoms, improve sexual function, and decrease pain during sexual intercourse long term (Cyr et al., 2022).

Counseling that explores relationship issues, changes in body image, and concerns related to vaginal intercourse can allow for the patient's expression of grief over the loss of normal sexual function, and referral to a mental health or sexual therapist may be of benefit (Malandrone et al., 2021). It is also important to address the ever-present fear of metastasis or disease recurrence. If needed, the choice of a personal caregiver should be carefully considered—it is important to understand that the patient's sexual partner may not always be the best choice. Indeed, some people have attributed significant negative changes in their sexual relationship to the participation of a sexual partner in postoperative wound care.

When diagnosed and treated early, vulvar cancer has a good prognosis, but unfortunately recurrence rates range from 12–37 percent, regardless of treatment regimens used (Committee on Gynecologic Practice, Society of Gynecologic Oncology, 2016, reaffirmed 2019; Zach et al., 2021). Most recurrences are diagnosed within 1 to 2 years of initial treatment, though recurrence 5 years or later after treatment has been noted (Abu-Rustum et al., 2024). Consequently, lifelong follow-up on a regular schedule is important. Many patients can return to their primary care clinicians for follow-up after surgical recovery and resolution of any postoperative wound healing complications. Vulvar cancer is thought to have a relatively slow rate of progression, so patients who have a good response to therapy and develop no new lesions at 6 and 12 months after treatment may be followed annually (Committee on Gynecologic Practice, Society of Gynecologic Oncology, 2016, reaffirmed 2019).

A comprehensive history and physical examination are standard components of follow-up care. New or persistent symptoms need to be reported promptly and evaluated carefully. Every follow-up visit should focus on the history of any new vulvar lesion, bladder function, bowel function, bone pain, and lower extremity lymphedema. After treatment, all patients should be taught how to perform a monthly self-examination of the vulva. Recurrent disease is always a possibility, and its early identification offers the best chance for effective treatment and survival (Abu-Rustum et al., 2024; Olawaiye, Cuello, & Rogers, 2021; Foundation on Women's Cancer, Society of Gynecologic Oncology, 2024).

Considerations for Specific Populations

Overall, cancer occurrence and mortality rates vary among racial and ethnic groups, which may be related to differences in risk factor exposure, decreased access to high-quality cancer care, and early detection and treatment of cancer. Disparities in cancer care have also been linked to socioeconomic status, educational level, and geographical locale (National Cancer Institute, 2024a). Recent research on vulvar cancer suggests that geographical region, age, stage, and type of treatment facility are associated with overall decreased survival (Gaulin et al., 2020; National Cancer Institute, 2024a). Survival may also be improved when care is received at certain facilities, such as National Cancer Institute–designated treatment centers where clinicians see a high volume of patients and treatment is guided by multidisciplinary teams (McDaniels-Davidson et al., 2022). Clinicians need to maintain vigilance in identification of characteristics that place individuals at risk for delayed diagnosis and poor treatment outcomes. If possible, referrals should be made to high-volume facilities that provide a multidisciplinary approach to vulvar cancer care. Due diligence is necessary to assure that all people diagnosed with HSIL, dVIN, or vulvar cancer achieve the best possible outcomes.

CERVICAL CANCER

Description of Cervical Cancer

Incidence and Prevalence

Globally, cervical cancer ranks as the fourth most common gynecologic malignancy, with an estimated 660,000 new cases diagnosed, and 350,000 deaths occurring, in 2022. Low- and middle-income countries carry the brunt of mortality with 94 percent of these deaths occurring amongst their communities (World Health Organization [WHO], n.d.). Worldwide, cervical cancer is the second most commonly diagnosed cancer and the second highest cause of cancer-related death among people with gynecologic organs who live in low-resource countries (Hull et al., 2020). Clearly, living in a low-resource country and being economically disadvantaged significantly increase a person's risks of developing cervical cancer and dying from it.

Annually in the United States, there are more than 13,000 new cases diagnosed, with approximately 4,200 deaths attributed to cervical cancer, or 2.3 per 100,000 individuals with a cervix (ACS, 2025a; NCI, 2023a). Although cervical cancer death rates in the United States have decreased by more than 50 percent over the past 30 years, mainly due to implementation of screening protocols, the overall death rates have not changed significantly in the past 15 years (ACS, 2020b). Today in the United States it is much more likely for a person to be diagnosed with cervical precancer than with invasive cervical cancer (ACS, 2025a). Early detection is key to minimizing mortality because people treated for localized (stage 1) lesions have a 5-year survival rate of 91.8 percent

(NCI, 2024b). In comparison, if the cancer is discovered in the regional lymph nodes, the 5-year survival rate drops to 56.3 percent, and if cancer is diagnosed at the metastasis stage, the survival rate decreases to 16.9 percent (NCI, 2024b).

Unfortunately, cervical cancer remains a disease of socioeconomic disparity in the United States. People who are Latiné or African American are more likely to be diagnosed with the disease and are more likely to die of it, compared to their white counterparts (ACS, 2025a). A review of the incidence of cervical cancer rates in the United States per 100,000 individuals with a cervix from 2012 to 2016 identified the risk percentiles for people of different race and ethnicity as follows: Asian/Pacific, 6.4; American Indian/Alaska Native, 7.9; white, 7.2; Black, 8.7; and Latiné, 9.3 (NCI, 2024b). The risk for people who identify with Asian/Pacific, American Indian/Alaska Native, or Latiné ethnicity may be underestimated due to the lack of a unified approach to understanding and accurately reporting race (Spencer et al., 2023). Higher incidence and mortality rates are indicative of barriers to health care, especially for people who are members of minoritized groups, those who have a lower socioeconomic status, and those who have recently immigrated to the United States. These communities are at higher risk because they may not have access to primary health care, adequate screening, or treatments for early precancerous cervical lesions (ACS, 2025a; CDC, n.d.-h). This disparity in access to care and subsequent treatment is experienced on a global scale, with statistics indicating that almost 90 percent of cervical cancer deaths occur in low- and middle-income countries (WHO, n.d.).

Etiology and Pathophysiology

Perpetual HPV infection is the most important causative agent in cervical carcinogenesis (NCI, 2020b; Okunade, 2020). This virus is detected in 99.7 percent of cervical cancers, and it is generally accepted that people must be infected by HPV before they develop cervical cancer (Okunade, 2020; NCI, 2020b). HPV is the most common STI worldwide (WHO, n.d.), and nearly all people who are sexually active will be infected with this virus at some point, with many individuals with a cervix experiencing repeated infections (ACS, 2020f; CDC, n.d.-b; Okunade, 2020; WHO, n.d.). Although HPV is considered an STI, it can be spread by skin-to-skin genital contact without intercourse. Most people with a cervix are infected shortly after beginning their first sexual relationship, with the highest prevalence seen in people younger than age 25. Thereafter, prevalence decreases rapidly, probably because of protection usage such as condoms, although condoms reduce but do not eliminate the risk of transmission (ACS, 2025a).

Despite the significant correlation between HPV infection and cervical cancer, 80 to 90 percent of infections are transient, sometimes causing only mild cytologic abnormalities, and they usually become undetectable within 1 to 2 years. A successful immune response results in viral control or clearance. When that does not occur, the oncogenic subtypes of HPV over a long period of time, estimated around 10 years, can create abnormal cellular change to the susceptible exposed columnar tissue of the transformation zone on the cervix (ACS, 2025a; CDC, n.d.-b; Okunade, 2020).

At least 250 genotypically distinct variants of HPV have been identified, approximately 40 of which will infect the epithelium of the skin or mucous membranes of the genital area (He et al., 2022). Genital HPV types can be divided into two broad categories based on their risk of oncogenesis. The low-risk HPV types include 6, 11, 40, 42, 43, 44, 55, 61, 81, 83 (Letafati et al., 2024). Types 6 and 11 are responsible for 90 percent of genital warts (condylomata acuminata) and low-grade cervical changes, such as mild dysplasia. Lesions due to low-risk HPV infections have a higher likelihood of regression and rarely progress to cancer (ACS, 2020f; CDC, 2024b). Nevertheless, approximately 20 to 56 percent of people infected with low-risk viruses have coinfection with high-risk HPV types (Wu et al., 2019). There are at least 13 genotypes that are known to cause persistent infection leading to high-grade cervical changes, such as moderate or severe dysplasia and neoplasia (Gong et al., 2021). Of these types, 16 and 18 are associated with 70 percent of diagnosed cervical cancer, and genotypes 31, 33, 35, 45, 52, and 58 are associated with another 20 percent of cases (Park et al., 2019). At the same time, these strains are frequently found to be the etiologic factor in minor lesions and mild dysplasia (**Table 28-2**).

HPVs are small, nonenveloped viruses containing 72 capsomers coating a genome of double-stranded circular DNA (Gearhart et al., 2020). The HPV genome has three regions:

- An early (E) region that codes for cellular transformation
- A late (L) region that codes for the structural proteins L1 and L2, which are responsible for creating the capsid
- A long control region that determines replication and gene function (Gearhart et al., 2020).

HPV types are differentiated by molecular methods according to genetic sequencing found on the outer capsid protein, L1. HPV infections begin developing when there is a break in the basal epithelium, and the virus enters and remains latent on a skin or mucosal surface. As infected well-differentiated keratinocytes leave the basal layer, the viral genes are activated and reproduce. The viral shredding then changes the epidermis and may result in warts. HPV viruses are specific to humans and have not been grown in vitro. Communicability is mainly through skin-to-skin rather than blood-borne contact and is assumed to be high secondary to the large numbers of new infections annually (CDC, n.d.-b; Gearhart et al., 2020). Cell-mediated immunity plays an

TABLE 28-2 Common HPV Types Associated With Benign and Malignant Disease

Risk	HPV Types	Manifestations
High risk	Types 16 and 18	Low-grade cervical changes High-grade cervical changes Cervical cancer Cancers of the vagina, vulva, anus, and penis
Low risk	Types 6 and 11	Benign low-grade cervical changes Genital warts

Data from American Cancer Society. (2019d). *HPV and HPV testing.* https://www.cancer.org/cancer/cancer-causes/infectious-agents/hpv/hpv-and-hpv-testing.html

Abbreviation: HPV, human papillomavirus.

important role in containing the infection; therefore, people with cell-mediated immunity deficiency are more prone to experience difficulty in treating HPV infections.

The major difference between low- and high-risk HPV types is that after infection is established, the low-risk HPV types are maintained as extrachromosomal DNA episomes, while the high-risk HPV genomes become integrated into the host cells' DNA in malignant lesions. Integration of the viral genome into the host cell genome is considered a hallmark of malignant transformation. High-risk HPV produces viral protein products (E6, E7) that bind and inactivate the host's tumor suppressor genes p53 and pRb. The inactivation of these genes blocks apoptosis (programmed cell death) and induces chromosomal abnormalities (ACS, 2020k; Gearhart et al., 2020).

Cervical cancer is characterized by a well-defined premalignant phase that can be identified through cytologic examination of exfoliated cells (Pap test) and confirmed on histologic examination. Premalignant changes can represent a spectrum of cervical abnormalities, which are referred to as squamous intraepithelial lesions (SIL) or cervical intraepithelial neoplasia (CIN). These early lesions form a continuum that is divided into low-grade or high-grade SIL or CIN 1, 2, and 3, which reflect the increasingly abnormal changes that occur in the cervical epithelium. Over time, the premalignant lesions can persist, regress, or progress to invasive malignancy. CIN 1 often regresses spontaneously, whereas CIN 2 and 3 are more likely to persist or progress. The premalignant changes usually occur in the metaplastic epithelium at the squamocolumnar junction. Unfortunately, cytologic and histologic examinations cannot reliably distinguish the few people with abnormal cytology who will progress to invasive cancer from the vast majority of people whose abnormalities will spontaneously regress (ACS, 2020f; Boardman & Matthews, 2025).

The latency period between HPV exposure and the development of cervical cancer is usually measured in years or decades. Longitudinal studies have shown that in untreated patients with carcinoma in situ lesions, 30 to 70 percent will develop invasive carcinoma over a period of 10 to 12 years. However, in less than 10 percent of patients, invasive lesions can develop in a period of less than 1 year (NCI, 2024b). The long natural history of this disease provides an opportunity to screen people for premalignant lesions, thereby preventing the lesions from evolving into cervical cancer (NCI, 2024b).

Two main types of cervical cancer are distinguished. The most common type is squamous cell carcinoma, which accounts for up to 90 percent of all cervical cancers. Squamous cell carcinoma arises from the squamous cells that cover the ectocervix (NCI, 2023a), and HPV 16 is implicated as the type most commonly associated with this type of cancer (Campos-Para et al., 2022). Adenocarcinoma, the second most common cervical cancer type, accounts for at least 10 percent of cervical cancer cases. It most often arises from the columnar epithelium—a group of mucus-producing glandular cells—located in the endocervix (NCI, 2023a) and has been associated most commonly with HPV 18, followed by HPV 16 (Campos-Para et al., 2022). An increase in the incidence of cervical adenocarcinomas has been observed during the past 20 to 30 years. Among people younger than age 35, the incidence more than doubled between 1970 and the mid-1980s. On rare occasions, cervical cancers have features of both squamous cell carcinoma and adenocarcinoma; these cases are called adenosquamous carcinomas or mixed carcinomas (ACS, 2020l).

Risk Factors Associated With Acquiring HPV

Age

Early age at first intercourse (age 18 years or younger) is a risk factor for HPV. It is believed the younger developing cervix is at a greater risk of being infected because of the normal physiologic process called squamous metaplasia. The process of squamous metaplasia occurs at the squamocolumnar junction, or transformation zone, where the more fragile columnar epithelial cells are replaced with hardier squamous epithelial cells. Squamous metaplasia is initiated by the eversion of the columnar epithelium onto the ectocervix, which occurs under the influence of estrogen and its ensuing exposure to the acidic vaginal pH. Although metaplasia may arise throughout the reproductive years, it is most active during adolescence and first pregnancy. Indeed, people whose first pregnancy occurs when they are younger than age 20 years are more likely to get cervical cancer in later life than people whose first pregnancy occurs at age 25 years or older (ACS, 2020f; Aggarwal & Ben Amor, 2023; Cooper & McCathran, 2023; NCI 2024b). Cells undergoing metaplasia are more vulnerable to carcinogenic agents, such as HPV.

The age of greatest risk, however, is midlife, when the majority of cervical cancer diagnoses are made. An estimated 15 percent of cases are diagnosed after age 65 years, with most occurring in people who have not participated in regular screening (ACS, 2020f).

Sexual Behavior

Having multiple sexual partners or having a partner with multiple sexual partners increases the risk of multiple exposures to HPV (ACS, 2020f; Okunade, 2020). Nevertheless, only a small proportion of people who become infected with HPV go on to develop cervical cancer (Okunade, 2020). Cofactors, such as smoking, are thought to play a contributing role in this evolution (CDC, n.d.-g; NCI, 2024b).

Smoking

Among people infected with HPV, current and former smokers have approximately 2 to 3 times the incidence of high-grade cervical intraepithelial lesions or invasive cancer. Passive smoking is also associated with increased risk, albeit to a lesser extent (ACS, 2020f; NCI, 2020a). People who smoke cigarettes are twice as likely as nonsmokers to develop cervical cancer. Smoking exposes the body to many carcinogens that affect more than just the lungs because carcinogens are absorbed by the lungs and carried in the bloodstream, thereby traveling throughout the body. Tobacco by-products have been found in the cervical mucus of people who smoke, and it is believed that these by-products damage the DNA in cervical cells. Smoking may also impair the immune response, thereby interfering with the body's ability to clear the HPV infection (ACS, 2020f; NCI, 2020b).

Immunosuppression

Patients who are immunocompromised from HIV, AIDS, or other causes (e.g., medications) have an increased prevalence and persistence of HPV infection. The immune system plays an important role in destroying cancer cells and slowing their growth and spread (ACS, 2020f). A precancerous lesion may develop more quickly into an invasive cancer if an individual is immunocompromised (ACS, 2020f). Indeed, invasive cervical cancer diagnosed in a person who is HIV positive is considered an acquired immunodeficiency syndrome–defining illness (Allredge et al., 2020).

Oral Contraceptives

The risk of cervical cancer doubles after 5 years of combined oral contraceptive (COC) use, but it returns to normal about 10 years following discontinuation of oral contraceptives (ACS, 2020f; NCI, 2024b). Interestingly, people who have used an intrauterine device (even for less than 1 year) appear to have a lower risk of developing cervical cancer (ACS, 2020f).

Although the connection between COCs and cervical cancer is not yet fully understood, it appears that the estrogenic effect of COCs may prevent the ectopy of the cervix from receding into the cervical canal, leaving the vulnerable area exposed. Moreover, COC users are less likely to use barrier protection, thereby increasing their risk of contracting HPV. Experts recommend that clinicians discuss the risks and benefits of COC use with people based on their individual history and risk factors (ACS, 2020f; Boardman & Matthews, 2025).

High Parity

Having had three or more full-term pregnancies has been associated with an increased risk for cervical cancer (ACS, 2020f; CDC, n.d.-h). Speculation for the causes of this relationship ranges to having had more unprotected sex and therefore more opportunities for HPV exposure, to the lower immunity state experienced during pregnancy coupled with hormonal changes that may facilitate cancer cell growth (ACS, 2020f).

Genetic Predisposition

Studies suggest that people whose mother or sisters have had cervical cancer are more likely to develop the disease. Twin studies also suggest that a familial susceptibility to cervical cancer is possible. Some researchers suspect a familial tendency is caused by an inherited condition that makes some people more susceptible to HPV infection than others (ACS, 2020f; Boardman & Matthews, 2025). Several genetic changes have been associated with cervical cancer. Indeed, changes in genes involved in apoptosis and gene repair have been suggested to explain why some people are not able to spontaneously clear HPV infection. Genetics, however, is estimated to affect less than 1 percent of cervical cancers (Boardman & Matthews, 2025).

Nutritional Status

Diets low in fruits and vegetables have been identified as potential contributing factors in the development of cervical cancer. Low levels of vitamins C and E, folate, and carotenoids have been linked to cervical cancer (ACS, 2020f; Ono et al., 2020). Decreased levels of folate and vitamin B_{12} might decrease immunocompetence in the cervical epithelium, which can play a role in the development of dysplasia (Silva et al., 2020). Further research is needed to clarify these relationships.

Poverty

Many people with a lower socioeconomic status or living in developing countries continue to lack ready access to adequate screening and treatment (ACS, 2020f; Hull et al., 2020).

Diethylstilbestrol

People whose parent took diethylstilbestrol (DES) during pregnancy are 40 times more likely to develop clear cell adenocarcinoma of the vagina and cervix than people who were not exposed to DES in utero. Clear cell adenocarcinoma is a rare form of vaginal and cervical cancer. The average age of people diagnosed with DES-related cervical cancer is 19 years. DES was removed from the market in 1971, so people who were exposed at age 19 years (or younger) are less likely to receive a diagnosis of cervical carcinoma. Nevertheless, it is not known how long they will remain at higher risk for contracting the disease (ACS, 2020f).

Infectious Agents

The specific role of herpes simplex virus 2 (HSV-2) and other infectious agents in the pathogenesis of cervical cancer remains unclear. Nevertheless, HSV-2 and *Chlamydia trachomatis* infections are known to be associated with a chronic inflammatory response and microulceration of the cervical epithelium. Such an inflammatory response is associated with the generation of free radicals, which play important roles in the initiation and progression of cancers (ACS, 2020f; Sausen et al., 2023). Free radicals directly damage DNA and DNA repair proteins and inhibit apoptosis, allowing the development of genetic instability (Alhmoud, 2020).

Clinical Presentation

Early cervical cancer is usually asymptomatic. As many as 20 percent of patients who have invasive cervical cancer are asymptomatic when the disease is diagnosed. If symptoms do occur, the most commonly noted are abnormal vaginal bleeding, such as postmenopausal bleeding, irregular menses, heavy menstrual flow, painless heavy menstrual bleeding, or most commonly postcoital bleeding. An abnormal vaginal discharge that is odiferous, watery, purulent, or mucoid may also be present. Late symptoms that suggest metastatic spread include bladder outlet or ureter obstruction causing loin pain from hydronephrosis; constipation; sciatica back pain due to pressure on nerve roots; pelvic pain; pain during intercourse; and leg swelling, often from deep vein thrombosis (ACS, 2019d; Boardman & Matthews, 2025; Burmeister, et al., 2022).

Assessment

History and Physical Examination

Key areas to cover in the history that can assist clinicians in identifying people at high risk for cervical cancer include the following (ACS, 2020f):

- Abnormal vaginal bleeding (intermenstrual or postcoital bleeding), unusual vaginal discharge, or dyspareunia
- Sexual history, including age at first intercourse, number of sexual partners in the past 6 months, number of lifetime partners, and presence of lesions in sexual partners
- Contraceptive history, including use of barrier methods
- HPV and other STIs in the patients and their partners
- Immunosuppression, including HIV infection
- Prior history of cancer or cancer therapy (e.g., radiation, chemotherapy, surgery)
- In utero DES exposure
- Date and result of the most recent Pap test
- Prior abnormal cervical cytology
- Menstrual history, including date of the last menstrual period
- Pregnancy history
- History of tobacco, drug, or alcohol use
- Family history of cervical cancer
- HPV immunization status

The physical examination should include a thorough pelvic, abdominal, inguinal lymph node, and rectal examination.

Cervical cancer usually begins around the cervical os. In its earliest stages, a cancerous cervix cannot be distinguished from a normal cervix. As the disease progresses, the cervix may appear abnormal, with gross erosion, ulcers, or a mass that bleeds easily on contact. In the late stages, an extensive, irregular, cauliflower-like growth may develop. The cervix may be hard and indurated, and its mobility may be restricted or lost. As the tumor enlarges, it grows by extending upward into the endometrial cavity, downward into the vagina, and laterally to the pelvic wall. It can invade the bladder and rectum directly. A bimanual examination can detect a mass or bleeding from tumor erosion.

Common sites for distant metastasis include the pelvic lymph nodes, liver, lungs, and bones (Boardman & Matthews, 2025). Metastasis to the liver may lead to findings of hepatomegaly. Leg edema is suggestive of tumor obstruction of the lymph or vascular systems. The triad findings of leg edema, pain, and hydronephrosis are indicative of spread to the pelvic wall (Boardman & Matthews, 2025).

Diagnostic Testing

Recommendations for cervical cancer screening continue to evolve. Research has demonstrated that 9 of 10 abnormal Pap tests will revert to normal. An intact immune system resolves approximately 90 percent of HPV infections (NCI, 2020b). The cost of treating precancerous cells or high-risk HPV infections that may spontaneously resolve without any intervention includes the anxiety of enduring more invasive and possibly painful testing procedures that have their own potential complications. The price of further diagnostic tests or interventions might also include a negative impact on future fertility and/or pregnancy (NCI, 2020b).

At the time of this book's publication, the most recent screening guidelines were published by the U.S. Preventive Services Task Force (USPSTF) in August 2018 and are in alignment with recommendations from the American College of Obstetricians and Gynecologists, the American Society for Colposcopy and Cervical Pathology, the American Cancer Society, and the American Society for Clinical Pathology. New screening guidelines are currently being developed and may be available following this edition's publication. It is important for clinicians to note that an individualized assessment of a person's risk profile, their subjective concerns, and assessment findings might justify an alternative treatment approach from current screening recommendations. The USPSTF reinforces this by pointing out that the recommendations do not apply to people who have previously been diagnosed with cervical cancer or a high-grade precancerous lesion, people who were exposed in utero to DES, and people who have a compromised immune system. In addition, recommendations for people aged 21 to 65 years apply regardless of HPV vaccination status or sexual history.

The 2018 USPSTF guidelines (**Table 28-3**) recognize the importance of HPV DNA testing, which was approved by the U.S. Food and Drug Administration (FDA) in 2014 as a replacement for cervical cytology testing (NCI, 2020c). Research has indicated that HPV DNA testing is more effective in detecting high-grade CIN and may be the most cost-effective and practical method of screening for people living in low-resource countries (WHO, 2021; Casas et al., 2022).

Over the past 10 years several changes in cervical cancer prevention, screening, and management have occurred, such as the increased use of liquid-based preparations for testing and co-testing (Pap test combined with high-risk HPV testing). The automated liquid-based Pap cytology has largely replaced conventional Pap tests. Although both tests appear to have similar efficacy for detecting cell abnormalities, the liquid-based testing enables the use of the same cell sample to test for high-risk types of HPV (NCI, n.d.-a).

Today there is a better understanding about the biology of HPV along with the approval and use of HPV vaccines. The terminology for histopathology has also changed during the past decade (Gadkari, Ravia, & Bhatia, 2022). For reporting results of cervical cytology, the Bethesda system was developed in 1988 to institute consistent terminology that ensured reliability between pathologists, laboratories, and clinicians. To ensure that the system reflects current research, revisions were made in 1991, 2001, and most recently in 2014 (Pangarkar, 2022).

TABLE 28-3 2018 USPSTF Cervical Cancer Screening Recommendations for Average-Risk Individuals

Age	Recommendation	Grade[a]
Younger than 21 years	No screening	D
Age 21 to 29 years	Screen with cervical cytology every 3 years	A
Age 30 to 65 years	Screen every 3 years with cervical cytology alone **or** Every 5 years with high-risk human papillomavirus (hrHPV) testing alone **or** Every 5 years with hrHPV testing in combination with cervical cytology (co-testing)	A
People older than age 65 who are not at risk and have had prior adequate screening	No screening	D
People who have had a hysterectomy with removal of the cervix and do not have a history of cervical cancer or a high-grade precancerous lesion	No screening	D

Data from US Preventive Services Task Force. (2018a). *Cervical cancer: Screening*. https://www.uspreventiveservicestaskforce.org/uspstf/recommendation/cervical-cancer-screening

[a]The USPSTF grade A indicates that the service is highly recommended. Grade D means that the USPSTF has recommended against the service because potential harm outweighs the benefit. Further information on grading is available on the USPSTF website (https://www.uspreventiveservicestaskforce.org/Page/Name/grade-definitions).

Cervical cytology requires a satisfactory specimen with at least 5,000 squamous cells for a liquid-based preparation and a minimum of 10 endocervical or squamous metaplastic cells (Pangarkar, 2022). Unsatisfactory specimens include those in which more than 75 percent of the epithelial cells are obscured, which may occur due to inflammation or blood (Sharma et al., 2020). The Bethesda system includes the general categories of "negative for intraepithelial lesion or malignancy," "epithelial cell abnormality," or "other," which may describe an unusual finding, such as endometrial cells that might require further investigation (Pangarkar, 2022). In people who are menstruating, it is normal to find exfoliated endometrial cells; however, the 2014 guidelines emphasize that benign-appearing endometrial cells for people aged 45 years and older need to be reported to alert practitioners about possible endometrial irregularities (Hernandez et al., 2020).

After ensuring an adequate specimen, the Bethesda system has an interpretation/result section that reports nonneoplastic findings (e.g., nonneoplastic cellular variations, reactive cellular changes, and glandular cells after hysterectomy) and identifies any organisms in the sample (e.g., *Candida*, *Trichomonas*, or cellular changes due to nonneoplastic viruses). The report then categorizes any epithelial cell abnormalities.

The Bethesda system considers abnormalities of squamous cells and glandular cells separately (**Table 28-4**). Squamous cells are found in the tissue that lines the ectocervix, whereas glandular cells line the endocervix. If there is an unusual or abnormal finding, the goal is to either document or rule out high-grade disease (CIN 3 or HSIL). This distinction is important because atypical glandular cells have an increased association with high-grade disease. Glandular cells are also specified according to cell type because treatment options may vary based on the type (Cianfrini et al., 2024).

Further Testing

Additional laboratory testing that might be indicated to rule out other causes of vaginal discharge or bleeding includes the following:

- STI testing: Chlamydia and gonorrhea are commonly encountered STIs that may produce symptoms similar to those of cervical cancer, namely dysuria, urinary frequency, vaginal discharge, and postcoital bleeding. Many other people who have chlamydia or gonorrhea are asymptomatic, however, so it is wise to test for HPV, chlamydia, and gonorrhea when a person presents with a vaginal discharge that has not resolved. Testing can be done using a single vaginal or cervical swab (CDC, 2019b).
- Wet mount preparation: People who have vulvovaginal candidiasis, bacterial vaginosis, or trichomoniasis can present with a variety of symptoms, including vaginal discharge, malodor, irritation, burning or itching, dysuria, and dyspareunia. Accurate identification of the pathogen requires microscopic examination of vaginal secretions. The microscopic examinations include a saline wet mount and a potassium hydroxide preparation (CDC, 2021a).
- Referral: People with suspicious lesions on physical examination require referral regardless of the cytology results (Boardman & Matthews, 2025). An abnormal Pap test may require a referral for colposcopic examination with a biopsy of the abnormal area.
- Endocervical curettage: A curette is inserted into the endocervical canal to remove tissue when the transformation zone is not visible. This procedure is aided by colposcopy.
- Cone biopsy: In this procedure, a cone-shaped tissue extending from the exocervix to the endocervical canal (including the transformation zone) is removed. The loop electrosurgical technique uses a wire hook heated by an electrical current to remove the tissue. A cold-knife biopsy uses either a surgical scalpel or a laser to remove tissue under anesthesia (ACS, 2020i).

In October 2019, the American Society for Colposcopy and Cervical Pathology and several other committed professional organizations developed *Risk-Based Management Consensus Guidelines* (American Society for Colposcopy and Cervical Pathology [ASCCP], 2019). The guidelines are designed to safely triage people with abnormal cervical cancer screening results. Research shows that risk-based management allows clinicians to better identify which patients will likely go on to develop precancer and which patients may be indicated to return to routine screening (ASCCP, 2019). These guidelines rely on individualized assessment of risk and take past history and current results into consideration. The estimation of risk uses newer technologies and will continue to be updated at a much more rapid rate than in the past, thereby adjusting to rapidly emerging science to keep the guidelines current. The American Society for Colposcopy and Cervical Pathology made the guidelines available in April 2020 on their website (https://www.asccp.org /Default.aspx).

Differential Diagnoses

Differential diagnoses for cervical cancer include the following conditions that must be ruled out prior to diagnosing cancer (Boardman & Matthews, 2025):

- Cervicitis (noninfectious related to trauma or chemical irritation; infectious related to STIs, such as chlamydia, *Neisseria gonorrhoeae*, HSV, and *Trichomonas*)
- Vaginitis
- Granulomatous (rare) or cervical polyps
- Pelvic inflammatory disease

Symptoms that are highly suggestive of cervical cancer may rarely be due to Paget disease, vaginal cancer, endometrial carcinoma, or primary myeloma.

Prevention

Primary Prevention

Since 2016, the only vaccine currently distributed in the United States for the prevention of cervical cancer is Human Papillomavirus 9-valent Vaccine Recombinant manufactured by Merck under the brand name Gardasil 9. This 9-valent (9vHPV) vaccine has replaced Cervarix, a bivalent (2vHPV) recombinant option, and its precursor, Gardasil, which was a quadrivalent (4vHPV) vaccine (CDC, 2024a). Gardasil 9 uses noninfectious virus-like particles prepared from the L1 capsid protein from HPV types 6, 11, 16, 18, 31, 33, 45, 52, and 58. This generates defensive, neutralizing antibodies to the aforementioned HPV types, providing protection from cervical, vulvar, vaginal, and anal cancer, as well as genital warts (condyloma acuminate) associated with HPV types 6 and 11 (Ashique et al., 2023).

The efficacy and safety of 9vHPV, which was licensed in 2014, was determined on data from seven prelicensure studies with

TABLE 28-4 2014 Bethesda Categories of Epithelial Cell Abnormalities

Category	Description
SQUAMOUS CELL	
ASC-US	Atypical squamous cells of undetermined significance. This term is used when the squamous cells do not appear completely normal, but it is not possible to determine the cause of the abnormal cells. Encompasses: infection with HPV; symptom of a benign growth (cyst or polyp); or low hormonal levels (seen in menopause). More testing such as HPV to be considered. An estimated 10–20% of people with ASC-UC may have CIN 2 or 3. An estimated 1 in 1,000 people with ASC-UC may have invasive cancer.
ASC-H	Atypical squamous cells—cannot exclude HSIL. May be precursor to cervical cancer if not treated. More testing is needed.
LSIL	Low-grade squamous intraepithelial lesion. Encompasses: • HPV transient infection • CIN 1 (mildly abnormal cells): Lesion involves the initial one third of the epithelial layer
HSIL	High-grade squamous intraepithelial lesion. Encompasses: • HPV persistent infection • Moderately abnormal cells (CIN 2) • Severely abnormal cells; includes carcinoma in situ (CIN 3)
Squamous carcinoma	Malignant cells penetrate the basement membrane of the cervical epithelium and infiltrate the stromal tissue (supporting tissue). In advanced cases, cancer may spread to adjacent organs such as the bladder or rectum, or to distant sites in the body via the bloodstream and lymphatic channels.
GLANDULAR CELL	
Atypical (Not otherwise Specified or Specify)	Endocervical cells Endometrial cells Glandular cells
Atypical (Favor neoplastic)	Endocervical cells Glandular cells
Endocervical adenocarcinoma in situ	Endocervical cells
Adenocarcinoma	Endocervical Endometrial Extrauterine Not otherwise specified (NOS)
OTHER	Specify other malignant neoplasms

Data from Pangarkar M. A. (2022). The Bethesda System for reporting cervical cytology. *CytoJournal*, 19, 28. https://doi.org/10.25259/CMAS_03_07_2021

Abbreviations: ASC-H, atypical squamous cells, cannot exclude HSIL; ASC-US, atypical squamous cells of undetermined significance; CIN, cervical intraepithelial neoplasia; HPV, human papillomavirus; HSIL, high-grade squamous intraepithelial neoplasia; LSIL, low-grade squamous intraepithelial neoplasia.

approximately 15,000 participants. Results indicated that the vaccine was well tolerated, with an adverse-effect profile similar to that of its precursor, 4vHPV (CDC, 2024a). Differences noted were more injection-site swelling and erythema and a higher spontaneous abortion rate than reported with the 4vHPV vaccine (although the spontaneous abortion rate was still within expectations for rates of early loss of pregnancy; therefore, there may not be a causal relationship).

Current recommendations from the Advisory Committee on Immunization Practices are to begin HPV immunization for people aged 11 or 12 years (or 9 years, if deemed necessary) and to follow a two-dose schedule (0, then 6 to 12 months) as long as the series is started between 9 and 14 years. For people beginning the series between the ages of 15 and 45, a three-dose schedule is recommended, spaced at 0, 2, 6 months (CDC, 2021b; CDC, 2021c). Early immunization, preferably in the teenage years, is important because the vaccine is most effective when administered before exposure to HPV and the body produces a more robust immune response when the vaccine is received at younger ages (ACS, 2024b). In a recent study of almost 1.7 million people, there was a nearly 90 percent reduction in cervical cancer incidence among people who received the vaccine prior to 17 years of age (Lei et al., 2020). Clearly, it is essential to vaccinate patients before they are potentially exposed to HPV. However, in 2018, the FDA did expand usage of Gardasil 9 to include people between the ages of 27 and 45 (Meites et al., 2019). This broadened expansion came with the realization that there was an estimated 90 percent prevention against persistent infection and disease caused by the HPV types in the vaccine.

People who already have abnormal cervical cytology results are still candidates for the vaccine because it does not treat current disease, but it will provide protection from infections caused by other HPV types. It is important to emphasize that vaccination does not eliminate the need for cervical cancer screening (CDC, 2024b). Following immunization, the identification and treatment of early precancerous lesions are critical to the prevention of cervical cancer. Screening is essential for both vaccinated and unvaccinated people (CDC, n.d.-h). Scheduling and keeping appointments for regular gynecologic examinations and Pap tests decreases the incidence and mortality of cervical cancer (NCI, 2020b). Abnormal changes in the cervix are readily detected by the Pap test and are easily cured before cancer develops. Preventive measures should include educating people that the risk of infection can be decreased by delaying the onset of sexual activity, decreasing the number of sexual partners, using condoms consistently, and eliminating tobacco use. Controversial, but reported in several studies, is also the protective effect of having a partner whose penis is circumcised (Punjani et al., 2022). Contraindications for receiving the vaccine include hypersensitive or severe allergic reactions to yeast or a previous dose of Gardasil 9.

The HPV vaccine is not recommended during pregnancy, but it may be given to patients who are breastfeeding (CDC, 2019a). ACOG recommends HPV vaccination for individuals who are breastfeeding and 26 years of age or younger (ACOG, 2020). People who have inadvertently received a first dose during pregnancy may be reassured that there is no evidence from clinical trials or through interim analysis of 5 years of pregnancy registry data that suggests the immunization increases the risk of adverse outcomes (CDC, 2019a; ACOG, 2020). Practitioners are requested to contact the appropriate manufacturers' registry to add to the knowledge base regarding safety during pregnancy (CDC, n.d.-f).

Management

The choice of treatment depends primarily on the stage of disease at the time of diagnosis, but other factors, such as a person's general health and preferences, should also be considered (ACS, 2020j). The quest to identify the cellular events that stimulate carcinogenesis continues because this understanding ultimately will enable better tumor classification and prognostication (Balasubramaniam et al., 2019). Current technology allows for analysis of DNA, RNA, and proteins; thus, genetic and molecular studies can be performed on blood and tissue samples obtained during operative evaluation and treatment of the cancer (Nikanjam, Kato, & Kurzrock, 2022). Findings from these studies will provide a path for the development of a classification system that is based on genomic and proteomic foundations.

Pharmacologic Treatment

A gynecologic oncologist will review several options, including participation in clinical trials, for people with locally advanced and advanced stages of cervical cancer (Abu-Rustum et al., 2023). When surgical options are limited, cervical cancer is treated with external beam radiation therapy (EBRT), intensity-modulated radiotherapy (IMRT), and/or brachytherapy (internal RT) (Burmeister et al., 2022). External-beam radiation therapy may be augmented with internal brachytherapy (Williamson et al., 2021). Adding chemotherapy as an adjunct has been shown to boost positive response to radiation. The use of platinum compounds (e.g., cisplatin) is standard treatment, followed by plant alkaloids (e.g., paclitaxel) and topoisomerase inhibitors (e.g., topotecan). Adding bevacizumab—a monoclonal antibody that inhibits angiogenesis and slows the growth of new blood vessels supplying cancer cells—appears to increase survival rate by 3.5 months without adversely affecting quality of life (Burmeister et al., 2022). A recent new adverse event associated with bevacizumab is the development of rectovaginal and vesicovaginal fistulas in patients who had previously received pelvic radiotherapy (Kim, Choi, et al., 2021). Despite this potential, adding bevacizumab with chemotherapy is considered first-line treatment for people experiencing recurrent or metastatic cervical carcinoma (Kim, Choi, et al., 2021).

First-line single agents include cisplatin and carboplatin. Metastatic or recurrent cervical cancer requires combination therapy, including the use of pembrolizumab (Monk et al., 2023; Abu-Rustum et al., 2023) or Atezolizumab (Oaknin, Gladieff, et al., 2024; NCCN 2024a). First-line preferred combination therapies include pembrolizumab/cisplatin/paclitaxel +/- bevacizumab, pembrolizumab/carboplatin/paclitaxel +/- bevacizumab, cisplatin/paclitaxel/bevacizumab, carboplatin/paclitaxel/bevacizumab, atezolizumab/cisplatin/paclitaxel/bevacizumab,andatezolizumab/carboplatin/paclitaxel/bevacizumab (Abu-Rustum et al., 2023).

Surgical Treatment

Cervical cancer is complex to stage and uses the FIGO and AJCC TNM systems. Results from physical exam, imaging test, biopsies, or other tests, such as cystoscopy and laparoscopy, are used to determine a clinical stage that helps determine treatment options (ACS, 2020b; NCI, 2024b). Treatment of precancerous lesions and carcinoma in situ (stage 0; Tis, N0, M0) includes cryosurgery or laser ablation to kill abnormal cells. Loop electrosurgical excision or cold-knife conization can be used for definitive treatment in people with early-stage IA1 (T1a1, N0, M0) who want to preserve fertility (ACS, 2020j; NCI, 2024b). After treatment, patients require lifelong surveillance at regular intervals. The clinician determines the timing and frequency of follow-up based on Pap test results and colposcopy examinations (NCI, 2020b).

Hysterectomy is a choice for stage IA1 cancers and some stage 0 disease if cone biopsy reveals positive margins. For cervical cancer stages IA2 (T1a2, N0, M0), IB (T1b, N0, M0N0M), and sometimes IIA (T2a, N0, M0), a radical hysterectomy removing the uterus, parametria and uterosacral ligaments, upper part of the vagina, and sometimes lymph nodes is indicated (NCI, 2024b). Postoperative complications associated with any pelvic surgery can include urinary incontinence, surgical wound infection, or deep vein thrombosis (Jing et al., 2022). Oftentimes, the ovaries and fallopian tubes are preserved. Patients might need emotional support for issues such as loss of fertility, possible need for a catheter because voiding can be difficult with the disruption of nerves, and concerns regarding sexuality. Clinicians can reassure patients that the clitoral area is not disturbed and that their ability to have sexual relations and achieve orgasm will remain intact (Abu-Rustum et al., 2023). Individuals and their partners may need counseling for feelings of loss or difficulty with intimacy.

A surgical option is available to people with IA2, IB, or IIA cervical cancer who want to preserve fertility and have lesions smaller than 2 cm. A trachelectomy removes the cervix and upper part of the vagina while preserving the body of the uterus (ACS, 2025b; NCI, 2020b). Patients who are not eligible for this procedure should be encouraged to consult with a reproductive specialist regarding embryo or oocyte cryopreservation prior to surgery.

Other options for people with stage IA2, IB, or IIA cancer include bypassing surgery and choosing external-beam pelvic radiation plus internal brachytherapy. When biopsies have positive margins, chemotherapy is added to the radiation therapy. Definitive radiation therapy has growing support in the literature (ACS, 2020i; Chino et al., 2020). Patients will still require reproductive counseling because radiation therapy has been associated with early menopause (ACS, 2024b).

Advanced-stage cervical cancers—that is, IIB (T2b, N0 M0), III (T3, N0, M0), or IVA (T4, N0, M0)—are usually not treated with surgery. Instead, external pelvic radiation with internal brachytherapy is combined with chemotherapy. Special attention is given to imaging studies (MRI, PET scan) to ascertain possible metastasis. The treatment of stage IVB (any T, any N, M1) cervical cancer is primarily palliative because cure is not possible. Palliative radiation may be used to control bleeding, pelvic pain, or urinary or bowel obstruction from pelvic disease. Current clinical trials are examining the efficacy of new chemotherapy regimens (ACS, 2020b; Abu-Rustum et al., 2023).

People with recurrent cervical cancer are candidates for total pelvic exenteration, which extends the removal of organs and tissues from the radical hysterectomy to include pelvic lymph node dissection and, depending on spread, removal of the bladder, vagina, rectum, and part of the colon. Emotional and physical recovery needs are extensive when such surgery is performed because the patient must learn to manage urostomy and colostomy sites and may have difficulty with edema in the legs from removal of lymph nodes. A new vagina may be surgically constructed and, if desired, a person can resume a satisfactory sex life (ACS, 2025b; Abu-Rustum et al., 2023).

Emerging Evidence That May Change Management

Screening Tests

Ongoing research into more specific screening tests and monitoring for disease progression is yielding promising results. HPV tests that identify the viral DNA, mRNA, or E6 and E7 oncoproteins found on oncogenic HPV types are already on the market (White et al., 2024). Although there are five FDA-approved tests for primary screening, four detect HPV DNA, and only Cobas and BD Onclarity are approved as a single test. Hybrid Capture [HC2], Cervista, and the Aptima HPV assay are used in co-testing. The Cobas HPV DNA test and the Aptima HPV assay detect 14 high-risk HPV types, including HPV 16 and 18 (White et al., 2024). These types of HPV detection tests have been shown to have higher sensitivity for identifying CIN 2/3 lesions and have great promise for communities with lower resources who do not have the infrastructure for analyzing cytology results (Mahajan et al., 2024).

Another area of investigation is changes in the levels of microRNA molecules in infected tissues, which might be exploited in monitoring for disease progression (NCI, 2020b).

Avoidance of unnecessary treatment is being addressed in current research studies. The ASCUS-LSIL Triage Study is trying to identify biomarkers that might predict whether a person's immune response will effectively clear low-grade cervical lesions. The Study to Understand Cervical Cancer Early Endpoints (SUCCEED) is seeking to elucidate the molecular distinctions that occur throughout each stage of cancer progression to identify biomarkers that might assist with management decisions (NCI, 2020b).

Therapeutic Vaccines

Vaccines for treating established high-grade cervical dysplasia by triggering the immune response are also under ongoing investigation. These DNA recombinant vaccines use the HPV 16 E7 antigen and the HPV 16 and HPV 18 E6 and E7 antigens to stimulate an immune response that has been shown to resect cervical tissue (NCI, 2020b).

Pharmacologic Therapy

Promising research into immunotherapy is examining alternatives for second-line therapies. Medications that block immunosuppressive checkpoints allow for an appropriate response to attacking cancer cells. Tumor cell antigens avoid immune detection through a costimulatory pathway primarily through programmed cell death protein-1 (PD-1) and cytotoxic T-lymphocyte protein-4 (CTLA-4). Infusing antibodies to antagonize the CTLA-4 immune checkpoint (ipilimumab) is continuing to be studied in clinical trials for both tolerance and efficacy (ACS, 2020c; Oaknin, Moore, et al., 2024). Pembrolizumab and Nivolumab, which bind to the PD-1 receptor on T cells have already been proven to be efficacious in chemotherapy regimens for cervical carcinoma (Monk et al., 2023; NCCN 2024a).

Researchers also continue to study the best doses and combinations of chemotherapeutic agents that are more effective and best tolerated. One area of interest is the use of plant extracts such as glycyrrhizic acid, which is derived from licorice, as antiviral agents (Bravo et al., 2023). Another curiosity under study is a nutritional supplement, active hexose correlated compound, which is derived from a Japanese mushroom and has shown promise in eradicating persistent HPV infection (Smith et al., 2022). Still another area of research is carrageenan, a compound extracted from seaweed and widely used for its gelatin effects in the food industry; it shows promise for inhibiting HPV as a topical microbicide (NCI, n.d.-b).

Patient Education

HPV vaccination guidance has changed significantly since 2011. The CDC's Advisory Committee on Immunization Practices (ACIP) recommended the 3-dose HPV series for only female children from 2008–2011. Then, from 2011–2016, it was recommended that all children receive the 3-dose series. In 2016, ACIP recommended vaccination before the age of 15 and with two doses (NCI, 2024c). Immunization rates for HPV in 2022 in adolescents 13–17 years old who received 1 or more HPV doses was 76 percent whereas 62.6 percent were up to date. HPV vaccination was lowest among teens who were uninsured and insured by Medicaid (Pingali, 2024). In the United States, HPV is the most common sexually transmitted infection (Reiter, Bustamante, & McRee, 2020) and clinicians play an important role in advocating for HPV vaccination and dispelling misinformation that vaccination encourages sexual activity or is not safe. Clinicians should adhere to ACIP guidelines and encourage their adolescent patients to receive HPV vaccination with other routine vaccinations such as tetanus, diphtheria, and acellular pertussis vaccine; and the quadrivalent meningococcal conjugate vaccine (Pingali et al., 2024).

People who have received the full HPV immunization series should be encouraged to engage in cervical cancer screening. Education and reeducation regarding the screening protocols, along with phone or letter reminders, are important to integrate into practice. When discussing an abnormal Pap test, clinicians need to be aware that precancerous lesions are often associated with a diagnosis of cancer. Clarifying misperceptions and education regarding the treatment protocols for early lesions can alleviate stress.

Finally, clinicians need to educate people on the association between HPV infection and cervical cancer and review STI prevention strategies and safe sex practices (CDC, n.d.-h). Young patients need to be advised of the importance of delaying the risk of HPV exposure through delaying the onset of sexual activity, decreasing the number of sexual partners, using condoms to decrease risk, and eliminating use of tobacco products. In the past, screening for cervical cancer was offered at intervals less than 3–5 years and was also an opportunity to offer chlamydia testing. Astute clinicians need to evaluate risk factors and educate patients on the need for sexually transmitted disease screening, even on visits not warranting cervical cancer screening.

Considerations for Specific Populations

Disparities in Screening

Studies have found that persons who are from minoritized groups, who live in rural areas, the Midwest or parts of the South, have less than a high school education, are of lower socioeconomic status, and are uninsured, underinsured, or insured by Medicaid face more barriers to screening than their counterparts which increases their risk of cervical cancer and morbidity and mortality associated with the disease (Johnson et al., 2020; ACSCAN, 2024). A history of sexual abuse can lead to stress with, and avoidance of, pelvic exams which in turn decreases cervical cancer screening in these individuals (Danan et al., 2022). Providing cervical cancer literacy education to high-risk groups is essential to eliminating these disparities. Sensitivity to potential avoidance of screening exams by offering a comfortable, trauma-informed environment and promoting simple choices, when possible, may assist with adherence (Kohler et al., 2021).

Treatment During Pregnancy

Cervical cancer is the most common gynecologic malignancy during pregnancy. Fortunately, most patients are diagnosed in stage I. No treatment is warranted for preinvasive lesions of the cervix during pregnancy, although expert colposcopy is recommended to exclude the possibility of invasive cervical cancer. Treatment of invasive cervical cancer depends on the stage of the cancer and the gestational age at diagnosis. When the cancer is diagnosed before fetal maturity, the traditional approach is to recommend immediate therapy appropriate for the stage of disease. Other reports suggest that if the cancer is in the early stages, delaying therapy may be a reasonable option to allow for improved fetal viability (NCI, 2020b; Abu-Rustum et al., 2023). Most experts advocate a cesarean birth at fetal viability with concurrent radical hysterectomy and pelvic node dissection (Abu-Rustum et al., 2023). Management of cervical cancer during pregnancy is a complex dilemma and requires a multidisciplinary approach.

ENDOMETRIAL CANCER

Description of Endometrial Cancer

The majority of cancers affecting the uterine corpus are adenocarcinomas affecting the endometrium (ACS, 2019h; NCI, 2025). Per the American Cancer Society, carcinoma of the endometrium is the most prevalent gynecologic malignancy and the fourth most common malignant neoplasm in people with a uterus in the United States, after breast, lung, and colon cancers (ACS, 2019h). However, when you adjust for the premenopausal hysterectomy rate, endometrial cancer is the second most common cancer overall in individuals born with gynecologic organs in the United States (Doll & Winn, 2019). Globally, endometrial cancer ranks as the 6th most common cancer for people with gynecologic organs and the 15th most common overall malignancy (Bray et al., 2024). Interestingly, the incidence of endometrial cancer is greater in high-resource countries than in low-resource countries, although the risk of dying from endometrial cancer is greater in the latter. It is theorized that the increased incidence observed in high-resource countries is due to the larger number of people who have a larger body size and who are physically inactive. Both obesity and physical inactivity are risk factors for endometrial cancer (NCI, 2025; Mazidimoradi et al., 2024).

In 2025, approximately 69,120 new cases of endometrial cancer and 13,860 deaths from endometrial cancer were estimated to occur in the United States (NCI, 2025) compared to 61,880 new cases and 12,160 deaths in 2015 (NCI, 2019). Between 2012–2021, the incident rate of this disease increased by 0.7 percent per year, and the death rate increased by an average of 1.5 percent each year from 2013–2022 (SEER, n.d.-b; NCI, 2025). Although the majority of sources state that the incidence of endometrial cancer is higher in white individuals than in Black individuals, these estimates do not take into account the higher rate of premenopausal hysterectomies in Black individuals compared to their white counterparts. When hysterectomy is adjusted for, research has elucidated a higher incidence of endometrial cancer in Black individuals since 2002 (Doll & Winn, 2019). Additionally, Black individuals have a 55 percent higher 5-year mortality risk compared to white individuals (Doll, Snyder, & Ford, 2018) and deaths were nearly twice as frequent when compared to any other racial or ethnic group (Whetstone et al., 2022).

Significant disparities in endometrial cancer diagnosis and treatment among different racial and ethnic groups exist. At diagnosis, advanced stage disease is more common in Black and Latiné individuals (Whetstone et al., 2022). Guideline-concordant diagnostic procedures are less likely to be used with Black patients (Whetstone et al., 2022). Non-endometrioid histology is known to be more aggressive and presents in 28 percent of Black patients compared to 10–11 percent of Latiné, Asian, and white patients (Doll, Snyder, & Ford 2018). A mortality gap exists between Black patients and white patients with high-risk histology; however, this gap is nonexistent in large studies of institutions where a large proportion of the patient population is Black (Doll, Snyder, & Ford 2018). In regard to treatment, Black and Latiné patients are less likely to receive a hysterectomy, surgery, definitive surgical management, lymph node sampling or lymph node dissection. These communities are also less likely to receive minimally invasive surgery. Black patients are less likely to receive chemotherapy and Black, Latiné, and Indigenous patients are less likely to have guideline-compliant treatment (Whetstone et al., 2022).

Considering the disparate treatment of endometrial cancer among various racial and ethnic groups when compared to white individuals, it is imperative to acknowledge race as a social construct unrelated to biology and to understand how racism leads to a multitude of poor outcomes stemming from the unequal allocation of opportunity and resources. As such, disparities in endometrial cancer morbidity and mortality are related to the sociopolitical climate, including racism, and cannot be largely attributed to high-risk histology in minoritized racial or ethnic groups (Doll, Snyder, & Ford, 2018).

Most diagnoses of endometrial cancer in the United States occur between the ages of 45 and 74 with a median age of diagnosis at 64 years (SEER, n.d.-b). Interestingly, the most common cause of death among people diagnosed with endometrial cancer is cardiovascular disease. Research has shown that there is a higher prevalence of cardiovascular disease in patients with endometrial cancer at the time of their diagnosis than their matched counterparts and this most likely reflects shared metabolic risk factors between the two diseases (Anderson et al., 2022).

Etiology and Pathophysiology

Endometrial cancer is sometimes classified into two types. Type I, or estrogen-dependent endometrial cancer, is the most common and is diagnosed in more than 75 percent of cases. It is caused by an excess of endogenous or exogenous estrogen unopposed by progesterone. Long-term unopposed estrogen exposure allows for continued endometrial growth and the development of hyperplasia with or without atypia. The resulting tumors are usually low grade and have a favorable prognosis. A phosphatase and tensin homolog (PTEN) genetic mutation is commonly seen in these types of endometrial cancers. Histologic types include endometrioid adenocarcinomas (most cases); adenosquamous tumors, which contain elements of both glandular and squamous epithelium; and other rare variants, such as ciliated carcinoma. These types of well-differentiated tumors usually limit their spread to the surface of the endometrium (ACS, 2019h; ACOG, 2015, reaffirmed 2020; NCI, 2024e). For endometrial cancer, grading is dependent on the organization of cancer cells into glands that resemble normal tissue. Grades 1 and 2 are associated with type 1 endometrial cancer (ACS, 2019h).

Type II endometrial cancer accounts for approximately 10 to 30 percent of cases, is more common in people of smaller body size, and is traditionally thought to be estrogen independent because the endometrium is generally atrophic or has polyps with this type of disease. These neoplasms consist of poorly differentiated prognostic cell types (such as papillary serous or clear cell tumors), which often present as aggressive, higher-grade tumors that are more often diagnosed at an advanced stage and have a high risk of metastases and mortality, regardless of stage at diagnosis (ACS, 2019h; ACOG, 2015, reaffirmed 2020; NCI, 2025; Ebring et al., 2023). Overexpression of oncogenes p53 and HER-2/neu are more common in these types of endometrial cancers (NCI, 2025). Approximately 4 percent of type II cancers are uterine carcinosarcomas, also known as malignant mixed mesodermal tumors or malignant mixed Müllerian tumors, which have characteristics of both sarcomas and endometrial carcinomas (ACS, 2019h). Type II cancers are at a higher grade of 3, meaning that less than 50 percent of the cancer cells are in glandular form with a large degree of disorganization (ACS, 2019h). Another type II endometrial cancer is uterine carcinosarcoma, formerly known as malignant mixed Müllerian tumors (MMMTs). Containing features of a sarcoma, this type of rare cancer is thought to occur by chance, although there have been cases of carcinosarcoma in people who also have Lynch syndrome, a genetic condition predisposing people to develop uterine cancer (Sia et al., 2023).

There is an acknowledgment that the inter-rater reliability for classifying endometrial cancers is only moderate (0.41 to 0.68) among pathologists. This has potentially led to either over- or undertreatment regimens that potentially impact the quality of life for people diagnosed with endometrial cancer. In a new era of genomics, researchers using the Cancer Genome Atlas have now identified four molecular subtype groups of endometrial cancer: POLE (polymerase epsilon), microsatellite instability hypermutated, copy number low, and copy number high (López-Reig et al., 2019).

Risk Factors

Endometrial carcinoma has been linked to a genetic predisposition for the disease. As many as 3 percent of diagnoses occur in people who have the autosomal dominant syndrome known as Lynch syndrome (also called hereditary nonpolyposis colorectal cancer) (Post et al., 2021) with a lifetime risk of 25–60 percent, depending on the variant (ACOG 2015, reaffirmed 2020). Lynch syndrome manifests as heritable mutations in a germ line affecting mismatch repair genes—MLH1, MSH2, MSH6, EPCAM, and PMS2 (Post et al., 2021). Endometrial cancer can occur earlier in individuals with Lynch syndrome, including those who are premenopausal, and the average age of diagnosis in this population is 47–55 years (Underkofler & Ring, 2023). This syndrome is associated with a 4–2 percent lifetime risk of developing ovarian cancer and a 52–82 percent lifetime risk of developing colon cancer (ACOG 2015, reaffirmed 2020). In the United States, the prevalence of Lynch syndrome is estimated to be 1 in 279 people (Medline Plus, 2021).

Cowden disease (also known as multiple hamartoma syndrome) is another autosomal dominant disorder that involves germ line mutations of the tumor suppressing the PTEN gene and is associated with increased lifetime risks for endometrial (5–10%), colon (9%), breast (25–50%) (ACOG 2015, reaffirmed 2020), and thyroid (35–38%) cancer (Pîrlog et al., 2024). It is a rare hereditary syndrome with a prevalence of 1 in 200,000 (ACOG, 2015, reaffirmed 2020).

Although the exact cause of endometrial cancer is unknown, the current understanding of risk factors helps to identify people at risk for type I endometrial cancer due to estrogen excess. Risk factors associated with exogenous sources of estrogen include the following:

- Estrogen therapy (ET): For people with a uterus, the risk of endometrial cancer associated with unopposed estrogen use for 5 or more years is 20 times higher, compared with the risk in individuals not taking ET. Adding progestogen therapy continuously or for at least 10 days per month significantly mitigates this risk (NCI, 2024e; ACOG, 2015, reaffirmed 2020). Guidelines from the American College of Obstetricians and Gynecologists continue to advise clinicians to limit ET for menopausal symptoms to the lowest effective dose and shortest duration. Treatment decisions need to be individualized according to severity of symptom concerns and an analysis of risk versus benefit, regardless of age (ACOG, 2015, reaffirmed 2020). The North American Menopause Society 2022 clinical guidelines indicate a positive benefit-to-risk ratio for using hormone therapy in people younger than age 60 or in those who are within 10 years of menopause and are experiencing vasomotor symptoms or who are at risk for bone loss (North American Menopause Society, 2022). Clinicians are encouraged to consider the formulation, type of hormone replacement, route, and dose to achieve a balance between benefits and risks.
- Selective estrogen receptor modifier: Tamoxifen (Nolvadex), when used for chemoprevention of breast cancer, increases the risk of endometrial cancer nearly fourfold for people aged 50 years and older (NCI, 2024e; ACOG, 2015, reaffirmed 2020). A selective estrogen receptor modulator (SERM), tamoxifen has site-specific activity in different tissues. It suppresses growth in breast tissue but stimulates growth of the endometrial lining (NCI, 2024e; ACOG, 2015, reaffirmed 2020). Raloxifene, another SERM, has not been associated as a risk factor for endometrial cancer. The potential risk of using ospemifene, a SERM approved for treatment of dyspareunia, needs further postmarket assessment (ACOG, 2015, reaffirmed 2020).

Risk factors associated with endogenous sources of estrogen include the following:

- Early menarche: Starting menstruation before age 12 increases the number of years during which the endometrium is exposed to estrogen (ACOG, 2015, reaffirmed 2020; NCI, 2024e).
- Late menopause: Menopause occurring after age 50 increases the duration of estrogen exposure (ACOG, 2015, reaffirmed 2020; NCI, 2024e).
- History of infertility or nulliparity: During pregnancy, the hormonal balance shifts toward more progesterone, which protects the uterine lining (endometrium) (ACS, 2025c). Progesterone seems to expedite removal of premalignant cells, and pregnancy creates a protective immunity-mediated effect (ACOG, 2015, reaffirmed 2020). Consequently, people who have had many pregnancies have a reduced risk of developing endometrial cancer, whereas people who are infertile or who have never been pregnant have an increased risk (ACOG, 2015, reaffirmed 2020; NCI, 2025). Late age for a last pregnancy (40 years or older) also has a protective effect by further decreasing estrogen exposure just prior to menopause.
- Larger body size: The majority of people who develop endometrial cancer tend to have a larger body size. There is a 200 to 400 percent linear increase in risk for people who have a larger amount of adipose tissue. People who are young and diagnosed with endometrial cancer are more likely to have more adiposity, be nulliparous, and have type I well-differentiated histology (ACOG, 2015, reaffirmed 2020). People who have larger amounts of adipose tissue have higher levels of endogenous estrogen as a result of the conversion of androstenedione to estrone and the aromatization of androgens to estradiol—both are processes that occur in peripheral adipose tissue (ACS, 2019h; ACOG, 2015, reaffirmed 2020; NCI, 2024e).
- Chronic anovulation: Anovulation is a common cause of infertility and may be attributable to several factors. One of the leading causes of chronic anovulation is polycystic ovary syndrome (PCOS). People with PCOS have excess androgens and elevated luteinizing hormone and normal or low follicle-stimulating hormone levels. They may also have elevated levels of free estrogen owing to the peripheral conversion of androgens to estrogens and the decreased production of sex hormone-binding globulin in the liver, which serves to increase the unopposed effects of estrogen over time (ACS, 2019h). Please refer to Chapter 26 for more information about PCOS.
- Diabetes: Type 2 diabetes and hypertension have been associated with increased adiposity and up to a threefold increased risk for endometrial cancer. People who have less adiposity and have diabetes also have an increased risk of endometrial cancer (ACS, 2019h; ACOG, 2015, reaffirmed 2020).
- High-fat diet: Consumption of a high-fat diet may lead to larger body size which is a well-documented risk factor for endometrial cancer. Some researchers believe that fatty foods may also have a direct effect on estrogen metabolism, thereby increasing the risk for endometrial cancer (ACS, 2019h).
- Ovarian cancer: Certain ovarian tumors, such as granulosa theca cell tumors, produce estrogen, thereby increasing a person's risk of developing endometrial cancer (ACS, 2019h).

Other risk factors for endometrial cancer include increased age, smoking (for type II cancers), sedentary lifestyle, history of pelvic radiation to treat another cancer, and endometrial hyperplasia.

Clinical Presentation

Endometrial cancer occurs most frequently in people who are postmenopausal. The average age at diagnosis is approximately 64 years (NCI, 2025), with 15 percent of people being diagnosed before age 50 and 5 percent before age 40 (ACOG, 2015, reaffirmed 2020). Younger people usually have specific risk factors, such as morbid obesity, chronic anovulation, and heredity syndromes. The most common symptom—present in 90 percent of people—is abnormal uterine bleeding. In people who are menstruating, this symptom can take the form of bleeding between periods or excessive, prolonged menstrual flow. In people who are postmenopausal, any bleeding is considered abnormal and should be evaluated (ACS, 2019h; ACOG, 2015, reaffirmed 2020; NCI, 2025). Advanced symptoms include pelvic pain, abdominal distention with or without pain, bloating, change in bowel or bladder pattern, and change in appetite (ACOG, 2015, reaffirmed 2020).

Assessment

History and Physical Examination

Key pieces of information that assist the clinician in identifying people at high risk for endometrial cancer include the character of the bleeding, the pattern of the flow, and the number of pads used when bleeding occurs. Inquire about accompanying problems (e.g., dyspareunia, pain, bladder or bowel problems); ask the person if they are experiencing any unusual vaginal discharge or if they have ever been diagnosed with an STI. Obtain a menstrual history and inquire if the person is taking any hormones. Ask about the possibility of pregnancy and whether they have experienced any symptoms of pregnancy (e.g., missed period, breast/chest tenderness, or nausea and vomiting). If they have previously been pregnant, obtain a pregnancy history in addition to medical and family histories. Be sure to ask the person if they have a personal or family history of breast, ovarian, endometrial, pancreatic, or colorectal cancer. Ask if they have experienced infertility problems or if they have a history of PCOS (ACS, 2019h; NCI, 2025).

The physical examination should include a thorough abdominal, inguinal lymph node, pelvic, vaginal, and rectal examination. Abnormal bleeding from the genital tract can occur from the vagina, cervix, uterus, or fallopian tubes. Inspect the external genitalia for lesions or atrophic vaginitis, which may be the cause of the bleeding. Perform a vaginal examination to determine whether the bleeding is caused by vaginal or cervical infection. Note the amount, color, consistency, and odor of the vaginal discharge; determine whether the cervix is friable or has an unusual discharge and examine the patient for cervical polyps.

Perform a bimanual examination. Palpate the cervix, which normally feels smooth, firm, evenly rounded, and mobile. Note any cervical motion tenderness. Next, palpate the uterus, ovaries, and inguinal lymph nodes. Note uterine size and contour. Endometrial cancer seldom causes much uterine enlargement, and any increase in size usually occurs slowly. Uterine fibroids usually feel firm and may make the uterus asymmetrical. Note any enlargement of the ovaries and lymph nodes. Lastly, perform a rectal examination to identify lesions or other abnormalities.

Metastatic spread of endometrial cancer occurs in a characteristic pattern, commonly to the pelvic and para-aortic nodes. Common sites for distant metastasis include the lungs, inguinal and supraclavicular lymph nodes, liver, bones, brain, and vagina (ACS, 2019h).

Diagnostic Testing

There is currently no screening test to detect endometrial cancer. In particular, a Pap test is not effective in detecting endometrial cancer. Nevertheless, the finding of atypical glandular cells in a postmenopausal person is suggestive of uterine malignancy and requires further investigation by transvaginal ultrasound or endometrial biopsy, as does any postmenopausal bleeding (NCI, 2025).

Transvaginal Ultrasound Transvaginal ultrasound is used as an adjunctive means of evaluation for endometrial hyperplasia and polyps, myomas, and structural abnormalities of the uterus. An endometrial thickness of 4 mm or less indicates that biopsy can be deferred. Because rare cases of type II endometrial cancer present with endometrial thickness of 3 mm or less, ongoing symptoms of bleeding require biopsy. Additionally, research has shown that relying on endometrial thickness measurement via ultrasound at the 5 mm threshold resulted in a 11.4 percent chance of not identifying endometrial carcinoma in Black patients. Given this new data, any postmenopausal person presenting with bleeding should have tissue sampling performed (Doll et al., 2024). Persistent bleeding in the face of a negative biopsy also requires further investigation. For people who are premenopausal, the value of imaging is questionable because the measurement of endometrial thickness is irrelevant (ACOG, 2015, reaffirmed 2020). The clinician must make a decision to biopsy based on the clinical presentation and symptoms.

Endometrial Biopsy Endometrial biopsy is an office procedure that is now the primary method for histologic sampling of the endometrium (Dermawan et al., 2019; ACOG, 2015, reaffirmed 2020). The biopsy is obtained with an endometrial suction catheter that is inserted through the cervix into the uterine cavity. Endometrial biopsy detects 80 to 90 percent of endometrial cancers if an adequate tissue sample is obtained. However, it is estimated that 36 percent of biopsies do not obtain an adequate amount of tissue for diagnosis (NCI, 2019). If the biopsy result fails to provide sufficient diagnostic information or if abnormal bleeding persists, a dilation and curettage (D & C) with a hysteroscopy is recommended (NCI, 2025; ACOG, 2015, reaffirmed 2020). Appendix 25-A outlines the steps in performing an endometrial biopsy.

Dilation and Curettage D & C is the gold standard for assessing uterine bleeding and diagnosing endometrial cancer. If endometrial biopsy findings are inadequate or negative with ongoing symptoms of bleeding, or if the endometrial thickness as assessed by transvaginal ultrasound is greater than 4 mm, or if a high degree of suspicion exists, the patient needs a D & C under anesthesia to exclude malignancy (NCI, 2025; ACOG, 2015, reaffirmed 2020).

Hysteroscopy Hysteroscopy is used in the office setting to directly visualize the uterine cavity. With this technique, a tiny telescope is introduced through the cervix into the uterus. After filling the uterus with saline, the practitioner can visualize and biopsy suspicious areas. Hysteroscopy is not required in conjunction with the D & C, but it is recommended because it provides the best opportunity to examine the endometrium and confirm premalignant endometrial lesions (ACOG, 2015, reaffirmed 2020).

CA-125 Levels Elevated CA-125 levels are associated with some endometrial cancers. Extremely high levels are suggestive of metastasis beyond the uterus. Evaluation of CA-125 is another assessment option for people where surgical risks outweigh the benefits of surgical intervention (ACS, 2019g).

Referral

People who are diagnosed with endometrial cancer require surgical staging. Exceptions would be in people whose surgical risks outweigh the benefits of surgical intervention and require assessment of potential metastasis sites with imaging

(CT, MRI, PET/CT). In any case, decisions made preoperatively are complex and best suited to physicians with advanced expertise in endometrial carcinoma. A referral to a gynecologic oncologist ensures a comprehensive evaluation of the need for preoperative imaging (CT, MRI, PET/CT), extent of comprehensive staging or debulking, and best treatment options (ACOG, 2015, reaffirmed 2020).

Differential Diagnoses

The differential diagnoses for genital bleeding depend on the clinical picture. Bleeding from the lower genital tract can occur from the vagina (carcinoma, lacerations, trauma, infections, or atrophic changes with age) or the cervix (cervicitis, STIs, polyps, or cervical carcinoma). It may also occur from the uterus (carcinoma, fibroids, polyps, pregnancy, or dysfunctional uterine bleeding) or the fallopian tubes (pelvic inflammatory disease, ectopic pregnancy). People with a uterus who are on hormone replacement therapy may experience breakthrough bleeding (NCI, 2019; Manley et al., 2024).

Management

Primary Prevention

Although most cases of endometrial cancer cannot be prevented, several factors are associated with a decreased incidence of endometrial cancer:

- COCs: The risk of endometrial hyperplasia is increased by the presence of unopposed estrogen. Thus, using a COC instead of an estrogen-only contraceptive prevents the proliferative effect of estrogen, thereby decreasing the risk of developing abnormal endometrial hyperplasia, which might eventually result in endometrial cancer (ACS, 2019h). The chance of developing endometrial cancer due to unopposed estrogen is related to both risk and duration, and it remains increased for years after stopping use of unopposed estrogen. These effects are ameliorated by adding progestins in the correct dose and duration (ACS, 2019h; NCI, 2024e). Other measures known to minimize risk include the use of depot medroxyprogesterone acetate and use of a levonorgestrel-releasing intrauterine device (ACS, 2019h).
- Physical activity: Studies investigating the relationship between physical activity and the risk of endometrial cancer have shown an associated 38–46 percent relative decrease in risk (NCI, 2024e). It is believed that physical activity modifies the risk of endometrial cancer by reducing adiposity, a known risk factor for endometrial cancer (NCI, 2024e).
- Diet factors: A number of observational studies have demonstrated that consumption of a diet low in saturated fats and high in fruits and vegetables is associated with a reduced risk of developing endometrial cancer (NCI, 2019). Some studies have also seen a protective correlation between caffeinated coffee intake and decreased incidence of endometrial cancer (American Society of Clinical Oncology, 2019).

Family history on either side of the family may determine if a person is at risk for hereditary endometrial cancer (Daly et al., 2023). People with a personal history of endometrial or Lynch syndrome-related cancer (e.g. ovarian, colorectal, pancreatic), strong family history of Lynch syndrome-related cancers, or family history of predisposing genetic mutations, should be referred for formal genetic counseling (Daly et al., 2023). It is important for clinicians to be familiar with Lynch syndrome and Cowden syndrome as each carry high lifetime risks, screening guidelines, and risk-reducing surgery recommendations that can decrease morbidity and mortality if followed. Patients with qualifying personal or family history, and those who were previously tested with a limited panel, should be offered large, multigene panel testing, given the number of genes discovered that can predispose to cancer. Hereditary endometrial cancer genes, their cumulative risks to age 80, and screening and management guidelines include (Daly et al., 2023):

- Lynch syndrome:
  - MLH1 (34–54%)
    - Screening with endometrial biopsy every 1–2 years starting at age 30–35 can be considered
    - Hysterectomy with bilateral salpingo-oophorectomy may be considered at 40 years
  - MSH2 and EPCAM (21–57%)
    - Screening with endometrial biopsy every 1–2 years starting at age 30–35 can be considered
    - Hysterectomy with bilateral salpingo-oophorectomy may be considered at 40 years
  - MSH6 (16–49%)
    - Screening with endometrial biopsy every 1–2 years starting at age 30–35 can be considered
    - Hysterectomy with bilateral salpingectomy may be considered starting at 40 years, with delayed bilateral oophorectomy starting at 50 years
  - PMS2 (13–26%)
    - Screening with endometrial biopsy every 1–2 years starting at age 30–35 can be considered
    - Hysterectomy with bilateral salpingo-oophorectomy may be considered starting at age 50 years
- Cowden syndrome
  - PTEN (28%)
    - Screening with endometrial biopsy every 1–2 years starting by age 35 can be considered
    - Consider hysterectomy upon completion of childbearing (Daly et al., 2023)

Referral to a genetic counselor or clinician certified in hereditary cancer genomics is necessary when personal or family history is concerning for a genetic predisposition. Patients with the following history concerning for hereditary ovarian cancer risk should be referred promptly (Daly et al., 2023):

Personal history of a Lynch syndrome–related cancer* and any of the following:

- Diagnosed < 50 years
- A Lynch syndrome–related cancer, synchronous or metachronous (regardless of age)
- One 1st-degree or 2nd-degree relative with a Lynch syndrome–related cancer diagnosed < 50 years
- ≥ Two 1st-degree or 2nd-degree relatives with a Lynch syndrome–related cancer (regardless of age)

Family history of any of the following:

- ≥ One 1st-degree relative with a colorectal cancer or endometrial cancer diagnosed < 50 years
- ≥ One 1st-degree relative with a colorectal cancer or endometrial cancer and a synchronous or metachronous Lynch syndrome–related cancer (regardless of age)

- ≥ Two 1st-degree or 2nd-degree relatives with Lynch syndrome–related cancers including ≥ 1 diagnosed < 50 years
- ≥ Three 1st-degree or 2nd-degree relatives with Lynch syndrome–related cancers (regardless of age)

** Sebaceous neoplasms, small bowel, ovarian, gastric, pancreatic, biliary tract, brain, bladder, urothelial, and adrenocortical cancers*

Controlling Other Risk Factors

People with PCOS need appropriate treatment to avoid the effect of unopposed estrogen on the uterus. People who are menopausal and have an intact uterus should avoid using unopposed estrogen to relieve menopausal symptoms. People with a history of breast or ovarian cancer or hereditary nonpolyposis colorectal cancer (HNPCC; Lynch syndrome) need to be closely monitored for endometrial cancer. The American Cancer Society recommends that people with or at increased risk for HNPCC should be offered annual testing for endometrial cancer with endometrial biopsy beginning at age 35. These patients should also be counseled about preventive measures, such as the option of prophylactic hysterectomy with bilateral salpingo-oophorectomy at the completion of childbearing (ACS, 2019a).

Secondary and Tertiary Management

Transvaginal ultrasound has not been shown to be beneficial in patients who have a hereditary predisposition, such as Lynch syndrome; however, endometrial biopsy is highly sensitive and specific and can be utilized every 1–2 years beginning at ages 30–35, depending on the variant (Abu-Rustum et al., 2025). Although total hysterectomy decreases the incidence of endometrial cancer, it does not reduce mortality from endometrial cancer and therefore can be considered as a risk-reducing option (Abu-Rustum et al., 2025).

The choice of treatment for endometrial cancer depends primarily on the type and stage of the disease, the level of differentiation, the person's overall health, and their personal preferences (Abu-Rustum et al., 2025). Treatment options for endometrial cancer include surgery, radiation therapy, chemotherapy, hormonal therapy, and biologic therapy. Chemotherapy may be used in recurrent or advanced cases of endometrial cancer (Abu-Rustum et al., 2025). Extensive clinical guidelines for the management of endometrial cancer are available at the National Comprehensive Cancer Network website (Abu-Rustum et al., 2025).

Surgery Comprehensive surgical staging is achieved through total abdominal hysterectomy with bilateral salpingo-oophorectomy and peritoneal washing for cytology. Ongoing research has indicated that people who are eligible may be treated safely with a laparoscopic approach. People with a larger body habitus and higher anesthesia risk may benefit from a robotic approach (Abu-Rustum et al., 2025). The preferred extent of pelvic and para-aortic lymphadenectomy is the subject of debate; some surgeons choose selective lymph node sampling versus full dissection. Studies to date have not fully resolved this issue, but multiple-site sampling has been associated with improved survival rates. Complete pelvic and para-aortic lymphadenectomy remains the standard (ACOG, 2015, reaffirmed 2020) and sentinel lymph node mapping is preferred (Abu-Rustum et al., 2025). Patients with localized disease are usually cured with surgery alone. In contrast, patients with myometrial invasion are usually treated with a combination of surgery, chemotherapy, and/or adjuvant radiation therapy (NCI, 2025). Clinicians should refer patients with a diagnosis of endometrial cancer to a gynecologic oncologist for management when possible (Hamilton et al., 2021). Careful staging guides therapy (NCI, 2025).

Staging The FIGO surgical staging system is used for staging endometrial cancer (**Table 28-5**). Additional pathological findings also guide treatment and prevent overtreatment. Less favorable prognosis findings include the following: hormone receptor status (progesterone receptor site levels greater than 100 are associated with 93 percent disease-free survival rate at 3 years as opposed to a 36 percent rate when levels are less than 100); myometrial invasion; vascular invasion; presence of aneuploidy; oncogene (mutated gene) expression; and the fraction of cells in S phase (the percentage of cells in a tumor that are in the phase of the cell cycle when DNA is synthesized) (NCI, 2025).

Radiation Therapy Radiation treatment is indicated for patients with grade 1 to 2 tumors with low-risk histology and can include postoperative vaginal brachytherapy or radiation therapy alone. For patients with grade 3 tumors, indicating high-risk histology, adjuvant radiation is offered with or without chemotherapy. Radiation treatments may be given externally (external-beam radiation or EBRT), via an intracavitary method (brachytherapy), or both (NCI, 2025). Vaginal brachytherapy has less gastrointestinal toxicity and is better tolerated by most people (ACOG, 2015, reaffirmed 2020). EBRT is associated with urinary and colorectal side effects, including urinary pain and urgency and diarrhea (ACS, 2022a). In general, EBRT is reserved for patients with FIGO stage IA, grade 3, FIGO stage IB, grade 1 or 2 disease with myoinvasive and high-risk factors (i.e., LVSI), stage IB with clear cell histology, or stage II, any grade (Harkenrider et al., 2023).

Pelvic radiation may also cause vaginal stenosis (narrowing of the vagina from scar tissue), which may make vaginal intercourse painful. The use of a vaginal dilator or having vaginal intercourse several times per week can help prevent scar tissue formation. Use of vaginal lubricants may also be helpful (ACOG, 2015, reaffirmed 2020; NCI, 2019).

Chemotherapy and Immunotherapy Chemotherapy combined with immunotherapy has been shown to improve outcomes for people with advanced endometrial cancer. In 2023, the addition of pembrolizumab to standard chemotherapy was shown to significantly increase progression-free survival when compared to chemotherapy alone (Eskander et al., 2023) and its use became a preferred 1st-line therapy for advanced stage endometrial cancer (Abu-Rustum et al., 2025). Additionally, the FDA approved the use of dostarlimab in combination with chemotherapy in 2023 (NCI, 2023b). The most common systemic therapy agents used for treatment in advanced stages include paclitaxel and carboplatin in combination with one of the following immunotherapy agents: pembrolizumab, dostarlimab, durvalumab, trastuzumab, and bevacizumab (Abu-Rustum et al., 2025).

Hormone Therapy People who are not candidates for surgery or radiation, such as those who have advanced disease and whose surgical risks outweigh the benefits or are unwilling to undergo more aggressive treatment, may opt for hormonal therapy (ACS, 2019c; ACOG, 2015, reaffirmed 2020). The hormonal agents most commonly used for this purpose are progestational

TABLE 28-5 2023 FIGO Staging for Carcinoma of the Corpus Uteri

FIGO Stage	Description
I	Tumor confined to the uterine corpus and ovary
IA	Disease limited to the endometrium OR nonaggressive histological type (i.e., low-grade endometrioid), with invasion of less than half of myometrium with no or focal LVSI OR good prognosis disease
IA1	Nonaggressive histological type limited to an endometrial polyp OR confined to the endometrium
IA2	Nonaggressive histological types involving less than half of the myometrium with no or focal LVSI
IA3	Low-grade endometrioid carcinomas limited to the uterus and ovary
IB	Nonaggressive histological types with invasion of half or more of the myometrium, and with no or focal LVSI
IC	Aggressive histological types limited to a polyp or confined to the endometrium
II	Invasion of cervical stroma without extrauterine extension OR with substantial LVSI OR aggressive histological types with myometrial invasion
IIA	Invasion of the cervical stroma of nonaggressive histological types
IIB	Substantial LVSI of nonaggressive histological types
IIC	Aggressive histological types with any myometrial involvement
III	Local and/or regional spread of the tumor of any histological subtype
IIIA	Invasion of uterine serosa, adnexa, or both by direct extension or metastasis
IIIA1	Spread to ovary or fallopian tube (except when meeting stage IA3 criteria)
IIIA2	Involvement of uterine subserosa or spread through the uterine serosa
IIIB	Metastasis or direct spread to the vagina and/or to the parametria or pelvic peritoneum
IIIB1	Metastasis or direct spread to the vagina and/or the parametria
IIIB2	Metastasis to the pelvic peritoneum
IIIC	Metastasis to the pelvic or para-aortic lymph nodes or both
IIIC1	Metastasis to the pelvic lymph nodes
IIIC1i	Micrometastasis
IIIC1ii	Macrometastasis
IIIC2	Metastasis to para-aortic lymph nodes up to the renal vessels, with or without metastasis to the pelvic lymph nodes
IIIC2i	Micrometastasis
IIIC2ii	Macrometastasis
IV	Spread to the bladder mucosa and/or intestinal mucosa and/or distance metastasis
IVA	Invasion of the bladder mucosa and/or the intestinal/bowel mucosa
IVB	Abdominal peritoneal metastasis beyond the pelvis
IVC	Distant metastasis, including metastasis to any extra- or intra-abdominal lymph nodes above the renal vessels, lungs, liver, brain, or bone

Reproduced from National Cancer Institute (2025). *Endometrial cancer treatment.* https://www.cancer.gov/types/uterine/hp/endometrial-treatment-pdq

Abbreviations: FIGO, International Federation of Gynecology and Obstetrics; LVSI, lymphovascular space invasion.

drugs such as medroxyprogesterone (Provera) and megestrol (Megace). Response to hormones reflects the presence and level of hormone receptors and the degree of tumor differentiation (ACS, 2019c; NCI, 2025). Preferred hormone therapy for recurrent or metastatic endometrial carcinoma is alternating Megace and Tamoxifen or using Everolimus and Letrozole. Alternatively, patients can alternate Provera and Tamoxifen (Abu-Rustum et al., 2025).

Follow-Up

An important part of the treatment plan is a specific schedule of follow-up visits after surgery, chemotherapy, or radiation therapy. Follow-up visits are scheduled every 3–6 months during the first 2–3 years, then every 6–12 months for up to 5 years, then annually (Abu-Rustum et al., 2025). Eighteen percent of patients will experience recurrence and most recurrences are found within the first 2 years after initial surgical treatment (Siegenthaler, 2022).

An examination of the abdomen and inguinal lymph nodes, along with speculum and rectovaginal examinations, should be done at each follow-up visit. History questions should focus on symptoms that might indicate cancer recurrence because most recurrences are discovered during evaluation of symptomatic patients. If the patient's symptoms or physical examination results suggest recurrent cancer, imaging tests (such as a CT scan or ultrasound), a CA-125 blood test, or biopsies should be ordered. Conversely, if no symptoms or physical examination abnormalities are identified, routine blood tests and imaging tests are not recommended (ACOG, 2015, reaffirmed 2020). Clinicians need to keep in mind that the greatest risk of death in endometrial cancer survivors is associated with noncancer causes, so it is very important to encourage patients to consume a healthy diet and adopt healthy lifestyle behaviors.

Emerging Evidence That May Change Management

People with advanced or recurrent endometrial cancer, in particular, can benefit greatly from enrollment in a clinical trial. Multiple trials, with enrollment depending on staging, are examining different chemotherapeutic regimens and use of biologic agents (e.g., atezolizumab, olaparib) most commonly as adjuncts to chemotherapy (Tillmanns et al., 2024). Other trials are researching the use of adjuvant radiotherapy in combination with chemotherapy to improve survival rates (NCI, n.d.-c). Research is ongoing to find the least toxic, most effective therapeutic regimens.

Patient Education

Clinicians need to educate their patients on the early symptoms of endometrial cancer and encourage them to report any postmenopausal bleeding promptly, and should provide education to young people about the relationship between high BMI and the risk for endometrial cancer. Clinicians need to keep in mind that most endometrial cancer survivors die due to noncancer causes (ACS, 2019h; Anderson et al., 2022; NCI, 2025). Encouraging a healthy weight, balanced diet, and healthy lifestyle behaviors is a crucial aspect of patient management.

Considerations for Specific Populations

People of childbearing age may be devastated at the loss of fertility upon receiving a diagnosis of endometrial cancer. It is important to appreciate that this type of cancer is rare in people who are in their reproductive years, and a careful diagnosis must consider differentiating diagnoses, such as other estrogen-related conditions including atypical hyperplasia, polycystic ovaries, or a granulosa cell tumor (ACS, 2019h). After the diagnosis is confirmed, some patients are candidates for more conservative, fertility-sparing treatment options. People who have grade 1, well-differentiated endometrioid endometrial carcinoma without myometrial invasion or metastasis may want to discuss these options with a specialist. After careful evaluation and consideration of the risk, these people may choose a hormonal treatment with a progestin or a gonadotropin-releasing hormone agonist (ACS, 2019c; ACOG, 2015, reaffirmed 2020; Emons & Grundker, 2021; Cavaliere et al., 2021). Most experts continue to recommend surgical management immediately following completion of childbearing.

Other people might be interested in ovarian preservation, which is not traditionally recommended at the time of a hysterectomy. The ovaries are potential sites for occult metastatic disease—a variant estimated to occur in 19 percent of people who are premenopausal at time of diagnosis with endometrial cancer—and the ongoing production of estrogen is a risk factor for reoccurrence (ACOG, 2015, reaffirmed 2020). It is important to again emphasize that clinicians need to discuss the risks and benefits of conservative treatment to help their patients make informed treatment decisions regarding the potential for ovarian preservation.

Finally, people who are premenopausal require evaluation for quality-of-life issues following surgical treatment for early-stage endometrial cancer. New evidence suggests that ET to treat menopausal symptoms might be a viable option for these people despite the conventional wisdom that exogenous estrogen is a potential risk factor for reoccurrence (ACOG, 2015, reaffirmed 2020). A trial involving 1,236 patients with endometrial cancer indicated no significant difference in reoccurrence rates between patients receiving estrogen and those receiving a placebo (ACOG, 2015, reaffirmed 2020). Although the trial closed early, the American College of Obstetricians and Gynecologists has determined that ET to manage menopausal symptoms is a reasonable option given appropriate counseling and monitoring.

OVARIAN CANCER

Description of Ovarian Cancer

Ovarian cancer designation now includes fallopian tube and primary peritoneal cancer and will mainly be referred to as just ovarian cancer in this section.

Ovarian cancer has the highest mortality rate of all gynecologic cancers and is the fifth leading cause of all cancer deaths among people with gynecologic organs (Somaseger et al., 2024). During 2024 in the United States, approximately 19,680 new cases of ovarian cancer were diagnosed, and 12,740 people died of ovarian cancer (NCI, n.d.-c). Ovarian cancer is rare and accounts for 1 percent of all new cancer diagnoses, 2.1 percent of all cancer deaths (SEER, n.d.-c). Twenty-three percent of all gynecologic cancers are ovarian/fallopian tube/peritoneal in origin and represent almost 50 percent of cancer deaths from gynecologic cancers (Somaseger et al., 2024).

Malignant tumors of the ovary can occur in people of all ages (Berek et al., 2021). Overall, advancing age is a significant risk factor in the development of ovarian cancer, with the risk increasing at menopause and continuing into a person's 80s (NCI, 2024f). The average age of people in the United States who are diagnosed with ovarian cancer is 63 years (SEER, n.d.-c; NCI 2024f), and primary diagnoses of ovarian cancer occur most commonly in people aged 55 to 64 years (NCI, 2024f). Ovarian cancer has the highest incidence in Indigenous communities, followed by white, Latiné, Asian/Pacific Islander, and Black communities (NCI, 2024f). White patients have the second-highest incidence and mortality which may be due to the 1 in 40 incidence of hereditary mutations (i.e., BRCA1, BRCA2) in the Ashkenazi Jewish population (Mei et al., 2023). Meta-analyses have shown that Black and other racially and ethnically minoritized communities are less likely to receive guideline-concordant care, are more likely to be uninsured or underinsured, and experience more barriers to accessing care, all of which are rooted in racism (Mei et al., 2023). Geographically, incidence rates are highest in high-income parts of the world, including North America and northern, central, and eastern Europe (Huang et al., 2022).

Ovarian cancer is commonly diagnosed in late stages primarily because of its vague early symptoms and lack of reliable screening methods. The prognosis for most people with ovarian cancer remains poor and is approximately 31 percent when diagnosed at a later stage (SEER, n.d.-c). The rate of ovarian cancer deaths has decreased by 40 percent in the past 50 years with the majority of this decline occurring since the mid-2000s and likely related to improved treatment as well as decreased incidence (Committee on Gynecologic Practice, Society of Gynecologic Oncology, 2019; ACS, 2024c). If the disease is confined to the ovary (stage I) at the time of diagnosis, the 5-year survival rate is 91.9 percent; however, only 19 percent of people have localized disease at the time of their diagnosis. Most people are initially diagnosed with stage III to IV ovarian cancer, and those with stage IV disease have a 5-year survival rate of just 31.4 percent (SEER, n.d.-c). Overall, the 5-year survival rate for ovarian cancer is 50.9 percent (SEER, n.d.-c). Clinical and technological advances in early detection are urgently needed to decrease the morbidity and mortality associated with this disease.

Etiology and Pathophysiology

Epithelial ovarian carcinomas are the most common type of ovarian cancer, accounting for approximately 85 to 90 percent of diagnoses (Committee on Gynecologic Practice, Society of Gynecologic Oncology, 2019; Somaseger et al., 2024). Epithelial cancers are classified by histology as serous, endometrioid, mucinous, or clear cell tumors. Serous carcinomas are the most common and account for about 60–75 percent of epithelial carcinomas of the ovary (De Decker at al., 2023).

Epithelial ovarian cancer is now further categorized into two distinct classifications that differ in terms of pathogenesis and prognosis. Type I tumors include low-grade serous, endometrioid, mucinous, or clear cell carcinomas. With the exception of clear cell tumors, which are considered high-grade, type I tumors usually are large cystic masses confined to one ovary and are thought to develop from benign lesions that progress to atypia and finally to low-grade invasive disease. Type I tumors rarely have p53 mutations and are relatively stable from a genetic standpoint. Epithelial tumors of low-malignancy potential (borderline malignant ovarian carcinoma) are usually found in younger people and are often confined to the ovary at diagnosis. When confined to the ovary, type I tumors have an excellent prognosis (Lisio et al., 2019; Berek et al., 2021).

Type II tumors include high-grade serous carcinosarcomas, high-grade endometrioid carcinomas, and undifferentiated carcinomas (Pavlik et al., 2020; Berek et al., 2021). Type II tumors involve both ovaries, are aggressive, and usually present as advanced disease. Genetically, mutation of the p53 tumor suppressor gene is common. This type of ovarian cancer is also linked with mutations of the tumor suppressor genes BRCA1 and BRCA2, which normally encode for proteins that function in the DNA repair process (Lisio et al., 2019). High-grade serous ovarian neoplasms are the most dominant form diagnosed clinically and account for 80 to 90 percent of all deaths from ovarian cancer (Lisio et al., 2019; Berek et al., 2021).

Nonepithelial ovarian cancer types tend to be less aggressive and include germ cell tumors and sex-cord stromal tumors. They represent a small portion of ovarian cancer incidence, with germ cell tumors accounting for 2.6 percent (Gica et al., 2022) and sex-cord stromal cell tumors accounting for 5–7 percent of ovarian cancers (Li, Li, & Jiang, 2024). Lastly, metastatic neoplasms that originate in the breast, lung, uterus, cervix, or gastrointestinal tract may invade and grow in ovarian tissue (Berek et al., 2021; Bourgioti, Konidari, & Moulopoulos, 2023).

Traditionally, the surface epithelium of the ovary was thought to be the primary site of ovarian malignancy (Somasegar et al., 2024), and some types of epithelial and nonepithelial ovarian cancers, such as germ cell tumors and sex-cord stromal tumors, arise from ovarian cells (Committee on Gynecologic Practice, Society of Gynecologic Oncology, 2019). However, recent research indicates that many types of ovarian tumors arise from nonovarian origins. For example, type I mucinous tumors may derive from metastatic intestinal tumors, and some forms of endometrioid and clear cell ovarian cancer may originate from tissue that has embedded on the ovary related to the process of endometriosis (Lisio et al., 2019; Berek et al., 2021).

Research indicates that neoplastic cells originating in the fallopian tubes are shed through the tubal fimbriae and disseminated onto the ovarian surface or peritoneum, where they then develop into type II serous epithelial malignancy. In people with genetic predisposition for ovarian cancer and those with sporadic forms, lesions have been found in the fallopian tubes that closely resemble ovarian serous carcinomas. The precursor lesions in the fallopian tube lack the normal cilia of fallopian tube cells, have p53 mutations, and are associated with BRCA1 and BRCA2 DNA repair mutations (Committee on Gynecologic Practice, Society of Gynecologic Oncology, 2019; Lisio et al., 2019). Migration of neoplastic cells from the tubal fimbriae has been proposed as the actual origin of up to 80 percent of serous epithelial ovarian cancers and may account for why most type II ovarian cancers present as advanced disease (Lisio et al., 2019; Berek et al., 2021).

High-grade serous epithelial ovarian cancer does not require the blood or lymphatic system to metastasize; there are no anatomical barriers that can restrict spread to nearby structures when tumor cells detach from either the surface of the ovary or from the fallopian tube through the process known as cancer seeding (Lisio et al., 2019; Parashar et al., 2020). Ovarian cancer typically spreads through direct extension to nearby organs within the peritoneal cavity, where cancer cells become implanted on the peritoneal surface, omentum, or pelvic or abdominal organs. Invasive spread to the regional iliac inguinal, para-aortic, and hypogastric lymph nodes may occur, and diaphragmatic and liver surface involvement is common (Lisio et al., 2019; NCI, n.d.-c; Berek et al., 2021). Up to 24 percent of people who appear to have stage I ovarian cancer already have lymph node metastasis. Lymph node involvement is found in the majority of people who undergo node dissection, and it is present in 73 percent of advanced cases (NCI, n.d.-c). A finding of ascites is also common and is thought to occur because of blockage to lymphatic drainage or tumor secretion of vasoactive substances (Lisio et al., 2019; NCI, n.d.-c).

Risk Factors

The most important risk factor for ovarian cancer is family history. Approximately 15 to 21 percent of ovarian cancers have hereditary causes. People with two or more first-degree relatives who have been diagnosed with ovarian cancer are at the highest risk (Lisio et al., 2019; NCI, n.d.-c; ACS, 2021b; Liu et al., 2024).

People with ovaries and who carry the BRCA1 or BRCA2 genetic mutation have an increased risk for hereditary ovarian cancer. People with a BRCA1 gene mutation have 39–58 percent absolute risk of ovarian cancer by age 80. For people with a BRCA2 mutation, the ovarian cancer absolute risk is 13–29 percent by age 80 (Liu et al., 2024). Ovarian cancers involving BRCA mutations are more likely to be high-grade type II serous cancers that occur at an earlier age (Lisio et al., 2019). BRCA mutations associated with the development of cancer occur slightly more often in specific populations such as those of Ashkenazi (eastern European) Jewish descent, French Canadians, and Icelanders (Berek et al., 2021; Fierheller et al., 2021; NCI, 2024f), although founder mutations also exist in other populations such as Mexican and West African communities (Fragoso-Ontiveros et al., 2019; NCI, 2024f). People with BRCA mutations have a high risk of breast cancer and carry other cancer risks, including pancreatic cancer, and melanoma (Liu et al., 2024).

People with a history of Lynch syndrome (HNPCC syndrome) have an increased risk of developing several cancers, including colorectal and ovarian cancer (Lisio et al., 2019; NCI, n.d.-c; Liu et al., 2024). People with this autosomal dominant hereditary condition have an approximate 1–38 percent absolute risk of developing ovarian cancer in their lifetime, depending on the variant (Liu et al., 2024). The majority of ovarian cancers linked with Lynch syndrome are type I endometrioid tumors (Lisio et al., 2019; Capasso et al., 2023).

Age is also a factor in the development of ovarian cancer. Ovarian germ cell cancer occurs mainly in people younger than 20 years, and borderline malignant tumors typically occur in people in their 30s and 40s. For sex-cord stromal tumors, peak incidence is for people in their 50s, and the incidence of epithelial serous carcinoma peaks for people in their 70s (Lisio et al., 2019; Berek et al., 2021; Liontos et al., 2021). In general, the risk of ovarian cancer increases with age, and half of all ovarian cancers are diagnosed in people older than age 60 (NCI, n.d.-c; Berek et al., 2021).

The risk of ovarian cancer has been linked to reproductive and hormonal factors. People who have never been pregnant have a higher risk of developing ovarian cancer than people who have gone through at least one full-term pregnancy, and each additional pregnancy may further reduce risk (Lisio et al., 2019; ACS, 2021b; NCI, n.d.-c).

People who have used postmenopausal hormone replacement therapy with either estrogen alone or estrogen–progesterone combinations have a higher risk of developing ovarian cancer. (Daly et al., 2023; ACS, 2021b). Conversely, risk decreases in people who have used oral contraceptives, with users or former users having up to a 30 percent lower risk, compared to people who have never used oral contraceptives. The degree of risk reduction varies with duration of use; people who have used oral contraceptives for more than 5 years have the most risk reduction (Lisio et al., 2019; NCI, n.d.-c; Arshadi et al., 2024). Breastfeeding is also believed to decrease the risk of ovarian cancer, with greater risk reduction associated with longer duration of breastfeeding (Lisio et al., 2019; Momenimovahed et al., 2019; NCI, n.d.-c).

A history of tubal ligation or previous salpingectomy is associated with a decreased risk of ovarian cancer (Berek et al., 2021; Somaseger et al., 2024). Bilateral salpingectomy has a greater risk reduction than tubal ligation and may reduce risk of ovarian cancer by up to 65 percent (ACOG 2019; Duus et al., 2023). Bilateral salpingectomy alone or salpingo-oophorectomy is associated with decreased risk of ovarian cancer, with bilateral salpingo-oophorectomy having the greatest amount of risk reduction at 96 percent compared to 65 percent (ACOG 2019; Steenbeek et al., 2021; NCI, n.d.-c). Because recent research indicates that the actual origin of many serous epithelial, endometrioid, and clear cell ovarian cancers is migration of precursor malignant cells from the epithelium of the fallopian tubes, it may explain the decreased risk of ovarian cancer associated with tubal ligation or removal (Lisio et al., 2019; Berek et al., 2021).

Other risk factors associated with ovarian cancer include increased adiposity and smoking. Larger body habitus is associated with a higher risk of developing ovarian cancer, although this risk is associated with specific types, such as borderline malignant tumors, endometrioid, clear cell, and mucinous cancers (Liu et al., 2023). Smoking is linked to an increased risk for the mucinous type of ovarian cancer and some studies have shown that it may decrease risk for clear cell, serous, and endometrioid ovarian cancer, although the data has not been statistically significant (Liu et al., 2024; Zhou et al., 2019).

Talcum powder is a silicate that is similar to asbestos, which is a known carcinogen. The use of talcum powder has been identified as a risk factor in the development of ovarian cancer, although research results regarding the use of talcum powder as a risk factor are mixed. Research evidence of dose response has also been inconsistent based on the difficulty of defining and measuring exposure. Data collection has been further hindered by the small number of people with reported exposures and the overall rarity of the disease (O'Brian et al., 2020).

Certain disease processes are also associated with an increased risk of ovarian cancer. For example, people with a diagnosis of endometriosis are at higher risk of clear cell, endometrioid or low-grade serous ovarian cancers (Sun & Liu, 2021), and although research evidence is less clear, those with polycystic ovarian syndrome may be at increased risk for serous borderline ovarian tumors (Frandsen et al., 2023).

Other factors, such as physical activity, use of specific drugs, and diet, have been studied in determination of ovarian cancer risk. Physical activity has been associated with a decreased risk of ovarian cancer (Lee, 2019). The general health benefits of exercise are well known, and reduction in adipose tissue with resulting reduction in chronic inflammation may be partially responsible for decreased risk (Tan et al. 2023). The roles of diet and infertility drug treatments in relation to ovarian cancer remain uncertain (Rizzuto, Behrens, & Smith 2019; ACS, 2021b).

Clinical Presentation

The majority of ovarian cancer cases are diagnosed when the disease has already reached an advanced stage and the chance for cure is significantly decreased (Togashi et al., 2020). Often referred to as a silent disease, ovarian cancer is associated with vague symptoms that offer only subtle signs of its presence, such as abdominal bloating and discomfort, difficulty eating, early satiety, and urinary symptoms all of which can be caused by many factors. Clinicians should suspect ovarian cancer particularly in postmenopausal patients who present with persistent or progressive symptoms (Lisio et al., 2019; Liu et al., 2024). Signs of advanced disease include a worsening of abdominal distention and discomfort from ascites, anorexia, nausea or vomiting, vaginal bleeding, tenesmus, back pain, unexplained weight loss, or respiratory symptoms from increased intra-abdominal pressure

TABLE 28-6 Clinical Presentation of Ovarian Cancer

Early Symptoms	Later Symptoms
Abdominal bloating/ discomfort	Ascites
Early satiety	Anorexia
Indigestion/dyspepsia	Nausea or vomiting
Fatigue/weakness	Tenesmus
Vague abdominal pain/ painful areas in abdomen on palpation	Distinct abdominal pain
Urinary frequency, pressure, or urge	Vaginal bleeding
Diarrhea or constipation	Unexplained weight loss
	Back pain
	Cough or dyspnea

or pleural effusion (Lisio et al., 2019; Berek et al., 2021). Paraneoplastic syndromes, such as cerebellar degeneration, Cushing's syndrome, hypercalcemia, and deep vein thromboses, can occur with ovarian cancers (Brown et al., 2022). **Table 28-6** identifies the early and late symptoms that may occur with ovarian cancer.

Assessment

History and Physical Examination

Obtaining a thorough history will assist in determining whether a person has an average or high risk of developing ovarian cancer (Committee on Gynecologic Practice, Society of Gynecologic Oncology, 2017, reaffirmed 2019). Evaluation should include a discussion of any presenting symptoms, assessment of risk factors for ovarian cancer, and a review of personal and family history for breast, gynecological, and colon cancer. It is important for the clinician to remember that detection of early-stage ovarian cancer results in improved survival (Committee on Gynecologic Practice, Society of Gynecologic Oncology, 2017, reaffirmed 2019). Stage and survival are not changed by reducing time to diagnosis in symptomatic ovarian cancer, owing to the fact that most of these cancers are advanced stage once symptoms are present (Dilley et al., 2020). The clinician should seek clarification of any report of persistent abdominal bloating, pelvic or abdominal pain, difficulty eating, or loss of appetite. While a person's description of these symptoms may be disregarded or attributed to normal processes such as irritable bowel syndrome, menstruation, or menopause, they significantly increase the likelihood of ovarian cancer. If present for greater than 12 days per month in the previous 12 months, these symptoms are suggestive of late-stage ovarian cancer, especially in postmenopausal patients (Committee on Gynecologic Practice, Society of Gynecologic Oncology, 2017, reaffirmed 2019).

If an ovarian malignancy is suspected, a complete physical examination, including a breast, bimanual pelvic, and rectal examination to palpate for tumors, is indicated (Berek et al., 2021; NCI, 2024f). A palpable pelvic mass in a person who is postmenopausal should be considered abnormal and evaluated further. If palpated, malignant tumors may be large, nodular, and characterized by decreased mobility (Poudel et al., 2022). The clinician should also assess for signs of paraneoplastic syndromes, such as deep vein thrombosis, signs of metastatic disease, including inguinal lymphadenopathy, and evidence of ascites and pleural effusions (Berek et al., 2021; Brown et al., 2022).

Diagnostic Testing

People with clinical signs and symptoms suggestive of ovarian cancer and those with a pelvic mass should undergo transvaginal ultrasound, which can assess ovarian size, shape, solid and cystic components, and vascularity, ascites, loculations, and may differentiate benign from malignant adnexal masses (Liberto et al., 2022). Further imaging studies, such as CT scan or MRI of the abdomen and pelvis with IV contrast may be indicated (Liu et al., 2024). Fine needle aspiration for tumor biopsy is not recommended for suspected early-stage disease because it may cause tumor cells to further disseminate into the peritoneal cavity and upstage the cancer (Liu et al., 2024). A mammogram should be considered, depending on the person's risks for breast cancer, and a colonoscopy may be indicated when history, signs, or symptoms are suggestive of colon cancer (Berek et al., 2021).

Laboratory testing should include a complete blood count and chemistry profile with liver function tests. Tumor biomarkers such as CA-125 and carcinoembryonic antigen (CEA) should be obtained. CA-125 is a glycoprotein that is found in the epithelium of the fallopian tubes and the ovary. High levels of CA-125, especially in combination with radiological testing, may indicate epithelial ovarian, fallopian tube, or peritoneal cancer, though elevations are seen more often in late-stage disease. Gastric or colon cancer with metastasis should be considered with elevations in CEA. Biomarkers for nonepithelial ovarian cancers include inhibin A/B for sex-cord stromal tumors, and lactate dehydrogenase (LDH), α fetoprotein and beta human chorionic gonadotropin for germ cell tumors (Lisio et al., 2019; Berek et al., 2021; Liu et al., 2024).

Differential Diagnoses

Differential diagnoses in the evaluation for ovarian cancer include gastrointestinal malignancy, uterine fibroid, ovarian torsion, embryologic remnants, ovarian cysts or benign tumors, ectopic pregnancy, tubo-ovarian abscess, inflammatory bowel disease, appendicitis, diverticulitis, peritoneal inclusion cyst, and endometriosis (Elsherif et al., 2022, Arora et al., 2025). It is important for the patient and their clinician to maintain a high level of suspicion when signs and symptoms of ovarian cancer are present. Factors that may indicate the presence of ovarian malignancy are age (younger for germ cell cancers and older for epithelial cancers), presence of bilateral masses, tumor fixation, presence of ascites, and elevated tumor markers (Berek et al., 2021).

Prevention

Primary Prevention

Preventive strategies for ovarian cancer start with a determination of whether a person is at average risk or high risk for ovarian cancer (Committee on Gynecologic Practice, Society of Gynecologic Oncology, 2017, reaffirmed 2019). Shared decision making between a patient and their clinician will facilitate an individualized approach to risk factor reduction according to a person's age, history, and reproductive choices. Childbearing, oral contraceptive use, and breastfeeding decrease ovarian cancer risk. It is reasonable to suggest that people with mutations in BRCA consider oral contraceptives for cancer prophylaxis; contraceptive use is associated with a 30 to 60 percent decrease in risk of ovarian cancer in this subset of patients (Liu et al., 2024). In addition, explaining that ovarian cancer risk can be decreased with modification of risk factors, such as increasing exercise, weight reduction, and smoking cessation, may be helpful.

Maternal or paternal family history may determine if a person is at risk for hereditary ovarian cancer (Abu-Rustum et al., 2025). People with a personal history of breast, ovarian, or Lynch syndrome–related cancer, strong family history of breast or ovarian cancer, or family history of predisposing genetic mutations, should be referred for formal genetic counseling (Berek et al., 2021; Abu-Rustum et al., 2025). It is important for clinicians to be familiar with hereditary cancer syndromes and mutations other than BRCA 1 and BRCA 2 as other variants also may have high lifetime risks, screening guidelines, and risk-reducing surgery recommendations that can decrease morbidity and mortality if followed. Patients who have only had BRCA 1 and BRCA 2 testing should be offered panel testing, given the number of genes discovered that can predispose to cancer. Other hereditary ovarian cancer genes, and their absolute risks, include (Abu-Rustum et al., 2025):

- ATM (2–3%)
- BRIP1 (5–15%)
- PALB2 (3–5%)
- RAD51C (10–15%)
- RAD51D 10–20%)
- ATM (2–3%)
- Lynch syndrome genes:
  - MLH1 (4–20%)
  - MSH2/EPCAM (8–38%)
  - MSH6 (< 1–13%)
  - PMS2 (1.3–3%)

Referral to a genetic counselor or clinician certified in hereditary cancer genomics is essential when personal or family history is concerning for a genetic predisposition. Patients with the following history concerning for hereditary ovarian cancer risk should be referred promptly (Abu-Rustum et al., 2025):

- Personal history of breast cancer with any of the following:
  - Age ≤ 50 years
  - Triple negative breast cancer
  - Multiple primary breast cancers (synchronous or metasynchronous)
  - Ashkenazi Jewish ancestry
- Family history of a 1st- or 2nd-degree relative with:
  - Breast cancer ≤ 50 years
  - Familial male breast cancer (any age)
  - Ovarian cancer (any age)
  - Pancreatic cancer
  - Prostate cancer, metastatic or high/very high-risk pathology
  - ≥ 3 diagnoses of breast and/or prostate cancer (any grade) on the same side of the family (includes the patient with breast cancer)

The purpose of genetic cancer counseling is to inform individuals of the biological, environmental, and genetic risks for cancer to empower them in making informed decisions about risk reduction and genetic testing (Daly et al., 2023). The clinician should explain why genetic counseling is being offered; the risks, limitations, and benefits of genetic testing; and options related to results (Committee on Gynecologic Practice, Society of Gynecologic Oncology, 2017, reaffirmed 2019). Further discussion may include potential reproductive, psychological, and familial implications. Patients may have to make childbearing decisions based on results. They may experience increased anxiety over potential outcomes, or they may feel burdened with informing significant others and family members (Committee on Gynecologic Practice, Society of Gynecologic Oncology, 2017, reaffirmed 2019; NCI, n.d.-c). Clinicians should recommend education and testing of all family members (also known as cascade testing) who have been diagnosed with cancer and those who are potentially affected by the results (Committee on Gynecologic Practice, Society of Gynecologic Oncology, 2017, reaffirmed 2019).

Bilateral salpingo-oophorectomy is associated with significantly reduced risk for breast, ovarian, fallopian tube, and peritoneal cancers and is recommended as a risk-reducing strategy for people who carry BRCA1 or BRCA2 mutations at 35–40 years and 40–45 years, respectively (Abu-Rustum et al., 2025). Patients with BRIP1, RAD51C, and RAD51D are recommended to have a risk-reducing bilateral salpingo-oophorectomy at 45–50 years. For carriers of PALB2, this surgery can be considered at 45–50 years (Abu-Rustum et al., 2025). Patients with the Lynch syndrome mutations MLH1 and MSH6 can consider hysterectomy (for endometrial cancer risk reduction) with salpingectomy at age 40 and delayed oophorectomy at age 50 (Daly et al., 2023). Patients who choose a risk-reducing bilateral salpingo-oophorectomy continue to have a risk of breast and peritoneal cancer (3–4%) and need to continue to be followed. Both tubes and ovaries should receive careful pathological examination at time of removal related to the 3.5–4.6 percent risk of occult cancer being present (Liu et al., 2022; Daly et al., 2023). Patients considering this option should receive education regarding the clinical effects of premature menopause, such as vasomotor symptoms, vaginal dryness, and dyspareunia (Arora et al., 2025). As an overall preventive strategy for ovarian cancer, the Committee on Gynecologic Practice, Society of Gynecologic Oncology (2019) now recommends that bilateral salpingectomy also be offered to people who are already undergoing hysterectomy for other indications.

Secondary and Tertiary Prevention

The USPSTF (2018b) and NCCN (2024c) recommends against screening for ovarian cancer in asymptomatic patients who are not at high risk for hereditary forms. Routine screening with pelvic examination, transvaginal ultrasound, and tumor markers, such as CA-125 alone or in combination, has not been shown to decrease the number of deaths from ovarian cancer in asymptomatic patients. These measures have led to false-positive results (44%), unnecessary surgery (up to 3.2%), and major surgical complications in people who do not have cancer (Berek et al., 2021; Liu et al., 2024).

CA-125 Testing

CA-125 is found in about 80 percent of epithelial ovarian cancers, but it is present in only 50 percent of early-stage cancers. Consequently, its measurement has limited use in early detection (Charkhchi et al., 2020). An elevation in CA-125 (greater than 35 units) is not specific for ovarian cancer and may be elevated in people with endometriosis, lung cancer, and chronic liver disease (Charkhchi et al., 2020). An extremely high CA-125 level may assist in the evaluation of people who present with signs and symptoms of ovarian cancer, and it may suggest whether further definitive testing is needed. The clinician must consider the cost-effectiveness and psychological benefits and drawbacks of using this diagnostic test for ovarian cancer because of the variations in interpretation of results, the lack of evidence on its overall effect on survival, and the potential harms of false-positive results (Charkhchi et al., 2020; Berek et al., 2021).

Continued research and development of reliable, cost-effective and easily accessible screening and early diagnostic methods are urgently needed; the ability to detect ovarian cancers, particularly type II tumors, before they metastasize is critical to improving survival. Future screening methods should focus on identifying the unique features of aggressive early-stage tumors and improving imaging methods to enable early and accurate detection (Charkhchi et al., 2020). Prevention strategies for ovarian cancer also need to focus on other types of ovarian tumors and their pathogenesis. For example, people with endometriosis are over 4 times more likely to develop ovarian cancer and establishing criteria for identifying and treating people with endometriosis may assist in decreasing the risk of some forms of ovarian cancer (Barnard et al., 2024).

Management

Referral

When the history and physical examination, laboratory, or imaging results are suspicious for ovarian cancer, the clinician should refer the patient to a gynecologic oncologist. Indicators for referral include persistent signs and symptoms, elevated CA-125 levels, presence of ascites, a nodular or fixed pelvic mass, and evidence of abdominal or distant metastasis (Arora et al., 2025). In patients who are premenopausal, treatments that lead to infertility and abrupt entry into menopause can be devastating. Clinicians should educate their patients about childbearing options prior to treatment, and referral to a fertility specialist or sex counselor may be indicated.

Operative procedures for ovarian cancer should be done by gynecologic oncologists trained to appropriately stage and debulk tumors. Optimally, treatment should occur in facilities that have large volumes of ovarian cancer cases and can offer multidisciplinary support services to maximize patient outcomes. Studies have shown that patients who receive care at low-volume centers receive 30 percent less guideline-recommended treatment and patients over the age of 65 with advanced-stage ovarian cancer receive treatment according to established guidelines less often than their younger counterparts. It is well known that suboptimal treatment is associated with lower survival rates (van Walree et al., 2020; Mei et al., 2023). Delivery of ovarian cancer care that follows current practice guidelines in facilities that treat larger case volumes can result in improved survival for people with ovarian cancer (Mei et al., 2023). It is therefore important for clinicians to discuss ovarian cancer treatment options in terms of availability, cost, distance, and personal choice with patients and their significant others to make the most appropriate referrals for treatment.

Surgery

Treatment of ovarian cancer depends on the type of tumor, stage, and the person's age, health, and preferences (NCI, 2024f). Surgical exploration with staging laparotomy is the first step in ovarian cancer treatment and is required to make a definitive diagnosis of cancer, stage the extent of the disease, and debulk (remove) all the visible tumors in the abdomen and pelvis. The goal of debulking is to leave tumor diameter and thickness less than 1 cm, which is referred to as optimal debulking. Patients whose tumors have been optimally debulked have better outcomes than those left with larger tumors after surgery (Liu et al., 2024). A total abdominal hysterectomy, bilateral salpingo-oophorectomy, omentectomy, pelvic and para-aortic lymph node sampling and dissection, scraping of the undersurface of the diaphragm, multiple peritoneal biopsies, and aspiration of ascites for cytology are all part of the standard surgical procedure (Berek et al., 2021; Liu et al., 2024). For patients who wish to maintain fertility and those with very early-stage I disease or tumors with low potential for malignancy, unilateral salpingo-oophorectomy with preservation of the uterus may be considered (Berek et al., 2021).

The FIGO staging system is used to provide important prognostic information that is used to determine treatment options (**Table 28-7**). Currently, the FIGO staging system combines classifications for ovarian, fallopian tube, and peritoneal cancer. Stage I cancer is still confined to the ovaries or fallopian tubes. At stage II, there is spread to the pelvic organs. In stage III, metastasis to the peritoneal cavity or retroperitoneal lymph nodes has occurred. At stage IV, the cancer has spread to distant sites, including the lungs and extra-abdominal lymph nodes. The end stage of ovarian cancer is characterized by bowel obstruction from metastatic tumors, which leads to end-stage cancer symptoms such as cachexia, malnutrition, and death (Lisio et al., 2019; Berek et al., 2021; Prat & FIGO Committee on Gynecologic Oncology, 2014).

Pharmacologic Management

With the advent of personalized cancer medicine, histopathological diagnosis of ovarian cancer is an important component of successful treatment. Ovarian tumors have distinct molecular characteristics depending on the tumor type, and they respond to chemotherapy differently (Prat & FIGO Committee on Gynecologic Oncology, 2014). Except for people with stage I disease who have been identified as having a greater than 95 percent chance of survival after comprehensive laparotomy, people in all other stages of disease are potential candidates for clinical trials and should be offered participation in them if they meet the selection criteria (Liu et al., 2024).

Patients surgically staged as 1A or 1B, and those with low-grade subtypes of ovarian cancer, require continued observation but no further treatment after surgical staging because 5-year survival is greater than 90 percent for this subgroup (Lisio et al., 2019; NCCN, 2024). Stage II to IV disease is treated with a combination of staging and debulking surgery followed by postoperative chemotherapy. Standard combination chemotherapy includes intravenous platinum and taxane-based compounds, which are given in three to six cycles (Lisio et al., 2019; Berek et al., 2021; NCI, n.d.-c; Liu et al., 2024).

The use of intraperitoneal chemotherapy in combination with intravenous chemotherapy may be given to people with stage II and III disease; it has been shown to improve the disease-free interval in people with stage III disease who have had optimal debulking (Lisio et al., 2019; NCI, n.d.-c; Liu et al., 2024). Intraperitoneal chemotherapy allows higher doses of chemotherapy to be applied directly to the area most commonly affected by cancer spread. People undergoing this therapy may experience peritoneal catheter complications such as pain, catheter

TABLE 28-7 FIGO Staging Classification for Cancer of the Ovary, Fallopian Tube, and Peritoneum

Stage	Characteristics
Stage I	Tumor confined to the ovaries or fallopian tube(s) IA: Tumor limited to one ovary (capsule intact) or fallopian tube; no tumor on ovarian or fallopian tube surface; no malignant cells in the ascites or peritoneal washings IB: Tumor limited to both ovaries (capsules intact) or fallopian tubes; no tumor on ovarian or fallopian tube surfaces; no malignant cells in the ascites or peritoneal washings IC: Tumor limited to one or both ovaries or fallopian tubes, with any of the following: • IC1: Surgical spill • IC2: Capsule ruptured before surgery or tumor on ovarian or fallopian tube surface • IC3: Malignant cells in the ascites or peritoneal washings
Stage II	Tumor involves one or both ovaries or fallopian tubes with pelvic extension (below pelvic brim) or primary peritoneal cancer IIA: Extension and/or implants on uterus and/or fallopian tubes and/or ovaries IIB: Extension to other pelvic intraperitoneal tissues
Stage III	Tumor involves one or both ovaries or fallopian tubes, or peritoneal cancer, with cytologically and histologically confirmed spread to the peritoneum outside the pelvis and/or metastasis to the retroperitoneal lymph nodes IIIA1: Positive retroperitoneal lymph nodes only (cytologically or histologically proven) • IIIA1(i): Metastasis up to 10 mm in greatest dimension • IIIA1(ii): Metastasis more than 10 mm in greatest dimension IIIA2: Microscopic extrapelvic (above the pelvic brim) peritoneal involvement with or without positive retroperitoneal lymph nodes IIIB: Macroscopic peritoneal metastasis beyond the pelvis up to 2 cm in greatest dimension, with or without metastasis to the retroperitoneal lymph nodes IIIC: Macroscopic peritoneal metastasis beyond the pelvis more than 2 cm in greatest dimension, with or without metastasis to the retroperitoneal lymph nodes (includes extension of tumor to capsule of liver and spleen without parenchymal involvement of either organ)
Stage IV	Distant metastasis excluding peritoneal metastases IVA: Pleural effusion with positive cytology IVB: Parenchymal metastases and metastases to extra-abdominal organs (including inguinal lymph nodes and lymph nodes outside of the abdominal cavity)

Reproduced from Prat, J., & FIGO Committee on Gynecologic Oncology. (2014). Staging classification for cancer of the ovary, fallopian tube, and peritoneum. *International Journal of Gynecology and Obstetrics, 124*(1), 1–5. https://doi.org/10.1016/j.ijgo.2013.10.001. Reprinted with permission from John Wiley and Sons.

Abbreviation: FIGO, International Federation of Gynecology and Obstetrics.

blockage, and other side effects including nausea and vomiting, neuropathy, fever, and infections (Liu et al., 2024). Currently, intraperitoneal chemotherapy is not recommended for people who have ovarian cancer in stages I or IV (Liu et al., 2024).

Alternative treatment regimens may be used in specific cases of ovarian cancer. People with bulky stage III or IV cancer, those with distant metastasis, and those who are too weak or ill for major surgery may be offered neoadjuvant therapy, which is typically chemotherapy given to reduce tumor burden prior to staging and debulking surgery. Patients receive three to four cycles of chemotherapy, which is then followed by a tumor reduction surgery. Standard treatment regimens of chemotherapy may then be considered (Lisio et al., 2019; Berek et al., 2021; Liu et al., 2024).

Approximately 80 percent of people with advanced disease who respond to first-line treatments have recurrence of disease. The prognosis is poor when the disease recurs in less than 6 months and for those whose disease continues to progress after two consecutive regimens of chemotherapy (Lisio et al., 2019; Berek et al., 2021; Liu et al., 2024). People with recurrence of disease or evidence of progression may be followed up with second-line approaches, such as additional debulking surgery, clinical trials, and different combinations and dosing of chemotherapeutic agents (Lisio et al., 2019; Berek et al., 2021; Liu et al., 2024). Response to further treatment is highly individualized, and recurrent ovarian cancer is not curable in the majority of people. The aim of further treatment is to maintain quality of life and to control symptoms of the disease (Berek et al., 2021).

Other Treatment Options

Inhibition of angiogenesis and DNA repair in cancer cells has been the focus in the development of new drug therapies in the treatment of ovarian cancer. Vascular endothelial growth factor (VEGF) plays a central role in angiogenesis of cancer cells, allowing for endothelial cell proliferation and microvessel formation (Yang & Cao, 2022). The anti-VEGF monoclonal antibody, bevacizumab, inhibits signaling pathways for angiogenesis, and use of the drug in combination with standard chemotherapy has improved the period of progression-free survival for some ovarian cancer patients. Bevacizumab may be used in combination with primary chemotherapy or in the treatment of recurrent disease (Berek et al., 2021; Mao, Seow, & Chen, 2022; Liu et al., 2024). Poly (ADP-ribose) polymerase (PARP) inhibitor drugs affect cancer cells' ability to repair DNA and continue to replicate. PARP inhibitor drugs have demonstrated benefit especially in ovarian cancer associated with BRCA mutations and tumors that test positive for homologous recombination deficiency (Berek et al., 2021; O'Malley et al., 2023). PARP inhibitors may be used for maintenance therapy to delay progression of ovarian cancer and retreatment with chemotherapy (O'Malley et al., 2023; Liu et al., 2024). Another consideration in the treatment of ovarian cancer is the use of radiation therapy. Total abdominal and pelvic radiation therapy is rarely used for the primary treatment of ovarian cancer and is not included in the recent guidelines for ovarian cancer, although palliative localized radiation therapy is an option for symptom control in people with recurrent advanced disease (Macchia et al., 2023; Liu et al., 2024).

Emerging Evidence That May Change Management

An important aim for ovarian cancer screening is the detection of highly sensitive biomarkers and specific gene mutations associated with tumors in early stage (Charkhchi et al., 2020; Liu et al., 2024). A step in this direction has been made with the development of a blood test that uses assays for protein biomarkers and genetic alterations through plasma DNA-based testing. The blood test may be able to identify the presence and origin of early-stage cancers, such as ovarian, liver, stomach, pancreas, and esophagus (Rahaman, Li, & Wong, 2021). Further research and application of this screening test to larger populations may have the potential to facilitate early detection and decrease mortality from many cancers that currently do not have screening tests available to individuals at average risk (Enroth et al., 2022).

Numerous genetic and molecular alterations have been identified in the specific subtypes of ovarian cancers cells (Liberto et al., 2022). Research into distinct cancer cell characteristics has led to the development of new molecularly targeted drugs that have lower toxicity than conventional chemotherapy and may positively affect clinical outcomes in ovarian cancer. As more is known about the mechanisms responsible for cancer growth and spread, additional recommendations for targeted drug therapies, such as VEGF angiogenesis inhibitors and PARP inhibitors, may be proposed. However, progress in the development of new treatments for ovarian cancer has been slow, related in part to identified molecular changes not being easily targeted with known inhibitors (Lisio et al., 2019). Continued research and development in precision medicine is needed to improve prognoses and quality of life for those with ovarian cancer (Lheureux, Braunstein, & Oza, 2019).

Patient Education

The clinician should start with a consideration of a person's risk for ovarian cancer when planning patient education at annual checkups. For those at average risk, discussion may include modification of environmental and lifestyle factors, such as increasing exercise, weight reduction, and smoking cessation. Because early detection of ovarian cancer is associated with improved outcomes, patients with both average and high risk should receive education on the typical early signs of ovarian cancer, such as loss of appetite, early satiety, abdominal bloating, pain, or urinary symptoms, especially if they are either persistent or progressive in nature. Patients with a personal or family history of ovarian and breast cancer should be referred for genetic counseling and receive education on the risks, benefits, and limitations of genetic screening (Lisio et al., 2019; Berek et al., 2021; NCCN 2024c). Those with a known mutation in ovarian cancer predisposition genes should receive education on the risk-reducing benefits of oral contraceptive therapy and bilateral salpingo-oophorectomy (Committee on Gynecologic Practice, Society of Gynecologic Oncology, 2019; Liu et al., 2024).

People who have been diagnosed with ovarian cancer may benefit from a greater understanding of their prognosis and potential treatment options and are likely to have opinions about the importance of quality of life versus length of life related to treatment (Shrestha et al., 2019). Although many people consider the progression-free interval to be the most important factor in determining their preferred treatment, some people are willing to accept a reduction in the time spent without progression in return for improvements in quality of life, side effects, and convenience (Wenzel et al., 2021). A survivorship care plan may be discussed and recommended as a means to improve care coordination, address continued educational needs, and reduce stress in some cancer survivors. Survivorship care plans may be most valuable for patients who want detailed information about their cancer; however, the clinician should also consider that some people prefer to avoid medical information as a means of reducing stress, depression, and physical discomfort (Kvale et al., 2024).

Post-Treatment Patient Education and Follow-Up

All people with any stage of ovarian cancer require clinical follow-up after their initial treatment (Liu et al., 2024). The objectives for follow-up include early recognition and management of treatment-related complications or signs and symptoms of recurrent disease, emotional support, and promotion of general well-being and a healthy lifestyle (Berek et al., 2021; ACS, 2022).

Most people have widespread disease at the time of diagnosis; however, the 5-year survival rate in people with ovarian cancer who are treated with first-line cytoreductive surgery and chemotherapy has increased to approximately 49 percent due to advances in systemic therapy. (Berek et al., 2021; Liu et al., 2024). As treatments that are more effective have become available, increasing numbers of people with advanced disease at diagnosis are achieving complete remission with initial surgery and chemotherapy. Unfortunately, up to 37 percent of people diagnosed with early-stage disease, and the majority of people with advanced epithelial cancer, experience recurrence within 5 years, with the median progression-free survival time being approximately 16 months (Berek et al., 2021; Levine et al., 2023).

The primary goal of follow-up care is the early identification of recurrence in hopes that additional treatment will offer the possibility of disease control. A therapeutic partnership between the clinician and the patient improves the likelihood that early, subtle signs of recurrence will be promptly reported and evaluated. Lifelong follow-up will be required at regularly scheduled intervals. Follow-up needs to be coordinated with the primary care provider and the gynecologic oncologist or medical and radiation oncologists. Patients are usually seen for follow-up every 2 to 4 months with a gradual increase to every 4 to 6 months for 2 years, and then annually after the 5th year (Berek et al., 2021; ACS, 2022; Liu et al., 2024).

Recurrence of disease is identified clinically through physical examination, an evaluation of new or returning symptoms, CA-125 measurements, or imaging (Berek et al, 2021; Liu et al., 2024). During each follow-up visit, history taking should include questions about changes in appetite, increase in abdominal size or mass, weight gain or loss, changes in bowel or bladder function, pelvic pain, and leg edema (ACS, 2022; Liu et al., 2024). A complete physical and pelvic examination should be performed (Berek et al., 2021). A rising CA-125 level is highly suggestive of recurrent disease, but clinicians should bear in mind that ovarian cancer may recur without a corresponding elevation in CA-125. In addition, people who had fertility-sparing surgery as their initial treatment should be followed with ultrasound examinations of the abdomen and pelvis and, if indicated, completion surgery should be considered (Liu et al., 2024).

The fear of recurrence is always present for a person who has been treated for ovarian cancer. Remission followed by recurrence and the need for retreatment keep patients in an ongoing state of uncertainty and anxiety. Even in people with a good prognosis, the fear of recurrence commonly persists for years after completion of definitive treatment and may surface at some follow-up appointments and not others. The person who reports symptoms should be seen promptly, even though the symptoms may be a result of sometimes minor, transient problems such as indigestion or a muscle strain. Each follow-up assessment must always include the consideration of the possibility of recurrent disease and the delayed effects of surgery, chemotherapy, and radiation therapy.

Special Considerations

Loss of fertility, hormonal changes, and the permanent physical changes that accompany major debulking surgery followed by chemotherapy add to the stress that the cancer diagnosis places on the patient's personal relationships and feelings of sexuality. Sexual functioning is an important component of quality of life. It involves physical, emotional, and social aspects, and many ovarian cancer survivors experience a decrease in sexual interest, activity, and enjoyment (Fischer, Marguerie, & Brotto, 2019; Kim et al., 2021; Logue et al., 2022). The clinician should be prepared to explore a person's concerns about sexuality and offer clinically informative advice and a referral to a family or sex counselor as indicated (Logue et al., 2022).

When the diagnosis of ovarian cancer is first received, people often feel isolated and wish to avoid others who have the disease, although later some people will seek relationships with others who have ovarian cancer in an effort to share the lived experience and find emotional support. People with ovarian cancer often will take control of their treatment by seeking out alternative and complementary therapies that they will combine with conventional treatment. Some people worry about passing a genetic predisposition for cancer on to their children. Quality of life and the meaning of life itself are important issues for ovarian cancer survivors. Relationships may be reevaluated in addition to personal beliefs about life, death, and spirituality. Psychological support and spiritual care are both integral aspects of achieving the best outcomes for people with ovarian cancer and should always be part of their treatment plan.

Goals for all people with a diagnosis of ovarian cancer include symptom management, supportive care, long-term wellness care, and referral to palliative care and hospice as indicated (Liu et al., 2024). Palliative care improves the quality of life for patients and their families when faced with life-threatening illness and can significantly reduce the cost of care (Haag et al., 2022; Liu et al., 2024). Palliative care focuses on maintaining quality of life through management of disturbing symptoms such as pain, nausea, respiratory symptoms, cancer-related fatigue, anxiety, and depression (Haag et al., 2022; Mah et al., 2024). In addition, hospice care and discussions about advance directives should be offered to patients and their families to facilitate end-of-life decisions in a time appropriate manner.

Clinicians should also consider the anxiety and stress experienced by caregivers of people with gynecologic cancer. Although caregivers often feel honored to care for their loved ones, changes in work schedules and financial concerns may be difficult. Reducing work schedules to provide care can affect the ability to pay for medications and supplies. Those with lower incomes are less able to afford resources that support patient needs, thus adding to stress and worry. In addition, caregivers may experience unmet individual psychosocial needs related to providing care 24 hours per day, 7 days per week. Caregivers need to know how to care for the patient and also need education and support in self-care. Clinicians may reduce caregiving burden by suggesting interventions that can provide low-cost assistance with patient care, such as home care services, respite care, and meals available through community agencies. A consult with social work may be beneficial in providing resources for financial aid, and referrals can also include dietician assistance and support from rehabilitation therapists as indicated (Temkin et al., 2022; Johnston et al., 2021). Other noted resources to offer patients and their partners include the following: American Cancer Society (www.cancer.org); Cancer Hope Network (www.cancerhopenetwork.org); National Comprehensive Cancer Network (www.nccn.org); and Cancer Support Community (www.cancersupportcommunity.org).

CONCLUSION

People with gynecologic cancer derive great benefit and support from the presence of consistent, sensitive clinicians who take their symptoms and concerns seriously and provide prompt, thorough follow-up that does not offer any false sense of reassurance or undue sense of alarm. Clinicians who provide a holistic and patient-centered approach to cancer care can improve quality of life and provide invaluable support to people in their experience of living with cancer.

References

Abu-Rustum, N. R., Yashar, C. M., Arend, R., Barber, E., Bradley, K., Brooks, R., Campos, S. M., Chino, J., Chon, H. S., Crispens, M. A., Damast, S., Fisher, C. M., Frederick, P., Gaffney, D. K., Gaillard, S., Giuntoli, R., Glaser, S., Holmes, J., Howitt, B. E., Lea, J., ... Espinosa, S. (2023). NCCN Guidelines® Insights: Cervical Cancer, Version 1.2024. *Journal of the National Comprehensive Cancer Network : JNCCN, 21*(12), 1224–1233. https://doi.org/10.6004/jnccn.2023.0062

Abu-Rustum, N. R., Yashar, C. M., Arend, R., Barber, E., Bradley, K., Brooks, R., Campos, S. M., Chino, J., Chon, H. S., Crispens, M. A., Damast, S., Fisher, C. M., Frederick, P., Gaffney, D. K., Gaillard, S., Giuntoli, R., II, Glaser, S., Holmes, J., Howitt, B. E., Kendra, K., ... Espinosa, S. (2024). Vulvar Cancer, Version 3.2024, NCCN Clinical Practice Guidelines in Oncology. *Journal of the National Comprehensive Cancer Network : JNCCN, 22*(2), 117–135. https://doi.org/10.6004/jnccn.2024.0013

Abu-Rustum, N. R., Campos, S. M., Amarnath, S., Arend, R., Barber, E., Bradley, K., Brooks, R., Chino, J., Chon, H. S., Crispens, M. A., Damast, S., Fisher, C. M., Frederick, P., Gaffney, D. K., Gaillard, S., Giuntoli, R., Glaser, S., Howitt, B. E., Landrum, L., Lea, J., ... Sambandam, V. (2025). NCCN Guidelines® Insights: Uterine Neoplasms, Version 3.2025. *Journal of the National Comprehensive Cancer Network : JNCCN, 23*(8), 284–291. https://doi.org/10.6004/jnccn.2025.0038

Adjei Boakye, E., McKinney, S. L., Whittington, K. D, Boyer V. E., Franca M. C., Lee, M., McKinnies, R. C., Collins, S. K., & Gerend, M. A. (2022). Association between sexual activity and human papillomavirus (HPV) vaccine initiation and completion among college students. *Vaccines (Basel), 10*(12), 2079. https://doi.org/10.3390/vaccines10122079. PMID: 36560489; PMCID: PMC9784235.

Aggarwal, P., & Ben Amor, A. (2023). Cervical ectropion. In *StatPearls*. https://www.ncbi.nlm.nih.gov/books/NBK560709/

Alhmoud, J. F., Woolley, J. F., Al Moustafa, A. E., & Malki, M. I. (2020). DNA damage/repair management in cancers. *Cancers (Basel), 12*(4), 1050. https://doi.org/10.3390/cancers12041050. PMID: 32340362; PMCID: PMC7226105.

Alldredge, J., Leaf, M. C., Patel, P., Coakley, K., Longoria, T., McLaren, C., & Randall, L. M. (2020). Prevalence and predictors of HIV screening in invasive cervical cancer: A 10 year cohort study. *International Journal of Gynecological Cancer, 30*(6), 772–776. https://doi.org/https://doi.org/10.1136/ijgc-2019-000909. Epub 2020 Mar 9. PMID: 32156714; PMCID: PMC7872791.

American Cancer Society. (2019a). *Can endometrial cancer be found early*? https://www.cancer.org/cancer/endometrial-cancer/detection-diagnosis-staging/detection.html

American Cancer Society. (2019c). *Hormone therapy for endometrial cancer*. https://www.cancer.org/cancer/endometrial-cancer/treating/hormone-therapy.html

American Cancer Society. (2019d). *HPV and HPV testing*. https://www.cancer.org/cancer/cancer-causes/infectious-agents/hpv/hpv-and-hpv-testing.html

American Cancer Society. (2019g). *Tests for endometrial cancer*. https://www.cancer.org/cancer/endometrial-cancer/detection-diagnosis-staging/how-diagnosed.html

American Cancer Society. (2019h). *What is endometrial cancer*? https://www.cancer.org/cancer/endometrial-cancer/about/what-is-endometrial-cancer.html

American Cancer Society. (2020a). *Cervical cancer stages*. https://www.cancer.org/cervical-cancer/detection-diagnosis-staging/staged.html

American Cancer Society. (2020b). *Chemotherapy for cervical cancer*. https://www.cancer.org/cancer/cervical-cancer/treating/chemotherapy.html

American Cancer Society. (2020c). *Immunotherapy for cervical cancer*. https://www.cancer.org/cancertypes/cervical-cancer/treating/immunotherapy.html

American Cancer Society. (2025a). *Key statistics for cervical cancer*. https://www.cancer .org/cancer/cervical-cancer/about/key-statistics.html

American Cancer Society. (2020f). *Risk factors for cervical cancer*. https://www.cancer.org/cancer/cervical-cancer/causes-risks-prevention/risk-factors.html

American Cancer Society. (2020i). *Tests for cervical cancer*. https://www.cancer.org/cancer/cervical-cancer/detection-diagnosis-staging/how-diagnosed.html

American Cancer Society. (2020j). *Treatment options for cervical cancer, by stage*. https://www.cancer.org/cancer/cervical-cancer/treating/by-stage.html

American Cancer Society. (2020k). *What causes cervical cancer*? https://www.cancer.org/cancer/cervical-cancer/causes-risks-prevention/what-causes.html

American Cancer Society. (202la). *What is cervical cancer*? https://www.cancer.org/cancer/cervical-cancer/prevention-and-early-detection/what-is-cervical-cancer.html

American Cancer Society. (2021b). *Ovarian cancer risk factors*. https://www.cancer.org/cancer/types/ovarian-cancer/causes-risks-prevention/risk-factors.html

American Cancer Society. (2022). *Understanding cancer: Oncogenes, tumor suppressor genes, and DNA repair genes*. https://www.cancer.org/cancer/understanding-cancer/genes-and-cancer/oncogenes-tumor-suppressor-genes.html

American Cancer Society. (2022a). *Radiation therapy for uterine sarcomas*. https://www.cancer.org/cancer/types/uterine-sarcoma/treating/radiation-therapy.html

American Cancer Society. (2024b). *Radiation therapy for cervical cancer*. https://www.cancer.org/cancer/types/cervical-cancer/treating/radiation.html

American Cancer Society. (2024c). *Ovarian cancer*. https://www.cancer.org/cancer/types/ovarian-cancer.html

American Cancer Society. (2025). *Key statistics for vulvar cancer*. https://www.cancer.org/cancer/types/vulvar-cancer/about/key-statistics.html

American Cancer Society. (2025b). *Surgery for cervical cancer*. https://www.cancer.org/cancer/cervical-cancer/treating/surgery.html

American Cancer Society. (2025c). *Endometrial Cancer Risk Factors*. https://www.cancer.org/cancer/types/endometrial-cancer/causes-risks-prevention/risk-factors.html

American Cancer Society Cancer Action Network (ACSCAN). (2024). *Just the facts: Cervical cancer disparities*. https://www.fightcancer.org/sites/default/files/just_the_facts_cervical_cancer_disparities_fact_sheet_final_2.21.24.pdf

American College of Obstetricians and Gynecologists. (2015, reaffirmed 2020). ACOG practice bulletin no. 149: Endometrial cancer. *Obstetrics & Gynecology, 125*(4), e1006–e1026. https://doi.org/10.1097/01.AOG.0000462977.61229.de

American College of Obstetricians and Gynecologists. (2018, reaffirmed 2024). *The utility of and indications for routine pelvic examination*. https://www.acog.org/clinical/clinical-guidance/committee-opinion/articles/2018/10/the-utility-of-and-indications-for-routine-pelvic-examination

American College of Obstetricians and Gynecologists. (2019). *Opportunistic salpingectomy as a strategy for epithelial ovarian cancer prevention*. https://www.acog.org/clinical/clinical-guidance/committee-opinion/articles/2019/04/opportunistic-salpingectomy-as-a-strategy-for-epithelial-ovarian-cancer-prevention

American College of Obstetricians and Gynecologists. (2020). *Human papillomavirus vaccination*. https://www.acog.org/clinical/clinical-guidance/committee-opinion/articles/2020/08/human-papillomavirus-vaccination#:~:text=Human%20papillomavirus%20vaccination%20is%20not,have%20not%20previously%20been%20vaccinated

American Joint Committee on Cancer. (2020). *What is cancer staging?* https://cancerstaging.org/references-tools/Pages/What-is-Cancer-Staging.aspx

American Society for Colposcopy and Cervical Pathology. (2019). *Risk-based management consensus guidelines*. http://www.asccp.org/consensus-guidelines

American Society of Clinical Oncology. (2019). *Uterine cancer: Statistics*. https://www.cancer.net/cancer-types/uterine-cancer/statistics

Anderson, C., Olshan, A. F., Bae-Jump, V. L., Brewster, W. R., Lund, J. L., & Nichols, H. B. (2022). Cardiovascular disease diagnoses among older women with endometrial cancer. *Gynecologic Oncology, 167*(1), 51–57. https://doi.org/10.1016/j.ygyno.2022.08.014. Epub 2022 Aug 22. PMID: 36008183.

Arora, T., Mullangi, S., Vadakekut, E. S., & Lekkala, M. R. (2025). Epithelial Ovarian Cancer. In *StatPearls*. StatPearls Publishing. https://www.ncbi.nlm.nih.gov/books/NBK567760/

Arshadi, M., Hesari, E., Ahmadinezhad, M., Yekta, E. M., Ebrahimi, F., Azizi, H., Esfarjani, S. V., Rostami, M., & Khodamoradi, F. (2024). The association between oral contraceptive pills and ovarian cancer risk: A systematic review and meta-analysis. *Bulletin du Cancer, 111*(10), 918–929. https://doi.org/10.1016/j.bulcan.2024.05.010. Epub 2024 Sep 10. PMID: 39261253.

Ashique, S., Hussain, A., Fatima, N., & Altamimi, M. A. (2023). HPV pathogenesis, various types of vaccines, safety concern, prophylactic and therapeutic applications to control cervical cancer, and future perspective. *Virusdisease, 34*(2), 1–19. https://doi.org/10.1007/s13337-023-00824-z. Epub ahead of print. PMID: 37363362; PMCID: PMC10208188.

Balasubramaniam, S. D., Balakrishnan, V., Oon, C. E., & Kaur, G. (2019). Key molecular events in cervical cancer development. *Medicina (Kaunas), 55*(7), 384. https://doi.org/10.3390/medicina55070384. PMID: 31319555; PMCID: PMC6681523.

Barnard, M. E., Farland, L. V., Yan, B., Wang, J., Trabert, B., Doherty, J. A., Meeks, H. D., Madsen, M., Guinto, E., Collin, L. J., Maurer, K. A., Page, J. M., Kiser, A. C., Varner, M. W., Allen-Brady, K., Pollack, A. Z., Peterson, K. R,. Peterson, C. M., & Schliep, K. C. (2024). Endometriosis typology and ovarian cancer risk. *JAMA, 332*(6), 482–489. https://doi.org/10.1001/jama.2024.9210. PMID: 39018030; PMCID: PMC11255975.

Berek, J. S., Renz, M., Kehoe, S., Kumar, L., & Friedlander, M. (2021). Cancer of the ovary, fallopian tube, and peritoneum: 2021 update. *International Federation of Gynaecology and Obstetrics, 155*(Suppl 1), 61–85. https://doi.org/10.1002/ijgo.13878. PMID: 34669199; PMCID: PMC9298325.

Boardman, C. H., & Matthews, K. J. (2025). Cervical cancer. *Medscape*. https://emedicine.medscape.com/article/253513-overview

Boonlikit, S., & Tangterdchanakit, P. (2024). Multicentricity and the risk of recurrence/persistence after laser vaporization for high-grade vulvar and vaginal intraepithelial neoplasia. *World Journal of Oncology, 15*(1), 90–99. https://doi.org/10.14740/wjon1743. Epub 2024 Jan 10. PMID: 38274717; PMCID: PMC10807919.

Bourgioti, C., Konidari, M., & Moulopoulos, L. A. (2023). Manifestations of ovarian cancer in relation to other pelvic diseases by MRI. *Cancers (Basel), 15*(7), 2106. https://doi.org/10.3390/cancers15072106. PMID: 37046767; PMCID: PMC10093428.

Bravo, V., Serrano, M., Duque, A., Ferragud, J., & Coronado, P. J. (2023). Glycyrrhizinic acid as an antiviral and anticancer agent in the treatment of human papillomavirus. *Journal of Personalized Medicine, 13*(12), 1639. https://doi.org/10.3390/jpm13121639. PMID: 38138866; PMCID: PMC10744776.

Bray, F., Laversanne, M., Sung, H., et al. (2024). Global cancer statistics 2022: GLOBOCAN estimates of incidence and mortality worldwide for 36 cancers in 185 countries. *CA: A Cancer Journal for Clinicians, 74*(3), 229–263. https://doi.org/10.332-2/caac.21834

Brown, A., McKenna, S., Forbes, D., & Harley, I. (2022). Paraneoplastic syndrome associated with gynaecological malignancy: A review of the evidence. *The Obstetrician & Gynaecologist, 24,* 137–142. https://doi.org/10.1111/tog.12804

Brusen Villadsen, A., Bundgaard-Nielsen, C., Ambühl, L., Tang Svendsen, M., Søkilde Pedersen, I., Stµhr Hansen, E., Baandrup, U., Blaakµr, J., & Sørensen, S. (2021). Prevalence and type distribution of human papillomavirus infections in Danish patients diagnosed with vulvar squamous cell tumors and precursors. *Gynecological Oncology Reports, 37,* 100828. https://doi.org/10.1016/j.gore.2021.100828. PMID: 34621943; PMCID: PMC8484492.

Bucchi, L., Pizzato, M., Rosso, S., & Ferretti, S. (2022). New insights into the epidemiology of vulvar cancer: Systematic literature review for an update of incidence and risk factors. *Cancers, 14*(2), 389. https://doi.org/10.3390/cancers14020389

Burmeister, C. A., Khan, S. F., Schäfer, G., Mbatani, N., Adams, T., Moodley, J., & Prince, S. (2022). Cervical cancer therapies: Current challenges and future perspectives. *Tumour Virus Research, 13,* 200238. https://doi.org/10.1016/j.tvr.2022.200238. Epub 2022 Apr 20. PMID: 35460940; PMCID: PMC9062473.

Campos-Parra, A. D., Pérez-Quintanilla, M., Martínez-Gutierrez, A. D., Pérez-Montiel, D., Coronel-Martínez, J., Millan-Catalan, O., De León, D. C., & Pérez-Plasencia, C. (2022). Molecular differences between squamous cell carcinoma and adenocarcinoma cervical cancer subtypes: Potential prognostic biomarkers. *Current Oncology (Toronto, Ont.), 29*(7), 4689–4702. https://doi.org/10.3390/curroncol29070372. PMID: 35877232; PMCID: PMC9322365.

Capasso, I., Santoro, A., Lucci Cordisco, E., Perrone, E., Tronconi, F., Catena, U., Zannoni, G. F., Scambia, G., Fanfani, F., Lorusso, D., & Duranti, S. (2023). Lynch syndrome and gynecologic tumors: Incidence, prophylaxis, and management of patients with cancer. *Cancers (Basel), 15*(5), 1400. https://doi.org/10.3390/cancers15051400. PMID: 36900193; PMCID: PMC10000861.

Caretto, A. A., Servillo, M., Tagliaferri, L., Lancellotta, V., Fragomeni, S. M., Garganese, G., Scambia, G., & Gentileschi, S. (2023). Secondary post-oncologic vulvar reconstruction—a simplified algorithm. *Frontiers in Oncology, 13,* 1195580. https://doi.org/10.3389/fonc.2023.1195580. PMID: 37409264; PMCID: PMC10318400

Caruso, G., Barcellini, A., Mazzeo, R., Gallo, R., Vitale, M. G., Passarelli, A., Mangili, G., Pignata, S., & Palaia, I. (2023). Vulvar Paget's disease: A systematic review of the MITO Rare Cancer Group. *Cancers (Basel), 15*(6), 1803. https://doi.org/10.3390/cancers15061803. PMID: 36980691; PMCID: PMC10046936.

Casas, C. P. R., Albuquerque, R. C. R., Loureiro, R. B., Gollner, A. M., Freitas, M. G., Duque, G. P. D. N., & Viscondi, J. Y. K. (2022). Cervical cancer screening in low- and middle-income countries: A systematic review of economic evaluation studies. *Clinics (Sao Paulo), 77,* 100080. https://doi.org/10.1016/j.clinsp.2022.100080. PMID: 35905574; PMCID: PMC9335392.

Cavaliere, A. F., Perelli, F., Zaami, S., D'Indinosante, M., Turrini, I., Giusti, M., Gullo, G., Vizzielli, G., Mattei, A., Scambia, G., Vidiri, A., & Signore, F. (2021). Fertility sparing treatments in endometrial cancer patients: The potential role of the new molecular classification. *International Journal of Molecular Sciences, 22*(22), 12248. https://doi.org/10.3390/ijms222212248. PMID: 34830129; PMCID: PMC8625356.

Centers for Disease Control and Prevention. (n.d.-b). *Basic information about HPV and cancer.* https://www.cdc.gov/cancer/hpv/basic_info/

Centers for Disease Control and Prevention. (n.d.-f). *Vaccine adverse event reporting system (VAERS).* http://www.cdc.gov/vaccinesafety/ensuringsafety/monitoring/vaers/index.html

Centers for Disease Control and Prevention. (n.d.-g). *What are the risk factors for cervical cancer?* https://www.cdc.gov/cancer/cervical/basic_info/risk_factors.htm

Centers for Disease Control and Prevention. (n.d.-h). *What can I do to reduce my risk of cervical cancer?* https://www.cdc.gov/cancer/cervical/basic_info/prevention .htm

Centers for Disease Control and Prevention. (2019a). *HPV (human papillomavirus) VIS.* https://www.cdc.gov/vaccines/hcp/vis/vis-statements/hpv.html

Centers for Disease Control and Prevention. (2019b). *Inside knowledge about gynecological cancer. Module 2: Cervical cancer.* https://web.archive.org/web/20190111054847/ https://www.cdc.gov/cancer/cervical/index.htm

Centers for Disease Control and Prevention. (2021a). *Diseases characterized by vulvovaginal itching, burning, irritation, odor, or discharge.* https://www.cdc.gov/std/treatment-guidelines/vaginal-discharge.htm

Centers for Disease Control and Prevention. (2021b). *Administering HPV vaccine.* https://www.cdc.gov/vaccines/vpd/hpv/hcp/administration.html#:~:text=A%20three%2Ddose%20series%20

Centers for Disease Control and Prevention. (2021c). *HPV vaccination recommendations.* https://www.cdc.gov/vaccines/vpd/hpv/hcp/administration.html#:~:text=A%20three%2Ddose%20series%20

Centers for Disease Control and Prevention. (2024a). *Human papillomavirus (HPV) vaccine safety.* https://www.cdc.gov/std/treatment-guidelines/vaginal-discharge.html

Centers for Disease Control and Prevention. (2024b). *Chapter 11: Human papillomavirus.* https://www.cdc.gov/pinkbook/hcp/table-of-contents/chapter-11-human-papillomavirus.html

Centers for Disease Control and Prevention. (2024c). *HPV associated cancers.* https://www.cdc.gov/united-states-cancer-statistics/publications/hpv-associated-cancers.html

Charkhchi, P., Cybulski, C., Gronwald, J., Wong, F. O., Narod, S. A., & Akbari, M. R. (2020). CA125 and ovarian cancer: A comprehensive review. *Cancers (Basel), 12*(12), 3730. https://doi.org/10.3390/cancers12123730. PMID: 33322519; PMCID: PMC7763876.

Chino, J., Annunziata, C. M., Beriwal, S., Bradfield, L., Erickson, B. A., Fields, E. C., Fitch, K., Harkenrider, M. M., Holschneider, C. H., Kamrava, M., Leung, E., Lin, L. L., Mayadev, J. S., Morcos, M., Nwachukwu, C., Petereit, D., & Viswanathan, A. N. (2020). Radiation therapy for cervical cancer: Executive summary of an ASTRO clinical practice guideline. *Practical Radiation Oncology, 10*(4), 220–234. https://doi.org/10.1016/j.prro.2020.04.002. Epub 2020 May 18. PMID: 32473857; PMCID: PMC8802172.

Chow, L., Tsui, B. Q., Bahrami, S., Masamed, R., Memarzadeh, S., Raman, S. S., & Patel, M. K. (2021). Gynecologic tumor board: A radiologist's guide to vulvar and vaginal malignancies. *Abdominal Radiology (New York), 46*(12), 5669–5686. https://doi.org/10.1007/s00261-021-03209-2. Epub 2021 Aug 25. PMID: 34435227; PMCID: PMC8590682.

Cianfrini, F., d'Amati, A., Arciuolo, D., Travaglino, A., D'Alessandris, N., Scaglione, G., Valente, M., Urtueta, B. P., Addante, F., Narducci, N., Angelico, G., Piermattei, A., Mulè, A., Santoro, A., Rossi, E. D., & Zannoni, G. F. (2024). Atypical glandular cells and predictive features of malignancy in Pap smears: A retrospective monocentric study. *Cytopathology, 35*(4), 473–480. https://doi.org/10.1111/cyt.13383. Epub 2024 Apr 30. PMID: 38686982.

Committee on Gynecologic Practice, Society of Gynecologic Oncology. (2016, reaffirmed 2019). Committee opinion no. 675: Management of vulvar intraepithelial neoplasia. *Obstetrics and Gynecology, 675*(3), e937–e938. https://doi.org/10.1097/AOG.0000000000001704

Committee on Gynecologic Practice, Society of Gynecologic Oncology. (2017, reaffirmed 2019). Committee opinion no. 693: Counseling about genetic testing and communication of genetic test results. *Obstetrics and Gynecology, 129*(4), e96–e101. https://doi.org/10.1097/AOG.0000000000002020

Committee on Gynecologic Practice, Society of Gynecologic Oncology. (2018). Committee opinion no. 754: The utility and indications for routine pelvic examination. *Obstetrics and Gynecology, 132*(14), e174–e186. https://doi.org/10.1097/AOG.0000000000002895

Committee on Gynecologic Practice, Society of Gynecologic Oncology. (2019). Committee opinion no. 774: Opportunistic salpingectomy as a strategy for epithelial ovarian cancer prevention. *Obstetrics and Gynecology, 133*(4), e279–e284. https://doi.org/10.1097/AOG.0000000000003164

Cooper, D., & McCathran, C. E. (2023). Cervical dysplasia. *StatPearls.* https://www.ncbi.nlm.nih.gov/books/NBK430859/

Cyr, M. P., Dostie, R., Camden, C., Dumoulin, C., Bessette, P., Pina, A., Gotlieb, W. H., Lapointe-Milot, K., Mayrand, M. H., & Morin, M. (2022). Improvements following multimodal pelvic floor physical therapy in gynecological cancer survivors suffering from pain during sexual intercourse: Results from a one-year follow-up mixed-method study. *PLoS One, 17*(1), e0262844. https://doi.org/10.1371/journal.pone.0262844. PMID: 35077479; PMCID: PMC8789131.

Daly, M. B., Pal, T., Maxwell, K. N., Churpek, J., Kohlmann, W., AlHilli, Z., Arun, B., Buys, S. S., Cheng, H., Domchek, S. M., Friedman, S., Giri, V., Goggins, M., Hagemann, A., Hendrix, A., Hutton, M. L., Karlan, B. Y., Kassem, N., Khan, S., Khoury, K., ... Darlow, S. D. (2023). NCCN Guidelines® Insights: Genetic/Familial High-Risk Assessment: Breast, Ovarian, and Pancreatic, Version 2.2024. *Journal of the National Comprehensive Cancer Network : JNCCN, 21*(10), 1000–1010. https://doi.org/10.6004/jnccn.2023.0051

Danan, E. R., Brunner, J., Bergman, A., Spoont, M., Chanfreau, C., Canelo, I., Krebs, E. E., & Yano, E. M. (2022). The relationship between sexual assault history and cervical cancer screening completion among women veterans in the Veterans Health Administration. *Journal of Women's Health (Larchmont), 31*(7), 1040–1047. https://doi.org/10.1089/jwh.2021.0237. Epub 2022 Jan 18. PMID: 35049381; PMCID: PMC9289070.

Dasgupta, S., Ewing-Graham, P. C., Swagemakers, S. M. A., van der Spe,k P. J., van Doorn, H. C., Noordhoek Hegt, V., Koljenović, S., & van Kemenade, F. J. (2020). Precursor lesions of vulvar squamous cell carcinoma—histology and biomarkers: A systematic review. *Critical Reviews in Oncology/Hematology, 147,* 102866. https://doi.org/10.1016/j.critrevonc.2020.102866. Epub 2020 Jan 15. PMID: 32058913.

De Decker, K., Wenzel, H. H. B., Bart, J., van der Aa, M. A., Kruitwagen, R. F. P. M., Nijman, H. W., & Kruse, A. J. (2023). Stage, treatment and survival of low-grade serous ovarian carcinoma in the Netherlands: A nationwide study. *Acta Obstetrica et Gynecologica Scandinavia, 102*(3), 246–256. https://doi.org/10.1111/aogs.14518. Epub 2023 Feb 3. PMID: 36734363; PMCID: PMC9951382.

Dermawan, J. K. T., Hur, C., Uberti, M. G., Flyckt, R., Falcone, T., Brainard, J., & Abdul-Karim, F. W. (2019). Thickened endometrium in postmenopausal women with an initial biopsy of limited, benign, surface endometrium: Clinical outcome and subsequent pathologic diagnosis. *International Journal of Gynecological*

Pathology, 38(4), 310–317. https://doi.org/10.1097/PGP.0000000000000525. PMID: 29750705.

Dilley, J., Burnell, M., Gentry-Maharaj, A., Ryan, A., Neophytou, C., Apostolidou, S., Karpinskyj, C., Kalsi, J., Mould, T., Woolas, R., Singh, N., Widschwendter, M., Fallowfield, L., Campbell, S., Skates, S. J., McGuire, A., Parmar, M., Jacobs, I., & Menon, U. (2020). Ovarian cancer symptoms, routes to diagnosis and survival—Population cohort study in the 'no screen' arm of the UK Collaborative Trial of Ovarian Cancer Screening (UKCTOCS). *Gynecologic Oncology, 158*(2), 316–322. https://doi.org/10.1016/j.ygyno.2020.05.002. Epub 2020 Jun 17. PMID: 32561125; PMCID: PMC7453382.

Doll, K. M., Pike, M., Alson, J., Williams, P., Carey, E., Stürmer, T., Wood, M., Marsh, E. E., Katz, R., & Robinson, W. R. (2024). Endometrial thickness as diagnostic triage for endometrial cancer among Black individuals. *JAMA Oncology, 10*(8), 1068–1076. https://doi.org/10.1001/jamaoncol.2024.1891. PMID: 38935372; PMCID: PMC11211989.

Doll, K. M., Snyder, C. R., & Ford, C. L. (2018). Endometrial cancer disparities: A race-conscious critique of the literature. *American Journal of Obstetrics and Gynecology, 218*(5), 474–482.e2. https://doi.org/10.1016/j.ajog.2017.09.016. Epub 2017 Sep 28. PMID: 28964822.

Doll, K. M., & Winn, A. N. (2019). Assessing endometrial cancer risk among US women: Long-term trends using hysterectomy-adjusted analysis. *American Journal of Obstetrics and Gynecology, 221*(4), 318.e1–318.e9. https://doi.org/10.1016/j.ajog.2019.05.024. Epub 2019 May 22. PMID: 31125544.

Duus, A. H., Zheng, G., Baandrup, L., Faber, M. T., & Kjær, S. K. (2023). Risk of ovarian cancer after salpingectomy and tubal ligation: Prospects on histology and time since the procedure. *Gynecologic Oncology, 177,* 125–131. https://doi.org/10.1016/j.ygyno.2023.08.016. Epub 2023 Sep 6. PMID: 37683548.

Ebring, C., Marlin, R., Macni, J., Vallard, A., Bergerac, S., Beaubrun-Renard, M., Joachim, C., & Jean-Laurent, M. (2023). Type II endometrial cancer: Incidence, overall and disease-free survival in Martinique. *PLoS One, 18*(3), e0278757. https://doi.org/10.1371/journal.pone.0278757. PMID: 36928660; PMCID: PMC10019642.

Elsherif, S. B., Agely, A., Gopireddy, D. R., Ganeshan, D., Hew, K. E., Sharma, S., & Lall, C. (2022). Mimics and pitfalls of primary ovarian malignancy imaging. *Tomography, 8*(1), 100–119. https://doi.org/10.3390/tomography8010009. PMID: 35076619; PMCID: PMC8788482.

Emons, G., & Gründker, C. (2021). The role of gonadotropin-releasing hormone (GnRH) in endometrial cancer. *Cells, 10*(2), 292. https://doi.org/10.3390/cells10020292. PMID: 33535622; PMCID: PMC7912811.

Enroth, S., Ivansson, E., Lindberg, J. H., Lycke, M., Bergman, J., Reneland, A., Stålberg, K., Sundfeldt, K., & Gyllensten, U. (2022). Data-driven analysis of a validated risk score for ovarian cancer identifies clinically distinct patterns during follow-up and treatment. *Communications Medicine (London), 2,* 124. https://doi.org/10.1038/s43856-022-00193-6. PMID: 36196264; PMCID: PMC9526736.

Eskander, R. N., Sill, M. W., Beffa, L., Moore, R. G., Hope, J. M., Musa, F. B., Mannel, R., Shahin, M. S., Cantuaria, G. H., Girda, E., Mathews, C., Kavecansky, J., Leath, C. A., 3rd, Gien, L. T., Hinchcliff, E. M., Lele, S. B., Landrum, L. M., Backes, F., O'Cearbhaill, R. E., Al Baghdadi, T., Hill, E. K., Thaker, P. H., John, V. S., Welch, S., Fader, A. N., Powell, M. A., & Aghajanian, C. (2023). Pembrolizumab plus chemotherapy in advanced endometrial cancer. *New England Journal of Medicine, 388*(23), 2159–2170. https://doi.org/10.1056/NEJMoa2302312. Epub 2023 Mar 27. PMID: 36972022; PMCID: PMC10351614.

Falcicchio, G., Vinci, L., Cicinelli, E., Loizzi, V., Arezzo, F., Silvestris, E., Resta, L., Serio, G., Cazzato, G., Mastronardi, M., Mongelli, M., Marinaccio, M., & Cormio, G. (2022). Vulvar malignant melanoma: A narrative review. *Cancers (Basel), 14*(21), 5217. https://doi.org/10.3390/cancers14215217. PMID: 36358637; PMCID: PMC9653566.

Fischer, O. J., Marguerie, M., & Brotto, L. A. (2019). Sexual function, quality of life, and experiences of women with ovarian cancer: A mixed-methods study. *Sexual Medicine, 7*(4), 530–539. https://doi.org/10.1016/j.esxm.2019.07.005. Epub 2019 Sep 7. PMID: 31501030; PMCID: PMC6963110.

Foundation on Women's Cancer, Society of Gynecologic Oncology (2024). *Vulvar cancer.* https://foundationforwomenscancer.org/gynecologic-cancers/gynecologic-cancer-types/vulvar-cancer/

Fragoso-Ontiveros, V., Velázquez-Aragón, J. A., Nuñez-Martínez, P. M., de la Luz Mejía-Aguayo, M., Vidal-Millán, S., Pedroza-Torres, A., Sánchez-Contreras, Y., Ramírez-Otero, M. A., Muñiz-Mendoza, R., Domínguez-Ortíz, J., Wegman-Ostrosky, T., Bargalló-Rocha, J. E., Gallardo-Rincón, D., Reynoso-Noveron, N., Arriaga-Canon, C., Meneses-García, A., Herrera-Montalvo, L. A., & Alvarez-Gomez, R. M. (2019). Mexican BRCA1 founder mutation: Shortening the gap in genetic assessment for hereditary breast and ovarian cancer patients. *PLoS One, 14*(9), e0222709. https://doi.org/10.1371/journal.pone.0222709. PMID: 31545835; PMCID: PMC6756553.

Frandsen, C. L. B., Svendsen, P. F., Nøhr, B., Viuff, J. H., Maltesen, T., Kjaer, S. K., & Jensen, A. (2023). Risk of epithelial ovarian tumors among women with polycystic ovary syndrome: A nationwide population-based cohort study. *International Journal of Cancer, 153*(5), 958–968. https://doi.org/10.1002/ijc.34574. Epub 2023 Jun 26. PMID: 37357906.

Gadkari, R., Ravi, R., & Bhatia, J. K. (2022). Cervical cancers: Varieties and the lower anogenital squamous terminology. *Cytojournal, 19,* 39. https://doi.org/10.25259/CMAS_03_14_2021. PMID: 35928526; PMCID: PMC9345096

Gaulin, N. B., Lesnock, J. L., Tian, C., Osei-Bonsu, K., Jacobs, A., Richard, S. D., Krivak, T. C., Miller, E. M., Shriver, C. D., Casablanca, Y., Maxwell, G. L., & Darcy, K. M. (2020). Survival disparities in vulvar cancer patients in Commission on Cancer®-accredited facilities. *Gynecologic Oncology, 157*(1), 136–145. https://doi.org/10.1016/j.ygyno.2019.11.025. Epub 2020 Jan 15. PMID: 31954540.

Gearhart, P. A., Randall, T. C., Buckley, R. M., & Higgins, R. V. (2020, February 20). Human papillomavirus. *Medscape.* https://emedicine.medscape.com/article/219110-overview#a3

Gică, N., Peltecu, G., Chirculescu, R., Gică, C., Stoicea, M. C., Serbanica, A. N., & Panaitescu, A. M. (2022). Ovarian germ cell tumors: Pictorial essay. *Diagnostics (Basel), 12*(9), 2050. https://doi.org/10.3390/diagnostics12092050. PMID: 36140449; PMCID: PMC9498179.

Gong, J., Zhang, G., Wang, W., Liang, L., Li, Q., Liu, M., Xue, L., & Tang, G. (2021). A simple and rapid diagnostic method for 13 types of high-risk human papillomavirus (HR-HPV) detection using CRISPR-Cas12a technology. *Scientific Reports, 11*(1), 12800. https://doi.org/10.1038/s41598-021-92329-2. PMID: 34140632; PMCID: PMC8211657

Goodman, A. (2021). Delay in diagnosis and increasing incidence of vulvar cancer: A root cause analysis. *Menopause, 28*(2), 111–112. https://doi.org/10.1097/GME.0000000000001723. PMID: 33399321.

Gupta, S., Ahuja, S., Kalwaniya, D. S., Shamsunder, S., & Solanki, S. (2024). Vulval premalignant lesions: A review article. *Obstetrics and Gynecology Science, 67*(2), 169–185. https://doi.org/10.5468/ogs.23274. Epub 2024 Jan 23. PMID: 38262367; PMCID: PMC10948211.

Haag, J. G., Adler, A. D., Sheeder, J., Brubaker, L. W., & Lefkowits, C. (2022). Patterns of palliative care referral in platinum resistant ovarian cancer demonstrate reactive rather than proactive approach. *Gynecologic Oncology Reports, 43,* 101053. https://doi.org/10.1016/j.gore.2022.101053. PMID: 35958954; PMCID: PMC9358431

Hafez, M., Tawfik, G., Yousef, R., Antar, S., Nazzal, A., Hosh, M., Warda, M., Leu, R., & Refky, B. (2022). Predicting causes of death among vulvar cancer patients; SEER database analysis. *International Journal of Cancer and Biomedical Research, 6,* 31–40. https://doi.org/10.21608/jcbr.2022.115165.1242

Hamilton, C. A., Pothuri, B., Arend, R. C., Backes, F. J., Gehrig, P. A., Soliman, P. T., Thompson, J. S., Urban, R. R., & Burke, W. M. (2021). Endometrial cancer: A society of gynecologic oncology evidence-based review and recommendations. *Gynecologic Oncology, 160*(3), 817–826. https://doi.org/10.1016/j.ygyno.2020.12.021. Epub 2021 Jan 27. PMID: 33516529.

Harkenrider, M. M., Abu-Rustum, N., Albuquerque, K., Bradfield, L., Bradley, K., Dolinar, E., Doll, C. M., Elshaikh, M., Frick, M. A., Gehrig, P. A., Han, K., Hathout, L., Jones, E., Klopp, A., Mourtada, F., Suneja, G., Wright, A. A., Yashar, C., & Erickson, B. A. (2023). Radiation therapy for endometrial cancer: An American Society for Radiation Oncology clinical practice guideline. *Practical Radiation Oncology, 13*(1), 41–65. https://doi.org/10.1016/j.prro.2022.09.002. Epub 2022 Oct 22. PMID: 36280107.

He, J., Li, Q., Hu, C., Peng, J., Ma, S., Song, Z., Liu, Y., Cui, Y., Deng, J., Wei, X., & Ding, X. (2022). Human papillomavirus 68 prevalence and genetic variability based on E6/E7 genes in Sichuan. *Virology, 567,* 15–25. https://doi.org/10.1016/j.virol.2021.11.015. Epub 2021 Dec 6. PMID: 34942562

Hernandez, A., Schatz-Siemers, N., Zhou, F., Brandler, T. C., Negron, R., Modi, L., Elgert, P. A., & Simsir, A. (2020). Reporting of benign endometrial cells in papanicolaou tests. *American Journal of Clinical Pathology, 154*(3), 381–386. https://doi.org/10.1093/ajcp/aqaa041. PMID: 32405650.

Huang, J., Chan, W. C., Ngai, C. H., Lok, V., Zhang, L., Lucero-Prisno, D. E., 3rd, Xu, W., Zheng, Z. J., Elcarte, E., Withers, M., & Wong, M. C. S., on behalf of Ncd Global Health Research Group of Association of Pacific Rim Universities Apru. (2022). Worldwide burden, risk factors, and temporal trends of ovarian cancer: A global study. *Cancers (Basel), 14*(9), 2230. https://doi.org/10.3390/cancers14092230. PMID: 35565359; PMCID: PMC9102475.

Hull, R., Mbele, M., Makhafola, T., Hicks, C., Wang, S. M., Reis, R. M., Mehrotra, R., Mkhize-Kwitshana, Z., Kibiki, G., Bates, D. O., & Dlamini, Z. (2020). Cervical cancer in low and middle-income countries. *Oncology Letters, 20*(3), 2058–2074. https://doi.org/10.3892/ol.2020.11754. Epub 2020 Jun 19. PMID: 32782524; PMCID: PMC7400218.

International Society for the Study of Vulvovaginal Disease (ISSVD). (2023). *Squamous cell carcinoma of the vulva (SSC).* https://www.issvd.org/application/files/7016/8254/7203/SquamousCellCarcinoma.pdf

Jaeger, A., Prieske, K., Mathey, S., Fischer, I., Vettorazzi, E., Kuerti, S., Reuter, S., Dieckmann, J., Schmalfeldt, B., & Woelber, L. (2022). Pelvic lymphadenectomy in vulvar cancer and its impact on prognosis and outcome. *Archives of gynecology and obstetrics, 305*(1), 233–240. https://doi.org/10.1007/s00404-021-06156-x

Jing, H., Xiuhong, W., Ying, Y., Xiyun, C., Deping, L., Changmei, S., Qi, W., Tao, P., & Yiyun, P. (2022). Complications of radical hysterectomy with pelvic lymph node dissection for cervical cancer: A 10-year single-centre clinical observational study. *BMC Cancer, 22*(1), 1286. https://doi.org/10.1186/s12885-022-10395-9. PMID: 36476575; PMCID: PMC9730609.

Johnson, N. L., Head, K. J., Scott, S. F., & Zimet, G. D. (2020). Persistent disparities in cervical cancer screening uptake: Knowledge and sociodemographic determinants of papanicolaou and human papillomavirus testing among women in the United States. *Public Health Reports, 135*(4), 483–491. https://doi

.org/10.1177/0033354920925094. Epub 2020 Jun 9. PMID: 32516053; PMCID: PMC7383763.

Johnston, E. A., Ibiebele, T. I., van der Pols, J. C., Webb, P. M., OPAL Study Group. (2021). Dietitian encounters after treatment for ovarian cancer. *Journal of Human Nutrition and Dietetics, 34*(6), 1053–1063. https://doi.org/10.1111/jhn.12898. Epub 2021 Apr 9. PMID: 33749900.

Kesić, V., Vieira-Baptista, P., & Stockdale, C. K. (2022). Early diagnostics of vulvar intraepithelial neoplasia. *Cancers (Basel), 14*(7), 1822. https://doi.org/10.3390/cancers14071822. PMID: 35406594; PMCID: PMC8997501.

Kim, J., Whitcomb, B. W., Kwan, B., Zava, D., Sluss, P. M., Dietz, A., Shliakhtsitsava, K., Romero, S. A. D., Natarajan, L., & Su, H. I. (2021). Psychosocial stress and ovarian function in adolescent and young adult cancer survivors. *Human Reproduction, 36*(2), 405–414. https://doi.org/10.1093/humrep/deaa313. PMID: 33279981; PMCID: PMC7829546.

Kim, N., Choi, S. H., Chang, J. S., Kim, Y. T., Kim, S. W., Kim, G. M., & Kim, Y. B. Use of bevacizumab before or after radiotherapy increases the risk of fistula formation in patients with cervical cancer. *International Journal of Gynecological Cancer, 31*(1), 59–65. https://doi.org/10.1136/ijgc-2020-002031. Epub 2020 Dec 3. PMID: 33273018.

Kohler, R. E., Roncarati, J. S., Aguiar, A., Chatterjee, P., Gaeta, J., Viswanath, K., & Henry, C. (2021). Trauma and cervical cancer screening among women experiencing homelessness: A call for trauma-informed care. *Women's Health (London), 17,* 17455065211029238. https://doi.org/10.1177/17455065211029238. PMID: 34225506; PMCID: PMC8264729.

Kvale, E., Phillips, F., Ghosh, S., Lea, J., Hoppenot, C., Costales, A., Sunde, J., Badr, H., Nwogu-Onyemkpa, E., Saleem, N., Ward, R., & Balasubramanian, B. (2024). Survivorship care for women living with ovarian cancer: Protocol for a randomized controlled trial. *JMIR Research Protocols, 13,* e48069. https://doi.org/10.2196/48069. PMID: 38335019; PMCID: PMC10891493.

Laganà, A. S., Garzon, S., Raffaelli, R., Ban Frangež, H., Lukanovič, D., & Franch,i M. (2021). Vaginal stenosis after cervical cancer treatments: Challenges for reconstructive surgery. *Journal of Investigative Surgery, 34*(7), 754–755. https://doi.org/10.1080/08941939.2019.1695987. Epub 2019 Dec 10. PMID: 31818165.

Lee, J. (2019). Physical activity, sitting time, and the risk of ovarian cancer: A brief research report employing a meta-analysis of existing. *Health Care for Women International, 40*(4), 433–458. https://doi.org/10.1080/07399332.2018.1505892. Epub 2018 Oct 25. PMID: 30358498.

Lei, J., Ploner, A., Elfström, K. M., Wang, J., Roth, A., Fang, F., Sundström, K., Dillner, J., & Sparén, P. (2020). HPV vaccination and the risk of invasive cervical cancer. *New England Journal of Medicine, 383*(14), 1340–1348. https://doi.org/10.1056/NEJMoa1917338. PMID: 32997908.

Letafati, A., Motlaghzadeh, S., Ardekani, O. S., Memarpour, B., Seyedi, S., Bahari, M., Farahani, A. V., Khoshravan, A., Sarrafzadeh, S., Vasmehjani, A. A., Pournaseri, M., Bahrami, Y., & Talebi, F. (2024). Uncommon high distribution of HPV-16, HPV-54, and HPV-56 in female referred to a laboratory in Karaj, Iran: Indications of a paradigm shift in HPV genotypes? *Virology Journal, 21*(1), 182. https://doi.org/10.1186/s12985-024-02457-0. PMID: 39123176; PMCID: PMC11316285

Levine, M. D., O'Malley, D. M., Haight, P. J., Senter, L., Wagner, V., Bixel, K. L., Cohn, D. E., Copeland, L. J., Cosgrove, C. M., McLaughlin, E. M., & Backes, F. J. (2023). Recurrence rate in early-stage epithelial ovarian cancer: Is there a role for upfront maintenance with PARP inhibitors in stages I and II? *Gynecologic Oncology Reports, 46,* 101173. https://doi.org/10.1016/j.gore.2023.101173. PMID: 37082521; PMCID: PMC10111944.

Lheureux, S., Braunstein, M., & Oza, A. M. (2019). Epithelial ovarian cancer: Evolution of management in the era of precision medicine. *CA: A Cancer Journal for Clinicians, 69*(4), 280–304. https://doi.org/10.3322/caac.21559. Epub 2019 May 17. PMID: 31099893.

Li, J., Li, J.,& Jiang, W. (2024). Effects of different surgical extents on prognosis of patients with malignant ovarian sex cord-stromal tumors: A retrospective cohort study. *Scientific Reports, 14*(1), 22630. https://doi.org/10.1038/s41598-024-67446-3. PMID: 39349505; PMCID: PMC11442459.

Liu, J., Berchuck, A., Backes, F. J., Cohen, J., Grisham, R., Leath, C. A., Martin, L., Matei, D., Miller, D. S., Robertson, S., Barroilhet, L., Uppal, S., Hendrickson, A. W., Gershenson, D. M., Gray, H. J., Hakam, A., Jain, A., Konecny, G. E., Moroney, J., Ratner, E., ... Armstrong, D. K. (2024). NCCN Guidelines® Insights: Ovarian Cancer/Fallopian Tube Cancer/Primary Peritoneal Cancer, Version 3.2024. *Journal of the National Comprehensive Cancer Network : JNCCN, 22*(8), 512–519. https://doi.org/10.6004/jnccn.2024.0052

Liberto, J. M., Chen, S. Y., Shih, I. M., Wang, T. H., Wang, T. L., & Pisanic, T. R., 2nd. (2022). Current and emerging methods for ovarian cancer screening and diagnostics: A comprehensive review. *Cancers (Basel), 14*(12), 2885. https://doi.org/10.3390/cancers14122885. PMID: 35740550; PMCID: PMC9221480.

Liontos, M., Papatheodoridi, A., Andrikopoulou, A., Thomakos, N., Haidopoulos, D., Rodolakis, A., Zagouri, F., Bamias, A., & Dimopoulos, M. A. (2021). Management of the elderly patients with high-grade serous ovarian cancer in the REAL-WORLD setting. *Current Oncology, 28*(2), 1143–1152. https://doi.org/10.3390/curroncol28020110. PMID: 33800101; PMCID: PMC8025751.

Lisio, M.-A., Fu, L., Goyeneche, A., Gao, Z., & Telleria, C. (2019). High-grade serous ovarian cancer: Basic sciences, clinical and therapeutic standpoints. *International Journal of Molecular Sciences, 20*(4), Article 952. https://doi.org/10.3390/ijms20040952

Liu, Y. L., Breen, K., Catchings, A., Ranganathan, M., Latham, A., Goldfrank, D. J., Grisham, R. N., Long Roche, K., Frey, M. K., Chi, D. S., Abu-Rustum, N., Aghajanian, C., Offit, K., & Stadler, Z. K. (2022). Risk-Reducing Bilateral Salpingo-Oophorectomy for Ovarian Cancer: A Review and Clinical Guide for Hereditary Predisposition Genes. *JCO oncology practice, 18*(3), 201–209. https://doi.org/10.1200/OP.21.00382

Liu, Y., Yang, J., Hilliard, T. S., Wang, Z., Johnson, J., Wang, W., Harper, E. I., Ott, C., O'Brien, C., Campbell, L., Crowley, B., Grisoli, S., Stavrou, N. M., Juncker-Jensen, A., & Stack, M. S. (2023). Host obesity alters the ovarian tumor immune microenvironment and impacts response to standard of care chemotherapy. *Journal of Experimental & Clinical Cancer Research, 42*(1), 165. https://doi.org/10.1186/s13046-023-02740-y. PMID: 37438818; PMCID: PMC10337170.

Logue, C. A., Pugh, J., Foden, P., Mahmood, R. D., Morgan, R. D., Mitchell, C., Hasan, J., Clamp, A. R., & Jayson, G. C. (2022). Psychosexual morbidity in women with ovarian cancer: Evaluation by germline BRCA gene mutational status. *Sexual Medicine, 10*(1), 100465. https://doi.org/10.1016/j.esxm.2021.100465. Epub 2021 Dec 15. PMID: 34922303; PMCID: PMC8847828.

López-Reig, R., Fernández-Serra, A., Romero, I., Zorrero, C., Illueca, C., García-Casado, Z., Poveda, A., & López-Guerrero, J. A. (2019). Prognostic classification of endometrial cancer using a molecular approach based on a twelve-gene NGS panel. *Scientific Reports, 9*(1), 18093. https://doi.org/10.1038/s41598-019-54624-x. PMID: 31792358; PMCID: PMC6889294.

Macchia, G., Titone, F., Restaino, S., Arcieri, M., Pellecchia, G., Andreetta, C., Driul, L., Vizzielli, G., & Pezzulla, D. (2023). Is it time to reassess the role of radiotherapy treatment in ovarian cancer? *Healthcare (Basel), 11*(17), 2413. https://doi.org/10.3390/healthcare11172413. PMID: 37685447; PMCID: PMC10486999

Mah, S. J., Carter Ramirez, D. M., Schnarr, K., Eiriksson, L. R., Gayowsky, A., & Seow, H. (2024). Timing of palliative care, end-of-life quality indicators, and health resource utilization. *JAMA Network Open, 7*(10), e2440977. https://doi.org/10.1001/jamanetworkopen.2024.40977. PMID: 39466244; PMCID: PMC11519754.

Malandrone, F., Bevilacqua, F., Merola, M., Gallio, N., Ostacoli, L., Carletto, S., & Benedetto, C. (2021). The impact of vulvar cancer on psychosocial and sexual functioning: A literature review. *Cancers (Basel), 14*(1), 63. https://doi.org/10.3390/cancers14010063. PMID: 35008225; PMCID: PMC8750175.

Manley, K., Hillard, T., Clark, J., Kumar, G., Morrison, J., Hamoda, H., Barber, K., Holloway, D., Middleton, B., Oyston, M., Pickering, M., Sassarini, J., & Williams, N. (2024). Management of unscheduled bleeding on HRT: A joint guideline on behalf of the British Menopause Society, Royal College Obstetricians and Gynaecologists, British Gynaecological Cancer Society, British Society for Gynaecological Endoscopy, Faculty of Sexual and Reproductive Health, Royal College of General Practitioners and Getting it Right First Time. *Post Reproductive Health, 30*(2), 95–116. https://doi.org/10.1177/20533691241254413. Epub 2024 May 14. PMID: 38743767.

Mao, C. L., Seow, K. M., & Chen, K. H. The utilization of bevacizumab in patients with advanced ovarian cancer: A systematic review of the mechanisms and effects. *International Journal of Molecular Sciences, 23*(13), 6911. https://doi.org/10.3390/ijms23136911. PMID: 35805914; PMCID: PMC9266930.

Mazidimoradi, A., Momenimovahed, Z., Khalajinia, Z., Allahqoli, L., Salehiniya, H., & Alkatout, I. (2024). The global incidence, mortality, and burden of uterine cancer in 2019 and correlation with SDI, tobacco, dietary risks, and metabolic risk factors: An ecological study. *Health Science Reports, 7*(1), e1835. https://doi.org/10.1002/hsr2.1835. PMID: 38274134; PMCID: PMC10808991.

McDaniels-Davidson, C., Feng, C. H., Martinez, M. E., Canchola, A. J., Gomez, S. L., Nodora, J. N., Patel, S. P., Mundt, A. J., & Mayadev, J. S. (2022). Improved survival in cervical cancer patients receiving care at National Cancer Institute-designated cancer centers. *Cancer, 128*(19), 3479–3486. https://doi.org/10.1002/cncr.34404. Epub 2022 Aug 2. PMID: 35917201; PMCID: PMC9544648.

Medline Plus. (2021). *Lynch syndrome.* https://medlineplus.gov/genetics/condition/lynch-syndrome/#frequency

Mei, S., Chelmow, D., Gecsi, K., Barkley, J., Barrows, E., Brooks, R., Huber-Keener, K., Jeudy, M., O'Hara, J. S., & Burke, W. (2023). Health disparities in ovarian cancer: Report from the Ovarian Cancer Evidence Review Conference. *Obstetrics and Gynecology, 142*(1), 196–210. https://doi.org/10.1097/AOG.0000000000005210. Epub 2023 Jun 7. PMID: 37348095; PMCID: PMC10278570.

Meites, E., Szilagyi, P. G., Chesson, H. W., Unger, E. R., Romero, J. R., & Markowitz, L. E. (2019). Human papillomavirus vaccination for adults: Updated recommendations of the Advisory Committee on Immunization Practices. *MMWR Morbidity and Mortality Weekly Report, 68,* 698–702. https://doi.org/http://dx.doi.org/10.15585/mmwr.mm6832a3

Memorial Sloan Kettering Cancer Center. (2024). *How to use a vaginal dilator.* https://www.mskcc.org/cancer-care/patient-education/how-use-vaginal-dilator

Momenimovahed, Z., Tiznobaik, A., Taheri, S., & Salehiniya, H. (2019). Ovarian cancer in the world: Epidemiology and risk factors. *International Journal of Women's Health, 11,* 287–299. https://doi.org/10.2147/IJWH.S197604. PMID: 31118829; PMCID: PMC6500433.

Monk, B.J., Colombo, N., Tewari, K. S., Dubot, C., Caceres, M. V., Hasegawa, K., Shapira-Frommer, R., Salman, P., Yañez, E., Gümüş, M., Olivera Hurtado de Mendoza, M., Samouëlian, V., Castonguay, V., Arkhipov, A., Tekin, C., Li, K., Keefe, S. M., Lorusso, D.; KEYNOTE-826 Investigators. First-line pembrolizumab + chemotherapy versus placebo + chemotherapy for persistent, recurrent, or metastatic cervical cancer: Final overall survival results of KEYNOTE-826. *Journal of Clinical Oncology, 41*(36), 5505–5511. https://doi.org/10.1200/JCO.23.00914. Epub 2023 Nov 1. PMID: 37910822.

National Cancer Institute. (n.d.-a). *HPV and Pap testing*. https://www.cancer.gov/types/cervical/pap-hpv-testing-fact-sheet

National Cancer Institute. (n.d.-b). *Human papillomavirus (HPV) vaccines*. https://www.cancer.gov/about-cancer/causes-prevention/risk/infectious-agents/hpv-vaccine-fact-sheet#q10

National Cancer Institute. (n.d.-c). *Ovarian, fallopian tube, and primary peritoneal cancer—health professional version*. https://www.cancer.gov/types/ovarian/hp

National Cancer Institute. (2019). *Endometrial cancer treatment (PDQ®)—health professional version*. https://www.cancer.gov/types/uterine/hp/endometrial-treatment-pdq#link/_430

National Cancer Institute. (2020a). *Vulvar cancer treatment (PDQ®)—health professional version*. https://www.cancer.gov/types/vulvar/hp/vulvar-treatment-pdq#_1

National Cancer Institute. (2020b). *HPV and cancer*. https://www.cancer.gov/about-cancer/causes-prevention/risk/infectious-agents/hpv-and-cancer

National Cancer Institute. (2020c). *ACS's updated cervical cancer screening guidelines explained*. https://www.cancer.gov/news-events/cancer-currents-blog/2020/cervical-cancer-screening-hpv-test-guideline

National Cancer Institute. (2023a). *What is cervical cancer?* https://www.cancer.gov/types/cervical#:~:text=Types%20of%20cervical%20cancer,rare%20type%20of%20cervical%20adenocarcinoma.

National Cancer Institute (2023b). *Immunotherapy's role in treatment endometrial cancer expected to grow*. https://www.cancer.gov/news-events/cancer-currents-blog/2023/immunotherapy-endometrial-cancer-pembrolizumab-dostarlimab

National Cancer Institute. (2024a). *Cancer disparities*. https://www.cancer.gov/about-cancer/understanding/disparities

National Cancer Institute (2024b). *Cervical cancer treatment by stage*. https://www.cancer.gov/types/cervical/treatment/by-stage

National Cancer Institute. (2024c). *Cancer Trends Progress Report: HPV vaccination*. https://progressreport.cancer.gov/prevention/hpv_immunization

National Cancer Institute. (2024e) *Endometrial cancer prevention*. https://www.cancer.gov/types/uterine/hp/endometrial-prevention-pdq

National Cancer Institute. (2024f). *Ovarian, fallopian tube, and primary peritoneal cancer—health professional version*. https://www.cancer.gov/types/ovarian/hp

National Cancer Institute. (2025). *Endometrial cancer treatment*. https://www.cancer.gov/types/uterine/hp/endometrial-treatment-pdq

Nica, A., Covens, A., Vicus, D., Kupets, R., Osborne, R., Cesari, M., & Gien, L. T. (2019). Sentinel lymph nodes in vulvar cancer: Management dilemmas in patients with positive nodes and larger tumors. *Gynecologic Oncology*, *152*(1), 94–100.

Nikanjam, M., Kato, S., & Kurzrock, R. (2022). Liquid biopsy: Current technology and clinical applications. *Journal of Hematology & Oncology, 15*(1), 131. https://doi.org/10.1186/s13045-022-01351-y. PMID: 36096847; PMCID: PMC9465933.

North American Menopause Society. (2022). The 2022 hormone therapy position statement of the North American Menopause Society. *Menopause, 29*(7), 767–794.

Oaknin, A., Gladieff, L., Martínez-García, J., Villacampa, G., Takekuma, M., De Giorgi, U., Lindemann, K., Woelber, L., Colombo, N., Duska, L., Leary, A., Godoy-Ortiz, A., Nishio, S., Angelergues, A., Rubio, M. J., Fariñas-Madrid, L., Yamaguchi, S., Lorusso, D., Ray-Coquard, I., Manso, L., Joly, F., Alarcón, J., Follana, P., Romero, I., Lebreton, C., Pérez-Fidalgo, J. A., Yunokawa, M., Dahlstrand, H., D'Hondt, V., Randall, L. M.; ENGOT-Cx10–GEICO 68-C–JGOG1084–GOG-3030 Investigators. (2024). Atezolizumab plus bevacizumab and chemotherapy for metastatic, persistent, or recurrent cervical cancer (BEATcc): A randomised, open-label, phase 3 trial. *Lancet, 403*(10421), 31–43. https://doi.org/10.1016/S0140-6736(23)02405-4. Epub 2023 Dec 1. PMID: 38048793.

Oaknin, A., Moore, K., Meyer, T., López-Picazo González, J., Devriese, L. A., Amin, A., Lao, C. D., Boni, V., Sharfman, W. H., Park, J. C., Tahara, M., Topalian, S. L., Magallanes, M., Molina Alavez, A., Khan, T. A., Copigneaux, C., Lee, M., Garnett-Benson, C., Wang, X., & Naumann, R. W. (2024). Nivolumab with or without ipilimumab in patients with recurrent or metastatic cervical cancer (CheckMate 358): A phase 1-2, open-label, multicohort trial. *The Lancet. Oncology, 25*(5), 588–602. https://doi.org/10.1016/S1470-2045(24)00088-3. Epub 2024 Apr 9. PMID: 38608691.

O'Brien, K. M., Tworoger, S. S., Harris, H. R., Anderson, G. L., Weinberg, C. R., Trabert, B., Kaunitz, A. M., D'Aloisio, A. A., Sandler, D. P., & Wentzensen, N. (2020). Association of powder use in the genital area with risk of ovarian cancer. *JAMA, 323*(1), 49–59. https://doi.org/10.1001/jama.2019.20079. PMID: 31910280; PMCID: PMC6990816.

Okunade, K. S. (2020). Human papillomavirus and cervical cancer. *Journal of Obstetrics and Gynaecology, 40*(5), 602–608. https://doi.org/10.1080/01443615.2019.1634030. Epub 2019 Sep 10. Erratum in: J Obstet Gynaecol. 2020 May;40(4):590. https://doi.org/10.1080/01443615.2020.1713592. PMID: 31500479; PMCID: PMC7062568

Olawaiye, A. B., Cuello, M. A., & Rogers, L. J. (2021). Cancer of the vulva: 2021 update. *International Journal of Gynecology & Obstetrics, 155*(Suppl. 1), 7–18. https://doi.org/10.1002/ijgo.13881

O'Malley, D. M., Krivak, T. C., Kabil, N., Munley, J., & Moore, K. N. (2023). PARP inhibitors in ovarian cancer: A review. *Targeted Oncology, 18*(4), 471–503. https://doi.org/10.1007/s11523-023-00970-w. Epub 2023 Jun 3. PMID: 37268756; PMCID: PMC10344972.

Ono, A., Koshiyama, M., Nakagawa, M., Watanabe, Y., Ikuta, E., Seki, K., & Oowaki, M. (2020). The preventive effect of dietary antioxidants on cervical cancer development. *Medicina (Kaunas), 56*(11), 604. https://doi.org/10.3390/medicina56110604. PMID: 33182663; PMCID: PMC7698010.

Páez López, G., Martínez Gil, S., Zannin Ferrero, A., Ramos Hernández, D.,& Caicedo Páez, L. M. (2024). Vulvar reconstruction with keystone flaps after radical vulvectomy. *Plastic and Reconstructive Surgery Global Open, 12*(7), e5965. https://doi.org/10.1097/GOX.0000000000005965. PMID: 38988479; PMCID: PMC11236388

Pangarkar, M. A. (2022). The Bethesda System for reporting cervical cytology. *Cytojournal, 19*, 28. https://doi.org/10.25259/CMAS_03_07_2021. PMID: 35673697; PMCID: PMC9168399.

Parashar, D., Nair, B., Geethadevi, A., George, J., Nair, A., Tsaih, S. W., Kadamberi, I. P., Gopinadhan Nair, G. K., Lu, Y., Ramchandran, R., Uyar, D. S., Rader, J. S., Ram, P. T., Mills, G. B., Pradeep, S., & Chaluvally-Raghavan P. (2020). Peritoneal spread of ovarian cancer harbors therapeutic vulnerabilities regulated by FOXM1 and EGFR/ERBB2 signaling. *Cancer Research, 80*(24), 5554–5568. https://doi.org/10.1158/0008-5472.CAN-19-3717. Epub 2020 Oct 21. PMID: 33087324; PMCID: PMC7744365.

Park, E., Kim, J. Y., Choi, S., Kim, D.S., & Oh, Y. L. (2019). Carcinogenic risk of human papillomavirus (HPV) genotypes and potential effects of HPV vaccines in Korea. *Scientific Reports, 9*(1), 12556. https://doi.org/10.1038/s41598-019-49060-w. PMID: 31467383; PMCID: PMC6715722 https://pubmed.ncbi.nlm.nih.gov/31467383/

Pavlik, E. J., Smith, C., Dennis, T. S., Harvey, E., Huang, B., Chen, Q., Piecoro, D. W., Burgess, B. T., McDowell, A., Gorski, J., Baldwin, L. A., Miller, R. W., DeSimone, C. P., Dietrich, C., 3rd, Gallion, H. H., Ueland, F. R., & van Nagell, J. R., Jr. (2020). Disease-specific survival of type I and type II epithelial ovarian cancers Stage challenges categorical assignments of indolence & aggressiveness. *Diagnostics (Basel), 10*(2), 56. https://doi.org/10.3390/diagnostics10020056. PMID: 31973035; PMCID: PMC7168156.

Pingali, C., Yankey, D., Chen, M., et al. (2024). National vaccination coverage among adolescents aged 13–17 years—National Immunization Survey-Teen, United States, 2023. *MMWR Morbidity and Mortality Weekly Report, 73*, 708–714. https://doi.org/http://dx.doi.org/10.15585/mmwr.mm7333a1

Pîrlog, L. M., Pătrăşcanu, A. A., Militaru, M. S., & Cătană, A. (2024). Insights into clinical disorders in Cowden syndrome: A comprehensive review. *Medicina (Kaunas), 60*(5), 767. https://doi.org/10.3390/medicina60050767. PMID: 38792950; PMCID: PMC11123368.

Post, C. C. B., Stelloo, E., Smit, V. T. H. B. M., Ruano, D., Tops, C. M., Vermij, L., Rutten, T. A., Jürgenliemk-Schulz, I. M., Lutgens, L. C. H. W., Jobsen, J. J., Nout, R. A., Crosbie, E. J., Powell, M. E., Mileshkin, L., Leary, A., Bessette, P., Putter, H., de Boer, S. M., Horeweg, N., Nielsen, M., Wezel, T. V., Bosse, T., & Creutzberg, C. L. (2021). Prevalence and prognosis of Lynch syndrome and sporadic mismatch repair deficiency in endometrial cancer. *Journal of the National Cancer Institute, 113*(9), 1212–1220. https://doi.org/10.1093/jnci/djab029. PMID: 33693762; PMCID: PMC8418420.

Poudel, D., Acharya, K., Poudel, N., Adhikari, A., Khaniya, B., & Maskey, S. (2022). Bilateral ovarian mucinous carcinoma (stage III) with omental involvement and incidental hydronephrosis: A rare case report. *International Journal of Surgery Case Reports, 97*, 107415. https://doi.org/10.1016/j.ijscr.2022.107415. Epub 2022 Jul 16. PMID: 35863287; PMCID: PMC9403200.

Pouwer, A. W., VAN DEN Einden, L. C. G., VAN DER Linden, M., Hehir-Kwa, J. Y., Yu, J., Hendriks, K. M., Kamping, E. J., Eijkelenboom, A., Massuger, L. F. A. G., Bulten, J., VAN Tilborg, A. A. G., DE Hullu, J. A., & Kuiper, R. P. (2020). Clonal relationship between lichen sclerosus, differentiated vulvar intra-epithelial neoplasia and non HPV-related vulvar squamous cell carcinoma. *Cancer Genomics Proteomics, 17*(2), 151–160. https://doi.org/10.21873/cgp.20175. PMID: 32108037; PMCID: PMC7078831.

Prat, J., & FIGO Committee on Gynecologic Oncology. (2014). Staging classification for cancer of the ovary, fallopian tube, and peritoneum. *International Journal of Gynecology and Obstetrics, 124*(1), 1–5. https://doi.org/10.1016/j.ijgo.2013.10.001

Proppe, L., Jaeger, A., Goy, Y., Petersen, C., Kruell, A., Prieske, K., Schmalfeldt, B., Mueller, V., & Woelber, L. (2024). Systematic review—Adjuvant radiotherapy of the vulva in primary vulvar cancer. *Gynecologic Oncology, 190*, 264–271. https://doi.org/10.1016/j.ygyno.2024.09.003. Epub 2024 Sep 11. PMID: 39265464.

Rahaman, S., Li, X., Yu, J., & Wong, K. C. (2021). CancerEMC: Frontline non-invasive cancer screening from circulating protein biomarkers and mutations in cell-free DNA. *Bioinformatics, 37*(19), 3319–3327. https://doi.org/10.1093/bioinformatics/btab044. PMID: 33515231.

Reiter, P. L., Bustamante, G., & McRee, A. L. (2020). HPV vaccine coverage and acceptability among a national sample of sexual minority women ages 18-45. *Vaccine, 38*(32), 4956–4963. https://doi.org/10.1016/j.vaccine.2020.06.001. Epub 2020 Jun 11. PMID: 32536546; PMCID: PMC7323872.

Rizzuto, I., Behrens, R. F., & Smith, L. A. (2019). Risk of ovarian cancer in women treated with ovarian stimulating drugs for infertility. *The Cochrane Database of Systematic Reviews, 6*(6), CD008215. https://doi.org/10.1002/14651858.CD008215.pub3. PMID: 31207666; PMCID: PMC6579663.

Sand, F. L., Nielsen, D. M. B., Frederiksen, M. H., Rasmussen, C. L., & Kjaer, S. K. (2019). The prognostic value of p16 and p53 expression for survival after vulvar cancer: A systematic review and meta-analysis. *Gynecologic Oncology, 152*(1), 208–217. https://doi.org/10.1016/j.ygyno.2018.10.015

Sausen, D. G., Shechter, O., Gallo, E. S., Dahari, H., & Borenstein, R. Herpes simplex virus, human papillomavirus, and cervical cancer: Overview, relationship, and treatment implications. *Cancers (Basel), 15*(14), 3692. https://doi.org/10.3390/cancers15143692. PMID: 37509353; PMCID: PMC10378257.

Sharma, R., Ambroise, M. M., Ramdas, A., & Ravichandran, K. (2020). Predictors of unsatisfactory conventional pap smears. *Journal of Midlife Health, 11*(4), 231–235. https://doi.org/10.4103/jmh.JMH_110_20. Epub 2021 Jan 21. PMID: 33767564; PMCID: PMC7978046.

Shrestha, A., Martin, C., Burton, M., Walters, S., Collins, K., & Wyld, L. (2019). Quality of life versus length of life considerations in cancer patients: A systematic literature review. *Psychooncology, 28*(7), 1367–1380. https://doi.org/10.1002/pon.5054. Epub 2019 May 15. PMID: 30838697; PMCID: PMC6619389.

Sia, T. Y., Gordhandas, S. B., Birsoy, O., Kemel, Y., Maio, A., Salo-Mullen, E., Sheehan, M., Hensley, M. L., Rubinstein, M., Makker, V., Grisham, R. N., O'Cearbhaill, R. E., Roche, K. L., Mueller, J. J., Leitao, M. M., Jr., Sonoda, Y., Chi, D. S., Abu-Rustum, N. R., Berger, M. F., Ellenson, L. H., Latham, A., Stadler, Z., Offit, K., Aghajanian, C., Weigelt, B., Mandelker, D., & Liu, Y. L. (2023). Germline drivers of gynecologic carcinosarcomas. *Gynecologic Oncology, 174,* 34–41. https://doi.org/10.1016/j.ygyno.2023.04.024. Epub 2023 May 5. PMID: 37149903; PMCID: PMC10330315.

Siegel, R. L., Miller, K. D., Wagle, N. S., & Jemal, A. (2023). Cancer statistics, 2023. *CA: A Cancer Journal for Clinicians, 73*(1), 17–48. https://doi.org/10.3322/caac.21763

Siegenthaler, F., Lindemann, K., Epstein, E., Rau, T. T., Nastic, D., Ghaderi, M., Rydberg, F., Mueller, M. D., Carlson, J., & Imboden, S. (2022). Time to first recurrence, pattern of recurrence, and survival after recurrence in endometrial cancer according to the molecular classification. *Gynecologic Oncology, 165*(2), 230–238. https://doi.org/10.1016/j.ygyno.2022.02.024. Epub 2022 Mar 8. PMID: 35277281.

Silva, N. N. T., Silva Santos, A. C., Carneiro, C. M., & Lima, A. A. (2020). Association of serum folate and vitamin B12 with pre-neoplastic cervical lesions. *Clinical Nutrition ESPEN, 38,* 223–228. https://doi.org/10.1016/j.clnesp.2020.04.007. Epub 2020 May 4. PMID: 32690162.

Smith, J. A., Gaikwad, A. A., Mathew, L., Rech, B., Faro, J. P., Lucci, J. A., 3rd, Bai, Y., Olsen, R. J., & Byrd, T. T. (2022). AHCC® supplementation to support immune function to clear persistent human papillomavirus infections. *Frontiers in Oncology, 12,* 881902. https://doi.org/10.3389/fonc.2022.881902. PMID: 35814366; PMCID: PMC9256908.

Society of Gynecologic Oncology. (2021). *Joint statement on the elimination of the human papillomavirus (HPV).* https://www.sgo.org/news/joint-statement-on-the-elimination-of-human-papillomavirus-hpv/

Somasegar, S., Reddy, R. A., Chow, S., Dorigo, O., Renz, M., & Karam, A. (2024). Trends in ovarian, fallopian tube, and primary peritoneal cancer incidence, mortality, and survival: A 15-year population-based analysis. *Gynecologic Oncology, 184,* 190–197. https://doi.org/10.1016/j.ygyno.2024.01.034. Epub 2024 Feb 7. PMID: 38330833.

Spencer, J. C., Kim, J. J., Tiro, J. A., Feldman, S. J., Kobrin, S. C., Skinner, C. S., Wang, L., McCarthy, A. M., Atlas, S. J., Pruitt, S. L., Silver, M. I., & Haas, J. S. (2023). Racial and ethnic disparities in cervical cancer screening from three U.S. healthcare settings. *American Journal of Preventive Medicine, 65*(4), 667–677. https://doi.org/10.1016/j.amepre.2023.04.016. Epub 2023 May 3. PMID: 37146839; PMCID: PMC11135625

Steenbeek, M. P., Harmsen, M. G., Hoogerbrugge, N., de Jong, M. A., Maas, A. H. E. M., Prins, J. B., Bulten, J., Teerenstra, S., van Bommel, M. H. D., van Doorn, H. C., Mourits, M. J. E., van Beurden, M., Zweemer, R. P., Gaarenstroom, K. N., Slangen, B. F. M., Brood-van Zanten, M. M. A., Vos, M. C., Piek, J. M. J., van Lonkhuijzen, L. R. C. W., Apperloo, M. J. A., Coppus, S. F. P. J., Massuger, L. F. A. G., IntHout, J., Hermens, R. P. M. G., & de Hullu, J. A. (2021). Association of salpingectomy with delayed oophorectomy versus salpingo-oophorectomy with quality of life in BRCA1/2 pathogenic variant carriers: A nonrandomized controlled trial. *JAMA Oncology, 7*(8), 1203–1212. https://doi.org/10.1001/jamaoncol.2021.1590. PMID: 34081085; PMCID: PMC8176392

Sun, Y., & Liu, G. (2021). Endometriosis-associated ovarian clear cell carcinoma: A special entity? *Journal of Cancer, 12*(22), 6773–6786. https://doi.org/10.7150/jca.61107. PMID: 34659566; PMCID: PMC8518018.

Surveillance, Epidemiology, and End Results Program (SEER). (n.d.-a). *Cancer stat facts: Vulvar cancer.* National Institutes of Health. https://seer.cancer.gov/statfacts/html/vulva.html

Surveillance, Epidemiology, and End Results Program (SEER). (n.d.-b). *Cancer stat facts: Uterine cancer.* National Institutes of Health. https://seer.cancer.gov/statfacts/html/corp.html

Surveillance, Epidemiology, and End Results Program (SEER). (n.d.-c). *Cancer stat facts: Ovarian cancer.* National Institutes of Health. https://seer.cancer.gov/statfacts/html/ovary.html

Tan, L., Yan, W., Yang, W., Kamionka, A., Lipowski, M., Zhao, Z., & Zhao, G. (2023). Effect of exercise on inflammatory markers in postmenopausal women with overweight and obesity: A systematic review and meta-analysis. *Experimental Gerontology, 183,* 112310. https://doi.org/10.1016/j.exger.2023.112310. Epub 2023 Oct 20. PMID: 37844768.

Temkin, S. M., Smeltzer, M. P., Dawkins, M. D., Boehmer, L. M., Senter, L., Black, D. R., Blank, S. V., Yemelyanova, A., Magliocco, A. M., Finkel, M. A., Moore, T. E., & Thaker, P. H. (2022). Improving the quality of care for patients with advanced epithelial ovarian cancer: Program components, implementation barriers, and recommendations. *Cancer, 128*(4), 654–664. https://doi.org/10.1002/cncr.34023. Epub 2021 Nov 17. PMID: 34787913; PMCID: PMC9298928.

Tillmanns, T., Masri, A., Stewart, C., Chase, D., Karnezis, A., Chen, L. M., & Urban, R. (2024). Advanced endometrial cancer—The next generation of treatment: A Society of Gynecologic Oncology Journal Club clinical commentary. *Gynecologic Oncology Reports, 55,* 101462. https://doi.org/10.1016/j.gore.2024.101462. PMID: 39210987; PMCID: PMC11357875.

Togashi, K., Ooyama, N., Enomoto, K., & Sato, H. (2020). A case report of advanced ovarian cancer detected due to an inguinal metastasis in the canal of Nuck. *International Journal of Surgery Case Reports, 66,* 277–282. https://doi.org/10.1016/j.ijscr.2019.12.021. Epub 2019 Dec 19. PMID: 31884264; PMCID: PMC6939067.

Underkofler, K. A., & Ring, K. L. (2023). Updates in gynecologic care for individuals with lynch syndrome. *Frontiers in Oncology, 13,* 1127683. https://doi.org/10.3389/fonc.2023.1127683. PMID: 36937421; PMCID: PMC10014618.

U.S. Preventive Services Task Force. (2018a). *Cervical cancer: Screening.* https://www.uspreventiveservicestaskforce.org/uspstf/recommendation/cervical-cancer-screening

U.S. Preventive Services Task Force. (2018b). Screening for ovarian cancer: US Preventive Services Task Force recommendation statement. *JAMA, 319*(6), 588–594. https://doi.org/10.1001/jama.2017.21926

van Walree, I. C., Bretveld, R., van Huis-Tanja, L. H., Louwers, J. A., Emmelot-Vonk, M. H., & Hamaker, M. E. (2020). Reasons for guideline non-adherence in older and younger women with advanced stage ovarian cancer. *Gynecologic Oncology, 157*(3), 593–598. https://doi.org/10.1016/j.ygyno.2020.03.005. Epub 2020 Mar 11. PMID: 32171566

Wang, T., Baloda, V., Harinath, L., Jones, T., Zhang, H., Bhargava, R., & Zhao, C. (2023). Clinicopathologic diagnosis of dVIN related vulvar squamous cell carcinoma: An extended appraisal from a tertiary women's hospital. *Gynecology and Obstetrics Clinical Medicine, 3*(1), 30–37, ISSN 2667-1646. https://doi.org/10.1016/j.gocm.2023.01.004.

Weinberg, D., & Gomez-Martinez, R. A. (2019). Vulvar cancer. *Obstetrics and Gynecology Clinics of North America, 46*(1), 125–135. https://doi.org/10.1016/j.ogc.2018.09.008

Wenzel, L., Osann, K., McKinney, C., Cella, D., Fulci, G., Scroggins, M. J., Lankes, H. A., Wang, V., Nephew, K. P., Maxwell, G. L., Mok, S. C., Conrads, T. P., Miller, A., Mannel, R. S., Gray, H. J., Hanjani, P., Huh, W. K., Spirtos, N., Leitao, M. M., Glaser, G., Sharma, S. K., Santin, A. D., Sperduto, P., Lele, S. B., Burger, R. A., Monk, B. J., & Birrer, M. (2021). Quality of life and adverse events: Prognostic relationships in long-term ovarian cancer survival. *Journal of the National Cancer Institute, 113*(10), 1369–1378. https://doi.org/10.1093/jnci/djab034. PMID: 33729494; PMCID: PMC8486331.

Whetstone, S., Burke, W., Sheth, S. S., Brooks, R., Cavens, A., Huber-Keener, K., Scott, D. M., Worly, B., & Chelmow, D. (2022). Health disparities in uterine cancer: Report from the Uterine Cancer Evidence Review Conference. *Obstetrics and Gynecology, 139*(4), 645–659. https://doi.org/10.1097/AOG.0000000000004710. Epub 2022 Mar 10. PMID: 35272301; PMCID: PMC8936152.

White, C., Reynolds, S., Murphy, K., Keegan, H., Naik, P., O'Brien, R., Pilkington, L., Sharkey Ochoa, I., Glesson, G., Russell, N., Nuttall, D., Tewari, P., Wright, F., O'Toole, S., Sharp, L., Flannelly, G., O'Leary, J. J., Martin, C. M.; CERVIVA the Irish Cervical Screening Research Consortium. Performance of the HPV E6/E7 mRNA Aptima HPV assay combined with partial genotyping compared with the HPV DNA Cobas 4800 HPV test for use in primary screening: Results from the CERVIVA HPV primary screening study in Ireland. *International Journal of Cancer, 154*(1), 53–64. https://doi.org/10.1002/ijc.34685. Epub 2023 Aug 26. PMID: 37632406.

Williamson, C. W., Liu, H. C., Mayadev, J., & Mell, L. K. (2021). Advances in external beam radiation therapy and brachytherapy for cervical cancer. *Clinical Oncology (Royal College of Radiologists), 33*(9), 567–578. https://doi.org/10.1016/j.clon.2021.06.012. Epub 2021 Jul 12. PMID: 34266728.

World Health Organization (WHO). (n.d.). *Cervical cancer.* https://www.who.int/health-topics/cervical-cancer#tab=tab_1

World Health Organization (WHO). (2021). *WHO recommends DNA testing as a first choice screening method for cervical cancer prevention.* https://www.who.int/europe/news-room/11-09-2021-who-recommends-dna-testing-as-a-first-choice-screening-method-for-cervical-cancer-prevention

Wu, P., Xiong, H., Yang, M., Li, L., Wu, P., Lazare, C., Cao, C., Gao, P., Meng, Y., Zhi, W., Lin, S., Hu, J., Wei, J., Ma, D., Liu, J., Yin, P., & Xing, H. (2019). Co-infections of HPV16/18 with other high-risk HPV types and the risk of cervical carcinogenesis:

A large population-based study. *Gynecologic Oncology, 155*(3), 436–443. https://doi.org/10.1016/j.ygyno.2019.10.003. Epub 2019 Oct 8. PMID: 31604662

Xing, D., & Fadare, O. (2021). Molecular events in the pathogenesis of vulvar squamous cell carcinoma. *Seminars in Diagnostic Pathology, 38*(1), 50–61. https://doi.org/10.1053/j.semdp.2020.09.010. Epub 2020 Sep 25. PMID: 33032902; PMCID: PMC7749059.

Yang, Y., & Cao, Y. (2022). The impact of VEGF on cancer metastasis and systemic disease. *Seminars in Cancer Biology, 86*(Pt 3), 251–261. https://doi.org/10.1016/j.semcancer.2022.03.011. Epub 2022 Mar 17. PMID: 35307547.

Zach, D., Åvall-Lundqvist, E., Falconer, H., Hellman, K., Johansson, H., & Flöter Rådestad, A. (2021). Patterns of recurrence and survival in vulvar cancer: A nationwide population-based study. *Gynecologic Oncology, 161*(3), 748–754. https://doi.org/10.1016/j.ygyno.2021.03.013. Epub 2021 Mar 16. PMID: 33736857.

Zhou, A., Minlikeeva, A. N., Khan, S., & Moysich, K. B. (2019). Association between cigarette smoking and histotype-specific epithelial ovarian cancer: A review of epidemiologic studies. *Cancer Epidemiology, Biomarkers, and Prevention, 28*(7), 1103–1116. https://doi.org/10.1158/1055-9965.EPI-18-1214. Epub 2019 May 1. PMID: 31043418; PMCID: PMC6606332.

CHAPTER 29

Acute and Chronic Pelvic Pain

Melissa Romero

INTRODUCTION

Concern about pelvic pain is the reason for 1 to 2 percent of all healthcare visits made by women in primary care settings (Thomas & Porter, 2023). Historically, when a person presented with pelvic or lower abdominal pain, the clinician automatically focused solely on the gynecologic organs, assuming they were the cause of the problem. This narrow clinical view risks categorizing normal physiologic processes as abnormal and encourages the use of surgical interventions because it assumes pathology. A number of causes of pelvic pain are unrelated to the gynecologic organs (Arnold et al., 2021; Frasca et al., 2023). Often pelvic pain is caused by multiple factors, requiring clinicians to take a multidisciplinary, holistic approach to its assessment and management. An appreciation for the intertwining influence of the mind and body during assessment and in planning interventions is important. This approach places the patient at the center of the management plan and respects their credibility as the authoritative knower.

This chapter addresses acute and chronic pelvic pain that is gynecologic in origin. Nongynecologic acute pelvic pain and chronic pelvic pain are addressed in the context of providing differential diagnoses for the clinician to consider during assessment and evaluation. There are numerous aspects of pelvic pain prevention, clinical presentation, assessment, and management that are specific to cisgender, transgender, and gender-diverse people who are assigned female at birth.

DESCRIPTION AND DEFINITION

Pelvic pain is a broad term encompassing a number of etiologies within or across body systems. Pelvic pain is divided into two types: acute and chronic, which can be cyclic or noncyclic and may or may not be related to gynecologic organs. It may be symptomatic of an underlying cause, or it can be a syndrome unto itself. Pelvic pain can be so severe that it adversely affects normal functioning, keeping a person from maintaining a normal lifestyle. Although seeking treatment for pelvic pain is one of the most common reasons patients come to a clinician for care, diagnosing its cause and prescribing the appropriate treatment is often difficult because of the complexity of the pathophysiology and the myriad contributing factors.

Acute Pelvic Pain

Acute pelvic pain is defined as intense, noncyclic pain that occurs in the pelvis or lower abdomen that has a duration of less than three months (Frasca et al., 2023). The pain is intense and is generally characterized as having a sudden onset, being sharp, and having a short duration (Rapkin et al., 2020). Onset of acute pelvic pain may result from gynecologic disorders, such as pelvic inflammatory disease (PID); ruptured ovarian cyst; ectopic pregnancy with rupture; or torsion of an ovarian cyst, ovary, or fallopian tube (Thomas & Porter, 2023). Pelvic inflammatory disease accounts for approximately 20 percent of acute pelvic pain, ovarian cysts account for approximately 40 percent, and adnexal torsion accounts for approximately 16 percent (Thomas & Porter, 2023). One defining characteristic of acute pelvic pain is that it typically resolves with treatment.

Visits to the emergency department by women of reproductive age commonly occur due to acute pelvic pain caused by PID and lower genital tract infections (e.g., cervicitis, candidiasis, Bartholin abscess) (Lipsky & Hart, 2023). Given that acute pelvic pain is often associated with an identifiable cause such as PID or ectopic pregnancy, an incorrect diagnosis can lead to serious sequelae, such as impaired fertility, chronic pelvic pain, increased risk of future ectopic pregnancies, and life-threatening conditions such as hemorrhagic ovarian cyst, ruptured ectopic pregnancy, and even death (Lipsky & Hart, 2023; Rapkin et al., 2020). In other instances, patients who present with concerns about acute pelvic pain may be experiencing an extrapelvic condition arising from vascular, musculoskeletal, neurologic, psychiatric, urinary, or gastrointestinal system disorders, including urgent conditions such as appendicitis and pyelonephritis (Frasca et al., 2023; Lipsky & Hart, 2023; Thomas & Porter, 2023).

Scope and Incidence of Acute Pelvic Pain

Acute pelvic pain is a common presenting symptom with more than one third of individuals during their reproductive years experiencing nonmenstrual-related pelvic pain (Lipsky & Hart, 2023; Shetty, 2023). In the outpatient gynecologic care setting, approximately 2 to 10 percent of patients present with acute pelvic pain annually and non-trauma related gynecologic emergencies represent a considerable portion of hospital emergency room visits (Cairns & Kang, 2023; Fauconnier et al., 2020; Shetty, 2023). The exact prevalence of emergency room visits for acute pelvic pain is unknown because the condition is included under the category of abdominal pain, although pelvic pain, when included as part of abdominal pain accounts for 5 to 10 percent of visits annually (Dewey & Wittrock, 2019). In nonpregnant patients, the most common causes of acute pelvic pain from gynecologic sources include pelvic inflammatory disease, ruptured ovarian cyst or adnexal torsion, and degeneration of uterine leiomyomas and in pregnant patients, the most common causes of acute pelvic pain from gynecologic sources include ectopic pregnancy, placental disorders, and spontaneous abortion (Basta Nikolic et al., 2021; Franco et al., 2023; Frasca et al., 2023). Symptoms may also originate from nongynecologic sources (e.g., gastrointestinal, vascular, musculoskeletal, neurologic, psychiatric, and urinary systems).

Etiology and Pathophysiology of Acute Pelvic Pain

Acute pelvic pain is associated with an abrupt onset, sudden increase and short duration of symptoms with autonomic nervous system responses that include nausea, emesis, and diaphoresis (Rapkin et al., 2020). Signs of inflammation and infection (i.e., leukocytosis and fever) may be present with symptoms arising from gynecologic, urologic, vascular, musculoskeletal, or gastrointestinal structures (Shetty, 2023). Although acute pelvic pain usually arises from gynecologic sources, the afferent visceral pain pathways include all of the structures within the pelvis (vagina, uterus, ovaries, fallopian tubes, urinary bladder, ureters, sigmoid colon, rectum, muscles, vascular structures). Therefore, when pain signals are initiated from inflammation, infection, ischemia of an organ, or through bleeding or distention, the source of the pain may be difficult to locate (Lipsky & Hart, 2023). A listing of differential diagnoses is outlined in **Table 29-1**.

Clinical Presentation of Acute Pelvic Pain

Pelvic pathology causing acute pain includes diffuse or lower abdominal pain, pelvic pain, or low back pain (Lipsky & Hart, 2023). Individuals with chronic pelvic pain may also develop an acute process, either secondary to the chronic pain condition or arising from a new source (Lipsky & Hart, 2023). More than one third of individuals of reproductive age assigned female at birth will experience nonmenstrual pelvic pain, and in nearly half of individuals with acute pelvic pain, their condition will be due to PID and lower genital tract infections (e.g., cervicitis, candidiasis, Bartholin abscess) (Lipsky & Hart, 2023).

Acute pelvic pain includes pain in the lower abdomen or pelvic region that is present for less than 3 months duration; it may or may not be recurrent or related to the menstrual cycle (Hoffman, 2020). The patient usually describes acute pelvic pain as having a rapid onset and sharp intensity. The discomfort may consist of colicky pain or it may come and go like menstrual cramps. Vital signs may be unstable because of the sharpness of the pain and/or because of hemodynamic instability in emergent situations. Nausea and vomiting may be present due to visceral or severe pain. Fever and chills are suggestive of an infectious process. The cause of acute pelvic pain must be quickly diagnosed because a delay can result in increased morbidity and death (Lipsky & Hart, 2023; Rapkin et al., 2020). If the patient is of reproductive age, the first priority is to rule out pregnancy.

Chronic Pelvic Pain

Chronic pelvic pain is described as noncyclic pain lasting more than 6 months (American College of Obstetricians and

TABLE 29-1 Differential Diagnoses for Acute and Chronic Pelvic Pain

Diagnoses of Gynecologic Origin	Nongynecologic Diagnoses
Endometriosis	**Gastrointestinal:**
Pelvic inflammatory disease (PID)	Irritable bowel syndrome (IBS)
Dysmenorrhea	Diverticular disease
Abdominal adhesions	Inflammatory bowel disease
Pelvic congestion syndrome	Constipation
Mittelschmerz	Bowel obstruction
Pelvic muscle trigger points	Appendicitis
Pelvic organ prolapse	Malignancy
Leaking or ruptured ovarian cyst	Colitis
Ovarian mass	Celiac disease
Ovarian remnant syndrome	**Urologic:**
Adenomyosis	Cystitis (interstitial, radiation)
Endometrial endocervical polyps	Urinary tract infection (acute or chronic)
Torsion of adnexa	Urinary retention
Tubo-ovarian abscess	Urinary tract stone
Leiomyomas	Pyelonephritis
Prolapsing leiomyoma	Urinary tract cancer
Ectopic pregnancy	**Musculoskeletal:**
Abortion, threatened or incomplete	Spondylosis
Outflow tract obstruction	Faulty posture, muscle strain
Intrauterine contraceptive device	Disc disease, vertebral compression
Reproductive tract cancer	Degenerative joint disease
Uterine atrophy from testosterone gender affirming hormone therapy	Hernia
	Abdominal wall trauma
	Coccydynia
	Myofascial pain
	Levator ani syndrome
	Peripartum pelvic pain
	Neurologic:
	Neurologic dysfunction
	Pelvic or abdominal wall nerve entrapment
	Pudendal neuralgia
	Piriformis syndrome
	Spinal cord or sacral nerve tumor
	Other:
	Aortic aneurysm
	Pelvic thrombophlebitis
	Acute porphyria
	Abdominal angina
	Psychiatric disorders
	Physical or sexual abuse
	Shingles

Data from Gershenson, D. M., Lentz, G. M., Valeu, F. A., & Lobo, R. A. (2022). *Comprehensive gynecology* (8th ed.). Elsevier; Hoffman, B. L. (2020). Pelvic pain. In B. L. Hoffman, J. O. Schorge, L. M. Halvorson, C. A. Hamid, M. M. Corton, & J. I. Schaffer (Eds.), *Williams gynecology* (4th ed., pp. 253–278). McGraw Hill Education; Lipsky, A., & Hart, D. (2023). Acute pelvic pain in women. In R. Walls (Ed.), *Rosen's emergency medicine: Concepts and clinical practice* (10th ed., pp. 257–262). Elsevier; Rapkin, A. J., Lee, E., & Nathan, L. (2020). Pelvic pain in dysmenorrhea. In J. S. Berek (Ed.)., *Berek and Novak's gynecology* (16th ed., pp. 251–278). Wolters Kluwer; Thomas, D. J., & Porter, B. O. (2023). Common reproductive system complaints. In L. M. Dunphy, J. E. Winland-Brown, Porter, B. O., & D. J. Thomas (Eds.), *Primary care: The art and science of advanced practice nursing: An interprofessional approach* (6th ed., pp. 749–759). F. A. Davis Company.

Gynecologists [ACOG], 2020). Some types of chronic pelvic pain are associated with normal physiologic functions, such as menstruation and childbearing. However, a number of nongynecologic causes of pelvic pain must also be considered. Although the anatomy affected by chronic pelvic pain generally includes areas below the umbilicus and within the pelvis, many authors include portions of the external genitalia (vulva, vagina) and components of the musculoskeletal system that are located near the pelvis (Arnold et al., 2021; Carey et al., 2017; Casanova et al., 2024; Hoffman et al., 2020; Lamvu et al., 2021; Quaghebeur et al., 2021; Rapkin et al., 2020; Wozniak, 2016). For the purposes of this chapter, chronic pelvic pain is defined as "pain symptoms perceived to originate from pelvic organs/structures typically lasting more than six months. It is often associated with negative cognitive, behavioral, sexual and emotional consequences as well as with symptoms suggestive of lower urinary tract, sexual, bowel, pelvic floor, myofascial, or gynecological dysfunction" (ACOG, 2020, pp. 744-746).

Scope and Incidence of Chronic Pelvic Pain

Chronic pelvic pain is a complex, multifactorial health condition that affects up to 26 percent of women worldwide with a prevalence of approximately 15 percent in the United States (ACOG, 2020; Ahangari, 2014; Lamvu et al., 2021; Latthe et al., 2006; Mathias et al., 1996; Wozniak, 2016). The condition affects individuals in all age groups, with ages ranging from 14 to 80 years (Ahangari, 2014). Symptoms tend to be prolonged, often lasting longer than 1 year and contribute significantly toward healthcare expenditures (Casanova et al., 2024; Lamvu et al., 2021; Mathias et al., 1996; Veasley et al., 2015).

Sexual and gender minoritized people experience disparate rates of chronic pelvic pain. In a longitudinal study of 6,150 young cisgender women in the United States identifying as completely heterosexual, lesbian, bisexual, or mostly heterosexual, researchers found that 50 percent of respondents reported experiencing symptoms of chronic pelvic pain and of those, 90 percent experienced pain for the past year. In comparison to completely heterosexual women, lesbian, bisexual, and mostly heterosexual women were at an increased risk for lifetime chronic pain and bisexual women experienced chronic pelvic that interfered with their social activities (Tabaac et al., 2022). Although data are extremely limited, prevalence rates of pelvic pain in transgender men and gender diverse (TGD) persons assigned female at birth who took testosterone ranged from 36 to 72 percent (Grimstad et al., 2023; Zwickl et al., 2023; Russell et al., 2023). Using online survey methods, Grimstad et al. (2020) found that of 183 TGD persons assigned female at birth who recently started taking testosterone, 69.4 percent experienced pelvic pain. In contrast, other researchers who examined the relationship between testosterone and chronic pelvic pain found different results (Shim et al., 2020; Tordoff et al., 2024). Tordoff et al. (2024) used online methods to survey 2,579 TGD persons assigned female at birth and found that 457 (18%) of participants experienced chronic pelvic pain and 21 percent of those taking testosterone reported their pain had decreased. In another study of 35 TGD adolescent and young adult persons assigned female at birth who experienced pelvic pain caused from dysmenorrhea, Shim et al. (2020) found that after starting testosterone, pelvic pain decreased in 8 out of 12 participants. The differences in results may be due to a lack of differentiation of types of pelvic pain noted within the studies, as testosterone may reduce dysmenorrhea but increase pain from atrophy of the gynecologic organs.

Patients with chronic pelvic pain often experience poor treatment outcomes when they receive traditional gynecologic and medical therapies and may endure multiple unsuccessful surgical procedures to treat pain (Lamvu et al., 2021; Rapkin et al., 2020). In comparison to those who do not have pelvic pain, those who experience pelvic pain are more likely to have had a laparoscopy, hysterectomy, and reduced quality of life (Brichant et al., 2018; Rapkin et al., 2020). In two studies that examined TGD persons assigned female at birth with a history of testosterone use who were seeking hysterectomies, researchers found that 51 to 58 percent reported experiencing intermittent or chronic pelvic pain (Ferrando et al., 2021; Grimstad et al., 2019).

Mathias et al. (1996) obtained estimates on the prevalence of chronic pelvic pain in U.S. women aged 18–50 years in 1994 (n = 5,263). Incidence rates were examined to determine whether there were associations between chronic pelvic pain and quality of life, with results describing $2.8 billion in direct care costs each year attributed to chronic pelvic pain (Mathias et al., 1996). The loss of daily functioning because of pelvic pain may result in work absenteeism and contribute to feelings of hopelessness, depression, anxiety, marital distress, and lack of interest in sexual intimacy (Arnold et al., 2021; Lamvu et al., 2021).

Etiology and Pathophysiology of Chronic Pelvic Pain

Unlike acute pelvic pain, chronic pelvic pain is more often a complex condition that overlaps with other types of nonpelvic pain disorders and comorbid conditions (Carey et al., 2017). For example, individuals with chronic pelvic pain often present with other conditions, some of which include, irritable bowel syndrome, interstitial cystitis, depression, abdominal wall or pelvic floor myofascial syndrome, and neuropathy (Arnold et al., 2021; Lamvu et al., 2021; Rapkin et al., 2020). Therefore, when undergoing medical or surgical interventions for gynecologic-associated pelvic pain, patients may experience only partial improvement in their symptoms if urologic, musculoskeletal, neurologic, psychiatric, and gastrointestinal components are missed during the initial assessment.

Chronic pelvic pain can originate from visceral sources, such as the gynecologic, genitourinary, or gastrointestinal tracts; from somatic sources, such as the pelvic bones, ligaments, muscles, and fascia; and from nerves within the abdomen and pelvis. The pain may also include central sensitization and/or psychologic components (Hoffman, 2020; Rapkin et al., 2020). For these reasons, a comprehensive review of body systems, including psychosocial history and thorough physical examination are essential components in the diagnostic approach to chronic pelvic pain. Somatic pain originates in muscles, joints, bones, or connective tissue and is often described as being either sharp, gnawing, aching, or cramping and is usually localized (Hoffman, 2020). Visceral pain arises from internal organs and is often associated with strong muscle contractions (Hoffman, 2020). This type of pain is transmitted through the sympathetic nervous system and is difficult to isolate. Stretching, distention, ischemia, or spasm of abdominal organs can stimulate visceral pain (Hoffman, 2020). The pain is usually described as being diffuse and poorly localized; it may be associated with autonomic phenomena, such as diaphoresis, nausea, and vomiting.

Inflammatory or nociceptive pain arises from damage or injury to tissue caused by physical and chemical agents and is a result of activation of nociceptors in a normally functioning nervous system (Armstrong & Herr, 2023). This type of pain alerts the sufferer to tissue injury and/or disease. When the noxious stimulus is removed, the activity of the sensory pain receptors (also known as nociceptors) quickly ceases (Hoffman, 2020). Nociceptive pain subsides with proper treatment and/or healing of the associated injury and/or disease.

Neuropathic pain is described as a complex type of pain that occurs in response to a lesion or dysfunction within the central or peripheral nervous system (International Association for the Study of Pain, 2021). Neuropathic pain occurs when noxious stimuli have sustained action, producing continuous central sensitization and loss of neuronal inhibition that becomes permanent (Hoffman, 2020). The result is an increased pain threshold and perception of pain that may seem disproportionate to the amount of coexisting disease. When neuropathic pain occurs in the context of chronic pelvic pain, it often presents as paresthesia or a burning type of pain. This phenomenon explains why it is not uncommon for patients to experience pain that is disproportionate to the amount of coexisting disease (Hoffman, 2020).

In addition to a thorough assessment of the pain symptomatology of chronic pelvic pain, the assessment should also include evaluation of multiple organ systems, previous treatments, including current and prior use of testosterone as part of gender-affirming treatment, ability to function and participate in daily activities, and psychological/psychosocial factors such as the ability to maintain satisfactory emotional and sexual relationships (Arnold et al., 2021; Krakowsky et al., 2022; Lamvu et al., 2021). Such factors are especially relevant in those with a history of sexual or physical abuse, post-traumatic stress, depression, or anxiety (Hassam et al., 2020; Lampe et al., 2000; Lamvu et al., 2021; Rapkin et al., 2020; Till et al., 2019; Wall et al., 2024). Hassam et al. (2020) performed an exploratory systematic review and meta-analysis and found that Australian women with a history of sexual assault were more likely to experience gynecologic morbidity, pelvic pain, dyspareunia, dysmenorrhea, abnormal menstrual bleeding, and urinary incontinence. In another study that used correlational analyses, Lampe et al. (2000) found that participants with chronic pelvic pain reported significantly higher levels of sexual victimization before 15 years of age, exposure to physical violence, and emotional neglect in comparison to a control group of participants who did not report pain. These findings do not diminish the need for accurate physical diagnosis, but they do emphasize the importance of proper recognition and assessment of functional ability and psychological factors because these have been found to be important components of treatment (Arnold et al., 2021; Lamvu et al., 2021).

The three most frequent findings obtained on laparoscopy for those with chronic pelvic pain are endometriosis (15 to 40%), adhesions (25%), and in 60 to 80 percent of cases, an absence of pathologic condition (Hoffman, 2020; Howard, 1993; Rapkin et al., 2020). Associations between pain location, severity and pathology have been inconsistent in cases where endometriosis and adhesions were identified using laparoscopy (Rapkin et al., 2020). Other benign gynecologic causes of pain include, but are not limited to, adenomyosis, ovarian cyst, uterine fibroids (leiomyomas), pelvic muscle trigger points, vulvodynia, chronic PID, ovarian remnant syndrome, and pelvic congestion syndrome (Eid et al., 2019; Carey et al., 2017; Hoffman, 2020; Lamvu et al., 2021). There are many nongynecologic conditions associated with chronic pelvic pain, some of which include irritable bowel syndrome, bladder pain syndrome/interstitial cystitis, pelvic floor or abdominal myofascial syndrome, depression, and neuropathy (Arnold et al., 2021; Carey et al., 2017; Hoffman, 2020; Rapkin et al., 2020).

The historical approach has been to link a single etiology to chronic pelvic pain and attempt to cure the patient by addressing the suspected cause. However, the etiology of chronic pelvic pain is now understood as being multifactorial and complex, and it may encompass one or more body systems (gastroenterologic, urologic, gynecologic, neurologic) in addition to psychosocial systems (Arnold et al., 2021; Carey et al., 2017; Hoffman, 2020; Lamvu et al., 2021; Rapkin et al., 2020). When more than one organ system is affected, they are thought to serve as independent pain generators, thus making symptom identification and diagnosis challenging (Lamvu et al., 2021).

The role of central sensitization—the idea that exposure to repeated stimuli over time leads to amplified perceptions of pain—is increasingly being recognized as an important factor underlying conditions associated with chronic pelvic pain (Arnold et al., 2021; Hoffman, 2020; Lamvu et al., 2021; Rapkin et al., 2020). In a cross-sectional cohort study, Ryan et al. (2022) found that participants with pelvic pain and central sensitization (self-reported via survey) were significantly more likely to score higher on surveys measuring irritable bowel syndrome; bladder pain syndrome; prolonged pain (longer than 2 years); and other pain symptoms involving the back, bladder, bowel, and vulva. Study participants also were more likely to report previous diagnoses of mental health disorders (Ryan et al., 2022). Although the pathophysiology remains unclear, experts agree that in many cases the condition includes elements of hyperesthesia, allodynia, musculoskeletal pain, and pelvic floor dysfunction; it is conceptualized as being a complex neuromuscular–psychosocial disorder that includes elements of chronic regional and/or functional somatic pain syndromes (Lamvu et al., 2021; Rapkin et al., 2020).

It can be challenging for generalists to properly evaluate and treat chronic pelvic pain due to the level of complexity associated with the condition. In addition, there are limited evidence-based therapies that are multimodal. Given the myriad etiologic aspects associated with chronic pelvic pain, the approach to health care for individuals with pelvic pain must be multifaceted. The process of determining etiologies associated with pelvic pain and developing a successful treatment plan is often difficult, time-consuming, and costly for the patient, and it is difficult and confusing, at best, for even the most experienced clinicians. Because of limited evidence-based interventions that address all aspects of the condition (medical, lifestyle, psychosocial), clinicians must take a multidisciplinary approach and identify and treat physical causes of pain and comorbid psychological conditions (e.g., endometriosis, pelvic floor muscle tenderness, interstitial cystitis, irritable bowel syndrome, depression, and/or other mood disorder) (Arnold et al., 2021; Ball & Khan, 2020; Hoffman, 2020; Lamvu et al., 2021; Rapkin et al., 2020).

Clinical Presentation of Chronic Pelvic Pain

Chronic pelvic pain is often classified as either gynecologic or nongynecologic. Categorizing the pain further into cyclic or noncyclic categories assists the clinician in determining whether the pain may be related to the menstrual cycle. Sometimes, however, cyclic pain has no relationship to the menstrual cycle and is totally unrelated to the pelvic organs. Refer to Chapters 24 and 27 for further information on conditions that cause cyclic gynecologic pain.

Individuals presenting with chronic pelvic pain often have had the pain for some time (at least 6 months) and may be reluctant to seek medical advice and disclose information about all aspects of their condition (Jarrell et al., 2018; Lamvu et al., 2021). They do not always appear to be experiencing the amount of distress that individuals with chronic pain often display. This affect may reflect the fact that these individuals have lived with the pain for so long that they have normalized it and, therefore, do not present as a typical patient suffering from significant pain. Frequently they will describe unrelenting pain and an inability to work or function at home. It is also not unusual to observe that a person has seen a variety of clinicians over several years with a variety of concerns, all of which center on the pelvic pain.

ASSESSMENT

A detailed history and physical examination are essential to make an accurate diagnosis. This is particularly important when dealing with both acute and chronic pelvic pain because the signs and symptoms of many gynecologic and nongynecologic etiologies may overlap (Frasca et al., 2023; Hoffman, 2020; Rapkin et al., 2020). It is essential for the practitioner to obtain a thorough history for an accurate assessment (Hoffman, 2020; Lamvu et al., 2021). The approach to assessment and diagnosis of pelvic pain needs to be systematic and detailed, and an appropriate treatment plan should be developed. Care must be taken during the first visit to validate the patient's symptoms and acknowledge their important role in the healthcare process. It is important to allow enough time during the visit and to extend to sequential visits if necessary so the patient can establish trust with the clinician and tell their story in its entirety (ACOG, 2020; Jarrell et al., 2018; Lamvu et al., 2021). Patients with acute pelvic pain require a timely diagnosis because delays in treatment may increase risks for morbidity and mortality (Rapkin et al., 2020).

The clinician should focus on obtaining a history that covers quality, onset, and location of pain in addition to radiation of pain, timing and duration of symptoms, and aggravating and alleviating factors. A review of the patient's gynecology history should include an inquiry about vaginal bleeding and/or discharge, sexually transmitted infections, sex partners, sexual abuse, menstrual cycle (number of bleeding days), last menstrual period, information about previous pregnancies, current pregnancy status, use of contraceptives, hormonal therapies as part of gender-affirming care, and menstrual products. Other questions in the history should be focused on GI symptoms (nausea, vomiting, anorexia, constipation, flatus, hematochezia), urinary symptoms (dysuria, urgency, hesitancy, frequency, hematuria), signs of infection (fever, chills), and symptoms of heavy internal bleeding (dizziness, syncope, abdominal distension and pain) (Frasca et al., 2023; Rapkin et al., 2020).

Focused questioning is important for obtaining an accurate history, and active listening is essential. Valuing the patient's description of pain and validating their feelings are paramount in developing trust and rapport. A holistic approach considers how the pain is affecting every facet of the patient's life. The multiple roles most people play are all altered by pain, and obtaining information about how the pain affects the individual person physically and emotionally, how it impacts activities of daily living, and how it changes relationships is important.

A pain history should be taken during the first visit, including the nature of each pain symptom (i.e., duration, location, radiation, severity, quality, aggravating and alleviating factors); the effects of the menstrual cycle, stress, work, exercise, intercourse, and orgasm on the pain; the context in which pain arose; the social and occupational toll of the pain; and prior or current opioid use (Rapkin et al., 2020).

The mnemonic OLD CAARTS can be used as an aid for performing a pain history:

O = Onset: When and how did the pain start?

L = Location: Specific location of the pain. Can you put a finger on it?

D = Duration: How long does it last?

C = Characteristics: What is the pain like—cramping, aching, stabbing, burning, tingling, itching, and so on?

A = Alleviating or aggravating factors: What makes the pain better (e.g., medication, position change, heat) and what makes it worse (e.g., specific activity, stress, menstrual cycle)?

A = Associated symptoms: Gynecologic (dyspareunia, dysmenorrhea, abnormal bleeding, discharge, infertility), gastrointestinal (constipation, diarrhea), genitourinary (dysuria, urgency, incontinence), and neurologic (specific nerve involvement).

R = Radiation: Does the pain move to other areas on your body?

T = Temporal: What time of day is the pain worse and better?

S = Severity (on a scale of 1 to 10) (Rapkin et al., 2020, p. 264).

The use of a pain rating scale may assist the clinician to comprehend the intensity of the patient's pain. Pain rating scales, such as numeric ranking scales, visual analog scales, and verbal descriptive scales, allow the patient to identify the severity of pain. If there is a language barrier related to culture or mental ability, the Wong-Baker FACES pain rating scale (smile to frown) may be helpful in conveying this information (Wong-Baker Faces Foundation, 2016).

Using a formatted, widely accepted pelvic pain assessment tool can be helpful in ensuring that all critical points are covered. The International Pelvic Pain Society (IPPS, 2021) provides an Initial Patient Survey for chronic pelvic pain that is completed by the patient prior to the first visit and another pelvic pain assessment form titled Follow-up Patient Survey is used to evaluate patient progress at subsequent visits after a treatment plan has been established. Both the Initial Patient Survey and the Follow-up Patient Survey can be downloaded from: https://www.pelvicpaineducation.com/.

A detailed obstetric and surgical history should be also obtained. Pregnancy, labor, and vaginal childbirth can damage the pelvic floor and lead to neuromuscular, symphyseal, and sacroiliac joint pain (Hoffman, 2020). Cesarean birth has been linked to lower abdominal wall pain and adhesions. The surgical history provides information about the person's risk for adhesions, peritoneal injuries, infections, and related diagnoses that may be responsible for the pain (e.g., endometriosis). In addition, information about prior surgeries for gynecologic conditions should be obtained (Hoffman, 2020).

An accurate and nonjudgmental sexual history is very important. Clinicians need to be unbiased and inquire about sexual orientation, gender identity, sex assigned at birth, gender-affirming treatment, number of sexual partners, preferences, ability to achieve orgasm, satisfaction with sexual relationships, history of sexually transmitted infections, and sexual triggers of pain (intercourse, menstruation, touch). Several researchers have identified associations between chronic pelvic pain and sexual, physical, and emotional abuse (Hassam et al., 2020; Krantz et al., 2019; Lampe et al., 2000; Lamvu et al., 2021; Poli-Neto et al., 2018). Unrecognized abuse may have serious or even deadly consequences (Lipsky & Hart, 2023). The reasons for these associations are unknown, and more research on this topic is needed. If the abuse is currently occurring, it is important that the patient be counseled appropriately and a trauma-informed approach to care utilized. Refer to Chapter 5 for more information on trauma-informed care. Obtaining a careful inventory of family relationships and intimate partner violence assessment is critically important. Please refer to the paragraph below and Chapters 15 and 16 for additional information on care for persons experiencing sexual assault or intimate partner violence.

With respect to psychological risk factors, individuals with chronic pelvic pain experience higher levels of anxiety and depression than those without (Siqueira-Campos et al., 2019). The Society of Obstetricians and Gynaecologists of Canada (Jarrell et al., 2018; Lamvu et al., 2021) provides a guideline with the following list of psychosocial domains that should be reviewed with patients during the initial history and subsequent visits:

a. the effect of pain on functional roles (e.g., disability in family, sexual, work, and recreational activities) and emotional functioning (e.g., anxiety about pain and depression secondary to pain)
b. pain coping style (e.g., ignoring the pain, becoming inactive, seeking emergency care)
c. pain modulators (e.g., stress)
d. quality of interactions with previous healthcare clinicians
e. mental health history
f. history of neglect or sexual, physical, or emotional abuse
g. substance use or abuse
h. social support.

Physical Examination

The physical examination gives the clinician an opportunity to connect information collected during the history to a focused examination and development of a differential diagnosis list. This process may provide a good understanding about underlying causes of pelvic pain. Always obtain baseline vital signs, including blood pressure, temperature, pulse, and respirations, prior to performing the physical examination.

Acute Pelvic Pain

For patients with acute pelvic pain, an abbreviated physical exam is performed (abdominal, pelvic, and other body systems depending on information obtained during the history) (Dewey et al., 2019). An assessment of general appearance (pallor, diaphoresis, level of agitation, and facial expression) provides the clinician with an initial interpretation of whether the clinical condition is urgent (Hoffman, 2020). Other symptoms that require urgent evaluation include fever, tachycardia, and hypotension; these could be signs of intraabdominal pathology. Prolonged fever suggests possible appendicitis, PID, peritonitis, pyelonephritis, and diverticulitis (Hoffman, 2020).

Examination of the abdomen is performed to assess for peritoneal symptoms, identify any painful areas and palpable masses (Dewey et al., 2019). The exam begins with a visual inspection, assessing for previous surgical scars, incisional hernias, and evidence of abdominal distention. Next, the abdomen is auscultated; high-pitched bowel sounds are associated with bowel obstruction. The abdomen is then palpated in all four quadrants with palpation beginning in the quadrants farthest away from any painful areas (Hoffman, 2020). Any rebound tenderness or guarding during the exam is associated with peritoneal irritation. During the abdominal exam, the Carnett test can be used to assess for anterior abdominal wall pain. Ask the patient to raise their head off the table while in the supine position and have them straight-raise their legs and then palpate the area. If the patient has tenderness to palpation, the source is most likely anterior abdominal wall pain instead of visceral pain (Arnold et al., 2021).

A pregnancy test is obtained on any patient with the potential to be pregnant, and a full pelvic exam with bimanual and speculum examination is performed in reproductive-aged individuals (Hoffman, 2020; Dewey et al., 2019). The exam may be modified in patients in their nonreproductive years depending on clinical information. The pelvic exam includes visualization of the external genitalia, speculum exam of the vagina, cervix, and bimanual exam of the uterus and adnexa. A rectal exam may be performed to evaluate pelvic masses and colorectal disease and a stool guaiac for occult blood can provide information if the patient has rectal bleeding or changes in bowel habits (Hoffman, 2020).

Chronic Pelvic Pain

The physical examination for a patient with chronic pelvic pain includes a general assessment of affect, mobility, and posture followed by visceral, musculoskeletal, and neurosensory assessments to locate painful areas (Lamvu et al., 2021). A bimanual and speculum exam is performed last to identify any tender areas, masses, lesions, abnormal discharge or bleeding. Because the examination may cause feelings of anxiety and stress, the patient needs to know that the examination can be halted at any time (Hoffman, 2020). Clinician education and training in trauma-informed care and pelvic musculature assessment is highly recommended to reduce patient anxiety, provide the patient with a sense of control, and to identify myofascial trigger points (Lamvu et al., 2021). A few examples of trauma-informed care that apply to chronic pelvic pain include: (a) obtaining consent before performing the exam; (b) having an assistant present during the exam; (c) offering a mirror to visualize the anatomy; (d) screening for trauma and abuse; (e) obtaining the history with the patient dressed; and (f) explaining what will take place during the exam and giving the patient the option for asking questions and choosing what will be done (Jarrell et al., 2018; Lamvu et al., 2021; Raja et al., 2015). Please refer to Chapter 5 and Chapter 9 for additional information.

Observe the patient's gait, posture, and positioning while standing and sitting. Patients with pain coming from the musculoskeletal system may present with a gait disturbance, changes in posture (lordosis with kyphosis), limb length discrepancy, range of motion restrictions, antalgic gait, asymmetry while sitting, and frequent positioning changes (Hoffman, 2020; Lamvu et al., 2018).

Next, palpate the musculature of the abdomen, lower back, and pelvic regions (sacroiliac joints and pubic symphysis) to identify trigger points or larger areas of pain (Lamvu et al., 2018). With the patient in a supine position, inspect the abdomen, noting any scars, auscultating for bowel sounds, percussing, and palpating for organomegaly. Perform the Carnett test by asking the patient to raise their head off the table and straight-raise their legs while palpating the area. If the patient has tenderness during palpation, the source is most likely anterior abdominal wall neuromuscular/myofascial pain (Arnold et al., 2021). Another test that is helpful in eliciting neuromuscular pain in the pelvic region in patients with chronic pelvic pain is the flexion, abduction, and external rotation (FABER) test. The examiner flexes the patient's leg into 45 degrees of flexion and externally rotates and abducts the leg so that it rests on the ankle of the contralateral leg (Arnold et al., 2021). In one study, a positive FABER (pelvic floor muscle tenderness) test was found in 85 percent of patients with chronic neuromuscular pelvic pain (Neville et al., 2012). Other tests that can be used to identify neuromuscular/myofascial pain syndromes are the iliopsoas and obturator tests. Exam findings that are suspicious for myofascial dysfunction include trigger point and widespread areas of tenderness, muscle hypertonicity (inability to relax), and increased pain with movement (flexion, extension, and rotation of lumbar region) (Lamvu et al., 2021).

Pain mapping may also aid in diagnosis and can be accomplished during this part of the physical examination. Pain mapping enables patients who feel that they hurt all over to identify the location of their pain. The mapping is performed by asking the patient to point to or specify the exact location of the pain or painful areas. It is helpful to have the patient use a diagram of the body to identify the locations. Aibel and Moldwin's (2023) Pelvic Pain Map is a valid and reliable tool that can be used to localize pelvic pain and identify pain distribution patterns.

The neurosensory exam includes identifying painful areas by lightly touching the skin on the abdomen, vulva, and perineum using a cotton-tipped applicator (Lamvu et al., 2021). This technique is used to identify allodynia (painful response to nonpainful stimuli), hyperalgesia (an amplified response to painful stimuli), and pain radiation patterns (Hoffman, 2020; Lamvu et al., 2021). The neurosensory exam is suspicious for neuropathy if the patient presents with allodynia or hyperalgesia and describes the pain as burning, pins and needles, or a cutting type of pain (Lamvu et al., 2021).

The pelvic examination should begin with visual inspection, making particular note of areas of dermatologic abnormalities or signs of infection. A one-handed, single-digit vaginal examination of the pelvis using the index finger of the dominant hand is a technique recommended to detect areas of tenderness (Hoffman, 2020; Lamvu et al., 2021). During the pelvic examination, pay particular attention to the patient's reaction when the vagina is palpated to observe for any evidence ofdiscomfort or muscle spasms resulting from pressure along the pelvic floor; this finding may be indicative of myofascial pain syndrome. Tenderness of the urethra or bladder may indicate involvement of the genitourinary system. Pain with deep palpation may indicate endometriosis, whereas cervical motion tenderness is suggestive of PID, adhesions, and other conditions. The speculum examination includes using a small speculum, lubrication and slow insertion as tolerated (Lamvu et al., 2021). The walls of the vagina and cervix should be inspected for abnormal discharge, bleeding, lesions, masses, ulcerations, or any other abnormalities (Hoffman, 2020). In transgender individuals taking testosterone, exam findings may include vaginal pain and bleeding during the exam due to tissue atrophy (Krakowsky et al., 2022), and a pediatric speculum with lubrication should be considered for patient comfort. Samples for wet prep and sexually transmitted infection screening may be obtained if applicable. A rectal examination can be included in the pelvic examination depending on symptoms. Information about pelvic floor anatomy can be found in Chapter 8, and additional guidelines for the pelvic examination are provided in Chapter 9. The International Pelvic Pain Society (IPPS, 2021) also developed a Pelvic Pain Assessment Form for Healthcare Professionals that can be used by clinicians to guide the physical exam. The assessment form can be downloaded from their website: https://www.pelvicpaineducation.com/.

Diagnostic Testing for Acute Pelvic Pain

Laboratory testing for acute pelvic pain includes the following:

- Complete blood count (CBC) with differential
- Type and cross if hemorrhage or surgery is expected
- Fibrinogen and bleeding panel to assess for disseminated intravascular coagulation (DIC) if profound bleeding or hemodynamically unstable
- Liver function tests, chemistries, coagulation studies with D-dimer level, and blood cultures if sepsis is suspected and/or hemodynamically unstable
- Vaginitis and STI screening. Serologic testing for syphilis (if applicable)
- Urinalysis and urine culture (when appropriate)
- Pregnancy testing (if appropriate)
- Vaginal smears or cultures to rule out infection (if applicable)
- Stool guaiac to evaluate gastrointestinal pathology (if applicable)
- Measures of gastrointestinal function (if applicable)

Data from Hoffman, B. L. (2020). Pelvic pain. In B. L. Hoffman, J. O. Schorge, L. M. Halvorson, C. A. Hamid, M. M. Corton, & J. I. Schaffer (Eds.), *Williams gynecology* (4th ed., pp. 253–278). McGraw Hill Education; Lipsky, A., & Hart, D. (2023). Acute pelvic pain in women. In R. Walls (Ed.), *Rosen's emergency medicine: Concepts and clinical practice* (10th ed., pp. 257–262). Elsevier; Rapkin, A. J., Lee, E., & Nathan, L. (2020). Pelvic pain in dysmenorrhea. In J. S. Berek (Ed.), *Berek and Novak's gynecology* (16th ed., pp. 251–278). Wolters Kluwer; Stratton, P., Sharp, H. T., & Eckler, K. (2023). Acute pelvic pain in nonpregnant adult females: Evaluation. *UpToDate*. https://www-uptodate-com.nmu.idm.oclc.org/contents/acute-pelvic-pain-in-nonpregnant-adult-females-evaluation?source=autocomplete&index=0~3&search=acute%20pelvic.

Radiologic testing should be based on findings obtained during the history and physical examination. Most patients who present to emergency departments with acute pelvic pain require imaging studies (Dewey & Wittrock, 2019). Sonography is preferred because it is noninvasive, inexpensive, readily available, quick to perform with little patient preparation and does not expose the patient to ionizing radiation (Basta Nikolic et al., 2021; Dewey & Wittrock, 2019; Franco et al., 2023; Hoffman, 2020). If the condition is suspected to be obstetric or gynecologic, transvaginal and/or transabdominal sonography are preferred as first-line modalities (Karena & Mehta, 2023). Ultrasound may be used to diagnose a variety of gynecologic conditions such as PID (if salpingitis is found), ruptured and/or hemorrhagic ovarian cyst, adnexal torsion, and tubo-ovarian abscess (Lipsky & Hart, 2023). Ultrasound may also be used to examine the appendix, although it is not as reliable as CT in making a diagnosis of appendicitis (Lipsky & Hart, 2023). CT is highly effective, but there are concerns about safety and overuse of this modality. CT is most often used if ultrasound findings are inconclusive, if a gastrointestinal or urinary condition is suspected, or if larger field of view is necessary (Basta Nikolic et al., 2021; Dewey & Wittrock, 2019; Franco et al., 2023; Hoffman, 2020). MRI is often used for young and pregnant patients and may be helpful if ultrasound is not diagnostic due to pelvic anatomy distortion which can occur in situations of patient obesity, large leiomyomas, tumor growth, and other conditions (Hoffman, 2020). Additional studies and surgery may need to be performed depending on the diagnosis. For instance, laparoscopy is used to treat appendicitis, ruptured ectopic pregnancy, adnexal torsion, and ruptured ovarian cyst with hemorrhage (Hoffman, 2020).

Diagnostic Testing for Chronic Pelvic Pain

Laboratory testing for individuals with chronic pelvic pain includes the following:

- Urinalysis and urine culture
- Pregnancy testing (if appropriate)
- Vaginitis and STI screening
- Stool guaiac to evaluate gastrointestinal pathology (if applicable)
- Endometrial biopsy if chronic abnormal bleeding and if aged > 45 years

Data from Hoffman, B. L. (2020). Pelvic pain. In B. L. Hoffman, J. O. Schorge, L. M. Halvorson, C. A. Hamid, M. M. Corton, & J. I. Schaffer (Eds.), *Williams gynecology* (4th ed., pp. 253–278). McGraw-Hill Education; Lamvu, G., Carrillo, J., Ouyang, C., & Rapkin, A. (2021). Chronic pelvic pain in women: A review. *Journal of the American Medical Association*, *325*(23), 2381–2391. https://doi.org/10.1001/jama.2021.2631; Rapkin, A. J., Lee, E., & Nathan, L. (2020). Pelvic pain in dysmenorrhea. In J. S. Berek (Ed.), *Berek and Novak's gynecology* (16th ed., pp. 251–278). Wolters Kluwer.

Diagnostic testing for chronic pelvic pain should be based on findings obtained during the history and physical examination. Transvaginal ultrasound is the most frequently utilized diagnostic test that is employed to evaluate chronic pelvic pain and provides real-time assessment of the pelvis. Sonography of the pelvis assists in identifying a variety of pathologies, including adenomyosis, myomas, and endometriosis (Hoffman, 2020). CT or MRI generally does not offer additional information and is reserved for symptoms that are concerning (Lamvu et al., 2021). Additional imaging studies may be performed if symptoms indicate the need for them. For example, a barium enema, flexible sigmoidoscopy, or colonoscopy may be performed if bowel symptoms are present. Flexible sigmoidoscopy and colonoscopy tests are preferred because they allow for direct inspection and biopsy of the mucosa, whereas barium enema is used to identify malignancy, lesions, diverticular disease, and inflammatory bowel disease (Hoffman, 2020). If pelvic congestion is suspected, transvaginal color Doppler ultrasound is the tool of choice and if urinary symptoms are primarily associated with the pelvic pain, a cystoscopy is performed (Hoffman, 2020). Laparoscopy, once considered the gold standard for evaluation of chronic pelvic pain (CPP) is now ordered when pelvic pathology cannot be detected by physical examination or other forms of testing (Hoffman, 2020; Lamvu et al., 2021). Laparoscopy allows for direct visualization and may enable diagnosis and treatment of intra-abdominal pathology, including endometriosis or pelvic adhesions. However, many patients will continue to have pain after surgery (Arnold et al., 2021; Lamvu et al., 2021; Rapkin et al., 2020).

DIFFERENTIAL DIAGNOSES

Pathology within systems (nongynecologic and gynecologic) needs to be considered when developing a list of differential diagnoses for pelvic pain. The clinician should be mindful that there may be more than one cause of pelvic pain and involvement of more than one body system. Table 29-1 lists differential diagnoses of pelvic pain organized by system.

Acute Pelvic Pain

Gynecologic Causes of Acute Pelvic Pain

Common causes of acute pelvic pain coming from gynecologic sources include threatened or incomplete abortion, ectopic pregnancy with rupture, pelvic inflammatory disease, leaking or ruptured ovarian cyst, adnexal torsion, and endometriosis (Dewey & Wittrock, 2019; Frasca et al., 2023; Lipsky & Hart, 2023; Mouri et al., 2024; Redinger & Nguyen, 2024). A threatened abortion or miscarriage occurs before 20 weeks of gestation and symptoms include vaginal bleeding and crampy suprapubic or low-back pain (Mouri et al., 2024). During the examination, the cervical os is closed and there is no evidence of explusion of pregnancy contents. Common causes of threatened abortion include minor falls or injuries, stress, or genetic abnormalities of the fetus. Patients presenting with threatened abortion receive hemoglobin and hematocrit testing, blood type and Rh status, and β-hCG level, and a transvaginal ultrasound is used to determine the location, viability, and gestational age of the yolk sac/fetus (Mouri et al., 2024). If the abortion is incomplete, the pregnancy contents will be visible through the cervical os during the examination and a pelvic ultrasound and pregnancy test will be used to confirm the diagnosis (Redinger & Nguyen, 2024). A complete abortion includes expulsion of all pregnancy tissue.

Ectopic pregnancy occurs when fetal implantation takes place in a location other than the uterine cavity (Gershenson et al., 2022). Most often, implantation occurs in the fallopian tube leading to dilation of the tube, which increases risks of rupture. If rupture occurs, symptoms may include generalized abdominal and pelvic pain with unstable vitals signs caused by bleeding, which can develop into hemoperitoneum (Frasca et al., 2023). Pelvic ultrasound is used for diagnosis (Lipsky & Hart, 2023). Refer to Chapter 19 for more information.

PID is caused by pelvic infection by *Neisseria gonococcus* or chlamydia, which are gram-negative and gram-positive bacteria (Dewey & Wittrock, 2019; Gershenson et al., 2022). Symptoms include acute pelvic pain, fever, adnexal/cervical motion tenderness, and nausea/vomiting with leukocytosis and elevated sedimentation rate; a marker of inflammation (Frasca et al., 2023). Tubo-ovarian abscess is a complication of PID that can be life-threatening if the abscess ruptures (Dewey & Wittrock, 2019; Dewey et al., 2019).

Ovarian cysts include functional (physiologic) and hemorrhagic types of cysts. Functional cysts (an ovarian follicle or corpus luteum) are produced and rupture each month during ovulation as part of the normal menstrual cycle. The pain is referred to as *mittelschmerz*, is self-limiting and mild to moderate in nature (Thomas & Porter, 2023). Hemorrhagic cysts can become pathological when the follicle does not release an ovum and continues to grow or if the corpus luteum fails to involute and grows (Rapkin et al., 2020). If the hemorrhagic cyst ruptures, significant blood loss (hemoperitoneum) may occur and prompt surgery is required for management (Dewey & Wittrock, 2019). Uncomplicated ruptured cysts can be managed with hospitalization, observation, and repeated imaging (Rapkin et al., 2020).

Adnexal torsion is defined as torsion (twisting) of the ovarian structures or fallopian tube (Hoffman et al., 2020). The pain is usually severe and continuous unless the torsion is intermittent, in which case the pain will wax and wane (Rapkin et al., 2020). The patient may have a palpable mass and direct and/or rebound tenderness with palpation on the affected side during the physical exam (Thomas & Porter, 2023). If tissue ischemia is prolonged, necrosis may develop and the patient will present with fever, tachycardia, and leukocytosis (Lipsky & Hart, 2023). Diagnosis is based on history, physical exam findings, and transvaginal ultrasound with color doppler (Frasca et al., 2023). Surgical diagnosis via laparoscopy or laparotomy is the best diagnostic indicator and is used for treatment (Lipsky & Hart, 2023).

Endometriosis occurs when endometrial tissue implants located outside the uterine cavity proliferate with each menstrual cycle, leading to inflammation, scarring, and adhesion formation, which increases the risk of developing chronic pelvic pain (Hoffman, 2020). Pelvic pain from endometriosis can be acute or chronic in nature. The most common symptoms of endometriosis include dysmenorrhea, dyspareunia, irregular bleeding, and infertility (Rapkin et al., 2020). Physical exam findings include tenderness in one or both lower abdominal quadrants, with uterosacral ligament tenderness or nodules (Frasca et al., 2023). Laparoscopy or laparotomy are used to confirm the diagnosis if ultrasound results are inconclusive (Frasca et al., 2023; Hoffman, 2020).

Table 29-2 lists common differential diagnoses related to acute pelvic pain of gynecologic origin, and **Table 29-3** lists common differential diagnoses of acute pelvic pain that are not related to a gynecologic problem.

Common Nongynecologic Causes of Acute Pelvic Pain

Although acute pelvic pain is most often caused from reproductive, urinary, or gastrointestinal conditions, other disorders from the musculoskeletal, vascular, psychologic, and neurologic systems may also cause or contribute to symptomatology (Frasca et al., 2023; Dewey & Wittrock, 2019; Dewey et al., 2019). The most common nongynecologic causes of acute pelvic pain are addressed here because they should be considered when the clinician is developing a list of differential diagnoses (refer to Table 29-2). An in-depth discussion is beyond the scope of this text; instead, the reader is referred to the appropriate references at the end of this chapter.

The most common nongynecologic causes of acute pelvic pain coming from the gastrointestinal and urinary tracts include appendicitis, acute diverticulitis, bowel obstruction, urinary tract stones, and cystitis/pyelonephritis (Dewey & Wittrock, 2019; Frasca et al., 2023; Lipsky & Hart, 2023; Rapkin et al., 2020). According to Dewey and Wittrock (2019), appendicitis is the most common gastrointestinal cause of acute pelvic pain that requires

TABLE 29-2 Acute Pelvic Pain of Gynecologic Origin: Common Differential Diagnoses and Signs, Symptoms, and Location of Pain

Condition	Symptoms and Signs	Diagnostics and Treatment
Abortion: Threatened or incomplete	Crampy suprapubic or low-back pain Vaginal bleeding present with or without clots—may be postcoital	Pregnancy test usually positive If infection: Elevated WBC and ESR Analgesics and counseling are provided for threatened abortion Incomplete abortion requires analgesia and manual or medical evacuation to remove pregnancy tissue
Ectopic pregnancy with rupture	Unilateral lower abdominal pain that is localized Pain with vomiting, rebound tenderness, or guarding are signs of rupture Amenorrhea, blood may be present in the vaginal vault or bleeding may be present Shoulder pain if hemoperitoneum PE may reveal tender pelvic or adnexal mass	May have very slight elevation of temperature ESR and WBC may be slightly elevated Serum β-hCG is positive (1 week after conception) Transvaginal ultrasound is used to diagnose Fluid resuscitation if necessary with surgical management
Pelvic inflammatory disease (PID)	Lower abdominal, uterine, adnexal, and cervical motion tenderness with purulent discharge Pain is often described as dull or achy and may radiate to back or upper thighs May have nausea and vomiting due to pain and low-grade fever	Laboratory confirmation of gonorrhea or chlamydia Elevated WBC and ESR Mild to moderate PID is treated with parenteral cephalosporin, oral doxycycline, and oral metronidazole Severe PID is treated with hospitalization and IV antibiotic therapy Sexual contacts are treated Tubo-ovarian abscess is a complication of PID that can be life-threatening if the abscess ruptures

(continues)

TABLE 29-2 Acute Pelvic Pain of Gynecologic Origin: Common Differential Diagnoses and Signs, Symptoms, and Location of Pain (*continued*)

Condition	Symptoms and Signs	Diagnostics and Treatment
Leaking or ruptured ovarian cyst	Functional cysts (follicle or corpus luteum) rupture with ovulation (mid-cycle). The pain is referred to as *mittelschmerz* and is self-limiting and mild to moderate in nature Hemorrhagic cysts occur when the follicle does not release an ovum and continues to grow and/or the corpus luteum fails to involute and grows. Rupture of a corpus luteum cysts can result in significant blood loss, hypovolemia, and hemoperitoneum. Most critical symptom is significant abdominal tenderness, often associated with rebound tenderness due to peritoneal irritation May be able to palpate a mass during the pelvic examination	Diagnosed via transvaginal ultrasound and blood tests Fluid resuscitation if needed with surgical management via laparoscopy or laparotomy
Adnexal torsion	Occurs from torsion (twisting) of ovarian structures or fallopian tube Results in ischemia with progressively severe pelvic pain Pain is usually severe and constant unless torsion is intermittent, in which case the pain will come and go Mild fever, tachycardia, and leukocytosis Mass and direct and rebound tenderness to palpation on affected side (lower quadrant) during PE	Challenging to diagnose with no definitive criteria for imaging—surgical diagnosis via laparoscopy or laparotomy is best Treated via surgery
Endometriosis	Endometrial tissue implants are located outside the uterine cavity and implants proliferate with each menstrual cycle, leading to inflammation, scarring, and adhesion formation Most common symptoms are dysmenorrhea, dyspareunia, irregular bleeding, and infertility PE findings: tenderness in lower abdominal quadrants, one or both, fixed uterus	Laparoscopy with biopsy is the gold standard for diagnosis Treatments vary depending upon whether fertility is desired or not. Combined oral contraceptives or other hormonal therapies, gonadotropin releasing hormone antagonists, and surgery are options, with symptomatic care measures NSAIDs Hysterectomy if conservative measures are not effective and fertility is not desired

Data from Gershenson, D. M., Lentz, G. M., Valeu, F. A., & Lobo, R. A. (2022). *Comprehensive gynecology* (8th ed.). Elsevier; Hoffman, B. L. (2020). Pelvic pain. In B. L. Hoffman, J. O. Schorge, L. M. Halvorson, C. A. Hamid, M. M. Corton, & J. I. Schaffer (Eds.), *Williams gynecology* (4th ed., pp. 253–278). McGraw Hill Education; Lipsky, A, & Hart, D. (2023). Acute pelvic pain in women. In R. Walls (Ed.), *Rosen's emergency medicine: Concepts and clinical practice* (10th ed., pp. 257–262). Elsevier; Rapkin, A. J., Lee, E., & Nathan, L. (2020). Pelvic pain in dysmenorrhea. In J. S. Berek (Ed.). *Berek and Novak's gynecology* (16th ed., pp. 251–278). Wolters Kluwer; Thomas, D. J., & Porter, B. O. (2023). Common reproductive system complaints. In L. M. Dunphy, J. E. Winland-Brown, Porter, B. O., & D. J. Thomas (Eds.), *Primary care: The art and science of advanced practice nursing: An interprofessional approach* (6th ed., pp. 749–759). F. A. Davis Company.

Abbreviations: ESR, erythrocyte sedimentation rate; hCG, human chorionic gonadotropin; PE, physical examination; WBC, white blood cell.

Note: For additional information on the following topics, please refer to the indicated chapters: abortion, Chapter 20; ectopic pregnancy, Chapters 33 and 34; pelvic inflammatory disease, Chapter 25; ovarian cysts, Chapter 28; adnexal torsion, Chapters 26 and 28; endometriosis, Chapters 25 and 28.

surgery. Symptoms are similar to those of pelvic inflammatory disease and include diffuse abdominal pain that localizes to the right lower quadrant (McBurney point) and nausea, anorexia, and vomiting (Thomas & Porter, 2023). During the examination, patients may have severe abdominal muscle guarding, rigidity, and rebound tenderness with positive iliopsoas, Rovsing's, and obturator signs (Frasca et al., 2023). If ultrasound results are inconclusive, CT with oral and IV contrast can be used for diagnosis as this test is highly sensitive and specific for appendicitis (Frasca et al., 2023).

Acute diverticulitis occurs when diverticula in the colon become inflamed and/or infected. Symptoms include severe crampy left lower quadrant pain, fever, abdominal bloating, constipation, and/or diarrhea (Rapkin et al., 2020). If the diverticulum forms an abscess, it may perforate and result in peritonitis with unstable vital signs, leukocytosis, abdominal

TABLE 29-3 Acute Pelvic Pain of Nongynecologic Origin: Common Differential Diagnoses, Signs, Symptoms, and Location of Pain

Condition (System)	Symptoms	Signs	Comment
Appendicitis (GI)	Initially diffuse epigastric and/or midabdominal pain, localizes to right lower quadrant Anorexia, nausea, vomiting	May have low-grade fever and chills High fever if ruptured Rebound tenderness/guarding over McBurney's point Iliopsoas sign[a] /obturator sign[b] Rovsing's sign[c] May observe leukocyte shift to left	May be confused with gastroenteritis, pelvic inflammatory disease, urinary tract infection, or ruptured ovarian cyst
Diverticulitis (GI)	Abdominal bloating, constipation, and/or diarrhea Severe LLQ pain	Distended abdomen with LLQ tenderness with palpation Localized rebound tenderness May palpate mass in LLQ Hypoactive bowel sounds May notice elevated WBC	Mimics IBS Fistulas can occur *Note:* Diverticulitis can present with perforations or abscesses that produce peritonitis
Bowel obstruction (GI)	Colicky abdominal pain Abdominal distention Vomiting Constipation	Bowel sounds are abnormal; at onset they are high pitched during pain and later will decrease and may be absent due to ischemia Elevated WBC and fever are noted as the condition progresses	
Urinary tract stone (renal and ureteral lithiasis) (GU)	Severe, colicky pain in suprapubic area and in pelvis Urinary frequency Dysuria Nausea, vomiting	Hematuria Flank and costovertebral angle pain—may extend to the groin and/or abdomen Fever and chills may be present	Can mimic ectopic pregnancy
Cystitis (GU)	Lower abdominal or pelvic pain usually midline Dysuria, urinary urgency and frequency	Urine dipstick positive for leukocyte esterase or nitrite Urine microscopy positive for bacteria and WBCs	

Data from Gershenson, D. M., Lentz, G. M., Valeu, F. A., & Lobo, R. A. (2022). *Comprehensive gynecology* (8th ed.). Elsevier; Hoffman, B. L. (2020). Pelvic pain. In B. L. Hoffman, J. O. Schorge, L. M. Halvorson, C. A. Hamid, M. M. Corton, & J. I. Schaffer (Eds.), *Williams gynecology* (4th ed., pp. 253–278). McGraw Hill Education; Lipsky, A., & Hart, D. (2023). Acute pelvic pain in women. In R. Walls (Ed.), *Rosen's emergency medicine: Concepts and clinical practice* (10th ed., pp. 257–262). Elsevier; Rapkin, A. J., Lee, E., & Nathan, L. (2020). Pelvic pain in dysmenorrhea. In J. S. Berek (Ed.). *Berek and Novak's gynecology* (16th ed., pp. 251–278). Wolters Kluwer; Thomas, D. J., & Porter, B. O. (2023). Common reproductive system complaints. In L. M. Dunphy, J. E. Winland-Brown, Porter, B. O., & D. J. Thomas (Eds.), *Primary care: The art and science of advanced practice nursing: An interprofessional approach* (6th ed., pp. 749–759). F. A. Davis Company.

Abbreviations: GI, gastrointestinal; GU, genitourinary; IBS, irritable bowel syndrome; LLQ, left lower quadrant; MU, musculoskeletal; RLQ, right lower quadrant; WBCs, white blood cells.

[a]Iliopsoas sign: Passively lift the patient's thigh against the examiner's hand above the knee. A positive sign is pain in the RLQ.

[b]Obturator sign: The patient passively flexes the right hip and knee and internally rotates the right leg at the hip. A positive sign is when the pain travels from the periumbilical region to the RLQ.

[c]Rovsing's sign: Pressing the LLQ produces pain in the RLQ when pressure is released.

Note: For additional information on cystitis, please refer to Chapter 23.

guarding, and left lower quadrant rebound tenderness. Partial or complete bowel obstruction is another cause of acute pelvic pain coming from the gastrointestinal tract. Symptoms include colicky abdominal pain followed by distension, vomiting, and anorexia with abnormal bowel sounds; at onset of symptoms bowel sounds may be high pitched and later become hypoactive and eventually may be absent due to ischemia (Rapkin et al., 2020). Patients will develop leukocytosis and fever as the condition progresses. Imaging to diagnose bowel obstruction includes an upright abdominal x-ray series and CT scan (Rapkin et al., 2020).

Urinary tract causes of acute pelvic pain include urinary tract stones (renal and ureteral lithiasis), and cystitis. Urinary tract infections are bacterial in nature and are most often caused by *Escherichia coli, Proteus, Klebsiella,* and *Pseudomonas* (Rapkin et al., 2020). Cystitis pain is usually dull, occurs in the suprapubic region, and is associated with urinary frequency, urgency, dysuria, and hematuria, whereas pyelonephritis is associated with flank and costovertebral area tenderness (Lipsky & Hart, 2023). Urinary tract infections are diagnosed through urinalysis and microscopy which, if positive for infection, reveals bacteria, red blood cells, leukocytes with or without leukocyte esterase and nitrites; a urine culture is also obtained to confirm the diagnosis (Rapkin et al., 2020). Urinary stone symptoms occur as a result of different processes; (1) stones in the kidney or ureter may temporarily block the flow of urine, leading to an increase in backflow pressure and (2) movement of the stone through the ureter can cause tissue damage, subsequently leading to inflammation. Symptoms can be severe and include colicky pain that exends from the costovertebral angle (CVA) to the groin and/or abdomen (Lipsky & Hart, 2023). A combination of urinalysis, CT, ultrasound, and/or intravenous pyelography are used to diagnose the condition (Rapkin et al., 2020). Fever and chills may occur with pyelonephritis (Lipsky & Hart, 2023).

Chronic Pelvic Pain

Gynecologic Causes of Chronic Pelvic Pain

The most common gynecologic findings identified by laparoscopy in patients with chronic pelvic pain are endometriosis and adhesions (Hoffman, 2020; Howard, 1993; Rapkin et al., 2020). Endometriosis typically causes a cyclical type of pelvic pain that occurs prior to and throughout menses (Rapkin et al., 2020). Pelvic adhesions are coarse bands of tissue that connect organs to other organs or to the abdominal wall in places where there should be no connection. Adhesions may result from previous surgery, intra-abdominal infection, radiation, chemical irritation, foreign body reaction, or endometriosis (Hoffman, 2020; Rapkin et al., 2020). Although adhesions and endometriosis are considered to be contributors to chronic pelvic pain, the relationship between pain and pathology remains inconsistent (Hoffman, 2020; Rapkin et al., 2020). For example, up to 43 percent of patients with endometriosis are asymptomatic, regardless of stage, and not all patients with adhesions experience pain (Rapkin et al., 2020). In those who experience pain caused by adhesions, symptoms most often occur with sudden movement, intercourse, or other intentional activities that stretch the peritoneum or affected area (Hoffman, 2020). Please refer to Chapters 24 and 27 for more information about endometriosis.

Surgical lysis is often used to treat adhesions. However, surgery may lead to further development of adhesions and increase the risk of bowel injury (Arnold et al., 2021; Hoffman, 2020; Rapkin et al., 2020). Findings from two randomized controlled trials that compared women who had undergone adhesiolysis with a control group who did not undergo surgery found no significant differences in pain levels at 1 year (Hoffman, 2020; Peters et al., 1992; Swank et al., 2003). Therefore, surgical lysis of adhesions is not recommended for routine management of chronic pelvic pain (ACOG, 2020). Other gynecologic causes of chronic pelvic pain include ovarian remnant, ovarian retention syndrome, pelvic congestion syndrome, pelvic relaxation causing prolapse of gynecologic organs (e.g., pelvic organ prolapse), subacute salpingo-oophoritis, and cancers of gynecologic origin. **Table 29-4** summarizes diagnosis and treatment recommendations related to chronic pelvic pain. Please refer to Chapters 8, 27, and 28 for more information about pelvic organ prolapse, subacute salpingo-oophoritis, and cancers of gynecologic origin, respectively.

Ovarian remnant syndrome and ovarian retention syndrome are two separate but similar etiologies that may cause or contribute to chronic pelvic pain. They produce almost the same symptoms and are diagnosed and managed similarly. Ovarian remnant syndrome occurs when some of the ovarian tissue is left behind after an oophorectomy, whereas ovarian retention syndrome occurs when an ovary is purposely left behind after gynecologic surgery (Hoffman, 2020; Rapkin et al., 2020).

Pelvic congestion syndrome is typically seen in parous women of reproductive age and it usually resolves with menopause (Hoffman, 2020; Rapkin et al., 2020). The pathophysiology involved is not fully understood but the syndrome is believed to result from compression of the left renal vein where the superior mesenteric artery originates (Rapkin et al., 2020).

Common Nongynecologic Causes of Chronic Pelvic Pain

In a number of instances, the cause of chronic pelvic pain is not primarily gynecologic in origin. More often, the condition is multifactorial in nature with at least one out of five patients diagnosed with irritable bowel syndrome (IBS), interstitial cystitis (painful bladder syndrome), pelvic floor muscle tenderness, and/or depression (Arnold et al., 2021). The more common nongynecologic causes are addressed here because they should be considered when the clinician is developing a list of differential diagnoses for chronic pelvic pain (refer to Table 29-4). An in-depth discussion is beyond the scope of this text; instead, the reader is referred to the appropriate references at the end of this chapter.

Irritable bowel syndrome (IBS) is the most common functional gastrointestinal disorder, and accounts for as many as 60 percent of referrals to gynecologists for complaints of chronic pelvic pain; patients who have had a hysterectomy for chronic pelvic pain are twice as likely to have IBS (Rapkin et al., 2020). In addition to IBS, other causes of bowel dysfunction must be ruled out, such as Crohn's disease, diverticulitis, celiac disease, lactose allergy, and chronic appendicitis. IBS is characterized by recurrent abdominal pain and altered bowel habits. Clinical features include shifting abdominal pain accompanied by constipation or diarrhea, or both. Bloating, nausea, and vomiting are also common symptoms. The pain may be identified in one quadrant of the abdomen but then relocate during the next attack. Typically, but not in all cases, defecation provides relief from the pain. Although the exact etiology of IBS is unknown, its cause is believed to involve "brain-gut" dysregulation which leads to disruptions in gastrointestinal motility, permeability, and sensitivity (Hoffman, 2020).

Myofascial pain originating from trigger points in skeletal muscle and neuropathic pain are now recognized as potential causes and/or contributing factors leading to chronic pelvic pain (ACOG, 2020; Arnold et al., 2021; Fuentes-Marquez et al., 2019; Hoffman, 2020; Lamvu et al., 2021; Rapkin et al., 2020). In a case-controlled study, women with chronic pelvic pain were found to have a significantly higher percentage of trigger points that reproduced symptoms, compared to women who did not have chronic pelvic pain. The chronic pelvic pain group also exhibited widespread pressure pain hyperalgesia with significantly lower pressure pain thresholds (Fuentes-Marquez et al., 2019). Specific muscle groups that tend to be affected include those of the anterior abdominal wall (rectus abdominis, oblique, and trans-versus abdominis) and pelvis (levator ani, coccygeus, obturator internus, and deep transverse perineal and piriformis). Levator ani syndrome results from trigger points leading to pain within the levator ani muscles, and symptoms from muscle spasms in this area include lower abdominal pain, chronic constipation, low back pain, and dyspareunia (Hoffman, 2020). Testing for Carnett's sign assists in making a diagnosis of abdominal wall pain and identifying trigger points (Arnold et al., 2021).

Interstitial cystitis (IC), which is also referred to as bladder pain disorder (BPD) and endometriosis are two conditions found

TABLE 29-4 Gynecologic Causes of Chronic Pelvic Pain: Signs, Symptoms, Diagnosis, and Management

Condition	Symptoms	Signs	Diagnosis	Management
Adhesions	Lower abdominal or pelvic pain that occurs or increases when the peritoneum or organ serosa is stretched Dyspareunia Pain may be aggravated by sudden movement	May elicit abdominal pain with light palpation Decreased motility of pelvic organs	Laparoscopy is the diagnostic tool of choice	Surgical lysis is not recommended for routine management. Only in rare cases after a thorough evaluation and failed medical therapy
Endometriosis	Endometrial tissue implants are located outside the uterine cavity and implants proliferate with each menstrual cycle, leading to inflammation, scarring, and adhesion formation Most common symptoms are dysmenorrhea, dyspareunia, irregular bleeding, and infertility	PE findings: tenderness in lower abdominal quadrants, one or both, fixed uterus	Laparoscopy with biopsy is the gold standard for diagnosis	Treatments vary depending upon whether fertility is desired or not. Combined oral contraceptives or other hormonal therapies, gonadotropin releasing hormone antagonists, and surgery are options, with symptomatic care measures NSAIDs. Hysterectomy if conservative measures are not effective and fertility is not desired
Ovarian remnant syndrome; ovarian retention syndrome	Symptoms begin 2 to 5 years after surgery. May have pelvic pain with ovulation or luteal phase. Pain as described may be associated with GI or GU symptoms	Tender pelvic mass identified during bimanual examination	Ultrasound is the primary test. Magnetic resonance imaging can be performed	Hormonal therapy is used to suppress tissue but cannot be used long term Surgical excision via laparotomy is most often required
Pelvic congestion syndrome	Pain begins with ovulation and continues until the end of menses More common in premenopausal, parous women. Resolves with menopause	Lower abdominal and back pain that increases after standing, dysmenorrhea, abnormal uterine bleeding, irritable bowel symptoms May be tender with direct palpation of the ovaries and surrounding areas Uterus is bulky when palpated, with enlarged ovaries	Transuterine venography or MRI are the primary methods used for diagnosis Laparoscopy is not a preferred method for diagnosing	Begin with the least invasive measures Hormonal suppression measures include progestin or GnRH agonist Ovarian vein embolization or ligation Hysterectomy with bilateral salpingo-oophorectomy after child-bearing should be the last resort

Data from Gershenson, D. M., Lentz, G. M., Valeu, F. A., & Lobo, R. A. (2022). *Comprehensive gynecology* (8th ed.). Elsevier; Hoffman, B. L. (2020). Pelvic pain. In B. L. Hoffman, J. O. Schorge, L. M. Halvorson, C. A. Hamid, M. M. Corton, & J. I. Schaffer (Eds.), *Williams gynecology* (4th ed., pp. 253–278). McGraw Hill Education; Lipsky, A., & Hart, D. (2023). Acute pelvic pain in women. In R. Walls (Ed.), *Rosen's emergency medicine: Concepts and clinical practice* (10th ed., pp. 257–262). Elsevier; Rapkin, A. J., Lee, E., & Nathan, L. (2020). Pelvic pain in dysmenorrhea. In J. S. Berek (Ed.). *Berek and Novak's gynecology* (16th ed., pp. 251–278). Wolters Kluwer; Thomas, D. J., & Porter, B. O. (2023). Common reproductive system complaints. In L. M. Dunphy, J. E. Winland-Brown, B. O. Porter, & D. J. Thomas (Eds.), *Primary care: The art and science of advanced practice nursing: An interprofessional approach* (6th ed.). F. A. Davis Company.

in 60 to 70 percent of patients with chronic pelvic pain (Arnold et al., 2021). Most individuals diagnosed with IC/BPD are assigned female at birth and are between 40 and 60 years of age (Rapkin et al., 2020). The condition is considered to be a clinical syndrome, consisting of a complex of symptoms (suprapubic, pelvic, urethral, vaginal, vulvar, or perineal pain with disabling urinary frequency, urgency, and nocturia) with occasional dysuria and hematuria (Rapkin et al., 2020). Symptom relief often occurs partially by emptying the bladder. Pain that is reproduced when palpating the anterior vaginal wall over the border of the bladder and suprapubic area is suggestive of the disorder (Rapkin et al., 2020). Urinalysis is typically normal. Diagnosis is made primarily through exclusion; a careful history is taken and physical exam and labs are used to document symptoms consistent with IC/BPD and exclude other conditions (American Urological Association [AUA], 2022). Cystoscopy and urodynamic studies are only considered when the diagnosis is in doubt or for unusual conditions (AUA, 2022). Because IC/BPD is common in patients with chronic pelvic pain, ACOG (2020) recommends screening patients for this condition with additional testing and referral for patients who screen positive. See Chapter 23 for more information.

Mood disorders and other psychological conditions are common in individuals who suffer from chronic pain with depression being frequently reported (Arnold et al., 2021; Hoffman, 2020; Lamvu et al., 2021; Rapkin et al., 2020; Till et al., 2019). Patients with chronic pelvic pain are also more likely to have experienced adverse experiences and abuse in childhood. In a case-control study of women with and without chronic pelvic pain, researchers found that those with chronic pelvic pain reported significantly higher levels of childhood abuse (physical, sexual, verbal, or emotional) compared with those who were in the control group (Krantz et al., 2019). Recommendations for treating psychosocial conditions in patients with chronic pelvic pain include screening for mood disorders (anxiety, depression) with referral if the screening is positive and pelvic floor physical therapy, sex therapy, and cognitive behavior therapy (ACOG, 2020). These therapies can be prescribed alone but are thought to work best in combination. When assessing the patient for psychosocial causes of pain, it is important to establish a nonjudgmental and supportive approach because historically, patients who presented with pelvic pain were often told it was all in their head, and no further assessment took place.

MANAGEMENT

Acute Pelvic Pain

Patients with suspected life-threatening gynecologic conditions such as appendicitis, adnexal torsion, and hemorrhagic ovarian cyst are hospitalized, stabilized, and antibiotics are given prior to undergoing surgery (Lipsky & Hart, 2023; Dewey et al., 2019). Emergent conditions in pregnant patients such as ruptured ectopic pregnancy, incomplete abortion with heavy bleeding, placental abruption or uterine rupture also require immediate surgical intervention (Lipsky & Hart, 2023; Dewey et al., 2019). Treatment for septic shock due to abdominal or urinary conditions such as complete bowel obstruction, urinary stones, diverticulitis with abscess, obstruction, fistula, or perforation, and pyelonephritis includes admission to the intensive care unit with referral to medical and surgical services as needed (Rapkin et al., 2020). Analgesia should be administered promptly for patients in significant pain to improve comfort and the reliability of the history and physical examination (Lipsky & Hart, 2023). Intravenous opioids (morphine, hydromorphone) can be given to patients with severe pain; the onset of action is rapid and these drugs are considered to be safe in pregnancy (Lipsky & Hart, 2023).

In patients without emergent or critical gynecologic diagnoses, a treatment plan is established with close follow-up and referral if necessary. Management for threatened abortion includes analgesia, close monitoring with serial β-hCG levels, Rho(D) immune globulin (RhoGAM; if the patient's blood is Rh negative), and a follow-up pelvic ultrasound (Mouri et al., 2024). Those who are at 20 weeks gestation (or at a stage of fetal viability per institutional guidelines) should receive referral to obstetric services for fetal monitoring prior to discharge (Lipsky & Hart, 2023). Treatment for incomplete abortion includes analgelsia and removal of pregnancy tissue via manual or medical evacuation (Redinger & Nguyen, 2024). Management for complete abortion includes observation and follow-up pelvic ultrasound to confirm that all pregnancy contents have been evacuated (Rapkin et al., 2020; Redinger & Nguyen, 2024). Ectopic pregnancies that have not ruptured are treated medically using methotrexate or surgically via laparoscopy (Rapkin et al., 2020). Patients presenting with leaking or ruptured uncomplicated ovarian cysts who are hemodynamically stable are hospitalized and observed with repeated pelvic ultrasounds (Rapkin et al., 2020). Management of mild to moderate cases of pelvic inflammatory disease includes treatment with antibiotics; those with severe infection will require hospitalization with fluids and IV antibiotics (Frasca et al., 2023; Thomas & Porter, 2023). Sexual partners are contacted for treatment. Treatment for endometriosis is covered under chronic pelvic pain nonpharmacologic and pharmacologic treatment. For additional information about treatment options for common, emergent, and non-emergent gynecological causes of acute pelvic pain, refer to Table 29-2.

Treatment of common, non-emergent, nongynecologic causes of pelvic pain such as partial bowel obstruction and acute diverticulitis without abscess, obstruction, fistula, or perforation includes hospitalization, IV fluids, and bowel rest, with oral fluid restriction and broad-spectrum IV antibiotics for those with diverticulitis and nasogastric suctioning for those with partial bowel obstruction (Rapkin et al., 2020). Urinary tract causes of acute pelvic pain such as cystitis and uncomplicated pyelonephritis are treated on an outpatient basis with oral hydration, analgesics, and antibiotics with follow-up urine culture sensitivities (Lipsky & Hart, 2023; Thomas & Porter, 2023). Management for urinary stones in patients who are acutely ill and/or present with obstruction of the urinary system includes hospitalization with IV fluids, analgesia, antibiotics, and surgery for stone removal, which may include lithotripsy or open surgery (Rapkin et al., 2020). Nonpregnant patients who are not acutely ill with small stones are treated on an outpatient basis with hydration, analgesia, antiemetics, and in some cases, medical therapy (Rapkin et al., 2020). For additional information about treatment options for common, emergent, and non-emergent non-gynecological causes of acute pelvic pain (APP), refer to Table 29-3.

Chronic Pelvic Pain

Nonpharmacologic Treatment

Chronic pelvic pain is a complex condition that can be debilitating and difficult to manage. Pain may come from more than one source; therefore, treatment should be multifaceted with an interdisciplinary team that may include primary care, gynecology, pain management, gastroenterology, urology, mental health, and physical therapy (ACOG, 2020; Arnold et al., 2021; Carey et al., 2017; Lamvu et al., 2021). It is very important for the patient to understand that a distinct diagnosis does not ensure that treatment will be curative; indeed, recurrence of symptoms is common. Instead, clinicians should provide education about the potential for pain generators arising from multiple systems (musculoskeletal, gynecologic, urologic, gastrointestinal) and the role of the central nervous system in pain sensitization, and encourage the patient to participate in shared decision making regarding appropriate treatment strategies, and develop long-term goals and expectations. This will ensure the best possible outcomes for the patient with chronic pelvic pain. Enlisting the patient's input in developing the treatment plan, and encouraging them to take an active role is critical to the success of the management plan. Treatment needs to be multidisciplinary and comprehensive, and may include a combination of pharmacologic, nonpharmacologic, and complementary approaches. The treatment plan is most often dictated by diagnoses and the goal is to manage pain and optimize function.

In reference to adolescents, clinicians should aggressively manage chronic pelvic pain to avoid long-term negative impacts on physical and emotional health, fertility, sexual function, and quality of life (Smorgick & As-Sanie, 2018). Because of their stages of emotional and physical development, adolescents pose challenges to clinicians that are different from those associated with patients in their 20s and beyond. Developing a rapport with any teenager may be the biggest challenge facing clinicians who work with members of this age group. Suggestions for developing rapport include maintaining eye contact, demonstrating a nonjudgmental attitude, treating the teen with respect, and providing undivided attention. It is important to validate symptoms and the feelings that are associated with them. It is also important to be familiar with state and local statutes regarding health care for minors. Many states have parental consent laws, with differing levels of exceptions for sexual and reproductive health care. Each practice needs to have its own policy that must follow the legal parameters already in place.

With respect to evaluation and treatment of chronic pelvic pain, evidence-based guides and/or algorithms can be used to help guide the management plan. An evaluation and treatment algorithm that was developed by Lamvu et al. (2022) is available at: https://www.pelvicpaineducation.com/healthcare-professionals.

Pelvic floor physical therapy, cognitive behavioral therapy, and sex therapy may be ordered alone or combination. These therapies are recommended as needed to manage myofascial and psychologic pain, in addition to dyspareunia (ACOG, 2020; Arnold et al., 2021; Lamvu et al., 2021). Physical therapy activities can be used to maintain tissue and joint flexibility; improve posture, body mechanics, strength, and coordination; reduce neuropathic pain, dyspareunia, and myofascial pain; and restore function (Rapkin et al., 2020). In patients who have myofascial pain symptoms, physical therapy with a focus on the pelvic floor muscles is considered to be a first-line therapy (ACOG, 2020; Grinberg et al., 2019; Lamvu et al., 2021; Wallace et al., 2019). Pelvic floor therapy involves a variety of modalities, including muscle training and strengthening exercises, acupressure/acupuncture, biofeedback, manual therapy, trigger point or myofascial release, and mobilization techniques (Carey et al., 2017; Hoffman, 2020). Results from a longitudinal, pilot randomized controlled trial, conducted by Grinberg et al. (2019) found that myofascial physical therapy with a focus on the pelvic floor was an effective treatment. Participants in the study experienced significant improvements in pain intensity, sensitivity to experimental pain tests, and anatomical, psychological, and social therapeutic effects (Grinberg et al., 2019).

Cognitive behavioral therapy (CBT) is an effective tool that can be used to develop pain coping strategies and can be implemented as a component of psychotherapy (ACOG, 2020). In addition to CBT, psychotherapy includes biofeedback, counseling, group therapy, and mindfulness strategies which can be used to promote a self-care management plan aimed to improve sleep quality, mood, interpersonal relationships, and coping mechanisms, and reduce environmental stressors (Hoffman et al., 2020; Lamvu et al., 2020). Sex therapy is also recommended for patients with female orgasmic disorder and myofascial pelvic pain (ACOG, 2020; Arnold et al., 2021). In a study of over 300 persons with chronic abdomino-pelvic pain, a pain management and sex therapy–derived model, referred to as ReConnect, was implemented to help patients return to sexual activity and manage relationships while living with chronic pain (Edwards et al., 2020). Findings from the study showed significant reductions in anxiety around sex and in pain interference during sexual activity. The researchers recommended using the ReConnect model to promote sexual activity goals in patients with chronic pain (Edwards et al., 2020).

Other nonpharmacologic treatments include trigger point injections, neuromodulation, acupuncture, and yoga. Trigger point injections of saline, local anesthetics, steroids, or opioids is recommended by ACOG (2020) to improve myofascial pelvic pain and improve functional ability. In a study of 68 individuals with myofascial pelvic pain who were refractory to conventional treatment, visual analog pain scores were compared before and after trigger point injection therapy for pelvic floor myofascial spasm (Fouad et al., 2017). The researchers found that 65 percent of women in the study experienced a significant reduction in pain scores. It remains unclear whether trigger point injections using botulinum toxin are effective; therefore, use of this therapy is reserved for people with myofascial pelvic pain that does not improve with physical therapy (Arnold et al., 2021).

Neuromodulation is an emerging therapy which includes delivering electrical stimulation to a sensory nerve (Hoffman, 2020; Xiang et al., 2022). The therapy is believed to alter nerve activity which leads to reduced nociceptive processing of pain (Hoffman, 2020). Delivery modalities include transcutaneous electric nerve stimulation (TENS), percutaneous tibial nerve stimulation (PTNS), intravaginal electric stimulation (IVES), or sacral neuromodulation. TENS includes using electrodes on the skin which deliver a low-voltage electric current and IVES uses an intravaginal probe which stimulates muscle contractions via electrical impulses (Hoffman, 2020). Several of these modalities are approved by the Food and Drug Administration (FDA) for a variety of urinary conditions, fecal incontinence, and pelvic floor rehabilitation (Hoffman, 2020). Results from a narrative review by Xiang et al. (2022) found that neuromodulation was effective in treating chronic pelvic pain with few adverse effects, although there was a noted lack of high-quality randomized controlled trials and long-term follow-up. Research evaluating the effectiveness of neuromodulation in treating chronic pelvic pain remains ongoing. Anesthetic nerve blocks targeting the pudendal, genitofemoral, and ilioinguinal nerves are also used to treat neuropathic pain with variable long-term success rates (Carey et al., 2017).

Acupuncture and yoga are currently recommended by ACOG (2000) as a treatment for managing chronic pelvic pain of musculoskeletal etiology. In a meta-analysis that included 17 randomized controlled trials and 1,400 patients (867 females and 588 males) that examined the analgesic effectiveness of acupuncture in treating chronic pelvic pain, Lin et al. (2023) found that after the intervention, total pain scores were significantly lower in the chronic pelvic pain group in comparison to the control group. The researchers concluded that acupuncture may be included as a pain management tool for chronic pelvic pain; even as a monotherapy (Lin et al., 2023). With respect to yoga, in a follow-up randomized case-control study, women with chronic pelvic pain who practiced yoga for 8 weeks demonstrated significantly lower pain intensity scores and quality of life scores that were significantly higher in comparison to a control group of women with chronic pelvic pain who received NSAIDS (Saxena et al., 2017).

Pharmacologic Treatment

There is a lack of high-quality evidence available to clinicians for prescribing medications for patients with chronic pelvic pain. Unfortunately, most clinical recommendations are based on Level B and C evidence and are the same as recommendations used to treat other chronic pain syndromes (Arnold et al., 2021; Lamvu et a., 2020). Current recommendations for pharmacologic treatment include condition-specific drugs, some of which include analgesics, hormone therapy, GI therapies, bladder instillations, antidepressants, anticonvulsants, and mood stabilizers (ACOG, 2020; Arnold et al., 2021; Hoffman, 2020; Lamvu et al., 2020; Rapkin et al., 2020). Oral analgesics include acetaminophen (Tylenol) or NSAIDs. NSAIDs are helpful is there is an inflammatory component to the pain; acetaminophen does not have anti-inflammatory properties but may be helpful in providing analgesia in patients who have allergies or an intolerance to NSAIDs (Hoffman, 2020). Opioids are not recommended for treatment of chronic pelvic pain and patients who are currently taking opioids should be slowly weaned (ACOG, 2020). Opioid prescribing increases risks for developing adverse effects, tolerance, risk of overdose, and dependency while avoiding addressing the underlying cause(s) of the condition (Arnold et al., 2021).

Hormonal therapy is recommended for patients with cyclic pelvic pain caused by gynecologic conditions (endometriosis, dysmenorrhea) and for nongynecologic conditions that are exacerbated with menstrual cycle fluctuations (Hoffman, 2020; Lamvu et al., 2021). Combined hormonal contraceptives (pills, vaginal ring, transdermal patch) are useful in providing relief from primary dysmenorrhea and endometriosis (Hoffman, 2020). Continuous use of oral contraceptives was found in a meta-analysis to be more effective in controlling dysmenorrhea than cyclic use (Damm et al., 2019). Other hormonal options include progestin-only contraceptives (progesterone pills, levonorgestrel-releasing intrauterine system, progestin-releasing implanted rods, intramuscular depomedroxyprogesterone and gonadotropin-releasing hormone (GnRH) agonists and antagonists (Hoffman, 2020).

If pelvic pain is neuropathic in origin, pharmacotherapy selective serotonergic reuptake inhibitors and tricyclic antidepressants may be helpful in improving mood, sleep quality, and neuropathic pain symptoms (ACOG, 2020; Lamvu et al., 2021). These agents are also useful in treating the depression that often accompanies chronic pain. Amitriptyline (Elavil) and nortriptyline (Pamelor) have well-documented efficacy in the treatment of neuropathic pain (Hoffman, 2020). SSRIs are not recommended unless they are used to treat an underlying anxiety or depression (Hoffman, 2020). Although there is inconsistent data on their effectiveness in treating chronic pain in patients with pelvic pain, anticonvulsants, gabapentin (Neurontin), and pregabalin (Lyrica) may be considered for treating neuropathic pain (ACOG, 2020). One randomized controlled trial that included 306 women with chronic pelvic pain found no evidence of significant improvements in pain relief after treatment with gabapentin (Horne et al., 2020). In addition, similar findings were discovered in a separate randomized controlled trial that examined 89 patients with vulvodynia (Brown et al., 2018). In contrast, in another randomized controlled trial, gabapentin was more effective than placebo in improving sexual function, although sexual function remained lower than the control group that included women who were pain-free (Bachman et al., 2019). If an infection has been confirmed as the source of chronic pelvic pain, antibiotics should be prescribed. The type and length of antibiotic treatment often depend on culture and sensitivity results from the infectious sources.

Surgical Treatment

Surgical interventions may be necessary in some people with chronic pelvic pain depending on their diagnosis. When endometriosis is present and is unresponsive to hormonal agents, excision of the endometrial tissue using laparoscopy may be performed (Rapkin et al., 2020). Routine use of surgical lysis to treat adhesions is not recommended by the ACOG (2020) or by the Agency for Healthcare Research and Quality (2010). Adhesiolysis is associated with poor outcomes in patients with chronic pelvic pain, including bowel injury and increased pain (Arnold et al., 2021). Other surgical procedures that involve nerve ablation or removal (uterosacral nerve ablation and presacral neurectomy) are no longer recommended. Presacral neurectomy is performed laparoscopically and includes removal of the presacral plexus, a group of nerves that sends pain signals from the uterus to the brain. The procedure requires a highly skilled surgeon because there are risks for injury to major blood vessels and the right ureter. Long-term side effects include constipation and urinary retention (Hoffman, 2020). One other type of nerve transection procedure, laparoscopic uterosacral nerve ablation, involves destruction of uterine nerves that pass through the uterosacral ligament.

Hysterectomy should be considered only in specific situations and after other treatment methods have failed. If the individual is of reproductive age, every attempt should be made to treat pain with nonsurgical methods before considering hysterectomy. Although 19 percent of hysterectomies are performed for treatment of pelvic pain, 30 percent of women seen in primary care clinics have already undergone a hysterectomy without relief of pelvic pain symptoms, and 5 percent may experience worsening pain (Rapkin et al., 2020). One exception to this is when hysterectomy is considered as part of gender-affirming care for transgender and gender diverse individuals. An interprofessional approach to pelvic pain treatment with a team that includes a gynecologist, physical therapist, and psychologist has been shown to reduce the frequency of hysterectomies and other surgical interventions as management for pelvic pain symptoms (Rapkin et al., 2020).

Complementary and Alternative Medicine

Complementary and alternative medicine (CAM) is quite popular and is widely accepted. It is important for the clinician to be knowledgeable about available CAM therapies and be ready to have a discussion with the patient to gain an understanding about the types of therapies they might favor. Complementary and alternative medicine may be an important component of the multifaceted approach needed to resolve symptomatology. Some examples of CAM treatments for pelvic pain include massage, meditation, guided imagery, cannabinoids, osteopathic manipulative treatment, movement-based therapy (tai-chi, yoga, qigong), herbal supplements, and dietary modifications (Hoffman, 2020; Srinivasan et al., 2020). In an observational study, Chao et al. (2015) found that more than half (51%) of women with chronic pelvic pain in the sample used acupuncture, herbs, and/or nutritional supplements regularly, and minimal side effects were reported.

In a Cochrane review, moderate evidence supported using Capsicum frutescens (cayenne) for low back pain (Srinivasan et al., 2020). Other herbs that demonstrated some effectiveness in treating low pain were *Harpagophytum procumbens* (devil's claw), *Salix alba* (white willow bark), *Symphytum officinale* L. (comfrey), *Solidago chilensis* (Brazilian arnica), and lavender essential oil (Srinivasan et al., 2020). Dietary modifications that are regarded as potentially beneficial for chronic pain are anti-inflammatory, gluten-free, Paleo, antioxidants, and low fermentable oligosaccharides, disaccharides, monosaccharides, and polyols (low FODMAP) (Hoffman, 2020).

The use of cannabinoids in treating chronic pain is controversial (Srinivasan et al., 2020). Results from a Cochrane review that studied double-blind randomized controlled trials, found that the benefits of cannabis as a medicine might have outweighed risks associated with use in patients with chronic neuropathic pain (Mücke et al., 2018). More long-term research on the topic is needed (Srinivasan et al., 2020). With regard to massage, pain causes muscular contraction; therefore, techniques that relax muscles may help reduce some types of chronic pelvic pain. Although these alternatives to allopathic procedures may hold promise in the future, there are no current evidence-based recommendations for their use in treating chronic pelvic pain. Prospective, randomized controlled studies examining the effectiveness of these therapies are needed (Srinivasan et al., 2020).

WHEN TO REFER

Acute Pelvic Pain

Patients presenting with potentially life-threatening conditions are stabilized and referred to an appropriate medical facility for surgical and medical treatment with follow-up after hospitalization (Lipsky & Hart, 2023; Rapkin et al., 2020). In patients without emergent conditions, close follow-up after treatment should be established to confirm resolution of symptoms. In most situations, if the diagnosis is accurate, timely, and treatment is appropriate, acute pelvic pain symptoms will resolve (Dewey et al., 2019). In these cases, no further evaluation or treatment is necessary.

Patients who continue to experience pain or develop new symptoms may require additional testing and treatment (Dewey et al., 2019). In some situations, the condition may be complex and referral to a specialist is recommended. It is important for clinicians to be aware that some patients presenting with acute pelvic pain from gynecologic and nongynecologic causes may eventually go on to develop chronic pelvic pain (Dewey & Wittrock, 2019; Hoffman, 2020). These patients will likely require referral using a multidisciplinary approach.

Chronic Pelvic Pain

In many cases, chronic pelvic pain involves clinical overlap of gynecologic, gastrointestinal, urologic, musculoskeletal, and psychological disorders; thus, it is important to utilize a multidisciplinary approach. Consequently, it is imperative that the clinician perform a comprehensive history and physical examination to determine a precise differential diagnosis and effective treatment. An effective treatment plan most often includes referral to an appropriate specialist in a gynecologic or nongynecologic arena.

In addition to using referral as part of establishing an initial treatment plan, clinicians may need to seek consultation with members of the interdisciplinary team and/or pain specialists if there is no improvement in symptoms or if treatment goals are not being met within a mutually agreed-upon time frame. A follow-up visit should take place 4 to 8 weeks after establishing a treatment plan. If there is satisfactory improvement and treatment goals are being met, follow-up can move to every 6 to 12 months. If the treatment plan is unsatisfactory and consultation with the team is required, follow-up visits should continue every 4 to 8 weeks until there is improvement (Lamvu et al., 2021).

CURRENT AND EMERGENT EVIDENCE FOR PRACTICE

There are a number of pharmacologic, nonpharmacologic, and complementary and alternative medicine therapies that are currently being tested or used as treatments for pelvic pain. Research on many of these therapies has been provided in this chapter:

- Herbal supplements
- Trigger point injections of pelvic floor and other areas
- Pelvic floor injection with botulinum toxin A
- Massage
- Cannabinoids
- Meditation and guided imagery
- Neuromodulation/nerve stimulation therapies
- Acupuncture/acupressure
- Myofascial release and pelvic floor muscle exercises
- Yoga
- Nutritional supplementation, including high-level antioxidants
- Movement-based therapy (tai-chi, yoga, qigong)
- Alpha-2-Macroglobulin (A2M)

CONSIDERATIONS FOR SPECIFIC POPULATIONS

Cultural Influences and Racial, Sex, and Gender Bias

Knowing and appreciating the cultural background of a patient is a significant component of providing culturally competent health care. Cultural and social stratification influences decision making for both patient and clinician, as well as the treatment options that are offered and accepted. Should the clinician be shaking hands, making eye contact, or addressing the patient directly? If their partner is present, does the couple's culture dictate that the clinician includes them in the conversation as well? How close should the clinician stand or sit when taking a history? These are all culturally significant questions to consider. In addition, individuals of different cultures may express pain differently (Sharma et al., 2020). Validating a patient's feelings and recognizing and appreciating their cultural and ethnic background are important not only in gaining trust and establishing rapport, but also in understanding the scope of the presented problem.

Culture can also affect an individual's beliefs about pain, symptom reporting, and coping strategies. Sharma et al. (2020) conducted a systematic review to evaluate the extent to which pain-related beliefs, appraisals, coping, and catastrophizing differed between countries, language groups, and country economy and found that in over half of the 10 studies that were included, mean scores for all of the variables differed significantly between people from different countries. These findings emphasize that the clinician must have a clear understanding about the impact of culture on pain-related beliefs, appraisals, catastrophizing, and coping strategies. Ultimately, communication between the patient and clinician is essential to accurately diagnose and create an appropriate patient-centered treatment plan.

In addition to cultural influences, it is important for clinicians to be aware of racial and sex/gender biases that center around pain. Disparities in the assessment and treatment of pain and pain burden within minoritized racial and ethnic groups has been documented (Meints et al., 2019). With respect to sex/gender bias, pain-related gender norms include stereotypical expectations about how men and women react to pain that are shared across cultures (Bernardes et al., 2024). Stereotypical expectations for men's behavior includes high levels of stoicism, pain tolerance, and avoiding talking about pain and for women, being more sensitive and willing to report pain and sometimes exaggerating or feigning the pain (Samulowitz et al., 2018). The International Association for the Study of Pain (Bernardes et al., 2024) provides a fact sheet that includes guidelines and recommendations that practitioners can use to raise awareness and reduce sex/gender biases in practice. The fact sheet is available in **Appendix 29-A.**

Pain is an intimate experience that only the person experiencing it can truly comprehend. Because pain is a subjective phenomenon, it should be reliably assessed from the patient's perspective. For this reason, it is very important for the clinician to carefully interview patients who present with pelvic pain to assess the impact that the pain may be having on their quality of life and ability to complete activities of daily living. Part of effective treatment may include working with the patient to identify how some of the activities can be accomplished.

References

Agency for Healthcare Research and Quality. (2010, October). *Effective health care program. Comparative effectiveness of treatments for noncyclic chronic pelvic pain in women.* Retrieved July 9, 2024, from https://effectivehealthcare.ahrq.gov/products/pelvic-pain/research-protocol

Ahangari, A. (2014). Prevalence of chronic pelvic pain among women: An updated review. *Pain Physician, 17,* E141–E147.

Aibel, K., & Moldwin, R. (2023). Validation of the 'pelvic pain map': a new self-assessment tool for chronic pelvic pain localisation. *British Journal of Urology International, 131*(6), 763–769. https://doi.org/10.1111/bju.15979

American College of Obstetricians and Gynecologists. (2020, March). Chronic pelvic pain. ACOG practice bulletin summary, number 218. *Obstetrics & Gynecology, 135*(3), 744–746. https://doi.org/10.1097/AOG.0000000000003717

American Urological Association. (2022). *Diagnosis and treatment of interstitial cystitis/bladder pain syndrome.* Retrieved July 25, 2024, from https://www.auanet.org/guidelines-and-quality/guidelines

Armstrong, S. A., & Herr, M. J. (2023, May). Physiology, nociception. *StatPearls.* Retrieved July 23, 2024 from https://pubmed.ncbi.nlm.nih.gov/31855389/

Arnold, M. J., Osgood, A. T., & Aust, A. (2021). Chronic pelvic pain in women: ACOG updates recommendations. *American Family Physician, 103*(3), 186–188.

Bachmann, G. A., Brown, C. S., Phillips, N. A., Rawlinson, L. A., Yu, X., Wood, R., Foster, D. C., & Gabapentin Study Group (2019). Effect of gabapentin on sexual function in vulvodynia: A randomized, placebo-controlled trial. *American Journal of Obstetrics and Gynecology, 220*(1), Article 89. https://doi.org/10.1016/j.ajog.2018.10.021

Ball, E., & Khan, K. S. (2020). Recent advances in understanding and managing chronic pelvic pain in women with special consideration to endometriosis. *F1000Research, 9*(83), 1–8. https://doi.org/10.12688/f1000research.20750.1

Basta Nikolic, M., Spasic, A., Hadnadjev Simonji, D., Stojanović, S., Nikolic, O., & Nikolic, D. (2021). Imaging of acute pelvic pain. *The British Journal of Radiology, 94*(1127), 1–13. https://doi.org/10.1259/bjr.20210281

Bernardes, S. F., Samulowitz, A., Karos, K., & Mogil, J. (2024, April). *Fact sheet: Sex/gender biases in pain research and clinical practice.* International Association for the Study of Pain. Retrieved on September 29, 2024, from https://www.iasp-pain.org/resources/fact-sheets/sex-gender-biases-in-pain-research-and-clinical-practice/

Brichant, G., Denef, M., Tebache, L., Poismans, G., Pinzauti, S., Dechenne, V., & Nisolle, M. (2018). Chronic pelvic pain and role of exploratory laparoscopy as a diagnostic and therapeutic tool: A retrospective observational study. *Gynecological Surgery, 15,* Article 13. https://doi.org/10.1186/s10397-018-1045-5

Brown, C. S., Bachmann, G. A., Wan, J., Foster, D. C., & Gabapentin (GABA) Study Group (2018). Gabapentin for the treatment of vulvodynia: A randomized controlled trial. *Obstetrics and Gynecology, 131*(6), 1000–1007. https://doi.org/10.1097/AOG.0000000000002617

Brown, K., Teach, S. J., & Wiley, J. F. (2024). Evaluation of acute pelvic pain in female children and adolescents. *UpToDate.* Retrieved July 9, 2024, from https://www-uptodate-com.nmu.idm.oclc.org/contents/evaluation-of-acute-pelvic-pain-in-female-children-andadolescents?search=pelvic%20pain%20in%20adolescents&source=search_result&selectedTitle=1%7E150&usage_type=default&display_rank=1

Cairns C., & Kang, K. (2023). *National hospital ambulatory medical care survey: 2021 emergency department summary tables.* Available from: https://ftp.cdc.gov/pub/Health_Statistics/NCHS/Dataset_Documentation/NHAMCS/doc21-ed-508.pdf

Carey, E. T., Till, S. R., & As-Sanie, S. (2017). Pharmacological management of chronic pelvic pain in women. *Drugs, 77*(3), 285–301. https://doi.org/10.1007/s40265-016-0687-8

Casanova, R., Goepfert, A. R., Hueppchen, N., Weiss, P. M., & Connolly, A. (2024). Beckmann and Ling's *Obstetrics and gynecology* (9th ed.). Wolters Kluwer.

Chao, M. T., Abercrombie, P. D., Nakagawa, S., Gregorich, S. E., Learman, L. A., & Kupperman, M. (2015). Prevalence and use of complementary health approaches among women with chronic pelvic pain in a prospective cohort study. *Pain Medicine, 16,* 328–340.

Chronic Pelvic Pain: ACOG Practice Bulletin, Number 218. (2020). *Obstetrics and gynecology, 135*(3), e98–e109. https://doi.org/10.1097/AOG.0000000000003716

Damm, T., Lamvu, G., Carrillo, J., Ouyang, C., & Feranec, J. (2019). Continuous versus cyclic combined hormonal contraceptives for treatment of dysmenorrhea: A systematic review. *Contraception: X, 1,* 1–7. https://doi.org/10.1016/j.conx.2019.100002

Dewey, K., & Wittrock, C. (2019). Acute pelvic pain. *Emergency Medicine Clinics of North America, 37*(2), 207–218.

Edwards, S., Mandeville, A., Petersen, K., Cambitzi, J., Williams, A. C. C., & Herron, K. (2020). 'ReConnect': a model for working with persistent pain patients on improving sexual relationships. *British Journal of Pain, 14*(2), 82–91. https://doi.org/10.1177/2049463719854972

Eid, S., Loukas, M., & Tubbs, S. (2019). Clinical anatomy of pelvic pain women: A gynecological perspective. *Clinical Anatomy, 32*(1), 151–155. https://doi.org/10.1002/ca.23270

Fauconnier, A., Provot, J., Le Creff, I., Boulkedid, R., Vendittelli, F., Doret-Dion, M., Sroussi, J., Giraudet, G., Jacobs, R., Bourret, A., Bauville, E., Carvalho, S., Tourette, C., Koskas, M., Akladios, C., Nisolle, M., Lejeune, C., Huchon, C., Alberti, C., Dumont, A., & Bouvier-Colle, M. H. (2020). A framework proposal for quality and safety measurement in gynecologic emergency care. *Obstetrics and Gynecology, 136*(5), 912–921. https://doi.org/10.1097/AOG.0000000000004132

Ferrando, C. A., Chapman, G., & Pollard, R. (2021). Preoperative pain symptoms and the incidence of endometriosis in transgender men undergoing hysterectomy for gender affirmation. *Journal of Minimally Invasive Gynecology, 28*(9), 1579–1584. https://doi.org/10.1016/j.jmig.2021.01.018

Fouad, L. S., Pettit, P. D., Threadcraft, M., Wells, A., Micallef, A., & Chen, A. H. (2017). Trigger point injections for pelvic floor myofascial spasms refractive to primary therapy. *Journal of Endometriosis and Pelvic Pain Disorders, 9*(2), 125–130. https://doi.org/10.5301/jeppd.500

Franco, P. N., García-Baizán, A., Aymerich, M., Maino, C., Frade-Santos, S., Ippolito, D., & Otero-García, M. (2023). Gynaecological causes of acute pelvic pain: Common and not-so-common imaging findings. *Life, 13*(10), 1–19. https://doi.org/10.3390/life13102025

Frasca, D. J., Jarrio, C. E., & Perdue, J. (2023). Evaluation of acute pelvic pain in women. *American Family Physician, 108*(2), 175–180.

Fuentes-Marquez, P., Valenza, M. C., Cabrera-Martos, I., Rios-Sanchez, A., & Ocon-Hernandez, O. (2019). Trigger points, pressure pain hyperalgesia, and mechano-sensitivity of neural tissue in women with chronic pelvic pain. *Pain Medicine, 20*, 5–13. https://doi.org/10.1093/pm/pnx206

Gershenson, D. M., Lentz, G. M., Valeu, F. A., & Lobo, R. A. (2022). *Comprehensive gynecology* (8th ed.). Elsevier.

Grimstad, F. W., Boskey, E., & Grey, M. (2020). New-onset abdominopelvic pain after initiation of testosterone therapy among trans-masculine persons: A community-based exploratory survey. *LGBT Health, 7*(5), 248–253. https://doi.org/10.1089/lgbt.2019.0258

Grimstad, F. W., Boskey, E. R., Clark, R. S., & Ferrando, C. A. (2023). Prevalence of pelvic pain in transgender individuals on testosterone. *The Journal of Sexual Medicine, 20*(12), 1459–1465. https://doi.org/10.1093/jsxmed/qdad135

Grimstad, F. W., Fowler, K. G., New, E. P., Ferrando, C. A., Pollard, R. R., Chapman, G., Gomez-Lobo, V., & Gray, M. (2019). Uterine pathology in transmasculine persons on testosterone: A retrospective multicenter case series. *American Journal of Obstetrics and Gynecology, 220*(3), 257.e1–257.e7. https://doi.org/10.1016/j.ajog.2018.12.021

Grinberg, K., Weissman-Fogel, I., Lowenstein, L., Abramov, L., & Granot, M. (2019). How does myofascial physical therapy attenuate pain in chronic pelvic pain syndrome? *Pain Research & Management, (2019)*, 1–11. https://doi.org/10.1155/2019/6091257

Hassam, T., Kelso, E., Chowdary, P., Yisma, E., Mol, B. W., & Han, A. (2020). Sexual assault as a risk factor for gynaecological morbidity: An exploratory systematic review and meta-analysis. *European Journal of Obstetrics, Gynecology, and Reproductive Biology, 255*, 222–230. https://doi.org/10.1016/j.ejogrb.2020.10.038

Hoffman, B. L. (2020). Pelvic pain. In B. L. Hoffman, J. O. Schorge, L. M. Halvorson, C. A. Hamid, M. M. Corton, & J. I. Schaffer (Eds.), *Williams gynecology* (4th ed., pp. 253–278). McGraw Hill Education.

Horne, A. W., Vincent, K., Hewitt, C. A., Middleton, L. J., Koscielniak, M., Szubert, W., Doust, A. M., & Daniels, J. P. (2020). Gabapentin for chronic pelvic pain in women (GaPP2): A multicenter randomized, double-blind, placebo-controlled trial. *Lancet, 396*(10255), 909–917. https://doi.org/10.1016/S0140-6736(20)31693-7

Howard, F. M. (1993). The role of laparoscopy in chronic pelvic pain: Promise and pitfalls. *Obstetrical and Gynecological Survey, 48*(6), 357–387.

International Association for the Study of Pain. (2021). *IASP terminology*. Retrieved July 26, 2024 from, https://www.iasp-pain.org/resources/terminology/

International Pelvic Pain Society. (2021, April). *Initial patient survey*. Retrieved July 24, 2024, from https://www.pelvicpaineducation.com/resources

International Pelvic Pain Society. (2021, June). *Follow-up patient survey*. Retrieved July 24, 2024, from https://www.pelvicpaineducation.com/resources

International Pelvic Pain Society. (2021, August). *Healthcare professional—Pelvic pain INITIAL assessment form*. Retrieved July 24, 2024, from https://www.pelvicpaineducation.com/healthcare-professionals

International Pelvic Pain Society. (2023). *Chronic pelvic pain*. Informational handout. Retrieved July 24, 2024, from https://www.pelvicpain.org/public/resources/educational-resources/informational-handouts

Jarrell, J. F., Vilos, G. A., Allaire, C., Burgess, S., Fortin, C., Gerwin, R., Lapensee, L., Lea, R. H., Leyland, N. A., Martyn, P., Shenassa, H., & Taenzer, P. (2018). No. 164-consensus guidelines for the management of chronic pelvic pain. *Journal of Obstetrics and Gynaecology Canada, 40*(11), e747–e787. https://doi.org/10.1016/j.jogc.2018.08.015

Karena, Z. V., & Mehta, A. D. (2023, August). Sonography female pelvic pathology assessment, protocols, and interpretation. In *StatPearls*. Retrieved July 23, 2024, from https://www.ncbi.nlm.nih.gov/books/NBK585034/

Krakowsky, Y., Potter, E., Hallarn, J., Monari, B., Wilcox, H., Bauer, G., Ravel, J., & Prodger, J. L. (2022). The effect of gender-affirming medical care on the vaginal and neovaginal microbiomes of transgender and gender-diverse people. *Frontiers in Cellular and Infection Microbiology, 11*, Article 769950. https://doi.org/10.3389/fcimb.2021.769950

Krantz, T. E., Andrews, N., Petersen, T. R., Dunivan, G. C., Montoya, M., Swanson, N., Wenzl, C. K., Zambrano, J. R., & Komesu, Y. M. (2019). Adverse childhood experiences among gynecology patients with chronic pelvic pain. *Obstetrics and Gynecology, 134*(5), 1087–1095. https://doi.org/10.1097/AOG.0000000000003533

Lampe, A., Sölder, E., Ennemoser, A., Schubert, C., Rumpold, G., & Söllner, W. (2000). Chronic pelvic pain and previous sexual abuse. *Obstetrics and Gynecology, 96*(6), 929–933. https://doi.org/10.1016/s0029-7844(00)01072-3

Lamvu, G., Carrillo, J., Witzeman, K., & Alappattu, M. (2018, March). Musculoskeletal considerations in female patients with chronic pelvic pain. *In Seminars in Reproductive Medicine, 36*(2), 107–115. Thieme Medical Publishers.

Lamvu, G., Antunez-Flores, O., Orady, M.E., & Schneider, B. (2020). Path to diagnosis and women's perspectives on the impact of endometriosis pain. *Journal of Endometriosis and Pelvic Pain Disorders, 12*, 16–25. https://doi.org/10.1177/2284026520903214

Lamvu, G., Carrillo, J., Ouyang, C., & Rapkin, A. (2021). Chronic pelvic pain in women: A review. *Journal of the American Medical Association, 325*(23), 2381–2391. https://doi.org/10.1001/jama.2021.2631

Latthe P, Latthe, M., Say, L., Gülmezoglu, M., & Khan K. S. (2006). WHO systematic review of prevalence of chronic pelvic pain: A neglected reproductive health morbidity. *BMC Public Health, 6*, 177. https://doi.org/10.1186/1471-2458-6-177

Lin, K. Y., Chang, Y. C., Lu, W. C., Kotha, P., Chen, Y. H., & Tu, C. H. (2023). Analgesic efficacy of acupuncture on chronic pelvic pain: A systemic review and meta-analysis study. *Healthcare, 11*(6), 1–16. https://doi.org/10.3390/healthcare11060830

Lipsky, A., & Hart, D. (2023). Acute pelvic pain. In R. Walls (Ed.), *Rosen's emergency medicine: Concepts and clinical practice* (10th ed., pp. 257–262). Elsevier.

Mathias, S. D., Kuppermann, M., Libermann, R. F., Lipschutz, R. C., & Steege, J. F. (1996). Chronic pelvic pain: Prevalence, health-related quality of life, and economic correlates. *Obstetrics & Gynecology, 87*(3), 321–327.

Meints, S. M., Cortes, A., Morais, C. A., Edwards, R. R. (2019). Racial and ethnic differences in the experience and treatment of noncancer pain. *Pain Management, 9*(3), 317–334. https://doi.org/10.2217/pmt-2018-0030

Mouri, M., Hall, H., & Rupp, T. J. (2024). Threatened miscarriage. In *StatPearls*. Retrieved September 29, 2024, from https://www.statpearls.com/point-of-care/30087

Mücke, M., Phillips, T., Radbruch, L., Petzke, F., & Häuser, W. (2018). Cannabis-based medicines for chronic neuropathic pain in adults. *Cochrane Database of Systematic Reviews*. https://doi.org/10.1002/14651858.CD012182.pub2

Neville, C. E., Fitzgerald, C. M., Mallinson, T., Badillo, S., Hynes, C., & Tu, F. (2012). A preliminary report of musculoskeletal dysfunction in female chronic pelvic pain: A blinded study of examination findings. *Journal of Bodywork and Movement Therapies, 16*(1), 50–56. https://doi.org/10.1016/j.jbmt.2011.06.002

Peters, A. A., Trimbos-Kemper, G. C., Admiraal, C., Trimbos, J. B., & Hermans, J. (1992). A randomized clinical trial on the benefit of adhesiolysis in patients with intraperitoneal adhesions and chronic pelvic pain. *British Journal of Obstetrics and Gynaecology, 99*(1), 59–62. https://doi.org/10.1111/j.1471-0528.1992.tb14394.x

Poli-Neto, O. B., Tawasha, K. A. S., Romão, A. P. M. S., Hisano, M. K., Moriyama, A., Candido-Dos-Reis, F. J., Rosa-E-Silva, J. C., & Nogueira, A. A. (2018). History of childhood maltreatment and symptoms of anxiety and depression in women with chronic pelvic pain. *Journal of Psychosomatic Obstetrics and Gynaecology, 39*(2), 83–89. https://doi.org/10.1080/0167482X.2017.1306515

Quaghebeur, J., Petros, P., Wyndaele, J. J., & De Wachter, S. (2021). Pelvic-floor function, dysfunction, and treatment. *European Journal of Obstetrics, Gynecology, and Reproductive Biology, 265*, 143–149. https://doi.org/10.1016/j.ejogrb.2021.08.026

Raja, S., Hasnain, M., Hoersch, M., Gove-Yin, S., & Rajagopalan, C. (2015). Trauma informed care in medicine: Current knowledge and future research directions. *Family & Community Health, 38*(3), 216–226. https://doi.org/10.1097/FCH.0000000000000071

Rapkin, A. J., Lee, E., & Nathan, L. (2020). Pelvic pain in dysmenorrhea. In J. S. Berek (Ed.), *Berek and Novak's gynecology* (16th ed., pp. 251–278). Wolters Kluwer.

Redinger, A., & Nguyen, H. (2024). Incomplete miscarriage. In *StatPearls*. Retrieved September 29, 2024, from https://www.statpearls.com/point-of-care/17039

Russell, C. B., Foxx, A., Liu, Y., & As-Sanie, S. (2023). Pelvic pain in the transgender-nonbinary population. *American Journal of Obstetrics and Gynecology, 228*(3), S857. https://doi.org./10.1016/j.ajog.2022.12.102

Ryan, A., Healey, M., Cheng, C., Dior, U., & Reddington, C. (2022). Central sensitisation in pelvic pain: A cohort study. *The Australian & New Zealand Journal of Obstetrics & Gynaecology, 62*(6), 868–874. https://doi.org/10.1111/ajo.13596

Samulowitz, A., Gremyr, I., Eriksson, E., & Hensing, G. (2018). "Brave men" and "emotional women": A theory-guided literature review on gender bias in health care and gendered norms towards patients with chronic pain. *Pain Research and Management, 2018*, Article 6358624. https://doi.org/10.1155/2018/6358624

Saxena, R., Gupta, M., Shankar, N., Jain, S., & Saxena, A. (2017). Effects of yogic intervention on pain scores and quality of life in females with chronic pelvic pain. *International Journal of Yoga, 10*(1), 9–15. https://doi.org/10.4103/0973-6131.186155

Sharma, S., Ferreira-Valente, A., de C Williams, A. C., Abbott, J. H., Pais-Ribeiro, J., & Jensen, M. P. (2020). Group differences between countries and between languages in pain-related beliefs, coping, and catastrophizing in chronic pain: A systematic review. *Pain Medicine, 21*(9), 1847–1862. https://doi.org/10.1093/pm/pnz373

Shetty, M. (2023). Acute pelvic pain: Role of imaging in the diagnosis and management. *Seminars in Ultrasound, CT, and MR, 44*(6), 491–500. https://doi.org/10.1053/j.sult.2023.10.004

Shim, J. Y., Laufer, M. R., & Grimstad, F. W. (2020). Dysmenorrhea and endometriosis in transgender adolescents. *Journal of Pediatric and Adolescent Gynecology, 33*(5), 524–528. https://doi.org/10.1016/j.jpag.2020.06.001

Siqueira-Campos, V. M. E., Da Luz, R. A., de Deus, J. M., Martinez, E. Z., & Conde, D. M. (2019). Anxiety and depression in women with and without chronic pelvic pain: Prevalence and associated factors. *Journal of Pain Research, 12*, 1223–1233. https://doi.org/10.2147/JPR.S195317

Smorgick, N., & As-Sanie, S. (2018). Pelvic pain in adolescents. *Seminars in Reproductive Medicine, 36*(2), 116–122. https://doi.org/10.1055/s-0038-1676088

Srinivasan, M., Torres, J. E., McGeary, D., & Nagpal, A. S. (2020). Complementary and alternative (CAM) treatment options for women with pelvic pain. *Current Physical Medicine and Rehabilitation Reports, 8*(3), 240–248. https://doi.org/10.1007/s40141-020-00264-6

Swank, D. J., Swank-Bordewijk, S. C., Hop, W. C., van Erp, W. F., Janssen, I. M., Bonjer, H. J., & Jeekel, J. (2003). Laparoscopic adhesiolysis in patients with chronic abdominal pain: A blinded randomised controlled multi-centre trial. *Lancet, 361*(9365), 1247–1251. https://doi.org/10.1016/s0140-6736(03)12979-0

Tabaac, A. R., Chwa, C., Sutter, M. E., Missmer, S. A., Boskey, E. R., Austin, S. B., Grimstad, F., & Charlton, B. M. (2022). Prevalence of chronic pelvic pain by sexual orientation in a large cohort of young women in the United States. *The Journal of Sexual Medicine, 19*(6), 1012–1023. https://doi.org/10.1016/j.jsxm.2022.03.606

Thomas, D. J., & Porter, B. O. (2023). Common reproductive system complaints. In L. M. Dunphy, J. E. Winland-Brown, B. O. Porter, & D. J. Thomas (Eds.), *Primary care: The art and science of advanced practice nursing: An interprofessional approach* (6th ed., pp. 749–759). F. A. Davis Company.

Till, S. R., As-Sanie, S., & Schrepf, A. (2019). Psychology of chronic pelvic pain: Prevalence, neurobiological vulnerabilities, and treatment. *Clinical Obstetrics and Gynecology, 62*(1), 22–36. https://doi.org/10.1097/GRF.0000000000000412

Tordoff, D. M., Lunn, M. R., Flentje, A., Atashroo, D., Chen, B., Dastur, Z., Lubensky, M. E., Capriotti, M., & Obedin-Maliver, J. (2024). Chronic pelvic pain among transgender men and gender diverse adults assigned female at birth. *Andrology*, 10.1111/andr.13703. Advance online publication. https://doi.org/10.1111/andr.13703

Veasley, C., Clare, D., Clauw, D. J., Cowley, T., Nguyen, R. H. N., Reinecke, P., Vernon, S. D., & Williams, D. A. (2015). Impact of chronic overlapping pain conditions on public health and the urgent need for safe and effective treatment: 2015 analysis and policy recommendations. *Chronic Pain Research Alliance*. Retrieved from https://www.chronicpainresearch.org/public/CPRA_WhitePaper_2015-FINAL-Digital.pdf

Wall, C. L., Carson, J., Brown, G., & Bailey, R. (2024): "It's a right pain in the pelvis!": Post-traumatic stress and post-traumatic growth in a sample of females experiencing chronic pelvic pain. *Women's Reproductive Health, 11*(3), 1–12. https://doi.org/10.1080/23293691.2024.2323737

Wallace, S. L., Miller, L. D., & Mishra, K. (2019). Pelvic floor physical therapy in the treatment of pelvic floor dysfunction in women. *Current Opinion in Obstetrics & Gynecology, 31*(6), 485–493. https://doi.org/10.1097/GCO.0000000000000584

Wong-Baker Faces Foundation. (2016). *Wong-Baker faces® pain rating scale*. Retrieved July 23, 2024, from https://wongbakerfaces.org/

Wozniak, S. (2016). Chronic pelvic pain. *Annals of Agricultural and Environmental Medicine, 23*(2), 223–226.

Xiang, H., Zhang, T., Al-Danakh, A., Yang, D., & Wang, L. (2022). Neuromodulation in chronic pelvic pain: A narrative review. *Pain and Therapy, 11*(3), 789–816. https://doi.org/10.1007/s40122-022-00405-w

Zwickl, S., Burchill, L., Wong, A. F. Q., Leemaqz, S. Y., Cook, T., Angus, L. M., Eshin, K., Elder, C. V., Grover, S. R., Zajac, J. D., & Cheung, A. S. (2023). Pelvic pain in transgender people using testosterone therapy. *LGBT Health, 10*(3), 179–190. https://doi.org/10.1089/lgbt.2022.0187

APPENDIX 29-A

International Association for the Study of Pain Fact Sheet (Bernardes et al., 2024)

FACT SHEET

Sex/Gender Biases in Pain Research and Clinical Practice

- **Sónia F. Bernardes, PhD:** Iscte-Lisbon University Institute, Department of Social and Organizational Psychology, Lisbon, Portugal.
- **Anke Samulowitz, PhD:** University of Gothenburg, School of Public Health and Community Medicine, Gothenburg, Sweden.
- **Kai Karos, PhD:** Maastricht University, Department of Clinical Psychological Science, Maastricht, Netherlands.
- **Jeffrey Mogil, PhD:** McGill University, Department of Psychology, Montreal, Canada.

What are sex/gender biases in pain research and clinical practice?

- Sex/gender biases describe a tendency to (un)favor a group of individuals over another based on their sex/gender categorization [1]. They reflect unjustified stereotypical preconceptions and prejudiced attitudes towards females/women, males/men, or gender-diverse people, that may lead to discriminatory actions. In patriarchal societies, such biases often reflect a tendency to favor males/men over females/women and gender-diverse people. They are culture-bound, contextual and intersect with other social positions and identities like age, ethnicity, sexual orientation and/or socioeconomic status.
- Sex/gender biases can be explicit (i.e., conscious) or implicit (i.e., unconscious). Explicit and implicit biases can be contradictory[1]. For example, health care professionals or researchers may be explicitly committed to egalitarian values but implicitly hold gender stereotypical beliefs that shape their clinical judgements or their conceptual/methodological approaches, respectively.
- Two main types of sex/gender biases can be found in the health field [2]:
- Disregarding real or potentially relevant sex/gender differences under the assumption that females/women and males/men are "the same" or have similar needs, e.g., when females/women are excluded from clinical trials under the assumption that findings may be generalizable from male/men samples.
- Assuming differences between the sexes/genders when similarities should be acknowledged, e.g., underassessing a woman's pain compared to a man's pain despite similar complaints and needs.

ARE THERE SEX/GENDER BIASES IN PAIN RESEARCH?

Sex biases in preclinical research:

- Preclinical studies of pain have been historically performed exclusively in male rodents (rats and mice), because of the fear that cycling gonadal hormones (i.e., estrogen and progesterone) would "complicate" things in females and lead to higher levels of variability in the data, necessitating the use of more animals and raising costs. This fear was shown to be unfounded in studies of pain [3] and in biomedicine more generally. If anything, it is male rodents that feature higher levels of variability.
- A review of preclinical research published in the journal Pain from 1996–2005 showed that 79% of studies featured the exclusive use of male rats/mice, with an additional 3% of studies not even specifying the sex of the research subject [3]. A similar review of Pain papers published in 2015 showed that nothing had changed over 20 years; again, 79% of studies used males only [4].
- This use of male rodents to model conditions overwhelmingly affecting women is clearly unethical. In response, funding agencies around the world are instituting sex-as-a-biological- variable (SABV) mandates, i.e., policies recognizing sex as a variable to consider in research design, analysis and reporting. At the National Institutes of Health in the U.S., such a mandate was announced in 2014 and went into effect in 2016 [5].
- A review of preclinical papers published in Pain from 2015– 2019 showed that by 2019, only 50% of papers used males only [6]. However, of 127 identified studies in which both sexes were tested, and the experimental manipulation was found to "work" in one sex but not the other, 72% of the time it worked in males but not females [6]. This suggest that the literature is now thoroughly biased such that findings in males generate hypotheses that are found to be true only in males. We are thus likely only at early stages of understanding female pain biology in animal models.

Sex/gender biases in clinical research:

- Most current pain theories do not integrate sex/gender factors and most pain research with humans does not analyze nor report sex/gender differences. A systematic review of publications in Pain from 2012-2021 concluded that less than 20% presented data disaggregated by sex [7].
- Although recent studies have a more balanced representation of the sexes [7], sampling bias can still be found. As females/women are more likely to seek support or attend pain clinics, there is an overrepresentation of females/women in clinical studies. Conversely, experimental studies have a higher proportion of males/men in their samples, as masculine-identifying individuals are more likely to volunteer for experimental pain studies [8].
- Assessment of demographic characteristics is still often unable to tap the diversity of the sexes and gender identities, going little beyond "female/woman, male/man, other". Furthermore, gender-diverse populations are often lumped together or excluded from the data analysis, contributing to their marginalization in knowledge production [8].
- Dominant stereotypical sex/gender binary views still shape most research conceptual assumptions and designs [8]. For example, within-sex variations in biological factors (e.g., sex hormones) that may be linked to pain experiences have been less investigated. Also, research has mostly been focused on traditional western conceptions of femininity and masculinity, sometimes seen as mutually exclusive, instead of coexisting within all human beings. Indeed, little pain research has explored the diversity and fluidity of femininities and masculinities, which are often shaped by situational cues and other social positions (e.g., age, culture, ethnicity, social class).

Are there sex/gender biases in clinical practice?

- Sex/gender biases can influence pain communication, assessment and treatment decisions occurring within clinical encounters. Many studies have shown sex/and gender biases in acute and chronic pain contexts.
- Regarding acute pain, various studies have been conducted in emergency medical settings and post-operative pain contexts:
- A scoping review of articles published from 1960-2021 on biases in emergency medical services (EMS) in the US [9] concluded that although women are quicker in recognizing the signs and symptoms of acute coronary syndromes (such as chest pain), they wait longer to access the EMS system after seeking help compared to men. However, there was no clear consensus on sex/gender biases in prehospital interventions for acute coronary syndrome (e.g., ECG, aspirin or nitroglycerin) nor prehospital pain management.
- A systematic review of studies on biases in post-operative pain and pain management published from 1992-2022 [10] showed women reported higher postoperative pain scores than men in most studies but received less pain medication than men in more than half the studies.
- Regarding chronic pain, a theory-driven review of quantitative and qualitative studies published from 2000-2015 on gender bias in pain care [11] showed that, compared to men, women more often:
- must struggle for their pain to be seen as legitimate in the context of clinical encounters: their pain is more psychologized, mistrusted and judged as unreliable depending on their appearances (e.g., looking too good or not looking good enough).
- receive more referrals to psychological treatments, less effective pain relief, fewer opioid analgesics, and more antidepressants.
- This review [11] also showed that pain-related gender norms - stereotypical expectations regarding how men and women are and should behave when in pain – may partially account for such sex/gender biases in clinical practices. Indeed, there are widely shared expectations across various cultures that, in public spaces such as the clinical encounter:
- men with chronic pain are stoic, autonomous, in control, pain tolerant, avoid talking about pain and seeking help. They are also expected to prioritize paid work over household duties.
- women with chronic pain are often described in comparison with men (andro-normativity), being perceived as more sensitive to pain, more willing to report pain and sometimes as hysterical, malingerers or feigning the pain. They are also expected to engage in self-care practices more than men.
- Although implicit prejudice (e.g., unconscious negative attitudes) may also be an underlying mechanism of sex/gender biases in clinical practices, it has been much less investigated. A scoping review of articles published between 2011 and 2021 on health professionals' unconscious bias in different regions of the world [12] showed that only 13% of studies focused on gender biases and a minority of those did so in pain contexts.
- Although many studies show biases against women in acute and chronic pain contexts, some studies suggest the absence of biases or even (although less frequently) biases against men. For example, a systematic review and meta-analysis [13] showed that, health care providers significantly underestimate patients' pain, especially when most of the patients in the study sample were males/men (vs. females/women). This suggests that sex/gender biases in clinical practice are variable and most likely context dependent [14].

How can we minimize sex/gender biases in pain research and clinical practice?

- To minimize sex/gender biases in pain research, researchers can familiarize themselves with existing guidelines and recommendations to integrate sex and gender in health (and pain) research, such as the:
- Sex- and Gender-Based Analysis (SGBA) approach of the CIHR Institute of Gender and Health.
- Sex and Gender Equity in Research (SAGER) Guidelines [15].
- recent recommendations by Keogh and Boerner [8] on how to embed and integrated sex and gender perspective in pain research.

- The Genderful Research Consortium Platform is an example of a particularly useful initiative that "provides an overview of key resources per stage of biomedical, clinical and public health research".
- As for clinical practice, the first step to counter sex/gender biases is to raise awareness about them. There is, however, a lack of effective evidence-based interventions to overcome or reduce gender biases in clinical practice in general [16].
- Nonetheless, some tools can be found that aim to facilitate this process in pain contexts, such as the "gender equality tool" [17] that supports the analysis of gendered and social processes in the clinical assessment of pain through questions addressed at workplaces and professionals directly.
- Increased awareness about sex/gender bias in clinical practice is an ongoing process and it is important that health care organisations, colleagues and every individual professional find procedures and routines for how to discuss explicit and not least implicit biases continuously.

References

Brewer MB. Intergroup discrimination: Ingroup love or outgroup hate? In CG Sibley, FK Barlow (eds.), The Cambridge Handbook of the Psychology of Prejudice. Cambridge: Cambridge University Press, 2017, pp. 90–110.

Risberg G, Johansson E, Hamberg K: A theoretical model for analyzing gender bias in medicine. Int J Equity Health 2009: 28, 1-8.

Mogil JS, Chanda ML: The case for the inclusion of female subjects in basic science studies of pain. Pain 2005; 117: 1-5.

Mogil JS. Equality need not be painful. Nature 2016; 535:S7.

Clayton JA, Collins, FS. Policy: NIH to balance sex in cell and animal studies. Nature 2014; 509 (7005): 282-283.

Mogil JS. Qualitative sex differences in pain processing: Emerging evidence of a biased literature. Nat Rev Neurosci 2020; 21: 353-365.

Plumb AN, Lesnak JB, Berardi G, Hayashi K. Janowski AJ, Smith AF, Bailey D, Kerkman C, Kienenberger Z, Martin B,; Patterson E, Van Roekel H, Vance CGT, Sluka A: Standing on the shoulders of bias: lack of transparency and reporting of critical rigor characteristics in pain research. PAIN 2023; 164(8): 1775-1782.

Keogh E, Boerner KE. Challenges with embedding an integrated sex and gender perspective into pain research: Recommendations and opportunities. Brain Behav Immun 2024;117:112–121.

Farcas AM, Joiner AP, Rudman JS, Ramesh K, Torres G, Crowe RP, Curtis T, Tripp R, Bowers K, von Isenburg M, Logan R, Coaxum L, Salazar G, Lozano M Jr, Page D, Haamid A. Disparities in Emergency Medical Services Care Delivery in the United States: A Scoping Review. Prehosp Emerg Care. 2023;27(8): 1058-1071.

Thurston KL, Zhang SJ, Wilbanks BA, Billings R, Aroke EN: A Systematic Review of Race, Sex, and Socioeconomic Status Differences in Postoperative Pain and Pain Management. J Perianesth Nurs. 2023;38(3):504-515.

Samulowitz A, Gremyr I, Eriksson E, Hensing G: "Brave men" and "emotional women#: A theory-guided literature review on gender bias in health care and gendered norms towards patients with chronic pain. Pain Res Manag 2018; ID6358624.

Meidert U, Dönnges G, Bucher T, Wieber F, Gerber-Grote A: Unconscious Bias among Health Professionals: A Scoping Review. Int J Environ Res Public Health. 2023 12;20(16):6569.

Ruben, MA, Blanch-Hartigan, D., & Shipert JC: To know another's pain: A meta-analysis of caregivers' and healthcare providers' pain assessment accuracy. Annals Behav Med 2018; 52 (8): 662-685.

Bernardes SF, Lima ML: On the contextual nature of sex-related biases in pain judgments: The effects of pain duration, patient's distress and judge's sex. Eur J Pain 2011; 15(9): 950–957.

Heidari S, Babor TF, De Castro P et al. Sex and Gender Equity in Research: rationale for the SAGER guidelines and recommended use. Res Integr Peer Rev 2016; 1, 2.

Alcalde-Rubio L., Hernandéz-Aguado I, Parker LA, Bueno-Vergara E, Chilet-Roselt E: Gender disparities in clinical practice: A there any solutions? Scoping review of interventions to overcome or reduce gender bias in clinical practice. Int J Equity Health 2020; 19: 166.

Hammarström A, Wiklund M, Stålnacke BM, Lehti A, Haukenes I, et al: Developing a Tool for Increasing the Awareness about Gendered and Intersectional Processes in the Clinical Assessment of Patients – A Study of Pain Rehabilitation. PLOS ONE 2016; 11(4): e0152735.

SECTION

4

Introduction to Prenatal and Postpartum Care

CHAPTER 30

Preconception Care

Jamie Pelaez
Ellen Solis

The editors would like to acknowledge Kathleen Danhausen and Amy Romano, the authors of "Preconception Care" for the 4th edition of *Gynecologic Health Care.*

INTRODUCTION

The preconception period is generally considered the 3- to 4-month window prior to conception. Maturation of egg and sperm occurs during this time, creating a sensitive period when DNA and other cell structures become prepared for rapid replication. The quality of the gametes can be impacted by parental age, nutritional status, cardiometabolic health, environmental exposures, and toxic stress via mechanisms now understood to relate to epigenetic changes (Raghuraman & Tuuli, 2021). This process results in the expression of genes that become the blueprint for fetal and placental development. Additionally, embryonic development, including the critical period of organogenesis, takes place before the placenta is fully formed. As a result, the early development of organs relies on the health of the endometrium, which is influenced directly by prepregnancy health and follicular quality. Whether individuals in the preconception phase recognize it or not, they have a window of opportunity to lay the foundation for a healthier pregnancy and better birth outcome. A growing body of research continues to suggest that prepregnancy health is a strong and reliable predictor of pregnancy outcomes (Wang et al., 2023).

The period before a planned pregnancy is also a time of significant psychosocial transition. When people are considering pregnancy or actively trying to conceive, they may seek information about fertility, conception, or pregnancy and begin making health and lifestyle changes (Harper et al., 2023). They may also think about long-term goals and plans and the potential impact of a child on their family, career, and sense of self.

Preconception care is the provision of health services and education before conception, with the aim of positively influencing the outcome of the future pregnancy. The movement within health care to improve preconception health emerged in the 1980s. Early efforts focused on the potential of preconception care and counseling to reduce birth defects, then later expanded to other fetal and newborn outcomes such as preterm birth and low birth weight (Harper et al., 2023). More recently, there has been a broader understanding that the preconception period influences the long-term health of the individual who carries the pregnancy, especially in people with preexisting chronic disease or those who are at risk for developing chronic disease under the "stressor" of pregnancy and birth.

Not all individuals who become pregnant identify as female or women; however, these terms are used in this chapter, especially when discussing research. Use of these terms is not meant to exclude people who do not identify as women, and where possible gender-inclusive language is used.

Challenges in Delivering Preconception Care

Many factors pose barriers to providing effective preconception health care. The most significant factor is the high likelihood of an unintended pregnancy. Although the rate has declined in recent years, 42 percent of pregnancies in the United States are still unplanned, and individuals of low socioeconomic status and women of color report unintended pregnancies at even higher rates (Haiman & Cubbin, 2023). The context and landscape of U.S. health care, especially for pregnant-capable people, also presents challenges to delivering preconception care. Preconception health is impacted by many social determinants and structures and lifestyle and behavioral health factors. To be able to implement the practices that will improve preconception health and well-being, such as tobacco cessation or chronic disease management, patients may need services and support well beyond a single clinical encounter. However, even when people are insured, health plans may cover preconception care as a single preventive care visit. Most people with low incomes cannot access Medicaid insurance unless they are pregnant, so they are at high risk of being uninsured before and between pregnancies. Patients may also not be eligible for other programs like food assistance and housing benefits, even though these programs would likely benefit outcomes if available.

Another barrier to preconception care is consumer perception. Even when individuals intend to become pregnant or hope for pregnancy, they may not know the value of preconception care or the most important lifestyle or behavioral changes to optimize their preconception health (Harper et al., 2023). Data from the Pregnancy Risk Assessment and Monitoring Survey (PRAMS) suggests that less than 30 percent of women present to health care for a dedicated preconception visit but the majority of women (66% as of 2020) have at least one healthcare visit within 12 months of conception (Stulberg et al., 2023). Pregnant-capable individuals also may not share their reproductive life goals or pregnancy intentions in healthcare encounters, so it may be challenging to identify people who are either at risk of pregnancy or may benefit from preconception care and counseling. Thus, every encounter with a reproductive-aged client may be viewed as an opportunity to address family planning and preconception care.

BOX 30-1 PATH Model

Primary questions:

1. Do you think you would like to have (more) children at some point?
2. When do you think that might be?
3. How important is it to you to prevent pregnancy (until then)?

Follow-up questions:

1. Since you said _____, would you like to talk about ways to be prepared for a healthy pregnancy?
2. Do you have a sense of what is important to you about your birth control?
3. How would that be for you?
4. Has that ever happened before?
5. How did you manage it?

Reproduced from Envision Sexual and Reproductive Health. (n.d.). *About PATH*. https://www.envisionsrh.com/about-path

Asking all reproductive-aged people at every health visit about their plans for future pregnancy has been proposed as a way to increase the receipt of preconception services and education. The One Key Question campaign advises healthcare providers to routinely ask all people of reproductive age, "Would you like to become pregnant in the next year?" (American College of Obstetricians and Gynecologists [ACOG], 2019a). However, pregnancy intention can be complex and often nonbinary (e.g., people may feel ambivalent to pregnancy). The PATH model (PA: pregnancy attitudes; T: timing; H: how important) is a shared decision-making framework that aims to facilitate conversations to help individuals gain clarity about their reproductive goals and plan education and services accordingly (refer to **Box 30-1**) (Geist et al., 2019). For example, some people may need both contraceptive and preconception counseling, depending on their motivation to prevent pregnancy. Though there is a lack of research evaluating the effectiveness of these interventions, qualitative research suggests high client satisfaction with this framework (Goodsmith et al., 2023). One Key Question and the PATH model are now considered standard of care.

Preconception Health Indicators

Many reproductive-aged individuals in the United States have significant risk factors for poor outcomes, and these outcomes can be improved with the optimization of pregnant-capable individuals' health prior to pregnancy (U.S. Department of Health and Human Services, 2024). The National Preconception Health and Healthcare Initiative is a public–private partnership convened by the Centers for Disease Control and Prevention (CDC) in 2003 to advance evidence, strategies, and innovations for improving wellness and reducing infant mortality through the promotion of preconception health. This group originally identified 45 core health indicators and developed a set of 10 condensed indicators to track and measure progress in improving the preconception health of American women. These indicators include the individual's access to care, intention to become pregnant, use of a folic-acid containing multivitamin, avoidance of tobacco, control/maintenance of mental health, metabolic health (glycemic control/healthy weight for them), absence or treatment of STIs, and avoidance of teratogens (Frayne et al., 2016).

The most current National Preconception Health and Healthcare Initiative data suggest that U.S. women have suboptimal preconception health, though these numbers vary by age, ethnicity, and region (Robbins et al., 2018). For example, while body mass index (BMI) is not a precise or generalizable marker of good health (Pearl & Puhl, 2018; Tomiyama et al., 2018), more than half of all women report a BMI greater than 30, with higher prevalence seen among women without insurance (61%). In addition, only half of all women report getting adequate weekly physical activity. The proportion of U.S. women who were told they had diabetes in 2013 to 2015 ranged from 2 percent in Utah to 5 percent in Alabama; women reporting a lifetime diagnosis of hypertension ranged from 7 percent in Minnesota to 19 percent in Mississippi. Women who are older, non-Hispanic Black, or do not have health insurance report more risk factors and fewer protective factors than other U.S. women. Overall, women in southern states have poorer health indicators (Robbins et al., 2018).

Goals of Preconception Care

The overall goal of preconception care and counseling is to begin pregnancy as healthy and prepared as possible, screen for risks and prevention opportunities, and put in place changes that can impact fertility or early fetoplacental development and maternal physiologic adaptation. The clinician approaches the encounter by asking a rhetorical question: If this individual became pregnant today, would I expect them to have a healthy pregnancy? If a resulting pregnancy would likely be higher risk, prevention opportunities may exist in the preconception period that mitigate these risks.

Preconception and prenatal health are impacted by both biological and social determinants. Biological factors include genetics, health history, and chronic or acute health conditions, while social determinants include work and family environments, support systems, experiences of poverty or racism and other forms of discrimination, and individual routines and behaviors. There is evidence that these nonclinical factors are the primary drivers of birth outcomes, especially with respect to preterm birth, low birth weight, and maternal morbidity and mortality (ACOG, 2024). Thus, preconception care requires an integrated approach that addresses both biological and social determinants of health.

THE APPROACH TO A PERSON HOPING TO BECOME PREGNANT IN THE NEXT YEAR

When developing a preconception care plan, it is important to elicit the patient's goals and preferences, identify knowledge gaps, and assess support systems. This will enable the provider to tailor education and recommendations based on assessment of lifestyle, social and behavioral factors, genetic history and risk factors, preventive health practices, partner's health and lifestyle, infection risk, and medications or conditions that may impact fertility or pregnancy. With this background, the provider can deliver individualized care and counseling to optimize pregnancy timing and outcome. **Box 30-2** provides an overview of the clinical content of preconception care and counseling.

BOX 30-2 Clinical Content of Preconception Care

One Key Question: Do you hope to become pregnant in the next year? If the answer is no, review contraceptive options and safer sexual practices. Refer to Chapter 13 for more information on contraceptive care.

For those who desire or are ambivalent toward pregnancy, do the following:

1. Obtain a medical history, with close attention to the following:
   a. History of chronic illness and medication use
   b. Current or past history of depression, anxiety, or psychosis; treatment history
   c. Prior pregnancy history
   d. Family history, especially thrombophilias or genetic abnormalities
   e. Psychosocial risks
      i. Interpersonal safety
      ii. Access to care
      iii. Financial resources
   f. Vaccination history
   g. Toxic exposures—occupational hazards, substance use, medication/supplement use
   h. Partner history, especially toxic exposures and family history of genetic abnormalities
2. Optimize current health:
   a. Provide counseling on optimal weight, adequate physical activity, healthy diet
   b. Assist in managing chronic health conditions (euglycemia, euthyroid, euthymic, normotensive, etc.)
   c. Review medications, optimize pregnancy safety profile
3. Provide fertility education:
   a. Tracking cycle, signs of ovulation and timing of intercourse
   b. Importance of tracking cycle and last menstrual period
   c. How long to try to become pregnant before seeking further evaluation
4. Provide education for a healthy pregnancy:
   a. Folate supplementation
   b. Immunizations
   c. Avoiding toxic exposures
      i. Environmental exposures
      ii. Medications and supplements
      iii. Alcohol, tobacco, and illicit drugs
   d. Avoiding infection
      i. Cytomegalovirus, toxoplasmosis, tuberculosis, malaria, Zika; depending on habitat and occupation
      ii. Safer sexual practices
   e. Importance of seeking medical care when pregnancy is suspected, especially women with chronic health conditions
   f. Regular dental care
5. Provide preconception interventions:
   a. Treat chronic and acute conditions as indicated
   b. Screen for and treat sexually transmitted infections
   c. Vaccination titers as indicated, offer immunizations
   d. Refer for genetic/carrier testing as desired
   e. Refer for psychosocial support as indicated
   f. Provide resources or referrals for smoking cessation, substance abuse treatment

Eliciting and Clarifying Goals and Preferences

Individuals presenting for preconception care may have different levels of intention and motivation for pregnancy. Do they have a preferred time frame for getting pregnant or specific goals they want to achieve before pregnancy? The provider can work with them to realign or prioritize goals based on information gleaned from the history and clinical examination. Beginning from the foundation of the individual's initial goals and motivations is a tactic to improve the relevance and effectiveness of behavior change counseling.

Assessing Knowledge and Support Systems

It is important to assess the patient's knowledge about fertility and conception and health behaviors that support healthy pregnancy. Many people lack basic information about fertility and conception, and most individuals trying to conceive report that their primary source of information surrounding preconception health and pregnancy is the internet (Hammarberg et al., 2017). Furthermore, a 2019 study assessing the accuracy of online information targeting couples trying to conceive reported a 60 percent accuracy rate of claims identified (Kedzior et al., 2019). This highlights the importance of assessing patient knowledge so that clinicians may tailor counseling and provide evidence-based resources.

ASSESSMENT AND COUNSELING RELATED TO LIFESTYLE AND BEHAVIORAL FACTORS

Nutrition

The individual's nutritional behaviors may be assessed through questioning or use of a validated assessment instrument, such as a food frequency questionnaire or 24-hour diet recall. An optimal preconception diet emphasizes whole foods and limits highly processed foods. Ample consumption of fruits, vegetables, nuts, legumes, and high-quality animal products supports fertility. For many years, the Mediterranean diet was hailed as the best diet for fertility. The Mediterranean diet is loosely defined as a diet high in plant-based proteins, produce, whole grains and fish, but recent research suggests that the inclusion of full-fat dairy and red meat further supports fertility outcomes (Kim et al., 2017; Moleshi et al., 2019). The most impactful dietary shift is the limitation of highly processed foods, which research currently suggests makes up over half of the average American's daily intake (Wolfson et al., 2025).

People face a range of challenges to improving nutritional habits, including poor availability of fresh foods (sometimes referred to as food deserts); low cost of processed food, compared with fresh food alternatives; perceived lack of time; and other barriers. Individualized programs that provide counseling, coaching, group support, and accountability can help with efforts to improve nutrition. Micronutrient supplementation is also recommended to provide the range of nutrients needed to support fertility and early pregnancy. Due to the increased micronutrient demands of pregnancy, individuals who avoid or limit animal-based produces should be encouraged to supplement with vitamin D_3, vitamin B_{12}, choline, and calcium (Hess et al., 2025).

BOX 30-3 Dietary Sources of Folate

Avocado
Brewer's yeast
Citrus fruit
Egg yolk
Leafy green vegetables
Legumes
Liver

Folate Supplementation

The months immediately preceding and following conception are critical for optimizing the development of the gamete and placenta. Folate (vitamin B_9) provides essential support to DNA replication and is involved in amino acid synthesis and vitamin metabolism. Folic acid is a synthetic source of folate that is found in vitamins and fortified foods. Adequate folate intake can decrease the risk of neural tube defects, including anencephaly, spina bifida, and encephalocele, by up to 70 percent (Viswanathan et al., 2017). Adequate preconception folic acid intake has also been linked to a decreased risk of preterm birth and newborns who have low birth weight or are small for gestational age, with no effect seen in women who started folate supplementation after conception. In addition, folate supplementation has been associated with decreased incidence of miscarriage, stillbirth, neonatal death, and childhood autism (Strøm et al., 2018; Levine et al., 2018). A 2023 systematic review of recently published research on folic acid supplementation to prevent neural tube defects concluded that the new evidence was consistent with previous findings suggesting large benefit and no associated harms (Viswanathan et al., 2023). Because folate is not synthesized by the body, it must be obtained through either diet (refer to **Box 30-3**) or supplementation.

Supplementation with 400 to 800 mcg of folate should begin at least 1 month prior to attempting conception and continue through the first trimester (U.S. Preventive Services Task Force [USPSTF], 2023; ACOG, 2019). Some studies have found better outcomes with multivitamin supplementation containing folic acid, compared to folic acid supplementation alone (X. Yang et al., 2016). It is reasonable to recommend a daily multivitamin or folate supplementation to all reproductive-aged women who are sexually active with men and not actively preventing pregnancy.

Some pregnant people are at higher risk of neural tube defects and need additional folate supplementation (refer to **Box 30-4**). These patients should supplement with 4 mg of folate daily starting 3 months prior to pregnancy (ACOG, 2017e). Those needing additional folate supplementation should not take extra prenatal vitamins due to the risk of vitamin toxicity (especially vitamin A); they should supplement with folic acid or methylated folate only.

BOX 30-4 Indications for Additional Folate Supplementation (4 mg Folate Daily)

Personal or family history of neural tube defects
Prior pregnancy complicated by neural tube defects
Partner with personal history or prior child with neural tube defects
Insulin-dependent diabetes
Taking valproate or carbamazepine

Both folate and folic acid must be further reduced to the compound L-5-methyltetrahydrofolate (L-methylfolate) to become metabolically active. The enzyme methylenetetrahydrofolate (MTHFR) is critical to this process, converting folic acid to methylfolate (Levin & Varga, 2016). However, approximately 20 percent of individuals in the United States have some deficiency of the MTHFR enzyme (up to 40% among white and Hispanic people) and may not receive adequate methylfolate from their folic acid supplementation, placing them at higher risk for recurrent pregnancy loss and neural tube defects (Levin & Varga, 2016; Y. Yang et al., 2016) Patients with a known MTHFR deficiency should supplement with 400 mcg methylfolate daily, with some recommendations shifting to suggest routine supplementation with the more bioavailable L-methylfolate instead of folic acid for all women (Levin & Varga, 2016; Naninck, Stijger, & Brouwer-Brolsma, 2019). Interestingly, supplementation with methylfolate has also been shown to reduce rates of perinatal depression (Freeman et al., 2019).

Exercise

During the preconception period, regular aerobic exercise is important to overall health and can improve fertility. At least 150 minutes of moderate to vigorous exercise weekly is recommended, or about 20 to 25 minutes daily, with continued regular exercise while pregnant to improve pregnancy outcomes.

Studies have demonstrated that exercise is associated with resumption of ovulation in individuals with anovulatory infertility or polycystic ovary syndrome (PCOS) (Hakimi & Cameron, 2017) and increased birth rates in patients experiencing infertility who are overweight or obese (Best et al., 2017). The likely mechanism is modulation of the hypothalamic–pituitary– gonadal (HPG) axis due to increased activity of the hypothalamic–pituitary–adrenal (HPA) axis.

For individuals who exercise heavily and/or are underweight, excessive exercise may disrupt ovulation. Counsel these patients to avoid vigorous exercise exceeding 60 minutes per day if they are concerned about the impact of exercise on fertility and note that moderate to vigorous exercise of 30 to 60 minutes daily is associated with improved pregnancy outcomes (Hakimi & Cameron, 2017).

Stress Management

Humans and other mammals have well-honed mechanisms to detect and respond to threats or other stressful stimuli by activating the HPA axis and other neuroendocrine circuits. These responses enable the body to address the threat or challenge and reestablish homeostatic equilibrium. In the case of extreme or chronic stress, the stress response does not resolve into a state of balance, neuroendocrine signaling remains in an altered state, and various negative health effects may result (Tufts University Health & Nutrition Letter, 2024). Excessive activation of the HPA axis is associated with altered functions of the hypothalamus, pituitary, and ovaries, and it is associated with reduced fertility and poor pregnancy outcome (Joseph & Whirledge, 2017; Lewinski & Brzozowska, 2023). High levels of salivary stress biomarkers are associated with a longer time to pregnancy for women trying to conceive and a twofold risk of infertility, compared with women who have low stress (Lewinski & Brzozowska, 2023).

The clinician may inquire about the individual's levels and sources of stress and assist them to reduce stress where possible, encouraging the use of adaptive techniques such as self-care, mindfulness, and social support to manage stress rather than maladaptive responses such as substance use, emotional eating, and social withdrawal.

Interpersonal Violence

Standard of care is to screen all patients for current and past intimate partner violence, sexual abuse, and sexual assault; this screening may be done on paper or in person (U.S. Preventive Services Task Force, 2024). Privacy and confidentiality must be ensured; clinicians must be aware of their state's mandated reporting requirements. Intimate partner violence may include physical injury or threat of injury, psychological abuse, sexual assault, progressive isolation, stalking, deprivation, intimidation, and reproductive coercion (ACOG, 2012a, reaffirmed 2019). Reproductive coercion includes attempts to pressure a person to become pregnant or interfere with contraception, whereas sexual coercion is pressuring a person into having sex without using physical force. The American College of Obstetricians and Gynecologists (ACOG) recommends including questions about reproductive coercion when screening patients for intimate partner violence (refer to **Box 30-5**) (ACOG, 2013a, reaffirmed 2019). Clinicians must also remain aware of signs that a person is a victim of human trafficking, including a partner who will not leave their side, a lack of identification documents, uncertainty as to their address or the current date or time, an inability to answer specific questions, and physical injuries in various stages of healing (Tracy & Macias-Konstantopoulos, 2017). If a patient discloses violence, coercion, or fear, assess their safety and provide community resources and intervention services. More information about identifying victims of human trafficking in the healthcare setting can be found in Chapter 16. Refer to Chapter 15 for additional information about intimate partner violence.

BOX 30-5 Screening Questions for Intimate Partner Violence and Reproductive Coercion

Has your current partner ever threatened you or made you feel afraid?

Has your partner ever hit, choked, or physically hurt you?

Has your partner ever forced you to do something sexually that you did not want to do?

Has your partner ever tried to get you pregnant when you did not want to become pregnant?

Are you worried that your partner will hurt you if you do not do what they want with the pregnancy?

Does your partner support your decision about when or if you want to become pregnant?

Data from American College of Obstetricians and Gynecologists. (2012a, reaffirmed 2022). ACOG committee opinion no. 518: Intimate partner violence. *Obstetrics & Gynecology, 119*(2 Pt. 1), 412–417. https://doi.org/10.1097/AOG.0b013e318249ff74; American College of Obstetricians and Gynecologists. (2013a, reaffirmed 2022). ACOG committee opinion no. 554: Reproductive and sexual coercion. *Obstetrics & Gynecology, 121*(2 Pt. 1), 411–415. https://doi.org/10.1097/01.AOG.0000426427.79586.3b

Environmental Exposures

Toxic environmental chemicals are ubiquitous, and preconception and prenatal exposure to these agents has been associated with a range of deleterious effects, including subfertility and infertility in all genders, spontaneous abortion, congenital anomalies, childhood cancers, and other risks across the life span. Many toxic environmental factors disproportionately affect vulnerable and underserved populations, contributing to health disparities.

Meaningful reductions in toxic exposures can be achieved only with policy and public health approaches. However, clinicians can screen for toxic exposures and help preconception clients take pragmatic steps to reduce exposures. Screening should include workplace environmental exposures from industries that expose workers to heavy metals, radiation, solvents, pesticides, and other toxic agents. The clinician may consider referral to an occupational medicine specialist to help the individual understand the specific risks and establish a plan to reduce exposures. General awareness of toxic agents specific to the geographic area or key local industries is helpful.

Counseling in the primary care setting aims to reduce modifiable sources of toxins, including diet and household items (ACOG, 2013b, reaffirmed 2024). Pesticide consumption can be reduced by eating organic foods and washing conventional produce before eating. If cost is a barrier, individuals can be counseled to buy seasonal and local foods when possible and prioritize switching to organic for the "dirty dozen" foods that have the highest pesticide use. The dirty dozen list and a list of "clean 15" conventional foods that are safe to consume are published annually by the Environmental Working Group (2025) (refer to **Box 30-6**).

Additional actions that individuals can take to reduce harmful exposures include reducing consumption of processed foods, avoiding fatty fish that are high in mercury (e.g., shark, swordfish, king mackerel, and tilefish), and using products that are free of bisphenol A (BPA). For example, individuals should switch to glass containers for food and beverage storage when possible. Counsel patients to avoid phthalates in common household and personal-care products, and to limit outdoor activity during

> **BOX 30-6 Fruits and Vegetables with the Highest and Lowest Concentration of Pesticides**
>
> **Dirty Dozen: Produce with the Highest Concentration of Pesticides**
>
> Apples
> Bell and hot peppers
> Blueberries
> Cherries
> Grapes
> Green beans
> Kale, collard, and mustard greens
> Nectarines
> Peaches
> Pears
> Spinach
> Strawberries
>
> **Clean Fifteen: Produce with the Lowest Concentration of Pesticides**
>
> Asparagus
> Avocados
> Cabbage
> Carrots
> Honeydew melon
> Kiwis
> Mangoes
> Mushrooms
> Onions
> Papayas
> Pineapple
> Sweet corn
> Sweet potatoes
> Sweet peas (frozen)
> Watermelon
>
> Data from Environmental Working Group. (2024). *Shopper's guide to pesticides in produce*. https://www.ewg.org/foodnews/

poor air quality days. prolonged outdoor exposure during poor air quality dates as both have been repeatedly associated with poor pregnancy and fertility outcomes. In addition to avoidance behaviors, people may increase beneficial environmental exposures that have health-promoting effects and can counteract toxic effects. These include intake of fresh fruit, vegetables, and unprocessed food and outdoor activity.

Substance Use

All patients should be screened at regular intervals for nicotine and unhealthy alcohol use, as well as recreational drugs, opioids, and other medications used for nonmedical purposes (ACOG, 2013b, reaffirmed 2024). Individuals with substance use disorders are more likely to have comorbid mental illness and are also more likely to report unintended pregnancies and STIs (MacAfee et al., 2018). In addition, tobacco, marijuana, opioid, and alcohol use disorders all increase the risk of infertility (Wright, 2017). The preconception period is an excellent time to encourage women to stop unhealthy substance use behaviors to improve their fertility and the health of their pregnancy and child. Regardless of their pregnancy intendedness, encourage those identified as being at risk for, or diagnosed with, a substance use disorder to seek treatment, and facilitate a referral for services if desired. Clinicians should have a working knowledge of recovery services and providers in their community.

Tobacco and Nicotine

Tobacco is the leading cause of preventable deaths in the United States (Centers for Disease Control and Prevention, 2024). Tobacco and nicotine use during pregnancy is clearly associated with increased maternal and infant morbidity, including miscarriage, growth restriction, stillbirth, placental abruption, placenta previa, and abnormal maternal thyroid function (ACOG, 2019a, reaffirmed 2024). Children exposed to tobacco in utero and after birth are at increased risk of sudden infant death syndrome, asthma, obesity, and infantile colic (USPSTF, 2021). Tobacco use has also been shown to decrease fertility rates and embryo quality among women using assisted reproductive technologies, and it is reasonable to assume this is the case among women seeking spontaneous conception (Amaral et al., 2019; Mínguez-Alarcon et al., 2018).

Pregnancy and the preconception period are often times when individuals are motivated to quit smoking; approximately half of women who report smoking prior to pregnancy quit by the third trimester (Rockhill et al., 2016). Pharmacologic treatment can improve rates of smoking cessation. Nicotine replacement therapy, bupropion (Wellbutrin), and varenicline (Chantix) are first-line treatment for tobacco use disorder, along with evidence-based behavioral therapies for people in the preconception phase. Medications for smoking cessation are not recommended in pregnancy due to an overall lack of safety data (USPSTF, 2021). Some individuals may turn to e-cigarettes (vaping) in an attempt to quit smoking; however, this system delivers other aerosolized chemicals in addition to nicotine and may be at least as harmful as cigarettes, if not more harmful (Kuehn, 2019). Recent research on the use of e-cigarettes has demonstrated detrimental effects on male and female fertility including lower levels of anti-Müllerian hormone, higher rates of spontaneous abortion and lower sperm concentration, motility, and morphology (Montjean et al., 2023). Clinicians should counsel all individuals using any amount or type of nicotine on the importance of cessation. Individuals hoping to become pregnant immediately may consider bupropion to support their efforts to quit; this antidepressant medication has been studied in pregnancy with no major risks identified (Turner et al., 2019).

Alcohol

The U.S. Preventive Services Task Force (USPSTF) recommends screening all adults for unhealthy alcohol use in primary care settings and providing those people who screen positive with brief counseling interventions (USPSTF, 2018a). Data from the Behavioral Risk Factor Surveillance System by the CDC suggests that 20.2 percent of reproductive-aged women in the United States binge drink (Luong et al., 2023). Preconception counseling includes the information that alcohol is a known teratogen, and its use in pregnancy is associated with growth restriction, stillbirth, and fetal alcohol spectrum disorders (Dejong et al., 2019). Even moderate amounts of alcohol consumption have been shown to impact the menstrual cycle and reproductive hormones. Given that alcohol offers no nutritional value, it is reasonable to recommend that patients avoid or significantly limit alcohol consumption if trying to conceive. Refer to Chapter 9 for further information on screening for alcohol misuse.

Marijuana

As marijuana becomes legalized in many states, more people are reporting its use. There is limited data on rates of marijuana use in the preconception and early pregnancy window, though it is estimated that 5 to 6 percent of pregnant individuals use marijuana. Recent studies on consumer perception suggest that the majority of marijuana users perceive little to no risk to the fetus despite literature suggesting otherwise (Goodin et al., 2025). Few data exist that provide an estimate of the perinatal risks of marijuana use, and no data provide insight into the relationship between outcomes and marijuana dosage, frequency, and gestational timing of use. Notably, two recent studies evaluating over 300,000 individuals demonstrated an increased risk of gestational hypertension, preeclampsia, and placental abruption in individuals who used marijuana in the first 14 weeks of pregnancy, suggesting a negative impact on placental development (Young-Wolff et al., 2024; Metz et al., 2023). Research is limited on the impact of marijuana on fertility. Recent animal studies have demonstrated an impact of THC on egg and sperm quality, though this has not yet been replicated in humans. Professional organizations recommend against the use of marijuana in pregnancy due to the lack of confidence in its safety (ACOG, 2017c; Foeller & Lyell, 2017).

Opioids

Opioid use in the general population and among pregnant people has grown significantly in the past decade. In 2023, the most recent year national data are available, over 81,000 Americans died from opioid overdose, and as of 2021 an estimated 2.5 million people experienced an opioid use disorder (Tanz et al., 2025). Opioid use disorder is treatable but generally requires long-term behavioral therapy, pharmacological treatment, and recovery support. Opioid use in pregnancy is not associated with any major teratogenic effects, but it has been linked to ventricular and atrial septal cardiac defects, oral clefts, and clubfoot (Lind et al., 2017). In addition, there are several maternal and neonatal complications associated with opioid use, including miscarriage, preeclampsia, preterm birth, newborns who have low birth weight or are small for gestational age, placental abruption, fetal death, and sudden infant death (Lind et al., 2017). Neonatal opioid withdrawal syndrome is commonly observed as neonates withdraw from opioid exposure.

Clinicians should screen everyone for opioid use; those with a positive screen should receive a brief intervention and referral to services as indicated (ACOG, 2017b, reaffirmed 2021). Treatment prior to pregnancy is optimal because withdrawal from opioids can precipitate miscarriage. Those with opioid use disorder are often treated with methadone or buprenorphine; this treatment may be continued in pregnancy and is considered preferable to medically supervised withdrawal due to the risk of relapse (approximately 60 to 90%) (ACOG, 2017b, reaffirmed 2021). Relapse brings risks of overdose; transmission of infectious diseases, such as HIV, hepatitis C, and STIs; poor adherence to prenatal care; and adverse maternal and neonatal outcomes. However, with intensive follow-up support, patients may safely withdraw from opioids prior to attempting pregnancy (Gennette, 2017).

ASSESSMENT OF GENETIC RISK

Inquire about personal and family histories of genetic and developmental abnormalities. For individuals at risk of conceiving a child with genetic defects, the preconception time is optimal for pursuing carrier screening for genetic conditions, which can inform their decisions about when and how to proceed with pregnancy. Refer to **Box 30-7** for carrier screening recommendations. If a person is found to be a carrier for a certain condition, their partner should be tested for carrier status. Carrier screening needs to be performed only once in a person's lifetime (ACOG, 2017a, reaffirmed 2023).

ASSESSMENT OF PREVENTIVE HEALTH PRACTICES

Immunizations

Vaccine-preventable illnesses can have a profound impact on maternal, fetal, and neonatal health; thus, the review of a person's immunization status is an important part of primary and preconception care. In particular, immunization with the measles–mumps–rubella (MMR) and hepatitis B vaccines prior to pregnancy is highly recommended. Other potential preconception immunizations include the following: human papillomavirus (HPV); varicella; influenza; tetanus, diphtheria, and pertussis; pneumococcal; hepatitis A; and meningococcal (Dudley, 2018). Refer to **Table 30-1** for an overview of recommended preconception vaccinations.

Measles, Mumps, and Rubella

Measles and rubella can have a devastating impact on a developing fetus. Measles during pregnancy can cause miscarriage, preterm birth, and low birth weight and rates in the United States are rising (CDC, 2025a). Maternal rubella infection during pregnancy is linked with miscarriage and intrauterine fetal demise, and congenital rubella infection is associated with cardiac and auditory defects and cataracts (CDC, 2025b). The MMR

BOX 30-7 Recommendations for Carrier Screening

Recommend carrier screening for patients with personal or family histories of the following conditions:

Canavan disease[a]
Cystic fibrosis
Familial dysautonomia[a]
Fragile X syndrome
Hemoglobinopathy
Spinal muscular atrophy
Tay-Sachs disease[a]

[a]Recommended for those of Ashkenazi Jewish descent.

TABLE 30-1 Recommended Vaccines for the Preconception Period

Vaccine	Population	Administration Considerations
Measles, mumps, rubella	All individuals without evidence of immunity.	Live vaccine: Avoid pregnancy for 4 weeks after vaccination. One- or two-dose series based on risk, with 4 weeks between doses.
Hepatitis B	Individuals at high risk: Those from countries with endemic hepatitis B infection; household and sexual contacts of people who have hepatitis B; individuals who use injection drugs; individuals with hepatitis C or HIV; individuals with sexual exposure risk; individuals who are immunocompromised; international travelers; prisoners; workers in health care, public safety, and institutions.	Minimum 1 month and may take up to 6 months to complete series, depending on vaccine type; vaccine series may continue during pregnancy. Combined hepatitis A and B series available.
Human papillomavirus	Individuals aged 26 years and younger.	Minimum 5 months to complete. Not recommended during pregnancy.
Influenza	All individuals.	Avoid in individuals with allergy to vaccine component, Guillain-Barré syndrome, or current moderate or severe illness.
Varicella	All individuals without evidence of immunity.	One month to complete series. Live vaccine: Avoid pregnancy for 4 weeks after vaccination.
Tetanus, diphtheria, and pertussis (Tdap)	All individuals who have not received the Tdap vaccine.	Vaccination in third trimester of pregnancy also recommended; client may wish to defer until pregnant.
Pneumococcal disease	Individuals at high risk: Those with chronic heart, liver, or lung disease (including asthma); diabetes; immunodeficiencies; immunosuppressive therapies; asplenia; hemoglobinopathies; cerebral spinal leaks; cochlear implants; cigarette smoking.	Minimum 1 month to complete series. Dose and series depends on risk factor.
Hepatitis A	Individuals at high risk: Travelers to endemic areas; exposure to individuals with hepatitis A infection or biological samples; homelessness; injection or noninjection drug use; those with chronic liver disease or clotting factor disorders.	Minimum 6 months and may take up to 18 months to complete, depending on vaccine type; vaccine series may continue during pregnancy. Combined hepatitis A and B series available.
Meningococcal disease	Individuals at high risk: Asplenia, including sickle cell disease; immunodeficiencies; complement factor deficiencies; eculizumab use; travel to hyperendemic regions; those living in dormitories or military barracks.	Vaccine schedule based on risk.
coronavirus disease (COVID-19)	All individuals who are pregnant or contemplating pregnancy	Vaccine schedule based on risk.

Note: Refer to CDC vaccine schedule for specific series dosing.

vaccine is part of the recommended childhood vaccine series and 97 percent efficacious; however, some people were not vaccinated in childhood or have experienced waning immunity. Thus, all individuals of childbearing age who are not pregnant should be screened for rubella immunity and offered vaccination if they are not immune. Because MMR is a live vaccine, it cannot be given during pregnancy due to the theoretical risk of infection with one of the live components of the vaccine. Advise patients to avoid pregnancy for 4 weeks following MMR vaccination. If a person inadvertently receives the MMR vaccine while pregnant, assure them that studies have not found an increased risk of adverse outcomes (CDC, 2025b).

Hepatitis B

Hepatitis B virus is present in blood, semen, and vaginal secretions, and transmission usually occurs through contact with infected wounds or needles, sexual contact, or blood transfusions (Nelson et al., 2016). The risk of perinatal transmission is high, especially if a person has chronic infection (5 to 10% risk of perinatal transmission) or experiences acute infection during the third trimester (60% risk of perinatal transmission) (Shao et al., 2017). The USPSTF recommends screening all pregnant women for hepatitis B at their first prenatal visit but recommends against universal screening of the general population (USPSTF, 2025). As part of preconception care, it is reasonable to screen those who are at high risk of contracting hepatitis B and have not been previously vaccinated; those from countries with endemic hepatitis B infection; household and sexual contacts of people who have hepatitis B; people who use injection drugs; people with hepatitis C or HIV; people with sexual exposure risk (e.g., multiple or nonmonogamous partners and those seeking STI testing or treatment); those who are immunocompromised; international travelers; prisoners; and workers in health care, public safety, and institutions (Nassar et al., 2023). These same individuals at high risk of contracting hepatitis B would benefit from the hepatitis B vaccine prior to pregnancy.

Human Papillomavirus

HPV is implicated in over 99 percent of cervical cancers as well as cancers of the vagina, vulva, anus, and oropharynx. The HPV vaccine significantly reduces the incidence of HPV and decreases the need for cervical procedures (e.g., loop electrosurgical excision procedure [LEEP]) which are associated with cervical incompetence, preterm birth, and labor dystocia (Dudley, 2018). The HPV vaccine is not recommended during pregnancy; however, studies have not found an increased risk of adverse pregnancy outcomes with inadvertent vaccination during pregnancy (Dousti et al., 2023). Currently it is recommended that adolescents receive a two-dose series of the HPV vaccine as part of their routine immunization schedule, with a catch-up series recommended for females through age 26 (Kim & Hunter, 2019). Thus, individuals aged 26 years and younger who have not been previously vaccinated or did not complete a valid vaccination series may be offered the HPV vaccine. For individuals aged 27 to 45 years, the decision to vaccinate would be based on the individual's preferences, considering their risk of new HPV infections and potential benefits of vaccination (ACOG, 2020). Vaccinating eligible individuals can prevent HPV-related cancers and reduce the need for procedures that may adversely affect pregnancy outcomes. Refer to Chapters 22 and 28 for additional information about HPV and associated cancers.

Varicella

Varicella, or chickenpox, is a common childhood virus that can be severe in adults and fatal in neonates. Individuals who acquire varicella during pregnancy can give birth to fetuses with neurological defects, microcephaly, limb and muscular atrophy, eye problems, scarring of the skin, and low birth weight (Dudley, 2018). A two-dose varicella vaccine series is part of the CDC-recommended childhood immunization schedule. Individuals with no history of infection or vaccination should receive the live varicella vaccine series prior to pregnancy and be counseled to avoid possible pregnancy for at least 1 month after each injection (Nassar et al., 2023). If individuals are inadvertently vaccinated during early pregnancy, no intervention is needed.

Influenza

Influenza during pregnancy is associated with serious health complications and increased rates of hospitalization (Grohskopf et al., 2018). Universal vaccination of pregnant people at all gestational ages is recommended to reduce the risk of complications and to possibly transmit passive immunity to the fetus (Grohskopf et al., 2018). Generally, the influenza vaccine is considered low risk, although, as in the general population, do not offer vaccination to those who have a history of severe allergic reaction to an influenza vaccine, current moderate to severe acute illness (with or without fever), or a history of Guillain-Barré syndrome (within 6 weeks after prior influenza vaccination). Few data exist on the safety of the influenza vaccine during the first trimester, so, if possible, preconception immunization is preferred to vaccination early in pregnancy (Grohskopf et al., 2018).

Tetanus, Diphtheria, and Pertussis

All patients who have not been vaccinated for tetanus, diphtheria, and pertussis (Tdap), or whose vaccination status is unknown, should receive a single dose of the Tdap vaccine (Nassar et al., 2023). In addition, it is recommended that every pregnant person receive a Tdap vaccine during every pregnancy between 27 and 36 weeks' gestation because it has been shown to decrease the risk of pertussis in infants. The vaccine is most effective at preventing infant pertussis when received during pregnancy instead of prior to or immediately following pregnancy (Baxter et al., 2017).

Pneumococcal Disease

Pneumonia, meningitis, and bacteremia are associated with the pneumococcal pneumoniae bacterium. These diseases carry a significant burden and additional complications in pregnancy. The CDC recommends that high-risk individuals be vaccinated. Risk factors include chronic heart, liver, or lung disease (including asthma); diabetes; cigarette smoking; immunodeficiencies; immunosuppressive therapies; asplenia; hemoglobinopathies; cerebral spinal leaks; and cochlear implants (Nassar et al., 2023).

Hepatitis A

Hepatitis A is an acute, self-limiting viral illness that can cause abdominal pain, jaundice, nausea, and fever. It is transmitted through the fecal–oral route through food and drink or close contact with infected persons. The CDC recommends that high-risk adults be vaccinated. These include travelers to endemic areas; exposure to individuals with hepatitis A infection (e.g., international adoptee) or biological samples; individuals experiencing homelessness; injection or noninjection drug use; and those with chronic liver disease or clotting factor disorders (Nelson et al., 2020).

Meningococcal Disease

Meningitis infection carries a high risk of morbidity and significant mortality. The CDC recommends that individuals at high risk be vaccinated. Risk factors include asplenia, including sickle cell disease; immunodeficiencies; complement factor deficiencies; eculizumab use; travel to hyperendemic regions; and those living in dormitories or military barracks (Nassar et al., 2023).

COVID-19

The CDC currently recommends that all pregnant people or those trying to conceive stay up-to-date with COVID-19 vaccination due to the increased risk for severe sickness during pregnancy.

Additionally, COVID-19 infection during pregnancy is associated with increased risk for hospitalization and ventilation, as well as increased risk of preterm birth and stillbirth. For those who have not been previously vaccinated, a two-shot mRNA series is recommended with doses at least two months apart. For those who have previously completed a multi-dose mRNA series, a single yearly vaccination is recommended (CDC, 2024). Studies have not found any association between COVID-19 vaccination and increased risks of miscarriage, birth defects or pregnancy complications (Fleming-Dutra et al., 2023; Prasad et al., 2022).

Dental Care and Hygiene

Periodontal disease, characterized by inflammation and infection of the gums and supporting structures of the teeth, has been associated with adverse pregnancy outcomes. Because pathogens from the oral cavity and inflammatory mediators are believed to enter the systemic circulation, it is believed that they may lead to reduced fertility and increased rates of preterm birth, low birth weight, and preeclampsia. A recent systematic review and meta-analysis reported higher rates of these outcomes in pregnant women with periodontal disease (Daalderop et al., 2018).

The effect of dental disease on pregnancy outcomes is modest and varies by population and study design; findings are also confounded by socioeconomic status, race and ethnicity, and maternal tobacco and drug use (Sanz & Kornman, 2013). Moreover, the treatment of periodontal disease in pregnancy has shown mixed results regarding birth outcomes with some studies suggesting reduction of risk and other studies finding no significant effect (Lopez et al., 2019). This may indicate that dental care during pregnancy is too late to modify the early gestational environment. However, it is reasonable to recommend regular dental care to all patients, especially those considering pregnancy within the next year, to improve maternal health status, minimize potential fetal exposure to procedural medications, and minimize childhood exposure to caries-producing bacteria transmitted from parent to child through common interactions (e.g., kissing, sharing spoons).

ASSESSMENT AND MANAGEMENT OF INFECTION RISK

Sexually Transmitted Infections

Untreated STIs can cause infertility and increase an individual's risk of contracting HIV (American College of Obstetricians and Gynecologists & Society for Maternal–Fetal Medicine, 2019). STIs are also associated with increased rates of preterm birth. All individuals should be offered routine screening and subsequent treatment per CDC guidelines as a part of preconception care. Patients diagnosed with STIs should be counseled on partner treatment, which may be facilitated if possible. Please refer to Chapter 22 for more information about STIs.

ASSESSMENT OF HEALTH CONDITIONS AND MEDICATIONS THAT MAY IMPACT FERTILITY OR PREGNANCY

As the rate of pregnancy rises among individuals older than 35, and as the general health of people in the United States worsens, the number of pregnant people with chronic diseases is increasing. Preconception care strategies for those with chronic illnesses include optimizing disease control in preparation for pregnancy, switching potentially teratogenic medications to those with a better safety profile in pregnancy, and/or prescribing effective contraception to avoid pregnancy.

Body Size

Research shows that individuals living in larger bodies have higher rates of anovulation, infertility, subfertility, and early miscarriage (Boxem et al., 2024). There is also an increased risk of pregnancies affected by congenital anomalies, including neural tube defects, cardiovascular anomalies, limb reduction defects, and cleft palate (Huang et al., 2017; Parnell et al., 2017). Two recent systematic reviews concluded that maternal obesity is associated with an increased risk of pregnancy-related morbidity including gestational diabetes, hypertensive disorders, large-for-gestational-age infants, delivery-related complications, metabolic syndrome, and preterm birth (Helsehurst et al., 2022; Weir et al., 2024). Pregnant people with larger bodies are also more likely to experience stillbirth, perinatal death, and infant death, with risk increasing as body size and gestational age increase. They are also at higher risk of birth trauma, postpartum hemorrhage, cesarean birth, and subsequent wound infection (Zhang et al., 2024), as well as postpartum venous thromboembolism (VTE), more breastfeeding difficulties, and higher rates of depression (Nommsen-Rivers et al., 2023).

However, it is critical to recognize that many of these poor outcomes are not solely attributable to body size itself. A growing body of evidence highlights the significant role of weight stigma and provider bias in shaping health outcomes for people living in larger bodies. Weight stigma in healthcare settings can lead to delayed or inadequate care, reduced patient trust, and avoidance of medical services, all of which may contribute to adverse pregnancy outcomes. Provider bias may also result in over-attribution of symptoms to weight, under-treatment of medical concerns, and less patient-centered communication. These systemic issues can compound the physiological risks associated with higher body weight, creating a cycle of disadvantage that is not biological in origin (Olson et al., 2024).

Counseling patients to optimize their health prior to pregnancy is complex because weight loss is challenging, and methods take months or years, if they work at all. This puts weight loss goals at odds with goals related to the timing of conception and potential waning fertility. There is also significant bias against people living in larger bodies in society and in health care. For these and many other reasons, body size may be a sensitive topic for patients. Clinicians should ask the patient for permission to discuss weight and BMI prior to initiating counseling. Recommendations must be personalized to address patient concerns and to work toward achievable goals (Olson et al., 2024).

Preconception counseling should focus on the promotion of fertility-supporting behaviors such as moderate physical activity, consuming a nutrient-dense diet, and minimizing chronic stress. Weight alone is a poor proxy for health and thus a holistic approach is needed to promote optimal cardiometabolic health in the preconception period. Furthermore, the quality of the diet and activity level influence overall health and fertility more directly than body size. Patients should be screened for nutritional deficiencies and excesses using a validated screening tool, such as a food frequency questionnaire or a 24-hour diet recall. If highly processed foods and/or added sugars are prevalent in the diet, counsel the patient to make substitutions, such as drinking water or seltzer instead of a soft drink with meals and having oatmeal instead of sugary cereal. Refer to the previous sections about nutrition and exercise in this chapter for additional guidelines.

Hypertension

Individuals with chronic hypertension are at greater risk of pregnancy complications, including preeclampsia, iatrogenic preterm birth, placental abruption, and growth-restricted fetuses. Moreover, pregnant individuals with chronic hypertension are 5 to 6 times more likely to experience cardiovascular accidents, pulmonary edema, and renal failure (ACOG, 2019c).

Preconception care for those with chronic hypertension includes gathering a history focused on past pregnancy outcomes, duration of hypertension, prior use of antihypertensive medications, and previous related complications, including transient ischemic attack or stroke (Chahine & Sibai, 2019). Hypertension that has been poorly controlled despite treatment requires evaluation for underlying cause. Laboratory testing is indicated to assess for conditions that are associated with chronic hypertension, such as diabetes, dyslipidemia, and thyroid dysfunction. Further testing may be indicated for individuals with a history of uncontrolled hypertension, including an echocardiogram, assessment of renal function with a serum creatinine and spot urine protein-to-creatinine ratio or 24-hour urine protein, and referral for evaluation of retinopathy (Chahine & Sibai, 2019).

First-line management for chronic hypertension involves lifestyle modification, including support for tobacco cessation, following the DASH (Dietary Approaches to Stop Hypertension) diet, and engaging in increased physical activity (Wenger, 2019). In addition to being effective at reducing systolic and diastolic blood pressure, these lifestyle improvements have a range of other positive effects for fertility, pregnancy, and long-term health.

People with chronic hypertension who are considering pregnancy or not using an effective method of contraception should avoid using certain antihypertensive medications. Angiotensin-converting enzyme (ACE) inhibitors and angiotensin receptor blockers are contraindicated in pregnancy due to the risk of fetal malformations and growth restriction (ACOG, 2019c). Labetalol and nifedipine are the preferred antihypertensive medications in pregnancy. Methyldopa may also be used, but it is generally considered less effective and has a greater side effect profile. If an ACE inhibitor must be used, consultation with a maternal–fetal medicine specialist is indicated. Avoiding smoking and excessive sodium and caffeine is recommended. Individuals with chronic hypertension are at risk of developing preeclampsia in subsequent pregnancies and starting low-dose aspirin between 12 and 16 weeks' gestation may decrease their risk of preeclampsia (ACOG, 2019c).

Diabetes

Pregestational diabetes carries significant increased risk for pregnancy, specifically when not well controlled. Those with pregestational diabetes (type 1 or type 2) are at significantly higher risk of preeclampsia, preterm birth, cesarean section, congenital anomalies, large for gestational age, stillbirth and NICU admission, compared with individuals diagnosed with gestational diabetes, though these two groups have similar rates of low APGAR scores and neonatal hypoglycemia (Malaza et al., 2022). Tight glycemic control prior to pregnancy is essential because fetal malformations occur in rates directly proportional to elevations in maternal hemoglobin A1C. These malformations include anencephaly, microcephaly, cardiac malformations, and caudal regression syndrome (American Diabetes Association, 2019). A hemoglobin A1C less than 6.5 percent is associated with the lowest risk of anomalies (American College of Obstetricians and Gynecologists & Society for Maternal–Fetal Medicine, 2019). All pregnant-capable people with diabetes should be educated on the risks of unplanned pregnancy in the context of poor glycemic control, the need to seek care immediately when they become pregnant, and the availability of effective contraception until they are ready for pregnancy. The American Diabetes Association Standards of Medical Care strongly recommends that preconception counseling be integrated into all primary care encounters with adolescent girls living with diabetes (American Diabetes Association, 2018). Preconception counseling resources aimed at adolescents are available through the American Diabetes Association (www.diabetes.org).

Preconception care for individuals with diabetes includes laboratory testing (hemoglobin A1C, thyroid-stimulating hormone [TSH], creatinine, and urine protein–creatinine ratio). Those with diabetes are at risk for vasculopathy, and pregnancy may cause the development or progression of diabetic retinopathy; a dilated eye examination is indicated prior to pregnancy (American Diabetes Association, 2019). Similarly, an electrocardiogram is recommended to assess for underlying cardiovascular damage (ACOG, 2019a). Review medications for comorbid conditions, such as hyperlipidemia or hypertension, and discontinue ACE inhibitors, angiotensin receptor blockers, and statins prior to pregnancy (American College of Obstetricians and Gynecologists & Society for Maternal–Fetal Medicine, 2019). Patients with diabetes are at risk of developing preeclampsia in subsequent pregnancies; starting low-dose aspirin between 12 and 16 weeks' gestation may decrease their risk of preeclampsia (ACOG, 2019b).

The first trimester of pregnancy is a time of increased insulin sensitivity, and individuals with preexisting diabetes, particularly type 1 diabetes, may need lower amounts of insulin to achieve target glycemic levels. Clinicians should counsel patients with preexisting type 1 and type 2 diabetes to check their fasting and postprandial blood sugars after pregnancy is confirmed and to seek health care as soon as possible for blood sugar monitoring and management (American Diabetes Association, 2019). Type 2 diabetes is often associated with larger body size. Counseling for patients with type 2 diabetes includes information on weight gain recommendations and the importance of diet and exercise in maintaining glucose control and optimizing pregnancy outcomes.

Polycystic Ovary Syndrome

PCOS is a leading cause of infertility. It is characterized by hyperandrogenism, ovulatory dysfunction, and polycystic ovaries. Clinicians should suspect PCOS in any patient reporting irregular menses and consider screening due to a high prevalence of infertility among individuals with PCOS. In the United States, there is a strong correlation between larger body size and PCOS; indeed, even modest weight loss has been shown to normalize ovulatory function, restore fertility, and decrease a person's risk for diabetes and cardiovascular disease. Inform patients with

PCOS that fertility assistance, particularly with ovulation induction medications, may be needed to achieve pregnancy. First-line medications for PCOS management in the context of desired conception include metformin and inositol, with recent systematic reviews demonstrating that inositol is not inferior to metformin in improving ovulatory cycles amongst this population, with fewer undesirable side effects (Greff et al., 2023). However, the goal of preconception care is to emphasize the importance of a healthy diet and exercise, and to promote other healthy preconception behaviors, such as smoking cessation and reduced alcohol use (ACOG, 2018c). Because of the association between PCOS and metabolic syndrome, screen patients with PCOS for type 2 diabetes (with tight glycemic control ideally established prior to pregnancy) and cardiovascular risk factors. Refer to Chapter 26 for more information about PCOS.

Thyroid Disease

The American Thyroid Association considers some individuals at higher risk of thyroid dysfunction during pregnancy and recommends preconception screening with a serum TSH (refer to **Box 30-8**). Hypothyroidism is defined as the presence of an elevated TSH level and a decreased T4 level; subclinical hypothyroidism is defined as a normal TSH level with a low T4 level. Untreated hypothyroidism during pregnancy is associated with adverse outcomes, including infertility, miscarriage, preeclampsia, preterm birth, placental abruption, and perinatal death, and potential cognitive impairments in offspring (Zhang et al., 2021).

BOX 30-8 Preconception Thyroid-Stimulating Hormone Screening Indications

- History of thyroid dysfunction
- Symptoms of thyroid dysfunction: Fatigue, constipation, cold intolerance, dry skin, weight gain, periorbital edema, hair loss, hoarseness, memory impairment, bradycardia, delayed relaxation of deep tendon reflexes
- Presence of a goiter
- Known thyroid antibody positive
- Age 30 years and older
- History of type 1 diabetes or other autoimmune disorder
- History of infertility, pregnancy loss, or preterm birth
- History of head or neck radiation or prior thyroid surgery
- Family history of autoimmune thyroid disease or thyroid dysfunction
- BMI greater than 40
- Use of amiodarone, lithium, or recent administration of iodinated radiologic contrast
- History of two or more prior pregnancies
- Residing in an area of moderate to severe iodine deficiency

Data from Alexander, E. K., Pearce, E. N., Brent, G. A., Brown, R. S., Chen, H., Dosiou, C., Grobman, W. A., Laurberg, P., Lazarus, J. H., Mandel, S. J., Peeters, R. P., & Sullivan, S. (2017). 2017 guidelines of the American Thyroid Association for the diagnosis and management of thyroid disease during pregnancy and the postpartum. *Thyroid, 27*(3), 315–389. https://doi.org/10.1089 /thy.2016.0457

Evaluation of TSH levels is recommended for pregnant-capable people seeking care for infertility, and levothyroxine (LT4) is indicated for individuals with overt hypothyroidism (Alexander et al., 2017). Insufficient evidence exists on whether to treat those with subclinical hypothyroidism who are attempting to conceive as recent systematic reviews have found no clear benefit (Maraka et al., 2016). Refer to Chapter 20 for additional information.

Levothyroxine, a synthetic version of the T4 hormone, is the recommended treatment, with therapy titrated to achieve TSH levels of 2.5 or lower (Alexander et al., 2017). The majority of patients with hypothyroidism will need levothyroxine dose increases during pregnancy. Usually, an empiric adjustment of 25 to 30 percent is recommended as soon as pregnancy is diagnosed, with instructions to immediately notify the healthcare provider for further testing and treatment. The American Thyroid Association recommends counseling individuals to increase their levothyroxine dosage by two tablets weekly upon a positive pregnancy test until they see a healthcare provider (Alexander et al., 2017).

Hyperthyroidism affects less than 0.5 percent of pregnancies, with the majority caused by Graves' disease (Kobaly & Mandel, 2019). Poorly controlled Graves' disease has been associated with pregnancy loss, hypertensive disorders of pregnancy, medically induced prematurity and associated low birth weight, intrauterine growth restriction, stillbirth, thyroid storm, and congestive heart failure (Kobaly & Mandel, 2019). Ideally, patients are euthyroid for several months before conceiving. Methimazole and propylthiouracil are commonly used to treat hyperthyroidism during pregnancy. However, both medications have been associated with birth defects. Studies have found that methimazole use during the first trimester is linked to a higher rate of birth defects, including facial dysmorphia, cutis aplasia, choanal and esophageal atresia, abdominal wall defects and ventricular septal defects (Seo et al., 2018). Propylthiouracil, once considered safe in pregnancy, has also been associated with birth defects, including facial and neck cysts and urinary tract abnormalities in males (Alexander et al., 2017). Additionally, propylthiouracil carries a risk of liver failure, leading the U.S. Food and Drug Administration to issue a black box warning (Alexander et al., 2017).

Recent studies suggest that propylthiouracil is associated with a lower risk of birth defects compared to methimazole (Zhang et al., 2023). During the preconception period, euthyroid patients with mild disease may discontinue medication through the first trimester, or they can switch to propylthiouracil in anticipation of pregnancy (Alexander et al., 2017; Kobaly & Mandel, 2019). Patients may also elect to undergo thyroidectomy or iodine ablation. If this course is chosen, they may be treated with levothyroxine and are ideally euthyroid prior to pregnancy. Avoiding pregnancy for 6 months after radioactive iodine ablation is recommended (Alexander et al., 2017; Kobaly & Mandel, 2019). Although individuals may be generally counseled on these options during the preconception period, their endocrinologist will be responsible for management decisions.

Seizure Disorder

More than 500,000 pregnant-capable people of childbearing age have epilepsy and take antiepileptic drugs as first-line treatment (Barnard & French, 2019). The goal of treatment during pregnancy is to minimize the risk of fetal medication exposure while ensuring that symptoms remain controlled. Seizures during pregnancy are dangerous for both the individual and the fetus, and they are associated with fetal hypoxia and bradycardia, preeclampsia, preterm labor, low birth weight, stillbirth, and developmental delays (Li & Meador, 2022). Additionally, pregnant people with epilepsy face increased risks of obstetric complications such as spontaneous abortion, antepartum hemorrhage, gestational hypertension, preeclampsia, breech position, induction of labor, cesarean delivery, and preterm birth (Li & Meador, 2022).

Several antiepileptic drugs are known teratogens. Valproic acid, phenobarbital, phenytoin, and carbamazepine (at doses greater than 700 mg/day) are associated with the highest risk of major congenital malformations (Bromley et al., 2017). Valproic acid and phenobarbital are associated with cardiac defects and oral clefts; valproic acid is significantly associated with neural tube defects. Long-term cognitive delays have been associated with valproic acid, phenobarbital, and phenytoin (Nucera et al., 2022). Polytherapy, especially regimens that include valproic acid and carbamazepine, is associated with greater malformations than monotherapies. Lamotrigine is associated with the lowest rates of malformations, especially at daily doses of 325 mg or less (Barnard & French, 2019; Bromley et al., 2017).

Optimally, individuals with epilepsy who desire pregnancy will discuss medication management during pregnancy with a neurologist. Valproic acid should generally be avoided unless there is no alternative. Monotherapy in the lowest therapeutic dose is recommended (American College of Obstetricians and Gynecologists & Society for Maternal–Fetal Medicine, 2019). Due to changes in drug metabolism during pregnancy, it can be difficult to maintain therapeutic drug levels, particularly for lamotrigine, which is the least teratogenic antiepileptic medication (Barnard & French, 2019). Counsel patients to seek care as soon as they discover they are pregnant because they must be monitored frequently during pregnancy. Folate has been found to mitigate the effects of antiepileptic drugs on a developing fetus, but only if this supplementation occurs prior to conception. In a survey of women who have epilepsy and are of childbearing age, almost 80 percent reported an unintended pregnancy (Herzog et al., 2017). Thus, all individuals who have epilepsy and reproductive potential should be counseled to take folate, regardless of their intentions for pregnancy.

Inherited Thrombophilias

Up to 2 percent of pregnant people will experience a VTE, and VTEs contribute to almost 10 percent of pregnancy-related deaths (ACOG, 2018e). Those with inherited thrombophilias are at higher risk of VTE. It is unclear whether individuals with inherited thrombophilias are at higher risk of other pregnancy-related complications, such as preeclampsia, growth restriction, placental abruption, and stillbirth; the primary benefit of screening for inherited thrombophilias in pregnancy is to reduce the risk of VTE and pulmonary embolism (ACOG, 2018e). Even if a causal link were established between thrombophilias and adverse perinatal outcomes, there is no evidence that treatment improves outcomes; thus, universal screening is not indicated.

Screening for thrombophilia (or referral to maternal–fetal medicine or hematology) is recommended in patients with a personal history of VTE or a first-degree relative with a high-risk thrombophilia (refer to **Box 30-9**) (American College of Obstetricians and Gynecologists & Society for Maternal–Fetal Medicine, 2019). Treatment during pregnancy is guided by estimated risk of VTE, with high-risk thrombophilias defined as having a 3 percent or greater risk of VTE in pregnancy. These include homozygous factor V Leiden and antithrombin, protein C, and protein S deficiencies (ACOG, 2018e). Low-molecular-weight heparin is recommended during pregnancy and for 6 weeks postpartum in women with high-risk thrombophilias and in individuals with low-risk thrombophilias with a personal or family history of VTE or other risk factors. This therapy should be started as soon as pregnancy is confirmed (ACOG, 2018e). Counsel patients who are on anticoagulation treatment with warfarin prior to pregnancy to switch to low-molecular-weight heparin by 6 weeks' gestation (American College of Obstetricians and Gynecologists & Society for Maternal–Fetal Medicine, 2019). The involvement of a hematologist or maternal–fetal medicine specialist can assist in the development of a plan for thromboprophylaxis during pregnancy.

BOX 30-9 Screening Tests to Perform for Individuals With a Personal History of Venous Thromboembolism or a First-Degree Relative With a High-Risk Thrombophilia

Factor V Leiden mutation
Prothrombin G20210A mutation
Antithrombin deficiency
Protein S deficiency
Protein C deficiency
Antiphospholipid antibodies

HIV

Individuals living with HIV need preconception counseling woven into all of their clinical encounters to minimize the risk of perinatal HIV infection. Preconception counseling includes how to reduce the risk of perinatal transmission, potential risks of antiretroviral medication on fetal development, and strategies to enhance overall health and well-being (ACOG, 2016, reaffirmed 2019). Individuals with HIV may have complicated social situations or medical comorbidities, including substance use, mental illness, or interpersonal violence, that require special attention. In general, a team-based approach to care is preferred; in the preconception planning period, this team may include an infectious disease specialist, perinatal care provider, maternal–fetal medicine specialist, primary care provider, social worker, and psychiatric provider, as needed.

Ideally, patients with HIV are stable on antiretroviral therapy and have an undetectable plasma viral load prior to attempting to conceive. Pregnant people with uncontrolled HIV or those who are not on antiretroviral therapy are at risk for poor perinatal outcomes, including preterm birth, newborns who have low birth weight or are small for gestational age, and perinatal fetal demise. Additionally, adverse pregnancy outcomes among HIV-positive people on antiretroviral therapy remain elevated when compared to HIV-negative people (Tukei et al., 2021). Individuals who are HIV positive, and those who are HIV negative but have a partner who is HIV positive, may benefit from fertility specialists and advanced reproductive technologies when and if they desire to have a child. Guidelines from ACOG and the American Society for Reproductive Medicine underscore the importance of treating HIV as a chronic illness that should not disqualify people from seeking or receiving fertility treatments (ACOG, 2016, reaffirmed 2019; Ethics Committee of American Society for Reproductive Medicine, 2015). Refer these couples to a specialist in infectious disease or reproductive endocrinology and infertility for counseling and to develop a plan of care. Unknown infertility will increase the number of attempts at conception and potential exposure to HIV if one partner is HIV negative; therefore, a basic evaluation for infertility may be recommended prior to the couple's attempts to conceive.

Mental Health Disorders

Most mental health disruptions and disorders in individuals emerge during the childbearing years, with peak incidence of depression, anxiety, bipolar disorder, and schizophrenia spectrum disorders between puberty and 40 years of age (Solmi et al., 2022). Clinicians should screen all patients for depression and other mental health disorders at primary care, well-person, and preconception visits (USPSTF, 2023). In a preconception mental health screening, ask about a family history of mood and psychotic disorders and a personal history of depression, psychosis, and mania (ACOG, 2019a, reaffirmed 2024). The USPSTF recommends using a validated instrument, such as the Edinburgh Postnatal Depression Scale or the Patient Health Questionnaire-9 (Maurer et al., 2018). Patients who screen positive should receive an in-depth psychiatric assessment to ensure accurate diagnosis; clinicians should be prepared to initiate treatment or facilitate a referral to a qualified professional, or both (Maurer et al., 2018; USPSTF, 2023). Refer to Chapter 9 for additional information about depression screening.

Many patients taking psychotropic medication (e.g., antidepressants, mood stabilizers, antipsychotics, stimulants) are justifiably concerned about the effects of these medications on a developing fetus and perinatal outcomes more generally. Unfortunately, the data pertaining to psychotropic medication use in pregnancy are complicated because it can be difficult to separate the effects of the disease itself from the effects of the medication. Many of the effects attributed to medication use are also found with untreated disease. Moreover, the confounding effects of age, parity, larger body size, tobacco and other substance use, the use of multiple psychotropic drugs, and other medical and behavioral comorbidities are difficult to control. In addition, patients may not take the medication as prescribed, which can inaccurately reflect the treatment effect in studies (Pavlik & Rosculet, 2020). The National Curriculum for Reproductive Psychiatry provides free resources and educational materials for clinicians on how to best approach risk conversations about psychiatric medications use in pregnancy. These resources can be found at https://ncrptraining.org/.

Ideally, patients are stable with or without medication for a period of time prior to attempting conception. Every person trying to decide whether to continue or discontinue medication therapy in pregnancy needs an individualized risk assessment, either from the clinician conducting the visit, a trained mental health professional, or as part of an interprofessional team with perinatal and mental healthcare providers. This risk assessment takes into account the frequency and severity of past episodes, the person's prior response to medications and psychotherapy, any prior attempts to discontinue medication, and their wishes regarding medication use in pregnancy (Chisolm & Payne, 2016; Meltzer-Brody & Jones, 2015). Counsel patients on the risk of relapse and subsequent occupational and personal burden (Thomson & Sharma, 2018). For patients with moderate to severe illness and a high probability of relapse, remaining on medication may be the best choice (Chisolm & Payne, 2016; Kimmel et al., 2018). Many people on psychotropic medications discontinue use upon finding out they are pregnant; part of preconception care involves making a plan for medication use or discontinuation and relapse prevention during pregnancy. For more information, refer to the discussion of psychotropic medications in pregnancy later in this section.

If a patient desires to discontinue or switch medications, these adjustments are best done prior to pregnancy to minimize fetal exposure to multiple medications, ensure adequate treatment response, and monitor for relapse. However, recent guidelines caution against discontinuing effective pharmacotherapy solely due to pregnancy, as this may increase the risk of relapse. A slow tapering of medication is recommended to avoid withdrawal symptoms (Kimmel et al., 2018). It may also be possible to use "drug holidays" strategically, depending on the mechanism and half-life of the medication. In these situations, the patient may, for example, take the medication Monday through Thursday and abstain Friday through Sunday. Those who desire to discontinue their medication can be counseled that reintroducing medication after the first trimester or immediately postpartum is possible if symptoms reemerge during pregnancy or as a strategy to prevent onset of symptoms postpartum. Behavioral therapies, such as cognitive behavioral therapy, are strongly recommended as an adjunct in pregnancy, especially for anyone considering medication discontinuation. These therapies provide effective nonpharmacologic options to manage symptoms and reduce relapse risk (Molenaar et al., 2020).

Perinatal mood disorders can become difficult to treat, especially postpartum. Sleep disruption and hormone fluctuations can contribute to severe mood symptoms and postpartum psychosis. All individuals with a risk for perinatal mood disorders should be followed closely through pregnancy and postpartum (Kimmel et al., 2018). Encourage patients, and ideally their partner and/or family members, to create a plan for relapse prevention and monitoring. This should attempt to optimize the protective factors and support systems, strategize for optimal sleep and nutrition practices, decrease stressors, and outline a plan for intervention if the individual or their family members identify a recurrence of symptoms. Psychiatric co-management is recommended for those with moderate to severe illness or those requiring multiple medications for optimal disease control (Kimmel et al., 2018).

Psychotropic Medications

Antidepressant Medications SSRIs are the most studied antidepressants in pregnancy and are considered first-line treatment in pregnancy for both depression and anxiety. The exception is paroxetine, which has been linked in some studies to an increased risk of cardiac defects (Kimmel et al., 2018). Several meta-analyses have found no increased risk of birth defects when SSRIs are taken in the first trimester; however, there may be a small increase in the incidence of rare defects (Turner et al., 2019). Bupropion is also generally considered safe in pregnancy (Lebin & Novick, 2022), although it may confer a small increased risk of cardiac defects when used in the first trimester. Data on tricyclic antidepressants are limited and conflicting, with most studies suggesting no increased risk of malformations (Turner et al., 2019).

Some studies have found associations between SSRI use and miscarriage, preterm birth, and newborns who are small for gestational age. However, depression has also been linked to those outcomes, so it is unclear whether those adverse outcomes are linked to the medication, the illness, or both (Kimmel et al., 2018). Most experts agree that there is a small increased absolute risk of persistent pulmonary hypertension in newborns exposed to SSRIs in utero (adjusted odds ratio of 1.28 for SSRIs vs. 1.14 for non-SSRIs); there is also a slight risk of medication withdrawal and poor neonatal adaptation syndrome (Kimmel et al., 2018). SNRIs have a similar safety profile as SSRIs (Kimmel et al., 2018). Very little data are available concerning the maternal and neonatal risks of tricyclic antidepressants, monoamine oxidase inhibitors, and trazodone.

Valproate and Carbamazepine Both valproate and carbamazepine are teratogenic, known to cause neural tube defects and developmental delays, and are not recommended for pregnant-capable individuals of childbearing age (Grande et al., 2016). Patients who remain on these medications in the first trimester should supplement with 4 mg of folic acid daily.

Lithium and Lamotrigine Lithium and lamotrigine have been shown to be relatively safe in pregnancy, although lithium is associated with a slight increase in the overall risk of cardiac anomalies (Shea et al., 2024).

Antipsychotic Medications There are significantly more safety data on the use of first-generation antipsychotics than second-generation (atypical) antipsychotics, and for this reason they are considered first-line treatment in pregnancy. In general, high-potency typical antipsychotics (e.g., haloperidol) are considered less teratogenic than low-potency typical antipsychotics (e.g., chlorpromazine) (Breadon & Kulkarni, 2019). Because few long-term studies have been conducted with children exposed to second-generation antipsychotics, ACOG does not currently recommend their use in pregnancy. For patients taking atypical antipsychotics who have an unplanned pregnancy, a risk and benefit analysis may suggest that continuation of the medication is superior to exposing the fetus to a second medication (ACOG, 2008, reaffirmed 2018). If a person has a history of poor response to first-generation antipsychotics or is at high risk of relapse with medication discontinuation, continuation of their current regime is recommended (Breadon & Kulkarni, 2019; Tosato et al., 2017).

More safety data are emerging as the better-tolerated second-generation antipsychotics become more widely used, and studies suggest that if a risk of major congenital malformations exists, it is slight (Clark & Wisner, 2018). Most recent data do not indicate any major teratogenic risk for atypical antipsychotics. An older but important systematic review found that fetuses exposed to second-generation antipsychotics had a greater incidence of malformations, compared to those who were not exposed, but there was no difference between those exposed to first- versus second-generation drugs (Coughlin et al., 2015; Tosato et al., 2017). Cardiac defects—primarily atrial and ventricular septal defects—are the primary malformation associated with antipsychotic exposure, and these defects are not considered major. A detection bias has been suggested because individuals exposed to these medications may receive more in-depth screening for fetal abnormalities than unexposed people (for example, echocardiograms may be recommended more frequently) (Tosato et al., 2017).

Attention Deficit Hyperactivity Disorder Medications

Stimulant medications are first-line treatment for attention deficit hyperactivity disorder (ADHD). These include methylphenidate (Ritalin) or amphetamine derivatives (Adderall, Vyvanse). The use of ADHD medication has not been linked to any significant adverse outcomes for the woman or infant. Emerging data suggest that infants gestationally exposed to amphetamine derivatives are at increased risk of central nervous system disorders (e.g., seizures), preterm birth, and NICU admission, but confounding factors in the literature include polypharmacy with other psychotropic medications (Jiang et al., 2019; Norby et al., 2017). Congenital malformations do not seem to be associated with medication exposure, although methylphenidate has been associated with an increased risk of miscarriage (Jiang et al., 2019; Norby et al., 2017). Long-term neurodevelopmental outcomes are unknown.

Bupropion is a nonstimulant medication that has been used to treat both depression and ADHD. It is reasonable to attempt treatment during pregnancy with bupropion alone; however, it is not as efficacious as stimulants in treating ADHD symptoms (Baker & Freeman, 2018). However, any new drug trial should ideally be done prior to pregnancy to ensure efficacy and avoid exposing the fetus to multiple medications.

ASSESSMENT AND COUNSELING RELATED TO PERINATAL HISTORY

Interpregnancy care encompasses postpartum, well-person, and primary care provided after and between pregnancies. Because complications in one pregnancy can signal risks for future pregnancies or long-term health issues, it is essential for clinicians to provide follow-up care that includes education, preventive strategies, and early interventions. **Table 30-2** outlines key counseling topics, summarizes the core content to address with patients, and highlights findings that may require more detailed history taking and targeted counseling.

Partner's Health and Lifestyle

Preconception clinical care, research, and recommendations have historically focused on the pregnant-capable person However, it is increasingly recognized that the health and lifestyle of the partner—regardless of gender—can significantly influence fertility, pregnancy outcomes, and the well-being of the pregnant person and fetus. Clinicians should routinely address the health of all partners, including those who do not identify as male, as part of comprehensive reproductive care.

Attention is increasingly being paid to the contribution of the male partner or donor of sperm to the overall health of the fetus, the pregnancy, and the pregnant person. The goals of preconception care for everyone are similar: to optimize outcomes of their reproductive and sexual choices, mitigate the negative consequences of unhealthy lifestyle behaviors, counsel on pregnancy timing, identify and address possible fertility issues, and support healthy pregnancies and postpartum periods for their partners and children (Wilkes, 2016). Clinicians should screen all patients for their reproductive intentions. This allows for the opportunity

TABLE 30-2 Assessment and Counseling Related to Perinatal History

Topic	Counseling Content	Findings Warranting Further Investigation and Specific Counseling
Interpregnancy Spacing	Optimal spacing is 18–60 months; short intervals linked to more adverse outcomes.	Spacing < 18 months; unintended pregnancies; lack of postpartum contraception.
History of Preterm Birth	Prior preterm birth increases risk; short intervals worsen the risk.	Short intervals after preterm birth; lack of awareness; desire for quick conception.
Miscarriage	Recurrent losses warrant evaluation; conditions like antiphospholipid syndrome (APS), diabetes, polycystic ovarian syndrome (PCOS) increase risk.	≥ 2 early losses; fetal loss > 10 weeks; uncontrolled diabetes; obesity; PCOS.
Cesarean Birth	Recommend ≥ 18 months between cesarean and next birth to reduce risks.	Short intervals post-cesarean; planning TOLAC with short spacing.
Gestational Diabetes	History increases type 2 diabetes risk; screen every 1–3 years.	No recent diabetes screening; larger body size; poor diet/exercise habits.
Preeclampsia	History increases recurrence risk; manage BP and consider aspirin.	Uncontrolled hypertension; use of unsafe antihypertensives; no aspirin plan.
Perinatal Mood Disorders	History increases recurrence; screen and stabilize before conception.	Untreated mood disorders; no mental health plan; not euthymic preconception.
Venous Thromboembolism (VTE)	History increases recurrence; evaluate for thrombophilia; prophylaxis needed.	No thrombophilia workup; no anticoagulation plan; unmanaged VTE history.
History of Neural Tube Defect or Genetic Disorder	Supplement folate preconception; refer for genetic counseling.	No folate supplementation; no genetic counseling after affected pregnancy.

Data from Information for interpregnancy spacing from: American College of Obstetricians and Gynecologists & Society for Maternal-Fetal Medicine, 2019, reaffirmed 2021; Tessema et al, 2021.

Information for History of Preterm Birth from Koullali et al., 2017; Leaverton et al., 2016.

Information for Miscarriage from: ACOG, 2018f, reaffirmed 2025; ACOG, 2012b, reaffirmed 2019; ACOG, 2012b, reaffirmed 2019.

Information for Cesarean Birth from: American College of Obstetricians and Gynecologists & Society for Maternal-Fetal Medicine, 2019; Adily et al., 2025.

Information for Gestational Diabetes from McCarthy et al., 2023; American College of Obstetricians and Gynecologists & Society for Maternal-Fetal Medicine, 2019.

Information for Preeclampsia from ACOG, 2019b.

Information for Perinatal Mood Disorders from Stevens et al., 2019; USPSTF, 2023.

Information for Venous Thromboembolism from ACOG, 2018d

Information for History of Neural Tube Defect or Genetic Disorders from U.S. Preventive Services Task Force 2017.

to focus the conversation on ways to prevent pregnancy, the potential consequences of unprotected sex, and to promote health through screening and counseling.

Personal and Family History

Several health conditions are associated with decreased sperm count and quality, including STIs, diabetes, body size, and varicocele. Screening for and managing these conditions can contribute to overall fertility and the health of a potential pregnancy. Screening and treatment for STIs should also include discussion of safer sex practices and the impact of STIs on potential pregnancy and fertility (Wilkes, 2016; Khalafalla et al., 2023). Those with diabetes and/or larger bodies can benefit from targeted counseling, as glycemic control not only improves sperm quality and quantity but also reduces erectile dysfunction (George et al., 2024). Surgical correction of varicocele can increase sperm count and is more cost-effective than many assisted reproductive technologies (Masson & Brannigan, 2014).

Medications for chronic or acute health conditions can impair libido, erectile and ejaculatory function, and spermatogenesis. These include nifedipine, spironolactone, steroids, testosterone, colchicine, SSRIs, cimetidine, tetracyclines, allopurinol, phenytoin, opiates, and ketoconazole (Wilkes, 2016).

Clinicians should obtain a genetic history, including any personal or family history of birth defects. Several genetic disorders can impact fertility, including cystic fibrosis, Klinefelter syndrome, Kartagener syndrome, and polycystic kidney disease. Moreover, increasing paternal age and an associated decline in sperm quality has been strongly linked with increased risks of schizophrenia and autism (Nybo Andersen & Urhoj, 2017). Discussion of possible risks of infertility, genetic abnormalities, or age-related declines in sperm quality may impact a person's reproductive life planning, and anticipatory guidance for the involvement of genetic counselors or fertility specialists may be indicated.

Lifestyle

Optimizing health—including tobacco cessation, depression screening and treatment, healthy nutrition, adequate physical activity, and safer sexual practices—is important for all individuals who may become parents or support a pregnancy. Clinicians should address these topics with all partners, regardless of gender, as their health and behaviors can influence fertility, pregnancy outcomes, and the well-being of the pregnant person and child.

Counseling about healthy lifestyle practices can have a meaningful impact on a person's ability to parent and partner to the fullest capacity. For example, improving awareness of the importance of smoking cessation, healthy nutrition, and physical fitness in pregnancy can enhance a partner's contribution to and support for a healthy pregnancy. Substance use can also impair fertility; tobacco, alcohol, marijuana, and cocaine have all been shown to affect spermatogenesis (Duca et al., 2019). Moreover, substance use may make it more difficult for a pregnant partner to change their own substance use behaviors, which has implications for fetal and childhood health.

Chronic occupational exposure to metals, lead, mercury, radiation, heat, solvents, pesticides, and endocrine disruptors can affect the quality and quantity of sperm and result in pregnancies complicated by miscarriage or birth defects. Material safety data sheets can be obtained for any chemical exposure at work and reviewed for potential reproductive toxicity. Recreational exposure to chemicals may also affect spermatogenesis; these could include stripping chemicals, degreasers, or non-water-based glues used in refinishing furniture, repairing cars, or building models. In addition, chemicals used in woodworking, painting, pottery, stained glass, and gun handling and cleaning may also present a reproductive hazard. Regular use of hot tubs may also decrease sperm count (Wilkes, 2016).

Wellness visits are also an opportunity to screen partners for interpersonal violence in past and current relationships and to promote healthy and consensual sexual behaviors. Nutritional education and promotion of physical activity are important components of overall health, may play a role in fertility, and contribute to a healthier pregnancy. Stress reduction and mental health promotion can improve a person's general and cardiovascular health and also contribute to child well-being and development. Partners may be referred to psychosocial services, including behavioral counseling, social support services, and partner and parenting support when indicated. Refer to Chapter 10 for more information on male and AMAB individual health.

CONCLUSION

The preconception period is an opportune time for people to implement lifestyle and health behavior changes that can impact their long-term health, their experience of pregnancy, and the health of their future children. Clinicians can guide patients with information, encouragement, and health care to optimize their preconception health, which may have a more profound impact on maternal–child health status than interventions initiated after the pregnancy is established.

References

Adily, P., Bettison, T., Lauer, M., Narayan, R., Mackie, A., Phipps, H., Berghella, V., Haghighi, M. M., Perren, K., Johnson, G., & de Vries, B. (2025). Interpregnancy interval and uterine rupture during a trial of labour after one previous caesarean delivery and no previous vaginal births: A retrospective population-based cohort study. *eClinicalMedicine, 80*, 103071. https://doi.org/10.1016/j.eclinm.2025.103071

Alexander, E. K., Pearce, E. N., Brent, G. A., Brown, R. S., Chen, H., Dosiou, C., Grobman, W. A., Laurberg, P., Lazarus, J. H., Mandel, S. J., Peeters, R. P., & Sullivan, S. (2017). 2017 guidelines of the American Thyroid Association for the diagnosis and management of thyroid disease during pregnancy and the postpartum. *Thyroid, 27*(3), 315–389. https://doi.org/10.1089/thy.2016.0457

Amaral, M. E. B., Ejzenberg, D., Wajman, D. S., Monteleone, P. A. A., Serafini, P., Soares, J. M., Jr., & Baracat, E. C. (2019). Risk factors for inadequate response to ovarian stimulation in assisted reproduction cycles: Systematic review. *Journal of Assisted Reproduction and Genetics, 36*(1), 19–28. https://doi.org/10.1007/s10815-018- 1324-0

American College of Obstetricians and Gynecologists. (2008, reaffirmed 2018). ACOG practice bulletin: Clinical management guidelines for obstetrician–gynecologists number 92: Use of psychiatric medications during pregnancy and lactation. *Obstetrics & Gynecology, 111*(4), 1001–1020. https://doi.org/10.1097/AOG.0b013e31816fd910

American College of Obstetricians and Gynecologists Committee Opinion No. 762: Prepregnancy Counseling. (2019). *Obstetrics and gynecology, 133*(1), e78–e89. https://doi.org/10.1097/AOG.0000000000003013

American College of Obstetricians and Gynecologists. (2012a, reaffirmed 2019). ACOG committee opinion no. 518: Intimate partner violence. *Obstetrics & Gynecology, 119*(2 Pt. 1), 412–417. https://doi.org/10.1097/AOG.0b013e318249ff74

American College of Obstetricians and Gynecologists. (2012b, reaffirmed 2019). Practice bulletin no. 132: Antiphospholipid syndrome. *Obstetrics & Gynecology, 120*(6), 1514–1521. https://doi.org/10.1097/01.AOG.0000423816.39542.0f

American College of Obstetricians and Gynecologists. (2013a, reaffirmed 2019). ACOG committee opinion no. 554: Reproductive and sexual coercion. *Obstetrics & Gynecology, 121*(2 Pt. 1), 411–415. https://doi.org/10.1097/01.AOG.0000426427.79586.3b

American College of Obstetricians and Gynecologists. (2013b, reaffirmed 2024). ACOG committee opinion no. 575: Exposure to toxic environmental agents. *Fertility and Sterility, 100*(4), 931–935. https://doi.org/10.1097/01.AOG.0000435416.21944.54

American College of Obstetricians and Gynecologists. (2016, reaffirmed 2019). Practice bulletin no. 167: Gynecologic care for women and adolescents with human immunodeficiency virus. *Obstetrics & Gynecology, 128*(4), e89–e110. https://doi.org/10.1097/AOG.0000000000001707

American College of Obstetricians and Gynecologists. (2017a, reaffirmed 2023). Committee opinion no. 691: Carrier screening for genetic conditions. *Obstetrics & Gynecology, 129*(3), e41–e55. https://doi.org/10.1097/AOG.0000000000001952

American College of Obstetricians and Gynecologists. (2017b, reaffirmed 2021). Committee opinion no. 711: Opioid use and opioid use disorder in pregnancy. *Obstetrics & Gynecology, 130*(2), e81–e94. https://doi.org/10.1097/AOG.0000000000002235

American College of Obstetricians and Gynecologists. (2017c). Committee opinion no. 722: Marijuana use during pregnancy and lactation. *Obstetrics & Gynecology, 130*(4), e205–e209. https://doi.org/10.1097/AOG.0000000000002354

American College of Obstetricians and Gynecologists. (2017e). Practice bulletin no. 187: Neural tube defects. *Obstetrics & Gynecology, 130*(6), e279–e290. https://doi.org/10.1097/AOG.0000000000002412

American College of Obstetricians and Gynecologists. (2018c). ACOG practice bulletin no. 194: Polycystic ovary syndrome. *Obstetrics & Gynecology, 131*(6), e157–e171. https://doi.org/10.1097/AOG.0000000000002656

American College of Obstetricians and Gynecologists. (2018d). ACOG practice bulletin no. 196: Thromboembolism in pregnancy. *Obstetrics & Gynecology, 132*(1), e1–e17. https://doi.org/10.1097/AOG.0000000000002706

American College of Obstetricians and Gynecologists. (2018e). ACOG practice bulletin no. 197: Inherited thrombophilias in pregnancy. *Obstetrics & Gynecology, 132*(1), e18–e34. https://doi.org/10.1097/AOG.0000000000002703

American College of Obstetricians and Gynecologists. (2018f). ACOG practice bulletin no. 200: Early pregnancy loss. *Obstetrics & Gynecology, 132*(5), e197–e207. https://doi.org/10.1097/AOG.0000000000002899

American College of Obstetricians and Gynecologists & Society for Maternal-Fetal Medicine. (2019). Interpregnancy care. *American Journal of Obstetrics and Gynecology, 220*(1), B2–B18. https://doi.org/10.1016/j.ajog.2018.11.1098

American College of Obstetricians and Gynecologists. (2019a, reaffirmed 2024). ACOG committee opinion no. 762: Prepregnancy counseling. *Obstetrics & Gynecology, 133*(1), e78–e89. https://doi.org/10.1097/AOG.0000000000003013

American College of Obstetricians and Gynecologists. (2019b). ACOG practice bulletin no. 202: Gestational hypertension and preeclampsia. *Obstetrics & Gynecology, 133*(1), e1–e25. https://doi.org/10.1097/AOG.0000000000003018

American College of Obstetricians and Gynecologists. (2019c). ACOG practice bulletin no. 203: Chronic hypertension in pregnancy. *Obstetrics & Gynecology, 133*(1), e26–e50. https://doi.org/10.1097/AOG.0000000000003020

American College of Obstetricians and Gynecologists. (2020). ACOG Committee Opinion No. 809: Human papillomavirus vaccination. *Obstetrics & Gynecology, 136*(2), e15–e21. https://www.acog.org/clinical/clinical-guidance/committee-opinion/articles/2020/08/human-papillomavirus-vaccination

American College of Obstetricians and Gynecologists. (2024). ACOG committee statement no. 10: Racial and ethnic inequities in obstetrics and gynecology. *Obstetrics & Gynecology, 144*(3), e62– e74. https://www.acog.org/clinical/clinical-guidance/committee-statement/articles/2024/09/racial-and-ethnic-inequities-in-obstetrics-and-gynecology

American Diabetes Association. (2018). Children and adolescents: Standards of medical care in diabetes [Suppl. 1]. *Diabetes Care, 41*, S126–S136. https://doi.org/10.2337/dc18-S012

American Diabetes Association. (2019). Management of diabetes in pregnancy: Standards of medical care in diabetes [Suppl. 1]. *Diabetes Care, 42*, S165–S172. https://doi.org/10.2337/dc19-S014

Baker, A. S., & Freeman, M. P. (2018). Management of attention deficit hyperactivity disorder during pregnancy. *Obstetrics and Gynecology Clinics of North America, 45*(3), 495–509. https://doi.org/10.1016/j.ogc.2018.04.010

Barnard, S., & French, J. (2019). Collaboration of care for women with epilepsy in their reproductive years. *Journal of Women's Health (2002), 28*(3), 339–345. https://doi.org/10.1089/jwh.2018.7506

Baxter, R., Bartlett, J., Fireman, B., Lewis, E., & Klein, N. P. (2017). Effectiveness of vaccination during pregnancy to prevent infant pertussis. *Pediatrics, 139*(5), e20164091. https://doi.org/10.1542/peds.2016-4091

Best, D., Avenell, A., & Bhattacharya, S. (2017). How effective are weight-loss interventions for improving fertility in women and men who are overweight or obese? A systematic review and meta-analysis of the evidence. *Human Reproduction Update, 23*(6), 681–705. https://doi.org/10.1093/humupd/dmx027

Boxem, A. J., Blaauwendraad, S. M., Mulders, A. G, Bekkers, E., Kruithof, C., Steegers, E., Gaillard, R. & Jaddoe, V. (2024). Preconception and early-pregnancy body mass index in women and men, time to pregnancy and risk of miscarriage. *JAMA Network Open. 7*(9), e2436157. doi:10.1001/jamanetworkopen.2024.36157

Breadon, C., & Kulkarni, J. (2019). An update on medication management of women with schizophrenia in pregnancy. *Expert Opinion on Pharmacotherapy, 20*(11), 1365–1376. https://doi.org/10.1080/14656566.2019.1612876

Bromley, R. L., Weston, J., & Marson, A. G. (2017). Maternal use of antiepileptic agents during pregnancy and major congenital malformations in children. *JAMA, 318*(17), 1700–1701. https://doi.org/10.1001/jama.2017.14485

Centers for Disease Control and Prevention. (2024). *COVID-19 vaccines while pregnant or breastfeeding*. https://www.cdc.gov/covid/vaccines/pregnant-or-breastfeeding.html

Centers for Disease Control and Prevention. (2024, May 15). National and state tobacco control program. U.S. Department of Health & Human Services. https://www.cdc.gov/tobacco/php/tobacco-control-programs/index.html

Centers for Disease Control and Prevention. (2025a). *Measles cases and outbreaks*. U.S. Department of Health & Human Services. https://www.cdc.gov/measles/data-research/index.html

Centers for Disease Control and Prevention. (2025b). *Rubella during pregnancy*. U.S. Department of Health & Human Services. Retrieved March 1, 2025, from https://www.cdc.gov/rubella/pregnancy/index.html

Chahine, K. M., & Sibai, B. M. (2019). Chronic hypertension in pregnancy: New concepts for classification and management. *American Journal of Perinatology, 36*(2), 161–168. https://doi.org/10.1055/s-0038-1666976

Chisolm, M. S., & Payne, J. L. (2016). Management of psychotropic drugs during pregnancy. *BMJ (Clinical research ed.), 532*, h5918. https://doi.org/10.1136/bmj.h5918

Clark, C. T., & Wisner, K. L. (2018). Treatment of peripartum bipolar disorder. *Obstetrics and Gynecology Clinics of North America, 45*(3), 403–417. https://doi.org/10.1016/j.ogc.2018.05.002

Coughlin, C. G., Blackwell, K. A., Bartley, C., Hay, M., Yonkers, K. A., & Bloch, M. H. (2015). Obstetric and neonatal outcomes after antipsychotic medication exposure in pregnancy. *Obstetrics and gynecology, 125*(5), 1224–1235. https://doi.org/10.1097/AOG.0000000000000759

Daalderop, L. A., Wieland, B. V., Tomsin, K., Reyes, L., Kramer, B. W., Vanter, V. C., & Spaanderman, M. E. A. (2018). Periodontal disease and pregnancy outcomes: Overview of systematic reviews. *Journal of Evidence-Based Dental Practice, 18*(1), 1–27. https://doi.org/10.1177/2380084417731097

Dejong, K., Olyaei, A., & Lo, J. O. (2019). Alcohol use in pregnancy. *Clinical Obstetrics and Gynecology, 62*(1), 142–155. https://doi.org/10.1097/GRF.0000000000000414

Dousti, R., Allahqoli, L., Ayar Kocaturk, A., & Hakimi, S. (2023). Can human papillomavirus vaccination during pregnancy result in miscarriage and stillbirth? A meta-analysis and systematic review. *European Journal of Midwifery, 7*(April), 1–6. https://doi.org/10.18332/ejm/161793

Duca, Y., Aversa, A., Condorelli, R. A., Calogero, A. E., & La Vignera, S. (2019). Substance abuse and male hypogonadism. *Journal of Clinical Medicine, 8*(5), 732. https:// doi.org/10.3390/jcm8050732

Dudley, M. Z. (2018). *The clinician's vaccine safety resource guide: Optimizing prevention of vaccine-preventable diseases across the lifespan*. Springer.

Environmental Working Group. (2025). *Shopper's guide to pesticides in produce*. https://www.ewg.org/foodnews/

Envision Sexual and Reproductive Health. (n.d.). *About PATH*. https://www.envisionsrh.com/about-path

Ethics Committee of American Society for Reproductive Medicine. (2015). Human immunodeficiency virus (HIV) and infertility treatment: A committee opinion. *Fertility and Sterility, 104*(1), e1–e8. https://doi.org/10.1016/j.fertnstert.2015.04.004

Fleming-Dutra, K. E., Zauche, L. H., Roper, L. E., Ellington, S. R., Olson, C. K., Sharma, A. J., Woodworth, K. R., Tepper, N., Havers, F., Oliver, S. E., Twentyman, E., & Jatlaoui, T. C. (2023). Safety and effectiveness of maternal COVID-19 vaccines among pregnant people and infants. *Obstetrics and Gynecology Clinics of North America, 50*(2), 279–297. https://doi.org/10.1016/j.ogc.2023.02.003

Foeller, M. E., & Lyell, D. J. (2017). Marijuana use in pregnancy: Concerns in an evolving era. *Journal of Midwifery & Women's Health, 62*(3), 363–367. https://doi.org/10.1111/jmwh.12631

Frayne, D. J., Verbiest, S., Chelmow, D., Clarke, H., Dunlop, A., Hosmer, J., Menard, M., Moos, M.-K., Ramos, D., Stuebe, A., & Zephyrin, L. (2016). Health care system measures to advance preconception wellness: Consensus recommendations of the clinical workgroup of the National Preconception Health and Health Care Initiative. *Obstetrics & Gynecology, 127*(5), 863–872. https://doi.org/10.1097/AOG.0000000000001379

Freeman, M. P., Savella, G. M., Church, T. R., Goez-Mogollon, L., Sosinsky, A. Z., Noe, O. B., Kaimal, A., & Cohen, L. S. (2019). A prenatal supplement with methylfolate for the treatment and prevention of depression in women trying to conceive and during pregnancy. *Annals of Clinical Psychiatry, 31*(1), 4–16. https://www.ncbi.nlm .nih.gov/pubmed/30699214

Geist, C., Aiken, A. R., Sanders, J. N., Everett, B. G., Myers, K., Cason, P., Simmons, R. G., & Turok, D. K. (2019). Beyond intent: Exploring the association of contraceptive choice with questions about pregnancy attitudes, timing and how important is pregnancy prevention (PATH) questions. *Contraception, 99*(1), 22–26. https://doi.org/10.1016/j.contraception.2018.08.014

Gennette, S. (2017). Detoxification from opiate drugs during pregnancy. *Obstetrics and Gynecology (New York), 130*(1), 216–216.

George, B. T., Jhancy, M., Dube, R., Kar, S. S., & Annamma, L. M. (2023). The molecular basis of male infertility in obesity: A literature review. *International Journal of Molecular Sciences, 25*(1), 179. https://doi.org/10.3390/ijms25010179

Goodin, A., Varma, D. S., Dhillon, K., Kaleem, S., Dubare, S., Jennings, A., Goldberger, B. A., & Roussos-Ross, K. (2025). Perception of Risks of Cannabis and Cannabidiol Use during Pregnancy: A Multi-Methods Study. *Medical cannabis and cannabinoids, 8*(1), 130–143. https://doi.org/10.1159/000546312

Goodsmith, N., Dossett, E. C., Gitlin, R., Fenwick, K., Ong, J. R., Hamilton, A., & Cordasco, K. M. (2023). Acceptability of reproductive goals assessment in public mental health care. *Health Services Research, 58*(2), 510–520. https://doi.org/10.1111/1475-6773.14111

Grande, I., Berk, M., Birmaher, B., & Vieta, E. (2016). Bipolar disorder. *Lancet, 387*(10027), 1561–1572. https://doi.org/10.1016/S0140-6736(15)00241-X

Greff, D., Juhász, A. E., Váncsa, S., Váradi, A., Sipos, Z., Szinte, J., Park, S., Hegyi, P., Nyirády, P., Ács, N., Várbíró, S., & Horváth, E. M. (2023). Inositol is an effective and safe treatment in polycystic ovary syndrome: A systematic review and meta-analysis of randomized controlled trials. *Reproductive Biology and Endocrinology: RB&E, 21*(1), 10. https://doi.org/10.1186/s12958-023-01055-z

Grohskopf, L. A., Sokolow, L. Z., Broder, K. R., Walter, E. B., Fry, A. M., & Jernigan, D. B. (2018). Prevention and control of seasonal influenza with vaccines: Recommendations of the advisory committee on immunization practices—United States, 2018–19 influenza season. *Morbidity and Mortality Weekly Report Recommendations and Reports, 67*(3), 1–20. https://doi.org/10.15585/mmwr.rr6703a1

Haiman, M. D., & Cubbin, C. (2023). Impact of Geography and Rurality on Preconception Health Status in the United States. *Preventing chronic disease, 20*, E101. https://doi.org/10.5888/pcd20.230104

Hakimi, O., & Cameron, L. C. (2017). Effect of exercise on ovulation: A systematic review. *Sports Medicine, 47*(8), 1555–1567. https://doi.org/10.1007/s40279-016-0669-8

Hammarberg, K., Zosel, R., Comoy, C., Robertson, S., Holden, C., Deeks, M., & Johnson, L. (2017). Fertility-related knowledge and information-seeking behaviour among people of reproductive age: a qualitative study. *Human Fertility, 20*(2), 88–95. https://doi.org/10.1080/14647273.2016.1245447

Harper, T., Kuohung, W., Sayres, L., Willis, M. D., & Wise, L. A. (2023). Optimizing preconception care and interventions for improved population health. *Fertility and Sterility, 120*(3), 438–448. https://doi.org/10.1016/j.fertnstert.2022.12.014

Herzog, A. G., Mandle, H. B., Cahill, K. E., Fowler, K. M., & Hauser, W. A. (2017). Predictors of unintended pregnancy in women with epilepsy. *Neurology, 88*(8), 728–733. https://doi.org/10.1212/WNL.0000000000003637

Heslehurst, N., Ngongalah, L., Bigirumurame, T., Nguyen, G., Odeniyi, A., Flynn, A., Smith, V., Crowe, L., Skidmore, B., Gaudet, L., Simon, A., & Hayes, L. (2022). Association between maternal adiposity measures and adverse maternal outcomes of pregnancy: Systematic review and meta-analysis. *Obesity Reviews: An Official Journal of the International Association for the Study of Obesity, 23*(7), e13449. https://doi.org/10.1111/obr.13449

Hess, J. M., Comeau, M. E., Smith, J. L., Swanson, K., & Anderson, C. M. (2025). Vegetarian diets during pregnancy: With supplementation, ovo-vegetarian, lacto-vegetarian, vegan, and pescatarian adaptations of U.S. Department of Agriculture food patterns can be nutritionally adequate. *Journal of the Academy of Nutrition and Dietetics, 125*(2), 204–216.e17. https://doi.org/10.1016/j.jand.2024.08.001

Huang, H. Y., Chen, H. L., & Feng, L. P. (2017). Maternal obesity and the risk of neural tube defects in offspring: A meta-analysis. *Obesity Research & Clinical Practice, 11*(2), 188–197. https://doi.org/10.1016/j.orcp.2016.04.005

Jiang, H. Y., Zhang, X., Jiang, C. M., & Fu, H. B. (2019). Maternal and neonatal outcomes after exposure to ADHD medication during pregnancy: A systematic review and meta-analysis. *Pharmacoepidemiology and Drug Safety, 28*(3), 288–295. https://doi.org/10.1002/pds.4716

Joseph, D. N., & Whirledge, S. (2017). Stress and the HPA axis: Balancing homeostasis and fertility. *International Journal of Molecular Sciences, 18*(10), 2224. https://doi.org/10.3390/ijms18102224

Kedzior, S. G. E., Bianco-Miotto, T., Breen, J., Diener, K. R., Donnelley, M., Dunning, K. R., Penno, M. A. S., Schjenken, J. E., Sharkey, D. J., Hodyl, N. A., Fullston, T., Gardiner, M., Brown, H. M., & Rumbold, A. R. (2019). It takes a community to conceive: An analysis of the scope, nature and accuracy of online sources of health information for couples trying to conceive. *Reproductive Biomedicine & Society Online, 9*, 48–63. https://doi.org/10.1016/j.rbms.2019.08.004

Khalafalla, K., El Ansari, W., Sengupta, P., Majzoub, A., Elbardisi, H., Canguven, O., El-Ansari, K., & Arafa, M. (2023). Are sexually transmitted infections associated with male infertility? A systematic review and in-depth evaluation of the evidence and mechanisms of action of 11 pathogens. *Arab Journal of Urology, 21*(4), 216–232. https://doi.org/10.1080/2090598X.2023.2218566

Kim, D. K., & Hunter, P. (2019). Recommended adult immunization schedule, United States, 2019. *Annals of Internal Medicine, 170*(3), 182–192. https://doi.org/10.7326/M18-3600

Kim, K., Wactawski-Wende, J., Michels, K. A., Plowden, T. C., Chalhoub, N., & Schisterman, E. F. (2017). Dairy food intake is associated with reproductive hormones and sporadic anovulation among healthy premenopausal women. *The Journal of Nutrition, 147*(2), 218–226. https://doi.org/10.3945/jn.116.241521

Kimmel, M. C., Cox, E., Schiller, C., Gettes, E., & Meltzer-Brody, S. (2018). Pharmacologic treatment of perinatal depression. *Obstetrics and Gynecology Clinics of North America, 45*(3), 419–440. https://doi.org/10.1016/j.ogc.2018.04.007

Kobaly, K., & Mandel, S. J. (2019). Hyperthyroidism and pregnancy. *Endocrinology and Metabolism Clinics of North America, 48*(3), 533–545. https://doi.org/10.1016/j.ecl.2019.05.002

Koullali, B., Kamphuis, E. I., Hof, M. H. P., Robertson, S. A., Pajkrt, E., de Groot, C. J. M., Mol, B. W. J., & Ravelli, A. C. J. (2017). The effect of interpregnancy interval on the recurrence rate of spontaneous preterm birth: A retrospective cohort study. *American Journal of Perinatology, 34*(2), 174–182. https://doi.org/10.1055/s-0036-1584896

Kuehn, B. (2019). Vaping and pregnancy. *JAMA, 321*(14), 1344. https://doi.org/10.1001/jama.2019.3424

Leaverton, A., Lopes, V., Vohr, B., Dailey, T., Phipps, M. G., & Allen, R. H. (2016). Postpartum contraception needs of women with preterm infants in the neonatal intensive care unit. *Journal of Perinatology, 36*(3), 186–189. https://doi.org/10.1038/jp.2015.174

Lebin, L. G., & Novick, A. M. (2022). Selective Serotonin Reuptake Inhibitors (SSRIs) in Pregnancy: An Updated Review on Risks to Mother, Fetus, and Child. *Current psychiatry reports, 24*(11), 687–695. https://doi.org/10.1007/s11920-022-01372-x

Levin, B. L., & Varga, E. (2016). MTHFR: Addressing genetic counseling dilemmas using evidence-based literature. *Journal of Genetic Counseling, 25*(5), 901–911. https://doi.org/10.1007/s10897-016-9956-7

Levine, S. Z., Kodesh, A., Viktorin, A., Smith, L., Uher, R., Reichenberg, A., & Sandin, S. (2018). Association of Maternal Use of Folic Acid and Multivitamin Supplements in the Periods Before and During Pregnancy With the Risk of Autism Spectrum Disorder in Offspring. *JAMA psychiatry, 75*(2), 176–184. https://doi.org/10.1001/jamapsychiatry.2017.4050

Lewinski A., & Brzozowska M. (2023). Female infertility as a result of stress-related hormonal changes. *GREM, 3*, 94–98. https://doi.org/10.53260/grem.22302035

Li, Y., & Meador, K. J. (2022). Epilepsy and pregnancy. *Continuum (Minneapolis, Minn.), 28*(1), 34–54. https://doi.org/10.1212/CON.0000000000001056

Lind, J. N., Interrante, J. D., Ailes, E. C., Gilboa, S. M., Khan, S., Frey, M. T., Dawson, A. L., Honein, M. A., Dowling, N. F., Razzaghi, H., Creanga, A. A., & Broussard, C. S. (2017). Maternal Use of Opioids During Pregnancy and Congenital Malformations: A Systematic Review. *Pediatrics, 139*(6), e20164131. https://doi.org/10.1542/peds.2016-4131

López, N. J., Uribe, S., Martinez, B., & Corrales, A. (2019). Effect of periodontal treatment in pregnancy on perinatal outcomes: A systematic review and meta-analysis. *Journal of Maternal-Fetal & Neonatal Medicine, 32*(19), 3355–3363. https://doi.org/10.1080/14767058.2019.1678142

Luong, J., Board, A., Gosdin, L., Dunkley, J., Thierry, J. M., Pitasi, M., & Kim, S. Y. (2023). Alcohol Use, Screening, and Brief Intervention Among Pregnant Persons - 24 U.S. Jurisdictions, 2017 and 2019. *MMWR. Morbidity and mortality weekly report, 72*(3), 55–62. https://doi.org/10.15585/mmwr.mm7203a2

MacAfee, L. K., Dalton, V., & Terplan, M. (2018). Pregnancy intention, risk perception, and contraceptive use in pregnant women who use drugs. *Journal of Addiction Medicine, 13*(3), 177–181. https://doi.org/10.1097/ADM.0000000000000471

Malaza, N., Masete, M., Adam, S., Dias, S., Nyawo, T., & Pheiffer, C. (2022). A systematic review to compare adverse pregnancy outcomes in women with pregestational diabetes and gestational diabetes. *International Journal of Environmental Research and Public Health, 19*(17), 10846. https://doi.org/10.3390/ijerph191710846

Maraka, S., Singh Ospina, N. M., O'Keeffe, D. T., Rodriguez-Gutierrez, R., Espinosa De Ycaza, A. E., Wi, C. I., Juhn, Y. J., Coddington, C. C., 3rd, Montori, V. M., & Stan, M. N. (2016). Effects of Levothyroxine Therapy on Pregnancy Outcomes in Women with Subclinical Hypothyroidism. *Thyroid : official journal of the American Thyroid Association, 26*(7), 980–986. https://doi.org/10.1089/thy.2016.0014

Masson, P., & Brannigan, R. E. (2014). The varicocele. *Urologic Clinics of North America, 41*(1), 129–144. https://doi.org/10.1016/j.ucl.2013.08.001

Maurer, D. M., Raymond, T. J., & Davis, B. N. (2018). Depression: Screening and diagnosis. *American Family Physician, 98*(8), 508–515.

McCarthy, K., Lui, S., Huynh, M., Kennedy, J., Chan, H., Mayer, V., Vieira, L., Tabaei, B., Howell, F., Lee, A., Van Wye, G., Howell, E., & Janevic, T. (2023). Influence of gestational diabetes mellitus on diabetes risk and glycemic control in a retrospective population-based cohort. *Diabetes care, 46*(8), 1483–1491. http://doi.org/10.2337/dc22-1676

Meltzer-Brody, S., & Jones, I. (2015). Optimizing the treatment of mood disorders in the perinatal period. *Dialogues in Clinical Neuroscience, 17*(2), 207–218.

Metz, M., Maurer, M., & Metz, M. (2023). Mast cell silencing: A novel therapeutic approach for urticaria and other mast cell–related diseases. *Allergy, 78*(1), 13–27. http://doi.org/10.1111/all.15850

Minguez-Alarcon, L., Chavarro, J. E., & Gaskins, A. J. (2018). Caffeine, alcohol, smoking, and reproductive outcomes among couples undergoing assisted reproductive technology treatments. *Fertility and Sterility, 110*(4), 587–592. https://doi.org/10.1016/j.fertnstert.2018.05.026

Molenaar, N., Brouwer, M., Burger, H., Kamperman, A., Bergink, V., Hoogendijk, W., Williams, A., Bockting, C. & Lambregtse-Van den Berg, M. (2020). Preventative cognitive therapy with antidepressant discontinuation during pregnancy: Results from a randomized controlled trial. *Journal of Clinical Psychiatry, 81*(4). https://doi.org/10.4088/JCP.19l13099.

Montjean, D., Godin Pagé, M. H., Bélanger, M. C., Benkhalifa, M., & Miron, P. (2023). An overview of e-cigarette impact on reproductive health. *Life, 13*(3), 827. https://doi.org/10.3390/life13030827

Moslehi, N., Mirmiran, P., Namazi, N., Azizi, F., & Tahmasebinejad, Z. (2019). Do dietary intakes influence the rate of decline in anti-Mullerian hormone among eumenorrheic women? A population-based prospective investigation. *Nutrition Journal, 18*(1), 1–9. https://doi.org/10.1186/s12937-019-0508-5

Naninck, E. F. G., Stijger, P. C., & Brouwer-Brolsma, E. M. (2019). The importance of maternal folate status for brain development and function of offspring. *Advances in Nutrition (Bethesda, Md.), 10*(3), 502–519. https://doi.org/10.1093/advances/nmy120

Nassar, A. H., Hobeika, E., Chamsy, D., El-Kak, F., & Usta, I. M. (2023). Vaccination in pregnancy. *International journal of gynaecology and obstetrics: the official organ of the International Federation of Gynaecology and Obstetrics, 162*(1), 18–23. https://doi.org/10.1002/ijgo.14876

Nelson, N. P., Easterbrook, P. J., & McMahon, B. J. (2016). Epidemiology of hepatitis B virus infection and impact of vaccination on disease. *Clinics in Liver Disease, 20*(4), 607–628. https://doi.org/10.1016/j.cld.2016.06.006

Nelson, N. P., Weng, M. K., Hofmeister, M. G., et al. (2020). Prevention of hepatitis A virus infection in the United States: Recommendations of the Advisory Committee on Immunization Practices, 2020. *MMWR Recommendations and Reports, 69*(RR-5), 1–38. https://doi.org/10.15585/mmwr.rr6905a1

Nommsen-Rivers, L.A., Cetinkaya, H. & Stuebe, A.M. (2023). Enabling Breastfeeding for Women with Obesity. *Curr Obstet Gynecol Rep 12*, 147–157. https://doi.org/10.1007/s13669-023-00365-8

Norby, U., Winbladh, B., & Kallen, K. (2017). Perinatal outcomes after treatment with ADHD medication during pregnancy. *Pediatrics, 140*(6), e20170747. https://doi.org/10.1542/peds.2017-0747

Nucera, B., Brigo, F., Trinka, E., & Kalss, G. (2022). Treatment and care of women with epilepsy before, during, and after pregnancy: a practical guide. *Therapeutic advances in neurological disorders, 15*, 17562864221101687. https://doi.org/10.1177/17562864221101687

Nybo Andersen, A.-M., & Urhoj, S. K. (2017). Is advanced paternal age a health risk for the offspring? *Fertility and Sterility, 107*(2), 312–318. https://doi.org/10.1016/j.fertnstert.2016.12.019

Olson, S. M., Muñoz, E. G., Solis, E. C., & Bradford, H. M. (2024). Mitigating weight bias in the clinical setting: A new approach to care. *Journal of Midwifery & Women's Health, 69*(2), 180–190. https://doi.org/10.1111/jmwh.13578

Parnell, A. S., Correa, A., & Reece, E. A. (2017). Pre-pregnancy obesity as a modifier of gestational diabetes and birth defects associations: A systematic review. *Maternal and Child Health Journal, 21*(5), 1105–1120. https://doi.org/10.1007/s10995-016-2209-4

Pavlik, L. B., & Rosculet, K. (2020). Maternal obesity and perinatal depression: An updated literature review. *Cureus (Palo Alto, CA), 12*(9), e10736. https://doi.org/10.7759/cureus.10736

Pearl, R. L., & Puhl, R. M. (2018). Weight bias internalization and health: A systematic review. *Obesity Reviews, 19*(8), 1141–1163. https://doi.org/10.1111/obr.12701

Prasad, S., Kalafat, E., Blakeway, H., Heath, P. T., Ladhani, S. N., Khalil, A., & von Dadelszen, P. (2022). Systematic review and meta-analysis of the effectiveness and perinatal outcomes of COVID-19 vaccination in pregnancy. *Nature Communications, 13*, 2414. https://doi.org/10.1038/s41467-022-30052-w

Raghuraman, N., & Tuuli, M. G. (2021). Preconception care as an opportunity to optimize pregnancy outcomes. *JAMA: The Journal of the American Medical Association, 326*(1), 79. https://doi.org/10.1001/jama.2020.27244

Robbins, C., Boulet, S. L., Morgan, I., D'Angelo, D. V., Zapata, L. B., Morrow, B., Sharma, A., & Kroelinger, C. D. (2018). Disparities in preconception health indicators—behavioral risk factor surveillance system, 2013–2015, and pregnancy risk assessment monitoring system, 2013–2014. *Morbidity and Mortality Weekly Report Surveillance Summaries, 67*(1), 1–16. https://doi.org/10.15585/mmwr.ss6701a1

Rockhill, K. M., Tong, V. T., Farr, S. L., Robbins, C. L., D'Angelo, D. V., & England, L. J. (2016). Postpartum smoking relapse after quitting during pregnancy: Pregnancy risk assessment monitoring system, 2000–2011. *Journal of Women's Health, 25*(5), 480–488. https://doi.org/10.1089/jwh.2015.5244

Seo, G. H., Kim, T. H., & Chung, J. H. (2018). Antithyroid drugs and congenital malformations: A nationwide Korean cohort study. *Annals of Internal Medicine, 168*(6), 405–413. https://doi.org/10.7326/M17-1398

Shao, Z., Al Tibi, M., & Wakim-Fleming, J. (2017). Update on viral hepatitis in pregnancy. *Cleveland Clinic Journal of Medicine, 84*(3), 202–206. https://doi.org/10.3949/ccjm.84a.15139

Shea, A., Jumah, N. A., Forte, M., Cantin, C., Bayrampour, H., Butler, K., Francoeur, D., Green, C., & Cook, J. (2024). Guideline no. 454: Identification and treatment of perinatal mood and anxiety disorders. *Journal of Obstetrics and Gynaecology Canada, 46*(10), Article 102696. https://doi.org/10.1016/j.jogc.2024.102696

Solmi, M., Radua, J., Olivola, M., Croce, E., Soardo, L., Salazar de Pablo, G., Il Shin, J., Kirkbride, J. B., Jones, P., Kim, J. H., Kim, J. Y., Carvalho, A. F., Seeman, M. V., Correll, C. U., & Fusar-Poli, P. (2022). Age at onset of mental disorders worldwide: large-scale meta-analysis of 192 epidemiological studies. *Molecular psychiatry, 27*(1), 281–295. https://doi.org/10.1038/s41380-021-01161-7

Stevens, A. W. M. M., Goossens, P. J. J., Knoppert-van der Klein, E. A. M., Draisma, S., Honig, A., & Kupka, R. W. (2019). Risk of recurrence of mood disorders during pregnancy and the impact of medication: A systematic review. *Journal of affective disorders, 249*, 96–103. https://doi.org/10.1016/j.jad.2019.02.018

Strøm, M., Granström, C., Lyall, K., Ascherio, A., & Olsen, S. F. (2018). Research letter: Folic acid supplementation and intake of folate in pregnancy in relation to offspring risk of autism spectrum disorder. *Psychological Medicine, 48*(6), 1048–1054. doi:10.1017/S0033291717002410

Stulberg, D. B., Schumm, L. P., Schueler, K., Giurcanu, M., & Peek, M. E. (2023). Preconception care utilization: Self-report versus claims-based measures among women with Medicaid. *PLOS Global Public Health, 3*(11). https://doi.org/10.1371/journal.pgph.0002592

Tanz, L. J., Miller, K. D., Dinwiddie, A. T., Gladden, R. M., Asher, A., Baldwin, G., Nesbit, B., & O'Donnell, J. (2025). Drug Overdose Deaths Involving Stimulants - United States, January 2018-June 2024. *MMWR. Morbidity and mortality weekly report, 74*(32), 491–499. https://doi.org/10.15585/mmwr.mm7432a1

Tessema, G. A., Marinovich, M. L., Håberg, S. E., Gissler, M., Mayo, J. A., Nassar, N., Ball, S., Betrán, A. P., Gebremedhin, A. T., de Klerk, N., Magnus, M. C., Marston, C., Regan, A. K., Shaw, G. M., Padula, A. M., & Pereira, G. (2021). Interpregnancy intervals and adverse birth outcomes in high-income countries: An international cohort study. *PLOS one, 16*(7), e0255000. https://doi.org/10.1371/journal.pone.0255000

Thomson, M., & Sharma, V. (2018). Weighing the risks: The management of bipolar disorder during pregnancy. *Current Psychiatry Reports, 20*(20). https://doi.org/10.1007/s11920-018-0882-2

Tomiyama, A. J., Carr, D., Granberg, E. M., Major, B., Robinson, E., Sutin, A. R., & Brewis, A. (2018). How and why weight stigma drives the obesity 'epidemic' and harms health. *BMC medicine, 16*(1), 123. https://doi.org/10.1186/s12916-018-1116-5

Tosato, S., Albert, U., Tomassi, S., Iasevoli, F., Carmassi, C., Ferrari, S., Nanni, M. G., Nivoli, A., Volpe, U., Atti, A. R., & Fiorillo, A. (2017). A systematized review of atypical antipsychotics in pregnant women: Balancing between risks of untreated illness and risks of drug-related adverse effects. *The Journal of Clinical Psychiatry, 78*(5), e477–e489. https://doi.org/10.4088/JCP.15r10483

Tracy, E. E., & Macias-Konstantopoulos, W. (2017). Identifying and assisting sexually exploited and trafficked patients seeking women's health care services. *Obstetrics & Gynecology, 130*(2), 443–453. https://doi.org/10.1097/AOG.0000000000002144

Tufts University Health & Nutrition Letter. (2024). Possible health effects of chronic stress. *Tufts University Health & Nutrition Letter, 42*(8), 3.

Tukei, V. J., Hoffman, H. J., Greenberg, L., Thabelo, R., Nchephe, M., Mots'oane, T., Masitha, M., Chabela, M., Mokone, M., Mofenson, L., Guay, L., & Tiam, A. (2021). Adverse pregnancy outcomes among HIV-positive women in the era of universal antiretroviral therapy remain elevated compared with HIV-negative women. *The Pediatric Infectious Disease Journal, 40*(9), 821–826. https://doi.org/10.1097/INF.0000000000003174

Turner, E., Jones, M., Vaz, L. R., & Coleman, T. (2019). Systematic review and meta-analysis to assess the safety of bupropion and varenicline in pregnancy. *Nicotine & Tobacco Research, 21*(8), 1001–1010. https://doi.org/10.1093/ntr/nty055

U.S. Department of Health and Human Services. (2024). *Healthy people 2030*. https://www.healthypeople.gov/2030/

U.S. Preventive Services Task Force. (2017). Folic acid supplementation for the prevention of neural tube defects: U.S. Preventive Services Task Force final recommendation statement. *JAMA, 317*(2), 183-189. https://doi .org/10.1001/jama.2016.19438

U.S. Preventive Services Task Force. (2018a). Screening and behavioral counseling interventions to reduce unhealthy alcohol use in adolescents and adults: U.S. Preventive Services Task Force final recommendation statement. *JAMA, 320*(18), 1899-1909. https://doi .org/10.1001/jama.2018.16789

U.S. Preventive Services Task Force. (2021). Interventions for tobacco smoking cessation in adults, including pregnant persons: Recommendation statement. https://www.uspreventiveservicestaskforce.org/uspstf/recommendation/tobacco-use-in-adults-and-pregnant-women-counseling-and-interventions

U.S. Preventive Services Task Force. (2023). Screening for depression and suicide risk in adults: U.S. Preventive Services Task Force Recommendation Statement. *JAMA, 329*(23), 2057–2067. https://doi.org/10.1001/jama.2023.9297

US Preventive Services Task Force, Barry, M. J., Nicholson, W. K., Silverstein, M., Chelmow, D., Coker, T. R., Davis, E. M., Donahue, K. E., Jaén, C. R., Li, L., Ogedegbe, G., Rao, G., Ruiz, J. M., Stevermer, J., Tsevat, J., Underwood, S. M., & Wong, J. B. (2023). Folic Acid Supplementation to Prevent Neural Tube Defects: US Preventive Services Task Force Reaffirmation Recommendation Statement. *JAMA, 330*(5), 454–459. https://doi.org/10.1001/jama.2023.12876

U.S. Preventive Services Task Force. (2024, October 29). *Draft recommendation statement: Intimate partner violence and caregiver abuse of older or vulnerable adults: Screening*. U.S. Preventive Services Task Force.

U.S. Preventive Services Task Force, Silverstein, M., Wong, J. B., Davis, E. M., Chelmow, D., Coker, T. R., Fernandez, A., Gibson, E., Jaén, C. R., Krousel-Wood, M., Lee, S., Nicholson, W. K., Rao, G., Ruiz, J. M., Stevermer, J., Tsevat, J., Underwood, S. M., & Wiehe, S. (2025). Screening for Syphilis Infection During Pregnancy: US Preventive Services Task Force Reaffirmation Recommendation Statement. *JAMA, 333*(22), 2006–2012. https://doi.org/10.1001/jama.2025.5009

Viswanathan, M., Treiman, K. A., Kish-Doto, J., Middleton, J. C., Coker-Schwimmer, E. J., & Nicholson, W. K. (2017). Folic acid supplementation for the prevention of neural tube defects: An updated evidence report and systematic review for the U.S. Preventive Services Task Force. *JAMA, 317*(2), 190–203. https://doi.org/10.1001/jama.2016.19193

Viswanathan, M., Urrutia, R. P., Hudson, K. N., Middleton, J. C., & Kahwati, L. C. (2023). Folic acid supplementation to prevent neural tube defects: Updated evidence report and systematic review for the U.S. Preventive Services Task Force. *JAMA, 330*(5), 460–466. https://doi.org/10.1001/jama.2023.9864

Wang, S., Mitsunami, M., Ortiz-Panozo, E., Leung, C. W., Manson, J. E., Rich-Edwards, J. W., & Chvarro, J. E. (2023). Prepregnancy healthy lifestyle and adverse pregnancy outcomes. *Obstetrics and Gynecology, 142*(6), 1278–1290. https://doi.org/10.1097/AOG.0000000000005346

Weir, T. L., Majumder, M., & Glastras, S. J. (2024). A systematic review of the effects of maternal obesity on neonatal outcomes in women with gestational diabetes. *Obesity Reviews: An Official Journal of the International Association for the Study of Obesity, 25*(7), e13747. https://doi.org/10.1111/obr.13747

Wenger N. K. (2019). Female-friendly focus: 2019 ACC/AHA Guideline on the primary prevention of cardiovascular disease. *Clinical Cardiology, 42*(8), 706–709. https://doi.org/10.1002/clc.23218

Wilkes, J. (2016). AAFP releases position paper on preconception care. *American Family Physician, 94*(6), 508–510.

Wolfson, J. A., Tucker, A. C., Leung, C. W., Rebholz, C. M., Garcia-Larsen, V., & Martinez-Steele, E. (2025). Trends in Adults' Intake of Un-processed/Minimally Processed, and Ultra-processed foods at Home and Away from Home in the United States from 2003-2018. *The Journal of nutrition, 155*(1), 280–292. https://doi.org/10.1016/j.tjnut.2024.10.048

Wright, T. E. (2017). Screening, brief intervention, and referral to treatment for opioid and other substance use during infertility treatment. *Fertility and Sterility, 108*(2), 214–221. https://doi.org/10.1016/j.fertnstert.2017.06.012

Yang, X., Chen, H., Du, Y., Wang, S., & Wang, Z. (2016). Periconceptional folic acid fortification for the risk of gestational hypertension and pre-eclampsia: A meta-analysis of prospective studies. *Maternal & Child Nutrition, 12*(4), 669–679. https://doi.org/10.1111/mcn.12209

Yang, Y., Luo, Y., Yuan, J., Tang, Y., Xiong, L., Xu, M., Rao, X., & Liu, H. (2016). Association between maternal, fetal and paternal MTHFR gene C677T and A1298C polymorphisms and risk of recurrent pregnancy loss: A comprehensive evaluation. *Archives of Gynecology and Obstetrics, 293*(6), 1197–1211. https://doi.org/10.1007/s00404-015-3944-2

Young-Wolff, K. C., Chi, F. W., Lapham, G. T., Alexeeff, S. E., Does, M. B., Ansley, D., & Campbell, C. I. (2024). Changes in Prenatal Cannabis Use Among Pregnant Individuals From 2012 to 2022. *Obstetrics and gynecology, 144*(4), e101–e104. https://doi.org/10.1097/AOG.0000000000005711

Zhang, L., Liu, Y., & Li, J. (2021). Preconception thyrotropin levels and risk of adverse pregnancy outcomes. *JAMA Network Open, 4*(8), e2118681.

Zhang, L., Liu, Y., & Li, J. (2023). Comparison of the safety between propylthiouracil and methimazole in the treatment of hyperthyroidism during pregnancy: A meta-analysis. *PLOS ONE, 18*(5), e0286097. https://doi.org/10.1371/journal.pone.0286097

Zhang, Y., Lu, M., Yi, Y., Xia, L., Zhang, R., Li, C., & Liu, P. (2024). Influence of maternal body mass index on pregnancy complications and outcomes: a systematic review and meta-analysis. *Frontiers in endocrinology, 15*, 1280692. https://doi.org/10.3389/fendo.2024.1280692

CHAPTER 31

Anatomic and Physiologic Adaptations of Normal Pregnancy

Andie Zengion

The editors would like to acknowledge Ellise Adams, the author of Anatomic and Physiologic Adaptations of Pregnancy for the 4th edition of Gynecologic Health Care.

INTRODUCTION

Pregnancy is a time of profound change, affecting nearly every organ system in the body, as well as emotional, social, economic, and role-related aspects of a person's life. This chapter explores the normal anatomic and physiologic adaptations of pregnancy using a body systems approach. While each system is discussed individually, it is important to understand that these changes are interconnected; hormonal and functional effects on one organ system often influence others. These adaptations support the increased metabolic demands of pregnancy, childbirth, and lactation, including the needs of the fetus. Understanding these physiologic changes helps clinicians provide informed care and empowers patients with knowledge about their own bodies. Many early signs and symptoms of pregnancy result from these adaptations and often prompt individuals to seek prenatal care (refer to **Table 31-1**). This chapter focuses specifically on the physical changes caused by pregnancy. Chapter 32 covers prenatal care more broadly. All pregnancy dates in this chapter are given in terms of gestational age—measured from the first day of the last menstrual period—rather than embryonic age, which starts from conception (typically around week 3 of the cycle). This is consistent with clinical practice in most settings. Pregnancy is confirmed by observing specific "positive signs," while other signs—classified as "presumptive" or "probable"—may suggest pregnancy but are not definitive, as they can result from other conditions (refer to Table 31-1).

Many of the changes described in this chapter are the result of the numerous hormonal changes observed in pregnancy. This begins with increased progesterone secreted by the ovarian corpus luteum and the early placenta. Estrogen and progesterone levels rise dramatically in early pregnancy and impact many organ systems. Human chorionic gonadotropin (HCG), produced by the early placenta, is used as a biomarker for probable diagnosis of pregnancy, but is also a hormone involved in a number of changes that occur in early pregnancy, including immune system modulation, and alteration of blood vessels to allow formation of the placenta (d'Hauterive et al., 2022). In addition, uterine responses to many hormones are modified throughout pregnancy: for instance, the uterus is less responsive in pregnancy to oxytocin, which is involved in stimulating uterine contractions. Oxytocin receptors are then upregulated as the pregnancy reaches the late third trimester (Kissler & Hurt, 2023).

BREAST CHANGES

Most organs of the body form during the fetal period and complete their maturation during puberty. This is not the case for the breast, which completes the development necessary to allow lactation to occur only if it is stimulated to do so by the hormones of pregnancy (Fu et al., 2020). Some of these hormones have been used therapeutically to promote lactogenesis in nongestational parents/caregivers, though rigorous examination of these protocols is not always available. In addition, transgender men who carry a pregnancy can undergo lactogenesis if they have tissue available to do so, but would need to continue avoidance of testosterone to breast/chestfeed (Farah et al., 2021). Testosterone may lower levels of prolactin, thus decreasing the milk supply (LactMed, 2022).

During pregnancy, changing hormone levels contribute to breast changes and development in preparation for lactation. Progesterone and prolactin are the major hormones that cause development of the mammary gland during pregnancy. Progesterone and prolactin promote breast changes and development, but rising levels of progesterone and estrogen also block prolactin's effects and prevent it from triggering milk production until after the birth of the placenta. The placenta's delivery is a stronger stimulus for milk production than the birth, and in fact, placental retention can prevent milk production (Farah et al., 2021). Milk production increases most dramatically in the days following placental expulsion as progesterone levels drop precipitously and the breast is stimulated, most effectively when the infant begins sucking, or when pumping is initiated (Geddes et al., 2021). During pregnancy, many people experience heaviness, fullness, and tenderness in the breast as proliferation occurs; these symptoms are among the early presumptive signs of pregnancy. The weight of the breasts also increases throughout pregnancy (Graham & Montgomery, 2019). Refer to Chapter 34 for more information about the process of lactation.

By the second trimester, the number of mammary alveoli and ducts increase, and branching of the ducts takes place (Graham & Montgomery, 2019). It is important to note that breast size does not correlate with the degree of milk production; smaller breast size is not correlated with reduced milk supply (Geddes et al., 2021). Nipples become more erect and may lengthen, and there is often an increase in the width of the areola. Increased activity of the sebaceous glands increases the size of the Montgomery tubercles, the

TABLE 31-1 Presumptive, Probable, and Positive Signs of Pregnancy

Sign	Clinical Findings
Presumptive (subjective signs)	Amenorrhea, nausea and vomiting, increased urinary frequency, excessive fatigue, breast tenderness, sensation of fetal movement (quickening), changes in skin pigmentation of the abdomen or face, and increased basal body temperature in the absence of infection
Probable (objective signs)	Softening of the cervix (Goodell sign) Bluepurple discoloration of the cervix (Chadwick sign) or labia Softening of the lower uterine segment (Hegar's sign) Uterine enlargement Irregular uterine contractions (Braxton Hicks contractions) (may be palpated beginning in the second trimester) Uterine soufflé (soft blowing sound due to blood pulsating through the placenta) Integumentary pigment changes Ballottement Palpable fetal outline Positive pregnancy test (not a definitive sign as HCG may be secreted by hydatidiform mole, choriocarcinoma, or with increased pituitary gonadotropins at menopause)
Positive (diagnostic)	Fetal heart tone auscultation Ultrasonographic visualization of the fetus or fetal cardiac motion

Data from Phillippi, J., & Kantrowitz-Gordon, I. (Ed.). (2023). Varney's Midwifery (7th ed.). Jones & Barrett Learning. Ch 19, Anatomy and Physiology of Pregnancy; El Hage, L., & Hatipoglu, B. (2021). Elevated hCG can be a benign finding in perimenopausal and postmenopausal women. Cleveland Clinic journal of medicine, 88(11), 635–639. https://doi.org/10.3949/ccjm.88a.18069; Oyatogun, O., Sandhu, M., Barata-Kirby, S., Tuller, E., & Schust, D. J. (2021). A rational diagnostic approach to the "phantom hCG" and other clinical scenarios in which a patient is thought to be pregnant but is not. Therapeutic advances in reproductive health, 15, 26334941211016412. https://doi.org/10.1177/26334941211016412

papules on the nipples that secrete fluid that lubricates the nipple during lactation. This fluid also provides an olfactory homing beacon to the newborn in lactation; newborns respond strongly to the scent of this fluid by increasing mouthing and other behaviors associated with successful lactation (Schaal et al., 2020). During pregnancy, the skin of the breast becomes thinner, and striae may develop on the surface of the breasts. The areolae often become more darkly pigmented in pregnancy. Nipples may increase in diameter and length (Geddes et al., 2021). Lactogenesis begins in the late first and early second trimesters when alveolar cells start to produce colostrum (Jozsa & Thistle, 2023).

REPRODUCTIVE SYSTEM CHANGES

Uterine Changes

During pregnancy, the uterus changes its proportions substantially, starting its dramatic growth within a week of conception as the anteroposterior diameter increases (Phillippi & Kantrowitz-Gordon, 2023). Around the same time, the uterine isthmus (lower segment) softens and becomes more compressible for about 2 weeks, from approximately 4–6 weeks of gestation. This is known as Hegar's sign and is considered a probable sign of pregnancy. Circulation to the mucosa, including in the vagina and over the cervix, increases rapidly, making the cervix softer (Goodell sign) and more bluish/purple (Chadwick sign, appears around 6–8 weeks), both considered probable signs of pregnancy (Gupta et al., 2024).

Each layer of the uterus undergoes marked change. Uterine volume increases from 10 mL to 5 L at term as a result of myocyte hyperplasia in early pregnancy and hypertrophy in late pregnancy. Myometrial cells develop increased amounts of the actin and myosin fibers that mediate contractility, as well as the mitochondria needed to fuel the substantial workload of labor and birth (McEvoy & Sabir, 2022). The myometrium, or muscular layer of the uterus, must both prepare for the aerobic work of birth and contracts irregularly to prepare for the task of fetal expulsion. However, it must also maintain a state of quiescence, minimizing contractile activity in order to prevent preterm birth. To prepare for labor, muscle fibers must realign themselves throughout pregnancy, and gap junctions must form to allow for increased contractility compared to the person's non-pregnant baseline. This process is still being understood, but is likely driven by placental steroidal hormones and inflammatory markers. As the pregnancy approaches term, receptors to oxytocin (the pituitary hormone which stimulates rhythmic uterine contraction) are upregulated, inflammatory markers increase, and substances which relax the myometrium (i.e., nitric oxide) decrease (Zangeneh & Hantoushzadeh, 2023). Alongside these cellular changes, the uterine wall thickens from 10 to 25 mm by 16 weeks' gestation. However, by term the uterine wall thins to 5 to 10 mm as a result of distention due to fetal growth (sometimes referred to as mechanical distention). The shape of the uterus also changes. The nonpregnant uterus is roughly pear-shaped. In early pregnancy, it becomes round but as it grows into the abdomen, the uterus elongates into a cylindrical shape (Cunningham et al., 2022).

While the myometrium and body of the uterus undergo the most dramatic visual transformation, the endometrium also changes radically during pregnancy. This process, called decidualization, begins in the latter half of every menstrual cycle. During decidualization the endometrium begins its early changes to become the decidua, which is a biochemically and vascularly specialized tissue capable of creating a placental interface and providing all necessary metabolic support to the fetus via the placenta. During the menstrual cycle, the endometrium undergoes remodeling of its vasculature to prepare for conception, and, should conception not occur, to minimize harms of menstrual cycle bleeding (e.g., reducing flow of blood). In early pregnancy, further changes occur, decreasing vascular resistance in these arteries and making them more permeable, which appears to be important for proper formation of the placenta (Massri et al., 2023). While conditions such as gestational diabetes and early pregnancy loss have many possible causes, it is likely that they and many other pregnancy complications have roots in dysfunction of decidualization (Ng et al., 2020).

The uterus is supported and held in place in the pelvis by a number of ligaments. The round ligament is cord-like in shape and radiates laterally from the sides of the uterus and through the inguinal canal, inserting on the labia majora and the pubic bone. These are not true ligaments but are actually comprised of, and behave like, smooth muscle. In other words, they are capable of spasm and contraction. Round ligament pain is common in pregnancy, especially in the early/mid-second trimester, and is the result of hypertrophy, stretching, and sometimes spasticity of this ligament (Buksh et al., 2023).

At conception, the uterus is a pelvic organ protected by the pubic bone, but the uterine fundus rises out of the pelvis into the abdomen as pregnancy progresses. At 12 weeks' gestation, the fundus is located at the level of the symphysis pubis. By 20 weeks' gestation, the fundus is typically at the same height as the umbilicus. Between 24–38 weeks, the fundus enlarges approximately 1 cm per week, and comparing the measurement of fundal height to weeks of gestation is used to assess growth of the fetus; when the gestational age in weeks and fundal height vary by 2–3 cm, fetal growth may be abnormal. In other words, if fundal height is larger than gestational age it may indicate excessive fetal growth, and a fundal height 2–3 cm smaller than gestational age may indicate fetal growth restriction. Uterine fibroids, multiple gestation, and the pregnant person's abdominal size may alter fundal height measurement (ACOG, 2021).

Blood flow to the uterus increases markedly throughout pregnancy. By term, the uterus receives approximately 800 mL of blood, or one-fifth of the pregnant person's circulating blood volume (Ng et al., 2020). During labor, each uterine contraction pushes additional blood into the pregnant person's circulation, increasing cardiac preload and output. In the immediate postpartum, the blood that was present in the uterus and placenta is autotransfused back into the pregnant person's circulation, increasing preload and cardiac output by up to 60–80 percent (Lau et al., 2024).

Uterine soufflé—a quiet swishing sound that reflects the pregnant person's pulse—is made by blood flow to the placenta. Occasionally, this may be auscultated while listening to the fetal heart rate via ultrasound, and can be mistaken for the fetal pulse (Cunningham et al., 2022).

Cervical Changes

The cervix undergoes numerous changes during pregnancy. The prepregnant cervix is firm to palpation and approximately 25 mm in length. The cervix is the cylindrical "neck" of the uterus connecting it with the vagina. The cervix is comprised largely of cartilage, and by smaller amounts of smooth muscle fibers, both of which experience a series of dramatic changes throughout pregnancy. The cervix produces mucous that plays a role in uterine and vaginal function, including facilitating conception (LaCroix et al., 2020). Once conception has occurred, composition of the cervical mucous changes to become thicker and stickier. The cervix has two openings, an internal os that communicates with the uterine cavity, and an external os that communicates with the vagina—with the possible effect of preventing entry of sperm and microbes into the uterine cavity. Cervical length is approximately 30–40 mm in most pregnant people. As mentioned above, the cervix also receives an increasing amount of blood flow, resulting in changes apparent upon visual inspection.

Beginning shortly after conception and throughout pregnancy, collagen fibers in the cervix change their alignment to support dilation of the cervix at term. The cervix grossly alters its orientation in pregnancy. For most of the pregnancy, the cervix is oriented such that it points roughly posteriorly. This displaces the weight of the fetus and other uterine contents, pressing obliquely instead of longitudinally on the cervix, which helps the cervix maintain its function of helping to retain the fetus within the uterus. By term, it shifts its position, with the internal os being oriented superior and posterior to the external os, so the weight of the fetus is now pushing along the axis of the cervix instead of perpendicular to it, helping it to dilate (Fidalgo et al., 2024).

The cervix undergoes several changes at the end of pregnancy. It softens as cervical collagen is broken down slowly by increasing levels of collagenase (Kissler & Hurt, 2023). At some point, the cervix enters the "ripening" phase, wherein the cervix undergoes more rapid softening, effacement (shortening), and dilation. This process is the result of multiple factors, including pressure of the fetal head, uterine contractions, physiologic inflammation, and both parental and fetal hormonal signaling (Fidalgo et al., 2024). The cervix also contains a small amount of smooth muscle oriented around its circumference that appears to begin contracting just prior to labor, before the rest of the uterus begins its contractions, to facilitate the ripening process (Kissler & Hurt, 2023).

Pressure exerted on the cervix by the fetal head and the overall weight of the uterus may also decrease oxygen supply and increase inflammatory processes that help stimulate labor (Kissler & Hurt, 2023). Hormonal changes around this time also influence the cervix. For instance, progesterone levels, which have remained high throughout pregnancy, continue at similar levels as cervical change and early labor begin but the dominant type of progesterone receptor in the uterus and cervical tissue begins to change. While the dominant progesterone receptor type during pregnancy (PR-B) suppresses contraction of the uterus, PR-B gives way to PR-A, which makes uterine contraction possible (Cope & Monsivais, 2022).

An ongoing difficulty in care of childbearing people is in prevention of preterm labor. Understanding of the cause and mechanism of preterm labor remains incomplete, but many factors, including infection and mechanical and psychosocial stress, all have been shown to play a role (Fidalgo et al., 2024).

Vaginal and Vulvar Changes

Mucosa throughout the body becomes hyperemic, which can lead to localized bleeding (e.g., nosebleeds, cervical spotting, bleeding gums, etc.). As noted above, the vulva and vagina become increasingly vascularized. Weight of the uterus decreases the rate of venous return in the pelvic vasculature, backing up into the vulva. This can lead to generalized edema and varicosities of the vulva (Gianella et al., 2022).

During pregnancy, the vaginal walls thicken, its smooth muscle hypertrophies, and rugae (vaginal folds) and other perineal structures may become more pronounced. Thickening of rugae increases the surface area of the vaginal mucosa, allowing for better stretching of the vagina when the fetus passes through it. Leukorrhea is common throughout pregnancy, especially in the second and third trimesters, and manifests as either a thin or thick, white or yellow discharge without itching or irritation (Phillippi & Kantrowitz-Gordon, 2023).

The vaginal microbiome is thought to play a major role in mitigating infection and dysbiosis of the vaginal flora has been linked with increased risk of preterm birth. Vaginal flora in term pregnancies show an increased prevalence of *Lactobacillus* spp., which is one of the most important normally occurring bacteria in the vaginal microbiome. Presence of other pathological organisms is correlated with preterm birth and intra-amniotic infection. Estrogen levels help maintain predominance of *Lactobacillus* spp. during pregnancy. When estrogen falls in the postpartum, it can lead to an increase in pathogenic species, increasing the risk of postpartum vaginal infections (Zhu et al., 2022).

Pelvic Floor Changes

Increasing levels of progesterone and the hormone relaxin (which increases in response to estrogen) during pregnancy soften the ligaments and muscles of the pelvic floor. Relaxin is produced in pregnancy by the placenta, corpus luteum, and endometrium, and "relaxes" ligaments and other musculoskeletal structures, musculature of the pelvic floor, likely because it alters production of collagen and extracellular matrix proteins (Fede et al., 2019). These muscles and ligaments are further stretched by the weight of the gravid uterus and during birth. Muscular weakness, tension, and anatomic changes in the pelvic floor occurring during pregnancy and birth may predispose people to urinary and fecal incontinence, hemorrhoids, dyspareunia, and other complications both during and after pregnancy. Diagnosis and early treatment of these conditions, especially in the postpartum, can play a major role in improving symptoms and quality of life (DeLancey et al., 2024).

INTEGUMENTARY SYSTEM CHANGES

During pregnancy, there is an increased activity of the sebaceous glands, with increased sweating. Production of melanin increases and causes hyperpigmentation in up to 90 percent of pregnant people. Melanocyte activation likely occurs in response to estrogen, progesterone, and increased levels of melanocyte-stimulating hormone (MSH). It is possible that MSH's increase is related to increased levels of adrenocorticotropin hormone (ACTH), which is secreted in very high levels in pregnancy and has a common precursor molecule (proopiomelanocortin) with MSH. Increased pigmentation is typically seen on the areola, genitalia, abdomen, and face (chloasma gravidarum), as well as in the form of the linea nigra—a dark line beginning at the umbilicus or near the sternal notch and continuing downward to the symphysis pubis and genitalia (Gupta et al., 2024).

Striae gravidarum or distensae (stretch marks in pregnancy) may appear on the breasts, abdomen, hips, and thighs due to thinning of elastin fibers in the skin (Gupta et al., 2024). These marks may be a deep red or purple color during pregnancy but typically fade to a color approaching the person's skin tone in the months following pregnancy.

Hair also appears thicker, both in terms of diameter of individual hairs and because the normal metabolism of hair (patterns of growth and shedding) is often paused; because of this, some people shed less hair in pregnancy than they normally do. People who have less shedding in pregnancy often undergo a sudden, marked increase in hair loss after pregnancy. Hair usually returns to its usual patterns of growth/shedding within a few months of pregnancy, but pigmentation may persist for longer or may not return to the original color (Gupta et al., 2024).

GASTROINTESTINAL CHANGES

Because of the effects of progesterone, peristalsis, gastric emptying, and the overall rate of gastrointestinal transit slow during pregnancy. These changes are responsible for many of the digestive side effects seen in pregnancy, including nausea, gastroesophageal reflux, constipation, and altered appetite. As is the case with the diaphragm and other organs that lie in the path of the growing uterus, the intestines may be displaced from their usual location. This can worsen constipation and may also make diagnosis of conditions such as appendicitis more difficult; the appendix may be displaced from the right lower quadrant, and pain symptoms may not present classically in pregnancy. During pregnancy, the gastric contents become more acidic, possibly worsening reflux symptoms (Kazma et al., 2020).

Oral health is impacted by the hormones of pregnancy, especially the gums. Gingival tissue has a strong response to both estrogen and progesterone, leading to a number of consequences: both hormones increase inflammatory markers in the gums, suppress certain aspects of the immune system, and alter the composition of the oral microbiome. Periodontal disease may arise or worsen during pregnancy and has been linked to increased incidence of adverse pregnancy outcomes, including pre-eclampsia, preterm labor/birth, and low birth weight (Wen et al., 2023).

CARDIOVASCULAR SYSTEM AND HEMATOLOGIC CHANGES

The heart, blood vessels, and hematologic markers all undergo significant changes during pregnancy.

The heart is displaced upward and to the left within the chest cavity by the pressure of the gravid uterus on the diaphragm. As pregnancy progresses, hypotension can result for some pregnant people due to compression of the inferior vena cava and aorta. Hemodynamic changes and anatomic changes also may alter vital signs in a pregnant person (**Table 31-2**).

Plasma volume increases by 30–50 percent, peaking around 24 weeks' gestation, although half of the total increase in cardiac output occurs by the eighth week of pregnancy (Kazma et al., 2020). The increase in blood volume improves blood flow to the vital organs and protects against excessive blood loss during birth. The volume of red blood cells increases by only 30 percent, leading to a relative physiologic dilutional anemia in pregnancy. Because of this, normal hemoglobin/hematocrit ranges are different in each trimester, relative to those for nonpregnant adults. While anemia can lead to clinically significant sequelae and increase risk of adverse birth outcomes, mild physiologic

TABLE 31-2 Vital Sign Changes in Pregnancy

Vital Sign	Changes in Pregnancy	Measurement Alterations in Pregnancy
Heart rate (HR) and heart sounds	Volume of the first heart sound may be increased with splitting Third heart sound may be detected Systolic murmurs may be detected HR increases by 15–25% beats/min beginning in 1st and peaking in 3rd trimester (Morton, 2021)	Palpate the maternal pulse when auscultating the fetal heart rate to be able to distinguish the two Systolic murmurs are generally best auscultated at the left lateral sternal border
Respiratory rate	Remains in normal range, though minute ventilation increases	None
BP	First trimester: Same as prepregnancy values Second trimester: Diastolic BP decreases to its nadir at 24–26 weeks due to peripheral vascular resistance Third trimester: Gradually returns to prepregnancy values	Auscultating blood pressure, rather than use of an automated device, is the gold standard for BP monitoring in pregnancy. Devices, including those used in clinic, should be recalibrated regularly. Home cuffs should be calibrated with clinical devices. Not all BP monitoring devices are validated for pregnancy. Measure BP while the person is sitting. If this is not possible, the left lateral position is preferred to avoid compression of the aorta.

Data from Blackburn, S. T. (2018). Maternal, fetal and neonatal, physiology: A clinical perspective (5th ed.). Saunders Elsevier; Jarvis, C. (2016). Physical examination and health assessment (7th ed.). Saunders Elsevier; Kazma et al., 2020; Phillippi & Kantrowitz-Gordon, 2023; Hurrell et al., 2022.

Abbreviation: BP, blood pressure.

hemodilutional anemia may be of benefit to the evolution of placental vascularity as well as fetal development. Hemoglobin that exceeds normal levels for pregnancy in the third trimester is, in fact, associated with increased rates of NICU admission. Elevated hemoglobin may reflect inadequate blood volume expansion and lead to increased viscosity of the blood, which can damage the placenta, impairing its function (Smith et al., 2022).

As blood volume increases by the third trimester, so does cardiac output. It increases by 30–45 percent, as a product of increased heart rate and increased contractility (Morton, 2021) and represents increased stress on the heart compared to the nonpregnant state. Increased blood flow may lead to systolic murmurs; these are generally considered benign, although diastolic or severe murmurs may be pathological (Kazma et al., 2020). Therefore, a pregnant person with cardiac disease may experience exacerbation and possibly become symptomatic even during the first trimester.

Systemic vascular resistance decreases in pregnancy as a consequence of widespread vasodilation, which is itself triggered by the actions of progesterone, nitric oxide and prostacyclin (Calimag-Loyola & Lerma, 2019). Due to activation of the renin-angiotensin-aldosterone (RAAS) system, water retention is increased, but this does not normally increase blood pressure due to vasodilation. Red blood cell mass also increases by as much as 50 percent, but often not to the extent that serum volume increases, leading to physiologic anemia in pregnancy (Calimag-Loyola & Lerma, 2019).

As the red blood cell volume increases, iron demands of the fetus also increase. Clotting factors increase as well, creating a risk for clotting events during pregnancy.

Systemic vascular resistance is reduced due to the effects of progesterone, prostaglandins, estrogen, and prolactin. This lowered systemic vascular resistance, in combination with inferior vena cava compression, is partly responsible for the dependent edema that occurs in pregnancy.

For most pregnant people, the changes that occur to the cardiovascular system are well tolerated and resolve in the postpartum period. However, it is important for clinicians to note that cardiovascular disease is a significant cause of both postpartum and long-term morbidity and mortality for birthing people, especially from communities that experience systemic health inequities and oppression (Gad et al., 2021).

RESPIRATORY SYSTEM CHANGES

One of progesterone's many actions in pregnancy is to stimulate respiratory activity, increasing respiratory rate, and minute ventilation. This leads to a mild respiratory alkalosis that is usually well compensated but means that the pregnant person is more at risk for complications from metabolic alkalosis, including diabetic ketoacidosis (Kazma et al., 2020). The metabolic demands of pregnancy increase oxygen consumption by 30%; this need is well met by the alterations in ventilation in most pregnant people but can represent significant physiologic strain in people with chronic pulmonary disease or other forms of respiratory compromise. Changes in breathing patterns and lung volumes are accompanied by alterations in the geometrical structure of the thoracic cage; these changes are primarily mediated by relaxin. The diameters of the rib cage expand, and the angle of the ribs shifts superiorly to accommodate the increasing size of the uterus. Compliance of the chest wall decreases slightly, and respiratory muscles undergo increased stretching (LoMauro & Aliverti, 2022).

Increased edema of the pharynx and larynx during pregnancy may cause respiratory congestion in some pregnant people. Blood vessels in the nose vasodilate, causing engorgement of the capillaries (Kazma et al., 2020). This may increase risk of benign nosebleeds during pregnancy.

IMMUNE SYSTEM CHANGES

The immune system is normally configured to attack tissue that is nonself, that is, tissue with a different cellular, genetic and metabolic makeup than the body's own. The fetus is genetically distinct from the pregnant person's body and is therefore nonself. In pregnancy, however, both the innate and adaptive immune systems' actions are modulated to create a state of immunotolerance, preventing the immune system from attacking the fetus. Progesterone plays a significant role in affecting these changes by altering the balance of various populations of T cells in the uterus and throughout the body, reducing aspects of the activity of natural killer cells, and generally reducing inflammation. This is one of the proposed reasons why certain types of autoimmune conditions become less active during pregnancy; progesterone may increase the population of the Th2 line of T cells, while many autoimmune diseases rely on activity of the Th1 line (Motomura et al. 2023).

The adaptive branch of the adult immune system uses major histocompatibility (MHC) molecules to recognize the body's own tissue and differentiate it from "foreign" tissue. Cells of the placental interface, called extravillous trophoblast cells, present a different profile of MHC molecules than other somatic cells (Mao et al., 2023), helping to make them more invisible to the parental immune system, but sometimes the pregnant person's body can form anti-fetal antibodies or fail to make the immune adaptations necessary for successful embryonic implantation or placentation. Immune rejection can therefore be etiologic in a variety of conditions such as miscarriage, infertility, and pre-eclampsia (Robertson et al., 2022; Jung et al., 2022).

It is important to understand that modification of the immune response begins prior to conception. Immune activity in the endometrium changes at the end of each luteal phase in anticipation of possible pregnancy, and there is a shift in populations of immune cells and inflammatory markers that assists in vascular remodeling as well as preparing the uterus to host the fetoplacental unit without attacking it (Motomura et al., 2023).

Though pregnant people are more at risk for certain types of infection, immune changes also protect the fetus from infection, and persistence of nonpregnant immune system function may be one of the mechanisms for miscarriage (Li et al., 2021). Leukocytosis occurs in pregnancy, with white blood cell counts increasing to as much as 14,000 to 17,000 cells/mm^3 of blood, but increased leukocytes correlate with this modified immune function, rather than heightened immune function overall.

These immune system alterations have a number of effects. Natural killer cells likely play a major role in remodeling the spiral arteries of the uterine decidua. This remodeling minimizes the ability of these arteries to vasoconstrict, which helps allow for adequate perfusion of the placenta (Robertson et al., 2022). A lack of adequate remodeling, in which parental arteries retain their ability to constrict, is linked to pre-eclampsia and poor placental perfusion.

RENAL SYSTEM CHANGES

From the beginning of pregnancy, renal function alters to meet the body's changing metabolic needs. In early pregnancy, the kidney maintains pH balance with the onset of low-level hyperventilation and mild respiratory alkalosis. It also responds to progesterone-mediated systemic vasodilation, increasing glomerular filtration rate (GFR) by 25 percent within 2 weeks of conception and by 50 percent overall by 12 weeks of gestation. These changes account for some of the urinary frequency and nocturia commonly experienced during pregnancy (Beers & Patel, 2020). This vasodilation results in activation of the renin-angiotensin-aldosterone system (RAAS), increasing total body water and contributing to increased body fluid volume by 6–8 L. At the same time, the body also becomes less sensitive to the effects of angiotensin II, allowing the RAAS to increase fluid volume but reducing its tendency to increase blood pressure (Calimag-Loyola & Lerma, 2019). As a result of increased renal blood flow, the kidneys increase in size (Beers & Patel, 2020).

Increased blood flow, glomerular permeability, and GFR alter both glomerular function and the composition of the urine. Glucose handling in particular is affected; more glucose passes through the glomerulus, and the tubules are able to reabsorb glucose less efficiently. As a consequence, mild glucosuria is normal in pregnancy and does not on its own represent diabetes (Calimag-Loyola & Lerma, 2019).

Once again, progesterone-mediated smooth muscle relaxation plays a major role in an organ change, in this case, dilation of the ureters, urethra, and bladder. This can result in stasis of urine and increased risk for stress incontinence and bladder infection (Beers & Patel, 2020). Dilation of the ureters and possible backflow of urine during pregnancy increase the risk for ascending infection, especially pyelonephritis.

MUSCULOSKELETAL SYSTEM CHANGES

Several musculoskeletal changes occur during pregnancy and are primarily related to the effects of progesterone, estrogen, and relaxin on ligaments and joints, as well as the increasing weight of the uterus. Particularly notable is the relaxation of ligaments and joints in the pelvis, which affect the pelvic floor musculature, as described earlier. The sacroiliac joint experiences increased mechanical stress during pregnancy and may separate, as is the case for the pubic symphysis (Vincent et al., 2019). Both of these changes can lead to pelvic pain, difficulty walking, sciatica, altered gait, and other issues. Noticeable alterations in posture manifest as lordosis and kyphosis; they are due to a shifting center of balance caused by the enlarging uterus.

ENDOCRINE SYSTEM CHANGES

As discussed, pregnancy is driven by a number of hormonal processes, yielding changes to the endocrine system. Trophic hormones found in nonpregnant people are secreted at different levels and sometimes from different sources in the pregnant person. For instance, in nonpregnant adults, gonadotropin-releasing hormone (GnRH) and corticotrophin-releasing hormone (CRH) are produced by the hypothalamus, and adrenocorticotrophic hormone (ACTH) is produced by the anterior pituitary. As such, much of the regulation of reproductive hormone function, including menstruation and expression of sex characteristics, is usually mediated by the hypothalamic–pituitary–adrenal/gonadal axes. In pregnancy, however, the placenta produces analogues of GnRH, CRH and ACTH, increasing the circulating levels of these hormones dramatically. ACTH, for instance, is 3 times higher than the levels seen in the nonpregnant person (Morton & Teasdale, 2022). These placental analogues have the same effect as their normal counterparts, but often have a shorter half-life.

The elevated CRH and ACTH, secreted by both the pregnant person and the placenta, are responsible for the cortisol elevation seen in pregnancy. This elevated cortisol may contribute to symptoms like fatigue and edema but appears to be necessary for fetal development and initiation of labor. This is interesting because both normal and pathologic stress responses involve increased levels of cortisol, and there is a large body of evidence demonstrating how stress in the pregnant person can contribute to adverse fetal outcomes to the extent that toxic stress has been described as a "developmental teratogen" (Bakhireva et al., 2024). More research is necessary to elucidate the role of stress and when it harms or protects the pregnancy.

Of the endocrine system alterations, changes in thyroid function are some of the most profound and necessary for fetal development, especially in early pregnancy. Until the fetus begins producing their own thyroid hormone, the pregnant person's thyroid is essential for fetal development and organogenesis. Both hyper- and hypothyroidisim in the pregnant person can result in abnormal fetal growth or miscarriage (Morton & Teasdale, 2022).

Because of the important role of thyroid hormone, iodine intake is a significant nutritional consideration for the pregnant person. When the fetus is able to produce their own thyroid hormone, iodine is transported transplacentally, drawing on the pregnant person's own iodine supply. If a pregnant person has limited iodine intake, fortified foods or other supplementation may be necessary (Morton & Teasdale, 2022).

A palpable, mild enlargement of the thyroid often occurs early in the first trimester. Thyroid-stimulating hormone levels decrease initially but return to normal by birth (ACOG, 2020). Thyroid hormone demand is high in pregnancy, but thyroid stimulating hormone (TSH), the pituitary trophic hormone responsible for stimulation of the active thyroid hormones T3 and T4, is secreted at lower levels during pregnancy. This occurs in large part because human chorionic gonadotropin (HCG) has TSH-like function and acts on the thyroid to increase production of T3 and T4 (Morton & Teasdale, 2022).

Glucose regulation, especially that involving insulin output and cellular insulin resistance, changes dramatically in order to adequately feed the fetus. As pregnancy progresses, the fetus requires more glucose and the pregnant person's body develops increasing levels of insulin resistance in order to make glucose more available to them. As insulin resistance increases, pancreatic beta cell hyperplasia occurs, increasing insulin production. This increased insulin output should happen by around 28–32 weeks; if it does not, gestational diabetes (GDM) develops (Kampmann et al., 2019).

While GDM has long been regarded as a pregnancy complication, it is important for the clinician to recognize that GDM is, for many childbearing people, an early manifestation of chronic beta cell impairment and insulin dysfunction. These issues increase the person's risk of both future diabetes and cardiovascular disease, and follow-up in the months and years after pregnancy should take this into account (Fu & Retnakaran, 2022).

The pituitary gland also grows larger and increases secretion of prolactin in preparation of lactation (Kazma et al., 2020). Lipid metabolism is also altered in pregnancy. The pregnant person generally gains adipose tissue in the first two trimesters and enters a catabolic phase in the third trimester, when lipolysis may increase. During this time, serum triglycerides and total cholesterol also increase. Adipose tissue produces hormones such as leptin (involved in regulating glucose and energy homeostasis) and adiponectin (which increases sensitivity to insulin) (Morton & Teasdale, 2022; Phillippi & Kantrowitz-Gordon, 2023).

NEUROLOGIC SYSTEM AND PSYCHOSOCIAL CHANGES

Changes to central nervous system vascularity, increased proportions of white matter and decreased proportions of gray matter, and hormonal alterations all have significant impacts on brain function. Neural plasticity (the ability of the brain to form new neural pathways, alter function, and adapt to its environment) is seen in all stages of the human life span, but is profound in pregnancy and the postpartum. Changes in activation in regions of the brain associated with caregiving and social connection are seen, as are alterations in motivation, executive function, and somatosensory perception. Some neurologic changes seem to target the parent's ability to perceive their own infant's signals and needs; these changes do not seem to predispose pregnant people to respond more to other infants' cues. Exposure to their own infant's cues stimulates the postpartum person's brain to activate its reward pathways (Barba-Müller et al., 2019). Many behavioral and neurologic alterations (increased appetite, response to stress, etc.) are influenced by various hormones, including prolactin and hormones secreted by the placenta (Behura et al., 2019; Kazma et al., 2020).

Postpartum people are at risk for either new or worsening mental health conditions during and after pregnancy (also refer to Chapter 34). Many factors play a role here; for example, social stress and breakdown of community structures, sleep alterations, systemic inequities (including disparities in rates of referral and treatment on the basis of structural racism), hormonal alterations, or nutritional deficiencies or imbalances (Haight et al., 2024; Rupanagunta et al., 2023), but pregnant and postpartum people are at significant risk for adverse mental health outcomes, and screening and treatment should be important priorities for their clinicians.

CONCLUSION

An understanding of the physiologic basis for the symptoms and changes a person's body undergoes during pregnancy can help demystify the process and empower clients and families. It is also important to understand that the experience of severe stress, both acutely and over time, impact the body's function, including in the context of pregnancy. Perinatal mortality rates for both the pregnant person and the neonate are much higher in communities of color, especially in Black and Indigenous populations in the United States, in a way that is not adequately explained by disparities in traditional social determinants of health (Riggan et al., 2021). While factors such as clinician bias, structural racism, and higher rates of medical trauma in marginalized groups contribute to adverse care outcomes and adverse client experience (Wang et al., 2021; Haight et al., 2024), an increasing body of research is illuminating mechanisms explaining how experiencing discrimination and systemic oppression changes the body. For example, weathering is the experience of chronic and severe stress, and allostatic load is a method for estimating the effects of this stress (Lueth et al., 2022; Riggan et al., 2021). Lueth and colleagues (2022) found that people with a significant allostatic load—and Black birthing people were the group with the highest rate of significant allostatic load—in the first trimester of pregnancy were more likely to experience adverse outcomes in pregnancy. Another study found that Black women who chronically experienced racism demonstrated alterations in DNA methylation, an epigenetic mechanism associated with increased rates of pathologic inflammation (Ruiz-Narváez, 2025). Pregnancy does not occur in a vacuum, and the stress that pregnant people and their communities experience affects the biologic changes caused by pregnancy. The clinician must consider both the physiology of pregnancy and the way the pregnant person's experiences in the world may shape this.

References

American College of Obstetricians & Gynecologists. (2020). Thyroid Disease in Pregnancy: ACOG Practice Bulletin, Number 223. *Obstetrics and gynecology, 135*(6), e261–e274. https://doi.org/10.1097/AOG.0000000000003893

American College of Obstetricians & Gynecologists. (2021). Fetal Growth Restriction: ACOG Practice Bulletin, Number 227. *Obstetrics and gynecology, 137*(2), e16–e28. https://doi.org/10.1097/AOG.0000000000004251

Bakhireva, L. N., Solomon, E., Roberts, M. H., Ma, X., Rai, R., Wiesel, A., Jacobson, S. W., Weinberg, J., & Milligan, E. D. (2024). Independent and combined effects of prenatal alcohol exposure and prenatal stress on fetal HPA axis development. *International Journal of Molecular Sciences, 25*(5), 2690. https://doi.org/10.3390/ijms25052690

Barba-Müller, E., Craddock, S., Carmona, S., & Hoekzema, E. (2019). Brain plasticity in pregnancy and the postpartum period: Links to maternal caregiving and mental health. *Archives of Women's Mental Health, 22*(2), 289–299. https://doi.org/10.1007/s00737-018-0889-z

Beers, K., & Patel, N. (2020). Kidney physiology in pregnancy. *Advances in Chronic Kidney Disease, 27*(6), 449–454.

Behura, S. K., Dhakal, P., Kelleher, A. M., Balboula, A., Patterson, A., & Spencer, T. E. (2019). The brain-placental axis: Therapeutic and pharmacological relevancy to pregnancy. *Pharmacological Research,* 149, 104468. https://doi.org/10.1016/j.phrs.2019.104468

Buksh, M. M., Al Naib, S., & Al Samaraee, A. (2023). Round ligament varicosity: A rare but important differential diagnosis of groin lumps during pregnancy. *British Journal of Hospital Medicine (London, England: 2005), 84*(5), 1–15. https://doi.org/10.12968/hmed.2022.0469

Calimag-Loyola, A. P. P., & Lerma, E. V. (2019). Renal complications during pregnancy: In the hypertension spectrum. *Disease-a-month: DM, 65*(2), 25–44. https://doi.org/10.1016/j.disamonth.2018.03.001

Cope, D. I., & Monsivais, D. (2022). Progesterone receptor signaling in the uterus is essential for pregnancy success. *Cells, 11*(9), 1474. https://doi.org/10.3390/cells11091474

Cunningham, F., Leveno, K. J., Dashe, J. S., Hoffman, B. L., Spong, C. Y., & Casey, B. M. (Eds.). (2022). *Williams Obstetrics* (26th ed.). McGraw Hill.

d'Hauterive, S. P., Close, R., Gridelet, V., Mawet, M., Nisolle, M., & Geenen, V. (2022). Human chorionic gonadotropin and early embryogenesis: Review. *International Journal of Molecular Sciences, 23*(3), 1380. https://doi.org/10.3390/ijms23031380

DeLancey, J. O. L., Masteling, M., Pipitone, F., LaCross, J., Mastrovito, S., & Ashton-Miller, J. A. (2024). Pelvic floor injury during vaginal birth is life-altering and preventable: What can we do about it? *American Journal of Obstetrics and Gynecology, 230*(3), 279–294.e2. https://doi.org/10.1016/j.ajog.2023.11.1253

Drugs and Lactation Database (LactMed®) [Internet]. Bethesda (MD): National Institute of Child Health and Human Development; 2006-. *Testosterone.* [Updated 2022 May 15]. Available from: https://www.ncbi.nlm.nih.gov/books/NBK501721/

El Hage, L., & Hatipoglu, B. (2021). Elevated hCG can be a benign finding in perimenopausal and postmenopausal women. *Cleveland Clinic Journal of Medicine, 88*(11), 635–639. https://doi.org/10.3949/ccjm.88a.18069

Farah, E., Barger, M. K., Klima, C., Rossman, B., & Hershberger, P. (2021). Impaired lactation: Review of delayed lactogenesis and insufficient lactation. *Journal of Midwifery & Women's Health, 66*(5), 631–640. https://doi.org/10.1111/jmwh.13274

Fede, C., Pirri, C., Fan, C., et al. (2019). Sensitivity of the fasciae to sex hormone levels: Modulation of collagen-I, collagen-III and fibrillin production. *PLoS One, 14*(9), e0223195. doi:10.1371/journal.pone.0223195

Fetal Growth Restriction: ACOG Practice Bulletin, Number 227. (2021). *Obstetrics and Gynecology, 137*(2), e16–e28. doi:10.1097/AOG.0000000000004251

Fidalgo, D. S., Jorge, R. M. N., Parente, M. P. L., Louwagie, E. M., Malanowska, E., Myers, K. M., & Oliveira, D. A. (2024). Pregnancy state before the onset of labor: A holistic mechanical perspective. *Biomechanics and Modeling in Mechanobiology, 23*(5), 1531–1550. https://doi.org/10.1007/s10237-024-01853-3

Fu, J., & Retnakaran, R. (2022). The life course perspective of gestational diabetes: An opportunity for the prevention of diabetes and heart disease in women. *EClinicalMedicine,* 45, 101294. https://doi.org/10.1016/j.eclinm.2022.101294

Fu, N. Y., Nolan, E., Lindeman, G. J., & Visvader, J. E. (2020). Stem cells and the differentiation hierarchy in mammary gland development. *Physiological Reviews, 100*(2), 489–523. https://doi.org/10.1152/physrev.00040.2018

Geddes, D. T., Gridneva, Z., Perrella, S. L., Mitoulas, L. R., Kent, J. C., Stinson, L. F., Lai, C. T., Sakalidis, V., Twigger, A. J., & Hartmann, P. E. (2021). 25 years of research in human lactation: From discovery to translation. *Nutrients, 13*(9), 3071. https://doi.org/10.3390/nu13093071

Gad, M. M., Elgendy, I. Y., Mahmoud, A. N., Saad, A. M., Isogai, T., Sande Mathias, I., Misbah Rameez, R., Chahine, J., Jneid, H., & Kapadia, S. R. (2021). Disparities in cardiovascular disease outcomes among pregnant and post-partum women. *Journal of the American Heart Association, 10*(1), e017832. https://doi.org/10.1161/JAHA.120.017832

Giannella, L., Montanari, M., Delli Carpini, G., Di Giuseppe, J., & Ciavattini, A. (2022). Huge vulvar varicosities in pregnancy: Case report and systematic review. *The Journal of International Medical Research, 50*(5), 3000605221097764. https://doi.org/10.1177/03000605221097764

Graham, G. A., & Montgomery, A. (2019). Breast anatomy and milk production. In S. H. Campbell, J. Jauwers, R. Mannel, & B. Specer (Eds.), *Interdisciplinary lactation care* (pp. 83–99). Jones & Bartlett Learning.

Gupta, S. N., Madke, B., Ganjre, S., Jawade, S., & Kondalkar, A. (2024). Cutaneous changes during pregnancy: A comprehensive review. *Cureus, 16*(9), e69986. https://doi.org/10.7759/cureus.69986

Haight, S. C., Daw, J. R., Martin, C. L., Sheffield-Abdullah, K., Verbiest, S., Pence, B. W., & Maselko, J. (2024). Racial and ethnic inequities in postpartum depressive symptoms, diagnosis, and care in 7 U.S. jurisdictions. *Health Affairs (Project Hope), 43*(4), 486–495. https://doi.org/10.1377/hlthaff.2023.01434

Hurrell, A., Webster, L., Chappell, L. C., & Shennan, A. H. (2022). The assessment of blood pressure in pregnant women: Pitfalls and novel approaches. *American Journal of Obstetrics and Gynecology, 226*(2S), S804–S818. https://doi.org/10.1016/j.ajog.2020.10.026

Jozsa, F., & Thistle, J. (2023). Anatomy, Colostrum. In *StatPearls*. StatPearls Publishing. https://www.ncbi.nlm.nih.gov/books/NBK513256/

Jung, E., Romero, R., Yeo, L., Gomez-Lopez, N., Chaemsaithong, P., Jaovisidha, A., Gotsch, F., & Erez, O. (2022). The etiology of preeclampsia. *American journal of obstetrics and gynecology, 226*(2S), S844–S866. https://doi.org/10.1016/j.ajog.2021.11.1356

Kampmann, U., Knorr, S., Fuglsang, J., & Ovesen, P. (2019). Determinants of maternal insulin resistance during pregnancy: An updated overview. *Journal of Diabetes Research*, 5320156. https://doi.org/10.1155/2019/5320156

Kazma, J. M., van den Anker, J., Allegaert, K., Dallmann, A., & Ahmadzia, H. K. (2020). Anatomical and physiological alterations of pregnancy. *Journal of Pharmacokinetics and Pharmacodynamics, 47*(4), 271–285. https://doi.org/10.1007/s10928-020-09677-1

Kissler, K., & Hurt, K. J. (2023). The pathophysiology of labor dystocia: Theme with variations. *Reproductive Sciences (Thousand Oaks, Calif.), 30*(3), 729–742. https://doi.org/10.1007/s43032-022-01018-6

Lacroix, G., Gouyer, V., Gottrand, F., & Desseyn, J. L. (2020). The cervicovaginal mucus barrier. *International Journal of Molecular Sciences, 21*(21), 8266. https://doi.org/10.3390/ijms21218266

Lau, E. S., Aggarwal, N. R., Briller, J. E., Crousillat, D. R., Economy, K. E., Harrington, C. M., Lindley, K. J., Malhamé, I., Mattina, D. J., Meng, M. L., Mohammed, S. F., Quesada, O., Scott, N. S., & ACC Cardiovascular Disease in Women Committee (2024). Recommendations for the management of high-risk cardiac delivery: ACC Cardiovascular Disease in Women Committee Panel. *JACC: Advances, 3*(4), 100901. https://doi.org/10.1016/j.jacadv.2024.100901

Li, W. X., Xu, X. H., & Jin, L. P. (2021). Regulation of the innate immune cells during pregnancy: An immune checkpoint perspective. *Journal of Cellular and Molecular Medicine, 25*(22), 10362–10375. https://doi.org/10.1111/jcmm.17022

LoMauro, A., & Aliverti, A. (2022). Respiratory physiology in pregnancy and assessment of pulmonary function: Best practice & research. *Clinical Obstetrics & Gynaecology, 85*(Pt A), 3–16. https://doi.org/10.1016/j.bpobgyn.2022.05.007

Lueth, A. J., Allshouse, A. A., Blue, N. M., Grobman, W. A., Levine, L. D., Simhan, H. N., Kim, J. K., Johnson, J., Wilson, F. A., Murtaugh, M., Silver, R. M., & National Institutes of Health (NIH), Eunice Kennedy Shriver National Institute of Child Health and Human Development (NICHD), Nulliparous Pregnancy Outcomes Study: Monitoring Mothers-to-Be (nuMoM2b), and National Heart, Lung, and Blood Institute (NHLBI) nuMoM2b Heart Health Study (nuMoM2b-HHS) (2022). Allostatic load and adverse pregnancy outcomes. *Obstetrics and Gynecology, 140*(6), 974–982. https://doi.org/10.1097/AOG.0000000000004971

Mao, J., Feng, Y., Zhu, X., & Ma, F. (2023). The molecular mechanisms of HLA-G regulatory function on immune cells during early pregnancy. *Biomolecules, 13*(8), 1213. https://doi.org/10.3390/biom13081213

Massri, N., Loia, R., Sones, J. L., Arora, R., & Douglas, N. C. (2023). Vascular changes in the cycling and early pregnant uterus. *JCI Insight, 8*(11), e163422. https://doi.org/10.1172/jci.insight.163422

McEvoy, A., & Sabir, S. (2022). Physiology, pregnancy contractions. In *StatPearls*. StatPearls Publishing. https://www.ncbi.nlm.nih.gov/books/NBK532927/

Morton A. (2021). Physiological changes and cardiovascular investigations in pregnancy. *Heart, Lung & Circulation, 30*(1), e6–e15. https://doi.org/10.1016/j.hlc.2020.10.001

Morton, A., & Teasdale, S. (2022). Physiological changes in pregnancy and their influence on the endocrine investigation. *Clinical Endocrinology, 96*(1), 3–11. https://doi.org/10.1111/cen.14624

Motomura, K., Miller, D., Galaz, J., Liu, T. N., Romero, R., & Gomez-Lopez, N. (2023). The effects of progesterone on immune cellular function at the maternal-fetal interface and in maternal circulation. *The Journal of Steroid Biochemistry and Molecular Biology,* 229, 106254. https://doi.org/10.1016/j.jsbmb.2023.106254

Ng, S. W., Norwitz, G. A., Pavlicev, M., Tilburgs, T., Simón, C., & Norwitz, E. R. (2020). Endometrial decidualization: The primary driver of pregnancy health. *International Journal of Molecular Sciences, 21*(11), 4092. https://doi.org/10.3390/ijms21114092

Oyatogun, O., Sandhu, M., Barata-Kirby, S., Tuller, E., & Schust, D. J. (2021). A rational diagnostic approach to the "phantom hCG" and other clinical scenarios in which a patient is thought to be pregnant but is not. *Therapeutic Advances in Reproductive Health,* 15, 26334941211016412. https://doi.org/10.1177/26334941211016412

Phillippi, J., & Kantrowitz-Gordon, I. (Eds.). (2023). *Chapter 19, Anatomy and Physiology of Pregnancy. Varney's Midwifery* (7th ed.). Jones & Barrett Learning.

Riggan, K. A., Gilbert, A., & Allyse, M. A. (2021). Acknowledging and Addressing Allostatic Load in Pregnancy Care. *Journal of racial and ethnic health disparities, 8*(1), 69–79. https://doi.org/10.1007/s40615-020-00757-z

Robertson, S. A., Moldenhauer, L. M., Green, E. S., Care, A. S., & Hull, M. L. (2022). Immune determinants of endometrial receptivity: A biological perspective. *Fertility and Sterility, 117*(6), 1107–1120. https://doi.org/10.1016/j.fertnstert.2022.04.023

Ruiz-Narváez, E. A., Cozier, Y., Zirpoli, G., Rosenberg, L., & Palmer, J. R. (2025). Perceived experiences of racism in relation to genome-wide DNA methylation and epigenetic aging in the Black Women's Health Study. *Journal of Racial and Ethnic Health Disparities, 12*(2), 754–763. https://doi.org/10.1007/s40615-024-01915-3

Rupanagunta, G. P., Nandave, M., Rawat, D., Upadhyay, J., Rashid, S., & Ansari, M. N. (2023). Postpartum depression: Aetiology, pathogenesis and the role of nutrients and dietary supplements in prevention and management. *Saudi Pharmaceutical Journal: SPJ: The Official Publication of the Saudi Pharmaceutical Society, 31*(7), 1274–1293. https://doi.org/10.1016/j.jsps.2023.05.008

Schaal, B., Saxton, T. K., Loos, H., Soussignan, R., & Durand, K. (2020). Olfaction scaffolds the developing human from neonate to adolescent and beyond. Philosophical Transactions of the Royal Society of London. *Series B, Biological Sciences, 375*(1800), 20190261. https://doi.org/10.1098/rstb.2019.0261

Smith, J. S., Bullens, L. M., van der Hout-van der Jagt, M. B., van Runnard Heimel, P. J., & Oei, S. G. (2022). Effect of intrapartum maternal hemoglobin on mode of delivery and short-term neonatal outcome: A systematic review. *Obstetrical & Gynecological Survey, 77*(10), 595–605. https://doi.org/10.1097/OGX.0000000000001074

Vincent, R., Blackburn, J., Wienecke, G., & Bautista, A. (2019). Sacroiliac joint pain in pregnancy: A case report. *A&A Practice, 13*(2), 51–53. https://doi.org/10.1213/XAA.0000000000000987

Wang, E., Glazer, K. B., Sofaer, S., Balbierz, A., & Howell, E. A. (2021). Racial and ethnic disparities in severe maternal morbidity: A qualitative study of women's experiences of peripartum care. *Women's Health Issues: Official Publication of the Jacobs Institute of Women's Health, 31*(1), 75–81. https://doi.org/10.1016/j.whi.2020.09.002

Wen, X., Fu, X., Zhao, C., Yang, L., & Huang, R. (2023). The bidirectional relationship between periodontal disease and pregnancy via the interaction of oral microorganisms, hormone and immune response. *Frontiers in Microbiology,* 14, 1070917. https://doi.org/10.3389/fmicb.2023.1070917

Zangeneh, F. Z., & Hantoushzadeh, S. (2023). The physiological basis with uterine myometrium contractions from electro-mechanical/hormonal myofibril function to the term and preterm labor. *Heliyon, 9*(11), e22259. https://doi.org/10.1016/j.heliyon.2023.e22259

Zhu, B., Tao, Z., Edupuganti, L., Serrano, M. G., & Buck, G. A. (2022). Roles of the microbiota of the female reproductive tract in gynecological and reproductive health. *Microbiology and Molecular Biology Reviews: MMBR, 86*(4), e0018121. https://doi.org/10.1128/mmbr.00181-21

CHAPTER 32

Overview of Prenatal Care

Susanrachel B. Condon

The editors acknowledge Julia C. Phillippi and Bethany Sanders, who were authors of a previous version of this chapter.

INTRODUCTION

Pregnancy may be one of the most significant events in the lives of individuals and their families. The United States currently faces multiple crises regarding reproductive health care, including access to both abortion and prenatal care, and rising maternal and neonatal morbidity and mortality. In 2024, the March of Dimes published a report on maternity care deserts in the United States, citing both geographic and social determinants of health as well as policies that contribute to rising death rates, particularly in communities of color (Archer, 2025). These include shortages of care providers, availability of clinics, travel time, and insurance access. Decision making and options for continuing or terminating a pregnancy have changed significantly in the United States since the *Dobbs v. Jackson Women's Health* ruling by the Supreme Court in 2022. Clinicians must be attentive to the statutes where they practice, but their priority should be providing ethical and evidence-based care. A reliable tool providing up-to-date information about abortion restrictions and bans can be found on the website for the Center for Reproductive Rights at https://reproductiverights.org/maps/abortion-laws-by-state/.

The purpose of this chapter is to furnish an up-to-date, early antepartum framework for clinicians who provide primary and gynecologic care. For more in-depth guidance on providing antepartum care, clinicians may consult midwifery and obstetric books such as *Varney's Midwifery,* 7th ed. (Phillippi & Kantrowitz-Gordon, 2023), *Prenatal and Postnatal Care: A Woman-Centered Approach* (Grace et al., 2023), and *Gabbe's Obstetrics: Normal and Problem Pregnancies,* 9th ed. (Landon et al., 2025). In addition, national, professional organizations such as the Association of Women's Health, Obstetric and Neonatal Nurses, the American College of Nurse-Midwives, and the American College of Obstetricians and Gynecologists issue practice bulletins and statements that synthesize current evidence for clinicians, and these references may be helpful in providing evidence-based prenatal care according to the most up-to-date standards. These are generally accessible on the internet.

Adequacy of prenatal care is considered by clinical and research authorities to be of paramount importance for healthy outcomes. However, controversy about what constitutes adequate prenatal care abounds. Some indices emphasize the number of visits while others consider the length of visits, overall quality of interactions, and continuity of care. Developing trust with clinicians encourages patients to return for routine care because they see the value in doing so.

Clinicians who do not attend births must ascertain the information needed to provide referrals for ongoing care based on the health of each individual, special characteristics of a given pregnancy, clinical practice philosophy, personal and cultural preferences, and preferred place of birth. One crucial component of quality care is listening attentively and respectfully.

Obtaining a thorough history using open-ended questions is the keystone of prenatal care. Clinicians must consider each individual's health literacy, the impact of social determinants of health, and must aspire to demonstrate cultural humility when offering first-trimester screening for genetic conditions, infections, and health challenges that may impact a pregnancy as it progresses.

MODELS OF AND APPROACHES TO PRENATAL CARE

Numerous innovations in approaches to prenatal care have emerged in recent decades. Models of group prenatal care, such as CenteringPregnancy™, may increase the appeal of attending regular visits, as they provide an opportunity for pregnant patients to engage socially with their peers. Group prenatal care has been found to offer consistent attendance and high patient satisfaction (Boothe et al., 2022). Attending group prenatal care increases attendance at postpartum visits and timely initiation of contraception for those who choose or need it (Heberlein et al., 2020).

Another important development is the conscientious integration of trauma-informed care. A history of trauma, adverse childhood events (ACE), economic hardship, housing and/or food insecurity, complex immigration status, racism, discrimination, intimate partner or interpersonal violence, substance use disorder, and social or family instability can impact well-being during pregnancy and clinical pregnancy outcomes (Racine et al., 2021). A prolonged physiologic stress response can impact multiple body systems, resulting in pregnancy complications and adverse health and psychosocial outcomes (Johnson et al., 2023). Examples of a trauma-informed care approach are shown in **Box 32-1**. For more information about providing trauma-informed care, refer to Chapter 5.

BOX 32-1 Approaches to Trauma-Informed Care (Adapted from Owens, 2022)

1. Ask open-ended questions.
   a. Are there any ongoing challenges you'd like to talk about today?
2. Encourage ongoing dialogue.
   a. I understand you'd like information about routine testing. We'll talk over tests ahead of the next visit so you have time to decide.
3. Express willingness to revisit a discussion at a later date.
   a. It sounds like you need more time to consider genetic testing. I'll give you some information to review and we can talk about it next time.
4. Avoid interpreting or telling people how they feel—ask.
   a. It sounds like you'd like some ongoing support between visits; do I have that right?
5. Request consent every time.
   a. May I assess your blood pressure?
6. Offer options whenever possible to promote autonomy.
   a. Would you prefer to sit up or lie down for the blood draw?
7. Avoid medical jargon.
   a. "The baby is growing nicely" rather than "your uterine size is consistent with your gestational age."

Data from Owens, L., Terrell, S., Low, L. K., Loder, C., Rhizal, D., Scheiman, L., & Seng, J. (2022). Universal precautions: the case for consistently trauma-informed reproductive healthcare. *American journal of obstetrics and gynecology, 226*(5), 671–677.

INITIAL PRENATAL VISIT

The initial prenatal visit usually includes dating and confirmation of the pregnancy with a urine or blood pregnancy test or auscultation of fetal heart tones, depending on the number of weeks gestation. These are followed by a comprehensive history and physical examination, decision making about laboratory studies and imaging, and anticipatory guidance about ongoing care.

DIAGNOSIS OF PREGNANCY

Information about the diagnosis of pregnancy, determination of location and viability, and compassionate discussions surrounding plans for pregnancy continuation, adoption, and abortion are discussed in Chapter 19.

ASSESSMENT

The first few prenatal visits should address the individual patient's needs and desires. Even if the patient plans to obtain and continue care at another location, careful assessment, discussion of preventative measures, and supportive counseling can improve self-efficacy and both short- and long-term health outcomes. Assessment should be comprehensive, including both psychosocial and clinical components. Subjective and objective information are used to develop a plan designed to optimize pregnancy outcomes through appropriate education, testing, services, and referrals.

Initial Prenatal Visit

Obtaining a thorough health history is an essential component of the initial prenatal visit. Because pregnancy may affect all aspects of health and well-being, the history should include an in-depth inquiry of overall health, obstetric, and gynecologic history in addition to information about family, social support, nutrition, occupation, and recreational activities. Critical components of the prenatal health history are highlighted below. Refer to Chapter 8 for basic elements of a health history.

Menstrual History

Gestational age refers to the length of pregnancy from the first day of the last menstrual period (LMP) and is described in weeks and days. The estimated date of birth (EDB) is approximately 280 days after the first day of the LMP. Data about the most recent, typical menstrual cycle are used for initial determination of gestational age and EDB (Phillippi & Kantrowitz-Gordon, 2023). Certainty regarding the LMP is needed to date the pregnancy, and adjustments should be made if cycles are greater or fewer than 28 days apart. This represents the mean for length of cycles ranging from 21 to 35 days. Ovulation and implantation days vary; therefore, though the EDB is referred to throughout pregnancy, the clinician may emphasize to the patient that it provides an approximation because just as the length of cycles may vary, the length of a term pregnancy ranges from 37 to 42 completed weeks (Phillipi & Kantrowitz-Gordon, 2023).

While the most valid pregnancy dating is obtained with first trimester ultrasound, it is important to ascertain the gestational age to determine when ultrasound will be accurate. This can be accomplished with a gestational wheel, web-based application, electronic health record calculator, and, for those with 28-day cycles, using Näegele's rule.

Näegele's rule, named for the 18th-century German obstetrician who developed the concept, is used to estimate the due date or date of birth (EDB) based on the assumption that the duration of pregnancy is 40 weeks or 280 days (Lawson, 2021). When using Näegele's rule, the clinician adds 7 days to the first day of the LMP, then subtracts 3 months (**Box 32-2**). If cycles are regular and slightly longer or shorter than 28 days, the EDB will need to be adjusted. A patient with 30-day cycles would have 2 days added to the calculated EDB, and a patient with 26-day cycles would have 2 days subtracted. If using a gestational wheel, software, or computer application, the clinician must ensure the version is accurate and accounts for a leap year when indicated.

Referral for ultrasound is indicated for those who are uncertain of their LMP. This may occur with people who do not track their cycles, those using contraception, when pregnancy is unplanned, or for those with conditions that affect menstruation such as polycystic ovary syndrome, eating disorders, lactational or idiopathic amenorrhea, and for those with low body fat.

The American College of Obstetricians & Gynecologists (ACOG), the American Institute of Ultrasound Medicine, and the Society for Materal-Fetal Medicine hold that early accurate dating improves outcomes and that first-trimester ultrasound dating is the optimal

> **BOX 32-2 Näegele's Rule**
>
> Example of using Näegele's rule to calculate an estimated date of birth from the date of the last menstrual period.
>
> LMP of 4/23
> + 7 days
> 4/30
> −3 months
> 1/30 January 30 (of following year)

means of confirming estimated due date. They recommend ultrasound examination for dating up to 13 6/7 weeks. (ACOG, 2022). Accurate dating assists clinicians in assessing for appropriate fetal growth, may reduce iatrogenic prematurity due to early induction of labor and may reduce still birth related to post-term pregnancy. Gestational age-appropriate care and anticipatory guidance for parents follows a well-dated pregnancy. Early ultrasound also distinguishes intrauterine versus ectopic pregnancy and singleton versus multiple gestation. Timely treatment of ectopic pregnancy is necessary to preserve health and reproductive capacity should future pregnancies be intended. If continuation of an intrauterine pregnancy is not desired, accurate dating is imperative to ensure timely referral for care in the best interest of the patient (ACOG, 2022).

Ultrasound guidelines state that either transvaginal or transabdominal ultrasound may be performed in the first trimester. Abdominal ultrasound is preferred when the uterine fundus is above the pubic symphysis. However, if transabdominal ultrasound is not definitive, a transvaginal approach should be used and the referring clinician should note this in the order as some imaging centers will not perform the transvaginal scan unless it is included. Given the invasive nature of a transvaginal ultrasound, clinicians should prepare patients with the rationale for transvaginal imaging, describe the procedure, and request consent for the referral. The accuracy of ultrasound dating declines as pregnancy progresses, so a timely referral is important (Rodgers et al., 2024).

Social History

A thorough social history provides an opportunity to learn more about patients and their lived experiences for the purpose of individualizing care, establishing a rapport, and addressing specific needs and risk factors. It is important to determine whether patients' households have adequate food, heat, and other resources such as transportation; if they do not, they should be referred to social services and community organizations for needed assistance. Follow-up is important to ensure the needed services are available and obtainable.

The social history should also include who lives with the patient, their religious affiliation (if any), gender identity and pronouns, sexual orientation, dietary choices and restrictions, physical exercise, general lifestyle, levels of stress, occupational hazards, and chemical exposure. Clinicians should address tobacco, alcohol, and substance use and abuse using a neutral tone and be prepared to offer referrals for smoking cessation and treatment (Fathi & Kathuria, 2023; Tarasi et al., 2022).

A pregnancy can strengthen or strain relationships. Patients should be asked about safety and their support systems and screened for intimate partner violence. If a patient lives in an insecure or dangerous environment, pregnancy may exacerbate tension and put the patient more at risk of harm. Pregnant adolescents should be screened for abuse. If physical and/or sexual abuse is a factor, it is the clinician's responsibility to follow state laws as mandated reporters. State by state rules regarding what must be reported either by statute or voluntarily can be found at https://mandatedreportertraining.com/resources/blog/which-states-have-mandatory-domestic-violence-reporting/. Refer to Chapter 15 for information regarding screening for intimate partner violence.

Race is socially constructed and impacts how people are perceived and treated, limiting access to the foundations of health equity. Systemic racism creates health disparities and impacts parental, fetal, and neonatal outcomes. Individuals who experience persistent racism are at higher risk for pregnancy complications and severe morbidity and mortality. This is especially true for Black and Indigenous people. Clinicians must be conscious of the impact of discrimination in the context of race, class, and religion and actively work to mitigate avoidable poor outcomes (van Daalen et al., 2022).

Contraceptive History

Obtaining a contraceptive history is important for patients with partners who can cause pregnancy. Patients who conceive while using oral contraceptives, injections, vaginal rings, or patches can rest assured that if they choose to continue their pregnancies, these methods rarely cause harm. Long-acting reversible contraceptive (LARC) use will require careful management. For example, implants have a failure rate of < 0.1 percent, usually due to use of medications that make the implant less effective or failure to replace the implant after 3 years. Implants should be removed when pregnancy occurs. Fewer than 1 percent of patients with copper intrauterine devices (IUD) and approximately 0.2 percent of patients with levonorgestrel devices experience pregnancy (Bahamondes et al., 2020). Removal of IUDs is recommended because pregnancy complications including pregnancy loss, preterm labor, and intra-amniotic infection are increased when they are left in place. Removal of an IUD can be done in the clinician's office, but the procedure may cause unintended pregnancy loss. When pregnancy does occur with LARC, patients should be referred for ultrasound to confirm the pregnancy is intrauterine. Ectopic pregnancy is slightly more common with LARC failure and must be treated without delay (Stabile et al., 2022). Clinicians should encourage ongoing condom use for those at risk for sexually transmitted infections.

Obstetric History

Information about previous pregnancies contributes to understanding both the individual's clinical and psychosocial stories. History of recurring spontaneous abortion, induced abortion, preterm birth, induction of labor, and vaginal versus cesarean birth may have a significant impact on guidance for the plan of care going forward. For each prior pregnancy, using a trauma-informed approach, the clinician asks about the year, gestational age at the time the pregnancy ended, and how the pregnancy ended. In addition, clinicians should inquire and about pregnancy, birth, or postpartum complications, including mental health difficulties (Moore et al., 2021).

ACOG and the Society for Maternal–Fetal Medicine concur that patients who are at increased risk for preeclampsia, particularly those with diabetes, chronic hypertension, renal disease, or autoimmune disorders, should take 81 mg of aspirin daily starting between 12 and 28 weeks, (but ideally by 16 weeks) and continuing until birth to reduce the risk of preeclampsia with the current pregnancy (ACOG, 2022).

In addition, those with one or more moderate risk factors may also consider taking low-dose aspirin daily to reduce the risk of developing preeclampsia. Moderate risk factors include Black race, nulliparity, living in a large body, family history of a mother or sibling with preeclampsia, low socioeconomic status, age 35 or older, previous adverse pregnancy outcome, previous small-for-gestational-age or low-birth-weight infant, or a more than 10-year interpregnancy interval. An increased prevalence of bleeding has not been associated with this protocol so discontinuing aspirin at term is not advised. While low-dose aspirin has been associated with decreased spontaneous abortion, fetal growth restriction, low birth weight, and still birth, prophylaxis is not recommended in the absence of risk factors for preeclampsia (ACOG, 2023).

Preterm birth accounts for 10 percent of all births and is the leading cause of neonatal mortality (ACOG, 2023). Patients with a history of previous preterm birth, defined as birth before 37.0 weeks gestation, should be followed by midwives, obstetrician gynecologists, or maternal–fetal medicine specialists for periodic ultrasound assessment of cervical length. Intramuscular 17-OHPC progesterone injections were used to prevent preterm birth until being withdrawn from the market by the Food & Drug Administration (FDA) in 2023. Patients with a history of preterm labor and/or birth may be concerned that this medication is no longer available. According to ACOG, vaginal progesterone may be considered as a treatment option for patients with a history of preterm birth, singleton gestation, and a shortened cervix but it has not been effective in preventing preterm birth without a shortened cervix and should not be considered as an equivalent alternative to progesterone injections (ACOG, 2023).

Patients with prior uterine surgeries including cesarean for a nonrecurring indication should be offered personalized counseling regarding the potential benefits and harms of vaginal versus cesarean birth. While this topic will be discussed during early prenatal care in the review of history and systems, in-depth discussion, counseling, and decision making may be planned for later in pregnancy. Patients should be given the most current available information about their options to inform their choices and time to consider them.

Mental Health History

Understanding a patient's mental health history and current status or diagnosis is essential to making a comprehensive plan to address psychosocial needs throughout and after pregnancy. Self-care, the assistance of friends and family, psychotherapy, and medications may be used to help patients manage the profound changes inherent in pregnancy and thrive through pregnancy and the postpartum period. Those with eating disorders or mood disorders such as depression and anxiety may benefit from cognitive behavioral therapy as an adjunct to or substitute for pharmacological treatment for mild to moderate symptoms (Shortis et al., 2020). There are other safe and effective therapeutic interventions for individuals who have experienced trauma, have post-traumatic stress disorder, or who fear of childbirth. Eye Movement Desensitization and Reprocessing Therapy (EMDR) has been effective in pregnant individuals who fear childbirth, as has Mindfulness Based Intervention (Abdolalipour et al., 2023; Baas et al., 2022; Baas et al., 2020).

Patients who need psychiatric medications beyond selective serotonin reuptake inhibitors should be given immediate psychiatric or psychopharmacologic referral to develop a plan that supports their mental health with minimal fetal effects.

Infectious Disease History

Several serious and potentially teratogenic infectious diseases have grown more common due to vaccine hesitancy, and childhood vaccination may or may not confer immunity into adulthood. Those who work with or live with young children may be more susceptible to exposure to infections such as rubeola (measles), rubella (German measles), and varicella (chicken pox). The live vaccines that prevent these infections are contraindicated during pregnancy. A history of prior infectious diseases, vaccinations, and current immunity is needed to establish risk and to plan for drawing titers and offering vaccines postpartum when indicated.

If a patient has traveled to areas where tuberculosis (TB) is endemic or has ever been exposed to tuberculosis, the QuantiFERON (QFT) blood test is used for diagnosis, even when the infection is latent. This test, which is superior to the tuberculin skin test, measures how well T cells release interferon-gamma in response to stimulation from *m. tuberculosis* peptide antigens. The CDC recommends QFT as an alternative to the tuberculin skin test. It may be included with a routine prenatal laboratory panel and is more convenient as it does not require a second visit as is needed to "read" the skin test result. Refer to current guidelines at https://www.cdc.gov/tb/hcp/testing-diagnosis/interferon-gamma-release-assay.html.

Appropriate vaccines should be offered during pregnancy (**Table 32-1**). The CDC updates the adult vaccine schedule often, and this information can be easily accessed on its website https://www.cdc.gov/vaccines/hcp/imz-schedules/adult-age.html (CDC, 2024).

Pregnancy decreases the immune response. For those with increased risk of exposure, TORCH screening is indicated. TORCH is an acronym for toxoplasmosis, rubella, cytomegalovirus, and herpes simplex. Other infections are also frequently considered part of the TORCH panel, including syphilis, hepatitis B, parvovirus, and varicella. Patients who garden or live with cats that go outdoors or live in homes with rodents can take precautions to decrease their risk of contracting toxoplasmosis, an infection that is transmitted through handling the feces of cats that hunt. Litter boxes should be changed (preferably daily) by someone other than the pregnant patient to prevent contact with the *Toxoplasma gondii* parasite. Wearing gloves while gardening and careful hand washing are also important. More information and patient handouts are available at the CDC website. Patients who are HIV positive may be more susceptible to TORCH infections (Batra et al., 2020).

Patients working in occupations that involve exposure to food-borne, droplet-borne, or body fluid-borne pathogens should employ universal precautions, use appropriate protective personal equipment, and practice rigorous handwashing. If exposed to infectious diseases, they should contact their clinicians or the appropriate staff to determine whether blood tests and immune globulin treatments are indicated.

TABLE 32-1 Vaccines in Pregnancy

Recommended During Each Pregnancy	Rationale	Timing
Influenza (flu)[a]	Pregnancy increases risk for complications.	When available
SARS-CoV-2 (COVID-19)	Pregnancy increases risk for complications.	When available
RSV	Recommend (Pfizer Abrysvo only)	Between weeks 32–36
Tetanus, diphtheria, acellular pertussis (TDaP)	Antibodies cross the placenta and decrease the risk of pertussis infection in the newborn and for the first 6 months of life.	Third trimester, ideally between gestational weeks 27–36
Advised With Elevated Risk	**Rationale**	**Timing**
Hepatitis B	Indications include risk of occupational exposure to blood, treatment for a sexually transmitted infection, more than one sexual partner in the past 6 months, recent intravenous drug use, and a sex partner who is HBsAg positive.	Three injections beginning at any point in pregnancy with the first 2 doses a month apart and the third 6 months later
Contraindicated	**Rationale**	
Measles, mumps, rubella (MMR)	This live virus vaccine has a (theoretical) risk to the fetus.	N/A
Varicella (Varivax)	This live virus vaccine has a (theoretical) risk to the fetus.	N/A

Data from Centers for Disease Control and Prevention. (2024). *Guidelines for vaccinating pregnant persons.* https://www.cdc.gov/vaccines-pregnancy/hcp/vaccination-guidelines/index.html.

Abbreviations: HBsAg, hepatitis B virus surface antigen; HBV, hepatitis B virus.

[a]Live attenuated influenza vaccine (LAIV, brand name FluMist) should not be given during pregnancy.

Screening for sexually transmitted infections (STIs) is routine in early pregnancy. A history of STIs, some of which are teratogenic or otherwise impact pregnancy outcomes, should be discussed in a respectful manner. Early treatment and careful planning are important. The type and timing of treatment for STIs may be different during pregnancy (Workowski & Bachmann, 2022). The most current guidelines can be located on the CDC website or their free mobile application.

Patients of Size

Being significantly overweight can predispose people to a range of pregnancy complications such as congenital fetal anomalies, cardiac dysfunction, obstructive sleep apnea (particularly in the third trimester), gestational diabetes, hypertensive disorders, and still birth. Patients who have undergone weight loss surgeries should be evaluated for nutritional deficiencies (ACOG, 2021).

The use of GLP-1 receptor agonists and glucagon-like peptide-1 receptor agonists has increased significantly. While it is advised that people avoid these medications when seeking pregnancy, unplanned pregnancies have occurred. It appears that weight loss drugs may decrease the effectiveness of hormonal contraceptives, though more research is needed. One early observational study found no major identifiable fetal abnormalities, but due to the recent rise in the use of these medications, it is too early to know about long-term adverse effects (Cesta et al., 2024).

Genetic History

The history should include family and genetic history of both parents if known. Patients who were adopted or are uncertain about their family history can report back if there is an opportunity to speak with relatives, or this information can be documented as unknown.

Substance Exposure Including Medications, Illicit Drugs, and Chemicals

The first 12 weeks of pregnancy are crucial for normal development. In the first 2 weeks after implantation, there is no shared blood supply. Minimal, accidental, or occasional exposure to drugs or toxic substances during this time poses little risk. This time is referred to as the "all or none period." Exposure to substances that impact implantation will result in pregnancy loss; exposure to most substances will do no harm (Mother to Baby, 2023).

In the embryonic period, from the third to the beginning of the ninth week, exposure to some chemicals can affect development of organs or entire systems. Due to tragic, historic errors in underestimating risk from exposure to medications in pregnancy, there is now a tendency to overestimate teratogenic harm (Shroukh et al., 2020). Assessment of exposure to drugs and chemicals can assist patients in avoiding toxins while continuing or adapting needed therapies (Sarayani et al., 2022).

Mother to Baby is an organization that provides evidence-based, accessible information about exposure to toxins and drugs for clinicians and the public. Their website is www.mothertobaby.org.

Prescription Medications

Safety data for medication use during pregnancy is limited, as little controlled research is performed with pregnant individuals for obvious ethical reasons. The FDA requires that labeling for all drugs follow the Pregnancy and Lactation Labeling Rule, which is designed to assist clinicians in discerning the known relative safety of prescription drugs during pregnancy and lactation based on available research. The same labeling is not required for over-the-counter medications. Each patient's prescription and over-the-counter medications should be reviewed for known risks during pregnancy. The benefits and potential harm of all medications should be considered with regard to clinical needs and patient experience and preferences. The harms of discontinuing some medications can outweigh their risks. For example, discontinuing an antidepressant may pose more harm than good. If a patient needs pharmacologic treatment for a health condition and the current drug has evidence of fetal toxicity, another class of drug with a different risk profile can usually serve as a substitute. Polypharmacy should be avoided if a single agent is appropriate and effective as this reduces fetal exposure (Anand et al., 2023; Subramanian et al., 2023). Changes in medication should be done with the patient as the driver in collaborative decision making, and specialists should be consulted as needed. **Box 32-3** provides resources for up-to-date information about medication use in pregnancy.

Recreational Drug Use and Substance Use Disorder

Pregnant individuals should be screened for cannabis, tobacco, alcohol, and illicit substance use. The history should include both current and past use of specific drugs, including heroin, cocaine, and other street drugs because those in recovery may be at risk for relapse. When obtaining a history, it is imperative that clinicians avoid using judgmental verbal or body language.

Legalization of recreational and medicinal cannabis use across the United States increases the likelihood of its use during pregnancy; however, there are no data that suggest whether cannabis can be used safely at this time. One large cohort study published in 2024 found an association with gestational hypertension, preeclampsia, weight gain outside of guidelines, and placental abruption (Young-Wolff et al., 2024).

Tobacco use has been proven harmful. In addition to contributing to low birth weight and preterm birth, smoking causes vasoconstriction and elevates blood pressure, decreases placental perfusion, and is associated with placental abruption (Cohn et al., 2023; Incognito et al., 2024).

The use of electronic cigarettes and vaping has increased significantly in the last decade. Marketing has suggested these nicotine delivery methods are less harmful to health than combustable cigarettes. E-cigarettes without nicotine contain chemicals that have not been adequately studied. The use of vaping products during pregnancy has been associated with fetal growth restriction (Wang et al., 2020).

It is the consensus of the Centers for Disease Control and Prevention and other health-related associations to recommend complete cessation of alcohol use during pregnancy, as no amount of alcohol consumption has been shown to be safe. Moderate alcohol use in pregnancy has been associated with poor perinatal outcomes and child developmental disorders (Oei et al., 2020).

Substance use disorder affects people of all geographic areas, ethnic, racial, and socioeconomic groups. In the past decade, prescribing narcotics to treat pain has increased dramatically in the United States. Use of these drugs often begins for legitimate, short-term, clinical reasons but too often progresses to dependence. It is well established that narcotics can have detrimental effects on a developing fetus and neonate. Although elimination of opioid use is a goal, rapid discontinuation can be harmful and may be associated with higher rates of relapse. Individuals who use opioids persistently will need interprofessional care that includes clinical treatment with opioid antagonist pharmacotherapy and support for any underlying conditions causing pain (ACOG, 2021). Therapeutic and recreational use of hallucinogens should be screened for, as use of lysergic acid, psilocybin, Methylenedioxymethamphetamine (MDMA), ketamine, and other drugs has increased dramatically. According to one study, hallucinogen use has nearly doubled in young adults between the ages of 19 and 30 from 2018 to 2021 (Keyes et al., 2023).

Patients with recent substance use can benefit from support, referrals, and follow-up to assist them in recovery. Although a toxicology screen can be performed, these require informed consent and have minimal value in detecting many substances, depending on how long their metabolites remain in body systems. While controversial, univeral screening is often recommended to mitigate persistent age, racial, and ethnic biases that prompt some clinicians to test disproportionately in non-white, younger, and low-income patients. This can have a profound impact on individuals and families when child protective services is summoned at the time of birth (Cohen et al., 2023).

The value of drug testing should be weighed against the importance of nurturing trust so patients feel supported and return for all prenatal visits. A compassionate approach is essential in helping patients access needed care and services. Patients with a history of substance use should be encouraged to use resources for support during pregnancy and parenting when indicated.

Chemical Exposure

The initial history should include travel with potential exposure to parasites, infectious disease, or recent immigrant status to determine whether referral to infectious disease specialists is warranted. In addition, clinicians should inquire about past or recent known exposure to chemicals/pesticides, solvents, heavy metals, fumes, dust, noise, radiation, or other hazards. The Occupational Safety and Health Administration mandates that the names and health effects of all work-related chemicals be made available to employees in the workplace via safety data sheets. This information may be found at https://www.osha.gov/.

BOX 32-3 Sources of Information About Medications in Pregnancy

- FDA-approved drug prescribing and labeling information
- https://www.nlm.nih.gov/toxnet/index.html
- Reprotox*: https://www.reprotox.org/
- https://mothertobaby.org/

Informing patients about relevant safety data sheets is a starting point for assessment of workplace chemical exposures.

Exposure to chemicals and dangerous substances may occur at work, at school or home, and while traveling. A summary of specific substances to be included in initial data gathering and discussion can be found in **Table 32-2**. Avoidance or mitigation of exposure to these toxic substances should be encouraged. The Program on Reproductive Health and the Environment provides up-to-date information on its website: https://prhe.ucsf.edu/. ACOG provides up-to-date guidance about exposure to toxic substances (ACOG, 2024). Clinicians should bear in mind that the risk of exposure is heightened in some communities and remains a significant social determinant of health (Morelli et al., 2017).

Safety

General Safety

All normal safety precautions are important to continue during pregnancy. For instance, seat belts should continue to be used throughout pregnancy, even though they may become uncomfortable. There are pregnancy seatbelt adapters on the market that are designed to improve comfort without compromising safety.

The physiologic changes of pregnancy may increase susceptibility to musculoskeletal injuries and falls. The hormone relaxin increases the elasticity of ligaments, thus destabilizing weight-bearing joints. Changes in weight distribution affect gait and may increase the risk of trips and falls. Diastasis recti is common and may compromise abdominal support for the lumbar spine. The rising uterus and plasma volume expansion contribute to shortness of breath. Poor sleep and insomnia can also contribute to injuries (Günal et al., 2022). Pregnant individuals may need to adapt their participation in activities that involve more than moderate exertion, risk of injury, or heat exhaustion. They should be encouraged to avoid overheating to avoid dizziness and therefore the risk of fainting or falling. Patients should use their judgment and comfort during exertion as a guide.

Occupational Safety

Sound body mechanics can prevent injury, and adjustments to the frequency and type of lifting and movement are advisable as pregnancy progresses. Pregnant individuals should not be required to perform job tasks that involve carrying heavy objects, sitting all day, or lifting from the floor or lifting above the head. Pregnancy is a hypercoagulable state. Prolonged sitting can increase the risk of developing a deep vein thrombosis. Inadequate bathroom breaks can increase the risk of urinary tract infection (Franco et al., 2020). Many people, especially those in low-paying jobs, experience pregnancy-related discrimination and may not want to disclose their health status to their employers (Mehra et al., 2023). Clinicians may need to advocate for patients who will need a note to adjust their work tasks.

Exercise

Exercise is important for cardiovascular, musculoskeletal, and mental health. Consistent physical activity has been found to decrease complications such as hypertensive disorders, gestational diabetes, and excessive weight gain. Both the World Health Organization and ACOG recommend healthy pregnant individuals engage in 150 minutes of moderate exercise weekly. Aerobic and resistance exercise with gradual warm-up and cool-down periods are advised. Pregnant patients should be encouraged to continue to perform moderate exercise as tolerated throughout pregnancy (Yang et al., 2022). Further, clinicians should encourage previously sedentary patients to engage in regular low-impact exercise several times weekly (Bull et al., 2020).

TABLE 32-2 Potentially Toxic Environmental Exposures

Substance	Potential Exposure	Potential Problem	Recommendations
Cigarette smoke including secondhand smoke	Lit cigarettes	Low birth weight, preterm birth	Leave the area Open a window
Lead	Older buildings with lead pipes, lead paint, hobbies using lead (stained glass, furniture restoration, ceramics)	Neurotoxin: Learning deficits, developmental delays	Do not disturb pre-1978 paint Run water 30 seconds in lead pipes Drink bottled water
Mercury	Fish: Swordfish, king mackerel, tilefish, shark, albacore tuna	Neurotoxin: Learning deficits, developmental delays	Avoid fish with high mercury levels and limit albacore tuna to 4 oz per week Check local fish safety advisories
Organic solvents	Occupations or hobbies involving adhesives, cleaning solvents, paints, resins, plastics, dyeing, and printing materials	Birth defects	Eliminate contact Ensure adequate ventilation Wear personal protection, such as gloves and mask

Data from Program on Reproductive Health and the Environment. (Updated 2024, March). *Clinical practice: Resources for health care professionals to promote environmental health.* University of California San Francisco, https://www.fda.gov/food/consumers/advice-about-eating-fish

PHYSICAL EXAMINATION

All individuals who are newly pregnant should be offered a complete, general, physical examination. In addition, there are three areas of concern to consider: dental care, cervical cancer screening, and abdominal palpation.

Dental Care

Consistent, personal dental hygiene is important during pregnancy. Patients should be advised that some bleeding while flossing may be a response to hormones of pregnancy and is not in and of itself alarming. The oral cavity serves as a bacterial reservoir and subclinical infection may contribute to serious prenatal complications. Hormonal changes may exacerbate periodontal disease, which has been associated with preterm birth and preeclampsia (Tsikoura et al., 2024; Machado et al., 2023). Some states cover the cost of basic dental care in pregnancy for low-income individuals (Adeniyi et al., 2020). A referral for hygiene and evaluation should be given to pregnant patients when dental care is due or overdue.

Cervical Cancer Screening

Cervical cancer screening guidelines should be adhered to. If a patient is under 21 years old the Pap test is not indicated. If the patient had a Pap test recently, cervical cancer screening may be deferred until at least 4 weeks postpartum or until next indicated according to the guidelines (USPSTF, n.d.). For more information on screening recommendations, refer to Chapter 9. Pap tests may be offered at the initial visit if there is a concern about a patient being lost to care. Speculum examinations are invasive and even when performed perfectly, Pap specimens may lack the endocervical component during pregnancy due to normal histological changes. Further, the increased vascularity of the cervix may cause bleeding even when the specimen is collected gently. Bleeding in early pregnancy may be alarming to patients, so anticipatory guidance is warranted. Colposcopy is the only acceptable procedure following a report of high-grade intraepithelial lesion (HSIL) during pregnancy. This result is consistent with significant cellular changes, suggestive of a pre-cancerous state. Unless a Pap result is HSIL, colposcopy can safely be deferred until a postpartum visit. If cervical cancer screening is not indicated, a speculum examination is unnecessary unless the patient is experiencing symptoms of a vaginal infection or requests one for another reason (Zagorianakou, et al., 2023).

Abdominal Examination

In a singleton pregnancy at 12 weeks gestation, the uterine fundus should be palpable abdominally, at the level of the symphysis pubis. At 16 weeks gestation, the fundus is expected to be midway between the symphysis and the umbilicus (**Figure 32-1**). Prior to 12 weeks gestation, a bimanual examination may be performed to estimate uterine size and to assess the adnexa for tenderness. If the patient will be undergoing first trimester ultrasound, this intrusive examination is unnecessary. Patients should be advised that the ultrasound examiner may suggest a transvaginal scan to better visualize the pelvic organs. If the uterine size does not match dating by LMP, ultrasound can identify an ectopic, nonviable, or multifetal pregnancy.

FIGURE 32-1 Approximate normal fundal heights during pregnancy.

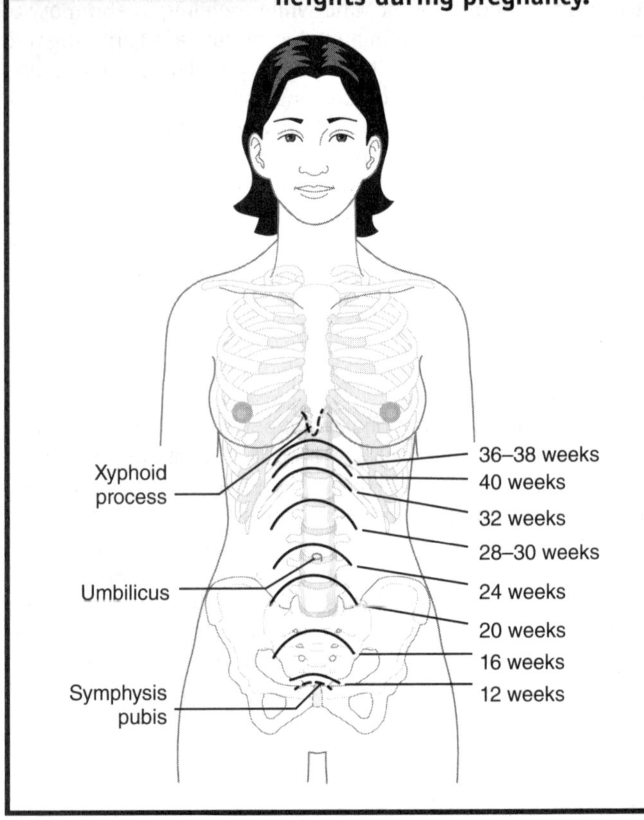

FIGURE 32-2 Handheld doppler.

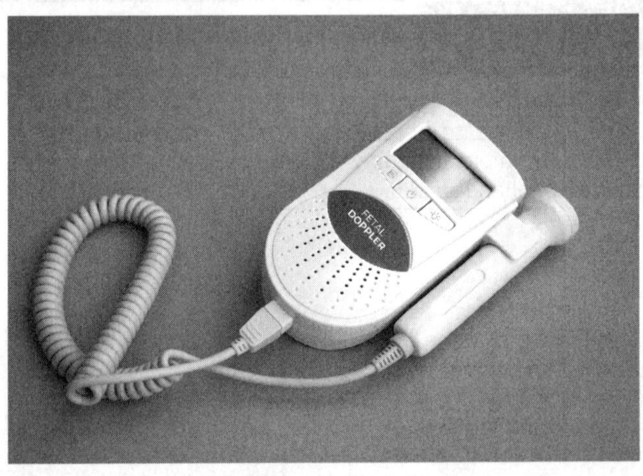

© samperix/Shutterstock

Fetal heart tones can be heard with a handheld doppler (**Figure 32-2**) as early as 10 to 12 weeks from the LMP or slightly later in patients of size. The examiner palpates the fundus of the uterus with the ulnar border of their hand and directs the doppler probe to scan systematically. The fetal heart tones are best heard by slowly rotating the probe to amplify the sound of the fetal heart valves clicking. The normal range for fetal heart tones is 110 to 160 beats per minute. Some dopplers display the heart rate, but these displays may not be reliable. The clinician can

TABLE 32-3 Laboratory Testing at the First Prenatal Visit

Test	Notes
Urinalysis	Baseline screening for protein and assessment of renal function
Urine Culture	Reduces perinatal complications
Blood Type ABO/Rh	Determine need for alloimmunization prophylaxis and documented in case blood transfusion is indicated
Antibody Screen	Baseline titer is used to monitor for changes
Complete Blood Count	Screens for anemia, infection, abnormal platelet count
Hepatitis B	To develop a plan of care to prevent transmission to fetus
Hepatitis C	Advised to screen for this under-reported condition
Human Immunodeficiency Virus	To develop a plan of care to prevent transmission to fetus
Rubella, Rubeola, Varicella Titers	To offer vaccination after birth
Quantiferon	Risk-based assessment, to monitor for comorbidities and develop an appropriate plan of care
Thyroid Stimulating Hormone	Optional, with family history Early diagnosis and treatment can reduce adverse outcomes
Syphilis	Recommended to treat and prevent fetal transmission
Chlamydia (NAAT preferred)	Recommended to prevent perinatal transmission for all at risk—diagnosis or another STI, new or multiple partners, commercial sex work, drug use, inconsistent or no condom use
Gonorrhea	Recommended for all at risk—diagnosis or another STI, new or multiple partners, commercial sex work, drug use, inconsistent or no condom use
Gestational Diabetes (Do not perform if patient has overt diabetes.)	Screening is usually performed at 28 weeks. Consider testing at entry to care if: BMI > 25, sedentary, previous GDM diagnosis, previous newborn weighing > 4,000 gm, first-degree relative with diabetes, polycystic ovary syndrome, race or ethnicity with high allostatic load, history of cardiovascular disease and/or hypertension

Data from Phillippi, J. C., & Kantrowitz-Gordon, I. (2023). Varney's midwifery (7th ed.). Jones & Bartlett Learning.

count the auscultated beats for 6 seconds and multiply by 10 several times to confirm an accurate heart rate. The sound produced by the umbilical cord, or funic sound, will have the same rate as the fetal heart but will sound "swishy." The parental heart rate can be heard through the placenta, and will also sound "swishy."

Laboratory Testing

Specific laboratory tests are usually performed during the initial prenatal visit (refer to **Table 32-3**). Although some tests are based on risk factors or patient preferences for testing, other tests are standard because they provide valuable information to guide care that improves parental, fetal, or newborn health. Essential tests should be performed at the initial prenatal visit to maximize the opportunity to intervene if there are concerning results. Each test and its purpose should be discussed with the patient. Questions should be answered honestly and consent should be obtained.

Genetic Screening

A variety of genetic and developmental tests are available in pregnancy, and these tests should be offered to all patients, regardless of their absolute risk for any given condition. These tests should be offered without coercion or judgment and with respect for the patient's autonomy to make genetic screening decisions. Insurance reimbursement varies and may be a consideration in decision making. If either parent has risk factors for genetic or developmental disorders, the patient may benefit from an early referral for genetic counseling or to a maternal–fetal medicine specialist. Although in-depth discussion of genetic testing is beyond the scope of this chapter, common tests are shown in **Tables 32-4** and **32-5** to facilitate understanding and enhance access to screening and diagnostic testing. Since these tests are usually performed at or after 10 weeks, an overview is provided, but it is recommended screening be discussed further and offered by midwives and obstetricians who are providing ongoing care.

Some patients will request genetic carrier screening. Several conditions are linked to genetic heritage. Testing for carrier status can be performed prior to pregnancy or at any time during pregnancy. As carrier status does not change, these tests do not need to be repeated for individual patients who have been tested in prior pregnancies, but new partner testing may be indicated. Clinicians who order these tests should be prepared to provide pre- and posttest counseling and referral to a genetic counselor when indicated.

TABLE 32-4 Genetic Disorders and Recommended Screening

Genetic Disorders	Offer Testing
Cystic Fibrosis	All individuals
Spinal Muscular Atrophy	All Individuals
Hemoglobinopathies Including Sickle Cell Disease	CBC results with RBC indices Consider automatic for those of African, Mediterranean, Middle Eastern, Southeast Asian, or West Indian descent
Canavan Disease	Ashkenazi Jewish
Familia Dysautonomia	Ashkenazi Jewish
Tay-Sach's Disease	Ashkenazi Jewish, French-Canadian, Cajun, or family history of Tay-Sach's
Fragile X Syndrome	Family history of intellectual disability, unexplained ovarian insufficiency

TABLE 32-5 Fetal Screening Tests

Screening Test	Components	Indicates Risk	Timing
Maternal serum screening	Free beta HCG, PAPP-A, AFP obtained from a finger stick	Trisomy 13, 18, 21	10–13 6/7 weeks
Nuchal translucency	Ultrasound measurement of the nuchal fold	Aneuploidy, fetal anomalies	10–13 6/7 weeks (ideally 11 weeks)
Noninvasive prenatal testing	Laboratory evaluation of cell-free fetal DNA in maternal serum obtained through venipuncture	Aneuploidy, limited fetal gene disorders	9–10 weeks until term
Quad screen	Serum screen of various markers from maternal serum obtained through venipuncture	Neural tube defects, trisomy 13, 18, 21	15–22 weeks
Anatomy scan	Ultrasound of fetus, umbilical cord, placenta, and measurement of amniotic fluid levels	Fetal structural anomalies in all body systems, aneuploidy	18–22 weeks

Data from Data from American College of Obstetricians and Gynecologists. (2020). ACOG Practice Bulletin No. 226: Screening for fetal chromosomal abnormalities (Reaffirmed 2024). https://www.acog.org/clinical/clinical-guidance/practice-bulletin/articles/2020/10/screening-for-fetal-chromosomal-abnormalities

Some patients will request screening for fetal chromosomal variations such as trisomy 21, trisomy 13, trisomy 18, and sex-linked chromosomal conditions such as Turner syndrome and Klinefelter syndrome. Testing for these conditions changes as technology advances and more choices become available. There are financial, ethical, social, and legal aspects of this kind of testing, an in-depth discussion of which is beyond the scope of this chapter.

Abnormal findings on one or more screening tests warrants referral for diagnostic testing, which is performed with chorionic villus sampling or amniocentesis. The screening tests are effective at detecting fetuses with genetic variations, but they can be associated with high rates of false-positive findings. Even if a low-risk patient has a positive screening test, the likelihood that the fetus has a genetic variation is small. Key points to consider when discussing genetic screening are presented in **Box 32-4**.

MANAGEMENT

Patient Education

Education is an essential component of prenatal care. It should be adapted in consideration of an individual's health literacy and social determinants of health such as access to nutritious food, exposure to environmental hazards, and personal safety. Priorities for the first visit include ensuring the patient has adequate resources and encouraging lifestyle modifications, when indicated. An unrushed initial visit should include general information on topics such as sexuality during pregnancy, oral hygiene,

BOX 32-4 Key Points in Offering Fetal Screening

- All patients should be offered screening tests for chromosomal variations and neural tube defects up to 20 weeks gestation.
- Screening does not diagnose anomalies; it indicates increased risk. Further testing is needed for diagnosis. Clinicians should ensure patients understand and accept this before they choose to undergo screening.
- Nondirective counseling should be used when discussing testing options and requesting consent.
- Patients may decline genetic and developmental screening and diagnostic tests for a variety of reasons, and their decisions are to be respected and documented.

exercise, safety adaptations for exercise, helmet and seat belt use, and avoidance of hot tubs and saunas. However, it is important to avoid overwhelming patients with information that can be discussed later, especially if pregnancy was not intended and they need time to absorb the news and consider their options.

Innovative approaches to patient education and communication, such as the Teach Back Method, and collaborative decision making have proven to result in excellent outcomes in various environments and populations.

In the Teach Back Method, the clinician asks open-ended questions, takes responsibility for clarity and accuracy, and invites patients to clarify or rephrase what was said to assess effectiveness. For instance, instead of asking "Do you understand?" using a warm and inquisitive tone, the clinician would say, "We talked about a lot of things, and I want to be sure I explained them clearly. Will you tell me what I said in your own words so I can be sure I was clear?" During this type of encounter, the clinician uses plain language instead of clinical jargon and may use decision aids or pictures to reinforce complex concepts.

Collaborative decision making involves carefully listening to a patient's perspective and preferences, providing information in a noncoercive manner, discussing available options for care, and offering adequate time for patients to select what is right for them.

All pregnant patients should be given information about when to call their clinicians without delay. Warning signs and symptoms of first-trimester complications include vaginal bleeding, abdominal pain, and persistent nausea and vomiting, which are reviewed later in this chapter.

The importance of giving reliable sources of evidence-based education during pregnancy cannot be overstated. The internet is fraught with easily accessed misinformation about pregnancy and birth. Patients should be directed to reliable sources of information and given links or QR codes regarding prenatal topics designed to be accessible to all, including those with low literacy or limited English proficiency. The Journal of Midwifery & Women's Health provides such a resource at their Ask the Midwife website, https://onlinelibrary.wiley.com/page/journal/15422011/homepage/ask-the-midwife. Clinicians should advise their patients to bring concerns they have about information on websites or social media platforms to their prenatal visits.

Nutritional Guidance

Nutritional assessment and counseling about weight gain are also components of comprehensive prenatal care. There is reason for concern about weight and weight gain in pregnancy (Golawski et al., 2023). However, it is necessary to bear in mind the increasingly problematic nature of relying on body mass index (BMI) as a primary indicator of overall health (Olson et al., 2024). An athletic patient with short stature who is very muscular may inaccurately skew toward being overweight or even obese on a BMI calculator—even with very low body fat—and people of size can be healthy. Consider diet, nutrition, and individual body composition. It is critical to emphasize the importance of nutrition over specific weight gain and to avoid language that engenders shame or blame (Cantor et al., 2021; Langley-Evans et al., 2022).

Detailed general information about nutrition and portion size should be included in comprehensive prenatal care. A balanced diet with an increase of approximately 350 calories per day after the first trimester, spread over three meals and two snacks daily, is recommended. The website MyPlate.gov (http://www.MyPlate.gov) is an excellent online resource from the United States Department of Agriculture. The Canadian government's equivalent, Food-Guide Canada (https://food-guide.canada.ca/en/), offers appealing videos with many examples of healthy, balanced meals and snacks.

All patients, and particularly those considered overweight or underweight at the beginning of pregnancy, should be encouraged to have a consultation with a dietician or nutritionist skilled in prenatal nutritional counseling. This is particularly important for individuals with dietary sensitivities, allergies, or restrictions.

The Special Supplemental Nutrition Program for Women, Infants, and Children, a federally operated assistance program, offers dietary counseling and provides vouchers for healthy foods for those living at or below a variable percentage of the federal poverty guidelines. The income and family size–based eligibility are determined annually and can be accessed at https://www.fns.usda.gov/wic. A generic prenatal vitamin and mineral supplement is recommended to ensure iron, folic acid, and vitamin needs are met. Patients may be counseled to take a docosahexaenoic acid (DHA) supplement during pregnancy, either as part of or in addition to a prenatal vitamin, because DHA has been shown to support fetal brain and eye development (Basak & Duttaroy, 2023). Food-based supplements may be less likely to lead to unpleasant side effects such as nausea and constipation. Food safety strategies for pregnancy are shown in **Table 32-6**.

Although there are no conclusive data on safe doses, caffeine increases parental catecholamine levels, so intake during pregnancy should be limited to approximately 200 mg daily, which is approximately equivalent to one 12-ounce cup of coffee (ACOG, 2023). Tapering consumption over several days to a week can help prevent withdrawal headaches. High doses of caffeine are associated with an increased risk of first-trimester pregnancy loss and pregnancy complications (Rohweder et al., 2023). So-called energy drinks containing caffeine are not recommended during pregnancy. According to the FDA, these beverages range from 50–350 mg of caffeine per 16 ounces. Nutritional supplements, beyond reputable prenatal vitamins, are not regulated by the FDA and may contain harmful or untested substances, so they should be avoided in pregnancy unless recommended or prescribed under the guidance of a knowledgeable clinician.

TABLE 32-6 Food Safety in Pregnancy

Wash Thoroughly Fruits and vegetables
Cook Thoroughly or Heat Until Steaming Prepackaged lunch meat, hot dogs, pâté, and meat spreads Eggs Meat (cook at least to medium) Fish and shellfish
Avoid Unpasteurized soft cheeses (e.g., Camembert), gorgonzola, Mexican cheeses (e.g., queso fresco) Unpasteurized milk and juices

Data from FoodSafety.gov. (2019). People at risk: Pregnant women. U. S. Department of Health and Human Services. https://www.foodsafety.gov/people-at-risk/pregnant-women

Common Discomforts in Early Pregnancy

Many individuals experience pregnancy-related discomforts due to both structural and physiologic changes. Though these are common, they may cause distress and should not be simply dismissed as "normal and temporary." Education about the cause, suggesting comfort measures, and offering referrals when indicated may provide both emotional support and relief. In addition, patients should be informed of warning signs to assist them in distinguishing between healthy adaptations to pregnancy and signs or symptoms of complications. Refer to Chapter 33 for more information. Nausea with or without vomiting, breast tenderness, and fatigue are three common discomforts that interfere with quality of life for extended periods of time, particularly in the first trimester.

Nausea and Vomiting

Many individuals experience some nausea with or without vomiting early in pregnancy. Typically, it begins as pregnancy hormone levels rise before 9 weeks, peaks at 12 weeks, and gradually subsides by 20 weeks. Symptoms range from mild queasiness to frequent vomiting at any time of day. A variety of strategies can be used to decrease symptoms. Although there is no evidence that any one treatment is effective for everyone, there are numerous lifestyle modifications and nonpharmacologic therapies that may provide some relief. These include eating five or six small meals throughout the day, consuming bland, lukewarm, or cold foods rather than spicy or hot foods, and having protein-rich snacks minutes before getting up in the morning. Because the iron in multivitamins may exacerbate nausea, patients may eliminate their full prenatal vitamin and take folic acid alone (at least 600 mcg/day) until their symptoms resolve. Triggers of nausea, such as noxious odors or cooking should be avoided when possible. Other commonly recommended remedies include acupressure bands, marketed as Sea Bands™, vitamin B_6, and ginger consumed in candies, tea, or carbonated soda. Ginger can also be taken in 250 mg capsules with a maximum daily dose of 1,000 mg (ACOG, 2024).

Fewer than 3 percent of patients experience severe and persistent nausea and vomiting, known as hyperemesis gravidarum, which results in dehydration, ketonuria, and a 5 percent or greater weight loss. Hyperemesis may persist throughout pregnancy. Those diagnosed with hyperemesis need in-depth assessment and treatment and often benefit from pharmacologic therapies and even hospitalization. Intravenous fluids can correct dehydration, but treatment should then focus on prevention of ongoing symptoms and further health deterioration. While several classes of medications can be utilized in the treatment of hyperemesis, referral is recommended as these patients should be followed closely. Some of the recommended medications may cause drowsiness and they should be prescribed with careful consideration of the patient's activities, responsibilities, and schedule. Medication interactions are common so polypharmacy should be practiced with caution. While a number of classes of medications, such as antihistamines, are used off label, the only FDA-approved pharmacologic treatment for pregnancy-related nausea and vomiting is doxylamine succinate/pyridoxine hydrochloride (brand names Bonjesta and Diclegis). Dosing starts with two tablets (10 mg each) at bedtime and can be increased up to four tablets per day (ACOG, 2024). If this regimen fails to control symptoms, multidrug treatment is indicated. Patients who have struggled with hyperemesis in past pregnancies may benefit from doxylamine succinate/pyridoxine hydrochloride treatment early in pregnancy to avert severe symptoms. Clinicians may need to obtain prior authorization to obtain insurance coverage for these treatments. Antiemetic suppositories may be used for patients who cannot tolerate oral treatment, though more research is needed to discern the safety of medications such as ondansetron (brand name Zofran) (Ashour, 2023).

Breast Tenderness

Breast tenderness is a common pregnancy symptom that may occur as early as 2 weeks after fertilization. Frequently it is the first symptom patients notice, even prior to a missed menstrual period. Increase in breast size and darkening of the areolae begin in the first trimester due to increased levels of progesterone and estrogen which prepare the breasts for lactation (Alex et al., 2020). Patients experiencing breast discomfort should wear a properly fitted, supportive bra, which may mean obtaining a maternity or nursing bra in a larger than usual size. Reassurance and education about anticipated changes as the body prepares for lactation provide an opportunity to begin education about the many benefits of breast/chestfeeding.

Fatigue

Growing a placenta is hard work and extreme fatigue is another common early pregnancy symptom that usually decreases after 12 weeks gestation (Effati-Daryani et al., 2021). However, reporting of fatigue should not be presumed normal and dismissed, as it may be related to serious health conditions. Screening for hypothyroidism, anemia, insomnia, depression, and other potential causes of fatigue is warranted. Assessment of thyroid function during pregnancy is complex but important since thyroid disorders can cause significant complications. When evaluating for thyroid disorders, clinicians should use thyroid stimulating hormone levels as the standard, utilizing a trimester-based laboratory value range, and may consider testing for Hashimoto thyroiditis by including thyroid peroxidase antibodies (Geno & Nerenz, 2022).

To screen for anemia, in addition to a complete blood count with differential, ferritin should be ordered. Patients with a history of anemia should be followed carefully and provided with culturally sensitive nutritional guidance. If patients are told which foods are iron rich but are not asked if they eat those foods, the intended guidance will fail. They should also be asked about avoidance of iron supplements because of unpleasant side effects such as nausea and constipation.

Obtaining adequate sleep can be a challenge during pregnancy for multiple reasons, including but not limited to anxiety and cognitive arousal, physical discomfort, restless leg syndrome and cramps, sleep apnea, shift work, tinnitus, the need to empty one's bladder, and caring for others. An interval history should explore inadequate or interrupted sleep patterns and remedies that have been tried. Common remedies that are generally considered safe include use of extra pillows, antihistamines, non-habit–forming sedatives with a low-risk profile (such as Unisom), chamomile tea, cognitive behavioral therapy, and guided meditation applications. Since lack of adequate sleep can cause significant quality-of-life disturbance and contributes to unsafe driving and decreased productivity, it should be taken seriously by clinicians during pregnancy. For a review of approaches to treatment for mood disorders, refer to the mental health section of this chapter (Felder et al., 2020). Patients with sleep disturbances should be encouraged to rest during the day as they are able. Notably, many patients will experience improvement during the second trimester and a return of fatigue at the end of pregnancy. Anticipatory guidance may prove reassuring.

FIRST-TRIMESTER BLEEDING AND EARLY PREGNANCY LOSS

Approximately 15–25 percent of pregnant individuals will experience vaginal bleeding in the first trimester (Sundermeye et al., 2023). Half of these bleeds will end in spontaneous abortion (Hendriks et al., 2019). Bleeding in pregnancy may cause anxiety, and patients benefit from prompt, compassionate care that includes a calm and thorough assessment. It is important to provide as much information as possible about the prognosis of the pregnancy and reasons for any needed referrals (Nord et al., 2022).

Subchorionic hematoma or hemorrhage occurs in the first trimester of up to 22 percent of pregnancies (Naz et al., 2022). The etiology is usually unknown, but such bleeds are thought to occur due to a regional separation of the chorion from the decidua (Naz et al., 2022). Outcomes vary widely, depending on the gestational age, size of the hemorrhage, and other factors (Naz et al., 2022).

Vaginal bleeding originates from the vagina, cervix, or uterus. The timing, amount, and color of blood may be useful in determining the site of bleeding. First-trimester bleeding may start as pink or red then taper to dark red or brown over hours or days. A single episode of painless spotting that is light and decreasing does not warrant further evaluation. Bright red or pink blood is suggestive of active bleeding; dark red or brown indicates the blood was expelled earlier and has oxidized. Light bleeding around the expected menstrual period, 4 weeks from the LMP, can be caused by implantation (Chandrakala & Reshmi, 2024). While parents may find it concerning, implantation bleeding is not clinically significant and requires no additional assessment, though reassurance is often appreciated. Patients who engage in penetrative sexual behaviors may experience cervical bleeding due to increased vascularity of the cervix. Saturated undergarments and pain warrant a prompt examination, laboratory studies, and ultrasound.

Examination should include blood pressure, pulse, and a gentle speculum examination to visualize the vagina and cervix to determine the color, amount, and origin of the blood. Bleeding of the cervix is common in pregnancy, but uterine bleeding through a dilated cervix likely signals impending pregnancy loss. Cervical motion tenderness, adnexal pain, or adnexal mass on bimanual examination suggest ectopic pregnancy, and an ultrasound should be performed without delay.

A quantitative, serum human chorionic gonadotropin (hCG) value that approximately doubles when repeated in 48 hours is suggestive of a viable pregnancy. If the hCG level is greater than 3,500 mIU per mL, a gestational sac will be visible on ultrasound 99 percent of the time (Park et al., 2023). Ultrasound is also used to confirm the location and viability of the pregnancy, especially after 6 weeks, when embryonic cardiac activity should be identifiable. When cardiac activity is not demonstrated, the ultrasound can be repeated in case the estimated due date was calculated inaccurately. If repeat ultrasound at least 11 days later does not find either cardiac activity or a fetal pole, then a diagnosis of inevitable abortion can be made with certainty (Park et al., 2023).

When transvaginal ultrasound confirms nonviability, the clinician should demonstrate compassion and engage in collaborative decision making about options. These are (1) awaiting spontaneous passage of the pregnancy, (2) taking a short course of misoprostol to hasten the process, or (3) undergoing a procedure (da Silva et al., 2023). Expectant care in a first-trimester loss has shown success rates ranging from 75–80 percent; however, more complete results occur with a procedure, which also lowers the risk of infection (Acharya et al., 2023). Other considerations in management of an early pregnancy loss include the option for analgesia, sedation, and comparably rapid completion of the abortion with a procedure versus the potential for more privacy and social support when passing the pregnancy at home. An unhurried discussion, with time for the patient to decide later and make necessary arrangements, provides an opportunity to reach a state of equipoise, where the outcomes will be the same, but the choice is made according to the patient's needs and preferences. Equipoise supports patient autonomy and self-efficacy, which may improve psychosocial outcomes with a pregnancy loss. Referral for the appropriate care option following decision making may expedite treatment and reduce stress and anxiety (Davies et al., 2021).

Patients who choose to await spontaneous abortion are advised to expect cramping and bleeding that resolves gradually after passage of a small mass of tissue. If spontaneous abortion does not occur within 2 weeks, patients experience extensive bleeding (saturating more than one pad per hour), feel faint or feverish, or have unacceptable pain, they will need further assessment and care. If a qualified clinician is not available, emergency departments are equipped to treat individuals experiencing complex pregnancy losses in states without abortion restrictions. If a patient lives in an area where treatment may be limited, unavailable, or refused, the referring clinician should facilitate access to care in an alternative setting without delay to the best of their ability. Delays in management of spontaneous abortion have led

TABLE 32-7 Terminology Distinguishing Types of Nonviable Pregnancies

Threatened Abortion	Vaginal bleeding and cramping in a viable pregnancy
Missed Abortion	Following pregnancy loss, products of conception are not expelled without intervention
Incomplete Abortion	Following pregnancy loss, partial products of conception are expelled, some are retained
Inevitable Abortion	Following pregnancy loss, vaginal bleeding and an open cervix are in evidence
Complete Spontaneous Abortion	All products of conception are expelled without intervention

to increased, avoidable morbidity and mortality as a result of state-level restrictions (Hamui et al., 2023).

Patients requesting treatment for early pregnancy loss are managed in the same manner as with abortions: with medication, manual vacuum aspiration, or dilation and curettage. Referrals from clinicians who do not offer abortion care should be based on patient history, urgency—as with impending hemorrhage or sepsis—distance to appropriate care, and patient preferences. These should be weighed carefully in order to ensure timely access to services with consideration for patient's travel time, means of transportation, and expenses.

Following a pregnancy loss, a clinical evaluation is encouraged to ensure physical and emotional healing and to assess the desire for contraception or preconceptual counseling when indicated. Timing for this evaluation can range from 2 weeks to 1 month, depending on the patient's overall health and concerns. Rh D immunoglobulin administration for patients who have Rh-negative blood and gestational partners with Rh-positive blood is no longer recommended. Research has demonstrated a very low risk of alloimmunization resulting from spontaneous pregnancy loss or induced abortion in the first 12 weeks (Horvath et al., 2023; Horvath et al., 2020; Wiebe et al., 2019). Classification of nonviable pregnancies is illustrated in **Table 32-7**.

BOX 32-5 Items to Provide After a Diagnosis of Pregnancy

- Prenatal vitamin prescription or recommendation
- Confirmation of pregnancy documentation for Women, Infants, and Children program and health insurance, if needed
- Laboratory order, if not drawn at clinic
- Information about the prenatal care schedule and answers to frequently asked questions
- Ultrasound order, if needed
- Other prescriptions, medications, or referrals, if needed

PLANNING FOR PREGNANCY CARE

A thorough history, appropriate physical examination, and laboratory reports should provide adequate data to determine the need for routine versus specialized care. In addition, clinicians who provide attentive care for the first few visits can ascertain whether patients have adequate support and resources, or if immediate referral for social services is warranted. Social services referrals can take time to coordinate and it is essential that those with urgent needs are not lost to care. Healthy individuals without additional risk factors may need time to consider other aspects of their care plan as well. Follow-up regarding the status of referrals for services or imaging should be added to the clinician's schedule.

Pregnant patients should leave their initial visits with the items listed in **Box 32-5**. A follow-up call or electronic portal message may be valuable to inquire whether the patient has additional questions or concerns.

Referral for Routine Prenatal Care

Although pregnancy is a physiologic state, it is also a transformative time, encompassing profound emotions and role change. Optimal pregnancy care requires a respectful approach that considers physical, social, and emotional needs. It can take time for patients to find the clinician or practice that is right for them. Referrals and recommendations for clinicians should be made intentionally, with an understanding of patients' priorities. Health records from the initial diagnostic visit should be sent to the chosen clinician as soon as possible. All patients should be supported in choosing a care provider who best meets their personal needs.

Early and consistent prenatal care can promote overall health, connect patients with valued resources, and offer education to prepare for birth, providing newborn care, and parenting. Individuals in demographic groups that have historically been marginalized or discriminated against may need additional assistance or information to find a provider they trust.

Many types of prenatal care clinicians with different knowledge, skills, and philosophies may be consulted for ongoing care (**Table 32-8**). Care led by midwives has been shown to yield superior outcomes for healthy individuals with uncomplicated pregnancies (Sakala et al., 2022). In some settings, midwives are members of teams that care for clinically complex individuals in collaboration with specialist physicians. Those who have substantial clinical risk factors may be best seen by an interprofessional team to provide a unified, multifaceted approach to a high-risk pregnancy (Task Force on Collaborative Practice, 2019).

Prenatal care and birth options vary locally, and individuals should select a provider and location they can easily access that is appropriate for their preferences and clinical needs. After a clinician is chosen and a records release is signed, the health

TABLE 32-8 Types of Clinicians Providing Prenatal Care in the United States

Type of Care Provider	Typical Birth Settings
Certified professional midwife (CPM)	Homes, birth centers
Certified nurse-midwife/certified midwife (CNM/CM)	Homes, birth centers, hospitals
Family practice physician	Birth centers, hospitals
Obstetrician/gynecologist	Hospitals
Maternal–fetal medicine specialist	Hospitals and tertiary-care hospitals

record from early care should be provided without delay. Preferred location for birth is a deeply personal choice and local regulations may influence options for choosing a clinician. Most births in the United States occur in hospitals. Freestanding birth centers and home birth are safe options for healthy individuals experiencing uncomplicated pregnancies when a licensed, qualified attendant with access to specialty care is available (MacDorman et al., 2020; Backes & Scrimshaw, 2020).

References

Abdolalipour, S., Charandabi, S. M. A., Mashayekh-Amiri, S., & Mirghafourvand, M. (2023). The effectiveness of mindfulness-based interventions on self-efficacy and fear of childbirth in pregnant women: A systematic review and meta-analyses. *Journal of Affective Disorders*, *333*, 257–270.

Acharya, A., Prabhu, A., Negi, S., Sharma, K., Dwivedi, R., & Athe, R. (2023). Spontaneous miscarriage/abortion in the first trimester and expectant management—a meta-analysis approach. *Przeglad menopauzalny/Menopause review*, *22*(3), 135–141. https://doi.org/10.5114/pm.2023.131307 Epub 2023 Sep 20. PMID: 37829272; PMCID: PMC10566328.

ACOG. (2021, reafffirmed 2024). Committee Opinion 832: Reducing Prenatal Exposure to Toxic Environmental Agents. https://www.acog.org/clinical/clinical-guidance/committee-opinion/articles/2021/07/reducing-prenatal-exposure-to-toxic-environmental-agents

Adeniyi, A. A., Laronde, D. M., Brondani, M., & Donnelly, L. (2020). Perspectives of socially disadvantaged women on oral healthcare during pregnancy. *Community Dental Health*, *37*(1), 39–44.

Alex, A., Bhandary, E., & McGuire, K. P. (2020). Anatomy and physiology of the breast during pregnancy and lactation. *Diseases of the Breast during During Pregnancy and Lactation*, 3–7.

American College of Obstetricians & Gynecologists Practice Advisory on Low Dose Aspirin Use for the Prevention of Preeclampsia and Related Morbity and Mortality. (Reaffirmed 2022). Available at: https://www.acog.org/clinical/clinical-guidance/practice-advisory/articles/2021/12/low-dose-aspirin-use-for-the-prevention-of-preeclampsia-and-related-morbidity-and-mortality

American College of Obstetricians & Gynecologists. (2017, reaffirmed 2022). Committee Opinion 700: Methods for Estimating the Due Date. Available at https://www.acog.org/clinical/clinical-guidance/committee-opinion/articles/2017/05/methods-for-estimating-the-due-date

American College of Obstetricians & Gynecologists. (2023). Updated Practice Advisory for the Use of Progesterone Supplementation for the Prevention of Recurrent Preterm Birth. https://www.acog.org/clinical/clinical-guidance/practice-advisory/articles/2023/04/updated-guidance-use-of-progesterone-supplementation-for-prevention-of-recurrent-preterm-birth

American College of Obstetricians & Gynecologists. (reaffirmed 2023). Committee Opinion 743: Low Dose Aspirin Use in Pregnancy. https://www.acog.org/clinical/clinical-guidance/committee-opinion/articles/2018/07/low-dose-aspirin-use-during-pregnancy

American College of Obstetricians & Gynecologists. Committee Opinion 711 (Reaffirmed 2021). Committee Opinion 711: Opioid Use and Opioid Use Disorder in Pregnancy. Available at: https://www.acog.org/clinical/clinical-guidance/committee-opinion/articles/2017/08/opioid-use-and-opioid-use-disorder-in-pregnancy

American College of Obstetricians & Gynecologists. (Reaffirmed 2023). Committee Opinion 462: Moderate Caffeine Consumption During Pregnancy. (Reaffirmed 2023) Available at: https://www.acog.org/clinical/clinical-guidance/committee-opinion/articles/2010/08/moderate-caffeine-consumption-during-pregnancy

American College of Obstetricians & Gynecologists. (Reaffirmed 2019). Task Force Guidelines. (reaffirmed 2019). Available at: https://www.acog.org/clinical/clinical-guidance/task-force-report/articles/2016/collaboration-in-practice-implementing-team-based-care

American College of Obstetricians & Gynecologists. (Replaces Practice Bulletin Number 156, December 2015. Reaffirmed 2021). Committee Opinion 230: 2021 https://www.acog.org/clinical/clinical-guidance/practice-bulletin/articles/2021/06/obesity-in-pregnancy

American College of Obstetricians & Gynecologists. (Replaces Practice Bulletin 153, Reaffirmed 2024). Practice Bulletin 189: Nausea & and Vomiting of Pregnancy. https://www.acog.org/clinical/clinical-guidance/practice-bulletin/articles/2018/01/nausea-and-vomiting-of-pregnancy

Anand, A., Phillips, K., Subramanian, A., Lee, S. I., Wang, Z., McCowan, R., ... & Azcoaga-Lorenzo, A. (2023). Prevalence of polypharmacy in pregnancy: A systematic review. *BMJ openOpen*, *13*(3), e067585.

Archer, R. E. (2025). Surviving in the midst of 'Nowhere': Disrupting the conceptualisation of a maternity care desert. *Sociology of Health & Illness*, *47*(1), e13847.

Ashour, A. M. (2023). Efficacy and safety of ondansetron for morning sickness in pregnancy: a A systematic review of clinical trials. *Frontiers in Pharmacology*, *14*, 1291235.

Baas, M. A. M., Van van Pampus, M. G., Stramrood, C. A. I., Dijksman, L. M., Vanhommerig, J. W., & de Jongh, A. (2022). Treatment of pregnant women with fear of childbirth using EMDR therapy: Results of a multi-center randomized controlled trial. *Frontiers in psychiatryPsychiatry*, *12*, 798249.

Baas, M. A., van Pampus, M. G., Braam, L., Stramrood, C. A., & de Jongh, A. (2020). The effects of PTSD treatment during pregnancy: Systematic review and case study. *European Journal of Psychotraumatology*, *11*(1), 1762310.

Backes, E. P., & Scrimshaw, S. C. (Eds.). (2020). *Birth settings in America: Outcomes, quality, access, and choice*. National Academies Press.

Bahamondes, L., Fernandes, A., Monteiro, I., & Bahamondes, M. V. (2020). Long-acting reversible contraceptive (LARCs) methods. *Best Practice & Research Clinical Obstetrics & Gynaecology*, *66*, 28–40.

Basak, S., & Duttaroy, A. K. (2023). Maternal PUFAs, placental epigenetics, and their relevance to fetal growth and brain development. *Reproductive Sciences*, *30*(2), 408–427.

Batra, P., Batra, M., & Singh, S. (2020). Epidemiology of TORCH infections and understanding the serology in their diagnosis. *Journal of Fetal Medicine*, *7*(1), 25–29.

Boothe, E., Olenderek, M., Noyola, M. C., Rushing, J., Allred, E., & Kaplan, S. (2022). Psychosocial outcomes of group prenatal care. *Journal of Public Health*, *30*(6), 1373-1380.

Bull, F. C., Al-Ansari, S. S., Biddle, S., Borodulin, K., Buman, M. P., Cardon, G., Carty, C., Chaput, J. P., Chastin, S., Chou, R., Dempsey, P. C., DiPietro, L., Ekelund, U., Firth, J., Friedenreich, C. M., Garcia, L., Gichu, M., Jago, R., Katzmarzyk, P. T., Lambert, E., ... Willumsen, J. F. (2020). World Health Organization 2020 guidelines on physical activity and sedentary behaviour. British journal of sports medicine, 54(24), 1451–1462. https://doi.org/10.1136/bjsports-2020-102955

Cantor, A. G., Jungbauer, R. M., McDonagh, M., Blazina, I., Marshall, N. E., Weeks, C., ... & Chou, R. (2021). Counseling and behavioral interventions for healthy weight and weight gain in pregnancy: Evidence report and systematic review for the U.S. Preventive Services Task Force. *Jama, 325*(20), 2094–2109.

Centers for Disease Control and Prevention. (2025, October 7). Healthcare professionals: Adult immunization schedule by age. https://www.cdc.gov/vaccines/hcp/imz-schedules/adult-age.html

Cesta, C. E., Rotem, R., Bateman, B. T., Chodick, G., Cohen, J. M., Furu, K., Gissler, M., Huybrechts, K. F., Kjerpeseth, L. J., Leinonen, M. K., Pazzagli, L., Zoega, H., Seely, E. W., Patorno, E., & Hernández-Díaz, S. (2024). Safety of GLP-1 Receptor agonists and other second-line antidiabetics in early pregnancy. *JAMA Internal Medicine, 184*(2), 144–152.

Chandrakala, S., & Reshmi, M. G. (2024) Maternal and fetal outcomes in women experiencing first trimester vaginal bleed: a multicentric approach. *International Journal of Reproduction, Contraception, Obstetrics and Gynecology, 13*(10), 2766.

Cohen, S., Nielsen, T., Chou, J. H., Hoeppner, B., Koenigs, K. J., Bernstein, S. N., Smith, N. A., Perlman, N., Sarathy, L., Wilens, T., Terplan, M., & Schiff, D. M. (2023). Disparities in Maternal-Infant Drug Testing, Social Work Assessment, and Custody at 5 Hospitals. *Academic pediatrics, 23*(6), 1268–1275. https://doi.org/10.1016/j.acap.2023.01.012

Cohn, A. M., Elmasry, H., Wild, R. C., Johnson, A. L., Abudayyeh, H., Kurti, A., & Coleman-Cowger, V. H. (2023). Birth outcomes associated with E-cigarette and non–E-Cigarette cigarette tobacco product use during pregnancy: an An examination of PATH Data Waves 1–5. *Nicotine and Tobacco Research, 25*(3), 444–452.

da Silva, T. M., de Araujo, M. A. G., Simões, A. C. Z., de Oliveira, R., de Medeiros, K. S., Sarmento, A. C., ... & Gonçalves, A. K. (2023). Efficacy, safety, and acceptability of misoprostol in the treatment of incomplete miscarriage: A systematic review and meta-analysis. *Revista Brasileira de Ginecologia e Obstetrícia/RBGO Gynecology and Obstetrics, 45*(12), e808–e817.

Davies, L., Beard, D., Cook, J. A., Price, A., Osbeck, I., & Toye, F. (2021). The challenge of equipoise in trials with a surgical and non-surgical comparison: a A qualitative synthesis using meta-ethnography. *Trials, 22,* 1–24.

Effati-Daryani, F., Mohammad-Alizadeh-Charandabi, S., Mohammadi, A., Zarei, S., & Mirghafourvand, M. (2021). Fatigue and sleep quality in different trimesters of pregnancy. *Sleep scienceScience, 14*(S 01), 69–74.

Fathi, J. T., & Kathuria, H. (2023). Tobacco prevalence and treatment. In *Lung Cancercancer: A comprehensive guide for the clinician* (pp. 49–69). Cham: Springer International Publishing.

Felder, J. N., Hartman, A. R., Epel, E. S., & Prather, A. A. (2020). Pregnant patient perceptions of provider detection and treatment of insomnia. *Behavioral Sleep Medicine 18*(6), 787–796. https://doi.org/10.1080/15402002.2019.1688153. Epub 2019 Nov 6. PMID: 31694403; PMCID: PMC7200275.

Franco, J., Morris, L., Lee, J., & Williams, J. C. (2020). The health care provider's role in securing work accommodations for pregnant and postpartum patients. *Journal of midwifery Midwifery & women's Women's healthHealth, 65*(4), 474–486.

Geno, K. A., & Nerenz, R. D. (2022). Evaluating thyroid function in pregnant women. *Critical reviews Reviews in Clinical Laboratory Sciences, 59*(7), 460–479.

Goławski, K., Giermaziak, W., Ciebiera, M., & Wojtyła, C. (2023). Excessive gestational weight gain and pregnancy outcomes. *Journal of Clinical Medicine, 12*(9), 3211.

Grace, K. T., Farley, C. L., Jeffers, N. K., & Tringali, T. (Eds.). (2023). *Prenatal and postnatal care: A Personwoman-centered Approachapproach.* John Wiley & Sons.

Günal, A., & Demirtürk, F. (2022). Occupational hazards, sleep quality and musculoskeletal problems of pregnant workers. *Journal of Obstetrics and Gynaecology, 42*(2), 215–219.

Hamui, R. M., Aquino, E. M., Menezes, G. M., Velho Barreto de Araújo, T., Seabra Soares de Britto e Alves, M. T., Valongueiro Alves, S., & Almeida, M. D. C. C. (2023). Delays in obtaining hospital care and abortion-related complications within a context of illegality. *Plos One, 18*(6), e0286982.

Heberlein, E., Smith, J., Willis, C., Hall, W., Covington-Kolb, S., & Crockett, A. (2020). The effects of CenteringPregnancy group prenatal care on postpartum visit attendance and contraception use. *Contraception, 102*(1), 46–51.

Hendriks, E., MacNaughton, H., & MacKenzie, M. C. (2019.) First trimester bleeding: evaluation Evaluation and management. *American fam Family physicianPhysician., 99*(3), 166–174.

Horvath, S., Huang, Z., Koelper, N. C., Martinez, C., Tsao, P. Y., Zhao, L., et al. (2023). Induced abortion and the risk of Rh sensitization. *JAMA, 330,* 1167–1174. https://doi.org/10.1001/jama.2023.16953

Horvath, S., Tsao, P., Huang, Z., Zhao, L., Du, Y., Sammel, M. D., et al. (2020). The concentration of fetal red blood cells in first-trimester pregnant women undergoing uterine aspiration is below the calculated threshold for Rh sensitization. *Contraception, 102,* 1–6. https://doi.org/10.1016/j.contraception.2020.02.011

Incognito, G. G., Grassi, L., & Palumbo, M. (2024). Use of cigarettes and heated tobacco products during pregnancy and maternal–fetal outcomes: a A retrospective, monocentric study. *Archives of Gynecology and Obstetrics, 309*(5), 1981–1989.

Johnson, S., Kasparian, N., Cullum, A, Flanagan, T., Ponting, C., Kowalewski, L., & Main, E. K. (2023). Addressing adverse childhood and adult experiences during prenatal care. *Obstetrics & Gynecology 141*(6) 1072–1087. | https://doi.org/10.1097/AOG.0000000000005199

Keyes, K. M., & Patrick, M. E. (2023). Hallucinogen use among young adults ages 19–30 in the United States: Changes from 2018 to 2021. *Addiction, 118*(12), 2449–2454. https://doi.org/10.1111/add.16259

Landon, M. B., Galan, H. L., Jauniaux, D. A., Berghella, V., Grobman, W. A., Kilpatrick, S. J., Cahill, A. G. (2025). *Gabbe's Obstetricsobstetrics: Normal and Problem problem Pregnanciespregnancies.,* (9th ed.). Elsevier.

Langley-Evans, S. C., Pearce, J., & Ellis, S. (2022). Overweight, obesity and excessive weight gain in pregnancy as risk factors for adverse pregnancy outcomes: A narrative review. *Journal of human nutrition and dieteticsDietetics, 35*(2), 250–264.

Lawson, G. W. (2021). Naegele's rule and the length of pregnancy - —A review. *Aust N Z JThe Australian and New Zealand Journal of Obstetrics & Gynaecology., Apr ;61*(2):), 177–182. https://doi.org/10.1111/ajo.13253. Epub 2020 Oct 20. PMID: 33079400.

MacDorman, M. F., Barnard-Mayers, R., & Declercq, E. (2022). United States community births increased by 20% from 2019 to 2020. *Birth, 49*(3), 559–568.

Machado, V.,; Ferreira, M.,; Lopes, L.,; Mendes, J. J.,; & Botelho, J. (2023). Adverse pregnancy outcomes and maternal periodontal disease: An overview on meta-analytic and methodological quality. *J. ournal of Clin. ical Med., icine, 12,* 3635.

Mehra, R., Alspaugh, A., Dunn, J. T., Franck, L. S., McLemore, M. R., Keene, D. E., ... & Ickovics, J. R. (2023). "'Oh gosh, why go? 'cause they are going to look at me and not hire": intersectional Intersectional experiences of black Black women navigating employment during pregnancy and parenting. *BMC pregnancy Pregnancy and childbirthChildbirth, 23*(1), 17.

Moore, J. E., McLemore, M. R., Glenn, N., & Zivin, K. (2021). Policy opportunities to improve prevention, diagnosis, and treatment of perinatal mental health conditions: Study examines policy opportunities to improve prevention, diagnosis, and treatment of perinatal mental health. *Health Affairs, 40*(10), 1534–1542.

Morelli, V., Ziegler, C., & Fawibe, O. (2017). Environmental justice and underserved communities. *Primary Care 44*, 155 – 170.

Mother To Baby | Fact Sheets (2023). *Critical Periods periods of Developmentdevelopment.* Organization of Teratology Information Specialists (OTIS). Available at: https://www.ncbi.nlm.nih.gov/books/NBK582659/

Naz, S., Irfan, S., Naru, T., & Malik, A. (2022). Subchorionic hematoma and pregnancy outcomes in patients with threatened miscarriage. *Pakistan jJournal of med Medical sciSciences 38*(3Part-I), 511–516. https://doi.org/10.12669/pjms.38.3.4283. PMID: 35480501; PMCID: PMC9002424.

Nord, G. A., Doty, A. M., Monick, A. J., McCarthy, D. M., Casten, R. J., Aldeen, A. Z., ... & Rising, K. L. (2022). Emergency medicine clinician experiences addressing uncertainty in first-trimester bleeding. *Journal of patient Patient experienceExperience, 9*, 23743735221140698.

Oei, J. L. (2020). Alcohol use in pregnancy and its impact on the mother and child. *Addiction, 115*(11), 2148–2163.

Olson, S. M., Muñoz, E. G., Solis, E. C., & Bradford, H. M. (2024). Mitigating weight bias in the clinical setting: a A new approach to care. *Journal of Midwifery & Women's Health, 69*(2), 180–190.

Owens, L., Terrell, S., Low, L. K., Loder, C., Rhizal, D., Scheiman, L., & Seng, J. (2022). Universal precautions: the The case for consistently trauma-informed reproductive healthcare. *American journal Journal of obstetrics Obstetrics and gynecology Gynecology, 226*(5), 671–677.

Park, K. E., Latack, K. R., Vestal, N. L., Ingles, S. A., Paulson, R. J., & Awadalla, M. S. (2023). Association of HCG level with ultrasound visualization of the gestational sac in early viable pregnancies. *Reproductive sciencesSciences, 30*(12), 3623–3628.

Phillippi, J., & Kantrowitz-Gordon, I. (2023). *Varney's midwifery.* (7th ed.). Jones & Bartlett Learning.

Racine, N., Ereyi-Osas, W., Killam, T., McDonald, S., & Madigan, S. (2021). Maternal-child health outcomes from pre- to post-implementation of a trauma-informed care initiative in the prenatal care setting: A retrospective study. *Children, 8*(11), 1061.

Rodgers, S. K., Horrow, M. M., Doubilet, P. M., Frates, M. C., Kennedy, A., Andreotti, R., & Strachowski, L. M. (2024). A lexicon for first-trimester US: Society of Radiologists in Ultrasound Consensus Conference recommendations. *Radiology, 312*(2), e240122.

Rohweder, R., de Oliveira Schmalfuss, T., dos Santos Borniger, D., Ferreira, C. Z., Zanardini, M. K., Lopes, G. P. T. F., ... & Fraga, L. R. (2023). Caffeine intake during pregnancy and adverse outcomes: An integrative review. *Reproductive toxicologyToxicology*, 108518.

Sakala, C., Hernández-Cancio, S., Mackay, E., & Wei, R. (2022). Improving our maternity care now through midwifery. *The Journal of Perinatal Education, 31*(4), 181.

Sarayani, A., Albogami, Y., Thai, T. N., Smolinski, N. E., Patel, P., Wang, Y., ... & Winterstein, A. G. (2022). Prenatal exposure to teratogenic medications in the era of risk evaluation and mitigation strategies. *American journal Journal of obstetrics Obstetrics and gynecologyGynecology, 227*(2), 263--e1.

Shortis, E., Warrington, D., & Whittaker, P. (2020). The efficacy of cognitive behavioral therapy for the treatment of antenatal depression: a A systematic review. *Journal of affective Affective disordersDisorders, 272*, 485–495.

Shroukh, W. A., Steinke, D. T., & Willis, S. C. (2020). Risk management of teratogenic medicines: a A systematic review. *Birth Defects Research, 112*(20), 1755–1786.

Stabile, G., Godina, C., Cracco, F., Mangino, F. P., Canton, M., Romano, F., & Ricci, G. (2022). Hysteroscopic removal of intrauterine device in early pregnancy. *BMC Women's Health, 22*(1), 425.

Subramanian, A., Azcoaga-Lorenzo, A., Anand, A., Phillips, K., Lee, S. I., Cockburn, N., ... & MuM-PreDiCT Group. (2023). Polypharmacy during pregnancy and associated risk factors: a A retrospective analysis of 577 medication exposures among 1.5 million pregnancies in the UK, 2000-2019. *BMC medicineMedicine, 21*(1), 21.

Sundermeyer, R. L., LeFevre, N., Kolker, A., & Williamson, B. (2023). Common Issues in Prenatal Care: First Trimester Bleeding. *FP Essentials (Online), 525*, 7.

Tarasi, B., Cornuz, J., Clair, C., & Baud, D. (2022). *Cigarette smoking during pregnancy and adverse perinatal outcomes: a A cross-sectional study over 10 years. BMC Public Health*, 22(1), 2403.

Tsikouras, P., Oikonomou, E., Nikolettos, K., Andreou, S., Kyriakou, D., Damaskos, C., ...& Nikolettos, N. (2024). the The impact of periodontal disease on preterm birth and preeclampsia. *Journal of Personalized Medicine, 14*(4), 345.

USPSTF. (n.d.). *Cervical cancer: Screening*. Recommendation: Cervical Cancer: Screening | United States Preventive Services Taskforce. https://www.uspreventiveservicestaskforce.org/uspstf/draft-update-summary/cervical-cancer-screening-adults-adolescents

van Daalen, K. R., Kaiser, J., Kebede, S., Cipriano, G., Maimouni, H., Olumese, E., Chui, A., Kuhn, I., & Oliver-Williams, C. (2022). Racial discrimination and adverse pregnancy outcomes: a A systematic review and meta-analysis. *BMJ Global Health, 7*(8), e009227. https://doi.org/10.1136/bmjgh-2022-009227. PMID: 35918071; PMCID: PMC9344988.

Wang, X., Lee, N. L., & Burstyn, I. (2020). Smoking and use of electronic cigarettes (vaping) in relation to preterm birth and small-for-gestational-age in a 2016 U.S. national sample. *Preventive medicineMedicine, 134*, 106041.

Wiebe, E. R., Campbell, M., Aiken, A. R., & Albert, A. (2019). Can we safely stop testing for Rh status and immunizing Rh-negative women having early abortions? A comparison of Rh alloimmunization in Canada and the Netherlands. *Contraception*, 100001. https://doi.org/10.1016/j.conx.2018.100001

Workowski, K. A., & Bachmann, L. H. (2022). Centers for Disease Control and Prevention's sexually transmitted diseases infection guidelines. *Clinical Infectious Diseases, 74* (Supplement_2), S89–S94.

Yang, X., Li, H., Zhao, Q., Han, R., Xiang, Z., & Gao, L. (2022). Clinical practice guidelines that address physical activity and exercise during pregnancy: a A systematic review. *Journal of midwifery Midwifery & women's Women's healthHealth, 67*(1), 53–68.

Young-Wolff, K. C., Adams, S. R., Alexeeff, S. E., Zhu, Y., Chojolan, E., Slama, N. E., ... & Avalos, L. A. (2024). Prenatal cannabis use and maternal pregnancy outcomes. *JAMA Internal Medicine, 184*(9), 1083–1093.

Zagorianakou, N., Mitrogiannis, I., Konis, K., Makrydimas, S., Mitrogiannis, L., & Makrydimas, G. (2023). The HPV-DNA Test in Pregnancy: A Review of the Literature. *Curēus (Palo Alto, CA), 15*(5), e38619. https://doi.org/10.7759/cureus.38619

CHAPTER 33

Common Complications of Pregnancy

Wendy R. Gibbons
Desiree M. Clement

The editors acknowledge Ellise D. Adams and Kerri Durnell Schuilling, who were authors of a previous version of this chapter.

With maternal mortality rates on the rise in the United States, it is important that clinicians screen for and recognize complications that commonly occur during pregnancy. This chapter focuses on the screening, diagnosis, and initial management of commonly seen conditions that may complicate pregnancy. Management of the conditions will include referral when appropriate for escalation of care needs. An overview of the normal anatomic and physiologic changes that occur during pregnancy is provided in Chapter 31.

There are numerous aspects of the complications of pregnancy, such as assessment and management, that are specific to people assigned female at birth. Not all individuals assigned female at birth identify as female or as a woman; however, terms such as "maternal" and "pregnant person" are used extensively in this chapter, in general, to refer to the gestational parent. The use of these gendered terms is not meant to exclude people who do not identify as women and seek care during pregnancy and birth. This chapter will cover a variety of complications that may be identified in pregnant people and influence the pregnancy outcomes—some complications that may be preexisting (infections), and some that arise as a result of the pregnancy.

INFECTIONS COMMONLY DIAGNOSED DURING PREGNANCY

During pregnancy, a person's immune system undergoes many changes; this has three distinct phases. After conception and in the first trimester there is a pro-inflammatory phase that prevents the rejection of the embryo; the pregnant person often struggles with general malaise as the body works to adapt to the presence of the fetus (Mor & Abrahams, 2023). Although these changes prevent fetal rejection, these changes also increase the risk of acquiring an infection that may be passed on to the fetus. The second phase is anti-inflammatory as the fetus grows and develops; prior to the onset of labor, the immune system returns to a pro-inflammatory state to facilitate the expulsion of the fetus and placenta (Mor & Abrahams, 2023). An important factor related to these changes is the passage of maternal antibodies across the placenta. Maternal immunoglobulin G (IgG) antibodies provide the fetus with passive immunity. Nevertheless, some viruses and bacteria can cross the placental barrier and can endanger the fetus; this mode of transmission is called vertical or perinatal transmission. Perinatal transmission describes the passage of an infectious agent from the pregnant person to their infant during pregnancy, birth, or lactation (HIVinfo@NIH.gov, 2024).

Urinary Tract Infections

Urinary tract infections are more likely to develop in people assigned female at birth (AFAB) than people assigned male at birth (AMAB) for a variety of reasons, anatomy being one of them. AFAB individuals tend to have a shorter urethra and the external one third of their urethra is exposed to vaginal and rectal orifices. Failure to fully empty the bladder and ease for potential bacterial transmission into the bladder from the vagina during coital activities may also cause infections (Wylie, 2023). If a person becomes pregnant, urinary frequency is also more common due to bladder compression from the gravid uterus, which is also a commonly reported discomfort of pregnancy.

Physiological changes of pregnancy occur, especially in response to progesterone which can lead to ureteral smooth muscle peristalsis and obstruction of the ureters that can predispose pregnant persons to UTIs (Wylie, 2023). Clinician awareness is critical for recognizing that urinary frequency is also a common symptom for an underlying urinary tract infection (UTI). Common symptoms for a potential urinary infection can include the presence of dysuria, hematuria, nocturia, suprapubic pressure, hematuria, urinary frequency, or urgency.

During the perinatal period, the majority of UTIs can be classified according to the site of infection: lower urinary tract infection (asymptomatic bacteriuria and symptomatic acute cystitis) or upper urinary tract infection (acute pyelonephritis) (Graseck et al., 2023; Wylie, 2023). *Escherichia coli* is the most identified bacterial pathogen found to be responsible for both asymptomatic and symptomatic bacteriuria (Graseck et al., 2023). Critical importance should be placed on the early recognition of UTIs and the potential for ASB to escalate from being a descending infection into the development of an ascending infection like acute pyelonephritis. Caution should be taken to identify UTIs early to avoid further development into acute pyelonephritis due to potential associated risks resulting in preterm birth (PTB), low birth weight, adult respiratory distress syndrome (ARDS), disseminated intravascular coagulation (DIC), and sepsis (Wylie, 2023). When considering the differential diagnoses with those presenting during pregnancy with urinary symptoms, a clinician should also rule out rupture of membranes and gestational diabetes (Graseck et al., 2023; Wylie, 2023).

Asymptomatic bacteriuria (ASB) screening is important as multiple studies have shown that even without urinary symptoms during pregnancy, significant bacterial counts have been found on laboratory tests (Wylie, 2023). Many cases of ASB are detected at the first prenatal visit (Wylie, 2023). ASB derives from normal flora ascending into the urinary tract from the vaginal, periurethral, or gastrointestinal tracts. When ASB is present, the bacteria will persist inside the urinary tract but without eliciting a sufficient response to signal to the body there are any urinary symptoms (Wylie, 2023). Due to the body's inability to send these urinary symptom signals, it has become an accepted clinical practice to screen urine for ASB at least once early in the pregnancy with a clean catch urine culture (Graseck et al., 2023). Treatment should include a 5- to 7-day course of targeted antibiotics for urine colony counts > 1,000,000 CFU/mL (Graseck et al., 2023).

Acute cystitis in pregnancy can present as an underlying urinary tract infection. As a clinician, it is crucial to differentiate between typical symptoms of pregnancy due to an expanding uterus versus the presence of urinary symptoms which can be suggestive for acute cystitis. A urine culture and urinalysis are helpful to further determine acute cystitis from ASB or typical symptoms of pregnancy. A positive urinalysis should be confirmed with a urine culture resulting at or greater than 1,000,000 CFU/mL followed by prescribed treatment with a 5- to 7-day course of targeted antibiotics that typically will include nitrofurantoin, beta-lactams, sulfonamides, and Fosfomycin (Graseck et al., 2023). Clinicians should avoid use of amoxicillin or ampicillin if needing to start empiric therapy before the culture and sensitivity results are received, due to the potential risks for *E. coli* resistance that can occur with these medications (Graseck et al., 2023).

Although acute urinary tract infections are commonly treated with quinolones and sulfonamides in nonpregnant persons, quinolones are not approved for use during pregnancy due to their potential teratogenic effect on fetal cartilage (Wylie, 2023). Sulfonamides also should be prescribed with caution due to their increased likelihood of causing hyperbilirubinemia in the neonate and, therefore, should also be avoided during the third trimester. Thus, some clinicians do not recommend prescribing a combination of trimethoprim/sulfamethoxazole during the first or third trimesters (Briggs et al., 2021).

Acute pyelonephritis may also occur during the perinatal period. Any pregnant person presenting with a temperature of 100.4 degrees Fahrenheit or 38 degrees Celsius or higher, upper urinary tract symptoms (flank pain or costovertebral angle tenderness), possible nausea and/or vomiting, and urine lab studies suggestive of a UTI are all suspect for a diagnosis of acute pyelonephritis (Graseck et al., 2023). Although acute pyelonephritis more commonly occurs during the second trimester, this infection can arise at any time throughout the pregnancy, along with there being a higher risk for potential occurrence, especially for anyone recently diagnosed with either ASB or acute cystitis. A history of multiple UTIs during pregnancy also places a pregnant person at higher risk for the development of acute pyelonephritis, which is one of the most common causes for hospitalization during pregnancy (Graseck et al., 2023). Therefore, repeating a urine culture after a UTI approximately 1–2 weeks after treatment completion or evaluating if symptoms have resolved is warranted by clinicians. Likewise, clinicians may consider initiating antimicrobial suppression therapy using a daily lower single dose with an antibiotic found to be susceptible for those pregnant persons experiencing recurrent UTIs for the prevention of acute pyelonephritis (Graseck et al., 2023). Acute pyelonephritis should be managed only in the inpatient setting with empiric antibiotics able to penetrate the renal tissue and organisms specifically identified on urine culture, due to the high-risk nature for developing severe complications leading to maternal or neonatal adverse outcomes (Graseck et al., 2023; Wylie, 2023). Further information about urinary tract infections can be found in Chapter 23.

Group B Streptococcus

Group B streptococcus (GBS), also known as *Streptococcus agalactiae*, is a gram-positive bacterium that is a normal component of the intestinal and vaginal microbiome in some people (Committee on Obstetric Practice, 2020). However, if it colonizes in the vagina or rectum of pregnant people, it can transition from a physiologic resident to a pathogenic bacterium; this colonization can be intermittent, transient, or persistent (CoOP, 2020). The transient nature of GBS colonization is why pregnant people need to be screened both in the first trimester (with a urine culture) and in the late third trimester (36–37 weeks) with a rectovaginal culture.

It is estimated that 50 percent of people who are pregnant and are colonized with GBS will transmit the bacteria to their newborns (Committee on Obstetric Practice, 2020). The presence of GBS during pregnancy is typically associated with increased UTIs, preterm labor (PTL), and preterm birth (PTB) (Committee on Obstetric Practice, 2020). Risks for transmission include maternal vaginal–rectal colonization during labor and birth, gestational age less than 37 weeks, extremely low birth weight, prolonged rupture of membranes, intra-amniotic infection, having a previous infant affected by GBS, and young maternal age (ACOG, 2019). Laboring people who are positive for GBS should receive care from a clinician equipped to provide intrapartum antibiotic prophylaxis during labor. People whose GBS status is unknown at the time of labor should be provided with intrapartum antibiotic prophylaxis if they have risk factors such as gestation less than 37 weeks, rupture of membranes for 18 hours or longer, maternal temperature of 100.4°F (38°C) or higher, or positive nucleic acid amplification test for GBS (Committee on Obstetric Practice, 2020). The only exception to receiving antibiotic prophylaxis in someone who has a positive prenatal GBS culture is an individual who undergoes cesarean birth prior to the onset of labor or rupture of membranes (Committee on Obstetric Practice, 2020).

GBS remains the number one cause of neonatal early-onset sepsis (occurring during the first week of life) and a significant cause of late-onset sepsis in young infants in the United States (Puopolo et al., 2019). The two most common types of GBS disease in newborns are early-onset disease, presenting in the first 7 days after birth, and late-onset disease (7 days post-birth to 2–3 months) (Committee on Obstetric Practice, 2020). To date, the only available effective strategy to prevent perinatal GBS early-onset disease is intrapartum antibiotic prophylaxis (Puopolo et al., 2019). Unfortunately, no effective approach to prevent late-onset disease is known. During the early newborn period, infants born to mothers who are GBS positive are at risk for developing pneumonia, septicemia, and meningitis. Newborn infections related to GBS can occur up to 12 weeks of age and may be associated with speech and language delays, spastic quadriplegia, blindness, deafness, seizures, and hydrocephalus (Committee on Obstetric Practice, 2020).

Listeriosis

Listeriosis is an infection caused by *Listeria monocytogenes,* a gram-positive bacterium that can contaminate many foods. If a person eats food contaminated with *Listeria*, they can become infected with the bacteria. Listeriosis is the third leading cause of death from foodborne illness in the United States (CDC, 2024n). Listeriosis infection is rare, but it can be profoundly serious especially for people who are immunocompromised or pregnant, and the incidence of listeriosis is approximately 13 times higher in pregnancy than in the general population (CDC, 2024n). If a pregnant person becomes infected with *Listeria,* even if the disease symptoms are mild, there is an association with stillbirth, preterm labor, and fetal infection (Wylie, 2023). Similar to GBS infection (with an early and late onset of disease) in the neonate, early onset *Listeria* disease is associated with diffuse sepsis with organ and CNS involvement. Early-onset listeriosis is associated with a high rate of stillbirth and neonatal mortality, and occurs more frequently in infants born preterm. Late-onset disease usually presents with meningitis and hydrocephalus; developmental delays are also commonly seen with late-onset neonatal listeriosis (Wylie, 2023).

Fetal and neonatal infection occurs when *Listeria* is disseminated to the placenta via maternal bacteremia. This placental "seeding" by *Listeria* can result in placental abscesses and fetal septicemia. The rate of fetal death is inversely proportional to the gestational age of maternal infection (Wylie, 2023). Diagnosis can be challenging for the obstetric provider because many pregnant people with the infections will be asymptomatic or present with mild symptoms (gastrointestinal or flu-like symptoms). If a person has a known exposure, a fever ≥ 100.6, and symptoms consistent with listeriosis, they should be tested (with blood cultures) and treated (Committee on Obstetric Practice, 2014, reaffirmed 2023). It is important to note to the laboratory performing the blood cultures to specifically assess for *Listeria* to ensure the bacteria is not mistaken as a contaminant. Treatment for listeriosis is high-dose intravenous ampicillin (at least 6 gms per day) for 14 days; gentamycin is often added because of its demonstrated synergism with ampicillin (Committee on Obstetric Practice, 2014, reaffirmed 2023). When a pregnant person is diagnosed with listeriosis, management and care should be coordinated with an infectious disease specialist.

Education and prevention are the most effective tools against *Listeria* infection. Education should begin with wellness visits and reinforced during prenatal care. Refrigeration does not kill *Listeria* but heating foods or meats prior to eating can kill the bacteria. Educate patients, especially pregnant people, about foods to avoid and alternatives to those foods (**Table 33-1**) (CDC, 2024f).

TORCH Infections

TORCH refers to the congenitally acquired infections of (T) toxoplasmosis, (O) other infections such as syphilis, hepatitis B, varicella, parvovirus, and zika, (R) rubella, (C) cytomegalovirus, and (H) herpes simplex (Jaan & Rajnik, 2023). This section discusses the potential implications and complications for a pregnancy complicated by a TORCH infection. Intrauterine transfer of these infections to the fetus can produce multiple symptoms when the infant is born. Risk factors include maternal lapsed immunizations; community, animal, and occupational exposures; and sexually transmitted infections (Jaan & Rajnik, 2023).

Toxoplasmosis

Toxoplasmosis is the illness caused by the parasite *Toxoplasma gondii*. Transmission occurs via three routes:

- Eating undercooked meat or shellfish or unwashed, contaminated fresh produce.
- Animal-to human: ingestion of parasite oocytes through contact with cat feces or contaminated soil.
- Congenital transmission: a newly infected pregnant person passes the infection to their fetus.

If a person with a healthy immune system becomes infected with toxoplasmosis, they may experience flu-like symptoms, swollen lymph nodes, muscle aches, or they may remain symptom-free. Pregnant people and people with a compromised immune system are at greatest risk for a more severe infection that can damage the brain, eyes, or other organs (CDC, 2024q). Parasitemia can occur after infection; in pregnant people, this parasitemia can seed the placenta and cause a fetal infection (ACOG, 2015, reaffirmed 2024). A new toxoplasmosis infection presents the most risk to the fetus when acquired in the first trimester. Congenital infection with toxoplasmosis typically presents with abnormal neurologic findings on prenatal ultrasound, including intracranial echogenic foci, ventriculomegaly, intracranial cysts, and periventricular echogenicities (Megli & Beigi, 2023). If toxoplasmosis is newly diagnosed in pregnancy, the pregnant person requires a multidisciplinary team to include a perinatologist, infectious disease specialist, and obstetrical care providers.

Routine screening for toxoplasmosis infection is not recommended; however, serologic testing may be done if a person is immunocompromised or has contact with outdoor cats (Megli & Beigi, 2023). Diagnosis is accomplished with serologic testing looking for rising levels of IgM and IgG maternal titers. Prevention strategies remain the key to managing toxoplasmosis infection in pregnancy:

- Clean areas and tools used to handle raw food with hot, soapy water after preparing each food item.
- Freeze meat for several days to a sub-zero temperature (0^0F) to reduce the chance of infection.
- Use a food thermometer to ensure food is cooked to a safe internal temperature (FoodSafety.gov, 2024).
- Wash fruits and vegetables using running water and produce wash.
- Do not eat unpasteurized dairy products or raw seafood or shellfish.
- Wear gloves when gardening or if handling any soil, sand, or cat litter (CDC, 2024q).

Parvovirus B19, Zika, Varicella, HIV

The clinical presentation of **Parvovirus B19** is known as Fifth disease. Parvovirus B19 only infects people; a person cannot acquire the infection from a dog or cat (CDC, 2024o). Parvovirus B19 spreads from person to person via respiratory droplets, blood products, or perinatally (pregnant person to fetus). Parvovirus B19 infection usually causes no symptoms or mild illness (flu-like symptoms, runny nose, rash, joint pain) in people who are otherwise healthy. The symptom most often associated with Parvovirus B19 illness is a red rash on the face or "slapped cheek"

TABLE 33-1 Making Safer Food Choices

Foods to Avoid	Instead Choose . . .
Raw or undercooked poultry or meat	Poultry and meat cooked to a safe internal temperature (FoodSafety.gov, 2024) using a food thermometer to check the temperature
Unheated deli meat, cold cuts, hot dogs, fermented or dry sausage	Deli meat, cold cuts, hot dogs, fermented or dry sausage that has been heated to 165⁰F or until steaming hot
Refrigerated pâté preprepared or meat spreads	Any meat spread or pâté in a sealed, airtight container that does not require refrigeration
Premade deli salads (coleslaw, potato salad, tuna salad, chicken salad, egg salad)	Homemade salads that are freshly made
Raw or undercooked sprouts	Heat sprouts (even for a salad) until steaming hot
Unwashed fruits and vegetables	Washed fruits and vegetables (cooked are the safest)
Pre-cut melon, especially at room temperature or warmer	Freshly cut melon, or cut melon kept refrigerated for fewer than 7 days
Unpasteurized or "freshly squeezed" juice or cider	Pasteurized juice or cider Heat unpasteurized juice or cider to a rolling boil for 1 minute.
Unpasteurized milk or dairy products made from raw milk	Pasteurized milk and dairy products made from pasteurized milk
Raw or undercooked eggs (runny yolks) or foods that may contain raw or undercooked eggs. (Caesar salad dressing, raw cookie dough, homemade eggnog, some mousse desserts)	Eggs that are cooked until the whites and yolks are firm (scrambled, hard boiled) Quiche or egg dishes cooked to 165⁰F
Raw or undercooked fish or seafood Refrigerated smoked seafood	Fish cooked to a safe internal temperature. Shellfish cooked until the shells open or until it is pearly white and opaque. Canned fish and seafood Smoked seafood in a sealed, airtight container that does not require refrigeration
Raw cookie dough or raw batter	Dough or batter that is labeled "edible" or "safe to eat"

Data from Centers for Disease Control and Prevention. (2024f, May 2). *Safer food choices for pregnant people*. U.S. Department of Health and Human Services. https://www.cdc.gov/food-safety/foods/pregnant-women.html

rash (CDC, 2024o). Most adults have already had a Parvovirus B19 infection and have existing immune protection.

If a person acquires a new infection with Parvovirus B19 during pregnancy, most of the time it will not affect the pregnancy or have long-term impacts on the fetus (CDC, 2024o). If a pregnant person is infected with Parvovirus B19, the transmission rate to the fetus ranges from 17–33 percent (ACOG, 2024b). Most cases of fetal infection will resolve without complication; however, there is a 5–10 percent risk of adverse fetal outcomes if the virus infects the fetus (ACOG, 2024b). The effects of Parvovirus B19 could include severe fetal anemia, hydrops fetalis, cardiomegaly, miscarriage, or impaired fetal growth (CDC, 2024p).

Routine screening for Parvovirus B19 during pregnancy is not recommended; however, it is important to obtain a thorough health, employment, and social history. People who are pregnant and are at greatest risk for contracting Parvovirus B19 are those who are immunocompromised, those exposed to school-age children, schoolteachers, and day care workers. Patients should be counseled to report any new exposures (children, co-workers) to their obstetrical providers. The best way to confirm the diagnosis of a maternal parvovirus infection is via serologic testing after a known or suspected exposure. The presence of IgM antibodies is confirmatory of a new, acute infection (refer to **Table 33-2**) (Megli & Beigi, 2023). If a new parvovirus infection is confirmed during pregnancy, the pregnant person should be referred to a perinatologist (maternal–fetal specialist) for serial ultrasound examinations to screen for hydrops, placentomegaly, and Doppler assessment of peak systolic fetal mid-cerebral artery (MCA) blood flow (Megli & Beigi, 2023).

All people who are pregnant should be taught methods to prevent Parvovirus B19 transmission.

- Stay up to date with immunizations.
- Practice good hygiene with shared items and surfaces (toys, computer keyboards, light switches).
- Cover coughs and sneezes.
- Additionally, if desired, use masks and physical distancing (CDC, 2024c).

Zika virus (ZIKV) is a zoonotic, RNA virus belonging to the *Flaviviridae* family. ZIKV was first identified in 1947 in a monkey

TABLE 33-2 Parvovirus Serology

IgM	IgG	Interpretation
Negative	Negative	No prior infection with Parvovirus B19
Negative	Positive	Previous infection, immune to parvovirus
Positive	Negative	New, acute infection
Positive	Positive	Subacute infection > 7, < 120 days ago

Reproduced from Megli, C., & Beigi, R. (2022). Maternal-fetal infections. In C. Lockwood, J. Copel, L. Dugoff, J. Louis, T. Moore, R. Silver, & R. Resnik (Eds.), Creasy & Resnik's maternal-fetal medicine (9th ed., pp. 959–972). Elsevier.

in Uganda and later in humans in 1952 (Megli & Beigi, 2023; World Health Organization, 2022). The virus gained global attention in 2014–2016 due to an epidemic in the Americas. This ZIKV outbreak resulted in an increase of travel-related cases in the United States; Puerto Rico, and the U.S. Virgin Islands also reported a widespread outbreak of ZIKV (CDC, 2024i). Zika has an incubation period of less than 14 days. Some people may be asymptomatic, but when symptoms are present, they can include fever, rash, headache, arthralgia, conjunctivitis, and muscle pain (CDC, 2024m).

Infection with ZIKV primarily occurs from a bite by an infected *Aedes* mosquito; ZIKV can also be transmitted through sexual contact, blood transfusion, and perinatally (Megli & Beigi, 2023). Both AFAB and AMAB individuals can pass ZIKV through sexual contact (vaginal, oral, anal, and sharing sex toys). ZIKV is generally only found in the blood through the first week of infection; however, the virus remains in semen for a longer period (CDC, 2024h). When ZIKV is transmitted perinatally, the virus can breach the placental barrier via an unknown mechanism, infecting the developing fetus (Megli & Beigi, 2023). Perinatal transmission of ZIKV can result in congenital Zika syndrome which is characterized by the following features:

- Microcephaly
- Hearing loss and vision problems
- Difficulty swallowing
- Congenital contractures and muscular hypertonia
- Subcortical calcifications

Not all infants born with congenital Zika syndrome will present with all these conditions. Some infants with known perinatal exposure may not have any of the features present at birth, but these infants can develop microcephaly and long-term health problems as they grow (CDC, 2024l).

If a pregnant person presents with symptoms suggestive of a ZIKV infection and has recently traveled to an area with endemic infection, nucleic acid amplification testing (NAAT) should be ordered. The CDC has guidelines and recommendations for ZIKV testing available for clinicians (CDC, 2024h). If ZIKV infection is suspected or confirmed, the pregnant person needs close follow up and surveillance with a perinatologist and serial growth ultrasounds (refer to **Table 33-3**). Treatment of ZIKV involves supportive and symptomatic care. The key to reducing perinatal ZIKV transmission is prevention and minimizing exposure: Encourage pregnant people to check the CDC's Travel Health Notices page (CDC, 2024r) prior to travel during pregnancy, wear protective clothing, use mosquito repellant, and avoid unprotected sex with people who have a known exposure to ZIKV (Megli & Beigi, 2023). People desiring a pregnancy who have a proven infection or known exposure should delay conception for at least 8 weeks after symptoms appear or 8 weeks after the last possible exposure (Megli & Beigi, 2023).

Varicella-zoster virus (VZV) is a DNA virus in the herpes group; it is highly contagious and easily transmissible by direct contact and respiratory droplets. Varicella, commonly known as chicken pox, causes a self-limited illness in children (CDC, 2024e). Among people in the United States of reproductive age, 96 to 99 percent are seropositive for VZV due to the widespread childhood vaccination program. This results in a low rate of VZV during pregnancy (approximately 1 to 5 cases per 10,000 pregnancies) (CDC, 2024e; Nielsen-Saines & Cambou, 2023). Although the risk of infection among pregnant adults versus nonpregnant adults overall is low, the risk for severe disease because of VZV has increased in people who are pregnant (Neilsen-Saines & Cambou, 2023).

Among pregnant people who get VZV, pneumonia is the most significant risk and complicates approximately 10–20 percent of maternal VZV infections. Smoking increases a person's risk of varicella pneumonia during pregnancy (Neilsen-Saines & Cambou, 2023). The greatest risk for VZV pneumonia occurs if a pregnant person contracts VZV in the third trimester. Prior to the use of anti-viral medications (acyclovir), maternal mortality rates for varicella pneumonia were as high as 35–40 percent (Pippen & Gibson, 2023). Varicella can be diagnosed in people who are pregnant through clinical findings, although PCR assay of vesicle fluid is also available. For people who are pregnant and do not have documented immunity to varicella, varicella-zoster immune globulin (VZIG) is indicated. The risk of a primary varicella infection is decreased if VZIG is administered within 96 hours of exposure, although this treatment may be effective up to 10 days following exposure (Phillippi & Kantrowitz-Gordon, 2024, pp. 845–847).

Perinatal transmission of VZV is rare, likely due to a person's pre existing vaccination or previous exposure to the illness. If a pregnant person contracts VZV, perinatal transmission occurs between 0.4 to 2.0 percent of the time and can have serious implications for fetal health (CDC, 2024e). Congenital VZV has been associated with spontaneous abortion, intrauterine fetal death (IUFD), fetal growth restriction (FGR), microcephaly, eye and limb malformations, ventriculomegaly, and echogenic foci in the liver (Neilsen-Saines & Cambou, 2023). Ultrasound and referral to a perinatologist should be utilized to monitor fetal growth and development if VZV is diagnosed during pregnancy. If a pregnant person develops a varicella rash 5 days before to 2 days after birth, the neonate is at risk for neonatal varicella; neonatal varicella raises the neonate's mortality risk as high as 30 percent. If VARIZIG is administered and intensive supportive care is provided, this can reduce the risk of neonatal mortality to about 7 percent (CDC, 2024e).

Varicella immunity status should be determined early in pregnancy either by medical history of the disease or a history of vaccination (Phillippi & Kantrowitz-Gordon, 2024, pp. 845–847). If both are negative, an IgG test can be done to determine immunity. All nonpregnant people of childbearing age should be screened for varicella (either the vaccine or prior infection).

TABLE 33-3 Guidelines for Zika Testing in Pregnant People

Asymptomatic Pregnant Patient	Traveled to an area with an active CDC Zika Travel Health Notice during pregnancy	Traveled to an area with current or past Zika transmission outside the United States	
	• NAAT testing may be considered up to 12 weeks after travel	• Routine testing is not recommended • If the decision is made to Zika test, NAAT testing can be done up to 12 weeks after travel	
Symptomatic Pregnant Patient	Lived in or traveled to an area with an active CDC Zika Travel Health Notice during pregnancy **OR** had sex during pregnancy with someone living in or with recent travel to an area with an active CDC Zika Travel Health Notice	Lived in or traveled to an area with current or past Zika virus transmission during pregnancy	Had sex during pregnancy with someone living in or with recent travel to an area with current or past Zika transmission
	• Specimens should be collected as soon as possible after onset of symptoms up to 12 weeks after symptom onset • Order dengue and Zika virus NAAT and IgM testing on a serum specimen • Order Zika virus NAAT on a urine specimen • If Zika NAAT is positive and the Zika IgM is negative, repeat NAAT test on newly extracted RNA from the same specimen to rule out false-positive results.	• Specimens should be collected as soon as possible after onset of symptoms up to 12 weeks after symptom onset • Order dengue and Zika virus NAAT on a serum specimen • Order Zika virus NAAT on a urine specimen • Perform IgM testing for dengue only • If dengue NAAT or IgM is positive, this is adequate evidence of dengue infection, and no further testing is indicated.	• Specimens should be collected as soon as possible after onset of symptoms up to 12 weeks after symptom onset • Only Zika NAAT should be performed • If Zika NAAT is positive and the Zika IgM is negative, repeat NAAT test on newly extracted RNA from the same specimen to rule out false-positive results.

Reproduced from Centers for Disease Control and Prevention. (2024h, May 15). Clinical testing and testing for zika virus disease. U.S. Department of Health and Human Services. https://www.cdc.gov/zika/hcp/diagnosis-testing/index.html

Anyone who is negative should be offered the vaccine; however, pregnancy should be delayed at least 1 month following vaccination (CDC, 2024e).

Human Immunodeficiency Virus (HIV) is included in the TORCH section because of the virus's ability to cause a perinatal infection. Fetal infection with HIV can occur transplacentally (during pregnancy) or during labor and birth when the neonate is exposed to the virus in the mother's blood or other body fluids. The first step for optimizing HIV management during pregnancy begins with screening pregnant people. All pregnant people should be screened for HIV at the first antepartum visit and again in the third trimester if the initial screen was negative. All pregnant people should be tested for HIV using an opt-out method (they can choose not to be tested); pregnant people should be informed that HIV testing is part of their routine screening, and no one should be tested without their knowledge (Committee on Obstetric Practice HIV Expert Work Group, 2018, reaffirmed 2024). If HIV test results are positive, the patient should be given the results in person along with a detailed discussion about the implications of HIV infection and risks of infection to the neonate. Newborns who contract HIV are at risk for failure to thrive, upper respiratory tract infections, chronic diarrhea, dermatitis, thrush, and other infections. Additionally, all pregnant people who are HIV positive can benefit from patient teaching related to adequate rest, stress reduction, and consumption of a diet rich in fruits, vegetables, antioxidants, and omega-3 fatty acids to complement their pharmacologic treatment.

Optimizing the health of the pregnant person and decreasing the risk of fetal/newborn transmission are goals of care for providers caring for people who are HIV positive. Pregnant people with a positive HIV test should have care that is co-managed with an HIV specialist, a perinatologist, and a pediatric/neonatology specialist. Anti-retroviral therapy (ART) should be utilized to minimize the risk of perinatal transmission. Ideally, a pregnant person with HIV can gain an undetectable viral load and a normal CD4 T-lymphocyte count. The blood tests should be ordered and followed by a provider who specializes in managing people with HIV. If a pregnant person has an undetectable viral load and normal CD4 count, the risk of transmission to the fetus/newborn is ≤ 1–2 percent. Vaginal birth is encouraged for people with undetectable viral loads and normal CD4 counts; cesarean delivery before rupture of membranes or the onset of labor has been shown to decrease the rate of transmission in people with viral loads ≥ 1,000 copies per milliliter. However, patient autonomy must be respected regarding the decision about the mode of delivery (Committee on Obstetric Practice HIV Expert Work Group, 2018, reaffirmed 2024).

Breastfeeding has also been documented as a route of neonatal transmission (Committee on Obstetric Practice HIV Expert Work Group, 2018, reaffirmed 2024). Most current recommendations regarding HIV-positive people still encourage formula feeding to eliminate the risk of transmission to the newborn; however, the CDC and the American Academy of Pediatrics (AAP) recently changed their positions on breastfeeding for HIV-positive people (CDC, 2023; Abuogi et al., 2024). While the risk will never be zero, when people maintain an undetectable viral load and continue their ART, the risk of transmission via breastfeeding is less than 1 percent (CDC, 2023; Abuogi et al., 2024). Pediatric and family practice providers should be ready to support lactation and breastfeeding in HIV-positive people.

Rubella

Rubella, also called German measles or 3-day measles, is caused by an RNA virus that is transmitted by contact with an infected person who spreads the virus by airborne droplets when coughing or sneezing. Typically, the infection is mild with a fever and a rash, although up to half of those who contract rubella have no symptoms (Phillippi & Kantrowitz-Gordon, 2024, pp. 845–847; CDC, 2024g). Rubella that occurs in pregnancy can have profoundly serious outcomes, including miscarriage, fetal death, or congenital rubella syndrome (CDC, 2024d).

Congenital rubella syndrome is an illness that results from rubella infection during pregnancy (National Library of Medicine, 2023). Infants with congenital rubella syndrome usually present with more than one sign or symptom consistent with congenital rubella infection, although hearing impairment is the most common single defect (National Library of Medicine, 2023). The more common consequences associated with congenital rubella syndrome (CRS) are ophthalmologic (cataracts, retinopathy, microphthalmos, congenital glaucoma), cardiac (patent ductus arteriosus, peripheral pulmonary artery stenosis), auditory (sensorineural health impairment), and neurologic (behavioral disorders, meningoencephalitis, intellectual disability) (CDC, 2024d). Symptoms in children exposed during pregnancy may be delayed for 2 to 4 years. Many children who have congenital rubella syndrome develop type 1 or type 2 diabetes mellitus later in childhood.

All people who are pregnant should undergo serologic screening for rubella immunity at the first prenatal visit unless they are known to be immune by documentation of vaccination with one dose of live rubella-containing vaccine, laboratory evidence of immunity, or laboratory confirmation of the disease. People who are pregnant and who have symptoms suggestive of rubella should have a viral culture, PCR, or IgM antibody testing. Fetal surveillance for a pregnant person with confirmed rubella illness includes ultrasound to determine fetal malformations and referral to a perinatologist, especially if the infection was contracted in the first half of pregnancy because congenital defects occur in approximately 85 percent of cases when infection occurs during the first 12 weeks of pregnancy (Phillippi & Kantrowitz-Gordon, 2024, pp. 845–847). The pregnant person needs to be advised of the risks of fetal infection, and the choice of pregnancy termination should be discussed. The risks of congenital infection decrease over the pregnancy and are rare after the 20th week of gestation.

People without immunity to rubella should be counseled to avoid exposure to infected individuals. The rubella vaccine should not be given to anyone who may be pregnant because it is a live, attenuated virus and therefore is not recommended during pregnancy. In contrast, rubella vaccination is recommended in the immediate postpartum period for people with nonimmune status. The clinician should explain the importance of avoiding pregnancy for 4 weeks following vaccination (CDC, 2024d).

Cytomegalovirus

Cytomegalovirus (CMV) is a member of the large family of DNA viruses known as Herpesviridae; thus, it is considered a herpes virus. Cytomegalovirus is the most common infectious cause of birth defects in the United States (CDC, 2024k). Like other herpes-type viruses, CMV can remain latent in a host's cells; reactivation of the virus can trigger reinfection (Neilsen-Saines & Cambou, 2023). People acquire CMV through close personal contact (sexual, contact with saliva or urine) since CMV is not a highly contagious virus. Household crowding, a factor for people with a lower socioeconomic status, promotes transmission of the virus. Horizontal transmission occurs when a person acquires CMV via a blood transfusion or organ transplant. Vertical or perinatal transmission can occur transplacentally, by exposure during delivery, or during lactation (Neilsen-Saines & Cambou, 2023). By age 40, over half of all adults have been infected with CMV (CDC, 2024k). People who are immunocompromised are particularly susceptible to CMV.

Fetuses exposed in the first 20 weeks of pregnancy are at greatest risk of developing congenital CMV. Congenital CMV can result in intellectual developmental disorders and cerebral palsy; however, hearing loss is the most common presentation (CDC, 2024k). Diminished hearing may only be present in one ear at birth but later can extend to the second ear. This is significant because the development of early language, communication, and social skills is affected by hearing loss (CDC, 2024k).

In the United States, 50–80 percent of adults have serologic evidence (positive IgG antibodies) of a previous CMV infection; however, this evidence of a previous infection is not necessarily protective against a reinfection or perinatal transmission (Neilsen-Saines & Cambou, 2023). The greatest risk of congenital infection is if the pregnant person experiences a primary CMV infection during the pregnancy. Pregnant people who experience a reactivated CMV infection are less likely to transmit the infection to their fetus or newborn. The greatest risk of perinatal transmission of CMV occurs when the maternal infection occurs in the third trimester; however, the risk for fetal injury is highest when maternal CMV infection occurs in the first trimester (Neilsen-Saines & Cambou, 2023). When suspicion of congenital CMV arises, ultrasound is used to identify fetal complications, such as abdominal and liver calcifications, hepatosplenomegaly, ascites, microcephaly, hydrops fetalis, and intrauterine growth restriction. Current recommendations for the diagnosis of fetal CMV infection are the use of polymerase chain reaction (PCR) or viral cultures (Neilsen-Saines & Cambou, 2023). Following confirmation of diagnosis, referral to a maternal–fetal specialist for co-management during the pregnancy is necessary. All pregnant people should be taught how to prevent CMV transmission. Good hand washing and hygienic practices with shared items, such as toys and hard surfaces, and distancing/masking when around people who are ill are the best forms of prevention.

Herpes Simplex Virus

Herpes simplex virus types 1 and 2 (HSV-1, HSV-2) can both infect the pregnant person; HSV-2 is the virus typically associated with genital herpes. After initial infection, HSV establishes latency in sacral ganglia and can cause lifelong infection; the virus is often transmitted in the absence of an active lesion (Hammad & Konje, 2021). While both types of the virus can be transmitted from the pregnant/birthing person to the neonate, HSV-2 is associated with poorer outcomes in the newborn (Hammad & Konje, 2021). Transplacental infection with HSV-2 is extremely rare; most often, the neonate becomes infected through contact with the virus during birth.

Herpes neonatorum, also known as neonatal herpes, is a serious viral infection in newborns. It is often acquired via asymptomatic viral shedding during birth. The greatest risk of transmission occurs when the pregnant person is diagnosed with a primary HSV infection in the third trimester. Generally, there is not sufficient time to develop and transplacentally transfer protective antibodies to the fetus. Newborn HSV transmission may be as high as 30–50 percent following a third-trimester primary infection; with recurrent HSV outbreaks, even in the third trimester, the transmission rate is as low as 1–3 percent (Hammad & Konje, 2021). Cesarean delivery should be considered for any person with an active lesion present with the onset of labor or after a primary HSV infection after 28 weeks (Hammad & Konje, 2021).

Late third trimester prophylactic antiviral therapy should be offered to anyone with a known history of HSV. Generally, pregnant people are treated with acyclovir (400 mg 3 times a day) or valacyclovir (500 mg twice a day). Providers should also document the absence of an active lesion at the time of labor.

Sexually Transmitted Infections During Pregnancy

Sexually transmitted infections (STIs) can create a serious risk to maternal and fetal health during pregnancy and to the newborn during the postpartum period. The identification of STIs early in pregnancy through appropriate screening and prompt treatment can minimize complications to the pregnant person, fetus, and neonate. Therefore, it is important to inquire about STIs with pregnant persons and their partners (Workowski et al., 2021). The following section details concerns specific to STIs in pregnancy. For detailed information about the screening, diagnosis, and management of STIs, please refer to Chapters 21 and 22. Two notable STIs, HIV and herpes simplex virus, are described earlier in this chapter.

Bacterial Vaginosis

Bacterial vaginosis (BV) is a condition that exists when there is an imbalance of bacteria in the vagina. BV is commonly found within the lower genital tract of pregnant people. Although BV is not classified as an STI, it is often associated with other STIs. Pregnant people who are symptomatic for BV (presence of vaginal thin milky discharge and/or a fishy odor) do necessitate further evaluation and treatment due to the potential association of BV with premature labor and premature rupture of membranes, intra-amniotic infection (IAI), and postpartum endometritis (Owens et al., 2020; Workowski et al., 2021). Currently, the research is not supportive of routine screening of BV when pregnant persons are asymptomatic, due to uncertainty with the benefits outweighing the risks that can occur with sampling and treatment (Owens et al., 2020; Workowski et al., 2021). When treating BV in pregnancy, there is no contraindication to either oral metronidazole or clindamycin; both have demonstrated safety and efficacy in pregnancy. Additionally, oral therapy has not demonstrated superior efficacy over topical (vaginal) therapy. Pregnant people may be treated with any of the topical or oral dosing regimens of either metronidazole or clindamycin (Workowski et al., 2021).

Trichomoniasis Vaginalis

Trichomonas vaginalis infection during pregnancy is associated with premature rupture of membranes, a two- to threefold increase in premature birth, and low birth weight in the newborn (Workowski et al., 2021). There is no recommended routine screening for trichomoniasis in people who are pregnant, although screening should occur upon symptom recognition. Trichomoniasis is characterized by a vaginal discharge that is profuse, frothy, and green in color; this discharge may also have a foul odor, especially after coitus. Many people will be asymptomatic. On exam, there is usually a copious amount of discharge on speculum exam and the vaginal pH is often elevated, although it may be less than 5. Pregnant people may be treated at any stage during pregnancy with one dose of metronidazole 2 grams orally. For a person who is lactating, an alternative treatment is metronidazole 400 mg 3 times daily for 7 days. Although several reported case series found no evidence of adverse effects in newborns exposed to metronidazole in breastmilk, some clinicians suggest suspending breastfeeding for 12 to 24 hours following treatment with the single-dose regimen (Briggs et al., 2021; Workowski et al., 2021).

Chlamydia

Chlamydia is caused by the bacterium *Chlamydia trachomatis* and often accompanies gonorrhea. Transmission to the newborn occurs during birth from exposure to the cervix of the infected pregnant person. Chlamydial infection can cause infertility, and during pregnancy it is associated with spontaneous abortion (SAB), ectopic pregnancy, premature rupture of membranes, intra-amniotic infection (IAI), postpartum endometritis, preterm birth (PTB), and stillbirth. A neonate who contracts chlamydia is 10 times more likely to die in the newborn period (CDC, 2024b). The neonate is at elevated risk for developing neonatal conjunctivitis 5 to 12 days after birth. Subacute, afebrile pneumonia can occur 1 to 3 months after birth (CDC, 2024b). All pregnant people should be screened at the first antepartum visit regardless of social history. Retesting should occur during the third trimester if the pregnant person is at an increased risk for STIs. People who are pregnant and test positive for chlamydia should be treated with azithromycin 1 gm orally in one dose, or amoxicillin 500 mg orally 3 times daily for 7 days. A test of cure should be done 3 to 4 weeks following treatment and again within 3 months (CDC, 2024b; Workowski et al., 2021).

Gonorrhea

Gonorrhea is a sexually transmitted bacterial infection caused by *Neisseria gonorrhoeae*. In pregnancy, gonorrhea infections are associated with ectopic pregnancy, preterm birth (PTB), premature rupture of membranes, intraamniotic infection (IAI), and fetal growth restriction. Transmission of the bacterium to the newborn occurs during exposure to the cervix of a person who is pregnant and has gonorrhea. Newborn illness usually occurs 2 to 5 days after birth and is manifested as ophthalmia neonatorum and sepsis (Workowski et al., 2021). All pregnant people should be screened for a gonorrheal infection at the first antepartum visit. If the risk for gonorrhea continues into the pregnancy, retesting should occur during the third trimester (Workowski et al., 2021). Gonorrhea during pregnancy is treated with ceftriaxone 500 mg in a single intramuscular dose. Do not treat for chlamydia unless a chlamydial infection has also been identified. If the pregnant person has a cephalosporin allergy or other concerns with this treatment, an infectious disease or STI treatment specialist should be consulted regarding management (Workowski et al., 2021). A test of cure should be conducted 3 to 4 weeks after completing treatment.

Human Papillomavirus

Human Papillomavirus (HPV) infection is characterized by the presence of precancerous genital lesions, sometimes called warts (Workowski et al., 2021). During pregnancy, these lesions can grow, proliferate, and become friable; this growth may be due to changes in immune response, hormones, and increased vaginal discharge contributing to a moist environment that can enhance the proliferation of HPV warts. Some lesions may grow quite large, to the point that obstruction of the introitus is possible. In rare instances, HPV types 6 and 11 can cause respiratory papillomatosis in the neonate and possible obstruction of the pharynx. However, in people with HPV, the presence of large perineal lesions is not an indication for cesarean birth unless there is complete obstruction of the introitus or there is risk of excessive bleeding (Workowski et al., 2021). Cesarean birth does not offset all possible means of transmission since HPV DNA has been detected in amniotic fluid and the placenta (Chilaka et al., 2021). Pregnant people should be counseled that there is a minimal risk for laryngeal warts in their newborn leading to respiratory papillomatosis (Workowski et al., 2021). Screening people who are pregnant for HPV in conjunction with cervical cancer screening is recommended at the same screening intervals as for people who are not pregnant. Treating HPV warts with podofilox, podophyllin, and sinecatechins is not appropriate in pregnancy (Workowski et al., 2021). There is limited data to support the use of imiquimod during pregnancy, so its use should be avoided (Briggs et al., 2021). Lesions during pregnancy should be observed closely, and treatment should be delayed until after birth because many lesions will resolve spontaneously.

Hepatitis B Virus

Hepatitis B virus (HBV) transmission to a fetus can occur during pregnancy, birth, and breastfeeding through exposure to bodily secretions such as vaginal fluid, amniotic fluid, blood, saliva, and breast milk. HBV infections during pregnancy have associated risks such as spontaneous abortion and premature birth. Due to HBV being highly transmissible, all pregnant persons should be tested during each pregnancy for the hepatitis B surface antigen (HBsAg) at their first prenatal visit regardless of prior testing or vaccine status (Workowski et al., 2021). Additionally, all pregnant persons should be tested for HBsAg again in the late third trimester or at delivery (Workowski et al., 2021). All pregnant persons whose test result is HBsAg positive should be tested for HBV DNA to further assess need for antiviral therapy, receive a hepatitis B vaccination, and be referred to a perinatology specialist, along with notification sent to their state and local perinatal hepatitis B prevention programs (Briggs et al., 2021; CDC, 2024a).

Perinatal transmission of HBV is preventable, with the highest risk for transmission at time of birth. Therefore, all neonates born to a pregnant person with HBV infection or who has a documented positive carrier status, regardless of the delivery mode, will require postexposure immunoprophylaxis to include an initial hepatitis B vaccine and hepatitis B immunoglobulin (HBIG) within 12 hours, and the initial bath as soon as the infant is stable following birth. Infants born to people who are HBsAg positive may continue to breastfeed (CDC, 2024a; Workowski et al., 2021).

Hepatitis C Virus

Hepatitis C Virus (HCV) antibody testing is recommended for all pregnant persons at their first prenatal visit, even though transmission to a fetus can be quite variable based on how much HCV is already present or if found to be concomitant with HIV. The highest risk for HCV transmission during pregnancy is mainly during labor or at time of birth, regardless of delivery method. Currently, there are no approved treatments available for prescribing HCV-positive pregnant persons to assist with decreasing risks of potential neonatal transmission (Committee on Clinical Practice Guidelines-Obstetrics, 2023; Workowski et al., 2021). If HCV antibody testing result is positive, then follow-up testing for HCV RNA needs to occur to assess level of disease. As part of the management plan, clinicians should make referrals to gastroenterology or infectious disease specialist and perinatology to assess for potential complications while also providing a risk and benefit discussion to begin planning for direct-acting antiviral treatment postpartum and after lactation completion (Committee on Clinical Practice Guidelines-Obstetrics, 2023; Workowski et al., 2021). Although there are no reports of HCV transmission through breast milk, clinicians should recommend avoiding breastfeeding for HCV-positive lactating persons if nipples become cracked or bleeding to prevent exposure (Workowski et al., 2021).

Syphilis

Syphilis is a systemic sexually transmitted infection, caused by *Treponema pallidum,* with further division into multiple stages based on clinical findings which can guide necessary treatment and follow-up (Workowski et al., 2021). These various stages of syphilis are known as primary, secondary, tertiary, and latent. Primary syphilis is often found at the site of infection as a solitary, painless ulcer called a chancre; but this stage can also present as multiple, painful, atypical-appearing lesions. Secondary syphilis symptoms often appear as a skin rash with multiple lesions found within the mouth or along the mucus membranes with accompanying lymphadenopathy present. Tertiary syphilis can include symptoms of gummatous lesions, tabes dorsalis, and general paresis along with cardiac involvement. Latent stages of syphilis are typically asymptomatic and more commonly detected with serologic testing alone (Workowski et al., 2021). At any stage of syphilis, the central nervous system can be infected, leading to neurosyphilis. A diagnosis of syphilis requires use of two serological tests for confirmation: a non-treponemal antibody test (using either a VDRL or RPR) and a treponemal test. A reactive (positive) non-treponemal test should always be followed with a treponemal test, which is mandated across most states (Workowski et al., 2021). Non-treponemal antibody tests can also be used for monitoring treatment response with syphilis.

The risks for perinatal transmission of syphilis are related to the stage of syphilis upon diagnosis. The highest risk for perinatal transmission occurs during the primary and secondary stages of syphilis. Due to these perinatal risks for transmission related to syphilis, recent recommendations are for all pregnant persons to receive serological testing at their first prenatal care visit, followed by universal rescreening during the third trimester and again at time of birth (ACOG, 2024a). When a syphilis diagnosis occurs during the second half of pregnancy, an ultrasound is recommended to further assess the fetus for signs of congenital syphilis: hepatomegaly, ascites, hydrops, fetal anemia, or a thickened placenta. Syphilis diagnosed during the second trimester is correlated with an increased risk for premature birth. Benzathine penicillin G is the only known effective treatment for syphilis during pregnancy and for any stage of syphilis that can also assist in the prevention of congenital syphilis; regardless of a reported penicillin allergy, a pregnant person will first require desensitization, followed by treatment (ACOG, 2024a; Workowski et al., 2021).

FIRST-TRIMESTER COMPLICATIONS

Hyperemesis Gravidarum

Hyperemesis gravidarum (HG), is a severe form of nausea and vomiting in pregnancy (NVP). NVP is experienced by approximately 70 percent of pregnant people; about 24 percent of pregnant people will be prescribed antiemetic medication. NVP is often referred to as a common discomfort of pregnancy. The etiology of NVP remains unknown but existing theories proposed include hormonal, evolutionary adaptation, and psychologic predisposition. People experiencing NVP often face bias and minimalization of their symptoms, resulting in many pregnant people feeling or being dismissed or undertreated (Committee on Obstetric Practice, 2018, reaffirmed 2024). The symptoms of NVP often begin in the first trimester and are associated with undernutrition and inability to tolerate prenatal vitamin supplements (Fejzo, 2024).

The incidence of HG is approximately 0.3 to 3.0 percent of all pregnancies (Committee on Obstetric Practice, 2018, reaffirmed 2024). Risk factors include an increased placental mass (molar pregnancy, multiple gestation), previous history of HG, history of motion sickness, migraine headaches, and a family history of HG (Committee on Obstetric Practice, 2018, reaffirmed 2024). There are no single diagnostic criteria for HG. The most associated criteria for a diagnosis of HG are persistent vomiting not due to other causes, large ketonuria, and an objective measure of weight loss (most often at least 5% of prepregnancy weight) (Committee on Obstetric Practice, 2018, reaffirmed 2024). Differential diagnoses include gastrointestinal conditions such as gastroenteritis, cholecystitis, pancreatitis, hepatitis, and appendicitis; genitourinary tract conditions such as pyelonephritis, uremia, and kidney stones; metabolic conditions such as diabetic ketoacidosis, Addison disease, hyper- or hypothyroidism, and porphyria; neurologic disorders such as vestibular lesions, migraine headaches, and tumors of the central nervous system; miscellaneous conditions such as drug intolerance or psychologic conditions; and pregnancy-related conditions such as preeclampsia (Committee on Obstetric Practice, 2018, reaffirmed 2024).

Pregnant people with HG report uncontrolled nausea and vomiting, anorexia, fatigue, loss of work, and difficulty managing activities of daily living. Recognition, acknowledgment, and education are key components to managing both NVP and HG; it is important not to dismiss patient symptoms as a normal adaptation of pregnancy. The primary goal in treatment of HG is to correct dehydration and electrolyte imbalance. Treatment may require hospitalization and include bed rest and fetal surveillance, improving/facilitating nutritional intake, intravenous fluids, antiemetics, and dietary counseling. Care may include referral to a maternal–fetal specialist as HG has been associated with poor pregnancy outcomes (**Box 33-1**) (Fejzo, 2024).

Vaginal Bleeding During Early Pregnancy

Vaginal bleeding occurring early during a pregnancy should always necessitate further evaluation by a perinatal care provider to promptly identify if there is also presence of other accompanying symptoms that may help distinguish between presence of simple vaginal spotting of pregnancy versus more potential

BOX 33-1 Pregnancy Complications Associated With Hyperemesis Gravidarum

Maternal

- Thyrotoxicosis
- Detached retinas
- Pneumothorax
- Esophageal tears
- Rib fractures
- Preeclampsia
- Thromboembolism
- Wernicke's encephalopathy
- Cardiac morbidity/mortality
- Hemorrhage
- Suicide
- Nutritional deficiencies
- Liver dysfunction
- Kidney dysfunction
- Placental dysfunction

Fetal

- Intrauterine fetal demise (IUFD)
- Termination of the pregnancy
- Abnormal brain growth
- Intracranial hemorrhage

Data from Fejzo, M. (2024). Hyperemesis gravidarum theories dispelled by recent research: A paradigm change for better care and outcomes. *Trends in Molecular Medicine, 30*(6), 530–540. https://doi.org/10.1016/j.molmed.2024.04.006

complexities of an early pregnancy loss, spontaneous abortion (SAB), ectopic (tubal) pregnancy, or a molar pregnancy (ACOG, 2018b/2022; ACOG, 2018c/2025). According to the American College of Obstetricians and Gynecologists, in clinical practice and often during the first trimester of pregnancy, the terms pregnancy loss, SAB, and miscarriage may often be used interchangeably, although they may have varying meanings (ACOG, 2018c/2025). Therefore, it is pertinent for clinicians to do a thorough medical history intake and examination. Ultrasonography and serum β-hCG are also useful in the evaluation process of the vaginal bleeding before making a final diagnosis.

Early Pregnancy Loss

Early pregnancy loss is defined as an intrauterine, nonviable pregnancy occurring before 12 6/7 weeks gestation. Diagnosis is confirmed through ultrasonography examination that demonstrates either absence of a gestational sac, presence of a gestational sac but without an embryo, or presence of a gestational sac with embryo but no evidence of fetal cardiac activity (ACOG, 2018c/2025). Early pregnancy loss can be common and accounts for approximately 10 percent of all pregnancies, and 50 percent of those losses when further evaluated are found to be attributed to chromosomal abnormalities (ACOG, 2018c/2025). Management options for an early pregnancy loss may include expectant management, medical treatment, or surgical evacuation (ACOG, 2018c/2025). Expectant management is typically only offered during the first trimester of pregnancy due to increased risk for hemorrhage or incomplete expulsion (ACOG, 2018c/2025).

Spontaneous Abortion

Spontaneous abortion (SAB) is defined as a pregnancy loss that occurs any time prior to 20 weeks gestation and happens naturally without any medical intervention. Ultrasonography, if available, is the preferred modality to verify the presence of a viable intrauterine gestation if there is no documentation this has been confirmed before (ACOG, 2018b/2022; ACOG, 2018c/2025). The following risk factors may place a person at higher risk for a potential SAB to occur: advancing maternal age; endocrine disorders (i.e., thyroid disease, diabetes mellitus, and polycystic ovarian syndrome); history of prior SABs; presence of viral or bacterial infections; a history of an anatomic reproductive disorder (i.e., uterine malformation); history of chronic diseases; and/or environmental toxin exposure (ACOG, 2018c/2025). There are multiple types of SABs that clinicians will need to differentiate between when making a diagnosis as to category type (refer to **Table 33-4**).

Diagnosis of an SAB or early pregnancy loss requires assessing uterine size by either physical examination or ultrasound, identifying if fetal heart tones are present by either doppler

TABLE 33-4 Types of Spontaneous Abortion

Type	Definition	Symptoms	Prognosis
Threatened	Symptoms of SAB present Products of conception intact	Minimal vaginal bleeding Abdominal cramping Uterine size is equal to dates Cervical os is closed	Possible pregnancy loss
Inevitable	Symptoms of SAB increased in severity, to include cervical dilation Products of conception intact	Moderate vaginal bleeding Moderate to severe uterine cramping Uterine size is equal to dates Cervical os is dilated	Poor
Incomplete	Symptoms of SAB present, to include cervical dilation Partial products of conception intact	Heavy vaginal bleeding Moderate to severe uterine cramping Uterine size is equal to dates Cervical os is dilated	Poor
Complete	Products of conception expelled in entirety following symptoms of SAB	Minimal vaginal bleeding Prior uterine cramping has subsided Uterus is prepregnancy size Cercival os is either closed or dilated	Pregnancy loss
Missed	Products of conception retained for up to 6 weeks following symptoms of SAB	Vaginal bleeding has occurred, subsided, and reoccurs No current uterine contractions, but there is a history of uterine cramping	Pregnancy loss
Recurrent	Three or more SABs occurring consecutively	Same as all previously listed types	Poor for maintaining future pregnancies without intervention; refer to assistive reproduction specialist

Abbreviations: SAB, spontaneous abortion.

auscultation or visualization with an ultrasound, examination of the cervical os to assess for dilation, and serial β-hCG measurements if below 13 weeks gestation. Differential diagnoses include reproductive cancers, ectopic pregnancy, and hydatidiform mole. Upon identification of symptoms related to SAB, referral to a physician for options with treatment management is appropriate. Follow-up management typically also includes confirmation of complete expulsion by ultrasound examination and/or will include serial serum β-hCG measurements to follow until down to undetectable levels (ACOG, 2018c/2025).

Rho (D) immune globulin (RhoGAM) administration following an SAB is indicated for women who have RhD-negative blood type. Any RhD-negative women who will be also undergoing surgical management for their SAB or an early pregnancy loss will need to receive Rho(D) immune globulin as prophylaxis because of the increased risk for alloimmunization present during surgical procedures (ACOG, 2018c/2025).

Ectopic Pregnancy

Ectopic pregnancy is the implantation of a fertilized ovum in locations other than the uterine cavity. The most common site of ectopic pregnancy is the fallopian tube (ACOG, 2018b/2022). Ectopic pregnancies carry significant risk for pregnancy loss, tubal rupture, excessive blood loss, and future infertility due to tubal scarring. Refer to **Box 33-2** for a summary of risk factors associated with an ectopic pregnancy.

Pelvic and abdominal pain and unexplained vaginal bleeding are the primary symptoms of ectopic pregnancy. The pain may be described as vague, sharp, diffuse, or unilateral. The person may have had a time of amenorrhea, and pregnancy may or may not already be diagnosed. A ruptured ectopic pregnancy is characterized by a sudden onset of vaginal bleeding and sharp, severe, unilateral abdominal pain. Following rupture, symptoms of significant blood loss and resulting shock may include hypotension, shoulder pain, and breast tenderness.

BOX 33-2 Risk Factors for Ectopic Pregnancy

- Previous ectopic pregnancy
- Any previous tubal surgery or tubal deformity
- History of ascending pelvic infection
- History of infertility
- Past or current use of intrauterine device[a]
- Assisted reproduction
- History of therapeutic abortion, especially with complications
- Age greater than 35 years (less significant risk factor)

Data from American College of Obstetricians and Gynecologists. (2019d). Tubal ectopic pregnancy: ACOG practice bulletin no. 193. https://www.acog.org/clinical/clinical-guidance/practice-bulletin/articles/2018/03/tubal-ectopic-pregnancy

[a]Because use of an intrauterine device decreases the risk of pregnancy, the risk of ectopic pregnancy is lower; however, if pregnancy occurs with an intrauterine device in place, there is a higher risk that it is an ectopic pregnancy (ACOG, 2018b).

Physical findings associated with ectopic pregnancy include cervical motion tenderness, a uterus that is not enlarged, adnexal mass, and adnexal tenderness. A transvaginal ultrasound evaluation is the minimum diagnostic evaluation of a suspected ectopic pregnancy, and it should be done by someone trained in obstetrical sonography. Often a serial hCG level is taken at the same time to confirm diagnosis. Management of an ectopic pregnancy should be by an obstetrician or maternal–fetal specialist. Differential diagnoses include appendicitis, pelvic inflammatory disease, bowel irritability or obstruction, cholecystitis, pyelonephritis, and ovarian torsion. However, all people who are sexually active and present with clinical signs and/or physical symptoms of ectopic pregnancy, such as abdominal pain and vaginal bleeding, should be screened for pregnancy regardless of whether they are using contraception (ACOG, 2018b/2022).

Management prior to a confirmed diagnosis includes close observation to avoid the medical emergency of tubal rupture. Early diagnosis also may facilitate the use of methotrexate to dissolve the products of conception and avoid tubal rupture. The presence of signs and symptoms of rupture requires prompt medical attention in an institution that is equipped with surgical capabilities. Close follow-up includes Rho(D) immune globulin (RhoGAM) administration when appropriate, monitoring β-hCG levels, emotional care due to pregnancy loss, and future fertility counseling.

Molar Pregnancy (Hydatidiform Mole)

Hydatidiform mole, often referred to as a molar pregnancy, is a form of gestational trophoblastic neoplasia which arises from abnormal proliferation of the placental tissue that is developing into benign tumors with a potential for metastasis (Soper, 2021). The most common presenting symptom of a molar pregnancy is early abnormal vaginal bleeding occurring in the first trimester, sometimes with reports of vaginal tissue passage that is described as "grapelike" in appearance (hydropic villi). Other potential associated signs or symptoms that may be encountered are uterine enlargement, sizing larger than suspected gestational dates, absence of fetal heart activity, abnormal elevation of β-hCG levels, hyperemesis gravidarum, or early onset of pregnancy-induced hypertension.

There are two types of molar pregnancies, partial and complete. In a partial molar pregnancy, there is presence of nonviable fetal tissue; alternately, with a complete molar pregnancy, there is no presence of fetal tissue (Soper, 2021). In a partial molar pregnancy, the patient may present with symptoms of a missed SAB with uterine size still as expected related to the last normal menstrual period. However, a complete molar pregnancy is a uterine size greater than expected related to the last normal menstrual period and vaginal bleeding accompanied with passage of grapelike villa. Increased incidence of complications is associated with a complete molar pregnancy. Pregnant persons at higher risk are age younger than 20 years or older than 40 years (Soper, 2021).

Patients with a molar pregnancy may experience the following symptoms: dark red or brown vaginal bleeding; abdominal tenderness, especially over the ovaries; severe nausea and vomiting persisting beyond 12 weeks gestation; extreme fatigue; pelvic pain; coughing and shortness of breath; hemoptysis; and weight loss. Symptoms of preeclampsia may develop prior to 24 weeks. Gathering careful objective data assists with the diagnosis of molar pregnancy. An ultrasound reveals a snowstorm pattern, lack of fetal parts, and lack of fetal movement. No fetal heart tones will be auscultated. Levels of β-hCG will be consistently high and rising.

Management requires a referral to a maternal–fetal specialist. If a malignancy is diagnosed, a referral to an oncologist is necessary. Evacuation of the molar tissue may be accomplished pharmacologically or surgically. Follow-up care will include monitoring β-hCG levels to determine if the levels are decreasing, contraception, consultation with a maternal–fetal specialist, avoidance of pregnancy for 6 to 12 months, and emotional care due to pregnancy loss (Soper, 2021).

SECOND-TRIMESTER COMPLICATIONS

The second trimester is typically a time when there is some resolution of the physical discomforts often associated with the first trimester. The period of organogenesis has passed, and the fetus continues to grow and develop at a rapid rate. Several of the complications can be identified during routine prenatal screening. ACOG (2016b, reaffirmed 2022) recommends a 20-week ultrasound during pregnancy to screen for fetal anatomy and growth, placental location, and cervical length. The goal of this section is to provide clinicians with the ability to identify potential complications, set care priorities, and develop an appropriate plan of care to optimize outcomes for the pregnant person and fetus/newborn.

Cervical Insufficiency

Cervical insufficiency is a term used to describe the inability of the uterine cervix to retain a pregnancy in the absence of signs and symptoms of labor or contractions during the second trimester (ACOG, 2014, reaffirmed 2024). A shortened cervix may be identified at the 20-week ultrasound, not diagnostic of cervical insufficiency, but is associated with preterm birth (ACOG, 2014, reaffirmed 2024). Diagnosis of cervical insufficiency is made with the clinical findings of painless cervical dilation after the first trimester followed by complete expulsion of the pregnancy in the second trimester. Risks for cervical insufficiency include a congenital disorder (hypoplastic cervix), surgical trauma (LEEP or conization cervical procedures), traumatic damage of the cervix (repeated cervical dilation), and inflammation that is often due to infection (Buhimschi et al., 2023).

Cervical insufficiency is not always present with clinical symptoms. If symptoms are present, they may include backache, uterine contractions, vaginal spotting, pelvic pressure, an increase in vaginal discharge, decrease in cervical length, and cervical dilation confirmed by speculum examination (ACOG, 2014, reaffirmed 2024). Management for cervical insufficiency includes referral to a maternal–fetal specialist. Cervical cerclage placement may be appropriate, particularly in people with a previous pregnancy loss due to cervical insufficiency (ACOG, 2014, reaffirmed 2024). Additionally, continued prenatal surveillance including serial transvaginal ultrasounds beginning at 16 weeks gestation may be indicated (ACOG, 2014, reaffirmed 2024).

Preterm Labor, Preterm Birth, and Preterm Prolonged Rupture of Membranes

Preterm labor (PTL) is defined as regular uterine contractions that result in cervical change (dilation, effacement, or both) occurring between 20 weeks and 36 weeks, 6 days; preterm birth (PTB) is a birth that occurs (for any reason) between 20 weeks and 36 weeks, 6 days. Prelabor rupture of membranes (PROM) is rupture of membranes prior to the onset of labor; when membranes rupture before labor and the gestation age is less than 37 weeks, a diagnosis of preterm premature rupture of membranes (PPROM) is made (ACOG, 2020).

Of note, 30 percent of cases of PTL will spontaneously resolve, and 50 percent of people hospitalized for PTL will deliver at term (ACOG, 2016a, reaffirmed 2022). According to the March of Dimes (2024), the PTB rate was 10.4 percent of all births in 2022; the southern United States had the highest rates of PTB in the country. Neonatal complications of PTB include respiratory distress syndrome, infection, intraventricular hemorrhage, necrotizing enterocolitis, and cognitive impairment/learning difficulties; PTB accounts for approximately 70 percent of neonatal deaths, 36 percent of infant deaths, and up to 50 percent of all neurodevelopmental impairments in children (ACOG, 2016a, reaffirmed 2022). Preterm birth may be either spontaneous or provider-initiated (usually due to maternal–fetal complications) (Buhimschi et al., 2023). Preterm birth remains an ongoing public health issue, and evidence is needed to support interventions used to delay birth and improve outcomes (March of Dimes, 2024).

There are no clear guidelines for identifying people who will give birth prematurely. Risk identification remains key to early intervention. The National Institutes of Child Health and Human Development (NICHD) (2023) note risk factors for PTL and PTB as:

- previous preterm labor and/or birth
- multiple gestation
- assisted reproductive technology
- reproductive tract anomalies
- infection
- very low or very high BMI prior to pregnancy
- short interval between pregnancies
- placental abnormalities
- hypertension
- diabetes mellitus (pre existing or gestational)
- smoking
- alcohol or drug use during pregnancy
- intimate partner violence

PTL, PTB, and PPROM may be caused by maternal factors, fetal factors, or both, including fetal growth restriction, placenta previa, preeclampsia, or placental abruption. Maternal infection and inflammation in the reproductive tract may be linked to 20 to 30 percent of all PTBs (Buhimschi et al., 2023). Despite all that is known about risk factors for PTL and PTB, many pregnant people with PPROM, PTL, and PTB have no identifiable risk factors. Pregnant people who are at risk for PPROM include those with a history of PPROM, amniotic infection, and risks associated with PTL. Referral to a maternal–fetal specialist is required upon recognition of PPROM.

Two evidence-based interventions have dramatically improved neonatal outcomes for preterm infants: antenatal corticosteroids and magnesium sulfate therapy for fetal neuroprophylaxis. Administration of antenatal corticosteroids is associated with lower rates of respiratory distress syndrome, intraventricular hemorrhage, and necrotizing enterocolitis in the preterm neonate. Betamethasone and dexamethasone are the two corticosteroids with the most evidentiary support for use in pregnant people in preterm labor. A single course of corticosteroids is recommended for pregnant people between 24 weeks and 34 weeks who are at risk of delivery within 7 days (ACOG, 2016, reaffirmed 2022). There is supporting evidence that the use of corticosteroids between 34 weeks and 36 weeks, 6 days decreases respiratory complications in late-preterm infants (ACOG, 2016, reaffirmed 2022). Magnesium sulfate administration reduces the severity and risk of cerebral palsy in infants born before 32 weeks; protocols for dosage and duration are developed by individual hospitals and should be grounded in the evidence (ACOG, 2016, reaffirmed 2022).

Tocolytic therapy may offer short-term prolongation of a person's pregnancy, primarily to allow for the pregnant person to receive antenatal corticosteroids and magnesium sulfate (if indicated). There is no evidence that supports the use of medication, bedrest, reduced sexual activity, and increased hydration to prolong pregnancy (ACOG, 2016, reaffirmed 2022). There are contraindications to tocolytic therapy: intrauterine fetal demise (IUFD), a lethal fetal anomaly, nonreassuring fetal status, severe pre eclampsia or eclampsia, intraamniotic infection, and/or maternal bleeding with hemodynamic instability. Any patient presenting with preterm labor or at risk for preterm birth must first be evaluated for any of these conditions prior to any tocolysis.

A person with a singleton pregnancy and a prior PTB that occurred spontaneously should be offered progesterone supplementation beginning at 18 to 24 weeks gestation and cervical length screening (ACOG 2023). Progesterone (P4) is essential for the establishment and maintenance of pregnancy. P4 maintains pregnancy, in part, by blocking labor. Interventions such as bed rest, reduced sexual activity, and increased hydration are not supported by evidence and should no longer be recommended (ACOG, 2016, reaffirmed 2022).

Risk assessment and prompt management of potential PTL may contribute to reduced incidence of PTB. Symptoms associated with PTL include menstrual-like uterine cramps; a low, dull backache and pelvic pressure prior to 36 weeks gestation that may be due to fetal descent; diarrhea; increased vaginal discharge; leakage of clear fluid from the vagina; and vaginal bleeding. If these symptoms are experienced, the clinician must refer the person to a maternal–fetal specialist and to a facility equipped for the care of preterm infants.

Gestational Diabetes Mellitus

Gestational diabetes mellitus (GDM) is one of the most common complications of pregnancy. It occurs when a carbohydrate intolerance develops during pregnancy, a time of metabolic alterations to support changes that are essential to provide adequate nutrients to the fetus to enable fetal growth and development. GDM affects 3–9 percent of all U.S. pregnancies (Committee on Obstetric Practice Bulletins-Obstetrics, 2018a, reaffirmed 2024). Due to gestational carbohydrate intolerance, persistent hyperglycemia develops between gestational weeks 20 and 30. There is an increased incidence of gestational diabetes among pregnant persons of Hispanic, African American, Native American, and Asian or Pacific Islander origin. Gestational diabetes risk factors are the same as for type 2 diabetes and include obesity, increased maternal age, and family history (**Table 33-5**) (Committee on Practice Bulletins-Obstetrics, 2018a, reaffirmed 2024). Pregnant persons who developed gestational diabetes in a prior pregnancy are at increased risk for gestational diabetes in subsequent pregnancies.

Pregnancy-associated complications with gestational diabetes include spontaneous abortion (SAB), pyelonephritis, PTL and PTB, polyhydramnios, pre eclampsia, and an increased rate of operative birth, particularly cesarean birth. Later life risks for the pregnant person, fetus, and newborn associated with gestational diabetes include stillbirth; macrosomia leading to increased risk for operative birth, shoulder dystocia, birth trauma, neonatal hypoglycemia, hyperbilirubinemia, hypocalcemia, polycythemia, and an increased risk for obesity and type 2 diabetes later in life (Committee on Practice Bulletins-Obstetrics, 2018a, reaffirmed 2024).

TABLE 33-5 Risk Factors for Gestational Diabetes

Demographic Characteristics	Medical and Family History	Previous Obstetric History
Advanced age (≥ 35) during pregnancy Member of a racial or ethnic group at increased risk for type 2 diabetes: • Hispanic/Latiné • Black/African American • Native American • South or East Asian • Pacific Islanders	Prepregnancy weight 110% or more of ideal body weight or body mass index (BMI) greater than 30 kg/m^2; significant weight gain in early adulthood or between pregnancies; or excessive gestational weight gain Physical inactivity History of abnormal glucose tolerance Current use of glucocorticoids Polycystic ovary syndrome Chronic hypertension HDL cholesterol < 35 mg/dL Triglycerides > 250 mg/dL A1C ≥ 5.7%, impaired glucose tolerance, or impaired fasting glucose on previous testing First-degree relative with diabetes	History of adverse pregnancy outcomes associated with gestational diabetes: • Infant more than 4,000 g at birth • Unexplained stillbirth • Infant with congenital anomalies • Previous gestational diabetes mellitus

Data from Committee on Practice Bulletins-Obstetrics. (2018a, reaffirmed 2024). *Gestational diabetes mellitus* [Practice Bulletin no. 190]. American College of Obstetricians and Gynecologists. https://www.acog.org/clinical/clinical-guidance/practice-bulletin/articles/2018/02/gestational-diabetes-mellitus

In 2021, the U.S. Preventive Services Task Force (USPSTF) recommended screening all pregnant persons for gestational diabetes between 24 and 28 weeks gestation (USPSTF, 2021). Pregnant people who are at higher risk for GDM should be screened during the first trimester (Table 33-5; **Box 33-3**) (Committee on Practice Bulletins-Obstetrics, 2018a, reaffirmed 2024). If the first-trimester screen is negative, it should be repeated at 24 to 28 weeks gestation (Committee on Practice Bulletins-Obstetrics, 2018a, reaffirmed 2024).

The most common approach to screening for gestational diabetes is to administer 50 gm oral glucose, followed by a 1-hour venous blood glucose test. Pregnant persons whose blood sugar is greater than 130 to 140 mg/dL should undergo a 3-hour glucose tolerance test with a 100 gm oral glucose dose. Diagnosis of gestational diabetes can be made with two elevated blood glucose values on the 3-hour glucose tolerance test **(Table 33-6).**

The goal of care is to normalize the level of glycemic control to the level of a nondiabetic pregnant person. Nutritional education, physical activity/exercise, and fetal surveillance are part of the standard of care for GDM. People with gestational diabetes who cannot be managed with diet therapy alone are considered to have a higher-risk pregnancy and should receive care either in collaboration with or through referral to a maternal–fetal specialist. Pharmacologic management should be considered for people who are unable to maintain their blood sugar with complementary care.

BOX 33-3 Early Screening Recommendations for Gestational Diabetes

Consider early testing for all pregnant people with a BMI > 25 or one of the following:

- Physical inactivity
- First-degree relative with diabetes
- Previous infant ≥4,000 g
- Previous GDM
- Hypertension
- Polycystic ovary syndrome
- HDL cholesterol < 35 mg/dL
- Triglycerides > 250 mg/dL
- A1C ≥ 5.7%, impaired glucose tolerance, or impaired fasting glucose on previous testing
- History of cardiovascular disease

Data from Committee on Practice Bulletins-Obstetrics. (2018a, reaffirmed 2024). *Gestational diabetes mellitus* [Practice Bulletin no. 190]. American College of Obstetricians and Gynecologists. https://www.acog.org/clinical/clinical-guidance/practice-bulletin/articles/2018/02/gestational-diabetes-mellitus

TABLE 33-6 Screening and Diagnostic Criteria for Gestational Diabetes

Organization	Plasma Glucose Diagnostic Values
American College of Obstetricians and Gynecologists	1. 50-gram glucose screening test: a. Gestational diabetes diagnosed if greater than 200 mg/dL. b. If greater than 140 mg/dL, move to 3-hour GTT. 2. Three-hour GTT at 24 to 28 weeks gestation. Gestational diabetes is diagnosed if two values are greater than the following threshold values: a. Carpenter–Coustan plasma or serum glucose level: Fasting, greater than 95 mg/dL; 1 hour, greater than 180 mg/dL; 2 hour, greater than 155 mg/dL; 3 hour, greater than 140 mg/dL. b. National Diabetes Data Group plasma level: Fasting, greater than 105 mg/dL; 1 hour, greater than 190 mg/dL; 2 hour, greater than 165 mg/dL; 3 hour, greater than 145 mg/dL
International Association of the Diabetes and Pregnancy Study Groups; American Diabetes Association	1. Measure fasting plasma glucose, HbA1c, or random plasma glucose of all pregnant persons or all high-risk pregnant persons at initial prenatal visit: a. Overt diabetes diagnosed: Fasting, 126 mg/dL or greater; HbA1c 6.5% or greater; random plasma glucose 200 mg/dL or greater that is subsequently confirmed via HbA1c or fasting blood glucose value. b. Gestational diabetes diagnosed: Fasting, 92 mg/dL or greater but less than 126 mg/dL. 2. If initial values do not detect overt diabetes or gestational diabetes, do 75-gram 2-hour GTT at 24 to 28 weeks gestation: a. Overt diabetes diagnosed: Fasting, 126 mg/dL or greater. b. Gestational diabetes diagnosed if one value is greater than the following threshold values: Fasting, greater than 92 mg/dL; 1-hour plasma glucose greater than 180 mg/dL; 2-hour plasma glucose greater than 153 mg/dL

Data from American College of Obstetricians and Gynecologists Committee on Obstetric Practice-Obstetrics. (2018a, reaffirmed 2024). *Gestational diabetes mellitus* [Practice Bulletin no. 190]; International Association of Diabetes and Pregnancy Study Groups Consensus Panel. (2010). International Association of Diabetes and Pregnancy Study Groups recommendations on the diagnosis and classification of hyperglycemia in pregnancy. *Diabetes Care, 33*(3), 676–682. https://doi.org/10.2337/dc09-1848.

Abbreviations: GTT, glucose tolerance test; HbA1c, glycated hemoglobin.

Fetal surveillance is recommended for all patients with pregestational diabetes and pregnant persons with gestational diabetes who have poor glycemic control (especially if requiring medication). If a person with gestational diabetes has good glycemic control, expectant management is used for labor and birth; however, if they have poor control and a suspected large for gestational age infant (> 4,500 g estimated fetal weight), cesarean birth may be recommended (Committee on Practice Bulletins-Obstetrics, 2018a, reaffirmed 2024).

Although gestational diabetes usually resolves after birth, up to one third of pregnant persons will have development of type 2 diabetes or impaired glucose metabolism at a postpartum screening (Committee on Practice Bulletins-Obstetrics, 2018a, reaffirmed 2024). Therefore, all people diagnosed with gestational diabetes should have a follow-up screen at 6–8 weeks postpartum with fasting glucose, and a 75 g, 2-hour oral glucose tolerance test. All people with gestational diabetes need to follow up with a primary care clinician for assessment and referral for medical therapy.

Alloimmunization During Pregnancy

Alloimmunization is defined as an immune response to antigens that are foreign and distinct from antigens on an individual's cells. During pregnancy, the most concerning type of alloimmunization is the immune-mediated response caused by maternal IgG antibodies crossing the placenta and specifically targeting fetal red blood cells. This occurs because the fetal red blood cells contain an antigen not found in the pregnant person. This maternal antibody response can lead to fetal red blood cell hemolysis and fetal anemia (Committee on Practice Bulletins-Obstetrics, 2018b, reaffirmed 2024). Many terminologies have been used to identify human blood groups, and therefore, to provide uniformity, a list of alternative names for antigens is used (often called Rh incompatibility). In a few cases the more commonly used name is provided, as with ABO and Rh, and specific subtypes use a second designation (Committee on Practice Bulletins-Obstetrics, 2018b, reaffirmed 2024). RhD is used to signify the erythrocyte antigen, and people who carry the RhD antigen are classified as Rh positive; those who do not are classified as Rh negative.

RhD alloimmunization occurs when a RhD-negative person is exposed to cells expressing the RhD antigen. Although the fetal and maternal blood circulations are separate, there is a possibility of mixing fetal and maternal blood during pregnancy due to miscarriage, ectopic pregnancy, antenatal bleeding, and during birth. Additional potential sensitizing events in RhD-negative persons during their pregnancy include chorionic villus sampling, amniocentesis, threatened miscarriage or miscarriage, antepartum hemorrhage, pregnancy termination, abdominal trauma, and external cephalic version (Committee on Practice Bulletins-Obstetrics, 2018b, reaffirmed 2024).

The risk of RhD alloimmunization occurs when an Rh-negative pregnant person carries an Rh-positive fetus; fetal red blood cells can enter maternal circulation triggering an immune response and causing the development of IgG antibodies to the Rh (D) antigen. Subsequent pregnancies with Rh-positive fetuses are then at risk when the IgG antibodies cross the placenta, attach to fetal cells, and cause hemolysis; such hemolysis may lead to erythroblastosis fetalis and stillbirth. The risk associated with Rh factor isoimmunization has significantly decreased since the late 1960s due to the development of Rho (D) immune globulin (RhoGAM), an anti-D immune globulin prophylaxis (Committee on Practice Bulletins-Obstetrics, 2018b, reaffirmed 2024). Prophylaxis with RhoGAM prevents development of the IgG antibodies. All pregnant people should be tested at the time of their first prenatal visit (for every pregnancy) for ABO blood group and RhD type, and they should be screened for the presence of erythrocyte antibodies (Committee on Practice Bulletins-Obstetrics, 2018b, reaffirmed 2024). RhoGAM should be administered by the 28th week of gestation to pregnant persons with a negative titer. A second dose of RhoGAM is administered within 72 hours of birth for mothers who give birth to Rh-positive infants. The American Association of Blood Banks also recommends repeating the antibody screening prior to the administration of anti-D immune globulin at 28 weeks gestation, at the time of birth, and postpartum (Committee on Practice Bulletins-Obstetrics, 2018b, reaffirmed 2024). Undiagnosed Rh alloimmunization carries a significant risk of perinatal mortality. All pregnant persons who are diagnosed with untreated alloimmunization need to be referred to a maternal–fetal specialist.

BLEEDING ASSESSMENT IN THE SECOND AND THIRD TRIMESTER OF PREGNANCY

Abnormal Placentation

Placenta previa occurs when the placenta implants in the lower segment of the uterus in a location that obstructs the cervical os. The terminology of placenta previa has changed because of the use of transvaginal ultrasound, which allows for a higher degree of accuracy in diagnosis (Hull et al., 2023). The NICHD recommended changing the definitions of placenta previa and low-lying placenta. A placenta that covers the cervical os to any degree (completely or close enough to cause bleeding during dilation or labor) is considered a placenta previa. A placenta that is 2 cm or more from the cervical os does not pose a risk for bleeding and should be considered normal. In many cases a placenta previa or low-lying placenta will resolve as the pregnancy progresses through a process called trophotropism (Hull et al., 2023). Placental location should be documented at the 20-week ultrasound.

Pregnant persons who are at increased risk for placenta previa include those with a history of placenta previa, history of cesarean birth, previous uterine surgeries, history of SAB or therapeutic abortion, age 35 years or older, history of multiple pregnancies, and history of smoking and cocaine abuse. Complications associated with placenta previa include abruptio placentae, placenta accreta, fetal malpresentation, postpartum hemorrhage, disseminated intravascular coagulation, infertility, and increased perinatal mortality. Painless vaginal bleeding is a hallmark sign of placenta previa. Bleeding may occur after 24 weeks gestation and is usually bright red, but it varies in amount. This is an important consideration anytime a pregnant patient presents with painless vaginal bleeding. Cervical exams or any kind of vaginal exam are contraindicated with all active vaginal bleeding until placental location can be verified. Pregnant people experiencing active bleeding may report fatigue and syncope. Symptoms of shock can occur with excessive bleeding.

Management depends on the extent of the placenta previa. In general, if bleeding occurs at or beyond 36 weeks, delivery is indicated. Antenatal corticosteroids should be ordered if the pregnant person is 34 weeks gestation or less. If a pregnant person has a placenta 2 cm or less from the cervical os, a cesarean delivery is planned by 36 weeks to avoid the risk of a sudden, excessive bleeding episode. No intervention is necessary if there is no bleeding, but patients need education regarding vaginal bleeding and when to seek care. Pregnant people diagnosed with placenta previa should be referred to a perinatologist (Hull et al., 2023).

Placenta Accreta Spectrum

Placenta accreta spectrum (PAS) (also known as morbidly adherent placenta), refers to a range of pathologic adherence of the placenta to the uterine lining. The incidence of PAS has increased from 1 in 4,017 in the 1980s to as high as 1 in 272 among delivered people in the United States by 2016 (ACOG, 2018, reaffirmed 2021). The increased incidence of PAS may be attributed to an increase in risk factors, notably the rise in the cesarean delivery rate (ACOG, 2018, reaffirmed 2021). Other risk factors include any previous uterine surgery, advanced maternal age, multiparity, Asherman syndrome, and placenta previa. Placental implantation over a previous uterine scar seems to increase the risk of PAS. The more cesarean births a person has had, the greater their risk for a morbidly adherent placenta.

PAS is classified by the depth of placental invasion in the uterine wall; this classification was developed by the International Federation of Obstetrics and Gynecology (FIGO) (Jauniaux et al., 2019). PAS grade 1 refers to superficial myometrial attachment; the villi penetrate beyond the normal fibrous boundary layer (Nitabuch layer) and attach to the myometrium (Gilner & Deshmukh, 2025; Hull et al., 2023). A grade 2 morbidly adherent placenta invades the myometrium, and PAS grade 3 describes placental invasion through the full thickness of the myometrium and into surrounding pelvic structures or tissues (bladder, bowel, pelvic organs). PAS grades 1, 2, and 3 replace the previous terminology of accreta, increta, and percreta (Gilner & Deshmukh, 2025). Please refer to **Figure 33-1**.

Diagnosis of PAS is done with an ultrasound exam in the second or third trimester, often at the 20-week ultrasound. Doppler flow imaging may detect a turbulent blood flow pattern around the implantation of the placenta. Anytime an ultrasound exam is inclusive or potentially suggestive of PAS, the pregnant person must be referred to a perinatologist for detailed imaging and planning for delivery. Sometimes magnetic resonance imaging (MRI) is ordered to confirm the diagnosis (ACOG, 2018, reaffirmed 2021). It is critical to diagnose PAS prenatally because hemorrhage at birth is anticipated in all cases of a morbidly adherent placenta. Management of PAS requires a multidisciplinary care team (e.g., obstetrician, anesthesiologist, perinatologist, pelvic surgeon specialist, urology, interventional radiology, neonatology, critical care experts) and delivery at a level III or IV care center (ACOG, 2018, reaffirmed 2021). There is often the need for a large volume blood transfusion at delivery. A cesarean delivery and hysterectomy are often planned when a person has a known morbidly adherent placenta (ACOG, 2018, reaffirmed 2021).

Placental Abruption

Placental abruption (also known as *abruptio placentae)* is the premature separation of the placenta from the uterine wall before birth, after 20 weeks gestation (Hull et al., 2023). Placental abruption can occur over a broad spectrum, from very minor degrees of separation with minor impact to maternal or fetal health to a major abruption associated with maternal and fetal morbidity and mortality (Hull et al., 2023). A placental abruption can be classified as obvious or occult. With an obvious placental abruption there is external, observable vaginal bleeding, whereas with an occult abruption, the separation of the placenta may occur at the central portion of the placenta rather than the edge of the placenta. Bleeding may be concealed by the fetal head (or other presenting part, such as the breech) if the presenting part is firmly applied to the cervical os.

FIGURE 33-1 Placenta accreta spectrum (PAS).

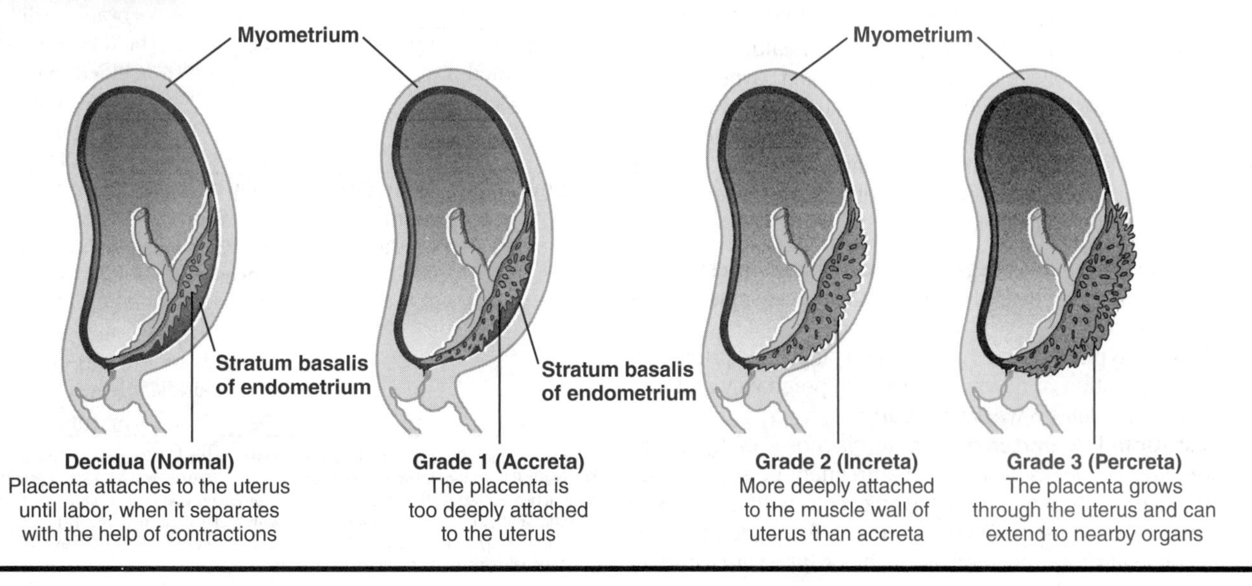

The most significant risk factor associated with placental abruption is an abruption in a previous pregnancy. Chronic hypertension increases abruption risk five fold; chronic hypertension with superimposed preeclampsia has an eight fold risk of abruption. Other risk factors include cigarette smoking (risk increases with the number of cigarettes smoked daily), substance abuse (a drug that causes vasospasm or hypertension [cocaine]), uterine fibroids, sudden uterine decompression (as in sudden rupture of membranes); abdominal trauma (motor vehicle accident, IPV) (Hull et al., 2023). The hemorrhage associated with placental abruption is a life-threatening complication for both the pregnant person and the fetus.

Painful, bright red vaginal bleeding and the sudden onset of sharp, localized abdominal pain are characteristics of a placental abruption; however, a person may also present with mild back pain, abdominal cramping, and minimal or no vaginal bleeding. Uterine tenderness may be both reported by the pregnant person and elicited by the clinician on abdominal examination. The pregnant person's abdomen (especially over the uterus) may be palpated as boardlike and firm. Fetal heart tones may be diminished or absent, and nonreassuring fetal status on ultrasound or electronic fetal monitoring may be noted. Initial assessment and management should focus on maternal hemodynamic status. Decisions regarding management and possible delivery depend on maternal–fetal status (Hull et al., 2023).

Suspicion of placental abruption requires referral to an obstetrician or maternal–fetal specialist because this condition is considered an emergent situation. The pregnant person with suspicion of a placental abruption should be cared for in a facility that can manage surgical intervention, manage a hypoxic newborn, and assist with maternal vascular support if necessary.

THIRD-TRIMESTER COMPLICATIONS

Hypertensive Disorders of Pregnancy

Hypertensive disorders of pregnancy (HDPs) continue to be a leading cause of maternal and neonatal mortality; HDPs complicate an estimated 2–8 percent of pregnancies worldwide. HDPs also account for a huge financial care burden for both pregnant people and their newborn infants (attributed to the care required for a preterm infant). Also, HDPs, particularly preeclampsia, can have negative long-term effects on a person's health.

The American College of Obstetricians and Gynecologists published practice bulletins that created straightforward definitions of hypertension in pregnancy, allowing healthcare clinicians worldwide to utilize the same phrasing and definitions (Committee on Practice Bulletins-Obstetrics, 2019; Committee on Practice Bulletins-Obstetrics, 2020).

- **Hypertension in pregnancy**: any blood pressure ≥ 140/90 mmHg measured on at least two occasions at least 4 hours apart.
- **Chronic hypertension**: hypertension diagnosed prior to 20 weeks gestation or newly diagnosed in pregnancy and persisting for at least 6 weeks postpartum.
- **Gestational hypertension**: new diagnosis of hypertension after 20 weeks gestation in a pregnant person with no evidence of proteinuria. Pregnant people with gestational hypertension must be followed closely for signs of evolving preeclampsia; additionally, if blood pressures remain elevated after 6 weeks postpartum, the diagnosis is changed to chronic hypertension.
- **Preeclampsia-eclampsia:** preeclampsia is new onset hypertension with proteinuria (or other symptoms). Eclampsia is the new onset of tonic-clonic, focal, or multifocal seizures in the absence of any previous known illness.
- **Chronic hypertension with superimposed preeclampsia:** preeclampsia is diagnosed in a person with chronic hypertension with new onset of proteinuria, neurologic symptoms, or laboratory values compatible with preeclampsia (thrombocytopenia, elevated liver transaminases, worsening renal function).

Chronic and Gestational Hypertension

Pregnant people with hypertension (chronic or gestational) should be managed with anti-hypertensive medications to optimize blood pressure (< 140/90), and to help reduce maternal and fetal morbidity and mortality. Angiotensin-converting enzyme (ACE) inhibitors and angiotensin receptor blockers (ARBs) should not be prescribed during pregnancy. If a person is taking one of these drugs prior to pregnancy, its use should be discontinued (refer to **Table 33-7** for medication and dosing recommendations) (Harper et al., 2025). Because pregnant people with

TABLE 33-7 Suggested Medication Management for Chronic Hypertension in Pregnancy

Medication	Dose	Frequency	Comments
Aspirin	81 mg	Daily	Initiate at 12 weeks and continue until delivery
Labetalol	Begin at 100 mg Can increase to 400 to 800 mg	Twice daily to 3 times a day	Maximum dose of 2,400 mg/day. Contraindicated with asthma, heart disease, heart block or bradycardia
Nifedipine, extended-release form	up to 120 mg daily	Usually once daily	The dose can be divided into twice daily dosing; avoid in people with tachycardia
Methyldopa	Up to 3,000 mg per day	Usually divided into 2 to 3 doses per day	Requires monitoring for hepatic dysfunction with liver function tests (alkaline phosphatase, aminotransferases, and bilirubin)

Data from Luger, R., & Kight, B. (2022). Hypertension in pregnancy. In *StatPearls*. StatPearls Publishing. https://www.ncbi.nlm.nih.gov/books/NBK430839/; Committee on Practice Bulletins-Obstetrics. (2020). *Gestational hypertension and preeclampsia* [Practice Bulletin no. 222]. American of Obstetricians and Gynecologists. https://www.acog.org/clinical/clinical-guidance/practice-bulletin/articles/2020/06/gestational-hypertension-and-preeclampsia hypertension are at a higher risk of developing preeclampsia, low-dose aspirin therapy should be started after 12 weeks gestation and continued until delivery (ACOG, 2020). Management for pregnant people with hypertension should also include consultation with a maternal–fetal medicine specialist.

Preeclampsia and Eclampsia

Preeclampsia is new onset of hypertension (≥ 140/90) most often occurring after 20 weeks of pregnancy and accompanied by a new onset of proteinuria (**Box 33-4**). **Eclampsia** is the new onset of tonic-clonic, focal, or multifocal seizures in the absence of any know previous illness or history such as epilepsy, cerebral infarction, intracranial hemorrhage, or drug use (Committee on Practice Bulletins-Obstetrics, 2020). High risk factors for preeclampsia include multifetal gestation, history of preeclampsia with a previous pregnancy, pre existing (chronic) hypertension, pregestational diabetes type 1 or 2, autoimmune disease (especially systemic lupus erythematosus or antiphospholipid syndrome), renal disease, assisted reproductive technology, and obstructive sleep apnea. Moderate risk factors for preeclampsia

BOX 33-4 Diagnosing Preeclampsia

Type	Signs and Symptoms
Preeclampsia	Blood pressure ≥ 140 mmHg systolic and ≥ 90 mmHg diastolic on two or more occasions at least 4 hours apart after 20 weeks gestation in a person with a previously normal blood pressure OR • Blood pressure ≥ 160 mmHg systolic or ≥110 diastolic AND **Proteinuria** • 300 mg or more in a 24-hour urine collection OR • Protein/creatinine ratio of 0.3 or higher
Preeclampsia exists in the absence of proteinuria if the person has	New onset of hypertension and any of the following: • Thrombocytopenia (platelet count < 100 $\times 10^9$/L • Renal insufficiency (serum creatinine > 1.1 mg/dL or doubling of serum creatinine in the absence of other kidney disease) • Impaired liver function, elevated liver transaminases at double normal values • Pulmonary edema • New onset headache unrelieved by medication • Visual disturbances

Preeclampsia with severe features	• Blood pressures ≥ 160 mmHg systolic or ≥ 110 mmHg diastolic on two occasions at least 4 hours apart
	• Thrombocytopenia, platelet count < 100 $\times 10^9$/L
	• Impaired liver function evidenced by
	  • Elevated liver transaminases at least double the normal values
	  • Right upper quadrant or epigastric pain unresponsive to medication
	• Renal insufficiency (serum creatinine > 1.1 mg/dL or doubling of serum creatinine in the absence of other kidney disease)
	• Pulmonary edema
	• New onset headache unrelieved by medication
	• Visual disturbances

Eclampsia	• New onset of tonic-clonic, focal, or multifocal seizures in the absence of other causative conditions Eclampsia is a severe manifestation of preeclampsia with potentially resulting sequalae: • Death of the pregnant or postpartum person (maternal mortality) • Hypoxia • Trauma • Aspiration pneumonia • Impaired memory or cognitive function • Posterior reversible encephalopathy syndrome Headache is considered the most common premonitory sign of potential eclampsia. Eclampsia is an emergent situation requiring prompt medical attention to include seizure precautions and immediate birth of the fetus.

Data from Committee on Practice Bulletins-Obstetrics. (2020). *Gestational hypertension and preeclampsia* [Practice Bulletin no. 222]. American of Obstetricians and Gynecologists. https://www.acog.org/clinical/clinical-guidance/practice-bulletin/articles/2020/06/gestational-hypertension-and-preeclampsia include nulliparity, age ≥ 35 years, BMI > 30, low socioeconomic status, > 10-year pregnancy interval, fetal growth restriction, African American race, a first-degree relative with preeclampsia, or previous adverse pregnancy outcome (Committee on Obstetric Practice-Obstetrics, 2018a, reaffirmed 2024; Luger & Kight, 2022). Preeclampsia is associated with both maternal and fetal complications. People with preeclampsia are at risk for renal and liver failure, disseminated intravascular coagulopathy, placental abruption, emergent operative birth, cardiovascular disease, stroke, and death. The fetus of a mother with preeclampsia may develop intrauterine growth restriction, oligohydramnios, fetal intolerance of labor, and preterm birth (and its associated complications).

People who are diagnosed with preeclampsia need referral to an obstetrician and a maternal–fetal specialist. A collaborative management plan can be developed and used; however, if the symptoms become severe, care should be turned over to a specialist. Hospitalization, increased maternal and fetal surveillance, pharmaceutical administration, and emergency birth may be necessary once preeclampsia is diagnosed (Harper et al., 2023). Pregnant people with severe features of preeclampsia must be treated with seizure prophylaxis that continues for 24 hours after birth; magnesium sulfate intravenous solution remains the preferred medication for preeclamptic seizure prophylaxis.

HELLP Syndrome

HELLP syndrome (**H**emolysis, **EL** elevated liver enzymes, and **LP** low platelets) is a severe form of preeclampsia and is associated with increased rates of maternal morbidity and mortality (Committee on Practice Bulletins-Obstetrics, 2020). It is characterized by hemolysis, elevated liver enzymes, and low platelet count. It is most often diagnosed in the third trimester, but in 30 percent of cases it is first expressed in the postpartum period (Committee on Practice Bulletins-Obstetrics, 2020). The main presenting symptoms are right upper quadrant pain and generalized malaise with nausea and vomiting. The serious risks associated with HELLP syndrome are hepatic rupture, disseminated intravascular coagulopathy, and eclampsia.

It is important to note that preeclampsia–eclampsia may develop as a new onset disease up to 6 weeks after birth. Postpartum patients may present to urgent care clinics or emergency departments reporting persistent headaches, and chest or abdominal discomfort with elevated blood pressures. Approximately 60 percent of patients with postpartum preeclampsia have not had any diagnosis of a hypertensive disorder during their pregnancies (Hauspurg & Jeyabalan, 2023). It is important for clinicians to ask about pregnancy history, manage hypertension, and implement seizure prophylaxis as appropriate when caring for people who may present with these symptoms.

Intrahepatic Cholestasis of Pregnancy

Intrahepatic cholestasis of pregnancy (ICP) is a poorly understood liver disorder generally occurring in the late second and early third trimester; the cause of ICP is thought to be multifactorial and possibly influenced by genetics, pregnancy hormones, and environmental factors. Pregnant people with ICP generally present with intractable pruritus, usually generalized, but most notably on the palms of the hands and the soles of the feet; the symptoms are usually worse at night. Pruritus is the hallmark sign, and it often occurs in the absence of a rash. Other symptoms could include nausea, anorexia, fatigue, right upper quadrant pain, dark urine, and pale stools (Pillarisetty & Sharma, 2023). In general, a person's physical examination is normal. Often, the only remarkable changes are scratch marks noted from intractable itching.

Maternal bile acids can cross the placenta and accumulate in the fetus and the amniotic fluid. This accumulation of bile acids in the fetus is most associated with adverse obstetric outcomes; adverse outcomes include preterm labor (potentially due to increased serum bile acids triggering prostaglandin release), fetal asphyxia events, meconium-stained amniotic fluid, and intrauterine fetal demise (IUFD) (Halscott & Vaught, 2023). Sudden IUFD is the most concerning and unpredictable risk of ICP and the risk of IUFD increases as maternal serum bile acid levels increase (Pillarisetty & Sharma, 2023).

Diagnosing ICP is based on patient symptoms and elevated serum bile acids (> 10 μmol/L), levels greater than 40 μmol/L indicate a severe form of the disease, increasing the likelihood of adverse outcomes including IUFD (Halscott & Vaught, 2023). It is important to note that pruritus often precedes lab abnormalities. If a patient presents with pruritus (especially palms of hands and soles of feet) and they have normal serum bile acids, the lab work should be repeated if the symptoms persist (Halscott & Vaught, 2023; Pillarisetty & Sharma, 2023).

Management for a person with ICP should include a consultation with a perinatologist and an obstetrician. The goal of care for ICP is to decrease the risks of perinatal morbidity and mortality and alleviate the symptoms for the pregnant person (Pillarisetty & Sharma, 2023). Ursodeoxycholic acid (UDCA) is the only drug or treatment that has consistently demonstrated the ability to improve symptoms for the pregnant person and lower serum bile acids (Halscott & Vaught, 2023). UDCA is usually initiated at a dose of 300 mg twice daily and may be increased to 3 times a day (Pillarisetty & Sharma, 2023). Twice weekly antenatal testing (biophysical profile and non-stress testing) is generally initiated at the time of diagnosis of ICP; however, reassuring testing does not preclude a sudden fetal demise. The mechanism of fetal death in people with ICP has been hypothesized to be related to a sudden fetal cardiac arrythmia triggered by elevated bile acids in the fetus. Hence, sudden IUFD can occur in the presence of reassuring antenatal testing (Committee on Obstetric Practice & Society of Maternal–Fetal Medicine, 2021, reaffirmed 2024). Early delivery is the only known intervention shown to significantly reduce the risk of IUFD in people with ICP.

Amniotic Fluid Disorders

Amniotic fluid (AF) is essential for maintenance of a stable uterine temperature and pressure, fetal lung development, adequate room for fetal movement and growth, cushioning to protect the fetus from trauma, and for its bacteriostatic properties which can help maintain a sterile intrauterine environment. In early pregnancy, AF arises as a transudate of the placenta. Later in pregnancy, AF production arises from the fetal lungs and fetal kidneys (Ross & Beall, 2023). Amniotic fluid is especially important to the growth and development of fetal lungs. Amniotic fluid volume (AFV) increases until about 34 weeks. The levels then remain relatively constant until term. The AFV then begins to steadily decrease after 40 weeks (Keilman & Shanks, 2022). Assessment of AFV is conducted by transabdominal ultrasound using measurements of either the maximum vertical pocket (MVP) (measuring the depth of the largest pocket of fluid) or the amniotic fluid index (AFI), dividing the uterus into four quadrants and adding the sum of the amniotic fluid pockets in each quadrant. When assessing AFV, any pocket of fluid may not contain a fetal body part or umbilical cord (Keilman & Shanks, 2022).

Oligohydramnios is defined as decreased amniotic fluid for gestational age; gestational age is a crucial factor in assessing AFV since fluid volume changes with gestational age (Keilman & Shanks, 2022). An MVP less than 2 or an AFI less than 5 are consistent with oligohydramnios; the measurement used may vary from one institution or practice to another (Keilman & Shanks, 2022).

Oligohydramnios is associated with many different conditions or complications of pregnancy including fetal, maternal, placental, and idiopathic (unknown or indeterminate cause) (**Table 33-8**) (Keilman & Shanks, 2022). Clinical signs of oligohydramnios include a fetus that is not ballotable, an easily outlined fetal body by abdominal palpation, and fundal height less than expected for gestation of pregnancy.

Once oligohydramnios is diagnosed, management includes weekly measurements of AFV and a weekly non-stress test. Fetal growth should also be followed on an ongoing basis. Depending on the gestation at diagnosis, the care of pregnant persons diagnosed with oligohydramnios can be managed by a perinatal care provider, although consultation with a perinatologist or maternal-fetal specialist is indicated due to the frequency of comorbid fetal growth disruption. Delivery at 37 weeks is usually indicated unless the cause is PPROM (Keilman & Shanks, 2022).

Polyhydramnios is an excessive amount of amniotic fluid (AFI), defined as an AFI of 25 cm or greater or MVP greater than 8 cm as observed by ultrasound (Hwang & Mahdy, 2023). Polyhydramnios is considered idiopathic in 50 to 60 percent of pregnant persons and is usually not evident until the third trimester. Idiopathic polyhydramnios is a diagnosis of exclusion after other causes or factors have been ruled out: multiple gestation, maternal hyperglycemia, decreased fetal swallowing, STIs, congenital infections, maternal or fetal anemia, alloimmunization, and fetal cardiac abnormalities (Hwang & Mahdy, 2023).

Polyhydramnios is usually suspected when uterine enlargement and fundal height are greater than expected for the weeks of gestation. Ultrasound confirmation is needed for the diagnosis of polyhydramnios. Additionally, ultrasound may be able to detect fetal or placental abnormalities contributing to the excessive amount of amniotic fluid (Hwang & Mahdy, 2023). If polyhydramnios is diagnosed, it is important to consult a perinatologist or maternal–fetal medicine specialist. Polyhydramnios can complicate fetal descent during labor and birth and may inhibit effective labor. Umbilical cord prolapse is more common in people experiencing polyhydramnios and ROM. Additionally, people with polyhydramnios are at an increased risk for postpartum hemorrhage due to the overdistention of the uterus (Boushra et al., 2023).

Peripartum Cardiomyopathy

Peripartum cardiomyopathy (PPCM) is a form of acute cardiac degeneration leading to clinical heart failure during pregnancy (usually in the late third trimester) or in the postpartum period (5 months). In some cases, PPCM can present earlier in pregnancy and up to a year postpartum (Arany, 2024; Mubarik et al., 2023). PPCM complicates approximately 1 in 2,000 births worldwide and is a significant cause of maternal mortality. In diagnosed cases of PPCM, 60 to 90 percent of cases presented after delivery (Arany, 2024). The underlying causes of PPCM are presently poorly understood but believed to be a confluence of several factors, including genetics, environmental, pre existing diseases, nutritional, immunologic, hemodynamic, and pregnancy risk factors (**Box 33-5**) (Mubarik et al., 2023; Arany, 2024).

The key to managing PPCM and reducing severe morbidity and mortality is recognition and diagnosis. PPCM is diagnosed

TABLE 33-8 Differential Diagnoses of Oligohydramnios

Fetal	Maternal	Placental
• Ruptured membranes • Genitourinary tract abnormalities • Post-term pregnancy • Fetal growth restriction • Chromosomal abnormalities • Fetal demise	• Hypertensive disorders including preeclampsia • Vascular disease • Thrombophilia • Maternal diabetes • ACE inhibitors • NSAID use • Cocaine use	• Abruption • Twin-to-twin transfusion syndrome

Data from Keilman, C. & Shanks, A. (2022, September 12). Oligohydramnios. In StatPearls. *StatPearls* Publishing. https://www.ncbi.nlm.nih.gov/books/NBK562326/

BOX 33-5 Risk Factors for Peripartum Cardiomyopathy

- Age 35 or greater
- High parity (3 or more pregnancies)
- High gravidity
- Multifetal gestations
- Tocolytic therapy
- Hypertension
- Cocaine use
- African descent (incidence is as high as 1 in 100 in some parts of Africa)

Data from Mubarik, A., Chippa, V. & Muhammad, I. (2023, August 8). Postpartum cardiomyopathy. In *StatPearls*. StatPearls Publishing. https://www.ncbi.nlm.nih.gov/books/NBK534770/; Arany, Z. (2024, January 10). Peripartum cardiomyopathy. *New England Journal of Medicine, 390*(2), 154–164. https://doi.org/ 10.1056/NEJMra2306667 in a person with a left ventricular ejection fraction (EF) of less than 45 percent in the absence of any previously diagnosed heart disease. Of note for clinicians in urgent care, emergency care, or general practice settings is that the presenting symptoms often mirror symptoms and discomforts associated with pregnancy and postpartum. Patients may present reporting symptoms associated with heart failure including fatigue, dyspnea (at rest and exacerbated with activity), orthopnea, pulmonary rales, diaphoresis, and edema. A B-type natriuretic protein (BNP) test in people with PPCM is elevated; the diagnosis is confirmed with an echocardiogram (Mubarik et al., 2023).

CONCLUSION

Complications of pregnancy, specifically HDPs, preterm birth, and GDM have long-term effects on a person's cardiometabolic health. There is a strong link between HDPs and dyslipidemia, chronic hypertension, increased risk for coronary vascular disease, heart failure, and stroke; additionally, a history of preeclampsia has been linked to an increased risk of early-onset (before age 65) risk of vascular dementia (Tong & Hastie 2024). Clinicians need to elicit a careful history of pregnancy for all people and recognize the need for specialized follow-up (e.g., cardiology) depending on the person's pregnancy history.

Effective care of a person who experiences complications during pregnancy includes taking a holistic approach, providing culturally competent, evidence-based care for the maternal–fetal dyad while providing educational and emotional support for the pregnant person and their family. Proactive risk screening can prevent some complications and allow for the prompt management of others. Clinicians who care for people who are experiencing complications during pregnancy can contribute significantly to positive outcomes by astute and accurate assessment and evaluation and making appropriate referrals to maternal–fetal specialists when complications arise.

References

Abuogi, L., Nobel, L., Smith, C. and the Committee on Pediatric and Adolescent HIV; Section on Breastfeeding. (2024). Infant feeding for persons living with and at risk for HIV in the United States: Clinical report. *Pediatrics, 153*(6), e22024066843. https://doi.org/10.1542/peds.2024-066843

American College of Obstetricians and Gynecologists. (2014, reaffirmed 2024). ACOG practice bulleting no. 142: *Cerclage for the management of cervical insufficiency.* https://www.acog.org/clinical/clinical-guidance/practice-bulletin/articles/2014/02/cerclage-for-the-management-of-cervical-insufficiency

American College of Obstetricians and Gynecologists. (2015, reaffirmed 2024). *Cytomegalovirus, Parvovirus B19, Varicella zoster, and toxoplasmosis* [Practice Bulletin no. 151]. https://www.acog.org/clinical/clinical-guidance/practice-bulletin/articles/2015/06/cytomegalovirus-parvovirus-b19-varicella-zoster-and-toxoplasmosis-in-pregnancy

American College of Obstetricians and Gynecologists. (2016a, reaffirmed 2022). *Management of preterm labor* [Practice Bulletin 171]. https://www.acog.org/clinical/clinical-guidance/practice-bulletin/articles/2016/10/management-of-preterm-labor

American College of Obstetricians and Gynecologists. (2016b, reaffirmed 2022). *Ultrasound in pregnancy* [Practice Bulletin 175]. https://www.acog.org/clinical/clinical-guidance/practice-bulletin/articles/2016/12/ultrasound-in-pregnancy

American College of Obstetricians and Gynecologists. (2018a, reaffirmed 2021). *Placenta accreta spectrum* [Obstetric Care Consensus 7]. https://www.acog.org/clinical/clinical-guidance/obstetric-care-consensus/articles/2018/12/placenta-accreta-spectrum

American College of Obstetricians and Gynecologists. (2018b, reaffirmed 2022). ACOG practice bulletin no. 193: Tubal ectopic pregnancy. *Obstetrics & Gynecology, 131*(3). https://doi.org /10.1097/AOG.0000000000003269

American College of Obstetricians and Gynecologists. (2018c, reaffirmed 2025). ACOG practice bulletin no. 200: Early pregnancy loss. *Obstetrics & Gynecology, 132,* e197–207. https://www.acog.org/clinical/clinical-guidance/practice-bulletin/articles/2018/11/early-pregnancy-loss

American College of Obstetricians and Gynecologists. (2019). *Preterm labor rupture of membranes* [Practice Bulletin no. 217]. https://www.acog.org/clinical/clinical-guidance/practice-bulletin/articles/2020/03/prelabor-rupture-of-membranes

American College of Obstetricians and Gynecologists. (2020). *Management of preterm labor.* [Practice Bulletin no. 171]. https://www.acog.org/clinical/clinical-guidance/practice-bulletin/articles/2016/10/management-of-preterm-labor

American College of Obstetricians and Gynecologists. (2023). *Updated clinical guidance for the use of progesterone supplementation for the prevention of recurrent preterm birth* [Practice Advisory]. https://www.acog.org/clinical/clinical-guidance/practice-advisory/articles/2023/04/updated-guidance-use-of-progesterone-supplementation-for-prevention-of-recurrent-preterm-birth

American College of Obstetricians and Gynecologists. (2024a, April). *Screening for syphilis in pregnancy.* [Practice Advisory]. https://www.acog.org/clinical/clinical-guidance/practice-advisory/articles/2024/04/screening-for-syphilis-in-pregnancy

American College of Obstetricians and Gynecologists. (2024b, August). *Increase in human Parvovirus B19 activity in the United States* [Practice Advisory]. https://www.acog.org/clinical/clinical-guidance/practice-advisory/articles/2024/08/increase-in-human-parvovirus-b19-activity-in-the-united-states

Arany, Z. (2024, January 10). Peripartum cardiomyopathy. *New England Journal of Medicine, 390*(2), 154–64. https://doi.org/10.1056/NEJMra2306667

Baer, R., Bandoli, G., Chambers, B., Chambers, C., Oltman, S., Rand, L., Ryckman, K., & Jelliffe-Pawlowski, L. (2019). Risk of preterm birth among women with a urinary tract infection by trimester of pregnancy [Suppl.]. *American Journal of Obstetrics & Gynecology, 220*(1), S433–S434. https://doi.org/10.1016/j.ajog.2018.11.675

Boushra, M., Stone, A., & Rathbun, K. (2023, May 8). Umbilical cord prolapse. In *StatPearls.* StatPearls Publishing. https://www.ncbi.nlm.nih.gov/books/NBK542241/#:~:text=Umbilical%20cord%20prolapse%20is%20when,not%20rapidly%20diagnosed%20and%20managed

Briggs, G. G., Freeman, R. K., Towers, C. V., & Forinash, A. B. (2021). *Briggs drugs in pregnancy and lactation: A reference guide to fetal and neonatal risk* (11th ed.). Lippincott Williams & Wilkins.

Buhimschi, C., Mesiano, S., & Muglia, L. (2023). Pathogenesis of spontaneous preterm birth. In C. Lockwood, J. Copel, L. Dugoff, J. Louis, T. Moore, R. Silver, & R. Resnik (Eds.), *Creasy & Resnik's maternal-fetal medicine* (9th ed., pp 102–126). Elsevier.

Centers for Disease Control and Prevention. (2023, December 18). *HIV and breastfeeding.* U.S. Department of Health and Human Services. https://www.cdc.gov/breastfeeding-special-circumstances/hcp/illnesses-conditions/hiv.html

Centers for Disease Control and Prevention. (2024a, February 9). *Clinical overview of perinatal Hepatitis B.* https://www.cdc.gov/hepatitis-b/hcp/perinatal-provider-overview/index.html

Centers for Disease Control and Prevention. (2024b, February 20). *About chlamydia.* U.S Department of Health and Human Services. https://www.cdc.gov/chlamydia/about/index.html

Centers for Disease Control and Prevention. (2024c, March 1). *Preventing respiratory illnesses.* U.S. Department of Health and Human Services. https://www.cdc.gov/respiratory-viruses/prevention/index.html

Centers for Disease Control and Prevention. (2024d, April 22). *Pregnancy and rubella.* U.S. Department of Health and Human Services. https://www.cdc.gov/rubella/pregnancy/index.html

Centers for Disease Control and Prevention. (2024e, April 24). *About chickenpox.* U.S. Department of Health and Human Services. https://www.cdc.gov/chickenpox/about/index.html

Centers for Disease Control and Prevention. (2024f, May 2). *Safer food choices for pregnant people.* U.S. Department of Health and Human Services. https://www.cdc.gov/food-safety/foods/pregnant-women.html

Centers for Disease Control and Prevention. (2024g, May 15). *Clinical overview of rubella.* U.S. Department of Health and Human Services. https://www.cdc.gov/rubella/hcp/clinical-overview/index.html

Centers for Disease Control and Prevention. (2024h, May 15). *Clinical testing and testing for zika virus disease.* U.S. Department of Health and Human Services. https://www.cdc.gov/zika/hcp/diagnosis-testing/index.html

Centers for Disease Control and Prevention. (2024i, May 15). *How zika spreads.* U.S. Department of Health and Human Services. https://www.cdc.gov/zika/causes/index.html

Centers for Disease Control and Prevention. (2024j, May 15). *Zika cases in the United States.* U.S. Department of Health and Human Services. https://www.cdc.gov/zika/zika-cases-us/index.html

Centers for Disease Control and Prevention. (2024k, May 30). *About cytomegalovirus (CMV) and congenital CMV infection.* U.S. Department of Health and Human Services. https://www.cdc.gov/cytomegalovirus/about/

Centers for Disease Control and Prevention. (2024l, May 31). *Congenital Zika syndrome and other birth defects.* U.S. Department of Health and Human Services. https://www.cdc.gov/zika/czs/index.html

Centers for Disease Control and Prevention. (2024m, May 31). *Zika symptoms and complications.* U.S. Department of Health and Human Services. https://www.cdc.gov/zika/signs-symptoms/index.html

Centers for Disease Control and Prevention. (2024n, August 2). *About Listeria infection.* U.S. Department of Health and Human Services. https://www.cdc.gov/listeria/about/#cdc_disease_basics_treatment-treatment

Centers for Disease Control and Prevention. (2024o, August 13). *Increase in human Parvovirus B19 activity in the United States.* U.S. Department of Health and Human Services. https://www.cdc.gov/han/2024/han00514.html

Centers for Disease Control and Prevention. (2024p, August 13). *Preventing Parvovirus B19.* U.S. Department of Health and Human Services. https://www.cdc.gov/parvovirus-b19/prevention-treatment/

Centers for Disease Control and Prevention. (2024q, September 10). *About toxoplasmosis.* U.S. Department of Health and Human Services. https://www.cdc.gov/toxoplasmosis/about/index.html

Centers for Disease Control and Prevention. (2024r, October 7). *Travel health notices.* U.S. Department of Health and Human Services. https://wwwnc.cdc.gov/travel/notices

Committee on Clinical Practice Guidelines-Obstetrics. (2023). *Viral Hepatitis in pregnancy* [Clinical Practice Guideline no. 6]. American College of Obstetricians and Gynecologists. https://www.acog.org/clinical/clinical-guidance/clinical-practice-guideline/articles/2023/09/viral-hepatitis-in-pregnancy

Chilaka, V. N., Navti, O. B., Al Beloushi, M., Ahmed, B., & Konje, J. C. (2021). Human papillomavirus (HPV) in pregnancy—An update. *European Journal of Obstetrics & Gynecology and Reproductive Biology, 264*, 340-348.

Committee on Obstetric Practice. (2014, reaffirmed 2023). *Management of pregnant women with presumptive exposure to Listeria monocytogenes* [Committee Opinion no. 614]. American College of Obstetricians and Gynecologists. https://www.acog.org/clinical/clinical-guidance/committee-opinion/articles/2014/12/management-of-pregnant-women-with-presumptive-exposure-to-listeria-monocytogenes

Committee on Obstetric Practice. (2018, reaffirmed 2024). *Nausea and vomiting of pregnancy* [Practice Bulletin no. 189]. American College of Obstetricians and Gynecologists. https://www.acog.org/clinical/clinical-guidance/practice-bulletin/articles/2018/01/nausea-and-vomiting-of-pregnancy

Committee on Obstetric Practice. (2020). *Prevention of group B streptococcal early-onset disease in newborns* [Committee Opinion no. 797]. American College of Obstetricians and Gynecologists. https://www.acog.org/clinical/clinical-guidance/committee-opinion/articles/2020/02/prevention-of-group-b-streptococcal-early-onset-disease-in-newborns

Committee on Obstetric Practice HIV Expert Work Group. (2018, reaffirmed 2024). *Labor and delivery management of women with human immunodeficiency virus infection* [Committee Opinion no. 751]. American College of Obstetricians and Gynecologists. https://www.acog.org/clinical/clinical-guidance/committee-opinion/articles/2018/09/labor-and-delivery-management-of-women-with-human-immunodeficiency-virus-infection

Committee on Obstetric Practice, Society for Maternal-Fetal Medicine. (2021, reaffirmed 2024). *Indications for outpatient antenatal fetal surveillance* [Committee Opinion no. 828]. American College of Obstetricians and Gynecologists. https://www.acog.org/clinical/clinical-guidance/committee-opinion/articles/2021/06/indications-for-outpatient-antenatal-fetal-surveillance

Committee on Practice Bulletins-Obstetrics. (2018a, reaffirmed 2024). *Gestational diabetes mellitus* [Practice Bulletin no. 190]. American College of Obstetricians and Gynecologists. https://www.acog.org/clinical/clinical-guidance/practice-bulletin/articles/2018/02/gestational-diabetes-mellitus

Committee on Practice Bulletins-Obstetrics. (2018b, reaffirmed 2024). *Management of alloimmunization during pregnancy* [Practice bulletin no. 192]. American College of Obstetricians and Gynecologists. https://www.acog.org/clinical/clinical-guidance/practice-bulletin/articles/2018/03/management-of-alloimmunization-during-pregnancy

Committee on Practice Bulletins-Obstetrics. (2019). *Chronic hypertension in pregnancy* [Practice Bulletin no. 203]. American College of Obstetricians and Gynecologists. https://www.acog.org/clinical/clinical-guidance/practice-bulletin/articles/2019/01/chronic-hypertension-in-pregnancy

Committee on Practice Bulletins-Obstetrics. (2020). *Gestational hypertension and preeclampsia* [Practice Bulletin no. 222]. American of Obstetricians and Gynecologists. https://www.acog.org/clinical/clinical-guidance/practice-bulletin/articles/2020/06/gestational-hypertension-and-preeclampsia

Fejzo, M. (2024). Hyperemesis gravidarum theories dispelled by recent research: A paradigm change for better care and outcomes. *Trends in Molecular Medicine, 30*(6), 530–540. https://doi.org/10.1016/j.molmed.2024.04.006

FoodSafety.gov. (2024). *Cook to a safe minimum internal temperature.* U.S. Department of Health and Human Services. https://www.foodsafety.gov/food-safety-charts/safe-minimum-internal-temperatures

Gestational Hypertension and Preeclampsia: ACOG Practice Bulletin, Number 222. (2020). *Obstetrics and gynecology, 135*(6), e237–e260. https://doi.org/10.1097/AOG.0000000000003891

Gilner, J., & Deshmukh, U. (2025). Evidence-based perioperative management of placenta accreta spectrum disorder. *Obstetrics and Gynecology, 145*(6), 595–610. https://doi.org/10.1097/AOG.0000000000005920

Graseck, A. S., Thompson, J. L., Bryant, A. S., Cahill, A. G., Silverman, N. S., & Turrentine, M. A. (2023). Urinary tract infections in pregnant individuals. *Obstetrics and Gynecology, 142*(2), 435–445.

Halscott, T., & Vaught, A. (2023). Diseases of the liver, biliary system, and pancreas. In C. Lockwood, J. Copel, L. Dugoff, J. Louis, T. Moore, R. Silver, & R. Resnik (Eds.), *Creasy & Resnik's maternal-fetal medicine* (9th ed., pp. 1257–1276). Elsevier.

Hammad, W. & Konje, J. (2021). Herpes simplex virus infection in pregnancy—An update. *European Journal of Obstetrics & Gynecology, 259,* 38–45. https://doi.org/10.1016/j.ejogrb.2021.01.055

Harper, L. M., Kuo, H. C., Boggess, K., Dugoff, L., Sibai, B., Lawrence, K., ... & Tita, A. T. (2025). Blood pressure control in pregnant patients with chronic hypertension and diabetes: should< 130/80 be the target? *American journal of obstetrics and gynecology, 232*(5), 482-e1.

Hauspurg, A., & Jeyabalan, A. (2023). Postpartum preeclampsia/eclampsia: Defining its place and management among the hypertensive disorders of pregnancy. *American Journal of Obstetrics & Gynecology, 226*(2S), S1211–S1221. https://doi.org/10.1016/j.ajog.2020.10.027

HIVinfo@NIH.gov. (2024). *Preventing perinatal transmission of HIV.* https://hivinfo.nih.gov/understanding-hiv/fact-sheets/preventing-perinatal-transmission-hiv

Hull, A., Resnik, R., & Silver, R. (2023). Placenta previa and accreta, vasa previa, subchorionic hemorrhage, and abruptio placentae. In C. Lockwood, J. Copel, L. Dugoff, J. Louis, T. Moore, R. Silver, & R. Resnik (Eds.), *Creasy & Resnik's maternal-fetal medicine* (9th ed., pp. 799–809). Elsevier.

Hwang, D., & Mahdy, H. (2023, February 20). Polyhydramnios. In *StatPearls.* StatPearls Publishing. https://www.ncbi.nlm.nih.gov/books/NBK562140/

International Association of Diabetes and Pregnancy Study Groups Consensus Panel. (2010). International Association of Diabetes and Pregnancy Study Groups recommendations on the diagnosis and classification of hyperglycemia in pregnancy. *Diabetes Care, 33*(3), 676–682. https://doi.org/10.2337/dc09-1848

Jaan, A., & Rajnik, M. (2023, July 17). TORCH complex. In *StatPearls.* StatPearls Publishing. https://www.ncbi.nlm.nih.gov/books/NBK560528/#:~:text=The%20term%20TORCH%20complex%20or,virus%20(HSV)%2C%20respectively.

Jauniaux, E., Ayres-de-Campos, D., Langhoff-Roos, J., Fox, K., Collins, S., & FIGO Placenta Accreta Diagnosis and Management Expert Consensus Panel. (2019). FIGO classification for the clinical diagnosis of placenta accreta spectrum disorders. *International Journal of Gynaecology and Obstetrics, 146*(1), 20–24. https://doi.org/10.1002/ijgo.12761

Keilman, C., & Shanks, A. (2022, September 12). Oligohydramnios. In *StatPearls.* StatPearls Publishing. https://www.ncbi.nlm.nih.gov/books/NBK562326/

Luger, R., & Kight, B. (2022, October 3). Hypertension in pregnancy. In *StatPearls.* StatPearls Publishing. https://www.ncbi.nlm.nih.gov/books/NBK430839/

March of Dimes. (2024). *2023 March of Dimes report card.* https://www.marchofdimes.org/peristats/assets/s3/reports/archives/March-of-Dimes-2024-Full-Report-Card.pdf

Megli, C., & Beigi, R. (2023). Maternal-fetal infections. In C. Lockwood, J. Copel, L. Dugoff, J. Louis, T. Moore, R. Silver, & R. Resnik (Eds.), *Creasy & Resnik's maternal-fetal medicine* (9th ed., pp. 959–972). Elsevier.

Mor, G., & Abrahams, V. (2023). Immunology of pregnancy. In C. Lockwood, J. Copel, L. Dugoff, J. Louis, T. Moore, R. Silver, & R. Resnik (Eds.), *Creasy & Resnik's maternal-fetal medicine* (9th ed., pp. 127–142). Elsevier.

Mubarik, A., Chippa, V., & Muhammad, I. (2023, August 8). Postpartum cardiomyopathy. In *StatPearls.* StatPearls Publishing. https://www.ncbi.nlm.nih.gov/books/NBK534770/

National Institutes of Child Health and Human Development. (2023, May 9). *What are risk factors for preterm labor and birth?* U.S. Department of Health and Human Services. https://www.nichd.nih.gov/health/topics/preterm/conditioninfo/who_risk

National Library of Medicine. (2023). Congenital rubella. *MedlinePlus.* U.S. Department of Health and Human Services, National Institutes of Health. https://medlineplus.gov/ency/article/001658.htm

Neilsen-Saines, K., & Cambou, M. (2023). Maternal and fetal viral infections. In C. Lockwood, J. Copel, L. Dugoff, J. Louis, T. Moore, R. Silver, & R. Resnik (Eds.), *Creasy & Resnik's maternal-fetal medicine* (9th ed., pp. 908–937). Elsevier.

Owens, D. K., Davidson, K. W., Krist, A. H., Barry, M. J., Cabana, M., Caughey, A. B., . . . & U.S. Preventive Services Task Force. (2020). Screening for bacterial vaginosis in pregnant persons to prevent preterm delivery: U.S. Preventive Services Task Force recommendation statement. *Journal of American Medical Association, 323*(13), 1286–1292.

Pillarisetty, L., & Sharma, A. (2023, June 4). Pregnancy intrahepatic cholestasis. In *StatPearls.* StatPearls Publishing. https://www.ncbi.nlm.nih.gov/books/NBK551503/

Phillippi, J., & Kantrowitz-Gordon, I. (2024). Varney's midwifery 7th ed. Jones & Bartlett Learning.

Pippin, J., & Gibson, K. (2023). Respiratory diseases in pregnancy. In C. Lockwood, J. Copel, L. Dugoff, J. Louis, T. Moore, R. Silver, & R. Resnik (Eds.), *Creasy & Resnik's maternal-fetal medicine* (9th ed., pp.1106–1131). Elsevier.

Puopolo, K. M., Lynfield, R., Cummings, J. J., AAP Committee on Fetus and Newborn, & AAP Committee on Infectious Diseases. (2019). *Management of infants at risk for group B streptococcal disease* [Clinical Report]. American Academy of Pediatrics. https://doi.org/10.1542/peds.2019-1881

Ross, M., & Beall, M. (2023) Amniotic fluid dynamics. In C. Lockwood, J. Copel, L. Dugoff, J. Louis, T. Moore, R. Silver, & R. Resnik (Eds.), *Creasy & Resnik's maternal-fetal medicine* (9th ed., pp. 66–71). Elsevier.

Soper, J. T. (2021). Gestational trophoblastic disease: Current evaluation and management. *Obstetrics & Gynecology, 137*(2), 355–370.

Tong, S., & Hastie, R. (2024). Preeclampsia and the risk of young-onset dementia. *JAMA Network Open, 7*(5), e2412780. https://doi.org/10.1001/jamanetworkopen.2024.12780

United States Preventative Services Task Force. (2021). *Gestational diabetes: Screening.* https://www.uspreventiveservicestaskforce.org/uspstf/recommendation/gestational-diabetes-screening

Workowski, K. A., Bachmann, L. H., Chan, P. A., Johnston, C. M., Muzny, C. A.,Park, I., Reno, H., Zenilman, J. M., & Bolan, G. A. (2021). Sexually Transmitted Infections Treatment Guidelines, 2021. *Morbidity and Mortality Weekly Recommendations and Reports, 70*(RR-4), 1–187. http://dx.doi.org/10.15585/mmwr.rr7004a1

World Health Organization. (2022, December 8). *Zika virus.* https://www.who.int/news-room/fact-sheets/detail/zika-virus

Wylie, B. (2023). Bacterial and parasitic infections in pregnancy. In C. Lockwood, J. Copel, L. Dugoff, J. Louis, T. Moore, R. Silver, & R. Resnik (Eds.), *Creasy & Resnik's maternal-fetal medicine* (9th ed., pp. 879–907). Elsevier.

CHAPTER 34

Overview of Postpartum Care

Deborah Brandt Karsnitz
Tia Andrighetti
Linda McDaniel
Elizabeth G. Munoz

The editors acknowledge Kelly Wilhite, who was an author on the previous version of this chapter.

The period following the birth of a newborn is known as the postpartum period or puerperium. Traditionally, the puerperium begins after the birth of the placenta and continues throughout 6 to 8 weeks postpartum. Designation of this particular time frame is attributed to the average time necessary for physiologic return to a nonpregnant state. However, postpartum restoration, both physical and emotional, is influenced by a variety of factors prompting individual differences within this time frame.

This chapter provides an overview of the normal physiologic and psychologic changes that occur as the body returns to a nonpregnant state. Selected postpartum complications are also discussed. To obtain an in-depth understanding of these topics, resources are provided at the end of this chapter.

POSTPARTUM PHYSIOLOGY

Many physiologic changes occur during the postpartum period as organ systems, structures, and hormonal balances return to their nonpregnant state. The puerperium begins immediately following the delivery of the placenta. Placental separation results in immediate physiologic events that promote hemostasis and initiate restoration to a nonpregnant state.

Hemostasis

Uterine contractions facilitate a shortening of myometrial fibers, which reduces uterine size and facilitates uterine compression to decrease bleeding. Increased blood volume, which was important during pregnancy, is no longer necessary. While some blood loss occurs during birth, 10 to 15 percent of blood volume is autotransfused. In addition, extracellular fluid is mobilized and returned to circulation. Coagulation changes initially increase dramatically then remain increased for 1 to 2 weeks postpartum. Total blood volume returns to a nonpregnant state by 1 week postpartum. However, increased venous diameter and decreased blood flow may take as long as 6 weeks to return. For this reason, postpartum patients have an elevated risk for thromboembolic events during the puerperium. Postpartum individuals' heart rates remain increased for approximately 1 hour after birth before returning to a nonpregnant rate, while blood pressure can remain slightly elevated for up to 4 days. Cardiac output is elevated after childbirth and remains somewhat elevated for approximately 1 week postpartum.

Uterus

Involution describes the process of the uterus returning to a nonpregnant state (approximately 100 gm or less). Involution of the uterus occurs through contraction of uterine smooth muscles, autolysis of excess tissue, regeneration of endometrial tissue (resulting in the shedding of decidual tissue), and regeneration of the placental site, leaving no scar behind. In most cases, the uterus becomes a pelvic organ by 10 to 14 days postpartum and is no longer palpable abdominally. The rate of uterine descent is typically 1 cm per day. The process for uterine restoration is usually completed by 6 weeks postpartum (refer to **Figure 34-1**).

Lochia

Lochia, the term used to denote vaginal discharge after birth, indicates the phases of restoration of the uterus and can vary in duration from 4 to 8 weeks. Because the amount of bleeding differs among individuals, it is important to note that a continuous decrease in lochia amount over time is an important consideration and stages of lochia do not always occur during specific time frames. Postpartum patients may experience a transient increase in lochia discharge (7 to 14 days), referred to as the release of the eschar or sloughing of the placental site. This should be short-lived and only last a few hours and then lochia should return to the pattern present prior to release of the eschar. **Table 34-1** identifies the postpartum stages of lochia.

Cervix

Following childbirth, the cervix is often soft, edematous, and sometimes bruised. Within several days, however, it begins to return to an altered nonpregnant state. By 1 week postpartum, the cervix is further restored, with the external os being approximately 1 cm dilated. The cervical os no longer resembles the nulliparous os (dimple) and now has the appearance of a slit.

Vagina

Following the birth of a newborn, the vagina can be bruised, edematous, and sometimes lacerated. The vaginal mucosa is

FIGURE 34-1 **Postpartum involution of the uterus.**

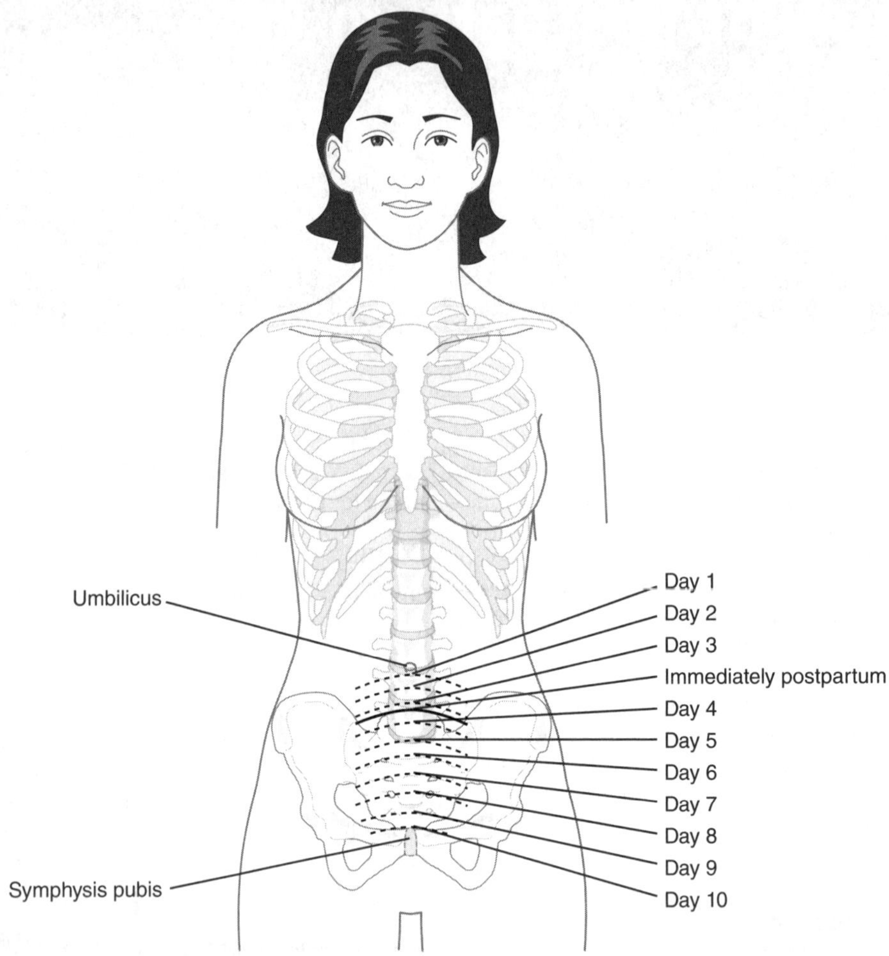

TABLE 34-1 **Ranges of Normal Postpartum Lochia**

Lochia Stage	Postpartum Days/Weeks	Lochia Color
Rubra	Days 2 to 7	Dark red
Serosa	Days 7 to 22	Lighter red
Alba	Days 14 to 42	White to yellow–white

Data from Azulay Chertok, I. R., & Wolf, J. H. (2019). Postpartum period and lactation physiology. In S. T. Blackburn (Ed.), *Maternal, fetal, and neonatal physiology: A clinical perspective* (5th ed., pp. 142–162). Saunders Elsevier.

smooth, rugae are absent, and tone is decreased. Within 3 to 4 weeks postpartum, the rugae are restored, although tone may remain decreased, improving over time but perhaps not to the same prepregnant tone.

Endocrine System

Expulsion of the placenta signals dramatic hormonal changes as blood levels of estrogen, progesterone, human placental lactogen, and human chorionic gonadotropin all decrease. These immediate changes initiate other systematic changes, including lactogenesis (process to begin developing the ability to produce milk) (King, 2023). Estrogen returns to its nonpregnant level within 1 to 2 weeks, and progesterone levels return to the nonpregnant state within 48 hours.

Pituitary

Follicle stimulating hormone (FSH) and luteinizing hormone (LH) levels remain low for 2 weeks postpartum, with a gradual rise to nonpregnant levels. Lactation, however, can interfere with the return of LH and FSH to nonpregnant levels. Subsequently, ovulation and return of menses vary in relation to frequency and duration of chest/breast feeding. Resumption of ovulation in individuals who are not breast/chestfeeding usually occurs at some point between 45 and 94 days postpartum. Although few individuals regain fertility by 2 weeks postpartum, contraception counseling should include postpartum hormonal influences, whether a patient is solely chest/breast feeding and how often, and other influential factors related to return of ovulation and fertility.

Renal System

Postpartum return of bladder tone and reduced dilation of the renal tract occur over a 6- to 8-week time frame or longer. Bladder displacement or trauma during labor and childbirth can predispose an individual to urinary tract infections.

Gastrointestinal System

Decrease in progesterone aids in the restoration of muscle tone, relieving reflux and constipation within 2 to 3 days postpartum. However, perineal trauma from childbirth, lack of fluids, or lack of mobility can result in continued constipation.

POSTPARTUM CARE

The postpartum period signifies the end of a pregnancy and the beginning of a new journey. Despite significant physiologic and emotional transitions, following discharge from a hospital the postpartum patient is typically not evaluated until 6 weeks postpartum. Yet, during the 6 weeks prior to the first postpartum visit, there is physical restoration, role attainment, and formation of new relationships. Postpartum individuals in the United States are rarely given more than 6 weeks of parental leave, and many do not receive pay during this time. Most individuals are expected to resume regular activity within a few weeks. Except for selected complications, postpartum research in the United States is limited.

The postpartum period is rich with cultural influences, beliefs, and traditions that impact restoration, recovery, role transitions, and family dynamics. A patient's cultural practices should be included in all aspects of health care and should guide assessment, management, and education. Expectations of recovery can differ and should be assessed prior to educating individuals and their families. Many traditions during the postpartum period influence diet and rest, as well as lactation and newborn care. Traditions are often intended to protect the postpartum individual from current and long-term illness. Family and/or female support is a central tenet in many cultural practices. As the new postpartum individual's needs are met, they are able to focus solely on the newborn.

POSTPARTUM ASSESSMENT

Because the early postpartum period is exemplified by abrupt and dramatic changes, postpartum patients must be reassured and educated regarding usual occurrences and their variances. Many factors can influence the duration of these changes, which vary depending on length of labor, type of birth, parity, and other circumstances. After individual needs are met and reassurance is provided, individuals can begin to fully focus on infant care, role adaptations, and eventual return to daily activity.

Adaptation

The process of adapting to a parenting role, whether or not it is the first time, differs for everyone. Although some individuals immediately take on this new role, others find a gradual transition more acceptable. Clinicians can help facilitate patients' transitions by listening to the birth story, filling in gaps when possible, and helping the family acclimate to a new situation (Mercer, 1985). Many births are different than imagined. Subsequently, the 'taking in' phase after childbirth helps the individual process the birth (Rubin, 1961), thereby allowing the person to gain an overall understanding of the birth experience. Eventually, the postpartum patient will move toward taking hold and begin self-recovery, care of the newborn, and attention to family (Rubin, 1961). Many family configurations are possible—single parent, biological parents, nonbiological parents, extended family, and more. For this reason, knowledge of family structure can facilitate meeting individual needs during the transition period.

Bonding, described by Klaus and Kennell (1976) as the early attachment formed during the first encounter between the postpartum person and infant, plays a significant role in the long-term emotional bond between them. Nevertheless, studies indicate bonding continues to develop over time and can include other family members (Amiel Castro et al., 2024).

Impaired bonding or an insecure attachment can have significant negative developmental consequences for the developing infant. Many factors can influence bonding. Patient bonding can be influenced by type of birth, medical problems, a lack of support, mental health conditions, or emotional factors (de Waal et al., 2024; Doyle et al., 2023). Parental anxiety can impair both antepartum and postpartum bonding (Macdonald et al., 2022). Additionally, infant temperament, medical conditions, or separation from parent(s) can delay infant bonding (de Waal et al., 2024; Doyle et al., 2023). Difficult births, long labors, cesarean birth, birth trauma, or postpartum pain have been noted to delay bonding and subsequent care of the infant (Altuntuğ et al., 2023; Dekel et al., 2019). In addition, infant cues, such as crying, arm waving, and facial expressions, impact the extent of bonding (Butti et al., 2018).

Immediately after birth, the release of oxytocin facilitates a peaceful, loving feeling that can influence the patient's reaction (Shorey et al., 2022; Walter et al., 2021). chest/breast feeding and various newborn sounds and behaviors also enable oxytocin release (Walter et al., 2021). Oxytocin can increase euphoria, decrease stress, and facilitate attachment (Shorey et al., 2022; Walter et al., 2021).

Skin-to-Skin Contact (Kangaroo Care)

When possible, skin-to-skin contact (SSC) between the infant and parent or caregiver should be encouraged and facilitated postpartum. The World Health Organization (WHO) recommends immediate and uninterrupted SSC following birth (UNICEF & World Health Organization [WHO], n.d.). SSC has been shown to induce a physiologic response in the newborn and is known to promote stabilization of infant breathing, heart rate, skin temperature, and blood glucose; it also influences the duration and frequency of chest/breast feeding (Lord et al., 2023). Furthermore, newborns are reported to cry less and have increased quiet sleep (Lord et al., 2023). The percentage of healthcare facilities promoting SSC continues to increase in the United States. In 2022 it was reported that 70 percent of newborns receive SSC after vaginal birth; however, this number is down from previous years (Centers for Disease Control and Prevention [CDC], 2022).

Family

A newborn may live with a variety of people who will raise and nurture them. Finding out who is involved in the pregnancy, birth, and childrearing will help the healthcare provider be inclusive of all families. Asking about how the family is adjusting and encouraging patience and grace between members will allow the whole family to adjust during the early postpartum period. Sibling adjustment to a newborn can be influenced by many factors, including family dynamics, culture, personality, gender, or interest. Age is not the significant factor it was once reported to be, nor do first siblings experience behavior regressions or long adjustment periods (Volling, 2012). Familiar lifestyle is altered, however, and there can be periods of behavioral exhibitions, such as mimicry of infant behaviors, toileting accidents, or even moments of aggression (Volling, 2012).

Helpful strategies involve family inclusion during prenatal visits, sibling involvement during infant care, alone time with siblings, and encouragement of other family members to include siblings while visiting.

POSTPARTUM EXAMINATIONS

Early postpartum assessment focuses on physiologic changes associated with return to the nonpregnant state. Some changes occur immediately after childbirth (first few days to 1 week), whereas others emerge over a longer period of time. Subjective assessment of the postpartum patient includes general overall feelings, orientation, comfort, sleep, nutrition, and emotions. Objective assessment includes examination of the patient's general appearance, vital signs, neurologic system, heart and lungs, breasts, gastrointestinal system, urinary system, perineal area, anal area, and lower extremities, as well as laboratory analysis if indicated.

The initial postpartum examination should include a review of systems and teaching components of early postpartum considerations, what to expect, duration of these changes, and when to call a clinician. Postpartum teaching should begin during prenatal care and continues throughout the puerperium. Postpartum teaching can also occur at various times, such as with a systems review or during an examination. In addition, all postpartum patients should receive a teaching booklet with clearly printed warning signs (when to call the clinician). **Table 34-2** illustrates common concerns in the early postpartum period.

Later postpartum examinations have similar components, but teaching will be different. Timing of postpartum exams really varies from practice to practice. ACOG recommends an early visit before 3 weeks postpartum and a later visit before 12 weeks postpartum (ACOG, 2025a). Most postpartum complications or concerns occur prior to 6 weeks and delayed assessment can prevent early identification and treatment, thereby increasing the risk of severe illness. Additionally, chest/breast feeding assessment and support can increase the duration of chest/breast feeding. **Table 34-3** highlights components of the early and later examinations.

Activity

Postpartum individuals should ambulate soon after birth, even if it is simply to get out of bed to void. In fact, encouragement of increased fluid intake and the need to keep the bladder empty can facilitate early ambulation. Fatigue is common, individualized, and can be increased after a long labor. The sooner activity increases, the sooner energy and strength will return and opportunities for thromboembolism will decrease. Patients recovering from a cesarean birth are encouraged to ambulate and can adjust activity as needed based on medical and surgical situation (American College of Obstetricians and Gynecologists [ACOG], 2020).

Clinicians should encourage postpartum exercise in a modified form soon after a vaginal birth. Walking is a great exercise that can improve mood and increase oxygen consumption and circulation. Patients can gauge uterine healing by lochia flow and adapt exercise or return to activity as needed. Too much activity can increase bleeding, but with rest, this aspect of healing should quickly return to normal.

Abdominal exercises will aid the restoration of abdominal muscle tone and can begin soon after a vaginal birth. Postpartum patients are encouraged to begin slowly and increase exercising abdominal muscles according to their comfort level and healing. Initial abdominal exercise involves lying flat with knees bent while raising the head slowly. As healing progresses, repetitions can increase and abdominal crunches can be added (ACOG, 2020).

Pelvic floor muscle exercises, also known as Kegel exercises, should begin during pregnancy and continue after a vaginal birth. This particular exercise not only strengthens and tightens vaginal tone but also increases urinary tone and circulation to the perineal area, thereby promoting healing (Anastasya Siregar, et al., 2024). Refer to Chapter 23 for more information on Kegel exercises.

Exercise capability differs among individuals and can depend on the prior level of proficiency. However, all healthy patients should be encouraged to exercise during pregnancy and resume their routine shortly after giving birth. It is important to teach warning signs related to exercise and to encourage patients to report increased bleeding, change in color of lochia, pain, shortness of breath, leg pain, or dizziness that persists. If they are breast/chestfeeding, patients may choose to feed prior to exercise for comfort. In addition, keeping hydrated is important (ACOG, 2020).

Sexuality

Traditionally, patients were told to not resume penetrative intercourse until after the 6-week postpartum examination. However, there is no evidence to support this instruction, which is most likely based on uterine healing. Many couples resume sexual intercourse by 1 month, and most by 2 months, with about 20 percent not having resumed intercourse by 3 months postpartum (Graziottin et al., 2024). Resuming intimacy is a personal choice and is associated with circumstances related to birth, recovery, emotional readiness (both partners), and physiologic comfort. Additionally, numerous factors can interfere with or delay the resumption of intercourse, such as fatigue, vaginal bleeding, perineal discomfort, decreased lubrication, diminished desire, leaking breasts, body image, and fear of subsequent pregnancy. Furthermore, resumption of intimacy may also be perceived as being in discordance with partner's desire (Graziottin, et al., 2024). Clinicians can help alleviate anxiety by discussing comfort measures, birth control, and other forms of intimacy. Postpartum individuals should be supported in their choice and encouraged to resume intercourse when they are ready, and they should recognize that time frames will vary.

TABLE 34-2 **Common Early Postpartum Concerns**

Condition	Etiology	Duration	Management	Notes
Afterbirth pains	Uterine contractions during involution	Immediate to several days	Empty bladder Prone position chest/breast feeding Analgesics	Pain increased if second or more births, and overdistended uterus (multiple gestation) Prone position keeps uterus contracted which decreases cramping chest/breast feeding may initially increase cramps Nonsteroidal anti-inflammatory drugs (NSAIDs) are particularly effective
Diuresis/ diaphoresis	Physiologic elimination of excess retained water through voiding and perspiration	Usually days 2 to 5, but may begin as early as 12 hours and last up to 21 days	Keep bladder empty Reassurance Comfort measures	Approximately 3,000 cc/day Frequent showers Wear natural fibers Dress in layers Drink to thirst
Constipation	Slowed motility during labor and birth Decreased intake during labor Elimination during birth	Up to 1 week	Encourage mobility Increase fluids Increase high-fiber foods Mild laxatives/stool softeners	Fear can play a role if the patient experienced a laceration or episiotomy; provider reassurance is helpful Take as directed
Hemorrhoids	Venous distention, common during pregnancy and may be exacerbated during childbirth	Most painful 24 to 48 hours postpartum but often remain present at varying degrees	Tucks or witch hazel compresses Ice packs Ointments (Preparation H) Anesthetic sprays Warm sitz baths Stool softeners/suppositories	Prevention by increasing fluids, fiber, mobility
Perineal discomfort	Secondary to laceration or episiotomy	Usually, 1 to 3 weeks	Decrease edema Ice packs initially (24 hours) Topical anesthetics Warm sitz baths Kegel exercises Witch hazel compresses Analgesics	Varies according to degree of laceration/episiotomy or if sutures were required Improve circulation
Breast engorgement	Increased vascularity and congestion as milk supply increases	Usually occurs 2 to 3 days after childbirth and lasts 24 to 48 hours	Lactating patients: Early initiation of breast/chestfeeding Frequent feeding Warmth/heat NSAIDs Nonlactating patients: Support/supportive bra Ice packs NSAIDs Application of cold cabbage leaves to breasts	Lactating: Encourage immediate breast/chestfeeding Avoid supplementation or pumping if possible Avoid expressing excessive milk Consider therapeutic breast massage Nonlactating: Encourage no stimulation of breast until milk reabsorbed

Data from Andrighetti, T. P., & Butler, J. M. (2024). Components of postnatal care. In K. T. Grace, C. L. Farley, N. K. Jeffers, & T Tringali (Eds.), *Prenatal and postnatal care: A woman-centered approach* (3rd ed., pp. 450–469). Wiley-Blackwell; Howe-Hayman, A. (2023). Postpartum care. In J. Phillippi & I. Kantorwitz-Gordon (Eds.), *Varney's midwifery* (7th ed., pp. 2258–2332). Jones & Bartlett Learning; King, T. L. (2023). Anatomy and physiology of postpartum. In J. Phillippi & I Kantorwitz-Gordon (Eds.), *Varney's midwifery* (7th ed., pp. 2230–2257). Jones & Bartlett Learning; Witt, A. M., Bolman, M., Kredit, S., & Vanic, A. (2016). Therapeutic breast massage in lactation for the management of engorgement, plugged ducts, and mastitis. *Journal of Human Lactation, 32*(1), 123–131. https://doi.org/10.1177/0890334415619439

TABLE 34-3 Postpartum Assessment

Initial Postpartum Examination	Subjective	Objective	Unusual Findings	Teaching
General	Well-being, emotions Ambulation Nutrition/fluids Rest Comfort Infant feeding Review birth story	Appearance Weight	Discomfort, pain Sadness Unable to ambulate No appetite Unable to rest	Ambulate often Drink when thirsty Sleep when infant sleeps Analgesics Infant feeding Formula: 2–3 hours Discuss birth experience
Vital signs	Breathing Shortness of breath	BP, temperature, pulse, respirations	BP > 140/90 mm Hg BP < 85/60 mm Hg Temperature > 38°C (100.4° F) Pulse >100 bpm	Signs and symptoms of infection
Neurologic	Orientation to time and place	Alert, oriented	Excessive drowsiness Headaches	Headache Analgesic effects Report blurred, double vision, spots before eyes
Cardiovascular	Chest pain or increased heart rate	Regular rate and rhythm	Noted chest pain Irregular rate and rhythm/tachycardia	Report shortness of breath, chest pain
Pulmonary	Breathing	Lungs clear	Shortness of breath	Report shortness of breath
Breasts	Pain, tenderness Milk production/colostrum Breast/chestfeeding frequency and duration Nipple tenderness	Soft: days 1–2 Fullness: days 3–4 Nipples: intact, erect	Engorgement Nipples: cracked, bleeding Nipples: inverted/flat	Frequent breast/chestfeeding Proper latch Binder or support if not breast/chestfeeding Analgesia
Genitourinary	Voiding amounts Frequency Pain or inability to void	Bladder nondistended No CVAT	Pain with urination Frequency with inability to void Positive CVAT Bladder distention	Increased voiding noted for 3–5 days postpartum Inability to void can be due to perineal edema Increase fluids
Gastrointestinal	Abdominal pain or tenderness Bowel movement	Abdomen nontender Bowel sounds present	Abdominal tenderness Lack of bowel sounds Constipation/lack of flatulence Nausea or vomiting	Stool softeners Ambulation Increase fiber Increase fluids
Uterus	Cramping, pain Bleeding amount/color	Size: involution as expected Firm without tenderness Lochia	Size greater than expected Soft, boggy Lochia: amount increased, clots Malodorous	Decreased activity Keep bladder empty Lie prone Heat pad Normal lochia progression
Perineum	Pain or tenderness	Intact	Erythema, edema	Ice or warm soaks, witch hazel Analgesics

Initial Postpartum Examination	Subjective	Objective	Unusual Findings	Teaching
Lower extremities	Able to ambulate Muscle soreness	Reflexes Some edema	Pain, erythema, or edema noted: generalized or local	Ambulate
Anus	Pain or tenderness, bleeding with bowel movement	Hemorrhoids	Hemorrhoids noted, edematous, bruised or bleeding	Hemorrhoid cream, tucks Stool softeners

First Few Weeks Exam and Later Examination	Subjective	Objective	Unusual Findings	Teaching
General	Well-being Mood: EPDS Activity Nutrition/fluids Rest Family adaptation Infant feeding Lochia Voiding/stooling Sexuality	Appearance EPDS score < 10	Signs and symptoms of postpartum depression or anxiety EPDS score ≥ 10 Decreased activity Decreased appetite Unable to rest chest/breast feeding concerns Increased bleeding Constipation	Discuss postpartum depression, anxiety Sleep when infant sleeps Family roles Infant feeding Review normal lochia progression Sexuality/ contraception
Vital signs	Breathing	Weight BP, temperature, pulse, respirations	BP $>$ 140/90 mm Hg BP $<$ 85/60 mm Hg Temperature $>$ 38°C (100.4° F) Pulse $>$ 100 bpm	Signs and symptoms of infection
Neurologic	Orientation to time and place	Alert, oriented	Headaches	Review tension headaches, analgesics Review warning signs of spots before the eyes and blurred vision
Cardiovascular	Palpitations	Regular rate and rhythm	Irregular rate and rhythm/ tachycardia	Report shortness of breath, or chest pain
Pulmonary	Breathing	Lungs clear	Shortness of breath	Report shortness of breath
Breasts	Lactation Nipple tenderness Breast infection	Soft (depending on last breastfeed) Nipples: intact, erect	Nipples: cracked, redness, bleeding Nipple *Candida* Mastitis Any lasting breast lump	Review chest/breast feeding schedule, signs and symptoms of mastitis or nipple *Candida*, pumping, and return to work Report any lasting breast lump
Abdomen/ gastrointestinal	Pain or tenderness Nausea or vomiting Bowel movement	Soft Diastasis recti Bowel sounds	Herniation Abdominal tenderness No bowel sounds Constipation	Abdominal exercises Stool softeners Fiber Fluids
Genitourinary	Voiding amounts/ frequency	Bladder nondistended No CVAT	Pain with urination Frequency with inability to void Positive CVAT Bladder distention	Signs and symptoms of urinary tract infection
Uterus	Lochia cessation Occurrence of menses since birth	Uterus not palpated abdominally	Palpation of uterus larger than expected for weeks postpartum Lochia still present	Activity level Contraception

(*continues*)

TABLE 34-3 Postpartum Assessment (*continued*)

Initial Postpartum Examination	Subjective	Objective	Unusual Findings	Teaching
Perineum	No pain or tenderness at laceration/ episiotomy site	Intact	Erythema, edema	
Vagina (6 weeks)	No discharge	Pink Consider assessing for vaginal tone		Kegel exercises as needed
Cervix		Pink, firm		
Sexuality	Resumption of sexual intercourse			Sexuality Resumption of fertility and family planning
Lower extremities	Pain, tenderness, edema	No edema or redness	Pain, erythema, or edema noted: generalized or local	Ambulate Signs and symptoms of thrombophlebitis
Anus	Pain or tenderness, bleeding with bowel movement	Hemorrhoids	Hemorrhoids noted; edematous, bruised or bleeding	Hemorrhoid cream, tucks Stool softeners Fiber Fluids

Data from Andrighetti, T. P., & Butler, J. M. (2024). Components of postnatal care. In K. T. Grace, C. L. Farley, N. K. Jeffers, & T. Tringali (Eds.), *Prenatal and postnatal care: A woman-centered approach* (3rd ed., pp. 450–469). Wiley-Blackwell. Permission conveyed through Copyright Clearance Center, Inc.; Wambach, K., & Spencer, B. (Eds.). (2021). *Breastfeeding and human lactation* (6th ed.). Jones & Bartlett Learning.

Abbreviations: BP, blood pressure; CVAT, costovertebral angle tenderness; EPDS, Edinburgh Postnatal Depression Scale.

Contraception

Contraceptive choices for postpartum patients require careful consideration and should be discussed at various times throughout pregnancy and postpartum. Contraceptive counseling should be offered to all pregnant-capable patients who do not desire conception during the postpartum period, including clients who are gender diverse. It is important to counsel transgender, gender diverse, and nonbinary patients that taking testosterone alone may not prevent pregnancy (Curtis et al., 2024). Discussion of different contraceptive options will give patients the opportunity to consider which choices best fit their lifestyles and circumstances. Nonhormonal methods, such as abstinence, withdrawal, condoms, or other barrier methods, can be used earlier in the postpartum period in patients who are breast/chestfeeding and in those who are not. Combined oral contraceptives and other combined methods are contraindicated until 21 days postpartum due to increased risk of venous thromboembolism (VTE) (Cason et al., 2023; Nguyen et al., 2024). Patients with risk factors for VTE should be further evaluated if they wish to use hormonal contraceptives. Intrauterine devices can be inserted immediately postpartum (within 10 minutes of birth of placenta) or after 4 weeks postpartum. Contraceptive options (type, efficacy, ease of use, lifestyle needs) will vary according to numerous factors.

Patients who are breast/chestfeeding frequently, without supplementation and without occurrence of menses after childbirth, experience a natural form of contraception known as lactation amenorrhea. With ideal use, the lactation amenorrhea method can be up to 98 percent effective for the first 6 months postpartum (Cason et al., 2023). Refer toChapter 13 for further information on ideal use requirements and methods.

Hormonal contraception while breast/chestfeeding remains controversial. The WHO (Nguyen et al., 2024) recommends that patients who choose to breastfeed/chestfeed do not use hormonal methods containing estrogen during the first 6 weeks (contraindicated) and up to 6 months (relative contraindication) postpartum. Other sources disagree, suggesting that although there is some risk, not enough research has been conducted to support strong restrictions. The Centers for Disease Control and Prevention (2016) recommends restriction of hormonal methods only during the first 3 weeks postpartum. Although past recommendations suggested initiation of progestin-only contraceptives after 4 to 6 weeks postpartum, there have been no reports to indicate adverse effects on lactation or newborn health. The Centers for Disease Control and Prevention (2016) supports initiation of such contraception during the first month postpartum because the benefits outweigh the risks.

Breast/Chestfeeding

For some patients, the method used to feed their infant can be a difficult decision. Consideration about the method of feeding should begin early during the prenatal period, with discussion continuing until the birth of the newborn and in the early postpartum period as needed. Evidence continues to showcase the benefits of breast/chestfeeding for both the birthing person and newborn. The U.S. Department of Health and Human Services has promoted breast/chestfeeding as a goal in the Healthy People initiative to improve health care. The Healthy People goals for 2030 include increased chest/breast feeding initiation and duration (HealthyPeople.gov, 2024). Furthermore, the American Academy of Pediatrics (AAP) supports breast/chestfeeding as the newborn feeding method of choice and recommends exclusive breast/chestfeeding for at least 6 months (2012). The AAP further recommends continued breast/chestfeeding with introduction of other foods for up to 1 year or more.

Breast/chestfeeding initiation rates have continuously improved from 73.9 percent in 2009 to 83.2 percent in 2019 (CDC, 2022). In addition, breast/chestfeeding continuation at 6 months has increased from 46 percent in 2009 to 55.8 percent, and chest/breast feeding at 1 year increased from 25 percent in 2009 to 35.9 percent in 2019 (CDC, 2022). The WHO and AAP recommend skin-to-skin contact immediately following birth for at least 1 hour to facilitate initiation of chest/breast feeding (Feldman-Winter & Goldsmith, 2016; Meek & Noble, 2022; UNICEF & WHO, n.d.).

The breast prepares for lactation throughout pregnancy, completing the task when the newborn begins to suckle. Hormones influence breast growth and development early in pregnancy (lactogenesis I), and patients can begin secreting colostrum between 12 and 16 hours after childbirth. Lactogenesis II (milk production) begins following delivery of the placenta, with subsequent decreases in progesterone and increases in prolactin being observed. Patients usually experience fullness in their breasts during this time (2 to 3 days postpartum) and colostrum can be expressed. Arrival of milk usually occurs between 32 and 96 hours postpartum.

Breast/chestfeeding should be initiated as soon as possible following the birth of a newborn. An earlier introduction of the newborn to breast/chestfeeding will increase the likelihood of milk production (Meek & Noble, 2022). Patients report feeling a let-down reflex (flow of milk), which occurs when the patient breastfeeds, holds, cuddles, or sometimes just thinks about the newborn. The let-down or milk ejection reflex occurs when oxytocin is released from the posterior pituitary gland, causing contraction of the myoepithelial cells and transport of the milk to the nipple. Prolactin levels increase with suckling and maintain lactation.

Correct latch and suck are very important for nipple integrity and continued nutritional intake. Newborns should be assessed for proper latch and swallowing to ensure they are getting milk. Patients (especially during the early postpartum) find supporting the breast assists with latch. The C hold (the patient's thumb placed above the areola and the index finger below the areola) assists the patient during attempts at latch and is helpful while learning to breastfeed/chestfeed. It is important to remind the patient to take precautions not to compress the nipple.

Positioning

Comfort and proper positioning of the newborn and the patient contribute to successful chest/breast feeding. Encourage the patient to choose a comfortable position using pillows or rolled blankets for support. Many different positions can facilitate effective breast/chestfeeding (**Table 34-4**). Teaching all positions allows the patient to choose which works best in different situations.

The cradle position (the most common position) involves the patient holding the infant in their arms with the baby facing the patient (stomach to stomach). The infant's head is higher than the hips, and the infant's nose is aligned with the patient's nipple, with chin placement below the nipple.

The cross-cradle position is similar to the cradle position, but the infant is held in the patient's opposite arm, with their hand holding the infant's head. This position is ideal for early breast/chestfeeding when a newborn needs better head control.

The clutch or football position allows the patient to use a pillow at their side to support the infant. The infant is placed on the pillow lying somewhat on the side, facing the patient's breast and tilted toward the breast. This position is excellent for a patient after cesarean birth and also allows for better infant head control.

The lying down position allows the patient to lie on their side and also place the infant on their side, facing the patient. A rolled blanket can help support the infant's back. This position is also helpful if a patient has experienced a cesarean birth.

Latch

When the patient is comfortable and has chosen a position, encourage them to bring the infant to their breast rather than bring their breast to the infant. The infant's nose should be aligned with their nipple as they support the breast and allow the infant to latch. Proper latch is demonstrated by the infant securing a large part of the areola, rather than just nipple, and by visualizing and hearing the infant swallow. The infant's lips should flare outward, and a seal should be formed around the breast. If smacking or clicking sounds are heard, reposition the latch. To break the seal (if repositioning is needed), the patient should place their index finger in the corner of the infant's mouth and apply mild downward pressure.

Table 34-5 identifies some items to be assessed regarding the infant's breast/chestfeeding behavior.

Milk Supply

Patients who choose breast/chestfeeding need education and support. Breast assessment is crucial to determine if a patient will need further assistance if choosing to breast/chestfeed. Whether the nipples are erect, flat, or inverted can impact the type of breast/chestfeeding support needed. Additionally, common misconceptions must be addressed. Breast size has no impact on breast/chestfeeding, but there are factors that can delay milk production (lactogenesis II). Specifically, lactogenesis can be affected by delayed initiation of breast/chestfeeding, ineffective suckling, cesarean birth, increased stress, and medical conditions, which in turn can impact successful continuation of chest/breast feeding (Graham & Montgomery, 2019; Meek & Noble, 2022). Additionally, much has been written about the correlation between delayed lactogenesis and chest/breast feeding initiation in patients living in bigger bodies. It is important to remember that patients who receive adequate and unbiased support are often successful in chest/breast feeding (Reichental et al., 2022).

While some patients experience decreased milk production, other patients have an overabundance of milk, which can lead to inadequate emptying or milk stasis. The let-down reflex in such a case can overwhelm the infant's ability to swallow or take in milk effectively. The infant will often make choking sounds, attempt to turn away, or detach from the breast. Also, the patient will have increased leaking, which may interfere with other activities. Evaluation includes newborn assessment for problems associated with swallowing (gastroesophageal reflux). Teaching includes position change, pumping or expression of milk

TABLE 34-4 Common Body Positions for chest/breast feeding

Position	Description	Advantages	Illustration
Cradle position	The infant is side lying, facing the patient, with the side of the head and body resting on the patient's forearm of the arm next to the breast to be used.	This is the most commonly used breast/chestfeeding position and tends to feel most natural for the patient. However, it offers the least amount of control over the infant's head.	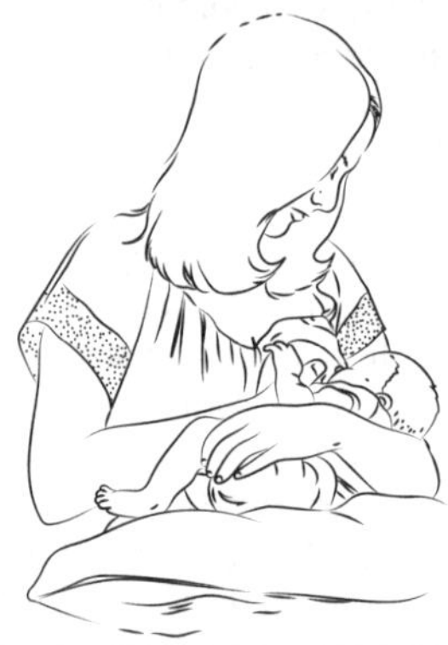
Cross-cradle posture	The infant is side lying, facing the patient, with the side resting on the patient's forearm of the arm on the opposite side of the breast being used.	This posture is considered especially useful for the patient of a newborn or preterm infant. It offers greater control over the infant's head.	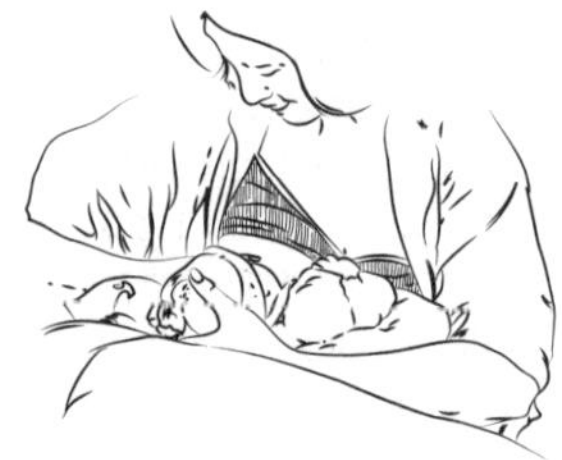
Football or clutch	In this sitting position, the infant lies on their back, curled between the side of the patient's chest and their arm. The infant's upper body is supported by the patient's forearm. The patient's hand supports the infant's neck and shoulders. The infant's hips are flexed up along the chair back or other surface that the patient is leaning against.	This position is helpful for patients after cesarean birth and those who have large pendulous breasts or are nursing multiple infants.	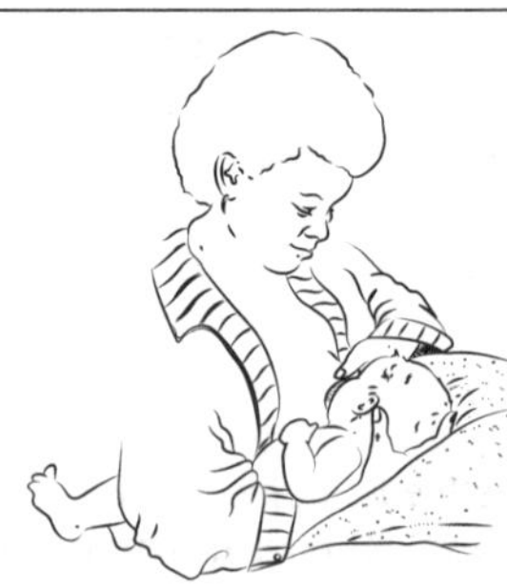
Semi reclining	The patient leans back, and the infant lies against their body in chest-to-chest contact, usually prone.	This is the most comfortable position for patients recovering from a cesarean birth, those who have large pendulous breasts, and those who choose to co-sleep with their infants.	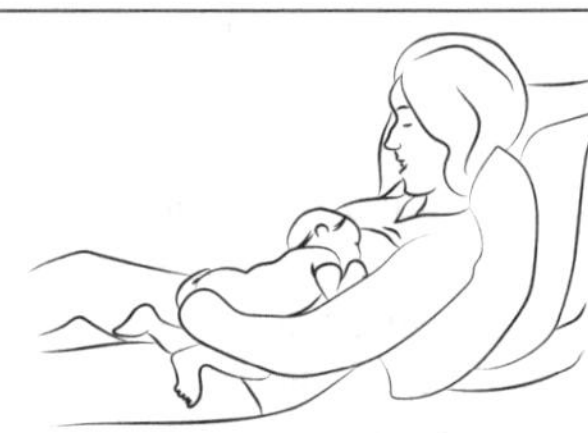
Side lying	The patient lies on their side. The infant is side lying, chest to chest with the patient. The patient's arm closest to the mattress supports the infant's back.	This position is helpful for patients who have had a cesarean birth or have large or pendulous breasts.	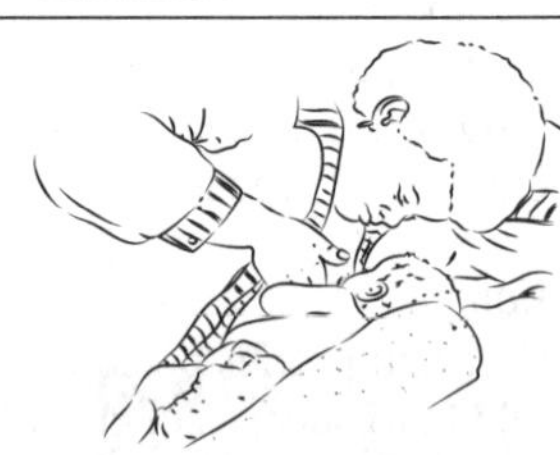
Australian or "laid back" method	The patient is "down under," lying on their back, with the infant supported on their chest.	This posture allows the infant to be in maximal control of the feeding and is especially valuable when the milk flow is faster than the infant can handle.	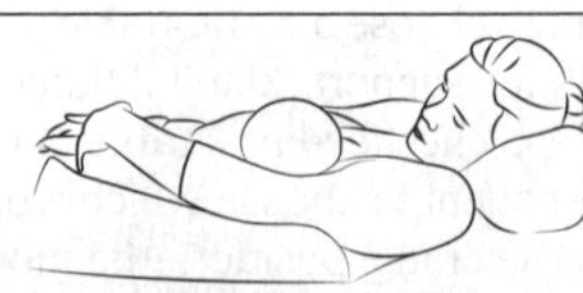

Reproduced from Campbell, S. H., Lauwers, J., Mannel, R., & Spencer, B. (Eds.). (2019). *Core curriculum for interdisciplinary lactation care*. Jones & Bartlett Learning.

TABLE 34-5 Chest/breast feeding Assessment of the Newborn

Assessment	Expected Findings	Provider Notes
Rooting	Infant turns face toward breast	Cue that infant is ready to feed Do not wait until infant cries
Latch	Jaw angled at 120–160°	Allows for better grasp of areola
	Tongue extends past lower gum	Better milk flow
	Audible or visible swallow	Indicates infant getting milk (should not hear smacking or clicking sound)
	Tight seal (tongue under breast, lips flanged)	Seal needs to be broken by placement of patient's index finger

to eliminate milk stasis, and use of one breast only for several feedings. If problems continue after a few weeks, pharmacologic assistance can be considered.

Galactagogues

There is a lack of evidence promoting effectiveness of specific pharmacologic or herbal remedies as treatments for decreased milk supply, although some common galactagogues have been used with some success. Pharmaceuticals such as metoclopramide (Reglan) and domperidone (Motilium) have been used to increase milk supply. Domperidone use results in a significantly improved milk supply; however, there is conflicting evidence about the possibility of QT segment elevation on electrocardiogram (McBride et al., 2021; Paul et al., 2015; Taylor et al., 2018). Metoclopramide, because it crosses the blood–brain barrier, may result in neurological side effects, including tardive dyskinesia if taken long term (Drugs and Lactation Database, 2018). Additionally, herbal remedies, such as fenugreek, may be used to increase milk supply and can be taken as capsules or tea (Khan et al., 2018; McBride et al., 2021).

BREAST/CHESTFEEDING COMPLICATIONS

Mastitis

Lactation mastitis—inflammation in an area of the breast—most commonly occurs during breast/chestfeeding within the first 2 months postpartum (Barker et al., 2020). Patients report unilateral localized erythema, breast tenderness, and warmth at the site, and they can present with accompanying fever and flu-like symptoms. Mastitis is usually short lived and should not interfere with breast/chestfeeding. Breast/chestfeeding continuation is encouraged and will usually aid recovery.

Mastitis can be infective or noninfective depending on the mode of occurrence. Plugged ducts or milk stasis is most often related to noninfective mastitis. Infective mastitis can occur secondary to entry of bacteria from nipple trauma/cracking, stress and fatigue, milk stasis, or sometimes without explanation. Bacteria causing this condition include *Staphylococcus aureus* (coagulase-negative *Staphylococcus* is most common), *Escherichia coli*, *Enterobacteriaceae*, *Mycobacterium tuberculosis*, and *Candida albicans*. Infective mastitis can occasionally occur in both breasts.

The incidence of mastitis is approximately 20 percent with a recurrence rate of 10 percent. Risk factors include stress and fatigue, cracked or fissured nipples, milk stasis/engorgement, breast trauma or restriction (too-tight bra), oversupply of milk, use of nipple shields, and attachment difficulties (Amir et al., 2014; Barker et al., 2020). Risk increases with a prior history of mastitis (Barker et al., 2020; Wambach, 2016). The presence of *S. aureus* on the breast or in the milk has also been implicated in mastitis (Amir et al., 2014).

Treatment includes continuation of breast/chestfeeding, increased rest, fluids, nutrition, application of moist heat, anti-inflammatory medications, and possible use of antibiotics. Standard treatment for lactation mastitis includes a penicillinase-resistant penicillin or cephalosporin (which eradicates *S. aureus*) for 10 to 14 days. Symptoms should resolve by 48 hours; if they do not, consider the possibility of methicillin-resistant *S. aureus* infection and obtain a milk culture (Amir et al., 2014; Barker et al., 2020).

Patients with mastitis should be encouraged to empty the breasts and maintain frequency of feedings. Altering the feeding schedule can increase the risk of milk stasis and subsequent mastitis. Likewise, proper latch will ensure nipple integrity.

Breast Abscess

Untreated mastitis or infection that does not respond to antibiotic therapy can result in a breast abscess (Barker et al., 2020). An abscess is a collection of pus (like a boil) that will most likely need to be incised and drained. Culture will determine the appropriate antibiotic treatment.

When abscess is present, breast/chestfeeding is encouraged, albeit usually on the unaffected breast. If treatment with drains or position of the abscess does not interfere with latch, infants can breastfeed/chestfeed on the affected breast. Additionally, expression or pumping of milk may be necessary.

Nipple Candidiasis

Candidiasis, commonly referred to as thrush, is caused by *C. albicans*, a fungus that thrives in a warm, moist environment, such as the infant's mouth or within the patient's nipples. Infant exposure can occur during vaginal birth and be subsequently transmitted to the patient's nipples while breast/chestfeeding. Nipple candidiasis generally occurs bilaterally and usually presents as a reddened area with satellite areas on the breast (Berens, 2019). Patients describe deep red coloration, burning, and shooting or stabbing pain in both nipples that occurs during and after breast/chestfeeding (Barrett et al., 2013; Berens, 2019). Patients or infants receiving antibiotic treatment are at risk of acquiring a yeast infection. Because this infection can pass between the patient and infant, both should be treated to eradicate the fungal infection (Wambach & Spencer, 2021).

The most common treatment for nipple candidiasis is application of nystatin (painted on the infant's tongue and in the oral cavity) after each breast/chestfeeding. Fluconazole (Diflucan) is prescribed for both the patient and infant if infection persists. Infants should receive treatment regardless of visualized thrush. Patients should also be assessed for a vaginal yeast infection and subsequently treated (Wambach & Spencer, 2021). For a more in-depth discussion of breast/chestfeeding, refer to the resources at the end of this chapter.

SELECTED POSTPARTUM COMPLICATIONS

Postpartum recovery is typically uneventful. Indeed, with proper nutrition, rest, and support, most individuals can return to daily activity without complication. However, complications do occasionally occur, and medical management is needed for recovery.

Puerperal Infection

Unfortunately, there are various definitions of childbirth-related infections, and none are universally used. Terms such as maternal sepsis, genital tract sepsis, puerperal fever, puerperal sepsis, and puerperal infection are often used interchangeably in the literature. The WHO defines puerperal sepsis as "infection of the genital tract occurring at any time between the rupture of the membranes (or labor) and the 42nd postpartum day in which two or more of the following are present: pelvic pain, fever, abnormal vaginal discharge, abnormal smell or odor to the discharge or delay in uterine involution" (WHO, 2015). Although commonly defined as an infection of the genital tract following childbirth, miscarriage, or termination, puerperal infections can occur secondary to dehydration, urinary or respiratory infections, and mastitis. Additionally, puerperal morbidity may be caused by cardiovascular or thromboembolic events, mood and anxiety disorders, or other medical conditions.

Historically, the lethal triad (hemorrhage, infection, and blood pressure) was the major cause of morbidity and mortality in postpartum women. Recent trends reflect that pregnancy-related sepsis continues to impact mortality (Liu, Wen et al., 2024). Infection after childbirth had significant consequences prior to the introduction of hand washing, aseptic techniques, and, eventually, antibiotics. Despite a generally decreased trend in puerperal genital tract infection in the 20th century and controlling for the increase due to the COVID-19 pandemic during 2020, infection remains a significant cause (12.8%) of pregnancy-related morbidity and mortality (Trost et al., 2024). Recent trends indicate an increase in puerperal morbidity and mortality from complications related to medical conditions within the first year after childbirth (Trost et al., 2024). In the past decade, the incidence of puerperal sepsis has increased in the United States while decreasing in many other countries (Liu, Wen et al., 2024). Although the reason for this increase might be better data recording or new classifications in data collection, it may also be related to increased obesity, surgical birth, chronic health problems, and access to care (Wisner, et al., 2024). While the complex immune response to infection in some individuals is not always an immediate consideration, given the severity of sepsis, vigilance is crucial. Suspicion of sepsis warrants immediate attention (Nieuwoudt et al., 2024). Physician consultation or referral is indicated for postpartum infection.

Most infections following vaginal birth are polymicrobial and occur at the placental site, laceration, or episiotomy. Abdominal wound infections occur after rupture of membranes and secondary to ascent of colonized bacteria. Common pathogens include those existing normally in the genital tract or bowel and others found on the skin surface, in the nasopharynx, or in the environment. Bacteria most often associated with puerperal infection include the following:

- Aerobes:
  - Gram-positive cocci—group A, B, and D streptococci: *Enterococcus*, *S. aureus*, *Staphylococcus epidermis*
  - Gram-negative bacteria: *E. coli*, *Klebsiella*, *Proteus* species
  - Gram-variable species: *Gardnerella vaginalis*
- Anaerobes:
  - Cocci: *Peptostreptococcus* and *Peptococcus* species
  - Others: *Clostridium*, *Bacteroides*, *Fusobacterium*, and *Mobiluncus* species

Cesarean birth, wound infection, pneumonia, and chronic health problems account for some of the most common risk factors for puerperal infection (Liu, Wen et al., 2024). Most postpartum infections occur within the first few weeks following childbirth, though patients are often not scheduled to return for a follow-up visit until 6 to 8 weeks. For this reason, some infections go unreported, or patients present to an emergency department for diagnosis and treatment (Liu, Wen et al., 2024).

Fever can occur from factors such as dehydration, engorgement, thrombophlebitis, or other infections unrelated to the genital tract. A fever spiking to 39°C (102.2° F), abruptly occurring within 24 hours after cesarean birth, may indicate group A *Streptococcus* infection (Karsnitz & McDaniel, 2024b). The most common puerperal conditions associated with fever are uterine infection, wound infection, mastitis, and urinary tract infection (Black et al., 2021).

Uterine Infection

Uterine infection (metritis) can occur in the endometrium (endometritis), myometrium (myometritis), and parametrium (endoparametritis) and is one of the more common infections diagnosed postpartum. Postpartum endometritis occurs in 1 to 3 percent of individuals without risk factors following vaginal birth, but this incidence rises dramatically to a 5- to 20-fold risk following cesarean birth (Taylor & Pillarisetty, 2022). The American College of Obstetricians and Gynecologists recommends a single dose of prophylactic antibiotics within 60 minutes prior to a cesarean birth (ACOG, 2007, reaffirmed 2018; ACOG, 2018b). Risk factors for uterine infection include cesarean birth, long labor, frequent vaginal examinations, prolonged rupture of membranes, internal uterine or fetal monitoring, instrumental birth, tissue trauma, traumatic birth, uterine exploration, postpartum hemorrhage, retained placental fragments, common medical conditions, larger body habitus, and low socioeconomic status.

Classic symptoms include persistent elevated temperature of 38–39°C (100.4–102.2°F) or higher depending on the type of infection, tachycardia, and uterine tenderness. Other symptoms (such as chills; malaise; pelvic pain on examination; scanty, odorless, or malodorous seropurulent lochia; and uterine subinvolution) can also occur. Onset and severity can occur in the early postpartum period (24 hours) to 2 to 3 weeks postpartum or longer depending on the type of causative organism.

In addition to physical examination, management includes laboratory analysis of urine and blood cultures, urinalysis, and a complete blood count. The white blood cell count can exceed 20,000 cells per mm^3. If lung infection is suspected, a chest radiograph should be included in the diagnostic process.

Broad-spectrum antimicrobial therapy is the treatment of choice for a uterine infection. Mild uterine infection following vaginal birth can be treated only with oral antibiotics, such as ampicillin (Principen) and gentamicin (Garamycin). Patients with moderate to severe uterine infections will be hospitalized for intravenous therapy. The gold standard for an intravenous regimen is clindamycin (Cleocin) and gentamicin (Garamycin) (Mackeen et al., 2015; Singh & Sethi, 2022). Nearly 90 percent of patients respond to treatment within 48 to 72 hours and may be discharged home after being afebrile for at least 24 hours (Mackeen et al., 2015). If left untreated, uterine infection can result in salpingitis, peritonitis, septic pelvic thrombophlebitis, or necrotizing fasciitis.

The incidence of uterine infection would decrease dramatically with a reduction in the number of cesarean births, in addition to improved obstetric management (prenatal infection surveillance and treatment), limiting the number of vaginal examinations during labor, and appropriate use of procedures such as internal monitoring, induction, episiotomy, rupture of membranes, and uterine manipulation (Karsnitz & McDaniel, 2024b). Administering a single dose of antimicrobials within 60 minutes prior to cesarean birth has been shown to decrease postpartum infection and is now standard practice. It has also been noted that vaginal cleansing with chlorhexidine prior to cesarean surgery reduced uterine infection (Haas et al., 2020).

Wound Infection

Puerperal wound infections can occur at the site of laceration or episiotomy (vaginal birth) or abdominal incision (after cesarean birth). Patients often report increased pain at the wound site with or without accompanying fever. Wound infections increase the likelihood of hospitalization and, like other puerperal infections, can interrupt or cause discontinuation of breast/chestfeeding and increase the cost of health care.

The National Inpatient Sample (2000–2020) showed a 3.5 percent postpartum infection rate with 0.3 percent incidence of wound infection (Liu, Friedman et al., 2024). Organisms often associated with wound infection include *S. aureus*, *Streptococcus*, and both aerobic and anaerobic bacilli.

Risk factors for wound infection are similar to those for uterine infection. Patients present with localized pain and erythema and edema present at the wound edges. At times, exudate and wound dehiscence may occur. Fever is often low grade, approximately 38.3°C (101°F). Dysuria can be secondary to perineal infection. Wound infection management depends on location and severity. Management for an infection occurring in a laceration or episiotomy can include suture removal, opening, debridement, and cleansing. Administration of a broad-spectrum antibiotic is indicated. Most perineal wounds do not need further repair unless third- or fourth-degree extension occurs (Liabsuetrakul et al., 2020). Abdominal wound infections require similar management with inclusion of antibiotics and occasionally drainage. If dehiscence occurs in an abdominal wound, repair may be necessary. Abdominal wound management can include daily debridement and packing depending on the severity of infection (Zuarez-Easton et al., 2017).

Urinary Tract Infection

Urinary tract infection is a common cause of puerperal morbidity (Mohr et al., 2022). Urinary stasis, which may result from multiple factors (e.g., decreased bladder tone, increased bladder volume, use of epidural anesthesia, inability to empty completely, pain or edema from perineal trauma, diabetes), increases the likelihood of infection. Patients receiving catheterization are also at increased risk for urinary tract infection. Common pathogens include *E. coli* (early postpartum, 90%), *Proteus mirabilis*, and *Klebsiella pneumoniae* (Karsnitz & McDaniel, 2024a). Bacteria that ascend into the kidney will result in pyelonephritis.

Symptoms of urinary tract infection include frequency, urgency, low abdominal pain, and dysuria, whereas symptoms of pyelonephritis include low-grade fever with spikes, flank pain, costovertebral angle tenderness, nausea, and vomiting. Diagnosis is made by urine culture, and postpartum management is the same as in patients who are not pregnant.

Uterine Subinvolution

Subinvolution occurs when uterine restoration is interrupted and unable to return (involute) to prepregnant size during the standard postpartum time frame. Typically, by 2 weeks postpartum the uterus should not be able to be palpated abdominally and should be located below the symphysis pubis. Subinvolution can be the result of inhibition of the myometrial fibers to contract effectively. Other causative factors may include retained placental fragments, infection, or myomata. Additionally, increased activity can slow uterine restoration. Placental site subinvolution occurs when the uteroplacental arteries do not close properly, filling with thrombi and delaying regeneration of the placental site. This condition has been identified as later causing hemorrhage, usually about 2 weeks postpartum (ACOG, 2017).

Symptoms often include reports of increased, continued bleeding and cessation and then return of bleeding. Subinvolution is noted on examination with presentation of a boggy, larger-than-expected uterus for that time period. If subinvolution occurs secondary to infection, along with increased size, uterine tenderness and malodorous lochia are usually present.

Management depends on the presenting symptoms. Increased or persistent bleeding requires ultrasound to assess for retained placental fragments. Ultrasound may not always show fragments, however, so occasionally uterine exploration is performed. If infection is suspected, treatment with broad-spectrum antibiotics is indicated. When there are no signs of placental fragments or infection, treatment with methylergonovine (Methergine) or ergonovine (Ergotrate) 0.2 mg orally, every 6 hours for 24 to 48 hours, is indicated. Patients are encouraged to rest, increase fluids and nutrients, and return for follow-up in 2 weeks.

Secondary (Delayed) Postpartum Hemorrhage

Postpartum hemorrhage remains a leading cause of morbidity and mortality despite advances in management and reductions in incidence during the 20th century (WHO, 2023). Postpartum hemorrhage is defined by blood loss exceeding or equal to 1,000 mL of cumulative blood loss associated with signs and symptoms of hypovolemia within the first 24 hours following childbirth (Wormer et al., 2024). Secondary postpartum hemorrhage is defined as increased bleeding occurring after the first 24 hours following childbirth and until 12 weeks postpartum (ACOG, 2017; WHO, 2023).

Risk factors for secondary postpartum hemorrhage are similar to those for immediate postpartum hemorrhage, including uterine atony, retained placental fragments, and infection. However, most cases occur secondary to subinvolution of the placental site (ACOG, 2017). Because patients without risk factors can experience a postpartum hemorrhage, national organizations encourage use of a risk assessment tool on admission and throughout labor, delivery, and postpartum to identify risk factors that develop during childbirth (ACOG, 2017). Additionally, patients who present with increased bleeding during the first week postpartum (days 2 to 5) should be evaluated for von Willebrand disease. This disease, which occurs when there is a deficiency of von Willebrand factor (a protein necessary for platelet adherence), affects 0.6 to 1.3 percent of women. Levels of von Willebrand factor increase during pregnancy and decrease postpartum, usually by 48 hours after childbirth (ACOG, 2025b). Patients with von Willebrand disease are at increased risk for secondary postpartum hemorrhage up to 4 months postpartum.

Signs and symptoms of secondary postpartum hemorrhage include increased or persistent heavy bleeding, cessation of bleeding followed by its sudden return, and possibly signs and symptoms of hypovolemia or shock. The shock index, a tool that predicts early hypovolemia by determining the ratio of heart rate to systemic blood pressure, can also be used to recognize adverse outcomes from postpartum blood loss and prompt initiation of treatment (Kohn et al., 2019). A sudden, transient episode of increased bleeding, usually 7 to 10 days postpartum, is related to sloughing of the eschar (placental site) and is not considered a postpartum hemorrhage.

Management of secondary postpartum hemorrhage includes ultrasound for detection of placental fragments (suction and evacuation if needed) and treatment with uterotonics or curettage. Uterotonics, such as ergonovine, methylergonovine, oxytocin, or a prostaglandin analog, are usually sufficient. Curettage is less likely to be performed due to the increased risk for perforation attributable to the soft nature of the puerperal uterine wall.

Puerperal Hematoma

Genital tract hematoma occurs when extravasated blood accumulates as a result of vascular trauma during birth or the birth procedure. Hematoma formation can also occur spontaneously. Puerperal hematoma occurs in approximately 1 in 700 to 4,000 births, usually presenting immediately or within several hours after birth (Janisiewicz, Mazurkiewicz, & Stefaniak, 2022). Vulvar hematomas usually stem from ruptured blood vessels, especially in the vulva, vagina, or broad ligament.

Risk factors for puerperal hematoma include instrumental or surgical birth and failure to discern or repair a torn vessel. Other risk factors include vulvovaginal varicosities, medical conditions, coagulopathies, preeclampsia, primiparity, multiple gestation, and prolonged labor.

Signs and symptoms include persistent bleeding despite a firm uterus; increased vulvar, vaginal, or rectal pain and pressure; and presentation of a fluctuant edema with bluish coloration. Increased lateral uterine or flank pain or signs and symptoms of shock necessitate assessment for broad ligament or subperitoneal hematoma.

Small hematoma formation can be expectantly managed by marking the affected area and observing for size increase. Moderate to large hematomas will usually need surgical incision and drainage.

Postpartum Venous Thrombophlebitis and Venous Thromboembolism (VTE)

The advent of early and frequent ambulation after birth dramatically decreased the incidence of puerperal thromboembolism. Despite this, VTE remains one of the leading causes of pregnancy-related morbidity and mortality (Friedman, 2021). Patients have a substantially increased risk of VTE in the 6 weeks following childbirth, especially in the first 3 weeks, where the risk is 20 to 37 times higher than usual (Friedman, 2021; Maughan et al., 2023). The incidence of puerperal morbidity and mortality from thromboembolism remains significant, and pulmonary embolism is responsible for 10–15 percent of deaths during pregnancy in high-income countries (Maughan et al., 2023).

A variety of risk factors contribute to thromboembolic events, including a history of thrombophlebitis, inherited thrombophilias, history of varicosities, surgical birth, larger body, advanced maternal age, smoking, antiphospholipid antibody syndrome, sickle cell disease, other comorbid illnesses and medical conditions. Slightly more than 50 percent of VTEs occur postpartum and the early weeks following childbirth present the greatest risk (ACOG, 2018a; Maughan et al., 2023). Patients are at increased risk for thromboembolic events during postpartum due to hypercoagulability, stasis, and vascular trauma (Virchow triad). Notably, hormonal effects from progesterone and venous pressure from the growing uterus increase the possibility of venous stasis. Birth-related risk factors include cesarean birth, operative vaginal birth, infection, vascular trauma, immobilization, and postpartum hemorrhage.

Signs and symptoms depend on the thromboembolic event. During the postpartum period, patients with superficial thrombophlebitis present with localized extremity pain, a firm cord-like structure, edema, erythema, and warmth at the site. Ultrasound is indicated to rule out underlying deep vein thrombosis (DVT). DVT often occurs with abrupt onset of severe leg pain, which worsens when ambulating or standing. Generalized edema of the entire leg is present, and patients may present with a slight temperature and mild tachycardia. There may or may not be localized tenderness and warmth at the site of the thrombosis. Positive Homan sign is no longer considered diagnostic of DVT because it could also indicate muscular strain (ACOG, 2007, reaffirmed, 2018; Maughan et al., 2023).

Laboratory analysis can include d-dimer studies. However, d-dimer levels can increase in pregnancy for several reasons, so they are not considered diagnostic. Nevertheless, a negative d-dimer result can be encouraging. Compression ultrasound of the proximal veins is considered the initial diagnostic study (Karsnitz & McDaniel, 2024a; Maughan et al., 2023).

Management for DVT includes anticoagulation therapy (for at least 6 months) and rest until symptoms resolve. After leg pain diminishes and most symptoms resolve, gradual ambulation can begin. Patients should be fitted for and taught proper use of compression stockings. Warfarin (Coumadin) can be used while chest/breast feeding. Other management includes nonsteroidal anti-inflammatory agents.

Postpartum Preeclampsia/Eclampsia and Late Preeclampsia

Preeclampsia is a hypertensive disorder that most commonly presents prenatally. It is typically characterized by hypertension and proteinuria and can range from mild to severe in presentation. Although less common, puerperal preeclampsia usually presents within 24 to 48 hours after birth, and late preeclampsia presents after 48 hours and before 4 months postpartum (ACOG, 2020). In developed countries, eclampsia occurs in 1.6 to 10 per 10,000 births (Bartal & Sibai, 2022).

Risk factors include current diagnosis of gestational hypertension or preeclampsia (the disease can worsen postpartum). Additionally, there is an increased risk of pulmonary edema from postpartum extravascular fluid shift, use of intravenous fluids during labor and birth, and renal dysfunction secondary to severe preeclampsia. Puerperal preeclampsia also increases the risk for eclampsia (seizures), thromboembolism, and stroke.

The presentation of preeclampsia is more subtle during the postpartum period than in its prenatal form. Patients typically present with headaches, visual changes, nausea and vomiting, and epigastric pain. Hypertension and proteinuria are not necessarily the primary signs of developing preeclampsia. Neurologic symptoms are more common postpartum (ACOG, 2020).

Management includes treatment with intravenous magnesium sulfate, other antihypertensive therapy, and hospitalization for at least 24 hours (Karsnitz & McDaniel, 2024a). Physician consultation is indicated for hypertension occurring postpartum. The consensus bundle for severe hypertension during pregnancy and postpartum developed by the National Partnership for Maternal Safety recommends notification and referral to a physician if blood pressure is 160 (systolic) and 110 (diastolic) (ACOG, 2020).

Postpartum Thyroiditis

Postpartum thyroiditis—that is, inflammation of the thyroid gland—can present any time during the first postpartum year (usually 1 to 4 months) as either hypothyroiditis or hyperthyroiditis or both, alternating from one to the other (ACOG, 2020; Rad & Deluxe, 2022). Overabundant release of thyroid hormones occurs initially (3 months postpartum), lasting 2 to 3 months, followed by insufficient release; thus, hyperthyroidism usually presents first. In contrast, hypothyroiditis usually occurs 4 to 8 months postpartum. The prevalence varies from 1.1 to 16.7 percent, although some cases may be unreported. Signs and symptoms are subtle and may not be readily recognized because manifestation of thyroiditis can mimic common postpartum occurrences (ACOG, 2020; Rad & Deluxe, 2022).

Risk factors include patients with autoimmune disorders, diabetes, or a history of thyroid dysfunction. The risk of this complication increases in patients with type 1 diabetes or family history (Rad & Deluxe, 2022). A positive thyroid antibody test during the first trimester is correlated with a nearly 50 percent risk of postpartum thyroiditis (Rad & Deluxe, 2022).

Signs and symptoms of hyperthyroiditis include fatigue, anxiety, palpitations, insomnia, irritability/nervousness, weight loss, and goiter. Signs and symptoms of hypothyroiditis include fatigue, inability to concentrate, depression, dry skin, constipation, weight gain, and goiter. Patients can experience dysphoria, which sometimes may lead to misdiagnosis of postpartum psychosis. Because some signs and symptoms of hyperthyroiditis and hypothyroiditis are similar to some mental health disorders, thyroid function studies are indicated when assessing patients for perinatal mood and anxiety disorders.

Laboratory analysis for hyperthyroiditis include thyroid-stimulating hormone (TSH; low levels), presence of thyroid peroxidase antibodies, and decreased TSH receptor antibodies. Diagnosis of hypothyroiditis includes TSH (elevated) and a positive test for antithyroid peroxidase antibodies.

Management depends on the phase and severity of symptoms. Beta blockers are the treatment of choice for hyperthyroiditis, whereas thyroid supplementation is prescribed for hypothyroiditis. chest/breast feeding need not be interrupted or discontinued during treatment.

Thyrotoxicosis (thyroid storm), a potentially life-threatening condition, can occur during the first month postpartum. Its onset is abrupt, short lived, and characterized by fever, nausea, vomiting, diarrhea, tachycardia, and tremor. Treatment is imperative and includes hydration and decrease of excessive circulating thyroid hormones (ACOG, 2020). Physician management is indicated.

Postpartum Mood and Anxiety Disorders

Postpartum mood and anxiety disorders (PMAD) are common complications of childbearing and can affect 10–20 percent of postpartum individuals, depending on the specific disorder and study (Garapati et al., 2023). Underlying mental health conditions account for a major factor in maternal mortality (Trost et al., 2024). A meta-analysis of 58 studies suggested a prevalence of 17 percent for postpartum depression in women without a previous history of depression. These findings are within the range of additional studies reporting on women with a history of depression (Shorey et al., 2018). Anxiety disorders, including generalized anxiety disorder, panic disorder, obsessive–compulsive disorder, and post-traumatic stress disorder, often accompany depression (3 out of 5) (Robbins et al., 2023). Prenatal anxiety has been associated with more than a twofold increase in postpartum depression within the first 6 months postpartum (Grigoriadis et al., 2018). The prevalence rate of diagnosis of either a mood or anxiety disorder during pregnancy and postpartum varies significantly and can be as high as 26 percent and 24 percent, respectively (Werner et al., 2024). Individuals with postpartum depression often report symptoms in the first few weeks, but their signs and symptoms can occur at various times throughout the first year after childbirth or at even more distant times (Slomian et al., 2019). Of particular note is the link between suicide and perinatal mood and anxiety disorders within 1 year postpartum, particularly at about 10 months (Gelabert et al., 2024).

The etiology of PMAD has not been settled, despite ongoing research in this area, but a combination of genetics and environmental factors is thought to influence its development. Recent discussion includes inflammation and immune disruption from normal pregnancy and comorbid illness (Drexhage et al., 2024). The hypothalamus–pituitary–adrenal axis and noradrenergic and serotonergic systems should work in harmony. When dysfunction occurs, PMAD can develop.

Risk factors for PMAD, along with physiologic changes after childbirth (hormonal, hypothalamus–pituitary–adrenal axis), include stressors such as social and economic influences, lack of sleep, demands of a new infant, role adaptation, and family needs (Karsnitz & McDaniel, 2024b). Additional factors include substance use, preterm birth, young maternal age, single-parent status, intimate partner violence, and comorbid illnesses. In particular, a personal or family history of mental illness or a personal history of postpartum mood or anxiety disorders increases risk (Karsnitz & McDaniel, 2024b).

Signs and symptoms vary according to severity and type of illness. People describe symptoms that range from mild to severe (an inability to perform daily activities or thoughts of harming oneself). Mental health stigma often inhibits patients from reporting these symptoms, however, so clinicians must be particularly aware of screening all patients. **Table 34-6** describes clinical presentations for PMAD.

Management depends on severity and/or comorbid illness. Diagnosis and treatment of PMAD can be complex. A team approach with a mental health specialist provides the best opportunity for appropriate care.

Screening

Assessment for PMAD should begin at the first prenatal visit and be ongoing throughout pregnancy and postpartum as indicated. The American College of Nurse-Midwives (2024) supports universal screening. Other professional organizations also fully support screening for depression. ACOG (2023), for example, identifies a need for screening at least once during the perinatal period (before 12 weeks postpartum). The U.S. Preventive Services Task Force (O'Connor et al., 2023) recommends screening for all adults—including pregnancy and the postpartum period. The American Association of Family Physicians follows the U.S. Preventive Services Task Force recommendations.

The Edinburgh Postnatal Depression Scale (EPDS), the most commonly used self-report screening tool, has been validated in numerous studies, is available in many languages, and is accessible without cost. The EPDS has a sensitivity of 86 percent and a specificity of 78 percent, with a positive predictive value of 73 percent (Cox et al., 1987). Other screening tools include the Generalized Anxiety Disorder 7 (GAD-7), Postpartum Depression Screening Scale (PDSS), the Patient Health Questionnaire (PHQ-9), the Beck Depression Inventory (BDI), and the Center for Epidemiological Studies' Depression

TABLE 34-6 Postpartum Mood and Anxiety Disorders: Clinical Presentations and Symptoms

Postpartum Mood Disorders

Blues (Symptoms Less Than 14 Days)	Depression	Psychosis
Tearful Irritability Mood swings Fatigue Appetite changes	Tearful Irritability or anger Mood swings Fatigue Lack of interest in the baby Sleep disturbances Appetite disturbances Guilt or shame Feelings of isolation Hopelessness Loss of pleasure Feelings of harming the baby or self	Hallucinations Delusions Inability to communicate Rapid mood change Paranoia Anxiety Inability to sleep Hyperactivity Disorganized thoughts

Postpartum Anxiety Disorders

Generalized Anxiety Disorder	Obsessive–Compulsive Disorder	Panic Disorder	Post-Traumatic Stress Disorder
Excessive worry Sleep disturbances/fatigue Appetite changes Feelings of dread Physical symptoms Restlessness Lack of concentration	Intrusive thoughts Checking Cleaning Hypervigilance of infant	Fear of dying Dizziness, shortness of breath Heart palpitations Feeling of impending doom Extreme anxiety Irritable bowel	Flashbacks or nightmares Anxiety Panic attack Powerlessness Increased arousal Avoidance of situations Detachment

Data from Karsnitz, D., & McDaniel, L. (2024). Common complications during the postnatal period. In K. T. Grace, C. Farley, N. Jeffers, & T. Tringali (Eds.), *Prenatal and postnatal care: A woman-centered approach* (3rd ed. pp. 626–644). Wiley-Blackwell.

Scale (CESD-R). Despite their ease of use and widespread availability, such self-report screening tools are generally underutilized.

Postpartum Blues

Many believe postpartum blues to be a mild form of postpartum depression. Postpartum blues affects nearly 80 percent of all postpartum people, is transient, and is short lived, occurring most often in the first 7 to 10 days postpartum. To counteract this condition, postpartum individuals should be encouraged to rest when possible, increase nutrition and fluids, get fresh air, and ask for family support.

Postpartum Depression

Postpartum depression can occur at any time within the first year postpartum but often presents at about 2 months postpartum. Because signs and symptoms of depression may mimic common prenatal occurrences (fatigue or sleep disturbance), depression can begin prenatally, only to become exacerbated in the early postpartum period. Signs and symptoms lasting longer than 2 weeks should be considered postpartum depression. Assessment should always include suicidal ideation or consideration of a plan to commit suicide.

Management includes treatment with antidepressants. First-line treatment consists of selective serotonin reuptake inhibitors (SSRIs). Additionally, cognitive behavioral therapy, interpersonal or group support therapy can be helpful. Of note, treatment with antidepressants could trigger a manic episode and subsequent psychosis in an individual with undiagnosed bipolar disorder (Sharma et al., 2024). For this reason, it is important to collaborate with a mental health clinician when caring for someone with postpartum depression (Garapati et al., 2023).

Postpartum Psychosis

Postpartum psychosis (also known as puerperal psychosis) can occur anytime within the first year postpartum. Although psychosis incidence can peak at about 4 weeks postpartum, it often presents early in the postpartum period (the first few days to 10 days after childbirth) and is usually abrupt in onset. Incidence is 1 to 2 per 1,000 postpartum individuals (Raza & Raza, 2022). Individuals with bipolar disorder or previous diagnosis of a mental health disorder are at increased risk for postpartum psychosis (Rommel et al., 2021). Other risk factors include sleep deprivation for an extended period (Raza & Raza, 2022). Postpartum psychosis can have devastating consequences, with an increased risk of suicide and infanticide. Suspicion of this condition warrants immediate referral for inpatient mental health treatment.

Generalized Anxiety Disorder

Generalized anxiety disorder can be difficult to diagnose during the postpartum period because extreme anxiety or worry (impacting daily activity) must occur for at least 6 months to warrant this diagnosis. According to previous studies, prevalence during the postpartum period is reported to be as high as 13 percent (Viswasam et al., 2019). Risk factors include past or present history of generalized anxiety disorder, family history of generalized anxiety disorder, life stressors, and the hormonal fluctuations associated with the postpartum period.

Pharmacologic treatment, as in depression, consists of SSRIs. Combined treatment with both pharmacologic therapy and psychotherapy can be most effective. Cognitive behavioral therapy and other therapies, such as exposure-based or mindfulness-based therapies, are often indicated to help identify triggers and subsequent coping mechanisms (Green et al., 2021).

Panic Disorder

Panic disorder is characterized by recurrent panic attacks occurring at any time with or without necessary triggers. The perinatal prevalence of this condition is 0.5 to 2.9 percent (Beck, 2021). Panic disorder impacts the person's quality of life, affecting both work and social events. Those experiencing panic disorder will often avoid an environment that can potentially trigger an attack. Hormonal fluctuations increase risk for exacerbations during postpartum.

Risk factors include hormonal influences, substance abuse, and stressful circumstances. Panic disorder is also a risk factor for postpartum depression (APA, 2022). Treatment includes psychotherapy and psychotropic agents.

Obsessive–Compulsive Disorder

Obsessive–compulsive disorder manifests as intrusive thoughts and ritualistic behaviors. A weighted perinatal prevalence of obsessive–compulsive disorder is 16.9 percent with a cumulative incidence of 5 percent by 4 weeks postpartum and 9 percent by 6 months postpartum (Fairbrother et al., 2021). Reports include an onslaught of disruptive thinking and a need to perform repetitive actions, such as cleaning, checking, and counting, to relieve stress. For most individuals these are minor disruptions, while others experience significant impairment (Drake et al., 2023). Some individuals report intrusive thoughts of harming their infant; others fail to report due to fear of misrepresentation. These thoughts are considered postpartum-specific intrusive thoughts (egodystonic) and should be differentiated from psychosis. Differentiation is considered when the person expresses self-awareness, disbelief that they could have this thought, and guilt (Fairbrother et al., 2022). Providers must include assessment for obsessive–compulsive disorder because individuals are not likely to express symptoms. Treatment includes psychotherapy and psychotropic agents.

Post-Traumatic Stress Disorder

Post-traumatic stress disorder occurs when an individual experiences a real or perceived threat of death to self or another, then is exposed to the same or a similar environment in which the trauma first occurred (APA, 2022). Individuals experiencing post-traumatic stress disorder report feelings of extreme fear and helplessness. Reporting of traumatic childbirth varies from 9 to 50 percent (Horsch et al., 2024). The estimated prevalence of postpartum post-traumatic stress disorder is 3 to 6 percent (Heyne et al., 2022).

Birth experiences and perceptions vary and can have long-term consequences. Post-traumatic stress disorder related to childbirth can result in attachment or relationship issues (Beck, 2023) and has been indicated in the development of postpartum depression. Debriefing or discussing events around childbirth can help with understanding specifics of the experience. Furthermore, examining aspects of the birth that are unclear can correct misinformation and give the person an opportunity to express any concerns or fears. Management includes treatment with SSRIs and psychotherapy (Nillni et al., 2018; Taylor et al., 2021).

Complementary Therapy

Complementary therapies can be used for PMAD. In particular, omega-3 fatty acid supplements, St. John's wort, and kava root can be helpful in patients with PMAD (Nillni et al., 2018; Taylor et al., 2021). Nevertheless, it is important to recognize that most complementary treatments are not evidence based. Furthermore, patients should be assessed for current use of any complementary therapies before beginning treatment. Teaching should include variations in strength, use of active ingredients, or ways in which substances are derived.

CONCLUSION

The postpartum period encompasses numerous physiological and psychological changes as individuals return to a prepregnant state and transition to a new or an additional role. The plans for interactions between new parents and members of the healthcare community in the United States do not fit well with this time frame because healthcare providers often do not communicate with their patients until 6 weeks postpartum. Postpartum complications usually occur before this 6-week visit, however, and breastfeeding is frequently discontinued prior to this visit. Clinicians have an opportunity to facilitate an uneventful recovery while employing judicious assessment for recognition of complications. Consideration of cultural influences, education, and team approach will impact treatment and promote long-term health care.

For additional resources on postpartum care, refer to **Box 34-1**.

BOX 34-1 Additional Resources About Postpartum Care

Postpartum Web Resources

Academy of Pediatrics information on breastfeeding: https://www.aap.org/en-us/advocacy-and-policy/aap-health-initiatives/Breastfeeding/Pages/default.aspx

Baby-Friendly USA: http://www.babyfriendlyusa.org

Birth Trauma Association: https://www.birthtraumaassociation.org/

Edinburgh Postnatal Depression Scale: https://nj.gov/health/fhs/maternalchild/documents/PPD-Edinburgh-Scale.pdf

La Leche League International: http://www.lalecheleague.org

MedlinePlus information about drugs, herbs, and supplements: http://www.nlm.nih.gov/medlineplus/druginformation.html

Postpartum Support International: http://www.postpartum.net

Maternal Patient Safety Bundles

Maternal Venous Thromboembolism: https://safehealthcareforeverywoman.org/patient-safety-bundles/maternal-venous-thromboembolism/

Perinatal Mental Health Conditions: https://saferbirth.org/psbs/perinatal-mental-health-conditions/

Postpartum Discharge Transition: https://saferbirth.org/psbs/postpartum-discharge-transition/

Sepsis in Obstetric Care: https://saferbirth.org/psbs/sepsis-in-obstetric-care/

Severe Hypertension in Pregnancy: https://safehealthcareforeverywoman.org/patient-safety-bundles/severe-hypertension-in-pregnancy/

References

Altuntuğ, K., Kiyak, S., & Ege, E. (2023). Relationship between birth memories and recall and perception of traumatic birth in women in the postpartum one-year period and affecting factors. *Current Psychology*, 1–9. https://doi.org/10.1007/s12144-023-04336-3

American Academy of Pediatrics. (2012). Breastfeeding and the use of human milk. *Pediatrics, 129*(3), 827–841.

American College of Nurse-Midwives. Position statement. *Mental health during childbirth and across the lifespan.* https://www.midwife.org/acnm/files/acnmlibrarydata/uploadfilename/000000000324/PS-Mental%20Health%20During%20Childbirth%20and%20Across%20Lifespan.pdf

American College of Obstetricians and Gynecologists. (2020). Physical activity and exercise during pregnancy and the postpartum period. Committee on Obstetric Practice: Committee opinion no. 804. *Obstetrics & Gynecology, 135*, e178–e188.

American College of Obstetricians and Gynecologists. (2020). Thyroid disease in pregnancy: Practice bulletin no. 223. *Obstetrics & Gynecology, 135*, e261–274.

American College of Obstetricians and Gynecologists. (2017). Postpartum hemorrhage: Practice bulletin no. 183. *Obstetrics & Gynecology, 130*(4), 168–186.

American College of Obstetricians and Gynecologists (ACOG). (2020). Gestational hypertension and preeclampsia: Practice bulletin no. 222. *Obstetrics and Gynecology, 135*(6), e237–e260.

American College of Obstetricians and Gynecologists. (2018a). Thromboembolism in pregnancy: Practice bulletin no. 196. *Obstetrics & Gynecology, 132*(1), e1–e17.

American College of Obstetricians and Gynecologists. (2018b). Use of prophylactic antibiotics in labor and delivery: Practice bulletin no. 199. *Obstetrics & Gynecology, 132*(3), e103–e119.

American College of Obstetricians and Gynecologists. (2007, reaffirmed 2018). Prevention of deep vein thromboembolism and pulmonary embolism: Practice bulletin no. 84. Obstetrics & Gynecology, 110, 429-440.

American College of Obstetricians and Gynecologists. (2023). Screening and diagnosis of mental health conditions during pregnancy and postpartum: ACOG clinical practice guideline no. 4. *Obstetrics & Gynecology. 141*(6), 1232–1261. PubMed doi:10.1097/AOG.0000000000005200

American College of Obstetricians and Gynecologists. (2025a). Optimizing Postpartum Care. Committee on Obstetric Practice: Committee opinion no. 736. *Obstetrics & Gynecology,* 131:e140–50.

American College of Obstetricians and Gynecologists. (2025b). Committee on Gynecologic Practice. Committee opinion no. 580: Von Willebrand disease in women. *Obstetrics & Gynecology, 122*, 1368–1373.

American Psychiatric Association (APA). (2022). *Diagnostic and statistical manual of mental disorders* (DSM-5-TR), (5th ed. Text Revision). American Psychiatric Association.

Amiel Castro, R. T., Pinard Anderman, C., O'Connor, T. G., Glover, V., & Kammerer, M. (2024). Maternal and paternal postpartum early mood and bonding. *Journal of Reproductive and Infant Psychology*, *42*(4), 741–752. https://doi.org10.1080/02646838.2022.2159351

Amir, L. H., Trupin, S., & Kvist, L. J. (2014). Diagnosis and treatment of mastitis in breastfeeding women. *Journal of Human Lactation, 30*, 10–13.

Anastasya Siregar, R., Sari Batubara, N., Heriansyah, R., Endang, T., Lubis, F., & Latifah Harahap, M. (2024). Knowledge of postpartum mothers about kegel exercises for perineal wound healing. *International Journal of Public Health Excellence, 3*(2), 656–665. https://doi.org10.55299/ijphe.v3i2.788

Andrighetti, T. P., & Butler, J. M. (2024). Components of postnatal care. In K. T. Grace, C. L. Farley, N. K. Jeffers, & T. Tringali (Eds.), *Prenatal and postnatal care: A woman-centered approach* (pp. 450–469). Wiley.

Azulay Chertok, I. R., & Wolf, J. H. (2019). Postpartum period and lactation physiology. In S. T. Blackburn (Ed.), *Maternal, fetal, and neonatal physiology: A clinical perspective* (5th ed., pp. 142–162). Saunders Elsevier.

Barker, M., Adelson, P., Peters, M., Steen, M. (2020). Probiotics and human lactational mastitis: A scoping review. *Women and Birth, 33*(6), e483–e491. https://doi.org/10.1016/j.wombi.2020.01.001

Barrett, M., Heller, M. M., Stone, H. F., & Murase, J. E. (2013). Dermatoses of the breast in lactation. *Dermatologic Therapy, 26*(4), 331–336.

Bartal, M. F., & Sibai, B. M. (2022). Eclampsia in the 21st Century. *American Journal of Obstetrics & Gynecology*, 226(2), S1237–S1253.

Beck, C. T. (2021). Postpartum onset of panic disorder: A metaphor analysis. *Archives of Psychiatric Nursing, 35*, 369–374.

Beck, C. T. (2023). Postpartum mood and anxiety disorders: A lexicon of methaphors. *Journal of Holistic Nursing, 41*(3), 246–255. https://doi.org/ 10.1177/08980101221097212

Berens, P. D. (2019). Breast pathology. In S. H. Campbell, J. Lauwers, R. Mannel, & B. Spencer (Eds.), *Core curriculum for interdisciplinary lactation care* (pp. 317–330). Jones & Bartlett Learning.

Black, C. M., Vesco, K. K., Mehta, V., Ohman-Strickland, P., Demissie, K., & Schneider, D. (2021). Hospital readmission following delivery with and without severe maternal morbidity. *Journal of Women's Health, 30*(12), 1736–1743. https://doi.org/10.1089/jwh.2020.8815

Butti, N., Montirosso, R., Borgatti, R., Urgesi, C. (2018). Maternal sensitivity is associated with configural processing of infant's cues in preterm and full-term mothers, *Early Human Development, 125,* 35–45.

Campbell, S. H., Lauwers, J., Mannel, R., & Spencer, B. (Eds.). (2019). *Core curriculum for interdisciplinary lactation care.* Jones & Bartlett Learning.

Cason, P., Cwiak, C., Edelman, A., & Kowal, D. (2023). *Contraceptive technology*. Jones & Bartlett Learning.

Centers for Disease Control and Prevention. (2016). U.S. medical eligibility criteria for contraceptive use, 2016. *Morbidity and Mortality Weekly Report, 65,* 1–108.

Centers for Disease Control and Prevention. (2022). *Breastfeeding report card.* https://www.cdc.gov/breastfeeding-data/breastfeeding-report-card/?CDC_AAref_Val=https://www.cdc.gov/breastfeeding/data/reportcard.htm

Centers for Disease Control and Prevention. (2022). *Maternity practices in infant nutrition and care (mPINC) 2022 national results report.* https://www.cdc.gov/breastfeeding/data/mpinc/national-report.html

Cox, J. L., Holden, J. M., & Sagovsky, R. (1987). Detection of postnatal depression: Development of the 10-item Edinburgh Postnatal Depression Scale. *British Journal of Psychiatry, 150*, 782–786.

Curtis, K. M., Nguyen, A. T., Tepper, N. K., et al. (2024). U.S. selected practice recommendations for contraceptive use, 2024. *Morbidity and Mortality Weekly Report. Recommendations and Reports, 73*(No. RR-3), 1–77. https://doi.org10.15585/mmwr.rr7303a1

de Waal, N., Lodder, P., Nyklíček, I., Hulsbosch, L. P., van den Heuvel, M. I., van der Gucht, K., de Caluwé, E., Pop, V. J. M., & Boekhorst, M. G. B. M. (2024). Trait mindfulness during pregnancy and maternal-infant bonding: Longitudinal associations with infant temperament and social-emotional development. *Early Human Development, 196,* 106082.

Dekel, S., Thiel, F., Dishy, G., & Ashenfarb, A. L. (2019). Is childbirth-induced PTSD associated with low maternal attachment? *Archives of Women's Mental Health, 22*(1), 119–122.

Doyle, F. L., Dickson, S. J., Eapen, V., Frisk, P. J., Kimonis, E. R., Hawes, D. J., Mul, C., Richmond, J. L., Mehta, D., & Dadds, M. R. (2023). Towards preventative psychiatry: Concurrent and longitudinal predictors of postnatal maternal-infant bonding. *Child Psychiatry & Human Development, 54,* 1723–1736. https:// doi.org/10.1007/s10578-022-01365-0

Drake, M. H., Friesen-Haarer, A. J., Ward, M. J., & Miller, M. L. (2023). Obsessive-compulsive disorder symptoms and intrusive thoughts in the postpartum period: Associations with trauma exposure and PTSD symptoms. *Stress & Health, 40*(2), e3316. https://doi.org/10.1002/smi.3316

Drexhage, H. A., Bergink, V., Poletti, S., Benedetti, F., & Osborne, L. M. (2024). Conventional and new immunotherapies for immune system dysregulation in postpartum mood disorders: Comparisons to immune system dysregulations in bipolar disorder, major depression and postpartum autoimmune thyroid disease. *Expert Review of Clinical Immunology, 21*(2), 113–135. https://doi.org/10.1080/1744666X.2024.2420053

Drugs and Lactation Database. (2018). *Metoclopramide*. National Library of Medicine.

Fairbrother, N., Collardeau, F., Albert, A. Y. K., Challacombe, F. L., Thordarson, D. S., Woody, S. R., & Janssen, P. A. (2021). High prevalence and incidence of obsessive-compulsive disorder among women across pregnancy and the postpartum. *The Journal of Clinical Psychiatry, 82*(2), 30368.

Fairbrother, N., Martin, R., & Challacombe, F. (2022). Unwanted, intrusive thoughts of infant-related harm. In A. Bramante, V. Brenna, C. Pariante, & M. Percudani (Eds.), *Key topics in perinatal mental health* (pp. 93–112). Springer Nature Switzerland AG. https://doi.org/10.1007/978-3-030-91832-3_6

Feldman-Winter, L., & Goldsmith, J. P. (2016). Safe sleep and skin-to-skin care in the neonatal period for healthy term newborns. *Pediatrics, 138*(3), e20161889. https://doi.org/10.1542/peds.2016-1889

Friedman, A., M. (2021). Obstetric venous thromboembolism prophylaxis, risk factors and outcomes. *Current Opinions in Obstetrics and Gynecology, 33*(5), 384–390. http://doi.org/10.1097/GCO.0000000000000733

Garapati, J., Jajoo, S., Aradhya, D., Reddy, L. S., Dahiphale, S. M., & Patel, D. J. (2023). Postpartum mood disorders: Insights into diagnosis, prevention, and treatment. *Cureus, 15*(7), e42107. https://doi.org/10.7759/cureus.42107

Gelabert, E., Plaza, A., Roca-Lecumberri, A., Bramante, A., Brenna, V., Garcia-Esteve, L., Lega, I., Subirà, S., Toscano, C., & Torres-Giménez, A. (2024). Suicide attempts during pregnancy and postpartum: A systematic review and meta-analysis. *Maternal and Child Health Journal, 28*(9), 1443–1453.

Graham, G. A., & Montgomery, A. (2019). Breast anatomy and milk production. In S. H. Campbell, J. Lauwers, R. Mannel, & B. Spencer (Eds.), *Core curriculum for interdisciplinary lactation care* (pp. 83–99). Jones & Bartlett Learning.

Graziottin, A., Di Simone, N., & Guarano, A. (2024). Postpartum care: clinical considerations for improving genital and sexual health. *European Journal of Obstetrics and Gynecology and Reproductive Biology, 296,* 250–257.

Green, S. M., Donegna, E., McCabe, R. E., Streiner, D. L., Furtado, M., Noble, L., Agako, A., & Frey, B. N. (2021). Cognitive behavior therapy for women with generalized anxiety disorder in the perinatal period: Impact on problematic behaviors. *Behavior Therapy*, 52(4), 907–916. https://doi.org/10.1016/j.beth.2020.11.004

Gregoiadis, S., Graves, L., Peer,M., Mamisashvili, L., Tomlinson, G., Vigod, S.N., Dennis, C.-L., Steiner, M., Cheung, A., Dawson, H., Rector, N.A., Guenette, M., & Richter, M., (2018). A systematic review and meta-analysis of the effets of antenatal anxiety on postpartum outcomes. Archives of Women's Mental Health, 22, 543-566. https://doi.org/10.1007/s00737-018-0930-2

Haas, D. M., Morgan, S., Contreras, K., & Kimball, S. (2020). Vaginal preparation with antiseptic solution before cesarean section for preventing postoperative infections. *Cochrane Database Systematic Review, 4,* CD007892. https://doi.org/10.1002/14651858.CD007892.pub7

HealthyPeople.gov. (2024). *Maternal, infant, and child health. MICH-15: Increase the proportion of infants who are breastfed exclusively through age 6 months.* U.S. Office of Disease Prevention and Health Promotion. https://odphp.health.gov/healthypeople/objectives-and-data/browse-objectives/infants/increase-proportion-infants-who-are-breastfed-exclusively-through-age-6-months-mich-15

Heyne, C., Kazmierczak, M., Souday, R., Horesh, D., Lambregtse-van den Berg, M., Weigl, T., Horsch, A., Oosterman, M., Dikmen-Yildez, P. & Garthus-Niegel, G. (2022). Prevalence and risk factors of birth-related posttraumatic stress among parents: A comparative systematic review and meta-analysis, *Clinical Psychology Review, 94,* 102157. https://doi.org/10.1016/j.cpr.2022.102157

Horsch, A., Garthus, S., Ayers, S., Chandra, P., Hartman, K., Vaisbuch, E., & Lalor, J. (2024). Childbirth-related posttraumatic stress disorder: Definition, risk factors, pathophysiology, diagnosis, prevention, and treatment. *American Journal of Obstetrics and Gynecology, 230*(3), S1116–S1127. https://doi.org/10.1016/j.ajog.2023.09.089

Janisiewicz, K., Mazurkiewicz, B., & Stefaniak, M. (2022). Vaginal haematoma as a postpartum complication: A case report. *Med Sci Pulse, 16*(4), 49–55. https://doi.org/10.5604/01.3001.0016.0922.

Kantrowitz-Gordon, I. (2019). Postpartum care. In T. L. King, M. C. Brucker, K. Osborne, & C. M. Jevitt (Eds.), *Varney's midwifery* (6th ed., pp. 1183–1216). Jones & Bartlett Learning.

Karsnitz, D. B., & McDaniel, L. R. (2024a). Postpartum complications. In J. Phillippi & I. Kantrowitz Gordon (Eds.), *Varney's midwifery* (7th ed., pp. 1489-1507). Jones & Bartlett.

Karsnitz, D., & McDaniel, L. (2024b). Common complications during the postnatal period. In K. T. Grace, C. Farley, N. Jeffers, & T. Tringali (Eds.), *Prenatal and postnatal care: A woman-centered approach* (3rd ed., pp. 626–644). Wiley-Blackwell.

Khan, T. M., Wu, D. B.-C., & Dolzhenko, A. V. (2018). Effectiveness of fenugreek as a galactagogue: A network meta-analysis. *Phytotherapy Research, 32*(3), 402–412.

King, T. L. (2023). Anatomy and physiology of postpartum. In J. Phillippi & I. Kantrowitz-Gordon (Eds.), *Varney's midwifery* (7th ed., pp. 2230–2257). Jones & Bartlett Learning.

Klaus, M. H., & Kennell, J. H. (1976). *Maternal–infant bonding: The impact of early separation or loss on family development.* Mosby.

Kohn, J. R., Dildy, G. A., & Eppes, C. S. (2019). Shock index and delta-shock index are superior to existing maternal early warning criteria to identify postpartum hemorrhage and need for intervention. *The Journal of Maternal–Fetal & Neonatal Medicine, 32*(8), 1238–1244.

Liabsuetrakul, T., Choobun, T., Peeyananjarassri, K., & Islam, O. M. (2020). Antibiotic prophylaxis for operative vaginal delivery. *Cochrane Database Systematic Review, 3,* CD004455. https://doi.org/10.1002/14651858.CD004455.pub5

Liu, L., Wen, T., Reddy, U., Mourad, R., Goffman, D., Nathan, L., Sheen, J., D'Alton, M. E., & Friedman, A. (2024). Risk factors, trends, and outcomes associated with postpartum sepsis readmissions. *Obstetrics & Gynecology, 143*, 346–354. https://doi.org/10.1097/AOG.0000000000005437

Liu, L. Y., Friedman, A. M., Goffman, D., Nathan, L., Sheen, J. J., Reddy, U. M., D'Alton, M. E., & Wen, T. (2024). Infection and Sepsis Trends during United States' Delivery Hospitalizations from 2000 to 2020. *American journal of perinatology, 41*(13), 1767–1778. https://doi.org/10.1055/s-0044-1780538

Lord, L. G., Harding, J. E., Crowther, C. A., & Lin, L. (2023). Skin-to-skin contact for the prevention of neonatal hypoglycaemia: A systematic review and meta-analysis. *BMC Pregnancy and Childbirth, 23,* 744. https:// doi.org/10.1186/s12884-023-06057-8

Mackeen, A. D., Packard, R. E., Ota, E., & Speer, L. (2015). Antibiotic regimens for postpartum endometritis. *Cochrane Database of Systematic Reviews, 2015*(2), CD001067. https://doi .org/10.1002/14651858.CD001067.pub3

Maughan, B. C., Marin, M., Han, J., Gibbins, K. J., Brixey, A. G., Caughey, A. B., Kline, J. A., & Jarman, A. F. (2023). *Venous thromboembolism during pregnancy and the postpartum period: Risk factors, diagnostic testing, and treatment.* PMC Home. https://pmc.ncbi.nlm.nih.gov/articles/PMC10042329/

McBride, G. M., Stevenson, R., Zizzo, G., Rumbold, A. R., Amir, L. H., Keir, A. K., & Grzeskowiak, L. E. (2021). Use and experiences of galactagogues while breastfeeding among Australian women. *PLoS One, 16*(7), e0254049.

Meek, J. Y., & Noble, L. (2022). Section on breastfeeding. Policy statement: Breastfeeding and the use of human milk. *Pediatrics, 150*(1), e2022057988

Mercer, R. T. (1985). The process of maternal role attainment over the first year. *Nursing Research, 34*(4), 198–204.

Mohamed-Ahmed, O., Hinshaw, K., & Knight, M. (2018). Operative vaginal delivery and post-partum infection. *Best Practice & Research Clinical Obstetrics & Gynaecology, 56*, 93–106. https://doi.org/10.1016/j.bpobgyn.2018.09.005

Mohr, S., Raio, L., Gobrecht-Keller, U., Imboden, S., Mueller, M. D., & Kuhn, A. (2022). Postpartum urinary retention: What are the sequelae? A long-term study and review of the literature. *International Urogynecology Journal*, *33,* 1601–1608. https://doi .org/10.1007/s00192-021-05074-5

Nguyen, A. T., Curtis, K. M., Tepper, N. K., Kortsmit, K., Brittain, A. W., Snyder, E. M., Cohen, M. A., Zapata, L. B., & Whiteman, M. K. (2024). U.S. Medical Eligibility Criteria for Contraceptive Use, 2024. *Morbidity and Mortality Weekly Report Recommendations and Reports, 73*(4), 1–126. https://doi.org/10.15585/mmwr.rr7304a1

Nieuwoudt, C., White, S., Heine, R., & Widelock, T. (2024). Maternal sepsis. *Clinical Obstetrics & Gynecology, 67,* 589–604. https://doi.org/10.1097/GRF .0000000000000881

Nillni, Y. I., Mehralizade, A., Mayer, L., & Milanovic, S. (2018). Treatment of depression, anxiety, and trauma-related disorders during the perinatal period: A systematic review. *Clinical Psychology Review,* 66, 136–148. https://doi.org/10.1016/j .cpr.2018.06.004

O'Connor, E., Henninger, M., Perdue, L. A., et al. (2023). *Screening for depression, anxiety, and suicide risk in adults: A systematic evidence review for the U.S. Preventive Services Task Force [Internet].* Agency for Healthcare Research and Quality (U.S).; 2023 Jun. (Evidence Synthesis, No. 223.) Chapter 1, Introduction. Available from: https://www.ncbi.nlm.nih.gov/books/NBK592808/

Paul, C., Zénut, M., Dorut, A., Coudoré, M.-A., Vein, J., Cardot, J.-M., & Balayssac, D. (2015). Use of domperidone as a galactagogue drug: A systematic review of the benefit-risk ratio. *Journal of Human Lactation, 31*(1), 57–63.

Rad, N. S., & Deluxe, L. (2022). Postpartum thyroiditis. In *StatPearls.* StatPearls Publishing. https://www.ncbi.nlm.nih.gov/books/NBK557646/

Raza, S. K., & Raza, S. (2022). Postpartum psychosis. In *StatPearls.* StatPearls Publishing

Reichental, Z. L., O'Brien, V. M., & O'Reilly, S. L. Interventions to support women with overweight or obesity or gestational diabetes mellitus to initiate and continue breastfeeding: Systematic review and meta-analysis. *Obesity Reviews, 23*(3), e13371. https://doi:10.1111/obr.13371

Robbins, C. L., Ko, J. Y., D'Angelo, D. V., Salvesen von Essen, B., Bish, C. L., Kroelinger, C. D., Trevendale, H. D., Warner, L., & Barfield, W. (2023). Timing of postpartum depressive symptoms. *Preventing Chronic Disease, 20,* 230107. https://doi .org/10.5888/pcd20.230107.

Rommel, A. S., Molenaar, N. M., Gilden, J., Kushner, S. A., Westerbeek, N. J., Kamperman, A. M., & Bergink, V. (2021). Long-term outcome of postpartum psychosis: A prospective clinical cohort study in 106 women. *International Journal of Bipolar Disorders, 9*(1), 31. https://doi.org/10.1186/ s40345-021-00236-2

Rubin, R. (1961). Basic maternal behavior. *Nursing Outlook, 9*(11), 683–686.

Sharma, V., Wood, K. N., Weaver, B., Mazmanian, D., & Thomson, M. (2024). Occurrence of postpartum manic or mixed episodes in women with bipolar I disorder: A systematic review and meta-analysis. *Bipolar Disorders*, 26(3), 240–248. https://doi.org/:10.1111/bdi.13405

Shorey, S., Chee, C. Y. I., Ng, E. D., Chan, Y. H., Tam, W. W. S., & Chong, Y. S. (2018). Prevalence and incidence of postpartum depression among healthy mothers: A systematic review and meta-analysis. *Journal of Psychiatric Research, 104*, 235–248.

Shorey, S., Rajesh Asurlekar, A., Shi Chua J., & Hsiu Kim Lim, L. (2022). Influence of oxytocin on parenting behaviors and parent-child bonding: A systematic review. *Developmental Psychobiology, 65,* e22359. https://doi.org/10.1002/dev.22359

Singh, N., & Sethi, A. (2022). Endometritis—diagnosis, treatment and its impact on fertility—a scoping review. *JBRA Assisted Reproduction, 26*(3), 538–546. https://doi .org/0.5935/1518-0557.20220015

Slomian, J., Honvo, G., Emonts, P., Reginster, J. Y., & Bruyére, O. (2019). Consequences of maternal postpartum depression: A systematic review of maternal and infant outcomes. *Women's Health, 15,* 1–55. https://doi.org/10.1177 /1745506519844044

Taylor, M. P. G., Sinclair, M., Gillen, P., McCullough, J. E. M, Miller, P. W, Farrell, D. P., Slater, P. F., Shaprio, E., & Klaus, P. (2021) Early psychological interventions for prevention and treatment of post-traumatic stress disorder (PTSD) and post-traumatic stress symptoms in post-partum women: A systematic review and meta-analysis. *PLoS ONE, 16*(11), e0258170. https://doi.org/10.1371/journal .pone.0258170

Taylor, A., Logan, G., Twells, L., & Newhook, A. (2018). Human milk expression after domperidone treatment in postpartum women: A systematic review and meta-analysis of randomized controlled trials. *Journal of Human Lactation, 35*(3), 501–509. https://doi.org/10.1177/0890334418812069

Taylor, M., & Pillarisetty L. S. (2022). Endometritis. In *StatPearls.* StatPearls Publishing. https://www.ncbi.nlm.nih.gov/books/NBK553124/

Trost, S. L., Busacker, A., Leonard, M., et al. (2024). *Pregnancy-related deaths: Data from maternal mortality review committees in 38 U.S. States, 2020.* Centers for Disease Control and Prevention, U.S. Department of Health and Human Services.

UNICEF & World Health Organization. (n.d.). *Baby friendly hospital initiative; ten steps to successful breastfeeding from UNICEF & the World Health Organization.* https:// www.unicef.org/documents/baby-friendly-hospital-initiative

Viswasam, K., Eslick G. D.., & Starcevic, V. (2019). Prevalence, onset and course of anxiety disorders during pregnancy: A systematic review and meta analysis. *Journal of Affective Disorders,* 255, 27–40. https://doi.org/10.1016/j.jad.2019 .05.016. Epub 2019 May 11. PMID: 31129461.

Volling, B. (2012). Family transitions following the birth of a sibling: An empirical review of changes in the firstborn's adjustment. *Psychological Bulletin, 138*(3), 497–528.

Walter, M. H., Abele, H., & Plappert, C. F. (2021). The role of oxytocin and the effect of stress during childbirth: Neurobiological basics and implications for mother and child. *Frontiers in Endocrinology,* 12. https://doi.org/10.3389/fendo.2021.742236

Wambach, K. (2016). Breast-related problems. In K. Wambach & J. Riordan (Eds.), *Breastfeeding and human lactation* (5th ed., pp. 291–324). Jones & Bartlett Learning.

Wambach, K., & Spencer, B. (Eds.). (2021). *Breastfeeding and human lactation* (6th ed.). Jones & Bartlett Learning.

Werner, E., Le, H-N., Babineau, V., & Grubb, M. (2024). Preventive interventions for perinatal mood and anxiety disorders: A review of selected programs. *Seminars in Perinatology*, *48*(6), 151944. https://doi.org/10.1016/j.semperi.2024.151944

Wisner, K. L., Murphy, C., Thomas, M. M. (2024). Prioritizing maternal mental health in addressing morbidity and mortality. *JAMA Psychiatry, 81*(5), 521–526. https://doi.org /10.1001/jamapsychiatry.2023.5648

Witt, A. M., Bolman, M., Kredit, S., & Vanic, A. (2016). Therapeutic breast massage in lactation for the management of engorgement, plugged ducts, and mastitis. *Journal of Human Lactation, 32*(1), 123–131. https://doi.org/10.1177 /0890334415619439

World Health Organization. (2015). *WHO recommendations for prevention and treatment of maternal peripartum infections.* https://www.ncbi.nlm.nih.gov/books /NBK327082/

World Health Organization. (2023). *A roadmap to combat postpartum haemorrhage between 2023 and 2030.* https://www.who.int/publications/i/item/9789240081802. https://www.who.int/publications/i/item/9789240081802

Wormer K. C., Jamil, R. T., & Bryant S. B. (2024). Postpartum hemorrhage. In *StatPearls.* StatPearls Publishing. https://www.ncbi.nlm.nih.gov/books/NBK499988/

Zuarez-Easton, S., Zafran, N., Garmi, G., & Salim, R. (2017). Postcesarean wound infection: Prevalence, impact, prevention, and management challenges. *International Journal of Women's Health, 9*, 81–88.

INDEX

Note: Boxes, figures, and tables are indicated with *b*, *f*, and *t* following the page numbers.

A

B

C

D

F

G

I

Q

T

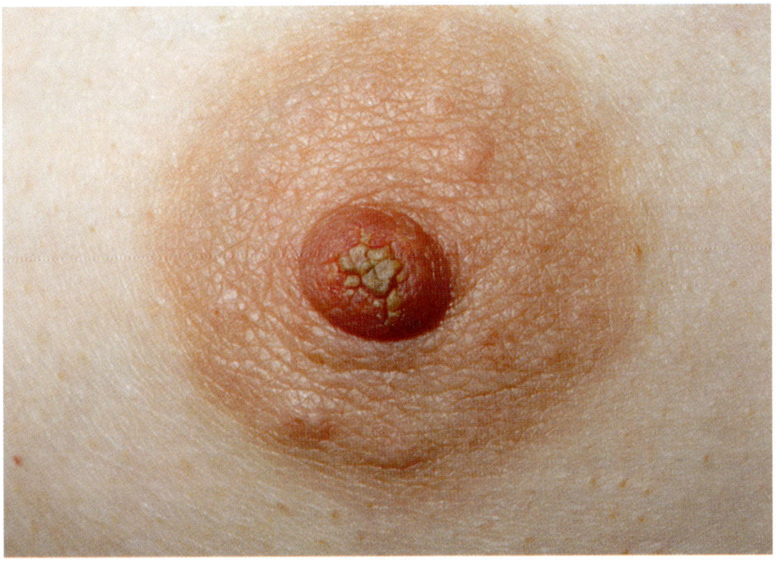

COLOR PLATE 1 An example of nipple discharge.

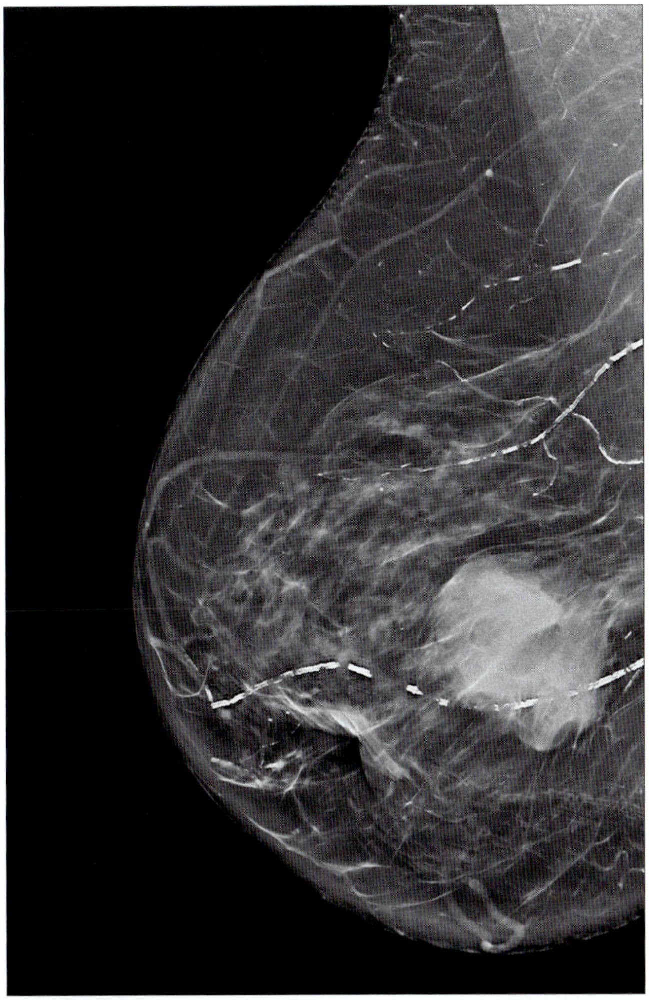

COLOR PLATE 2 An example of breast masses as visualized by mammography.

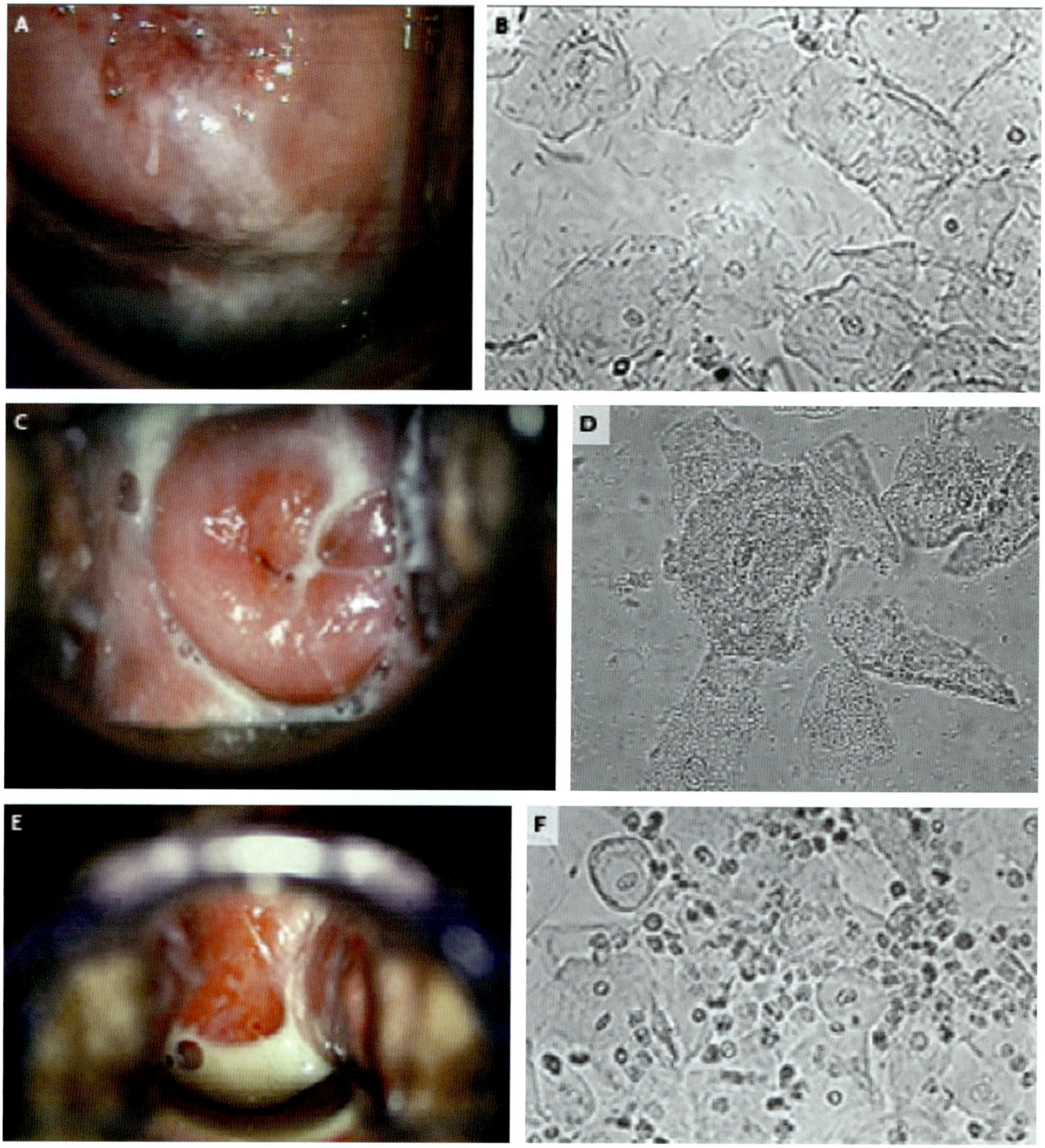

COLOR PLATE 3 Comparison of discharge and microscopy for normal discharge, bacterial vaginosis (BV), and desquamative inflammatory vaginitis (DIV).

Reproduced from Paavonen, J., & Brunham, R. C. (2018). Bacterial Vaginosis and Desquamative Inflammatory Vaginitis. *The New England journal of medicine, 379*(23), 2246–2254. https://doi.org/10.1056/NEJMra1808418.

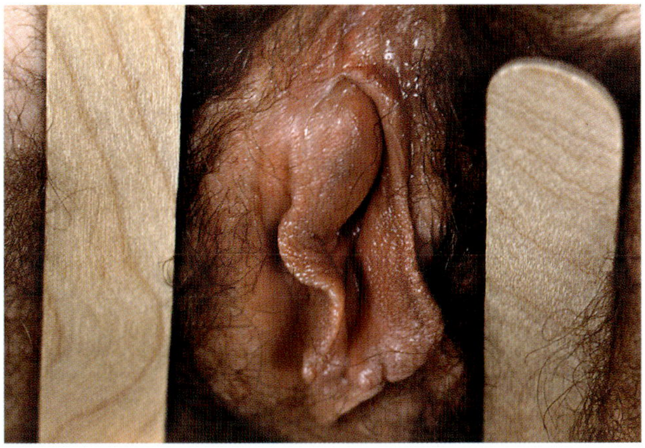

COLOR PLATE 4 Vestibular gland cyst.
Courtesy of CDC/Susan Lindsley.

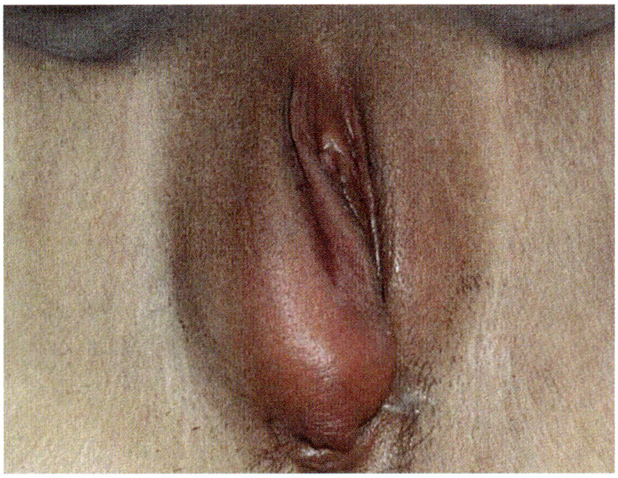

COLOR PLATE 5 Vestibular gland abcess.
Reproduced from Ozdegirmenci, O., Kayikcioglu, F., & Haberal, A. (2009). Prospective randomized study of marsupialization versus silver nitrate application in the management of Bartholin gland cysts and abscesses. *Journal of Minimally Invasive Gynecology, 16*(2), 149–152. Copyright 2009, with permission from Elsevier.

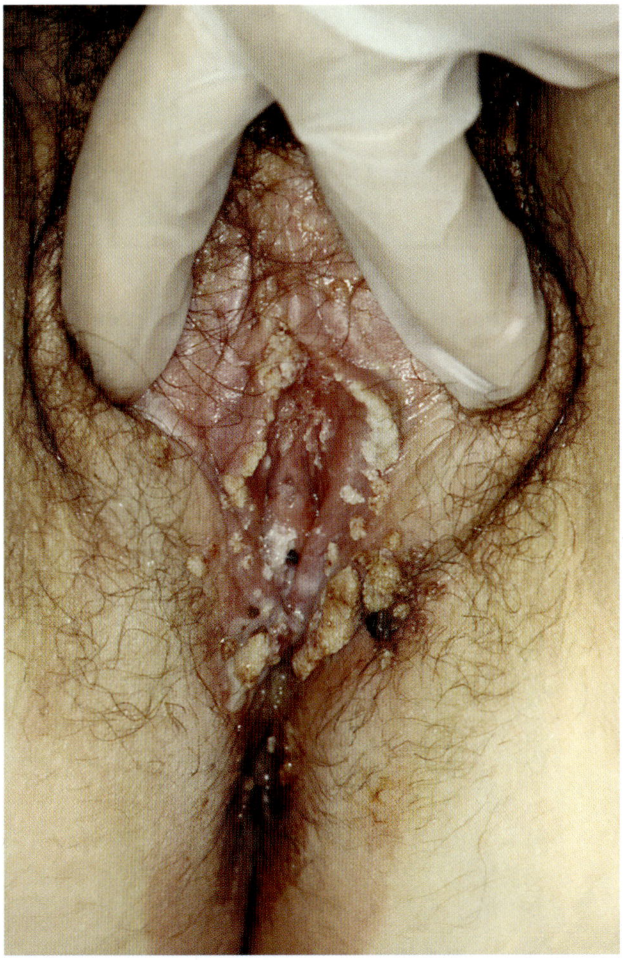

COLOR PLATE 6 Genital warts.
Courtesy of CDC/Joe Millar.

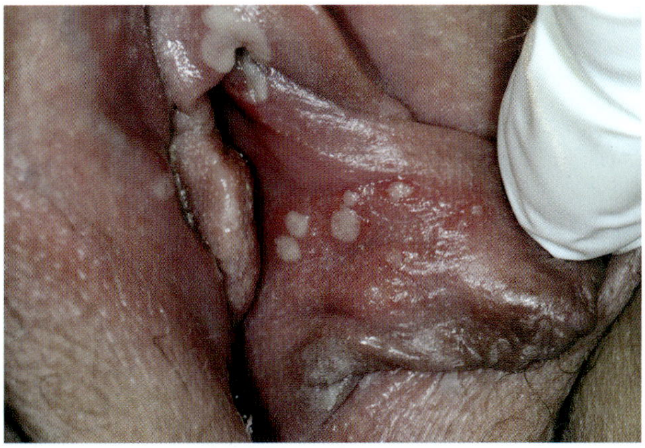

COLOR PLATE 7 Genital herpes lesions.
© Dr P. Marazzi/Science Source

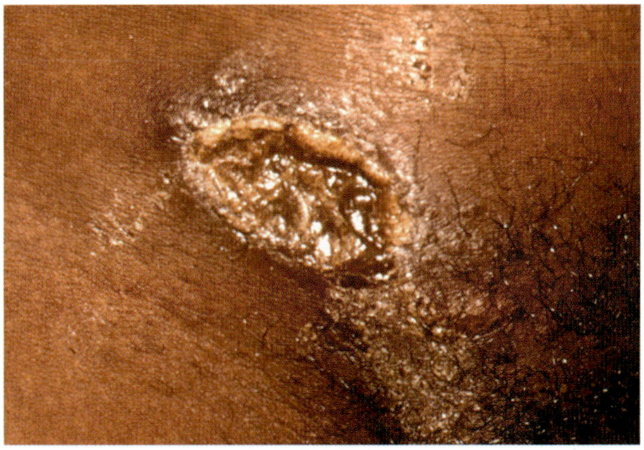

COLOR PLATE 8 Chancroid lesion.
Courtesy of CDC/J. Pledger.

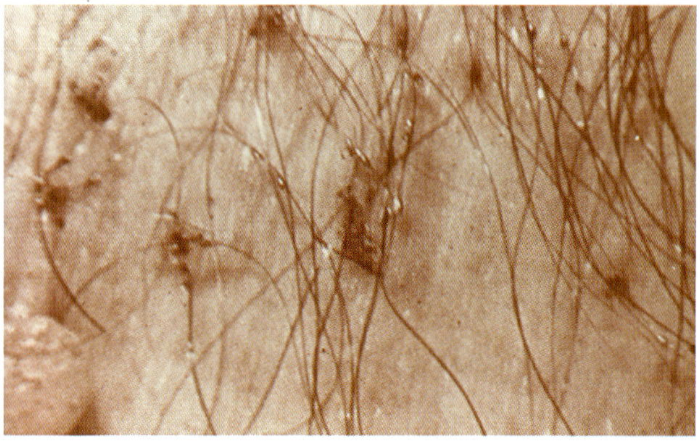

COLOR PLATE 9 Pediculosis pubis.
Courtesy of CDC/Joe Miller.

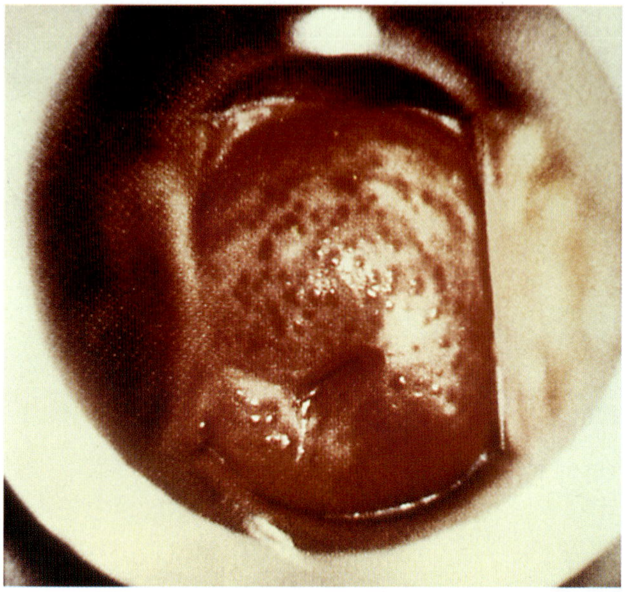

COLOR PLATE 10 Cervical petechiae observed with trichomoniasis.
Courtesy of CDC.

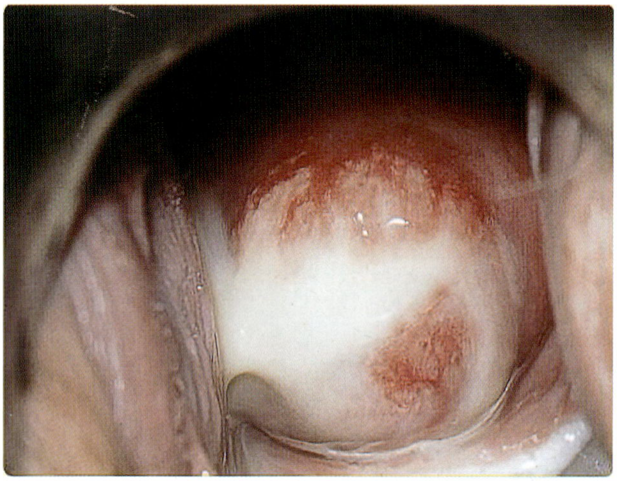

COLOR PLATE 11 Chlamydial mucopurulent discharge.
Reproduced from Aidsfonds. *SOA Chlamydia trachomatis female*. https://commons.wikimedia.org/w/index.php?curid=45718. It is licensed under the Creative Commons Attribution-Share Alike 3.0 Unported license. (https://creativecommons.org/licenses/by-sa/3.0/deed.en)

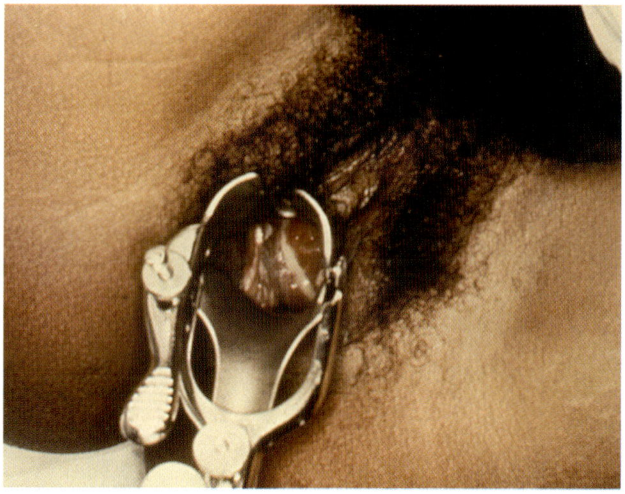

COLOR PLATE 12 Gonorrheal mucopurulent discharge.
Courtesy of CDC.

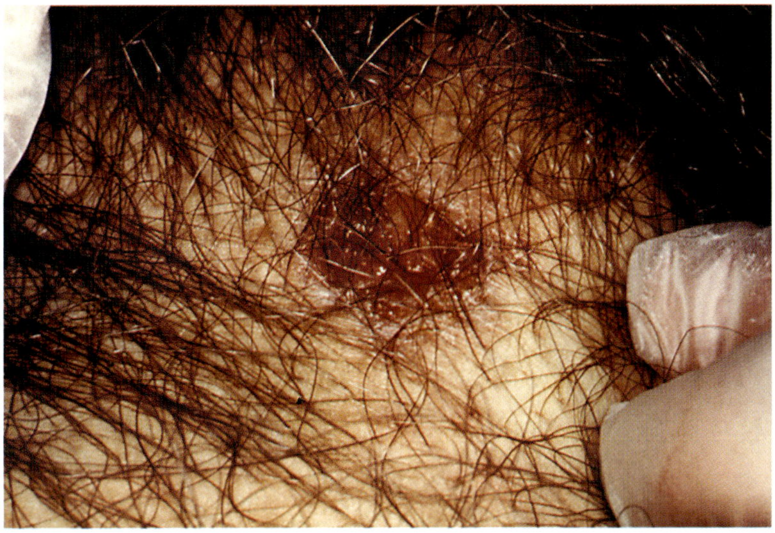

COLOR PLATE 13A Syphilitic chancre (primary syphilis).
Courtesy of CDC/Joe Miller/Dr. N.J. Fiumara.

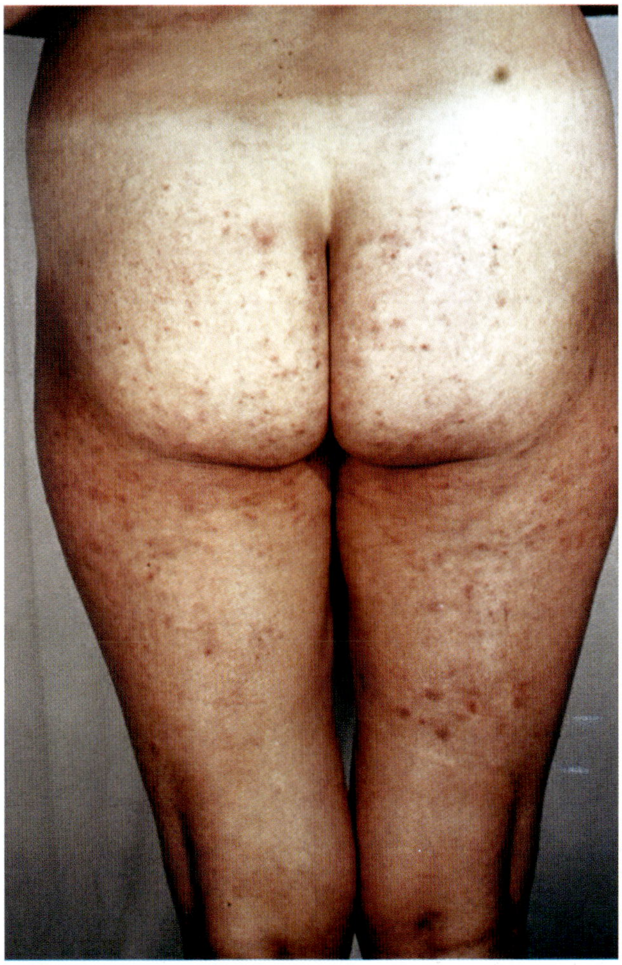

COLOR PLATE 13B Syphilitic rash(secondary syphilis).
Courtesy of CDC/J. Pledger, BSS, VD.

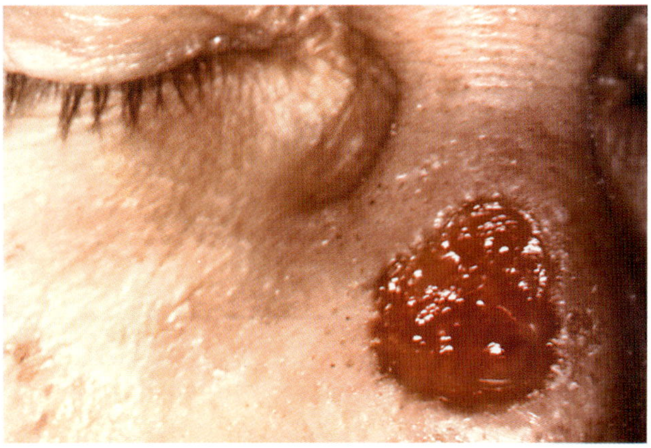

COLOR PLATE 13C A gumma, which is a soft noncancerous growth resulting from the tertiary stage of syphilis.
Courtesy of CDC/J. Pledger.

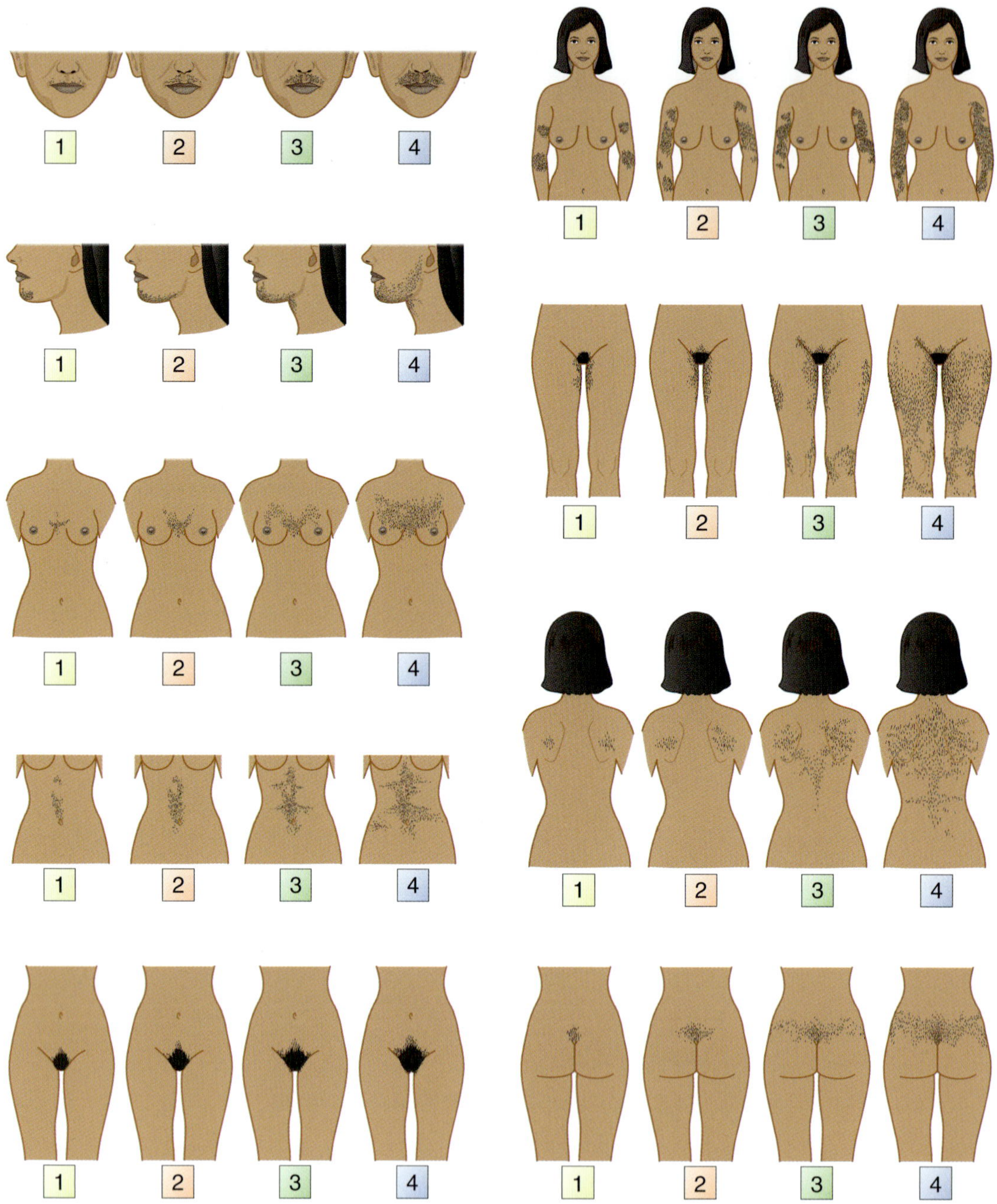

COLOR PLATE 14 Modified Ferriman–Gallwey hirsutism scale. This is a visual method of scoring hair growth in women, modified from the original scale reported by Ferriman and Gallwey in 1961. Each of the nine areas is given a score ranging from 0 (no hair) to 4 (extensive terminal hair). The scores for each of the nine areas are totaled, and a score of 8 or greater indicates hirsutism. Factors that affect body hair distribution and amount, such as genetic and hormonal influences, should be considered.

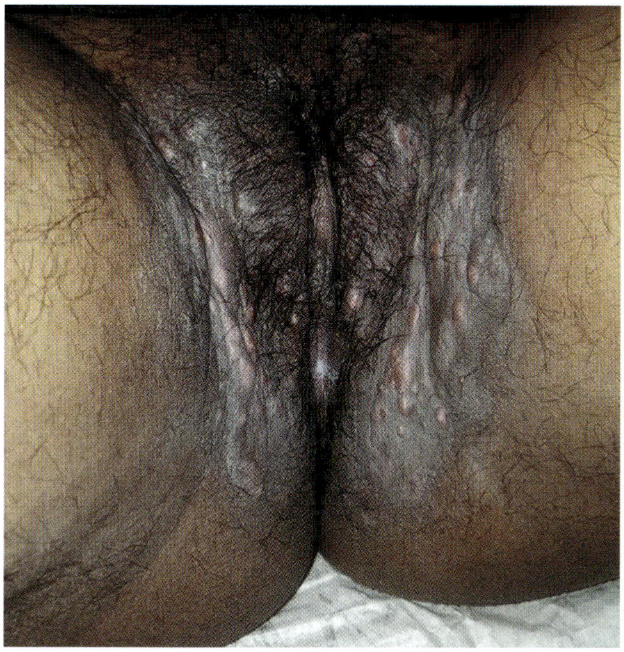

COLOR PLATE 15 Genital hidradenitis suppurativa.
© Rasika Pereir/Medical Images

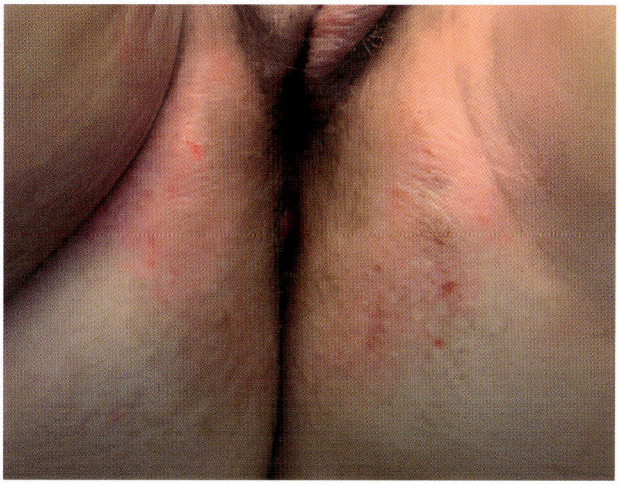

COLOR PLATE 16 Irritant contact dermatitis.
Reproduced from Dermatitis © 2010 American Contact Dermatitis Society.

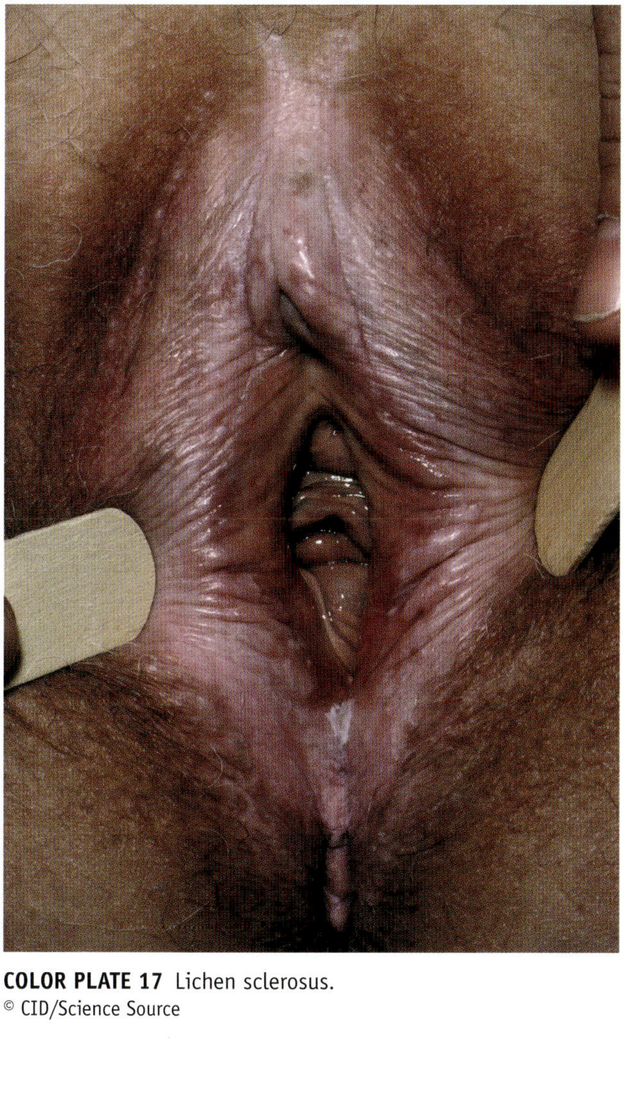

COLOR PLATE 17 Lichen sclerosus.
© CID/Science Source

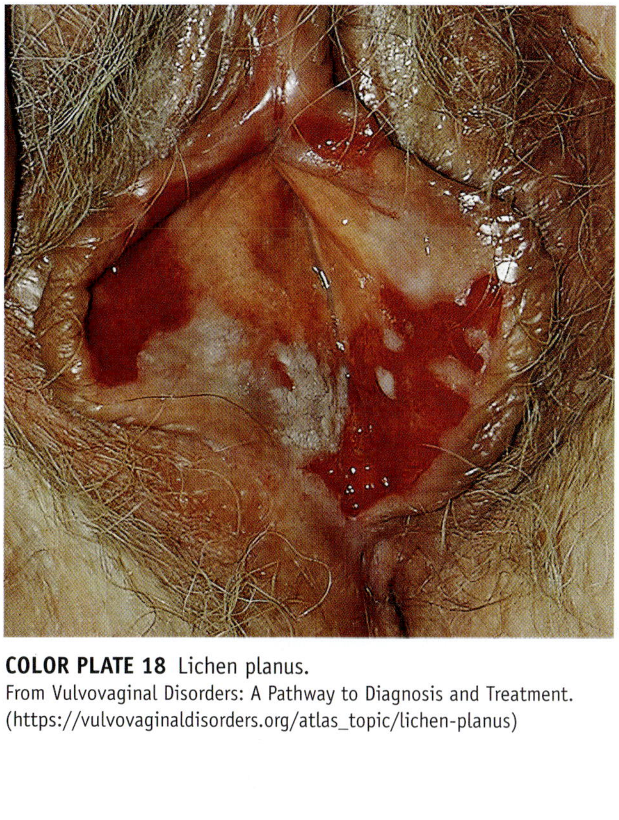

COLOR PLATE 18 Lichen planus.
From Vulvovaginal Disorders: A Pathway to Diagnosis and Treatment.
(https://vulvovaginaldisorders.org/atlas_topic/lichen-planus)

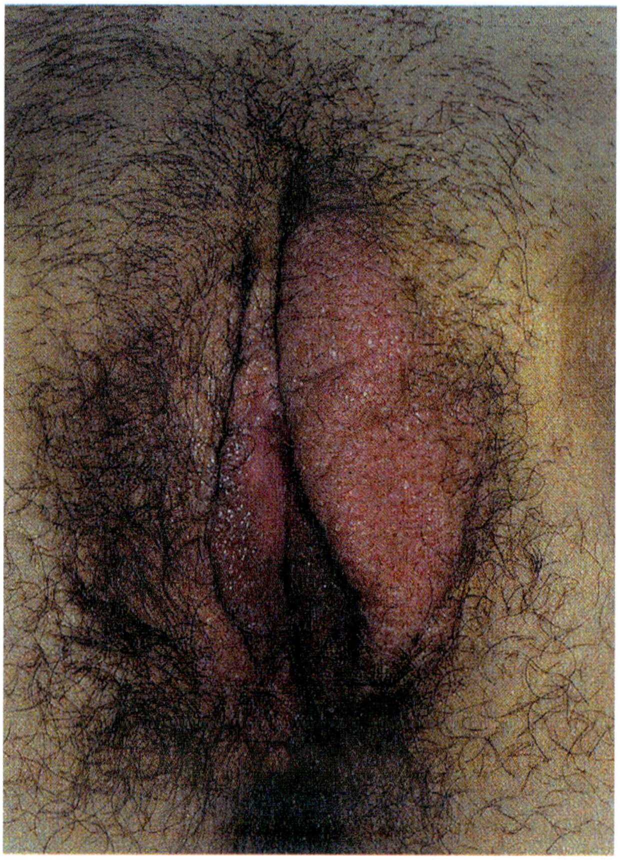

COLOR PLATE 19 Lichen simplex chronicus.
Reproduced from Stewart, K. M. (2010). Clinical care of vulvar pruritis, with emphasis on one common cause, lichen simplex chronicus. *Dermatologic Clinics, 28*(4), 669–680. Copyright 2010. Used with permission from Elsevier.

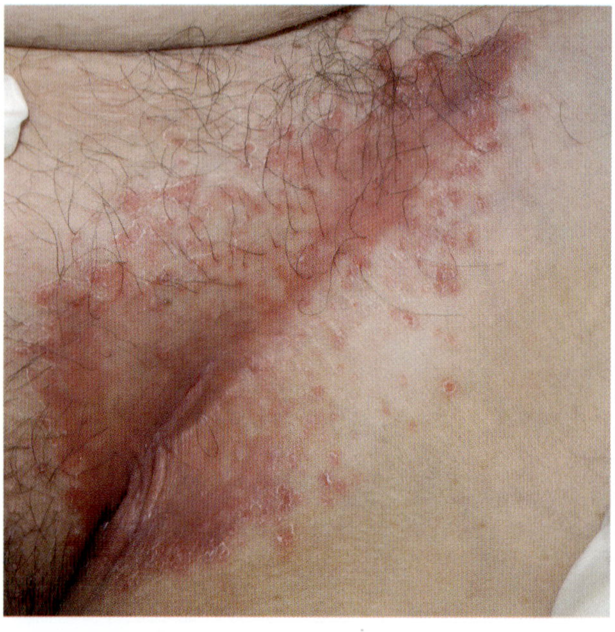

COLOR PLATE 20 Genital psoriasis.
© SCIENCE PHOTO LIBRARY/Science Source

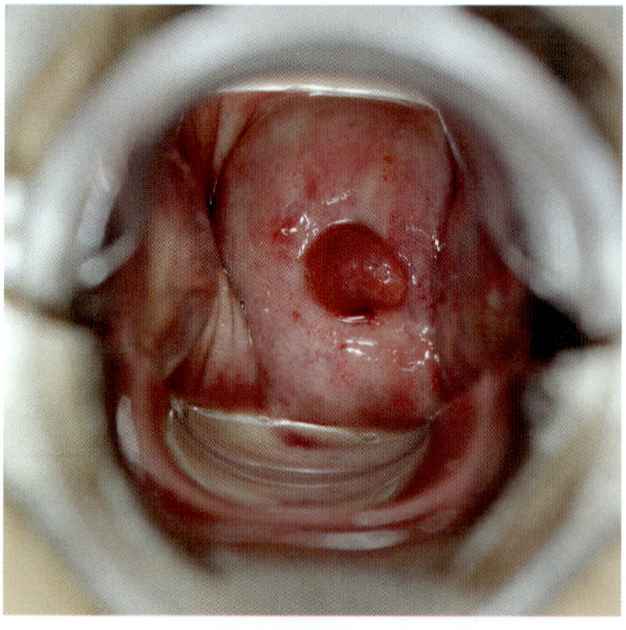

COLOR PLATE 21 Cervical polyp.
© Dr P. Marazzi/Science Source